Example of Nursing Process Displays

Example of Nursing Process and . . .

Clinical pharmacology
and nursing management

Roberta Todd Spencer, R.N., M.S.

Emeritus Associate Professor
Department of Nursing
State University of New York College at Plattsburgh
Plattsburgh, New York

Lynn Wemett Nichols, B.S.N., M.S.N.

Associate Professor
Department of Nursing
State University of New York College at Plattsburgh
Plattsburgh, New York

Gladys B. Lipkin, R.N., C.S., M.S., F.A.A.N.

Nurse Psychotherapist in Private Practice
Childbirth (Lamaze) Instructor; Lecturer
Bayside, New York

Helen Sabo Henderson, B.S.N., M.ED.

Emeritus Associate Professor
Department of Nursing
State University of New York College at Plattsburgh
Plattsburgh, New York

Frances M. West, R.N., M.S.N.

Vice-President, Patient Services Division
Champlain Valley Physicians Hospital Medical
    Center
Plattsburgh, New York

Contributors

Mary X. Britten, ED.D., R.N.
Associate Dean and Associate Professor
Decker School of Nursing
State University of New York at Binghamton
Binghamton, New York

Frances R. Brown, PH.D., R.N.
Assistant Professor
Decker School of Nursing
State University of New York at Binghamton
Binghamton, New York

Martha Fortune, R.N., M.S.
Hospice Nurse
Visiting Nurse Service of New York
New York, New York

Patricia Hryzak Lind, R.N., M.S.
Director of Nursing Operations, Analysis, and
    Evaluation
Strong Memorial Hospital
Rochester, New York

Charlotte Shimmons Torres, ED.D., R.N., C.S.
Assistant Professor
University of Rochester School of Nursing
Rochester, New York

Clinical pharmacology and nursing management

Fourth edition

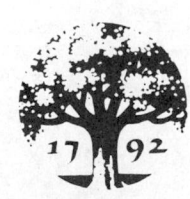

J. B. Lippincott Company
Philadelphia

Acquisitions Editor: Ellen M. Campbell
Developmental Editor: Marian Bellus
Project Editor: Amy P. Jirsa
Indexer: Maria Coughlin
Design Coordinator: Kathy Kelley-Luedtke
Interior Designer: Anne O'Donnell
Cover Photo: Steve Weinrebe
Cover Designer: Louis Fuiano
Production Manager: Helen Ewan
Production Coordinator: Maura C. Murphy, Kathryn Rule
Compositor: Circle Graphics
Printer/Binder: Courier/Westford
Cover Printer: Lehigh Press

4th Edition

6 5 4 3 2 1

Library of Congress Cataloging-in-Publication Data

Clinical pharmacology and nursing management / Roberta Todd Spencer
    . . . [et al.]. — 4th ed.
      p.   cm.
    Includes bibliographical references and index.
    ISBN 0-397-54935-0
    1. Pharmacology.   2. Nursing.   I. Spencer, Roberta Todd.
    [DNLM: 1. Pharmacology, Clinical—nurses' instruction.   QV 38
C6415]
    RM300.C526   1993
    615'1'024613—dc20
    DNLM/DLC
    for Library of Congress   92-20818
                                                                        CIP

Any procedure or practice described in this book should be applied by the healthcare practitioner under appropriate supervision in accordance with professional standards of care used with regard to the unique circumstances that apply in each practice situation. Care has been taken to confirm the accuracy of information presented and to describe generally accepted practices. However, the authors, editors, and publisher cannot accept any responsibility for errors or omissions or for any consequences from application of the information in this book and make no warranty express or implied, with respect to the contents of the book. Every effort has been made to ensure drug selections and dosages are in accordance with current recommendations and practice. Because of ongoing research, changes in government regulations and the constant flow of information on drug therapy, reactions and interactions, the reader is cautioned to check the package insert for each drug for indications, dosages, warnings and precautions, particularly if the drug is new or infrequently used.

The publisher wishes to acknowledge the following persons at Kentmere Nursing Care Center in Wilmington, Delaware, for their kind assistance in obtaining photographs in Chapter 13: Judy Loringer, Elva Mitchell, Ellen Pindus Kurtz, and Louise Jackson.

Dedication

The meaning of the word *dedication* may include setting apart and devoting to a special purpose or addressing to another as a token of respect or affection. In accord with these definitions, we would like to once more dedicate this volume to nursing clients, through its use by students and faculty of schools of nursing and practicing nurses, and to our families and friends, with thanks for their understanding and support.

Contributors' chapters

The following is a list of the chapters written by each author. An asterisk (*) indicates chapters authored by more than one contributor.

Mary X. Britten
Chapter 37

Frances R. Brown
Chapter 21

Martha Fortune
*Chapter 19, Appendix**

Helen Sabo Henderson
Chapters 11 and 26

Patricia Hryzak Lind
Chapter 17

Gladys B. Lipkin
Chapters 16, 35, 36, 38, and 41–46

Lynn Wemett Nichols
*Chapters 9, 27, 28, 39, 47–49, and 50**

Roberta Todd Spencer
Chapters 1–4, 7, 8, 10, 13, 14, 20, 22–25, 29–34, 40, 50, 51–54, Appendix**

Charlotte Shimmons Torres
Chapter 18

Frances M. West
Chapters 5, 6, 12, and 15

Consultants for
the fourth edition

Virginia Birnie, R.N., B.SC.N.
Professor
Okanagan College
School of Nursing
Kelowna, British Columbia, Canada

Regina Stanback-Stroud, R.N., M.S.H.R.
Professor
Health Sciences Department
Rancho Santiago College
Santa Ana, California

Janet L. Stewart, R.N., B.S.N., M.N.ED.
Instructor
The Western Pennsylvania Hospital
School of Nursing
Pittsburgh, Pennsylvania

Barbara L. MacDermott, M.S., R.N.
Assistant Dean and Associate Professor
Syracuse University College of Nursing
Syracuse, New York

Maxine C. Mott, R.N., B.N., M.ED.
Instructor
Department of Nursing and Allied Health
Mount Royal College
Calgary, Alberta, Canada

Sandra Clark, R.N., M.S.N.
Assistant Professor
Armstrong State College
School of Nursing
Savannah, Georgia

Preface

Clinical Pharmacology and Nursing Management was originally conceived when we, as nursing instructors, had difficulty selecting a suitable pharmacology textbook for our students because no one volume seemed to present all aspects of the discipline pertinent to nursing. Most texts handled one or more facets of the subject well but omitted or slighted others. We also recognized that there seemed to be a considerable body of knowledge about the nursing aspects of pharmacology that did not appear at all in the standard references. In this fourth edition of *Clinical Pharmacology and Nursing Management* we have refined, updated, and expanded our original concept of providing all the nursing aspects of pharmacology in a concise and readable style.

Purpose

Our intent is to provide a useful textbook for nursing students who are beginning the study of pharmacology. Our objective is to produce a text that presents (1) the concepts necessary for good judgment in the use of chemical agents, (2) a theoretical base for the skills required to administer medications, and (3) a ready reference for drug data required most frequently by nurses. We address the social use and abuse of chemicals, toxicology, and the medicinal use of drugs across a broad spectrum of health-care situations.

Structure

The text is divided into 14 sections. *Unit One*, Introduction to Pharmacology, presents a brief history of the discipline and discusses its relationship to nursing, describes legal controls over drug production and use and harmful effects of chemical exposure, presents the nursing process as it pertains to pharmacotherapeutics, and suggests approaches helpful to the study of pharmacology. *Unit Two*, Therapy With Drugs, discusses concepts underlying the medicinal use of drugs, including pharmacodynamics and pharmacokinetics, interaction of drugs and food and psychosocial aspects of drug use, and describes currently used drug preparations. A theoretical base for the skills relevant to the administration of medications is offered in *Unit Three*.

A variety of considerations is treated in *Unit Four*, Special Considerations in Drug Therapy. This unit includes individual chapters on maternal, pediatric, and gerontologic care as well as unique chapters on drug therapy in community health nursing and self-medication with over-the-counter drugs.

Units Five through Fourteen present information on drugs in current use, including discussions of major drug classifications and data on specific medicinal agents. Included in these sections are the physiology and the pathophysiology of the particular body system being discussed, and their relevance to medication. In most cases, the discussion of drugs is broken down into pharmacodynamics, pharmacokinetics, therapeutic uses, adverse reactions, and precautions and contraindications.

Nursing process content

Specific nursing information has been worked into the design of the book so that it is easy to find. Most chapters—and all within the drug family unit—have sections called Nursing Management. These sections are further broken down into sections entitled Nursing Implications and Nursing Process. New for this edition is the delineation of collaborative problems, which are listed following the nursing diagnoses wherever applicable. A checklist of nursing actions provides a quick review, in imperative (command) form, of the important nursing actions. The wellness/illness continuum is evident throughout the book, especially in some of the client education sections.

In addition, the nursing process as it pertains to pharmacotherapeutics is presented in Chapter 3. The responsibilities of the nurse are defined broadly, encompassing those responsibilities inherent in the evolving roles of primary-care provider and client advocate.

Pedagogical features

Learning Experiences and Enrichment Experiences. Experiential materials that promote or enrich the student's learning are suggested at strategic points in the text and in the Student Workbook. Some may form the basis for group field trips or class discussion. Others may be pursued by the individual. Not all of these experiences will be possible in any given setting, but all are designed to increase the reader's awareness of the pervasiveness of chemical use and the implications of pharmacologic issues in nursing practice.

Review Displays. As in the previous edition, review materials and information to be emphasized have been set off from the text, in this edition in screened displays rather than boxes.

Drug Tables. These provide at-a-glance specifics for individual drugs. Each group of drugs displayed is discussed in terms of their pharmacodynamics, dosage and route of administration, therapeutic uses, adverse reactions, and precautions and contraindications.

Examples of Nursing Process. Case studies are presented with related care plans as examples of the nursing care of clients undergoing drug therapy.

Illustrations. Using photos and drawings, both nursing actions involved in the administration of medications and concepts of chemical structure and action are illustrated.

Glossary. The glossary, consisting of over 350 common drug-related terms, is intended to be a useful reference to the student.

Appendix. The Appendix has been expanded for this edition to include more materials for easy reference.

References and Bibliography. In each chapter, these provide sources for text information and resources for additional information.

New features for the fourth edition

- Two new displays have been added to this edition:
  Focus Boxes. These give the reader an overview of the similarities *and* the

differences between the individual drugs in a pharmacologic class in a readable and concise format.

Issues in Drug Therapy Boxes. These present discussion of some of the current topics that have arisen in connection with the use of a particular drug or group of drugs.

- More information for easy reference is provided in the drug tables:

  The FDA Pregnancy Category, where assigned

  Canadian Trade Names, where appropriate

- Updated drug information throughout the text and drug tables

- Delineation of collaborative problems, listed separately in the nursing process sections

- Index entries re-designed to give more information at a glance: generic drug names in boldface, trade names in small caps, Canadian trade names followed by (Can). The designations *t*, *f*, and *d* direct the reader to the specific type of discussion: table, figure, or display.

Ancillaries

Also available with the fourth edition of *Clinical Pharmacology and Nursing Management* are the *Student Workbook*, the *Instructor's Manual*, and a Computer Test Bank.

The *Student Workbook* enables the student to follow the text chapter by chapter. A variety of materials is used to supplement learning, including some of the Learning Experiences presented in the text in the previous edition. The *Instructor's Manual* provides each chapter with a list of concepts with which the text deals, and from which program-specific objectives can be derived. In this way learning objectives can be tailored specifically to the program of study pursued by the reader. The Computer Test Bank provides NCLEX-style test items, to assist both the faculty and the student in effectively measuring learning.

We believe that we have produced a package that will give a practical background in pharmacology to all nursing students and will provide an easy reference for special nursing needs.

The Authors

About the factual content of this textbook

The authors, contributors, and editors of this book have expended considerable time and effort to ensure that the facts and opinions offered in the text and tables of this book are in accordance with official standards and with the consensus of foremost authorities at the time of publication.

However, drug therapy is a very dynamic branch of medicine, marked by the continual marketing of new drugs and the discontinuation and withdrawal (often without notice) of older drug products. In addition, the Food and Drug Administration (FDA) constantly orders changes in the labeling of even well-established drug products, on the basis of ongoing studies of their safety and efficacy. For this reason, no claims are made that statements made here concerning the current status of these drugs will continue to reflect the views of the drug industry or the FDA or that the data presented in tabular form are, or will remain, complete and correct in every detail.

The most important aspect of this problem lies in the area of dosage recommendations. Every effort has been made to check that statements made in the tables are, within the limits of space, precisely correct. However, dosage schedules are frequently ordered changed in accordance with accumulating clinical experience.

For this reason, we urge that *before administering any drug, you check the manufacturer's latest dosage recommendations* as presented in the package insert that accompanies each unit of every drug product.

Acknowledgments

The preparation of a textbook requires the involvement of many people who support and complement the work of the authors. This book is no exception. It would be impossible to name everyone who contributed to its publication. However, we would like to acknowledge, with gratitude, the following contributions to this fourth edition:

Contributors: Mary Britten, Frances Brown, Patricia Hryzak Lind, Martha Fortune, and Charlotte Torres

Editors: Ellen Campbell, Margaret Belcher, Marian Bellus, Amy Jirsa, and Kathy Kelley-Luedtke

Contents

2

Therapy with drugs   57

5

Drugs that affect the nervous system 313

6

Drugs affecting the cardiovascular system   531

7

Drugs affecting the gastrointestinal system 651

8

Drugs affecting the endocrine system 719

43 Drugs used to treat infections caused by viruses and fungi 1068

44 Drugs used to control vector-borne diseases, and protozoan, helminthic, and ectoparasitic infections 1093

45 Antipyretics 1130

46 Agents used in debridement of wounds 1141

47 Anti-inflammatory and related agents 1147

12

Drugs affecting neoplastic disease 1177

48 Chemotherapeutic agents: Alkylating agents and antimetabolites 1178

Clinical pharmacology and nursing management

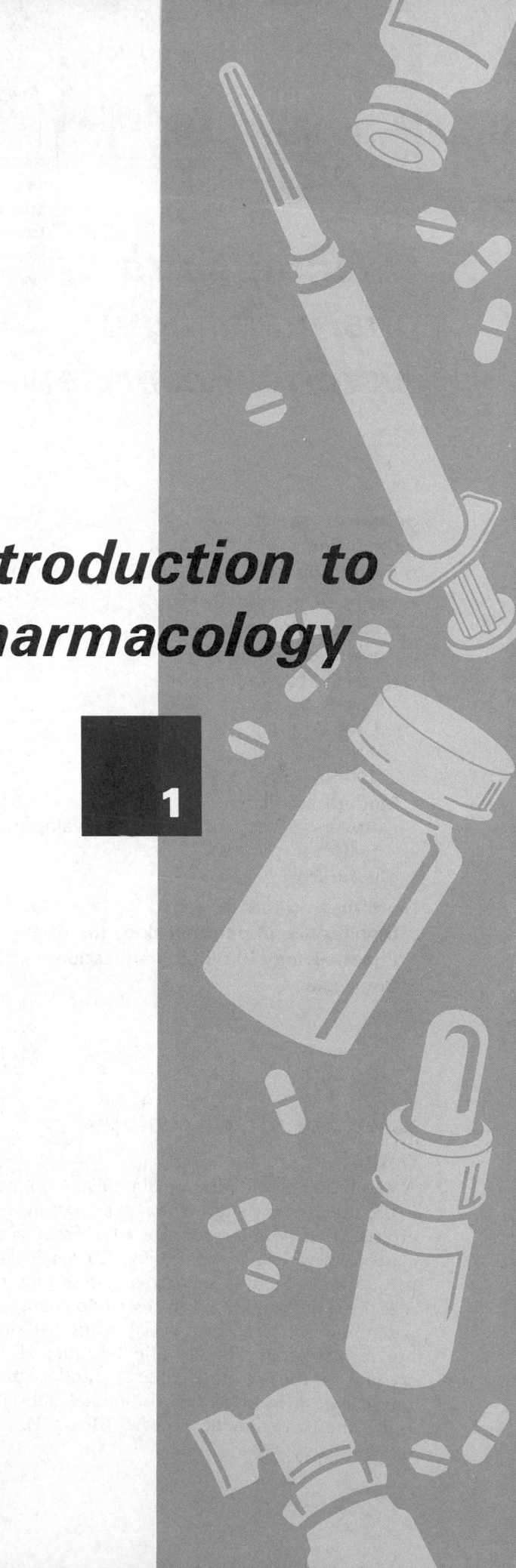

Introduction to pharmacology

1

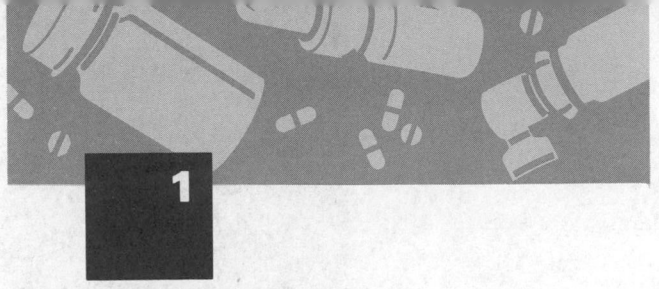

1

Orientation to pharmacology: historical overview

Box 1-1. What is pharmacology?

Pharmacology is the study of the effects of chemical substances on living tissue, including:

- The study of medicinal drugs
- The study of chemicals with toxic properties
- The study of the use of chemicals for psychotropic or social purposes

Scope of pharmacology

Definition

A widely accepted definition of pharmacology is that it is the science of drugs—their preparation, use, and effects. The popular concept that pharmacology is concerned with medicinal drugs, in particular those prescribed by a physician to treat illness, fails to recognize the significance of nonprescription drugs, such as patent medicines, and the social drugs: caffeine, alcohol, nicotine, and tobacco. The definition also fails to account for the use of illegal drugs, and it ignores the physiologic effects of environmental substances to which the body may be exposed (Box 1-1).

A broader definition of pharmacology is the study of the effect of chemical substances on living tissues (Leake, 1975). Under this increasingly popular definition, the discipline is considered to be concerned with the identification and use of all chemical substances that affect living organisms. Within this broad definition, drugs are defined as chemicals that affect living tissues. The study of pharmacology encompasses not only all medicinal effects but also the impact of social drugs, poisons, pharmacologically active foods, and pollutants.

An interdisciplinary study

Chemistry is the traditional scientific discipline most closely related to pharmacology. Chemical analysis is essential to the identification of active drug substances. Inorganic, organic, and molecular chemistry and biochemistry are all involved in the study of drug properties. The chemist determines the relation of molecular structure to biologic activity, modifies chemicals so as to change their drug properties, and synthesizes new molecules to be used as drugs.

Botany, geology, microbiology, genetics, nutrition, and both animal and human physiology also contribute to the process of identifying active drug substances. Modern drugs are derived from many sources: minerals, plants, microbial cultures, and animal and human tissues. Their extraction and manufacture depend on knowledge of these sciences, as well as chemistry. In addition, the principles and techniques of medicine and veterinary science are essential to the study of the action of chemicals in living animals. The dependence of pharmacology on the material sciences (*ie*, those dealing with material phenomena) is fairly obvious. More obscure, perhaps, are the social ramifications of drug use.

Drugs have played a role in the religious practices of many cultures. Sacramental wine, the "sacred" mushroom, and peyote have all had their ritualistic uses. In many societies, the use of drugs has been linked to and largely controlled by the priestly caste. However, from the peace pipe of the American Indians to the champagne of modern weddings, nonreligious rites and ceremonies also have involved the

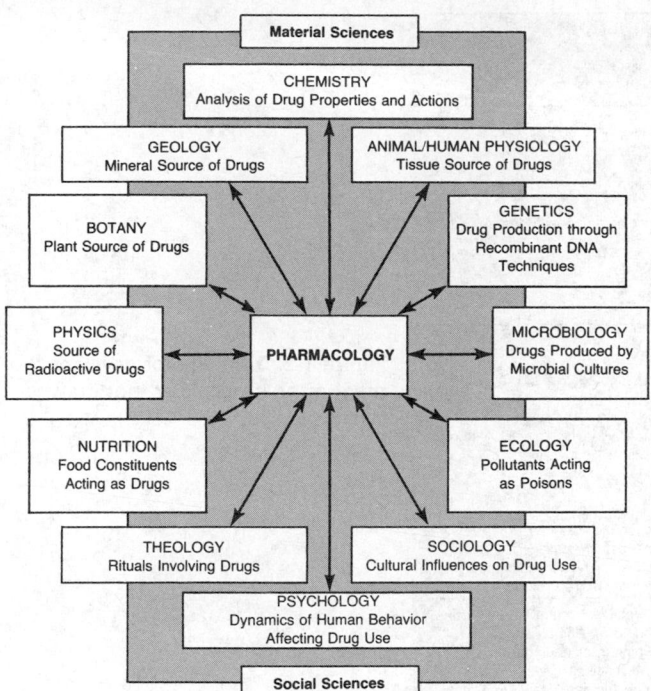

Figure 1-1. The scope of pharmacology.

use of drugs. Cultural influence is a powerful factor that affects attitudes toward and practices of drug use.

Because drugs are used for both social and medicinal purposes, psychological dynamics, social customs, religious practices, and legal controls influence individual and group drug practices. In modern times, a multitude of psychotropic (mind-altering) chemicals have been developed that can change human behavior, release inhibitions, and alter mental functions. These effects pose difficult moral and ethical problems. The study of pharmacology, therefore, involves the social, as well as the biologic, sciences.

In its broadest sense, then, pharmacology is an interdisciplinary study; it crosses the boundaries of the physical, biologic, and social sciences. It involves knowledge of body functions, the nature of matter, pollution, foods, and human behavior. A comprehensive study of the subject requires a multidisciplinary background (Fig. 1-1).

History of pharmacology

Prehistoric/primitive era

Pharmacology is one of the oldest sciences known to humans (Fig. 1-2). Natural substances used in healing were often discovered by chance trial and error. The resulting knowledge was transmitted from generation to generation through oral communication. The first person who tasted a strange plant in the hope that it was nutritious was conducting an experiment in both nutrition and pharmacology. If the plant proved nontoxic, nourishment might be extracted from it. If it was

poisonous, illness or death could result. In addition to gaining knowledge in nutrition, slowly people were realizing the harmful and healing capabilities of some of these plants.

Information about pharmacologically active substances abounds in the tribal traditions of prehistoric and ancient cultures. Every known culture used certain active substances and materials for their effects on living beings. Herbal remedies used on humans and animals are a part of the knowledge of every culture. This knowledge is often quite sophisticated and includes the use of chemicals that modern medicine has only recently begun to produce and use in therapy. Indeed, the therapeutic potential of the medicinal information contained in such folklore has not been exhausted. Through scientific analysis and testing, drug industries continue to develop new and useful drugs from the traditional remedies of various cultural groups.

Salt is one chemical long recognized as being essential to health. Some of the earliest known trade routes were developed to meet the need for this substance by populations located far from the sea or from natural deposits of the mineral. Alcohol, another drug substance known and used by most cultures, had particular value as a tranquilizer and anesthetic. Alcohol is a chemical that arises from the fermentation of carbohydrate foods. Most cultures have developed characteristic alcoholic beverages derived from local foods: grapes (from which wine is made), potatoes (vodka), rice (saki), and other sweet or starchy materials.

The need for mood-altering drugs was not completely met by alcohol alone. The variety of psychotropics that have been used in various cultures includes marijuana, opium, coca, tobacco, peyote, coffee, tea, pituri, fly agaric, caapi, chocolate, kava, and betel. There are few, if any, people in the world who lack drugs that ease the difficulties of life or allow a temporary escape from the problems of daily existence.

Another class of drugs used by certain cultures was useful in hunting animals. Smeared on arrowheads and other hunting implements, these substances were toxic and were used to stun or kill animals. Such poisons were sometimes used in warfare against other enemy tribes. South American Indians used curare in this way.

Still other drugs were used specifically for medicinal effects. Most early civilizations understood the use of laxatives and emetics.* Herbs such as rauwolfia were useful in cardiovascular and psychiatric illness. Folk remedies included practices such as poulticing with mouldy bread (a crude application of topical antibiotic). Most of the remedies used were mixtures of substances in which one or more active ingredients was accompanied by many others that were totally ineffec-

---

*Substances that induce vomiting.

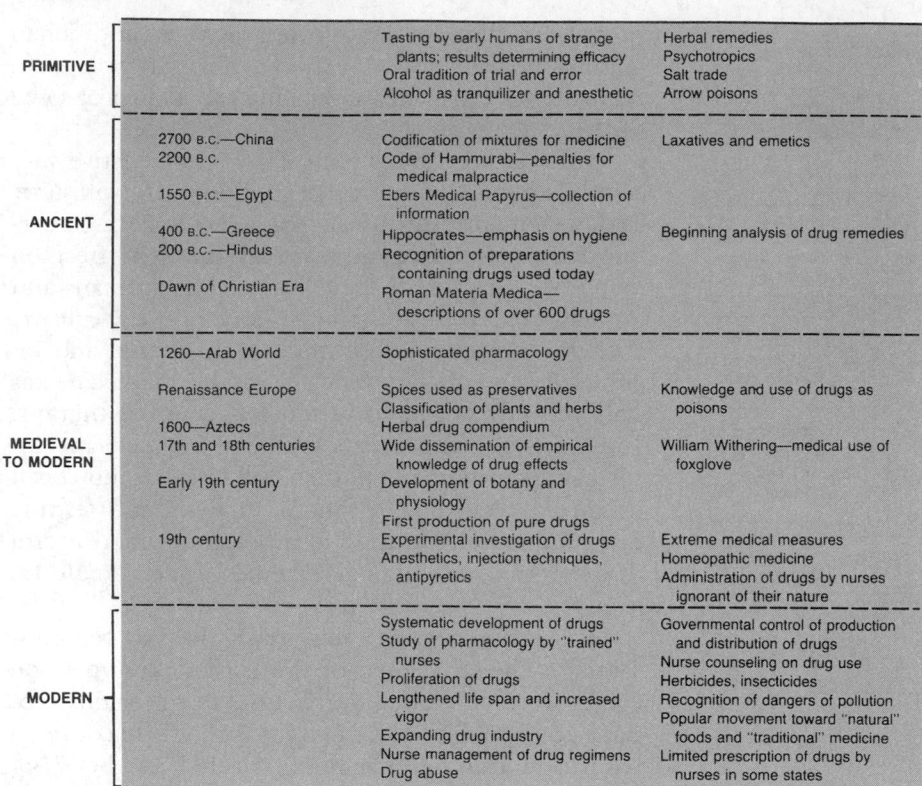

PRIMITIVE		Tasting by early humans of strange plants; results determining efficacy	Herbal remedies
		Oral tradition of trial and error	Psychotropics
		Alcohol as tranquilizer and anesthetic	Salt trade
			Arrow poisons
ANCIENT	2700 B.C.—China	Codification of mixtures for medicine	Laxatives and emetics
	2200 B.C.	Code of Hammurabi—penalties for medical malpractice	
	1550 B.C.—Egypt	Ebers Medical Papyrus—collection of information	
	400 B.C.—Greece	Hippocrates—emphasis on hygiene	Beginning analysis of drug remedies
	200 B.C.—Hindus	Recognition of preparations containing drugs used today	
	Dawn of Christian Era	Roman Materia Medica—descriptions of over 600 drugs	
MEDIEVAL TO MODERN	1260—Arab World	Sophisticated pharmacology	
	Renaissance Europe	Spices used as preservatives	Knowledge and use of drugs as poisons
		Classification of plants and herbs	
	1600—Aztecs	Herbal drug compendium	
	17th and 18th centuries	Wide dissemination of empirical knowledge of drug effects	William Withering—medical use of foxglove
	Early 19th century	Development of botany and physiology	
		First production of pure drugs	
	19th century	Experimental investigation of drugs	Extreme medical measures
		Anesthetics, injection techniques, antipyretics	Homeopathic medicine
			Administration of drugs by nurses ignorant of their nature
MODERN		Systematic development of drugs	Governmental control of production and distribution of drugs
		Study of pharmacology by "trained" nurses	Nurse counseling on drug use
		Proliferation of drugs	Herbicides, insecticides
		Lengthened life span and increased vigor	Recognition of dangers of pollution
		Expanding drug industry	Popular movement toward "natural" foods and "traditional" medicine
		Nurse management of drug regimens	Limited prescription of drugs by nurses in some states
		Drug abuse	

Figure 1-2. Time line of development of pharmacology (not drawn to scale).

tive except as placebos (pharmacologically inactive substances that cause changes in the body by the power of suggestion).

Ancient civilizations

One of the earliest collections of information about drugs was a codification of mixtures for medicinal use that appeared in China about 2700 B.C. A textbook of medicine dating from the same period recommended drugs such as ephedra, rhubarb, and senna, which are still in use today. Remedies no longer recognized as effective include rhinoceros horn (a reputed aphrodisiac), pomegranate, and animal excreta. Ginseng, a favorite remedy mentioned in the text, has been investigated recently for possible therapeutic use as an antidepressant (Fig. 1-2).

Another early collection of information about drugs is the Ebers Medical Papyrus of Egypt, which dates from about 1550 B.C. This manuscript is evidence of a beginning standardization of drug preparations as early as the second millenium B.C. The Egyptians were interested particularly in preservative substances that could be used to prevent decay of the body after death; however, the Papyrus also included substances used to treat the living. In this early era of pharmacology, the use of chemical substances was shrouded in mystery, a closely guarded secret of the priestly caste.

In southwest Asia, the Sumerians of the third millenium B.C. knew about hyssop and beer. The Code of Hammurabi (about 2000 B.C.) listed penalties for medical malpractice, recognizing the role of physicians in successfully—or unsuccessfully—treating disease. As in many early civilizations, drug use in Sumer was regulated by the priests. Hindu pharmacology, dating from about 200 B.C., recognized such preparations as colchicum, gentian, castor beans, and digitalis—all of which contain drugs used in current medical practice. Flavoring agents such as anise and caraway also were believed to have medicinal properties.

Greco-Roman civilization incorporated the use of many drugs in its medical practice. Although Hippocrates' treatment of disease included few drugs, emphasizing instead hygienic regimens, the analysis of remedies began soon after his time. A pupil of Aristotle collected data on about 500 drugs. By Nero's reign, about 600 substances were listed in the Roman Materia Medica.

Medieval to modern times

During the Middle Ages, drug use in Europe returned to a primitive empiricism in which people relied on experience, rather than scientific principles, as a basis for knowledge. However, herbs were cultivated in the gardens of monasteries for their medicinal properties, and the harmful effects of certain substances such as mushrooms and smutty rye were recognized. Isolated centers of learning preserved some of the older knowledge, and indigenous drug lore was exploited. A few new remedies were developed such as the ashes of sponges for goiter and the use of alcohol as an antiseptic.

In the Arab world, the science of pharmacology continued to advance. A compendium appearing in 1260 listed drugs such as ergot, borax, quicksilver, and cinnabar. The knowledge was systematized, and meticulous care was exercised in compounding drugs. Arabian practice of pharmacology reached a comparatively high level of sophistication.

The Renaissance

As it had done in many areas of inquiry in Europe, the Renaissance brought to pharmacology renewed interest and expansion of study. Much of the impetus for exploration during this era arose from the need for spices, which were valuable for their preservative and medicinal properties. During this time, plants and herbs were classified, the relation of dose to toxicity was recognized, and the beginnings of empirical chemistry fostered the use of pure chemical agents as drugs. These happy developments were accompanied by a darker side of the science—the use of poisons for homicide. Political assassination by poison was epitomized by the activities of the Borgia family in Italy.

Latin America

In the New World, the people of Latin America had accumulated considerable drug knowledge. An Aztec herbal compendium is known from the mid-16th century. These New World natives used coca, chili, balsam, castor oil, jalop, sarsaparilla, tobacco, and an oxytocic* (cihuapatli) called "woman's medicine." They also employed hallucinogens such as mushrooms, peyote, and morning glory in their religious rites. Latin American natives used quinine and curare, the former to treat fevers, the latter as an arrow poison.

17th and 18th centuries

During the 17th and 18th centuries, empiric knowledge of drug effects continued to grow steadily and became more widely disseminated as world travel and trade developed. The stimulating properties of tea, coffee, and cacao were recognized. Quinine from the New World, ginseng from China, and cassein, cinchona, and ipecac from India were added to the compendia of the "civilized" world. In the late 18th century, the medicinal uses of foxglove were described by an English physician, William Withering. (The leaves of foxglove are a source of digitalis, a heart stimulant.) The Royal Society of London fostered scientific investigation in many areas significant to the emerging science of pharmacology. Drugs were highly regarded and widely used by physicians and lay persons alike.

19th century

From antiquity to the 19th century, knowledge of drugs had derived from empiric observations. Crude preparations characterized by multiple ingredients

*A drug that stimulates contraction of the uterus.

were used in the treatment of disease. This was to change in the 19th century with the use of experimental investigations concerning the site and mode of actions of drugs. Such investigations had not been possible until the scientific method of inquiry was developed as a means of analyzing, classifying, and systematizing knowledge.

The growing science of chemistry made it possible to extract the active ingredients of medicines for study under controlled conditions. In the early 19th century, the active ingredients of opium, colchicum, and other drugs were isolated. For the first time, morphine, colchicine, strychnine, caffeine, quinine, and similar chemicals were available in pure form. Simultaneously, the development of botany and physiology enabled pharmacologists to discover new active drugs in plant life and to study the action of pure drugs in the body. As quantitative chemistry and systematic biology were established, a modern science of pharmacology began to emerge.

During the 19th century the fundamental problems of pharmacology were recognized:

- Dose—effect relationships
- Processes involved in absorption, distribution, chemical transformation, and excretion of drugs
- Localization of the site of action of the drug
- Specific mechanisms of drug action
- Relationship between chemical makeup and biologic activity of substances

The emphasis of 19th century pharmacology was on the organ and tissue effects of chemicals. Among the discoveries of this period were anesthetics, injection techniques, and antipyretic analgesics (medicine to treat fever and pain), such as aspirin.

Medical therapy during this era was characterized by extreme measures designed to force the body to resume normal functions. Patients were subjected to violent purges, sweating, emetics, and bloodletting. Under these conditions, the treatment was often more harmful to the patient than the disease it was intended to cure. In reaction to this situation, there arose a system of medicinal therapy called *homeopathic medicine* that was based upon crude drugs used in markedly reduced (diluted) dosages. Homeopathy was concerned with helping the body to heal itself. Although the very weak medicinal preparations administered by homeopathics may not have accomplished a therapeutic purpose, neither did they do any harm, and the sympathetic support of the physician undoubtedly aided the natural recuperative powers of the body. Homeopathy provided an alternative to the heroic medicine of the era, and is still practiced in some areas.

Modern medicine

Since the 19th century and particularly in the middle to late 20th century, pharmacology has been transformed into a complex science associated with a burgeoning drug industry. Purified chemicals are prepared from all conceivable natural materials: mineral, plant, and animal tissues and microbial cultures. Increasingly, drugs are developed, modified, and tailor-made through chemical synthesis. Our compendium of drugs is vast and includes both therapeutic medications and mind-altering compounds. Virtually every body function can be enhanced, suppressed, or manipulated by chemical means. A multitude of anti-infective agents now controls bacterial infections that in the past killed many people of all ages. The use of drugs has enabled modern medicine to lengthen the human life span and increase vigor during the additional years.

Adverse effects of chemical development

The ready availability of chemicals with powerful effects on the mind and body has caused an increasing problem of drug abuse. Psychotropic drugs appear initially to relieve the stresses of modern living. However, they also cause chemical dependence and acute overdose—catastrophic conditions that are very difficult to treat.

Modern technology has also developed a multitude of chemical substances for use by industry and agriculture in producing material products. These agents include herbicides, insecticides, fuels, solvents, and a bewildering variety of toxins that permeate our environment. Exposure to pollutants is associated with an increasing incidence of cancer, allergy, and poisoning.

Return to nature

One reaction to the artificiality of modern life is the resurgence of interest in nature, including natural foods and "traditional" medicine. Virtually all people have retained some of the herbal folklore used by earlier generations of their cultural group. In some cases, the legacy is well preserved and is used extensively; in others only fragments remain, and the practical knowledge necessary for safe use of native remedies has been lost. Individuals and groups interested in historic preservation of this information are actively investigating folk practices and publishing their findings. Many of these people use and teach herbal medical techniques. Others view this fund of knowledge as a broad base for further research and development of new drugs (Aikman, 1977).

The future

Many problems still challenge the medical and pharmaceutical sciences. Viral and fungal infections often do not respond well to currently available medicines. A more precise control of the immune system could prevent or control allergy, autoimmune diseases, and transplant rejection. Babies with genetic diseases are living longer but as yet we cannot restore them to full health. Gene therapy, now in the early experimental

stages, may someday accomplish this. However, therapeutic agents powerful enough to produce such miracles are also likely to cause many harmful effects.

The proper use of drugs and chemicals is a major problem of modern civilization. We should balance the use of drugs to ameliorate illness and suffering with controls that minimize the danger of toxicity and user dependence. We should promote the best quality of life without poisoning ourselves and the environment. It is unlikely that we can return to the past when our exposure to chemicals was limited to those contained in natural substances. It is far more likely that humans will continue to produce more chemicals in their quest for progress. The importance of pharmacology as a guide to the wise use of chemical substances will increase proportionately. It will remain a critical area of study for future generations.

Enrichment experience 1-1

Interview an older relative or friend to explore the experiences he or she has had with drug use throughout the life span. Ask questions about traditional family remedies, patent medicines, prescription drugs, and nonmedicinal drugs (alcohol, nicotine, caffeine, and so forth.) If the relative remembers prohibition, find out how he or she felt about this attempt to control the use of alcohol. How does this attitude compare with the person's viewpoint of the decriminalization of marijuana?

Compare your findings with those of your classmates. What cultural contexts are reflected in the drug practices reported? Are the attitudes expressed similar or dissimilar? Do the data offer any clues to factors influencing these attitudes? How do the attitudes of older adults compare with those of young people today?

■ Summary

Pharmacology is the study of the effects of chemical substances on living tissues. It is one of the oldest sciences known to humankind. Originally it was part of a trial-and-error method of survival; modern pharmacology is more sophisticated, though not perfected.

Every culture has studied plants and has developed a system of medicine founded on the use of plants. Many of these ancient herbs and chemicals are still used; many others have been revived in modern medicine.

Pharmacology is an interdisciplinary study, involving all sciences in an amalgam of physical (*ie*, material) and social knowledge. Pharmacology presents a challenge for the present and the future to balance the use of drugs to prevent or ameliorate illness with the least danger of toxicity and user dependence.

Nursing implications
Significance of pharmacology in nursing
The administration of drugs was one of the first medical functions delegated by doctors to nurses. Initially, medication was very tightly controlled by the physician. The nurse was often ignorant of the nature of the drugs that would be given to the client. With time, increasing responsibility was given to the nurse, who was expected to exercise judgment in the management of drug therapy. This required an understanding of drug action and the ability to detect both therapeutic and adverse reactions in the client. In the practice of modern medicine, increasing latitude is given to nurses to modify drug regimens in accordance with protocols developed jointly with the medical profession. Nurses are now expected to counsel clients on the management of their drug regimens for optimal effect. Eventually, nursing practice will involve the prescribing of medications. Some states already allow this in selected client situations. Thus, the once dependent nursing function related to prescribed drug therapy is developing a new, independent dimension.

Nurses have always counseled people about the use of nonprescription drugs. With the proliferation of chemical substances in modern technology, this teaching has expanded to include poison control, nonmedicinal use of drugs, and drug abuse and addiction. This function has become very important for the promotion of health and the prevention of drug-related disease.

The role of the nurse in the prevention of drug-related problems in healthy clients primarily involves public health nursing, occupational health nursing, and individual office practice. The nurse is concerned with the health impact of environmental pollutants and health aspects of social, medicinal, and illegal drug use. The function of the nurse is mainly educational. A major concern is teaching the population at large how to avoid drug hazards and prevent chemically-induced disease. The nurse also may contribute to the body of knowledge applicable in the prevention of illness by gathering pertinent data on the effects on humans of environmental chemicals and medicinal agents.

Early detection of drug-related problems in otherwise healthy clients involves case finding and referral. The nurse seeks early evidence of drug-related problems such as dependence, toxicity, or adverse reactions from the use of drugs (medicinal or nonmedicinal), and detrimental effects of exposure to chemicals. The nurse works with clients to improve self-care practices and, when necessary, refers the individual to a proper source for treatment.

When caring for clients with acute health needs, the nurse usually administers required medications. This function is far more demanding than in the past because of the proliferation of new drug agents and the complexities of multiple-drug therapy. The safety and efficacy of drug therapy at this level depends upon an assessment of the client's response to the treatment agents employed. The nurse must detect early signs and symptoms of toxicity, adverse reactions, and drug interactions (as well as therapeutic response), and work closely with the physician to revise the drug regimen for optimal effect.

During convalescence, clients require education and assistance to resume control of life and to maximize health potential. Continuity of nursing care is promoted by referral to community nursing services prior to the time of discharge from acute care facilities. In many cases, long-term use of drugs is necessary to control chronic disease processes. The client must be taught to manage the drug regimen, as well as other aspects of self-care.

It is apparent that there are few, if any, areas of nursing where a knowledge of pharmacology is not needed. Beginning students must learn the rudiments of the science and acquire the skills whereby this basic knowledge may be developed continually throughout their nursing careers.

Pharmacology in nursing education
The study of pharmacology has long been a required part of nursing education. When physicians began to delegate to nurses the responsibility of monitoring client response to drug therapy, the study of pharmacology was incorporated into the curricula of nursing schools. Courses emphasized memorization of drug information and rigid adherence to rituals of medication administration designed to ensure accurate drug dose delivered to the client. Lectures often were delivered by physicians, and the skills necessary for the delivery of drug doses were taught in laboratory courses dealing with "nursing arts" or "fundamentals of nursing."

In the mid-20th century, the evolution of nursing education from training programs to educational curricula gained momentum, and the responsibility for instruction was assumed by nurse educators. During this period, most schools developed integrated curricula in which content previously taught in isolated discrete courses (pathology, pharmacology, clinical psychomotor skills, ethics) was incorporated as themes in standard nursing courses. Because of the vastly increased knowledge that relates to drugs, students were no longer required to memorize isolated drug facts but were encouraged to learn information pertinent to the drug regimens of their clients. It was expected that through such a program students would encounter a representative variety of medicines.

Integrated curricula are still used by some schools of nursing; however, many nurse educators have become dissatisfied with this organization of content. They believe that too little time is devoted to discrete areas of content, and that students often fail to acquire a comprehensive base of knowledge. To meet this need, many schools have created separate courses in subjects such as pathophysiology and pharmacology.

Introductory courses in pharmacology need to emphasize scholarly skills required for continued study, processes by which chemicals affect living matter, and basic knowledge about major drug groups. Such courses lay the foundation for growth and learning throughout the student's nursing career.

Conclusion

The nurse applies knowledge and skills from many fields to help the client develop and implement a plan of care that will achieve optimal therapeutic effect. Within this context, the use of drugs to prolong life span and alleviate suffering poses problems of value judgments related to the quality of life. As in other aspects of health care, the nurse should respect the client's interest in self-determination. The passive recipient role of the past has been replaced by the active involvement of the client (or family) in determining the therapy to be chosen and the regimen through which it will be carried out.

Overall, the role of nursing in relation to pharmacology is to promote responsible use of chemicals to enhance health while at the same time minimize the detrimental effects of such use. This requires some knowledge in virtually all fields in the physical and social sciences in addition to knowledge of issues in ethics and law that pertain to nursing roles. In carrying out drug therapy, nurses must be skilled in practical technical procedures required to handle, control, and administer drugs safely. They must be able to work cooperatively with others to develop plans and regimens for the use of drugs in a manner acceptable to the client, physician, and society at large. The supervision and administration of medicinal therapy is an art as well as a science.

References

Aikman L. (1977). Nature's healing arts: From folk medicine to modern drugs. In *Folk medicine: An enduring art.* Washington, DC: National Geographic Society.

Leake CD. (1975). *An historical account of pharmacology to the twentieth century*, p 3. Springfield, IL: Charles C Thomas.

Bibliography

Coulter CR. (1986). *Portraits of homeopathic medicines.* Washington, DC: Wehawken Book Co.

Krantz JC. (1967). *Profiles of medical science and inspired moments.* Baltimore: John D Lucas.

Li CP. (1974). *Chinese herbal medicine.* (Pub. No. NIH75-732). Washington, DC: United States Department of Health, Education and Welfare.

Mann RD. (1984). *Modern drug use.* Boston: MTP Press, Ltd.

Navarra T. (1990). Drug therapy: The history of a love affair. *American Journal of Nursing 90*, 91.

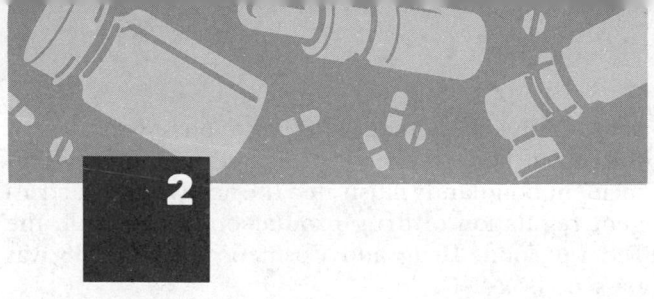

2

Standards and controls

Just as every society has discovered and used pharmacologically active substances (see Chapter 1), so has each society developed controls on their use. The earliest limitations of drug use were from religious practices and social mores. For example, in primitive societies, the use of substances affecting the central nervous system was often restricted to religious rituals. The effects of the substances were treated as mystical or spiritual experiences. Poisons used for killing animals were carefully applied to the hunting tools in ceremonial fashion. Drug use thereby became sacred; casual use was forbidden. Certain practices were outlawed by taboos; breaking taboos could bring severe punishment.

Although formal legislation provides restrictions in most modern societies, religious and social controls continue to influence the use of chemicals. For example, some contemporary religious denominations prohibit the use of alcohol. By social custom, drinking is more acceptable in the afternoon and evening hours than in the early morning. Social mores can be more effective than government laws in influencing behavior, as was illustrated by the failure of prohibition to eliminate drinking in the United States in the 1920s.

Many modern societies have elaborate and strict legislative controls governing drug use. Laws in most countries restrict the production, distribution, prescription, and administration of drugs. A large number of medicinal substances are not legally available to the general population except through licensed health professionals. However, certain groups of people who advocate permissiveness in the use of active substances oppose these controls. Illicit production and illegal diversion of pharmaceuticals provide large quantities of drugs to individuals and members of subcultures who value the drug "experience" and habitually use and abuse pharmacologically active chemicals.

Drug controls

Formal controls on the use of active substances range from the policies of individual institutions to governmental legislation. Attempts are made at the international, national, state or provincial, and local levels to control drugs legally. Further constraints in health care settings become institutional policies. Generally, restrictions become more severe as the unit becomes smaller, with each organization abiding by the restrictions of the larger units of which it is a part while adding to the constraints and specifying in greater detail the procedures for enforcement.

International controls

International drug controls are based on treaty agreements among national governments established through diplomatic conferences. These agreements have been concerned mainly with controlling substance abuse but there is a growing interest in promoting consumer safety through the development of standards for drug purity, nomenclature, labeling, and statistics. Under present conventions (the Single Convention on Narcotic Drugs), several bodies within the United Nations are involved in drug control. The Commission on Narcotic Drugs is authorized to make recommendations for the implementation of the provisions of the convention and to amend it when necessary. An expert body, the International Narcotics Control Board, was created to supervise the workings of the treaties regarding both licit and illicit drug trade. In addition, there are three secretariats within the United Nations involved with control of substance abuse: The United Nations Division of Narcotic Drugs, The International Narcotics Control Board Secretariat, and the World Health Organization Drug Dependence and Alcoholism Secretariat. In the absence of administrative or judicial structures for enforcement at this level, controls are dependent upon voluntary cooperation among nations.

National controls

Legislative guidelines for drug controls are largely at the national level. The severity and complexity of these laws vary from country to country and are not necessarily correlated. Countries with the most severe penalties for infractions may make fewer distinctions and exceptions in their laws. Penalties for drug infractions in many countries are much more severe than in the United States. For example, possession of marijuana, considered a misdemeanor in many states, is punishable by long prison sentences in some European countries.

Legislation in the United States

Early legislation

In the United States, federal legislation began with the 1906 passage of the Food, Drug and Cosmetic Act. This law was largely concerned with the purity of food but it did designate official standards for drugs (*The United States Pharmacopeia* and *The National Formulary*), empowering the federal government with enforcement. The law required that the strength and purity of drugs conform to the claims made for them by manufacturers and that labels indicate the kinds and amounts of narcotic ingredients in preparations.

Since the passage of the Food, Drug and Cosmetic Act, a number of new laws have extended federal drug controls. The first of these, the Shirley Amendment of 1912, prohibited fraudulent therapeutic claims. Though this measure implied that drug producers would be required to prove the efficacy of a remedy, enforcement was ineffective and for decades drug advertisements continued to claim wide-ranging benefits from the use of medicines, though there was little or no evidence to prove these claims.

In 1914, the first federal controls on habit-forming drugs were established. The Harrison Narcotic Act classified certain drugs believed to be habit-forming as *narcotics* and regulated their importation, manufacture, sale, and use. Included in this category were marijuana, opium, cocaine, and all their compounds and derivatives, as well as certain synthetic analgesics. Although this legislation has been superseded by the Controlled Substances Act of 1970, it remains historically significant because it was the first narcotic control act passed by any nation.

Food, Drug and Cosmetic Act of 1938

In the 1930s, more than 100 people died as a result of ingesting a solution of the antibacterial drug sulfanilamide that had been prepared with a toxic sol-vent, diethylene glycol. The poisonous properties of the vehicle had not been investigated prior to use. This incident poignantly illustrated the need for more stringent regulation of drug production. As a result, the Federal Food, Drug and Cosmetic Act of 1938 was passed (Box 2-1).

This law provided for government approval of new drugs as safe before they could enter interstate commerce. The law also specified requirements for labeling and conferred official status on drugs listed in the *Homeopathic Pharmacopoeia of the United States*.

In 1945, the Food, Drug and Cosmetic Act of 1938 was amended by a law that provided for certification of certain drugs through testing by the Food and Drug Administration (FDA) of each batch produced. This measure opened the door for involvement of the government in the direct supervision and inspection of production of pharmaceuticals.

Box 2-1. Provisions of the Federal Food, Drug, and Cosmetic Act of 1938

1. Standards acceptable for drug preparations include those outlined in *The United States Pharmacopeia*, *The National Formulary*, or the *Homeopathic Pharmacopoeia of the United States*.
2. Before new drugs may be marketed outside the state of origin, the preparation must be approved by the FDA as safe for use as recommended by the manufacturer.
3. Labels on drugs must conform to the following specifications:
   a. Contents of the preparation must be accurately stated.
   b. The official or (for nonofficial drugs) usual name of the drug(s) must be specified.
   c. The presence of certain substances (alcohol, bromides, atropine, digitalis, and others) must be indicated, and quantity and proportion specified.
   d. The presence of all habit-forming drugs must be noted, with a statement warning of their habit-forming potential.
   e. The name and address of the manufacturer, packer, or distributor must be included.
   f. Adequate directions for use and warnings against unsafe use must be included. Recommendations must be for dosage levels and frequency that are not dangerous to health.
   g. New drugs not yet approved for interstate commerce must bear the statement: "Caution: New Drug—Limited by Federal Law to Investigational Use."
   h. Statements on the label must not be false or misleading in any way.

Prescription and nonprescription drugs

The Durham-Humphrey Amendment of 1952 distinguished between prescription (legend) and nonprescription (over-the-counter) drugs, and specified procedures governing the distribution of prescription drugs. As a result of the power given to it by this law, the FDA has classified most of the efficacious therapeutic drugs (which, because of their potency, tend to be somewhat toxic) as legend drugs (Box 2-2).

Safety and effectiveness

In the 1950s, the public became increasingly aware of the potential for harm of many drug substances. The deleterious effects of drugs were publicized widely in the media. Two incidents of particular concern involved medicinal preparations. The Salk vaccine, the first drug available for immunization against poliomyelitis, was rushed into production in 1954 in an attempt to forestall the usual summer epidemic of this dreaded disease. One or more batches of the drug appeared to have been inadequately attenuated (weakened), and over 200 cases of permanent paralysis developed in recipients. The drug thalidomide, an antiemetic sedative that had been widely used in Europe to treat nausea and vomiting during pregnancy, proved to be teratogenic (harmful to the developing fetus). Numerous children afflicted with phocomelia (congenital absence or severe deformity of the limbs) were born to mothers who received the drug during early pregnancy. During this same period, problems arising from widespread abuse of both legal and illegal drugs were extensively publicized by the news media. As a result, a growing number of people became cautious about the use of any drug. Many joined the movement to "natural living," some embracing traditional herbal medicine in preference to pharmaceuticals. Media exposés of the huge profits earned by drug companies provided impetus for new drug legislation, culminating in the 1962 passage of the Kefauver-Harris Amendment to the Food and Drug Act.

The Kefauver-Harris Amendment attempts to provide assurance of the safety and effectiveness of drugs, and improve communication of necessary information about drugs (Box 2-3). It delegates broad powers to the FDA to regulate the manufacturing, distribution, and sale of drugs.

Effectiveness of therapeutic claims

The National Research Council of the National Academy of Sciences evaluates data supporting therapeutic claims for the FDA, rating effectiveness according to the following scale:

- *Ineffective:* There is no substantial evidence of effectiveness.
- *Ineffective as a fixed combination:* The product is not effective in fixed dosage combinations for reasons of safety or because one or more components lack substantial evidence of effectiveness.
- *Possibly effective:* Effectiveness might be shown eventually, but at the present time little evidence of efficacy is available.

Box 2-2. Provisions of the Durham-Humphrey Amendment of 1952

1. The dispensing of certain (legend) drugs by the pharmacist is limited to prescription by licensed health professionals. Prescriptions may be written or, for certain drugs, can be verbal (oral or telephone). Substances classified as legend drugs include:
   a. Hypnotic, narcotic, or habit-forming drugs and their derivatives
   b. Drugs considered unsafe for unsupervised use because of their toxicity or the method by which they are administered
   c. New drugs considered unsafe for use by lay persons or those limited to investigational use
2. Refilling of prescriptions without authorization of the prescriber is prohibited.
3. Drugs limited to prescription use must be labeled "Caution: Federal Law prohibits dispensing without prescription."

Box 2-3. Provisions of the Kefauver-Harris Amendment of 1962

1. The Food and Drug Administration was empowered to supervise drug production to ensure good manufacturing practices. Included are requirements for:
   a. Annual registration of individuals and firms involved in the drug industry
   b. Inspection of every registered establishment at least every 2 years
   c. Withdrawal of approval of drugs when substantial doubt arises as to their safety or effectiveness
2. Statements in advertisements of prescription drugs must be truthful as to effectiveness, side-effects, and contraindications.
3. Manufacturers must report adverse reactions attributed to new drugs and antibiotics promptly to the government.
4. The effectiveness of new drugs must be established by substantial evidence before marketing.
5. Safety and effectiveness of all antibiotics for human use must be certified by the government.
6. Official names for drugs are to be established by the FDA.
7. Greater controls are to be exercised over investigational drugs, including adequate preclinical studies before testing on human subjects.

- *Probably effective:* Some evidence of effectiveness is available but it is insufficient to establish drug effectiveness.
- *Effective:* There is substantial evidence of effectiveness.
- *Effective but:* Although effective, there is a qualification or restriction imposed on the drug until completion of further studies, or the drug is effective for some recommended uses but not for all and hence a change in labeling is required.

Data acceptable as evidence of efficacy must be derived from well controlled scientific and clinical investigations by qualified experts. Observations or testimonials based on inadequate controls are not acceptable. Once evaluated, a drug must include its official rating on its label.

The federal government also collects data on reactions to drug therapy. Reports from health care professionals are accepted by the Division of Epidemiology and Drug Experience (HFD-210), FDA, 5600 Fishers Lane, Rockville, MD 20857 (see Appendix for Drug

Experience Report). Forms for the submission of reports are included in copies of the *FDA Drug Bulletin*, a publication of the United States Department of Health and Human Services. Reports from health care providers, especially physicians, have led to changes in the labeling of drugs by revealing adverse reactions not previously reported by manufacturers.

Legal requirements for safeguards during the development and production of drugs have tremendous impact on the drug industry (Fig. 2-1). The development of a new drug now takes 7–10 years and usually costs over $25 million. Approximately nine substances are investigated and rejected for every drug that is accepted. The return on research and development investments, estimated at 5% yearly, is inadequate to offset inflation. Such economic pressures can seriously inhibit drug research. Many small firms have discontinued their research and development programs. During the 1970s, declines in investments in the United States and increases in expenditures abroad indicated a flow of capital out of this country. By 1980, the number of new drugs developed yearly in the

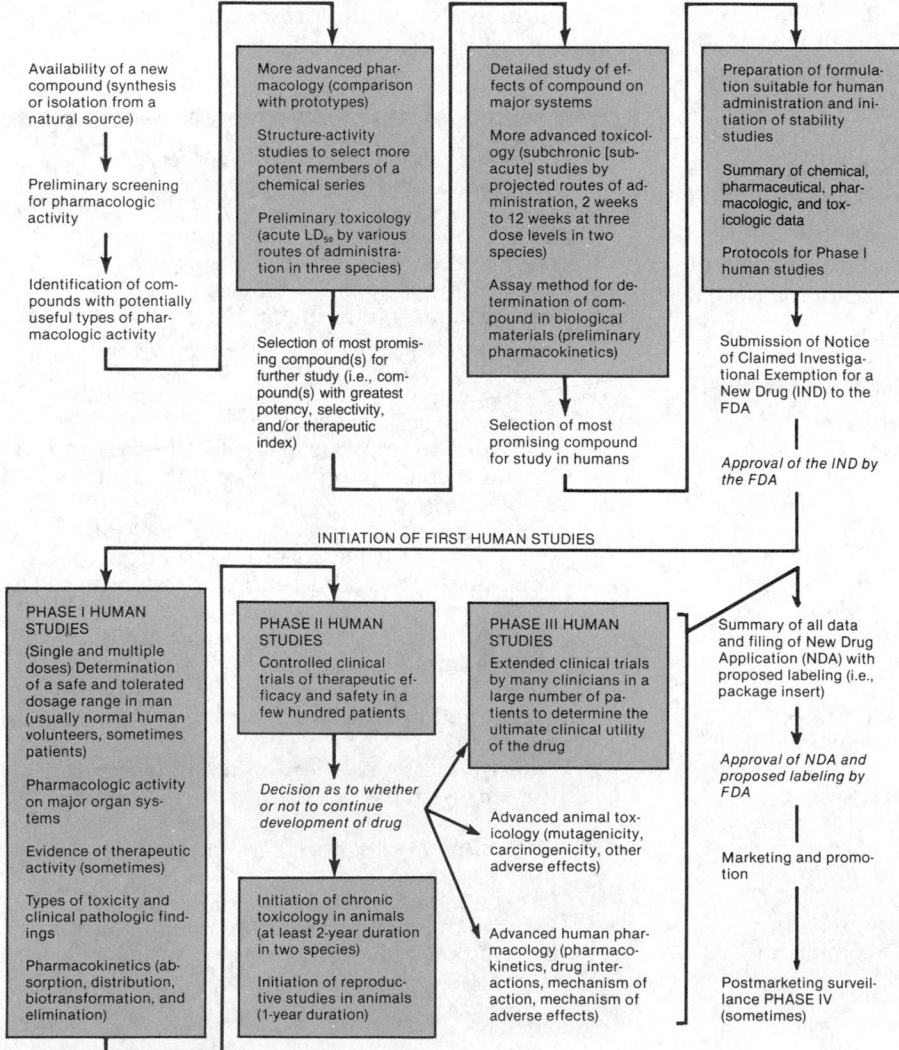

Figure 2-1. Steps in the development of new drugs illustrate some reasons for the high expense of drug research and for the long delays before drugs reach the market. (Bezoid C: The Future of Pharmaceuticals, p 9. New York, John Wiley and Sons, 1981; after Standaert FG: Department of Pharmacology, Georgetown University Schools of Medicine and Dentistry, Washington, DC.)

United States had declined to about 17, compared with 50–60 prior to 1962. Research and development were limited mainly to large companies in foreign countries, and the flow of new drugs into domestic markets slowed to a trickle. Since 1980, however, this trend has been reversed somewhat through streamlining of the Federal FDA testing and approval processes. More recently, in the case of drugs for the treatment of devastating conditions such as Alzheimer's disease or AIDS, large scale human trials have been allowed much earlier in the testing processes.

Drug abuse and drug dependence

In the 1960s, increasing public concern about the problems of drug abuse and drug dependence led to the passage of the Comprehensive Drug Abuse Prevention and Control Act of 1970 (also known as the Controlled Substances Act). This legislation not only outlined strict controls on the manufacture and distribution of habit-forming drugs, but it also established government programs to promote the prevention and treatment of drug dependence (Box 2-4).

Although specific procedures for the control of harmful drugs may be spelled out in more detail by state legislation, the Controlled Substances Act provides a basis in federal law for at least minimal administration of these regulations. Under this law, possession of a controlled substance without a written prescription is unlawful. Exceptions for possession are made to licensed personnel only when necessary for medical practice. Nurses and other professionals handling controlled substances such as narcotics must keep accurate, detailed records that account for each dose of these drugs. It is a crime to transfer any drug listed in schedules II, III, or IV to persons other than the client for whom the drug was ordered or prescribed. In many states, narcotics must not be administered except under the direction of a professional (physician or dentist) licensed to prescribe them. Unused narcotics must be returned to the source from which they were obtained (*eg*, the pharmacy) or to an office of the state agency responsible for narcotic regulation. Violation of the Controlled Substances Act is punishable by fine, imprisonment, or (for health professionals) revocation of the license to practice. Enforcement of the Controlled Substances Act is delegated to the Drug Enforcement Administration in the Department of Justice.

Legislation in Canada

Canadian drug laws include the Canadian Food and Drugs Act (originally passed in 1953 and amended yearly) and the Canadian Narcotic Control Act of 1961 (amended periodically).

The Canadian Food and Drugs Act provides for regulation of the manufacture and sale of drug substances (Box 2-5). Sale of drugs that are contaminated, adulterated, or unsafe for use is prohibited. Labels must not be false, misleading, or deceptive. Drugs must comply with the proposed standards under which they are sold or standards outlined in specific pharmacopeiae. No food, drug, cosmetic, or device may be advertised or sold as a treatment, prevention, or cure for alcoholism, arteriosclerosis, or cancer. The law provides for government supervision of the process and conditions of manufacture of some drugs. The act classifies drugs into groups with various degrees of control over distribution and sale. It also outlines requirements for labeling, proof of appropriate drug release from oral dose forms, and governmental powers to control the marketing of drugs in accordance with proof of effectiveness and safety.

The Canadian Narcotic Control Act of 1961 restricts the sale, possession, and use of opiates, coca, and marijuana. Amendments to the act have extended its controls to methadone. The law restricts possession of these drugs to authorized persons: licensed dealers, health care professionals, persons licensed to work with these materials for scientific purposes, members of the Royal Canadian Mounted Police (when necessary in connection with their employment), and persons for whom a narcotic drug is prescribed. Persons in possession of these drugs must ensure their security, promptly report any loss or theft, and maintain complete records of the disposition of the drugs. Narcotic drugs may be dispensed only upon prescription and must be labeled with the symbol *N*. Administration of The Canadian Narcotic Control Act is delegated by the Department of National Health and Welfare to the Royal Canadian Mounted Police.

Legal possession of narcotics by a nurse is limited to times when a drug is administered to a client according to a physician's order; when the nurse is acting as the custodian of narcotics in a health care agency; or when a narcotic has been prescribed for medical treatment of the nurse.

State controls

State laws regulating drugs must be compatible with federal laws. They may not refute any federal restrictions but may impose additional ones. The regulations of some states specify in great detail the procedures required for compliance with drug control legislation.

Some states have laws regulating the sale of drugs not controlled by federal legislation. For example, laws controlling the sale and use of alcoholic beverages vary from state to state as do the legal penalties for the possession, use, or sale of illegal drugs such as marijuana. Many states impose restrictions, similar to the national restrictions on opiates, on additional drugs, notably the barbiturates. In practical terms, this means that the specific drugs that have to be "counted" periodically in health care institutions vary from state to state. As evidence accumulates about the habit-forming potential of newer drugs such as diazepam and

Box 2-4. Provisions of the Controlled Substances Act of 1970

1. Definitions of drug dependence were established as follows:
   a. *Drug-dependent person:* "A person who is using a controlled substance (as defined in the Controlled Substances Act) and who is in a state of psychic or physical dependence, or both, arising from the use of that substance on a continuous basis. Drug dependence is characterized by behavioral and other responses, which include a strong compulsion to take the substance on a continuous basis in order to experience its psychic effects or to avoid the discomfort caused by its absence."
   b. *Drug addict:* "Any individual who habitually uses any narcotic drug so as to endanger the public morals, health, safety, or welfare, or who is so far addicted to the use of narcotic drugs as to have lost the power of self-control with reference to his addiction."
2. Funds were provided for:
   a. The development and dissemination of educational material on drug use and abuse
   b. The development and evaluation of programs for drug abuse education
   c. The development of treatment programs for drug-dependent persons
3. The Secretary of Health, Education and Welfare (now Health and Human Resources) was directed to work with professional groups to develop guidelines for treating narcotic addicts.
4. A Commission of Marihuana* and Drug Abuse was established to study marijuana use and abuse.
5. The authority and responsibility for drug controls by federal agencies was redistributed in the following manner:
   a. The responsibility for enforcing drug controls was transferred from the Treasury Department to the Department of Justice, under the Attorney General.
   b. The Department of Health, Education and Welfare was assigned responsibility for scientific evaluation of drugs and for final decisions on which drugs should be controlled.
6. All persons involved in experimentation with or the manufacturing and sale of controlled drugs were required to register with the Bureau of Narcotics and Dangerous Drugs. Controls were imposed to guard against diversion of controlled substances to unauthorized channels.
7. Controlled drugs were classified according to the following schedules:
   a. Schedule I: drugs that currently do not have accepted medical use, have a high potential for abuse, and lack accepted safety measures for use (*eg*, LSD, peyote, heroin)
   b. Schedule II: drugs that have medical use and a high potential for abuse; those that tend to cause severe dependence (*eg*, morphine, secobarbital, amphetamines, methadone)
   c. Schedule III: drugs used in medical practice with less potential for abuse than schedule II drugs; those that tend to cause moderate or low physical dependence or high psychologic dependence (*eg*, nalorphine, drug combinations containing small amounts of narcotics such as codeine)
   d. Schedule IV: drugs that have medical use and lower potential for abuse than schedule III drugs; those that tend to cause limited physical or psychologic dependence (*eg*, meprobamate, chlordiazepoxide, diazepam)
   e. Schedule V: drugs that have medical use and lower potential for abuse than schedule IV drugs; those that tend to cause less physical or psychologic dependence (*eg*, mixtures of limited quantities of narcotics such as cough syrups containing codeine)
8. Prescriptions of controlled drugs were regulated as follows:
   a. Each prescription must include recipient's full name and address, the date, and the name, address, registration number, and signature of the practitioner issuing it.
   b. Prescriptions dispensed to nonhospitalized clients must be labeled with date of filling, pharmacy name and address, serial number of prescription, prescribing practitioner's name, directions for use, and cautionary statements.
   c. Prescriptions for schedule II drugs can be filled only once; refills are prohibited; for hospitalized patients, not more than 7 days' supply may be dispensed at one time. Possession of schedule II drugs by institutionalized patients prior to administration is prohibited.
   d. Prescriptions for schedule III and IV drugs are limited to five refills. These prescriptions expire 6 months after the date of issue. For hospitalized patients not more than a 33 days' supply or 100 dosage units (whichever is less) is to be dispensed at one time and possession by the institutionalized patient prior to administration is prohibited.
   e. Prescriptions for schedule V drugs can be refilled as authorized on the prescription.
   f. Records of the recipient and dispensing of controlled drugs must be kept (and made available to authorized persons) by pharmacists for a period of at least 2 years.

*The alternative spelling of marijuana was used in the legislation.

Box 2-5. Major Provisions of the Canadian Food and Drugs Act

1. The sale of contaminated, adulterated, or unsafe drugs is prohibited.
2. The sale of drugs whose labels are false, misleading, or deceptive is prohibited.
3. Drugs must comply with professed standards under which they are sold, or the standards prescribed by recognized pharmacopeiae and formularies. Recognized compendia include *Pharmacopoeia Internationalis, The British Pharmacopoeia, The United States Pharmacopeia, Pharmacopée Française, The Canadian Formulary,* the *British Pharmaceutical Codex,* and the *Compendium of Pharmaceuticals and Specialties.*
4. The process and conditions of manufacture of such drugs as parenteral and radioactive preparations must be approved before the medicines may be sold.
5. Safety approval of batches is required for such drugs as arsphenamines and sensitivity disks and tablets.
6. The sale of certain drugs (*eg* thalidomide) can be forbidden absolutely.
7. Certain drugs such as antibiotics, hormones, and tranquilizers can be sold only on prescription; refills must be specified by the prescriber and are limited to a period of 6 months. The symbol PR must be placed on containers of these drugs to designate that a prescription is required.
8. Certain drugs (amphetamines, barbiturates, methaqualone, pentazocine, and phenmetrazine) are termed *controlled*; prescriptions cannot be refilled unless the refills are ordered on the original prescription, with specific directions for time intervals between refills.
9. The prescription of certain drugs is limited to use in specific conditions unless special permission is obtained. Such "designated" drugs include amphetamines and metrazines. Their uses are limited to the treatment of narcolepsy, hyperkinesis in children, minimal brain dysfunction, epilepsy, parkinsonism, and anesthesia-induced shock.
10. The sale of hallucinogens is prohibited but research on them is allowed by qualified investigators authorized by the Minister of Health and Welfare.
11. Sample drugs may be distributed only to duly licensed individuals (physicians, dentists, or pharmacists).
12. Prescription and controlled drugs cannot be advertised to the general public.
13. The information required to be on the labels of drugs is delineated.
14. Specific regulations to control the safety and efficacy of certain drugs or drug doses are described.

---

pentazocine, more drugs are likely to be added to these lists.

In many states, drug control agencies spell out in detail the procedures required for compliance. Their regulations may specify such things as the number of locks required on narcotic storage areas in hospital units; the number of people allowed access to such storage areas; the information required on controlled drug records; and even the type of signature required on drug count sheets. To administer state regulations, agents inspect establishments handling controlled substances. These inspections may be more frequent than federal inspections and are usually at times other than those conducted by federal officials.

Local regulations

County and town (borough) regulations of drugs usually involve restrictions on the sale or use of alcohol or tobacco. Some areas (so-called dry towns or counties) prohibit the sale of alcoholic beverages. In a few areas, the sale of cigarettes and other tobacco products is forbidden. In the opinion of the author, these restrictions rarely are effective in controlling the use of these substances because the substances are readily available in nearby towns or counties.

Institutional controls

The policies of health care institutions on the handling and control of drug substances may vary greatly. They must conform to federal, state, and local regulations in effect at any given time. Institutional policies generally are more restrictive than these governmental controls. They are designed to prevent health problems stemming from drug use and to minimize technical violations of existing drug controls. For example, many health care institutions adopt policies requiring periodic renewal of orders for drugs not controlled by state or federal law. Commonly, orders for antibiotics or corticosteroids are discontinued automatically after a certain number of days of treatment (often 10–14 days). Such policies help to prevent problems of drug-resistant infections or toxic syndromes that tend to develop with prolonged medication regimens. Physicians may continue medication by renewing the order but it is less likely that drug treatment will be inadvertently prolonged. As another example, in states with laws requiring a renewal of narcotic orders for hospitalized patients every 72 hours, hospital policy may require renewal every other day. This prevents lapsing of the order, which could occur with a 3-day renewal policy if a physician orders the drug early in the first day but renews it at a later hour on the third day.

Individual control

At a personal and family level, client practices influence drug use greatly. These are established in accord with personal beliefs about and attitudes toward drug use. By giving or withholding consent to treatment and by complying or not complying with the drug regimen, the individual exerts the final control on drug use.

■ **Summary**

All societies develop controls of drug use. The earliest controls from religious practices and social mores continue to influence the use of chemicals today. Formal controls range from simple institutional policies to government legislation (local, state, provincial, national, and international). Generally, restrictions become more severe as the unit of administration becomes smaller. In the long run, the client has final control over personal drug use.

Nursing implications

Nurses must be familiar with regulations affecting drug use in the particular area in which they practice. When moving from one legal jurisdiction to another, the nurse should study information about current laws in the new area. If this material is not available in public or health care institution libraries, it may be obtained from the institution pharmacy or directly from the state drug control agency.

Practicing nurses can keep informed on changes in state regulations through consultation with officials from the state regulatory agency. In-service programs for staff personnel in health care agencies should be held periodically to reinforce and update employee knowledge of regulatory requirements. As part of their educative function, state officials may be willing to participate in such programs. Nurses also must know the policies of the institution or agency in which they work. Policies may vary greatly from institution to institution.

Nurses must abide by the drug control laws within their professional practices. When advising clients on the use of drugs, they must not recommend the use of illegal substances or provide drugs for clients' use without the proper authorization (order or prescription). The security of drugs must be maintained at all times to prevent diversion to unauthorized persons. For example, in health care institutions, medications are commonly locked during storage; some drugs must be kept under double locks. While handling medications, the nurse should keep unlocked drugs under direct observation and control. Careful records must be maintained of the disposition of each dose of certain drugs such as opiates. Similar precautions must be maintained in the community setting (Schaffner & Dietrich, 1986). Although nurses are involved in the handling and administration of controlled substances

when functioning as health care professionals, this privilege does not extend to their nonprofessionals lives. When not necessary for professional practice, the possession of such drugs or drug paraphernalia without a personal prescription is as much of a crime for the nurse as for any lay citizen. In addition to the usual penalties for such a drug offense, the nurse's license to practice may be suspended or revoked.

The client has final control on drug use; it is the client who gives or withholds consent to treatment and who finally determines compliance. Therefore, it is especially important for health care personnel to ascertain the client's drug attitudes and practices during assessment; to tailor the regimen of care accordingly (or explain carefully the need to change old habits); and to give clear explanations and descriptions of drug regimens. The nurse must respect the competent client's refusal of treatment including drug therapy.

Learning experience 2-1

Examine the policy and procedure manuals at a hospital or nursing home to determine drug controls in effect in that health care setting. Compare these requirements with those imposed by the state or provincial government. Which policies represent controls that are stricter than state or provincial requirements? Are any of them required by county or town ordinance? Pay particular attention to policies regarding automatic expiration of drug orders, security measures for controlled drugs, and recording of the disposition of narcotics.

Drug standards

Standards are the yardsticks by which drug preparations are judged. In primitive societies, the potency and safety of drug preparations depended on the skill of the preparer. Techniques for preparing and handling potions were transmitted by word of mouth through an apprentice system. The practitioner had no way to purify preparations and few methods for measuring their potency. Modern technology provides elaborate techniques for determining the chemical composition and biologic effects of drugs, and for defining standards of purity and efficacy.

Role functions related to drug use, which are largely established by law, are discussed in Chapter 13.

Standards for drug quality are generally established and enforced by the government. Many standards are outlined in the official pharmacopeiae (in the United States, *The United States Pharmacopeia and National Formulary*). Others are established by bureaucratic regulation.

Medicines can vary considerably in their purity,

Table 2-1. Properties of drugs controlled by standards of quality

Property	Summary of pertinent information
Purity	1. A truly pure drug contains only one specific chemical agent. Pure drugs are rarely attainable. 2. Additives may be needed to facilitate formulation or manipulate absorption. 3. Dusts or other contaminants from the environment may enter the substance. 4. The kind and concentration of extraneous substances allowed are specified by standards of purity.
Potency	1. Potency is generally dependent on the concentration of active drug in the medicinal preparation. 2. When active ingredients are unknown, potency is measured by testing in animals (bioassay). 3. When active ingredients are known, potency is measured by chemical assay.
Bioavailability	1. The degree that a drug can be absorbed and transported by the body to its active site determines bioavailability. 2. Factors influencing bioavailability include particle size, crystalline structure, solubility, and polarity. 3. Blood or tissue concentrations at a specified time following administration are commonly used to measure bioavailability.
Efficacy	1. The effectiveness of the drug in promoting desirable clinical changes is called efficacy. 2. Objective measures are rarely available for determining efficacy; data are usually interpreted subjectively. 3. Double-blind studies are needed to establish efficacy as distinguished from placebo effect.
Safety/toxicity	1. The incidence and severity of adverse reactions attributable to the use of a drug determines the safety of that drug. 2. No active chemical is free of toxicity. 3. The difference between therapeutic and toxic dosages determines the margin of safety of a substance. 4. When considering use of a drug, its adverse reactions must be weighed against its benefits.

strength, bioavailability, efficacy, and safety or toxicity. To be effective, standards for these or other properties must provide a method for measuring the attribute to be evaluated, as well as an acceptable level or range for these measurements. These standards are discussed in the following text and summarized in Table 2-1.

Purity

A truly pure drug is one that contains only one specific chemical agent and no contaminating ingredients. Few substances sold on the open market approach this level of purity. (Interestingly, the white dextrose sugar available in grocery stores is one that does.)

Impurities from the raw materials used for manufacturing drugs often remain in medicinal materials. Even if a pure substance is developed during the production process, it may be necessary to add other ingredients to the chemical to facilitate formulation of a dose form or to manipulate the absorption process. Such additives include solvents, fillers, disintegrators, buffers, waxes, dyes, inks, and plastics. In addition, dusts and other contaminants from the environment of the production plant may find their way into a batch of drugs. Standards for purity, therefore, rarely require that the substance in question be 100% drug chemical. Instead, they tend to specify the type and concentration of extraneous substances allowed to be present in the drug product.

Potency

The strength (potency) of a drug is measured by assay techniques. Chemical analysis is used when possible to determine the ingredients present in a preparation

and their relative amounts. Chemical analysis cannot be applied to preparations whose active ingredients are unknown, or if there are no available techniques for measuring those ingredients. In such cases, the relative strengths of various preparations are determined by testing in laboratory animals. Standards are established by specifying a definite, measurable effect on a suitable laboratory animal as the "unit" of measurement (bioassay). When reliable chemical tests become available for drugs measured by bioassay, chemical analysis is usually adopted and the substance is labeled in terms of absolute measure of the active ingredient. Common drugs still marketed in preparations whose strengths are measured in biologic units include insulin and heparin. Penicillin, which was originally assayed biologically, is now usually measured in milligram doses.

Bioavailability

Bioavailability is the degree to which a drug can be absorbed and transported by the body to its site of action. It may be influenced by particle size, crystalline structure, solubility, and polarity of the drug compound. Bioavailability is commonly measured by blood or tissue concentration of the drug at a specified time following administration of a dose. In the past, bioavailability has not been well standardized. However, a concerted effort is now being made by scientists, drug manufacturers, and government agencies to develop reliable tests of this property. Mass spectrometry, presently used most commonly for the study of physiologic biochemistry, is one promising technique.

Efficacy

Efficacy, the effectiveness of a drug in treatment, is difficult to measure in absolute terms. Animal studies provide some objective data for certain drugs. Clinical trials compare the clinical progress of people given the drug against that of others given placebos or against reference standards. Such trials must be carefully controlled to generate reliable data. Because clinical status is not always measurable in objective terms, and the desirability of various clinical responses involves value judgments, interpretation of such data is, by necessity, often subjective.

Safety/toxicity

Safety (or its opposite, toxicity) is measured by the incidence and severity of reported adverse reactions following the use of a drug. As with efficacy, controlled tests are required to generate data pertinent to this quality. Some harmful effects (*eg*, carcinogenicity) may not appear in the recipient until considerable time has elapsed. For this reason, a complete assessment of safety or toxicity is not always possible before a new medicine is marketed. Safety standards are in the process of evolution. They are being continuously clarified as the deficiencies of past standards become apparent and new techniques for measurement are developed.

Testing procedures

Standards for drug quality depend on testing procedures. Insofar as possible, these tests should be quick, easy to perform, economical, and valid for the uses of the drug substance to be tested (Table 2-2). Chemical assays, when available, are usually economical in cost and time. Bioassays are more costly and time-consuming. Clinical trials tend to be both expensive and lengthy. Tests for efficacy and safety performed on animals or other laboratory models may not be valid as possible human responses. For example, a test for mutagenicity performed on bacterial cultures (the Ames test) is believed to reflect carcinogenicity in humans. However, the degree to which it actually does so has not been proven conclusively.

■ Summary

Drug preparations are evaluated in the light of standards for purity, potency, bioavailability, efficacy, and safety or toxicity. Procedures for testing drugs may involve chemical assay, bioassay, or trials on laboratory models, animals, and human subjects. When available, chemical assays tend to be the most reasonable of the three tests. Not only are they highly valid, but they also are the least costly and time-consuming to perform.

Nursing implications

To interpret drug data intelligently, nurses must be familiar with the significance of each property and the limitations of the testing procedures used to measure it. Generally, pure drugs are more easily controlled in terms of dosage, and they generate fewer side-effects. Bioavailability may vary from one trade name preparation to another of the same generic drug; low bioavailability may lead to treatment failure.

Nurses must evaluate therapeutic response in clients receiving medication. Response not related to placebo effect (a response to *any* treatment received with an expectation of improvement) reflects the drug's efficacy. Adverse or toxic effects must be monitored also, especially when drugs used have a narrow margin of safety (low therapeutic index). The earlier adverse reactions are diagnosed, the easier it is to treat them.

Nurses are sometimes involved in clinical trials of experimental drugs on human subjects. In such a situation, meticulous assessment of clients is required: 1) to protect clients from serious harm stemming from their exposure to unproven drugs; and 2) to generate valid data for evaluation of the experimental drugs. Usually, in clinical trials, some clients are given the active drug while others receive a placebo or reference standard. Before giving permission to be included in a clinical trial of this sort, clients must be aware that they may be given an inactive substance instead of the experimental drug. Neither the subjects nor the staff conducting the trials know which clients receive which

Table 2-2. Advantages and disadvantages of testing procedures for drug quality

Test	Advantage	Disadvantage
Ideal test	*Quick, easy to perform, economical, valid*	
Chemical assays	Usually objective, reasonable in time and cost involvement	Results are not always available.
Bioassays	Allow assessment of potency of substances of unknown composition	Tests are costly and time-consuming.
Tests on animals or lab models	Pose no risk to human subjects	Results may not be valid in humans.
Clinical trials	Yield data relative to effects on human subjects	Tests are expensive, lengthy, and involve risk to human subjects.

substance (hence the *double-blind* designation applied to such trials). Security of the information identifying the experimental and control subjects must be maintained until data collection is complete or else the validity of the results may be compromised.

References

Schaffner AT, Dieterich D. (1986). Streetwise narcotic safety: Precautions in home care. *American Journal of Nursing, 86,* 707–708.

Bibliography

Food and Drugs Act and Regulation, 1972, with Amendments to Food and Drugs Act and Regulation to January 1982.

(1982). Department of National Health and Welfare. Ottawa: Queen's Printer and Controller of Stationery.

Kleist T. (1986). Biotech rules receive scrutiny. *Science News, 130,* 71.

Lasagna L. (1983). Discovering adverse drug reactions. *JAMA, 249,* 2224.

Narcotic Control Act and the Narcotic Control Regulations. (1982). Department of National Health and Welfare. Ottawa: Queen's Printer and Controller of Stationery.

Navarra T. (1990). Drug therapy: The history of a love affair. *American Journal of Nursing 90,* 91.

Ninety-first Congress. Public Law 91–513. (1972). Washington, DC: US Government Printing Office.

*Silverman A, Lee PR. (1974). *Pills, profits and politics.* Los Angeles: University of California Press.

*Recommended for further reading.

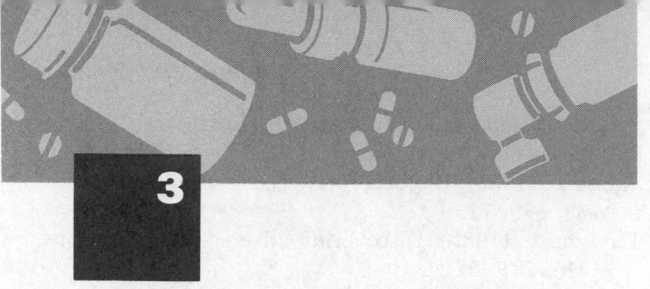

3

Nursing process in the management of clients with drug-related problems

Assessment
  Data base
    History
    Physical examination
  Analysis
    Contraindications
    Precautions
    Drug interactions
    Adverse reactions
    Tolerance and dependence
    Compliance ability
    Need for teaching
Nursing diagnosis
Planning
Intervention
Evaluation

The primary concern of nurses is the health care of individual clients and families. It is important that nurses understand the impact of exposure to chemicals—both medicinal and nonmedicinal—on health. Medicinal substances include prescription and over-the-counter drugs, and home and herbal remedies. Nonmedicinal substances that can affect health include social and illegal drugs, pollutants, and poisons. The nurse uses the nursing process to promote optimal response to chemicals; to decrease the risk of adverse reactions; and to assist clients in achieving optimal health through the proper use of drugs.

This chapter deals primarily with the nursing process, which treats human responses to changes in health status, specifically, the independent function of the nurse in treating clients receiving prescription drugs. Dependent nursing functions related to drug therapy are numerous, and responsibilities relating to them may be critical, particularly in institutional settings. However, these aspects of care are addressed in Chapter 13, Basic Principles of Medication.

The nursing process provides the framework for logical, scientific problem solving in nursing care. This process involves the following steps: assessment, diagnosis, planning, intervention, and evaluation (Box 3-1). The same process is applicable to the care of clients receiving prescription medications, to those using nonprescription drugs, and to those exposed to nonmedicinal chemicals.

Assessment

Data base

History

Initial assessment of the client who is to receive drug therapy involves taking a drug history and evaluating the client's physical and psychological responses to previous drug exposure. The scope of the drug history varies with the setting and situation. A complete history includes the following: 1) data about the chemicals to which the client is currently exposed; 2) chemical use and contacts in the past; 3) responses to drug use and chemical exposure; 4) practices for handling and storing chemical materials; 5) precautions for minimizing the risk of poisoning or other adverse reactions; 6) problems perceived by the client as being chemically related; and 7) the client's attitude toward the use of chemicals including drugs. In a given situation, the particular aspects to be included depend on the circumstances. For example, when treating a client for drug overdose, the most important information to obtain is what substance or substances the individual took. Most other data are irrelevant until the emergency situation is resolved. Data about the conditions of drug storage may not be pertinent in an institutional setting but would be in the home. Information related to self-dosage might not be pertinent in settings where medications are administered by professionals. Occupational exposure would be important when assessing noninstitutionalized adults.

The nurse should consider such questions as the following: What drugs have been used in the past? For what purposes? How frequently? In what dosages? With what success? What problems occurred? Which drugs were prescribed by a physician or dentist? Which were self-prescribed? What nonmedicinal drugs has the client used in the past or is using currently? How often? In what quantities? What happens when habitual use of a substance is interrupted? Use of alcohol, tobacco, caffeine, and illegal substances should be assessed specifically.

Box 3-1. The nursing process in drug therapy

1. Assessment
   a. Drug history (specific aspects vary with the situation)
      (1) Previous drug use
         (a) Prescription drugs ordered to treat illness
         (b) Self-prescribed drug substances
         (c) Nonmedicinal drugs and chemicals
         (d) Drugs taken within the recent past
      (2) Responses to drug use
         (a) Therapeutic response
         (b) Adverse reactions
         (c) Idiosyncratic reactions
         (d) Allergic reactions
         (e) Tolerance and dependence
      (3) Family history of unusual drug reactions
         (a) Idiosyncratic
         (b) Allergic
      (4) Attitudes toward drugs and their use
   b. Analysis
      (1) Identification of contraindications for drug use, or factors indicating the need for unusual caution
      (2) Evaluation of the risk of undesirable drug interactions
      (3) Assessment of physical and psychologic responses to previous drug exposure
      (4) Comparison of drug data and client data to identify potential problems in the planned drug regimen
      (5) Evaluation of factors affecting administration of drugs or self-medication by the client
      (6) Comparison of the client's knowledge base with the knowledge needed for optimal participation in the drug regimen
      (7) Evaluation of the client's attitude toward drug use.
2. Nursing Diagnosis
   a. Identification of actual problems arising from the drug regimen
   b. Identification of potential problems arising from the drug regimen
3. Planning
   a. Objectives of nursing care
      (1) Prevention of drug-related problems
      (2) Amelioration of symptoms
      (3) Correction of abnormal states
      (4) Improvement of function
   b. Goals
      (1) Minimization of side-effects
      (2) Prevention of drug dependence
      (3) Prompt detection and treatment of adverse reactions to drugs
      (4) Withdrawal from a dependency-producing chemical
      (5) Reduction in (or promotion of) drug use
4. Intervention
   a. Psychologic care measures
   b. Physical care measures
   c. Consultation with physician or pharmacist regarding changes in the drug regimen
   d. Client teaching
5. Evaluation
   a. Collection of evaluative data
   b. Comparison of evaluative data with predetermined, measurable criteria for success

Clients may be reluctant to give information about social or illegal use of drugs. If questions relating to specific drugs are left until near the end of the interview, the client may have developed enough trust in the nurse to provide candid answers. The sequential listing of drugs should proceed from medicinal substances and generally accepted drug practices to more sensitive topics, leaving illegal and generally unacceptable drug practices to the last. Throughout the interview, the nurse should maintain a uniform, matter-of-fact, nonjudgmental demeanor. Some clients might respond more freely if they are asked to complete a written questionnaire.

How does the client feel about the use of drugs? The client's expressed attitude should be compared with the nurse's objective assessment of the client's emotional response during the taking of the drug history. Heavy use of or dependence on drugs may not be admitted freely, owing to the social stigma attached to such behavior.

The nursing history also should thoroughly explore allergies and diseases that have affected the client. The drugs used and the symptoms for which they were taken offer clues to previous and present illnesses. Much of this data also appears in the general nursing history and may be duplicated by the physician. Comparison of the nursing and medical histories often reveals discrepancies indicating that one or both histories may be incomplete or inaccurate. Clients may relate information to the nurse that they would hesitate to reveal to the physician about alterations of drug dosage schedules, use of proprietary drugs, obsolete prescriptions, home remedies, "borrowed" prescriptions, or drugs ordered by other physicians.

Physical examination

During examination of the client, the nurse should be alert to findings related to previous exposure to drugs or reactions to present medications. If a new drug regimen or a change in drug orders is anticipated, specific data pertinent to the substances involved should be gathered.

The data may include contraindications for the use of specific drugs. These must always be reported to the physician responsible for prescribing drugs. Although the primary responsibility for determining the appropriateness of the prescription rests with the physician, the nurse who is aware of a contraindication and does not inform the physician will share the blame if harm results.

Analysis

Data from the history and examination are analyzed to determine actual and potential problems related to drug use. Conditions or circumstances that are contraindications for drugs in use or under consideration and factors requiring dosage alterations or precautionary measures should be identified. Although the primary responsibility for these safeguards rests with the physician, the nurse is also responsible for evaluating the risks involved in administration of specific drugs. The nurse should also consider whether the client needs assistance in carrying out the prescribed drug regimen, how the client's attitude is likely to influence the use of drugs, and if there is a need for teaching related to the drug regimen.

Contraindications

Certain conditions often preclude the use of specific drugs. The contraindications are listed among the data in drug references. Predisposition to serious adverse reactions common to the drug, specific disease conditions, organ impairment, and pregnancy and lactation are frequently cited as contraindications. Pertinent drug data and assessment data should be compared to determine whether the drugs in question are likely to be safe for the client to use.

Precautions

Persons with impaired organ systems involved in the metabolism and excretion of drugs may require reduced doses or preferential selection of drugs that are eliminated by the system or systems in best condition. The nurse should compare the assessment data with the pharmacokinetics* of the medications to determine whether the client is likely to have difficulty in eliminating drugs. Medications that may remain in the body longer than usual and pose a risk of toxicity should be identified.

Specific precautions are also listed in data on drugs. The client's data base should be compared with data on the medications to determine what precautions are needed to safeguard the client. As an example, glucocorticoids are not administered for long periods to individuals with a history of exposure to tuberculosis unless prophylactic antimycobacterial drugs

*These are the processes by which chemicals enter the body, circulate through the tissues, are stored and metabolized by the body, and are subsequently eliminated through excretory pathways.

are administered to prevent active infection. A client with a history of arrested tuberculosis or a positive tuberculin or tine test reaction would be at risk for active infection if prednisone were prescribed without concurrent anti-infective treatment.

Drug interactions

Certain drug combinations pose obvious risks of adverse interactions. If the list of substances to be considered is long, analysis by a pharmacist may be required. Drugs that have been taken in the recent past, as well as current medications, must be included because residues of drugs previously used may interact with newly prescribed medications.

Adverse reactions

Information regarding usual response to drugs should be studied to determine whether the client has experienced adverse reactions such as allergies, toxicities, or failure of therapeutic effect. When the client's history is negative but there is a positive family history, this should be considered as suggestive of potential problems. Responses to drugs are affected by body metabolism, biochemistry, integrity of organ function, and allergic tendencies. These variables are heavily influenced by genetic factors, and a family history of adverse reactions to certain chemicals should alert health care personnel to increased risk of adverse reactions if these or related compounds are prescribed.

Tolerance and dependence

Data on response to drugs should be evaluated for evidence of tolerance or dependence. Either one can affect the client's response to related substances and influence the choice of drugs appropriate for treatment. Clients with an existing dependence will experience alterations in function if drugs are withdrawn. For those who have recovered from dependence, repeated use of the substances involved may cause renewed dependence.

Compliance ability

Factors influencing the ability of the client to carry out a prescribed regimen include emotional acceptance of the need for drug therapy; financial resources to pay for the prescriptions; physical and mental abilities necessary for proper administration of medications; knowledge of what constitutes appropriate self-care; and functional capacity to make adjustments required for management of the regimen. The success of a drug program may hinge on obscure data such as difficulty in swallowing or inability to manipulate bottle caps or medication syringes.

Need for teaching

As soon as drug therapy is prescribed, the nurse should compare the client's knowledge about the drugs involved with the knowledge required for carrying out the desired regimen. Discrepancies between

(Text continues on p. 27)

Model nursing care plan illustrating use of the nursing process

ASSESSMENT

Selected data from the nursing history and examination

The client, Thomas, is a 17-year-old high school student with retinitis following thermal injury to both eyes resulting from an attempt to view an eclipse of the sun through sunglasses. The physician has prescribed prednisone, 40 mg every other day. The drug treatment is expected to last for 6 months to 1 year. Thomas' growth and development is essentially normal. He is 5 feet 6 inches tall and weighs 150 pounds. (His father and older brother are both over 6 feet tall.) Thomas denies taking drugs except for a daily multivitamin table (maintenance strength) and an occasional dose of aspirin (10 grains) for minor aches and pains, mainly headaches. He has had no allergic or other adverse reactions to drugs; family history is also negative for drug reactions. One aunt has diabetes mellitus. Thomas states that he "eats everything and likes food from fast food restaurants (hamburgers and milk shakes)."

Thomas likes sail boating and spends much time studying and playing the saxophone. He does not engage in competitive sports but participates regularly in extracurricular activities (club and social events) at school. He also is active in the "big brother" program of the local boys' club. His "little brother" has been ill recently and is being treated for tuberculosis.

Thomas states that the physician discussed prednisone treatment with him and his parents, and he understands that the drug may limit further growth in height. He remarks, "That is a small price to pay to safeguard my sight." He also states that he knows nothing about prednisone except that it will help to limit his loss of vision.

Selected data on prednisone from drug references

Prednisone is a glucocorticoid anti-inflammatory drug used to control harmful inflammation and minimize scar formation. Usual adult dosage is 5–60 mg daily; alternate-day regimens usually provide for 2 days' dosage to be taken as a single dose every other day. The drug is dispensed as oral tablets. It is metabolized by the liver and excreted through the kidneys.

Side-effects and toxic effects of prednisone include the following:

Fluid and electrolyte imbalance (retention of sodium and water and depletion of body potassium)
Hypertension related to hypervolemia
Hyperglycemia (diabetes mellitus in susceptible individuals)
Peptic ulcers in susceptible individuals
Changes in fat distribution (sometimes causing "moon face" or "buffalo hump")
Negative nitrogen balance (protein loss, striae, skeletal muscle atrophy, and osteoporosis)
Immunosuppression
Inhibition of cell division (stunting of growth, delayed healing)
Increased coagulability of blood (with increased risk or thromboemboli)
Central nervous system stimulation
Inhibition of the pituitary secretion of corticotropin causing adrenal atrophy

Among the precautions and contraindications are the following:

Glucocorticoids are contraindicated for growing children unless the benefits of therapy outweigh the risk of stunting of growth.
Individuals with a history of exposure to tuberculosis should be given concomitant anti-mycobacterial therapy.
Recipients with diabetes mellitus should be monitored carefully for glucose imbalance and those at high risk for this disease should be monitored for signs and symptoms of diabetes mellitus.
Prophylactic antiulcer therapy should be considered for individuals susceptible to peptic ulcer.

Analysis

Because Thomas has not yet completed his adolescent growth spurt, the administration of prednisone may prevent him from attaining the maximum height he otherwise would. Thomas has discussed this with the physician and his parents and has accepted it as necessary for the protection of his sight. However, this may be only the first of several factors disturbing to his self-image. As drug therapy progresses, changes characteristic of glucocorticoid excess (so-called cushingoid appearance) are likely to develop. In addition to his altered physical appearance, Thomas may find his emotional affect changing in inappropriate ways in response to the stimulating effects of the drug.

Prednisone treatment will reduce Thomas' natural protection against infection. He also has had a recent exposure to tuberculosis and could be harboring an initial infection.

The ulcerogenic property of prednisone will act synergistically with that of aspirin to increase Thomas' risk of peptic ulcer.

(Continued)

Model nursing care plan illustrating use of the nursing process (continued)

Because of a family history of diabetes mellitus, Thomas is at increased risk for the development of this disease while on prednisone treatment. Other adverse reactions likely to develop as a result of the drug regimen include hypertension, hypokalemia, which predisposes to constipation, and weakening of the bones.

Because his muscles will tend to atrophy and weaken, Thomas may have problems with muscle coordination. If an accident occurs, his weakened bones would be more vulnerable than normally to fractures. Fat embolus, a complication of long-bone fractures, could be especially serious in Thomas because of the increased coagulability of his blood. Healing of wounds will be delayed. Therefore, Thomas is at increased risk for accidental injury and for complications of such injuries.

Prednisone is stimulating to the central nervous system and may cause difficulty in sleeping, especially on the day the medication is taken.

Thomas will be receiving glucocorticoid therapy in large doses for a prolonged period of time. Because prednisone inhibits pituitary production of ACTH, atrophy of the adrenal glands will probably occur. This produces a physiologic dependence on the drug and reduces the body's compensatory response to stress.

Thomas' health care practices appear to have been adequate but will need to be changed to help prevent complications from the drug therapy. He knows little about the drug he will receive.

NURSING DIAGNOSIS Nursing diagnoses arising from the preceding analysis include:*

1. Situational low self-esteem related to physical and mental changes secondary to prednisone therapy
2. High risk for infection related to altered immune response secondary to prednisone therapy
3. Fluid volume excess related to sodium and water retention secondary to prednisone therapy.
4. Constipation related to hypokalemia secondary to prednisone therapy
5. High risk for injury related to musculoskeletal changes secondary to prednisone therapy
6. Sleep pattern disturbance related to central nervous system stimulation secondary to prednisone therapy
7. Pain: epigastric discomfort related to hyperacidity secondary to use of prednisone and aspirin
8. Knowledge deficit concerning:
   a. Adverse reactions likely to develop with prednisone therapy
   b. Hygiene measures to decrease the risk of adverse reactions
   c. Health supervision and monitoring
   d. Management of the dosage regimen

PLANNING **Objective of nursing care**
1. Maintenance of positive self-image
   Goals:
   a. Continued participation by Thomas in social activities appropriate to his age and comparable to his former activities
   b. Maintenance of a positive self-concept throughout drug therapy
2. Freedom from serious infection
   Goals:
   a. Knowledge of risk factors that are associated with potential for infection are demonstrated by Thomas
   b. Precautions to prevent infection are practiced by Thomas
3. Maintenance of normal fluid and electrolyte balance and nutrient metabolism
   Goals:
   a. Maintenance of normal sodium and water balance
   b. Knowledge of causative factors and methods of preventing edema are demonstrated by Thomas
4. Prevention of constipation; Prompt treatment of constipation should it develop
   Goals:
   a. Absence of discomfort from fecal elimination
   b. Prompt resolution of constipation, should it develop
5. Prevention of serious injury especially skeletal fractures
   Goals:
   a. Promotion of muscle and bone strength through establishment of a regular exercise regimen.
   b. Increase in Thomas' safety awareness and improvement in his safety practices

*Collaborative problems that should be differentiated from the nursing diagnoses include the following: Potential complications: cardiac/vascular, hyperglycemia, hypernatremia, hypokalemia, immunodeficiency, GI bleeding, pathologic fractures.

(Continued)

Model nursing care plan illustrating use of the nursing process (continued)

6. Maintenance of adequate rest and sleep
   Goal:
   a. Maintenance of average daily sleep equal to Thomas' usual duration of sleep
7. Prevention/prompt treatment of epigastric discomfort (heartburn)
   Goals:
   a. Absence of heartburn
   b. Prompt treatment of heartburn should it occur
8. Knowledge deficit: inadequate information about:
   a. Adverse reactions likely to develop with prednisone therapy
   b. Hygienic measures to decrease the risk of adverse reactions
   c. Health supervision and monitoring
   d. Management of the dosage regimen

INTERVENTIONS

In relation to Nursing Diagnosis 1

1. Establish good rapport with Thomas, conveying warm acceptance of him as a person.
2. Compliment him appropriately on his appearance and accomplishments.
3. Refer him for advice concerning personal grooming and attire if changes in appearance cause a decrease in physical attractiveness (*eg*, hair styling to minimize the round appearance of the face, clothes that will make body contours appear more normal).
4. Encourage Thomas to continue to socialize with classmates and friends.

In relation to Nursing Diagnosis 2

1. Caution Thomas to avoid exposure to infectious illness while on prednisone therapy.
2. Advise Thomas to treat minor wounds carefully to prevent the development of infection.
3. Teach Thomas hand-washing and avoidance of contact with brother's sputum, towels, or other contaminated objects

In relation to Nursing Diagnosis 3

1. Recommend foods high in potassium.
2. Teach Thomas how to reduce sodium intake; suggest herbs and spices as seasoning substitutes.

In relation to Nursing Diagnosis 4

1. Teach Thomas measures to prevent constipation including use of nonirritating foods that are rich in potassium.
2. Advise Thomas to use a mild laxative such as milk of magnesia to relieve constipation, if it develops.

In relation to Nursing Diagnosis 5

1. Advise Thomas to engage in regular exercise (such as walking) that involves weight bearing to stimulate bone regeneration.
2. Caution Thomas to avoid hazardous activities and to seek help when engaging in activities requiring muscular strength to maintain safety (*eg*, he probably should not sail his boat alone, but should take a companion along who can help maneuver the equipment).

In relation to Nursing Diagnosis 6

1. Teach Thomas techniques to promote rest and sleep.

In relation to Nursing Diagnosis 7

1. Teach Thomas the following adjustments in self-care:
   a. Substitution of acetaminophen (a nonulcerogenic analgesic) for aspirin for the treatment of minor aches and pains
   b. Elimination of gastric irritants from the diet
   c. Use of an antacid containing calcium salt for occasional heartburn
   d. The need to report persistent heartburn to his doctor

In relation to Nursing Diagnosis 8

1. Teach Thomas the following adjustments in self-care:
   a. Diet limited in sodium, moderate in calories, and rich in protein, potassium, and calcium
   b. Stress-management techniques to prevent sudden increases in stress for which the body might be unable to compensate
   c. The importance of wearing a medical identification device stating that he is receiving prednisone medication

(Continued)

Model nursing care plan illustrating use of the nursing process (continued)

2. Teach Thomas signs and symptoms of glucocorticoid excess:
   a. Those that are acceptable, such as changes in appearance and mild central nervous system stimulation
   b. Those that are unacceptable and must be reported to the physician for treatment such as persistent or marked hyperglycemia, pronounced weakness, and bone pain
3. Warn Thomas neither to discontinue medication nor to reduce its dosage without first consulting his physician.

EVALUATION

Criteria for evaluation	**Evaluative data**
In relation to Nursing Diagnosis 1	
1. In discussions with the nurse, after 3 months of drug therapy, Thomas will report no net decrease in the number of social contacts with his age peers.	During a visit with the nurse 3 months after initiation of drug therapy, Thomas described his social life as being "as active as ever."
2. Thomas will continue to maintain a neat, wellgroomed appearance.	Thomas' appearance during this visit showed some cushingoid changes, but he was wellgroomed and well dressed.
3. Thomas will continue to exhibit good posture and maintain eye contact when conversing with the nurse.	Thomas sat erectly and maintained eye contact with the nurse.
4. When Thomas speaks about himself, positive comments will outnumber negative ones.	During the interview, Thomas made one negative comment about himself and two positive ones.
In relation to Nursing Diagnosis 2	
1. Thomas will seek early medical attention and treatment for infectious illness.	Thomas had no infectious illnesses during the first 3 months of drug therapy.
2. Minor wounds will heal without developing purulent drainage.	Thomas reported that he had sustained two minor injuries: a knife cut to his hand and contusions and abrasions from a fall from his bicycle; each had healed with no signs of infection.
In relation to Nursing Diagnosis 3	
1. Edema will not develop to a significant degree.	Thomas shows little or no swelling of soft tissues at his weekly visits.
2. Thomas' diet reflects his understanding of the role of sodium in development of fluid retention.	Diet as recorded by Thomas is low in salt.
In relation to Nursing Diagnosis 4	
1. By the third week of therapy, Thomas will state that he has no discomfort with fecal elimination.	Three weeks after the initiation of therapy, Thomas stated "I have no problem with constipation."
2. If constipation occurs, it will be promptly relieved by the use of a laxative.	During the third visit with the nurse, Thomas stated he had used milk of magnesia once at bedtime, and that evacuation the next morning relieved his discomfort.
In relation to Nursing Diagnosis 5	
1. By the fourth week of therapy, Thomas will describe his exercise regimen; this should involve daily activity that requires weight bearing.	Two weeks after the initiation of drug therapy, Thomas reported to the nurse that he had begun swimming regularly at the local YMCA pool. The nurse pointed out that swimming does not involve weight bearing. Two weeks later, Thomas reported walking daily one-half mile each way to and from school.
2. Thomas will describe appropriate safety practices as taught by the nurse.	On the fourth weekly visit following initiation of drug therapy, Thomas was able to describe accurately the recommendations of the nurse.

(Continued)

Model nursing care plan illustrating use of the nursing process (continued)

Criteria for Evaluation	Evaluative Data
3. Thomas will report appropriate changes in his safety practices.	On this visit, Thomas stated that he took a companion with him (his father or his best friend) when he went sailing. He also stated he was using special kitchen devices to immobilize food he wished to cut to minimize the risk of injury.
In relation to Nursing Diagnosis 6 1. Total sleep over a 2-day span will equal twice the usual daily sleep duration prior to initiation of prednisone therapy.	On the fourth weekly visit with the nurse, Thomas reported that his sleep on the night following medication with prednisone usually lasted 5 hours. On alternate days, sleep usually lasted 9 hours. Thomas normally sleeps 7½ hours per day. This criterion has not been met.
In relation to Nursing Diagnosis 7 1. By the third weekly visit with the nurse, Thomas will report that he has purchased acetaminophen to use as a substitute for aspirin.	During the third weekly visit, Thomas stated that he has purchased a supply of acetaminophen but has not yet needed to use any.
2. By the third weekly visit with the nurse, Thomas will identify foods that act as gastric irritants that he has eliminated from the diet.	During the third weekly visit, Thomas reported that he has had to eliminate highly spiced pizza and spaghetti sauce from his diet.
3. Thomas' complaints of epigastric discomfort will decline from the second weekly visit to the 3-month visit.	On the second weekly visit Thomas reported four episodes of epigastric discomfort (heartburn). During the 3-month visit, he reported only one episode the previous week. He stated that he uses Tums (a calcium salt antacid) to relieve heartburn.
In relation to Nursing Diagnosis 8 1. By the third weekly visit with the nurse, Thomas will be able to describe accurately (with appropriate rationale) the recommendations regarding diet, signs and symptoms that should be reported to the physician, and measures to control and manage stress.	During the third weekly visit, Thomas successfully described the recommendations for self-care.
2. By the first weekly visit with the nurse, Thomas will be wearing an appropriate medical identification device.	On the first weekly visit, Thomas was carrying a wallet card indicating that he was receiving prednisone. He had ordered a Medic-Alert bracelet but it had not yet arrived.

the two indicate a need for teaching. All clients need to understand the plan of care but those who are to manage their drug regimens independently need more detailed teaching than do the more dependent clients in institutional settings.

Finally, a client's attitude toward drug use and the influence it has exerted on past use of drugs should be considered. Either a reluctance to take drugs or an undue reliance on drug use may interfere with optimal drug therapy. A client's expressed attitude should be compared with the nurse's objective assessment of the client's emotional responses during the taking of the drug history. Proper assessment of clients' attitudes toward drugs can guide nurses in selecting an appropriate psychological approach to their drug regimens and in identifying needs for teaching.

Nursing diagnosis

A nursing diagnosis can be defined as an actual or potential health problem that focuses upon the *human response* of an individual or group and for which the nurse is responsible and accountable for identifying and treating *independently* (Alfaro, 1990, p 66).

In nursing pharmacology, nursing diagnoses identify undesirable changes in the client secondary to drug therapy that can be treated by nursing measures. Some examples of appropriate diagnoses are as follows: constipation secondary to iron therapy; noncompliance related to fear of stimulant drug use; and anxiety related to knowledge deficit concerning anticoagulant therapy. In each of these nursing diagnoses the diagnostic statement identifies a problem and a cause that are amenable to nursing intervention.

In the course of developing the appropriate nursing diagnoses, the assessment data may indicate an actual or potential health problem (complication) that focuses upon the *pathophysiologic response* of the body and for which interventions must be carried out *in collaboration with the physician* (Alfaro, 1990, p 66). Some examples of collaborative problems include pneumothorax secondary to chest tube; cardiac arrythmias secondary to potasssium deficiency; and hypertension related to amphetamine therapy. As these complications require intervention in collaboration with a physician, they will be identified in this text as collaborative problems and will be listed separately from the nursing diagnoses.

The list of official nursing diagnoses of the North American Nursing Diagnosis Association (NANDA) is shown on the end page.

Planning

Objectives of nursing care in drug therapy are, for the most part, to enhance drug action, prevent drug-related problems, ameliorate symptoms of adverse reactions, correct abnormal states, and improve function. Specific goals could be to minimize side-effects, prevent drug dependence, promptly detect and treat adverse reactions, promote withdrawal from a dependency-producing chemical, reduce or promote drug use (depending on the client's attitudes and needs), and educate clients to manage their drug regimens independently.

Intervention

Nursing interventions include psychological and physical care measures to reduce the need for drugs; to enhance the effectiveness of the drug regimen; and to prevent or ameliorate adverse reactions to medications. In addition, nurses may influence the drug regimen by suggesting to physicians or requesting from them orders for drugs that they believe are appropriate. Teaching clients about medications is another primary concern. This education may be designed to help clients derive the greatest benefit from the drug regimen while in an acute care setting, or it may be designed to prepare them or their families to manage their drug regimens at home.

Table 3-1. Examples of evaluative data and criteria

Criteria	Evaluation
For client receiving iron	
Stools will be soft and client will state that defecation is free of discomfort.	Soft, formed stool is passed after breakfast. Client states that there was "no problem with bowel elimination today."
For client on anticoagulant therapy	
Client will wear a medical identification device warning of anticoagulant use.	Client reports that Medic-Alert tag bearing the words "on anticoagulant therapy" is worn constantly; appropriate Medic-Alert bracelet is observed on client's wrist.
For client on diuretic therapy	
Client will take medication regularly as shown by a tablet count within two of the appropriate number when prescription is half used.	Tablet count on the 15th day of use of a new prescription was 16 (amount dispensed—30; prescribed dosage—1 tablet daily).

Evaluation

The success of nursing intervention should be measured by comparing client data following the administration of care to predetermined criteria established as goals in the planning stage. Skill in the development of appropriate criteria is acquired with experience in the field. If criteria are stated in measurable terms, progress can be assessed even when the criteria are not fully met. Some examples of evaluate data and criteria for success are given in Table 3-1.

■ Summary

The nursing process is applicable to all nursing care situations. The nurse should diagnose (or rule out) problems arising from exposure to toxins, drug treatment regimens, and inappropriate use or abuse of drugs. Goals are to eliminate inappropriate use of drugs; to promptly detect and treat adverse reactions to therapeutic drugs; and to teach clients to appropriately manage their self-care as it relates to drugs. Evaluation requires ongoing monitoring of clients for drug effects.

Learning experience 3-1

While caring for clients in the clinical laboratory, integrate pharmacologic aspects into your care plan at every step in the process. Compare the drug regimen of your client with those of others who are treated for the same or similar conditions. Can you provide reasonable rationales for differences in the drug regimens?

Reference

*Alfaro RA. (1990). *Applying nursing diagnosis and nursing process: A step-by-step guide*, 2nd ed. Philadelphia: JB Lippincott Co.

Bibliography

*Carpenito LJ. (1992). *Nursing diagnosis: Application to clinical practice*, 4th ed. Philadelphia: JB Lippincott Co.

*Recommended for further reading.

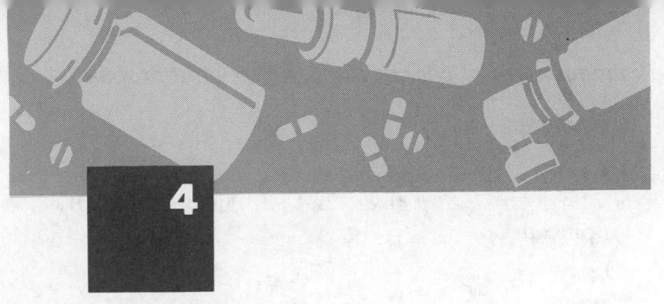

4

Development of a knowledge base in pharmacology

Before applying pharmacology in nursing practice, a nurse must master knowledge relevant to the activities of chemicals in the body. An understanding of the general mechanisms influencing drug absorption, transport, metabolism, excretion (pharmacokinetics), and drug effects (pharmacodynamics) is essential for good judgment in the management of drug therapy. The student must also practice the techniques of drug administration to ensure accurate, safe, and effective delivery of the prescribed medication to the proper body tissues. Once the basic skills and knowledge are acquired, the nurse is ready to begin practice with clients (Box 4-1).

A personal drug file

The number of drugs in present use is too vast for anyone to memorize. It is absolutely vital, however, that the nurse know the facts pertaining to any and all drugs a particular client is using. Before undertaking the care of any client, the nurse should look up drugs in a reliable source. Many nursing students then find it helpful to write out the essential facts on paper or file cards. (The act of copying data is a useful technique for those individuals who learn effectively through kinesthetic nerve pathways.) These cards or sheets can be carried into the clinical setting for ready reference (Fig. 4-1).

If drug information is recorded on individual cards or sheets (excluding specifics relative to the current client), it becomes suitable for inclusion in a personal file that can be used by the nurse in future situations. Pulling a file card on a drug used in the past for other patients can reduce the time required to prepare for care. Ready made drug cards are also available for purchase from several publishers; these could serve as basic references and as a nucleus around which to build a personal collection.

The student will find that drugs used frequently will soon become familiar. It is important to learn thoroughly the basic drugs in common use because there is no substitute for a well stocked memory. In the pressures of the clinical situation, time to look up needed information is sometimes limited.

It is recommended that some classification system be developed to facilitate retrieval of data in personal files. For example, drugs may be grouped according to physiologic action or filed alphabetically according to generic names. As new drugs are developed and others fall into disuse, the personal file can be modified.

Data pertaining to specific drugs should include drug name and family; physiologic actions; therapeutic uses; adverse effects; data about administration, metabolism, and elimination; and nursing implications (Box 4-2).

Box 4-1. Requirements for safe management of drug therapy

- Understanding of pharmacokinetics and pharmacodynamics
- Techniques of drug administration

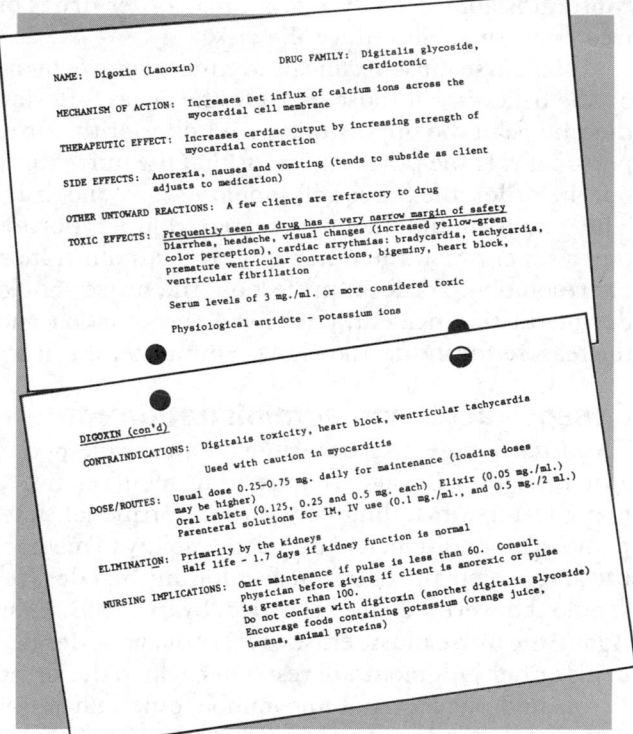

Figure 4-1. A sample drug summary as it might look if the notes were typed on a card that can be but put in the nurse's pocket.

Name of drug

The name by which the drug is ordered may be one of several types: trade name, generic name, chemical name, or generally recognized abbreviation (see Table 8-1; these names and abbreviations are discussed in Chapter 8). All names by which a drug is known in the local health community should be recorded.

Drug family

Drugs may be classified in many ways and any one substance may belong to more than one drug "family," depending on the classification used. Thus, a drug may be designated by its chemical derivation (heavy metals, xanthines, steroids, phenothiazines, and so forth); mechanism of action (central nervous system depressant, anticholinergic, anti-inflammatory, and so forth); or route of administration (inhalant, oral, parenteral, and so forth). The student must know the general properties and characteristics of each classification. Terms used to describe drugs on reference entries should indicate the nature of the substance as succinctly as possible. For example, hydroxyzine (Atarax, Vistaril) might be described as a piperazine-derivative antihistamine used as an antiemetic, antipruritic, tranquilizer, and sedative. Atropine is a belladonna alkaloid that can be described as anticholinergic, antispasmodic, anhidrotic, and mydriatic. These terms, although not adequate for comprehensive de-

scription of the drug, do give the student clues concerning the drug's physiologic action, side effects, and toxicity.

Desired physiologic effects

The desired physiologic (therapeutic) effect should include information that will indicate the mechanism of action of the drug. It is not sufficient to say that a drug is a laxative: Does the drug act by lubrication, stimulation, saline catharsis, alteration of surface tension, or formation of bulk in the stool? In the case of analgesics, pain relief may be accomplished by antagonism of prostaglandins, central nervous system depression, inhibition of inflammation, neutralization of acid (in the stomach), vasodilation (in angina), or muscle relaxation. To make sound judgments, the nurse must understand how a medication affects function at the cellular or molecular level if possible.

Side effects

Side effects of a drug are physiologic effects exerted by the chemical that are not related to the desired therapeutic effect. They may be desirable or undesirable. A side effect in one clinical situation might be the desired therapeutic effect in another and vice versa. Side effects of drugs may be myriad. It is important that the nurse be familiar with serious side effects (no matter how rare) and commonly occurring side effects (no matter how benign). When rare but clinically insignificant side effects cause concern to a client, reference to a comprehensive drug source book will usually clarify their relation to the drug regimen. Virtually all drugs have side effects. The number and range of side effects may indicate the relative toxicity of a given medication.

Adverse reactions

Adverse reactions include any undesirable effect apparent in the recipient. They may be paradoxic (opposite to the desired effect), allergic, or extraneous.

Box 4-2. Elements of a drug file summary

- Names of the drug
- Drug families to which the chemical belongs
- Desired physiologic effect
- Common or serious side effects
- Other adverse reactions
- Toxic effects
- Contraindications
- Usual dosage range and routes of administration
- Elimination
- Nursing implications

Those unusual effects seen in certain clients because of individual differences are labeled *idiosyncratic*. Paradoxic reactions are sometimes related to the age of the client. Allergic and idiosyncratic responses are often due to genetic factors and tend to be familial. When giving drug histories, clients may label all adverse reactions "allergic" because this potentially lethal reaction is accepted more readily and regarded more seriously by health care personnel than other, more benign reactions.

An important adverse effect is interference in embryonic development when used during pregnancy. The federal Food and Drug Administration has begun an effort to classify drugs on a scale that indicates risk during pregnancy. Doubt has been cast on the validity of the Food and Drug Administration pregnancy categories by a critique published by a group of clinical teratologists in Canada (Friedman et al, 1990). At this stage of development, it is difficult to evaluate the reliability and validity of present rating systems. In the absence of a readily available, clearly defined, and widely accepted rating scale, the Food and Drug Administration categories will be included in the drug data of this text. The reader should bear in mind that ratings may change in the near future as techniques for assessing relative risks to the fetus are refined (see Chapter 16 for a more detailed discussion of ratings of risks to the fetus of drugs administered to the mother.)

Toxic effects

Toxic effects are those that involve an excessive drug effect. They tend to be exaggerations of therapeutic effects or side effects. For example, toxicity from a central nervous system depressant used for sedation may induce a coma. If the depressant is an opiate, which acts as a miotic, the pupils are reduced to pinpoint size. The margin of safety between therapeutic and toxic doses varies greatly but any substance that is physiologically potent enough to produce therapeutic effects is also given the proper circumstances, potentially harmful to the body. Toxic symptoms may appear in clients receiving doses well within the usual dosage range because drug response, metabolism, and excretion vary greatly from person to person. If an antidote or emergency treatment is recommended for toxicity, it should be included among the data.

Contraindications

Contraindications are those conditions or symptoms that alert the health care practitioner to the potential dangers of the drug. For example, glaucoma is a contraindication for anticholinergics (anticholinergics dilate the pupils and may precipitate an acute episode of glaucoma). However, physicians may with good reason order drugs when contraindications are present. In these situations, the nurses should question the physicians for clarification to be sure they are aware of the contraindications. The physician may order drugs or treatment that will reduce the risk.

The nurse must decline to administer any drug he or she believes will cause harm to the client, offering the physician the opportunity to administer the drug personally. If the physician insists that the nurse carry out the order, the nurse still should *not* give the drug. The matter should then be referred to supervisors or other superiors in the nursing service administration for resolution. For legal protection, the nurse should document the incident, describing the situation and the reasons for the decision not to administer the drug.

Dosage range and administration route

The usual dosage must be included for each method of administration. Dosages require adjustment relative to many factors, including body mass, nutritional state, pathologic condition, and the client's ability to metabolize and excrete the drug. Orders for unusual dosages should be verified and clarified by the physician. Again, the nurse must refuse to carry out an order that in his or her judgment will result in harm to the client. Errors in dosage are not uncommon, especially in the case of verbal orders, and it is the nurse's responsibility to alert the physician to the possibility of error.

Elimination

The nurse must be aware of the physiologic mechanisms by which a drug is inactivated and eliminated from the body. The efficiency of these processes affects the efficacy and potential for toxicity of a given medication. Many drugs are deactivated by microsomal enzymes in the liver and excreted by the kidneys. Clients with abnormal function of these organs are at increased risk for complications related to the use of these drugs.

Nursing implications

Nursing implications encompass anything relative to drug use that influences and affects nursing care. These may include timing of doses, special techniques for administration, precautions necessary prior to administration, assessment of toxicity and side effects, the potential for tolerance or addiction, legal constraints on the use of the drug, and so forth. Only in recent years have nursing implications appeared in drug reference sources to a significant extent. This is an area of nursing knowledge that needs further development. The student would be wise to enter under this category verbal information gleaned from experienced nurses, as well as data from published sources.

■ **Summary**
Before administering a drug, the nurse must know certain information about the substance: its names, drug family or families, desired effects and mechanism of action, side effects, ad-

verse reactions, toxic effects, contraindications, dosage range and administration route, elimination, and nursing implications. The development of a personal file of drug cards or sheets is recommended for the beginning student.

Sources of drug information

There is no single source that will provide all the drug information needed by the nurse in a given clinical situation. The student must become familiar with a variety of publications, using each for the particular information it best provides. When evaluating references the following questions should be considered:

What is the source of the data? How accurate is it? Does the author represent any particular point of view or have a vested interest in the effect the information may have on the reader?

For whom is the information written? Material published for physicians or pharmacists may assume knowledge that the nurse lacks or emphasize aspects of limited use to the nurse while omitting others of particular value in nursing practice.

Is pertinent data readily available and generally understandable? Appropriate organization and indexing assist the nurse in locating information; clear, concise writing is essential. Print should be large enough for easy reading.

How pertinent is the material to nursing? The best source will include comprehensive information relative to nursing practice but will not contain irrelevant material.

Is the information up to date? Textbook material may be 2 or more years old when first published. Journal articles tend to involve several months of preparation. The frequency of revision and updating of pharmacopeiae and subscription services affects the usefulness of their data.

Is availability of the reference limited by its cost? Price influences which references individuals, institutions, and libraries will purchase. A hospital may choose an inexpensive volume for nursing unit libraries rather than a superior but more costly subscription service.

Is the format of the publication appropriate and convenient? Pocket-sized volumes are useful for clinical reference; looseleaf formats with discrete entries facilitate updating of material.

The student will find that no single volume will qualify as ideal. Often more than one reference must be consulted. Types of publications include pharmacopeiae, textbooks, specialized books, journals, subscription services, and literature from pharmaceutical firms.

Pharmacopeiae (Compendia)

Pharmacopeiae are collections of drug data considered standard by the group developing them (medical or pharmaceutical societies or government task forces), or by some other authority. In most modern countries, one or more pharmacopeiae are adopted by governmental action to indicate that country's "official" drugs. In the United States, an official drug is one that is included in *The United States Pharmacopeia & National Formulary (USP & NF)*. This publication has been designated by law as the official compendium. In the United Kingdom, official drugs are listed in *The British Pharmacopoeia (BP)*. Canada uses *The Canadian Formulary*, as well as *USP & NF* and *BP*. Pharmacopeiae are written by committees of experts (pharmacologists, physicians, and pharmacists) designated by sponsoring government or private agencies. They usually include information vital to the preparation, compounding, and dispensing of drugs (Table 4-1). Revised periodically (often every 5 years), new editions of pharmacopeiae exclude previously listed drugs that have fallen into disuse or disrepute while adding new drugs considered acceptable. The information in official pharmacopeiae is more useful to pharmacists than to other health care personnel because there is little medical and no nursing information incorporated in them. One or more official pharmacopeiae are usually available in college libraries and hospital pharmacies. Certain nonofficial compendia do include medical information and are consulted regularly by health care professionals (see Table 4-1).

Textbooks

Textbooks are written for students of nursing, medicine, or pharmacy. Traditional nursing textbooks provide a general background in pharmacology; specific instruction on the preparation and administration of drugs; and drug data on medications in common use. They function, therefore, not only as textbooks on nursing functions but also as reference sources for drug information. Drugs described in these sources include traditional remedies, as well as newer drugs whose patents and copyrights are still in force.

Nursing textbooks are usually available in college and hospital libraries; a nurse may purchase one as a student and may keep an up-to-date text in a personal library.

Medical textbooks are written for medical students and physicians and emphasize therapeutic considerations in the prescribing of drugs. Most include detailed discussions and comprehensive data concerning drug action, pharmacokinetics, drugs in common use, and the treatment of poisoning. These texts tend to be

(*Text continues on p. 36*)

Table 4-1. Drug compendia

Title	Author(s)	Publication data	Authority	Contents
Official pharmacopeiae				
The United States Pharmacopeia XXI & National Formulary XVI (U.S.P. & N.F.)	Committee of Revision of the United States Pharmacopeial Convention, Inc. (outstanding pharmacists, physicians, and pharmacologists who donate their services to the convention)	1990; published about every 5 years, with supplements as needed, by the Board of Trustees of the United States Pharmacopeia Convention, Inc. Rockville, MD	Adopted as official by the United States Congress in the Federal Food, Drug and Cosmetic Act of 1906	Single drugs of proved therapeutic value and low toxicity (whose method of preparation and content are not secret) are described as to source; physical and chemical properties; standards for identity, strength, and purity; method of storage; and dosage range for therapeutic use. Drugs may be deleted when they are supplanted by newer or better drugs, or when there is a high incidence of toxic reactions after extensive use. Listings are according to official name.
The British Pharmacopoeia, 13th ed. (B.P.)	The British Pharmacopoeia Commission	1988; published about every 5 years by the Medicines Commission for Her Majesty's Stationery Office	Adopted by Parliament by the Medical Act of 1968 for use in the United Kingdom; also adopted by some members of the British Commonwealth	Similar to *U.S.P. & N.F.*
British Pharmaceutical Codex	Department of Pharmaceutical Sciences, Pharmaceutical Society of Great Britain	1984; published by the Council of the Pharmaceutical Society of Great Britain	Adopted by the United Kingdom and some units of the British Commonwealth	Contains drugs listed in B.P., as well as descriptions of the actions and uses of other drugs
Martindale's The Extra Pharmacopeia	James Reynolds, ed.	1989; published by Pharmaceutical Press, London	The expertise of the Royal Pharmaceutical Society of Great Britain	Drug monographs, formulas of proprietary medicines, and directory of manufacturers
The European Pharmacopoeia (E.P.)		Published under a convention signed by the governments of Belgium, France, West Germany, Italy, Luxembourg, the Netherlands, Switzerland, and the United Kingdom	Adopted by cooperating countries by a resolution of a committee of the Council of Europe in 1972	Monographs on articles used in medical practice
The International Pharmacopoeia, 2nd ed.	Committee of World Health Organization	1980; published by the United Nations	Used by the United Nations to encourage development of pharmacopeiae and the standardization of drugs worldwide; no official status except when adopted by authority of individual nations	Published in English, French, and Spanish; nomenclature is Latin

(Continued)

Table 4-1. Drug compendia (Continued)

Title	Author(s)	Publication data	Authority	Contents
Nonofficial compendia				
Drug information (92, 93, 94, and so on)	Gerald K. McEvoy, ed.	Published annually by the American Hospital Formulary Service under the authority of the American Society of Hospital Pharmacies	The expertise of the members of the American Society of Hospital Pharmacies	Information on classes of drugs as well as monographs on individual preparations
Drug Evaluations	American Medical Association Department of Drugs	W.B. Saunders Co., Philadelphia	The expertise of the members of the American Medical Association	Evaluations of information on virtually all therapeutic agents in the official compendia as well as new single-entity drugs and mixtures, arranged according to therapeutic category
The British National Formulary (B.N.F.)	The Joint Formulary Committee of the British Medical Association and the Pharmaceutical Society of Great Britain		The expertise of the British Medical Association and the Pharmaceutical Society of Great Britain	Detailed descriptions of the properties, actions, and uses of most preparations in current use in medical practice; it contains useful information on the relative therapeutic value of different remedies in a pocket-size book for ready reference
U.S.P. Dispensing Information (D.I.)	Committee of Revision of the United States Pharmacopeial Convention	Published annually and updated bimonthly by the Board of Trustees of the United States Pharmacopeia, New York	The expertise of the members of the Committee of Revision of the United States Pharmacopeial Convention	Information pertinent to the dispensing and administration of common drugs and jargon-free guidelines that may be made available to consumers of drugs by health care professionals
Facts and Comparisons	B. Olin, ed.	Updated monthly; J.B. Lippincott Co., Philadelphia	No official status	Drug monographs and product listings
Compendium of Pharmaceuticals and Specialties	Carmen Krogh, ed.	Published yearly by the Canadian Pharmaceutical Association	The expertise of the members of the Canadian Pharmaceutical Association	Drug monographs, charts, and clinical guidelines
Remington's Pharmaceutical Sciences	Arthur Osol, ed.	Mack Publishing Co., Easton, PA	No official status	Comprehensive data on almost all drugs and chemicals used today in medicine and pharmacy, classified according to therapeutic use as well as chemical structure. Commentaries on official drugs listed in the *U.S.P. & N.F., B.P., The International Pharmacopoeia*, and other current reference sources are included

excellent sources of background information concerning physiologic dynamics of drug therapy and adverse reactions to medication. They do not apply this information to nursing practice. Examples of medical textbooks are *Goodman and Gilman's The Pharmacological Basis of Therapeutics, 8th ed.* by Gilman, et al, and *Goth's Medical Pharmacology, 12th ed.* by Clark.

Books written for pharmacy students emphasize information needed for accurate compounding and dispensing of drugs, as well as the clinical applications of drug treatments. Chemical data concerning drugs are very extensive, and information about compatibility and interactions is detailed (see Remington's *Pharmaceutical Sciences*, Table 4-1). Pharmacy textbooks are not generally available except in the libraries of colleges with pharmacy students.

Journals

Journals are an important source of information when a specific topic is to be researched in detail. Journals in the fields of nursing, medicine, and nutrition are particularly valuable. Pertinent articles may be located through the appropriate indices: *Index Medicus* and *Cumulative Index to Nursing and Allied Health Literature*.

A survey of the literature should begin with the most recent publications and continue backward until the relevant material appears to be exhausted. This time period will vary with the topic but usually includes at least 5 years.

Nurses will wish to read regularly those periodicals most pertinent to their areas of practice. Many nursing journals feature departments that publish drug information on a regular basis. In addition, articles dealing with special drug problems appear from time to time. Although journal articles may be written several months in advance of publication, they still tend to be more up-to-date than books.

Journals limited to drug information are also available for general use. They may be published monthly or biweekly (see *The Medical Letter on Drugs and Therapeutics* in the Bibliography section).

Subscription services

Subscription services are designed to provide current drug information for health care agencies. They provide a basic text (sometimes in looseleaf format) and regularly publish revisions to be incorporated in the reference volumes. The drug data tend to be detailed and comprehensive. However, the material is organized according to therapeutic use, and pages may not be numbered consecutively, presenting difficulties in locating needed information efficiently. These services also tend to be expensive and because of their cost are not generally available. However, many hospital pharmacies maintain one copy, and some college libraries also subscribe. Three major subscription services are *Drug Information*, published by the American Hospital Formulary Service by the authority of the American Society of Hospital Pharmacies, *Compendium and Pharmaceuticals*, published by the Canadian Pharmaceutical Association, and *Facts and Comparisons*, published by JB Lippincott Co.

Package inserts and the *Physicians' Desk Reference*

Pharmaceutical firms publish a great deal of information about their medicinal products. Content of this material is controlled, in part, by national legislation, which forbids claims of therapeutic efficacy not supported by research data and requires inclusion of certain information concerning drug toxicity, side effects, and adverse reactions. Within these constraints, however, drug firms can and do slant the descriptive material to promote the use of their products. The information must be interpreted with this bias in mind. Data concerning individual drugs usually are included as a package insert when the medicine is marketed. These brochures are written for prescribing physicians and assume that the reader has a wide background of knowledge in pharmacology. For this reason, references and allusions may seem cryptic to the nonphysician reader.

The most widely used drug information reference in the United States, the *Physicians' Desk Reference (PDR)*, consists of a compilation of selected package inserts, arranged by drug manufacturers and trade names. Drug firms are charged for the listings by the publisher, who then distributes the book to physicians. The volume is revised yearly (supplements are published during the year). Its most valuable uses are in identifying the generic drug contained in new trade name preparations and in identifying nonlabeled drugs by the physical appearance of their dosage forms (through its section containing color photographs of various drugs). It is often the only easily available source listing a new proprietary drug. Once the generic constituent of a drug is identified, however, the reader is likely to find data in other references that are more objective and more comprehensive than that offered by the *PDR*.

The pharmacist

Inevitably, situations will arise in which needed information cannot be obtained from the available publications. The nurse should then consult with the pharmacist who dispensed the drug. The pharmacist may be able to supply a brochure or other information on the preparation. As an expert in the field of drug therapy, the pharmacist is a valuable member of the health team and should be involved in client care in ways other than as a consultant of last resort (see Chapter 13 on role functions of the pharmacist). However, it is important that the nurse not waste the pharmacist's time by requesting information available from other sources.

Drug firms

When information about drugs is required that cannot be obtained from any other source, the pharmaceutical manufacturer may be contacted directly by telephone. Most firms either maintain a toll-free number or will accept collect calls. There may be different listings for general product, medical, and pharmaceutical information; for reporting of side effects; and for after-hour emergencies. Current telephone numbers may be obtained from the telephone company's information service or from listings in the *PDR* or the *Compendium and Pharmaceuticals*.

Supplementary information

The student should become familiar with as wide a range of references as possible. Each nurse will adopt sources that are found to be useful and convenient but should guard against undue reliance on any one reference for information. Periodic consultation of supplementary sources will help prevent a systematic bias in the selection of data that will then influence a nursing judgment. In this as well as in other areas of nursing expertise, the student is advised to develop sound habits of scholarship.

■ Summary

It is necessary for nursing students to learn about the general mechanisms of drug action and to practice the techniques of drug administration before they are ready to apply pharmacology to clinical practice. It is helpful to have a personal drug file that includes the name of the drug, drug family, desired therapeutic effects, side effects, adverse reactions, toxic effects, contraindications, dosage range and administration route, drug elimination, and nursing implications. The file should be kept up to date. A card or paper can be pulled from the file with information concerning the drug a specific patient is using.

There is no single source that can provide all this information. The nurse should become familiar with many sources of information: pharmacopeiae, textbooks, journals, subscription services, pharmaceutical firms, and the pharmacist. The student is advised to acquire sound habits of scholarship from which to develop and maintain an adequate, up-to-date knowledge base.

Nursing implications

Safe, effective nursing care involves not only the accurate administration of medications but also the exercise of sound judgment to minimize the risks of drug use and to maximize therapeutic benefits. Nursing judgments must be based on pharmacologic facts. Nurses should have a broad background of knowledge in this discipline, and they must be able to supplement this base by locating additional data when required by the clinical situation. Data acquisition must be efficiently performed because time is limited in most clinical settings.

Nurse practitioners should allocate time for the regular study of drug data, focusing on the drugs encountered in their particular clinical setting. All available references should be used, and new publications should be explored as they appear. The mass of material is expanding so rapidly that computers increasingly are being relied on for quick retrieval of pertinent information. In the meantime, only continuing study will enable a nurse to maintain safe drug therapy practice.

Learning experience 4-1

Prepare an outline of essential information for a drug ordered for a client or acquaintance. Use at least five references, including (if possible) *Drug Information, Facts and Comparisons,* or *Compendium of Pharmaceutical and Specialities*; a nursing textbook on pharmacology; a medical textbook on pharmacology; and the *Physician's Desk Reference*.

It is apparent that one can never be certain to have all the facts (even the known facts) about all the drugs used in work with clients. The nurse should not be discouraged, however, since the client is a factor equal in importance to the drugs in the therapeutic situation. Begin by observing and assessing the client. First, make observations that are pertinent to therapeutic and adverse reactions to the specific drugs involved. For example, clients on antihypertensive drugs should have their blood pressures checked regularly. A drop toward normal indicates a therapeutic response. Hypotension, or a rapid drop, accompanied by symptoms suggestive of hypovolemic shock, warn of toxicity. Even without using a sphygmomanometer, blood pressure may be estimated by palpating the pulse; the amplitude of the pulse reflects systolic pressure. Many specific observations are recommended for certain drugs (*eg*, pulse rate for digitalis preparations, respiratory rate for narcotics).

In addition to individual assessments required by specific drugs, a global assessment should be made. This may be done quickly. Posture and activity, skin color, facial expression, vocal expression, and the general impression from listening to and viewing the client will provide many clues to changes that may be drug-related. Any unusual or unexpected changes in emotional affect, physiologic function, mental ability, or comfort levels should be investigated with that possibility in mind. The nurse who checks to see if the client's signs and symptoms might be drug-related may diagnose many adverse reactions to medications that otherwise would remain undetected.

References

Friedman JM, et al. (1990). Potential human teratogenicity of frequently prescribed drugs. *Obstet Gynecol 75(4)*, 594–599 (April).

Bibliography

American Medical Association, Dept. of Drugs, Division of Drugs and Technology. (1986).

American Medical Association Staff. (1989). *The American Medical Association Encyclopedia of Medicine.* New York: Random House.

AMA drug evaluations, 6th ed. Philadelphia: WB Saunders.

Appelt GD, Appelt JM. (1988). *Therapeutic pharmacology.* Philadelphia: Lea and Febiger.

Clark, et al. (1988). *Goth's medical pharmacology*, 12 ed. St. Louis: C V Mosby.

*Gilman AG, et al, eds. (1990). *Goodman and Gilman's the pharmacological basis* of therapeutics, 8th ed. New York: Pergamon Press.

Handbook of nonprescription drugs, 8th ed. (1986). Washington, DC: American Pharmaceutical Association.

*Krogh CME, ed. *Compendium of pharmaceuticals and specialties.* Ottawa: Canadian Pharmaceutical Association. (Published yearly)

Long JW. (1988). *The essential guide to prescription drugs.* New York: Harper and Row.

*Loebl S, Spratto G, Woods LH. (1989). *The nurse's drug handbook,* 5th ed. New York: John Wiley & Sons.

*McEvoy GK, ed. (1991). *Drug information 91.* Bethesda: American Hospital Formulary Service. (Published yearly with quarterly updates)

The medical letter on drugs and therapeutics. (Med Let Drug Ther; a biweekly newsletter, New Rochelle)

Medicines Commission for Her Majesty's Stationery Office. (1980). Cambridge: University Printer House. (With yearly addenda)

National Health Service (Great Britain). *Prescribers' Journal* (A bimonthly publication, London)

Olin BR, ed. *Drug facts and comparisons.* Philadelphia: JB Lippincott. (Published yearly with monthly updates)

Osol A, ed. (1985). *Remington's pharmaceutical sciences,* 17th ed. Easton, PA: Mack.

Physicians' desk reference. (1992). Oradell, NJ: Medical Economics Books.

The United States pharmacopeia & national formulary (U.S.P. and N.F.). (1989). Rockville, MD: The U.S. Pharmacopeia.

USAN and the USP dictionary of drug names. Washington, DC: US Pharmacopeial Convention.

Windholz M, ed. (1989). *Merck index: An encyclopedia of chemicals and drugs,* 11th ed. Rahway, NJ: Merck Publishing.

*Recommended for further reading.

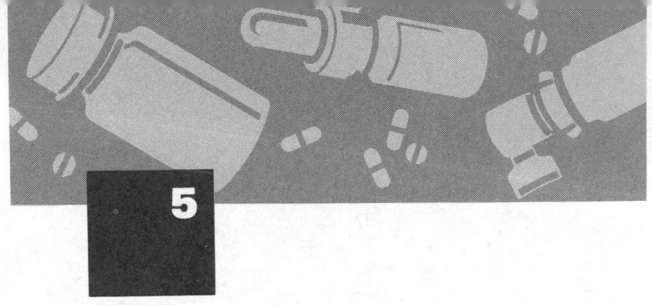

5

Toxicology

The science of toxicology can be defined as the study of the effects of chemicals on biologic systems with emphasis on the mechanisms of harmful effects of chemicals and the conditions under which harmful effects occur.

Although toxicology embraces a variety of specialized fields, three branches—environmental, economic, and forensic—are recognized as the major divisions of this science.

Environmental toxicology is concerned with a wide range of toxic agents that influence the health and safety of people in their work environment, in the atmosphere, and in the nutrients ingested through food and drink. Environmental toxicology also studies the effects on the human organism of exposure to toxic elements. *Economic toxicology* deals with the effects of toxic chemicals on species of plants and animals that have little or no economic value. Study in this area has led to the development of insecticides, food additives, food preservatives, and pesticides. *Forensic toxicology* studies relate the degree of damage to human beings caused by exposure to specific quantities of a toxic substance. This branch of toxicology also deals with legal issues related to chemically-induced illness or death. In all three divisions of this field, scientists are able to study the effect of toxic substances on humans, their environment, and all living creatures. Toxicology has enabled scientists to determine the fine line between a therapeutic chemical agent and a lethal chemical dose.

Access routes of toxic substances

The degree of a chemical substance's toxicity to humans is determined by the nature of the substance, the dose, the susceptibility of the individual, biologic factors, genetic factors, and the route of the poison's administration. Toxins come in contact with the human organism through a variety of routes, which include the percutaneous, gastrointestinal (GI), inhalation, and parenteral routes (Fig. 5-1).

Percutaneous route

Humans are most commonly exposed to toxins of all kinds through percutaneous, or skin, contact. Toxic matter penetrates the skin at different rates of time depending upon the nature of the substance. For example, gases generally pass freely through the skin, and liquids move across the membrane with less ease, whereas solids that are insoluble in water are least likely to penetrate the epidermal tissue.

Loomis (1974) points out that a variety of factors such as pH, extent of ionization, molecular size, and water and lipid solubility are all involved with the transfer of chemicals through the skin. Local factors, such as temperature and blood flow to the site, will influence the rate of absorption and, therefore,

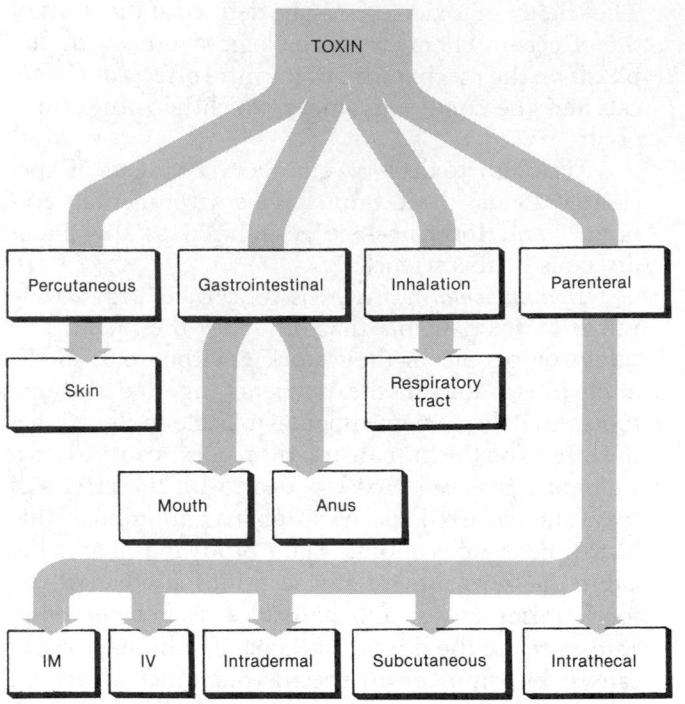

Figure 5-1. Routes by which toxins come in contact with human organisms.

the percutaneous toxicity of potent chemicals (see Fig. 5-1).

Gastrointestinal route

Poisons can enter the body through the GI tract; this means that substances can enter either through the mouth or through the anus. The level of toxicity depends on the amount of substance absorbed from the mouth or GI tract. Chemicals tend to cause local irritation and tissue destruction before exerting a systemic effect. The toxicity of orally ingested chemicals also depends on preexisting conditions in the GI tract. For example, toxic substances taken when there is food in the stomach tend to be less potent than those taken when the stomach is empty. An additional factor influencing the toxic action of chemicals in the GI tract is the nature of preexisting stomach secretions and the presence of hydrochloric acid. The pH of stomach contents will be influenced by the toxin and can result in damage to the mucosal cell lining of the stomach and intestines.

Parenteral route

Entry by the parenteral route refers to the introduction of substances into the body by means of injections, thereby circumventing body orifices. The most common parenteral routes of administration include intramuscular, intravenous, intradermal, intrathecal, and subcutaneous. Because these methods bypass the body's protective membranes, their potential for creating toxic levels is greater. Because high concentrations of a chemical can be produced rapidly by parenteral administration of medication, caution and the careful

calculation of doses are essential to avoid unintentional poisoning.

Inhalation route

Finally, humans are exposed to chemical toxins in the atmosphere that enter the body through inhalation.

In 1989, nearly 20,500 exposures to fumes, gases, and vapors, which required medical attention, were reported according to the American Association of Poison Control Centers (Table 5-1). To enter the respiratory tract, poisons must be in the form of gases or particulate matter that is not filtered out in the airway passages. To protect the public from potential hazards in the atmosphere, governmental regulatory agencies, such as the Environmental Protection Agency, Nuclear Regulatory Commission, and the Occupational Safety and Health Administration set standards, conduct research, and enforce regulations on environmental and occupational health.

Scope of poisoning

Litovitz, reporting annual poison exposure rates from the American Association of Poison Control Centers National Data System, notes that while 1,581,540 were reported by participating poison centers, it is estimated that there were in excess of 2.1 million exposures in the United States in 1989. For this period, the total number of deaths reported as a consequence of human poison was 590. Of this number, 76% of adult (>17 years old) deaths were intentional. Nearly 92% of the reported human exposures occurred in the home,

Table 5-1. 1989 Profile of exposure cases by generic category, by age (pharmaceutical and nonpharmaceutical)

| | Number of exposures | | |
Category	<6 Years	>6+ Years	Total*
Household cleaning substances	101,553	57,943	160,652
Analgesics	85,507	73,706	160,591
Cosmetics/personal care products	108,582	20,949	130,207
Plants, paint, stripping agents	84,295	15,729	100,704
Cough/cold preparations	68,916	21,444	90,798
Bites/envenomations	13,295	44,891	58,750
Hydrocarbons	29,231	28,883	58,616
Topicals	45,742	10,849	56,920
Foreign Bodies/toys	43,652	12,322	56,356
Chemicals	19,512	32,812	53,011
Sedatives/hypnotics/antipsychotics	7,965	42,094	50,833
Antimicrobials	32,296	17,552	50,236
Food poisoning	13,029	34,694	48,336
Insecticides/pesticides	25,025	22,650	48,283
Alcohols	17,741	25,296	43,539
Vitamins	34,147	6,613	40,922
Gastrointestinal preparations	26,314	6,101	32,616
Arts/crafts/office supplies	22,180	5,760	28,127
Antidepressants	3,284	21,375	25,029
Antihistamines	11,805	12,381	24,377
Hormones	15,822	4,832	20,794
Fumes/gases/vapors	2,207	17,884	20,437
Cardiovascular drugs	9,981	10,174	20,311
Screens/stimulants/street drugs	4,710	15,032	20,023
Adhesives/glues	9,702	7,813	17,682
Electrolytes/minerals	10,657	3,181	13,951
Deodorizers	12,433	1,385	13,896
Asthma therapies	6,579	6,153	12,828
Polishes/waxes	10,295	1,364	11,762

*Numbers listed in the less than 6 and 6+ columns do not equal the total poison exposure experience since data was also collected in "unknown" categories.

Source: Adapted from Litovitz TL, Schmitz BF, Bailey KM. (1990). 1989 Annual Report of the American Association of Poison Control Center National Data Collection System. *Am J Emerg Med, 8 (5)*, pp 407–428.

with 61% of overall exposures occurring in children under the age of six (Litovitz, Schmitz, & Bailey, 1990).

Table 5-1 identifies the total number of cases of substance exposure reported to poison control centers in 1989 by age. Table 5-2 describes exposure categories with the largest number of deaths in 1989.

Causes of poisoning

Although childproof containers have been credited with producing a decline in the incidence of deaths of children under 5 years of age, statistics indicate that over one-half of the deaths in this age group involve medical products. Analgesics and antipyretics remain the leading medicinal ingestants most frequently encountered in poisoning emergencies. Goldfrank (1990) notes that of the more than 20,000 different pharmaceutical products available on the market today, fewer than 20 products (excluding alcohol) account for nearly 90% of the reported nonaccidental toxic ingestions. Of the nonaccidental ingestions, the drugs encountered with the greatest frequency include amphetamines, antidepressants, barbiturates, benzodiazepines, cocaine, opioids, and analgesics (ASA, acetaminophen). Data reported in 1989 by the American Association of Poison Control Centers show similar trends in the reported incidents of improper exposure to plants, pesticides, household products, medications, and cosmetics. Table 5-3 identifies the frequency of plant exposures reported in the 1989 data.

Poison management

The basic steps in poison management are to provide first aid, remove and eliminate the poison, administer an antidote, and prevent future poisoning. These steps are addressed in this chapter.

Exposure to toxic levels of chemical agents, whether intentional or accidental, remains a commonly encountered emergency that requires accurate knowledge and an immediate response. This is especially likely in medical emergencies involving children under 5 years of age.

Table 5-2. Exposure categories with largest number of deaths in 1989

Category	Number of exposures		Number of deaths
	<6 Years	>6+ Years	
Antidepressants	3,284	21,375	140
Analgesics	85,507	73,706	126
Stimulants/street drugs	4,710	15,032	64
Sedatives/hypnotics	7,965	42,094	78
Cardiovascular drugs	9,981	10,174	70
Alcohol	17,741	25,296	53
Gases and fumes (CO_2, CO, Cl)	2,207	17,884	46
Asthma therapies	6,579	6,153	34
Hydrocarbons (gasoline, turpentine, benzene)	29,231	28,882	31
Chemicals	19,512	32,812	27
Cleaning substances	101,553	57,943	25
Pesticides	25,025	22,650	14

Source: Adapted from Litovitz TL, Schmitz BF, Bailey KM. (1990). 1989 Annual Report of the American Association of Poison Control Centers National Data Collection System. *Am J Emerg Med, 8 (5),* p 429.

Information

The science of toxicology and techniques used in current practice when intervening in chemical emergencies are constantly evolving. Therefore, it is essential that anyone attempting remediation in a chemical emergency apply the most current first-aid practices and treatment.

Poison control centers

The most reliable information about poisoning emergencies is generally available through an established network of regional poison control centers. At present, there are over 600 poison centers across the United States. Canada and Mexico also have such centers. These centers maintain information hot-lines 24 hours a day and serve as resources for emergency medical advice about poison treatment.

A list of centers in the United States can be obtained from the Director, National Clearinghouse for Poison Control Centers, Food and Drug Administration, United States Department of Health and Human Services, Bethesda, MD 20016, or from the State Coordinator of Poison Control Centers. The front of most telephone books lists local poison information centers with emergency numbers. Lists are also given in *Taber's Cyclopedic Medical Dictionary* (including centers in Canadian provinces and Mexico) and in the *Physicians' Desk Reference.* However, because telephone numbers may change, these reference works do not always contain the latest information.

Poisondex

Poison control centers use a variety of reference sources when responding to inquiries. A computerized information retrieval system that contains emergency poison management information is available. This microfiche data base is known as Poisondex Information System. The system contains the world's most complete listing of product ingredients. Updated every 3 months, Poisondex is one of the most accurate

Table 5-3. Reported frequency of plant exposures by plant type, 1989

Common name	Botanical name	Poisonous part	Exposure frequency
Philodendron	Philodendron spp.	All	6,361
Dumbcane	Dieffenbachia spp.	All	4,049
Poinsettia	Euphorbia pulcherrima	Sap, berries	3,080
Holly	Llex spp.	Fruit, leaves	2,397
Poison ivy	Toxicodendron radicans	All	1,694
Pothos, devil's ivy	Scindapsus aureus	Leaves	1,512
Yew	Taxus spp.	All	1,416
Pokeweed, inkberry	Phytolacca americana	All	1,290
Climbing nightshade	Solanum dulcamara	All	934
Rhododendron, azalea	Rhododendron spp.	All	914

Source: Adapted from Litovitz TL, Schmitz BF, Bailey KM. (1990). 1989 Annual Report of the American Association of Poison Control Centers National Data Collection System. *Am J Emerg Med, 8 (5),* p 429.

resources available for poison emergencies. Other similar resources are Drugdex Information System and Identidex.

First aid for acute poisoning or exposure

The nurse may be present at the telephone or in the emergency room when a poison crisis arises. Although each situation requires a slightly different approach, in general, management of poisoned or exposed patients requires specific first-aid measures. Remaining calm is a priority.

Initial telephone contact

It is very important that telephone intervention defuses the crisis and avoids panic. Questioning and repeating instructions in a calm, clear manner is essential. The following principles are recommended when the initial contact is made by telephone:

1. Treat the victim, not the poison. The most significant question to ask is, "What is the condition of the victim?" No matter what the type of poisoning, if the victim is not breathing and is not responsive, basic life-support measures should be started immediately. Resuscitation should continue until breathing is well established. Once the victim is stabilized, intervention for the poison can be determined.
2. Obtain such basic information as name, weight, age, address, and telephone number.
3. Obtain a poison history, including the type of poison, route of entry, and amount. It is estimated that 50% of the data taken during a poison crisis may be inaccurate. This fact necessitates a telephone follow-up to ensure compliance with emergency instructions, the condition of the client, and repetition of instructions about first-aid measures, if the initial information was inaccurate.
4. Assess the victim's condition for respiratory problems and shock. Instruct the caller to implement measures to resuscitate the victim and stabilize his or her immediate condition, provided the caller has the skills required to carry out the resuscitation. Try to determine if the situation is life-threatening, stable, nonthreatening, or if hospitalization is required. The interviewer should be aware that objectivity is lost in a telephone assessment.
5. Take steps to intervene based on the victim's condition and the route of the poison's entry.
   a. If the poison was *ingested*, and the victim is alert and able to swallow, give milk or water to dilute the swallowed material. Never give liquid to an unconscious person. Be certain that a gag reflex is present when considering emesis. Unless contraindicated, emesis may be induced on the recommendation of a poison control center. Syrup of ipecac is the method of choice to induce emesis (Box 5-1). Syrup of ipecac is contraindicated if strychnine, petroleum distillates, or corrosives such as lye or strong acids have been ingested; if the patient is seizing; or if there is cirrhosis or thrombocytopenia present.
   b. If the poison was *inhaled*, remove the victim to fresh air. A common toxic situation in the home involves the inhalation of poisonous fumes resulting from the interaction of bleaches and ammonia in the diaper pail.
   c. If *skin contamination* occurs, flood the skin with water for 2–3 minutes. Placing the victim under a shower is the best method. However, other systems of flushing water over the patient can be used in emergencies. Speed in applying water and washing away the chemical is very important. Remove the affected apparel when the patient is under the stream of water. After flooding the skin, gently wash the exposed part with soap and water.
   d. If the *eyes* are contaminated, irrigate them copiously with lukewarm water for 15 minutes. You may have to hold the eyelids open to wash the eyes thoroughly. Do not use chemicals, such as eye drops.
6. If the victim's condition warrants emergency room treatment, calmly direct the caller to the nearest facility. Advise the caller to bring along anything that may be helpful in determining the kind of poisoning and the amount of poison used, such as the bottle of pills or vomitus, if the victim has vomited.
7. Follow-up contact must be made to evaluate the

Box 5-1. Syrup of ipecac: doses for inducing emesis

Pediatric

Age 6 to 12 months, administer 10 ml orally; age over 1 year, administer 15 ml orally, followed by 1–2 glassfuls of whatever fluid the child will tolerate (ipecac is not effective on an empty stomach). It is important to maintain activity level. Results should occur within 30 min.

Adult

Administer 30 ml. The same procedure as above is applied to the adult victim.

outcome, especially if the poisoning did not seem serious enough to warrant emergency room treatment. (The Rocky Mountain Poison Control Center in Denver, CO, recommends 1-hour, 4-hour, and 24-hour follow-up telephone calls.) Part of this follow-up care includes counseling to prevent further poisoning incidents (Box 5-2).

Initial emergency room contact

There are times when the initial contact with a client is made in the emergency room. In this case, hospital personnel can make firsthand assessments, which are easier than telephone contacts. Conversely, because the client may not have received previous first-aid care, treatment often has been delayed and interventions similar to those described in the first aid section are used.

1. Evaluate the client's general condition for adequate ventilation and presence of shock.
2. Initiate life-support measures as indicated.
3. Decontaminate the skin if appropriate, being careful to protect emergency personnel in the process.
4. Obtain a complete history from the client or family when possible.

Patient evaluation

After first aid has been given and a complete history obtained, further evaluation of the client's condition is made to determine what the next steps in treatment are. Suggestions for this are given in Box 5-3. Decisions about the use of each of these approaches to treatment require careful assessment based on specific criteria.

Administering an antidote

Selecting an appropriate antidote that forces excretion, promotes adsorption, or implements the mechanical removal of the toxic chemical depends on the toxicity of the agent ingested and the condition of the patient. By definition, an *antidote* is an agent that counteracts the action of a poison. There are several mechanisms of action known:

- The antidote may form an inert complex with the toxin, which will then be excreted.
- The antidote may enhance the detoxification of a poison.
- The antidote may slow down conversion of a poison to a more toxic material.
- The antidote may compete with or block essential receptor sites that mediate toxic effects of poisons.

It is estimated that specific antidotes are available for less than 2% of all poisonous substances. The antidotes listed on the labels that appear on caustic household chemical products are frequently incorrect. For instance, the use of a weak acid such as lemon juice is often suggested to neutralize the poison or the caustic substance. This procedure is now thought to be potentially harmful by some experts because of the exothermic heat reaction caused in the neutralization process. The United States Consumer Product Safety Commission, which is responsible for first aid antidotal labeling of poisonous household products, is attempting to ensure accurate information on product labels. Poisondex is the most reliable source of information for selecting the correct antidote for a diagnosed poison. Experts suggest that emergency rooms maintain a cyanide kit that contains clear instructions for use and is packaged according to the order in which its contents should be used. A number of other materials

---

Box 5-2. Outline of first-aid measures by telephone

- Treat the victim, not the poison.
- Obtain basic information: telephone number, name, weight, age, and address.
- Obtain a poison history: type of poison, route of entry, and amount.
- Assess the client's condition and evaluate if the condition is life-threatening.
- Intervene, taking steps based on the client's condition and the route of the poison's entry.
- Direct the caller to the nearest facility if the victim's condition warrants emergency room treatment.
- Follow up to evaluate outcome and begin poison prevention education.

Box 5-3. Further evaluation for acute poisoning or exposure

1. Can further absorption be prevented, and by what methods?
   a. Skin decontamination
   b. Emesis
   c. Lavage
   d. Charcoal
   e. Cathartic
2. Can enhanced excretion of the poison be achieved?
   a. Forced diuresis
   b. Peritoneal dialysis
   c. Hemodialysis
   d. Exchange transfusion
   e. Hemoperfusion
3. Can symptoms be treated with specific physiologic antagonists (antidotes)?

suggested for use in poison emergencies are listed in Box 5-4.

The list, which is not complete, gives only the basic supplies. Other emergency drugs and specific protocols to be used in the treatment of poisons are available through poison control centers and the Poisondex microfiche system.

Box 5-4. Emergency room antidote supplies

acetylcysteine (Mucomyst)

activated charcoal, U.S.P. and N.F. (medicinal charcoal, active carbon)

ammonium chloride

amyl nitrite, U.S.P. and N.F.

Antivenins

ascorbic acid

atropine

botulinal antitoxin

Cyanide kit

deferoxamine (desferrioxamine, Desferal)

dimercaprol, U.S.P. and N.F., B.P. (BAL)

diphenhydramine hydrochloride, U.S.P. and N.F. (Benadryl)

edetate calcium disodium, U.S.P. and N.F. (Calcium Disodium Versenate, CaEDTA)

ethanol

glucagon

ipecac syrup

magnesium sulfate, U.S.P. and N.F., B.P. (Epsom salt)

methylene blue

naloxone hydrochloride, U.S.P. and N.F. (Narcan)

Non-oil cathartics

oxygen

penicillamine (Cuprimine)

physostigmine salicylate, U.S.P. and N.F. (Antilirium)

pralidoxime chloride, U.S.P. and N.F. (Protopam, 2-PAM)

sodium sulfate, U.S.P. and N.F., B.P. (Glauber's salt)

sorbitol

syrup of ipecac, U.S.P. and N.F.; ipecacuanha, B.P.

Vasopressors

vitamin K_1

Eliminating the poison

Some of the first steps in first aid are to remove and eliminate the poison. If the route of the poisoning was percutaneous, it is necessary to flood the skin or eyes with water. Other steps commonly used in eliminating the poison include emesis, lavage, adsorption by activated charcoal, and cathartics. As mentioned above in "Initial telephone contact," more active steps may be required, such as forced diuresis, peritoneal dialysis, hemodialysis, exchange transfusion, or hemoperfusion. These steps would be taken only after thorough evaluation by a physician.

Emesis

Experts are divided about recommending emesis as the treatment of choice. Vomiting is generally believed to be superior to lavage when there are no contraindications. Most clinicians consider emesis to be contraindicated if any of the following conditions are present:

- Ingestion of volatile hydrocarbons
- Ingestion of corrosives (strong acids or bases)
- Coma, convulsions, loss of gag reflex
- Frank shock
- Strychnine poisoning

Syrup of ipecac is the preferred method for inducing emesis. The dosage and procedure for its use are discussed earlier in this chapter.

Lavage

Gastric lavage is used to evacuate the stomach's contents when emesis is contraindicated but when the removal of gastric content is considered safe and necessary. This procedure, referred to by lay persons as "pumping the stomach," must be performed only by trained personnel. Because all of the toxin is not usually removed by lavage, further absorption of poison must be prevented.

Activated charcoal

Several ingestants can be adsorbed by activated charcoal, which is a black, powdery substance that is tasteless, odorless, and nontoxic to humans.

Contraindications to the use of activated charcoal are minimal and include the presence of caustic acids or alkalis, ileus, and in patients with an unprotected airway for whom aspiration is a risk. Some of the substances adsorbed by activated charcoal include atropine, barbiturates, narcotics, alcohol, salicylates, strychnine, digitalis, phenothiazines, penicillin, and benzodiazepines. Because activated charcoal will inactivate syrup of ipecac, it is best to administer activated charcoal after emesis. The desired dose is mixed with water and/or a cathartic in a 1:4 or 1:8 charcoal-to-liquid ratio forming a slurry (Box 5-5). It is administered orally or through an orogastric tube. The exact dose is not critical because it is a nontoxic substance.

Box 5-5. Activated charcoal doses

Dose for adult and child

Initial dose: 1 g/kg body weight or 10:1 ratio of activated charcoal: drug, whichever is greater. Following massive ingestions, 2 g/kg may be indicated; however, it may be difficult to administer doses in excess of 100 g.

Repetitive doses

0.5–1 g/kg body weight every 2–6 h tailored to the dose and dosage form of drug ingested (larger doses and shorter dosing intervals may occasionally be indicated). Note: Do not use repetitive doses of cathartics routinely.

Procedure

1. Add 4–8 parts of water to chosen quantity of activated charcoal, if in powdered form. This will form a transiently stable slurry that the patient can drink or have placed down an orogastric hose.
2. The activated charcoal can be given in a mixture with the chosen cathartic.
3. If the patient vomits the dose, it should be repeated. Smaller, more frequent, or continuous nasogastric administration may be better tolerated. An antiemetic is sometimes needed.
4. Repetitive doses are probably useful for drugs with a small volume of distribution, low plasma protein binding, biliary or gastric secretion, or active metabolites that recirculate.

Source: Flomenbaum NE, et al. General management of the poisoned or overdosed patient. In *Goldfrank's toxicologic emergencies*, 4th ed. 1990, p 10.

Shortly after the administration of charcoal, it is removed by lavage.

Cathartics

Cathartics are often used to facilitate the rapid transport of ingestants through the GI tract. This process decreases the absorption of ingestants. The use of oil-based cathartics is discouraged due to their potential for causing aspiration pneumonitis. Magnesium-based cathartics are contraindicated when the patient is in renal failure. Clinicians commonly use magnesium (2–4 hours), the remaining dose may be given or withheld. Magnesium sulfate and syrup of ipecac are emergency drugs that should be kept in every household at all times for the first-aid treatment of poisons when use is recommended by a poison control center or medically knowledgeable personnel.

Poison prevention

An informed and aware public is essential to reduce the incidence of toxicologic emergencies. Poison control centers provide an assortment of tools that can be used by nurses in a variety of clinical settings. Because a significant number of poisonings occur in children under 5 years of age, pediatric nurses in clinics and physicians' offices could be a major force in educating parents of young children about ways to decrease accidental poisoning. Many poison control centers can provide information, such as check sheets for poison-proofing a home, first-aid measures, tips on how to prevent childhood poisonings, lists of household items that are toxic to children, and other teaching materials useful for public education. Health education materials for poison prevention, such as the comic book *Dennis the Menace Takes a Poke at Poison* and the "Officer-Ugg" or "Mr. Yuk" stickers are attractive aids to use with the high risk preschool age group.

Community health nurses have an ideal opportunity to demonstrate poison control and safety measures to families in the home. For example, the skull-and-crossbones symbol for poison, which is required on the labels of toxic household products, can be pointed out to children on an exploratory poison-proofing adventure through their home. The consciousness-raising efforts of all health care professionals with parents and children can reduce the chances of accidental poisoning. Knowledge of the resources available in a community to cope with toxicologic emergencies, client education, accurate first-aid knowledge, and supportive care are essential for therapeutic intervention during a poison crisis.

Experts recommend that parents be taught the principles for preventing childhood poisonings (Box 5-6).

■ Summary

Toxins come in contact with the human body through a variety of routes, including percutaneous, GI, parenteral, and inhalation. Such a poisoning emergency requires accurate knowledge and quick responses. People who participate in such emergencies need up-to-date information from a poison control center or Poisondex. Calmness is of primary importance in the initial contact with a poisoned victim or the parent of a poisoned child. The second goal is to treat the victim and not the poison. Other steps include the use of an antidote and the dilution, removal, and elimination of the poison. Common ways to achieve the removal and elimination are emesis, lavage, activated charcoal, and cathartics. Finally, the key component in the treatment for poisoning is prevention through education.

Box 5-6. Household principles for preventing childhood poisoning

1. Keep all medications and toxic products in original containers.
2. Keep childproof caps on toxic products if children live in the home or are frequent visitors.
3. Keep all medications, including vitamins, out of the reach of children, in a locked chest.
4. Keep household chemical products out of the reach of children.
5. Do not treat medicines as candy.
6. Do not take or give medicine in the dark.
7. Read labels carefully before using drugs or toxic products.
8. Keep emergency poison control telephone numbers handy.
9. Have emergency drugs in the home—syrup of ipecac and Epsom salts.
10. Use toxic chemical products in a well ventilated area.
11. Do not mix common household cleaning products.
12. Destroy all old medications.
13. Destroy unused medications by incineration, flushing down toilet or washing down sink, rather than by throwing in trash.
14. Use childproof containers when available.
15. Identify any poisonous houseplants, and keep seeds, bulbs, leaves, and fruits of such plants away from children.

Lead poisoning

Lead poisoning remains a major type of poisoning in the United States.

Exposure to lead in the environment is generally unavoidable. As a heavy metal, lead (Pb) is present in the environment from automobile emissions, in water supplies, and from industrial emissions. In addition, household paint used before 1940 contains lead; tobacco and foodstuffs contain lead, usually as a result of processing any pesticide residues; newspaper print, ceramic glazes, decals used to decorate glass, and urban dust contain quantities of lead. Therefore, the amount of the lead to which anyone may be exposed is variable. Lead in any amount has no positive function in the body.

The inhalation or ingestion of lead is of particular concern with children between the ages of 12 and 36 months when the practice of mouthing foreign, nonnutritive substances is most common, thus increasing the potential for lead exposure. A family history of lead poisoning and the presence of pica (the ingestion of nonfood products) in children of this age group would indicate that such children are at risk for an increased lead burden. In adults, lead poisoning usually results from environment or occupational exposure. Children absorb nearly 50% of lead that has been ingested. It is estimated that 4% of U.S. children under 5 years old have elevated lead levels of 30 mg/dl or greater (Goldfrank, Osborn, & Hartnett, 1990, p 628.)

Pathophysiology

How much lead is absorbed into the body depends on the child's general nutritional state, age (younger children absorb lead more than older children), and the size of the lead particles absorbed. The lead level determined through serum analysis represents the balance between the lead that is present in the body's bones and tissues and that which is excreted. Lead absorbed in the bloodstream may be deposited in the kidney, the brain, or the bone marrow. Because of its chemical similarity to iron, lead may displace the iron in red blood cells and lead to anemia. Other body systems affected by lead absorption include the GI tract and the reproductive, immune, endocrine, and cardiovascular systems.

Signs and symptoms

An early sign of lead poisoning (*plumbism*) is an elevated free erythrocyte protoporphyrin (FEP) level. The FEP represents the final link in hemoglobin synthesis and normally is at a blood level of 50 or below. When the FEP and iron combine, a red blood cell is formed. The relationship between iron and lead and hemoglobin synthesis is significant in screening and diagnosing plumbism. If the body is deficient in iron, the FEP level will be elevated. A lack of available iron results from poor nutrition, malabsorption, blood loss, or displacement of iron by the chemically similar element lead. Free erythrocyte protoporphyrin levels approaching 200 generally indicate anemia. Levels higher than 200 are caused by lead poisoning.

Symptoms of lead poisoning may range from none to serious ones that reflect the site of tissue absorption of the lead. In mild plumbism, fatigue, mood swings, loss of appetite, malaise, pallor, restless sleep, irritable behavior, and developmental delays may be noted. Complaints of vomiting, abdominal pain, ataxia, weakness, clumsiness, alterations in the level of consciousness, and acute encephalopathy indicate serious lead poisoning.

A positive diagnosis of plumbism exists when:

- Two successive venous Pb levels are ≥70 µg/dl with or without symptoms
- FEP is ≥250 µg/dl and venous Pb level is 50 µg/dl with or without symptoms
- FEP is >109 µg/dl and there is an elevated venous Pb level of ≥30 µg/dl with symptoms
- Venous Pb level is >49 µg/dl with symptoms

and there is evidence of toxicity, such as abnormal FEP and positive results from provocative chelation (Preventing lead poisoning in young children, 1978, p 1)

Interventions

Treatment of lead poisoning should take into account the chronic nature of the disease. Although therapeutic interventions may be successful in removing lead from the soft tissues of the body, deposits in the bone are not mobilized for excretion. As long as the lead is contained within the bone tissue, little danger exists. Such a situation, however, requires long-term monitoring due to the possibility of a gradual and intermittent release of lead from the bones into the bloodstream. It is not yet known if long-range neuropsychiatric pathologies accompany chronic exposure.

The most successful intervention reflects prompt diagnosis and treatment of an acute toxic incident, removal of the toxin from the client's environment, and the education of family members about the cause of the illness and ways to control exposure and prevent pica. In addition, a successful intervention involves the strict enforcement of environmental standards requiring de-leading homes in high-risk categories.

Chelation therapy is used to mobilize the lead for potential excretion. Three agents used for this purpose are edetate calcium disodium (CaEDTA), D-penicillamine (PCA), and 2,3-dimercaptopropanol or British anti-lewisite (BAL). Table 5-4 identifies the schedule for chelation based on symptoms and documented lead levels.

The FDA has recently approved the first oral medication for treatment of severe lead poisoning in children. Succimer (Chemet) is recommended for a course of 19 days in children with blood levels greater than 45 mg/dl.

Because the process of chelation has a potentially toxic effect on the kidney, patients need to be well hydrated and to have their renal function monitored throughout the treatment. Because this therapy can also deplete the body's calcium, the patient must be monitored for signs of hypocalcemia.

The anemia that frequently accompanies plumbism must also be treated but iron-replacement therapy is contraindicated during the process of chelation. Children frequently remain on long-term iron therapy once treatment for toxicity has been completed.

Chelation is a painful experience for the child who receives intramuscular injections of the chelating agents. Chelating agents, therefore, are usually prepared with procaine to minimize the discomfort.

Prevention

Prevention of additional exposure to lead usually requires collaboration by several agencies. Guidelines are delineated by local agencies for the required environmental investigations and interventions. Permanent removal of hazards in the home is of primary importance, especially when pica is present. Once the home has been de-leaded, soil and dust may continue to recontaminate the child. A supportive attitude on the part of the health care providers is essential to assist families in dealing with the consequences of this chronic disease.

Enrichment experience 5-1

Investigate the incidence of lead poisoning in your community. What populations are at risk of being in contact with toxic levels of lead? What other heavy metal toxins are present in your locality? How are hazardous waste materials disposed of in your community?

Mercury poisoning

Methylmercury, an organic compound, is one of the most potent toxins in the environment. Its effects on the human organism are usually permanent, causing irreversible damage to the central nervous system (CNS). Inorganic mercury (Hg) in the form of mercury salts (such as mercuric chloride) is less hazardous because of its low solubility, although it is known to be toxic to the kidneys. Contamination of the environment originates largely from industrial and geologic sources of pollution in the water supply. The greatest source of industrial pollution is a result of inappropriate use of ethyl and methyl (organic compounds) mercury in fungicides. They enter the food chain when used as a seed and grain chemical protector. Chemical contamination of the water supply occurs when these toxic compounds become a part of the food chain for marine life.

The uptake of mercury by fresh-water fish may also be enhanced. Acid rain leaches metals from the soil and contaminates the fresh water. Action of microorganisms found at the bottom of fresh water bodies may interact chemically to change inorganic mercury to the organic form, methylmercury.

Pathophysiology

Absorption of mercury may occur through the respiratory tract, the GI tract, or the skin. If inhaled, it is oxidized in the blood and may be deposited in the brain. When ingested, it may be absorbed and found in various concentrations in the pancreas, kidney, liver, spleen, blood, bone marrow, mucosa of mouth and respiratory tract, skin, brain, and lungs. It is excreted mainly through the renal and GI systems. It is not readily eliminated from the tissues of the body and is detectable for years after treatment.

Table 5-4. Choice of chelation therapy based on symptoms and blood-level concentration

Clinical Presentation	Treatment	Comments
Symptomatic: encephalopathy present	BAL 450 mg/m²/d CaNa₂-EDTA 1,500 mg/m²/d	Start with BAL 75 mg/m² IM every 4 h. After 4 h start continuous infusion of CaNa₂-EDTA 1,500 mg/m²/d. Therapy with BAL and CaNa₂-EDTA should be continued for 5 days. Interrupt therapy for 2 days. Treat for 5 additional days, including BAL if blood Pb remains high. Other cycles may be needed depending on blood Pb rebound.
Symptomatic: encephalopathy absent	BAL 300 mg/m²/d CaNa₂-EDTA 1,000 mg/m²/d	Start with BAL 50 mg/m² IM every 4 h. After 4 h start CaNa₂-EDTA 1,000 mg/m²/d, preferably by continuous infusion, or in divided doses IV (through a heparin lock). Therapy with CaNa₂-EDTA should be continued for 5 days. BAL may be discontinued after 3 days if blood Pb<50 µg/dl. Interrupt therapy for 2 days. Treat for 5 additional days, including BAL if blood Pb remains >50 µg/dL. Repeated cycles may be needed depending on blood Pb rebound.
Asymptomatic before treatment, measure venous blood lead Blood Pb: ≥ 70 µg/dL	BAL 300 mg/m²/d CaNa₂-EDTA 1,000 mg/m²/d	Start with BAL 50 mg/m² IM every 4 h. After 4 h start CaNa₂-EDTA continuous infusion, or in divided doses IV (through a heparin lock). Treatment with CaNa₂-EDTA should be continued for 5 days. BAL may be discontinued after 3 days if blood Pb <50 µg/dL. Other cycles may be needed depending on blood Pb rebound.
Blood Pb: 56–69 µg/dL	CaNa₂-EDTA 1,000 mg/m²/d	CaNa₂-EDTA for 5 days, preferably by continuous infusion, or in divided doses (through a heparin lock). Alternatively, if lead exposure is controlled, CaNa₂-EDTA may be given as a single daily outpatient dose IM or IV. Other cycles may be needed depending on blood Pb rebound.
Blood Pb: 25–55 µg/dL Perform CaNa₂-EDTA provocation test to assess lead excretion ratio (µg Pb/mg EDTA) If ratio >0.70	CaNa₂-EDTA 1,000 mg/m²/d	Treat for 5 days IV or IM, as above.
If ratio 0.60–0.69 Age <3 years of age	CaNa₂-EDTA 1,000 mg/m²/d	Treat for 3 days IV or IM, as above.
Age >3 years of age	No treatment	Repeat blood Pb and EP, and CaNa₂-EDTA provocation test periodically.
If ratio <0.60	No treatment	Repeat blood Pb and EP, and CaNa₂-EDTA provocation test periodically.

From Piomelli S, Rosen JF, Chisolm, JJ, Graef JW: (1984). Management of childhood lead poisoning. *J Pediatr, 105*, 527.

Signs and symptoms

The toxicity of any chemical is affected by its physical properties since they determine the degree to which the substance affects man and the environment. A chemical may exist as a volatile gas or may be soluble under certain conditions. The vapors of mercury are highly toxic to the brain, penetrating the tissue 10 times more readily than do other forms. Poisoning by mercury vapors presents with symptoms of CNS disturbances. The individual will show signs of psychological disturbance such as anxiety, mood swings, irritability, and excessive shyness. Changes in appetite, complaints of insomnia, and weight loss may also be present.

Methylmercury poisoning presents with symptoms of CNS damage. Complaints are of hearing loss, motor deficits, numbness and tingling in fingers and toes, tunnel vision, loss of position sense, exaggerated deep tendon reflexes, spasticity, and muscle rigidity. Ethylmercury poisoning is indicated by muscle tenderness, tremor, dysphagia, pink skin (acrodynia), desquamation of the palms and soles of the feet (if direct skin contact occurs), fatigability, and optic atrophy. Renal and GI symptoms may also be present in ethylmercury poisoning. They include polyuria, increased blood urea nitrogen, oliguria, hematuria, albuminuria, nausea, vomiting, and abdominal cramps.

Interventions

The World Health Organization has indicated that acceptable daily intake from additive, nutritional, or residue sources of mercury is 5 µg/kg/d. The minimum toxic dose for methylmercury is 0.35 mg for a 70-kg man.

Acute exposure to inorganic mercury may respond to chelation therapy with dimercaprol, which offers protection against kidney damage. Organic methylmercury poisoning does not respond well to treatment of any kind, and prevention becomes the only real option.

Toxins in the hospital environment

Surgical hazards

Operating room exposure to hazardous vapors from anesthesia gases and chemical fixation agents places hospital personnel at considerable health risk. Although the therapeutic use of anesthetics is recognized (see Chapter 24), employee exposure to nitrous oxide (N_2O) and halothane in the ambient air has been related to an increased incidence of cancer, spontaneous abortions, stillbirths, birth defects, and hepatic and renal diseases. Alterations in psychomotor skills have also been noted to occur at certain levels of exposure.

Nitrous oxide and halothane gases are rapidly absorbed into the bloodstream on inhalation and deposited in body tissues. Minimizing employee risks of exposure requires adherence to the National Institute of Occupational Safety and Health (NIOSH) standards, which recommend specific operating room ventilation exhaust systems. Exposure limits defined by National Institute of Occupational Safety and Health indicate that 25 parts per million time-weighted average for nitrous oxide and 2 parts per million per hour of exposure for halothane are the maximum permissible doses.

The use of methylmethacrylate represents another potential hazard for operating room personnel.

This substance is compounded from a liquid and a powder during a surgical procedure just prior to its use to bond implanted prostheses. It has been associated with certain other patient complications, including cardiac arrest, blood and air emboli, and acute hypotension.

Employees exposed to the vapors of methylmethacrylate may experience local irritation of the respiratory mucosa and may face an increased risk of cancer.

Prevention of toxic levels of exposure is the key to reducing hazards in the work environment. Periodic screening, monitoring ambient air concentrations, and using appropriate ventilation and exhaust techniques for toxic gases will greatly enhance the safety of these work settings.

Chemical sterilants

Ethylene oxide (EtO) is a colorless gas that can be found as a liquid or vapor and has an etherlike odor. In the hospital setting, it is used for its sterilant properties with items that cannot withstand steam or the intense heat of sterilization. It is highly toxic to patients and personnel if inhaled or absorbed systemically, or if it has been in contact with skin or mucous membranes.

Symptoms of exposure include the following: initial eye, nose, throat, and respiratory tract irritation; headache, nausea, vomiting, dyspnea, pulmonary edema, and weakness, with continued exposure; burns and irritation from skin contact; potential carcinoma with long-term contamination; and possible reproductive complications, chromosomal aberrations, and mutagenic changes in short-term, high-concentration exposure.

Certain safety precautions are recommended when using EtO:

- EtO is a flammable liquid and is potentially explosive when exposed to air. Store away from heat, in appropriate containers, and in a well ventilated area.
- Avoid creating sparks when manipulating containers.
- Use in a properly ventilated area that allows for direct venting of gas to the outside.
- Do not exceed permissible levels of exposure as established by the Occupational Safety and Health Administration of 1 parts per million per 8 hours time-weighted average in airborne concentrations. Short-term exposure should not exceed 10 parts per million of air averaged over a 15-minute period.
- When unloading a sterilizer using EtO, open the sterilizer door 2–4 inches immediately after the cycle is completed. (This is not necessary if the sterilizer has a purge system.) Remain out of the room for at least 15 minutes after opening the door.

- EtO is often used to sterilize kidney dialyzers. If there is sufficient residual chemical remaining in the equipment, it may be toxic to the patients. Symptoms of an allergic reaction would be present. In addition, severe chest, head, and back pain may be experienced.
- Allow for adequate aeration of EtO sterilized equipment.

Chemical disinfectants

There are five categories of chemical disinfectant: alcohols, halogens (chlorine, iodophor), phenols, quaternary ammonium compounds, and aldehydes (glutaraldehyde, formaldehyde). The aldehydes pose the greatest toxic risk from exposure.

Glutaraldehyde ($C_5H_8O_2$) is an unstable chemical that may cause burns of the skin and mucous membranes on contact. It also corrodes and stains high carbon metals, leaving a residue on some. It is, therefore, unsuitable for cleaning certain instruments.

Formaldehyde (CH_2O) is a highly corrosive chemical frequently used to disinfect dialysis machines. On contact with the skin, dermatitis may occur; it also irritates the mucous membranes of the eye, nose, and upper respiratory tract. Chemical peritonitis may result if the formaldehyde is not thoroughly rinsed from the dialysis machines. Patients would complain of a smothering, burning sensation and a strange taste in the mouth. Residual build-up of formaldehyde could also lead to symptoms of neurologic and metabolic disturbances, hemolysis, and anticoagulation problems.

Chemotherapy

It is generally recognized that a significant number of cytotoxic drugs are carcinogenic or mutagenic in studies of animals and have similar effects in man. These chemotherapeutic agents are incapable of differentiating between healthy and diseased cells and are developed for the express purpose of causing cell death.

Until recently, the risks associated with preparing, administering, and disposing of antineoplastic agents went unnoticed. Although definitive scientific studies are pending, organizations including the Oncology Nursing Society, the National Institutes of Health, and the National Cancer Institute, and hospital pharmacy groups have published guidelines designed to provide direction for safe procedures when handling these substances. The toxic effects of antineoplastic drugs are discussed in Chapters 48 and 49. The present discussion will address the potential hazards associated with handling the products and by-products of chemotherapy.

Inadvertent exposure during drug preparation or administration may occur through inhalation of an aerosolized drug, direct skin contact as a result of spills, leaks, or dressing contamination, and patient excretions of a specific drug. Contact with improperly disposed hazardous waste products from drug preparation and administration may also occur. Personnel who are exposed to cytotoxic drugs as a result of inadequate safety precautions may experience symptoms of hair loss, itching, nausea, lightheadedness, dizziness, headache, or coughing.

It is recommended that antineoplastic drugs be prepared by qualified personnel using a class II, type B biologic safety cabinet with vertical-exhaust air flow. Protective outer garments are necessary. Preparation, decontamination, and disposal procedures require that the work area and the contaminated products comply with standards for clean-up and disposal of hazardous wastes.

The Oncology Nursing Society established guidelines for nursing practice in cancer chemotherapy. These recommendations indicate policies to be followed by specially prepared nurses to ensure client and nurse safety. Two potential adverse client responses are highlighted: extravasation* and anaphylaxis. Table 5-5 identifies whether specific drugs are vesicant/irritants or nonvesicants. Table 5-6 lists antidotes empirically recommended at this time and thought to be useful for treating an area of extravasation.

The potential for an allergic reaction should be anticipated and the necessary emergency equipment made available. It is important to note that an allergic response may occur at any time, whether or not the client has ever shown any prior sensitivity to a given drug.

■ Summary

Client and employee potential for exposure to hazards in the workplace is present in the chemicals used to sanitize and sterilize the environment and equipment, in building materials, and in gases used in diagnostic and treatment procedures. Scientific research is inconclusive in many respects as to the type and amount of real risk from exposure to these agents. Yet the prudent course would seem to indicate that caution, respect, and continued research direct the nurse's actions with regard to his or her own safety and that of the patient.

Nursing management

Nursing implications

Nurses are taking significant roles in the field of toxicology. Poison prevention, education, and implementation for treatment are major areas in which nurses can have an impact on health care.

---

* Leakage of a vesicant or irritant drug into the subcutaneous tissue.

Table 5-5. Vesicant/irritant and nonvesicant cancer chemotherapeutic drugs

Generic name	Trade or other name
Vesicant drugs (commercial agents)	
dactinomycin	Actinomycin D
dacarbazine	Dtic-Dome
daunomycin	Cerubidine
doxorubicin	Adriamycin
mithramycin	Mithracin
mitomycin C	Mutamycin
estramustine phosphate	Estracyte
mechlorethamine	Nitrogen mustard
vinblastine	Velban
vincristine	Oncovin
Vesicant drugs (investigational agents)	
amsacrine	M-AMSA
bisantrene	
maytansine	
pyrazofurin	Pyrazomycin
vindesine	Eldisine
Irritant agents	
carmustine	BiCNU
etoposide	VP-16-213 Vepesid
streptozocin	Zanosar
teniposide*	VM-26
mitoguazone*	Methyl-GAG
Nonvesicant agents	
bleomycin†	Blenoxane
cyclophosphamide	Cytoxan
cytarabine	ARA-C
floxuridine	FUDR
fluorouracil†	5-FU
tegafur	Ftorafur
methotrexate	
cisplatin‡	Platinol
thiotepa	
mitoxantrone	
asparaginase	Elspar
thioguanine injection	

Definitions: **Vesicant:** a cancer chemotherapeutic agent capable of causing or forming a blister or causing tissue destruction; **Irritant:** a cancer chemotherapeutic agent capable of producing venous pain at the site or along the vein, with or without an inflammatory reaction; **Extravasation:** the leakage of a vesicant or irritant drug into the subcutaneous tissue that is capable of causing pain, necrosis, or sloughing of the tissue.

* Investigational drug now in clinical trials.

† Occasionally causes mild phlebitis.

‡ Single case report each of cellulitis and fibrosis. (1980) (*Cancer Treat Rep 64 [10]*, 1162–1163.)

(*Cancer chemotherapy: Guidelines and recommendations for nursing education and practice,* p 15. (1984). Pittsburgh: Oncology Nursing Society.)

Nurses are now active in poison control centers and are responsible for responding to calls from the community about first-aid measures; providing information about product contents to identify toxins; and educating the public and health care professionals about poison control and safety. Because many nurses involved in the field of toxicology feel there is a need for specialization, they are designing a curriculum to prepare toxicology clinicians.

Nursing process

Assessment In a toxicologic emergency, obtaining a poison history immediately is essential. Assessment factors should include the following:

- Physiologic parameters, including cardiac and respiratory status, mental status, level of consciousness, and neurologic status
- Poison history, including assessment of first-aid measures implemented, as well as type, amount, and route of poisoning
- Psychological support needs appropriate to the nature of the emergency for patient and family

Once the poisoning emergency is resolved, assess educational needs to prevent recurrence.

Nursing diagnosis Nursing diagnoses relate to the specific agent affecting the client and its physiologic effects. Examples include the following:

Ineffective breathing patterns related to CNS depression secondary to sedative overdose
Altered tissue perfusion: hypotensive shock related to depressant overdose
Impaired tissue integrity related to chemical burns by corrosive substances
High risk for aspiration related to emesis or gastric lavage
Anxiety related to CNS overactivity secondary to stimulant overdose

A collaborative problem that should be differentiated from the nursing diagnoses is

Potential complication: neurologic/sensory related to plumbism.

If toxicity is related to a suicidal episode, additional diagnoses may include:

Ineffective individual coping
Hopelessness
Situational low self-esteem
Body image disturbance

Many clients will exhibit a

Knowledge deficit regarding poisoning and poison prevention.

Planning Appropriate nursing goals are to maintain vital functions, prevent continued absorption of toxic materials, prevent aspiration during emetic therapy or lavage procedures, reduce fear or anxiety, prevent or minimize permanent tissue damage, and educate the client concerning poison prevention. In cases of attempted suicide, the client should be given psychological counseling to improve his or her coping skills and self-image.

Intervention Nurses are often involved in answering calls to poison control centers. It should be assumed

Table 5-6. Antidotes for vesicant/irritant drugs

Drug classification	Specific agent	Local antidote	Positive effect — Animal studies	Positive effect — Clinical case reports	Antidote preparation	Method of administration	Comments
Alkylating Agent	mechlorethamine (Nitrogen mustard)	Isotonic sodium thiosulfate 1 g/10 ml (manufacturer's recommendations)	None	Yes	Mix 4 ml of 10% Na thiosulfate with 6 ml sterile water for injection (1/6 molar solution results).	1. Injection 5–6 ml (0.2–0.24 g) IV through the existing line and SQ into the extravasated site with multiple injections. 2. Repeat dosing SQ over the next several hours. 3. Apply cold compresses. 4. No total dose established	1. *Action:* chemical neutralization 2. Initiate treatment immediately and liberally.
	mitomycin C (Mutamycin)	Topical DMSO (RIMSO)	Yes	None	1–2 ml of 1 mmol DMSO 50%–100%	1. Apply topically one time to the site.	1. ACTION: carrier solvent or oxygen radical 2. Probably not effective for distal or delayed ulcers. 3. Initiate treatment immediately.
Plant Alkaloids	vinblastine (Velban) vincristine (Oncovin) vindesine (Eldisine) teniposide (VM-26)	hyaluronidase (Wydase) 150 U/ml (manufacturer's recommendations)	Yes	None	Add 1 ml USP sodium chloride (150 U/ml results).	1. Inject 1–6 ml (150–900 U) SQ into the extravasated site with multiple injections. 2. Repeat dosing SQ over the next several hours. 3. Apply *warm* compresses. 4. No total dose established	1. *Action:* enhances adsorption and dispersion of the extravasated drug. 2. Corticosteroids and topical cooling appear to worsen toxicity. 3. Warm compresses increase systemic absorption of the drug.
	etoposide (VP-16-213 Vepesid)	hyaluronidase (Wydase) 150 U/ml	Yes	None			
Anthracycline Antibiotics	doxorubicin (Adriamycin) daunomycin (Cerubidine)	Topical cooling	Yes	Yes	Topical cooling may be achieved using —ice packs —cooling pad with	1. Cooling of site to patient tolerance for 24 hours. 2. Elevate and rest	1. Application of cold compresses inhibit cytotoxicity of drug.

(Continued)

Table 5-6. Antidotes for vesicant/irritant drugs (Continued)

Drug classification	Specific agent	Local antidote	Positive effect		Antidote preparation	Method of administration	Comments
			Animal studies	Clinical case reports			
					ice water circulating —cryogel packs changed frequently	extremity 24–48 hours then resume normal activity as tolerated. 3. If pain, erythema, or swelling persist beyond 48 hours, refer patient immediately to plastic surgeon for consultation. Surgical debridement may be necessary; however, only one-third of vesicant extravastions lead to ulceration.	2. Some studies suggest a role for topical dimethyl sulfoxide (DMSO) while others show no benefit or delayed healing. 3. Local singular injection of low doses (less than 50 mg) soluble hydrocortisone may still be beneficial. Avoid multiple injections into site.
	bisantrene	sodium bicarbonate 1 mEq/1 ml (premixed)	Yes	Yes	Mix equal parts of 1 mEq/ml sodium bicarbonate with sterile normal saline (1:1 solution). Resulting solution is 0.5 mEq/ml.	1. Inject 2–6 ml (1–3 mEq) IV through the existing line and SQ into the extravasated site with multiple injections. 2. Apply cold compresses. 3. Total dose not to exceed 10 ml or 0.5 mEq/ml solution (5 mEq)	1. *Action:* chemical activation 2. Dilute bicarbonate chemically degrades the drug.

(Cancer Chemotherapy Guidelines. *Module V: Recommendations for the Management of Extravasation and Anaphylaxis*, p 8 [1988]. Pittsburgh: Oncology Nursing Society.)

Example of nursing process and drug overdose

A 30-year-old, single woman, accompanied by a boyfriend, presents in the emergency department after having reportedly ingested 100 tablets of diazepam (Valium) 10 mg. She is crying and complaining of pain in the right nostril, which is swollen and draining. She has a history of depression.

Assessment data	Nursing diagnosis	Intervention	Goals and outcome criteria
History of depressant overdose	High risk for ineffective breathing pattern; apnea related to CNS depression secondary to diazepam overdose	**Prepare** equipment for emergency resuscitation if hypopnea develops. **Prepare** for gastric lavage; position client to prevent aspiration during procedure.	Adequate respirations will be maintained; signs and symptoms of hypoxemia will not develop.
History of drug overdose; weeping	Ineffective individual coping	**Provide** a nonthreatening environment; maintain a nonjudgmental attitude. **Assist** client to identify stressors and alternative techniques for dealing with them. **Encourage** client to verbalize needs. **Locate** resources to ensure follow-up care for psychological needs.	The client will be able to identify stressors related to suicide attempt or accept counseling follow-up.

that callers reporting an incidence of poisoning or overdose are likely to be emotionally distraught. The name and address of the caller should be obtained first so help can be sent, in case the call is interrupted. The nurse follows protocols regarding advice to the caller, depending on the toxic substance involved. In most cases, the victim should be seen in an acute care facility following first aid. If possible, the package containing the toxic substance should be brought with the victim.

Priority is given to maintaining the victim's vital functions until his or her condition is stabilized. It may be necessary to administer emetics or gastric lavage, during which time the client should be positioned to avoid aspiration of stomach contents. Seizure precautions should be implemented.

The nurse should interview the client or family to determine exactly what toxin is involved and, if possible, the quantity to which the victim has been exposed. Medical management depends on the client's condition and the toxin involved.

Both client and family need emotional support during the acute treatment phase. Victims affected by CNS stimulants or hallucinogens need a nonthreatening environment and protection from extraneous stimuli. These clients should not be left alone. Therapeutic communication is helpful in "talking down" clients who are experiencing "bad trips" from stimulants such as hallucinogens.

When the victim's condition stabilizes, the need for poison prevention education, or for referral for psychological counseling, should be determined and follow-up care ensured.

Evaluation Data required for evaluation include serial observations of vital signs, the emotional reactions of the victim and family, the occurrence or absence of signs and symptoms of permanent tissue damage following the toxic episode, and a determination of whether the overdose or poisoning is a recurrence. (See Example of Nursing Process and Drug Overdose.)

References

Goldfrank L. (1990). Overview: General management and diagnostic tools. *Goldfrank's toxicologic emergencies*, 4th ed. Norwalk, CT: Appleton & Lange.

Goldfrank L, Osborn H, Hartnett L. (1990). Lead. *Goldfrank's toxicologic emergencies*, 4th ed. Norwalk, CT: Appleton & Lange.

Investigation of risks and hazards associated with hemodialysis devices. (1980). Washington, DC: FDA, Public Health Service, US DHEW.

Litovitz T, Schmitz B, Bailey K. (1990). 1989 Annual Report of the American Association of Poison Control Centers National Collection System. *Am J Emerg Med, 8,* 394–397.

Loomis T. (1974). *Essentials of toxicology*, 2nd ed. Philadelphia: Lea & Febiger.

Bibliography

Gilman AG, Goodman LS, Rall TW, Murad F. (1990). *Goodman and Gilman's the pharmacological basis of therapeutics*, 8th ed. New York: Pergamon Press.

Goldfrank L. (1990). Overview: General management and diagnostic tools. *Goldfrank's toxicologic emergencies*, 4th ed. Norwalk, CT: Appleton & Lange.

Goldfrank L, Osborn H, Hartnett L. (1990). Lead. *Goldfrank's toxicologic emergencies*, 4th ed. Norwalk, CT: Appleton & Lange.

Williams DR, Halstead BW. (1982–1983). Chelating agents in medicine. *J Toxicol Clin Toxicol, 19*, 1081–1115.

Therapy
with drugs

2

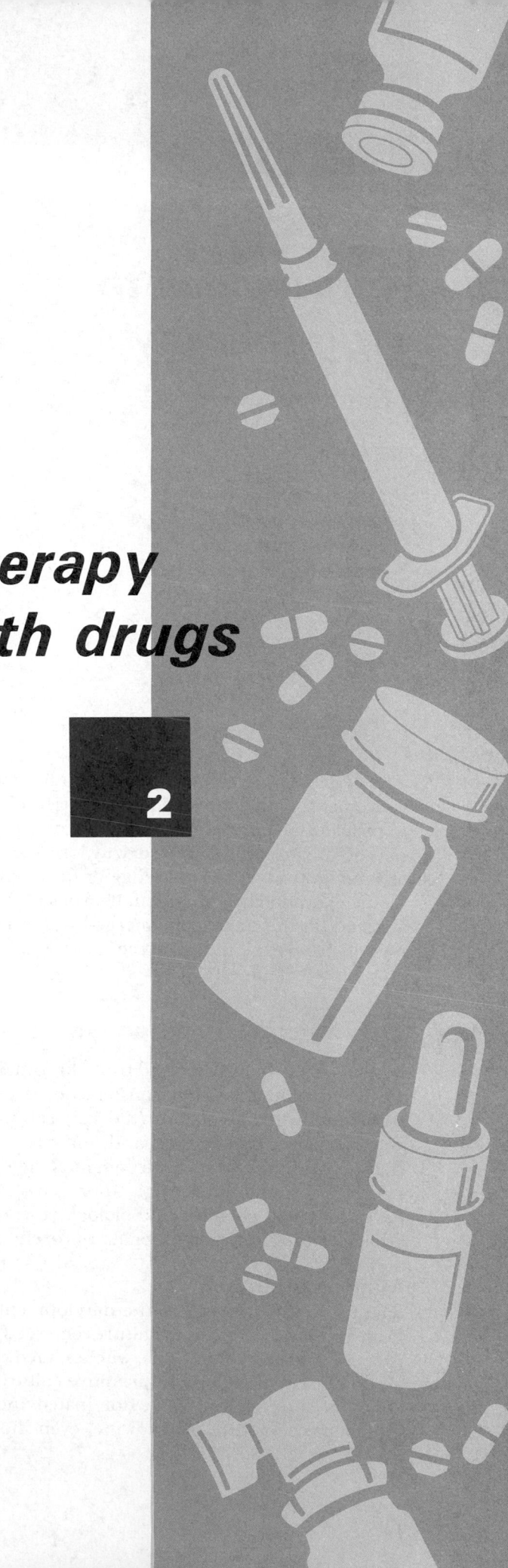

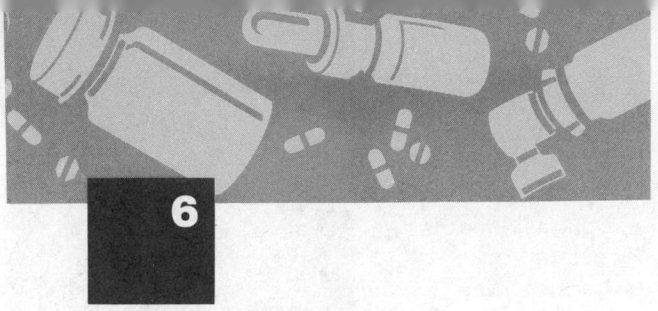

6

Approaches to drug therapy

The development of medicine parallels humanity's advancements in the application of the scientific method to problems in our natural environment. The uniqueness of human culture allowed drug lore to accumulate as families passed on knowledge of healing remedies from generation to generation. Pharmacology became a science as this knowledge merged with information derived from explorations in the concepts of cause and effect (see Chapter 1).

Three major approaches

Modern drug therapy evolved from three major areas: 1) the development and transmission of oral tribal traditions in drug folklore (the magical approach); 2) experience, observation, and analysis of cultural traditions in the use of environmental elements (the empirical protopharmacologic approach); and 3) the development of chemical and biologic research methodologies (the scientific rational approach; Box 6-1).

Magical approach

The use of medicines and the development of basic health customs in different cultures emerged from the practices of spiritual persons, witches, medicine men, and other tribal leaders. In primitive cultures, beliefs about the supernatural forces dominated understanding about the nature of medicine, even though religion, magic, and medicine were intertwined. Chauncey Leake (1975, p 26) reports that these (uses of magic) reflected the wishful effort to achieve what was desired from the unknown surrounding powers of good and evil, either by shamanistically propitiating angry forces, driving out or frightening away evil influences, or cajoling indifferent fateful powers for benefit, individually in sickness, or tribally in epidemics. In the absence of any clear knowledge of the causes of infections or metabolic diseases, this recourse to magic was reasonable.

This lack of knowledge about cause and effect allowed people to become victims of superstition and fear. Ritual and magical were major controlling forces in early Egyptian medicine. Medicines were composed frequently of many elements compounded for a single remedy. These elements were animal, vegetable, or mineral drugs and were combined with religious rituals in most healing practices. Demonic possession was thought to be the cause of illness and magical remedy was its only cure.

It is difficult to separate the influence of magic from the development of empirical science. The belief in magic inhibited progress toward a scientific rational approach to medicine, while at the same time, it facilitated the experimental use of natural elements. Merchant exchanges among Egypt, Crete, the Aegean Islands, Sicily, and Italy during the pre-Hippocratean period (before 6th century B.C.) influenced the evolution of empirical healing practices. Recorded evidence indicates that attributing natural rather than supernatural or magical causes to occurrences probably began during this period. Imported substances found in the Egyptian pharmacopeia included saffron and sage from the isle of Crete, spices and perfumes from Arabia, and cinnamon from China. Minerals and metals such as copper, alum, carbon, and antimony were also prevalent (Lyons & Petrucelli, 1978, p 97).

The Greeks combined philosophic inquiry and empirical practices in their medical teaching and healing strategies through small gatherings of scientists, philosophers, and itinerant medical practitioners. Thales (640?–546 B.C.), known as the "Father of Science," sought to discover nonmagical or religious causes for natural events. The Greek philosopher/scientist Hippocrates (about 460–370 B.C.) supported the evolution of the rational approach to solving medical questions (Lyons & Petrucelli, 1978, p 215).

By 146 B.C., Rome began to emerge as the center of medicine, albeit greatly influenced by the spread of Greek practices known to date (Lyons & Petrucelli, 1978, p 231). The Roman Caius Pliny the Elder (A.D. 23–79) was noted for his "Historia Naturalis," which contained extensive writings on all available information in the fields of physics, anatomy, biology, food, magic, folklore, history, plants, and medicine. It recorded important information on the history of ancient civilization and reflected early attempts to use medicines based on experimentation. Pliny credits a variety of forces with the discovery of the medicinal value of certain remedies—notably divine revelation, dreams, and change (Thorndike, 1929, p 56).

Empirical approach

Empiricism as an approach to pharmacology attempted to relate drug use to experience. Empirics believed that certain substances were useful in specific circumstances but they were not able to account rationally for the therapeutic effectiveness of those substances. In ancient Egypt, the pharmacists were responsible for gathering, categorizing, evaluating, preparing, and preserving the various elements commonly used as medicines. Physicians turned to the pharmacist to compound drug preparations for use by patients. Some 200 drugs are known to have been used by the ancient Egyptians. These remedies were probably plant, mineral, or animal materials, which, having been ingested at one time or another, were known to have produced certain effects. From those observations, an empirical approach to drug use developed—an approach based on experience.

The empirics of the Roman Empire held that all things were discovered by experience. They rejected reason as a criterion of validity. They further believed that there was no systematic order in the discovery of medicines, attributing the discovery of remedies to dreams and chance (Thorndike, 1929, pp 155–157).

Antidotes I. Galen (circa A.D. 129–200), a Greek physician in the Roman Empire, was credited with bridging the gap between magic, empiricism, and a more rational approach to medical care. He was a meticulous observer who carefully noted in his travels the pharmacologic use of plants and minerals. He was an advocate of the humoral theory, which proposed that imbalances in the body's phlegm, yellow bile, black bile, and blood were the cause of illness. Galen was most noted for his extensive use of medicinal plants, blending remedies from several agents by correlating them with the properties of the four humors and their characteristics of hot/cold/moist/dry (Lyons & Petrucelli, 1978, p 251). He used systematic methods to describe the use of plants, animals, and minerals as remedies and is believed to have pioneered experimental physiology (Leake, 1975, pp 66–67). His writings influenced medicine until the 16th century.

For centuries, efforts were made to mold empirical protopharmacology into a systematic compilation of information on known remedies throughout the world. The 17th and 18th centuries were characterized by attempts to develop a quantitative methodology. The science of pharmacology emerged from the development of chemistry and biology into genuine quantitative sciences in the late 18th and early 19th centuries.

Rational approach

Empirical protopharmacology led to a rational approach to thought at the end of the 18th century. The rational approach depended on the development of procedures for the methodologic evaluation of crude drugs and chemical compounds. Decisions about the rational use of drugs could be made once science was able to provide answers to questions regarding the chemical and biologic effects of various compounds on other substances.

Systematic experimentation with drugs developed slowly. Observations from early experiments on the biologic activities of crude drug preparations led to the recognition of toxic properties. The foundation of the modern science of pharmacology began in the 19th century. In the first half of the century, biologically active agents of crude drugs, formerly used empirically, were isolated in chemically pure form. The latter half of the 19th century saw rapid success in the use of quantitative and qualitative chemical analysis.

Much of this foundation was laid by François Magendie (1783–1855) and his pupils. As a result of their work, specific problems related to the science were defined using the rational approach to problem-solving methodology in pharmacology. They include the following (Leake, 1975, p 123):

- The dose-effect relationship of a drug
- Time and chemical factors involved in absorption, distribution, chemical transformation, and removal of a drug into and out of living material
- Localization of the site of action of a drug
- Scientific mechanism of action of a drug
- Relation between the chemical constitution of a drug and its biologic activity

The rational approach to drug therapy now relies on the process of biologic assay in pharmacologic research and includes efforts by chemists, pharmacologists, and clinicians. Bioassay procedures are used to standardize the biologic properties of drugs. Biologic assay can be defined as the estimation of the potency of a drug or other substance by comparison of its biochemical, pharmacological, or toxic effects on animals against those of a reference standard. Today the standardization of drugs is accomplished by the study of their physical and chemical properties and through bioassay techniques.

■ Summary

Modern drug therapy developed from three major areas: oral tribal traditions in folklore, cultural traditions, and the employment of chemical and biologic methodologies. Lack of knowledge about cause and effect gave rise to a magical approach to healing—superstition, fear, or wishful thinking concerning use of natural products and persons involved with healing. The empirical approach arose from this as it became clear that certain substances were useful in particular circumstances. These substances were used even though the healer did not know why the substance was helpful. Some systematic methods evolved under empiricism. The rational approach appeared at the end of the 18th century as science developed a methodologic evaluation of crude drugs and chemical compounds. Systematic experimentation developed slowly, eventually leading to the problem-solving methodology of modern pharmacology. The biologic approach now relies on bioassay.

Nursing management

Nursing implications

Health care practices today continue to reflect magical, empirical, and rational orientations in client and health care provider behaviors. In modern health care delivery, clients are increasingly involved in establishing a diagnosis, as well as in providing input into the decision-making process for treatment. The self-care movement in the United States is attracting participants rapidly, and trends toward holistic health care represent the consumer's interest in becoming an active member of the health care team.

As health care providers internalize the concepts inherent in the holistic health movement, new problems arise. Until recently, clients generally pursued health care only after illness or incapacitation had taken place. They sought medical care to be given something to cure the malady or to relieve its symptoms. With health care delivery increasingly moving toward primary care in ambulatory settings today, clients experience frustration when they do not receive medication. Many clients hope that the prescription will be the cure—the magical approach. The magical powers of medicine are further exemplified through the use of placebos. A visit to the physician is often considered wasted or unacceptable unless a prescription is written.

Physicians often prescribe medications and use devices in the delivery of health care on an empirical basis only. For example, the intrauterine device has long been used without a clear understanding of how it actually prevents pregnancy, although there are a number of theories regarding its mechanism of action. Diethylstilbestrol, aspirin, and antihistamines are examples of drugs whose mechanisms of action are still questionable or not fully understood.

Empirical evidence also serves as a basis for the continued use of home remedies in the face of information that contradicts their therapeutic value. This is evident in practices that are peculiar to a specific cultural or ethnic population.

Scientific investigations using rational approaches underlie the development of many modern drugs.

Learning experience 6-1

1. Interview a friend or family member to explore his or her beliefs about the use of medications and personal drug habits related to the taking of prescribed medicines. Explore the following questions in your interview:
   a. What was the presenting problem?
   b. What interventions, if any, did the individual try prior to seeking medical advice?
   c. How did he or she approach the health care provider to resolve a problem?
   d. How did he or she comply with the recommended regimen for taking the medication?
   e. What approaches to the use of pharmacologic agents are you able to identify in this interview?
2. Interview friends or peers to solicit information regarding health-seeking practices that reflect an empirical orientation.
3. Explore the availability of folk remedies or herbal products found in a health food store and identify the rationale for use of the specific products.

The pharmaceutical chemist determines the molecular properties associated with therapeutic action and side effects, and may construct a drug with the most desirable combinations of these properties.

Client education. Historically, clients have not been socialized to be good consumers of health care and to participate actively in their treatment regimens. Although it appears that this has been changing in recent years, nurses continue to serve an important role—as practitioner, school nurse, and community health nurse—in educating clients to be informed health care consumers and in promoting a wellness rather than an illness orientation to health care.

References

Leake CD. (1975). *An historical account of pharmacology to the 20th century*. Springfield, IL: Charles C Thomas.
Lyons A, Petrucelli RJ. (1978). *Medicine: An illustrated history*. New York: Harry N Abrams.
Thorndike L. (1929). *A history of magic and rxperimental science: During the first thirteen centuries of our era, vol 1*. New York: Columbia University Press.

Bibliography

Gilman AG, et al, eds. (1990). *The pharmacological basis of therapeutics*, 8th ed. New York: Pergamon Press.
Thorndike L. (1963). *Science and thought in the fifteenth century*. New York: Hafner Press.

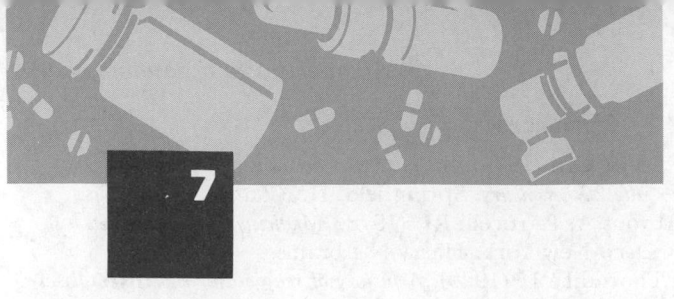

7

Pharmacodynamics and pharmacokinetics

Pharmacodynamics
  Alteration of cellular environments
  Alteration of genetic material
  Provision of substrate material
  Alteration of the speed of cell functions
    Receptor theory of drug action
  Agonist/antagonist interaction
  Nursing management
Pharmacokinetics
  Drug absorption
    Mechanisms of absorption
    Routes of absorption
  Drug distribution
    The blood-brain barrier
    Tissue trapping
    Movement of drugs across membranes
  Drug biotransformation
    Biotransformation by the liver
    Factors in biotransformation
  Drug excretion
    Excretion processes
  Interaction of pharmacokinetic processes
  Nursing management

To exert effects on the body, drugs must reach target tissues in suitable forms and in sufficient concentrations to initiate specific changes. The processes by which drugs are distributed within the body are termed *pharmacokinetics*; the processes by which they subsequently influence cell physiology are called *pharmacodynamics*. The study of these subjects is concerned with the response of tissues to chemicals and with the absorption, distribution, biotransformation, and excretion of drugs within the body. Individual physiology must be considered. The body is not a passive recipient of chemicals; it is actively involved in all the above processes (Box 7-1).

Pharmacodynamics

In the tissues, drugs may act either to change the environment of the cell or to alter the rate of cell functions. Some drugs act by destroying or inhibiting the growth of foreign organisms or rapidly proliferating (malignant) cells. Other drugs may protect cells from the influence of physical or chemical agents; promote cell function by providing substances needed for metabolism; or speed up or slow down cell processes. Drugs cannot, however, alter the nature of cell function. Research presently in progress is aimed at changing the genetic material within cells to prevent or treat inherited conditions stemming from abnormal genes.

Alteration of cellular environments

Drugs change the environment of body cells by either physical or chemical processes. Physical actions may involve all the processes of physics from lubrication to ionizing radiation (Table 7-1). Individual drugs may exert more than one effect. For example, many lubricants also impose a lipid barrier between tissues to which they are applied and irritating substances. The chemical environment of cells is changed when drugs react with other chemicals, producing changes in the constituents of body fluids (Table 7-2). Drugs that affect body chemistry also may act by more than one mechanism. For example, electrolytes such as chlorides not only change serum levels of individual ions but also influence the *p*H of body fluids. A drug may act both physically and chemically, as do intravenous (IV) fluids that influence serum osmotic pressure and chemical makeup of the blood.

Alteration of genetic material

Researchers hope to correct genetic defects by introducing into the cells normal genes produced by recombinant gene processes. In some instances, viral or other molecular particles are used as carriers of the genes. Reports from initial clinical trials are promising but no investigators to date claim the achievement of a usable drug.

> **Box 7-1. Definitions**
>
> *Pharmacodynamics*—the processes by which drugs influence cell physiology
>
> *Pharmacokinetics*—the processes by which drugs are distributed within the body

Table 7-1. Processes by which drugs alter the physics of cell environments

Process	Examples
Imposition of barriers	Application of petroleum jelly to skin of diaper area of babies to prevent contact with urine
	Application of tincture of benzoin to skin to protect it from friction of sheets or clothing
	Sunscreen lotions applied to prevent sunburn
Lubrication	Mineral oil administered by mouth to facilitate passage of feces
	Cornstarch applied to skin folds to reduce friction
Osmosis	Saline catharsis
	Mannitol administered intravenously to stimulate osmotic diuresis
	Saturated magnesium sulfate soaks used to reduce tissue edema
	Intravenous injection of magnesium sulfate to reduce cerebral edema
Adsorption	Kaopectate administered to absorb toxins that cause diarrhea
	Activated charcoal given orally to reduce the absorption of harmful chemicals in cases of poisoning
Alteration of surface tension	Surfactant stool softeners
	Quaternary compounds used as antiseptic cleansers
Ionizing radiation	Radioactive tracers used in diagnostic tests
	Radioactive iodine used to ablate thyroid tissue in hyperthyroidism

Provision of substrate material

Many chemicals that act as substrate for metabolism are classified as nutrients and are not considered to be true drugs. However, because they affect living tissue, they fall under the general classification of drugs. Recent findings by nutritional researchers indicate that food constituents such as amino acids are pharmacologically active. Increasingly, specific nutrients are formulated as drugs and used for pharmacologic effect.

Alteration of the speed of cell functions

Drugs that alter cell function interact with one or more structures of the cell. Such interactions may be general, altering cell membranes or cellular processes, or they may be specific, affecting specialized regions of the cell. General mechanisms of drug-cell interaction include interference with or facilitation of cell membrane functions and alteration of metabolic processes (Table 7-3). The specialized cellular structures with which some drugs interact are called *receptors*.

Receptor theory of drug action

According to the receptor theory of drug action, specific macromolecules in cells interact with certain chemicals because of the nature of their respective three-dimensional structures. If three or more sites on the molecular surfaces match in such a way as to promote chemical bonding, the drug attaches to the cellular structure. These drugs are visualized as "fitting" the receptor as a key fits a lock. Receptors are most often cellular proteins or nucleic acids but can also be enzymes, carbohydrate residues, and lipids.

A drug that directly alters the functional properties of the receptor with which it interacts is termed an *agonist*. To function as an agonist, a chemical must have an *affinity* for the target tissue (a propensity to locate at the receptor site) and *efficacy* (the ability to initiate biologic activity). According to the receptor theory of drug action, the agonist forms bonds with the receptor on at least three sites, locking the two molecules together. (Attachment at one site would allow the two

Table 7-2. Processes by which drugs alter the chemistry of cell environments

Process	Examples
Alteration of pH	Antacids given to neutralize excess stomach acidity
	Vinegar douches to inhibit bacterial/fungal growth in the vagina
Inactivation of toxins and poisons	Antitoxin used to treat diphtheria
	In opiate poisoning, potassium permanganate gastric lavages to precipitate the opiate, thus reducing absorption
Alteration of body fluid chemistry	Intravenous fluid and electrolyte therapy
	Heparin anticoagulation

Table 7-3. General processes of drug-cell interaction

Process	Examples
Facilitation of membrane transport	Insulin administered to promote cell utilization of glucose
Inhibition of membrane function	Reduction of nerve and muscle irritability by ionized calcium salts in the treatment of tetany
	General anesthetics that reduce the permeability of nerve cell membranes, depressing their function and causing unconsciousness
Support of energy metabolism	Oxygen administered to sustain energy metabolism
	Glucose administered to correct hypoglycemia
Inhibition of energy metabolism	Cyanide that poisons by inactivating mitochondrial cytochrome oxidases
Precipitation of cellular protein	Alcohol used as an antiseptic

substances to rotate around the single bond; attachment at two sites allows hingelike movement of the two molecules; attachment at three sites produces a rigid bond.)

The electromagnetic forces produced by these bonds tend to distort the molecular configuration of the receptor molecule, changing its biochemical properties. It is believed that some receptor molecules extend from the outside of the cell membrane to the inside. Occupation of the exterior site by an agonist distorts the portion of the molecule on the interior surface of the cell membrane, altering its ability to interact with intracellular compounds, including enzymes active in metabolic processes (Fig. 7-1).

Receptors are believed to have evolved for the purpose of interacting with endogenous biologic compounds. Some of these compounds have been identified and studied. For example, certain brain enkephalins and endorphins interact with opiate receptors on nerve cells, causing the same reduction of pain and emotional euphoria characteristic of opiate administration. These chemicals are released from the brain as a result of various stimuli, including vigorous exercise such as jogging and the expectation that pain will be relieved because some therapeutic action has been taken (*placebo effect*).

Receptors themselves are subject to external influences. Continued stimulation may result in a decrease in receptor response. This process is termed *desensitization*; the end state is termed *refractoriness*. Desensitization involves a reduction in the number of receptors on cell membranes or a change in existing receptors. If a chronic level of receptor stimulation is reduced, a state of supersensitivity or hyperreactivity may develop. This effect reflects a restoration of receptors to a responsive state or the synthesis of additional receptors.

A drug is usually classified according to its most prominent effect, its most usual therapeutic effect, or the actions thought to be the basis of these effects. This practice tends to obscure the fact that every drug produces a spectrum of effects. When a drug is administered for a single purpose, the extraneous results are termed *side effects*. Side effects may be desirable and helpful, neutral in nature, or undesirable and potentially dangerous. The relationship between the dosages required to produce a therapeutic response and those that produce adverse reactions is termed *therapeutic index*, *margin of safety*, or *specificity* (Box 7-2). No

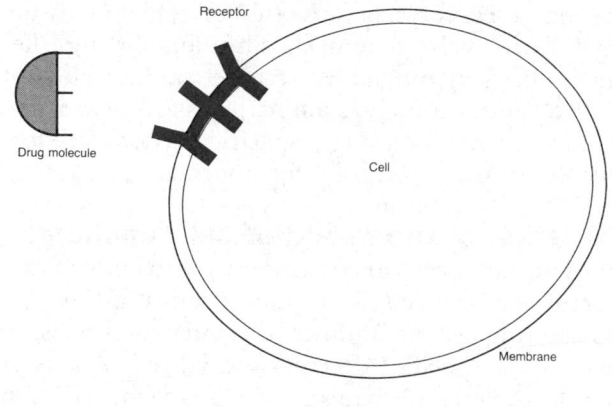

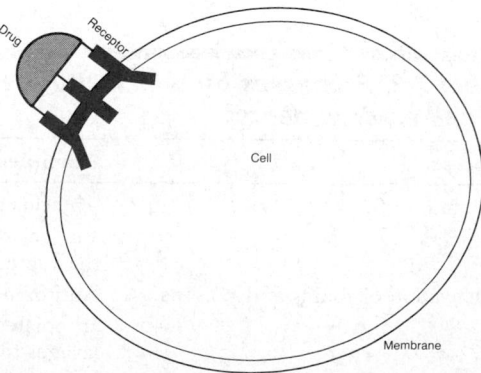

Figure 7-1. The interaction of a drug with a target cell at the cell receptor site. The distortion of the receptor molecule alters its function within the cell.

Box 7-2. Terms used to indicate the relationship between therapeutic and toxic dosages

Therapeutic index

The number indicating the ratio between lethal dose or toxic dose and effective dose. Therapeutic index is computed according to the following formula:

$$TI = \frac{LD_{50} \text{ or } TD_{50}}{ED_{50}}$$

TI equals therapeutic index; LD_{50} is the dose producing death in 50% of test animals, ED_{50} is the dose producing the desired therapeutic effect in 50% of test animals, and TD_{50} is the dose producing toxic symptoms in human subjects.

Margin of safety

The relative distance between therapeutic and toxic dosage ranges. Drugs with a high therapeutic index are said to have a wide safety range, those with a low therapeutic index a narrow safety range.

Specificity

The relative degree to which a drug produces a desired therapeutic effect without producing undesired (side-) effects. Generally, the more specific a drug is, the greater its therapeutic index and the wider its margin of safety.

---

drug produces only a single effect, and few are selective enough to be described as specific.

Therapeutic indices are derived from animal research and clinical trials in humans during the development of new drugs by pharmaceutical firms. A single drug may have several therapeutic indices, one for each therapeutic effect under investigation. Although these indices are not always applicable to human populations, they do give an indication of the relative safety of the drug.

Agonist/antagonist interaction

Antagonists are drugs that reduce the physiologic effect of other drugs. They are often used as antidotes for drug toxicity.

The site of action of an antagonist may be the same as that of the agonist (*eg*, a cell receptor site), or it may be at a distinctly different anatomic site. For example, anticholinesterase insecticides and nerve gas inhibit the enzyme that breaks down acetylcholine at synapses and neuromuscular junctions. As a result, acetylcho-

line persists and continues to stimulate the nerves and muscles upon whose receptors it acts; seizures is one of its effects. Atropine relieves these seizures and other manifestations of anticholinesterase toxicity but not by exerting any effect on either the anticholinesterase or the excess acetylcholine. Instead, it blocks the nerve and cell receptors which are stimulated by acetylcholine.

The action of atropine is an example of *competitive inhibition*. The agonist and antagonist bind with the receptor equally well, and compete for occupation of the receptor site. When the agonist binds more tightly to the receptor than the antagonist, the action of the antagonist is relatively weak. When the antagonist binds more tightly than the agonist to the receptor, the action of the antagonist is relatively strong. Some antagonists are degraded or excreted more rapidly than the agonists they oppose. Therefore, their actions are short-lived and they must be administered repeatedly to prevent the recurrence of toxic signs and symptoms.

■ Summary

Drugs either change the cellular environment or alter the rate of cellular function. Changes in environment are brought about by either physical action or chemical reactions. A drug may have one action or both actions. Drugs interact with one or more cellular structures to alter cell functions. Interactions may be general or specific. The specialized structures with which some drugs interact are called *receptors*. Receptors are most often cellular proteins or nucleic acids. A drug that directly alters the functional properties of the receptor with which it interacts is termed an *agonist*. A compound inhibiting the action of an agonist is called an *antagonist*. Continual stimulation of a receptor may result in desensitization, a decrease in receptor response. If the stimulating drug is then removed, a state of supersensitivity or hyperreactivity may develop.

A drug is usually classified according to its most prominent effect but every drug produces a spectrum of effects.

Learning experience 7-1

Select one of the following drugs to study: atropine, secobarbital, warfarin. Look up the drug you select to determine the specific mechanism of action. Can you explain how the drug's action determines therapeutic effect? Side effects? Toxic manifestations? Compare the action of the drug with that of antidotes and/or corrective treatment of toxicity.

Box 7-3. Mechanisms of absorption

I. Passive transport mechanism
   A. Transport through open passageways
      1. Blood vessels
      2. Lymph vessels
      3. Interstitial space
      4. Pores
   B. Lipid membrane diffusion
   C. Pinocytosis
II. Active transport mechanism: Carrier mechanisms

Nursing management

A knowledge of drug action provides helpful guidelines for monitoring client response to drugs and for corrective action to treat adverse drug reactions. The mechanism of action of a drug implies its therapeutic uses, side effects, and toxic manifestations. A global assessment of the client should be carried out regularly and frequently to detect changes attributable to drug action. Corrective actions to control harmful effects are effective to the degree that they reverse or delay the drug's action. Sound nursing judgments are best made with an understanding of pharmacodynamics at the cellular and molecular level.

Pharmacokinetics

The effect of drugs is markedly influenced by their form and concentration in the tissues. The study of absorption, distribution, transformation, and excretion of drugs in the body is termed *pharmacokinetics*.

Drug absorption

Drugs applied for their local effect usually act superficially on the surface. Most drugs, however, must penetrate the body to be effective. If a systemic effect is desired, the drug enters the blood and is distributed widely throughout body tissues. Absorption of chemicals conforms to the scientific laws affecting the kinetics of matter. It strongly influences the efficacy and toxicity of drugs.

Mechanisms of absorption

Chemicals migrate through tissues by water or lipid transport and by active transport mechanisms (Box 7-3). Water-soluble drugs are carried by body fluids wherever the passageways (blood vessels, lymph vessels, interstitial spaces, or pores in membranes) are large enough to allow penetration by solute particles. Where membranes whose pores are impermeable to the solute separate compartments, the drug molecule may cross by diffusion, pinocytosis, or active transport (Fig. 7-2). Diffusion requires dissolution in the lipid portion of the membrane and is available only to nonpolar, or nonionized, particles. It requires no energy but is dependent on concentration gradients from one side of the membrane to the other. Passive mechanisms of transport operate in both directions across membranes. Speed of transfer is dependent on and directly related to the degree of dissolution, drug concentration, and the area of membrane-drug exposure. Active transport mechanisms can transfer molecules against concentration gradients but they require the expenditure of energy to accomplish this work. Both passive and active transport mechanisms play a role in excretion as well as absorption of drugs (Table 7-4).

The rate of active transport is limited by the capacity of the carrier mechanism. Below the level at which the carrier mechanism is saturated, the rate of transfer is proportional to drug concentration. Passive diffusion is inversely related to the degree of ionization (and hence polarization) of the drug chemical. Both dissolution and ionization are affected by pH values in body solutions.

Routes of absorption

There are several routes by which drugs may be absorbed into the body: skin, mucous membranes, oral ingestion, inhalation, and injection.

Skin

The skin is less permeable to chemicals than most other ports of entry. Because the epidermis acts as a

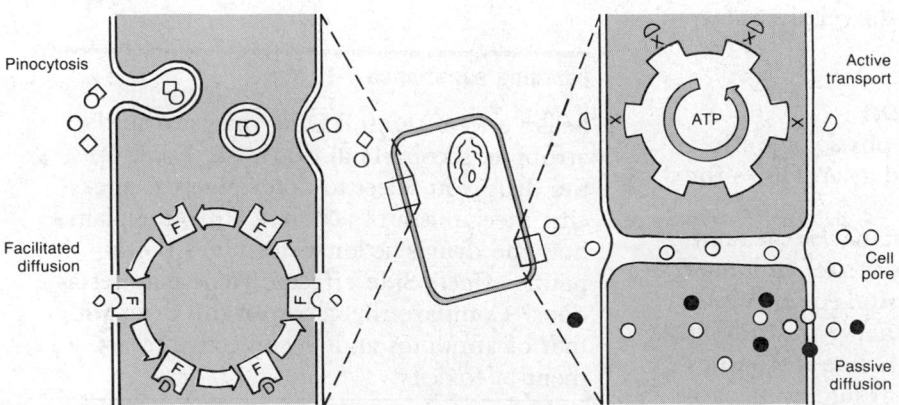

Figure 7-2. Schematic view of physiologic membranes and mechanisms of drug passage.

Table 7-4. Comparison of passive and active processes of drug absorption, distribution, and excretion

Passive mechanisms	Active transport
Rate of transfer is proportional to concentration gradient between the compartments involved.	Rate of transfer is proportional to concentration of drug available until carrier mechanism is saturated, beyond which point rate of transfer cannot increase.
Capacity of the system is limited only by the area of the membrane.	Capacity of the system is limited by the number of carrier units.
Drug molecules move from regions of relatively high concentrations to areas of relatively low concentrations.	The system can work against the concentration gradient.
Molecules move across membrane in both directions.	The system is generally a "one-way" transport process.
The process does not require energy (other than the kinetic energy of Brownian movement).	The process consumes energy because of the work done by the carrier.
Many kinds of molecules can diffuse, usually determined by the size of the molecule. Drugs that are capable of existing in both a charged and noncharged form approach an equilibrium state primarily by transfer of the noncharged particles across the membrane.	The system is structure specific, that is, designed to transport only a specific or similar chemical structure(s). Similar structures compete for transport.

lipid barrier, only lipid-soluble substances are absorbed through the intact skin. Abraded skin permits penetration by a greater variety of substances because the dermis is freely permeable to many solutes. Hair follicles and other dermal structures alter absorption rate, and the skin can also metabolize (biodegrade) drugs. The skin does not present a uniform barrier to drug absorption (Raloff, 1988; see Box 7-4).

Most drugs applied to the skin are topical remedies employed for a local effect. Historically, when systemic absorption was desired, the medicinal chemical was suspended in an oily vehicle and rubbed into the skin, a process known as *unction*. Metallic salts were administered by unction for the treatment of disease, including syphilis. The transdermal route has been consistently used for over-the-counter remedies containing methyl salicylate (oil of wintergreen.) (The salicylate is systemically absorbed, and can provide an effective dose of analgesic drug for the relief of arthritic pain.) For some time, this method of administration was seldom used for prescription drugs.

However, topical preparations of vasodilators, estrogens, and antiemetics have recently been marketed. There seems to be renewed interest in the transdermal route for systemic medication.

Systemic toxicity can occur when substances are absorbed through the skin. Salicylate poisoning has been reported with overuse of the nonprescription arthritis preparations described above. Oily solutions of insecticides are known to have caused poisoning by skin contact alone. The drug hexachlorophene, used widely at one time for skin cleansing and for treatment of acne, was proven to be absorbed from the skin in sufficient quantity to cause neurotoxicity. Because of this risk, it can no longer be purchased without a physician's prescription.

Mucous membranes

Many drugs are applied to mucous membranes for local effect. However, lipid-soluble drugs capable of traversing the mucous and capillary membranes can be absorbed directly into the circulation when applied to the mucosa. Where blood vessels are close to the surface, absorption is rapid. This route of administration provides a prompt systemic effect without injection. It can be used when the substance to be given would be destroyed by the digestive process, when the patient is unconscious, or when nausea and vomiting preclude ingestion of medications (Table 7-5). Application of drugs to mucous membranes may produce toxic symptoms if absorption is very rapid (Leavitt & Zweifler, 1988). Mucous membranes commonly used for administration of drugs include the sublingual, buccal, nasal, conjunctival, vaginal, and rectal mucosae.

Box 7-4. Drug absorption by the skin

- Skin is less permeable than other ports of entry.
- Only lipid-soluble substances are absorbed through intact skin.
- Hairy skin absorbs chemicals faster than hairless skin.
- Abraded skin permits penetration by a greater variety of substances.
- Most drugs applied to the skin are topical for local effect.
- The transdermal route is sometimes used for systemic drugs.
- Systemic toxicity can occur when substances are absorbed by the skin.

Table 7-5. Drugs commonly administered by application to mucous membranes

Site of membrane	Examples
Sublingual	Nitroglycerin used for rapid relief of anginal symptoms.
	Isoproterenol used to dilate the bronchi in asthma.
Buccal	Pitocin administered to stimulate uterine contractions during labor and delivery.
Nasal	Pitressin insufflations used for the control of diabetes insipidus.
	Decongestant nose drops (administered for local effect but drugs can be absorbed causing systemic side-effects).
	Cocaine "sniffed" by addicts for psychoactive effect.
Conjunctival	Miotic, mydriatic, or anti-inflammatory drops (administered for local effect but drugs can be absorbed from conjunctiva, lining of the tear duct, or nasal mucosa, causing systemic side-effects).
Vaginal	Estrogenic creams administered topically to alleviate atrophic vaginitis (can be absorbed by vaginal mucosa of the recipient or the genital tissues of male sex partner, causing systemic effects in either).
Rectal	Bisacodyl suppositories to relieve constipation by local stimulation of reflex peristalsis; aspirin suppositories to reduce fever by systemic action.

Many drugs administered topically by application to mucous membranes are irritating, and the mucosa can be injured if a site is used repeatedly. Following drug absorption, the site should be rinsed with water to remove residues of the drug formulation. If drugs are given regularly by this route, sites should be rotated if possible (Box 7-5).

Oral ingestion

Because it is comfortable, convenient, and economic, the oral route is used for administration of many medications. Drugs to be swallowed may be prepared as solutions, suspensions, powders, tablets, or capsules. Ingested chemicals must be resistant to degradation by the digestive process. Although a few drugs may be administered for a local effect within the gastrointestinal tract (laxatives, antacids, adsorbent antidiarrheals), most are given with the expectation of systemic effect.

Intestinal absorption. A few drugs are rapidly absorbed by a discrete segment of the intestine. These small areas of gut contain carrier substances that move specific chemicals through the membrane by active transport. Substances known to be absorbed by this process include the nutrients sodium, potassium, vitamins, amino acids, simple sugars, uracil, and thymine; bile salts; and the drugs 5-fluorouracil and 5-bromouracil.

Intestinal absorption of most drugs is dependent on passive diffusion. The rate of absorption is, therefore, influenced by dissolution and ionization of the drug. Solubility of the preparation depends on particle size and chemical form of the drug. Solid dosage forms such as tablet or capsule must first disintegrate to expose large surface areas of the chemical to the gastric or intestinal juices. As the drug deaggregates, it begins to dissolve in the fluid medium. Drug forms that ionize readily (usually salts) go into solution more rapidly than nonelectrolytes. To facilitate dissolution, disintegrators and chemical buffers may be added to the formulation. Disintegrators are relatively inert substances (such as starch) that dissolve readily, causing the solid drug to fragment rapidly when moistened. Buffers promote immediate dissolution during the initial stages of disintegration without significantly changing the pH of gastric or intestinal fluids (Figs. 7-3 and 7-4).

Because they are largely nonionized in the acid medium of gastric secretions, drugs that are acidic in nature are absorbed rapidly by the gastric mucosa. Basic drugs normally remain ionized in this compartment and are not absorbed until they reach the intestines where the pH is higher. The presence in the stomach of foods or antacids that raise the pH tends to retard absorption of acid drugs and may initiate absorption of basic drugs in this organ.

Though absorption of some drugs may be delayed by foods, overall drug uptake is usually maximal regardless of the timing of drug dose in relation to meals because of the large surface area for absorption provided by the gut and the long time required for intestinal transit. Immediate absorption is not always desirable because blood concentrations may rise rapidly

Box 7-5. Drug absorption by mucous membrane

- Routes of absorption are sublingual, buccal, nasal, conjunctival, vaginal, and rectal.
- Drugs are absorbed directly into the circulation.
- These rates allow rapid absorption.
- Uses of these routes include administration of drugs in the following situations:
  The oral route cannot be used.
  The drug would be destroyed by the digestive process.

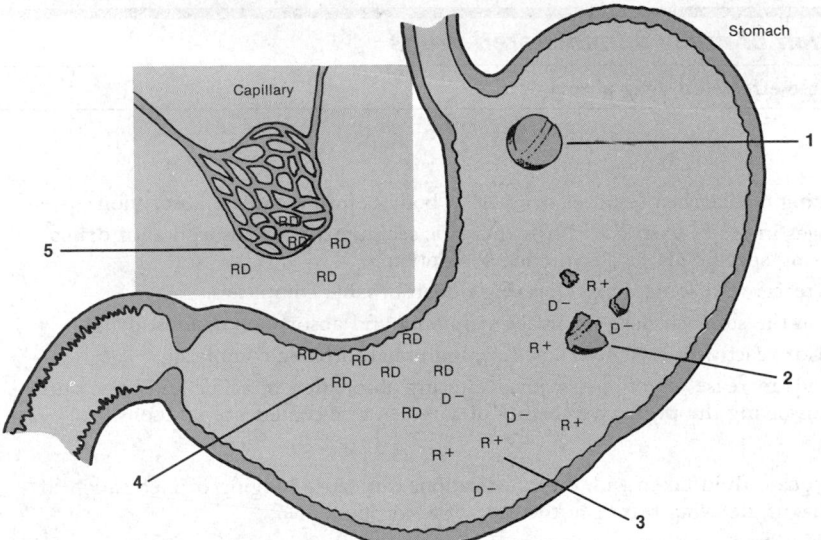

Figure 7-3. Steps in the absorption of solid tablets, acid salts: (*1*) Solid tablet enters stomach. (*2*) Tablet begins to disintegrate. Base buffer in tablet promotes dissolution. (*3*) Charged ions diffuse into the large pool of stomach juices whose pH has not been raised by small amount of buffer in tablet. (*4*) In acid medium, ions reunite forming nonpolarized compound. (*5*) Nonpolarized particles diffuse readily through lipid membranes. (*D*, drug radical; *R*, nondrug radical)

enough to reach toxic levels. Prolonging absorption time also produces a steadier serum drug level.

The rate of drug absorption is influenced by the speed of transit through the tract. Rapid stomach emptying accelerates absorption of basic drugs because they more rapidly reach the small intestine where they are then absorbed. Acidic drugs may not be completely absorbed in the stomach if they are propelled prematurely from that organ. Generally, drugs ingested with food are absorbed more slowly and gradually than are drugs taken on an empty stomach.

Abnormal digestion and drug absorption. Abnormal digestion can markedly affect absorption of drugs from the digestive tract. Achlorhydria (absence of hydrochloric acid in the stomach) retards gastric absorption of acid drugs and dissolution of basic drugs. Deficiencies of pancreatic and intestinal secretions may completely prevent the dissolution of enteric-coated

tablets, causing them to be excreted unabsorbed in the feces. (Enteric coatings are designed to disintegrate only in the small intestine.) Vomiting or diarrhea tends to propel drugs from the tract before absorption can be completed (Table 7-6).

Manipulation of drug absorption. Mixing drugs with food can impair absorption if the drug forms a nonabsorbable complex with elements in the food. For example, tetracycline combines chemically with polyvalent cations (calcium, magnesium, iron, aluminum) to form complexes that cannot be broken down by the digestive process but are excreted unabsorbed in the feces. For this reason, these drugs must be administered on an empty stomach. Neither food nor antacid drugs (many of which contain polyvalent cations) can be taken within 2 hours before and 1 hour after medication if the drug is to be absorbed properly.

Absorption of oral drugs can be manipulated

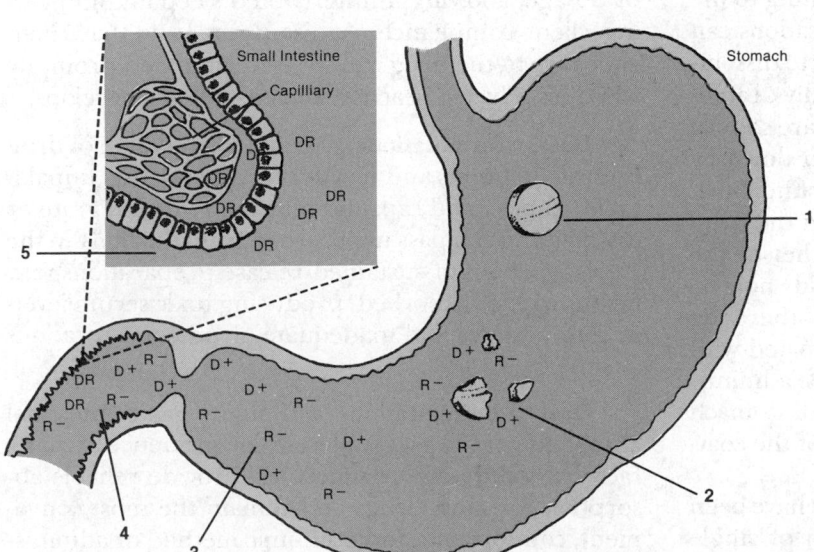

Figure 7-4. Steps in the absorption of solid tablets, basic salts: (*1*) Solid tablet enters stomach. (*2*) Tablet begins to disintegrate. Acid medium of stomach favors rapid dissolution of basic salts. (*3*) Ions remain dissociated in low pH of stomach. (*4*) Pancreatic juice enters duodenum, raising pH. Drug ions reunite, forming nonpolarized compound. (*5*) Nonpolarized particles diffuse readily through lipid membranes. (*D*, drug radical; *R*, nondrug radical)

Table 7-6. Factors influencing absorption of orally administered drugs

Factors	Possible effects on drug absorption
Client-related factors	
State of digestive function	
Peristalsis	Vomiting or diarrhea removes drug from body before complete absorption.
Secretions	Changes in *p*H of gastric acid or pancreatic secretions alter absorption of drugs requiring specific *p*H or enzyme for absorption.
Presence of food in the tract	Food reacts with some drugs, forming nonabsorbable complexes.
	Food in the stomach delays stomach emptying and absorption of most drugs.
Presence of antacids in the stomach	Antacids react with certain drugs, forming nonabsorbable complexes.
	Antacids increase *p*H of gastric juice, altering absorption of acidic and basic salts and dissolving the protective coating of some enteric-coated preparations.
Method of taking drug	
Fluid intake	Inadequate fluid taken with oral medications can cause lodging of medication in esophagus, delaying transit to the area of absorption.
Crushing, chewing tablets	Crushing and chewing reduce particle size and tend to accelerate absorption. They may also disrupt enteric coating, releasing drugs inappropriately in the stomach (gastric irritation or destruction of the drug may occur).
Medication-related factors	
Formulation of dosage form	
Physical state of drug	Amorphic drugs dissolve more rapidly than crystals and are absorbed more rapidly.
	Solutions are absorbed more rapidly than solid drugs, powders more rapidly than tablets.
Inactive ingredients in formulation	Disintegrators and buffers accelerate absorption.
Enteric coating	Enteric coating delays dissolution of drug until it reaches intestine, retarding absorption.

through changes in the formulation of the medicine. Solutions are absorbed most rapidly, then powers, capsules, tablets, and enteric-coated tablets, in descending order. Blending the active drug with a readily soluble, pharmacologically inactive substance accelerates disintegration of a tablet. Chemical buffers can also accelerate dissolution of the drug.

Some medications should not be liberated in the stomach, either because the acid juices chemically destroy the drug, or because the drug is irritating to the gastric mucosa. Solid forms of these medications can be coated with a substance which is resistant to dissolution by the gastric juices but which will readily disintegrate in the small intestines. Some coatings are soluble only in a basic medium; others are broken down by digestive enzymes specific to the small intestine. Such an *enteric coating* provides a barrier between the drug and the stomach, preventing damage to either by the other. Enteric-coated preparations should not be crushed because this procedures liberates the drug prematurely in the stomach. Medications coated with an acid-resistant substance should also not be administered with drugs or foods that raise the *p*H of stomach contents, since this could cause dissolution of the coating in the stomach.

Special (sustained-release) formulations have been developed to prolong the period of action of single dosage forms. These preparations contain two or more forms of a drug with different absorption times. To prolong absorption, the drug may be encapsulated, enteric coated, or combined with waxes or fats, ion-exchange resins, colloids, or porous plastics. Sometimes a tablet is prepared in a manner that retards disintegration. Many sustained-release preparations incorporate an initial "dose" that is rapidly absorbed to achieve a minimally effective serum level promptly. Sustained-released formulations reduce the frequency of dosage, allowing uninterrupted sleep and improving client compliance. A disadvantage is that client exposure to the drug cannot be terminated promptly when an adverse reaction such as allergy develops.

Dosage formulations. No one formulation of drug is ideal. Solutions and powders are frequently unpalatable. Tablets and capsules may fail to disintegrate or dissolve and can pass unabsorbed from the body in the stools. Portions of sustained-release preparations may be improperly absorbed, producing toxic serum levels at certain times and inadequate blood concentrations at others.

Oral administration. Although gastrointestinal absorption of drugs is subject to the influence of many factors, oral dosage regimens do provide reliable absorption for most drugs and remain the most convenient, comfortable, and economic method of administering systemic drugs (Box 7-6).

Box 7-6. Drug absorption following oral administration

- Oral ingestion is the most convenient, comfortable, and economical method of administering systemic drugs.
- Ingested chemicals must be resistant to degradation by the digestive process and liver metabolism.
- The rate of drug absorption is influenced by the speed of transit through the tract.
- Abnormal digestion can markedly affect absorption of drugs.
- Some foods impair absorption of certain drugs.
- Absorption of drugs can be manipulated through changes in the formulation of the medicine.
- Drugs that are not to be liberated in the stomach are enteric-coated.
- Sustained-release formulations prolong the period of action.
- The absorption of drugs is influenced by their acidity or alkalinity and the pH of the gastrointestinal contents.

Inhalation

The lungs provide a large surface for absorption of gaseous chemicals. The total blood volume traverses the lungs, and rich capillary networks close to the alveolar surface provide a ready reservoir for drug absorption. Inhaled compounds diffuse rapidly from the alveolar space to the bloodstream. Because absorption of inhalant drugs is not compromised by circulatory shock, this route is sometimes used in emergency situations.

To be tolerated by the lungs, substances administered by inhalation must not interfere with respiration (*ie*, oxygen and carbon dioxide gas exchange). Therefore, drugs for inhalation must be prepared in the forms of gases or fine mists. Most mists (aerosols) are generated from aqueous solutions but sometimes a solid drug in the form of fine powder is employed (Table 7-7). Devices used to propel medications into the alveolar tree include pressure tanks for dispensing gases, ultrasonic or nebulizer mist generators, and hand-operated inhalers.

Drugs requiring the use of respirators are usually administered by respiratory therapists, the acknowledged experts in the management of these machines. Because the inhalant anesthetics have a narrow safety margin, their use is reserved for physicians and qualified nurse anesthetists. Nurses are commonly responsible only for administering oxygen, drugs delivered by hand-operated inhalers, and aromatic spirits of ammonia, a first-aid remedy for fainting (Box 7-7).

Injection

Systemic drugs can be injected into various tissues of the body when other routes of administration are inappropriate or contraindicated. This method of administration provides more rapid absorption than either topical application or ingestion. Drugs may be injected into virtually every tissue except bone (Table 7-8).

When local rather than systemic effects are desired, drugs are injected directly into or near the target tissue. Medicines may also be delivered to divisions of the body by means of extracorporeal perfusion or intra-arterial infusion. In all of these methods except extracorporeal perfusion, the drugs eventually escape from the target tissues and are absorbed by the general circulation. Their concentration in the general tissues, however, is lower than otherwise possible because their diffusion gradients flow from target tissue to blood rather than the reverse.

Systemic drugs are commonly injected into subcutaneous tissues, muscles, or veins. Absorption and distribution are most rapid from veins, then from muscles, and, slowest of all, from subcutaneous tissue. Risk of tissue damage by the drug is greatest with subcutaneous injection. Muscle tissue tolerates many irritating substances that cannot be administered by hypodermic (injection beneath the skin). Some substances that are too irritating for intramuscular use can be administered intravenously, although they tend to induce phlebitis.

Because of the speed of distribution, the IV route has the greatest potential for serious toxicity and infection. Doses cannot be retrieved nor absorption delayed because absorption and distribution are virtually immediate. The absorption of drugs administered subcutaneously and intramuscularly can be slowed by constricting or occluding blood vessels in the area, thus

Box 7-7. Drug absorption by inhalation

- Substances administered by inhalation must not interfere with respiration.
- Drugs for inhalation must be prepared in the form of gases or fine mists.
- Devices that propel medications into the alveolar tree include pressure tanks, ultrasonic and nebulizer mist generators, and hand-operated inhalers.
- Drugs requiring the use of respirators are usually administered by respiratory therapists.
- Inhalant anesthetics are administered only by physicians and qualified nurse anesthetists.
- Nurses are responsible for administering oxygen, drugs delivered by hand-operated inhalers, and aromatic spirits of ammonia.

Table 7-7. Substances commonly absorbed by inhalation

Drug agent	Physical form(s)	Effect(s)
Therapeutic agents		
Oxygen	Gas	Enhancement of oxygen transport to the tissues in hypoxia
Anesthetics: ether, nitrous oxide, halothane	Gases and volatile liquids	Loss of consciousness and insensitivity to pain during surgery
Cromolyn	Aqueous solutions and dry powder	Prevention of asthma by inhibition of release of autocoids such as histamine
Mucolytics: acetylcysteine (Mucomyst), deoxyribonuclease	Aqueous solutions	Thinning of respiratory secretions
Bronchodilators: epinephrine	Aqueous solutions	Bronchodilation, central nervous system stimulation
Aromatic spirits of ammonia	Volatile drug in aqueous solution	Respiratory stimulation, elevation of blood pressure
Pollutants and substances of abuse		
Carbon tetrachloride, paint thinner, industrial solvents, glue	Volatile liquids and volatile substances in solution	Intoxication, emotional disturbance, hallucinations (with chronic exposure, liver damage)
Anesthetics: ether, nitrous oxide, halothane (Fluothane) inhaled by OR staff	Gases and volatile liquids	Excitation, emotional disturbance, unconsciousness (in the case of chronic exposure to Fluothane: increased risk of birth defects and spontaneous abortion)
Poisons		
Carbon monoxide	Gas	Hypoxia and asphyxiation

reducing local circulation. Among the techniques available are applications of cold (ice packs), local injection of epinephrine, or the intermittent application of a tourniquet (if the injection site is in an extremity).

Absorption from subcutaneous sites. Drugs deposited in subcutaneous tissue are normally in aqueous solution. Depot preparations* and irritating drugs usually are not administered by this route because they tend to cause tissue damage, including the formation of sterile abscesses and sloughing. Volumes up to 1 ml can be administered in a single injection to most adults with minimal discomfort. To reach the bloodstream, they must traverse the extracellular compartment to a capillary and diffuse across the blood vessel membrane. Movement through the tissues is impeded by the presence of hyaluronic acid, an adhesive that cements the cells together. For this reason and because the blood supply to subcutaneous tissue is relatively poor, absorption is relatively slow. If peripheral circulation is impaired (as in shock), the drug may remain in the tissue site for prolonged periods.

When rapid absorption of large amounts of fluid by the subcutaneous route is desired, hyaluronidase (an enzyme that breaks down hyaluronic acid) can be administered into the injection site. This medication is often prescribed when fluids are ordered by hyperdermoclysis. As the tissue hyaluronic acid decreases, passageways become available between the cells, allowing rapid dispersal of the fluid through tissue planes.

When small amounts of medicine are administered subcutaneously, massage of the tissue site after injection accelerates absorption.

Absorption from muscle sites. Drugs administered intramuscularly include solutions, suspensions, and complexes of drugs and various inactive substances that alter the rate of absorption. Ingredients of intramuscular medications include oils and other irritating chemicals, which are not well tolerated by subcutaneous tissue and which might be dangerous if injected directly into veins. Volumes that may be injected safely and comfortably vary with the mass of tissue available at the injection site. In the author's experience, volumes up to 2 ml are easily tolerated; volumes up to 5 ml are sometimes injected into large muscles of adult clients.

As with subcutaneous injection, drugs administered intramuscularly must reach a capillary and diffuse through the blood vessel wall. Muscle tissue, however, is more richly supplied with blood vessels and the journey is relatively short. Movement through the tissues is accelerated by massage of the injection site and

*Drugs formulated by combination with substances such as oils that delay absorption.

Table 7-8. Routes for drug delivery by injection

Route	Site of drug delivery
For systemic effect	
Subcutaneous	Subcutaneous tissue or pocket
Intramuscular	Muscle tissue
Intravenous	Venous blood
Central venous catheter	Superior vena cava or right atrium of the heart (used when solutions must be rapidly diluted to prevent damage to the blood)
For local effect	
Intradermal	Skin
Intra-articular	Joint space
Intrathecal	Cerebrospinal fluid
Intraperitoneal	Peritoneal cavity
Intrapleural	Pleural cavity
Intra-arterial	Arterial blood (used when drug effect at high or toxic levels is desired in a localized area)
Extracorporeal perfusion	Isolated circulation of a segment of the body, commonly an extremity (drug and blood circulate through a perfusion circuit; drug may be removed and fresh blood infused when procedure is completed)
Epidural	Spinal nerves or a segment of the spinal cord

exercise of the muscles containing the drug. Hence, the more active the muscle used for injection, the more rapid is absorption.

When gradual absorption of an intramuscular medication is desired, substances are added to the drug that form nonabsorbable or poorly absorbed complexes. Such preparations provide a depot of drug in the tissues that dissipates gradually as biochemical processes in the tissues break down the complex. Depot medications decrease the number of injections required to provide a supply of drug over a prolonged time, and sustain a more steady blood level of drug than repeated injections.

Intravenous injection. Intravenous injection delivers chemicals directly into the vascular system, thus reducing time for onset of action to a minimum. In general, only aqueous solutions may be administered by IV injection. One exception is the IV administration of fat emulsion during parenteral feeding (hyperalimentation). As mentioned previously, drugs administered intravenously are potentially toxic. Blood levels rise rapidly, and the drug cannot be retrieved once it has been administered. Intravenous lines are a very reliable route for drug delivery in very ill patients and when peripheral circulation is compromised.

To reduce toxicity, it is important to control the speed with which the drug is delivered into veins. This may be accomplished by slow infusion over a period of time. When a bolus of drug is to be administered (IV "push"), it must be injected slowly, usually over a period of minutes.

Irritating drugs are best tolerated when injected by the IV route. They require gradual administration to minimize vein irritation, which can cause inflammation and subsequent loss of the IV site (Box 7-8).

Drug distribution

When a systemic effect is desired, the drug enters the blood through absorption and is then distributed throughout body tissues. Drugs pass more readily between the intravascular and interstitial compartments than between other compartments of the body. The vascular membrane offers little resistance to dissolved particles unless they are of large (colloid) size or they are bound to serum proteins. The leakiness of the blood vessel wall may be due to the nature of the intracellular cement in that tissue or the presence of water-filled microapertures (pores).

The speed of distribution can be measured in terms of *distribution half-life*, which is the time required for blood levels of the drug to drop by half because of migration into tissues, including tissue depots.

Assuming free movement of drug from blood vessel to extracellular fluid, the concentration of drug at any specific site would depend on the following:

- Density of blood vessels in the tissue
- Degree of local vasodilation or vasoconstriction
- Rate of general circulation of the blood

Tissues with a minimal blood supply, such as bone or the middle ear, are relatively poorly perfused, and delivery of adequate drug concentrations is difficult. Factors influencing tissue distribution of drugs include exercise and warming or chilling, which change local circulation dynamics; and changes in cardiac pumping, blood pressure, and blood volume, which impair or enhance general circulation.

Box 7-8. Drug absorption by injection

- Injection of drugs allows administration of systemic drugs when other routes of administration are inappropriate or contraindicated.
- Injection provides more rapid absorption than either topical application or ingestion.
- Drugs may be injected into virtually every tissue except bone.
- In all methods except extracorporeal perfusion, the drugs eventually escape the target tissues and are absorbed by general circulation.
- Systemic drugs are commonly injected into subcutaneous tissues, muscles, or veins.
- Drugs deposited in subcutaneous tissue are normally in aqueous solution form.
- Drug absorption in subcutaneous tissues is relatively slow. The drug may remain in the tissue site for prolonged periods if there is impaired peripheral circulation. When small amounts are administered, massage after injection accelerates absorption.
- Risk of tissue damage is greatest with subcutaneous injections.

- Drugs administered intramuscularly include solutions, suspensions, and complexes of drugs with various inactive substances.
- The more active the muscle used for injection, the more rapid the absorption. Massage accelerates absorption.
- Muscle tissue tolerates many irritating substances that cannot be administered subcutaneously.
- Some substances that are too irritating for intramuscular use can be administered intravenously (although they tend to induce phlebitis).
- Intravenous injections deliver chemicals directly into the vascular system and are the most rapid form of injection. They are potent and potentially toxic. The drug cannot be retrieved and its effect cannot be delayed once it is administered. To reduce toxicity, the speed of delivery of the drug can be controlled.
- Intravenous lines are a reliable route for drug delivery to very ill patients and when peripheral circulation is compromised.

Because drugs cross lipid membranes by means of diffusion, the movement of chemicals is in both directions. Drugs administered by injection, therefore, may appear in the intestinal secretions, sputum, saliva, semen, breast milk, and vaginal secretions, having diffused outward from the blood vessel to those compartments. Volatile substances such as alcohol are excreted by the lungs by this mechanism (Box 7-9).

Movement of drugs to and from the vascular compartment is not entirely free, however. Certain tissues pose barriers to drug passage, whereas other tissues tend to trap drugs in various ways.

Box 7-9. Factors that influence tissue distribution of drugs

- Exercise, warming, and chilling change local circulation dynamics.
- Changes in cardiac pumping, blood pressure, and blood volume alter general circulation.
- The chemical nature of the drug influences passage through tissue barriers and storage in tissue depots.

The blood-brain barrier

Transcapillary exchange within the central nervous system is highly selective. Water soluble nutrients and metabolites pass through readily but larger water soluble molecules penetrate little or not at all. The blood-brain barrier is believed to be due to the compact organization of a one-cell thick lining of the inner walls of cerebral capillaries. The spaces between these cells is filled by proteins that virtually occlude the openings (pores) that would otherwise allow entrance to large molecules. Fat soluble compounds can cross this barrier by dissolving in the lipid portion of endothelial cell membranes (Box 7-10).

The blood-brain barrier is an important protective mechanism because it safeguards the brain from ready disturbance by chemical changes in body fluids. It poses problems, however, when drugs must be delivered to central nervous tissue. In some cases, such as dopamine, a pro-drug (L-dopa) can be developed that is capable of crossing the blood-brain barrier. Once inside the brain, the pro-drug is transformed by metabolic processes into the desired pharmaceutical agent. Other approaches that remain experimental include joining a drug to a fat soluble chemical producing a fat soluble drug complex; linking a drug to an antibody which is then absorbed by the capillary cell and transported to the brain; and using chemicals that open the

Box 7-10. The blood-brain barrier

- The blood-brain barrier is a compact layer of cells that line the cerebral capillary.
- The blood-brain barrier acts to exclude certain chemicals from the brain.
- The blood-brain barrier is an important protective mechanism for the brain.
- The blood-brain barrier can prevent therapeutic drugs from reaching the central nervous tissues.
- Very small molecules and fat-soluble substances cross the blood-brain barrier more readily than do large molecules and water-soluble compounds.

Box 7-11. Tissue trapping

- Certain tissues bind or collect drugs, rendering them inactive (bound drug).
- When drugs leave the tissue-binding site, they again become physiologically active (free drug).
- Drugs, endogenous chemicals, and drug metabolites often compete for binding sites and can displace each other from them. This process is the cause of many drug interactions.

pores in the cerebral capillary wall (Brownlee, 1990). Sometimes drugs must be injected intrathecally to bypass the blood-brain barrier.

For some time, a similar barrier was hypothesized for the placenta. Later studies of the effects of maternal drugs upon the fetus indicated, however, that the placenta acts as a simple lipoidal membrane and is not highly selective.

Tissue trapping

Certain tissues bind or collect drugs temporarily or permanently, converting them to inactive forms. Until these storage depots are saturated, the level of free drug available for pharmaceutical effect may remain low. Some drugs bind with specific tissues in the body. Metallic ions tend to be deposited in bone, and hydrocarbons in fatty tissue. Iodine is stored in the thyroid, and B complex vitamins in the liver.

Plasma proteins bind many substances. Acidic drugs and endogenous bilirubin bind with albumin; basic drugs bind to a_1-acid glycoproteins.

Below the saturation level, stored (bound) drug and free drug maintain a dynamic equilibrium between their levels. If this is disturbed, the drug moves freely from one form to the other to establish a new balance. In the interval between dosages and after administration is discontinued, the chemical moves from the storage depot into the serum as free drug, thus prolonging the physiologic effects.

Drugs, endogenous chemicals, and drug metabolites often compete for binding sites and can displace each other from them. This process is the cause of many drug interactions requiring adjustment of dosages when two drugs sharing the same binding sites are administered together (Box 7-11).

Movement of drugs across membranes

Not all drugs cross the membranes dividing body compartments with equal facility. A few drugs cannot cross the vascular wall. Others (*eg*, bromides) cannot cross cell membranes. Many drugs cannot penetrate the blood-brain barrier. The cells that secrete milk, tears, saliva, sweat, bile, joint fluid, and gastric, pancreatic, and intestinal juices are permeable to some substances but not to others. Although it is not highly selective, the placenta does exclude some substances. Exudates and capsules around abscesses or tumors are barriers of particular significance for antibiotic and antineoplastic chemotherapy. Though blood is the most efficient vehicle for transporting drugs to tissue sites, there are many mechanisms operating to produce differential distribution. Many substances disseminate unevenly throughout the body, and concentration of a drug may vary markedly from one organ to another. Moreover, the tissue to be treated by the medicine is not necessarily the area that will attain the highest concentration of the drug.

Drug biotransformation

Within the tissues, drugs, like other chemicals, are subject to multiple biochemical processes by which they are changed to different compounds. Most of these metabolic processes are mediated by enzymes. The products of these reactions (metabolites) have properties different from those of the original drugs. Their biologic activity may be increased, decreased, or eliminated (Table 7-9). Lipid-soluble compounds may become water-soluble substances. As such, their molecules often polarize (acquire electric charges on their surfaces), and they tend to ionize (split into charged particles). The general trend of these metabolic processes is to render foreign chemicals less biologically active, less prone to tissue binding, and easier to excrete. Overall, biotransformation serves to break down, detoxify, and remove from the body biologically active chemicals.

A variety of chemical processes are involved in biotransformation: oxidation, reduction, hydrolysis, and synthesis. Multiple enzymes may be involved in each type of reaction. For example, oxidative enzymes include oxidases, peroxidases, dehydrogenases, and transaminases. Examples of synthetic processes are alkylation, acetylation, methylation, and conjugation

Table 7-9. Examples of changes in pharmacologic action produced by biotransformation

Drug	Type of transformation	Metabolite
L-dopa (inactive pro-drug)	activation (by brain tissue)	dopamine (active neurotransmitter)
fluoroacetic acid	toxication (by citric acid cycle)	fluorocitric acid (toxic rodenticide)
codeine (narcotic analgesic)	toxication (by the liver)	morphine (more potent narcotic analgesic)
heroin (narcotic analgesic)	alteration with unchanged activity (by liver)	morphine (narcotic analgesic)
epinephrine (sympathetic hormone)	partial deactivation (by liver)	metanephrine (less potent sympathomimetic)
cyanide (a poison disruptive of internal respiration)	detoxification by inactivation (by liver)	thiocyanate (pharmacologically inactive compound)

with glucuronic or mercapturic acid. Each class of reaction has its favored substrate (*ie*, water-soluble compounds are frequently oxidized), and each produces characteristic changes (as conjugation increases water solubility; Box 7-12).

Metabolic pathways for the transformation of drugs may be serial or parallel. In serial transformation, a given molecule undergoes several changes, one after the other:

$$A \rightarrow B \rightarrow C \rightarrow D$$

Parallel transformation indicates that a given substance may undergo several kinds of changes yielding different products:

$$A \rightarrow B$$
$$A \rightarrow C$$
$$A \rightarrow D$$

By either pathway, a single compound gives rise to several different metabolites. Generally a number of metabolites are produced as a given drug is broken down by the body.

Though knowledge of biotransformation has increased rapidly in recent years, metabolic processes are extremely complex, and much remains to be explored.

Box 7-12. Chemical processes involved in biotransformation

1. Oxidation
2. Reduction
3. Hydrolysis
4. Synthesis
   a. Alkylation
   b. Acetylation
   c. Methylation
   d. Conjugation with glucuronic acid
   e. Conjugation with mercapturic acid

Biotransformation by the liver

Virtually every tissue in the body is capable of biotransformation. Biochemical processes of this type have been described in the lungs, blood, skin, and brain. However, the liver is by far the most important organ performing this function. This biochemical powerhouse is the major site for oxidation and reduction reactions. Hydrolysis and conjugation also occur at significant rates. Lipid-soluble compounds, a class that includes many important drugs, are transformed by microsomal enzymes in the endoplasmic reticulum of liver cells. This arrangement is fortuitous because it protects the body from many toxic substances ingested with food. Much of the material absorbed by the intestinal tract enters the portal circulation, which traverses the liver before mixing with the general circulation. This "first pass" through the liver allows for degradation of harmful chemicals before they are widely distributed in the tissues.

Factors in biotransformation

Factors influencing the biotransformation of drugs include genetic differences, physiologic status, and environmental factors (Box 7-13).

Genetic factors

Genetic influences include species, sex, and familial traits. Enzyme systems involved in biotransformation in one species may be completely absent in others. This is the reason certain animals thrive on foods that are lethal to other species. These differences limit the ability to generalize to humans the results of pharmaceutical research involving animals.

Males of certain species of rats have greater capacity to degrade certain chemicals than females of the same species. The reverse is true in other species. These differences may reflect differences in the genes located on the X and Y chromosomes. Because each enzyme relates to a specific gene on a chromosome, metabolic patterns are more likely to be similar within families than between unrelated individuals.

An important principle of genetic influence on

Box 7-13. Factors in biotransformation

Genetic Differences

Species
Sex
Familial traits

Physiologic Status

Age
Hormone status (including pregnancy)
Nutrition
Disease

Environmental Factors

Stress
Radiation
Effect of chemicals
All of these factors can operate to increase or decrease biotransformation. Each individual metabolizes chemicals in a unique way.

---

biotransformation is that *each individual, by virtue of a unique genetic makeup, will metabolize chemicals in a unique way.*

Physiologic factors

Physiologic factors influencing biotransformation include age, hormone status (including effects of pregnancy), nutrition, and disease. Very young children have not yet developed full capacity to metabolize chemicals. Their immature metabolisms are not capable of handling either the range or total quantity of chemicals that adult systems can. Aged adults also have a limited capacity to handle drugs. Although impaired excretory capacity is one reason for this decrease, reduction in biotransformation also plays a role. To what degree this loss can be attributed to natural aging or to disease and decreased nutrition is not known.

Hormones are degraded by the same metabolic processes as drugs. To some degree, these compounds compete with each other in biotransformation. Either may also stimulate or inhibit certain metabolic pathways, altering the capacity of the system. Influences of hormones on drug metabolism may underlie the observed fluctuations of drug efficacy and toxicity with diurnal rhythms.

As with all body processes, drug metabolism is dependent on adequate nutrition for proper cell function and generation of biochemicals. The enzymes involved in biotransformation are protein substances and cannot be produced optimally in malnourished individuals. Some foods also may influence enzyme activity because many nutrients are metabolized by biotransformation systems.

Any disease that impairs organ function can interfere with drug metabolism. Liver pathology has the greatest potential for limiting biotransformation. Individuals with impaired liver function often are unable to handle normal doses of drugs, and certain drugs can be toxic in any amount.

Environmental factors

Environmental factors may operate either to decrease or to increase biotransformation. Stress affects metabolism by altering hormone levels and neural activity in the body. Toxic influences such as ionizing irradiation or poisons that impair tissue function can reduce biotransformation. Cigarette smoking is known to enhance the hepatic metabolism of many drugs. An important mechanism by which environmental agents affect drug metabolism is alteration in the rate of microsomal enzyme activity.

Certain chemicals affect the liver enzymes, either stimulating or inhibiting their function. A few exhibit a diphasic effect, initially decreasing, then later increasing enzyme activity. Enzyme inducers stimulate proliferation of the endoplasmic reticulum; an increase in microsomal protein content indicates hyperplasia of the structures involved in biotransformation. Many chemicals affecting the microsomal enzyme system are drugs. With repeated doses, a drug may stimulate the enzyme pathways for its own metabolism, resulting in an apparent decline in potency of succeeding doses. Enzyme induction or inhibition underlies many drug-drug interactions in which one drug appears to increase or decrease the effect of a second.

Drug excretion

Drugs are excreted from the body in the form of both intact molecules and metabolites. Pathways for elimination include respiration, urination, fecal elimination, and exocrine secretion. Efficient excretion of drugs is dependent upon proper functioning of the physiologic systems involved with general excretion: the cardiovascular system (required to transport wastes to the organs of excretion), lungs, kidneys, liver, intestines, and sweat, salivary, and mammary glands.

The rate of removal of drug from the body is termed *clearance. Half-life* ($t_{1/2}$) is another term frequently used to estimate how fast a drug leaves the body. By definition, half-life is the length of time necessary for the concentration of drug in a specific area of the body to decrease by one-half. Both clearance and half-life vary greatly from one drug to another. For example, in humans, penicillin has a serum half-life of less than 1 hour, whereas that of digitoxin is approximately 1 week. The rate of excretion varies with concentration and increases gradually as serum levels rise. A steady state is reached when the rate of excretion reaches the rate at which drug enters the system. If the rate of loss fails to equalize with the rate of absorption, serum drug levels will continue to rise gradually, a phenomenon called *cumulation*.

Owing to their long half-lives, certain drugs such as digitalis tend to cumulate in most recipients, posing an increased risk of toxicity. A second factor influencing the appearance of adverse reactions is the margin of safety. The narrower the margin of safety, the more likely it is that clinical signs of toxicity will appear. Drugs like digitalis, which have both a long half-life and a narrow margin of safety, are most likely to produce toxic reactions and are often described as *cumulative*. To avoid toxicity, the serum levels of cumulative drugs should be allowed to rise gradually. Loading doses (high initial doses used to saturate tissue depots) are unwise except in cases where a prompt therapeutic response is critical.

When administration of a drug is discontinued, the rate of excretion declines in exponential proportion to the declining serum levels (Fig. 7-5). The serum half-life of many drugs is about 6 hours or less. Thus, 2–3 days are generally sufficient to eliminate significant levels of these drugs from the serum. Drugs with longer half-lives may require 2 weeks for dissipation. A few drugs with large storage depots remain in the body for much longer periods.

Excretion processes

The most important route for excretion of drugs is via the urine. However, the lungs, intestinal tract, and exocrine glands can excrete some substances (Box 7-14).

Lungs

The lungs are the favored route for excretion of gaseous and volatile compounds. Agents that are adminis-

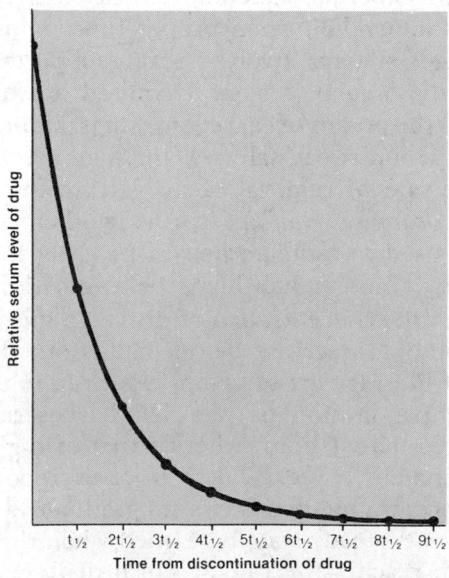

Figure 7-5. General pattern of drug elimination.

> ### Box 7-14. Excretion of drugs
>
> *Pathways*—respiration, urination, fecal elimination, and exocrine secretion
>
> *Physiologic systems*—cardiovascular system, lungs, kidneys, liver, intestines, and sweat, salivary, and mammary glands

tered by inhalation such as general anesthetics are largely eliminated by this route. In addition, ingested substances such as ethanol may diffuse from the blood into the lungs and be subsequently exhaled. Excreted alcohol is the source of breath odor characteristic of individuals who are drinking alcoholic beverages. Respiratory excretion may cause damage to the lungs, as is seen in kerosene poisoning. Excretion of this hydrocarbon through the lungs causes a lipoidal pneumonia that can be life-threatening.

Support and stimulation of respiration promote the excretion of volatile drugs. This is the principle underlying the effectiveness of postoperative "stir-up" regimens used in surgical recovery rooms. Stimulation alone does not change the level of brain function, which is controlled by drug levels in the central nervous system. Repeated deep breathing by the patient, however, does accelerate excretion of these volatile gases, hastening the return to full consciousness.

By their presence in air exhaled from postoperative patients, anesthetic gases pollute the ambient air in recovery suites. Unless these areas are well ventilated, hospital personnel can experience vertigo or syncope due to inhalation of these gases. The staff should avoid close face-to-face contact with patients because this increases exposure.

Exocrine glands

Exocrine glands excrete lipid-soluble drugs that cross cell membranes readily. Excretion of chemicals in the saliva often causes characteristic tastes in the mouth. If the saliva is swallowed, the drug will not be lost from the body but may reenter it by intestinal absorption. Sweat containing drug chemicals sometimes alters body odor, and evaporation of perspiration from the skin leaves a film (frost) of solid drug that can irritate the skin. This is relatively rare and occurs mainly in toxic states when drug levels are very high. Elimination of drugs through the mammary glands of a nursing mother is a matter of special concern because the chemicals may be absorbed by the nursing infant. Normally, exocrine glands do not eliminate large quantities of drugs from the body. They can become important pathways for excretion if a primary excretory system (such as the kidneys) is not functioning properly.

Kidneys

The kidneys are by far the most important organs for the excretion of drugs. Most water-soluble compounds of low relative molecular mass ($M_r < 100$), are eliminated in the urine. Soluble drugs with small molecules filter freely through the glomerular membrane. The proportion that remains in the urine depends on the level of passive and active reabsorption and active secretion by the renal tubule. Ionized (polar) compounds tend to become trapped in the urine because they do not readily diffuse back through the lipid membrane of the tubule to the blood.

Urinary excretion can be influenced by the rate of glomerular filtration, changes in urinary pH, and competition for reabsorption. As the volume of urine increases, the filtrate passes through the tubule more quickly, and less time is available for reabsorption. This effect is exploited in the treatment of poisoning by the use of forced diuresis. Alterations in pH influence ionization of drugs in the urine, minimizing or enhancing the "trapping" effect of polarization of chemicals in the filtrate. The more acidic the urine, the more rapid the elimination of basic drugs. Acid drugs are more readily excreted in basic urine. If a drug (such as penicillin) is actively secreted by the renal tubule, the administration of a compound that competes for the active transport mechanism (such as probenecid) will reduce excretion.

Renal failure greatly prolongs the serum half-life of most drugs. Dosages of therapeutic agents must be reduced and intervals between drug dosages lengthened in clients with poor kidney function. If the client is treated by dialysis, drugs removed by the dialysis process should be administered after the treatment.

Liver and intestines

Drugs or drug metabolites with a relative molecular mass greater than 100 (such as glucuronides) are excreted largely by the biliary system. All the drug secreted by the liver is not eliminated at once; a portion is reabsorbed in the intestinal tract. This enterohepatic cycle allows only a portion of bile constituents to escape in the feces, producing a gradual elimination. Excretion of such drugs can be hastened by the administration of laxatives or cathartics to stimulate peristalsis and reduce bowel transit time.

Interaction of pharmacokinetic processes

Once a drug enters the body, the processes of absorption, distribution, transformation, and excretion are carried out simultaneously. Therefore, the quantity and distribution of drug in various compartments are constantly changing. The relationships between these processes and their effect on drug levels are illustrated schematically in Figure 7-6.

Movement of drugs into and out of storage areas affects plasma half-life and can produce biphasic and

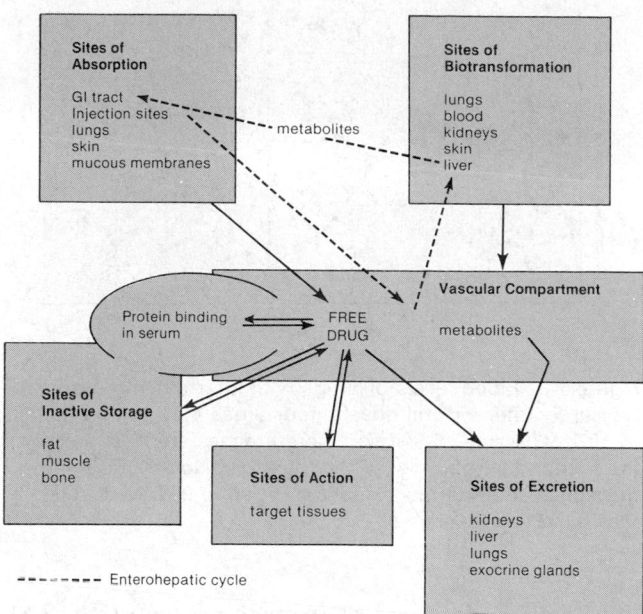

Figure 7-6. Body processes affecting drug distribution.

triphasic half-life times. Initial $t_{1/2}$ is shorter than $t_{1/2}$ after saturation of storage depots. Plasma $t_{1/2}$ is increased by movement of drug out of storage depots after intake is discontinued. When storage depots are exhausted, plasma $t_{1/2}$ may drop.

Regimens for drug administration are designed to maintain a steady state of drug within the therapeutic range. Single doses of medication produce blood and tissue levels similar to the curves shown in Figure 7-7. Repeated doses are required to raise drug concentra-

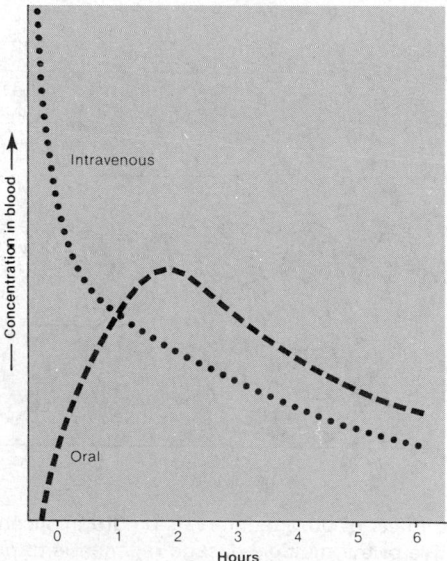

Figure 7-7. Drug levels following single dose administration. The figure demonstrates the time course for drug in blood following oral and intravenous doses. (Dashed line: Oral drug; dotted line: IV drug.)

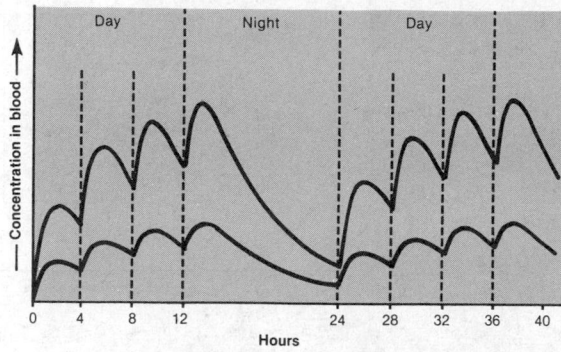

Figure 7-8. Blood levels of drugs with intermittent dosage. A typical regimen or oral dosage four times a day on a schedule of 10-2-6-10 or 9-1-5-9. Two different doses are illustrated over the first and second day of the regimen. (Notari BE: Biopharmaceutics and Pharmacokinetics. 4th ed, p 254. New York, Marcel Dekker, 1987.)

tions as free drug is lost from the system (Fig. 7-8). Frequency of dosing also affects drug concentrations (Fig. 7-9). When constant blood levels are required, a continuous IV infusion is generally preferred (Fig. 7-10).

■ Summary

Blood levels of drugs are affected by rates of absorption, storage in inactive tissue depots, biotransformation, and excretion. Each of these processes is subject to the influence of genetic, physiologic, and environmental factors. Tissue concentration of drugs, therefore, can vary greatly from individual to individual and from time to time within the same individual.

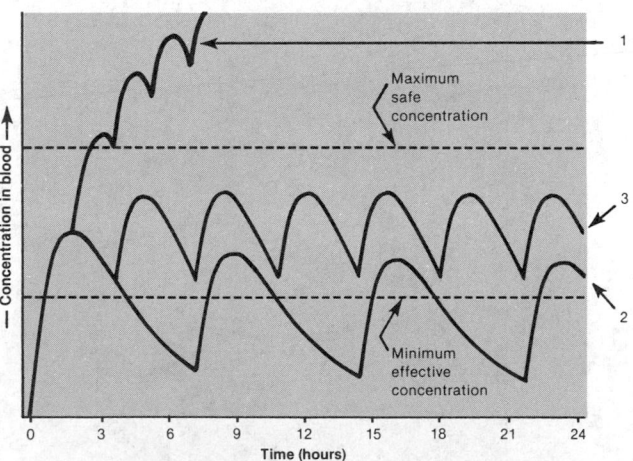

Figure 7-9. Effect of dosage intervals on drug concentration. The objective of the multiple-dosage regimen is to maintain the patient's blood level with maximum and minimum concentrations as shown in the figure. The dosage interval is too short in *curve 1*, too long in *curve 2*, and ideal in *curve 3*. The initial dose used for this simulation is 33% more than the maintenance dose. (Notari BE: Biopharmaceutics and Pharmacokinetics, 4th ed, p 248. New York, Marcel Dekker, 1987.)

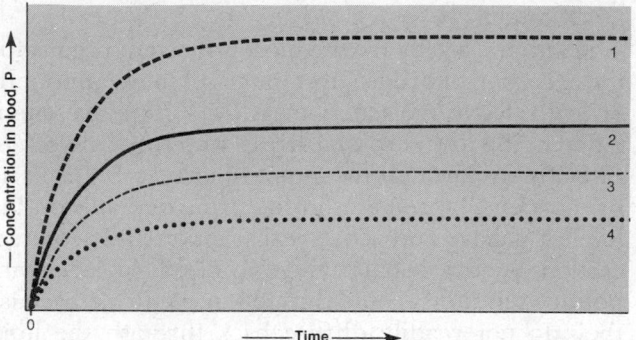

Figure 7-10. Blood concentrations following intravenous infusion. Steady-state blood levels achieved by constant-rate intravenous infusion of drug. The steady-state levels are proportional to the infusion as follows: 10 (*curve 1*), 6.6 (*curve 2*), 5 (*curve 3*), and 3.3 (*curve 4*). (Notari BE: Biopharmaceutics and Pharmacokinetics, 3rd ed, p 100. New York, Marcel Dekker, 1980.)

Learning experience 7-2

Investigate the pharmacokinetic processes by which the following drugs are absorbed, distributed, metabolized, and excreted by the body: glucose administered intravenously, halothane administered by inhalation, sulfamethoxazole administered by mouth, and chlorpromazine administered intramuscularly. What can you deduce about risk factors for toxicity, nursing measures to prevent adverse reactions, and emergency treatment for harmful reactions from this information?

Nursing management

The way in which a given drug is absorbed, distributed, metabolized, and excreted by the body markedly changes its potency, efficacy, and toxicity. Not only must nurses understand the pharmacokinetic processes influencing drug concentration, but they also must monitor clients carefully for responses to drugs that may indicate individual differences in the way their bodies transport, metabolize, and eliminate those drugs. Assessments should be global and carried out at regular and frequent intervals.

When drugs are secreted in saliva, the client needs frequent oral hygiene. In toxic states, both oral hygiene and bathing should be carried out more often.

References

Brownlee S. (1990). Blitzing the defense. *US News and World Report, October 15,* 100.

Leavitt A, Zweifler A. (1988). Nifedipine, hypotension and myocardial injury (letter). *Ann Intern Med, 108,* 305 (February).

Raloff J. (1988). Hairy portals for toxic chemicals. *Science News, 133*, 407 (June 25).

Bibliography

*Conn PM, Gebhart GF. (1989). General principles of drug action and pharmacokinetics. *Essentials of pharmacology*, chap. 1. Philadelphia: FA Davis Co.

*Notari RE. (1987). *Biopharmaceutics and pharmacokinetics*, 4th ed. New York: Marcel Dekker.

Sexually transmitted anticancer drug. (1986). *Science News, 130*, 105.

*Weiss R. (1989). Delivering the goods. *Science News 133*, 360 (June 4).

*Recommended for further reading.

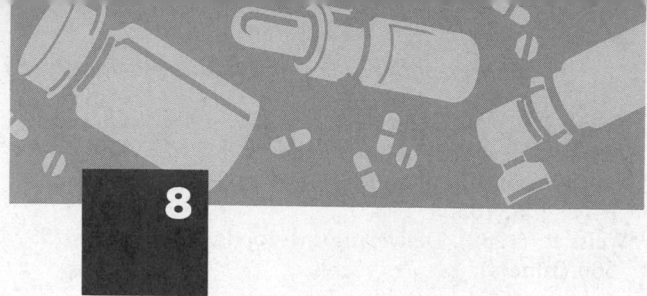

Drug preparations

Substances used for a pharmacologic effect must usually undergo some kind of preparation before medicinal use. Rarely, if ever, are the raw materials containing pharmacologically active chemicals found in a chemically pure form. To eliminate extraneous substances, the active chemical is usually extracted from the raw source, purified, and incorporated in a formulation designed to deliver the drug to the appropriate tissues.

Drug nomenclature

A single drug may be designated by a number of names: chemical, generic, official, and proprietary (or trade). It may also be identified as a member of a number of drug families (Box 8-1).

Chemical name

The chemical name of a drug indicates its atomic and molecular structure. It may be given as a chemical formula or accompanied by a diagram of its structure. These names are of particular interest to the chemist and research pharmacist. They are written without capitalization. Chemical names are often so long and complicated that they are unsuitable for general use. For example, one common drug's chemical name is acetylsalicylic acid ($C_6H_4COOHOCOCH_3$), and its chemical structure is diagrammed as follows:

$$
\begin{array}{c}
O \\
\parallel \\
O-C-CH_3 \\
COOH
\end{array}
$$

Generic name

By strict definition, the term *generic* should designate a chemical derivation. However, in common usage, it is used to denote the nonproprietary name of a compound used medicinally. For clarity and convenience, generic names should be both concise and distinctive. These names are often proposed by the company that first develops the drug. Like chemical names, generic names are not capitalized. Following our example, the generic name for acetylsalicylic acid is aspirin. In the United States, a generic name or U.S. Adopted Name, is selected by the U.S. Adopted Name Council, a body sponsored by the American Medical Association, the U.S. Pharmacopeial Convention, Inc., and the American Pharmaceutical Association in consultation with a representative of the U.S. Food and Drug Administration.

Official name

Official names are those adopted by bodies authorized to do so by a governing body. In the United States, these names are chosen by a Committee of Revision of the U.S. Pharmacopeial Convention, made up of pharmacists, physicians, and pharmacologists who donate their services. An official name may be identical to the generic name of the drug and is not capitalized. Official names are found in the *U.S. Pharmacopeia and National Formulary (USP & NF)*.

Trade name

Trademarks, trade names, brand names, and proprietary names are interchangeable terms used to identify the drugs manufactured by various drug companies. Thus, a specific generic drug may have many different trade names. The symbol ™ after the trade name indicates that the trade name is registered, and its use is restricted to the manufacturer who owns it. Although all trade name preparations of a particular generic or official drug must contain the indicated drug chemical, formulations may vary in the type and number of additives used.

Trade names may be chosen to denote the drug's chemical structure; to identify the company responsible for manufacturing the drug; or to represent some property of the drug. Names are easily confused if a number of different drugs bear similar names because of a similarity in chemical makeup or medicinal properties, or if different drugs are given similar names indicative of the company of origin.

There are many different trade names for our example, aspirin including: Arthritis Pain Formula, Ascriptin, Bayer Aspirin, Bufferin, Easprin, and Zorprin. Trade names are capitalized.

Abbreviations

Drugs in frequent use may be ordered by abbreviated names adopted for expediency. These vary from locality to locality and are rarely standardized or authorized by any official procedure. Most frequently, abbreviations are acronyms containing the initial letters of a multiword name (*eg*, MOM for milk of magnesia) or prominent letters from the generic name (*eg*, HCTZ for hydrochlorothiazide). An abbreviation often used to designate aspirin is ASA. Abbreviations should not be used unless they have been formally adopted and standardized in the written policies of an institution.

Table 8-1 illustrates nonproprietary (official, generic, chemical) and trade (proprietary, brand, trademark) names.

Drug families

Drugs with similar characteristics are often grouped together in families. The family name may denote chemical structure (*eg*, barbiturate), mode of action (*eg*, antacid), physiologic action (*eg*, diuretic), or therapeutic effect (*eg*, anticonvulsant, analgesic). One drug may be listed under more than one classification. Again, using our previous example, aspirin is an analgesic, antipyretic, and anti-inflammatory drug, which acts as a prostaglandin inhibitor (Box 8-2).

■ Summary

For pharmacologic use, drugs are listed according to chemical name, generic name, official name, and trade name. Chemical names denote the atomic and molecular structure. Generic names are concise names adopted for perma-

Table 8-1. Examples of names given common drugs

Generic name	Chemical name	Trade name(s)	Commonly used abbreviation
aspirin	acetylsalicylic acid	Ecotrin, Bufferin	ASA
milk of magnesia	magnesium hydroxide	Phillips' Milk of Magnesia	MOM
tetracycline	hydrochloride of 4-(dimethylamino)-1,4,4a,5,5a,6,11,12a-octahydro-3,6,10,12,12a-pentahydroxy-6-methyl-1,11-dioxa-2-napthacenecarboxamide	Achromycin, Tetracyn, Panmycin	
prednisone	11β,17,21-trihydroxypregna-1,4-diene-3-20-dione	Deltasone, Meticorten	
repository corticotropin injection	adrenocorticotropic hormone	Cortigel, Cortrophin gel	ACTH
chlorothiazide	6-chloro-2*H*-1,2,4-benzothiadiazine-7-sulfonamide 1,1-dioxide	Diuril	CTZ
chlorthalidone	2-chloro-5-(2,3-dihydro-1-hydroxy-3-oxo-1*H*-isoindol-1-yl) benzenesulfonamide	Hygroton	
hydrochlorothiazide	6-chloro-3,4-dihydro-2*H*-1,2,4-Benzothiadiazine-7-sulfonamide 1,1-dioxide	Esidrix, HydroDiuril, Oretic	HCTZ
ethacrynic acid	[2,3,-dichloro-4(2-methylene-1-oxobutyl)-phenoxy] acetic acid	Edecrin	

Box 8-2. Drug families

Chemical structure (*eg*, barbiturates, phenols, aminoglycosides)

Mode of action (*eg*, antacid, central nervous system stimulant)

Physiologic action (*eg*, diuretic, anticholinergic)

Therapeutic effect (*eg*, anticonvulsant, analgesic)

nent use. Official names are those authorized by governmental units for use in official compendia; they may be the same as the generic name. Trade names indicate preparations manufactured by a specific pharmaceutical firm. Acronym abbreviations usually are unauthorized and may vary from place to place. Drug families are groups of drugs with similar chemistry, action, or effect. A single drug may belong to several drug families.

Nursing management

Nursing implications

In institutional practice, nurses usually prepare and administer medication doses. Errors may arise because drug orders may be inaccurately transcribed, or there may be an inconsistency in drug name use by physicians and pharmacists. Nurses should actively participate in the development of institutional policies and procedures governing the use of drug names. Accuracy in prescribing, transcribing, and administration should be given priority. It may be advisable to require the use of official or generic names. If acronym abbreviations are in common usage, written policies should clearly identify appropriate abbreviations and their meanings.

When preparing doses of drugs for clients, nurses must adhere to procedures that promote accurate identification of drug agents prior to administration. If names used for prescription and those on drug labels are not the same, the nurse must verify that the two names refer to identical drugs before the medication can be given.

Nursing process: problems related to self-medicating clients

Assessment When taking a drug history, the nurse must be careful to identify accurately the substances used by a client. The label attached to the medication container usually identifies the active drug or drugs in the preparation. If it does not or if the label is illegible, the nurse should contact the pharmacist directly to

determine the therapeutic agent or agents. The list of drugs taken should be examined to make sure there are no duplicate orders. Prescriptions written by different physicians may refer to the same drug under different names, or may denote two different drugs with similar action that should not be taken concurrently. In such cases, the client may be taking both preparations and experiencing symptoms of overdose. Sometimes, when a drug is discontinued, the client will return to a previous prescription of the same drug by a different name, thus continuing the medication without the physician's knowledge.

Nursing diagnosis The nursing diagnosis most likely to be made for self-medicating clients is knowledge deficit relating to prescription drugs and their use in the medical treatment regimen. Other nursing diagnoses depend upon the drug involved. The undesirable effect on the client may be:

> Impaired tissue integrity
> Altered nutrition: less than body requirements
> Fluid volume deficit or fluid volume excess
> Impaired physical mobility,

or any one of numerous other effects of inappropriate medication. The cause may be overmedication, inadequate dosage, or inappropriate medication.

Planning The goal of nursing care is to educate the client so that management of self-medication will improve.

Intervention A teaching plan appropriate to the client's needs should be prepared. The nurse may need to consult with the physician or pharmacist to clarify the drug regimen. The client should be taught clearly what drugs have been prescribed and how to use them. The nurse should assist the client to the limit of his or her expertise and serve as a resource person when additional information is required.

Evaluation The client's ability to carry out the drug regimen accurately and his or her response to the drug regimen should improve after the teaching plan

Enrichment experience 8-1

List drug abbreviations noted on patients' charts and Cardexes in a medical unit within a health care facility. Compare this list with those abbreviations noted in two other specialty units (*eg*, pediatrics, maternity, or psychiatric unit). Fill in the correct generic or brand name for each abbreviation. Ask a colleague to do the same, then compare responses. Consider the professional and legal implications if you were unable to identify a drug correctly.

is completed. Data required for evaluation include the incidence or absence of errors in self-medication by the client.

Sources of drugs

Drugs are developed from a wealth of natural resources, including plants, animal tissues, organic and inorganic minerals, and chemical synthesis.

Plant kingdom

Plants were one of the earliest sources of therapeutic agents. Seeds, bark, roots, stems, fruit, and sap were all used for medicinal purposes. Because most of these preparations contained inert ingredients or multiple active ingredients, they were called *crude drugs*. As extraction of the active ingredients from plants was developed and refined, *pure drugs* emerged from the plant kingdom.

Animal kingdom

Animal tissues have also been used to produce crude drugs (eg, liver extract). In modern practice, most tissues are refined to a considerable degree. (In place of liver extract, a pure form of cyanocobalamin, or vitamin B_{12}, is now used.) Animals are the source of drugs such as hormones (eg, insulin from the pancreases of pigs and cows) and vitamins (eg, vitamins A and D from fish oil). Slaughter is not always necessary, for example, vaccines may be produced from cultures grown in eggs, and antitoxins from horse serum. Animals contribute further by serving as subjects in the early stages of drug research and development.

Mineral resources

Commonly used mineral products include metallic and nonmetallic compounds, acids, bases, and salts. Coal tar is a source of many drugs such as sulfonamides and salicylates.

Synthetic chemicals

Substances that do not occur naturally may be developed in a pure form in laboratories. Sophisticated equipment and highly skilled personnel are required for this operation. Except for simple substances, such as inorganic salts, complete synthesis of a drug is relatively rare. More commonly, a substance derived from natural sources will be manipulated chemically to produce an improved drug with increased specificity or reduced toxicity. A promising development in laboratory production of drugs is the use of genetic engineering involving recombinant DNA techniques. Although manmade, these preparations would incorporate biologic components such as genes, viruses, or protein fragments (Table 8-2).

■ **Summary**

Drugs may be derived from plants, animals, and mineral resources; they may also be produced synthetically in the laboratory. At present, many drugs of natural origin are altered chemically to produce semisynthetic drugs with more desirable medicinal properties.

Nursing management

Nursing process

Assessment When gathering a history from a client, the nurse should ask specifically about intolerance of or allergy to drugs, foods, and other substances. A complete list of medicines used by the client should also be made. Any allergies and intolerances should be compared to the sources of drugs currently in use or to others likely to be ordered.

Nursing diagnosis Clients allergic to plants, animals, or pollens may react adversely to medications derived from related plants or animals. For example, clients allergic to fish are at increased risk of adverse reaction to protamine, which is derived from fish tissues. Some clients experience toxic effects from dosages well within the normal therapeutic range. Others will not react therapeutically unless they receive higher than normal amounts of drug. (See Chapters 4 and 9 for other types of adverse reactions.)

Planning Goals of nursing care are to prevent adverse drug reactions, and promptly detect and treat adverse reactions should they occur.

Table 8-2. Sources of drugs

Source	Example	Summary of pertinent information
Plant kingdom	Opium poppy: morphine	Any part of plant may be useful. Plant may be used whole or active ingredients extracted.
Animal kingdom	Pancreas: insulin	Drugs are tested on animals. Biologic constituents of animals are used to make drugs for treatment and prevention of disease.
Mineral resources	Coal tar: aspirin	Metallic and nonmetallic minerals, acids, bases and salts are used.
Synthetic chemicals	Oral contraceptives	Pure drugs are produced. Natural drugs are improved by modification. Recombinant DNA techniques produce drugs by genetic engineering.

Intervention Medications likely to produce an adverse reaction should not be administered without consultation with the physician, who may change the drug order or take precautions to reduce the severity of harmful reactions. Clients known to be allergic to certain drugs (or sources of drugs) should be warned to inform medical personnel of such problems. The wearing of a medical identification device listing the problem should be recommended.

Evaluation Data required for evaluation include the absence or incidence of adverse reactions, and the severity of reactions that may occur.

Drug constituents

A medicinal preparation is made up of one or more active ingredients and various additives chosen to alter certain properties of the final formulation.

Active ingredients

The active ingredients of a preparation are responsible for producing desired effects. Pharmacologic agents vary considerably in their chemical structure and are systematically classified according to their chemical properties. Major classes include salts, alkaloids, glycosides, polypeptides, and steroids. When a preparation contains only one active ingredient, it is known by the name of that substance. Combinations of more than one ingredient are rarely used for prescription drugs but are common among nonprescription preparations. As a matter of convenience, multidrug combinations are often known by their trade names.

Salts are compounds consisting of a positive ion other than hydrogen and a negative ion other than hydroxyl. Solid salts tend to form crystals; in solution, a certain proportion of their molecules separate, releasing ions that are electrically charged and (often) chemically active. Pharmacologic activity is usually confined to either the cation (positively charged ion) or the anion (negatively charged ion). Compounds that contain drug ions with like charges tend to be chemically compatible, whereas drug ions of unlike charges tend to form inactive precipitates when combined.

A major drug source is the salts formed when *alkaloids* react with acids. Alkaloids are organic compounds that contain nitrogen and have a basic *p*H. They are found in the seeds, roots, leaves, or bark of certain plants (*eg,* the opium poppy, tobacco, cinchona bark). Examples of drugs derived from alkaloids are atropine (a powerful anticholinergic), opiates such as codeine and morphine, and strychnine, a dangerous poison. Most drugs whose names end in "ine" are alkaloid derivatives.

Glycosides are substances derived from plants that, when hydrolyzed, yield a sugar and one or more additional products. Sugars derived from glycosides are usually glucose (from glucosides) or galactose (from galactosides). A major family of glycoside drugs is that of digitalis, a cardiotonic derived from foxglove plants.

Polypeptides are protein in nature and tend to be high molecular weight compounds. Although their molecules do not ionize, they usually are amphoteric (*ie,* they exhibit electric charges at two or more sites on the molecule). Polypeptides used for a systemic effect must be administered parenterally because they are easily hydrolyzed by proteases in the digestive tract. Many enzymes (*eg,* pancrelipase) and hormones (*eg,* insulin) are polypeptides.

Steroids are compounds that contain a characteristic structure composed of one pentagonal and three hexagonal carbon rings:

Naturally occurring compounds having a steroid nucleus include cholesterol and the adrenocortical hormones. Steroids used as drugs include estrogen, testosterone, cortisone, and the digitalis glycosides. These medications are usually unaffected by digestion and may be administered orally.

Additives

Among the substances commonly added to drug formulations are vehicles, fillers, binders, disintegrators, lubricants, flavorings, dyes, and preservatives. Each is used to impart a desired property to the medicinal preparation. Additives must be nontoxic and compatible with the active drug, as well as each of the other additives.

Vehicles are substances added to a formulation to carry the active ingredient by giving it form and substance. Common vehicles include water, oils, syrups, and other solvents; and cocoa butter, petrolatum, and other solids. Vehicles may have a significant effect on the physical and chemical properties of the drug.

Fillers are powders (*eg,* dextrose, lactose, starch) added to dry drugs to provide bulk needed for producing solid preparations of uniform dose. Most fillers are relatively inert. Hydrophobic fillers (fillers which do not dissolve readily in water) are sometimes used to delay the dissolution of the medication, thereby achieving a timed-release effect. Some people may be intolerant of certain fillers (*eg,* lactase-deficient individuals experience digestive upsets when given lactose).

Diluents are substances that increase the bulk of the formulation, thus reducing the concentration of the active ingredient. Both vehicles and fillers act as diluents.

Binders are substances added to solid formulations to improve the cohesiveness of dry ingredients, which facilitates shaping into durable dose forms. Dextrose and lactose act as binders. *Disintegrators* (eg, starch) facilitate disaggregation and dissolution when solid medications are placed in water. *Lubricants* (eg, talc, stearates, hydrogenated vegetable oils) prevent tablets and caplets from adhering to compression machinery during the production of solid dose forms.

Flavorings are substances added to formulations (usually liquids or chewable tablets) to improve palatability. Common agents are cherry, raspberry, chocolate, and licorice syrup.

Dyes are added to formulations to make products more attractive and to facilitate identification of drugs involved in overdose or poisoning. Colors used in drugs, foods, and cosmetics are under careful scrutiny by the U.S. Food and Drug Administration. Some dyes (eg, certain reds) have been banned as carcinogenic.

Tartrazine (Food and Drug Administration Yellow No. 5) is known to cause allergic reactions in sensitive individuals (mainly asthmatics prone to nasal polyps who are allergic to aspirin; see Table 8-3).

Nursing management

Nursing process: unexpected response to drugs

Assessment When compiling a drug history, trade and generic names should be recorded. If the client has used more than one trade name preparation of a generic drug, the time intervals of their use should be logged. Client response to the drug regimen should be carefully appraised. Data on client response to drug therapy should be compared with the drug history to

Table 8-3. Constituents of drugs

	Form	Examples	Points of interest
Active ingredients			
Responsible for producing the action of the drug *Categorized according to physical and chemical properties*	Salts	morphine sulfate, potassium chloride	Ionize when placed in solution
	Alkaloids	nicotine, atropine	Contain nitrogen Are basic in nature Form salts when they react with acids Are a major source of drugs Have names ending in "ine"
	Glycosides	digitalis	Yield glucose or carbohydrate-containing molecules
	Polypeptides	insulin	Include high molecular weight proteins Are destroyed by the digestive process Include enzymes and hormones
Additives			
Impart desired characteristics to drug formulations *Must be compatible with the active ingredient and with each other*	Vehicles	water, oils, cocoa butter, petrolatum	Give form and substance to the preparations May change the physical and chemical properties of a preparation
	Fillers	dextrose, lactose, starch	Are relatively inert May alter dissolution of the active principle Can cause adverse reactions in recipients
	Diluents	vehicles and fillers	Reduce the concentration of the active ingredient
	Binders	dextrose, lactose	Improve cohesiveness of the dry ingredients
	Disintegrators	starch	Facilitate disaggregation and dissolution of solid preparations
	Flavorings	cherry, raspberry, or licorice syrups	Improve palatability
	Dyes	tartrazine (FDA Yellow No. 5)	Make products attractive Facilitate identification of drugs May cause adverse reactions in recipients

ascertain whether response to different trade name drugs is quantitatively or qualitatively different. Because trade name formulations of a given drug may vary in the salt of the drug used and in the additives, bioavailability, therapeutic response, and adverse reactions may also vary. Allergic responses to one or more additives may also occur.

Nursing diagnosis Whenever possible, a nursing diagnosis of adverse drug reaction should indicate the nature of the response and the specific formulations that trigger it. For example, a client who has recently ingested a drink containing caffeine may become agitated if a central nervous system stimulant is administered.

Planning The goal of nursing care is to alleviate the adverse signs and symptoms and/or to adjust the medication regimen for optimum response.

Intervention Nursing measures to relieve the signs and symptoms of unavoidable adverse reactions are appropriate. In collaboration with the physician or pharmacist and the client, the nurse determines which of the drugs used produced optimum response. An appropriate drug regimen is devised. The nurse then prepares a teaching plan appropriate to the individual client. Trade name preparations that produce an optimum response should be identified.

Evaluation Data required for evaluation include signs and symptoms indicating the client's response to nursing measures and/or changes in the drug regimen.

Nursing process: risk of accidental poisoning

Assessment Identify drugs listed in the drug history that pose significant risk of accidental ingestion.

Drugs that resemble candy in flavor or color, and those that are advertised as pleasant-tasting, pose the greatest risk. Ascertain whether the drugs are accessible to children or other individuals who might take them inappropriately.

Nursing diagnosis An appropriate nursing diagnosis would be high risk for injury related to accidental poisoning secondary to (name the drug) ingestion.

Planning Nursing goals include prevention of accidental poisoning.

Intervention A teaching plan is prepared and implemented. Clients should be taught to keep drugs in secure places that are not accessible to children or other individuals who might take them inappropriately.

Evaluation Data required for evaluation include the absence or incidence of accidental poisoning involving the client's drugs.

Types of preparations

Pharmaceutical preparations are available in a variety of formulations designed to facilitate the administration of the drug. The therapeutic effects of the drug's active ingredients are often determined by the type of preparation and its dosage. Factors that influence formulation include the route to be used for administration, the rapidity of response desired, suitability for the client, acceptability by the recipient, and the specific properties of the drug itself (*eg*, solubility, stability, and bioavailability).

Solids

Tablets are small disklike masses of medicinal powder that have been compressed sufficiently to maintain their shape. The term *pill* is sometimes used to refer to spheric or pellet-shaped tablets. Most tablets and pills are administered orally.

Various types of tablets include the following: 1) *buccal*, designed to be held in the mouth between the cheek and gum until dissolved and absorbed; 2) *coated*, containing an outside layer usually of sugar or chocolate; 3) *effervescent*, containing a mixture of sodium bicarbonate and an acidulant, such as citric acid, that generates carbon dioxide when added to water; 4) *enteric-coated*, containing an outside layer that does not dissolve until the tablet reaches the small intestine; 5) *sublingual*, designed to be placed beneath the tongue until dissolved and absorbed; and 6) *prolonged-action* or *timed-release*, designed to be released and absorbed in stages or gradually over time. Tablets that resemble capsules in shape are sometimes called *caplets*.

Hard compressed tablets do not dissolve readily. Because solubility affects bioavailability, the degree to which tablets disintegrate and dissolve is tested during manufacture. As tablets (particularly pills) age, they tend to dry out (become "case-hardened") and become less soluble.

Capsules are gelatin cases used to enclose solid drugs. Capsules melt and release their drugs very quickly after ingestion. If the capsule contains powder, the drug tends to dissolve and be absorbed rapidly. In a capsule that contains beads, some are enteric-coated, causing a *sustained-release (prolonged action, timed-release)* effect. Capsules are more easily tampered with after manufacturing than are caplets. Sustained release capsules containing pellets that release their drugs at different times are still widely used.

Troches (lozenges) are discoid or cylindric medications consisting chiefly of medicinal powder, sugar, and mucilage. They are designed to be placed in a body cavity for absorption by the mucous membrane. Lozenges are oral preparations; troches may be oral or vaginal.

Pellets are small pills or balls of medication. Currently, pellets are made of materials that are absorbed slowly from muscle or subcutaneous tissue after surgical implantation.

Needles are long, thin cylinders; like pellets, they are surgically implanted for sustained-release effect.

Patches resemble adherent dressings in appearance. On the inner surface is an adhesive rim surrounding a central area. The drug may be imbedded in either the adhesive ring or in the central area. When applied to the skin, the medication is released gradually and absorbed transdermally.

Powders are measured doses of solid medication in powder form. They are usually dissolved in water before ingestion.

Granules are dry medications that resemble powders in appearance but whose particles are larger than those in powders. Granules may be prepared as single-dose packets or packaged in bulk.

Dusts are very fine powders. They may be applied topically to the skin or mucous membranes, or administered by inhalation (*eg*, cromolyn administered by inhalation to control asthma).

Semisolids

Suppositories are cylindrical or cone-shaped medications whose vehicles (*eg*, cocoa butter) melt at body temperature. They are molded to conform to the contours of body cavities, such as the rectum, vagina, or urethra.

Pastes are thick, gelatinous substances usually intended for topical application to the skin. Vehicles and fillers used in pastes include oils, waxes, and starch.

Ointments are fatty, soft substances applied to the skin or eyes. Ointments may be nonwater soluble (based on petrolatum, lard, or lanolin) or water soluble. Other terms synonymous with ointment are *salve, unction, and unguent.*

Creams are topic preparations whose consistency is less viscous than ointments but more viscous than lotions. Creams tend to hold their shape when undisturbed but can be easily spread.

Foams are mixtures of finely dispersed gas bubbles interspersed in a liquid (*eg*, contraceptive vaginal foams).

Liquids

Lotions are liquids with a creamy consistency that are applied topically to the skin (*eg*, calamine lotion).

Solutions are mixtures of two or more substances dissolved in another substance. In solutions, the molecules of each solute disperse homogenously but do not change chemically. Although solutions may be either gaseous, liquid, or solid, medicinal solutions are mainly liquids. Various solutions may be administered orally, rectally, topically, by injection, or by inhalation. They are also instilled in the eye, nose, and ear and used as sprays or irrigations.

Liniments are liquids containing an alcoholic, oily, or soapy vehicle. They are rubbed on the skin and usually act as counterirritants.

Elixirs are clear liquids containing water, alcohol, sweeteners, and flavors (*eg*, elixir of phenobarbital). They are usually administered orally.

Tinctures are alcoholic extracts of vegetable or animal substances (*eg*, tincture of belladonna, tincture of benzoin). Tinctures may be administered topically or orally. The usual dose of an oral tincture is 1 dram (1 teaspoon). Potent drugs are dispensed as 10% concentrations, less potent drugs as 20%. Tinctures often contain tannic acid.

Extracts are concentrated solutions prepared by dissolving the active principle of a substance in alcohol or water and evaporating part or all of the solvent. The drug is then dissolved or diluted with an alcoholic solvent. The strength of an extract is usually several times stronger than the crude drug. *Fluid extracts* are alcoholic solutions of 100% concentration (*ie*, each milliliter of solution contains 1 g of pure drug).

Aromatic waters are saturated aqueous solutions of volatile substances (*eg*, spearmint oil, peppermint oil).

Syrups are solutions of sugar and water, usually flavored, to which a drug is added. Syrups are used for palatability, especially in pediatric medications (*eg*, syrup of ipecac).

Suspensions are mixtures of a solid and liquid in which the solid particles do not dissolve. *Gels* and *magmas* are viscous suspensions of mineral precipitates in water (*eg*, aluminum hydroxide gel, milk of magnesia). These mixtures tend to separate upon standing and must be shaken well before use.

Oils are viscous, greasy liquids that are insoluble in water. There are two types: volatile and fixed. Volatile oils evaporate easily, leaving no greasy residue; fixed oils do not evaporate readily. Oils may act as drug agents (*eg*, castor oil) or may be used as vehicles to dissolve other drugs (*eg*, pitressin tannate in oil).

Emulsions are mixtures of two liquids (usually oil and water) that are not mutually soluble. When thoroughly shaken, the oil will divide into globules that disperse throughout the mixture. Emulsions tend to separate upon standing but can be stabilized by the addition of an agent that reduces surface tension. Medications dispensed in the form of emulsions may contain oils of low palatability. The emulsion alters the greasy consistency of the substance and tends to disguise its taste.

Nursing management

The modern drug industry produces a vast array of medicinal preparations designed to cure or ameliorate the symptoms of virtually every ailment. Pharmaceutical companies rely heavily on advertising and promotional techniques to influence physicians and consumers to use their products. Nurses must be familiar with the various formulations of drugs to collaborate effectively with physicians in developing a suitable regimen of prescription drugs, and to guide clients in appropriate selection of nonprescription remedies.

The formulation of a drug influences its safety, acceptability, and efficacy. When problems arise in the use of a particular preparation, substitution of another preparation of the same drug may sometimes be appropriate. However, certain substitutions may be hazardous. For example, care must be exercised when a preparation designed for one route of administration is ordered to be given by a different route. Many intravenous solutions are too irritating to be infused subcutaneously or intramuscularly. Solutions intended for subcutaneous or intramuscular injection often cannot be given intravenously because they are too concentrated, or because they contain ingredients such as lipids that would be harmful, even lethal, if administered intravenously. Occasionally, injectable solutions are administered by inhalation but solutions prepared for inhalation administration are not appropriate for injection. Some injectable drugs may be effective when administered orally but others may be degraded by the digestive process. Nurses should be able to suggest acceptable alternatives to a physician and recognize the potential for harm from an inappropriate drug order.

Checklist of nursing actions

☐ When taking a drug history, identify all medications accurately by both generic and trade names.

☐ Assess client response to medications.

☐ Identify intolerances of or allergies to drugs manifested by the client.

☐ Analyze the drug history to detect possible duplication of drug preparations and multiple prescriptions for similar drugs.

☐ To identify adverse drug reactions, compare client's signs and symptoms with usual adverse reactions caused by preparations in current use by the client.

☐ Compare the chronology of the client's signs and symptoms with the chronology of drug use to identify unusual drug reactions.

☐ Consult with physicians and pharmacists as necessary to clarify the drug regimen and to develop a regimen tailored to meet the client's needs.

☐ Teach clients appropriate information about their drug regimen.

☐ Serve as a resource person to obtain further information about drugs for the client.

☐ When administering medication, identify all drugs accurately before delivering them to the client.

☐ Participate in developing institutional policies and procedures that promote accuracy in medication.

☐ Promote the development of written policies that define common abbreviations used for drug names.

☐ Consult with the physician for a change in orders prior to administering drugs identified as posing for the client a high risk of adverse reaction.

☐ Teach clients who are allergic to drugs to inform medical personnel of this fact and to wear a medical identification device that lists the allergies.

☐ Teach clients the necessary precautions to prevent poisoning from accidental ingestion of drugs.

Bibliography

Glanze WD. (1990). *Mosby's medical and nursing dictionary,* 3rd ed. St. Louis: CV Mosby.

Osol O, ed. (1987). *Remington's pharmaceutical sciences,* 15th ed. Philadelphia: FA Davis.

Thomas L, ed. (1985). *Taber's cyclopedic medical dictionary.* Philadelphia: FA Davis.

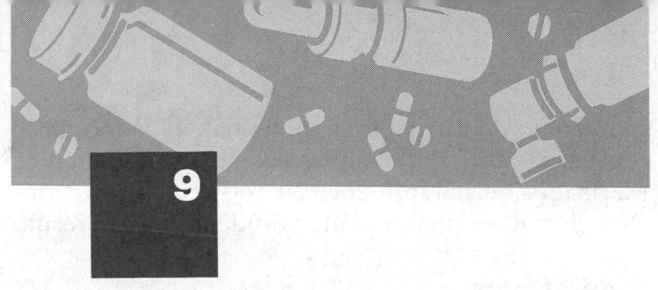

Drug reactions and interactions

Adverse reactions for drugs
  Toxic reactions
  Side effects
  Allergic reactions
  Idiosyncratic reactions
  Chain reactions
  Cumulative reactions
  Tolerance and dependence
Mechanism of drug interaction
  Absorption
    Direct interaction of drugs
    Dissolution rate changes
    Avoiding interactions during absorption
  Distribution
    Displacement
  Biotransformation
    Inhibition of metabolism
    Acceleration of metabolism
    Drugs involved in both inhibition
      and acceleration
  Excretion
    Weak acid interactions
    Weak base interactions
  Clinically desirable interactions
  Nursing management
    Nursing implications
    Nursing process

Every physiologically active drug has the potential to cause an undesirable reaction that may induce illness in the recipient. Such a condition is called *iatrogenic* (arising from the treatment). Adverse reactions are of many types and include toxic reactions, side effects, allergic reactions, idiosyncratic reactions, chain reactions, cumulative reactions, tolerance and dependence, and detrimental drug interactions.

For identification of common reactions to a specific drug, it is often necessary for the drug to have been in therapeutic use for 10–20 years. Even then, some problems may not be recognized as being drug-related. For example, aspirin was widely used for decades before its detrimental effects were acknowledged.

When an interactant chemical modifies the therapeutic results that have been anticipated with a drug, a drug interaction has occurred. This interactant may be another drug or some combination of drugs, natural or artificial chemical components of the diet, pollutant chemicals from the environment, endogenous body chemicals, or chemicals used for diagnostic laboratory tests (Box 9-1).

Chances of a drug interaction increase with the number of drugs the patient is taking, or when the client consults more than one physician and a variety of medications are prescribed. In one study, the pharmacy profiles of 1,825 surgical patients were reviewed (21,888 patient days and 15,527 medication exposures). At least one potential drug interaction was found in 17% (310) of the patients. Interactions occurred at the rate of one for every 59 patient days. Digoxin and cimetidine were the potential interacting drugs in about 90% of the cases (Durrence et al, 1985, pp 1553–1554).

Drug interactions are varied (Fig. 9-1). They may be beneficial or detrimental and may vary from person to person. They may be of major clinical significance or of no clinical significance at all. They may affect absorption, distribution, biotransformation (metabolism), or excretion of drugs.

Long lists of reported drug interactions have been generated in recent years. However, many are based on insufficient data, observation of a limited number of patients, or animal data alone. The best way to be prepared is to understand the basic mechanisms of drug interactions.

Both detrimental and beneficial drug interactions are discussed in this chapter. However, interactions that might be called pharmaceutical interactions (*ie*, those that occur with two drugs in an infusion solution) are not discussed in this chapter.

Box 9-1. Chemical interactants

- Another drug
- A combination of drugs
- Nature chemical components of the diet
- Artificial chemical components of the diet
- Pollutant chemicals from the environment
- Endogenous body chemicals
- Chemicals used for diagnostic laboratory tests

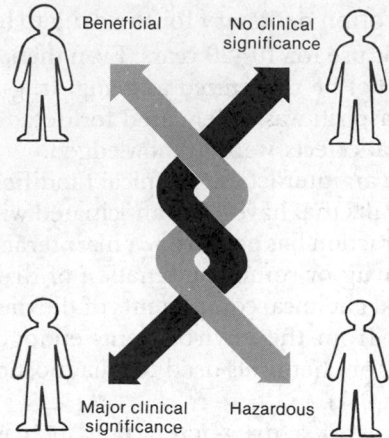

Beneficial No clinical significance

Major clinical significance Hazardous

Figure 9-1. Drug interactions may vary.

Adverse reactions to drugs

Adverse reactions to drugs take varying lengths of time to develop. Some become apparent immediately, while others may require weeks or months to appear. Their severity may range from mild to catastrophic. Any body tissue or organ can be affected. The variety manifested is suggested by the examples in Table 9-1. Table 9-2 details the signs and symptoms of some adverse drug reactions.

Clients receiving relatively new drugs are particularly vulnerable to unexpected complications. The newer the drug, the greater the risk of unknown danger. However, adverse reactions to drugs that have been well tolerated for extended periods of time can occur, owing to changes in the ability of the client to metabolize or excrete the drug or because of intercurrent illness. Slow accumulation of some drugs produces delayed toxicity. Intermittent use of a medication fosters the development of allergic hypersensitivity. For these reasons, adverse reactions may occur at any time during a course of treatment.

Toxic reactions

Although all of the reactions identified as adverse reactions could be termed toxic in the general sense of the word (*ie*, exerting deleterious effects), toxic states are defined more narrowly here. They refer to those effects characteristic of high doses of the drug. These effects may occur due to excessive dosage of the drug or from hyperresponsiveness to the drug.

The likelihood of toxicity is inversely related to the safety margin of a substance (*eg*, it is rarely seen with drugs such as water-soluble vitamins, which must be administered in huge doses to precipitate harmful effects). When drugs with a narrow safety margin, such as digitalis or insulin, are used the therapy must be closely monitored and carefully managed to avoid toxicity. Some drugs have no safety margin and are dangerous in therapeutic doses. No useful drug is completely devoid of toxic potential. If a substance is effective, it either changes physiologic function or exerts an external influence on body function. If this change reaches sufficient magnitude, harm can result.

Side effects

Side effects are those actions of a drug that are not specifically desired in a treatment situation. No drugs exert a single effect on the body; rather, a spectrum of multiple effects occurs. A substance administered in one instance for a particular purpose may be used in another for a different effect. Which of the actions are termed therapeutic and which are deemed side effects depends on the situation. Side effects are not all undesirable; many drugs are chosen for prescription to exploit their desirable side effects. For example, diazepam (Valium) is both a tranquilizer and a skeletal muscle relaxant. When administered to reduce anxiety, its relaxant properties are considered side effects. When used to treat low-back pain, tranquilization is considered a side effect. In the latter instance, the side effect is usually considered helpful because the client often has difficulty adjusting to the immobility and pain associated with the disorder.

Among common undesirable side effects from drugs are nausea, vomiting, skin rashes, electrolyte imbalance, and changes in the level of consciousness or emotional affect. Side effects can be mild or they can be severe and life-threatening. The less serious ones are often undiagnosed and in long-term drug therapy may persist as troublesome and distressing conditions that are refractory to treatment.

Allergic reactions

Allergic reactions to drugs are the result of the body's immunologic response to a drug following previous exposure to that same drug. Allergic reactions do not occur during the first exposure to a drug. This does not mean that the patient with an allergic reaction to a penicillin, for example, will be able to document having received penicillin at an earlier time. Persons may be exposed unknowingly to penicillins through food since these drugs are often used in the treatment of the animals that are the sources of milk or meat.

Allergic reactions to drugs account for up to 10% of all drug reactions. An allergic reaction may be triggered by the drug in its unchanged form, by a drug metabolite, or by supposedly inert ingredients used in drug manufacture. Injected penicillins have been primary offenders in allergic reactions to drugs.

Allergic reactions may be evidenced by a variety of symptoms. A common reaction is urticaria (hives), the appearance of intensely pruritic wheals or welts on the skin. The wheals are irregularly shaped, circumscribed elevations that are white in the center with a pale red periphery, and vary in size.

Allergic reactions involving the cardiovascular and

Table 9-1. Drug-induced health problems

Condition	Examples of drugs involved
Acid/base imbalance	aspirin (toxic doses), antacids, diuretics
Electrolyte imbalance*	
Hypernatremia	hypertonic saline infusions, sodium citrate, sodium penicillin (large doses), sodium phosphate, oral electrolyte solutions, sodium bicarbonate, cholestyramine, lithium, demeclocycline, methylflurane, amphotericin B, propoxyphene, isophosphamide, povidone/iodine, lactulose, estrogens, glycyrrhizic acid (in licorice)
Hyponatremia	laxatives, hypertonic phosphate enemas, adrenocorticotropin, amphotericin B, polymyxin B, thiazide diuretics, ethacrynic acid, furosemide, lithium, mannitol, vincristine, cyclophosphamide, clorpropamide, tolbutamide, ibuprofen, clomipramine, amitriptyline, thioridazine, thiothixine, tranylcypromine, carbamazepine, chlorthalidone, cyclothiazide, clonidine, nicotine, morphine, barbiturates, oxytocin, thiazides, amiloride, captopril
Hyperkalemia	Intravenous solutions containing potassium, potassium chloride (as medication or salt substitute), oral rehydration solutions, potassium penicillin (IV), triamterene, amiloride, spironolactone, indomethacin, captopril, heparin, barbiturates, heroin, phencyclidine, amphetamines, succinylcholine, digoxin (toxic doses), arginine, amiloride
Hypokalemia	Laxatives, hypertonic enemas, amphotericin B, polymyxin B, outdated tetracyclines, gentamicin/cephalexin, prostaglandin F_2, neomycin, corticosteroids (oral, intravenous, nasal spray), glycyrrhizic acid (licorice), carbenoxolone, gentamicin, L-dopa, thiazide diuretics, furosemide, ethacrynic acid, penicillin, ampicillin, carbenicillin, nafcillin, ticarcillin, barium, salbutamol, terbutaline, lithium
Hypercalcemia	Intravenous lipid emulsion, large doses of vitamin D and calcium, vitamin D alone, vitamin A, furosemide, thiazides, chlorthalidone, lithium, tamoxifen, estrogens, large doses of antacids accompanied by large intake of milk
Hypocalcemia	heparin, phosphate (oral, rectal or intravenous), magnesium sulfate, colchicine, propylthiouracil, furosemide, calcitonin, mithramycin, glutethamide, aspirin, estrogens (in individuals with breast cancer), neomycin, streptozocin
Hypermagnesemia	Magnesium-containing laxatives or enemas, magnesium sulfate, magnesium-containing antacids, magnesium citrate, lithium
Hypomagnesemia	gentamicin, tobramycin, capreomycin, neomycin, carbenicillin, cisplatin, amphotericin B, polymyxin B, digitalis, diuretics, laxatives, and purgatives
Hyperphosphatemia	intravenous phosphate, phosphate-containing laxatives and enemas
Hypophosphatemia	Aluminum-containing antacids, thiazide diuretics, androgens, corticosteroids, glucagon, epinephrine, gastrin, mannitol, hyperalimentation solutions
Delayed healing	corticosteroids, antineoplastics
Skin disorders	
Dermatoses (rashes)	penicillin, streptomycin, sulfonamides, chlorpromazine, bromides, thiazide diuretics
Acne	Corticosteroids, androgenic hormones
Photosensitivity	hydroxyzine, tetracycline, griseofulvin
Pseudoporphyria (blistering)	naproxin
Urticaria (hives)	Sulfonamides, procaine, procaine penicillin
Arthralgia	amphotericin B, carbamazepine
Serum sickness	Sulfonamides, penicillin, streptomycin, thiouracil derivatives
Increased risk of infection	Immunosuppressants (cyclosporin, corticosteroids), antineoplastics
Superinfection	Broad-spectrum and anti-infectives
Lupus-like reaction	vancomycin
Anaphylaxis	Penicillins, cephalosporins, aminoglycosides, tetracyclines, nitrofurantoin, amphotericin B, sulfonamides, iodides and iodinated radiopaque dyes, bromsulphthalein, dehydrochloric acid, blood and blood products, sera, bupivacaine, lidocaine, procaine, tetracaine, allergenic extracts, insect venoms, adriamycin, bleomycin, cisplatin, cyclophosphamide, asparaginase, mephalen, tolmetin, zomespin, histamine, adrenocorticotropin, aspirin, codeine, morphine, dextran, thiazides, hydralazine, meprobamate, succinylcholine, tubocurarine

(Continued)

Table 9-1. Drug-induced health problems (Continued)

Condition	Examples of drugs involved
Myelosuppression (leukopenia, thrombocytopenia, anemia, pancytopenia)	allopurinol, amoxapine, aminopyrine, phenylbutazone, choramphenicol, antineoplastics, thiazides, sulindac, ranitidine, ethosuximide
Malignant neoplasms	Alkylating antineoplastics, radioactive drugs (therapeutic doses), psoralen (administered with ultraviolet light in PUVA treatment), tar (topical), arsenic
Central nervous system changes	
Headache	ranitidine, thyroid hormone, corticosteroids, oral contraceptives, tetracycline, vitamin A (overdose)
Change in mood	Narcotics, sedatives, tranquilizers, CNS stimulants, corticosteroids, thyroid hormone, ibuprofen
Confusion	cimetidine, ranitidine (also seen often in the elderly receiving multiple drugs)
Insomnia	Nonsteriodal anti-inflammatory drugs, caffeine, amphetamines, cocaine, corticosteroids, decongestants
Aseptic meningitis	ibuprofen
Oversedation	Narcotic analgesics, antihistamines
Hyperkinesis	Decongestants, vasopressors
Symptoms of psychosis	Corticosteroids, thyroid hormone, amphetamines, LSD, alcohol, phenylbutazone, acetaminophen
Nystagmus	phenytoin
Dystonia	Antiemetics, phenothiazines, amoxipine, trazodone
Guillain-Barré syndrome	Viral vaccines such as flu vaccine
Seizures	amoxapine, meperidine
Intellectual impairment	Antineoplastic drugs (CNS prophylaxis in childhood leukemia)
Neuroleptic malignant syndrome	metaclopramide, antipsychotic drugs
Tinnitus/hearing loss	Aminoglycosides, aspirin, naprosyn, fenoprofen, ibuprofen, quinine, chloramphenicol, erythromycin, ethacrynic acid, furosemide
Change in smell	chlorpheniramine
Change in taste	ampicillin, tetracycline, griseofulvin, carbamazepine
Visual loss	oxygen (in newborns), corticosteroids
Conjunctivitis	potassium iodide
Irritated eyelids	Iodides, halides
Black deposits in the conjunctiva	Tetracyclines, epinephrine eye drops
Peripheral neuropathy	cisplatin, alcohol (prolonged use)
Carpal tunnel syndrome	trancypromine, danazol
Cardiovascular changes	
Hypertension	cisplatin, glycyrrhizic acid (in licorice), intravenous fluids (given to excess), vasopressors (epinephrine, norepinephrine)
Congestive heart failure	Beta blockers, piroxicam, intravenous fluids (given to excess)
Cardiac dysrhythmias	epinephrine, drugs affecting potassium levels such as thiazides, antiarrhythmic drugs such as quinidine
Raynaud's phenomenon (vasospasm and pain on exposure to cold)	imipramine, vinblastine, bleomycin, nicotine
Gangrene of an extremity	propranolol, ergotamine
Reye's syndrome	aspirin (in children with viral infections), insecticides
Changes in the blood	
Decreased platelet aggregation	aspirin (low doses), nonsteroidal anti-inflammatories
Hemolysis	Incompatible blood, sulfonamides, methyldopa
Thrombi and thrombo-embolism	Corticosteroids, oral contraceptives
Gastrointestinal changes	
Anorexia, nausea, vomiting	Occurs in low incidences with virtually any drug; in high incidences with meperidine and antineoplastic drugs
Dental caries	Sugar-sweetened formulations
Stomatitis	Antineoplastic drugs
Irritation or bleeding	Nonsteroidal anti-inflammatory drugs including aspirin, corticosteroids, antineoplastic drugs

(Continued)

Table 9-1. Drug-induced health problems (Continued)

Condition	Examples of drugs involved
Peptic ulcers	Nonsteroidal anti-inflammatory drugs including aspirin and auranofin, Corticosteroids
Gastric rupture	sodium bicarbonate (used as an antacid)
Liver impairment	acetaminophen, alcohol, chloroform, primaxin, anabolic male hormones
Pancreatitis	alcohol (prolonged use), sulindac
Appendicitis	barium
Constipation	Narcotic analgesics, anticholinergics
Intestinal obstruction	Enteric-coated tablets
Diarrhea	Broad-spectrum antibiotics, lactulose, anticholinesterases
Starch peritonitis	Starch applied to surgical gloves before sterilization and inadequately removed before surgery.
Respiratory changes	
Bronchial asthma	Nonsteroidal anti-inflammatory drugs including aspirin, tartrazine (a yellow dye used to color many medications)
Pneumonitis	methotrexate
Kidney impairment	tolectin, aminoglycosides, nonsteroidal anti-inflammatory drugs, phenacetin, sulfonamides
Reproductive changes	
Gynecomastia	metronidazole
Impotence/anorgasmia/decreased libido	Antihypertensives, female sex hormones when administered to males
Precocious puberty	Sex hormones, Philips corona ointment (applied topically in infancy)
Gonadal atrophy/infertility	Alkylating antineoplastic drugs, procarbazine
Birth defects	alcohol, bendectine, thalidomide, carbohydrates (when they cause prolonged hyperglycemia during pregnancy), phenytoin, trimethadione, ethosuximide, carbarmazepine, valproic acid
Changes in hair	
Loss	Alkylating antineoplastic drugs, terfenadine, trimethadione
Hirsutism	phenytoin, carbamazepine
Changes in distribution	Sex hormones of the opposite sex
Hypoglycemia	insulin, oral hypoglycemics, sulfonamides
Hyperglycemia	adrenocorticotropin, somatotropin, corticosteroids
Cushing's syndrome	Corticosteroids
Dependence addiction/habituation (with withdrawal syndrome)	Narcotic analgesics, tranquilizers, barbiturates, cocaine, amphetamines, tricyclic antidepressants, antihypertensives
Organ atrophy	Corticosteroids

*Adapted from Nanji AA. (1983). Drug-induced electrolyte disorders. *Drug Intell Clin Pharm, 17,* 177.

respiratory systems are life-threatening. This type of reaction is called *anaphylactic shock.* Anaphylactic shock is a systemic reaction characterized by dyspnea and respiratory difficulty (related to bronchospasm and laryngeal edema), cough, cyanosis, angioedema, sometimes urticaria, pulse variations, hypotension, sometimes convulsions, unconsciousness, and acute cardiovascular collapse. The reaction is primarily caused by contraction of smooth muscles and increased vascular permeability.

Treatment of allergic reactions depends on their severity. One drug used to treat urticaria is the antihistamine diphenhydramine (Benadryl). Drugs used to treat anaphylactic shock include epinephrine, antihistamines, and bronchodilators.

Allergic reactions to drugs are more common in people with a history of allergies. This does not neces-sarily mean a history of allergies to drugs; it could mean a history of food allergies. Allergic tendencies are also familial, and a family history of allergies to drugs may be significant. See Chapter 35 for further discussion of allergic reactions.

Idiosyncratic reactions

Idiosyncratic reactions are defined as genetically de-termined, unexpected responses to a drug. They can be very serious. The response may take the form of extreme sensitivity to low doses or extreme insensitivity to high doses of the drug. Sometimes the reaction takes the form of a paradoxic response—an effect opposite to that desired. Identification and treatment of idiosyncra-tic reactions frequently depend on the alertness of the health care personnel caring for the client.

An example of an idiosyncratic reaction is the he-

Table 9-2. Signs and symptoms of common adverse drug reactions

Reaction	Signs and symptoms
Allergy	
Anaphylaxis	Any organ can be affected, including the central nervous system, gastrointestinal system, bone marrow, and liver, with signs and symptoms similar to those listed below for these systems.
Anaphylaxis	Itching of palms, chin, throat; a sensation of swelling in the throat; apprehension, lacrimation, wheezing, dyspnea, hypotension, and cardiovascular collapse
Arthralgia	Joint pain, difficulty in ambulation, impaired manual dexterity
Skin eruption	Erythema, itching, rash
Bone marrow suppression	
Anemia	Weakness, dyspnea, headaches, syncope, unusual tiredness or weakness
Leukopenia	Fever, chills, sore throat, dry nonproductive cough, malaise, redness or pain in a body area
Thrombocytopenia	Petechiae, ecchymoses, unusual bleeding following minor trauma or from mucous membranes, hemorrhage
Central nervous system disturbances	
Confusion	Forgetfulness, disorientation, inappropriate verbal responses, anxiety
Excitation	Restlessness, talkativeness, irritability, insomnia, anxiety
Sedation	Sleepiness, lethargy, coma
Gastrointestinal irritation or bleeding	
	Dysphagia, anorexia, stomatitis (dryness or cracking of lips, swelling and redness of mouth tissues, soreness to burning pain of mouth tissues, mouth odor), nausea, vomiting, abdominal pain, bloody or black tarry stools, diarrhea
Hepatotoxicity	
	Anorexia, malaise, fatigue, nausea, jaundice, fever, hepatic tenderness, enlargement of the liver, elevated serum glutamic oxaloacetic transaminase, elevated alkaline phosphatase, dark urine, light-colored stools
Nephrotoxicity	
	Decrease in urination (oliguria to anuria); edema; unusual weight gain; hematuria, albuminuria, or crystalluria; progressive azotemia
Ototoxicity	
	Abnormal ringing or other noises in the ear (tinnitus), increased sensitivity to noise, difficulty in understanding speech, audiograms showing loss of perception, particularly of high tones

molytic anemia seen in 10% of black males when they receive primaquine. These clients have an inherited deficiency in an enzyme called erythrocytic glucose-6-phosphate dehydrogenase. Without this enzyme, in the presence of primaquine, metabolic processes in erythrocytes are diminished, vital functions can no longer be carried out, and alterations in the cell membranes result in lysis of the cells. This sensitivity of erythrocytes to primaquine is also seen in Greeks and Iranians.

Chain reactions

Medications are often added to a regimen to control side effects of other drugs. This can initiate a chain reaction, which greatly increases the number of substances administered to the client. For example, when cortisone is required to treat a serious inflammatory condition, it can cause hypertension, ulcers, diabetes, and a reactivation of arrested tuberculosis. The client may require diuretics, antacids or histamine$_2$-receptor antagonists, insulin, or an antituberculous agent. If isoniazid is chosen as the antimycobacterial, vitamin B$_6$

may be prescribed to prevent a deficiency state, which can be induced by this drug. If the antacid Amphojel is recommended, the client may require a stool softener. Thus, the initiation of cortisone therapy can result in the prescription of six or more additional drugs (Fig. 9-2). Such proliferation of drug use causes a geometric increase in the risk of undesirable interactions.

Cumulative reactions

Drugs accumulate in the body whenever the dosage exceeds the amount the body can eliminate through metabolism or excretion. Because the efficiency of these processes is influenced by many extraneous factors, accumulation can occur unexpectedly and despite constant dosage regimens. There may be no discernible effect until drug concentrations reach toxic levels. This is most apt to happen when the therapeutic margin of safety is narrow or the medication is taken over a long time. Drugs such as digitalis, to which both conditions apply, frequently cause deleterious cumulative reactions.

In recent years, techniques for measuring serum

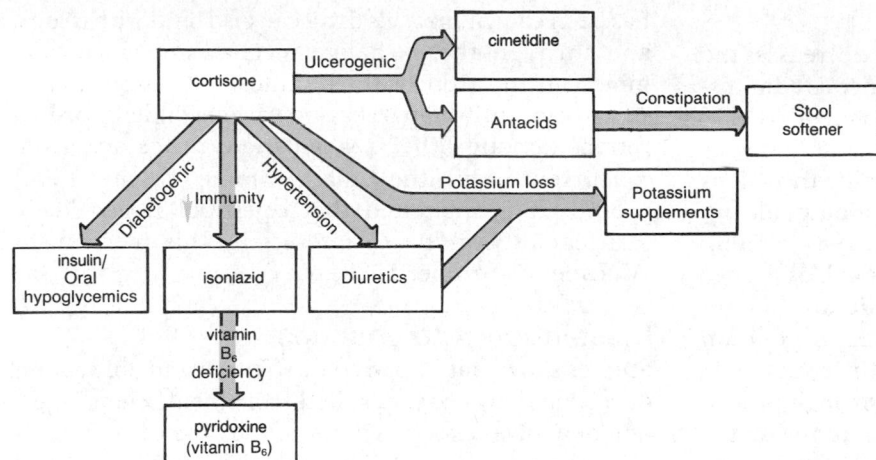

Figure 9-2. Multiple drug prescriptions stemming from the prescription of cortisone therapy.

levels of many drugs have been developed. These are very useful not only when toxicity is suspected but also in optimizing doses for therapeutic efficacy. They are expensive, however. Development of a simple, inexpensive monitoring technique would be extremely useful in maintaining long-term treatment regimens with minimal risk of cumulative reactions.

Tolerance and dependence

Habitual use of drugs may create a tolerance not only to the drug in use but also to other related drugs. This is not a pathologic condition because the client develops no signs or symptoms of illness when taking the drugs. However, as long as the tolerance persists, the client will not respond appropriately to subsequent administration of either the drug involved or related substances that exhibit cross-tolerance to it.

Habitual use of drugs can also produce physical dependence. The dependent individual will develop signs and symptoms of illness when the drug is withdrawn. Withdrawal is always uncomfortable and can be dangerous.

Many substances induce both tolerance and physical dependence. Individuals who have been given heavy doses of opioid analgesics over a prolonged time sometimes exhibit withdrawal and cross-tolerance to other central nervous system depressants. If depressants are required for treatment, large doses may be necessary to achieve the desired response. The risk of adverse reactions is thereby increased because tolerance may be greater for some drug effects than for others.

Mechanisms of drug interaction

The mechanisms usually responsible for the adverse effects associated with drug interactions are those in which one drug affects the absorption, distribution, biotransformation, or excretion of another drug (Box 9-2).

Absorption

Interactions during the absorptive phase result in an increase or decrease in either the relative rate of absorption, the total amount of drug that is absorbed, or both. A drug may be absorbed so slowly that it never reaches effective serum levels, that the rate of onset of the drug may be greatly delayed when prompt relief of acute symptoms (*eg*, pain) is needed, or that an effect of the drug may be unduly prolonged.

Learning experience 9-1

In clinical laboratory, select a client receiving multiple therapeutic drugs. *Prior to* investigating these drugs, assess the client's condition. List subjective complaints and objective signs that are problematic. Look up the drugs included in the client's medication regimen, noting adverse reactions they can cause. How many of your client's signs and symptoms could be caused by medication? Plan nursing interventions to eliminate or alleviate these problems.

Box 9-2. Mechanisms of drug interactions

1. Absorption
   a. Direct interaction of drugs
   b. Dissolution rate changes
2. Distribution
   a. Displacement through drug competition for protein-binding sites
   b. Displacement of natural body chemicals
3. Biotransformation
   a. Inhibition of metabolism
   b. Acceleration of metabolism
4. Excretion
   a. Various influences on renal excretion

Direct interaction of drugs

An example of an interaction that decreases the amount of drug absorbed is the simultaneous administration of the salts of divalent or trivalent metals (Ca^{2+}, Mg^{2+}, Al^{3+}) and tetracycline antibiotics. Simultaneous use of tetracycline and products containing those ions (*eg*, antacids and laxatives) or foods containing calcium should be avoided (D'Arcy & McElnay, 1987, p 609).

The tetracycline forms relatively insoluble chelates with metallic ions, such as calcium, magnesium, aluminum, iron (*eg*, ferrous sulfate), and zinc. Aluminum ions form the most stable complex with tetracycline.

Tetracycline is probably absorbed through passive diffusion and, apparently, the formation of the metallic complex interferes with the passage of the tetracycline molecule through the gut wall. The formation of the metallic complex is dependent on *p*H. At low *p*H, there is little complex formed; at high *p*H, the amount of complex increases.

The amount of calcium present in whole milk, buttermilk, and cottage cheese is sufficient to interfere with tetracycline absorption. Calcium phosphate cannot be used as the filler in tetracycline capsules because it interferes with tetracycline absorption.

The size of the available surface area in an empty stomach, as opposed to one filled with food, will also influence the dissolution and absorption processes of drugs. (See Chapter 10 for more information on food and drug interactions). The absorption of several other drugs is reduced by simultaneous administration of antacids. Besides the tetracycline antibiotics, drugs also affected include isoniazid, phenytoin, digoxin, chloroquine, cimetidine, quinidine, and nonsteroidal anti-inflammatory drugs. Increased gastric *p*H due to antacids has been shown to increase the absorption rate of enteric-coated aspirin and the sulphonamides. It is likely that there would be increased absorption of some enteric-coated drugs when they are administered with an antacid because one form of enteric coatings is designed to be insoluble at acidic *p*H and to dissolve as the *p*H is raised.

Sucralfate (Carafate) is a complex aluminum hydroxide salt of a sulphated disaccharide, which is an antiulcer agent. It probably facilitates the healing of the ulcer by binding to proteins in the ulcer base to form a chemical barrier between the ulcer and acid, pepsin, and bile. It has been reported to reduce phenytoin absorption by 20% (McInnes & Brodie, 1988, p 87).

A final example of an action that can affect absorption involves cholestyramine (Questran). This is an antilipemic that is not absorbed from the gastrointestinal tract. Cholestyramine is used to lower plasma low density lipoproteins and cholesterol in patients with type II hyperlipoproteinemia. It exchanges chloride ions for bile acids, which it binds into an insoluble complex that is subsequently excreted in the feces. It has been shown that this drug can also bind with drugs, and through the exchange mechanism, cholestyramine can interfere with the intestinal absorption of thyroxine, anticoagulants, and various digitalis preparations (among others) when these drugs are given concurrently with the cholestyramine (Levine, 1990, p 309). It is suggested that colestipol is less likely than cholestyramine to interact by this mechanism (McInnes & Brodie, 1988, p 87).

Dissolution rate changes

Studies show that impaired dissolution and absorption of certain drugs have resulted from insufficient ingestion of a solvent such as water at the time the drug was administered. Antibiotics, namely amoxicillin and penicillin, have demonstrated significantly low levels in serum when they were administered with small quantities (1–1½ ounces) of water. These findings support the need for an adequate intake of fluid (8 ounces for adults) to promote the disintegration and absorption processes of the drug's active ingredients.

The release of active ingredients is affected by the type of preparation. The commonly advertised chewable tablets must be chewed adequately because chewable tablets may not contain certain disintegration agents to maximize the dissolution process. Swallowing the tablet whole may interfere with the absorption process.

The dissolution rate of a drug will change when a drug is adsorbed onto the surface of a solid. Thus, administration of a kaolin-pectin suspension (*eg*, Kaopectate, an adsorbent antidiarrheal) and clindamycin will reduce the absorption rate of the clindamycin. However, the clindamycin is apparently well enough absorbed that all of the clindamycin will eventually be physiologically available. That is, the total amount of clindamycin absorbed is not decreased. However, administration of kaolin-pectin suspension will inhibit both the amount and the rate of digoxin and tetracycline absorption.

Drugs that affect gastrointestinal motility may have effects on absorption by changing residence time of the drug at the site of dissolution. Foods or drugs may hasten or delay gastric emptying and may hasten or delay the absorption of another drug. Metoclopramide (Reglan) stimulates gastric emptying and has been shown to increase the absorption rates of acetaminophen, levodopa, and lithium.

However, metoclopramide has been shown to reduce serum digoxin concentration when it is coadministered with slowly dissolving digoxin tablets. Absorption may be decreased. It is felt that this interaction can probably be minimized by the use of rapidly dissolving digoxin preparations such as Lanoxin tablets or Lanoxicaps.

Propantheline has anticholinergic activity and reduces gastrointestinal motility and stomach-emptying rate. With the administration of propantheline, there was increased absorption of digoxin with one form of digoxin but no effect was noted with two other forms of digoxin (Welling, 1984). Codeine, morphine sulfate, atropine, and chloroquine are known to delay gastric emptying and to depress the rate of absorption of other drugs (Levine, 1990, p 312).

Poorly soluble drugs pass into the intestine where they may slowly dissolve over a period of hours (*eg*, griseofulvin dissolves over 20–30 hours). The serum levels of orally administered griseofulvin may be lowered to clinically ineffective levels by the concurrent administration of phenobarbital. One suggested explanation is that phenobarbital may decrease the transit time in that section of the intestine from which griseofulvin is maximally absorbed by stimulating bile secretion, which, in turn, stimulates peristalsis (McInnes & Brodie, 1988, p 87).

Avoiding interactions during absorption

Most authorities agree that most drug interactions during the absorptive phase can be avoided or significantly reduced by not giving the drugs simultaneously. The doses of the two interactant drugs can be separated by 3 or 4 hours (D'Arcy & McElnay, 1987, p 610).

Distribution

Many drugs are transported to their sites of metabolism bound to plasma proteins, primarily albumin. Drugs may be bound to binding sites in the tissues, as well as being bound within the plasma. Drugs are in equilibrium with their binding sites. If free drug is removed (*eg*, by glomerular filtration), then bound drug will dissociate from its binding sites. It is generally accepted that the bound fraction is devoid of pharmacologic activity and the therapeutically important concentration is that of the free, unbound drug.

Displacement

Drug competition for protein-binding sites

Bound drug concentration depends on the amount of binding materials present in both plasma and tissues and the affinity of the drug for the binding sites on these materials.

In the past, it was recognized that drugs could be displaced from their binding sites by other drugs, and this phenomenon was considered to be a very important reason for drug-drug interactions. It is now felt that the importance of *in vivo* protein-binding displacement interactions has been exaggerated.

Certain drugs do indeed compete with other drugs for drug-binding sites on albumin and can displace albumin-bound drugs. However, the body's clearance rate for drugs is proportional to the fraction of drug unbound in the plasma. After displacement, the drug's rate of clearance is increased. In most cases, the compensatory increase in clearance reduces the transient increase in free drug concentration to proportions that are not of clinical importance.

Secondary mechanisms

Because free drug concentration often remains unchanged after protein-binding displacement, there should be no major drug interactions where displacement alone is responsible. To date, interactions considered to be due to displacement probably are due to a second interaction mechanism.

Phenylbutazone will cause an increased anticoagulant response when given concurrently with warfarin. Normally 98% of warfarin is bound. Therefore, if binding is reduced to 96%, the pharmacologically active concentration of warfarin goes from 2% to 4% (*ie*, is doubled), and hemorrhagic crises have occurred. This effect occurs within hours or days of starting the drug combination and is reversed if the second drug is withdrawn. Whereas this interaction was felt to be due to displacement at first, now it is felt that a more plausible mechanism is the inhibited metabolism of warfarin isomers that is induced by phenylbutazone (McInnes & Brodie, 1988, pp 91–92). Inhibition of metabolism increases circulating anticoagulant levels.

Sodium valproate will cause a rise in free phenytoin concentration when the two are given concurrently and signs of intoxication may occur. When sodium valproate is introduced in a patient with epilepsy who is already established on phenytoin, serum phenytoin concentrations usually decrease but free drug levels may increase by up to 50%–100%. The rise in free phenytoin concentration is partly due to displacement of phenytoin from tissue binding sites but inhibition of phenytoin metabolism is the more important mechanism (McInnes & Brodie, 1988, p 95).

Another example of an interaction caused by displacement and a second mechanism is the interaction between methotrexate and aspirin. Methotrexate is displaced by aspirin. A second mechanism operates simultaneously. Methotrexate and aspirin (or its metabolites) are excreted primarily by the kidney. Aspirin competes with and inhibits the renal secretion of methotrexate, resulting in an increase in the serum methotrexate level. These interactions can lead to evidence of hematopoietic toxicity to methotrexate because there is a narrow margin between the therapeutic and toxic effects of methotrexate (McInnes & Brodie, 1988, p 96).

Tissue-binding displacement has more potential for adverse effects than does plasma protein-binding displacement. However, to date, laboratory methods have not been available to study this mechanism thoroughly.

Displacement of natural body chemicals

Another type of displacement can occur. Many natural body chemicals (such as thyroxine, norepinephrine, and bilirubin) are stored in various depots in the body.

Many drugs displace these endogenous chemicals from their storage sites. The effects of ephedrine, amphetamines, and reserpine are attributed, in part, to their ability to displace norepinephrine from its storage areas (Craig, 1990, p 843).

Biotransformation

Inhibition of metabolism

Many drugs must be metabolized, usually by the liver, before they are excreted from the body, usually through the kidneys. The hepatic mono-oxygenase enzyme system is involved in the biotransformation of a great many lipid-soluble therapeutic agents. The drug circulates through the liver and enzymes gradually convert it to water-soluble metabolites. The metabolites may continue to be pharmacologically active or they may be inactive.

One drug may inhibit the metabolism of another drug or of a hormone, neurotransmitter, or other endogenous compounds. This means it can block or slow the metabolic breakdown of these substances, thus increasing their plasma concentration, possibly to the point of toxicity. Drugs that reduce the metabolism of others are called *inhibitors* (Box 9-3).

Inhibition usually arises from competition between one drug and an interacting drug for the active site on an enzyme. Drug metabolizing enzymes are present in multiple forms (*ie*, there are at least 15 forms of cytochrome P-450). Drugs may be metabolized by more than one form of an enzyme. Inhibition of metabolism occurs only if both drugs bind to the active site of the same form of the enzyme. Inhibition may be the purpose of drug administration, as when allopurinol (xanthine oxidase inhibitor) inhibits the oxidation of purine to uric acid, or when a cholinesterase inhibitor increases the effectiveness of acetylcholine at neuromuscular junctions.

However, metabolic inhibition may also result in unwanted effects.

Monoamine oxidase (MAO) inhibitors include isocarboxazid, pargyline, phenelzine, and tranylcypromine. In the 1960s, MAO inhibitor therapy was widely employed in patients undergoing antidepressive treatment. Current use of these inhibitors is more limited. The therapeutic effect of these inhibitors is due, in part, to their ability to inhibit the enzyme MAO, which normally metabolizes catecholamines such as norepinephrine. If the enzyme MAO is inhibited, the body will store more norepinephrine than usual at receptor sites in adrenergic neurons. A patient taking an MAO inhibitor should not take another drug that might release this norepinephrine. Indirect-acting sympathomimetics, such as amphetamines, might release the norepinephrine and cause severe headache, hypertensive crisis, cardiac dysrhythmias, or intracranial bleeding from the release of excess norepinephrine.

Some interacting sympathomimetics, such as ephedrine, phenylephrine, and phenylpropanolamine, are found in nonprescription medications, including diet pills and cold, sinus, and hay fever remedies. Some nonprescription medications that have caused cardiovascular complications when taken with MAO inhibitors include Robitussin-PE (contains phenylephrine); Vicks Formula 44D Decongestant Cough Mixture (contains pseudoephedrine); CoTylenol (contains pseudoephedrine); and Alka-Seltzer Plus Cold Medicine (contains phenylpropanolamine).

Tyramine is a substance that is ordinarily harmless because it is rapidly oxidized by MAO but it may cause toxic reactions in patients who receive MAO inhibitors. Tyramine is found in many foods. Earlier lists of forbidden foods are now felt to have been unnecessarily restrictive. Red wine (like Chianti), fava beans, and broad bean pods are still strictly prohibited. Any food that is aged, fermented, overripe, spoiled, or simply old should be avoided. Cheeses like Camembert, cheddar, Stilton, and Roquefort are still usually mentioned as to be avoided. Foods now considered safe, if eaten in moderation, include very fresh cheeses, sour cream, yogurt, cream cheese, cottage cheese, ricotta cheese, pickled herring, sausage, and chopped liver. Likewise, alcoholic beverages other than red wine are apparently safe in moderate amounts. When the tyramine is not oxidized, it is freely absorbed and able to reach the adrenergic nerve endings through the circulating blood. Here there is an accumulation of norepinephrine due to the preceding effect of the MAO inhibitor. Tyramine causes the release of this surplus norepinephrine, resulting in the cardiovascular complications mentioned earlier. Fatal cerebral hemorrhages have occurred (Levine, 1990, p 281).

More commonly prescribed enzyme inhibitors include erythromycin, cimetidine, sodium valproate, propoxyphene, oral contraceptives, propranolol, and some tricyclic antidepressants, phenothiazines, and sulphonamides.

A significant amount of oral digoxin is normally inactivated by intestinal bacteria. Administering erythromycin to the patient on digoxin has increased

---

Box 9-3. Enzyme inhibitors

- erythromycin
- cimetidine
- sodium valproate
- propoxyphene
- oral contraceptives
- propranolol
- certain tricyclic antidepressants, phenothiazines, sulphonamides

serum concentration of active digoxin by up to 100%. Apparently, the erythromycin reduces the population of bacteria that inactivate the digoxin. With the rise in serum levels of digoxin, there is the increased likelihood for digoxin toxicity (Raasch, 1987, p 71). Erythromycin metabolites form a stable complex with hepatic enzymes and this results in a slowed metabolic rate of warfarin, theophylline, and carbamazepine with possible toxic symptoms from them (Raasch, 1987, p 70).

Cimetidine (Tagamet), an H_2-receptor antagonist, is a potent inhibitor of hepatic enzyme activity. The results are delayed clearance and increased effects of diazepam, chlordiazepoxide, carbamazepine, theophylline, chlormethiazole, labetalol, warfarin, phenytoin, and propranolol. With warfarin, phenytoin, and carbamazepine, serious unwanted effects are likely (McInnes & Brodie, 1988, p 91). Another H_2-receptor antagonist, ranitidine, has a lesser inhibitory effect which is unlikely to have clinical relevance. Certain drugs are metabolized through glucuronide conjugation and this process is not altered by cimetidine. Therefore, cimetidine is unlikely to affect lorazepam (Ativan), oxazepam (Serax), and temazepam (Restoril).

Acceleration of metabolism

The amount of hepatic drug-metabolizing enzymes may be increased by compounds that stimulate their synthesis. Several hundred compounds have been identified as being able to induce the synthesis of these enzymes (Box 9-4).

These compounds are known as *inducers*. The most powerful inducers include rifampicin, phenytoin, carbamazepine, primidone, griseofulvin, and cigarette smoke. The compound that is the inducer may cause a drug administered concurrently to be metabolized and excreted faster than normal, thus reducing its effects.

Smoking appears to quicken the metabolism of several drugs by stimulating hepatic drug-metabolizing enzymes. Studies suggest the polycyclic hydrocarbons in the cigarette smoke increase the activity of the enzymes. This action can lower blood levels and reduce therapeutic effects of the drug involved. The enzyme-inducing effect appears to be very long-lasting, persisting for up to 3 months after the individual has ceased smoking. There also appears to be a relationship between the number of cigarettes smoked per day and the significance of the smoking-drug interactions. Heavy smokers (20 or more cigarettes per day) tend to manifest interactions with drugs more often than those smoking fewer cigarettes. Reports show lowered blood levels of phenacetin, theophylline, imipramine, antipyrine, and pentazocine in smokers. Reports also show reduced pharmacological effect in smokers of pentazocine, chlorpromazine, diazepam, chlordiazepoxide, and propoxyphene (Craig & Stitzel, 1990, p 53).

Phenytoin and other enzyme-inducing anticonvulsants enhance the metabolic elimination of hydrocortisone, dexamethasone, prednisolone, and methylprednisolone. Adding such a drug to the regimen of a steroid-dependent asthmatic has significantly worsened the asthma (McInnes & Brodie, 1988, p 89).

Long-term treatment with enzyme-inducing anticonvulsants of women on oral contraceptives increases the incidence of cycle disturbances and of contraceptive failure. Furthermore, conventional doses of estrogens may be ineffective in relieving postmenopausal symptoms in patients taking anticonvulsants. The mechanism appears to involve a substantial increase in the clearance of ethinyl estradiol without much change in the clearance of the progestagen (McInnes & Brodie, 1988, p 89).

In opiate-dependent patients treated with methadone, introduction of rifampicin for tuberculosis treatment has resulted in symptoms of withdrawal. Rifampicin decreases plasma concentrations of methadone and increases the urinary excretion of its major pyrrolidine metabolite (McInnes & Brodie, 1988, p. 89).

Drugs involved in both inhibition and acceleration

Some drugs are commonly involved in interactions due to both inhibition and acceleration.

Drugs which inhibit warfarin metabolism include disulfiram, metronidazole, allopurinol, tricyclic antidepressants, clofibrate, phenylbutazone, chloramphenicol, propoxyphene, and some sulphonamide preparations, such as co-trimoxazole (trimethoprim plus sulphamethoxazole). Inhibition of metabolism increases circulating anticoagulant levels and hemorrhage may occur.

Because of the concept of enzyme induction, administering barbiturates, rifampicin, dichloralphenazone, or carbamazepine to the patient on warfarin will cause an increased metabolism of warfarin. Therefore, higher doses of warfarin are required for suitable anticoagulant activity. A hemorrhagic crisis can then occur if the maintenance dose of the anticoagulant is not

---

Box 9-4. Enzyme inducers

- rifampin
- phenytoin
- carbamazepine
- primidone
- griseofulvin
- cigarette smoke

lowered when the interactant agent is withdrawn from the therapeutic regimen.

Other drugs commonly involved in both inhibition and acceleration reactions include theophylline, sulphonylureas, cyclosporin, ethanol and sulfinpyrazone (Table 9-3).

Excretion

Most drugs and drug metabolites are excreted through active and passive mechanisms by the kidney. The hepatobiliary route of excretion is important for some drugs, including ampicillin, digitoxin, and glutethimide. Drugs are also excreted to a lesser and more variable extent by the lungs, through the skin, and in saliva, breast milk, and sweat.

Excretion by the kidney occurs at a rate proportional to the amount of drug present in the body, by passive glomerular filtration of the fraction of the drug not bound to plasma proteins, or by active tubular secretion, using one carrier mechanism for weak acids and another carrier mechanism for weak bases. The main location of the secretion of drugs is the proximal convoluted tubule.

Any change in the pH of the urine will influence the excretion process. Changes in the urinary flow rate will affect both the process of reabsorption and the pH and, thus, influence the excretion of drugs through the kidney. Although there are hundreds of possible drug interactions during excretion, only a few of them have been found to be clinically significant. The drug interactions that seem to be the most important during the excretory phase involve certain diuretics, probenecid, and quinidine.

Changes in urinary pH could be induced by sodium bicarbonate (alkalizer), ammonium chloride (acidifier), long-term, high-dose antacid therapy, acetazolamide (alkalizer), and thiazide diuretics.

Most drugs are weak organic acids or bases. It is usually the ionized portion of the drug molecule that is water soluble and can thus be excreted by the kidney. If the urine has a pH at which the drug is primarily present in the ionized form, the possibility of passive reabsorption is reduced. If it has a pH at which the drug is not ionized, the possibility of passive reabsorption is enhanced. Weak acids are excreted more rapidly in alkaline urine; weak bases are excreted more rapidly in acid urine. In an alkaline urine, weak bases will be more nonionized and less water soluble, while acidic drugs will be more ionized and thus more prone to excretion. Alkalinization of urine increases the rate of excretion of acidic drugs (*eg*, acetazolamide, phenobarbital, salicylates, sulfonamides). Likewise, acidification of urine increases urinary excretion of basic drugs (*eg*, amphetamines, quinidine, tricyclic antidepressants).

By contrast, acidification of urine may decrease urinary excretion of acidic drugs, and alkalinization of urine may decrease urinary excretion of basic drugs.

Weak acid interactions

Interference in the urinary excretion of drugs is important if the fraction of the drug excreted unchanged is large. Furosemide is a weak acid, and 90% of the absorbed fraction is eliminated by the kidney in unchanged form. Both indomethacin and aspirin weaken the diuresis obtained with furosemide if they are used with furosemide. The mechanism for the indomethacin-furosemide interaction is not fully established. Observations to date indicate the furosemide-aspirin interaction relates to competition for the same carrier mechanism in the tubular cell.

Long-term thiazide therapy reduces renal lithium clearance. Lithium and diuretics have been indicated for use together with lithium-induced nephrogenic diabetes insipidus or with the combination of endogenous depression and heart failure. Therefore, lithium concentration should be carefully monitored if these drugs are combined, and the lithium dose will probably need to be reduced.

Probenecid is a benzoic acid derivative. Its urico-

Table 9-3. Examples of drug interactions related to biotransformation

Inhibition of metabolism

Inhibitor	Metabolism inhibited
MAO inhibitors	amphetamines, ephedrine, phenylephrine, phenylpropanolamine, tyramine
erythromycin	digoxin, warfarin, theophylline, carbamazepine
cimetidine	diazepam, chlordiazepoxide, carbamazepine, theophylline, chlormethiazole, labetalol, warfarin, phenytoin, propranolol

Acceleration of metabolism

Inducer	Metabolism accelerated
smoking	phenacetin, theophylline, imipramine, antipyrine, pentazocine, chlorpromazine, diazepam, chlordiazepoxide, propoxyphene
phenytoin	hydrocortisone, dexamethasone, prednisolone, methylprednisolone
rifampicin	methadone

suric action is related to its ability to block the carrier-mediated transport of many weak organic acids from and into the tubular lumen. It promotes the excretion of uric acid by blocking its reabsorption through the tubular epithelium. It blocks the tubular excretion of many acid drugs but few of the interactions are of clinical concern, either because the interacting drug has a wide margin of safety or because there are no clinical indications to combine the drugs. However, probenecid should not be combined with salicylates because they antagonize the uricosuric effect of probenecid. Probenecid actively competes with the penicillins for the renal transport process and diminishes their secretion. The result of concurrent administration of penicillin and probenecid is higher and more sustained serum antibiotic levels. This principle has been applied deliberately by combining ampicillin, amoxicillin, or procaine penicillin G with probenecid in the treatment of gonorrhea and other severe infections (Craig, 1990, p 664).

Aspirin has been shown to compete with methotrexate for tubular excretion (as discussed under displacement), resulting in increased methotrexate concentrations and adverse effects.

Weak base interactions

Quinidine raises serum digoxin levels in about 90% of patients using the combination of digoxin and quinidine. The extent of the rise in serum digoxin is related to the dose of quinidine. Two different mechanisms seem to be involved in this interaction. Quinidine apparently displaces digoxin from peripheral tissue-binding sites in striated muscle without affecting binding to cardiac receptors, and competes with digoxin for carrier-mediated excretion mechanisms in the proximal tubule. By these mechanisms, digoxin levels may be elevated to twice the normal level, which may bring it into the toxic serum range. The patient may manifest toxicity with cardiac arrhythmias and the other usual symptoms of digitalis toxicity (McInnes & Brodie, 1988, p 95).

Clinically desirable interactions

In discussing mechanisms of drug interactions, the emphasis has been on problems created by drug combinations during the processes of absorption, distribution, biotransformation, and excretion (Table 9-4). However, drugs are also used concurrently to enhance their clinical effect. "A desirable drug interaction is defined as either a beneficial drug effect that is enhanced or a detrimental drug effect that is mitigated by the concomitant use of another drug" (Caranosos, Stewart, & Cluff, 1985, p 73).

When the combined effects of two drugs acting simultaneously are greater than the algebraic sum of the individual effects of these drugs, it is said the drugs are acting synergistically. The antimicrobial combination of sulfamethoxazole and trimethoprim is an example of synergism. This combination blocks two steps in the process of the bacterial synthesis of folic acid. Trimethoprim inhibits the bacterial enzyme called dihydrofolate reductase. Sulfamethoxazole blocks the synthesis of dihydrofolate by inhibiting bacterial utilization of para-aminobenzoic acid to form dihydropteroic acid (Caranosos & Stewart, 1985, pp 72–73).

The combination of trimethoprim and sulfamethoxazole is marketed as Bactrim, Septra, and others, and can be constituted with 80 mg trimethoprim and 400 mg sulfamethoxazole or 160 mg trimethoprim and 400 mg sulfamethoxazole. The combination works well with aerobic gram-negative bacteria and also some gram-positive organisms and the protozoal organism, *Pneumocystis carinii*.

The combined use of penicillin and an aminoglycoside to treat enterococcal infections is another example of a beneficial drug interaction. The intact cell wall of enterococci is impermeable to the aminoglycosides. Penicillin, as an inhibitor of cell-wall synthesis, permits the uptake of aminoglycosides. The combination of penicillin and gentamicin is being used in enterococcal endocarditis and meningitis.

A combination of carbidopa and levodopa has proven helpful in the management of Parkinson's disease. It was found that levodopa, when used alone to treat Parkinson's disease, was rapidly decarboxylated to dopamine by peripheral dopa decarboxylase. To ensure that an adequate amount of levodopa reached and crossed the blood-brain barrier, large doses had to be administered, which frequently produced undesirable adverse effects. Carbidopa is a peripheral dopa decarboxylase inhibitor. When these two drugs are given concurrently, decarboxylation of levodopa in peripheral tissues is diminished. This produces higher levodopa plasma concentrations and a prolonged half-life, which allows more levodopa to cross the blood-brain barrier. The dose of levodopa can be reduced, and, thus, adverse effects are eliminated or significantly diminished.

The combination of carbidopa and levodopa is marketed as Sinemet. Sinemet 10/100 contains 10 mg of carbidopa and 100 mg of levodopa. Sinemet 25/250 and 25/100 are also available.

The combination of aluminum hydroxide and magnesium hydroxide (as in Maalox, Gelusil, and Mylanta) is a common and useful drug interaction. Aluminum hydroxide is constipating, and magnesium hydroxide has a laxative effect. The purpose of combining the two agents is to have one cancel out the undesirable effect of the other. Magnesium hydroxide is fact-acting and aluminum hydroxide is slow-acting, so the combination also increases total buffering time.

■ Summary

Adverse reactions to drugs are of many types and include toxic reactions, side effects, allergic reactions, idiosyncratic reactions, chain reac-

Table 9-4. Examples of drug interaction

Drug	Other drug	Mechanism	Possible outcome	Nursing interventions
Tetracyclines	Antacids containing aluminum, calcium, or magnesium	Decreased absorption of tetracycline	Decreased anti-infective effect	Give antacid 3 hours after tetracycline preparation.
digoxin	quinidine	Displacement of digoxin from peripheral tissue-binding sites and reduced digoxin excretion	Digoxin toxicity	Monitor serum levels of digoxin. Observe for signs and symptoms of digoxin toxicity.
cimetidine (Tagamet)	phenytoin (Dilantin)	Cimetidine inhibits hepatic enzyme activity so that metabolism of phenytoin is inhibited	Phenytoin toxicity	Monitor serum levels of phenytoin. Observe for signs and symptoms of phenytoin toxicity.
cholestyramine	thyroxine, anti-coagulants, digitalis preparations	Decreased absorption of thyroxine and other affected drugs	Decreased effectiveness of bound drug	Give all medications 1 hour before cholestyramine or 4 hours after cholestyramine. Assess cardiac glycoside level if both drugs are used.
Penicillins	probenecid	Decreased excretion of penicillin	Higher and more sustained serum antibiotic level	No action necessary. This principle is applied deliberately to treat gonorrhea and other serious infections.

tions, cumulative reactions, and tolerance and dependence. Identification of the most common reactions to a specific drug takes 10–20 years of widespread use and study of the drug. Drug interactions may be either detrimental or beneficial and may affect absorption, distribution, biotransformation, or excretion of drugs. Drug interactions may be of major clinical significance or of no clinical significance at all. It would be impossible to memorize all potential adverse reactions and interactions of any given drug and this mandates that the nurse understand that there are potential problems related to any drug regimen. Based on this understanding, the nurse should be responsible to regularly refer to pharmacology texts and references for current information on specific drugs about adverse reactions and interactions.

Nursing management

Nursing implications

As the health care practitioner with the closest and most prolonged contact with the client, the nurse bears a heavy responsibility for protecting the client from drug reactions and interactions.

Nursing process

Assessment It is essential to include a detailed medication history as part of the nursing history. Through this assessment process, the nurse can help identify clients who are at high risk for adverse reactions and drug interactions. Many people (either by personal choice or medical necessity) are under treatment by two or more physicians at the same time. This situation can result in drug reactions or interactions because each physician is unaware of the other's medication regimen.

In taking the client's history, the nurse should elicit information about the existence and management of other temporary or permanent medical or dental problems. He or she should include information about drugs presently in use, as well as drugs taken within the preceding 2 weeks. The nurse also should inquire fully about the use of over-the-counter preparations (specifically vitamin and mineral preparations, analgesics, antihistamines, antacids, antidiarrheals, cough preparations, laxatives, and sedatives).

Allergic and other adverse reactions to medication should be explored. The usual dose required when drugs are used (as compared with the usual therapeutic range) may indicate the client's responsiveness to drugs in general. Factors influencing the risk of toxic reactions include age, body size, hepatic function, and renal function. Clients at increased risk for drug-induced problems are the very thin or very obese, the very young or very old, individuals with a history of allergy, individuals with renal or hepatic impairment, and those with a history of previous drug-related problems.

Since various components of the diet can have an influence on drug therapy (see Chapter 10), the history should cover the nature of dietary habits. The use of habitual agents (coffee, tobacco, and alcohol) should be examined.

Hospitalized clients should be closely monitored for drug effects. In addition to observing the degree of therapeutic response, the nurse should watch for side effects characteristic of specific drugs.

Observations must be recorded and reported promptly and in detail. Unusual complaints by the client should be heeded. Even if the complaint does not fit the nurse's knowledge of effects of the specific drug, there is the potential for a complaint to be an idiosyncratic reaction or an as yet unrecognized effect of the drug. Special attention must be paid to the client using multiple drugs, particularly as drugs are being added to or discontinued from the regimen. (See Table 9-2 for signs and symptoms of common adverse drug reactions.)

To be able to assess and evaluate the client for drug effects, nurses must be informed about the drugs they are administering. One major problem in controlling adverse reactions and interactions is recognizing their occurrence. Professional responsibility for updating personal knowledge about drugs cannot be overemphasized. Physicians, nurses, and pharmacists should be involved together in conferences and workshops on pharmacology; drug administration must be viewed as a shared responsibility. Resource material for drug information must be readily available for health care providers.

To prevent overdosage, the nurse must evaluate the physician's order against recommended dosage ranges, administer the medicines accurately, and support the physiologic processes whereby the client's body distributes, metabolizes, and excretes the drugs. The nurse should work with the physician to adjust the drug regimen for optimum effect. Any individual drug dose deemed harmful to the client should be withheld until the physician can be consulted.

In some settings, the nurse may find that a computerized drug-interaction screening program exists to help prevent adverse reactions and drug interactions. During a 100-day study period in one such program, over 100 potential, clinically significant reactions were identified. Of these, 49% involved antacids, 22% warfarin, 13% digoxin, and 8% other agents (Greenlaw, 1981, p 519). In a second setting, the drugs most responsible for potential interactions included aspirin, steroids, digoxin, propranolol, phenytoin, aminophylline, prochlorperazine, quinidine, and penicillin.

Analysis The nurse compares information on the client with data about the drugs prescribed to determine the risk of problems stemming from the drug regimen. Both actual (existing) problems and the degree of risk for future reactions should be considered.

Nursing diagnosis In making their diagnoses, nurses should be able to identify the client's adverse responses, their causes, and the drug or drugs to which they are related.

Planning The goals are to reduce the risk of adverse reaction and to detect and treat promptly any reactions that may develop. Measurable criteria for evaluation should be developed during the planning stage.

Intervention The nurse must be prepared to counteract harmful drug effects when they occur. For this reason, hazardous drugs are administered only in hospitals or other health care institutions where definitive treatment is readily available. When drug therapy is begun, the antidote (if any) should be at hand. Emergency drugs and equipment also must be available. The health care staff must be proficient in the treatment of such emergencies as respiratory or cardiac arrests and anaphylaxis.

Disease syndromes arising from drug therapy require treatment by the physician. Such drug-induced conditions as peptic ulcers, Cushing's syndrome, and aplastic anemia do not significantly differ from comparable states that occur naturally. If the offending drug cannot be discontinued, the condition may be somewhat resistant to treatment and require more vigorous treatment. The client will need skilled nursing care to assist in the control of symptoms until the offending drug can be withdrawn and the iatrogenic disease resolved.

Nursing management of any client must include teaching the client about any prescribed medication. The client should know why the drug is being taken, how the drug works, what its expected effects should be, and what its possible adverse effects are. The client needs to know how to take the drug correctly to avoid potential interactions; the amount and kind of solution to take with the drug (*eg*, milk, water); the proper method of ingestion (*eg*, chewable versus swallowing whole); and the amount and kind of food, if any, to take with the drug. Clients should be aware of significant signs and symptoms pertinent to the drugs they are receiving. They should be encouraged to report any unusual response so that it may be evaluated in relation to the medications prescribed. The emphasis in health teaching should be on the right of the client to be informed about his or her condition and its management.

The nurse can assist the client who experiences common drug-related problems (Table 9-5).

Anorexia, nausea, and vomiting. Drugs administered systemically often inhibit appetite or cause nausea or vomiting. The nurse should eliminate any noxious stimuli that will contribute to these symptoms. As much as possible, clients should be spared unpleasant sights, sounds, and odors. Rapid motion that tends to initiate nausea should be avoided. Food should be served in attractive surroundings and in small quantities. To increase intake, between-meal snacks may be offered. When antiemetics are prescribed, they are

Table 9-5. Nursing approaches to common problems related to drug therapy

Problem	Nursing interventions
Anorexia, nausea, vomiting	Serve attractive meals containing foods preferred by the client.
	Administer antiemetics prior to mealtime.
Postural hypotension	Maintain adequate hydration.
	Instruct client to change position slowly.
Itching	Teach client to apply pressure rather than scratch the itching areas.
	Keep affected areas cool.
	Identify and eliminate the offending drug to prevent more serious allergic reactions.
Alterations in bowel function	
Constipation	Maintain adequate hydration.
	Encourage eating of foods rich in fiber and those with laxative substances, if allowed.
	Encourage exercise, if allowed.
	Help the client establish regular patterns of elimination.
Diarrhea	Counsel client to eliminate irritating foods from the diet.
	Recommend tea and astringent berries, if allowed.
	Reduce stressors affecting the client.
Mental and emotional changes	Identify and eliminate the offending drug, if possible.
	Counsel client and family regarding the iatrogenic nature of the changes and techniques for managing functional and interpersonal problems resulting from them.

more effective if administered prophylactically before meals than if given therapeutically after nausea and vomiting have developed. The client may tolerate food brought in from home when institutional food is unappealing. If this is not possible, the nurse should ascertain what foods have been used by the client in the past when difficulty in eating has been experienced, and arrange for these foods to be served.

Postural hypotension. Many drugs used for long-term treatment cause postural hypotension by impairing the normal vasoconstriction response to changes in position as a person rises. In this condition, rapid movement causes vertigo or a feeling of faintness. The client should be instructed to rise gradually, sitting for a time before standing, to provide time for adaptation. To prevent falls, an assistant should accompany the client while ambulating. Ample fluids should be taken to maintain hydration because hypovolemia accentuates the problem.

Itching. Itching is a major symptom of allergic hypersensitivity. When hypersensitivity is suspected, the physician must be notified immediately. Usually, another drug will be substituted for the offending medication. Occasionally, there is no therapeutic alternative, and therapy must be continued. Antihistamines may be prescribed to reduce the allergic response. Several nursing actions help to ameliorate the itching. The client should be taught to press on the affected areas rather than scratch them. Pressure inhibits the transmission of sensation, whereas scratching contributes to inflammation and increases itching. Overheating (warm clothing and bed covers) stimulates itching and is to be avoided. Cold compresses applied locally reduce discomfort. Cold reduces sensation and can even produce numbness. Distraction also reduces the client's perception of itching. Caution should be exercised when attempting to use this technique. Many clients will believe their symptoms are not being taken seriously if they are aware of the attempts to distract them. They may feel it is believed that the symptom is not real, but "all in their head."

Altered bowel function. Disturbances in the function of the lower digestive tract are frequent side effects

Table 9-6. Examples of foods affecting gastrointestinal motility

Laxative foods	Foods acting as stool softeners	Antidiarrheal foods
Rhubarb	Whole-grain cereals	Tea
Prunes	Fruits and vegetables, especially when served raw	Blackberries
Pears		Elderberries
Raisins		Blueberries
Coffee		

of medication. Either constipation or diarrhea may occur. Both conditions are uncomfortable and potentially dangerous. (Examples of foods to be avoided or used in these conditions are listed in Table 9-6.) To ameliorate constipation, the nurse should encourage a greater intake of dietary fiber, full hydration, increased ambulation, and prompt defecation when the urge is felt. A stool softener may be recommended. Diarrhea is treated by medications such as Kaopectate or Lomotil; laxative foods should be avoided. Hydration must be adequate to replace fluids lost in the stools. (Nursing care in altered bowel function is discussed in detail in Chapter 31.)

Mental and emotional changes. Drugs affect central nervous system function by a number of mechanisms. Some stimulate or inhibit nerve cells. Others alter fluid and electrolyte balance or reduce cell nutrition or oxygenation. Drugs may produce euphoria, depression, loss of inhibitions, drowsiness, increased or decreased libido, confusion, and excitement. Adverse reactions can mimic neuroses, psychoses, or senility. Often such symptoms are treated by the addition of antipsychotics to the drug regimen. A more rational approach would be to search for the causes of the client's change in condition. If medication is the cause, the drug regimen should be altered.

Evaluation In addition to measuring the client's progress toward meeting the established criteria, evaluation should assess the client for further drug reactions.

Checklist of nursing actions

Before initiating a medication regimen

☐ Take a complete drug history, which should include all drugs currently and recently used, as well as a personal and family history of unusual or adverse reactions to medications.

☐ Assess the client for symptoms of adverse drug reactions.

☐ Compare the client data with data about the drugs ordered by the physician.

☐ Identify potential problems related to the drug regimen.

☐ Employ nursing measures to reduce the need for medication, to reduce the risk of adverse reaction, to detect adverse reactions promptly, and to ameliorate symptoms that may develop.

☐ When necessary, consult with the physician for a change in the medication order, or for orders for medical treatment of adverse reactions.

Throughout drug therapy

☐ Maintain ongoing assessment of client's responses to medication.

☐ Take appropriate action if a delayed adverse reaction to medication develops.

References

Caranosos GJ, Stewart RB, Cluff LE. (1985). Clinically desirable drug interactions. *Annu Rev Pharmacol Toxicol, 25,* 67–95.

Craig CR, Stitzel RE. (1990). *Modern pharmacology,* 3rd ed. Boston: Little, Brown and Co.

D'Arcy PF, McElnay JC. (1987). Drug-antacid interactions: Assessment of clinical importance. *Drug Intelligence and Clinical Pharmacy, 21,* 607–617.

Durrence CW III, DiPiro JT, May R, Nesbit RR Jr, Sisley JF, Cooper JW. (1985). Potential drug interactions in surgical patients. *Am J Hosp Pharm, 42,* 1553–1556.

Greenlaw CW. (1981). Evaluation of a computerized drug interaction screening system. *Am J Hosp Pharm, 38,* 517–521.

Hussar DA. (1986). Drug interactions—another good reason for checking and rechecking before you administer medications. *Nursing, 16(8),* 34–40.

Levine RR. (1990). *Pharmacology: Drug actions and reactions,* 4th ed. Boston: Little, Brown and Co.

McInnes GT, Brodie MJ. (1988). Drug interactions that matter: A critical reappraisal. *Drugs, 36,* 83–110.

Nanji AA. (1983). Drug-induced electrolyte disorders. *Drug Intelligence and Clinical Pharmacy, 17,* 176–181.

Raasch RH. (1987). Interactions of oral antibiotics and common chronic medications. *Geriatrics, 42(1),* 69–74.

Welling PG. (1984). Interactions affecting drug absorption. *Clin Pharmacokinet, 9(5),* 404–434.

Bibliography

Baciewicz AM, Self TH, Bekemeyer WB. (1987). Update on rifampin drug drug interactions. *Arch Intern Med, 147,* 565–568.

Carson JL, Strom BL, Soper KA, West SL, Morse ML. (1987). The association of nonsteroidal anti-inflammatory drugs with upper gastrointestinal tract bleeding. *Arch Intern Med, 147,* 85–88.

Dayton MT, Kleckner SC, Brown DK. (1987). Peptic ulcer perforation associated with steroid use. *Arch Surg, 122,* 376–380.

*Hansten PD. (1985). *Drug interactions,* 5th ed. Philadelphia: Lea and Febiger.

*Hansten PD. (1988). Drug interactions: Decision support tables. In *Applied therapeutics: Clinical use of drugs.* St. Louis: Applied Therapeutics for Clinical Pharmacist Service.

Harrison W, et al. (1989). MAOIs and hypertensive crises: The role of OTC drugs. *J Clin Psychiatry, 50,* 64–65.

Hospitalizations from adverse drug reactions. (1987). *Nurses Drug Alert, 11(2),* 15–16.

Mackowiak PA. (1987). Drug fever: Mechanisms, maxims, and misconceptions. *Am J Med Sci, 294(4),* 275–286.

*Mathewson K. (1989). Drug interactions. *Critical Care Nurse, 9(4),* 84–92.

Newton M, et al. (1987). General treatment of poisoning of household products and medications. *Journal of Emergency Nursing, 13,* 16–26.

*Recommended for further reading.

*Rizack M. (1989). *The medical letter handbook of adverse drug interactions*. New Rochelle, NY: The Medical Letter.

Scheller MS, Sears KL. (1987). Postoperative neurological dysfunction associated with preoperative administration of metoclopramide. *Anesth Analg, 66*, 274–276.

Stark BJ, Earl HS, Gross GN, Lumry WR, Goodman EL,

Sullivan TJ. (1987). Acute and chronic desensitization of penicillin-allergic patients using oral penicillin. *J Allergy Clin Immunol, 79*, 523–532.

Sullivan TJ, Bachmann KA. (1990). Method for assessing the probability of toxicity from drug interactions having a pharmacokinetic basis. *Clin Pharm, 9*, 136–139.

Thurkauf GE. (1987). Acetaminophen overdose. *Critical Care Nurse, 7*, 20–29.

*Recommended for further reading.

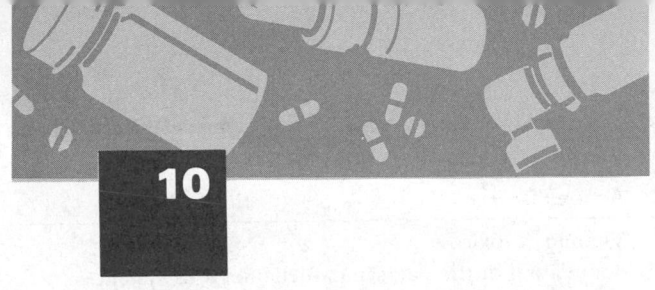

10

Interactions between food and medications

Foods* may alter the action of drugs in two ways: intrinsic pharmacologic properties of the food may antagonize or accentuate the action of the drug; or the food may change the pharmacokinetics of the drug. Conversely, medications may affect the absorption and metabolism of foods.

*When the word *food* is used throughout this chapter, it refers to both food and beverage substances.

Pharmacologic properties of food
Toxins
Natural poisons are found in both plant and animal tissues. These toxins operate as a survival factor because organisms containing them are less likely to be consumed by predators as food. However, various animals including man have developed detoxification systems that help protect them from certain toxins. Unless the substances are too concentrated, or large quantities of the food are consumed in a short time, the poisonous substance is degraded as rapidly as it is absorbed.

Historically, people have used the process of trial and error to determine which nutritive substances in the environment were safe to use as foods. Foods containing dangerous levels of active chemicals were usually classified as nonfoods or were prescribed by the imposition of a taboo. For example, Eskimos have long avoided consumption of polar bear liver, which contains toxic levels of vitamin A. Certain mushrooms are poisonous and must be carefully differentiated from nonpoisonous species that are also highly nutritious. Grains that become moldy can cause disease (see Table 10-1). In some instances, methods to detoxify foods have enabled populations to eat things known to be harmful in their natural states. As with the cassava root (from which tapioca is made), the plant is usually macerated and soaked in water, a process that dissolves and removes water-soluble toxins.

Contrary to the prevailing belief that commonly used foods have no harmful substances, many foods contain low concentrations of one or more toxins. Normally, these foods cause no adverse reactions. Only when used in excess or when eaten by people unusually sensitive to the toxic component do these foods cause difficulties. In some food sources, the concentration of chemicals is uneven with certain tissues containing toxic amounts, while the parts used for food have tolerable levels. For example, rhubarb leaves are highly toxic. Fatalities have resulted from attempts to use them as dietary greens, whereas the stalks may be stewed to make a safe piquant fruit sauce.

White potatoes, a traditional staple in the American diet, contain at least 150 potential toxins including solanin, oxalate, arsenic, tannin, and nitrate. The toxins are concentrated in the sprouts and so these parts should not be consumed. Other pharmacologic agents found in foods include goiterogens (found in many vegetables and fruits); oxalic acid (certain greens, rhubarb); astringents (tea, berries); intestinal irritants (pears, prunes); lactobacilli (yogurt, sour milk, buttermilk); phytates (cereals); avidin (egg whites); citral (orange peel); thiaminase (seafood, certain fruits and vegetables); lathyrogens (legumes); and mineral oil (low-calorie dietetic salad dressings). Although these chemicals sometimes exert beneficial effects in the body, they have the potential for causing

Table 10-1. Selected foods containing toxins

Food	Toxin	Action/effect
Polar bear liver	Vitamin A	Vitamin A toxicosis
Poisonous mushrooms	Muscarine	Stimulation of the parasympathetic nervous system
Grains (usually rye) infected with "rust" fungi	Ergot and LSD	Peripheral vasoconstriction and gangrene, central nervous system changes and hallucinations
Moldy grains and peanuts	Aflatoxins	Enteritis and liver damage, increased risk of cancer
Cassava, fruit pits and seeds	Cyanide	Asphyxiation by interference with cellular use of oxygen
Rhubarb leaves	Oxalic acid	Intestinal irritation, acidosis, renal stones

health problems, such as goiter, urinary tract stones, constipation, and specific nutritional deficiencies. Certain indigestible sugars (trioses found in beans) promote bacterial growth and fermentation in the intestine, causing excessive flatus (see Table 10-2).

Other foods that have potential for harm include:

- Refined sugar, which increases the risk of obesity, diabetes mellitus, heart disease, dental caries, and B vitamin deficiency
- Milk (Cerrato, 1987), which aggravates rheumatoid arthritis
- Cereals such as wheat, oats, rye (Cerrato, 1987), which can trigger joint problems in some arthritics
- Chocolate (Phillips, 1987), which increases acid reflux into the esophagus by relaxing the cardiac sphincter of the stomach

So many foods contain carcinogens that an official of the federal Food and Drug Administration (FDA) has stated that the threat of cancer stemming from food outweighs that of pesticides or other contaminants, naming fats, beer, bread, yogurt, mushrooms, cinnamon, and nutmeg as specific offenders (Rubin, 1990).

Certain adverse effects of foods are attributed to allergic sensitivity in the consumer. For example, the mechanism by which foods exacerbate rheumatoid arthritis are suspected to be of this nature. Although *any* body tissue can be affected by allergy, bronchial constriction (asthma) and skin rashes are the most well known reactions. Among the foods most frequently recognized as common allergens are seafood, nuts, cow's milk, acid fruits, and wheat. However, *any* food can cause an allergic reaction in *certain* individuals (Box 10-1).

Protectants

Certain foods have the reputation for exerting protectant effects against diseases. At one time, it was believed that drinking large quantities of citrus juice would protect against the common cold. Although some components of these foods (the fluid and vitamin C) are now believed to relieve symptoms of the disease, research indicates that they neither prevent the infection nor shorten its duration. Garlic has long enjoyed a reputation as being "good for the health." Its active oils are now thought to inhibit some of the processes underlying cardiovascular disease. Ironically, these active components are not retained in garlic extracts sold as "health foods." Other research indicates that milk (and other protein foods rich in tryptophan), mackerel, tuna, rainbow trout, sardines, broccoli, cabbage, and cauliflower confer specific health benefits on those who consume them regularly. Tryptophan stimulates the brain's production of serotonin and acts to reduce pain and promote sleep (see Chapter 50). The fish listed above contain eicosopentaenoic acid, which acts as an anti-inflammatory and reduces the signs and symptoms of psoriasis (Bittiner & Cartwright, 1988; Cerrato, 1987). The cruciferous vegetables (broccoli, cabbage, and cauliflower) contain as yet unidentified agents that decrease the risk of cancer (Cerrato, 1987; Fackelmann, 1990).

Foods containing lactobacilli (unpasteurized buttermilk, yogurt, cottage cheese) help replenish the normal level of intestinal lactobacilli in people taking broad spectrum antibacterial medication. A lack of such acid-producing bacilli in the gut increases susceptibility to infection by yeasts and other microorganisms that are resistant to the anti-infective agent.

In addition to chemicals recognized as drug agents, many nutritive components of foods have nutrients with pharmacologic properties. The electrolyte sodium promotes water retention and adequate blood pressure. Potassium, in conjunction with calcium, controls the force of cardiac contraction and the duration of systole and diastole. Fiber softens the stool and stimulates peristalsis. Sugars hydrate the stool by osmosis. The nature of the residues of nutrient metabolism (the "ash") affects the chemical balance of the

Box 10-1. Potential for allergic reaction to food

Any body tissue can be affected.
Any food can cause allergy in *some* person.

Table 10-2. Pharmacologic properties of common foods

Food	Active component	Action/effect
Potatoes	Solanin, oxalate, arsenic, tannin, nitrate	When consumed in normal quantities, none; in large quantities, all act as poisons
Rutabagas, turnips, cabbage, kale, rape, Chinese cabbage, Brussel sprouts, broccoli, kohlrabi, peaches, raisins, lettuce, celery, radishes, green peppers	Goitrogens	Inhibition of thyroid function
Spinach, beet tops, Swiss chard, lamb's quarters, poke, purslane, rhubarb	Oxalic acid	Decrease in intestinal absorption of calcium; laxative
Tea	Tannin	Astringent and antidiarrheal; animal and human data indicate that tannin is carcinogenic
Berries	Various astringents	Astringent and antidiarrheal
Bran	Fiber	Laxative
Pears, prunes	Sugars and intestinal irritants	Laxative (sugars pull water into the gut osmotically; irritants stimulate peristalsis)
Sour milk, yogurt	Lactobacilli	Maintainance of the natural flora of the digestive tract
Wheat, sesame seed, soybeans	Phytates	Binding of zinc, calcium, and other minerals, decreasing their absorption in the intestines
Raw egg whites	Avidin	Binding of biotin, decreasing its absorption
Orange peel	Citral	Antagonism of vitamin A
Blackberries, black currants, red beets, brussels sprouts, red cabbage, raw fish, sea food	Thiaminase	Destruction of thiamine
Legumes	Lathyrogens	Changes in collagen maturation and subsequent skeletal and skin abnormalities, (in animals) dissecting aneurysms
"Diet" salad dressings	Mineral oil	Interference with intestinal absorption of fat-soluble vitamins
Pickles, ham, bacon, saltine crackers, potato chips	Sodium	Water retention, rise in blood pressure
Soups, bananas, orange juice, apricots, animal products	Potassium	Increased relaxation of cardiac muscle during diastole; reduction of force of cardiac muscle contraction during systole
Beans	Trioses (nondigestible sugars)	Increased fermentation and gas production in the gut
Cranberries, plums, prunes, meats, cereals	Acid salts (in metabolic residue)	Decreased pH of urine
Milk, most fruits and vegetables	Alkaline salts (in metabolic residues)	Increased pH of urine
	Tryptophan	Increases brain levels of serotonin; decreases pain and promotes sleep
Beverages	Water	(In large quantities) water diuresis
Citrus fruits	Fluid, vitamin C	Reduced symptoms of the common cold
Garlic	Oils	Inhibition of coagulation, reduction of blood levels of low-density lipoproteins, increased levels of high-density lipoproteins

body. Acid ash foods tend to lower body pH and alkaline ash foods tend to raise it. Even plain water can alter body function by stimulating diuresis (see Table 10-2). In excess, the "protective" properties of food can also cause problems. For example, cranberry juice, which acidifies the urine and reduces the risk of calcium stone formation and infection in the urinary tract, increases the risk of uric acid and oxalate formation. The amount of these "protective" nutrients tolerated by different people can vary considerably. For example, individuals with renal impairment cannot tolerate a normal intake of potassium because it cannot be excreted at the usual rate and tends to accumulate to toxic levels.

■ Summary
All foods contain chemicals that affect body tissues and processes. Many contain nonnutritive chemicals that are pharmacologically active. Some of these components exert beneficial ef-

fects, whereas others cause adverse reactions. In some foods, toxins are present in such low concentrations that they produce no noticeable effects. In others, levels are so high that they must be reduced by special treatment before the food can be safely used. Substances containing high levels of toxins that cannot be removed are not normally classified as foods. Pharmacologic actions of food may strengthen or weaken the actions of medicinal substances used concurrently.

Nursing management

Nursing process

Assessment A complete history should include usual dietary intake, and food intolerances and allergies. Food preferences should also be noted. These data should be compared with evidence of health problems and the medical regimen. Analysis may indicate actual or potential problems related to the diet.

Nursing diagnosis Nursing diagnoses likely to be made include:

> Constipation related to high intake of tea and berries
> Diarrhea related to high intake of rhubarb (prunes, bran)
> Pain: abdominal discomfort and flatulence related to high intake of baked beans
> Fluid volume deficit related to osmotic diuresis secondary to high intake of sugar

A common collaborative problem that should be differentiated from the nursing diagnoses is

> Potential complication: goiter related to high intake of foods containing thyroid inhibitors.

Planning Common goals include moderation in consumption of individual foods, use of a wide variety of foods, and avoidance of dietary components to which the client reacts adversely. If signs and symptoms of food toxicity or allergy are present, the goal is their reduction or elimination.

Intervention A major function of nurses is to teach clients about the toxic potential of food. The nurse is not an expert in nutrition or pharmacognosy* and may be unable to answer specific questions about novel foods. However, clients should be advised to use caution and consult with experts in this field (or the fields of botany, horticulture, or conservation) to ascertain the potential for toxicity of unusual foods. The best safeguard against common food toxins is a varied diet and moderate consumption. If the diet is voluntarily restricted, the client should be encouraged to try new

*The science dealing with medicinal properties of natural materials.

dishes and to use a variety of foods. When dietary components cause actual or potential health problems, the nurse can assist the client in planning attractive menus, which include the protective foods specifically needed and exclude the harmful ones. Referral to a nutritionist may be helpful.

Allergic individuals should be encouraged to monitor food intake so as to identify the specific foods causing sensitivity. Infrequently, allergic reactions are manifested by rarely recognized syndromes such as irritability and headache (cerebral reaction) or abdominal pain and diarrhea (intestinal reaction). Although it may be helpful to inform these clients about foods with a high potential for antigenicity, these foods should not be excluded from the diet if the individual does not react to them. Often the nurse can help the client identify harmful foods not considered previously as allergenic and determine which foods contain the offending substance or its chemical relatives. Once offending foods are identified, the client should read the labels of processed foods carefully so as to avoid them. Unfortunately, preservatives and additives are not always listed on food labels.

Clients who are institutionalized rely on the dietary and nursing personnel to protect them from foods that affect them adversely. The nurse should monitor the food served and confer with the dietitian to plan an optimum diet. The nurse should also monitor foods brought in by visitors to verify that there are no undesirable components.

Foods may be used to alleviate or prevent certain problems. For example, constipation may be eased if the client ingests laxative foods. Prunes are not the only agent suitable for this; they are often disliked, particularly by children. Pears, raisins, raw fruits and vegetables, and bran may also be used. Prunes may be better tolerated if the juice is frozen and served as a "popsicle."

Evaluation The occurrence of adverse reactions attributable to foods should be monitored. The results are judged in relation to previously developed criteria.

Checklist of nursing actions

☐ Teach clients about the medicinal properties and toxic potential of food.
☐ Advise clients to eat a variety of foods in moderate amounts.
☐ Refer clients to nutritionists or pharmacognosists when further information is needed.

Food additives

The use of food additives is not new. For centuries, salt, vinegar, sugar, spices, herbs, alcohol, and smoke have been used as natural preservatives and flavorings for foods. Modern technology has vastly expanded this repertoire by producing over 3,000 new natural and artificial additives (Jacobson, 1985, p 181), which are used to enhance the color, taste, texture, convenience, and stability of foods. Emulsifiers retard drying of baked goods; preservatives inhibit bacterial growth in processed meats; antioxidants lengthen shelf-life of many foods; stabilizers prevent the formation of ice crystals in ice cream; and vitamins and minerals enhance the nutritional value of dietary staples. Without the use of additives to retard spoilage, extend shelf-life, and enhance flavor, food products would not only be more expensive but also less varied.

Government testing

About 400 additives approved for use by the federal FDA are listed on the generally regarded as safe (GRAS) list. Many of these substances have not been tested for toxicity but have been accepted because of their long history of use without any apparent adverse effects. Only since 1960 has the FDA required that new additives be tested for safety before being added to the list. Nevertheless, over the past 50 years, more than 25 chemicals have been removed from the GRAS list and banned by the federal government as unsafe (Jacobson, 1985, p 184). Among these were artificial colors: Red #2 (which until its banning in 1976 was the most widely used food coloring in the U.S.); Violet #1; butter yellow; and agene and dulcin. A committee of scientists has been appointed to review the safety of GRAS compounds but progress has been slow. Some recommendations approving additives have been made obsolete by subsequent toxicity studies, and inappropriate recommendations are not always revised.

For this reason, many substances on the GRAS list may still have a potential for toxicity.

Research by others

Jacobson (1985) has classified food additives according to their apparent safety. Additives considered safe include preservatives such as inhibitors of microbial growth (vinegar, salt) and antioxidants (vitamin K, vitamin C); conditioners such as emulsifiers and thickeners (citric acid, gelatin, dextrin, glycerin); bleaches (benzoyl peroxide, chlorine dioxide); coloring agents (beta-carotene, caramel); flavoring agents (caramel, vanillin, glycine); and an effervescent (carbon dioxide). Some of these substances are naturally occurring compounds with a long history of use. Others are relatively new products of advanced chemical technology (see Table 10-3 for examples of safe additives).

Some additives long considered safe now are known to cause adverse reactions in certain situations. Vitamin A and its precursor, beta-carotene, are essential nutrients used in foods to fortify their nutritional content and add color. Because so many foods have been treated in this way, A vitaminosis has become one of the more common food toxicities. Excesses of vitamin A are teratogenic and neurotoxic. Beta-carotene does not cause toxicity but it can temporarily color the skin yellow.

Certain additives are safe for most people but can be harmful to others. Sulfites and tartrazine produce allergic sensitivity in some individuals; and lactose causes intestinal upset in populations with a lactase deficiency. Caffeine is dangerous to pregnant women because it can cause birth defects, and is harmful to

Table 10-3. Some food additives deemed safe

Additive	Function	Use
Acetic acid (vinegar)	Preserve, flavor, acidify foods	Pickles, preserved meats
Agar	Conditions (prevents drying)	Icings
	Stabilizes	Ice cream, jam, whipped cream
Alpha tocopherol	Preservative (antioxidant)	Fats and oils
Amylases	Conditioner	Bread
Ascorbic acid	Antioxidant	Processed meats, frozen fruits
Beta-carotene	Coloring agent	Fats (margarine, butter), coffee "creamers," milk, cake mixes, toppings
Calcium compounds	Conditioners	A variety of foods
Caramel	Conditioner and coloring agent	Carbonated beverages, candy, baked goods, soy sauces, syrups, beers, whiskies
Casein	Conditioner	Ice cream and other frozen desserts
Carbon dioxide	Effervescent	Carbonated soft drinks
Gelatin	Thickener	Ice cream, yogurt, cheese spreads, beverages
Lecithin	Preservative (antioxidant) and emulsifier	Margarine, chocolate, ice cream, baked goods
Proteases (meat tenderizer)	Tenderizer	Meat
Vanillin (vanilla)	Flavoring agent	Ice cream, cakes, chocolate, and other sweet foods

(Data from Jacobson F. [1985]. *The complete eater's digest and nutrition scoreboard.* Garden City, NJ: Anchor Press.)

children, who are intolerant of its central nervous system stimulation.

Other additives are well tolerated in moderation but cause adverse effects when taken in excess. Included in this group are the natural sweeteners dextrose, fructose, and corn syrup; all are refined sugars that provide additional calories but have no other nutrients. When taken in excess, they contribute to obesity and B vitamin deficiencies, disturb glucose balance in diabetics, and contribute to high levels of blood cholesterol. Fructose and the poorly absorbed sweeteners, sorbitol and mannitol, are associated with increased risk of cataract formation when taken in large quantities. (See Table 10-4 for food additives now considered questionable.)

Jacobson advises avoiding additives whose risk–benefit ratio appears to be unfavorable. Yet, many harmful substances are still listed on the FDA GRAS list. This is largely because studies to validate research findings are time-consuming and because powerful food manufacturing lobbies often exert countervailing influences. Some additives have been associated with increased risk of malignant tumors in animal studies (*eg*, saccharin) but they have yet to be stricken from the GRAS list despite the 1958 Delaney Amendment requiring that carcinogenic substances be removed from the market. In 1970, the artificial sweetener cyclamate

was banned in the United States once it was proven carcinogenic. However, it is still available in Canada (see Table 10-5).

Dr. Ben Feingold has suggested that food additives, especially dyes and flavorings, may contribute to childhood hyperkinesis and learning disabilities. Dr. Feingold has reported considerable success in treating children with a restricted diet limiting exposure to food additives. Attempts to duplicate this success by other investigators have not been successful, and the treatment remains controversial. Nevertheless, some additives can affect the nervous system. Caffeine is a potent central nervous system stimulant. Nitrates and nitrites act as vasodilators and can precipitate migraine headaches. Monosodium glutamate (MSG, Accent) is reported to have produced brain damage in mice and monkeys. Preliminary reports of adverse reaction to aspartame (NutraSweet) indicate that this compound may be neurotoxic. A nonseptic encephalitis can also result from ingestion of chemicals to which the consumer has an allergic hypersensitivity.

Allergic reactions to additives vary depending on the antigenicity of the substance and the consumer's proclivity toward allergic reaction. Tartrazine (Yellow No. 5) and sulfites (used as preservatives for salad greens and in some alcoholic beverages) can cause attacks of severe respiratory distress in asthmatic con-

Table 10-4. Some food additives of questionable safety

Additive	Function	Possible toxicity
Aluminum compounds	Leavening agents	High aluminum intake and aluminum deposits in the brain are associated with several forms of senility.
Aspartame	Sweetener	When metabolized, aspartame releases phenylalanine, an amino acid harmful to phenylketonurics. The additive may be neurotoxic. In some studies, malignant brain tumors developed in test animals. Dizziness, headaches, and seizures have been reported by consumers.
Carrageenan	Conditioner	The additive has caused ulcers of the colon in test animals. It may cause necrotizing enterocolitis in premature infants.
Dextrose	Sweetener	Refined sugars promote tooth decay and add empty calories to food.
Glycyrrhizin	Flavoring	In susceptible individuals, ammonium glycyrrhizin caused hypertension, fatigue, edema, headache, and congestive heart failure.
Hydroxylated lethicin	Emulsifier and antioxidant	This additive has not been adequately tested for toxic effects.
Monosodium glutamate	Flavor intensifier	This additive is the cause of "Chinese restaurant syndrome" (burning sensations in the back of the neck and forearms, tightness of the chest, and headaches). Infant test animals given large amounts of MSG suffered damage to the hypothalamus and retina.
Iodine compounds	Conditioners, coloring agents (Red No. 3)	Adult diets are likely to contain iodine in ample amounts. Excesses can inhibit thyroid function and cause goiter.
Smoke flavoring	Flavoring agent	Although probably less carcinogenic than natural smoke, this partially purified smoke product has not been tested adequately for toxic effects.
Tragacanth gum	Thickening agent	This additive has not been adequately tested for toxicity.

(Data from Jacobson F. [1985]. *The complete eater's digest and nutrition scoreboard.* Garden City, NJ: Anchor Press.)

Table 10-5. Some food additives to avoid

Additive	Use	Reasons for avoidance
Artificial dyes	Coloring agents	Many dyes previously considered safe have been found to be carcinogenic. Most still on the market have not been tested adequately for safety.
Butylated hydroxyanisole (BHA)	Preservative	In a Japanese study, malignant tumors developed in the forestomachs of the test animals. Behavioral changes in test animals have been reported. Occasional allergic reactions have been reported in consumers.
Caffeine	Flavoring agent (?)*	Caffeine is a central nervous system stimulant that is addictive. It is suspected of acting as a mutagen and teratogen and is a causative factor in fibrocystic disease.
Cyclamate	Sweetener	Cyclamate is carcinogenic and may cause inheritable genetic damage.
Saccharin	Sweetener	Animal studies indicate that saccharin promotes the development of bladder cancer; in humans, it increases the risk of bladder cancer by 60%.
Sodium nitrites	Preservative (meats)	In large amounts, nitrites cause methemoglobinemia, which can be fatal. In combination with food, they form nitrosamines, which are potent carcinogens.
Sulfiting agents	Preservatives	These food additives have caused serious, sometimes fatal, allergic reactions in asthmatic individuals.
Tartrazine (Yellow No. 5)	Coloring agent	Tartrazine can cause acute allergic reactions in individuals with atopic allergy who are sensitive to aspirin.
Xylitol	Sweetener	Some animal studies have shown that xylitol is carcinogenic.

(Data from Jacobson F. [1985]. *The complete eater's digest and nutrition scoreboard.* Garden City, NJ: Anchor Press.)
*Studies do not support claims of flavor enhancement.

sumers. Other additives with a high potential for triggering allergy include corn products (syrup, starch, oil); wheat (flour thickeners); chocolate; and butylated hydroxytoluene (BHT, a preservative). Even additives generally considered nonallergenic, such as soybeans (oil, vegetable protein concentrate), can precipitate reactions in certain individuals.

■ Summary

Food additives are credited with significantly contributing to the abundant supply and infinite variety characteristic of American foods. They lengthen shelf-life and enable manufacturers to market many time-saving and labor-saving prepared foods. However, some additives are also implicated in the increased incidence of malignant tumors, birth defects, dangerous allergic reactions, and other health problems. At best, they are a mixed blessing.

Nursing management

Nursing implications

As professionals, nurses should seek to influence the enactment and enforcement of laws governing food additives. Carcinogens and other substances harmful to large numbers of people should be eliminated from the food supply. A requirement that food processors

Learning experience 10-1

While caring for a client taking multiple prescription and/or nonprescription medications, analyze the client's diet and medical regimen for potential food–drug interactions. Does your physical assessment data include signs and symptoms of these interactions? Are there other adverse signs and symptoms that could indicate unusual interactions? Include in your care plan measures to alleviate or eliminate undesirable food–drug interactions.

list all ingredients on the product label, including additives, would enable consumers to identify foods that are unsuitable to them because of individual sensitivity or other health problems. Nurses should also actively participate in educating the public regarding additives and their risks.

Nursing process

Assessment Data required include the client's usual diet and food preferences, history of adverse reactions to foods containing additives, and current signs and symptoms of such reactions. The client data should be compared with information about the potential danger of various additives.

Nursing diagnosis Nursing diagnoses identify adverse reactions to foods and the specific additives in foods responsible for sensitivities. For example:

> *Impaired gas exchange: acute asthma related to exposure to tartrazine (Yellow No. 5); contributing factor, allergic hypersensitivity to tartrazine*
> *Diarrhea related to high intake of saccharin*
> *Diarrhea related to exposure to soy protein; contributing factor, allergic hypersensitivity to soybeans*

Planning The goals are to alleviate or eliminate signs and symptoms of existing reactions; to reduce risk of adverse reaction to additives; and to maintain adequate nutrition. Measurable criteria for evaluation should be developed in the planning stage.

Intervention Nursing measures to alleviate signs and symptoms of adverse reactions should be implemented. The nurse may assist the client in identifying reactions to food additives. Clients often have difficulty interpreting labels and identifying various names used for specific additives. Nurses may also assist clients in planning nutritious, varied meals despite the need to avoid many commercially prepared foods. Some people who habitually use convenience foods (which frequently contain additives) may need lessons in how to cook "from scratch." Referral to a nutritionist or dietitian may be helpful.

Evaluation Data required for evaluation include the frequency and severity of signs and symptoms attributable to exposure to food additives; comments by the client indicating satisfaction with the diet; and evidence of nutritional status after a period of compliance with the diet.

Alteration of drug effect by food
Modification of drug pharmacokinetics
Absorption

The presence or absence of food in the intestinal tract influences the absorption of drugs administered orally. Absorption may be completely blocked when food and drug combine to carry the drug out of the system in the feces. For example, the charcoal present in charbroiled or burned foods adsorbs drug molecules, preventing them from crossing the intestinal mucosa. By a different process, tetracycline and related antibiotics combine chemically with divalent and trivalent cations (calcium, magnesium, iron, aluminum), forming a nonabsorbable complex. Similarly, the phytates in cereals inhibit the absorption of calcium, magnesium, potassium, iron, and zinc (components of many nutritional supplements). Although

heat tends to destroy phytic acid, cooking or baking does not necessarily prevent this complexation.

Absorption of drugs may be altered mechanically by the presence of food in the stomach at the time of medication. Once the drug mixes with the food mass, its exposure to the surface of the intestinal mucosa is reduced, thereby delaying or reducing its absorption. The presence of food in the tract also slows transit time, causing further delay in absorption. Slow absorption is often desirable because it minimizes fluctuations in drug blood levels. However, reduction in absorption lessens the efficacy of the drug. Because absorption may be erratic, it is difficult to compensate by adjusting the dosage. In contrast, certain drugs are absorbed more quickly and completely when mixed with food. For example, griseofulvin absorption is enhanced by the presence of fat in the intestinal tract.

Dissolution of a drug chemical is affected by the temperature of stomach contents. Dissolution (and subsequently absorption) proceeds more rapidly in warm temperatures than in cold. When rapid action is desired, administering a warm beverage with the medication is sometimes helpful.

The absorption of salts often is influenced by the pH of the gastrointestinal (GI) tract. Acid salts diffuse through the intestinal membrane more rapidly in the acid medium of the stomach. Basic salts are absorbed more rapidly in the small intestine where the pH is normally much higher. Coating a medication with a substance that does not dissolve in acid media, but does dissolve in basic media, allows the medication to pass through the stomach intact. This is one form of enteric coating. An increase in intragastric pH will enhance dissolution of this type of enteric coating and may release the drug prematurely in the stomach. Food in the stomach often raises the intragastric pH from two (the usual pH of stomach hydrochloric acid) to five. Because protein is amphoteric and can neutralize acids, a protein-rich feeding is most likely to produce this effect. An increase in stomach pH can also affect the absorption of acidic and basic salts. The dissolution of acidic salts in the stomach would be enhanced but absorption would be inhibited. The dissolution of basic salts would be inhibited but absorption of that part of the medication that does dissolve would be accelerated.

Excretion

The kidneys are the primary route for excretion of drugs and their metabolites. Excretion of acidic and basic salts varies depending on urinary pH. Because they are more soluble and more highly ionized in an acid medium, basic drugs are excreted more readily in acid urine. The reverse is true of acidic drugs. For this reason, excretion of basic drugs is enhanced by the consumption of acid ash foods, whereas excretion of acidic drugs is enhanced by the consumption of alkaline ash foods. (Further discussion on absorption, dis tribution, metabolism, and excretion processes can be found in Chapter 7.)

Modification of drug action

Some food components have been found to modify the action of certain drugs at the cellular level. For example, high carbohydrate, low protein meals increase the likelihood of toxicity (muscular dyskinesia) in clients receiving levodopa for the treatment of Parkinson's disease (Wurtman & Caballero, 1988). Levodopa's therapeutic action is inhibited by high levels of pyridoxine (vitamin B_6). Vitamin K reduces the effectiveness of warfarin anticoagulants by competing for access to receptors on liver cells that produce prothrombin. Because both of these vitamins are essential nutrients, they should not be wholly eliminated from the diet. The amounts taken in the diet should be the same each day to maintain a constant level in the body. The drug dosage can then be adjusted to compensate for the presence of antagonistic nutrients.

Two electrolytes influence the action of heart muscle and the effect of digitalis medications. Potassium decreases the force of contraction and prolongs diastole. Calcium increases the force of contraction and prolongs systole. Potassium antagonizes the action of cardiotonic drugs derived from digitalis, whereas calcium mimics and enhances their actions. Potassium is considered to be the physiologic antagonist for digitalis. It moderates adverse reactions, as well as therapeutic response to these drugs. Because digitalis has a narrow margin of safety, adequate potassium levels are a vital safeguard against digitalis toxicity. Hyperkalemia and either hypercalcemia or hypocalcemia are relatively uncommon but hypokalemia occurs frequently in individuals who lose excessive potassium from the intestinal tract (in diarrhea, excessive enemas, or laxative overuse) or from the urinary tract (with potassium-wasting diuretics or increased levels of corticosteroids). For these reasons, this interaction is important to remember during treatment for heart failure.

A further illustration of the complexity of food–drug interactions is the amino acid tyrosine, which is normally metabolized to tyramine (a pressor amine) and subsequently oxidized to form other, less active, metabolites. When an individual is treated for depression with monoamine oxidase inhibitors, the metabolic process that normally degrades tyramine is inhibited. If large amounts of tyrosine are ingested in foods, tyramine rapidly accumulates in the tissues. Its effects are so pronounced that a life-threatening hypertensive crisis can occur. Foods containing high levels of tyrosine include aged cheeses, fava beans, broad bean pods, red wines, salami, bologna, sausage, and chicken livers (Lippman, 1987). These foods should be eliminated from the diet when monoamine oxidase inhibitors are prescribed.

■ Summary

Foods may influence the action of drugs by altering their pharmacokinetics or pharmacodynamics. Foods may slow, accelerate, or reduce drug absorption. Renal excretion may be enhanced or inhibited by the effects of foods on the pH of urine. Foods that alter the action of a drug may contain nutrient or pharmacologic components that either mimic or antagonize the effects at the cell level. Some foods inhibit drug action by competitive inhibition. Food–drug interaction can involve alteration of complex enzymatic metabolic processes.

Nursing management

Nursing process

Assessment   To effectively medicate a client, a complete history must include a dietary history. The nurse should inquire specifically about foods known to affect the pharmacokinetics or pharmacodynamics of the prescribed drugs.

Nursing diagnosis   Nursing diagnoses identify actual or potential adverse interactions between foods and drugs.

Planning   The goals are to reduce the risk of adverse food–drug interactions and to diagnose and treat these interactions promptly should they develop.

Intervention   Clients are counseled to eliminate from the diet those foods that pose a risk of adverse interaction with their drugs or to control the amount and timing of their ingestion so as to eliminate or minimize the risk of interaction.

Evaluation   Data required for evaluation include signs and symptoms of therapeutic response to medications and incidence or absence of adverse reaction due to food–drug interaction.

Example of a problem related to adsorption of antihypertensive drug by a food component (charcoal)

Assessment   Data required include serial blood pressure readings, the components of the drug regimen, and a history of events associated with fluctuations in therapeutic response to antihypertensive medication. These are compared to identify food components that might impair drug absorption.

Nursing diagnosis   A possible diagnosis is altered tissue perfusion: episodic hypertension related to impaired absorption of benazopril medication secondary to concurrent ingestion of charbroiled foods.

Planning   The goal of care is to reduce the incidence of hypertensive episodes by reducing or eliminating periodic drug adsorption by charcoal.

Intervention A teaching plan that assists the client in reducing the incidence of drug adsorption by charcoal in foods should be planned and executed. Charbroiled foods should not be eaten during the period from 2 hours prior to medication until 1 hour afterward.

Evaluation Data required for evaluation include serial blood pressure readings.

Example of a problem related to altered digoxin action due to nutritional (potassium) deficiency

Assessment The required client data are the drug regimen, usual dietary habits, current state of nutrition, and signs and symptoms of drug toxicity. These should be compared with information on the properties of prescribed medications, in this case, digoxin and hydrochlorothiazide. Digoxin has a narrow margin of safety; its physiologic action is inhibited by potassium. A dose of digoxin that is appropriate for a client whose nutrition is adequate may produce toxic symptoms if blood potassium levels decline. Hydrochlorothiazide accelerates renal excretion of potassium and can cause hypokalemia.

Nursing diagnosis A possible diagnosis is pain: nausea related to potassium deficiency during digitalis therapy secondary to use of potassium wasting diuretics.

Planning The goal of care is to reduce the risk of nausea caused by digoxin toxicity by maintaining normal levels of potassium.

Intervention The client should be taught the nature of the potential problem and be advised to use potassium-rich foods daily. If the client is dependent on the care of others, potassium-rich foods should be offered frequently. If serum potassium levels are measured, results should be monitored.

Evaluation Data are required on the signs and symptoms of hypokalemia and digitalis toxicity.

Nutritional changes induced by medications

Drugs influencing gastrointestinal function

A number of drugs are capable of altering GI function in ways that affect nutrition. Drugs used to treat diseases of this system generally improve function and increase the absorption of nutrients. For example, digestants (hydrochloric acid, bile salts, enzymes) improve the chemical processes of digestion in persons with deficiencies of these substances. Antidiarrheals slow passage of intestinal contents and reduce the loss of nutrients by abnormally frequent defecations. Certain antibiotics are used to treat enteric infections and restore the system to normal function. Metoclopramide, a stimulant of small bowel peristalsis, is also sometimes employed to promote digestion. In these situations, medications improve digestion and nutrition.

Antiemetics are another class of drugs that enhance GI function by acting on the vomiting center in the central nervous system. By inhibiting this reflex, these drugs decrease nausea and promote the ingestion and retention of food. A derivative of marijuana, tetrahydrocannabinol, is now used to treat severe nausea and vomiting.

A few drugs used to treat intestinal ailments impair one or more digestive functions. For example, histamine$_2$ (H$_2$) receptor antagonists (cimetidine, ranitidine) raise stomach pH and can impair absorption of both iron and vitamin B$_{12}$, whose absorption is facilitated by gastric acidity. Adsorbents in antidiarrheals tend to hold nutrients, as well as irritants, on their molecules and carry them out of the system unabsorbed. Antibiotics acting locally in the gut can eliminate many protective organisms in the normal flora, causing a superinfection such as candidiasis, which because of sore mouth and throat and intestinal discomfort reduces food intake and overall nutrition. Emetics used to induce vomiting to remove ingested poisons also empty the stomach of any food that is present. Excessive use of laxatives or enemas reduces intestinal transit time and absorption of nutrients, notably potassium. (See Chapters 30 and 31 for detailed discussion of GI drugs.)

Other therapeutic agents

Medications intended to treat parenteral diseases also affect GI function. Anorexia, nausea, and vomiting are common adverse reactions to drugs. Oral drugs that irritate the GI mucosa can cause anorexia or nausea soon after administration. Other drugs cause intestinal upset whether administered by mouth or by injection. For example, one of the first toxic symptoms of the cardiotonic drug digitalis (which has a narrow safety margin) is loss of appetite. Intestinal mycotic infection is a common adverse reaction to broad spectrum antibiotics administered parenterally. Chemotherapeutic agents used to treat cancer frequently impair food ingestion and digestion because they damage the intestinal mucosa. Drug-induced nutritional impairment often retards recovery and can threaten life if allowed to progress.

By more subtle mechanisms, drugs may influence the way in which the body handles nutrients. Some oral medications combine with food in the intestinal tract to form nonabsorbable complexes. (See example of tetracycline discussed above.) Ion exchange resins administered to reduce reabsorption of cholesterol in the gut also inhibit the reabsorption of nutrients secreted in bile. Ion exchange resins should be administered between meals to minimize binding of nutrients in ingested food but the effect on nutrients within the enterohepatic circulation occurs regardless of the timing of medication. Specific active transport systems involved in nutrient absorption are sometimes inhibited by drugs. For example, riboflavin absorption in the small intestine is impaired by antipsychotic drugs such as chlorpromazine and tricyclic antidepressants, which interfere with the phosphorylation of this nutrient.

Drugs can influence the transport, storage, and metabolism of nutrients. Many drug-induced nutritional deficiencies are caused by the inhibition or induction of enzymes involved in the transformation (activation or degradation) of nutrients. Renal elimination of minerals such as sodium, potassium, calcium, magnesium, and other trace minerals is altered by diuretics. In most cases, elimination is increased but certain diuretics increase potassium reabsorption and conserve this nutrient (see Table 10-6). A few drugs increase internal concentrations of these electrolytes by stimulating inappropriate antidiuretic hormone secretion, diluting body fluids.

Drugs may also increase the body's need for a nutrient. For example, alcohol increases the need for the B vitamins involved in energy metabolism. Oral contraceptives increase the need for certain vitamins, possibly by inhibiting their action at the cellular level. Coumarin anticoagulants complete with vitamin K for receptor sites on liver cells involved in the production of prothrombin. Although this is the desired therapeutic effect, an excess of this drug can cause serious bleeding.

Epidemiology of drug-induced nutritional deficiency

In developed countries, nutritional deficiencies from inadequate diet occur less frequently than overnutrition. However, nutritional impairment from drug regimens is not rare. The incidence of such problems is directly related to the use of medications associated with "modern" medicine. The nutrient involved most frequently in single deficiencies is folic acid. Other B vitamins (pyridoxine and cyanocobalamin) are also affected by several drugs. The use of anticonvulsants is associated with impairment of vitamin D and calcium nutrition. Serious malnutrition frequently develops during cancer chemotherapy. Overuse of alcohol and other drugs is a major cause of malnutrition. Except in the case of marijuana, which stimulates the appetite, drug dependence tends to inhibit appetite and reduce food intake. In addition, alcohol damages the liver and reduces the organ's ability to store nutrients.

There are many risk factors for developing drug-induced nutritional deficiencies. Preexisting marginal or deficient nutrition, whether caused by disease, poverty, ignorance, or custom, is a predisposing factor. Certain climates affect nutritional needs; for example, more calories are required in cold weather than in hot, and more dietary vitamin D is needed in areas with little sunshine. Many physiologic states increase nutritional needs. These include hypermetabolic states, such as pregnancy, lactation, and rapid growth during childhood and adolescence. Vigorous exercise and other stressors also increase nutritional requirements. Certain genetic traits, such as lack of enzymes for degrading drugs or enzymes involved in nutrient metabolism, make other individuals vulnerable. Drug dependence and exposure to pollutants may enhance a food–drug interaction. Other risk factors include the use of oral contraceptives, anorexia, malabsorption, and maldigestion.

Medical factors predisposing to drug-induced deficiencies include illness, the type of drugs used for treatment, the duration of drug treatment, and the use of dialysis. Chronic diseases, especially those affecting the intestinal tract, tend to compromise nutrition. The use of certain drugs (antineoplastic chemotherapeutic agents, oral contraceptives, ion exchange resins) pose an increased risk. Lengthy medication regimens are more likely to cause serious nutritional problems than short-term therapy. Dialysis removes some nutrients from the blood. In addition, choice of physician can be a factor since some medical practioners are more knowledgeable about nutritional needs and drug-induced deficiencies than others.

■ **Summary**
Drugs may alter nutritional status by all of the mechanisms that underlie food–drug interaction. These include changes in absorption, activation, transport and tissue binding; moderation of the mechanisms of nutrition at the cellular level; and changes in the processes by which nutrients are metabolized, degraded, and excreted. Moreover, by influencing intestinal function, drugs may either enhance or impair the absorption of food, thus changing the general level of nutrition. Nearly every discrete nutrient may be influenced by some drug. A few drugs affect multiple nutrients. Food–drug interactions are frequently seen in drug dependence, use of oral contraceptives, anticonvulsant therapy, and antineoplastic chemotherapy. The risk of drug-induced nutritional deficiencies is increased when pretreatment nutrition is marginal or inadequate, during hypermetabolic states, during certain disease conditions, when digestive function is compromised, and when lengthy drug treatment is required.

(Text continues on p. 122)

Table 10-6. Selected drugs that tend to promote nutrient deficiency

Nutrient / Drugs	Vitamin A	Thiamin	Riboflavin	Folate	Vitamin B6	Vitamin B12	Niacin	Vitamin C	Vitamin D	Vitamin E	Vitamin K	Na	K	Ca	Mg	Fe	P	Cu	Zn
Alcohols																			
ethanol	X	X	X	X	X	X	X	X			X				X				X
Anesthetics																			
nitrous oxide						X		X											
Anorectics								X											
Antacids																			
Al, Mg salts								X									X		
Na$_2$CO$_3$				X															
Antiarrhythmics																			
quinidine								X					X						
Anticoagulants																			
warfarin											X								
Anticonvulsants				X		X		X	X					X					
Antidepressants																			
Tricyclics			X																
Antihypertensives																			
hydralazine					X														
Anti-infectives																			
pentamidine				X				X											
tetracycline								X											
neomycin	X					X		X			X	X		X					
gentamicin												X	X						
amphotericin B												X	X		X				
trimethoprim				X				X						X					
isoniazide					X		X	X								X			
cycloserine				X	X			X								X			
PAS				X		X													
rifampin				X				X	X					X					
pyrimethamine				X															

Anti-inflammatories
sulfasalazine
colchicine
Salicylates
Antilipemics
cholestyramine
colestipol
Antineoplastics
methotrexate
cyclophosphamide
vincristine
cisplatin
5-FU, 6-mercaptopurine
Anti-Parkinson agents
levodopa
Acids
boric acid
Histamine₂ receptor antagonists
Chelators
penicillamine
Diuretics (potassium sparing)
Diuretics (potassium wasting)
Hormones
Contraceptives
Glucocorticoids
Hypoglycemics (oral)
Laxatives
mineral oil
phenophthalein
calomel
Minerals
Calcium
potassium chloride
Sedatives
chloral hydrate
Sunscreens

(Data from Roe DA. [1985]. *Drug-induced nutritional deficiencies.* Westport, CT: AVI Publishing Co.)

Nursing management

Nursing process

Assessment To diagnose actual or potential nutritional problems, clients should be assessed for their state of nutrition and risk factors for deficiencies. The history should include a complete appraisal of drug use, food preferences, and a retrospective food history (usually for 24 hours). When necessary, this may be supplemented by a food diary. Previous illnesses and their treatments should also be listed. Other risk factors should also be determined.

Physical examination should include specific evaluation for nutritional deficiencies. Neurologic abnormalities or dermatitis may indicate a lack of B vitamins; visual changes, a lack of vitamin A; bone pain and skeletal abnormalities, a lack of vitamin D and calcium; and abnormal bleeding, a lack of vitamin K metabolism. Diarrhea usually denotes malabsorption. Weakness, fatigue, pallor, and tachycardia accompany anemia caused by folate or vitamin B_{12} deficiency. Growth retardation in children and weight loss occur with inadequate calorie or protein nutrition. (See Table 10-7 for symptoms associated with drug-induced nutritional deficiencies.) The nurse should focus on early changes arising from malnutrition so that problems may be detected before true deficiency syndromes develop.

The data base should be examined in relation to drug treatment regimens to determine the presence or the risk of drug-induced impairment of nutrition. In complex situations, the nurse should consult with a dietitian or nutritionist for assistance in diagnosis.

Nursing diagnosis Examples of appropriate diagnoses include

> *Altered nutrition: less than body requirements: inadequate intake of food related to nausea secondary to antineoplastic therapy*
> *Altered nutrition: less than body requirements: deficiencies of vitamins C and B complex and minerals calcium, iron, copper, and zinc related to increased tissue needs secondary to use of oral contraceptives*
> *Altered nutrition: less than body requirements related to liver dysfunction secondary to alcoholism*

Planning Usual goals are to correct existing nutritional problems or reduce the risk of drug-induced problems. Short-term goals include increasing oral in-

Table 10-7. Signs and symptoms of drug-induced nutritional deficiencies

Signs and symptoms	Nutritional deficiency
Decreased night vision, "dry eye"	vitamin A
Weakness, palpitations, tachycardia, pallor, shortness of breath	cyanocobalamine (vitamin B_{12}), pyridoxine, folic acid, iron or copper
Neutropenia, leukopenia	copper
Sore tongue	riboflavin, niacin, cyanocobalamine (vitamin B_{12})
Pain in lower extremities	pyridoxine (vitamin B_6)
Peripheral nervous system changes (paresthesia, hyperesthesia, weakness)	thiamine
Dermatitis	
Light-exposed areas	niacin
Face and scalp	pyridoxine
Abnormal bleeding	
Gums, subcutaneous (petechiae)	ascorbic acid (vitamin C)
Wounds, urinary or gastrointestinal tract	vitamin K
Bone pain, difficulty in ambulation	vitamin D or calcium
Weakness, constipation	potassium
Mental symptoms	
Depression	thiamine, niacin, pyridoxine
Irritability	thiamine, folic acid
Failure to concentrate	thiamine
Memory defects	thiamine, niacin
Lassitude	niacin
Apprehension	niacin
Insomnia	folic acid, pantothenic acid
Hypotension	sodium
Poor wound healing	zinc

gestion of nutrients likely to be deficient; promoting optimum function of the digestive tract; timing administration of drugs to minimize the risk of interaction within the GI tract; reducing risk factors such as stress; and teaching the client the measures required to maintain nutrition during self-care.

Intervention The diets of institutionalized clients should be monitored by the nurse to ensure that a variety of foods that contain the most vital nutrients are offered. To determine optimum diet, the client should confer with the dietitian. If the client is anorexic or nauseated, nursing measures to reduce these symptoms are required. If antiemetics or metoclopramide are ordered, doses should be timed for peak effect at mealtimes. If necessary, the physician may be consulted about ordering such drugs.

The nurse should develop and implement a teaching plan to help the client understand the nutritional problem and the food–drug interactions involved. The nurse can then devise a program for reducing the risk of deficiencies that is compatible with the client's lifestyle. If nutritional problems occur or worsen, the physician may be consulted about possible changes in the drug regimen.

Evaluation The client should be monitored for signs and symptoms of nutritional impairment, using predetermined criteria for evaluation.

Checklist of nursing actions

☐ Monitor the diets of institutionalized clients to ensure adequate nutrition.

☐ Use nursing measures to reduce nausea and anorexia.

☐ Administer prescribed antiemetic and antinauseant medications before meals.

☐ Teach clients about drug effects that affect food intake.

☐ When nausea is refractory, consult with the physician regarding possible changes in the drug regimen to reduce iatrogenic nausea and vomiting.

References

Bittiner S, Cartwright I, et al. (1988). A double-blind randomized, placebo-controlled trial of fish oil in psoriasis. *Lancet 1*, 378 (February 20).

Cerrato PL. (1987). What diet can do for your arthritis patient. *RN, 50(9)*, 69–71

Fackelmann KA. (1990). Cabbage chemical may bar breast cancer. *Science News, 137*, 375.

Jacobson MF. (1985). *The complete eater's digest and nutrition scoreboard*, p 181. Garden City, NY: Anchor Press.

Lippman S. (1987). Practical MAOI food and drug avoidances (letter). *Psychosomatics, 28*, 591 (November).

Phillips P. (1987). Chocolate not so sweet in esophagitis. *Medical Tribune, 28*, 11 (October 7).

Rubin R. (1990). Forget additives: It's the food that causes cancer. *Syracuse Herald-Journal, (February 20)*, A1, A10.

Wurtman R, Caballero B. (1988). Facilitation of levodopa-induced dyskinesias by dietary carbohydrates. *N Engl J Med 319(19)*, 1288 (November 10).

Bibliography

*Cerrato PL. (1986). Does your patient's food affect his mood? *RN, 49(3)*, 62–64.

Chinese salted fish linked to cancer. (1985). *Science News, 127*, 404.

*Mayer J, ed. *Tufts University Diet & Nutrition Letter*. A monthly periodical first published in March 1982).

The power of garlic. (1985). *University of California, Berkeley Wellness Letter, 2(1)*, 7. Rock-a-bye nutrients. (1984). *Science News, 126*, 360.

Roe D. (1985). *Drug-induced nutritional deficiencies*. Westport, CT: AVI Publishing Co.

Shultz CM. (1986). Sulfite sensitivity. *American Journal of Nursing, 86*, 914.

Silberner J. (1985). Broccoli pills? *Science News, 127*, 237.

*Worthington-Roberts BS. (1981). *Contemporary developments in nutrition*. St. Louis: CV Mosby.

*Recommended for further reading.

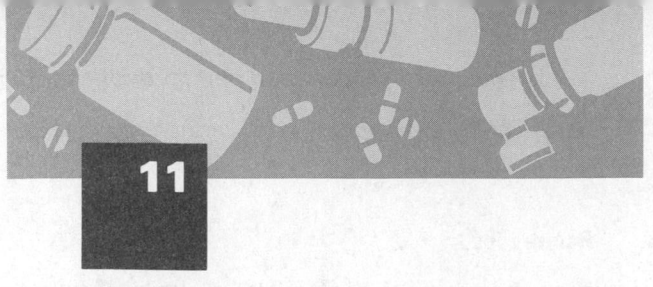

11

Psychological aspects of drug therapy

Each person has a unique response to drugs that develops through years of conditioning and is so intrinsic that it rarely enters the level of awareness. However, this response is important because of its impact on safe and effective drug use.

When a drug is administered to a client, an action–reaction process is initiated. Just as people react to the actions of other people in daily living, they also react to the administration of drugs. The action or response to medication is both physiologic and psychological; the psychological influences the physiologic.

Physiologic factors known to modify drug action are tolerance, cumulation, temperature, pregnancy, age, dosage, disease, route of administration, and other drugs. Psychological response can affect or be affected by all of these factors (Box 11-1).

In conjunction with pharmacodynamic action, the psychological response can influence the effectiveness of a drug by enhancing, negating, or producing an adverse reaction (Fig. 11-1). This explains why no two individuals react in exactly the same way to an identical medication given in an identical dosage. This chapter discusses various factors that play a part in behavioral responses.

Behavioral responses to drugs

Attitudes

Where are attitudes acquired? First, a person's genetic makeup influences his or her perception of and interaction with the environment. The next dominant factors are family, culture, education, religion, socioeconomic status, and health. These factors combine with genetic makeup to mold the individual.

Attitudes and patterns of behavior develop through this prolonged series of social experiences. It is not the aging process *per se* that influences attitudes but the social experiences that occur throughout that process. Although generally not part of conscious recall, early experiences with drug therapy continue to influence response at later stages of development.

Motivation

Motivation can be described as drive, incentive, and need. Drive stems from psychological and biologic needs and is geared toward activating behavior. An incentive directs the behavior toward achievement of a specific goal (satisfaction of need). Incentives are learned over time through interactions with others and with the environment.

Specific behavior used to satisfy need or pleasure is repeated and, thus, reinforced. This behavior may evolve through trial and error or through direct imitation of others. Therefore, motivation is associated with need, incentive, and drive in the client's response to drugs and drug taking.

Meaning attached to drugs

The meaning or significance the drug or drug taking has for the client affects response to drug treatment. It is necessary, therefore, for the nurse to be aware of and correctly identify the client's emotional state, in addition to his or her health-illness status. Feelings of dependency, anger, resentment, hostility, security, well-being, and anxiety can contribute to the client's response to a particular medication or to medication in general (Box 11-2).

Dependency

All of us experience feelings of dependency in the course of living. Some individuals respond to all experiences in this manner. Such a client is known as a *dependent personality*. Unable to use skills to meet his or her own needs independently, the individual may use other people, alcohol, or drugs to overcome this weakness, thus, eliciting temporary feelings of power and security. However, the use of a crutch may create an

Box 11-1. Physiologic factors modifying drug action

- Tolerance
- Cumulation
- Temperature
- Pregnancy
- Age
- Dosage
- Disease
- Route of administration
- Other drugs
- Psychological factors

Box 11-2. Behavioral responses to drugs

- Dependency
- Emotional states: Resentment, anger, hostility; security and well-being; anxiety and image
- Compliance, noncompliance, overcompliance

ever-expanding circle, leading to a dependence on larger or stronger amounts of a drug (Fig. 11-2). By virtue of their positions as authority figures and decision-makers, health care professionals sometimes foster these feelings of dependency in their clients.

Resentment, anger, and hostility

A dependent personality may also resent and be hostile toward significant others, including members of the health care team. These angry feelings arise with the change in health status and the alterations in daily living. Underlying the angry response may be feelings of powerlessness in controlling one's body or one's life. This can be true especially when the client's needs are being met through dependence on a drug, alcohol, or the sick role. The conflict that arises over attaining physical health and meeting dependency needs may result in adverse reactions to medication and an increase in physical symptoms (Fig. 11-3). Just as the appropriate mental state or belief in the therapeutic benefits of a drug will enhance the drug's effectiveness, so can anger and hostility reduce or negate its effectiveness.

If the client uses the sick role to gain attention or control of others, the drug therapy may well be sabotaged by the patient or family. For such a client, the degree of satisfaction experienced from maintaining this role far outweighs the possible benefits of the drug. The client is not inclined to jeopardize his or her position by getting well and losing these secondary benefits of being sick. Likewise, the family may focus on the client to escape acknowledging or working on difficulties in family roles and relationships. If the patient were to get well, family members would need to find another focus or be confronted with their own unsatisfactory and usually dysfunctional relationships. This constitutes too great a threat to maintaining family unity and, as such, is avoided by preventing the client from getting well.

If such is the case, the patient may take the drug but develop other symptoms or become increasingly ill; take enough of the drug to feel somewhat better without having to give up the sick role; or refuse to take the drug at all (Fig. 11-4). Family members may forget to administer the drug or purchase it, may tell the client that he or she is well enough to do without the drug, or criticize the health care providers and even the health care system itself.

Anger has been found to have a strong motivating effect on behavior. The resulting behavioral activities can be either passively or actively hostile. The nurse should be well aware of the strong anger response as individuals feel less control over their bodies and their lives.

Security and well-being

Other individuals gain a feeling of security or well-being from a daily intake of particular medications, which may be prescribed or sold over the counter. These individuals view medications as basically helpful. However, some of these same people do not view

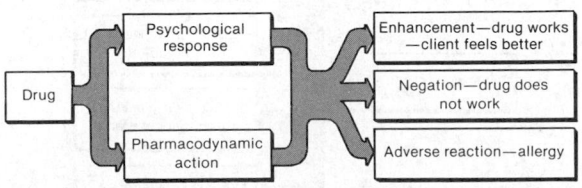

Figure 11-1. The effectiveness of a drug is influenced by psychological response and pharmacodynamic actions.

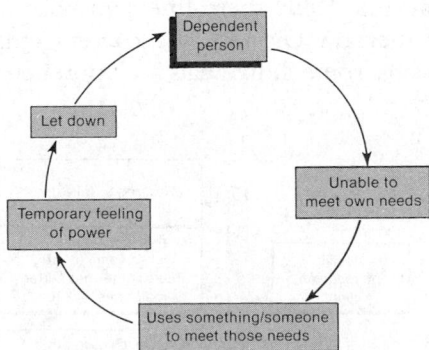

Figure 11-2. The dependent person's use of a crutch may create a repetitious cycle.

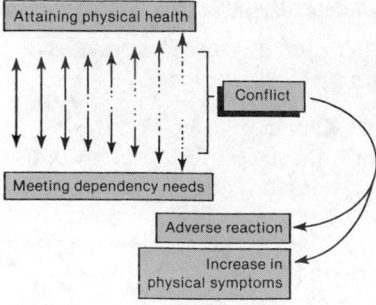

Figure 11-3. The hostile and resentful client's conflicts influence drug effectiveness.

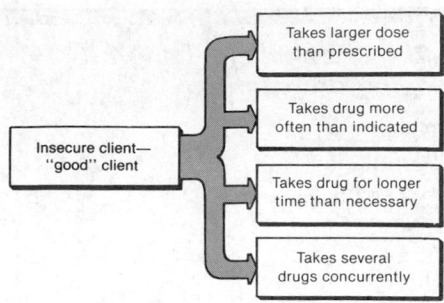

Figure 11-5. The insecure client response.

over-the-counter preparations as drugs. Vitamin C (to prevent colds), aspirin (for a variety of symptoms), or daily laxatives are a few of the commonly overused products. There are other prescribed medications that give a feeling of security, even when causing adverse reactions. One of the most common is digitoxin. The individual may suffer from digitoxin toxicity, yet would not consider contacting the physician or stopping the drug until extremely ill. Belief in the health professionals and efficacy of the drug regimen is so ingrained that the client does not link harmful reactions to such helpful drugs.

Similarly, we have known of "good" patients who have mistakenly been given a drug intended for another patient. The need to be accepted and cared for and to conform is so strong that they would not think of questioning a new or different medication. Some individuals undermine the therapeutic effectiveness of a drug by taking it more often than indicated, by taking the drug for a longer time than is necessary, or by taking several drugs concurrently without any knowledge of drug interaction (Fig. 11-5).

Anxiety and image
Conversely, there are those individuals who need to maintain an image of themselves as being strong. They resent being sick and fear dependency on drugs and other people. Resentment and fear can lead the client to strike out in anger. Often, such attitudes center around role change or loss of role function. These individuals may deny their illness and deny the need for drug therapy. Or, with the current emphasis on natural foods, some individuals are apprehensive about

taking anything into their bodies that may be potentially harmful or may upset the body's balance. Society's strong value on attractive bodies causes even more fear of the deleterious side effects of some medications.

Some of the fears held about drugs pertain to tolerance, addiction, routes of administration, sexual impotence, increased or decreased sexual desires, and side effects of radiation. These fears are seldom talked about but become firmly established and remain hidden in the client's mind, causing anxiety. Here there is potential for the client to undermine the effectiveness of drug therapy by taking a smaller dosage than prescribed, by taking the drug less often than needed, by discontinuing the drug before the course of therapy is completed, or by refusing to take the drug at all (Fig. 11-6).

Power of suggestion
The power of faith, along with a biologic readiness, has led to some spectacular results. This faith can be a religious one or it can be faith in a person, a particular drug, or the health care system in general. A case in point is laetrile, which engendered much controversy over its allegedly beneficial effects. Its effectiveness in the treatment of cancer has not been validated and, in fact, has been repudiated by most researchers. Some clients and their families, however, vouch for its curative power.

Drugs also tend to be more effective when the patient has been assured consistently of the benefits of the drug and has a positive attitude toward health personnel and the health care system.

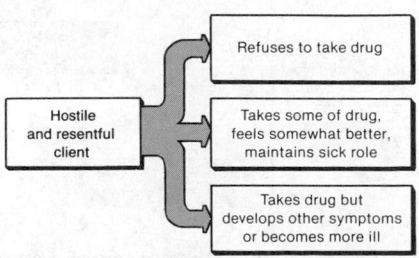

Figure 11-4. The hostile and resentful client response.

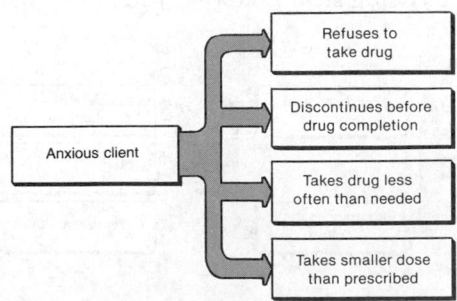

Figure 11-6. The anxious client response.

Positive response

Enhancing drug effectiveness is manifested by a positive response beyond what is usually expected. When penicillin was first marketed, it was hailed as a wonder drug with unlimited therapeutic benefit. People still view antibiotics in this light, although with more caution because of adverse side effects. The power of suggestion strongly affects the therapeutic value of a drug.

Placebos are pharmacologically inert substances administered for positive responses in the absence of direct chemical activity. They are given in the form of distilled water, normal saline, or sugar. The client believes, however, that a drug has been administered and experiences relief. The mechanisms by which this psychological response triggers physiologic effects are not well understood. In the case of placebos for pain, there is a growing belief among researchers that production of endorphins in the brain is stimulated through this treatment. Placebos have been highly effective in alleviating pain and anxiety, sleeplessness, and allergic reactions. They also can enhance the action of other drugs. Nevertheless, consideration must be given to the ethical aspects of administering something different from what the clients thinks they are receiving.

Adverse response

The power of suggestion can also cause adverse reactions. There are occasions when individuals complain of nausea, itching, or headaches shortly after taking one drug that resembled another drug that had produced such symptoms in the past. Or, the patient has symptoms similar to those of a friend or relative on the same drug. The expectation that a drug will produce a specific reaction can, in fact, produce such a reaction. Some health care providers have erroneously used this as a reason not to educate clients about the adverse reactions and side effects of drugs. The nurse is cautioned to thoroughly investigate any claim of hypersensitivity or other adverse reactions. Whether psychological or physiologic in origin, the results can be disastrous.

Type of illness

The type of illness affects the psychological response of the patient to treatment. If it is a chronic illness with a prognosis for minimal or no recovery, the response will be different from that of an acute short-term illness with prospects for a quick recovery. In other words, it is easier for an individual to respond positively when the course of the illness is short and drug therapy is brief.

Often in chronic illness and especially with a terminal disease, Kübler-Ross's stages in dying are seen: denial, anger, bargaining, depression, and acceptance (Kübler-Ross, 1973). The mechanism of denial is often used. Components of it may be found throughout the course of the illness but it is strongest during the first stage. As mentioned previously, denial of illness may lead to denial of treatment. Sometimes this individual, in a state of defiance or self-aggression, will refuse further drug therapy. A behavioral response of this kind may actually grow out of a fear of dependency or of pain, a need to regain some control over one's life, or a fear of dying. In the other stages, the client may refuse drug therapy because of a feeling of hopelessness and helplessness during depression or from anger and the need to strike out at others in the environment. Refusing to go along with the prescribed regimen is an attempt to lessen the psychological pain.

The nurse's behavioral response

Drug response is also affected by the behavioral response of the nurse who administers the drug (see below and Fig. 11-7). The nurse's attitude toward the client and the drug can create either a positive or a negative setting. It has been estimated that the nurse's attitude can increase the effectiveness of a drug by as much as 40%. For example, a caring individual who can instill feelings of trust can increase compliance when working with schizophrenic clients. This trust is important in overcoming a client's lack of confidence in the drug therapy.

Nursing actions have the potential for increasing drug effectiveness. The degree of effectiveness achieved will depend on the nurse's

- Knowledge of the pathologic process of the disease
- Knowledge of the drug administered
- Skill in using this knowledge in interaction with the client and family

Behavioral factors

The nurse's own sets of attitudes, emotions, and drives are developed and reinforced through a life time of social experiences. In approaching clients to adminis-

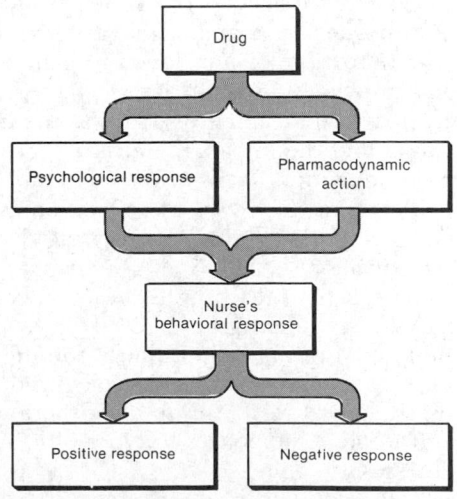

Figure 11-7. The nurse's behavioral response further influences drug effectiveness.

ter a drug, nurses should be aware of their own values and attitudes toward the drug and their emotional response toward the client. Part of this encompasses perception of role, function, and satisfaction of personal need. A particular style of interaction with clients is assumed according to the nurse's own needs. It could be any of a multitude of needs: a need to act out the role of unchallenged authority figure; a need to exert control over others; a need to evade responsibility; a need to be considered efficient; or a need to be a mothering figure. An awareness of one's own responses is an ongoing part of nursing care. Periodic self-evaluation enables the nurse to monitor his or her own actions by asking: Do I voice rejection of the drug's beneficial properties? Do I get angry at the client's refusal to take a medication? Do I project defiance at being questioned about a drug, or show pity or rejection for the client?

Nurses, as potentiators of drug effectiveness, must recognize their own feelings and attitudes and must be alert in identifying the client's ability to cope. The observant nurse, recognizing emotional factors, uses knowledge and skill in reinforcing positive responses to drug therapy and in helping the client develop acceptable alternative responses. The course of drug therapy is affected positively when the client has faith in the efficacy of the drug and faith in the power of health personnel to help (Box 11-3).

Box 11-3. Nurses as potentiators of drug effectiveness

For maximum effectiveness, the nurse should:

- Understand the relationship between physical and psychological responses
- Recognize the influence of attitudes and values on the response to drug therapy
- Develop an awareness of his or her own attitudes to drugs and client response
- Use knowledge of motivation in planning and implementing care
- Identify the meaning of drugs to the individual and the impact the ensuing feelings have on drug effectiveness
- Understand the power of suggestion in enhancing, decreasing, or negating drug effectiveness
- Initiate patient teaching from initial contact through discharge
- Be knowledgeable about drugs administered, and observant of physiologic and psychological responses to drug therapy
- Differentiate responses to types of illnesses.

Learning experience 11-1

With another student, role play a client in the following situations. Each of you take turns as nurse and as client.

- An individual recently diagnosed as having cancer, with chemotherapy scheduled within the week
- An individual with moderate hypertension, who must take an antihypertensive for the rest of his or her life
- An individual on a course of antibiotic for acute ear infection, with the original dosage given intramuscularly
- An individual on a mild analgesic for monthly discomfort of menstruation

For each situation, identify your responses to the drug therapy. What attitudes affect your responses? Does the length of time, degree of threat to life, type of medication, or route of administration influence your behavior? Identify those differences of attitudes and feelings when taking on the client role as opposed to the nurse role.

Summary

Each person has a unique response to drugs. Both physiologic and psychological factors modify drug action. Attitudes are influenced by genetic makeup and dominant environmental pressures. Motivation, including drive, incentive, and need, further influence the client's response to drugs. The client also attaches a particular significance to drugs. Drug taking may bring out feelings of dependency, anger, resentment, hostility, security, well-being, and anxiety. The power of suggestion may lead to a positive or adverse response. The type of illness plays a large part in the client's response to drug taking, whether the illness is short-term or terminal. Finally, the behavior of the nurse toward the drug and drug taking can strengthen, modify, or alter the client's response. The psychological factors that modify drug action may also influence the degree of compliance with the drug regimen.

Nursing management

As nurses go through each step of the nursing process during the administration of drugs, they should be aware of psychological factors and plan accordingly when developing interventions.

Nursing process

Assessment   Part of the assessment should include an evaluation of the client's attitude toward drugs and drug taking. By identifying the meaning the drug has for the client, the nurse is able to take actions that promote client compliance. Use of such data leads to an accurate diagnosis of problem areas in following a drug regimen.

Nursing diagnosis   Problem areas arise from a client's refusal to take a drug, or from a drug's inappropriate use, whether decreased or increased. Problems may also occur with those clients who comply too readily. There are situations where the client should question continued use of a drug, or specific dosages. Possible nursing diagnoses include:

> Noncompliance (refusal to take the drug or overmedication) related to unmet dependency needs, to fear of loss of control, or to lack of knowledge about drug action.
> Knowledge deficit regarding drug action.

Planning   A plan of care specific to the client's needs might include such goals as appropriate use of drugs, an increased awareness of behavior, and an improved response to drugs.

Intervention   Interventions for the noncompliant client would include client education, as well as identification and exploration of feelings and attitudes. Helping the client identify whatever feelings are aroused and to verbalize these feelings can help that person understand or become more aware of his or her behavior. Often individuals are not aware of their responses because attitudes toward drug taking accumulate over the years. It is beneficial for these clients to actively explore their behaviors with a concerned, nonjudgmental nurse.

Effective nursing care includes the client in decision making, always making sure that the goals of both nurse and client are congruent. It also includes identifying areas of responsibility for both client and nurse. Such nursing judgments reflect an awareness of the degree of client self-care or nursing care that will be needed. Otherwise, the effectiveness of the drug therapy can be undermined.

If the nurse feels a strong emotional response while administering a drug or initiating other treatment, it is an indicator that a personal value, belief, or attitude has been triggered. This influences the nurse's behavior toward the client, which may elicit a particular psychological response from the client.

Identifying each new medication and the expected effects is one way of involving the client in the drug regimen. Alerting the client to potential side effects and risks is another. Finding out how much clients know and understand about the prescribed drugs through discussion opens the way for further education or for correcting misinformation.

Evaluation   In evaluating the effect of medication on the client, the nurse should again be aware of psychological factors. Does further work need to be done to change these factors? Do problems lie with the client, the nurse, or the family? These factors need to be addressed repeatedly if optimal effectiveness in drug therapy is to be achieved.

References

Kübler-Ross E. (1973). Letter to a nurse about dying. *Nursing 73*, 3(11).

Bibliography

Irons P. (1978). *Psychotropic drugs and nursing interventions*, chap. 1. New York: McGraw-Hill.
Perry SW, Heidrich G. (1981). Placebo response: Myth and matter. *American Journal of Nursing, 81*, 720–725.
Selander S, Miller W. (1985). Prolixin group. *Psychosoc Nurs Ment Health Serv, 23(11)*, 17.
Smayak S. (1982). Schizophrenic outpatients and the problem of compliance: A nurse's view. *The schizophrenic outpatient, 1(2)*, 10–12.
Stanitus M, Ryan J. (1982). Noncompliance, an unacceptable diagnosis? *American Journal of Nursing, 82*, 941–942.
Wilson R, Elmassian B. (1981). Endorphins. *American Journal of Nursing, 81*, 722–725.

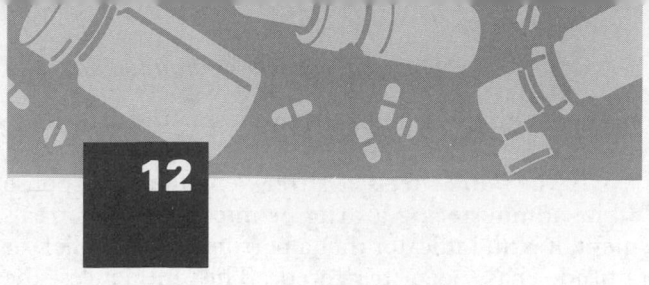

Cultural aspects of drug therapy

12

Sociopolitical influences on Western culture in recent decades have generated renewed interest in naturalism, ecology, and the study of different cultural heritages. The desire to exert more responsibility and control over one's body and lifestyle has led to a resurgence in self-care practices. These self-treatments frequently reflect health care practices influenced by folk remedies and the use of medicinal plants for maintaining health and treating common illnesses. In addition, the depersonalization frequently experienced in today's technologically oriented medical care delivery system may serve as an impetus to examine more traditional alternatives.

The rich variety of ethnic backgrounds in the United States has resulted in a wealth of ethnocultural folk practices that have been passed on from generation to generation. Each of the four major ethnic population subgroups in American society (black, Hispanic, Asian, and Native American) has culturally diverse practices that influence beliefs and interventions related to health and illness (Spector, 1991, pp 171–257).

Choices between ethnomedical options and medical interventions of Western science vary across ethnic groups; these choices are not subject to consistent application from one experience to another. At any given time, treatment may reflect exclusive use of traditional herbal remedies, a combination of ritual and prayer with the use of vegetable drugs, the custom of adhering to dietary and environmental guidelines, or the application of Western medical practices alone or as an adjunct to folk practices. From the traditions noted in folklore for the use of medicinal plants, to the recent scientific studies of the effects certain botanical drugs have in regulating or diminishing the body's response to diseases, a merging of folk beliefs, art, and science is reviving the efficacy of nature's botanical drugs. The science of ethnopharmacology attempts to bridge the gap between traditional uses of medicinal plants and their appropriate role in today's health care practice (Box 12-1).

Ethnomedicine

Factors that influence choices of cures are bound to cultural beliefs about the causes of illness. Ethnomedicine sees the ill client as a composite of psychosocial, cultural, physiologic, and spiritual forces that interact with the environment. This view contrasts with Western medical practices, which diagnose disease by categorizing the pathophysiologic deviations in body systems exhibited as symptoms of illness. The holistic approach of ethnomedicine may be considered an appealing departure from the Western rationale. Exploration of folk beliefs and practices in the black, Hispanic, Asian, and Native American populations reveals cross-cultural similarities in responses to illness. Traditional views consider a response to illness in relation to the spiritual and ritualistic practices that are basic to the religious expressions of the population (Box 12-2). Illness response is also considered in relation to expressions of discontinuity between existing sociocultural norms and the manner in which illness and therapeutic practices have been expressed from generation to generation (Fabrega and Silver, 1973, pp 5–6).

The following discussion intends to represent a composite of known beliefs and folk practices evident in the cultures of different ethnic populations. It is not meant to stereotype various groups; rather, it attempts to develop a historical perspective by describing how culturally diverse individuals are influenced in the ways they deal with health and illness. Indeed, as people migrated from the Far East, Middle East, Europe, and Africa over centuries, customs and practices blended, accounting for the threads of similarity that cross cultural boundaries.

Cross-cultural similarities and distinctions reveal epidemiologic differences in morbidity for a particular problem. This fact may be indicative of the culturally

---

Box 12-1. Variety of treatment regimens

- Use of traditional herbal remedies exclusively
- Combination of ritual and prayer with use of vegetable drugs
- Use of Western medical practices exclusively
- Use of Western medical practices as an adjunct to folk practices
- Adherence to dietary and environmental guidelines

---

specific significance placed on certain disease-related problems. Thus, the same problem may be selectively attended to in culturally unique ways. Etiologic factors do not dictate consistent responses. What may be considered problematic in one situation is ignored in another. The various responses may stem from cultural value orientation and the degree to which a specific condition is endemic to a population. What is commonplace and unavoidable may be considered insignificant; what is unacceptable symptomatic behavior, regardless of the cause, may be denied (Spector, 1979, pp 86–87). Therefore, societal differences in the style of health and illness care practices influence both the degree to which an individual is aware of body symptoms and the decision to act on these symptoms.

Black Americans

Health and illness beliefs

The black population in the U.S. is estimated at more than 30 million, according to the U.S. Department of Commerce (1990, Statistical Abstract of the United States, p 12).

Black people in North America often carry the traditional beliefs of their African heritage (Jacques, 1976, pp 115–124). Health beliefs are congruent with the holistic principles of ethnomedicine (*ie*, health denotes harmony with nature of the body, mind, and spirit). Illness is seen as a state of disharmony that

---

Box 12-2. Determination of health and illness practices of all ethnic groups

- Cross-cultural influences
- Socioeconomic status
- Language facility
- Strength and significance of kinship ties
- Degree to which one accepts beliefs and values of the dominant culture

---

results from natural causes or divine punishment. The desire to restore harmony and thereby the sense of self is the focal point of black folk practices. The individual, the family, and the community are essential interactive and supportive components of the health-belief model.

Survival depends on restoring and maintaining balance and harmony. The practices common to the art of healing and restoring balance stem from a fundamental belief that such power is a divine gift from God. Traditional healing practices may include treatments with herbs, seeking advice from voodoo practitioners, and rituals that have been known empirically to restore health. Folk practices of Native Americans and colonial Europeans have also been integrated into current ethnomedical rituals. Specific forms of healing include use of home remedies, seeking medical advice from a physician, and spiritual healing.

Remedies

No universal rules for selecting the most appropriate provider or efficacious form of intervention exist. In fact, simultaneous use of a variety of practitioners is not uncommon (Snow, 1977, pp 19–95). For example, a family member, friend, or neighbor may possess the gift of healing. Usually, the self-treatment practices recommended through this lay referral system must be exhausted before the initiation of any further consultation. If the client knows and trusts these practitioners, more timely consultation with a physician is likely.

Home remedies and medicines that are natural (made from plants) are important aspects of the treatment process (Table 12-1). The first line of intervention is generally prayer, alone or in conjunction with rituals, and the practice of laying on of hands. Magic rituals frequently include wearing charms or amulets to protect against evil spirits and disease. Folk practices that have withstood the test of generations provide reasonable interventions and comfort measures. For example, the use of hot baths and warm compresses for rheumatism and the use of herbal teas for respiratory illnesses have been validated by their positive results. Frequently, kitchen condiments are used to prepare home remedies. Substances such as lemon, vinegar, honey, saltpeter, alum, salt, baking soda, and Epsom salt are familiar ingredients in folk remedies. Goldenrod, peppermint, sassafras, parsley, yarrow, and rabbit tobacco are a few of the herbs used as medicinal ingredients. Table 12-1 explores the use of home remedies for various illnesses in the black American community.

Members of the black community in the U.S. are well versed in the use of home remedies, and reliance on them reflects a belief in their curative properties. Recognizing, valuing, and accommodating the personal choices of clients who seek care from the modern health care delivery system, while simultaneously

Table 12-1. Common illnesses and home remedies used among Black Americans

Common illness	Home remedy	Preparation
Cold, congestion	Hot toddy	Hot drink prepared with tea, lemon, honey, peppermint, alcoholic beverage
	Vicks Vaporub	As rub, sometimes swallowed
	Hot camphorated oil	Rub hot oil on chest and wrap in warm flannel
	Hot lemon, water, honey	Blended with garlic, onion, parsley, water and drunk
Fevers	Onions	Raw onions on the feet, wrapped in a warm blanket
	Herbs	Herbal teas
Worms	Turpentine, sugar	Mixed together and taken orally
Wound infection/ inflammation	Poultices: potato	Sliced or grated raw potatoes placed in a bag and applied to affected area; as the potatoes rot, the area improves, probably as a result of the mold produced as potatoes spoil
	Cornmeal and peach leaves	Cooked peach leaves with cornmeal are placed in cloth and applied to area inflamed; a fermentation process creates enzymes that are bactericidal
Open wounds	Ground bluestone	This mineral is crushed and applied to wound; it is believed to prevent inflammation
	Salt pork	Placed on cloth and applied to affected area
	Sour milk and stale bread	Milk is poured onto stale bread, wrapped in cloth, and placed on area
Boils	Raw egg shell skin	White skin of egg shell is placed on boil, bringing it to a head

(Spector R. [1979]. *Cultural diversity in health and illness*, pp 236–238. New York: Appleton-Century-Crofts.)

practicing folk medicine, are likely to facilitate a return to harmony in the mind, body, and soul of the client.

Hispanic Americans

The U.S. Department of Commerce estimates that nearly 20 million Hispanic Americans live in this country (1990, Statistical Abstract of the United States, p 14). Eighty percent of the Hispanic population consist of Mexican, Puerto Rican, and Cuban Americans. The remaining 20% have their origins in other Spanish-speaking regions, such as Central and South America (Spector, 1991, p 213 and Delgado, 1980, pp 26–32). In the following discussion, the cultural factors related to health care in the Hispanic population focus on beliefs and practices of Mexican American and Puerto Rican cultural groups.

Health and illness beliefs

Health and illness practices indigenous to Hispanics, as with other ethnic groups, are socially and culturally determined. The acceptance or rejection of traditional folk beliefs depends on the individual's cross-cultural influences, socioeconomic status, language facility, strength and significance of kinship ties, and the degree to which the individual subscribes to the beliefs and values of the dominant population group (Dorsey and Jackson, 1976, pp 41–80). Hispanic cultural influences include European, Spanish, South American, and Indian folk beliefs (including Mayan, Aztec, and other Native American beliefs). The use of folk healers, medicinal herbs, and magic, accompanied by religious ritual and ceremonies, is representative of the rich and varied customs known to the Hispanic people.

Fatalism is a dominant characteristic of the belief system. A healthy state of being exists when the psychosocial, biologic, and spiritual natures are holistically balanced in relation to the environment. Hispanics believe that God is responsible for allowing health or illness to occur. The state of wellness may be seen as a matter of good luck, as a reward for good behavior, or as a blessing from God. The use of prayers, the use of herbs and spices, the wearing of religious objects such as medals, and the maintenance of a balance in diet and physical activity are seen as appropriate ways to prevent evil or poor health.

For Hispanic Americans, maintaining a balance between "hot" and "cold" forces is important to promote wellness. Illness is often categorized as either hot or cold, and the required treatment is determined by the use or removal of hot or cold elements to counterbalance the disease type. To restore the body's balance, hot diseases require cold treatments and vice versa. Classification of diseases also reflects imbalances between wet and dry elements. The characterization of body fluids reflects these attitudes (Spector, 1991, pp 214–215):

Blood: hot/wet

Yellow bile: hot/dry

Black bile: cold/dry

Phlegm: cold/wet

An example of this belief is the use of chili, considered a hot substance, to treat pneumonia, a cold dis-

Table 12-2. Classification of emotional illness in segments of the Hispanic population

Disease type	Common cause	Specific diseases
Mental illness	Heredity	Epilepsy (*epilepsia*)
		Mental retardation (*inocencia*)
	Hex	Witchcraft (*hechiceria*)
		Evil eye (*mal ojo*)
	Derangement caused by worry	Pressure (*congoja*)
		Anxiety (*tirisia*)
	Derangement caused by fright	Nervous breakdown (*ataque de nervios*)
		Hysteria (*histeria*)
	Derangement caused from a blow to the head	Craziness (*locura*)
		Amnesia (*amnesia*)
Moral illness	Vice	User of drugs (*drogadicto*)
		User of marijuana (*marijuanero*)
	Weakness of character	Alcoholism (*alcoholismo*)
		Kleptomania (*cleptomania*)
	Emotions	Jealousy (*celos*)
		Rage (*coraje*)

(Kay M. [1977]. Health and illness in a Mexican American barrio. In Bauwens E, cd. *Ethnic medicine in the Southwest*, pp 126–127. Tucson: University of Arizona Press.)

ease. Other rules adhered to for maintaining balance include getting the head wet to avoid a sore throat from wet feet, the abstinence from pork (a cold food) after childbirth (a hot experience), the use of penicillin (a hot drug) to treat pneumonia (a cold disease; Kay, 1977, pp 99–166).

Illnesses (*enfermedad*) generally are classified as physical in nature when they have to do with the body and natural when they have to do with emotional or natural forces. Symptoms of physical illness may include fever (*calentura*), pain (*dolor*), nausea or vomiting (*basca*), cough (*tos*), or rash (*erupcion*). Physical illness is thought of as benign or mild, temporary, or grave.

Hispanic Americans tend to categorize emotional illnesses as either mental or moral. Table 12-2 classifies these illnesses and includes specific diseases in each category.

The range of diseases recognized by an individual and the choice of interventions depend on the degree of acculturation in white American society. It is important to remember that folk beliefs and traditional ethnopharmacologic practices may be person-specific. What may be common practice for treating an illness in one family may be contraindicated, or simply unheard of, in another. However, the practices that are consistent among Hispanic people can be studied and understood by those outside the culture.

In addition to physical or emotional illnesses that result from body imbalances, external supernatural or magic causes, envy, or intense emotional states, a fifth cause exists. This category reflects the belief that dislocation of body parts can cause illness. For example, a depressed anterior fontanelle in an infant is believed to be caused by touching the area (usually by medical personnel). Therefore, when examining an infant, the practitioner should be alert to this interpretation. Recognizing the interrelationships between folk beliefs and traditional health and illness practices is essential to understanding the cultural implications of drug use chosen to remedy disease.

Remedies

Assessing an illness to determine its identity and seriousness is a systematic, almost scientific, practice carried out by Hispanic women. They methodically consider signs and symptoms and balance them against what is believed to be health. A strong dichotomy between biophysical and supernatural illnesses does not seem to exist in Hispanic ethnomedical practices. Folk illnesses tend to represent the core group of ailments, but it is not uncommon to mix remedies that may be magical and biophysical to cure a single illness. Hispanic ethnopharmacology is notably more complementary to, rather than competitive with, Western medical practices. Table 12-3 identifies the core groups of the more commonly used botanical remedies and the conditions for which they are used.

The consideration of appropriate treatment follows identification of the specific illness. Three options commonly are available: home remedies (*remedio caseros*), which use medicinal vegetables and herbs; over-the-counter patent medicines, such as Alka Seltzer, Pepto-Bismol, or aspirin; and physician-prescribed medications. Herbs may be collected, dried, and stored by individual households, or they may be purchased in local herb stores. Most remedies are used

Table 12-3. Ethnopharmacologic treatments for common illnesses

Spanish name	English name	Botanical name	Ailments treated (usually in teas)
Manzanilla	Camomile	*Matricaria chamomilla*	Cure colic; soothe nausea, vomiting, cramps; alleviate mild vaginal or throat infection; cure *susto* (fright)
Savila	Aloe vera	*Aloe barbadensis* / *Aloe vera*	Treat burns, infected wounds, ulcers, acne, diabetes, constipation
Ruda	Rue	*Ruta graveolens*	Used in heated oil to treat earache; to treat upset stomach; to induce menstruation; to decrease postpartum pain
Yerba aniz	Anise	*Pimpinella anisum*	Mild sedative; to treat constipation; to treat stomach cramps; to cure *susto*
Yerba buena	Spearmint	*Mentha spicata*	Cure for colic, nervousness, colds, stomach upset, intestinal parasites, menstrual cramps
Estafiate	Wormwood	*Artemisia absinthium*	Treat flatulence, diarrhea, colic, nausea, stomach ache
Te de naranjo	Orange leaves	*Citrus aurantium*	Sedative; treat nervousness, colic, menstrual cramps
Albacar	Sweet basil	*Osimum basilicum*	To cure *susto*; used to ward off evil spirits; treat infections, insomnia, sores
Oregano	Oregano	*Monarda menthaefolia*	Treat colds, coughs, congestion, sore throat
Ajo	Garlic	*Allium sativum*	Treat insect bite, insomnia, toothache, earache
Canela	Cinnamon	*Pulchea orodata*	Cough
Romero	Rosemary	*Rosemarinus officinalis*	To induce menstruation
Borraja	Borage	*Borago officinalis*	Cough; to induce menstruation
Cenizo	Purple sage	*Leucophyllum texanum*	Stomach ache, whooping cough
Rosa de castillo	Rose	*Rosa centifolia*	Purge; to induce menstruation
Marijuana	Marijuana	*Cannabis sativa*	Nervousness

in the form of teas, infusions, or poultices to cure mild illnesses. Digestive problems may be relieved by drinking a mild mint tea. Colic may be treated with anise, rosemary, or camomile tea. A cough may be treated with oregano tea.

Ailments with a core group common to folk illnesses are stomach ache, menstrual disturbances, pneumonia, sores, and whooping cough (Trotter, 1981, pp 216–221). Ethnopharmacologic treatments used by Hispanic populations to cure these conditions are applied in a variety of forms, either as a single agent or as a combination of ingredients in a designated preparation.

Remedies used to cure stomach aches are usually prepared as teas that include wormwood, rue, sweet basil, cinnamon, purple sage, horehound, and coriander, as well as the ingredients already mentioned. Garlic is sometimes eaten raw for this problem, and a poultice made of bloodworm, egg mixture, corn tortilla, or other food mixtures may be applied to the stomach for relief (Trotter, pp 216–221, 1981).

Menstrual disturbances may be treated with a tea brewed from borage, bush pepper, rosemary, camomile, rose petals (rue), or cinnamon and aspirin. Sores are treated with remedies prepared in baths, including olive oil, sunflower, and copperleaf. Sores may also be cured by using herbs prepared in poultices that use sweet basil, onion, swallow wort, gum plant, or sunflower oil and butter (Trotter, 1981, pp 216–221).

Black burro's milk or teas brewed from purple sage are believed to be useful in treating whooping cough. Pneumonia may be treated with teas made from mallow or mint (Trotter, 1981, pp 216–221).

With options from both ethnomedicine and conventional medicine, the choice of remedies seems to be influenced by several factors, including one's personal experience, the severity of the illness, and the degree to which symptoms are accommodated in known folk-treatment modalities.

Puerto Rican Americans

The Puerto Rican concepts of disease etiology are similar to those of other Hispanic peoples. Puerto Ricans share the Hispanic belief in the doctrine of hot and cold.

Health and illness beliefs

Puerto Rican Americans credit metaphysical forces in the form of supernatural spirits with causing psychosomatic or incurable illnesses. This belief stems from a "personalistic" concept of disease etiology. The view that health is a state of equilibrium, with illness resulting from physical causes or conditions, reflects the "naturalistic" concept of disease etiology subscribed to by Puerto Rican people. Maintaining a balance between hot and cold is characteristic of the naturalistic belief system.

Remedies

The naturalistic view of disease posits that ailments, foods, and medicines or herbs have cold or hot properties. The hot or cold characteristics do not necessarily denote actual physical temperature, color, or shape.

Treatments for hot or cold illnesses require selection of substances that counterbalance the hot or cold quality of the disease. Common cold conditions, such as respiratory infections or menstruation, require hot remedies, such as chocolate or alcohol, and spicy or hot foods, such as onions or garlic. Hot conditions, including ulcers, constipation, or diarrhea, respond to treatment with cold or cool substances, such as fruits. Table 12-4 identifies the hot, cool, and cold classifications of body conditions, herbs and medicines, and foods.

The practitioner should be aware of and be sensitive to these cultural practices. Table 12-5 describes conditions and the behavioral characteristics of clients who believe in the naturalistic approach. A client who seeks a solution to health problems may use resources from both traditional and conventional health care delivery systems.

Asian Americans

Americans of Asian descent have their roots in Japan, the Philippines, Korea, Laos, Hawaii, China, Cambodia, Vietnam, and Thailand. The total Asian–American population is estimated to be about 3.5 million.

Folk medicine practices and traditional beliefs about health and illness are similar because of common influences from ancient philosophies and practices shared by most Asian cultures. These practices include meditation, special nutritional programs, herbology, and martial arts. A major difference between Eastern and Western cultures is the practice of health promotion and illness prevention. Asians practice prevention, whereas Western European concepts of health care emphasize illness intervention and treatment. These different values are reflected in varying degrees in the U.S. Many Chinese people who emigrated from their country in the 1920s still practice traditional healing and prevention and continue to influence family health practices. First- and second-generation Asian Americans blend Western medicine with aspects of traditional folk beliefs as part of their new lifestyle in the U.S.

Health and illness beliefs

For Asian Americans, harmony with nature is essential for physical and spiritual well-being. Universal balance depends on harmony between the elemental forces of fire, water, wood, earth, and metal. These forces are continuously interacting, creating the natural balance of elements in the world (Campbell and Chang, 1973, pp 245–247).

Table 12-4. The hot–cold classification among Puerto Rican Americans

	Frio (cold)	Fresco (cool)	Caliente (hot)
Illnesses or bodily conditions	Arthritis		Constipation
	Colds		Diarrhea
	Frialdad del estomago (cold stomach)		Rashes
	Menstrual period		Tenesmus (*pujo*)
	Pain in the joints		Ulcers
	Pasmo (shaky, chills)		
Medicines and herbs		Bicarbonate of soda	Anise
		Linden flowers (*flor de tilo*)	Aspirin
		Mannitol (*mana de Manito*)	Castor oil
		Mastic bark (*almacigo*)	Cinnamon
		$MgCO_3$ (*magnesia boba*)	Cod liver oil
		Milk of magnesia	Fe tablets
		Nightshade (*yerba mora*)	Penicillin
		Orange-flower water (*agua de azahar*)	Rue (*ruda*)
		Sage	Vitamins
Foods	Avocados	Barley water	Alcoholic beverages
	Bananas	Bottled milk	Chili peppers
	Coconut	Chicken	Chocolate
	Lima beans	Fruits	Coffee
	Sugar cane	Honey	Corn meal
	White beans	Raisins	Evaporated milk
		Salt-cod (*bacalao*)	Garlic
		Watercress	Kidney beans
			Onions
			Peas
			Tobacco

(Harwood A. [1971]. The hot–cold theory of disease: Implications for treatment of Puerto Rican patients. *JAMA, 216*[7], 1153–1158. Copyright 1971, American Medical Association.)

Table 12-5. Behavioral characteristics of patients who adhere to the hot–cold theory

Patient's condition	Behavioral characteristics
Common cold, arthritis, joint pains	Patient will not take cold-classified foods or medications but will accept those classified as hot
Diarrhea, rash, ulcers	Patient will not take hot-classified medications and uses cool substances as therapy
Requires a diuretic as part of a treatment regimen and has been told to supplement potassium intake by eating bananas, oranges, raisins, or dried fruit	Patient will not eat these cold-classified foods with a cold or other cold-classified condition (for female patients this includes the menses)
Requires penicillin or any other hot medication, particularly on an ongoing basis	Patient will stop taking hot medicine when suffering any hot-classified symptom (*eg*, diarrhea, constipation, rash)
Infant requires formula, which contains hot-classified evaporated milk	Mother will put baby on cold-classified whole milk or will, after feeding formula, "refresh" the baby's stomach with various cool substances, some of which are diuretic
Pregnant	Woman avoids hot medicine and hot foods and takes cool medicine frequently
Postpartum and during menstruation	Woman avoids cool foods and medicines, particularly those that are acidic

(Harwood A. [1971]. The hot–cold theory of disease: Implications for treatment of Puerto Rican patients. *JAMA, 216*[7], 1153–1158. Copyright 1971, American Medical Association.)

Regulating these universal elements are two forces believed responsible for maintaining physical and spiritual harmony in the body, the yin and the yang. The characteristics of yin and yang are described in Table 12-6. These forces provide the energy for monitoring control over the cosmos. Imbalance between yin and yang is thought to be the cause of physical disease or natural disaster (Chow, 1976, p 104).

Chinese physicians receive payment for their efforts to promote health and maintain the body's state of balance. Illness is viewed as a failure by the physician, who is not likely to collect a fee for treatment. Therapeutic options available to the traditional Chinese physician include prescribing herbs, meditation,

Table 12-6. Characteristics of the yin and yang forces

Yin	Yang
Female	Male
Negative energy	Positive energy
Emptiness	Fullness
Darkness	Light
Cold	Warm
Inside of the body	Surface of the body
Front of the body	Back of the body
Body organs: heart, liver, lungs, kidney, spleen	Body organs: stomach, small and large intestines, gallbladder, bladder
Winter and spring diseases	Summer and fall diseases
Control body pulses	Control body pulses
Stores essential life strength	Protects body from outside attacks
Certain foods (*eg*, watercress, winter melon)	Certain foods (*eg*, ginger root, chicken)

exercise, nutritional changes, or acupuncture. Potential body imbalances may be diagnosed through inspection (glossoscopy) of the client's external appearance, a history-taking or assessment of the problem through interviewing (anamnesis), palpation of deep and superficial pulses (sphygmology) to determine the severity of the condition, or use of the auditory and olfactory senses (osphretic) to determine the general condition of the individual (Chow, 1976, p 104). The treatments recommended may require consultation with an herbalist, a spiritual healer, an acupuncturist, or a Western physician.

The importance of health maintenance as the focal point of the Chinese health care system is based on the belief that the body is a gift from one's ancestors and, as such, should be revered and maintained in good repair throughout the life cycle.

Remedies

Maintaining or restoring yin and yang uses the principles of energy flow and balance of the vital organs of the body for health. If the practices discussed previously are insufficient to prevent illness, herbology is used to bolster the body's natural healing forces. Vegetable medicines enjoy a long and significant history in the traditions of Chinese folk remedies. Knowledge about the usefulness of specific agents for healing has been handed down through generations. This knowledge has been systematically studied, observed, experimented with, theorized about, and recorded. The earliest recordings of medicinal herb use are believed to be about 2000 years old. Since 1949, scientific analysis of Chinese medicinal herbs has isolated several valuable chemically active compounds (Li, 1974, p 99). Some of these herbs are identified in Table 12-7. The classification of the herbs is based on their active phar-

(Text continues on p. 139)

Table 12-7. Pharmacology of traditional Chinese herbs

Chinese name	Botanical name	Plant family and plant part used	Active ingredients	Properties/actions
Huai-niu-hsi or *Sun-niu-hsi*	*Achyranthes bidentata*	Amarantaceae	Calcium oxalate crystal, saponin, oleonolic acid, glucuronic acid, k-salt ash	Decreases blood pressure, peristalsis of the duodenum; causes strong uterine contractions in high doses; in alkaloid form, causes blood hemolysis and denatures protein
Fw-tze or *Wu-tow*	*Aconitum carmichaeli*	Ranunculaceae	Alkaloids of aconine and aconitine	Pain killer
Pin-liang-hua or *Fu-she-tsao*	*Adonis amurensis*	Ranunculaceae: whole plant	Cymarin	Slightly toxic, bitter taste; direct action on cardiac muscle, causing contractions, dilation of coronary blood vessels to increase blood flow; useful as diuretic and tranquilizer
Che-hsi	*Alsima plantago-aqua-tica*	Alismataceae: tuber stem with partial root	Volatile oil, plant sterols, alkaloids, resins, proteins, fatty acids, sugars	Nontoxic, slightly bitter taste; antibacterial agent; lowers blood pressure, blood glucose, and serum cholesterol
Tang-Kuei	*Angelica sinensis*	Umbellifera: main and branch roots	Angelicone, angelic acid, vitamin E, sucrose	Dried roots are sweet, aromatic; prepared in water extract—causes uterine contractions; prepared in ethyl alcohol—causes uterine muscles to relax; reverses vitamin E deficiency symptoms; produces calming effect on cerebral nerves
Tung-Kua or *Tung-Kua-jen*	*Benincasa hispida*	Cucurbitaceae: seed meal, whole plant	Urease, hispidamin, purine, trigonelline	Nontoxic; diuretic; treatment of coughs in infants
Chia-hu	*Bupleurum chinese*	Umbelliferae: dried root	Fatty oils, lignoceric acid, volatile oils	Nontoxic, slightly bitter taste; reduces fever; in extract preparation, used to treat malaria
Hung-hua	*Carthamus tinctorius*	Compositae: flower	Carthamiolin (after chemical treatment)	Nontoxic, slightly bitter taste; used as wound treatment that decreases pain and helps healing
Chi-kow or *Chi-shih*	*Citrus aurantium* (bitter-orange)	Rutaceae: fruit, leaves	Aurantiamanic acid, hesperidin, organic acids, linonene, vitamin C	Aids digestion, decreases gas pain by antispasmodic action; sedative
Shau-chu-yu	*Cornus officinalis*	Cornaceae: dried fruit	Cornin, garlic acid, malic acid, vitamin A, saponin, tannin	Chewy, acidic, slightly bitter taste; diuretic action; decreases blood pressure
Yan-hu-so	*Corydalis bulbosa*	Papaveraceae: tuber	Corydaline, protopine, corybulbine, captisine	Odorless, bitter taste, slightly toxic; improves circulation; reduces pain; tranquilizing effects
Pa-tou	*Croton tiglium*	Euphorbiaceae: dried seeds	Crotin, alkaloids, fatty acids, protein ash	Very toxic; strong cathartic that irritates skin and mucous membrane
Yu-chin	*Curcuma aromatica*	Zingiberaceae: tuber stem, root ends	Camphene, camphor, curcumene	Slightly aromatic; used to treat epileptic convulsions and circulatory disorders

(Continued)

Table 12-7. Pharmacology of traditional Chinese herbs (Continued)

Chinese name	Botanical name	Plant family and plant part used	Active ingredients	Properties/actions
Shan-yao	*Dioscorea batatas*	Dioscoreaceae: tuber roots, tubers above ground	Starch with amylase, saponin, allatonin, mucin	In dried powdered form, used as soothing paste for external application
Kan-sui	*Euphorbia sieboldiana*	Euphorbiaceae: tuber root	Palmitic acid, citric acid, oxalic acid, tannin, resin, glucose, sucrose, starch	Toxic, bitter taste, strong odor; used to treat edema, constipation
Kan-tsao	*Glycyrrhiza uralensis*	Leguminosae: root, lower stem	Glycyramarin, liquiritin, mannitol, glucose, starch, sucrose	Mild odor, sweet taste; an additive for herbal remedies; acts like adrenocortical hormones; used to treat duodenal and stomach ulcers
Shib-chi-ching or *Tung-ching*	*liex chinensis*	Aquifoliaceae: seed, leaves, bark	Tannin, volatile oil	Low toxicity; antiseptic agent used locally to treat burns
Mao-tung-ching	*liex pubescens*	Aquifoliaceae: roots, leaves	Theobromine, ilicin	Nontoxic, slightly bitter taste; acts on coronary artery by reducing blood pressure, increasing flow to cardiac muscle
Chuan-chiung	*Ligusticum wallichii*	Umbelliferae: underground tuber stem	Alkaloid, lactone derivative, ferulic acid	Bitter taste, aromatic; used to treat local pain and swelling; extract preparation used to control central nervous system activities
Hou-pu	*Magnolia officinalis*	Magnoliaceae	Alkaloids, saponin, volatile oil	Slightly bitter taste, aromatic; for treatment of respiratory tract
Chuan-lien-pi	*Melia toosendan*	Meliaceae: stems, bark, roots	Margosine, neutral resins, tannin	Very bitter taste; used to treat parasites
Pe-hua-she-shih-tsao	*Oldenlandia diffusa*	Rubiaceae: whole plant	Hydrocarbons, ureolic acid, stigmasterol, β-sitosterol, *p*-hydroxycinnamic acid	Used as diuretic, anti-infective; to treat heat stroke
Pe-shou	*Paeonia lactiflora*	Ranunculaeae: dried root	Volatile oil, benzoic acid, paeoniflorin, paeonol, paeonine, tannin, fatty oil, resin, starch	Odorless, slightly bitter taste; used as general tonic
Jen-seng	*Panax ginseng*	Araliaceae: dried root	Triterpenic saponosides, essential oils, a triester, panaxatriol	Regulates blood pressure; stimulates central nervous system; counteracts fevers; useful as general tonic to produce long life, strength, and happiness
Huang-pai or *Huang-pi-show*	*Phellodendron chinese*	Rutaceae: inside layer of dried tree bark	Berberine, palmatine, phellodendrine, magnoflorine, obakunone, dictamnolide	Bitter taste, slight odor; decreases fever in the treatment of dysentery; used to treat jaundice
Pan-hsia	*Pinellia ternata*	Araceae: tuber stem	β-sitosterolglucoside, choline, volatile oil, sterols, saponin, starch, fatty acid	Essentially tasteless, odorless; used for respiratory congestion; for relief of gas pain and vomiting during pregnancy
Fu-lin	*Poria cocos*	Polyporaceae: fungal growth on the roots of old pine trees	Pachymic acid, polysaccharide, ergosterol, choline, phospholipids, proteins, resins, fats, enzymes	Diuretic used to treat edema; soothes coughs; used as a tranquilizer

(Continued)

Table 12-7. Pharmacology of traditional Chinese herbs (Continued)

Chinese name	Botanical name	Plant family and plant part used	Active ingredients	Properties/actions
Tao-jen	*Prunus persica*	Rosaceae: dried seeds	Fatty oil, amygdalin	Nontoxic, slightly bitter taste; mild cathartic; used to treat general digestive tract problems
Di-huang	*Rehmannia glutinosa*	Scrophutariaceae: tuber root	Mannitol, glucose, rehumannin	Odorless, sweet taste; decreases fever; diuretic action; decreases blood sugar
Ta-huang	*Rheum tanguticum*	Polygonaceae: dried root stem	Glucosides, tannin, quinone derivatives, resins, dextrin, starch, sugar	Aromatic, bitter taste; used to treat occasional constipation
Dan-seng	*Salvia miltiorrhiza*	Labiatae: dried root	Tanshinone I, II, cryptotanshinone	Slight odor, mildly bitter taste; used to treat insomnia; circulatory problems; enlargement of the liver or spleen; hypertension
Di-yu	*Sanguisorba officinalis*	Rosaceae: tuber root	Tannin, sanguisorbin	Slight odor, slightly bitter taste; used to stop bleeding; externally used to treat burns, insect, or snake bites
Mu-hsiang	*Saussurea lappa*	Compositae: dried root	Volatile oil, resin, sugars, camphorene, saussurine, philladrene	Strong taste, aromatic; general health tonic
Huang-chen	*Scutellaria baicalensis*	Labiatal	Baicalin, wogonin	Odorless, bitter taste; reduces fever; diuretic action; prevents miscarriages; decreases blood pressure; increases blood sugar
Pu-kung-yin or *Kung-yin*	*Taraxacum mongolicum*	Compositae: whole plant, roots	Taraxacin, choline, taraxacerin, pectinum	Used to treat external wounds
Lang-yu	*Ulmus parvifolia*	Urticaceae	Starch, tannin, ergosterol, sterols	Nontoxic, bitter taste; external dressing for wounds
Chiang or *Kan-Chiang*	*Zingiber officinale*	Zingiberaceae: underground stem	Volatile oils, resin, zingirol, starch	Hot taste

macologic ingredients. The most common types of ingredients include volatile oils, resins, alkaloids, glycosides, and fixed oils (Lewin, 1990, p 588). Each component is classified as follows:

- Volatile oils, called ethereal or essential oils, are odorous ingredients that evaporate
- Resins are chemical ingredients that include esters, alcohols, and tannols
- Alkaloids are alkaline, organic ingredients
- Glycosides are compounds containing both carbohydrate and non-carbohydrate components
- Fixed oils are long-chain fatty acids and alcohols

Additional herbal plants and their toxic effects on various body systems are discussed later in this chapter. (See also Table 12-10.)

Cultivation of herbs is supported by the Chinese government, and techniques for growing and harvesting are explicit. The potency and usefulness of herbs are influenced by whatever part of the plant is collected, the life cycle of the plant at the time of harvest, the time of day and the season of the harvest, and the processing the plant must undergo (Li, 1974, p 7).

The cleaning process is important to ensure efficacy, increase or decrease potency, reduce toxicity, and enhance storage. It is common for a client to present a prescription for a specific remedy to the herbalist, who measures out the required ingredients and directs the client to prepare the herb by boiling it for a prescribed amount of time in a nonmetal container. It is then drunk as an extract or tea.

Treatment of body imbalances may also be carried out through a practice known as *moxibustion*, which is the custom of applying heat to traditional acupuncture points using the burning herb moxa (*Artemisia vulgaris*). Potency of the herb is determined by its age; it is thought to be most effective if older than 9 years

(Chow, 1976, p 107). Acupuncture is viewed as a cold treatment, whereas moxibustion is a hot treatment.

Native Americans

The Native American population in the U.S. is estimated to include about 200 tribes, in addition to the Eskimo and Aleutian peoples. Tribes with significant populations include the Navaho, Cherokee, Sioux, Chippewa, Pueblo, Lumbee, Hopi, Choctaw, Apache, Iroquois, Zuni, and Creek (Joe, Gallerito, and Pino, 1976, p 81). Each Native American community is unique in its cultural beliefs and language; therefore, discussion intended to represent an overview of popular traditional practices runs the risk of misrepresenting or stereotyping the entire population. The following information is intended to identify a cross-section of traditional beliefs and folk practices (though they may be characteristic of some tribes, but not of others).

As aborigines, Native Americans survived in harsh regions of the country through their understanding of the environment. The Spanish, Mexicans, and Europeans influenced their type of existence, which originally included gathering wild plants and hunting animals for food. Later, Native Americans developed an agricultural livelihood. As the Europeans began to colonize North America, Native Americans increasingly migrated West; California, Oklahoma, Arizona, and New Mexico have the largest numbers of Native Americans today (Scott, Camazine, and Bye, 1980, pp 355–356).

Health and illness beliefs

The theme of total harmony with nature is fundamental to Native American beliefs about health. The human body is both one with and interdependent with the universe. Health for the individual depends on maintaining a state of equilibrium among the physical body, the mind, and the environment. Health practices reflect this holistic approach to health and illness.

Illness is generally believed to be purposeful. It is accepted as a fact of life that happens in relation to a past or future event. One must deal with the external event rather than the illness itself to effect improvement. States of health or illness result from variations in the balance between positive and negative body energies and are thought to be controlled by spiritual means. Methods of intervention depend on a fundamental belief in the principle of cause and effect.

A state of unhappiness, sickness, or imbalance may result from several factors, such as tampering with the spirits, a disruption in the elements of nature, neglecting or misusing ceremonial rituals, or witchcraft (Spector, 1991, pp 337–338). The method of healing is determined traditionally by the medicine man, whose role is to diagnose and recommend the appropriate intervention. The diagnostic phase requires identification of the spiritual cause of an illness by using medication, herbs, and divination. Treatment is accomplished with chants determined through divination.

Divination is practiced in three ways: stargazing, hand trembling, and listening (Spector, 1991, p 339). Recommendations are then made to correct the illness. Treatment may include heat, herbs, sweat baths, massage, exercise, diet changes, or other interventions performed in a curing ceremony.

Diagnosis through stargazing is a learned ritual. Beams of light are believed to determine both the reason for the problem and the prognosis for recovery. Prayers ask the star spirit to identify the cause of an illness. Singing is a part of this ceremony.

In the hand trembling ritual, the diagnostician's hands move while chanting. As the practitioner thinks of a variety of diseases, he moves his hands in a set pattern. An involuntary change in his hand motions indicates he has thought of the correct disease.

The third type of divination practiced by some tribes is listening. The ceremony resembles stargazing, except that the diagnosis is heard rather than seen. Certain sounds represent specific ailments.

Diagnosis of an illness involves a consultation among the entire family and the medicine man that focuses on the condition of the person and the treatment necessary for recovery. Whether an ailment is caused by a breach of tribal taboos or by sorcery, the psychological influence of ceremonies and rituals for curing is significant to the family. These traditions provide personal attention, often for several days, which inspires faith in the predictions made by the medicine man.

Prevention of illness is also valued. Methods used to maintain health include wearing charms, purification through sweat baths, protection from extremes of temperature, dancing, and using herbal decoctions.

Remedies

Traditional folk practices reflected the belief that a person is one with nature. The practice of total body purification, achieved through immersion in water or other rituals, was believed essential to restoring or maintaining harmony. As hunters, gatherers, and farmers, Native Americans developed knowledge about the local vegetation. This information became an integral part of their health-belief system, and herbs were used in purification and healing rituals. Minor illnesses with obvious causes were treated by empirically validated folk remedies. When the ailment was thought to be of supernatural origin, the tribe-specific remedies would be sought from the medicine man. The contributions of Native American practices to the development of pharmacology are seen in the inclusion of more than 200 botanical medicines indigenous to different tribes in various editions of *The United States Pharmacopeia and National Formulary* and other drug directories (Chandler, Freeman, and Hooper, 1979, pp 49–68).

Experts in the medicinal use of native plants or animals were usually herbalists. Herbalists were different from medicine men, though both were believed to have healing powers. Superstition was a factor in determining who was gifted with healing powers. A common practice in herbal medicine was the application of the doctrine of signatures, which was a belief in the principles of "like cures like." Under the doctrine, the selection of a particular plant may be based on its odor, shape, or color. For example, the dandelion stem contains a "milk" that is used to stimulate increased lactation; red plants may be used for blood-related problems; and yellow plants are appropriate in the treatment of jaundice (Chandler, Freeman, and Hooper, 1979, pp 49–68). Numerous species of medicinal herbs are still commonly used by Native Americans. Table 12-8 identifies several ailments and their corresponding folk remedies.

The process of herb collection is prescribed and is based on cultural beliefs and values. Efficacy of an herb depends on collecting rituals that take into account the season of the year, time of day, direction of the sunlight, and phase of the plant life cycle. Autumn is generally thought to be the best time to harvest herbs for drying. The remedial power of a plant is believed to be the result of solar energy, with the early morning rays being the strongest. Therefore, a plant part with the benefit of an eastern exposure is preferable. Respect for nature requires use of only what is essential.

The traditional ways of coping with health and illness remain the first course of action for Native Americans, who have a rich heritage based on respect for self, others, and nature. The isolation and deprivation caused by the conflict of these values with Western values in medical care are taking their toll. The knowledge of traditional medicine is slowly being lost, as access to and availability of culturally supportive programs are limited.

White Americans of European descent

Health and illness beliefs

For white Americans of European descent, home treatments are often the front-line interventions used before seeking help from a modern health care practitioner. Traditional remedies practiced by white Americans of European descent for health maintenance, health promotion, or the treatment of an ailment are based on the magical or empirically validated wisdom of ancestors. These cures are frequently practiced in combination with religious rituals or spiritual ceremonies. For example, an American of Catholic French Canadian descent may wear camphor around the neck for protection from evil spirits, recite prayers for good health, or place a gold wedding ring on an infected eye and make the sign of the cross three times as a treatment for the problem (Spector, 1991, pp 33).

Table 12-8. Herbal remedies used by Native Americans for common ailments

Ailment	Herbal remedy	Plant part used	Active ingredients	Preparations
Skin wounds, cuts, sores	Balsam fir	Gum, underbark	Tannins and oleoresins have astringent and antiseptic properties	Underbark used as dressing; gum or saliva mixed with bark after chewing applied to affected area
	Spruce	Bark		
	Pine	Bark		
	Juniper	Bark		
Bleeding wounds	Tobacco plant	Leaves	Tannins provide mild antiseptic, astringent action	Cuts covered with leaves
	Spikenard			
	Pokeweed			
Infected cuts and burns	Birch	Bark	Methyl salicylate; alkaloids have antibacterial action	Poultice applied to area
	Bloodroot	Bark		Underbark applied to wound
	Balsam fir	Underbark	Tannins and volatile oils have astringent, antiseptic, and odor-masking properties	
	Cedar	Underbark		
Headache	Skunk cabbage	Plant	Tannins, aloe–emodin, chrysophanole, rheine	Snuff prepared from dried plant parts
	Rhubarb	Root		
	Buttercup	Leaves		
Cough	Wild cherry	Bark	Volatile oils have analgesic, diaphoretic, and stimulant properties	Expectorant made from tea
Constipation	Butternut	Bark	Contains irritant substances	Teas
	Dock	Root		
Nausea	Bittersweet	Root	Solanine, solanaceous alkaloids	Teas
Stomach ache	Milkweed	Root	Cyanogenetic glycosides, volatile oils, parasorbinic acid, malic acid, sugars	Teas, syrups, extracts
	Mountain ash	Fruit		
	Birch	Inside bark		
Decreased lactation	Dandelion, *Euphorbia* species	Milky latex in leaves, roots	Flavonoids, amino acids, alkanes, triterpenoids, alkaloids	Toxic; sometimes ingested after giving birth; also applied topically to nipples of breasts

Remedies

Remedies often represent rational approaches to uncomplicated problems. Household products, herbal teas, and patent medicines are familiar products used in home treatments (*eg,* salt-water gargle used for a sore throat, Vicks Vaporub applied to the nostrils to treat congestion, or cough syrup made from honey and whiskey). Applying cold wet tea bags to a sunburned eyelid and using baking soda and water for indigestion are also common home remedies (Spector, 1991, p 33–37).

Ethnopharmacology

"Ethnopharmacology is a multidisciplinary area of research concerned with the observation, description, and investigation of indigenous drugs and their biological activities" (Rivier and Bruhn, 1976, p 1). The outcome of this scientific research can be a better understanding of the usefulness of herbs in the treatment of certain diseases. Experimentation may yield information about the chemical structure of the biologically active components of plants. Such data could aid in the synthesis of effective vegetable drugs. For example, empirical evidence based on traditional folk remedies may suggest that an extract of a substance is therapeutic, whereas use of the isolated active ingredient could be toxic. Scientific investigation also could help standardize doses and specify the types of preparations that would produce more predictable outcomes. It is thought that some of the side effects of chemically active synthetic products could be more easily controlled or decreased by using medicinal plants (Thomson, 1976, pp 2–4). The significance of ethnopharmacology is underscored by the fact that the active ingredients in nearly half of the prescribed medicines used in the U.S. within the last few decades were natural (Chandler, Freeman, and Hooper, 1979, pp 49-68). In addition, it has been estimated that one in seven plants has potential medicinal powers, depending on proper selection and preparation (Schauenberger and Paris, 1977, p 12).

Several medicinal plants and herbal remedies have been discussed in relation to the cultural–ethnic value system in which they are used. Recognition of the active ingredients contained in the plants offers information about their potential use in health care delivery. As noted earlier, plants may contain vitamins essential for good health, nitrogenous organic compounds (alkaloids) that act on the vascular and central nervous systems, antibiotics that attack microorganisms, and essential oils, heterosides (glucides or sugars), acids, or minerals that interact chemically to affect certain body organs selectively (Schauenberger and Paris, 1977, pp 13–14). The chemical properties, drug action, and folk use of several medicinal plants are described in Table 12-9.

In addition to the herbs identified in Table 12-9, several other medicinal plants are significant. The purple foxglove (*Digitalis purpurea*) has been recognized for its effectiveness as a diuretic in the treatment of certain forms of heart failure. Its active ingredients include the glycosides digitalin, gitoxin, and digitoxin, which act on the cardiac muscle. The potency and potential for toxicity in the use of this herb are well recognized (Schauenberger and Paris, 1977, p 188). Other plants used in the treatment of various heart ailments include hawthorn (*Crataegus oxyacantha*), which contains flavonoids and leucoanthocyanidins; American hellebore (*Veratrum viride*), which contains a glycoside and alkaloids and has hypotensive actions; and rauwolfia (*Rauwolfia serpentina*), the main ingredient of which (reserpine) has hypotensive and sedative action (Thomson, 1976, pp 31–34).

Several medicinal plants have been experimented with as cancer cures. These include American mandrake root (*Atropa mandragora*), meadow saffron or autumn crocus (*Colchicum autumnale*), and periwinkle (*Catharanthus roseus*). Mandrake contains a highly irritating resin that has been used by Native Americans as a purgative, an emetic, and as a treatment for condyloma acuminatum (venereal warts). The latter is the only officially recognized use of this medicinal plant today (Thomson, 1976, pp 45–47). Meadow saffron contains the active ingredient colchicine, which prevents the division of cells. It is highly toxic and has been used historically in the treatment of certain forms of leukemia, as well as to alleviate the pain of acute gout and arthritis (Schauenberger and Paris, 1977, p 31). Periwinkle contains the two alkaloids vinblastine and vincristine, which are used to treat malignant conditions in which the proliferation of white cells is significant.

Many medicinal plants are recognized for their soothing qualities. The opium poppy (*Papaver somniferum*) is one of the oldest and best known of the pain-relieving herbs. This plant is chemically complex, with more than 25 alkaloids, fatty oils, lecithin, and albumin. The pain-relieving and sedative qualities of the opium poppy are found in its morphine and narcotine alkaloids (Schauenberger and Paris, 1977, p 48). Henbane (*Hyoscyamus niger*), common lettuce (*Lactuca virosa*), and cocaine, an alkaloid from the leaves of the *Erythroxylon coca* plant, are also used to reduce pain or to promote sedation. Henbane is a toxic plant with the active ingredients of several alkaloids, including scopolamine, hyoscyamine, and atropine. Its pharmacologic properties produce analgesia and sedation (Schauenberger and Paris, 1977, p 39).

Cocaine is one of the oldest known anesthetics. It was the first effective local anesthetic. Today, it is more commonly used as a topical anesthetic in certain clinical procedures or for minor surgery of the eye, nose, ear, throat, rectum, or vagina. Folk use of cocaine in general tonics was common because the alkaloids acted

Table 12-9. Common medicinal plants

Herb (part used)	Botanical name	Properties	Active components	Folk uses
Alfalfa, lucerne (leaves, seeds)	*Medicago sativa*	Antihemorrhagic, antianemic, nutritive, stimulant	Leaves contain vitamins A, C, D, E, K, calcium, potassium, iron, phosphorus	Healing ointment, arthritis, strength giving
Aloe (leaves)	*Aloe vera*	Laxative	Arthracenosides	Externally for healing wounds and treatment of burns; internally for chronic constipation
Anise (seed)	*Pimpinella anisum*	Diuretic, gastric stimulant, relieves flatulence and cramps, galactogenic	Essential oils of anethole and estragol, fatty oil, choline	Dry cough, flatulence
Bayberry (bark)	*Myrica carolinensis*	Emetic, general stimulant, astringent	Tannin	Gargle, mouth rinse for bleeding gums, douche
Blessed thistle	*Cnicus benedictus*	Appetite stimulant, diaphoretic, emetic, expectorant, diuretic (in high doses—causes burns of esophagus and mouth and may cause diarrhea)	Tannin, mucilage, essential oil, sesquiterpenoid lactone	Digestive problems, reduces fevers, breaks up congestion
Bugleweed (flowers)	*Ajuga reptans*	Astringent, tranquilizer, sedative	Tannin	Treatment of sore throat, coughs, appetite stimulant, relieves pulmonary bleeding
Catnip, wild catmint (leaves)	*Nepeta cataria*	Antidiarrhetic, diaphoretic, antispasmodic	Essential oil with thymol, caroacrol, nepetol, nepetalactone	Chronic bronchitis, diarrhea
Camomile (whole plant)	*Anthemis nobilis*	Antispasmodic, gastric stimulant	Chamazulene, coumarin, flavonic heterosides	Internally for migraines, gastric cramps, anxiety; externally for treatment of wounds, ulcers, conjunctivitis
Cayenne pepper (fruit, seeds)	*Capsicum frutescens*	Stimulant irritant, toxic in large doses	Aromaticamide, capsaicine, capsanthine	Stimulant, burn treatment wound treatment, relief of toothaches
Chestnut—(horse fruit, bark)	*Aesculus hippocastanum*	Narcotic, astringent, outer skin of fruit is toxic	Saponins, tannins, glycoside, flavones	Fluid extract of fruit used for sun protection, bark used for fevers
Chicory, wild succory (root, leaves)	*Chichorium intybus*	Tonic, diuretic, gastric stimulant, cholagogic, laxative	Inulin, intybin	Digestive tract problems, gout, stimulate bile secretion
Comfrey	*Symphytum officinale*	Emollient, sedation, wound healing	Allantoin, alkaloid, consolidine, choline, tannin, sugar, mucilage, starch, asparagine	Poultice for treatment of wounds, ulcers, cuts; gargle for tonsillitis
Dandelion (root)	*Taraxacum officinale*	Diuretic, gastric stimulant, tonic, cholagogic (inducing flow of bile)	Lactupicrine, tannin, inulin	Frequently found in patent medicines; treatment of liver and kidney disorders
Elder (bark, flowers)	*Sambucus nigra*	Mucilage, diaphoretic, antispasmodic	Terpenes, glucoside, mucilage, tannin	Used for fevers, chills; gargles for tonsilitis, pharyngitis
Ergot (fungus, not an herb)	*Claviceps purpurea*	Sedative, uterine stimulant	Ergotoxine, ergotamine	Menstrual problems, hemorrhage, migraine headache
Eucalyptus (leaves)	*Eucalyptus globulus*	Antibiotic, respiratory disinfectant, antimuculatic	Tannin, flavonoid pigment, bitter resin, essential oils	Decreases respiratory secretions, cough suppression, topical treatment for wounds

(Continued)

Table 12-9. Common medicinal plants (*Continued*)

Herb (part used)	Botanical name	Properties	Active components	Folk uses
Fennel (seeds)	*Foeniculum vulgare*	Stimulant, gastric stimulant, diuretic, antispasmodic, carminative, expectorant	Essential oils with anethole, fenchone, fatty oil	Enhances lactation; for treatment of colic, flatulence, gout
Garlic (juices)	*Allium sativum*	Mucosal irritant, vermifuge, antispasmodic, intestinal antiseptic, diuretic, expectorant, antihypertensive	Essential oil of allicine, allyl sulfide, enzymes, vitamins A, B_1, B_2, nicotylamide	Cold treatment, antiseptic, diuretic
Ginseng	*Panax ginseng*	Febrifuge, decreases cholesterol level, CNS stimulant	Essential oils, panaxatriol, saponosides	Tonic, weak aphrodisiac, blood pressure regulation
Goldenrod (leaves)	*Solidago virgaurea*	Stimulant, diuretic, expectorant, antidiarrhetic, would healing properties, aromatic	Saponin, flavonoids, essential oil, tannin, bitter compound	Treatment of kidney disorders, treatment of rheumatism, general discomfort, sore throat, eczema
Grapevine (leaves, roots)	*Vitis vinifera*	Laxative, diuretic	Potassium bitartrate, calcium bitartrate	Heart tonic
Hollyhock	*Althea rosea*	Diuretic	Mucilage, pectin, sugar	Chest problems
Horehound	*Marrubium vulgare*	Expectorant	Marrubine, tannin, essential oil	Respiratory problems, gastrointestinal disorders
Hound's-tongue (roots, aerial parts)	*Cynoglossum officinale*	Antidiarrhetic, toxic to some animals	Tannin, alkaloids	Diarrhea treatment
Ivy (leaves)	*Hedera helix*	Antispasmodic, berries are toxic, irritant	Saponin, hederagenine, acid	Treatment of rhinitis, cataracts
Juniper (berries)	*Juniperus communis*	Gastric tonic, diuretic	Essential oil containing alphapinene, cadinene, camphene, terpineol, organic acids, sugar	Stomach tonic, enhances appetite and digestion, diuretic, disinfectant of urinary tract
Licorice (root)	*Glycyrrhiza glabra*	Demulcent, expectorant, antispasmodic, diuretic	Saponoside, glycyrrhizin, flavonoids, steroid hormones	Soothes cough, prevents thirst, treatment of stomach ulcers
Lily of the valley (flowers)	*Convallaria majalis*	Powerful cardiotonic, antispasmodic, purgative, diuretic	Cardenolides, saponoside	Headaches, treatment of heart conditions, but may be toxic
Mandrake (roots)	*Atropa mandragora*	Diuretic, sedative, mydriatic	Alkaloids, scopolamine and hyoscyamine	Fertility aid
Marigold (leaves, flowers)	*Calendula officinalis*	Choleretic, antiphlogistic, vulnerary properties, diaphoretic	Resin, essential oil, saponin	Relief of muscle tension, enhances wound healing
Mistletoe (leaves)	*Viscum album*	Peripheral vasodilator, diuretic, hypotensive, narcotic, antispasmodic, toxic in large doses, cardiotonic	Saponoside, amyrines, viscotoxin	Treatment of hysteria, epilepsy, relieves menstrual cramps, sleeping agent
Mullein (flowers)	*Verbascum thapsus*	Expectorant, soothing gargle	Saponins, lanceolate	Smoked as decongestant, sedative as tea
Mustard (whole plant)	*Sisymbrium officinale*	Sedative, gastric stimulant, diuretic, cooling	Sulphur compounds, cardenolides	Purgative, expectorant, treatment of hoarseness
Nightshade (leaves, roots)	*Atropa belladonna*	Highly toxic, spasmolytic, sedative, diuretic, mydriatic	Hyoscyamine, scopolamine	Stimulates circulation, treatment of eye diseases, decreases smooth muscle activity
Parsley (seeds, leaves)	*Petroselinum crispum*	Diuretic, gastric stimulant, carminative, expectorant	Essential oil with apiol and myristicin, flavones, apiine, pinene, vitamin C	Jaundice, coughs, asthma, amenorrhea, dysmenorrhea, conjunctivitis

(Continued)

Table 12-9. Common medicinal plants (Continued)

Herb (part used)	Botanical name	Properties	Active components	Folk uses
Peppermint (leaves)	*Mentha piperita*	Antispasmodic, carminative, tonic, stimulant, aromatic	Essential oil with menthol menthone, jasmone, alcohol, aldehydes, tannins	Nervousness, insomnia, cramps, dizziness, coughs
Rosemary (leaves)	*Rosemarinus officinalis*	Stimulant, antispasmodic, stimulates bile secretion (toxic in large quantities), astringent	Essential oil with eucalyptol, borneol, ester, pinene	External: in ointment, to soothe rheumatism, sprains, wounds, bruises, eczema; internal: gastric stimulant, relieves flatulence, stimulates bile release from gallbladder, relieves colic
Saffron (flowers)	*Crocus sativus*	Appetite stimulant, regulates menstruation, sedative, diaphoretic	Glycoside (picrocrocine)	Amenorrhea, hysteria, used as an abortive agent, dysmenorrhea
Sarsaparilla (roots)	*Smilax regelii*	Enhances metabolism, enhances absorption, diuretic	Saponosides, essential oil, resin	Skin disorders, reheumatism
Slippery elm (bark)	*Ulmus fulva*	Tonic, astringent	Tannin, mucilage	Soothes stomach; diuretic, diaphoretic, antidiarrhea agent
Soapwort (rhizone, leaves, roots)	*Saponaria officionalis*	Purgative, expectorant, diuretic, detergent	Saponin (saporubine), saponarin, vitamin C	Relief of cough, congestion; to loosen secretions
Sweet violet (flowers)	*Viola odorata*	Expectorant, soothes coughs, antihypertensive	Saponins, alkaloid, aromatic compounds	Expectorants for treating respiratory disorders, purgative, emetic
Thyme (garden)	*Thymus vulgaris*	Antiseptic, deodorant, vermifuge, carminative	Essential oil, tannin, antibiotic and bitter compounds	External: liniment for wounds, in compresses, and as gargle; internal: antidiarrhetic, soothes bronchitis, laryngitis, relief of gastritis, cramps
White willow (bark, leaves)	*Salix alba*	Tonic, febrifuge, antirheumatismal	Glycosides of salicine and salicortine, tannin	To reduce fevers
Woodruff (dried seeds)	*Asperula odorata*	Deodorant, anticoagulant	Coumarin, dicumarol, aromatic compounds	Flavoring wine, to scent linen, blood purifier
Yarrow, milfoil (whole plant)	*Achillea millefolium*	Tonic, antiseptic, astringent, carminative, gastric stimulant, relieves cramps	Essential oils of eucalyptol, proazulene, achilleine	Used for anorexia, dyspepsia

(Leek C. [1975]. *Herbs: Medicine and mysticism*. Chicago: Henry Regnery; Schauenberg P, Paris F. [1977]. *Guide to medicinal plants*. New Cannaan, CT: Keats Publishing.)

as central nervous system stimulants (Turner, Ma, and Elsokly, 1981, p 293).

Lettuce (*Lactuca virosa*) is a toxic plant that contains several chemically active elements found in the bitter white latex that is exuded when the plant is cut. The latex in dried form is brown and contains the bitter compounds lactupicrine and lactucine, which have hypnotic and sedative actions and have been used in lozenges for the relief of coughs (Schauenberger and Paris, 1977, p 177).

See Table 12-10 for identification of additional herbal plants and their toxic effects on various body systems.

Preparation and use of herbs

Ethnopharmacology is the study of the proper collection, use, and storage of medicinal plants. Often, the clearly recommended rules for plant collection are based on the plant part that contains the vegetable drugs. For example, to avoid insect infestation, flowers are best when collected immediately on opening; drying should be done in an airy, dry, dark environment. Leaves are gathered for drying before and during the flowering season; larger leaves are hung, whereas smaller ones are laid out in a dry, airy place. Seeds require little special treatment. They do well if simply

(Text continues on p. 150)

Table 12-10. A systems-oriented approach to herbal toxicities

Herb name	Botanical name	Pharmacologic principle	Herbalist's use	Clinical effects	Toxicity	Miscellaneous
Central nervous system						
African yohimbe bark	*Corynanthe yohimbe*	Yohimbine	Stimulant achrodisiac	Hallucinogen	Increased BP, fatigue, abdominal distress, weakness, paralysis	Smoke or tea
Broom, Scotch broom	*Cytisus scoparius*	Cytisine, scarparin, sarothamonine hydroxytyramine, sparteine, genisteine	Relaxant	Sedative-hypnotic	Vomiting	Smoke, diuretic, cathartic, emetic
California poppy	*Eschscholtzia californica*	Alkaloids, tryamine and glycosides, coptisine, sanguinarine	Euphoriant	Euphoriant		Marijuana substitute poppy family (opioids)
Cinnamon	*Cinnamon camphora*	Tannin, mannitol, essential oil	Stimulant, carminative, astringent	Stimulant	Local irritant to skin or eye; nausea, vomiting, renal genitourinary irritation	Bark is smoked
Darniana	*Turnera diffusa aphrodsiaca*	Volatile oil, resin, tannin, damianin	Stimulant, purgative, aphrodisiac	Stimulant, purgative, aphrodisiac	Genitourinary irritation	Liquid, pill, smoke; may exacerbate preexisting UTI
Hops	*Humulus lupulus*	Lupulinic acid, lupulon, humulene oil	Sedative, antiseptic	Sedative	?Hemolysis	Not wild hops (*Byronia speciesis* toxic); fruit of plant used as tonic for dyspnea, diuresis
Hydrangea	*Hydrangea peniculata*	Hydragin (glycoside), saponin, cyanogenic glycoside	Stimulant, carminative	Stimulant	Dizziness, chest pain, nausea, vomiting	Decrease bladder calculi, treatment of cystitis, marijuana substitute; smoke
Kava-Kava	*Piper methysticum*	Arylethylene pyrone, flavokawain, methysticin, dihydromethysticin, kawain	Sedative	Sedative, hallucinogen	Yellow pigmented skin lesions; sedation	Drowsiness, pigmented lesions, diuretic, genitourinary antiseptic
Kola nut, gotu cola	*Cola nitida*	Caffeine, theobromine, kola catechin (tannin)	Stimulant, diuretic, astringent	Stimulant, decreases fatigue	Insomnia, anxiety, tachycardia, increase symptoms of peptic ulcer disease	Smoke, tea, capsules
Lobelia	*Lobelia inflata*	Lobeline, atropine, scopolamine, pyrridines	Stimulant, depressant	Euphoriant, antichol inergic	Nausea, vomiting, headache, convulsion, coma; ?hepatotoxin	Marijuana substitute

Common name	Scientific name	Constituents	Use	Action	Toxic effects	Form/comments
Mate	*Ilex paraguayensis*	Caffeine; ?phyrrolizidine alkaloids	Stimulant, diuretic	hallucinogen, laxative, diuretic, diaphoretic	Caffeinism, veno-occlusive disease	Smoke, tea, capsules
Mormon tea	*Ephedra nevadensis*	Ephedrine	Stimulant, asthma, rheumatism, syphilis, fever	Stimulant, sympathomimetic	Hypertension, tachycardia	Tea
Morning glory	*Ipomea purpurea*	Resin, lysergic acid amide	Hallucinogen, purgative	Hallucinogen	Nausea, diarrhea, confusion, coma	Marijuana-like effect
Nutmeg, Mace	*Myristica fragrans*	Myristicin (volatile oil), nutmeg oil, elemicin, eugenol	Hallucinogen, GI disorders, rheumatism, emmenagogue, abortifacient, aphrodisiac	Vomiting	Nausea, vomiting, hypothermia, chest pain, dizziness, headache	Myristicin converted to MMDA; elemicin converted to TMA
Passion flower	*Passiflora caerulea*	Cyanogenic glycosides, harmine alkaloids	Hallucinogen	Hallucinogen, stimulant	Convulsions, decreased blood pressure, temperature, respiratory rate	No report of cyanide poisoning; smoke, tea, capsules
Periwinkle	*Catharanthus roseus*	Indole alkaloids, vinca alkaloids	Euphoriant	Hallucinogen, dry mouth	Drowsiness, nausea, ataxia, hepatotoxicity, seizures, decreased bowel sounds, alopecia	Smoke, tea
Prickly poppy	*Argemone mexicana*	Isoquinolone alkaloids, protopine, berberine	Euphoriant		Visual difficulties, nausea, vomiting, diarrhea	Smoke seeds
Snake root	*Rauwolfia serpentine*	Reserpine, other alkaloids	Tranquilizer, decreases blood pressure	Decreased blood pressure	Bradycardia, coma, diarrhea, dizziness, hypotension, miosis, nasal congestion	
Thorn apple (sacred datura, jimson weed)	*Datura stramonium*	Atropine, hyoscyamine, scopolamine	Hallucinogen, asthma, dyspepsia	Anticholinergic syndrome	Anticholinergic syndrome, contact dermatitis	Smoke, tea, seeds
Tobacco	*Nicotiana species*	Nicotine	Stimulant	Stimulant	Nicotine syndrome	Cigarettes
Valerian (garden heliotrope)	*Valeriana edulis V. officianelias*	Valerine alkaloids and glycosides	Tranquilizer	Tranquilizer	Vomiting, drowsiness	Cigarettes
Wild lettuce	*Lactuca sativa*	Lactucarine nitrates; ?hyoscyamine	Depressant; ?opium substitute; cough medicine, relaxant	Sedative		In cattle, *L. scariola* causes emphysema after eating immature plants
Wormwood	*Artemisia absinthium*	Absinthol, volatile oil	Relaxant	Sedative, analgesic	Seizures, coma	Smoke, tea; use dried leaves and flowering tops

(Continued)

Table 12-10. A systems-oriented approach to herbal toxicities (Continued)

Herb name	Botanical name	Pharmacologic principle	Herbalist's use	Clinical effects	Toxicity	Miscellaneous
Cardiovascular system						
Buchu	*Barosma betulina*	Diosphenol (volatile oil)	Diuretic, also genitourinary uses	Diuretic	Nausea, vomiting	
Foxglove	*D. purpurea* *D. lanata*	Digitoxin, digoxin, gitoxin	Heart stimulant	Cardioactive	Vomiting, bradycardia, dysrhythmia	
Hellebore	*Veratrum viride* *V. album*	Steroidal glycolalkaloids, aconitine veratrum, veratrine, veratrosine	Decreased blood pressure, toxemia of pregnancy	Cardioactive	Vomiting, bradycardia, hypotension	Decreases in blood pressure and heart rate
Oleander	*Herium oleander*	Oleendroside, other cardioactive glycosides; ?nerioside	heart stimulant	Cardioactive	Vomiting, diarrhea	Dried root and rhizomes used in tea or made into tincture enemas
Gastrointestinal system						
Black cohosh	*Cimicifuga species*	Cimicifugin (resin)	Dyspepsia	Dyspepsia, cathartic, emetic	Nausea, vomiting	
Caraway	*Carum carvi*	Carvone (ketone), terpene (volatile oil), calcium oxalate	Colic	Carminative, flavoring agent	Nausea, vomiting, CNS depression	
Cardamom	*Ellettaria cardemonum* *Amonum cardemonum*	Cardemom	Condiment	Carminative, purgative	Nausea, vomiting, diarrhea	
Castor bean	*Ricinus communis*	Castor oil (fixed oil), lectin (ricin)	Laxative, cathartic		Nausea, vomiting, bleeding	Phytotoxin, protoplasmic poison
Coconut	*Cocos rufícera*	Trilaurin	Antihelminthic	Cathartic	Diarrhea	
Dandelion	*Taraxacum officinale*	Taraxacerin (resin)	Dyspepsia, diuretic	May stimulate gastric secretion	Vomiting	High in vitamin A, C, and niacin; protein, fat, iron
Gentian	*Gentiana lutea*	Gentiopicrin (glycoside)	Stomachic	Stimulates gastric secretion	Nausea, vomiting	?Malaria
Golden seal	*Hydrastis canadensis*	Hydrastine, berberine	Dyspepsia, stop postpartum bleeding	Nausea, vomiting	Nausea, vomiting, paresthesia, hypertension, CNS stimulant, respiratory failure	Fatalities; used to mask EMIT urine; toxicology screen for opioids

Common name	Scientific name	Active ingredient				
Ipecac	*Cephaelis acuminata* / *C. ipecacuerha*	Emetine, cephaline	Emetic	Emetic		Wound care
Jalap	*Exagonium purga* / Conquer root	Jalapin glycoside (resin), convolvulin	Cathartic	Watery diarrhea	Volume depletion, excessive catharsis	
Olive oil	*Olea europoea*	Olein (fixed oil)	Laxative	Emollient	Diarrhea	
Peanut oil	*Arachis hypogaea*	Olein	Laxative	Demulcent	Diarrhea	Increases serum cholesterol
Senna	*Cassia acutifolia* / *C. angustifolia*	Anthraquinones	Laxative	Watery diarrhea	Abdominal pain	
Respiratory system						
Grindelia	*Grindelia camporum* / *G. humilis* / *G. squarrosa*	Balsamic resin	Expectorant, asthma, bronchitis, mild sedative	Drowsiness, decreases heart rate, mydriasis, increases blood pressure, stimulate expectoration	Renal toxicity; ?selenium; cardiotoxicity	
Jimson weed	(See CNS system)		Asthma	Bronchodilation	(See CNS system)	
Lobelia	(See CNS system)		Asthma, expectorant			
Miscellaneous: metabolic, hepatic, and hematologic						
Heliotrope	*Crotalaria spectabulis*	Pyrrolizidine			Hepatic veno-occlusive disease, hepatic and pancreatic tumors	
Rattlebox	*Heliotropium europeaum*					
Groundsel						
Viper's bugloss						
Gordolobo	*Senecio species* / *Echium plantagineum*					
Ipecac	*Cephaelis* / *C. ipecacuenha*	Cephaeline, emetine	Edema, stress	Emetic		
Pennyroyal oil	*Hedeoma pulegioides*	Pulegone	Abortifacient	menstrual bleeding	Hepatotoxicity	Seizures, GI bleeding
Periwinkle			Hypoglycemic	(See CNS system)		

(Adapted from Lewin NA, Howland M, Goldfrank LR. (1990). Herbal preparations. In *Goldfrank's Toxicologic Emergencies*, 4th ed, pp 589–593. Norwalk, CT: Appleton & Lange.

allowed to air-dry. The whole plant is cleaned of dead foliage or soil and dried by hanging in well spread bundles. The bark and roots of a plant are best when young plants are used. The process involves washing, cutting into small pieces, then drying. After cleaning, fruit is dried in a low-temperature oven over a prescribed period of time (Schauenberger and Paris, 1977, pp 15–17).

Dried plants may be used for medicinal purposes in various ways. The most common practice is in the form of a tisane. The recipe for a tisane is specific and contains several elements (Schauenberger and Paris, 1977, pp 15–17):

- The basic remedy (which may have two or more ingredients)
- The adjuvant (to balance or enhance the effect of the basic remedy)
- The complement (added to enhance texture or appearance)
- The correctos (usually aromatic compounds to enhance flavor)

The active ingredients of the plants may be preserved in several ways until they are needed for a tisane: in dried powdered form, as a fluid, or as a solid (pill or suppository form). The methods used to prepare the tisane depend on the physical nature of the ingredients. For example, if the vegetable drug contains mucilage, a *maceration* is made; a maceration is an aqueous extraction of the product that has been soaking in cold water for 2 to 12 hours. If the flowers, seeds, or leaves of the plant contain the medicinal ingredient, an *infusion* is made by pouring boiling water on the plant parts. This plant steeps in a covered container for 5 to 15 minutes before it is filtered. When the vegetable drug is found in the bark, stems, or roots of a plant, a *decoction* is prepared by soaking the parts in cold water and then bringing them to a boil gradually. This mixture is cooked for 5 to 20 minutes, depending on the texture of the ingredients used.

Folk practices that use medicinal plants are complex processes that require accurate knowledge for safe use. In the traditional use of herbal remedies, empirical evidence of efficacy was sufficient to sustain the practice of using plants in the treatment of illness.

Applications of ethnopharmacology

Increasing awareness of the cultures of developing countries has focused attention on the use of traditional medicines. Scientists have begun to explore the rational use of medicinal plants within the context of the cultural system in which they are used. This study may lead to further documentation of the pharmaceutical efficacy of certain herbs, the psychosocial value of indigenous cultural healing practices, and the interdependence of mind, body, and the environment for healthy behavior. Penso reports that the use of medicinal plants in the industrialized countries of the world is generally confined to self-treatment with familial folk remedies, whereas in developing countries it is estimated that 90% of therapeutic interventions use vegetable medicines as a basis for therapy. Medicinal plants also compose the raw materials for the synthesis of pure chemical derivatives in the developing nations (Penso, 1980, p 183).

In 1978, the World Health Organization (WHO) set forth criteria for the study and documentation of medicinal plants in the developing countries of the world. The WHO recognized the necessity of using indigenous treatments in the provision of health care. It became important, therefore, to have accurate information about the actual use of botanical medicines in a given region, accompanied by any available scientific data on their pharmaceutical efficacy. The WHO attempted to standardize data gathering and investigations. As a result, the WHO has clarified the definition of medicinal plants and vegetable drugs and has established a procedure for the "botanical and ethnopharmacognostic investigation of a plant used in traditional medicine" (Penso, 1980, pp 186–188). A medicinal plant is defined as "any plant which in one or more of its organs contains substances that can be used for therapeutic purposes or which are precursors for chemopharmaceutical semisynthesis." The term *vegetable drug* refers to "the part of the medicinal plant used for therapeutic purposes" (Penso, 1980, p 184).

The format delineated for the investigation of these traditional medicines contains seven major categories: general information, ecological investigation, botanical investigation, information on the genuine therapeutic activity, other relevant observations, and identification of the plant (Penso, 1980, pp 186–188). The suggested format and criteria for description in each category are delineated by the WHO as follows:

Form for the botanical and ethnopharmacognostic investigation of a plant used in traditional medicine
General information
    Investigating team
        Organization to which attached
        Names of team members
    Person who obtained the plant (name and address)
    Local correspondents
        Healer (name and address)
        Interpreter (name and address)
    Local population
        Ethnographic data
        Ethnologic data
        Linguistic data
Ecological investigation
    Geographical investigation
        Country
        Region
        Locality

Place plant obtained
Climate
Geological investigation
  Type of soil
  Altitude
  Hydrology
  Other plants found in association
Botanical investigation
  General
    Inventory number
    Source of plant
    Vernacular name
    Translation and meaning of vernacular name
    Plant cultivated or picked in the wild state
    Size of plant population
    Extent of availability
    Prospects for expansion
  Description of the plant in the ground
    Type
    General appearance
    Morphologic description
  Preliminary classification
    Time of harvesting
    Conditions of harvesting
    Part collected
    Morphologic description
  Sampling
    Specimen for herbarium
    Specimens for research (quantity)
    Packaging
Pharmacognostic investigation
  Reasons why the plant is regarded as medicinal
    Tradition
    From healer's personal experience
    From its "signature"
  Harvesting or gathering of the plant
    Time of year
    Time of day
    Conditions
    Parts used
    Storage
  The drug
    Treatment of the plant to convert it into a drug
    Appearance of the drug
    Morphologic description
    Storage
  Dose forms used (describe preparation technique)
    Natural drug
    Crushed drug
    Powder
    Juice
    Extract obtained by infusion
    Extract obtained by maceration
    Extract obtained by decoction

Distillates
Soft pastes
Solid preparations
Other preparations
Method of use
  External use
    Poultice
    Liniment
    Lotion
    Other local applications
    Baths
  Internal use
    Chewing
    Ingestion
    Enema
    Inhalation
    Other routes
Therapeutic indications
  Treatment of specific pathology
  Dosage
Information on genuine therapeutic activity
  Information collected on the spot
  Personal observations
Any other information or observations
  Taxonomy study
    Order
    Family
    Genus
    Species
    Variety
  Person who identifies the plant

■ Summary

Health habits and health-seeking behavior are a function of environmental, economic, and cultural background for every individual. What we believe and are taught in the context of our growth and development is heavily influenced by family practices and historical patterns. Differences and similarities in health practices exist among each of the major population groups in the U.S.; the remedies considered therapeutic and the health or illness strategies applied are often steeped in tradition.

Plants and plant derivatives often contain chemically active elements that are found to be or thought to be therapeutic. Medicinal plants are known to play a significant role in the health practices of a number of cultural groups.

Nursing management

Nursing implications

Nursing education provides general knowledge about the impact of diverse cultural attitudes on individuals who enter the health care delivery system. However, the development of sensitivity to and respect for the unique beliefs of different ethnic and cultural groups is something the individual nurse must explore and internalize. Whether cultural beliefs are founded in the realm of magic, spiritualism, empiricism, or rational science, they represent humanity's struggle to come to terms with the limits of the human condition and the complexity of the environment. The nurse should be cautioned to assess each client as a unique individual and not ascribe generalized characteristics based on cultural background. The understanding of different value systems should not result in cultural stereotyping.

Nursing practice requires careful objective assessment of a client's health beliefs, traditional practices, and cultural realities to adjust interventions so that they are not antagonistic to the client's value system. The outcome of nursing interventions should facilitate social and psychological support for the client throughout the health care delivery system; it should recognize the value of traditional folk practices to a person's overall well-being. Therapy that accommodates a client's belief in traditional rituals is likely to encourage compliance and decrease the potential for cultural dissonance or the disenfranchisement of any ethnic group from the health care system.

Clients should be advised of the potential for chemical interactions between traditional home remedies and modern scientific prescriptions and should be encouraged to consider the possible harm that may result if therapies are mixed. Alternative forms of healing must be recognized, however. With this recognition may come the preliminary steps to bridging the gap between the scientific rationalism of medical practices and the consumer's culture-dependent beliefs about wellness and illness.

References

Campbell T, Chang B. (1973). Health care of the Chinese in America. *Nurs Outlook*, *21*(4), 245–247.

Chandler RF, Freeman L, Hooper S. (1979). Herbal remedies of the maritime Indians. J Ethnopharmacol, 1(1), 49–68.

Chow E. (1976). Cultural health traditions: Asian perspectives. In Branch M, Paxton P, eds. *Providing safe nursing care for ethnic people of color*, pp 104–107. New York: Appleton-Century-Crofts.

Delgado M. (1980). Providing child care for Hispanic families. *Young Children, Sept 80*, 26–32.

Dorsey P, Jackson H. (1976). Cultural health traditions: The Latino/Chicano perspective. In Branch M, Paxton P, eds. *Providing safe nursing care for ethnic people of color*, pp 41–80. New York: Appleton-Century-Crofts.

Fabrega H, Silver D. (1973). *Illness and shamanistic curing in Zinacantan, an ethnomedical analysis*. Stanford: Stanford University Press.

Jacques G. (1976). Cultural health traditions: A black perspective. In Branch M, Paxton P, eds. *Providing safe nursing care for ethnic people of color*, pp 115–124. New York: Appleton-Century-Crofts.

Joe J, Gallerito C, Pino J. (1976). Cultural health traditions: American Indian perspectives. In Branch M, Paxton P, eds. *Providing safe nursing care for ethnic people of color*, p 87. New York: Appleton-Century-Crofts.

Kay M. (1977). Health and illness in a Mexican American barrio. In Bauwens E, ed. *Ethnic medicine in the Southwest*, pp 99–166. Tucson: University of Arizona Press.

Lewin NA, Howland M, Goldfrank LR. (1990). Herbal preparations. In Goldfrank et al: *Goldfrank's Toxicologic Emergencies*, 4th ed. Norwalk, CT: Appleton & Lange, p 588.

Li CP. (1974). Chinese herbal medicine. *USDHEW Publication (NIH) 75–732*. Washington, DC: Public Health Service.

Penso G. (1980). The role of WHO in the selection and characterization of medicinal plants (vegetable drugs). *J Ethnopharmacol*, 2(2), 183.

River L, Bruhn J. (1979). Editorial. *J Ethnopharmacol*, 1(1), 1.

Schauenberger P, Paris F. (1977). *Guide to medicinal plants*. New Canaan, CT: Keats Publishing.

Scott A, Camazine S, Bye R. (1980). A study of the medical ethnobotany of the Zuni Indians of New Mexico. *J Ethnopharmacol*, 2(4), 365–366.

Snow L. (1977). Popular medicine in a black neighborhood. In Bauwens E, ed. *Ethnic medicine in the southwest*, pp 19–95. Tucson: University of Arizona Press.

Spector R. (1991). *Cultural diversity in health and illness*, 3rd ed. New York: Appleton-Century-Crofts.

Statistical Abstract of the United States. (1990). National Data Book. US Department of Commerce, pp 12, 14, 19.

Thomson W. (1976). *Herbs that heal*. New York: Charles Scribner's Sons.

Trotter RT II. (1981). Folk remedies as indicators of common illnesses: Examples from the United States–Mexico border. *J Ethnopharmacol*, 4(2), 216–221.

Turner CE, Ma C, Elsokly M. (1981). Constituents of *Erythoxylon coca* II: Gas-chromatographic analysis of cocaine and other alkaloids in coca leaves. *J Ethnopharmacol*, 3, 293.

Bibliography

Albert-Puleo M. (1980). Fennel and anise as estrogenic agents. *J Ethnopharmacol*, 2(4), 337–344.

Ayensu E. (1978). *Medicinal plants of west Africa*. Algonac, MI: Reference Publications.

Bauwens E, ed. (1977). *Ethnic medicine in the southwest*. Tucson: University of Arizona Press.

Bernardi B. (1980). An anthropological approach: The problem of plants in traditional medicine. *J Ethnopharmacol*, 2(2), 95–98.

Delgado M. (1980). Providing child care for Hispanic families. *Young Children, Sept 80*, 26–32.

Delgado M. (1979). Puerto Rican folk healers in the big cities. *Forum on Medicine*, 2(12), 784–792.

Fairbairn JW. (1980). Perspectives in research on the active principle of traditional herbal medicine. A botanical approach: Identification and supply of herbs. *J Ethnopharmacol, 2*(2), 99–104.

Farnsworth N. (1980). The development of pharmacological and chemical research for application to traditional medicine in developing countries. *J Ethnopharmacol, 2*(2), 173–181.

Harwood A. (1971). The hot–cold theory of disease: Implications for treatment of Puerto Rican patients. *JAMA, 216*(7), 1154–1155.

Larkin T. (1983). Herbs are often more toxic than magical. *FDA Consumer*. Depart of Health Human Services Publication No. (FDA) 86–1112. Rockville, MD.

Leek C. (1975). Herbs: Medicine and mysticism.

USDHEW Publication (NIH) 75–732. Washington, DC: Public Health Service.

Lewin NA, Howland M, Goldfrank LR. (1990). Herbal Preparations. In Goldfrank et al: *Goldfrank's Toxicologic Emergencies*, 4th ed. Norwalk, CT: Appleton & Lange, p 588.

Lonnelle A. (1977). *Nature's healing arts: From folk medicine to modern drugs*. Washington, DC: National Geographic Society.

Simmonite W, Culpeper N. (1957). *The Simmonite-Culpeper herbal remedies*. London: W Foulsham.

Sussman LK. (1980). Herbal medicine on Mauritius. *J Ethnopharmacol, 2*(3), 259–278.

Administration
of medications

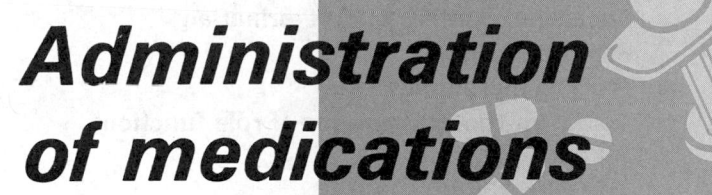

3

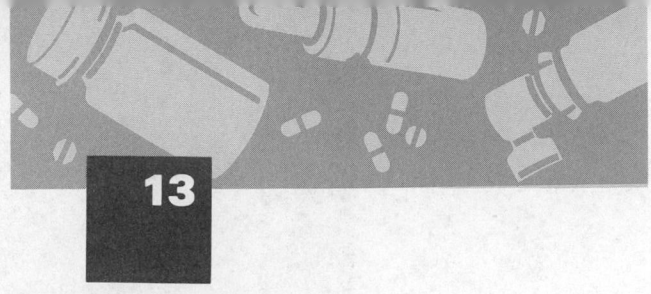

13

Basic principles of medication

Drug therapy is the use of chemical agents to bring about a desired change in a person (Fig. 13-1). Initially, someone has to decide that the use of drugs is appropriate. The recommendation of a specific substance with directions for its use is called a *prescription*. Next, the required chemical is compounded or prepared. Most modern drugs are compounded in factories that employ large-scale production techniques. Distribution of a supply of drug is termed *dispensing*. From such supplies, individual doses must be measured and delivered to the tissues of the client to be treated. Finally, an assessment of the effects of the drug must be made.

In the past, one person customarily assumed complete responsibility for drug treatment. Healers gathered medicinal substances themselves, prepared the dose, administered it to the client, monitored the drug's effects, and cared for the client until the situation was resolved. Today, for situations in which folk medicines are being used, the entire process may still be controlled by nonprofessionals—the person who seeks relief, relatives or acquaintances, and folk herbalists.

When over-the-counter (OTC) preparations are employed, the consumer controls all steps in the process except for compounding and dispensing, which are carried out by the drug industry and the pharmacist, respectively. With this limited number of substances for which no prescription is required, consumers can determine their need for the drugs, purchase them over the counter, administer the drug to themselves, and monitor the results. Only if some adverse reaction occurs must the consumer seek professional treatment. The vast majority of pharmaceuticals, however, are considered too dangerous for unsupervised lay use. Modern medical care is characterized by complexity and specialization. Drug therapy is no exception. Many people are involved in the various processes required for the manufacture, distribution, prescription, administration, and monitoring of drugs used to treat human diseases.

Role functions related to drug therapy

Within the formal health care system, stringent control is exercised over those who carry out the various steps in the process of drug therapy. Among the health care professionals who can be involved in this process are pharmacists, physicians and dentists, physician's assistants, nurses, and technicians (*eg*, respiratory therapists; Table 13-1).

Pharmacist
The preparation and distribution of drugs, whether carried out in a drug factory, a drugstore, or an institutional pharmacy, require the knowledge and expertise of trained professionals. The pharmacist is the profes-

Table 13-1. Role functions related to drug therapy and nursing implications

Role and setting	Responsibilities	Nursing implications
Pharmacist	Is licensed to compound and dispense drugs	
Laboratory of drug firm	Develops manufacturing processes for converting raw materials to dose forms; works with clients in test situations	Nurses have little contact with pharmacists in such settings
Retail drugstore; pharmacy of health care agency	Dispenses drugs; stores drugs properly; may mix solutions; monitors drug therapy; educates clients	Nurses and pharmacists work cooperatively through consultation
Physician, dentist, veterinarian	Determines state of health; identifies disease process; determines treatment; writes prescriptions; modifies treatment regimen; diagnoses and treats significant drug reactions; has the legal right to compound, dispense, and administer drugs	Nurses assess clients, administer drugs, evaluate treatment, monitor client response, educate clients; they also consult with the physician about client response to drugs and changes in the regimen to improve that response
Paraprofessionals		
Physician's assistant	Prescribes drug therapy in certain situations*	It is usually unwise for nurses to accept and carry out orders by a physician's assistant without verification by attending physician unless this is specifically allowed by state regulations
Practical or vocational nurse	Administers drugs†	Nurses provide assistance and supervision; nurses are responsible for competence
Respiratory therapist	Administers most substances given by inhalation other than anesthetics; expert with machines that deliver drugs to lungs	Nurses should be aware of drug administration and monitor client response
Ward clerk, ward manager	Fulfills clerical functions (transcribing of orders, ordering drugs, collecting information on allergies)	Nurses have final responsibility for these activities and must be sure they are properly carried out
Pharmacy clerk	Performs clerical tasks in large pharmacies	Nurses should take action if clerks are observed carrying out responsibilities reserved for professional practitioners
Nurse in institutional setting	Carries out every aspect of drug treatment except prescribing and dispensing; in the latter two areas, the nurse verifies the accuracy of actions taken by other professionals	
Nurse practitioner	All of the above, plus (in some states) is allowed limited prescription privileges	

*Legal status varies from state to state.

†Originally limited to chronic care facilities or private-duty situations; many acute care settings now assign such duties to technical personnel.

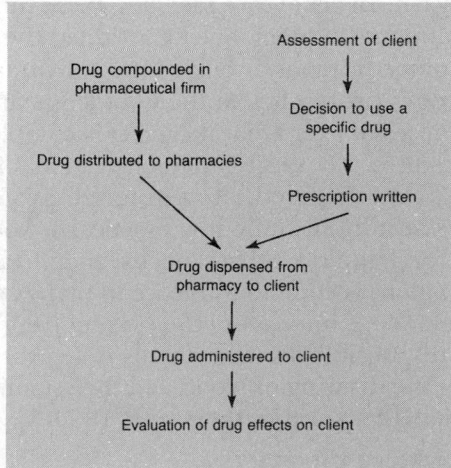

Figure 13-1. Series of events in drug therapy.

sional who is licensed to compound and dispense drugs. The pharmacist's education involves a detailed study of drugs, their chemical, physical, therapeutic, and toxic properties, and the precautions required for their safe use. Pharmacists work in many settings, from the laboratories of drug firms to the pharmacies of health care agencies and the retail drugstore. The nurse works with these professionals primarily in the last two settings.

Pharmacists employed by large drug firms develop manufacturing processes to convert raw medicinal materials into suitable dose units. They work with clients primarily in experimental situations that involve human testing of new substances for treatment.

Pharmacists who work in health care agencies or drugstores are less frequently involved in the compounding of drugs because most drugs arrive from the manufacturer ready for consumption. Pharmacists may have to add solvent to substances that deteriorate after dissolution or mix solutions for intravenous infusion, but these processing procedures are usually a minor part of the preparation. Proper storage of drugs under safe and secure conditions is an important part of their responsibility. Much of a pharmacist's time, however, is usually spent dispensing drugs, or packaging individual prescriptions with appropriate labels that indicate directions for their use.

A recent trend has established an expanding clinical role for pharmacists in the initial selection and monitoring of drug therapy. In institutional settings, this role may include computation of dosages (including loading doses) and adjustments in dosages based on serum drug concentrations and pharmacokinetic principles. These professionals are eminently qualified to recognize actual and potential problems related to drug interactions, toxicities, and adverse reactions. Increasingly, pharmacists are involved in client education and professional consultation with nurses and physicians about drug therapy. These broad clinical roles are also apparent in retail drug stores, where it is common for pharmacists to maintain drug "profiles" (histories) for each client to whom prescription drugs are dispensed. These profiles enable the pharmacist to advise clients about measures to enhance the therapeutic effects of the drug and reduce the risk of adverse reactions. When data on the profiles alert the pharmacist to potentially harmful drug interactions, the physician is consulted for a change in prescription.

Physician, dentist, and veterinarian

Diagnosis of diseases and drug prescription are limited by law in many states to the physician, dentist, or veterinarian. Within the appropriate parameters of the field, each professional is responsible for determining the state of the subject's health (human or animal), identifying disease processes, and determining what treatment is required. When drug therapy is appropriate, the professional writes a prescription or order for the desired preparation. In accordance with this order, the pharmacist dispenses the drug to the client or to the person responsible for the client's care. The professional who prescribes the drug also is responsible for modifying the treatment regimen as necessary and diagnosing and treating significant drug reactions, including toxicity. Physicians, dentists, and veterinarians retain the legal right to compound, dispense, and administer drugs when appropriate.

Paraprofessionals

The extension of medication privileges to paraprofessionals is recent. This trend may well continue. The right of technical personnel to prescribe or administer drugs may be specified by law. The drugs to be used and the situations appropriate for implementation by the paraprofessional are usually precisely defined.

Pharmacy technician

Often, technically trained personnel are assigned to large pharmacies to assist in the nonprofessional activities necessary for the administration of this busy department. In a few hospitals, technicians also administer certain medications such as scheduled antibiotics (Pharmacy techs, 1990). The pharmacist bears the responsibility for tasks he or she delegates to these staff members.

Physician's assistant

The legal status of the physician's assistant varies from state to state, but in many areas this health care practitioner is expected to prescribe drug therapy in certain situations following established protocols. A legal controversy has arisen over the advisability of this practice. Because the right to diagnose and prescribe is limited by law to the physician or dentist, the propriety of delegating this responsibility to a technician has been challenged. In some cases, in institutional settings, nurses have refused to follow the orders of a physician's assistant. The nurses have argued that nursing practice and licensing regulations designate only physicians and dentists as professionals whose prescriptions they may carry out. Moreover, the physician's assistant may have less professional training and experience than the nurse. Nurses fear they will be held responsible for administering drugs without proper authority, should the legality of the practice be challenged in court. The safety of the practice probably depends on the degree of supervision exercised over the assistant by the physician, a factor that can vary greatly according to circumstances.

Practical or vocational nurse

Until recently, the administration of drugs by registered practical and vocational nurses was limited to chronic care facilities or private duty care, in which the nurse functioned under the direct supervision of the physician. In acute care facilities, these nurses are more and more frequently being assigned the administration of medications, provided the individual nurse demonstrates proficiency in the knowledge and skills deemed necessary for accurate and safe completion of the procedure. (A similar demonstration of proficiency is also required of registered professional nurses.) The administration by practical or vocational nurses of oral, topical, subcutaneous, and intramuscular medications is common practice in many agencies. Controversy continues about the current trend to add to these responsibilities intravenous (IV) procedures, including the drawing of blood and the establishment of IV lines (LPNs widen their role, 1990).

Respiratory therapist

Other than anesthetics, most substances given by inhalation are administered by respiratory therapists. This practitioner is a recognized expert in the use of the special machines employed to deliver such drugs to the lungs. Drugs administered by inhalation include gases (air, oxygen), humidifiers (saline solution), mucolytics (acetylcysteine), and decongestants (terbutaline, metaproterenol). These substances are readily absorbed from the alveolar membrane and may produce systemic side effects.

Ward clerk and ward manager

Certain clerical aspects of drug therapy are often delegated to nonprofessional members of the unit staff. The transcription of orders, preparation of medication Kardex or treatment sheets, ordering of drugs from the pharmacy, and collection of information about clients' allergies to drugs are activities most often assigned to these assistants. The use of such personnel can increase the efficiency of the hospital staff.

Professional nurses

The traditional role of the professional nurse in drug therapy in institutional settings is to administer medications prescribed by the physician. In its broadest sense, the term *administration* includes all activities related to safe drug use. Assessing the risk to a client of a new drug order, delivering the drug dose to the proper body tissues, assessing the client's response to drug therapy, treating adverse reactions to drugs, consulting with the physician about adjusting the prescribed regimen, and educating the client about the proper use of drug substances are all the nurse's responsibilities. Thus, the nurse is directly concerned with every aspect of drug treatment. Even in the areas of prescribing and dispensing, the nurse verifies the accuracy of the actions taken by other professionals.

Trends in the assignment of role functions

Prescription

Traditionally, the right to diagnose disease and prescribe treatment has been reserved for licensed physicians and dentists. In more recent times, physicians have sometimes delegated the choice of drug regimen to an assistant (physician's assistant or nurse practitioner). However, such prescriptions or orders must be countersigned by the physician.

There is a trend toward granting limited prescribing privileges to health care professionals other than physicians. Factors that contribute to this trend include better educational preparation of these professionals (pharmacists, physician's assistants, and nurses), increased pressures for containment of health care costs, and the decontrol of increasing numbers of prescription drugs by reclassification as OTC medications. (Unfortunately, many insurance companies that pay for prescription drugs no longer pay for them when they are given OTC status.) It has been argued that consumers who understand the drug regimens recommended by their physicians are capable of managing their own care over the long term, with the guidance and assistance of other health care professionals (Rx-to-OTC trend fuels nurse prescribing debate, 1983).

A number of states have granted limited prescription privileges to nurses. These privileges are usually granted only to nurses with advanced credentials, such as certified nurse practitioners, and are often limited to specific drugs and approved protocols. In some cases, nurses who prescribe must be supervised by physician overseers. Whether other states will follow these precedents and to what degree the privilege of prescription will be extended depends on the future expansion of the nurse's role into areas previously reserved for the physician.

Physician's assistants may also be given broader choices of drug treatment. Technically, assistants are under the direction and supervision of the physicians who employ them. In actual practice, they assess clients and prescribe treatment (in accordance with standard protocols) with a minimum of physician involvement. In health care institutions, they renew medication orders and may order other drugs.

In the community setting, pharmacists have long recommended appropriate OTC preparations for the treatment of minor or self-limiting conditions. With the recent decontrol of certain prescription drugs to OTC status, the number and effectiveness of agents available for such treatment have increased. Such consultations constitute a kind of primary care. If they are to continue and expand, they should be granted legal status.

Compounding

Most drugs used as therapeutic agents are compounded by pharmaceutical firms in a factory setting. These firms supply convenient standardized dose forms of relatively pure drugs. However, the right to compound is retained by both physicians and pharmacists. Although unusual, the use of a medication prepared by one of these professionals is perfectly legal. At least one specialty pharmacy compounds drugs into forms particularly suited to individuals who cannot or do not choose to take the form provided by the drug manufacturer (Designer meds, 1989).

Dispensing

Only physicians, dentists, and pharmacists have the legal right to dispense drugs for the treatment of human disease. Nurses are not trained to dispense and cannot legally undertake this function.

Administration

At one time, physicians jealously guarded their prerogative to administer drug dosages. In recent decades, however, the trend has moved toward involving more members of the health care team in the delivery of medicines to clients.

When nurses were first delegated this task, they were not informed what substances were being used, since medicines were identified by number rather than by name. Gradually, nurses were given more responsibility and authority in drug therapy. Today, hospital nurses are expected to administer oral and topical drugs, as well as parenteral drugs, including those injected directly into the vascular system. In many institutions, the management of IV therapy is recognized as a nursing specialty that requires advanced training. Oncology nurses sometimes administer intra-arterial or intrathecal medication. The administration of anesthesia by nurses is restricted legally to specially qualified individuals. In other settings, such as physicians' offices, specialty functions include intralesional injection and the administration of hazardous drugs, such as allergenic extracts.

Only recently has anyone other than a nurse or physician been allowed to administer medicines in acute health care institutions. Because the administration of drugs by vocational or practical nurses and respiratory therapists has proved efficient and relatively safe, it is likely that technical personnel will increasingly be used for this purpose. With proper training, physiotherapists could administer muscle relaxants or analgesics before treatment, and laboratory technicians could administer many diagnostic agents.

In the community setting, clients (or their lay caregivers) often are responsible for administering medications. A strong trend is developing toward providing home health care for people with serious or terminal illness. Clients discharged from acute care settings to home care may have complex medication regimens. They often receive parenteral drugs by injection or infusion, which can include infusion through an implantable central venous or epidural line. Their lay caregivers must be taught the techniques necessary for safe, effective drug administration.

In health care institutions, self-medication is less likely, although clients may be allowed to administer some of their own drugs. Topical preparations, such as ointments or lotions, commonly are left at the bedside for the client's use. Drugs such as cough syrups, antacids, and nitroglycerin also may be left at the bedside, provided the physician writes an order to this effect. Proposals that clients be given total responsibility for self-medication in these settings have not always been well received, probably because physicians and nurses fear losing control over drug supplies and are concerned over a potential increase in medication. Clients may practice self-medication to learn the management of long-term medication regimens before discharge from acute care settings. Clients also manage opioid medication of acute pain by means of equipment that allows dosage up to but not beyond the maximum prescribed by the physician; this procedure is termed *patient controlled analgesia* (PCA) (Declaration of independence, 1985). An accurate record must be kept of medication, specifying the drug, route, and time of administration. Client response to medication (both therapeutic and adverse) must also be documented. The form of the medication record varies from agency to agency.

Nursing management

Nursing implications

The trend toward delegating professional functions to personnel with less than professional preparation is not without risk. The safety of such practices depends on proper training and adequate supervision.

Nurses must be familiar with current state laws about prescriptions and should consult with their state nurses' association for recommendations about the legal status of prescriptions issued by nonphysicians, such as physician's assistants and pharmacists. Unless the status of the physician's assistant is legally clarified by state law, it is probably unwise to accept and carry out an order by such a practitioner without verification by the attending physician. When verification is omitted, the nurse may have no legal protection should a malpractice suit result from administration of a drug. Regardless of legal status, the nurse should not hesitate to consult with the physician about orders that are questionable.

When vocational or practical nurses, aides, and ward managers or clerks are assigned tasks related to drug therapy, the responsibility for their actions remains with the professional nurse. Nurses must allocate sufficient time and energy to properly train and supervise the personnel who operate under their jurisdiction.

Nurses must also resist attempts to assign to personnel functions beyond the scope of their competence. Inappropriate responsibilities are sometimes delegated to ward clerks or pharmacy clerks. Nurses should protest such practices and work to strengthen institutional controls on role functions. The proper procedure is to document incidents that cause concern and present recommendations for administrative action through the existing chain of command to nursing service administration. Recommendations should be supported by evidence documenting the problem and a rationale for the need for change.

An example of inappropriate use of professional nurses is the request that supervising nurses dispense a supply of drugs from the institution's pharmacy "when necessary." This practice is most likely to occur in smaller health care institutions when not enough pharmacists to staff this department are available on a 24-hour basis. Because nurses do not receive the specialized training required for dispensing, and they are not licensed to do so, they should not accept such assignments. The issue may be resolved by calling in the pharmacist when needed or by securing drugs from a commercial pharmacy. Single doses may legally be administered by the nurse from supplies in the pharmacy, as from any stock bottle.

Nursing process

Assessment Before administering any medication, the nurse should determine whether the client has any risk factors that may be contraindications for the prescribed drug. The drug order also should be assessed to verify that it completely and appropriately relates both to the client's condition and to reference data that concern the usual protocols for use of the medication.

Nursing diagnosis Nursing diagnoses relate to client problems that complicate the implementation of the drug regimen. For example, the client may have difficulty swallowing oral drugs, or tissue perfusion may be inadequate for absorption of subcutaneous or intramuscular injections. Clients also may lack any knowledge about the drug regimen.

Planning The goal of care is to resolve problems related to drug therapy.

Intervention When a problem with the drug order or with client factors that contraindicate a drug arises, the nurse must consult with the physician. If such consultation resolves the nurse's concern about the order, the drug may be given, following the procedures adopted by the health care agency.

When drugs are ordered in a health care institution, certain clerical procedures are carried out to obtain the drug and to ensure its delivery to the client. The nurse usually is responsible for accurately transcribing drug orders and obtaining supplies from the pharmacy. The legal responsibility for these functions remains that of the nurse, although these actual tasks may be delegated to a ward secretary or another member of the staff. If these tasks are delegated, the nurse must be given adequate time to properly supervise the work.

Administration. In most health care institutions, the nurse (professional, practical, or vocational) is responsible for delivering drug doses to clients or residents. Opinion is divided on whether only professional nurses should administer doses. Licensed practical or vocational nurses are taught the procedures of drug administration and perform them well in selected situations. Some health care agencies are considering delegating the dosing procedure to technicians with even less preparation in health sciences. Once the client's condition is properly assessed and the decision is made to give a particular drug, preparing the dose is primarily a matter of accuracy. The major concern is that the correct drug be given to the right person, at the right time, by the right route, in the right amount. This process is facilitated by modern drug systems using unit dose forms.

It could be argued that dosing is a technical procedure that can be carried out by people with limited preparation. However, the delivery of doses is not the simple activity it appears to be. For example, problems in administering the dose often exist. Clients with impaired gag reflexes may aspirate oral drugs if special precautions are not taken; injection sites must be chosen to facilitate appropriate absorption. Psychological factors that influence clients' response to drugs are greatly altered by the manner in which they are given the medications. The attitude and skill of the person who administers the dose can markedly enhance or diminish the client's response. For this reason, the person who gives medication to a client should have the appropriate training and experience. Another argument for having professional nurses retain the function of administering drug doses, especially in acute care situations, is that a client's condition may change in the interim between professional assessment and technical administration of medicines. The nurse in this case could reconsider the decision to give a drug, whereas technicians may not detect the significant change. A minor argument in this controversy is that nurses who are not involved in drug administration may become less aware of the drug regimens of individual clients. (Techniques for delivery of drug doses are discussed in the next chapter.)

In addition to carrying out the drug orders of the physician, the nurse also influences the drug regimen in other ways. Nurses may suggest to physicians or request from them orders for drugs that they think are appropriate. Nursing care includes psychological and physical care measures to reduce the need for drugs and enhance the effectiveness of the drug regimen.

Client education. In the past, clients often have been kept relatively uninformed about the drugs prescribed for their medical treatment. Owing to the proliferation of therapeutic agents and the increasing frequency of multiple drug use, such a policy is no longer safe. Clients must be informed about their drug regimens so that they can cooperate intelligently in their own treatment. Teaching clients about medications is a primary concern of the nurse. This education may be aimed at helping clients derive the greatest benefit from the drug regimen while in the acute care setting, or it may be designed to prepare them to manage their own drug regimens after discharge.

Nurses provide appropriate information to the client about drugs and medication regimens. They assist clients in integrating their drug regimens into their daily routines and lifestyles. These nursing functions apply to OTC preparations and nonmedicinal drugs, as well as to prescription medications. Proper instruction about drugs may reduce the client's need for drugs or enhance the effect of those taken. In addition, clients need reassurance about minor side effects and techniques for minimizing them. Clients should learn the precautions necessary for accurately preparing and administering drugs. They also must be taught the significant indicators of adverse reactions, including toxicity, to judge when it is appropriate to contact their physician and whether to suspend drug doses pending changes in their regimen.

Effective client education requires that the nurse be knowledgeable about drugs and drug therapy and be skilled in teaching techniques. In addition to offering clients accurate pharmacologic information, nurses must be able to judge clients' readiness to learn and to choose appropriate teaching approaches and materials.

Documentation. All data pertinent to medication procedures and client response to drugs must be entered on the client's chart. It is important that the information recorded be precise and accurate. All doses should be entered with complete details, including name of the drug, dose, route of administration, and the exact time when it was given. The common practice of charting a dose as if it had been given precisely at the time scheduled, when drugs are actually administered as much as 20 to 30 minutes before or after the hour, is potentially dangerous. It might be crucial in some instances to be able to ascertain whether a drug ordered for 10 AM was actually given at 9:30 AM or 10:30 AM. Moreover, the reliability of the chart as legal evidence is placed in question when such careless charting practices become evident in court.

An accurate chart is an invaluable tool in assessing clients for drug-related problems. It provides the data needed to establish relationships between medication and the emergence of signs and symptoms of adverse reactions. It can establish whether the desired therapeutic response is occurring. Accumulated data in charts are also a valuable resource for research by health care professionals.

Evaluation   The professional nurse assesses, reports, and records the client's response to drug therapy. This monitoring is a most critical responsibility.

The quantity of drugs prescribed for the client is only an educated approximation based on the physician's estimate of the client's needs (Box 13-1). In accordance with the client's size, age, health status, and drug history, the physician selects an agent and a drug dosage likely to accomplish the desired therapeutic result. Whether the anticipated effect will in fact occur is not known until the client's response is evaluated. A number of factors can influence the result:

- The dose actually administered to the client may not correspond exactly to the order written by the physician. In manufacturing doses, drug

---

Box 13-1. Factors that can influence end results of drug therapy

- The dose administered may not correspond exactly to the written order.
- Absorption may be different from that anticipated.
- The drug may be transported or stored in unanticipated ways.
- The drug may be used by the body at a different rate of speed from that anticipated.
- Excretion of the drug may vary.
- An altered state of health may change the effects of the drug.
- Allergic reactions may occur.

---

firms are allowed to deviate from the designated dose level, often as much as 10%. When fractional doses must be prepared, a further deviation up to 10% may be acceptable. This deviation is dictated by the limitations of measuring devices and the inexactitude of mathematical computations used in converting from one measurement system to another. In extreme instances, when both deviations are maximum, the actual dose given may be as much as 20% above or below the dose that the physician ordered.

- The recipient of the drug may absorb more slowly or more rapidly than anticipated. Occasionally, the dose may not be absorbed at all.
- The drug may be transported or stored in the body of the recipient in unexpected ways, causing more or less of the drug than anticipated to be available to metabolic processes.
- Owing to individual differences in metabolism and enzyme systems, the recipient may use the drug more or less rapidly than expected.
- Excretion of the drug may vary owing to abnormal function of the organs involved in degrading and eliminating the drug.
- An altered state of health may change the recipient's sensitivity to the effects of the drug.
- Allergic manifestation may alter the drug's effect or cause harmful reactions in the recipient.

The initial administration of a drug involves giving an approximate dose to a client whose physiologic response to the substance is at best estimated and at worst completely unknown. Physicians are aware of these uncertainties in therapy and rely on the client or nurse to report significant data about the client's response; using this information, they can make necessary adjustments and refinements in the drug regimen to achieve the desired therapeutic results.

In assessing the client's response to therapy, the nurse must verify the improvement that is expected from drug action and detect adverse reactions. The nurse must judge which data require medical interaction and should be reported to the physician and which indicate minor responses amenable to nursing interaction. Assessment of a client's response to drug therapy must be carried out systematically and conscientiously. In the acute care setting, the nurse is responsible for recording these evaluations and promptly reporting data useful to other health personnel involved in the client's care. Tailoring the medical regimen to the client's specific needs depends on adequate assessment of the drug therapy. Because they are the professionals who have the most frequent contact with clients, nurses are responsible for observing and reporting clients' responses to drugs. In this way, nurses can determine the drugs' therapeutic effects, side effects, and any adverse reactions. The nurse determines when the physician should be consulted and may temporarily suspend the drug regimen or initiate emergency action when required. Sound professional judgment is required for this critical aspect of drug therapy.

As the responsibility for administering drugs is disbursed among various health care personnel, the risk of inadequate assessment of a client's response is increased. It is vital that nurses be aware of all drugs taken by the client, that they evaluate the client regularly and comprehensively for therapeutic response and adverse reactions, and that they intervene when necessary to ensure optimal drug therapy.

Evaluation of drug-related care must consider not only client outcomes but also the proper implementation of nursing intervention. In other words, the nurse must ask if the nursing plan was implemented as projected and if the interventions produced the desired effect. To determine the accuracy and consistency with which the nursing plan was carried out, the nurse should consider such questions as: Was a proper drug history taken? Were the effects of the drug treatment assessed regularly and systematically? Was the physician consulted when appropriate? Were the prescribed drugs delivered to the client accurately? Were nursing measures designed to augment the drug treatment or reduce side effects carried out as ordered? Was the teaching program implemented as planned? To determine the results in terms of the client's outcome, appropriate questions might be: Did the client's symptoms subside? Were side effects detected and controlled? Were acute reactions treated appropriately? Did the client demonstrate an adequate understanding of the prescribed drug regimen? Did the client emotionally accept the treatment plan? Did the client comply with the prescribed regimen at home? Did the client consult with the physician appropriately? Data accumulated during this evaluation are incorporated in the assessment phase of the nursing process as care is continued.

Delivery of drug doses

Once it has been decided that a particular dose of medication should be taken by the client, the skill with which the medication is prepared and administered becomes of paramount importance. No matter who prepares the dose or where it is administered, the accuracy of five factors must be ensured: the right drug, the right dose, the right client, the right route, and the right time (Box 13-2).

The right drug

To ensure that the *right drug* is used, the package label, the cardex, and medication card or sheet must be checked and double-checked (Fig. 13-2). Nurses should prepare the medications they give; they should not deliver to clients medication doses prepared by someone else. The person who administers the medication is held responsible. If a client questions the medication, recheck the order, label, and medication card. A mentally alert client will notice a change in medication or may mention problems that have arisen from the medication. Never ignore these statements and questions.

All doses are best prepared from the original container. It is impossible to read the package label as recommended if the medicine has been removed from the original container. Medicine should never be poured in the dark, nor should medication be taken in the dark. Good illumination is necessary for positive identification. The labels must be read three times.

Clients should be cautioned about the use of nonlabeled pillboxes, such as the decorative dispensers advertised for purses. The practice of mixing supplies of several tablets or capsules in a single container from which doses are selected on the basis of appearance alone is to be discouraged (Fig. 13-3).

The right dose

To obtain the *right dose*, the medicine must be carefully measured (Fig. 13-4). Measurement is fairly easy with dry medicines prepared as capsules or tablets. If half of a tablet is required, scored tablets may be cut into two pieces with a knife edge or folded in clean paper and broken with the fingers (Fig. 13-5). No attempt should be made to split nonscored tablets or divide the

---

Box 13-2. The five "rights" of medication

1. The RIGHT drug
2. The RIGHT dose
3. The RIGHT client
4. The RIGHT route
5. The RIGHT time

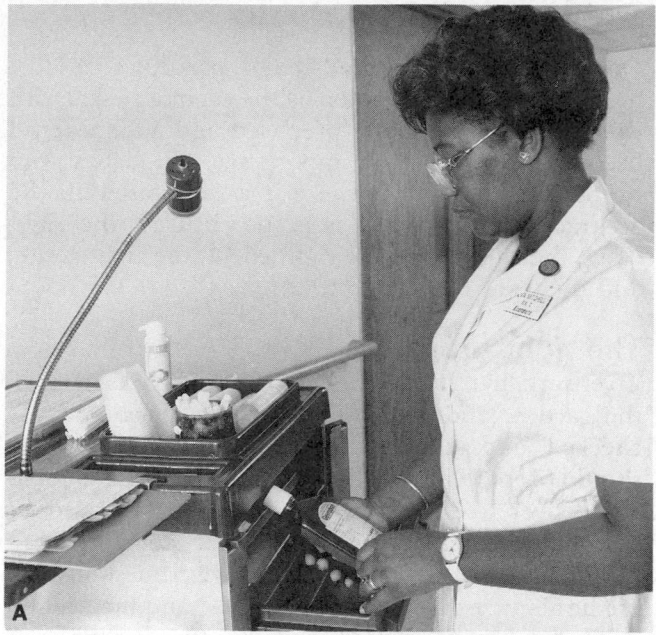

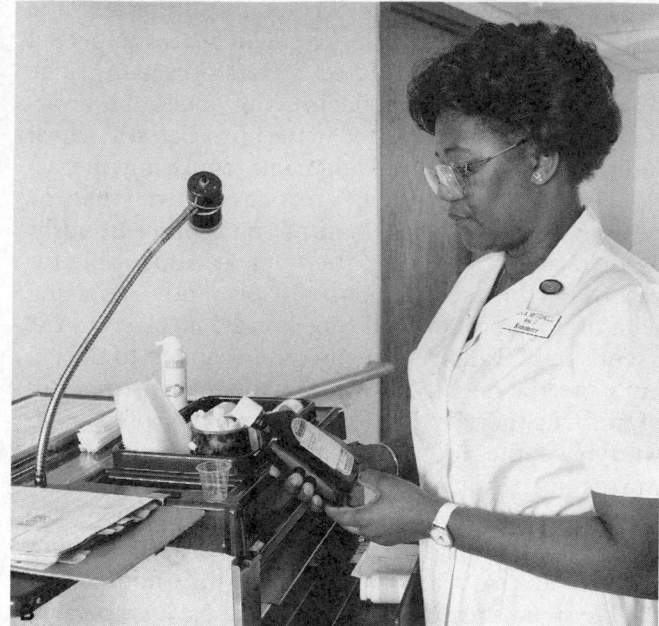

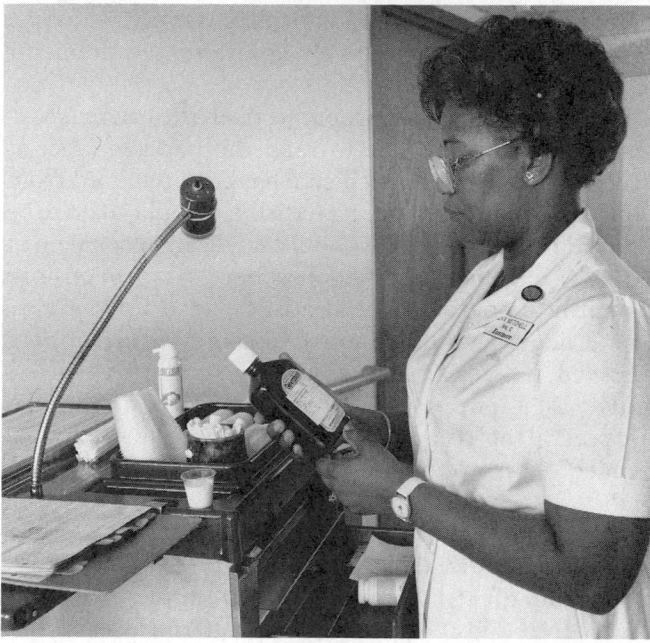

Figure 13-2. Medication labels should be checked (*A*) when removed from the shelf; (*B*) before pouring or measuring; (*C*) when returned to the shelf. Copyright © B. Proud

dose of a single capsule. When tablets are split, the two halves are given in successive doses, so that any deviation from the prescribed dose due to uneven breakage is leveled out as quickly as possible. It is not wise to break all the tablets available and mix the halves. Though this method may appear efficient and convenient, undue fluctuation in the doses is likely. For example, all the larger halves may be taken first, causing overmedication during the first half of the course of treatment and undermedication during the second half.

Liquids should be measured in a container with a scale that provides a mark for the required dose. Inexpensive plastic medicine "glasses" or spoons may be purchased for accurate measurement of liquids. If these are not available, kitchen measuring spoons are preferable to spoons used at the table, which may vary considerably in volume. Some liquid medicines are marketed with a measuring utensil, such as a scaled dropper. Figure 13-6 illustrates several measuring devices for liquids; Figure 13-7 illustrates the correct method for measuring liquids in a cup.

The right client

Making sure that the *right client* receives the right drug is rarely a problem outside of institutions. Relatives and lay attendants are likely to know the recipient very well. However, medicines recommended or prescribed for one person are sometimes offered or given to another. This practice can be dangerous. Even if both

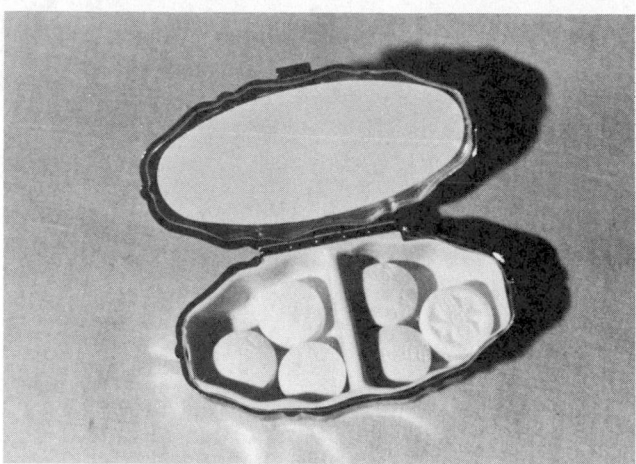

Figure 13-3. Decorative pillboxes can be lethal. This pillbox contains Fiorinal and Tylenol, which are both headache medications but of different compositions and strengths. See Chapter 18 for suggestions on handling drug dosages at home.

people are suffering from the same medical condition, a drug suitable for one person may be totally unsuitable for the other. Drugs should be given only to the person for whom they are prescribed or recommended.

Within single households or family groups, it is sometimes necessary to medicate several members for an identical condition. For example, contagious illness is likely to be shared in such close groups. Related members may be subject to familial ailments and respond similarly to drugs. Even in these situations, the physician should be consulted before using one person's prescription for another. The drug best suited for one person may be ineffective or even dangerous when given to another. If a physician does wish to treat more than one person with a drug, it is preferable to write individual prescriptions for each. In the rare situation that involves dosing of more than one person from a single drug supply, written records should be kept to ensure accurate medication. Figure 13-8 illustrates how nurses in an agency identify clients by checking their identification bracelets.

The right route

The *right route* must be used for drug delivery. Outside of health care institutions, most medicines are taken orally or by topical application. The client must clearly understand how the drug is to be taken. Sublingual or chewable tablets should not be swallowed whole. If swallowing is difficult, oral drugs should be crushed or taken in liquid form. However, sustained-release oral products, which are being used to a greater extent in therapy, must not be crushed.

Clients who must use parenteral drugs require careful training in injection techniques. Procedures

for application of topical drugs should also be demonstrated to clients and practiced by them.

Nurses in institutions must be aware of the usual routes for administering medications. Giving medication by the wrong route can cause death. The person who administers the drug is held responsible. The nurse should check the physician's orders and the cardex to verify the medication route. If the route specified is not in accord with that recommended for the drug preparation, the physician should be alerted.

The right time

The *right time* for drug administration is not usually indicated by the physician as clock time. Instead, the physician indicates the number of times a day a drug is to be given, the hourly interval between doses, or the relation of the dose to the client's activity patterns. For example, drugs may be taken before or after meals, on arising or retiring, or every 4 hours, 6 hours, or 12 hours. Clients should establish the times for taking drugs in accordance with their daily routine. Clients

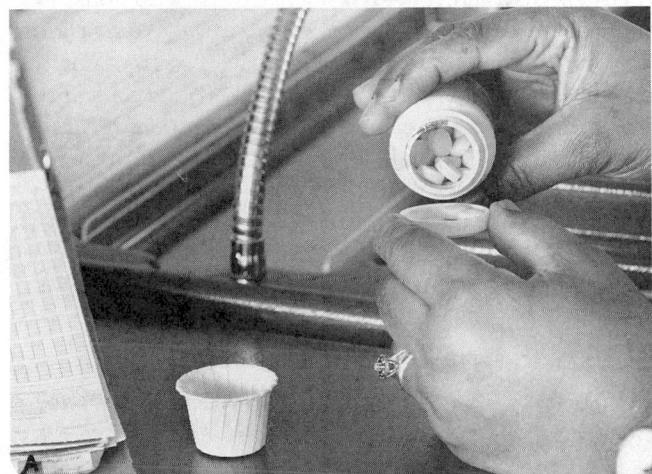

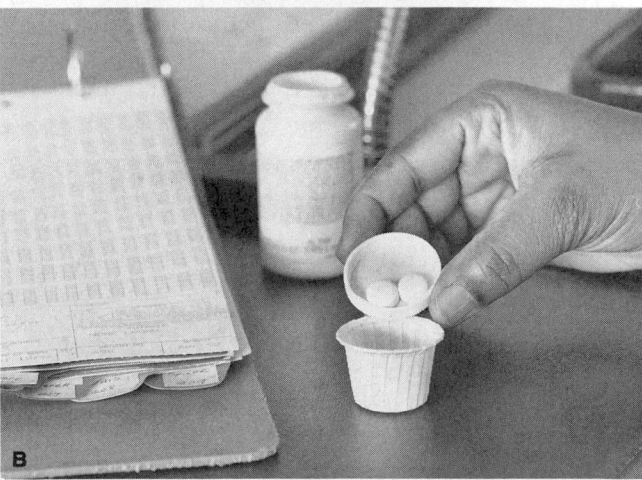

Figure 13-4. The proper technique for pouring solid drugs, such as capsules and tablets. To minimize handling of drugs, the required number of units in the dose are first (*A*) poured into the container's cap and then (*B*) poured from the cap to the medication cup. Copyright © B. Proud

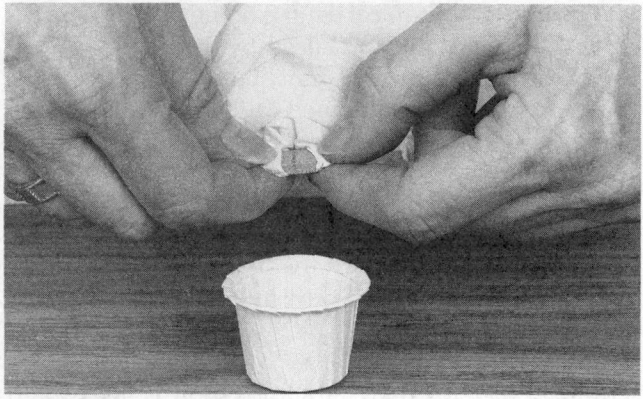

Figure 13-5. Scored tablets can be split by exerting digital pressure on each side of the slot. Fold tissue or paper towel around the tablet to avoid contact between hands and medication. This procedure is easiest with large tablets. Small tablets, which provide too little leverage for the fingers, may be cut with a knife, or the slot may be punctured by an unused injection needle. Copyright © B. Proud

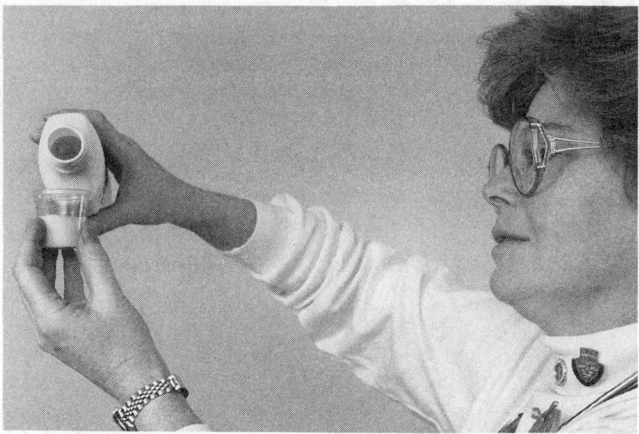

Figure 13-7. To pour a liquid medication, the nurse places a thumbnail at the marking on the medication glass to indicate the dose ordered for the client. The glass and medication bottle are held at eye level so that the meniscus is clearly visible, and the bottle label faces inward so that the solution does not drip on the label. Copyright © B. Proud

with poor time orientation, short-term memory defects, or distracting activity schedules need some system for guiding them in self-medication. Many clients find it helpful to dispense the doses required for the day at one time, labeling each dose with the data or day of the week and the hour it is to be taken. Nursing personnel in hospitals and other institutions set up routines for intervals and times for medication. However, each medication nurse must be familiar with classes of medications and the appropriate times for administering them.

Nursing management of drug therapy for institutionalized clients

Personnel involved in medication delivery

The current trend toward self-medication by clients is best illustrated by health-related facilities, where clients have been controlling their drug regimens for

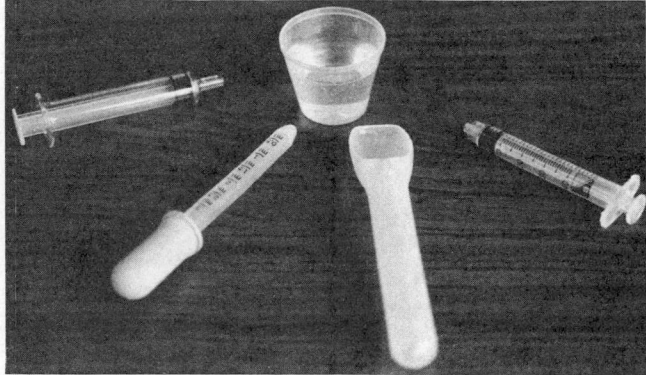

Figure 13-6. Devices used to measure liquid medication accurately: (*left to right*) oral syringe, dropper, medicine cup, spoonlike device, injection syringe without needle.

some time. Acute care agencies have been slower to adopt this practice, even in situations in which clients are alert, responsible, and energetic enough to take their own drugs. In these institutions, however, self-medication may be started before discharge as part of client education in the management of the medical regime at home. For the most part, however, medicines are controlled and administered by the nursing staff, and the system that is used varies, depending on the organizational pattern of the nursing service (Fig. 13-9).

When total client care is given by one person, such as with a private duty nurse, it is desirable that this person administer the client's medications for the entire work shift. In primary nursing, one nurse controls all care but shares caregiving activities with other staff members. Either the primary or an associate nurse may administer drugs in this system. When team nursing is the pattern of care, a variety of assignment patterns may be used. Qualified team members may be assigned to give medications to clients whose care is their responsibility. Clients assigned to aides or (in some institutions) practical or vocational nurses must be assigned to qualified personnel for medication. Often one team member is assigned to medicate all clients cared for by the team. In units with functional assignments, one nurse administers drugs to all clients in the unit; usually this is the only duty assigned to this nurse.

From the standpoint of continuity and comprehensiveness of a client's care, it is desirable to have medications administered by the nurse most familiar with the client. Such a method of assignment involves many people in the handling of drugs. In a typical nursing unit, medication activities are limited to a small room centrally located in the unit and to the medication cart, which moves from client unit to client unit. Use of these areas by many people results in congestion and confusion. Accuracy, efficiency, and drug security are difficult to maintain. Indeed, in some states regulations prohibit the use of the narcotic key by anyone other than the staff member responsible for controlled drug security and require that drugs be recounted each time a different person takes the key. To avoid these problems, many institutions use some form of functional assignment for medications.

Under the functional method, one nurse per unit or team is assigned to give drugs to all clients cared for by that unit or team. In some cases, one nurse is assigned to administer "routine" drugs (those given repeatedly at regular intervals) and another staff member gives all other medications (such as one-time-only doses or drugs given as needed to control symptoms). Such a system divides the work load (which may be too great for one person) and reduces the number of interruptions of "routine" medications. It also usually shortens the intervals between requests by clients for symptom-relieving drugs and their delivery.

Policies about who is allowed to give drugs vary from institution to institution. It is increasingly recognized that basic nursing education cannot provide the beginning practitioner with a high degree of skill in all procedures of all specialties in practice. Some acute care facilities restrict medication assignments to registered professional nurses who have demonstrated proficiency in these skills. Staff members are required to pass a proficiency test or complete a special course of study before they are allowed to administer drugs.

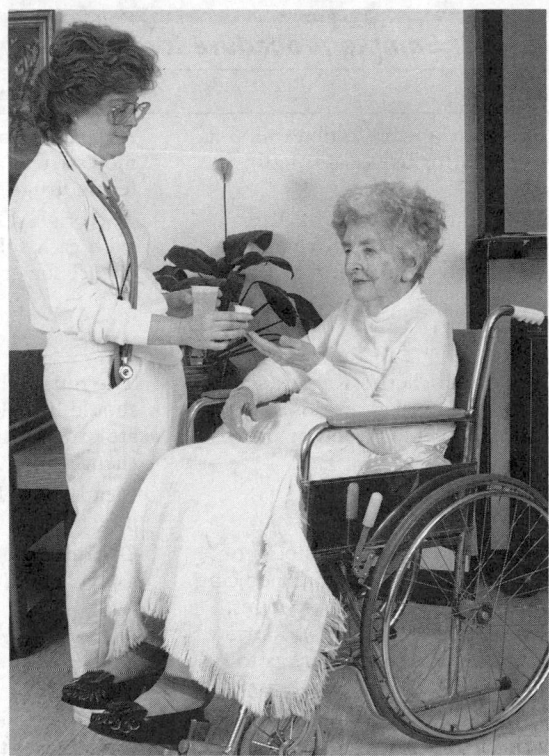

Figure 13-9. In residential institutions the procedure for administering medications is more flexible. Here the nurse administers medications in the day room. Copyright © B. Proud

Certain procedures, usually IV medication, may be restricted to specially trained staff members. Hospitals may allow approved licensed practical or vocational nurses to give medications in selected situations. In skilled nursing facilities, medications usually are administered by practical or vocational nurses.

No matter what method of assignment is used or what the criteria are for personnel, standard procedures are adopted for the administration of medications. Two systems can be used, one relying on medication cards and another using medication carts. The system using medication carts is outlined in Table 13-2. Drugs for either system may be dispensed in stock bottles or packaged in unit doses. The trend is moving toward unit-dose packaging and individual client supplies.

Medication procedures used in institutions

Elaborate procedures have been developed for the delivery of drug doses in institutions. Ritualistic precautions are taken to ensure accuracy and avoid errors. Despite these precautions, medication errors continue to be a serious problem in many institutions for many reasons. Probably the most significant is the tendency for practitioners to depart from routine precautions to one or the other extreme, either ignoring the details of

(Text continues on p. 170)

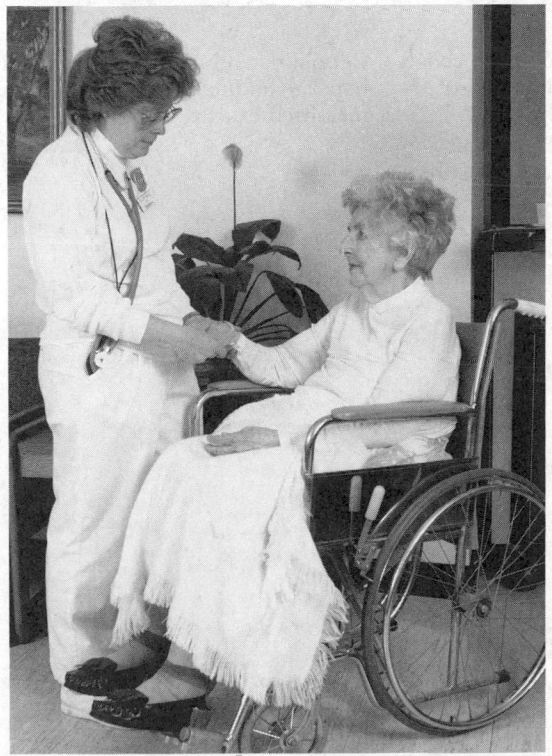

Figure 13-8. The client's name on his or her identification bracelet is checked with the name on the medication card in the nurse's hand. This check is essential to avoid errors.

Table 13-2. Sample procedure for administering medications using a medication cart

Action	Rationale (underlying principles)	Additional information
1. Inspect drug cart to determine its readiness for use (Fig. 13-10).	A neat, completely stocked cart promotes safety and efficiency in administering drugs.	
2. Verify Kardex listings of drugs to be given with master drug sheet or original physician's orders.	The original order is most reliable. With each subsequent transcription the chance for error increases.	Drugs given by one nurse during a complete 8-hour shift may be administered after a single complete verification. The original order sheets should be checked at regular intervals, preferably once every 24 hours.
3. Check each client's Kardex sheets for possible errors in doses, drug incompatibilities, or other problems.	The nurse who is administering drugs should be able to identify inappropriate orders and potential harm to the client	Inappropriate orders must be questioned. The dose should be omitted if likely to harm the client.
4. Wash your hands.	Clean hands help prevent cross-infection.	
5. If necessary, replenish stocks on the cart (*eg*, medications, medicine cups, syringes, alcohol sponges, gloves, lubricant, straws). Retrieve from the refrigerator drugs to be administered within the hour.	Organization of work promotes efficiency and saves times.	
6. Move cart to a position in or near room of first client to be medicated (Fig. 13-11).	Working close to the client being served saves time and energy.	
7. "Pour" each medication for the client as follows:		
a. Select the correct drug from stock in client's drawer (first label reading; see Fig. 13-2A).	Repeated reading of labels promotes accuracy.	Read label carefully each time. Concentrate on the task at hand.
b. Reread label (second label reading; see Fig. 13-2B), comparing to Kardex entry (Fig. 13-12).		
c. Compute the dose.	The volume of drug poured must contain a dose equal to or within 10% of the dose ordered by the physician.	Certain dangerous drugs (*eg*, insulin, heparin, antineoplastic drugs) must be measured exactly.
d. Measure the correct dose. For oral administration: pour the number of pills, capsules, or tablets, or the liquid measure of the preparation required into a medicine cup (see Figs. 13-4 and 13-7). If too much liquid is poured, discard the excess. Extra pills, capsules, or tablets may be returned to the drug container. Do not touch medicines with your fingers. For injections: using sterile aseptic technique, draw up the required volume of solution, adjusting amount exactly before removing needle from vial. For topical applications: select the tube, bottle, or jar needed. Place suppositories in medicine cup.	To minimize the chance of infection, cleanliness or sterility of drugs must be maintained.	
e. Place drug on top of cart next to Kardex sheet.	Drugs should be labeled for positive identification at all times.	A visible mark should be made on Kardex sheet to denote drugs that have been poured.

(Continued)

Table 13-2. Sample procedure for administering medications using a medication cart *(Continued)*

Action	Rationale (underlying principles)	Additional information
f. Reread the label on the drug container (third label reading; see Fig. 13-2C).	Repeated reading of labels helps prevent errors.	Read the label carefully. Concentrate on the task at hand.
g. Return unused drug to stock.	Control of clutter helps reduce confusion that can contribute to errors.	
8. Repeat step 7 until all drugs to be given to one client are poured. Dry drugs that you are sure will be given to the client may be combined in one cup. Controlled substances, any drug that may be refused by the client, or drugs that are administered based on the client's immediate condition should be kept separate.	Unnecessary use of multiple medicine cups are costly and inefficient. Excessive numbers of drug containers may contribute to clutter and confusion.	The label of the drug container should be read carefully three times each time a dose is poured.
9. Lock the medicine cart and remove the key.	To minimize the chance of abusive or erroneous use of drugs, security must be maintained at all times.	
10. Reread the client's name on Kardex sheet. Carry medications directly to the client. Read the client's identification band.	Careful identification procedures help prevent errors.	If the client is not wearing an identification band, ask, "Would you mind telling me your name?"
11. Observe the client for symptoms of adverse reactions to medication.	The dose should be omitted if likely to harm the client.	Specific observations to be made depend on the drugs involved.
12. If all is well, administer the drugs. Oral drugs: make sure the client has swallowed the medicines. Injection: place the syringe in a protected area to prevent accidental needle puncture. Topical applications: cover or cap drug container. Leave the client comfortable.	Oral: drugs may remain in the mouth to fall out or be removed later and lost. Injection: accidental needle "sticks" may cause serious illness. Topical drugs: proper storage conditions help preserve drugs.	Save any drugs that are not administered for proper disposal.
13. If necessary, wash your hands.	Clean hands help prevent cross-infection.	
14. Return to cart. Chart the drugs given on Kardex sheet. Make a note of observations that should be recorded in the client's chart.	Accurate charting is needed to guide the physician's treatment and nursing care. It is also necessary if the chart is to be used as a source of legal information in court. Written notes are more reliable than mental notes.	Chart the actual time the drugs were given, not the time for which they were scheduled.
15. Repeat steps 7 through 14 for each client in turn, moving cart from area to area as necessary.	Organization of work contributes to efficiency and saves time and energy.	
16. Return cart to medication room. Dispose of waste and used equipment. Leave cart clean and orderly.	A clean, neat cart will be needed for subsequent use.	Controlled drugs that have not been administered must be secured and returned to the pharmacy. Noncontrolled drugs may be discarded, preferably in an incinerator.
17. Take nursing notes to charting area and make appropriate entries in client's records.	Accurate charting is needed to guide the physician's treatment and nursing care. It is also necessary if the chart is used as a source of legal information in court.	Report orally any information of immediate importance.
18. At appropriate time intervals, evaluate the client's responses to drug doses administered.	Accurate evaluation of client's responses is needed to guide management of treatment regimen.	

prescribed routines ("cutting corners") or depending slavishly on ritual without exercising judgment. The careful observation of routine precautions does provide many safeguards to avoid error, but the principles that underlie steps in the routine must be clearly understood. Adherence to the principles guides the practitioner when deviation from the set routine is necessary.

A common medication procedure is described in Table 13-2. Details of procedures may vary from institution to institution, but the fundamental principles remain the same. For example, to ensure that the correct drug is given, drugs should be identified with a correctly written label at all steps in the procedure. This principle underlies the following rules followed by most institutions:

- Drug containers are labeled only in the pharmacy by the pharmacist. If a label becomes soiled or illegible, the container should be returned to the pharmacy for relabeling.
- If several drugs to be given to one client are poured out, they may be placed in one cup provided that the names of all the drugs are indicated in some way. If the client does not take all of the drugs mixed in this way, all must be discarded and the required drugs repoured, because individual drugs cannot be identified by appearance alone for removal from the group.
- Narcotics must always be identified by a written label. Because narcotics must be carefully accounted for, they are usually returned to the hospital pharmacy if they have been poured and subsequently not used.

The student should study the procedure example carefully to learn the fundamental principles. Steps or specifics of the procedure should not be memorized because they may vary from situation to situation. Instead, a capacity to evaluate the principles underlying a given procedure should be developed so that revisions may be suggested or adaptations safely made to improve practice in any particular situation.

Medication errors

Causes

Despite the elaborate rituals used for administering drugs, medication errors continue to be a serious problem in many institutions. Statistics on errors vary and are affected in part by the criteria used to determine what is an error. Allowable margins are often arbitrarily determined in relation to the five *rights* of correct administration. There is no question of error when a drug is administered to the wrong client, or when the wrong medication is given. The use of an inappropriate route is not always so clearly delineated. It may be difficult to determine whether a drug that a

physician had ordered to be given subcutaneously was actually delivered to muscle tissue because the needle selected was disproportionately long for a client's thin layer of subcutaneous tissue. Inadvertent IV injection may be difficult to substantiate if it was caused by shifting of the position of the needle tip in the tissues during the drug's injection. Most institutions have clear policies that require a written physician's order for the injection of a drug previously given by mouth. Guidelines may be less definite about changing a parenteral to an oral order when a client regains the ability to ingest medication. In such situations, errors of routes of administration tend to be underreported. Errors in timing, on the other hand, are often overreported. Definitions of such errors tend to be narrow, often specifying that medications given more than 20 or 30 minutes before or after the designated hour are in error. The validity of this timetable is questionable, because the actual hours are assigned arbitrarily by the nursing staff and the intent of the physician's order may be carried out properly with much greater tolerance for deviation.

For most drugs, a deviation of as much as 10% is allowed between the dose ordered and the dose received by the client. Some of the discrepancy arises from the conversion of doses from one system of measurement to another. True discrepancies arise when the physician's order specifies doses that cannot be measured precisely by the tools available to the nurse in charge of medication. Certain drugs, such as antineoplastics, insulin, and heparin, are considered so potentially dangerous that doses are expected to be more exact and the 10% deviation is not allowed.

Although medication error statistics must be interpreted in relation to recording procedures and criteria, potentially harmful errors occur too frequently in health care institutions. Mistakes in drug administration may arise at any step in the process from the physician's order to the delivery of the dose to the client. The following discussion considers possible sources of errors and the precautions that can help prevent them (Box 13-3).

Recording and transcribing orders

Whenever possible, orders should be written by the physician. Telephone orders and verbal orders under certain circumstances (*eg*, if the physician is scrubbed for a surgical procedure) may be written by a nurse, provided they are countersigned by the physician as soon as possible. Exceptions in some states are orders for schedule II controlled substances, which cannot be transmitted legally by telephone. The nurse who takes a spoken order should always read it back to the physician for verification. If pronunciation is unclear, the drug name should be spelled out to ensure accuracy. Drug orders should always include the name of the client, the name of the drug, the dose, the route of administration, and the frequency or timing of doses.

Box 13-3. Sources of medication errors and precautions

Inaccurate recording and transcribing of order

1. Orders should be written by the physician.
2. Some telephone and verbal orders may be written by a nurse provided they are countersigned by the physician as soon as possible.
3. The nurse who takes a verbal order should read it back to the physician.
4. Drug names should be spelled out if they are unclear.
5. Drug orders should include name of client, name of drug, dose, route of administration, and frequency or timing of doses.
6. If any part of order seems inappropriate, the physician should be contacted and given opportunity to make corrections.

Unclear or erroneous labeling of drugs

1. Discrepancies in terms (*eg*, generic and trade name) must be clarified. Nurse may add equivalent terms in parentheses on medication card or cardex.
2. Liquid medicine bottles should be held with label facing the palm of hand to prevent soilage of label.
3. If labels are damaged, bottles must be returned to the pharmacy for relabeling.

Misidentification of client

1. If no identification band is present, the client is asked to give his or her name; the client's name is not used.
2. A method that encourages cooperation rather than causes sarcasm or confusion should be used.
3. Clients who are unable to respond with their names should wear a visible name label at all times.
4. Recent photographs of the client are useful in some institutions.

Incomplete delivery of drugs

1. Injection sites that will give good absorption must be selected.

2. Drugs are best given by IV route to clients in shock.
3. Topical drugs must contact the affected tissue.
4. Topical applications must be protected from friction that will remove them.
5. With oral administration, swallowing of the medicine must be verified and adequate amounts of fluid given.
6. With clients who have problems swallowing, the nurse should inspect the client's mouth after administration to be sure the medicine was swallowed.
7. Solid medications (excluding sustained-release preparations) can be crushed for ease in swallowing, or liquid preparations can be given.
8. If the client is truly incompetent, medications may have to be forced. This action jeopardizes the nurse–patient relationship.

Verification errors

1. The nurse must make a conscious effort to concentrate on thorough verification of orders.
2. Written materials must be compared; reliance on memory is risky.
3. Dose must be labeled for identification between pouring and administration.

Use of inaccurate knowledge or inadequate knowledge base

1. Reliance on memory should be eliminated whenever possible.
2. Facts should be verified in reference sources.

Time and performance pressures

1. Work load should be appropriate for the skill and efficiency of the medication nurse.
2. Creative approaches and sound nursing judgment are needed to maintain accuracy and efficiency.

The nurse should ask the physician to verify the route desired if no route has been specified. Although physicians have a tendency to omit the route when oral drugs are ordered, it is not safe to assume that the oral route was intended. Policies that govern the role of student nurses in taking verbal orders vary from agency to agency. In general, a licensed nurse (instructor or staff member) listens to the orders with the student and cosigns the order written by the student. As with all verbal orders, the physician must countersign the order written by the nurse as soon as possible.

The handwriting of many physicians is not legible.

If doubt about any element of a drug order exists, oral verification must be sought from the doctor involved. Written orders also occasionally contain errors in dose, drug form, or other elements. If any part of the order appears inappropriate, the physician should be contacted and given the opportunity to correct any mistakes that may have been made.

Labeling of drugs

Pharmacy labels on drug containers may not use the same terms as the physician's order. For example, the physician may have ordered the drug by its trade

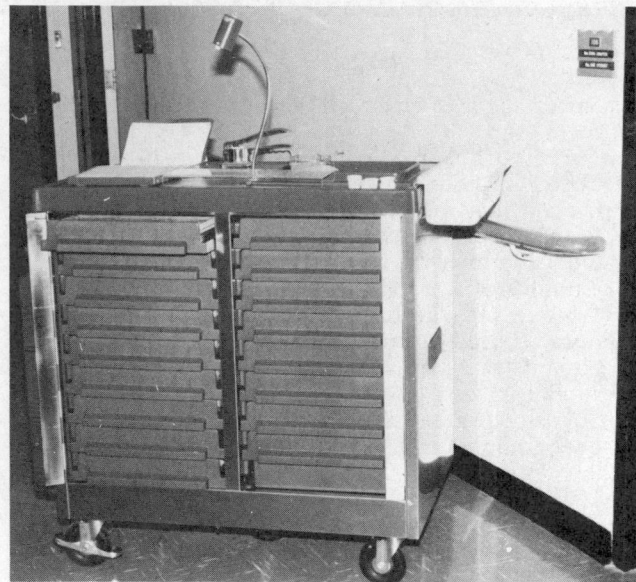

Figure 13-10. This newly acquired medication cart is about to be put to use. Notice the Kardex, the lamp for easier reading, and the pill crusher in the background (described in next chapter). Each client's drugs are kept in an individual drawer in the medication cart. Copyright © B. Proud

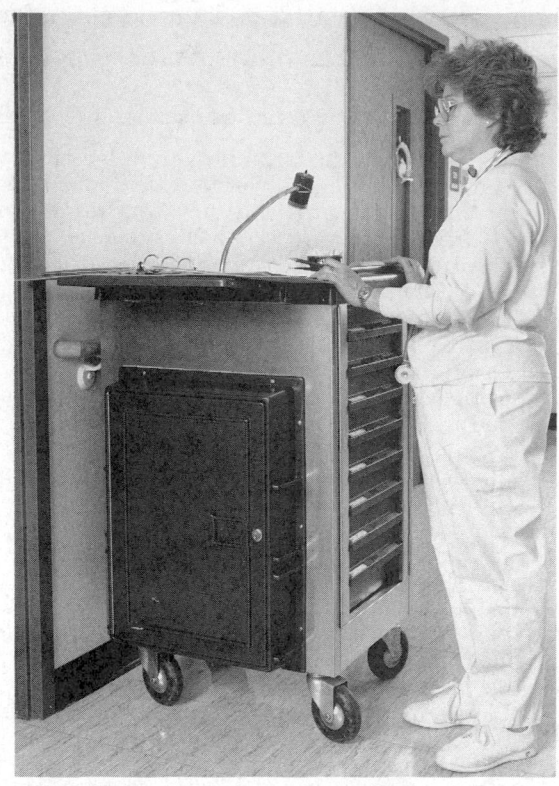

Figure 13-11. The medication cart and Kardex are taken to each client's room. The cart is stored between uses in a locked room near the nurse's station. Copyright © B. Proud

name, but the pharmacy dispensed it by its generic name. Most pharmacists label preparations with metric doses, whereas some physicians still employ apothecary doses. Discrepancies in terms must be reconciled. After verifying the drug name or dose, the nurse may add the terms used on the pharmacy label to the entry on the medication record and Kardex. Such additions are usually enclosed in parentheses.

Labels on liquid drugs may become soiled if the solution drips on the label during pouring. To keep the label clean, the nurse should hold the bottle with its label facing the palm of the hand while measuring the

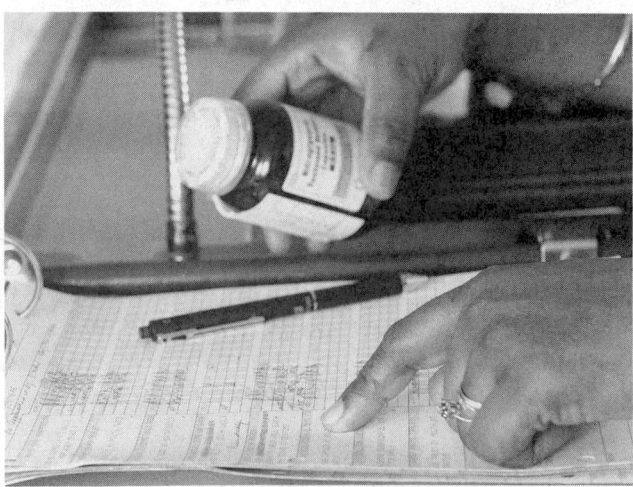

Figure 13-12. The nurse carefully checks the medication he or she will give with the Kardex. Copyright © B. Proud

drug. If labels are damaged or soiled, the bottle should be returned to the pharmacy for relabeling.

Identification of the client

Occasionally, a client who requires medication is not wearing an identification band. The band may have been removed temporarily to facilitate IV infusion or some other procedure, or it may have been removed permanently owing to the client's allergic hypersensitivity to its materials. In these situations, it is best to ask the client his or her name. Do not ask, "Is your name John Doe?" Clients who do not understand what has been said may answer affirmatively merely to acknowledge the communication. Misunderstandings of this type are especially likely during night and early morning hours, when clients are sleepy and are not using their hearing aids or eyeglasses. If a client is unfamiliar to the nurse, he or she may be asked, "What is your name?" This question may evoke a facetious answer or provoke unwillingness to respond if the client believes that the nurse should know him or her. In such cases, the question, "Would you mind telling me your name?" is usually more effective. It invites the client to cooperate in the identification ritual without implying that the nurse has forgotten the previous contacts.

Clients who are unable to respond with their

names owing to disorientation, expressive aphasia, or an altered level of consciousness should wear a visible name label at all times. When the standard device is unsuitable, ingenuity may be required to devise a satisfactory substitute. Only as a last resort, and only as a temporary measure, should the nurse rely on personal identification by staff members.

In long-term care facilities, resident rather than client status should be promoted for clients. Some institutions of this kind do not use any identification tags. Although the relative stability of resident and staff population reduces the risk of mistakes in identification, the danger of errors is not eliminated. Recent photographs of clients are useful for identification. The development of reliable and satisfactory identification procedures within this context is a challenge for creative nursing personnel.

Incomplete delivery of drugs

Drugs must reach the site of action to be effective. For many reasons, some or all of the dose given to the client may fail to complete this journey. Problems may be due to factors beyond the control of the nurse, such as malabsorption in the intestine, poor circulation in the injection site, or abnormally rapid metabolism and excretion. However, other problems stem from lack of skill in delivery techniques.

Injection of parenteral drugs must deliver the medication to tissues with adequate perfusion if the substance is to be absorbed rapidly into the systemic circulation. Selection of poor injection sites, such as edematous, hypoxic, or scar tissue, causes inadequate or delayed absorption. When clients are in shock, drugs are best administered intravenously. Intravenous lines established for the purpose of medication are often vital to proper treatment of the seriously ill or injured client. Intramuscular or subcutaneous injections should not be given to such clients until circulation has been restored to an adequate level.

Topical drugs must contact the affected tissue to exert a therapeutic effect. The presence of tissue debris or excessive exudate in a wound may prevent any response to local medication. Crusts or scales impose a similar barrier to topical applications. Once applied properly, topical applications must be protected from friction or other physical forces that remove them prematurely from the site. Judicious use of materials or devices such as dressings, stockingettes, plastic sheeting, or cradles can accomplish this protection.

When giving drugs orally, the nurse should make certain that the medicine is swallowed along with adequate amounts of an appropriate fluid to propel the dose into the stomach. Clients who experience mechanical difficulty in swallowing or impaired levels of consciousness may not "get the medication down" quickly or easily. For such clients, the nurse should inspect the mouth carefully after giving drugs orally to make sure the tablet or capsule has actually left the mouth. Solid medicines that remain in the oral cavity often appear hours later in the bedding or on the floor after they have fallen from the client's mouth. This problem may be solved by crushing the solid medication before its administration or by substituting a liquid preparation. Again, it is imperative to avoid crushing oral sustained-release preparations.

Occasionally clients deliberately refuse to swallow drugs or spit out drugs placed in the mouth. Others hide solid medications in the mouth and remove them after the nurse has left. Suicidal clients have been known to accumulate a lethal cache of drugs by saving doses retrieved in this way. With some clients, such behavior stems from belligerence or hostility toward the staff, which, in turn, is the outward expression of natural and normal psychological responses to illness, such as anxiety or despair. Clients with ambivalent feelings may accept liquid medications given by mouth. Open recognition of the client's right to refuse treatment, including medication, may resolve the conflict. Continued rejection of vital treatment raises difficult issues for the health care team.

If the client is truly incompetent (for such reasons as his or her status as a minor, delirium, or mental impairment), the health care team may resort to forced administration of drugs. Such action is apt to destroy all semblance of a therapeutic nurse–client relationship. The nurse should strive to maintain and convey to the client a basic attitude of caring and of helping the client to accept help. A show of force (*eg*, bringing two or more staff members to the bedside) may discourage active resistance; if possible, open conflict and physical struggle should be avoided. Many thorny legal and ethical questions arise when treatment is imposed on an unwilling client. In most situations, the issues are not black or white but some shade of gray. For example, few would question the need to administer glucose or glucagon by force to a belligerent client whose resistance stems from a temporary hypoglycemic state. Differences of opinion are far more likely when clients whose mental competence is uncertain resist treatment. In some cases, a legal determination of competence may have been made; in most instances, it has not. Such decisions may afford a measure of legal protection to the nurse (clients may charge staff members who assist in forced treatment with assault and battery), but rarely if ever do they resolve all moral issues. The nurse is confronted with many difficult ethical questions while caring for a resistant client.

Verification errors

Medication procedures customarily include a number of steps designed to detect errors so that they can be corrected before the drug is administered to a client. These steps include 1) comparison of the orders on the medication Kardex with the original orders written by the physician, 2) comparison of the client's name on written records with the name tag, and 3) repeated reading of drug labels. These routines tend to become rituals and often are carried out automatically, with little attention to or perception of their significance. The pouring of drugs is monotonous. If the nurse allows habit to control behavior, the motions of checking may be carried out without integration of the sensory stimuli that enter the brain. It is possible to "scan" a drug label without comprehending what the eyes have seen. The likelihood of such mechanical behavior is greater if the attention is allowed to wander. Interruptions and distractions must be eliminated as much as possible. The nurse must make a conscious effort to concentrate on the task at hand if routine checks are to be effective.

When data are compared for accuracy, reliance on memory is risky. Printed materials must be placed side by side for comparison. In practical terms, therefore, the medication card or Kardex sheet must be viewed simultaneously with the physician's order sheet. The medication card should be placed next to the client's name tag to verify identification. If any interval between pouring and administering the drug exists, the dose must be labeled for complete and certain identification. Careful observance of such practices helps ensure accuracy during the administration of drugs.

Use of inaccurate or inadequate knowledge base

Relying solely on memory about facts necessary for the safe use of all drugs should be avoided whenever possible. Pharmacologic information needed by the medication nurse has expanded so rapidly in recent years that it is unrealistic to expect anyone to remember all the facts needed every time. Knowledge frequently used is retained in reliable detail and may safely be used without verification. Any information that is not used regularly tends to be forgotten, and the details that are recalled are not reliable. Although a well stocked memory is a valuable resource, any fact about which the nurse is unsure must be verified in reference sources, which should be provided for this purpose. Useful references include encyclopedic volumes that contain drug data, charts that provide accurate metric-apothecary equivalents, compatibility tables that warn against incompatible drug mixtures, and any other visual materials considered appropriate to a given situation. It is much safer (and may be quicker) to look up such information than to attempt to recall it.

Time performance pressures on the medicator

The sheer number of doses to be given in a limited time span may preclude the careful attention to detail necessary to eliminate errors. Time is needed for such tasks as gathering basic drug data, careful reading of labels, and checking of clients' identification. Only practiced and efficient nurses can maintain the pace required in many situations. Less skilled personnel either "cut corners" (eliminate some of the steps) or fall hopelessly behind schedule (an error in itself).

In some situations, the administration of routine medications is subject to interruption for the administration of drugs ordered to be given at indeterminate times. This indeterminate scheduling includes doses to be administered when needed (PRN), immediately (STAT), or at a time determined by other circumstances (*eg,* a preoperative medication to be given "on call," depending on when the operating suite is available). Personnel other than the medicator responsible for routine drugs may be assigned to administer these drugs; as a result, the number of people who use the medication room and have access to controlled drugs is doubled, factors that tend to compromise security and increase the distractions and confusion in the medication area.

Clearly, the problem of medication errors is complex and its resolution difficult. Creative approaches and sound nursing judgment are needed to establish reliable procedures and precautions for accurate and effective drug therapy in a given situation. No perfect procedure and no one right way can be recommended.

Reporting an error

If an error in the medication procedure occurs, the nurse must report it immediately. When a nurse believes that the medication given was not in keeping with one of the *rights* (*ie,* the wrong drug, the wrong dose, the wrong client, the wrong route, or the wrong time), it is necessary to report it. In this way, the nurse and, more important, the client is protected. The medication error may be harmless, or it may pose serious threat to the client. Fast reporting of medication errors means that emergency measures can be taken and undesirable complications prevented.

References

Anderson K, Poole C. (1983). Self-administered medication on a postpartum unit. *Am J Nurs, 83,* 1178–1180.

Declaration of independence. (1985). *Nursing 85, 15*(4), 9.

Designer meds. (1989). *American Journal of Nursing, 89,* 1606.

LPNs widen their role; disagreement grows. (1990). *American Journal of Nursing, 90*(2), 16.

New system lets patients self-administer narcotics. (1983). *Nursing 83, 13*(1), 25.

Patients medicating themselves? (1983). *RN, 46*(3), 83.

Pharmacy techs are training for a bigger role. (1990). *RN, 53*(1), 16.

Rx-to-OTC trend fuels nurse prescribing debate. (1983). *RN, 46*(2), 15–17.

Bibliography

Arbeiter J. (1988). The safe way to work with the pharmacy. *RN, 51*(10), 91–92.

Carr DS. (1989). New strategies for avoiding medication errors. *Nursing 89, 19*(8), 39–45.

Casey A. (1985). Get it on tape. *Nursing 85, 15*(8), 64.

Chambers JK. (1987). Medications card. *Nursing 87, 17*(1), 92.

Clayton M. (1987). The right way to prevent medication errors. *RN, 17*(6), 30–31.

Cobb MD. (1990). Dealing fairly with medication errors. *Nursing 90, 20*(3), 42.

*Cohen MR. Medication errors. (A regular feature published monthly.) *Nursing*.

Cohen MR, Wieland K. (1988). What's in a name? *Nursing 88, 18*(9), 86.

*Cushing M. (1986). Drug errors can be bitter pills. *American Journal of Nursing, 86*, 895.

Cushing M. (1986). Who transcribed that order? *American Journal of Nursing, 86*, 1107.

Davis NM, Cohen ME. (1989). Today's poisons: How to keep them from killing your patients. *Nursing 89, 19*(1), 51.

Dispensing after hours. (1990). *Nursing 90, 20*(10), 102.

Drugs in litigation. (1988). Charlottesville, VA: The Michie Co.

Hull RL. (1987). Prospective changes in drug administration. *Nursing 87, 17*(1), 54–57.

*Labar C. (1986). Filling in the blanks on prescription writing. *American Journal of Nursing, 86*(1), 30–33.

Legal question: Question of competence. (1989). *Nursing 89, 19*(5), 28–29.

McGovern K. (1988). Ten golden rules for administering drugs safely. *Nursing 88, 18*(8), 34–41.

Moree NA. (1985). On patients and drug regimens. *American Journal of Nursing, 85*, 51.

The patient and 3-D. (1988). *Nursing 88, 18*(2), 19.

Unusual dosage. (1990). *Nursing 90, 20*(9), 25.

*Recommended for further reading.

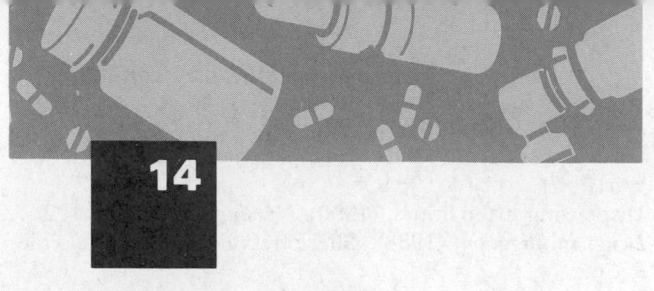

14

Special skills related to drug administration

Effective drug therapy depends on the delivery of accurate doses of active chemicals to the body tissues at the appropriate site of action for the drug involved. To complete this process successfully, the nurse must master certain technical skills. These skills are proper storage and handling of drugs, command of the language used in drug therapy, accurate computation of drug doses, and techniques used in delivering drugs by specific routes to specific sites.

Storage and handling of drugs

Preservation

Drug substances require careful storage and handling to maintain their safety and potency. All medicines should be kept in a special place and secured from access by unauthorized people. To preserve most drugs, storage areas should be kept cool and dry. Chemical deterioration is hastened by heat, moisture, and, in some cases, light. Water can dissolve solid drugs, and heat can melt the waxy bases of suppositories and ointments. Sterile substances must be protected from bacterial contamination. Stocks should be inspected periodically, and any drugs whose recommended shelf-life has expired or that have changed in appearance, indicating possible deterioration, should be discarded. Besides providing the proper conditions for preserving chemicals, storage areas should be kept clean and orderly.

Containers

Drugs are best kept in their original containers. Labeling is more accurate because copying may result in transcription errors. Original containers are effective in protecting their contents, for example, light-sensitive compounds are packaged in amber bottles or containers that filter out much of the harmful radiation. Transferral of sterile substances from container to container should be kept to a minimum because it increases the probability of contamination.

When drugs are handled, the container should be protected from soiling so that the label may remain legible as long as possible. Safe drug use requires that medicines have clear, accurate labels at all times.

Childproof caps

Many drugs are currently dispensed in containers with special childproof caps. These caps require relatively complex manipulation before they can be opened. This increases the time required for children to gain access to the drug and reduces the chances of accidental ingestion before detection. Although these special containers have lowered the incidence of drug poisoning in children, they are very difficult to open for clients with impaired manual dexterity or grip. Regular, easily opened containers can be requested at the time the medicine is dispensed but special precautions must be taken to prevent access by children if child-proof containers are not used.

Tamperproof packaging

Several incidents of lethal cyanide poisoning from over-the-counter analgesics occurred in the United States during the early 1980s. It is believed that poison was added to analgesic capsules once they had reached store shelves. To prevent these problems today, manufacturers package many drugs in tamper-resistant, sealed containers. Tamper-resistant containers typically have an aluminum foil inner seal together with either a plastic outer ring around the cap, or a shrink-seal, full-package cellophane wrapper. Some preparations are packaged as unit doses in individually sealed pouches.

The U.S. Pharmacopeial Convention has published a pamphlet designed to assist drug users in detecting tampering (Tips against tampering, 1991). The user is advised to inspect the preparation carefully for the following: a discrepancy between the lot number on the container and that on the outer wrapping or box; any breaks, cracks, or holes in the outer wrapping or protective cover or seal; indications that the outer covering may have been disturbed, unwrapped, or replaced; distortions or stretching of the shrink band around the top of the bottle; slits in or retaping of the shrink band; looseness of the bottle cap; bits of paper or glue on the rim of the bottle indicating that a seal may have been removed; discoloration or disarray of the cotton plug or filler; overfilling or underfilling of the bottle; and unusual appearance of the medication. Liquids should be checked for color, thickness, clarity, sediment, and odor. Tablets are suspect if they do not display the normal properties of color, shininess, smoothness, size or thickness, printing, taste, or odor. Capsules should be checked for dents, cracks, surface dullness or fingerprints; variations in printing, color, size, or length; and unusual odor. The protective seal on ophthalmic preparations (required to ensure sterility) should be intact. Tubes of topical medications should also be properly sealed and the bottom of the tube uniformly crimped, sealed, and clean in appearance. Ointments should be of uniform consistency, smooth, and not gritty (Box 14-1).

Whenever a medicine or its package appears unusual, the drug should be returned to the pharmacy that dispensed it. If tampering is evident, the pharmacist can report it to the Drug Product Problem Reporting Program, which is coordinated by the federal Food and Drug Administration in cooperation with the U.S. Pharmacopeia and the American Society of Hospital Pharmacists.

Storage in the home

In the home, drugs should be kept under lock and key wherever feasible. The standard bathroom medicine chest is not appropriate for two reasons: it rarely has a

---

Box 14-1. Clues to tampering

- Discrepancy between lot numbers on container and numbers on outer wrapping or box
- Breaks, cracks, or holes in outer wrapping, cover, or seal
- Disturbance in outer covering
- Distorted or stretched shrink band around top of bottle
- Slits in or retaping of shrink band
- Looseness of bottle cap
- Glue or paper fragments on rim of an unsealed bottle
- Discolored or disarrayed cotton plug
- Overfilled or underfilled container
- Unusual appearance of medication
- Unusual odor or taste of medication
- Broken seals on tops of tubes or bottles

---

lock, and the atmosphere in a bathroom is often excessively humid for proper drug storage. A locked container in the bedroom or linen closet would be better. Suppositories and multiple-dose, injectable drugs should be refrigerated; they should be enclosed in plastic or other airtight containers to protect them from humidity and food residues. Locking refrigerated drugs is rarely practical but the drugs should be placed where least accessible to children. Drugs should not be placed near the coils of the refrigerator because freezing may damage them.

Storage in institutions

In health care institutions, most nursing units have a medication room in which all drugs are prepared for use. At the very least, a locked cabinet is needed for storing medicines. Narcotic and other legally restricted drugs should be kept in a special locked compartment. (Many states specify that such drugs be kept under double lock.)

Stock drugs are those supplied in bulk to the nursing unit. All clients' doses are measured from this single supply. Stock preparations for internal use should be kept separate from preparations for external use. Although a few drugs still may be provided in stock bottles, most are presently dispensed in smaller quantities for the specific client. This system requires that each client's drugs be kept in a separate area. Typically, drug carts or cabinets provide a drawer for each client's supply. If drugs are charged to the client when dispensed, unused supplies must be returned to the pharmacy for crediting. Borrowing doses from one client's supply for use by another should be avoided because it increases the risk of error and, if different brand name drugs have been ordered, bioavailability may differ. When it is necessary, repayment (in drugs or credit) should be made.

Refrigerators are standard equipment in most medication rooms. Drugs that require refrigeration include suppositories with low melting temperatures, insulin, sera, vaccines, and certain antibiotics. To prevent contamination of medicines, food should not be stored in these areas.

If labels become soiled or illegible, the medicines should be returned to pharmacy for relabeling. In the institutional setting, nurses should not label or relabel drug containers.

Medication rooms and narcotic cabinets should be kept locked whenever they are not in use. Ideally, the key to the supply of controlled drugs remains in the possession of one nurse, the one who signed for the drugs at the beginning of the work shift. The common practices of propping open medicine-room doors and lending narcotic keys to fellow workers tend to break down the secure control of drug supplies and may allow unauthorized access to harmful substances (Box 14-2).

Insulin

The storage of insulin presents a special problem. Because this drug is dispensed in multiple-dose, sterile vials, bacterial contamination is possible owing to mul-

tiple punctures and prolonged time of use. Refrigeration would minimize the risk of bacterial growth; however, insulin should be administered at room temperature to reduce the risk of lipoatrophy or lipohypertrophy at the sites of injection. A preservative is added to insulin formulation to retard microbial growth. It is now recommended that vials in current use be kept at room temperature. Before use, vials should be inspected carefully for changes in color or clarity that might indicate bacterial contamination. If the appearance of the solution is abnormal, the vial should be discarded.

If insulin is found to have been refrigerated, the vial to be used should be removed to room temperature at least 1 hour before the dose must be administered.

Learning the language

For convenience and to save time, physicians use a system of abbreviations when writing drug orders and prescriptions. The same abbreviations are used by health care personnel who dispense and administer drugs. The nurse must know the terminology used in the setting of his or her practice if drugs are to be given accurately and efficiently.

Certain abbreviations are so common that they are

Box 14-2. Nursing implications in safe storage and handling of drugs

1. Preservation requires proper conditions to maintain chemical potency and safety.
   a. Heat, moisture, and light hasten chemical deterioration.
   b. Water dissolves solid drugs.
   c. Heat melts waxy bases of suppositories and ointments.
   d. Bacteria will invade sterile substances that are not protected.
2. Storage areas should be kept clean, orderly, cool, and dry.
3. All medications should be kept in a specific place and secured from access by unauthorized personnel.
4. Stocks should be inspected periodically and deteriorated or outdated medicines discarded.
5. Drugs should be kept in their original containers.
6. When drugs are handled, the labels should be protected from soiling.
7. Medicines must have clear, accurate labels at all times.
8. If childproof containers are not appropriate, the request should be made at the time the medicine is dispensed.
9. These are considerations for insulin storage:
   a. Store vials at room temperature.
   b. Do not expose to direct sun.
   c. Do not heat vials in hot water.
10. Drugs in the home should be kept under lock and key, wherever feasible.
11. Drugs should not be stored in the bathroom; they are too easily accessible to children, and the atmosphere is too humid.
12. Suppositories and multiple-dose injectable drugs should be refrigerated.
13. In the institutional medication room, a locked cabinet is necessary for storing medication.
14. In health care institutions, narcotic and legally restricted drugs must be kept in a special, locked compartment; some states specify a double lock for these drugs.
15. Medication rooms and narcotic cabinets should be kept locked.
16. The key should be controlled by one nurse— the one who signs for the drugs when the shift begins.
17. Stock preparations for internal use should be kept separate from preparations for external use.
18. Each client's drugs should be kept in a separate area, such as drug carts or cabinets.
19. Unused supplies for each client must be returned to the pharmacy for crediting to the client's account.
20. Avoid borrowing from one client's supply for use by another.
21. Drugs to be kept in the refrigerator in medication rooms are suppositories with low melting temperatures, insulins, sera, vaccines, and certain antibiotics.
22. Food should not be stored in medication refrigerators.

generally recognized and accepted (Tables 14-1 and 14-2). These should be memorized by the practitioner. Sometimes abbreviations that are not generally accepted are used habitually in a particular institution. These must be specified by written policy as required by the Joint Commission on Accreditation of Hospitals (Cohen, 1987) so there is no question of their meaning. A comprehensive policy should list and define all abbreviations acceptable for use in an institution. Certain abbreviations that are easily misread or misinterpreted should *not* be used (Table 14-3). Abbreviations not included on official lists should be questioned consistently for clarification until they are incorporated into the written policy. Assuming the meaning of an order leaves a nurse liable to error and legally vulnerable.

Physicians' orders for medication

Proper orders for medication convey clear directions that specify the client to be medicated, the chemical to be used, the dose to be given, the route of administration, and the timing of drug doses. The procedure used depends on the setting and the situation. Orders may be written for medications to be administered once only, repeatedly at designated time intervals, or when needed. One-time doses may be ordered to be given immediately (stat); at a designated hour in the future; when indicated by the physician at some time in the future (on call); or only if needed (SOS). Drugs to be administered repeatedly may be ordered at specified hourly intervals (*eg*, q3h, q4h, q6h), in relation to activity patterns (ac, pc, hs), or the number of doses per day may be indicated (bid, tid, qid). Standing orders are the usual orders that physicians wish to have carried out on clients in designated situations, unless specifically countermanded. For example, a physician might wish all clients receiving parenteral fluids by hypodermoclysis to have hyaluronidase added to the infusion. Standing orders are limited to the clients of the physician writing the order and should always be available in written form to the nurse carrying out the orders. Protocols are standing orders that outline the steps to be taken in a given situation and the criteria for identifying the situation (*eg*, regular insulin coverage q6h in accord with urine glucose tests: trace or $+1$, no insulin; $2+$, 5 units; $3+$, 10 units; $4+$, 15 units).

Institutional settings

In institutional settings, physicians' orders may be recorded on a special sheet on the client's chart or in a special drug order book. These orders are then re-layed to the pharmacist and the nursing staff for their action. The nurse (or ward secretary) who transcribes orders must read and copy the information accurately. The order must not be changed in any way. If there is reason to think that an error has been made, the physician should be consulted.

If, after consulting the physician, the nurse decides that the order as transmitted is likely to harm the client, he or she must decline to carry it out, in which case the physician must be notified. In this situation, a conflict between physician and nurse can develop; a suggestion by the nurse that the physician prepare and administer the dose personally may resolve it. (A nurse who questions the safety of an order may wish to consult a pharmacology reference and/or experienced colleagues before refusing to carry out a medication order, particularly if he or she is a new practitioner or is working in an unfamiliar clinical situation.)

When the transcription is completed, this fact should be noted on the order sheet. The written record of orders provides legal protection for everyone involved in the use of medicines—the nurse, physician, pharmacist, and client.

Verbal orders may be necessary in emergencies, when the physician is in sterile garb, or when an oral or telephone order is needed. These orders are written by the nurse on the usual record, with a notation that it was an oral or telephone order. The nurse should sign the entry after entering the physician's name. Such orders must be countersigned by the physician as soon as possible.

Verbal orders place the nurse in legal jeopardy if the physician fails to verify the order. The nurse rather than the physician may be held liable for harm caused to the client as a result of the drug order. If the physician repudiates the order, the nurse might even be charged with practicing medicine without a license. Verbal orders should be avoided whenever possible. When unavoidable, the physician should countersign them promptly.

Prescriptions

Drug orders for clients outside health care institutions are written as prescriptions. Drugs deemed by the Food and Drug Administration or Health Protection Branch to require a physician's supervision for their effective and safe use ("legend" drugs) can be obtained only by prescription. Prescriptions are written directions for the dispensing of drugs by a pharmacist. They are composed of the following parts: The *superscription* includes the client's name, age, address, the date, and the symbol Rx (*recipe*, which means in Latin "take thou"). The *inscription* supplies the name of the drug, the dosage form, and amount of the dose. In the *subscription*, directions are given to the pharmacist about preparing the drug and the number of doses to dispense. The *signature* is headed by the abbreviation S or *Sig* (*signa*, which means in Latin "write on the label"). Following this are directions for the client and

Table 14-1. Abbreviations and symbols for orders, prescriptions, and labels

Abbreviation	Meaning	Derivation (Latin or Greek)	Abbreviation	Meaning	Derivation (Latin or Greek)
aa	of each	*ana*	O S	left eye	*oculus sinister*
a c	before meals	*ante cibum*	OTC	over the counter	
ad	to, up to	*ad*	O U	each eye	*oculus uterque*
ad lib	as freely as desired	*ad libitum*	oz	ounce	*uncia*
Aq	water	*aqua*	PB	piggy back	
Aq dest	distilled water	*aqua destillata*	p c	after meals	*post cibum*
b i d	two times a day	*bis in die*	per	through or by	*per*
b i n	two times a night	*bis in nocte*	Pil	pill	*pilula*
c or c̄	with	*cum*	P O	by mouth	*per os*
caps	capsule	*capsula*	P R N	when required	*pro re nata*
comp	compound	*compositus*	*q d	every day	*quaque die*
D₅W	5% dextrose in water		q h	every hour	*quaque hora*
dil	dilute	*dilue*	q 2 h	every two hours	
elix	elixir	*elixir*	q 3 h	every three hours	
ext	extract	*extractum*	q 4 h	every four hours (and so on for any hourly interval)	
fld or Fl	fluid	*fluidus*			
Ft	make	*fiat*			
g, gm	gram	*gramma*	q i d	four times a day	*quater in die*
gr	grain	*granum*	q s	sufficient quantity	*quantum satis*
gtt	drop	*gutta*	R	right	
H	hypodermic		Rₓ	take thou	*recipe*
h	hour	*hora*	s or s̄	without	*sine*
h s	at bedtime	*hora somni*	S or Sig	write (on the label)	*signa*
I M	intramuscularly		S C	subcutaneously	
I V	intravenously		S L	beneath the tongue	*sub linguam*
L	left		Sol	solution	
M	mix	*misce*	S O S	if necessary (once only)	*si opus sit*
μ or min	minim	*minimum*	sp	spirit	*spiritus*
μg or mcg	microgram		ss or s̄s̄	one half	*semis*
mEq	millequivalent		stat	immediately	*statim*
mg	milligram		Syr	syrup	*syrupus*
mist or mixt	mixture	*mixtura*	t i d	three times a day	*ter in die*
ml	milliliter		t i n	three times a night	*ter in nocte*
Noct	at night	*nocte*	TO	telephone order	
non repetat	do not repeat	*non repetatur*	tr or tinct	tincture	*tinctura*
NS	normal saline (0.9% sodium chloride)		*U	unit	
½NS	0.45% sodium chloride		ung	ointment	*unguentum*
O	pint	*octarius*	×	times	
O D	right eye	*oculus dexter*	vin	wine	*vinum*
*o d	every day	*omni die*	VO	verbal order	
*o h	every hour	*omni hora*	>	more than	
ol	oil	*oleum*	<	less than	
o m	every morning	*omni mane*	=	equal to	
*o n	every night	*omni nocte*	↑,↗	increase, increasing	
os	mouth	*os*	↓,↙	decrease, decreasing	

*Abbreviations that are *not* recommended because they are easily misread or misinterpreted. Daily, nightly, hourly and unit should be written out.

Table 14-2. Commonly used abbreviations for drug names

Abbreviation	Drug
ASA	Aspirin (acetylsalicylic acid)
CO_2	Carbon dioxide
$FeSO_4$	Iron sulfate
KCl	Potassium chloride
$MgSO_4$	Magnesium sulfate
MO	Mineral oil
MOM	Milk of magnesia
m s	Morphine sulfate
O_2	Oxygen
SSE	Soap suds enema
SSKI	Saturated solution of potassium iodide
TWE	Tap water enema

Box 14-3. Parts of a prescription

Superscription: Patient's name, age, and address; the date and symbol *Rx*

Inscription: Name of drug, dosage form, and amount of dose

Subscription: Directions to pharmacist about preparing the drug and number of doses to dispense

Signature: An abbreviation *S* or *Sig*, followed by directions for the client and name of the drug to be placed on label

the name of the drug to be placed on the label. Although it was once considered advantageous to keep the client in ignorance about the drugs prescribed, today it is considered the consumer's right to have this information (Box 14-3).

In addition, prescriptions may designate whether a generic drug equivalent may be dispensed and the number of refills allowed. The physician's name, address, and telephone number are usually printed on the prescription blank. The physician must sign the prescription. If a drug listed in the Controlled Substances Act is included in the prescription, the physician's registry number must also be added.

An example of a prescription is shown in Figure 14-1.

Computation of drug doses

To compute drug doses and measure medication accurately, the nurse must understand several systems of measurement. Systems commonly used today have developed at different periods of time. The earliest measures used were defined in commonly available units—

the human hand, finger, foot, arm-span, pace, handful, a grain of wheat. Although they provided a rough approximation of quantity, such methods obviously varied with the size of the person or the grain sample used as a standard. Specifying the individual (often the reigning king) whose anatomic measures were to be adapted helped refine the system. Eventually, standard measures became generally accepted, although confusing variations tended to persist (*eg*, a ton varies depending on whether it is measured by troy or avoirdupois weight). Measurement systems that evolved from these historic models tend to be cumbersome to use. Any elementary school child struggling to convert inches to feet and feet to miles can testify to the complex mathematical computations necessary.

It was not until the late 18th century that a deliberate attempt was made to devise a system of weights and measures that would provide not only a single, unalterable standard but also a mathematical scale that would make computation relatively easy. The international standard (SI or metric) system developed as a result. Although it was adopted early by the scientific community, its acceptance by commerce and industry has been more gradual. Presently, most nations of the world either have adopted or are in the process of converting to the metric system as the official standard

Table 14-3. Abbreviations to avoid because they are easily misread or misinterpreted

Abbreviation	Drug	Misinterpretation
ARA-A	vidarabine	cytarabine (ARA-C)
CPZ	compazine	chlorpromazine
DIG	digoxin	digitoxin
HCl	hydrochloric acid	potassium chloride (KCl)
HCTZ	hydrochlorothiazide	hydrocortisone (HCT)
MTX	methotrexate	mustargen (mechlorethamine HCl)
MVI	Multiple vitamins *without* fat/soluble vitamins	Multivitamins *with* fat-soluble vitamins

Adapted from Cohen MR. (1987). Play it safe: Don't use these abbreviations. *Nursing 87, 17(7)*, 46–47.

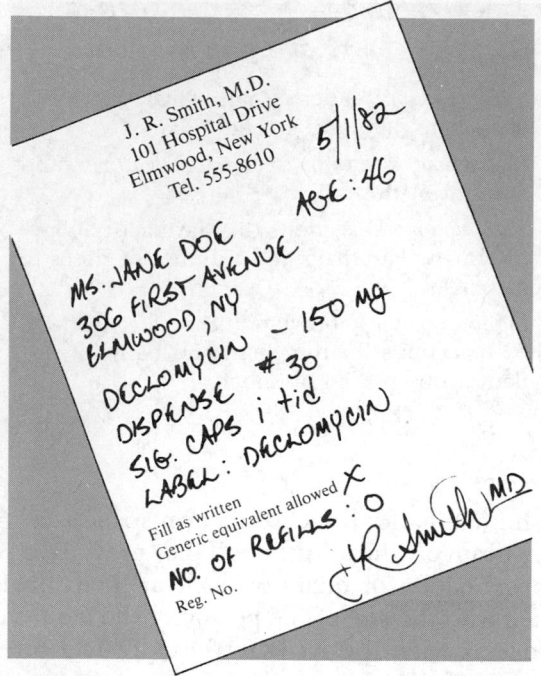

Figure 14-1. Sample of a completed prescription.

of measurement. The United States is a conspicuous exception. To date, Congress has recommended but not required the adoption of the metric system.

The metric system is used most often for drug therapy in institutional settings, although the apothecary system is also used occasionally. When a medicine is to be self-administered, the household system is sometimes used. In Canada only the international standard (metric) system is used.

The metric system

The basic unit of length in the metric system is the meter, which represents one ten-millionth of a quarter of the earth's circumference measured across the pole (Table 14-4). The standard of measurement for this length is a platinum bar deposited in the French Archives, which serves as a model for meter measures intended for actual use. Duplicates of the measure

used as working standards are retained by the governments of participating nations. Conditions such as temperature, which affect the volume of these models, are held constant when measures are taken. The meter is approximately 1 yard long, measuring about 39.37 inches. The designated unit for capacity or volume is the liter and that for weight is the gram. These units bear a specific relationship to the meter.

To facilitate computation, basic measures in the system may be either subdivided or multiplied by 10, 100, 1,000, or other multiples of ten. Greek or Latin prefixes designate the degree of subdivision or multiplication. *Deci* means ten, thus a *decimeter* is one-tenth of a meter; a *deciliter*, one-tenth of a liter; a *decigram*, one-tenth of a gram; *kilo* means one thousand, thus a kilometer equals 1,000 meters, a *kiloliter*, 1,000 liters, and a *kilogram*, 1,000 grams. The prefixes used and their relation to the unit in question are illustrated in Table 14-5.

The metric unit of capacity, the liter (litre), is defined as the contents of a cube whose sides measure 1 dm (10 cm). Originally intended to be exactly the same as the cubic decimeter, the liter actually varies slightly from this quantity because of the intricacies of measurement. This variation is so small that it is important only in precise measurements. In practice, however, the liter is considered equal to the cubic decimeter. Corresponding units of capacity and cubic linear measurement, such as the milliliter and cubic centimeter, are also treated as equivalent (Table 14-6).

The metric unit of weight, the gram, is defined as the weight of 1 milliliter (ml) of distilled water at 4°C. Kilograms, grams, milligrams, and micrograms are the related units commonly used in health work. Other quantities are expressed as multiples or decimals of these measures. For example, a centigram would be expressed as 10 milligrams (mg) or 0.01 gram (g) (Table 14-7).

The metric system has many advantages. All standard units bear a simple relationship to the fundamental unit and to each other. The use of decimal multiples simplifies mathematical computation and conversion from one unit to another.

Table 14-4. Metric linear measurements

Abbreviation	Unit of measurement	Relation to meter	Nonmetric approximation
μm	Micrometer	1/1,000,000 meter (m)	1/26,000 inch (in)
mm	Millimeter	1/1,000 meter (m)	1/26 inch (in)
cm	Centimeter	1/100 meter (m)	0.39 inch (in)
dm	Decimeter	1/10 meter (m)	3.9 inches (in)
m	Meter		39 inches (in)
dkm	Decameter	10 meters (m)	33 feet (ft)
hm	Hectometer	100 meters (m)	328 feet (ft)
km	Kilometer	1,000 meters (m)	5/8 mile

Table 14-5. Subdivisions of the metric system

Prefix	Meaning	Example(s)	Nonmetric equivalent
Kilo	1,000	1 kilogram = 1,000 grams (g)	2.2 pounds (lb) or 35.2 ounces (oz)
Hecto	100	1 hectogram = 100 grams (g)	3.5 ounces (oz)
Deca	10	1 decaliter = 10 liters (L)	2.6 gallons (gal)
	1	1 gram	about 1/30 oz
		1 liter	about 1 quart (qt)
		1 meter	about 39 inches (in)
Deci	0.1	1 deciliter = 0.1 liter (L)	about 3 1/3 ounces (oz)
Centi	0.01	1 centimeter = 0.01 meter (m)	about 1/2 inch (in)
Milli	0.001	1 milligram = 0.001 gram (g)	grains (gr) 1/60
Micro	0.000001 (10^{-6})	1 microgram = 0.000001 gram (g)	grains (gr) 1/60,000
		1 micrometer = 0.000001 meter (m)	about 1/30,000 inch (in)
Nano	0.000000001 (10^{-9})	1 nanogram = 0.000000001 gram (g)	grains (gr) 1/60,000,000
Pico	0.000000000001 (10^{-12})	1 picogram = 0.000000000001 gram (g)	grains (gr) 1/60,000,000,000

Table 14-6. Metric capacity measurements

Abbreviation	Unit of measurement*	Relation to liter	Approximate cubic metric equivalent
ml	milliliter	1/1,000 liter (L)	1 cubic centimeter (cc)
cl	centiliter	1/100 liter (L)	10 cubic centimeters (cc)
dl	deciliter	1/10 liter (L)	100 cubic centimeters (cc)
L	liter	1 liter (L)	1,000 cubic centimeters (cc)

*Units containing multiple liters (decaliter, and so on) are not in common usage.

Table 14-7. Metric weight measures

Abbreviation	Unit of measurement	Relation to gram	Nonmetric approximation
pg	picogram	0.000000000001 gram (g)	grain (gr) 1/60,000,000,000
ng	nanogram	0.000000001 gram (g)	grain (gr) 1/60,000,000
mcg	microgram	0.000001 gram (g)	grain (gr) 1/60,000
mg	milligram	0.001 gram (g)	grain (gr) 1/60
cg	centigram	0.01 gram (g)	grain (gr) 1/6
dg	decigram	0.1 gram (g)	grains (gr) iss
g or gm	gram	1 gram (g)	grains (gr) xv
dkg	decagram	10 grams (g)	1/3 ounce (oz)
hg	hectogram	100 grams (g)	3 1/2 ounces (oz)
kg	kilogram	1,000 grams (g)	2.2 pounds (lb)

Household measures

To lay people, household measurements are the most familiar system of measuring. This system uses quantities handled in familiar household containers, such as teaspoons, cups, pints, and quarts. However, not all common utensils found in the home are equal in measure. Teaspoons and cups vary in size. Scales on pint and quart containers may be inaccurate. Canning jars usually are not calibrated at all. Moreover, it makes a difference how a dry substance is measured. The amounts in a level, rounded, and heaping spoonful vary greatly. Experienced cooks recognize the value of standard measuring tools and the need to level off measurements. A client who measures potent drugs for self-treatment should exercise just as much care.

In the United States, a standard cup contains 8 ounces of volume. Special measuring spoons are available in sets which include 1/8-teaspoon, 1/4-teaspoon, 1/2-teaspoon, and 1-teaspoon sizes. Directions on liquid prescriptions used in the home commonly designate

Table 14-8. Household measurements of fluid volume

Abbreviation	Quantity	Recommended tool for measurement
t or ts	1 teaspoon (4–5 ml)	The teaspoon from a standard set of measuring spoons used for cooking
T or Tb	1 tablespoon (3 teaspoons, 12–16 ml)	If available, a tablespoon from a standard set of measuring spoons used for cooking or three standard teaspoons
oz	1 fluid ounce (2 tablespoons, 30–32 ml)	Measure as above for one tablespoon, or use a standard medication cup (plastic cups are available and relatively inexpensive)
c	1 cup; 1 glass (8 fluid ounces, 240 ml)	A translucent measuring cup
gtt	1 drop (0.06–0.07 ml for watery liquids)	The dropper dispensed with the specific medication to be taken.* (Most liquid medications measured in this unit are packaged with droppers.)

*The size of a drop varies with the density and viscosity of the liquid and the size and configuration of the dropper tip.

Table 14-9. Apothecary measurements

Symbol/abbreviation	Quantity	Recommended tool for measurement
Units of weight		
gr	grain	Apothecary balance scales (rarely needed because medicines measured in grains are almost universally prepared in small dose forms, such as tablets, capsules, or liquid preparations measured by volume)
ʒ	dram (60 grains or gr lx)	Apothecary balance scales
℥	ounce (480 grains or gr xxd)	Apothecary balance scales
Fluid (volume) measure		
min	minim	Minim glass
fʒ	fluidram (60 minims or min lx)	Minim glass, fluid ounce measure, or standard calibrated medicine glass
f℥	fluid ounce (8 fluidrams or Fʒviii, 480 minims or μxxd)	Fluid ounce measure or standard calibrated medicine glass
pt	pint (16 fluid ounces or ℥xvi)	Standard calibrated graduate or pitcher
qt	quart (2 pints or pt)	Standard calibrated graduate or pitcher
gal	gallon (4 quarts or qt)	Standard calibrated graduate or pitcher

household measurements, such as a *teaspoon* or a *cup*. Clients should be directed to use standard measuring utensils to determine the correct amounts. Typical household measurements and recommended utensils for measuring them are listed in Table 14-8.

Apothecary system

The apothecary system of measurement was introduced into the United States from England during the colonial era. It was the prevailing system for medications until recent times. Although the current trend is toward adopting the metric system, apothecary doses are still sometimes used, particularly by older physicians.

The basic unit of weight in the apothecary system, the grain, originally meant the weight of one grain of wheat. Other units of weight derived from the grain are the dram, the ounce, and the pound. The unit of fluid measurement, the minim, is approximately the quantity of water that would weigh a grain. Fluid measures derived from the minim include the fluidram,

fluid ounce, pint, quart, and gallon. Distinctive symbols are used for the apothecary units of measurement (Table 14-9).

When symbols are used, the quantity is expressed as a small Roman numeral placed after the symbol. For example, one grain is written as gr i; 10 minims as min x. Arabic numerals are used to express most fractions, although ½ is often abbreviated *ss* (*semis*, Latin for one-half).

Table 14-10. Approximate equivalents for household measures

Household measure	Equivalent
1 drop	1 minim (min)
1 teaspoon	1 dram (dr) or 4–5 ml
1 dessertspoon	2 drams (dr) or 9 ml
1 tablespoon	½ ounce (oz) or 15 ml
1 teacupful	6 ounces (oz) or 180 ml
1 cup or glassful	8 ounces (oz) or 240 ml

Conversion from one measurement system to another

As long as the use of household and apothecary measurements persists in the health care system, nurses must be proficient in converting values from one system to another. As noted above, equivalents are not exact, only approximations. A study of the metric–apothecary table reveals many discrepancies (Tables 14-10 and 14-11). For example, if 1 fl oz is equivalent to 30 cc, 1 qt (32 oz) is more nearly 960 cc than the 1 liter (1,000 cc), which is given as its equivalent. Using the equivalent 1½ gr to 100 mg, a grain would be equivalent to 66.7 mg, a considerable variance from the 60 mg listed in many charts. In actual practice, equivalents of 60, 64, 65, or 66⅔ mg are all used for converting grains to milligrams (or the reverse procedure)

Table 14-11. Approximate equivalents for metric and apothecary measures

Metric measure	Apothecary equivalent	Metric measure	Apothecary equivalent
Weight		**Weight**	
0.1 mg	grain (gr) 1/600	2 g	grains (gr) xxx
0.12 mg	grain (gr) 1/500	3 g	grains (gr) vl
0.15 mg	grain (gr) 1/400	4 g	grains (gr) lx
0.2 mg	grain (gr) 1/300	5 g	grains (gr) lxxv
0.25 mg	grain (gr) 1/250	6 g	grains (gr) xc
0.3 mg	grain (gr) 1/200	7.5 g	drams (ʒ) ii
0.4 mg	grain (gr) 1/150	10 g	drams (ʒ) iiss
0.5 mg	grain (gr) 1/120	15 g	drams (ʒ) iv
0.6 mg	grain (gr) 1/100	30 g	ounce (oz or ʒ) i
0.8 mg	grain (gr) 1/80	**Capacity**	
1 mg	grain (gr) 1/60	0.03 ml	min (♏) ss
1.2 mg	grain (gr) 1/50	0.05 ml	min (♏) 3/4
1.5 mg	grain (gr) 1/40	0.06 ml	min (♏) i
2 mg	grain (gr) 1/30	0.1 ml	min (♏) iss
3 mg	grain (gr) 1/20	0.2 ml	min (♏) iii
4 mg	grain (gr) 1/15	0.25 ml	min (♏) iv
5 mg	grain (gr) 1/12	0.3 ml	min (♏) v
6 mg	grain (gr) 1/10	0.5 ml	min (♏) viii
8 mg	grain (gr) 1/8	0.6 ml	min (♏) x
10 mg	grain (gr) 1/6	0.75 ml	min (♏) xii
12 mg (0.012 g)	grain (gr) 1/5	1 ml	minims (♏) xv or xvi
15 mg (0.015 g)	grain (gr) 1/4	2 ml	minims (♏) xxx
20 mg (0.02 g)	grain (gr) 1/3	3 ml	minims (♏) vl
25 mg (0.025 g)	grain (gr) 3/8	4 ml	fluidram (fʒ) i
30 mg (0.03 g)	grain (gr) ss	5 ml	fluidrams (fʒ) 1¼
40 mg (0.04 g)	grain (gr) 2/3	8 ml	fluidrams (fʒ) ii
50 mg (0.05 g)	grain (gr) 3/4	10 ml	fluidrams (fʒ) iiss
60 mg (0.06 g)	grain (gr) i	15 ml	fluidrams (fʒ) iv
75 mg (0.075 g)	grain (gr) 1¼		fluid ounce (fʒ) ss
100 mg (0.1 g)	grain (gr) iss	30 ml	fluid ounce (ʒ) i
125 mg (0.125 g)	grains (gr) ii	50 ml	fluid ounce (fʒ) 1¾
150 mg (0.15 g)	grains (gr) iiss	90 ml	fluid ounces (fʒ) iii
200 mg (0.2 g)	grains (gr) iii	100 ml	fluid ounces (fʒ) iiiss
250 mg (0.25 g)	grains (gr) iv	120 ml	fluid ounces (fʒ) iv
300 mg (0.3 g)	grains (gr) v	200 ml	fluid ounces (fʒ) vii
400 mg (0.4 g)	grains (gr) vi	250 ml	fluid ounces (fʒ) viii
500 mg (0.5 g)	grains (gr) viiss	500 ml	1 pint (pt)
600 mg (0.6 g)	grains (gr) x	750 ml	1½ pints (pt)
750 mg (0.75 g)	grains (gr) xii	1,000 ml	1 quart (qt)
1 g	grains (gr) xv		
1.5 g	grains (gr) xxii		

(Table 14-12). The practitioner can choose the equivalent that allows easy computation without generating fractions or involved decimals. Although the freedom to choose an equivalent is convenient, the nurse must bear in mind the error that is always introduced by this process and should keep the number of conversions to a minimum.

Conversion computation

The most reliable way to convert a quantity from one system of measurement to another is to look up its equivalent on an accurate conversion table. The accuracy of any table should be verified before it is used. Printing errors sometimes occur. Because most tables are incomplete or abbreviated, the specific quantity in question may not be listed. Multiplication or division using the appropriate equivalent will be necessary. Examples of such computations are listed below:

A physician orders aspirin, gr x to be given. The stock bottle of aspirin contains 300-mg tablets of aspirin. Either convert the apothecary measurement to metric or the metric to apothecary. Using the equivalent gr i equals 60 mg, multiply the grains ordered by 60 to find out how many milligrams of drug have been ordered:

$$\text{gr x} \times 60 = 600 \text{ mg ordered}$$

Thus, the client should be given two 300-mg tablets of aspirin. Using the equivalent 60 mg equals 1 gr, you may convert 300 mg to grains to find out how many grains are contained in each tablet:

$$300 \text{ mg} \div 60 = \text{gr v per tablet}$$

Again, the same answer is obtained (two 300-mg aspirin tablets). Any other milligram equivalent for 1

Table 14-12. Deviant equivalents commonly used for conversion computations*

Metric	Apothecary
Weight	
60, 64, 65, or 66⅔ mg	grain (gr) i
300, 325 mg	grains (gr) v
600 or 650 mg	grains (gr) x
Liquid	
1 ml	drops (gtt) xv or xvi†; minims (♏) xv or xvi
4 or 5 ml	dram (ʒ) i
240 or 250 ml	ounces (oz or ℥) viii
480 or 500 ml	1 pint

*When official conversion factors have been adopted by a health care institution or system, they should be used by the nurse.

†The standard drop should not be confused with the size of a drop in an intravenous administration set. Although some sets use a drop equivalent to 1/15 ml, others use drops of other sizes (eg, 1/20, or 1/20 ml). The drop factor is included in the package label information and must be used to compute intravenous flow rates.

Box 14-4. Use of ratios to compute conversions

Physician's order: aspirin, gr ×
Preparation on hand: aspirin, 300-mg tablets
Solutions:

1. gr ordered : mg ordered :: gr i : mg in gr i
   gr ordered : mg ordered :: gr i : 60 mg
   10 : × :: gr i : 60 mg
   (multiply the means and extremes)
   1 × = 10 × 60
   × = 600 mg ordered
2. mg/tablet : gr/tablet :: mg/gr i : gr i
   mg/tablet : gr/tablet :: 60 mg : gr i
   300 mg : × :: 60 mg : 1
   60 × = 1 × 300
   × = 300/60
   × = 5 gr per tablet

gr (64, 65, or 66⅔) would complicate the computation needlessly. This type of problem can also be solved by using ratios (Box 14-4).

Although frequently used equivalents will be memorized, it is best to check a table of equivalents to be certain, especially if conversion skills are infrequently used. Confusion of equivalents is common and can have disastrous consequences for the client. An accurate table of equivalents should be readily available in all areas where medications are prepared. Pocket-sized plastic cards with abbreviated tables of equivalents for personal use are available at no cost from several U.S. pharmaceutical manufacturers.

In preparing medications, it is common practice to equate drops and minims, drams and teaspoons, and grams and milliliters. These are not equal measures. A minim is a specific quantity, whereas the size of drops varies in accordance with several factors: the viscosity of the liquid; the size, composition, and configuration of the dropper used; and the angle at which the dropper is held. The standard teaspoon is not equal to a dram (6 t are considered equivalent to 1 oz, whereas 8 dr equal 1 oz). Only in the case of water is a milliliter equivalent to a gram. The more the density of a substance differs from that of water, the greater the deviation in measurement if milliliters are equated with grams. Although significant clinical problems do not appear to arise often as a consequence of such practices, in part this is due to the dose safety margin characteristic of most drugs. Also, most of the solids involved are crystalline substances that are fairly close to water in density. The nurse must recognize the error inherent in such practices and should use the indicated measure whenever possible.

A variety of containers are useful for accurate measurement of drugs (see Fig. 13-6, p 165). Unfortunately, equipment available in health care institutions may not facilitate strict accuracy in measurement. Apothecary scales and minim glasses, once standard equipment in medication areas, are rarely provided in modern institutions. Graduated containers also are unlikely to be readily available.

The nurse often must function as well as possible with the tools at hand. The standard medicine glass is scaled to measure household, apothecary, and metric units of an ounce, or parts of an ounce. Smaller quantities may be measured with the minim or milliliter scale on injection syringes. Graduated specimen jars (*eg*, sterile urine specimen containers) provide a metric scale for 100–200-ml quantities. Stainless steel graduates measuring liter quantities may be available from a centralized supply department. If possible, employ a scale that measures the particular units being used, thereby avoiding conversions. For example, measure drams on the dram scale on a medicine glass; do not convert to milliliters. If a measuring device is provided with the drug, use it. For example, liquids prescribed in small volumes are often packaged with a special dropper scaled for precise measurement. If makeshift measurements or involved conversions are frequently necessary, the nurse should initiate appropriate changes to eliminate them. New equipment, new prescription policies, or a change in medication dosage form may be needed.

Computation of doses

Traditional medication practices have required the nurse to compute drug doses frequently. A variety of formulas have been used to expedite computations, and the practitioner has been required to choose the correct formula before carrying out the appropriate arithmetic. In most health care settings today, drugs are dispensed in appropriate dosage forms so that computation is rarely necessary. What is needed in this context is a single method adaptable for many different computations. The following formula is appropriate for this purpose:

$$\frac{\text{dose ordered}}{\text{dose on hand}} \times \text{volume on hand}$$

$$= \text{volume to be administered*}$$

The *dose ordered* is the amount of pure drug

*The formula can be derived mathematically from the following ratio:
dose ordered : dose on hand :: volume to be administered : volume on hand

$$\frac{\text{dose ordered}}{\text{dose on hand}} = \frac{\text{volume to be administered}}{\text{volume on hand}}$$

$$\frac{\text{dose ordered}}{\text{dose on hand}} \times \text{volume on hand}$$

$$= \text{volume to be administered}$$

Box 14-5. Formula for computing drug dose

$$\frac{\text{dose ordered}}{\text{dose on hand}} \times \text{volume on hand}$$

$$= \text{volume to be administered}$$

---

needed by the client (the weight of dry drug or the volume of liquid drug ordered by the physician). The *dose on hand* represents the amount (weight or volume) of pure drug present in the unit supplied. This may be expressed on the label as the contents of one tablet or capsule, or the amount of drug per volume measure of a liquid drug. The *volume on hand* is the volume of drug that contains the dose on hand. For dry drugs, this is apt to be one tablet or capsule. For liquids, it may be a milliliter or some other capacity measure, depending on the label. The *volume to be administered* tells the nurse how much to measure out for the *client*. This is always expressed in the same units as the volume on hand, be it tablets, capsules, milliliters, or drams (Box 14-5).

If the units of measurement for dose ordered and dose on hand differ, a conversion must be made so that both measures are identical. The formula may be adapted for a multitude of operations, *eg*:

$$\frac{\text{milligrams ordered}}{\text{milligrams per capsule}} \times 1 \text{ capsule}$$

$$= \text{number of capsules to give}$$

$$\frac{\text{units ordered}}{\text{units per ml}} \times 1 \text{ ml}$$

$$= \text{number (or part) of a milliliter to give}$$

If a container label gives the amount of drug in a multiple number of volume units, it is not necessary to compute the amount of drug per unit. For example, Vistaril labels commonly express the concentration as 50 mg per 2 ml. Substitute the formula as follows:

$$\frac{\text{milligrams ordered}}{50 \text{ mg}} \times 2 \text{ ml}$$

$$= \text{milliliters to give}$$

The dose on hand and the volume on hand should correspond to the information on the drug label.

In some situations, the computation is fairly evident. For example, if the physician has ordered 500 mg of erythromycin, and the drug preparation is labeled 250 mg per capsule, the nurse probably will not need to write out the formula to know that two capsules should be given. However, the formula should be used in situations more conducive to error, such as the following example:

The physician orders 0.125 mg of digoxin to be given. The only preparation of digoxin tablets available contains 0.25 mg per tablet. A cursory visual inspection might suggest that five tablets should be given (125 is 5 times 25). Careful use of the formula reveals the correct answer:

$$\frac{0.125 \text{ mg}}{0.25 \text{ mg}} \times 1 \text{ tablet}$$

$$= \text{number of tablets to give}$$

Because quantities and measures in the fraction must be similar, zeros are added to correct the dissimilarity in numbers:

$$\frac{0.125 \text{ mg}}{0.250 \text{ mg}} \times 1 \text{ tablet}$$

$$= \text{number of tablets to give}$$

The correct answer, ½ tablet, becomes clear. If five tablets had been given, the patient would have received 10 times the ordered dose.

If scored tablets are supplied, one may be broken and half a tablet given. No other fractions of tablets can be given accurately. Capsules cannot be divided. If the answer to a computation does not "come out even," the nurse must decide if the amount that can be given (in whole capsules or whole and half tablets) is close enough to the amount ordered to be allowable. A deviation within 10% is allowable for most but not all drugs. (Particularly hazardous drugs, such as antineoplastics, heparin, and insulin, must be measured exactly.)

Example The physician orders 600 mg of aspirin. The stock bottle contains tablets labeled 325 mg. Substitute the formula as follows:

$$\frac{600 \text{ mg}}{325 \text{ mg}} \times 1 \text{ tablet} = 1\frac{275}{325} \text{ tablets}$$

The closest measure the nurse can give is two tablets. These contain, according to their label, 650 mg of drug. Because 10% deviation from 600 mg includes a range of 540 mg to 660 mg, the two-tablet dosage lies within this range and, therefore, can be given. Such deviations often result from using different conversion equivalents. For example, the physician in this case may have wished to give gr x of aspirin. Using a conversion of 300 mg to gr v, an order for 600 mg was written. The 325-mg tablet is also considered equivalent to gr v of drug by a different equivalent.

Liquid volume

The universal formula can also be used to compute liquid volumes to be administered.

Example The physician orders 250 mg of an antibiotic to be given in suspension form. The label on the medication bottle states that 5 ml contain 125 mg of the drug.

$$\frac{\text{dose ordered}}{\text{dose on hand}} \times \text{volume on hand}$$

$$= \text{volume to give}$$

$$\frac{250 \text{ mg}}{125 \text{ mg}} \times 5 \text{ ml} = 10 \text{ ml to give}$$

Example A preoperative order for atropine 0.4 mg intramuscularly is written by the anesthesiologist. The only atropine vial on hand contains 0.3 mg per milliliter.

$$\frac{\text{dose ordered}}{\text{dose on hand}} \times \text{volume on hand}$$

$$= \text{volume to give}$$

$$\frac{0.4 \text{ mg}}{0.3 \text{ mg}} \times 1 \text{ ml} = \text{⁴/₃ ml or } 1\text{⅓ ml to give}$$

In this case, because scales on IM syringes do not measure fractional parts of a milliliter, the fraction may be converted to a decimal:

$$1\text{⅓ ml} = 1.3333 \text{ or } 1.3 \text{ ml to give}$$

An alternate method is to convert 1⅓ ml to minims and use the minim scale on the syringe. Either 15 min or 16 min are considered equivalent to 1 ml. Using the equivalent of 16 will generate a new fraction or decimal, whereas using 15 will provide an answer in whole numbers:

$$\text{If } 1 \text{ ml} = 15 \text{ min,}$$

$$1\text{⅓ ml} = 1\text{⅓} \times 15 = 20 \text{ min to give}$$

Insulin doses

Most insulin preparations in common use are marketed as solutions containing 100 units per ml (or cc). Special insulin syringes calibrated in units for use with *this "standard" strength* solution simplify measurement. The number of units in the dose can be read directly from the scale on the syringe. These 100 unit syringes *cannot* be used for any other strength solution if the dose is to be measured by the scale on the syringe.

Insulin in "nonstandard" strengths are marketed for special purposes. Solutions with 200 or 500 units/ml are available for measuring very large doses and 40 units/ml insulin allows for more accuracy when measuring very small doses. Unless special insulin syringes, calibrated for the specific strength solution, are available, these solutions are best measured in "tuberculin" syringes (long slender syringes with 0.01 or 0.02

ml calibrations.) The standard formula may be used to compute dosage in milliliters.

Example The physician orders 12 units of insulin to be given from a supply of 40-unit insulin. There are no 40-unit insulin syringes available.

$$\frac{\text{dose ordered}}{\text{dose on hand}} \times \text{volume on hand}$$

$$= \text{volume to give}$$

$$\frac{12 \text{ units}}{40 \text{ units}} \times 1 \text{ ml} = 0.3 \text{ ml to give}$$

Using a syringe calibrated in hundredths of a milliliter, draw up 0.30 ml to administer.

Example The physician orders 240 units of NPH insulin (U-200) SC daily.

$$\frac{\text{dose ordered}}{\text{dose on hand}} \times \text{volume on hand}$$

$$= \text{volume to give}$$

$$\frac{240 \text{ units}}{200 \text{ units}} \times 1 \text{ ml} = 1.2 \text{ ml to give}$$

A 2-ml or 3-ml syringe would be used to measure the dose. The measurement should be as exact as possible for insulin has a narrow safety margin. (This is an unusually large dose but might be required for a client resistant to insulin.)

Example Administer 15 units of U-100 insulin. (The U-100 insulin syringe stocked by the institution has a scale that measures accurately only even units [*ie*, 2, 4, 6, and so forth]).

$$\frac{\text{dose ordered}}{\text{dose on hand}} \times \text{volume on hand}$$

$$= \text{volume to give}$$

$$\frac{15 \text{ units}}{100 \text{ units}} \times 1 \text{ ml} = 0.15 \text{ ml to give}$$

Using a tuberculin syringe, draw up solution to the 0.15-ml mark. (As this example illustrates, U-100 insulin may be measured directly on the scale of the tuberculin syringe because one-hundredth [0.01] ml contains 1 unit.)

In general, however, syringes specific for the use intended should be employed to minimize the risk of error.

Preparing solutions

Solutions are commonly prepared by diluting a given weight of dry drug or volume of liquid drug by sufficient solvent (usually water) to obtain the desired volume of solution. Solution strengths are commonly expressed as either percentages or ratios. The meaning of these terms is arbitrarily defined as follows.

Percentages indicate the number of units of weight of dry drug (or volume of liquid drug) per 100 units of solution. The volume unit used for the solution must correspond to the weight unit equivalent for water. That is, if the drug is measured in grams, the volume unit must be milliliters because 1 g of water equals 1 ml. In the apothecary system, grains are considered equivalent to minims, drams to fluidrams, and ounces to fluid ounces. Thus, a 10% solution could be expressed as follows:

10 g of dry drug dissolved in sufficient water to make 100 ml of solution,
OR
gr x of dry drug dissolved in sufficient water to make 100 min of solution,
OR
10 oz of dry drug dissolved in sufficient water to make 100 fl oz of solution.
OR
10 fl oz of liquid drug diluted with enough water to make 100 fl oz of solution.

Ratios indicate the number of parts of drug (dry weight or liquid measure) per part of solution (comparable liquid measure). A 1 : 1,000 solution contains one part of drug per 1,000 parts of solution and could be interpreted as follows:

1 g of dry drug dissolved in sufficient water to make 1,000 ml of solution,
OR
gr i of dry drug dissolved in sufficient water to make 1,000 min of solution,
OR
1 fl dr of liquid drug dissolved in sufficient water to make 1,000 fl dr of solution.

Notice that the drug is not added to a given volume of solvent because this will not yield an accurate measurement of solution in most cases. Adding a given weight of dry drug to 1,000 ml of water is likely to produce more than 1,000 ml of solution. In a few cases (notably alcohol mixed with water), the combination of substances produces a decrease in volume. A solution is always prepared by dissolving a given quantity of drug in "a volume of solvent sufficient to produce" the desired volume of solution.

Occasionally, a concentrated stock solution is used to prepare diluted solutions of drugs. This can be accomplished by first computing the amount of pure drug needed to prepare the desired solution and then using this quantity as the "dosage ordered" in the universal formula to determine the volume of stock drug needed.

Example Prepare 1 liter of 2% potassium permanganate solution from a 40% stock solution.

If a 2% solution contains, by definition, 2 g of drug

in 100 ml of solution, 20 g of drug would be needed to prepare 1,000 ml or 1 liter of solution.

Therefore the "dose ordered" is 20 g. (This can also be computed by setting up a ratio*.)

The stock solution contains 40%, or 40 g, of drug per 100 ml of solution.

$$\frac{\text{dose ordered}}{\text{dose on hand}} \times \text{volume on hand}$$

$$= \text{volume to use}$$

$$\frac{20 \text{ g}}{40 \text{ g}} \times 100 \text{ ml} = \frac{1}{2} \times 100$$

$$= 50 \text{ ml to use}$$

To prepare the solution, 50 ml of stock solution should be measured into a liter container and enough water added to make 1,000 ml (1 liter) of solution.

Preparing fractional doses from solid drugs

Though rarely necessary, it is possible to prepare fractional doses from a dry drug (powder or tablet), provided the drug is readily soluble. This is feasible only if the solution form is appropriate to give and reasonably palatable to the client. The volume of solution to be prepared depends on the amount needed and also on a measure that makes computation of the dose easy.

Example The physician has ordered 20 mEq of K-lyte to be administered orally. The label on the K-lyte package indicates that each tablet contains 25 mEq and is to be dissolved completely in 3–4 ounces of water just before administration.

If the nurse elects to prepare a 100 ml ($3\frac{1}{3}$ oz) solution from the tablet, the drug will be sufficiently diluted, and a number convenient for computation will be provided.

$$\frac{\text{dose ordered}}{\text{dose on hand}} \times \text{volume on hand}$$

$$= \text{volume to give}$$

$$\frac{20 \text{ mEq}}{25 \text{ mEq}} \times 100 \text{ ml} = \frac{4}{5} \text{ of } 100$$

$$= 80 \text{ ml to give}$$

Because the tablet is to be dissolved at the bedside, the nurse will need a container (*eg*, a sterile urine

---

*pure drug in volume ordered : volume ordered :: pure drug in desired solution : volume in desired solution

2% (by definition) = 2 g drug in 100 ml of solution

x = pure drug needed to make the ordered volume of solution

x:1000 :: 2:100

100x = 2000

x = 20 g of pure drug needed (or "dose ordered")

Learning experience 14-1

Examine the tools available in the hospital or nursing home for measuring drugs. Are these adequate for accurate preparation of doses? What additional tools would you recommend?

specimen container) to measure the tablet solution and a container (*eg* a 1-oz medicine cup) to measure the amount to be discarded. At the bedside, the tablet is dissolved in sufficient water to produce 100 ml of solution. The solution is stirred until the tablet is completely dissolved, 20 ml are removed by pouring into the smaller scaled container, and the remaining 80 ml are administered.

Verifying computed dosage

Most medications are dispensed in forms that provide the correct dosage in one or two units. That is, only one or two tablets or capsules are normally required for a single medication. Liquid preparations are also often labeled in quantities appropriate for single doses. For this reason, whenever a dosage computation yields an unusual answer (Box 14-6), the answer is suspect. The computations should be checked carefully for errors. The first time such a drug is given, it is wise to have another nurse verify the accuracy of the dosage.

Medication of children often requires computation of fractional doses. These dosages should also be verified (see Chapter 17).

Nurses who administer drugs must be able to compute accurately, and measure without error. Mistakes may be very harmful to clients, and can be fatal.

Occupational hazards related to drug administration

Exposure to drugs, including the preparation and administration of drug dosages, increases the risk of certain health problems in the health care practitioner. These conditions include chemical dependence, adverse reactions to contact with toxic substances, anti-

---

Box 14-6. Unusual drug dosages that require verification

- Fractional parts of a tablet other than $\frac{1}{2}$
- Three or more tablets or capsules
- More than 2 ml of injectable solution
- More than 1 unit dose of liquid oral medication
- More than 1 ounce of liquid oral medication

Box 14-7. Occupational hazards related to drug administration

- Chemical dependence
- Adverse reaction to toxic substances
- Antibiotic-resistant infections
- Blood-borne infection
- Allergy

biotic-resistant infections, blood-borne infection, and allergic sensitivity to drug agents (Box 14-7).

Chemical dependence

Both the medical and the nursing professions are at increased risk for developing dependence on psychoactive drugs. Factors contributing to the high incidence of dependence include knowledge about the effects of central nervous drugs, easy access to psychoactive substances, and conditioning through clinical experience to regard these drugs as appropriate agents for the treatment of pain or depression. A reluctance to confront dependent colleagues contributes to delay in treatment.

Adverse reaction to toxic substances

Some drugs are toxic in therapeutic concentrations, so that contact during preparation of doses must be avoided. For example, alkylating antineoplastics, are caustic to the skin. Oncology nurses who administer these drugs frequently must take special precautions (*eg*, wearing rubber gloves) to prevent contact. Another toxic drug is fluothane, an inhalant anesthetic. Chronic exposure to this gas is known to increase the risk of abortion in female members of operating room staffs. Atropine can cause visual symptoms. If, when preparing injections of this drug, the nurse's hands become contaminated, small amounts of the solution may be transferred inadvertently to an eye, causing pupil dilation and blurred vision. Nurses should avoid inhalation of drug powers. Serious lung malfunction and asphyxiation have occurred from inhalation of the bulk laxative, methylcellulose (Table 14-13).

Table 14-13. Selected substances used in health care that frequently affect personnel

Substance/drug	Effect on personnel (protective measures*)
Antineoplastic drugs	
Alkylating agents/anti-metabolites	Irritation at contact sites
	Allergy
	Dizziness, headache, coughing, nausea, hair loss
	Mutagenic changes, increased risk of miscarriage (pregnant women and nursing mothers should avoid all contact; doses should be prepared under vertical laminar flow hoods*)
Anesthetics	
fluothane	Psychomotor impairment, vertigo, fainting
	Increased risk of miscarriage (operating rooms and recovery rooms should be ventilated by efficient scavanger units)
Sterilizing agent	
Ethylene oxide	Anemia, nausea, vomiting, diarrhea, headache, irritation at contact sites
	Possibly carcinogenic, mutagenic and teratogenic (personnel responsible for gas sterilization require special training in ventilating units and handling articles exposed to ethylene oxide)
Anticholinergics	
Atropine	(Upon eye contact) blurred vision, widely dilated pupil
Antibiotics	
Broad-spectrum agents	Normal microbial flora becomes antibiotic-resistant
Human blood	Exposure to blood-borne infection such as acquired immunodeficiency syndrome, and hepatitis B virus
	(Precautions include careful disposal of contaminated equipment, universal blood/body fluid precautions, avoidance of "sticks" by used needles)

*For detailed precautions, see Jacobson. (1990). Hospital hazards: Part two: How to protect yourself. *Am J Nurs 90*, *20(4)*, 48–53 (April).

Antibiotic-resistant infections

Infectious organisms present in health care institutions may become resistant to antibiotics if these treatment agents are allowed to pollute the environment. Nurses whose clothing or skin contacts antibiotics tend to develop a flora of resistant organisms. As a result, those nurses and their families are at increased risk for infections caused by antibiotic-resistant staphylococcus organisms.

Blood-borne infections

Equipment used to administer medications parenterally is universally contaminated with the client's body fluids. Health care personnel accidentally injured by used equipment, such as needles, become inoculated with any systemic infectious agents harbored by the client. Infections known to be transmitted in this way include hepatitis and acquired immunodeficiency syndrome. These diseases are serious and can be fatal.

To minimize the risk of transmission of blood-borne disease to health care personnel, used equipment is deposited directly into special containers. Equipment should be handled as little as possible and used needles should *not* be recapped.

Allergy

Contact with even minute quantities of chemicals while handling drugs may induce an allergy to these substances. Drugs known to be allergenic, such as penicillin, are frequent offenders, but a nurse with a tendency toward allergy could develop antibodies to any chemical agent.

Nursing implications

To decrease the risk of occupational illness from drug administration, nurses should adhere to policies and practices designed to control contact with medications and contaminated injection equipment. For example, the nurse should take care not to scatter or inhale powders and granules. When preparing medications, spillage into the environment and personal contact should be avoided. If drugs are spilled, they should be cleaned up immediately and discarded into trash that will be incinerated.

Used injection equipment should be handled carefully to prevent needle sticks. Used needles should *not* be recapped but deposited into special receptacles which are subsequently incinerated.

All discarded drugs (except controlled drugs which are returned to the pharmacy for disposal) should be incinerated.

References

*Cohen MR. (1987). Play it safe: Don't use these abbreviations. *Nursing 87* 17(7), 46–47.

Tips against tampering. (1991). Rockville: The United States Pharmacopeial Convention.

Bibliography

Cartier A, et al. (1987). Occupational asthma in nurses handling psyllium-containing laxatives. *Clinical Allergy* 17, 1–6 (January).

Craft K. (1990). Do you really know how to handle sharps? *RN, 53(8),* 33–35 (August).

Gingrich MM. (1990). Should you take zidovudine after a needle stick? *Nursing 90(9),* 18–21.

If you're exposed to blood or body fluids. (1988). *RN 51,* 14–15 (September).

*Impaired nurses. (1986). *Nursing 86, 16(1),* 78.

*Jacobson E. (1990). Hospital hazards: Part two; how to protect yourself. *Am J Nurs 90(4),* 48–53.

*Kirkman-Liff B, Dandoy S. (1984). Hepatitis B: What price exposure? *American Journal of Nursing, 84,* 988–989.

Millam D. (1990). Avoiding needle-stick injuries. *Nursing 90(1),* 61–63 (January).

Steer clear of ribavirin. (1988). *Nursing 88 18(12),* 11–12.

* Recommended for further reading.

Special considerations in drug therapy

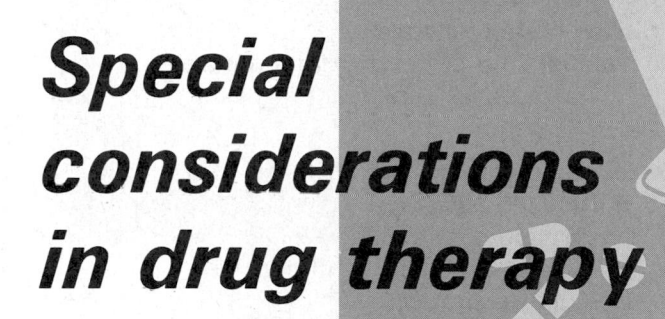

4

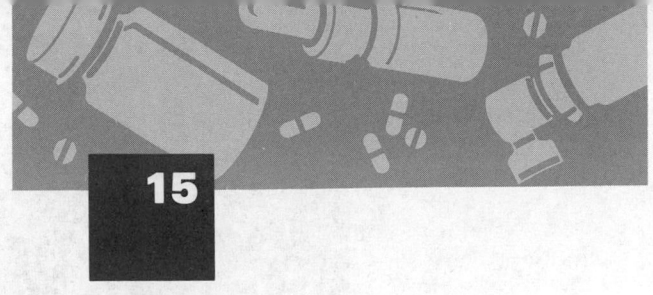

15

Substance abuse

Throughout history, societies have been affected by the use of pharmacologically active substances for non-therapeutic or "recreational" purposes. Substance abusers are broadly defined as people who use psycho-active products without medical sanction or who use such substances contrary to cultural norms. Tradi-tionally, the abuse of substances was motivated by their therapeutic qualities, such as relieving pain or altering mood. Today, motivating factors include curiosity, peer pressure, pain relief, anxiety, fatigue, pleasure, and escape from boredom.

Modern society is particularly burdened by drug-related problems. The scenario of substance abuse is complex; different people respond differently, from casual experimentation to addiction. The type of psy-choactive agent, the socioeconomic sphere (including peers, family, and community), and individual person-ality traits are all factors that influence a person's sus-ceptibility to substance abuse.

Nature of dependence and addiction

Definition of terms

To recognize and help substance abusers, one must first understand the terms and use of psychoactive substances in a nontherapeutic way. *Abuse* is a self-directed use of chemical substances for nontherapeu-tic purposes that does not comply with approved social and cultural norms. Extended use tends to interfere with one's biologic, psychological, and social health. On the other hand, *addiction* is a behavioral state charac-terized by loss of ability to control a drive or craving. Daily life tends to be dominated by the psychoactive agent.

When a person responds to a chemical substance by continuous or sporadic use to experience its phar-macologic effects, the person is said to be *dependent* on the drug. Two types of dependency exist: *psychological* and *physical*. The first is a compulsion to use a sub-stance on a continuous or sporadic basis to achieve a desired outcome, for example, to avoid anxiety or to feel pleasure. Physical dependence is characterized by an altered physiologic state from continuous use of the psychoactive agent. If the chemical substance is not maintained, a drug-specific withdrawal or abstinence syndrome results.

When a person needs to increase the amount of a drug to achieve the same effects experienced from a previously smaller dose, that person is said to have developed a *tolerance* to the substance. Tolerance also exists when a specific dose produces a reduced phar-macologic effect (either intensity or duration) after repeated use. Tolerance does not necessarily mean that physical dependence is also present.

The diagnosis of substance abuse requires typ-

Enrichment experience 15-1

Contact your regional office of the Drug Enforcement Administration to obtain in-formation about current rates of substance abuse in your community.

---

ically three criteria from the list identified in Table 15-1 in accordance with the *Diagnostic and Statistical Manual of Mental Disorders (DSM-IIIR)*.

Circles of dependence

With substance abuse, human behavior generally reflects a stereotypic pattern of social learning and reinforcement. The consequences of substance use or abuse reinforce and maintain the behavior. When drug use produces pleasurable effects, or a "high," drug use is positively reinforced. Drug use may also be "negatively reinforced" when it alleviates some unpleasant event, such as high stress or severe pain. In either case, the use of chemical substances conforms to a behavioral pattern in which environmental stimuli reinforce and intensify the behavior. The behavior involved in substance abuse becomes a vicious circle. The person who is vulnerable tries to cope with disequilibrium in social, psychological, biologic, or environmental influences, but adaptive responses fail to restore balance. The cycles reflected in drug dependence and addiction may be pharmacologic, cerebral, social, or psychological in nature (Fig. 15-1).

The circle of pharmacologic dependence or addiction occurs when tolerance to and physical dependence on a drug exist. The drug creates metabolic changes commonly exhibited in the symptoms of with-

Table 15-1. Diagnostic criteria for substance dependence*

Frequent preoccupation with seeking or taking substance

Substance often taken in larger amounts or a longer period of time than the individual intended

Tolerance develops

Withdrawal symptoms

The substance is taken to relieve or avoid withdrawal symptoms

Persistent desire or repeated efforts to cut down or control substance use

Person shows frequent intoxication or withdrawal symptoms when expected to fulfill social or occupational obligations or when substance use is hazardous

Important social, occupational, or recreational activity is given up or reduced because of its incompatibility with the use of the substance

Continuation of substance use despite a persistent social, occupational, psychological, or physical problem that it causes or exacerbates

* The diagnosis of substance abuse requires at least three of the above criteria. (From American Psychiatric Association. [1987]. *Diagnostic and statistical manual of mental disorders*, 3rd ed, rev. Washington, DC: American Psychiatric Press.)

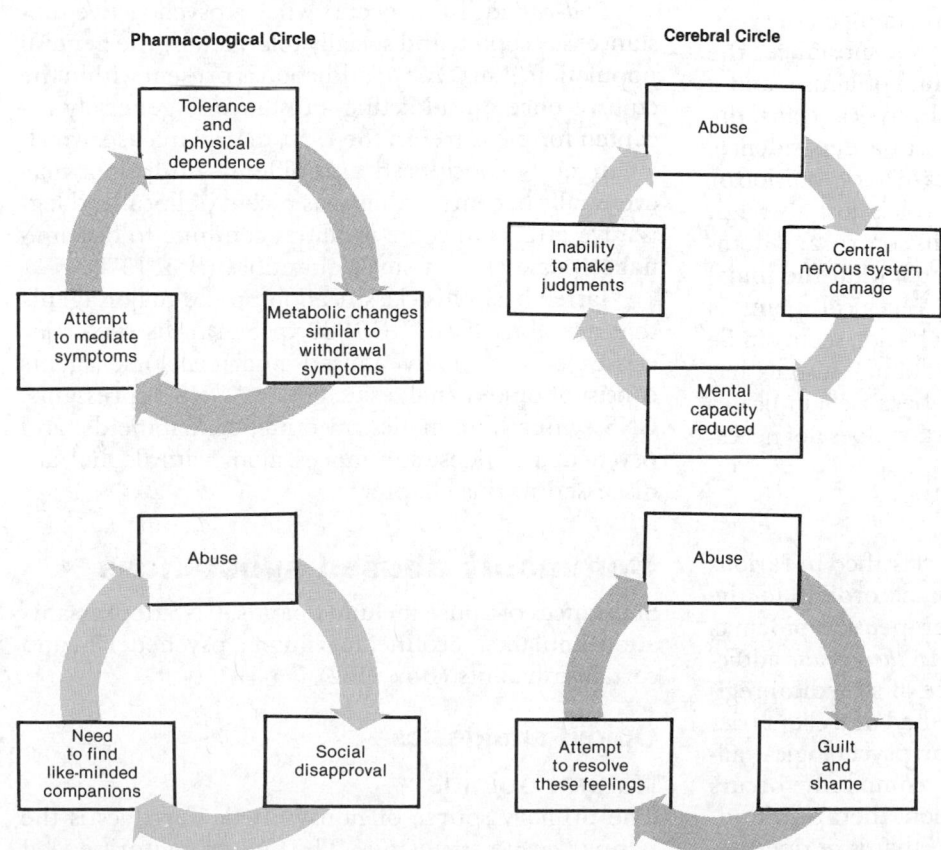

Pharmacological Circle

Tolerance and physical dependence → Metabolic changes similar to withdrawal symptoms → Attempt to mediate symptoms →

Cerebral Circle

Abuse → Central nervous system damage → Mental capacity reduced → Inability to make judgments →

Social Circle

Abuse → Social disapproval → Need to find like-minded companions →

Psychological Circle

Abuse → Guilt and shame → Attempt to resolve these feelings →

Figure 15-1. Cycles of dependence.

drawal. To mediate these symptoms, the drug must be taken again, thus reinforcing the circle.

The cerebral circle is the result of central nervous system (CNS) damage from excessive drug use. The damage occurs in the form of reduced mental capacity for regulating and controlling behavior, including a person's inability to make judgments about the drug-taking behavior.

The social consequences of the abuse reinforce and maintain drug use. The general social disapproval of drug abuse creates a need to find companions whose moral and social expectations tolerate or reinforce the habit of taking drugs.

In the psychological circle, unpleasant feelings, such as guilt and shame, that result from substance abuse are resolved by taking more drugs.

Whichever circle exists—and several may exist simultaneously—the pattern of behavior can be seen as predictable and self-perpetuating. Unless intervention is offered, the dependence or addiction worsens.

Relationship of potency and nature of dependence

A positive relationship exists between drug potency and the nature of addiction. The more potent a dependence-producing agent is and the more pleasure it produces, the more rapidly the addiction develops (Glatt, 1977, p 1). During the initial period of drug abuse, the user is capable of controlling consumption and the degree of intoxication. Depending on the variation in the addictive quality of the substance, the intensity, pattern, and length of time of abuse, and a person's specific psychological and physical traits, the abuse of a substance can progress to a dependence, which then shows the characteristics of a compulsion or craving. Once the power of control is lost through continued abuse, the addiction gains control and dominates the life of the user. No matter what the initial reason for the addiction, once a critical point is reached, the resultant addictive behavior seems to be independent of the original motivation. This fact has implications for treatment models, because it indicates that removing the "causes" of addiction does not necessarily result in recovery.

Classifications

Dependence and addiction can be classified in various ways. Bejerot classified addiction according to the manner in which it is acquired: therapeutic, epidemic, or endemic (Bejerot, 1977, p 69). In *therapeutic* addiction, the addiction is a consequence of a medical regimen (iatrogenic) or it is self-established (the client tries to treat his or her own physical or psychological ailments). This type of addiction commonly occurs among health personnel. In addition, therapeutic addiction is usually not "contagious," that is, it does not involve others.

Epidemic addiction is the most prevalent type in the

Box 15-1. Classification of addiction according to its acquisition

1. Therapeutic
   a. Consequence of medical regimen or established through self-treatment
   b. Most commonly occurs among health personnel
   c. Usually is not "contagious"
2. Epidemic
   a. Most common type in Western world
   b. Characterized by direct personal involvement between an established abuser and a novice
   c. Abusers tend to use more than one drug simultaneously
3. Endemic
   a. Psychoactive substance becomes accepted and socially tolerated by general population

(Based on Bejerot N. [1977]. The nature of addiction. In Glatt MM, ed. *Drug dependence: Current problems and issues*, pp 69–78. Baltimore: University Park Press.)

Western world. It is characterized by direct personal involvement between an established abuser and a novice. Epidemic abusers tend to use more than one substance simultaneously.

Endemic addiction occurs when a psychoactive substance is accepted and socially tolerated by the general population. This type of addiction is present within the culture once an addicting substance is generally accepted for pleasure. In the U.S., marijuana use, which is currently considered an epidemic addiction, may eventually become endemic as recent political and legislative efforts in some localities continue to decriminalize possession of small quantities (Box 15-1).

Jaffee bases his classification on the major agents that are abused (Jaffe, 1980, p 544). His six major classes of commonly abused pharmacologic agents consist of opioid analgesics, general CNS depressants, CNS sympathomimetics, nicotine, cannabinoids, and psychedelics. These substances, along with alcohol, are discussed in this chapter.

Commonly abused substances

Substances of abuse include opioids, CNS depressants and stimulants, nicotine, marijuana, psychedelics, and certain inhalants (Box 15-2).

Opioid analgesics

Natural opioids

The primary source of nonsynthetic narcotics is the poppy *Papaver somniferum*. The milk from unripe seed pods is collected and dried to form raw opium. Several substances are extracted from opium, two of which fall into the major chemical groups: phenanthrene and benzylisoquinoline. Analgesics and cough suppressants of the phenanthrene group include morphine, codeine, and thebaine; substances in the benzylisoquinoline group do not have the morphinelike effects of the former and are non-narcotic. Papaverine and noscapine are the major natural alkaloids of the benzylisoquinoline group. Phenanthrenes include opioid narcotics (Table 15-2); their therapeutic use as analgesics is discussed in Chapter 24.

Morphine, codeine, and thebaine are all extracted from opium, although morphine constitutes the major component in opium (4%–21%). Codeine concentrations in raw opium range from 0.7% to 2.5%. Thebaine is only a minor component of raw opium, but it acts as a stimulant instead of a depressant.

Morphine

Morphine is one of the most potent pain-relieving drugs available. A bitter-tasting odorless substance, it is marketed in several forms, including injectable preparations, syrups, and hypodermic tablets. Because morphine is so potent, dependence and tolerance develop rapidly. In street slang, morphine is known as "cube," "hocus," "first line," and "morf."

Codeine

Codeine can occur naturally in opium, or it can be produced from morphine. It is marketed in injectable and tablet form for the relief of mild to moderate pain, as well as in liquid form as an antitussive.

Semisynthetics and synthetics

In addition to natural opioid drugs, several commonly abused semisynthetic and synthetic substances are derived from components of opium or synthesized in the laboratory. Heroin, oxycodone (Percodan), meperidine (Demerol), and hydromorphone (Dilaudid) are

the more common semisynthetic drugs derived from opium chemicals.

Synthetic narcotics in common use include meperidine (Demerol), methadone (Dolophine, Amidone), levorphanol (Levo-Dromoran), alphaprodine (Nisentil), and anileridine (Leritine), to name a few. All of these synthetic narcotics have effects similar to those of morphine, although they vary in potency and in the duration of their action.

Heroin

Heroin in its pure state is a white bitter-tasting powder. Street (illicit) heroin is processed and diluted with quinine, starch, sugar, or powdered milk. Illicit heroin is sold in a 100-mg "bag," which usually contains less than 10% heroin. Heroin has a variety of street names, such as "scag," "smack," "junk," "horse," "H," and "brown sugar."

Hydromorphone

Hydromorphone (Dilaudid) is produced in both tablet and injectable forms. It is two to eight times more potent than morphine in relieving pain, but it is shorter acting and produces greater sedation than morphine.

Oxycodone

Oxycodone, the narcotic ingredient in Percodan and Percocet, is a semisynthetic narcotic derived from thebaine. Produced in tablet form, it is an effective pain reliever. Though similar to codeine, oxycodone is more potent and also leads to dependence. When used illicitly, tablets are dissolved, filtered, then injected intravenously, or "mainlined."

Meperidine

Meperidine (Demerol) is a widely used effective narcotic analgesic. The drug is marketed as oral tablets, an elixir, and an injectable substance. It is used most frequently as an illicit drug in its injectable form.

Methadone

Methadone (Dolophine) was first synthesized as a morphine substitute when morphine was in short supply during World War II. Methadone is available in tablet and injectable forms. The pharmacologic action of this drug is similar to heroin and morphine. Originally, methadone was used as an analgesic; however, since the 1960s it has been more commonly used in drug treatment programs for the detoxification of heroin addicts and in methadone maintenance programs.

Designer drugs

The term *designer drug* refers to chemical analogues derived from known controlled substances. These analogues have a risk of abuse because they are usually more potent and less expensive than the original drug. In the late 1970s, designer drugs, developed to look like and mimic the effects of heroin, appeared in California. The substances were derived from the drug

Table 15-2. Opioid analgesics

Drug name	Preparations	Additional information
Natural opioids		
Morphine	White crystals, injectable forms, hypodermic tablets	One of the most potent pain-relieving drugs available
		Bitter tasting, odorless
		Dependence and tolerance develop rapidly
Codeine	Injectable and tablet forms, liquid for antitussive action	Relief of moderate pain
Semisynthetic and synthetics		
Heroin	Bag of powder diluted with quinine, starch, sugar, or powdered milk	White, bitter tasting
		Similar in pharmacologic action to morphine
Hydromorphone (Dilaudid)	Tablet and injectable forms	2 to 8 times more effective than morphine
		Shorter-acting and more sedative effect than morphine
Thebaine (Percodan)	Tablet form; illicitly, tablets are dissolved and injected IV	Relief of pain
		More potent than codeine
		Leads to dependence
Meperidine (Demerol)	Tablets, elixir, injectable form	Widely used, effective narcotic analgesic
Methadone (Dolophine)	Tablet, liquid, and injectable forms	Similar in pharmacologic action to heroin and morphine
		Originally an analgesic agent
		Commonly used now in drug treatment programs
Oxymorphone (Numorphan)	Injectable solution or rectal suppository	As potent as morphine
Levorphanol tartrate (Levodromoran)	Oral or parenteral preparation	May produce less nausea and vomiting than morphine
Paregoric (Parepectolin)	Liquid tincture	Limited use as antidiarrheal agent
Diphenoxylate (in Lomotil)	Tablet and liquid, contains atropine	Definite constipating effect
Fentanyl (Sublimaze)	IV injectable	Used only for anesthesia
Propoxyphene (Darvon)	Oral preparation	More potent than morphine
		Related to methadone
		Relief of pain

fentanyl citrate (Sublimaze or Innovar), known as China White and new heroin. They were synthesized in clandestine labs by slightly altering the molecular structure of fentanyl, creating designer opiates known chemically as MPPP or MPTP. Both drugs were found to produce Parkinson-like symptoms in some users. Amphetamine modification has produced two other popular designer drugs known as MDMA, called Ecstasy, and MDE, called Eve.

In 1986, MDMA and other controlled substance analogues were placed on schedule I of the Controlled Substances Act under the Controlled Substance Analogue Enforcement Act, Anti-Drug Abuse Act of 1986 (Public Law 99-570). Drugs included under schedule I have a high potential for abuse. No acceptable use is recognized for them in the U.S. However, they may be acquired for use in approved research protocols. Additional legislative efforts are being addressed to make the manufacture and distribution of designer drugs illegal.

General pharmacologic effects. Opioid analgesics have been effective for relieving intense pain. They are also commonly used to treat diarrhea and suppress coughs.

These drugs cause short-lived euphoria, drowsiness, lethargy, decreased physical activity, pin-point pupils, decreased vision, and constipation. In large doses, they may induce sleep, nausea, vomiting, and even respiratory depression.

In nontherapeutic abuse, these drugs are administered orally, by sniffing, by smoking, or, for more immediate effects, by subcutaneous ("skin popping") or intravenous ("mainlining") injection. Rapid intravenous (IV) injection of a narcotic tends to produce warm flushed skin and a lower abdominal sensation that resembles an orgasm in quality and intensity. This sensation is termed "rush," "thrill," or "kick." Complications secondary to narcotic abuse include malnutrition, infections, untreated injuries or diseases, skin abscesses, endocarditis, and hepatitis.

Chapter 24 details other information about opioids, such as pharmacokinetics, pharmacodynamics, therapeutic uses, and nursing management.

Tolerance and dependence. Tolerance to opioid analgesics occurs at different degrees of pharmacologic potency. Opioid tolerance is characterized by a generalized decrease in the normal action of the drug in depressing the CNS. The amount of a drug necessary for a lethal dose is also significantly increased.

Physical dependence usually develops in proportion to the intensity and amount of alteration that has occurred in the CNS. In general, the withdrawal symptoms are characteristic of rebound activity in the physiologic systems most affected by the chemical substance.

The opiate withdrawal syndrome is visually dramatic to the observer and briefly disabling to the addict; however, provided general physical health is intact, it is probably less life-threatening than the withdrawal syndromes of other drug groups. Symptoms of opiate withdrawal usually develop from 2 to 48 hours after abstaining from drug use. They tend to peak within 72 hours.

Four phases of the syndrome represent accelerating intensity of the withdrawal process. The first phase is characterized by diaphoresis, generalized anxiety, insomnia, lacrimation, yawning, and rhinorrhea. The second phase is characterized by piloerection, abdominal cramps, mydriasis, arthralgia, muscle twitching, and myalgia. The third phase of the withdrawal syndrome is characterized by nausea, vomiting, anorexia, elevated temperature, blood pressure, and pulse, and extreme restlessness. Symptoms characteristic of the fourth phase include diarrhea, fetal position, hyperglycemia, vomiting, dehydration, chills that alternate with diaphoresis and flushing, and insistent drug-demanding behavior. The symptoms are immediately reversible by administration of an opiate. Without any treatment, all toxic symptoms should disappear in 7 to 10 days.

Treatment. The Food and Drug Administration (FDA) has detailed the legal protocol for treating drug-dependent people addicted to opioid substances. Although detoxification without drugs ("cold turkey") has been done, medically supervised withdrawal is available in federally designated treatment programs in which methadone is used. Methadone may also be administered by a physician to a drug-dependent person hospitalized for an illness not related to the addiction.

The FDA stipulates legal use of methadone only for detoxification, maintenance, or analgesia. According to its regulations, *detoxification* is defined as the use of methadone for medically supervised withdrawal from physical dependence on opiate drugs. Detoxification must be completed within a 21-day period.

FDA regulations define *maintenance* as the use of methadone as an oral substitute for morphinelike drugs and heroin for more than 21 days. Methadone may also be used for analgesia when clients in advanced stages of illness suffer from intractable pain. When methadone is used to treat hospitalized users, complications that result from drug interactions may precipitate the withdrawal syndrome, which can happen with pentazocine (Talwin), a narcotic antagonist.

Symptoms of methadone overdose include miosis, decreased respiratory rate, hypotension, drowsiness, bradycardia, hypothermia, and coma. In acute methadone overdose, pulmonary edema and renal failure can result. The treatment of choice in acute methadone overdose is naloxone hydrochloride (Narcan). When the possibility of multiple drug abuse exists, it is necessary to avoid opiate antagonists, such as nalorphine (Nalline) or levallorphan tartrate (Lorfan), which may cause respiratory depression. Therefore, when the causative agent of respiratory depression in a situation that involves acute overdose is unclear, naloxone is the antidote of choice.

General central nervous system depressants

The psychoactive substances considered to be general CNS depressants are barbiturates, related sedative–hypnotics, benzodiazepines, and alcohol. Medically, CNS depressants have traditionally been used to treat insomnia and to relieve tension, irritability, and anxiety. When used in high doses, they tend to produce alcoholic-like intoxication. These substances are discussed in detail in Chapter 24.

Barbiturates

In street jargon, barbiturates are called "barbs," "blue devils," "downers," "green dragons," "goofballs," "yellow jackets," "nimbies," "pink ladies," "rainbows," "red devils," "reds," and "stumblers." Table 15-3 categorizes common barbiturates and trade names according to the duration of their actions.

The pharmacologic effects of barbiturates range from calming anxiety after low doses to progressive stages of sedation, sleep, and coma as a result of larger doses. Death may result from cardiovascular and respiratory complications.

Ultrashort-acting barbiturates have rapid onset and cause anesthesia within minutes after IV infusion, although their action is brief. In the short- to intermediate-acting category are pentobarbital (Nembutal), amobarbital (Amytal), and secobarbital (Seconal), the most abused depressants. These drugs are generally prescribed for sedation and begin to take effect within 15 to 40 minutes. Their pharmacologic action can last up to 6 hours. The long-acting barbiturates are used as hypnotics, anticonvulsants, and sedatives. Their onset of action is slow, up to 1 hour, with a

Table 15-3. Barbiturates and duration of action

Very short acting	Short to intermediate acting	Long acting
Hexobarbital (Sombulex)	Amobarbital (Amytal)	Phenobarbital (Luminal)
Methohexital sodium (Brevital)	Aprobarbital (Alurate)	Mephobarbital (Mebaral)
Thiamylal sodium (Surital)	Butabarbital sodium (Butisol)	Metharbital (Gemonil)
Thiopental sodium (Pentothal)	Pentobarbital sodium (Nembutal)	
	Secobarbital (Seconal)	
	Talbutal (Lotusate)	

duration up to 16 hours. The slow onset of their action makes these long-acting depressants less attractive to abusers.

Barbiturates come in a variety of forms and in mixtures combined with other pharmacologic agents. They are available in powdered form for injection, as tablets, capsules, drops, syrups, elixirs, or suppositories.

Sedative–hypnotics

Pharmacologic substances in this category are used primarily to treat insomnia and anxiety. Table 15-4 identifies the more common drugs in this category that are used and abused.

Chloral hydrate

The oldest of the hypnotic drugs, chloral hydrate has been a popular sedative and sleep-inducing drug. It is available in capsules and in liquid form. The drug has a bitter caustic taste and a sharp, slightly acrid odor. When combined with alcohol, chloral hydrate is toxic.

Ethchlorvynol

Ethchlorvynol (Placidyl) is a sedative–hypnotic drug with rapid onset of effect and short duration. It is supplied in capsule form.

Glutethimide

Glutethimide (Doriden) is a CNS depressant used to produce sedation. The onset of the drug's action occurs in about 30 minutes, and its action is of long duration (4–8 hour). Glutethimide is available in capsule and tablet form. Slang terms include "cibas" or "CD."

Meprobamate

Meprobamate (Miltown, Equanil) is a CNS depressant commonly used for its anti-anxiety properties, including muscle relaxation. Drug action is rapid in onset and of short duration. Its pharmacologic properties closely resemble those of intermediate-acting barbiturates. Meprobamate is supplied in tablet form.

Methaqualone

Methaqualone (Quaalude, Sopor) is a commonly abused drug. It is used for its sedative–hypnotic, antispasmodic, anticonvulsant, local anesthetic, antitus-

sive, and mild antihistaminic qualities. The drug is supplied in tablet form. In street jargon, methaqualone is called "quads," "soapers," or "sopes."

Methyprylon

Methyprylon (Noludar) is a CNS depressant that produces a hypnotic effect similar to secobarbital. It is available in tablet and capsule preparations.

Paraldehyde

Paraldehyde (Paral), a rapidly acting hypnotic, is supplied as a colorless liquid with an unpleasant taste and strong odor. Because it decomposes to form acetic acid when exposed to air and light, paraldehyde is stored in air-tight amber containers. The drug possesses anticonvulsant properties and has been used chiefly to treat alcohol abstinence syndromes. Paraldehyde's unpleasant taste and odor make it an unlikely drug of abuse.

Benzodiazepines

Benzodiazepines (CNS depressants) produce sedation, prevent convulsions, relieve tension, suppress anxiety, and alleviate muscle spasms. Benzodiazepines include chlordiazepoxide (Librium), clonazepam (Clonopin), clorazepate dipotassium (Tranxene), diazepam (Valium), flurazepam hydrochloride (Dalmane), and oxazepam (Serax). Newer short-acting benzodiazepines include lorazepam (Ativan), triazolam (Halcion), and alprazolam (Xanax).

Drug action tends to be long-acting with relatively slow onset. In addition to previously identified drug actions, benzodiazepines are used to treat alcohol withdrawal syndrome. The drugs are supplied in tablets, capsules, liquids, and injectable preparations. Benzodiazepines are discussed in more detail in Chapter 26.

All benzodiazepines are comparable, but diazepam (Valium), which is one of the drugs prescribed most often in the U.S., stands out as the most frequently abused drug in this category.

General pharmacologic effects. Symptoms of depressant intoxication resemble alcoholic intoxication. In therapeutic use, depressants may decrease inhibitions, which can produce a short-term sense of eupho-

Table 15-4. Nonbarbiturate sedative–hypnotics

Drug name	Preparations	Additional information
chloral hydrate	Capsule and liquid	Popular sedative and sleep-inducing drug
		Combination with alcohol very toxic
ethchlorvynol (Placidyl)	Capsule	Also effective anticonvulsant and muscle relaxant
		Drug action is rapid and of short duration
glutethimide (Doriden)	Capsule and tablet	Onset of action is about 30 min and is of long duration (4–8 hr)
meprobamate (Equanil, Miltown)	Tablet	Muscle relaxant; antianxiety agent
		Anticonvulsant properties
methaqualone (Quaalude, Sopor)	Tablet	Used also as antispasmodic, anticonvulsant, local anesthetic, antitussive, and mild antihistaminic
methyprylon (Noludar)	Tablet and capsule	
paraldehyde (Paral)	Colorless liquid	Has been used chiefly in treatment of alcohol abstinence syndromes
		Unpleasant taste and strong odor make it an unlikely drug to abuse.

ria. Acute depressant intoxication is characterized by decreased mental acuity and physical activity, slurred speech, impaired thinking with poor judgment, poor memory, and limited attention span. With lowered inhibition, some basic personality traits may become exaggerated. Labile mood swings and release of aggressive or combative impulses can occur. The intoxicated person may appear unkempt and exhibit bizarre, paranoid, or even suicidal behavior.

Chronic abuse of depressants results in progressive neurologic changes. Symptoms of chronic intoxication include diplopia, nystagmus, thick slurred speech, vertigo, strabismus, positive Romberg's sign, dysmetria, ataxic gait, decreased superficial and deep tendon reflexes, and hypotonia.

In cases of overdose, neurologic functioning and the CNS are affected by progressive depression, exhibited as confusion, somnolence, and coma. At this stage, arousal is difficult; response to painful stimuli may be lacking, culminating in respiratory depression, shock, and death (Khantzian, McKenna, 1979, p 363).

Complications secondary to parenteral use of depressants include skin rashes, tetanus, sterile abscesses, bacterial endocarditis, and serum hepatitis.

Tolerance and dependence. Because tolerance to depressants occurs rapidly, the capacity to consume greater doses increases at the same time that the range between an intoxicating and a fatal dose decreases. Excessive and prolonged abuse of depressants leads to physical and psychological dependence. Abruptly ceasing or significantly decreasing the amount of depressant results in a withdrawal syndrome more severe than a narcotic withdrawal syndrome. Accordingly, withdrawal should be carried out under medical supervision. Figure 15-2 illustrates the overall abstinence syndrome commonly seen in depressant drug addiction. Withdrawal symptoms range from anxiety, tremor, insomnia, and weakness in mild cases to delirium and grand mal seizures in more severe cases.

Symptoms of abstinence are evident within 24 hours after the drug is discontinued. Symptoms from short-acting barbiturates usually peak in 2 to 3 days. These include nausea, vomiting, anxiety, restlessness, weakness, abdominal cramps, and orthostatic hypotension. Hyperactive blink and deep tendon reflexes may also be present. If seizures occur, they do so during peak symptom time. Without complications, withdrawal runs its course in a week. Symptoms of abstinence from long-acting depressants peak more slowly. Seizures may develop within 24 to 72 hours after the drug is discontinued. Delirium and hallucinations may

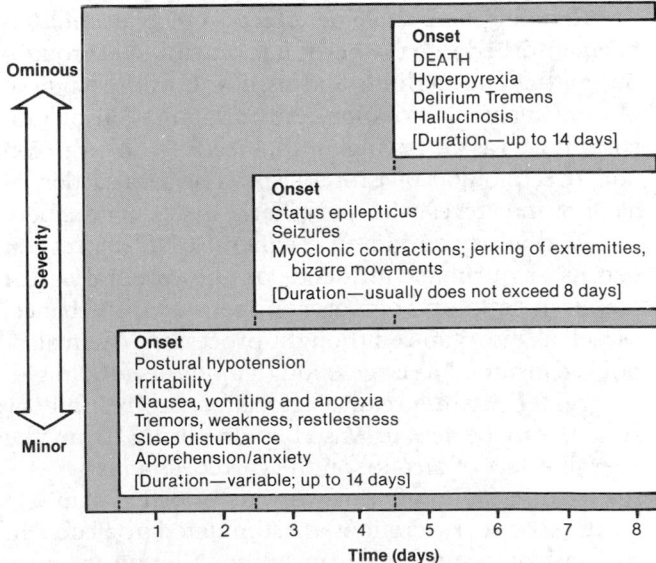

Figure 15-2. The barbiturate abstinence syndrome: onset, duration, and severity. (Khantzian EJ, McKenna GJ. [1979]. Acute toxic and withdrawal reactions associated with drug use and abuse. *Ann Intern Med, 90,* 361–372.)

develop between 3 to 8 days in the withdrawal process. Agitation and hyperthermia may accompany delirium and lead to eventual cardiovascular collapse and death.

Treatment. The life-threatening potential of the abstinence syndrome requires gradual controlled withdrawal using drugs that can stabilize and gradually detoxify the user from the addictive substance. Phenobarbital has become the substance of choice to carry out this process, with generally successful results (Khantzian, McKenna, 1979, p 363).

The phenobarbital-substitution technique can be used to treat benzodiazepine addiction, but the symptoms of abstinence and withdrawal tend to be delayed when compared to those with short-acting barbiturates. Because symptoms tend to peak between days 5 and 9, treatment should be extended.

Alcohol

Alcoholism is considered one of the most serious public health problems in the U.S. It is estimated that two-thirds of all Americans occasionally use alcohol. Excluding nicotine, alcohol is the most abused drug available to the public. An estimated 15.1 million alcoholics live in the U.S. today.

Based on descriptions from the National Institute on Alcohol Abuse and Alcoholism and the National Council on Alcoholism, a person is considered an alcoholic when alcohol is used to such an extent that it negatively influences or interferes with the activities of daily living in any of the following areas: physical health, emotional health, social health, or employment. Addictive drinking is characterized by an overall loss of control that manifests itself behaviorally as preoccupation, compulsiveness, and the tendency to relapse.

General pharmacologic effects. Once alcohol has been absorbed into the body, it is distributed throughout all the body's fluids and tissues. Local reaction to alcohol includes irritation and inflammation of mucosa. It acts as an astringent that leads to dehydration and precipitation of protoplasm. The local action of alcohol interferes with peripheral nerve conduction.

Alcohol is considered a general CNS depressant because its primary influence on the cerebral cortex results in symptoms of motor and sensory disturbance, as well as disorganized thought processes. When alcohol is consumed in large enough amounts (400 mg/dl or greater), its depressive effects on the respiratory system can be lethal. Vasodilation results from the overall effect of alcohol on the cardiovascular system, the manifestation of which is warm flushed skin.

Gastric acid secretions are stimulated by alcohol in the gastrointestinal (GI) tract. Immoderate use may lead to diarrhea or constipation. If large enough quantities are consumed, secretory and motor function of the GI tract are greatly diminished, causing delayed absorption and pylorospasm accompanied by vomiting. Pancreatitis may also occur.

Alcohol interferes with liver function, resulting in accumulation of fat in the liver, the development of alcoholic hepatitis, and possible progression into cirrhosis (Wooddell, 1979b, p 16).

The extent of the physiologic and psychological damage to the human being caused by alcohol abuse is more complex and extensive than this brief description indicates. The National Institute on Alcohol Abuse and Alcoholism is an excellent source of more information.

Chapter 24 details the pharmacodynamics, pharmacotherapeutics, adverse reactions, therapeutic uses of alcohol, precautions and contraindications, and drug interactions. It also discusses nursing management of medicinal alcohol.

The average adult is capable of metabolizing about 10 ml of alcohol per hour. This rate of absorption from the stomach is influenced by the type and dilution of the alcohol used, by the amount of time taken to ingest the substance, and by the presence or absence of food in the stomach. After absorption, the concentration of alcohol in the blood provides an indication of the degree of intoxication (Fig. 15-3). When blood alcohol levels reach 0.05%, a person's behavior is likely to be less inhibited, judgment may be impaired, and mood is generally carefree. Most states recognize a blood alcohol level of 0.10% as legal evidence of intoxication. At this level, motor coordination is impaired. When the blood alcohol level approaches 0.40%, coma occurs; at 0.50%, respiratory failure causes death.

Tolerance and dependence. Repeated use increases the body's capacity to metabolize alcohol, thereby requiring higher doses to achieve intoxication.

Physical dependence develops when the concentration of alcohol is chronically maintained at high levels. Abrupt cessation results in classic withdrawal symptoms known as *alcohol withdrawal syndrome.*

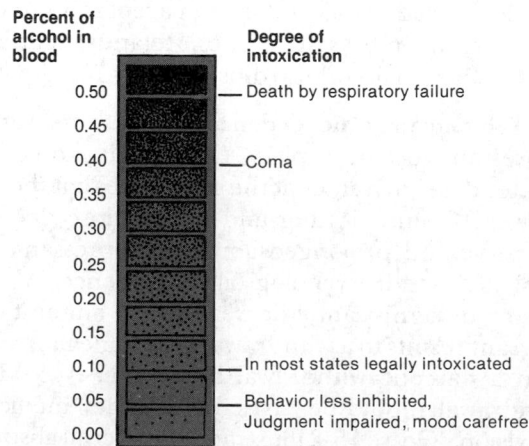

Figure 15-3. Degree of intoxication by blood alcohol levels.

Chronic alcohol intoxication over long periods of time results in adaptive neurophysiologic changes. Alteration of nervous pathways takes place, so that once alcohol consumption is stopped, a rebound hyperacuity of all senses ensues; that is, tactile, visual, and auditory responses become oversensitive.

Abstinence is followed by three usually predictable stages in the classic withdrawal syndrome (Box 15-3).

Delirium tremens (DTs) can occur from 3 days to 2 weeks after alcohol consumption ceases. High fever, exhaustion, nausea and vomiting, hyperventilation, and seizures also occur. Death can result from secondary complications of DTs. The mortality rate from DTs ranges from 4% to 20%. If death does not occur, the process of detoxification may last from 5 to 7 days (Ritchie, 1980, p 388).

Treatment. The primary goal of alcohol detoxification programs is to prevent or minimize symptoms of the abstinence syndrome. Most treatment programs use some form of drug therapy as part of the detoxification process. Paraldehyde (discussed earlier) has been used with some success; however, its irritating caustic nature and questionable effect on the liver do not make it a popular drug of choice. Phenytoin (Dilantin) is frequently used with clients who have a history of seizures. Benzodiazepines—in particular, chlordiazepoxide (Librium) and diazepam (Valium)—are, however, the most commonly used drugs for detoxification (Ritchie, 1980, p 388).

In addition to drug therapy, diets high in calories, proteins, and fluids are encouraged. Rehabilitating the alcoholic usually involves group counseling and self-help groups, such as Alcoholics Anonymous.

Disulfiram (Antabuse) is also sometimes used to augment rehabilitation. This drug significantly alters the intermediary metabolism of alcohol and, when taken in the presence of alcohol, greatly increases acetaldehyde concentration in the body. The drug's action creates respiratory depression, cardiovascular collapse, acute congestive heart failure, convulsions, unconsciousness, and possible death. Usually taken in the morning, Antabuse sensitizes the person to alcohol for 6 to 12 hours. It must never be administered without the client's knowledge. Persons who take disulfiram must avoid contact with *any* form of alcohol, including aftershave lotion, alcohol used in products for back rubs, or alcohol in sauces and fermented vinegar (Wooddell, 1979a, p 27).

Central nervous system sympathomimetics (adrenergics)

The CNS sympathomimetic group of psychoactive substances includes amphetamines and cocaine. In therapeutic doses, CNS stimulants suppress appetite, elevate mood, produce insomnia, and create a feeling of increased energy and hyperactivity; in addition, anxiety, apprehension, and irritability sometimes occur.

Stimulants are taken orally or intravenously. When taken intravenously, drug effects are intensified and produce abrupt sensations alternately called "rush" or "flash." Stimulants are referred to as "speed," "crank," "double cross," "uppers," "ups," "pep pill," "lightning," and "truck drivers." Table 15-5 includes additional slang terms used for the principle amphetamines available in the U.S. When taken orally, the onset of drug action usually takes place within 30 minutes and is of long duration. Several other stimulants and amphetamine-related stimulants are methylphenidate hydrochloride (Ritalin), benzphetamine hydrochloride (Didrex), chlorphentermine hydrochloride (Pre-Sate), clortermine hydrochloride (Voranil), diethylpropion hydrochloride (Tenuate, Tepanil), fenfluramine hydrochloride (Pondimin), mazindol (Sanorex), pemoline (Cylert), phendimetrazine (Plegine, Melfiat, Bacarate, Statobex, Tanorex, Trimstat, Trimtabs, Phenazine, Phendiat), phenmetrazine hydrochloride (Preludin), and phentermine (Ionamin, Wilpowr).

Amphetamines

Amphetamines are psychostimulant drugs that were originally used as nasal decongestants and appetite suppressants and for the treatment of narcolepsy. These drugs (primarily Ritalin) continue to be used to treat children who exhibit hyperkinetic behavior or

---

Box 15-3. Stages in the classic alcohol withdrawal syndrome

Stage I develops about 8 hours after abstinence or significant reduction in the use of alcohol. Symptoms at this stage include complaints of nausea, tremor, jittery feeling, headache, and anxiety.

Stage II occurs from 8 to 24 hours into withdrawal. Hyperactivity is evident with more severe tremor, increased nervousness, and irritability. The sufferer may be easily startled, feel restless, and complain of insomnia with nightmares, as well as visual, tactile, or auditory hallucinations. Seizures most likely occur during this stage.

Stage III presents with delirium tremens (DTs). DTs are a pathologic state of consciousness that results from interference with brain metabolism, causing confusion and disorientation.*

*(Wooddell WJ. [1979]. The alcohol withdrawal syndrome. *Family and Community Health*, 2, 23.)

Table 15-5. Principal amphetamines available in the U.S.

Generic name	Trade name	Street slang
amphetamine complex (amphetamine and D-amphetamine resin)	Biphetamine	
amphetamine combined	Obetrol, Delcobese	
D-amphetamine plus amobarbital	Dexamyl	
D-amphetamine plus prochlorperazine	Eskatrol	
dextroamphetamine sulfate	Dexadrine, Ferndex	Dexies, oranges, orange hearts
dextroamphetamine hydrochloride	Daro	
dextroamphetamine tannate	Obotan	
methamphetamine hydrochloride (desoxy-ephedrine hydrochloride)	Desoxyn, Methampex	Meth, crystal whites, speed
racemic amphetamine sulfate	Benzedrine	Bennies, peaches

brain damage. It may seem paradoxical, but amphetamines act as calming agents in children without neurologic deficits who are being treated for hyperactivity.

Many people become amphetamine abusers unwittingly. Dieters use amphetamines to lose weight; college students take them to stay awake for examinations; truck drivers are notorious for using amphetamines to stay awake on the road.

Cocaine

Cocaine is an alkaloid derived from the leaves of the South American coca plant. Cocaine, the strongest natural stimulant available, has the ability to block nerve conduction after local application. Drug action on the CNS initially affects the cortex. This effect creates restlessness, excitement, intense euphoria, and heightened mental acuity. Therapeutic use of cocaine is restricted to ear, nose, and throat surgery. It is also frequently found in the Brompton cocktail, a mixture used in cancer therapy for intractable pain. (People with known sensitivity to Novocaine, Xylocaine, or other local anesthetics may have similar adverse reactions to cocaine.)

Within the last few years, cocaine has become a popular recreational drug. Recent estimates indicate that more than 25 million people have tried cocaine, of whom 2 to 3 million have become compulsive users (Tarr and Macklin, 1987, p 322).

Between 1985 and 1988, the number of cocaine-related emergency department visits increased by 354% (DHHS, 1991, p 2). The Drug Abuse Warning Network (DAWN) notes that cocaine-related deaths in emergency departments rose from 628 in 1984 to 2,163 in 1988 (DHHS, 1991, p 115).

Cocaine is sold on the street as a crystalline powder that usually contains only 5% to 10% pure cocaine; the remainder is made up of white powders, such as procaine, lactose, and lidocaine. It is taken by IV injection or sniffing ("snorting"). Injection produces intense euphoria with accompanying elevation in heart rate, body temperature, and blood pressure. When used nasally, cocaine causes vasoconstriction, resulting in inflammation of the nasal mucosa and possible perforation of the nasal septum.

Another method of cocaine ingestion is "freebasing," in which cocaine is purified of its contaminants through heat processing with a solvent such as ether. This method has been linked to an increase in the number of people who experience signs of systemic toxicity.

Freebasing has been refined recently, creating a highly purified, inexpensive variety of cocaine known as "crack." The rapid popularity of crack is cause for concern because of the drug's ability to quickly promote dependency and addiction. The drug's purity and its route of administration make it especially attractive to drug users. Crack is found in small chips or "rocks" that are smoked. The impact of smoking crack reaches the brain within 8 seconds, producing euphoria followed by depression. The cycle of intense highs and crashing depressions reinforces the user's need for increasing the frequency of use. As a stimulant, crack creates paranoia, as well as increased anxiety and freneticism.

Street slang refers to cocaine as "snow," "Big C," "coke," "flake," "gold dust," "nose candy," "rock," and "white." Table 15-6 compares the characteristics of cocaine and crack.

Another variation of a smokable methamphetamine stimulant has been noted in Hawaii and on the West Coast of the U.S. Gaining in popularity because

Table 15-6. Characteristics of cocaine and crack

Characteristics	Cocaine	Crack
Primary route	Snort (nasal)	Inhaled by smoking
Onset of effects	1–3 minutes	4–6 seconds
Duration	20–30 minutes	5–7 minutes
Relative purity	5%–25%	90%

of its persistent stimulating effect is "ice." The "high" that it produces may last up to 24 hours and can lead to significant acute psychotic episodes.

General pharmacologic effects. Amphetamines and related stimulants raise systolic and diastolic blood pressure and increase pulse pressure. High doses can provoke tachycardia and tachyarrhythmia. Absorption is sometimes interfered with as a result of slow peristalsis, which leads to slow gastric emptying and constipation. Metabolic rate and oxygen consumption increase, and symptoms of pronounced CNS stimulation (discussed previously) are evident. Protracted use of stimulants leads to a period known as "crashing," characterized by depression and extended restless sleep.

A toxic dose of stimulants leads to symptoms of anxiety, agitation, fever, and insomnia. Some users react with panic or delirium. Excessive cardiovascular stimulation leads to headache, diaphoresis, nausea, vomiting, diarrhea, increased heart rate with palpitations and arrhythmia, hypertensive crises, and abdominal cramps. Death may result under conditions of extreme heat or excessive physical activity (Morgan, 1979, p 7).

Further toxic symptoms of chronic high-dose stimulant abuse include compulsive and repetitive body movements, bruxism, and facial grimacing. The initial sense of well-being is often replaced with violent, angry, and aggressive behavior. Paranoia and delusions are common, and hallucinations may be present.

Tolerance and dependence. Tolerance to these stimulants develops rapidly, increasing the risk of a toxic reaction. Experts debate whether tolerance to cocaine exists and tend to conclude that it does not. Stimulant withdrawal symptoms are less severe than from CNS depressants.

Gross physiologic changes do not occur during withdrawal from amphetamines. The abstinence syndrome with stimulants is much less dramatic than with opiates or barbiturates. However, the pattern of behavior consists of prolonged lethargy, sleep disturbance, and depression. Withdrawal does not produce life-threatening physiologic side effects.

Treatment. Toxic manifestations of chronic stimulant abuse, exhibited as psychotic reactions, can be treated with phenothiazines or antipsychotic agents, such as haloperidol. If severe amphetamine withdrawal symptoms occur in the form of depression, they can be treated with tricyclic antidepressants.

More detailed information on cocaine, as well as the nursing management for the therapeutic use of cocaine and for cocaine abuse appears in Chapter 23.

Nicotine

Nicotine, the active ingredient in tobacco, is considered the most widespread, costly, and physically addicting substance of abuse in the U.S. Despite extensive campaigns to educate the public about the harmful effects of smoking, it is estimated that 51.1 million adults in the U.S. are dependent on nicotine. Some 340,000 deaths result annually from diseases related to smoking, including lung and heart diseases and cancer (Gunby, 1988, p 2811).

General pharmacologic effects. Nicotine causes complex changes in the body, with both stimulant and depressant phases of action. The nicotine-stimulated release of epinephrine from the adrenal medulla accelerates heart rate and elevates blood pressure. Small amounts of nicotine stimulate the ganglion cells of the peripheral nervous system, whereas larger doses first stimulate then block transmissions.

The CNS is greatly stimulated by nicotine, which can provoke respiratory excitation and vomiting. Cardiovascular system reflexes to nicotine include vasoconstriction, tachycardia, and an increased cardiac workload and output. Stimulation of the parasympathetic nervous system increases tone and motor activity in the GI tract, resulting in occasional diarrhea.

Tolerance and dependence. Tolerance and dependence develop with chronic use of nicotine. On withdrawal, smokers experience such symptoms as irritability, hostility, depression, and difficulty in concentrating. These symptoms can last for several days after cessation of smoking but resolve themselves without drug therapy. Nursing management for the prevention and reduction of nicotine use appears in Chapter 22, as well as information on pharmacokinetics, pharmacodynamics, adverse reactions, and drug interactions of nicotine.

Cannabinoids

It is speculated that cannabis (marijuana) is ranked as the fourth most abused drug in our society after nicotine, alcohol, and caffeine. It is recognized as the most widely used illicit drug, though, over the past decade, overall use has declined as a consequence of intensive public education. Cannabis is a plant found in the temperate and tropical zones of the world. The pharmacologically active constituent of cannabis is delta-9-tetrahydrocannabinol (Δ^9-THC). All parts of the plant contain cannabinoids, but the flowering tops have the highest concentration. Cannabis grown in the U.S. is less potent than that found in more tropical regions. Concentrations of psychoactive ingredients may range from 0.2% to 2%; Mexican cannabis contains higher concentrations, whereas Jamaican varieties, which have more flowering tops, have a THC concentration that ranges from 4% to 8%.

Cannabis is sold on the drug market primarily as marijuana, hashish, or hashish oil. Marijuana, which resembles tobacco, is made by drying and chopping the leaves and tops of the cannabis plant. It is smoked in cigarette form ("joints") or through pipes, or it may be ingested. In street jargon, marijuana is known as "Acapulco gold," "gold," "gage," "grass," "hay," "hemp," "J," "Jane," "Mary Jane," "Panama red," "pot," "reefer," "smoke," and "weed."

Hashish, the dried resinous secretions from cannabis flowers, is significantly more potent than marijuana. The THC content of hashish may range from 5% to 12%. It is referred to as "hash," "Kif," "black Russian," "quarter moon," or "soles." Hashish is smoked or ingested.

Hashish oil is a concentrated form of cannabis produced by a repeated extraction process that results in a dark viscous oil that contains from 20% to 60% THC. A few drops are usually placed on cigarettes and smoked; it can also be mixed with less potent marijuana to enhance the quality of the "smoke." Less common is oral ingestion.

General pharmacologic effects. Cannabis in low doses tends to produce euphoria and a sense of well-being, followed by a dreamy state of total relaxation. Sensory perceptions are altered and enhanced; time and space seem to expand. Visual, auditory, and tactile senses are enhanced. Taste is more acute, and frequent food cravings occur ("munchies").

In moderate doses, reactions to THC are intensified, exhibited as rapid emotional changes, impaired memory, short or dulled attention span, and alterations in self-image. Toxic doses may result in panic reaction, hallucinations, loss of personal identity, delusions, and psychosis. Symptoms disappear when the drug is eliminated from the body.

Somatic effects of cannabis include stimulation of the cardiovascular system, including increased heart rate and blood pressure and markedly injected conjunctivae. Other characteristic symptoms include dry mouth, giddiness, loss of coordination, and cold extremities.

Tolerance and dependence. It is not clear how or whether one develops a tolerance to cannabis. Some evidence supports the existence of withdrawal symptoms in chronic heavy users; however, no pattern of physical dependence has been well defined. Some users do report abstinence symptoms, including loss of sleep, irritability, restlessness, decreased appetite, weight loss, hyperactivity, and diaphoresis.

Therapeutic use. Although the use of cannabis is increasingly becoming a part of our lives, little undisputed knowledge about the real hazards of cannabis and its potential therapeutic value exists. Under investigation are the effects of marijuana on the lungs, the fetus, the chromosomes, and reproduction. Because cannabis decreases intraocular pressure, it has been used experimentally to treat glaucoma. THC has been approved by the FDA under the trade name Marinol (dronabinol) for use with cancer clients who are undergoing chemotherapy; for these clients, it has been suc-cessful in alleviating the incapacitating nausea and vomiting that often accompany chemotherapy.

Psychedelics

Psychedelic drugs, which include hallucinogens, psychotomimetics, and psychotogens, are so called because they are capable of inducing a "psychedelic state" that results in the distortion of objectively perceived reality. Psychedelics can induce altered thoughts, perceptions, and feelings that are not experienced in any normal state of sleep or alertness. Effects of psychedelics are unpredictable, and responses may vary with each use.

Hallucinogens

Hallucinogens in common use include mescaline and peyote, psilocybin, psilocin, lysergic acid diethylamide (LSD), 2,5-dimethoxy-4-methylamphetamine (STP, DOM), dimethyltryptamine (DMT), diethyltryptamine (DET), 2,5-dimethoxy-4-methylamphetamine (DOE), 3-methoxy-4,5-ethylenedioxyamphetamine (MMDA), and phencyclidine (PCP).

Mescaline is derived from the peyote cactus (*Lophophora williamsii*) found in Mexico. Although it is also produced synthetically, in natural form, mescaline is produced by slicing the peyote cactus buttons into discs and drying them. The discs are chewed or ground into a powder and ingested. The powder is sometimes made into a tea to make it more palatable.

Mescaline is called "beans," "buttons," "cactus," "mesc," or "mescal." An oral dose of 350 to 500 mg produces psychedelic responses, including hallucinations and illusions. Onset of action varies from 1 to 3 hours and lasts from 4 to 12 hours.

Psilocybin and psilocin are natural drugs derived from the mushroom *Psilocybe mexicana*. The drugs can also be manufactured synthetically. The dose necessary to produce a psychedelic "trip" varies from 6 to 50 mg. Onset of drug action occurs within one-half hour, with symptoms of dizziness, anxiety, and nausea, and progresses to increased diaphoresis, impaired thought control, and enhanced auditory and visual sensitivity. The duration of the drug's effects varies from 4 to 12 hours and ends in a quiescent phase, when headache, tiredness, and lethargy occur. Street slang for these substances includes the terms "magic mushrooms" and "mushrooms."

The hallucinogen LSD is produced from lysergic acid, a natural fungus found in rye. Psychoactive drug experiences vary, reflecting the user's setting and personality. On a "good trip," the most common effects are visual-perceptual changes in light, color, texture, and shape. Time and space also seem altered. The user may experience delusions of grandeur, feelings of omnipotence, or a sense of loss of control. "Bad trips" result in intense anxiety, fear, and traumatic visions.

LSD is a highly potent, colorless, tasteless, odorless substance usually found in tablet forms. Amounts as small as ¹/₇₀₀ millionth of a person's body weight can produce a psychedelic experience. LSD is 100 times as potent as psilocybin and 4,000 times as potent as mescaline.

The psychedelic experience with LSD has three stages:

1. Some discomfort may result from symptoms of CNS overactivity, including anxiety and nausea; this stage may last for 1 hour.
2. The actual psychedelic experience lasts from 6 to 12 hours.
3. Waves of normal consciousness begin to occur; stage 3 ends with feelings of fatigue and relaxation.

Flashbacks of the psychedelic experience may recur at any time from 12 to 18 months later.

When sold in thin squares of gelatin, LSD is called "window pane"; when sold on small pieces of paper impregnated with the substance, it is known as "blotter acid." Other street jargon for LSD includes "acid," "beast," "blue heaven," "brown dots," "California sunshine," "chocolate chips," "haze," "mellow yellows," "orange mushrooms," "orange wedges," "paper acid," "sugar," "sunshine," "white lightning," and "yellows." See also Chapter 23 for more information on hallucinogens.

Psychotomimetics

STP or DOM is a semisynthetic substance in the psychotomimetic group of hallucinogens. It not only produces hallucinations but also has many of the same effects as amphetamines; it is chemically related to mescaline and amphetamines.

The chemical, 2,5-dimethoxy-4-methylamphetamine, became a popular street drug under the name STP, which stands for "serenity, tranquility, and peace." One effect of the drug is uncontrolled psychic energy with perceptual distortions. STP is much less potent than LSD, but about 100 times more potent than mescaline. Duration of action is extended.

Psychotogens

DMT is found in plants indigenous to South America and the West Indies. It can also be chemically synthesized. DET is produced synthetically. These drugs have a brief psychedelic action of 30 minutes, creating a rapid onset of autonomic effects and hallucinations that sometimes result in a panic reaction. DMT and DET are available in a liquid form that is applied to cigarettes, marijuana, or parsley and then smoked.

MMDA is chemically related to STP, mescaline, and amphetamines, producing stimulant effects and a sense of well-being. It is available as a powder, tablet, or liquid and may be taken orally, snorted, or injected intravenously. In street jargon, MMDA is known as "the love drug."

General pharmacologic effects. Hallucinogens stimulate the peripheral sympathetic nervous system, resulting in dilated pupils, elevations in heart rate, blood pressure, and body temperature, changes in simple reflex thresholds, muscular weakness, tremor, and nausea.

During the psychedelic experience, visual illusions and perceptual changes take place, and synesthesia is not uncommon. The user's subjective experience of time passing is seriously disrupted. The user often experiences labile mood swings and a sense of boundary disintegration.

Tolerance and dependence. Although the repeated use of hallucinogens produces a high degree of tolerance to the behavioral effects of the chemicals, normal sensitivities return after the drug is discontinued. Because no withdrawal syndrome is apparent when these substances are discontinued, it can be concluded that hallucinogens do not produce physical dependence.

Treatment. With psychedelic drugs, treatment is most commonly required when acute toxic reactions precipitate psychotic episodes. Continuous orientation and reassurance are frequently successful in "talking down" a user who is experiencing a "bad trip." When these methods are unsuccessful, pentobarbital is usually effective.

Other substances of abuse

Phencyclidine

When phencyclidine (PCP) was discovered in 1957, the drug was recognized to have amphetamine- and anesthetic-like properties. It was marketed as Sernyl and used as a human anesthetic. Frequent negative reactions resulted in its discontinuation as a drug for humans. Renamed Sernylan, it is currently used by veterinarians. Phencyclidine is easily manufactured and has become a popular drug of abuse, frequently being passed off as THC or mescaline.

Routes of administration include smoking—a treated marijuana cigarette ("Kay Jay")—or snorting. PCP is a white crystalline solid in pure form, which can be dissolved in water or alcohol for administration. Common street names include "angel dust," "peace pill," "surfer," "killer weed," "hog," "DOA" (dead on arrival), "rocket fuel," and "elephant tranquilizer." The popularity of PCP is declining overall. However, some major cities have not noted such a decline in use. The result of PCP abuse is frequently seen in emergency departments as bizarre behavior or unexplained psychosis.

PCP produces depressant and stimulant effects. Symptoms of intoxication with doses as low as 5 mg include drowsiness, ataxia, nystagmus, flushing, agitation, hyperreflexia, diaphoresis, miotic pupils, catatonic rigidity, and excitability. Moderate doses from

5 to 10 mg produce stupor, coma, vomiting, fever, repetitive motor activity, and myoclonia. High doses of 10 mg or more result in prolonged coma, which can last from 12 hours to several days. In addition, flushing, fever, diaphoresis, and vomiting may increase. Convulsions, lack of peripheral sensations, and hypertension complete the clinical picture of PCP poisoning.

Treatment. Opinions vary about what the safest intervention in PCP intoxication is. Generally accepted treatment includes gastric lavage, urine acidification, and use of diazepam for sedation, if required. If a combination anxiety–depression reaction occurs, haloperidol is preferred to diazepam.

Although PCP is removed from the body in 3 or 4 days, residual psychotic reaction may persist. The effects of chronic long-term use are unknown. It is thought that intellectual functioning may be dulled, resulting in a "burned out" personality.

Inhalants (toxic vapors)

The practice of inhaling toxic vapors ("sniffing") has decreased in popularity among adolescents. Glue is the most frequently used inhalant in this group. Gasoline vapors, paint thinner, aerosol sprays, and solvents, such as toluene, also lead to intoxication. Symptoms range from disorientation to coma after prolonged exposure.

The recent popularity of volatile nitrites is becoming a public health concern. Snorting volatile liquid nitrites is legal because they are marketed as room deodorizers. Referred to as "poppers" because of the sound created by crushing the capsules before inhaling the fumes, these products are sold under such names as "Ban Apple Gas," "Toilet Water," "Bullet," "Rush," and "Heart-On."

Adverse reactions to chronic use are not yet known. Contents of these products vary, but common effects of inhaling them include lightheadedness, weakness, delirium, nausea, headache, syncope, hypotension, vasoconstriction, and tachycardia.

Substance control

The federal government passed the Controlled Substances Act in 1970 to implement control mechanisms for the manufacturing, obtaining, and selling of specific substances listed in the act. The mechanisms set forth are restrictions on distribution, registration of handlers, restrictions on dispensing, requirements for record keeping, conditions for drug storage, criminal penalties for illicit trafficking, limitations on imports and exports, quotas on manufacturing, and reports of transactions to the government. A composite of controlled substances, their uses, and their effects can be found in Table 15-7.

Recognizing the impact of substance abuse in the work force, the federal government initiated legislation directed at employers. The 1988 legislation (Drug-Free Workplace Act of 1988) addresses the obligation of employers who hold federal government contracts to provide employees with specific information and education related to drug abuse. The requirements stipulated by the act include the necessity of imposing discipline or rehabilitation on employees affected under the act.

Drug abuse and AIDS

No discussion about substance abuse would be complete without focusing attention on the connection between the consequences of substance abuse and abusive lifestyles and the international human immunodeficiency virus (HIV) epidemic. The needle-sharing practices of addicts are recognized as the principal connection between IV drug abusers and transmission of blood-borne pathogens such as HIV, hepatitis, and bacterial endocarditis. Once addicts are infected with HIV, whether or not they develop acquired immunodeficiency syndrome (AIDS), a significant reservoir exists for transmission to other IV drug abusers and to their non–drug-abusing adult sexual partners and, consequently, to the pediatric population.

It is estimated that 25% of AIDS cases in the U.S. are related to needle sharing among drug abusers (Donahue, 1990). Eighty percent of pediatric AIDS cases result from an IV drug-abusing parent.

Opiates, heroin, and cocaine are the most intravenously abused drugs. The Centers for Disease Control estimates that, in the U.S., 28% of AIDS clients are IV drug abusers. Recent studies also note that abuse substances may suppress immune functions, leaving the individual ill prepared to resist or fight opportunistic infections that are associated with HIV.

Drug abuse treatment facilities and public health officials are focusing HIV infection prevention programs on promoting risk-reduction measures. Risk-reduction measures among IV drug abusers include decreasing the number of sexual partners, using latex condoms during all sexual encounters, and eliminating needle sharing. With the AIDS epidemic, the number of IV drug abusers who are seeking treatment for substance abuse has significantly increased. Entry into drug treatment is becoming a viable strategy to address the escalating number of IV drug abusers who are falling victim to AIDS.

■ Summary

The abuse of substances has a major impact on the biologic and psychosocial aspects of the individual and society. While education and attention have made strides in the fight against drugs over the last decade, abuse of psychoactive substances remains a significant problem throughout the U.S.

(Text continues on p. 212)

Table 15-7. Controlled substances: uses and effects

Drug name	Often prescribed brand names	Medical uses	Physical dependence	Potential psychological dependence	Tolerance	Duration of effects (in hours)	Usual methods of administration	Possible effects	Effects of overdose	Withdrawal syndrome
Narcotics										
opium	Dover's powder, Paregoric	Analgesic, antidiarrheal	High	High	Yes	3–6	Oral, smoked	Euphoria, drowsiness, respiratory depression, constricted pupils, nausea	Slow and shallow breathing, clammy skin, convulsions, coma, possible death	Watery eyes, runny nose, yawning, loss of appetite, irritability, tremors, panic, chills and sweating, cramps, nausea
morphine	Morphine	Analgesic	High	High	Yes	3–6	Injected, smoked			
codeine	Codeine	Analgesic, antitussive	Moderate	Moderate	Yes	3–6	Oral, injected			
heroin	None	None	High	High	Yes	3–6	Injected, sniffed			
meperidine (Pethidine)	Demerol, Pethadol	Analgesic	High	High	Yes	3–6	Oral, injected			
methadone	Dolophine, Methadone, Methadose	Analgesic, heroin substitute	High	High	Yes	12–24	Oral, injected			
Other narcotics	Dilaudid, Leritine, Numorphan, Percodan	analgesic, antidiarrheal, antitussive	High	High	Yes	3–6	Oral, injected			
Depressants										
chloral hydrate	Noctec, Somnos	Hypnotic	Moderate	Moderate	Probable	5–8	Oral	Slurred speech, disorientation, drunken behavior without odor of alcohol	Shallow respiration, cold and clammy skin, dilated pupils, weak and rapid pulse, coma, possible death	Anxiety, insomnia, tremors, delirium, convulsions, possible death
barbiturates	Amytal, Butisol, Nembutal, Phenobarbital, Seconal, Tuinal	Anesthetic, anticonvulsant, sedative	High	High	Yes	1–16	Oral, injected			

(Continued)

Table 15-7. Controlled substances: uses and effects (Continued)

Drug name	Often prescribed brand names	Medical uses	Physical dependence	Potential psychological dependence	Tolerance	Duration of effects (in hours)	Usual methods of administration	Possible effects	Effects of overdose	Withdrawal syndrome
glutethimide	Doriden	Sedative, sleep-inducer	High	High	Yes	4–8	Oral			
methaqualone	Optimil, Parest, Quaalude, Somnafac, Sopor	Sedative, sleep-inducer	High	High	Yes	4–8	Oral			
benzodiazepines	Ativan, Dalmane, Diazepam, Librium, Xanax, Serax, Valium, Tranxexe, Verstran, Versed, Halcion, Paxipam, Restoril	Antianxiety, anticonvulsant, sedative, hypnotic	Low	Low	Yes	4–8	Oral			
Other depressants	Equanii, Miltown, Noludar, Placidyl, Valmid	Antianxiety, sedative, hypnotic	Moderate	Moderate	Yes	4–8	Oral			
Stimulants cocaine*	Cocaine	Local anesthetic	Possible	High	Yes	2	Injected, sniffed	Increased alertness, excitation, euphoria, dilated pupils, increased pulse rate and BP, insomnia, loss of appetite	Agitation, increase in body temperature, hallucinations, convulsions, possible death	Apathy, long periods of sleep, irritability, depression, disorientation
amphetamines	Benzedrine, Biphetamine, Desoxyn, Dexedrine	Hyperkinesic, narcolepsy, weight control	Possible	High	Yes	2–4	Oral, injected			
phenmetrazine	Preludin	Weight control	Possible	High	Yes	2–4	Oral			
methylphenidate	Ritalin	Hyperkinesic	Possible	High	Yes	2–4	Oral			

Drug	Trade or Other Names	Medical Uses	Physical Dependence	Psychological Dependence	Tolerance	Duration (hours)	Usual Method	Possible Effects	Effects of Overdose	Withdrawal Syndrome
Other stimulants	Bacarate, Cylert, Didrex, Ionamin, Plegine, Pondimin, Presate, Sanorex, Voranil	Weight control	Possible	Possible	Yes	2–4	Oral			
Hallucinogens										
LSD	Acid, Microdot	None	None	Unknown	Yes	8–12	Oral	Illusions and hallucinations (with exception of MDA); poor perception of time and distance	Longer, more intense "trips," psychosis, possible death	Withdrawal syndrome not reported
mescaline and peyote	Mesc, buttons, cactus	None	None	Unknown	Yes	8–12	Oral			
amphetamine variants	2,5-DMA, PMA, STP, MDA, MDMA, TMA, DOM, DOB	None	Unknown	Unknown	Yes	Variable	Oral, injected			
phencyclidine	PCP, angel dust, hog	None	Unknown	High	Yes	Days	Smoked, oral, injected			
phencyclidine analogues	PCE, PCP, TCP	None	Unknown	High	Yes	Days	Smoked, oral, injected, sniffed			
Other hallucinogens	bufotenine, ibogaine, DMT, DET, psilocybin, psilocyn	None	None	Unknown	Possible	Variable				
Cannabis										
marijuana	None	None‡	Degree unknown	Moderate	Yes	2–4	Oral, smoked	Euphoria, relaxed inhibitions, increased appetite, disoriented behavior	Fatigue, paranoia, possible psychosis	Insomnia, hyperactivity, and decreased appetite reported in a limited number of users
hashish										
hashish oil										

*Designated a narcotic under the Controlled Substances Act.

†Designated a depressant under the Controlled Substances Act.

‡Medical use of cannabis has been approved to use in treatment of nausea and vomiting for cancer patients who are undergoing chemotherapy. (Drug Enforcement Administration. [1975]. *Drugs of abuse.* Washington, DC: U.S. Department of Justice.)

Recognizing the signs, symptoms, and interventions appropriate to treat substance abuse requires an understanding about the cycles of dependence, the pharmacologic effects of drugs, and treatment modalities available.

Nursing management

Nursing implications

The nursing care needs of a client who willfully or indiscriminately abuses potentially harmful drugs are vast. Recognizing one's own values and attitudes about substance abuse is fundamental in establishing a therapeutic relationship. In addition, accurate information about current trends in substance abuse, including an understanding of the legal issues that define the scope of the problem, facilitates nursing care.

Nurses have the opportunity to provide health information about the long-range and immediate risks to clients' biologic, psychological, and social health status in any area of nursing practice. Information is most effective when received at an early age, with emphasis on maintaining a healthy body. Schools have been instrumental in giving children accurate information about the hazards and risks of substance abuse, such as cigarette smoking. School nurses have the opportunity to collaborate with health educators to convey age-appropriate information in creative ways. Making literature available to clients can also offer people at any age an opportunity to assess choices of lifestyles and risks to health, such as the use of drugs, alcohol, or nicotine. Creating healthy attitudes about how to treat one's body may be a key to developing less self-destructive behaviors. In addition, the substance abuse habits of significant others are of particular importance to adolescents. Nurses should encourage parents to be aware of how their behavior influences their children.

Recognition can help nurses assess their client's problems. Familiarity with the physiologic, psychological, and social changes that result from abuse of stimulants, depressants, analgesics, and hallucinogens helps identify abusers or clients who could compromise their course of treatment in an acute setting. Accurate nursing histories need to take into account a client's susceptibility to exacerbating a previously resolved drug problem by using therapeutic doses of drugs to treat a current medical condition. Drug interactions or hypersensitivity to anesthetics can occur in some clients.

Helping clients cope with treatment regimens in acute and long-term rehabilitation programs is an-

---

Learning experience 15-1

Investigate the policies and procedures for monitoring controlled substances in various health care delivery systems. Identify standards for monitoring these practices.

---

other significant role of the nurse. Counseling and supportive interventions for the secondary symptoms of chronic substance abuse (*eg*, malnutrition and its accompanying skin and immune system responses, skin infections, and hepatitis from the use of contaminated drug paraphernalia) facilitate the client's recovery.

During the acute drug reaction period, managing the client's physical and behavioral action can be demanding. A generally calm, soothing, one-to-one interaction in an environment in which stimuli are minimal is usually effective. The nurse should also be able to recognize the client's overall condition and implement emergency procedures to reverse toxic reactions.

Encouraging clients to use community resources for rehabilitation requires adequate knowledge about the goals and criteria for acceptance in a specific program, so that the client's needs are addressed appropriately. Some organizations have outreach workers available to assist clients in acute distress and to establish contact with clients before their discharge from the acute care setting.

Many complex and sometimes obscure reasons why a client may decide to change habits that have compromised his or her health can be found. It may take repeated drug-induced crises or a serious jeopardy in health from excessive alcohol consumption or cigarette smoking before a client is ready to change. Whatever the motivation, a supportive nonjudgmental nurse–counselor is in a position to provide the impetus for change through education.

Nursing process

Assessment Overall assessment of the client's status should include all aspects of the following functional health patterns:

- Health perception/health management (awareness of current health status, factors that influence health behavior, overall history of health practices)
- Physiologic homeostasis (physical examination and general description of the client, including assessment of cardiovascular, neurologic, respiratory, mental, musculoskeletal, integumentary, and GI systems)
- Elimination (daily bowel and bladder habits)
- Nutrition and metabolic condition (appetite, weight, height, normal nutritional intake, status of mucous membrane, dental needs)
- Activity/exercise (usual level of activity, impact of present illness on activities of daily living)
- Sleep/rest (usual sleep patterns, use of sleeping aids)
- Cognitive and perceptual conditions (level of understanding, ability to comprehend, sensory responses and deficits, presence of pain or discomfort)

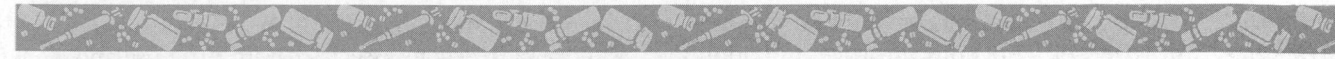

Example of nursing process and alcohol abuse

A 45-year-old female is admitted to the hospital with a primary diagnosis of GI bleeding secondary to alcohol abuse. She presents as a confused, somewhat restless patient who is experiencing periodic hallucinations. No family members accompany the client, although she is married. Her physical appearance is that of an undernourished, unkempt woman with dermatitis and petechiae on the face and arms. A strong alcohol odor is evident.

Assessment data	Nursing diagnosis	Intervention	Goals and outcome criteria
Alcohol odor Bleeding attributed to alcohol abuse Hallucinations Restlessness Confusion	Altered perception: hallucinations related to CNS overactivity due to alcohol withdrawal	Arrange for someone to remain with the client at all times. Furnish the client with information about her surroundings, explaining that unreal sensory perceptions are the result of drug withdrawal. Offer emotional support and reassurance that the abnormal sensations will not persist indefinitely.	The client will accept the explanation of hallucinations; she will not experience panic.
Alcohol abuse	Ineffective individual coping related to alcohol abuse	When the client's condition is stabilized, explore with her the patterns of and reasons for her alcohol abuse. Advise the client of the risks of continued alcohol use. Advise the client about community resources available for assistance should she decide to decrease her use of alcohol (*eg,* Alcoholics Anonymous, community treatment programs, and so forth). Teach the client alternative coping techniques for stressful situations.	The client will accept the need to decrease her reliance on alcohol; she will contact a source of help before discharge from the hospital.

- Self-perception/self-concept (general appearance, body image, sense of control)
- Roles and relationships (support systems, family constellation, sick role, communication skills, interpersonal relationships)
- Sexuality and reproductive status (reproductive history, incidence of sexual abuse or trauma, history of sexually transmitted diseases)
- Coping and stress tolerance (recent significant life changes, situational and maturational changes, coping strategies used—positive/ negative)
- Values and beliefs (religious preference, source of strength, life goals, health beliefs)

Nursing diagnosis Nursing diagnoses that should be considered are the following:

> *Ineffective individual coping*
> *Self-esteem disturbance*
> *Body image disturbance*
> *Altered nutrition: less than body requirements, related to alcoholic gastritis*
> *Ineffective breathing pattern*
> *Sensory/perceptual alterations: visual, auditory, or tactile hallucinations*
> *Pain: paresthesia related to peripheral neuropathy*
> *Knowledge deficit related to substance abuse*

Planning Nursing care goals are to improve coping strategies, improve self-concept, improve nutrition and weight gain, decrease or eliminate hallucinations, eliminate or alleviate pain, and educate client about substance abuse.

Interventions When drugs produce a medical crisis, as in overdose, the focus of immediate care is on maintaining vital functions and homeostasis. When CNS depressants are involved, a primary concern is to support respiration; mechanical respiratory assistance may be required. In stimulant abuse, the client may be at risk for hyperpyrexia; fever may require cooling blankets or other antipyretic treatment. Hallucinogens can cause accidental injury as a result of misperceptions or panic; emotional support and reassurance are vital nursing actions. Withdrawal from habitual use of depressants can also produce hallucinations and seizures. During such crises, clients require continuous monitoring and individual care.

Follow-up care involves measures to correct nutritional deficits, counseling about substance abuse, and referral to treatment programs or self-help groups, such as Alcoholics Anonymous, for long-term help.

Evaluation Data required for evaluation relate to coping strategies employed by the client (including absence or recurrence of substance abuse), communications about self-concept (including verbal comments and body language), weight gain, absence or presence of overt signs and symptoms of malnutrition, absence or presence of hallucinations, complaints of pain, and client ability to repeat information conveyed during teaching sessions (see the Example of Nursing Process and Alcohol Abuse).

References

Bejerot N. (1977). The nature of addiction. In Glatt MM, ed. *Drug dependence*, p 69. Baltimore: University Park Press.

Centers for Disease Control. (1989, September). *HIV/AIDS surveillance report.*

Department of Health and Human Services. (1986). *Statistical series semiannual report trend data Jul-Dec 1985*, series G, no 17. Washington, DC: Alcohol, Drug Abuse, and Mental Health Administration.

Donahoe R. (1990). Drugs of abuse and AIDS: Causes for the connection. In Pham P, Rice K, eds. *NIDA Research Monograph 96*. Rockville, MD: Department of Health and Human Services.

Gunby P. (1988). Surgeon General emphasizes nicotine addiction in annual report on tobacco use, consequences. *JAMA, 259*(19), 28.

Harris L. (1989). Problems of drug dependence. *Monograph Series 95*. Rockville, MD: National Institute on Drug Abuse Research.

Jaffee J. (1985). Drug addiction and drug abuse. In Gilman AG, et al, eds. *Goodman and Gilman's the pharmacological basis of therapeutics*, 8th ed, pp 532–581. New York: Pergamon Press.

Khantzian EJ, McKenna GJ. (1979). Acute toxic and withdrawal reactions associated with drug use and abuse. *Ann Intern Med, 90*, 361–363.

National Institute on Alcohol Abuse and Alcoholism. (1990). *Alcohol alert, #10* (October). Rockville, MD: Department of Health and Human Services.

National Institute on Drug Abuse. (1991). *Drug abuse and drug abuse research III* (DHSS Publication No. ADM 91–1704). Washington, DC: U.S. Government Printing Office.

National Institute on Drug Abuse. (1986). *Drug abuse statistics 1985: Population estimates*. Washington, DC: Alcohol, Drug Abuse, and Mental Health Administration.

National Institute on Drug Abuse. (1981). *National survey on drug abuse*. Washington, DC: Alcohol, Drug Abuse, and Mental Health Administration.

Pham P, Rice K, eds. (1990). Drugs of abuse: Chemistry, pharmacology, immunology and AIDS. *NIDA Research Monograph 96*. Rockville, MD: Department of Health and Human Services.

Tarr J, Macklin M. (1987). Cocaine. *Pediatr Clin North Am, 34*(2), 319–331.

Bibliography

American Psychiatric Association. (1987). *Diagnostic categories from the DSM-1112*. Washington, DC: American Psychiatric Press.

Department of Health and Human Services. (1991). *Drug abuse and drug research III* (DHHS Publication No. ADM 91–1704). Washington, DC: U.S. Government Printing Office.

Drug Enforcement Administration. (1975). *Drugs of abuse*. Washington DC: US Department of Justice.

Facts on alcoholism and alcohol-related problems. (1984). New York: National Council on Alcoholism.

Ford M, Hoffman R, Goldfrank L. (1990). Opioids and designer drugs. *Emerg Med Clin North Am, 8*(3), 495–511.

Giannini AJ, Slaby A, ed. (1989). *Drugs of abuse*. Oradell, NJ: Medical Economics Co.

Harris L. (1989). Problems of drug dependence. *Monograph Series 95*. Rockville, MD: National Institute on Drug Abuse Research.

Henderson GL. (1988). Designer drugs: Past history and future prospects. *J Forensic Sci 33*(2), 569–575.

Jekel J, Allen D. (1987). Trends in drug abuse in the mid-1980s. *Yale J Biol Med, 60*.

Martinez R. (1990). Alcoholism and society. *Emerg Med Clin North Am, 8*(4), 903–912.

National Institute on Drug Abuse. (1979). *Drug abuse prevention: For your community* (USDHEW Publication No. ADM 78–586). Washington, DC: U.S. Government Printing Office.

National Institute on Drug Abuse. (1979). *A woman's choice: Deciding about drugs* (USDHEW Publication No. ADM 79–820). Washington, DC: U.S. Government Printing Office.

National Institute on Drug Abuse Research. Monograph Series 95. "Problems of Drug Dependence," Harris (1989), Rockville, MD.

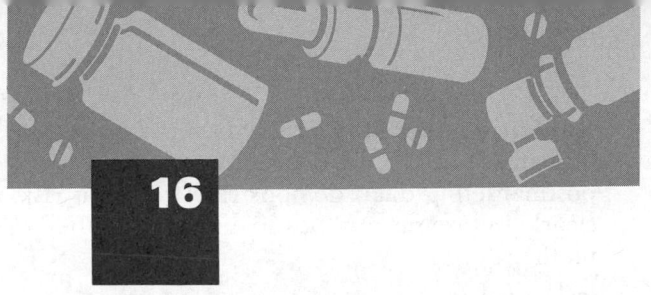

16

Drug therapy in maternal care

Drug use in pregnancy

From the beginning of pregnancy, the fate of the fetus is tied to that of its mother. Whatever physical agents affect the mother's body may affect the fetus. Any substance that she ingests, inhales, or receives parenterally may pass through the placenta to her baby unless it is destroyed or changed on its passage. The rate and mechanism of entry is important because a low degree of permeability increases the chance of undesirable agents being inactivated, whereas a high degree of permeability encourages passage. Substances that contain fat-soluble undissociated molecules at physiologic pH ranges are likely to pass through the placenta immediately. The molecular weight of drugs taken by the mother is also important; those less than 600 pass easily, whereas those greater than 1,000 find the placenta almost impermeable.

Substances that cross the placenta usually reach concentrations in the fetus that are 50% to 100% of the concentrations in the mother. A few drugs reach higher levels in the fetus when it excretes the drugs into the amniotic fluid then later swallows and recirculates them. The waste products from the fetus return to the mother through the two umbilical arteries, which pass through the placenta to the mother. This return of wastes (particularly toxic products) may be slow because many of the fetal systems involved in detoxification are not fully developed.

The five major considerations to be used in the evaluation of possible harm to the fetus from any substance are listed in Box 16-1.

When a drug ordered for the gravida can possibly cause adverse effects in the fetus, the substitution of another medication should be considered. The Food and Drug Administration (FDA) has actually approved only one prescription drug for use during pregnancy: ritodrine (a neurotransmitter that interrupts premature labor). A combination of doxylamine and pyridoxine, known as Bendectin, has been involved in several long court cases concerning the possibility that

---

Box 16-1. Considerations in evaluating a substance's fetal harm

The amount of the substance that can be expected to reach the embryo or fetus

The gestational age of the embryo or fetus at the time of administration

The duration of the exposure

The genotypes of the mother and embryo or fetus

The expected effects on the embryo or fetus of this substance when combined with other agents in the mother's body

---

birth defects resulted from its prenatal use for morning sickness (Haire, 1987). Physicians are not prevented from prescribing drugs not specifically approved for use during pregnancy. However, the mother must be given information about the potential effects before its use to meet the restrictions of "informed consent."

Approval by the FDA of medications for pregnant women does not guarantee the drug's safety for the mother or baby. It only means that, in the opinion of the FDA, the benefits to be gained by using the drug outweigh the possible risks.

Information gathered by the FDA may cause withdrawal of prior approval. For example, diazepam was reevaluated as unacceptable as an antianxiety drug for women in labor because of the adverse effects on the neonate (Haire, 1987).

FDA pregnancy category ratings for drugs

The FDA has developed a "use-in-pregnancy" rating, limited to drugs for which information is available, on the fetal risk vs. potential maternal benefits of various drugs. The ratings and their interpretations are as follows:

A: Well controlled studies in pregnant women do not demonstrate fetal risk from the drug in question.

B: No evidence of risk from the drug in human studies or animal studies is negative.

C: Risk from the drug cannot be ruled out since human studies are lacking and animal studies are either lacking or demonstrate fetal risk. However, potential benefits may justify the potential risk.

D: Positive evidence of risk from the drug exists as demonstrated by investigation or postmarketing data. However, potential benefits may outweigh the potential risk.

X: Contraindicated in pregnancy. Animal or human studies of the drug (investigational or postmarketing data) demonstrate fetal that risk clearly outweighs any possible benefit to the mother.

The FDA pregnancy categories are used when available throughout this book since pregnant women may require medication for conditions related or unrelated to pregnancy. Knowledge of pregnancy category ratings helps health providers compare the hazard of administering a drug that may place the fetus or neonate at risk with the drug's potential benefit to the mother.

TERIS and Canadian ratings

An automated teratology resource known as TERIS was developed in Canada, rating the human teratogenicity (birth defect) dangers of 157 drugs frequently prescribed for outpatients in the United States. Of the agents that had sufficient information to be rated, 92.5% were found to demonstrate minimal teratogenic risk. The information on 83 of the agents was compared to that presented in the FDA pregnancy categories (Friedman, et al, 1990).

The Canadian researchers believe that any information on risks needs to be modified for all the conditions of exposure, such as dose, route, and timing, to be valid. They disagree with the FDA classifications that combine risk and quality data in a single interpretation for client counseling. Canadians do not offer this type of counseling. They use their own rating system only after the client has been exposed to a particular drug, at which time the teratogenic risk to the fetus is considered.

Nonmedical factors that affect pregnancy

Maternal nutrition

One of the first considerations during pregnancy is maternal nutrition. The mother must have a sufficient intake of high-quality foods to encourage proper growth and development of the fetus and placenta. The old fears about maternal obesity that led to severe caloric restrictions have proved detrimental to the fetus. Inadequate nutrition prevents the increase in maternal blood volume needed to vascularize the uterus properly. Without this increase in blood flow, the necessary nutrients cannot be carried to the fetus in sufficient quantity to sustain proper growth. The food ingested by the mother must also be as free of contaminants as possible.

Nausea and vomiting are common during the early weeks of pregnancy, affecting 50% to 90% of all pregnant women. If possible, these should be controlled by diet—dry crackers eaten before arising in the morning and several small easily digested meals during the day. Clients on salt-restricted diets should be instructed to eat unsalted crackers. Antiemetic drugs are generally not used because their safety during pregnancy has not been established. Dietary and nursing measures are safer routes to combat nausea and vomiting.

During pregnancy, the mother's body prepares for lactation by storing fat that will provide the enormous amount of energy required for breast-feeding. Winick notes that preparation for lactation takes precedence over fetal growth because lactation takes biologic precedence; the widespread manufacture and use of infant formula is a recent historical phenomenon (Winick, 1981). Drugs or toxic substances that are fat soluble are thought to penetrate the placental barrier with greater ease.

Nutrients

In response to her body's need to deposit fat, the mother's appetite increases, as does her absorption of iron and calcium. If food supplies are inadequate, the fetus's growth suffers. If the mother eats properly, she will probably gain 25 lb or more during the course of pregnancy. Ideally, the neonate should weigh about 8 lb; therefore, the mother should have a daily increase of about 300 to 500 calories, with higher intake necessary if she was underweight before pregnancy. Even overweight women should be instructed to gain at least 15 lb during pregnancy. This gain is important to prevent low infant birth weights, which have a negative effect on the development and survival of neonates.

The source of the additional 300 to 500 calories consumed daily by the mother, although important, is not essential to the fetus. If maternal intake is largely carbohydrate rather than protein, the mother's own muscle tissue breaks down to provide the necessary amino acids for the fetus. Whenever possible, the maternal protein intake should increase by 30 g a day so that her own body is protected and fetal growth ensured.

Because the maternal blood volume increases during pregnancy and the fetus has to develop its own blood, the need for *iron* becomes pronounced. It can be met through the dietary intake of red meats, beans, dried fruits, and fortified grain products. If these are unavailable in sufficient quantity, supplementary iron should be taken.

Folic acid, a B vitamin rarely available in sufficient amounts in the diet, must be supplemented to ensure proper cell division of the uterus and of the fetus. A study that ran from 1983 to 1991 demonstrated that the intake of folic acid from the time of conception markedly lessened the risk of giving birth to babies with neural tube defects. This benefit was found to be true even in 72% of nearly 1,200 women who had previous children with this problem; recurrence would have been expected at a rate 10 times higher than in the general population (Wald, 1991).

Calcium is another important mineral that must be available for the fetus's proper skeletal development. To meet the combined needs of the gravida and the fetus, 1,200 mg of calcium per day are needed. Women who smoke may require an even higher level, because smoking may cause loss of calcium from the mother's bones. Calcium absorption is decreased if phosphorus intake is too high (as when the intake of nuts and grains is excessive). This decrease may cause an electrolyte imbalance and is an important point to make when teaching pregnant mothers about nutrition. It may be necessary to supplement calcium if the mother's diet does not contain adequate levels of dairy products.

Learning experience 16-1

A pregnant woman is admitted to the labor area, requesting medication. The cervix is 100% effaced and dilated 4 cm; the fetus is not engaged. Discuss nursing measures you can use to help her control the pain of labor.

Ingested contaminants

Alcohol ingestion

Alcohol is considered by some experts to be the most common teratogen that affects humans (Zamula, 1989, pp 9, 10). About 30% to 45% of pregnant women who ingest six mixed drinks or six cans of beer a day throughout pregnancy (the equivalent of 3 oz absolute alcohol or ethanol per day) can be expected to deliver infants with full-blown fetal alcohol syndrome (FAS; Fetal Alcohol Syndrome, 1990, pp 1–4). This condition is characterized by mental and growth retardation, central nervous system (CNS) problems, behavioral and developmental abnormalities, and heart, limb, and facial defects. It has surpassed Down's syndrome and spina bifida to become the leading cause of mental retardation in the U.S. (Fetal Alcohol Syndrome, 1990, pp 1–4).

It is estimated that between one in 500 (0.2%) to one in 1,000 (0.1%) live births in the U.S. involve children with FAS. Siblings of an FAS child are 100 to 400 times more likely to have FAS than children in the general population.

Fetal alcohol effects, a milder disorder found in children of mothers who do not ingest alcohol as heavily, are noted in at least five or ten times as many children as those who suffer from FAS. It has been reported that 25% of children born in communities in which alcoholism is epidemic may exhibit signs of fetal alcohol effects.

Because no minimum safe level for maternal alcohol ingestion has been set, the Surgeon General of the U.S. and the National Council on Alcoholism both recommend that a woman should abstain from drinking alcoholic beverages from the time that she actively seeks to conceive. No matter what stage she has reached in her pregnancy, she should stop, or at least decrease her intake as much as possible, to try to limit the damage to her fetus.

Referrals for professional counseling should be made if the alcoholic mother seems amenable or if she is unable to reduce her liquor consumption. If detoxification is indicated, it must be done in the hospital to monitor the effects of alcohol withdrawal on the fetus as well as the mother. When medications to control maternal withdrawal symptoms or to treat the alcoholism are prescribed, the possibility of placental transfer must be considered, as well as the effects of teratogenicity or carcinogenicity on the fetus. For example, researchers believe that maternal barbiturate sedation may increase the child's risk of developing cancer when older. Antabuse, helpful in treating alcoholics because it makes them physically ill if they drink, is contraindicated because it affects the pregnancy by inhibiting enzymes. Librium and Valium, frequently used in alcohol detoxification programs, are also contraindicated owing to their possible teratogenic effects. The mother who is undergoing treatment requires emotional as well as physical help.

In the past, alcohol was used as a tocolytic drug. Ritodrine has replaced it, however, and women are advised not to use alcohol because of its possible adverse effects on the fetus (see Chapter 24 for a more detailed discussion of alcohol).

Caffeine ingestion

Women who consume more than 300 mg of caffeine per day appear to have higher incidences of first trimester spontaneous abortions, stillbirths, and premature births (Morris & Weinstein, 1981, p 607; Worthington-Roberts & Weigle, 1983, p 21). Clients should be reminded that caffeine is present in coffee, tea, cocoa, chocolate, and some sodas. Prescription and over-the-counter (OTC) drugs should be checked for caffeine content (Brooton & Jordon, 1983).

Inhaled contaminants

Just as maternal food ingestion affects the fetus, so do the substances that she inhales. Respiratory functions in the pregnant woman change. The tidal volume increases about 40%, but the vital capacity and respiratory rates remain at about the prepregnancy levels. Inspiration increases, whereas the expiratory reserve decreases, so that the lung shows greater deflation after expiration. Both the residual and total lung volumes are reduced.

The alveolar tension of inhaled substances is normally diluted by the residual air volume in the lungs. Because pregnancy results in a decreased reservoir of air to dilute the inhaled air, contaminants are not weakened to the extent that they would have been before pregnancy. This fact places the mother who breathes impure air at risk for hypoxia, and, depending on the ability of the substance to cross the placenta, the inhalant may adversely affect her fetus. The stage of fetal development may determine how the same compound affects different cells, causing teratogenesis in immature embryonic cells and carcinogenesis in mature cells.

Cigarette smoke

One of the most common air contaminants is cigarette smoke. Its effect on the fetus has been noted for several years. Babies with low weight for gestational age are born twice as frequently to women who smoke compared to nonsmokers. These babies have smaller livers and have a higher rate of hypoglycemia (blood glucose levels below 30 mg/dl place the infant at risk for permanent brain damage). One study indicated a 35% increase in the risk of death near the time of birth among offspring of women who smoke (Clark & Hager, 1984).

The placenta seems vulnerable to maternal smoking, with higher incidences of abruptio, previa, and bleeding that occurs early or late in pregnancy. Long-term studies of children born to smoking mothers suggest adverse effects on growth, intelligence, and behavior. Retardation is associated with heavy smoking and may be due to chronic fetal hypoxia. Children born of mothers who smoked during pregnancy are at a 30% higher risk of developing leukemia and lymphoma than those born of nonsmoking mothers. It is estimated that 6% of childhood cancers and 17% of acute lymphatic leukemia cases may be related to maternal smoking. In children exposed only to paternal smoking during the pregnancy, the risk is 20% higher for development of leukemia, lymphoma, and brain cancer than in unexposed children. This information suggests that paternal smoking may have a genetic effect on sperm cells. Future studies will examine this relationship as well as the adverse effects related to postbirth exposure to cigarette smoke (Greater risk of cancer, 1991).

Carbon monoxide is one component of cigarette smoke. Normally, pregnant women show a 50% increase in endogenous CO production during pregnancy. Smoking not only increases the maternal CO level, but it increases the amount that crosses the placental barrier. The increased CO level interferes with the oxygenation of fetal tissue. If CO poisoning develops, neurologic sequelae may become evident in the child.

In addition to carbon monoxide, cigarettes contain tar and nicotine, which are being studied for teratogenicity and carcinogenicity in the fetus. Nicotine is known to increase body heat production by 10% to 15%. Whether or not a woman smokes, her basal body temperature increases by 0.3 to 0.6°C after ovulation. This elevation of temperature is maintained halfway through the pregnancy, after which it returns to a normal level. Because excessive heat is known to cause adverse fetal reactions, the mother may be placing the fetus at additional risk by raising her body heat production through smoking.

Anesthetic gases

Anesthetic gases are an occupational hazard for health care personnel. Anesthetists have a 38% abortion rate and operating room nurses a 30% rate (general duty nurses have an abortion rate of 10%). In one study of 24 women who worked with anesthetic gases, 31 pregnancies were documented. Of these, ten resulted in normal pregnancies, ten ended in spontaneous abortions, nine in pathologic pregnancies, and two in premature deliveries. One gas, halothane, which is a fluorinated hydrocarbon, has been closely linked with spontaneous abortions among female anesthetists.

Reproductive hazards from anesthetic gases are posed for families of the health care professional, since the gases are highly lipophilic and may be excreted in the breath of anesthetists up to 30 hours after their last exposure. Therefore, a pregnant woman in contact with the anesthetist may unknowingly be at risk (Moses, 1987, p 153).

The effects of exposure to the toxic and mutagenic effects of cytotoxic and antineoplastic drugs can be moderated if vertical-flow or biologic safety cabinets are used (horizontal laminar-flow hoods are not protective) and if the care provider uses personal protective equipment and is not a smoker. Testing of urine to detect mutagenicity may not be of sufficient sensitivity to detect low-level exposure and should not be relied on for that purpose (Moses, 1987, p 154).

Under the New York State Right to Know Law, workers, including nurses, are entitled to know of any hazardous substances that exist in their workplace at the present time or any time since 1980. A written request must be submitted to the employer, who must then provide the information within 72 hours, excluding weekends and holidays. Records of employees exposed to hazards must be kept by the employer for 40 years wherever federal statutes and regulations are in effect and must include information about the substance. This information, which is enforced by the New York State Attorney General, must be available to present or former employees, designated physicians, as well as the Commissioner of Health (Mancino, 1987, pp 8–9).

Radiotherapy

Nurses who care for any client who is receiving radiation therapy should use radiation precautions, including the wearing of a monitoring device or a lead-lined apron while involved in direct care or standing behind a portable shield when providing indirect care. Exposure can be minimized by planning efficiency in care ahead of time, working quickly, leaving the room as soon as possible, and caring for specimens in shielded containers. Pregnant nurses should not care for clients with radioactive sources (Jones, et al, 1987, p 46).

Industrial chemicals

Industrial chemicals inhaled by pregnant workers can be deadly. Of 95 women who died of beryllium poisoning, 66% were pregnant. Beryllium has also been found in the urine of children whose mothers were exposed to this chemical. Other inhalants known to cause teratogenicity include benzine, carbon tetrachloride, oxides of nitrogen, paraquat, polychlorinated biphenyls, Malathion, cyanides, and formaldehyde.

Illegal substances

Marijuana is known to impair DNA and RNA formation and therefore should be avoided during pregnancy. It may also decrease maternal oxygenation, making less oxygen available to the fetus.

Snorting cocaine, which permits inhalation of this strong vasoconstrictor, can cause the pregnant woman to develop seizures, hypertension, cardiac arrhythmia, respiratory arrest, and cardiac failure. Abruptio placentae due to clot formation behind the placenta may also occur and may result in fetal death (Acker, et al, 1983, p 220).

Electromagnetic radiation

Video display terminals have been introduced in the U.S. with very low frequency (VLF) levels of electromagnetic radiation. Swedish regulations go even further, reducing radiation to extremely low frequency emissions (ELF). Some American companies are incorporating these new guidelines in the production of their newer models of computers, televisions, and other electrical devices. Utility power lines and electrical devices used at home or in the workplace are suspected by some researchers of causing problems in pregnancy and increasing cancer rates.

Medications

Maternal medication

Pregnant women are susceptible to medical disorders found in the general population. If treatment depends on medications, the additional risk of the effects of the drugs on the fetus, as well as the mother, must be considered. Owing to increases in maternal blood and plasma volumes during pregnancy, the concentration of maternal serum protein is lower. Therefore, the capacity of the protein to bind any drugs in the maternal system is lowered, thereby leaving more drugs free to be transferred through the placenta.

Medication may be needed to treat a maternal condition throughout pregnancy and during lactation. The effects on the fetus may be different from those on the neonate. Table 16-1 compares fetal risk from medication given during pregnancy with neonatal risk during lactation.

Pharmacokinetics. Many drugs are metabolized in the liver. However, during pregnancy the hepatic

(Text continues on p. 224)

Table 16-1. Comparative effects of drugs on fetus and breast-fed neonate

Pharmacologic class	Fetal risk	Breast-feeding data
Antihistamines		
brompheniramine	Congenital defects	Single adverse report, therefore considered contraindicated by one manufacturer
buclizine (also antiemetic)	Teratogenic in animals; contraindicated in early pregnancy by manufacturer	No data available
chlorpheniramine (also antiemetic)	Possible malformations; more data needed to assess risk	No data available
cimetidine (H_2-receptor antagonist)	Crosses placenta at term but no adverse effects noted	Potential adverse effects on infant (gastric acidity, CNS stimulation), therefore contraindicated
cyclizine (also antiemetic)	Teratogenic in animals but apparently not in humans	No data available
diphenhydramine	No evidence of large numbers of major or minor malformations, but actual risk associated with individual cases needs further assessment	Manufacturer says contraindicated during lactation; American Academy of Pediatrics (AAP) says it is acceptable
doxylamine (also antiemetic)	Possible association with risk, including skeletal, cardiac, cleft palate, and lip	No data available
hydroxyzine (also tranquilizer)	Manufacturer says contraindicated in early pregnancy; seems safe in labor to relieve anxiety	No data available
meclizine (also antiemetic)	No evidence of large numbers of major or minor malformations, but actual risk associated with individual cases needs further assessment	No data available
pheniramine	Possible association with respiratory, eye, and ear problems	No data available
promethazine (also antiemetic)	No association between use in pregnancy and malformations; when used in labor may impair platelet aggregation in neonate, but less in mother; watch for bleeding in newborn	Accurate assessment not available owing to rapid metabolism
ranitidine (H_2-receptor antagonist)	Use in labor to prevent gastric acid aspiration does not appear to cause neonatal problems	Contraindicated since it decreases gastric acidity
trimeprazine	No evidence of large numbers of major or minor malformations, but actual risk associated with individual cases needs further assessment	Excreted in breast milk at levels too low to produce effects in baby; considered acceptable while breast-feeding by AAP
tripelennamine	No evidence of association with major or minor malformations	Manufacturer says contraindicated during lactation; AAP says it is acceptable
Anti-infectives		
Aminoglycosides		
gentamycin (antibiotic)	Possibility of eighth cranial nerve toxicity. Possible neuromuscular effect with MgSO	No data available
kanamicin (antibiotic)	Reports of eighth cranial nerve damage; ototoxicity with hearing losses reported	May affect bowel flora, may interfere with diagnostic culture results, may cause other adverse effects
neomycin (antibiotic)	Potential for eighth cranial nerve toxicity	No data available
streptomycin (antibiotic)	Ototoxicity and eighth cranial nerve toxicity have been reported	May affect bowel flora, may interfere with diagnostic culture results, may cause other adverse effects
Antifungals		
amphotericin B (antibiotic)	No negative reports	No data available
griseofulvin	Embryotoxic and teratogenic in animals; human data unavailable	No data available
miconazole (antibiotic)	Topical use not associated with congenital malformations; IV effects unknown	No data available
Cephalosporins		
cephalexin cephalothin	No defects or toxicity reported	May affect bowel flora, may interfere with diagnostic culture results, may cause other adverse effects

(Continued)

Table 16-1. Comparative effects of drugs on fetus and breast-fed neonate (Continued)

Pharmacologic class	Fetal risk	Breast-feeding data
Penicillins		
amoxicillin ampicillin oxacillin penicillin G penicillin V	No relationship to major or minor malformations	May affect bowel flora, may interfere with diagnostic culture results, may cause other adverse effects (allergy, sensitization)
Tetracyclines		
tetracycline (and others in this class)	Adverse effects on teeth and bones; congenital defects; possible association between minor malformations and tetracycline, major and minor malformations between demeclocycline and oxytetracycline	May affect bowel flora, may interfere with diagnostic culture results, may cause other adverse effects; remote possibility of dental staining and inadequate bone growth
Antiviral		
acyclovir	No controlled study available	No data available
amantadine	Animal studies: embryotoxic, teratogenic in animals in high doses	Potential for vomiting, skin rash, urinary retention; hence, contraindicated
Sulfonomides		
sulfapyridine	No relationship to major or minor malformations; has potential for toxicity in newborn; therefore, should not be administered near term	Apparently no risk to healthy, full-term newborn; do not administer if neonate is premature, has hyperbilirubinemia or glucose-6-phosphate dehydrogenase deficiency
Urinary germicides		
nalidixic acid	No defects due to the use of the drug observed	One case of hemolytic anemia in neonate with glucose-6-phosphate dehydrogenase deficiency reported
nitrofurantoin	No reports of congenital defects; however, manufacturer cautions against use near term since it may cause hemolytic anemia if neonate's red blood cells are deficient in reduced glutathione, or if neonate has glucose-6-phosphate dehydrogenase deficiency	Infants with glucose-6-phosphate dehydrogenase deficiency may develop hemolytic anemia
Autonomics		
Parasympathomimetics (cholinergics)		
neostigmine	No defects reported	Insufficient data
Parasympatholytics (anticholinergic)		
atropine	No relationship to major or minor malformations noted	No adverse effects reported
belladonna	Associated with malformations when administered in first trimester	No adverse effects reported
scopolamine	No relationship to malformations; however, when given at term, may cause fetal tachycardia, decreased heart rate, deceleration, and variability	No adverse effects reported
Sympathomimetics (adrenergic)		
albuterol (tocolytic)	No relationship to congenital anomalies reported, even with continuous IV for 17 weeks to prevent premature labor; may cause fetal tachycardia, hypoglycemia, and increased serum insulin (can be prevented with glucose); lower risk of respiratory distress syndrome	No data available
ephedrine	Some association of first trimester use with minor defects, inguinal hernias, clubfoot; may cause fetal tachycardia and beat-to-beat variability	One case of irritability, disturbed sleep, and excessive crying reported (reversed within 12 hours after breast-feeding stopped)
epinephrine	Some association of first trimester use with major and minor defects	No data available

(Continued)

Table 16-1. Comparative effects of drugs on fetus and breast-fed neonate (Continued)

Pharmacologic class	Fetal risk	Breast-feeding data
ritodrine (tocolytic)	Manufacturer says contraindicated before 29th week of gestation; fetal heart rate may increase to 200/min; ketoacidosis with fetal death has occurred; lower risk of respiratory distress syndrome	No data available
Sympatholytics (β-adrenergic blockers)		
acebutolol (cardioselective)	No malformations reported; should be observed for β-blockade if used near delivery (blood pressure and heart rate down); no data about use in first trimester or long-term exposure	Observe for signs or symptoms of β-blockade
atenolol (cardioselective)	Resembles acebutolol but lower birth weight	Resembles acebutolol; considered acceptable for breast-feeding by AAP
metoprolol (cardioselective)	Resembles acebutolol	Resembles atenolol
propranolol (nonselective)	Oxytocic effects after IV or extra-amniotic injections or high oral doses; may be related to intrauterine growth retardation; fetal and neonatal toxicity may occur; observe for β-blockade if used near delivery; no data on long-term exposure	Resembles atenolol
Cholesterol-lowering agents		
lovastatin	Contraindicated in pregnancy because cholesterol is needed for the synthesis of steroids and cell membranes essential for fetal development	Manufacturer says it is contraindicated
Coagulant/anticoagulant		
Anticoagulants		
coumarin derivatives	Multiple defects noted, with 30% of the infants born with abnormalities	Only warfarin and dicumarol (bishydroxycoumarin) considered acceptable with breast-feeding
heparin	No links with congenital defects reported; may cause indirect adverse effects on fetus, including lethal problems	Not excreted in breast milk
Thrombolytics		
streptokinase	No association with congenital defects	No data available
Cardiovascular drugs		
Cardiac drugs		
digitalis, digitoxin, digoxin (cardiac glycosides)	No association with congenital defects	Digoxin only cardiac glycoside reported as excreted in breast milk; considered acceptable for breast-feeding by AAP
quinidine (antiarrhythmic)	No association with congenital defects; has been used to treat fetal tachyarrhythmia	Excreted in breast milk; considered acceptable for breast-feeding by AAP
Antihypertensives		
acebutolol, atenolol, metoprolol, propranolol discussed previously		
Central nervous system drugs		
Analgesics and antipyretics		
acetaminophen	Appears safe for short-term use in therapeutic dosage range; no association with large categories of major or minor malformations; may be associated with congenital dislocation of the hip and club foot	Excreted in breast milk; considered acceptable for breast-feeding by AAP
aspirin	Increased perinatal mortality, intrauterine growth retardation, antepartum hemorrhage or bleeding complications after birth	Potential risk of adverse effects on platelet function

(Continued)

Table 16-1. Comparative effects of drugs on fetus and breast-fed neonate (Continued)

Pharmacologic class	Fetal risk	Breast-feeding data
Narcotic analgesics		
codeine	Not associated with large categories of major or minor malformations; however, first trimester use is linked to some defects, including respiratory defects; second trimester use is linked to alimentary tract defects; use in labor is linked to respiratory depression in the newborn	In breast milk in small amounts; considered acceptable for use while breast-feeding by AAP
meperidine	Not associated with large categories of major or minor malformations; use in labor linked to respiratory depression in the newborn	In breast milk, decreasing after 24 hours; considered acceptable for use while breast-feeding by AAP
Narcotic antagonists		
levallorphan nalorphine	Must be used with caution since its effectiveness in reducing respiratory depression in newborn is questioned; may actually increase the depression if not given in proper ratio to the amount of narcotic administered	No data available
naloxone	Should not be given before delivery, unless definite evidence of narcotic toxicity is present	No data available
Nonsteroidal anti-inflammatory drugs		
ibuprofen	No association with congenital defects reported; however, theoretic possibility of constriction *in utero* of ductus arteriosus	Considered safe while breast-feeding by AAP
indomethacin (analgesic and tocolytic)	May cause premature closure of ductus arteriosus when used in pregnancy; a few defects reported	Too little data available
Anticonvulsants		
bromides (also sedative)	No association with large categories of major or minor malformations; however, may be related to congenital defects (more data needed); newborns exposed *in utero* should be monitored for serum bromide concentrations	Contraindicated for mothers taking medications that contain bromide (intake of 5.4 g/day leads to rash, weakness, absence of cry)
carbamazepine (tricyclic)	Anomalies that have been observed may be due to the disease process (epilepsy) rather than to the medication; more data needed; this drug has been prescribed as the drug of choice for women who may become pregnant, requiring anticonvulsant therapy for the first time	Considered safe while breast-feeding by AAP
magnesium sulfate (also cathartic, tocolytic)	No association with congenital defects; should not be given with aminoglycoside antibiotics, since the combination may cause neonatal respiratory depression; if magnesium sulfate is given near delivery, neonate should be observed for signs of neurologic depression	Considered safe while breast-feeding by AAP
phenobarbital (also sedative)	May result in minor congenital defects, addiction, hemorrhage at birth; should be used at lowest possible effective dose to control epileptic seizures; does not appear to cause defects when used by nonepileptic mothers	Infant should be watched for sedation, and phenobarbital levels should be monitored to prevent toxicity; considered safe while breast-feeding by AAP. One case of methemoglobinemia reported
phenytoin	Fetal hydantoin syndrome may occur in varying degrees, causing craniofacial and/or limb malformations; teratogen effects vary; may also be a human transplacental carcinogen, with the possibility of tumor development occurring several years later; hemorrhages may occur within 24 hours after birth and may cause death; regardless of these adverse effects, it may be necessary to administer to the mother to prevent convulsions	Keeping the maternal level within the therapeutic range should not increase the risk to the infant; considered safe while breast-feeding by AAP; one case of methemoglobinemia reported

(Continued)

Table 16-1. Comparative effects of drugs on fetus and breast-fed neonate (Continued)

Pharmacologic class	Fetal risk	Breast-feeding data
primidone (structural analog of phenobarbital)	Anomalies similar to those in fetal hydantoin syndrome; hemorrhages may occur, as well as tumors; hyperactivity may also be present	The conversion of primidone to phenobarbital may lead to sedative effects in the infant; considered safe while breast-feeding by AAP
valproic acid	Anomalies similar to those in fetal hydantoin syndrome	No association with adverse effects; considered safe while breast-feeding by AAP
Antidepressants		
amitriptyline	Possibility of limb reduction anomalies	Considered safe while breast-feeding by AAP
imipramine	Symptoms of withdrawal in neonate may occur; not a major cause of congenital limb anomalies	Considered safe while breast-feeding by AAP
nortriptyline	Reports of limb reduction anomalies; observe neonate for urinary retention	Effects of chronic exposure unknown
Tranquilizers		
chlorpromazine (propylamino phenothiazine)	Possibility of delayed ocular damage; use during labor should be discouraged owing to possibly dangerous drop in maternal blood pressure	Observe breast-fed infant for sedation, lethargy; considered safe while breast-feeding by AAP
lithium	Possible association with congenital defects, particularly of the cardiovascular system; frequent reports of toxicity in the newborn, becoming normal within 1 or 2 weeks	Effects of long-term exposure unknown; considered safe while breast-feeding by AAP, but manufacturer says it should not be used
Sedatives and hypnotics		
amobarbital (barbiturate)	Possibility of congenital defects	No data available
chlordiazepoxide (benzodiazepine)	High potential for severe congenital anomalies but not linked to large classes of malformations	No data available
diazepam	Greater incidence of oral defects, inguinal hernia; use during labor does not seem harmful	May accumulate in breast-fed neonates, so should not be used while breast-feeding
ethanol	Teratogenic effects leading to fetal alcohol syndrome associated with as little as 1 oz of absolute alcohol daily (two drinks); growth retardation also associated with alcohol withdrawal; alcohol combined with hydantoin may be carcinogenic *in utero* and require long-term follow up	Considered safe while breast-feeding by AAP, even though adverse effects have been noted, including drowsiness, diaphoresis, sedation, weakness, decrease in linear growth, abnormal weight gain
Diuretics		
acetazolamide (carbonic anhydrase inhibitor)	No association with congenital defects or to large categories of major or minor defects reported	Watch for suppression of lactation; no data available
furosemide	Can be used to assess fetal kidney functions during pregnancy; should not be used during pregnancy except for treatment of maternal cardiovascular disorders	Manufacturer says breast-feeding should be discontinued if drug is used

blood flow does not increase, so that a minimal centrilobular bile stasis in the liver occurs. Therefore, drugs may be broken down more slowly. On the other hand, the kidneys may excrete drugs more rapidly as a result of the increased renal perfusion and glomerular filtration that occurs during pregnancy.

As discussed earlier, the lower the molecular weight of a substance, the greater the chance that it will travel through the placenta. Most drugs, which have a molecular weight of 250 to 500, can penetrate the trophoblast, connective, and endothelial tissues that divide the circulatory systems of mother and fetus. The changes in the placenta during the third trimester add to the probability of drug transfer through the placenta. According to Rayburn and Zuspan, some of the drugs that cross the placenta within minutes after administration to the mother include ampicillin, penicillin G, cephalothin, kanamycin, tetracycline, sulfonamides, streptomycin, diazepam, phenytoin, barbiturates, ethanol, meperidine, salicylate, lidocaine, mepivacaine, bupivacaine, and propranolol (Rayburn & Zuspan, 1980, p 115).

Some substances undergo metabolic changes through oxidation, reduction, dealkylation, or synthesis before crossing the placenta. Certain drugs are known to inhibit or increase the placental enzymes needed for their conversion or for transport mechanisms. Some evidence suggests that most carcinogenic drugs undergo oxidation to cross the placenta. Researchers are investigating whether this action lowers the resistance of the child to cancer in later life.

Once drugs have passed over to the fetal side of the placenta, they travel through the umbilical vein to the fetal liver by way of the portal vein. Some go through the liver to the ductus venosus in the right side of the heart. Traveling through the pathways that are less resistant, the drug-laden blood reaches the brain and heart. From there, more than 50% of the blood goes to the umbilical arteries, then to the placenta, returning to the maternal circulation. The remaining blood diffuses through the fetus. Because the level of protein available to bind drugs is lower in the fetus than in the mother, more of the drug is free to remain in fetal tissues. This process probably increases with gestational age, and some tissues are more receptive than others to certain drugs.

Intervention in maternal medical problems

Medications used to ensure the health of the mother must be evaluated for possible toxic effects at various stages of fetal development (Tables 16-2 and 16-3). Those used during the first 14 to 17 days of gestation (fertilization and implantation) must not interfere with cell division, or the pregnancy will end with the products of conception reabsorbed or expelled. Medications used between the 18th and 55th days after conception must not interfere with organ differentiation, or teratogenic effects will occur (Zacharius, 1983). Ongoing monitoring and evaluation of drugs are important, with reporting of possible teratogenic effects to the FDA for correlation with other consumer information.

Chronic maternal medical problems may escalate during pregnancy or may necessitate changes in maternal medications known to affect the fetus. Other maternal conditions may be associated only with pregnancy, requiring medical management to safeguard the physical status of mother and fetus. Maternal illness may be well controlled before pregnancy, but health may deteriorate with the imposition of the additional burden of pregnancy. Medication taken to keep the condition under control may have to be changed completely or given in a different dosage. A brief discussion of some of these conditions follows.

Hypertension and pregnancy

Hypertensive women may become pregnant, or pregnancy-induced hypertension (PIH) may occur in women with previously normal blood pressure. In either situation, it is important to diagnose and treat the client properly because PIH is the third leading cause of maternal deaths in the U.S. PIH can be anticipated in 5% to 7% of pregnancies, a figure that jumps to 25% to 35% for those with chronic hypertension (Hoffmaster, 1983). About one-third of PIH clients have a recurrence during a future pregnancy, possibly indicating an underlying latent essential hypertension.

Salt restriction and the use of diuretics are no longer considered advisable. The weight reduction or control that was formerly advised for PIH is now thought to add to fetal problems associated with low birth weights. However, diet is essential, with the recommendation that the woman have a high intake (75–80 g) of protein and a normal intake (2.5–7.0 g) of sodium each day. (Even in the presence of edema, 2.0–4.0 g of salt should be taken daily, with fluids at 6 to 8 glasses per day.)

Using medications to regulate PIH is controversial. Clients who took antihypertensive drugs before pregnancy may continue to take them, because the risk of abruptio placentae is greater if PIH is superimposed on hypertension. Sudden discontinuation of diuretics in the second to third trimesters may lead to rebound edema, with a 10- to 14-pound weight gain within a week. All medications should be decreased to the lowest possible effective dose, with a combination of hydralazine and methyldopa preferred for maximum efficacy and fewer side effects (Table 16-4). Methyldopa alone may lead to maternal sedation, a rare hemolytic anemia, and a positive Coombs's test. Hydralazine may cause maternal tachycardia and headaches. Fetal effects for both drugs are negligible. Nifedipine, a calcium channel-blocking agent, appears to be helpful in the treatment of PIH, particularly for severe preeclampsia. Few neonatal complications have been noted with its use, and maternal side effects appear to be minor: hot flushes and headaches controlled with the use of analgesics. In some instances, intravenous (IV) magnesium sulfate is given before the nifedipine, then stopped 24 hours after the blood pressure is stabilized. Nifedipine can then be administered orally as long as needed (Fenakel, 1991).

Various β-blockers are being studied for their effect on pregnancy. β-Adrenergic blocking agents have been reported to cause fetal growth retardation, neonatal respiratory distress, hypoglycemia, and bradycardia. Discontinuation of the drug a day before delivery prevents it from remaining in the neonate. The baby should be observed for signs of distress in the nursery.

A study in 1991 found that 60 to 150 mg of aspirin taken daily in the last two trimesters of pregnancy helped prevent PIH in 65% of the participants and reduced the number of births of severely low weight babies by 44%. The aspirin selectively inhibits synthesis of platelet thromboxane A_2. At the low dose, it did not cause maternal or fetal bleeding. Higher doses of aspirin are not appropriate and are contra-

(*Text continues on p. 228*)

Table 16-2. Reported effects of drug exposure on the fetus

Drug name	First trimester effects	Second and third trimester effects
Analgesics		
acetaminophen	None known	None known
Narcotics	None known	Depression, withdrawal
Salicylates	Frequent reports, none proved	Prolonged pregnancy and labor, hemorrhage
Anesthetics		
General	Anomalies, abortion	Depression
Local	None known	Bradycardia, seizures
Anorexics		
amphetamine	Anomalies	Irritable, poor feeding
phenmetrazine	Skeletal anomalies	Unknown
Anti-infection agents		
Aminoglycosides	Skeletal anomalies	Nephrotoxic, ototoxic
Cephalosporins	None known	Decreased positive cultures
chloramphenicol	None known	"Grey baby" syndrome (?)
clindamycin	None known	Unknown
erythromycin	None known	None known
ethambutol	None known	None known
ethionamide	Anomalies	None known
isoniazid	None known	None known
metronidazole	? Mutagenesis or carcinogenesis	None known
Penicillins	None known	None known; positive cultures
rifampin	None known	None known
sulfonamides	None known	Hemolytic anemia, thrombocytopenia, hyperbilirubinemia
Tetracyclines	Impaired bone growth	Bone growth, stained teeth (enamel hypoplasia)
D-penicillamine	Connective tissue disorder	None known
Anticoagulants		
coumadin/warfarin	Nasal hypoplasia, abnormal epiphyseal stippling	Hemorrhage, stillbirth
heparin	None known	Hemorrhage at placental site with possible stillbirth
Anticonvulsants		
Barbiturates	Anomalies (?)	Bleeding, withdrawal
carbamazepine	Anomalies	Bleeding withdrawal
clonazepam	Facial cleft	Withdrawal, depression
ethosuximide	None known	None known
phenytoin	Intrauterine growth retardation (IUGR), craniofacial abnormalities, hypoplasia of phalanges	Hemorrhage ⎫
primidone	Same as barbiturates	Hemorrhage ⎬ Depletion of Vitamin K– dependent clotting factor
trimethadione	IUGR, mental retardation, facial dysmorphogenesis	Hemorrhage ⎭
valproic acid	Spina bifida	Unknown
Cancer chemotherapy		
Alkylating agents	Abortion, anomalies	Hypoplastic gonads, growth delay
Antimetabolites Folic acid analogues	Abortion, IUGR cranial anomalies	Hypoplastic gonads, growth delay
Pyrimidine analogues arabineside	Abortion	Hypoplastic gonads, growth delay
Purine analogues (cytosine, 5-FU)	Abortion	Hypoplastic gonads, growth delay

(Continued)

Table 16-2. Reported effects of drug exposure on the fetus (*Continued*)

Drug name	First trimester effects	Second and third trimester effects
Antibiotics (actinomycin)	Abortion	Hypoplastic gonads, growth delay
Vinca alkaloids	Abortion	Hypoplastic gonads, growth delay
Hormones	(See *Hormones* below)	
Cardiovascular drugs		
Antihypertensives—		
alpha methyldopa	None known	Hemolytic anemia, ileus
guanethidine	None known	None known
hydralazine	None known	Tachycardia
propranolol	None known	Bradycardia, hypoglycemia, IUGR with chronic use
reserpine	None known	Lethargy
β-sympathomimetics	None known	Tachycardia
digitalis preparations	None known	Bradycardia
Cold and cough preparations		
Antihistamines	None known	None known
Cough suppressants	None known	None known
Decongestants	None known	None known
Expectorants	Fetal goiter	None known
Diuretics		
furosemide	None known	Death from sudden hypoperfusion
thiazides	None known	Thrombocytopenia, hypokalemia, hyperbilirubinemia, hyponatremia
Fertility drugs		
clomiphene	Chromosomal anomalies (?)	Unknown
Hormones		
Androgens	Masculinization (female fetus)	Adrenal suppression (?)
Corticosteroids	Cleft in animals, not in humans	Growth delay
Estrogens	Cardiovascular anomalies	None known
Progestins	Limb and cardiovascular anomalies	None known
Hypoglycemics		
insulin	None known	Hypoglycemia (unlikely)
Sulfonylureas	Anomalies	Suppressed insulin secretion
Laxatives		
bisacodyl	None known	None known
dioctyl sodium sulfosuccinate	None known	None known
mineral oil	Decreased vitamin absorption	None known
milk of magnesia	None known	None known
Psychoactive drugs		
Antidepressants/tricyclics	CNS (?) limb defects	None known
Benzodiazepines	Facial clefts; cardiac	Depression
hydroxyzine	None known	None known
meprobamate	Facial clefts	None known
Phenothiazines	None known	None known
Sedatives	None known	Depression
thalidomide	Phocomelia	None known
lithium	Cardiac abnormalities	None known

(*Continued*)

Table 16-2. Reported effects of drug exposure on the fetus (Continued)

Drug name	First trimester effects	Second and third trimester effects
Thyroid drugs		
Antithyroid agents		
I-131	Goiter, abortion, anomalies	Goiter, airway obstruction, hypothyroid, mental retardation
PTU	None known	Same
tapazole	Aplasia cutis	Same, aplasia cutis
thyroid USP	Dose not cross	None known
Tocolytics		
alcohol (ethanol)	Fetal alcohol syndrome	Intoxication, hypotonia, lethargy
magnesium sulfate	None known	Hypermagnesemia, respiratory depression
β-sympathomimetics	None known	Tachycardia
Vaginal preparations		
Antifungal agents	None known	None known
podophyllin	Mutagenesis (?)	Laryngeal polyps (?) CNS effects (?)
Vitamins (high doses)		
A	Renal anomalies	None known
B	None known	None known
C	None known	Scurvy after delivery
D	Mental retardation	None known
E	None known	None known
K	None known	Hemorrhage if deficiency

(Adapted from Ians JD, Rayburn EF. [1980]. Drug use during pregnancy. *Perinatal Press, 4,* 134.)

indicated during antiplatelet therapy (Imperiale, 1991, pp 260–264).

Diabetes and pregnancy

Maternal hyperglycemia acts as a teratogenic agent during the first trimester of pregnancy, resulting in congenital malformations, including neural tube defects, caudal regression syndrome, atrial and ventricular septal defects, and holoprosencephaly (Eriksson, et al, 1983, p 32). If present in the second or third trimesters, it may lead to babies that are larger for

Table 16-3. Drugs that exert a pronounced effect on the fetus when administered during pregnancy

Receptive tissue	Specific drugs
Heart	digoxin, phenytoin, isotretinoin
Skeleton	tetracycline, warfarin
Red blood cells	Sulfonamides
Central nervous system	diazepam, ethanol, narcotics
Platelets	aspirin
Adrenal gland	Sex steroids, phenytoin
Müllerian duct / Vagina	diethylstilbestrol, gentamycin, kanamycin (aminoglycosides)
Otic nerve	streptomycin
Brain, ears	isotretinoin

gestational age, with hypoglycemia, hypokalemia, and respiratory problems.

Women who have diabetes before pregnancy should have complete control of their blood glucose levels before conceiving. Glucose crosses the placenta, but insulin does not. The fetus starts to manufacture insulin at about the 12th week of pregnancy. By the 28th week, it produces sufficient insulin to keep its blood glucose at a normal level. The excess glucose received from the mother results in hypertrophy of the beta cells in the fetal pancreas. The fetus produces the additional insulin needed because of the excess glucose received from the mother. Fetal glycogen and fat stores then increase, leading to fetal obesity.

The most effective way to evaluate maternal glucose levels is by home blood glucose monitoring (HBGM). Although it requires compliance, HBGM is usually more acceptable to clients than urine monitoring (Good-Anderson, 1983, p 89). Tests should be conducted on fasting and postprandial blood. Ideally, blood sugar levels should be maintained at 60 to 90 mg/dl before meals, and less than 120 mg/dl 2 hours after meals. For people with type I diabetes, insulin requirements may change, with a need for larger amounts and different types than administered previously. More frequent blood glucose testing may also be necessary. Three well balanced meals are needed each day, plus snacks (particularly at bedtime) to maintain the proper blood glucose level.

Table 16-4. Drugs useful in pregnancy-induced hypertension

Drug name	Preparation(s) and usual dosage	Mechanism of action	Additional information
hydralazine (Apresoline)	*Oral:* 10 mg tid; may be increased to 50 mg qid *IM/IV:* 20–40 mg	Direct vasodilator; increases cardiac output by reducing peripheral resistance; increases heart rate	May cause nasal congestion, maternal dizziness, headache, flushing, sodium retention, flushing, palpitations, angina, vomiting, diarrhea, hypoxia in fetus
methyldopa (Aldomet)	*Oral:* 250 mg tid; may be increased to 500 mg qid	Stimulates central inhibitory α-adrenergic receptors	May cause sodium retention, constipation, drowsiness; suspension form contains sodium bisulfite and may cause a severe allergic reaction
magnesium sulfate	*IM:* 4–5 g of 50% solution in each buttock *IV:* 4 g in 250 ml D5W	Anticonvulsant for prevention and control of seizures in preeclampsia and eclampsia	May relax smooth muscle to extent that blood pressure decreases; may cause drowsiness, sweating, decreased or no reflexes, oliguria, circulatory collapse, respiratory paralysis; magnesium toxicity may appear in the neonate
thiopental sodium (Pentothal)	*IV:* 75–125 mg	Anticonvulsant	Respiratory and/or myocardial depression; cardiac arrhythmia; respiratory depression in fetus; have emergency equipment available for resuscitation
furosemide (Lasix)	*Oral:* 20–80 mg bid *IV:* 20–40 mg	Loop diuretic	Use only to treat maternal pulmonary edema or congestive heart failure; fetus in danger of being compromised owing to decreased placental perfusion
nitroprusside (Nitropress)	*IV:* 0.5–10 µg/kg/min (usually 3 µg/kg/min) supplied in 50-mg vial for IV use, dissolve in 2–3 ml of 5% dextrose in water; this concentrated solution is further diluted in 250 ml or 500 ml of D5W; solution must be wrapped in opaque binding because it deteriorates when exposed to light	Peripheral vasodilator; reduces peripheral resistance; immediate acting; action ends when IV infusion is discontinued	Nitroprusside is converted to cyanogen and subsequently thiocyanate; may result in lethal level in fetus; use should be restricted to cases unresponsive to other therapy; used only until blood pressure decreases, then a safer drug is substituted
nifedipine (Procardia)	*Oral:* 10–20 mg tid or qid; not more than 180 mg/day or 30 mg per single dose	Calcium channel blocker; peripheral vasodilator (dilates peripheral arterioles), reduces peripheral resistance; modest fall (5–10 mm Hg systolic) in blood pressure; decreased platelet aggregation, possible increase in bleeding time; onset of action: 10 min. Peak: 30 min.	Minor side effects reported to date: hot flushes, headaches; potential side effects: cardiac dysrhythmia, hypotension; use in pregnancy only if potential benefit justifies potential risk to fetus (increase in fetal resorption, lower fetal weight, increase in stunted forms and fetal deaths, lowered neonatal survival—all noted in animal studies, that used 3–10 times maximum recommended human dose; no human studies done); increased effects of hypertensive drugs; limit caffeine consumption

The client's emotional needs must be considered, since pregnancy and the stringent requirements for glucose control may increase the level of stress. The incorporation of exercise, rest, and psychosocial support are important factors to consider in meeting the needs of the client (Leff, 1991, pp 83–87).

To maintain control of blood glucose, pregnant diabetics have had to rely on multiple injections of insulin, using short- or intermediate-acting insulin, according to the glucose level shown by HBGM or monitoring of the diabetic urine. A continuous subcutaneous insulin infusion pump is believed to provide greater control of the maternal glucose level. It can be programmed to deliver insulin in small amounts throughout the day, along with larger doses preprandially.

Insulin requirements may vary considerably during pregnancy. During early gestation, the need may be decreased because of the lowered caloric intake due to nausea, and in the third trimester due to placental insufficiency. During the second trimester, the insulin may need to be more than doubled.

Insulin requirements of laboring women are met

according to the client's needs. After delivery, the amount needed drops precipitously. By the third post-partum day, only two-thirds of the prepregnancy dose is required. Usually, the dose at the end of the first postpartum week is the same as before pregnancy (Rayburn & Lavin, 1986, p 566).

The American Diabetes Association has provided a position statement on gestational diabetes mellitus, defined as carbohydrate intolerance of variable severity with onset or first recognition during the present pregnancy. The association recommends that all pregnant women who have not demonstrated a glucose intolerance before the 24th week of pregnancy have a screening glucose load between the 24th and 28th weeks. The definitive diagnosis is made if two or more of the venous plasma glucose concentrations meet or exceed the following levels: fasting, 105 mg/dl; 1 hour, 190 mg/dl; 2 hours, 165 mg/dl. Fasting levels above 105 mg/dl or postprandial levels above 120 mg/dl result in the greatest risk for intrauterine or neonatal death. Mothers who maintain normal glucose levels, with optimal obstetric care, place the fetus at lower risk than do those who are uncontrolled. One study reported a 16% increase in the risk of noninsulin dependent diabetes with each successive pregnancy (Kritz-Silverstein, 1989, p 1214–1219).

Any degree of gestational diabetes places the fetus at significant risk for macrosomia, hypoglycemia, hypocalcemia, and hyperbilirubinemia. Monitoring of maternal capillary blood or venous plasma for increased fasting or postprandial glucose levels is imperative. (Monitoring of maternal urinary glucose is no longer considered adequate.) Insulin may be ordered if diet does not control the glucose level, using only highly purified human insulin (a recombinant DNA product) with self-monitoring of blood glucose.

The American Diabetes Association also believes that breast-feeding should be encouraged in women with gestational diabetes. It advises that these women should be further evaluated at the first postpartum visit by having a 2-hour oral glucose tolerance with a 75 g glucose load, and that they should be followed carefully to ensure early detection of diabetes in the future.

Cardiovascular disease and pregnancy

The well controlled cardiac client may require changes in medication during pregnancy to protect the fetus. Propranolol, an effective β-blocker, may have been used to control hypertension and tachyarrhythmia but has the potential to induce premature labor or result in neonatal problems (Livingston, et al, 1982). Procainamide and disopyramide, used in the treatment of arrhythmia, should be avoided in pregnancy because of their potential to initiate uterine contractions. Warfarin (Coumadin), which is used as an anticoagulant, is also contraindicated in pregnancy because it may re-

sult in CNS abnormalities in the neonate or lead to stillbirth. Diuretics such as thiazides or furosemide may result in maternal hypovolemia that reduces placental perfusion, causing low–birth-weight infants. They may also cause symptomatic hyponatremia in the newborn. Therefore, diuretics are restricted to those gravidae with congestive heart failure or pulmonary edema.

Some cardiovascular medications can be safely used during pregnancy. They include quinidine (antiarrhythmic; 200–400 mg po qid) and digoxin (cardiac glycoside useful in congestive heart failure; 0.125–0.75 mg po daily). Some sodium restriction may be necessary for clients with fluid retention. If a thiazide diuretic has been used before pregnancy, it has to be tapered off carefully to prevent rebound edema. Thiazide diuretics may lead to thrombocytopenia and electrolyte disturbances in mother and fetus and therefore should not be administered (Rayburn & Lavin, 1986, pp 565–569).

If the pregnant client requires digitalization, an initial dose of digoxin 0.25 mg may be administered IV, repeated at 4- to 6-hour intervals until a dose of 0.75 to 1.0 mg has been reached. Oral digoxin may be the preferred route, with the administration of 1.25 to 1.5 mg in divided doses. The maintenance dose is 0.25 to 0.5 mg daily. The digoxin levels should be checked on a monthly basis. Side effects may include nausea and vomiting, headaches, and neurologic problems. Arrhythmia may occur and can be controlled with a β-adrenergic blocker, chiefly propranolol (Rayburn & Lavin, 1986, p 568), if the maternal good outweighs the risks to the fetus.

Rho(D)-negative women and pregnancy

Diagnosis and treatment of isoimmunization of Rh negative women during pregnancy is discussed in Chapter 36.

Cancer and pregnancy

Cancer is not a common complication of pregnancy; it occurs once in 1,008 pregnancies (Donegan, 1983, p 194). The most common cancers during pregnancy are breast, uterus, cervix, ovary, lymphomas, and colorectum. The depression of cellular immunity and suppressor T cells is necessary to prevent rejection of the fetus as foreign tissue. This action is also assumed to favor the growth of neoplastic disease.

Stages I and II of Hodgkin's disease can be treated with irradiation if the abdomen is shielded. However, as the fetus ascends in the abdomen, it is more difficult to shield the fetus properly. The exposure to the fundus at 16 weeks of pregnancy is about .104 rad, increasing to 1 rad at 30 weeks. If abdominal nodes are involved early in pregnancy, particularly in the first 10 weeks, termination may be necessary because of the potentially teratogenic effects of the chemotherapy. The same drugs used later in pregnancy may not affect the baby. Pregnancy is not advised for 2 years after treatment, because 80% of recurrences tend to happen during this span of time.

Any breast mass found in pregnant or lactating women should be diagnosed quickly, using a needle aspiration under local anesthesia. (Radioisotope scans should not be used because of possible danger to the fetus.) Treatment during pregnancy starts with a modified radical mastectomy, with removal of the breast and axillary lymph nodes. The risk of spontaneous abortion during the procedure is 1%. Radiation therapy cannot be used because of danger to the fetus.

If nodal metastasis has occurred during the first trimester of pregnancy and chemotherapy is ordered, the client may require a therapeutic abortion because of the probable teratogenic effects of the drugs. Cancers diagnosed nearer to term may also require chemotherapy, but treatment may be delayed until after delivery (Sahni, et al, 1981, p 167).

Carcinoma of the cervix is not influenced by endocrine changes, and the client may be followed carefully during pregnancy with vaginal examinations, Pap smears, colposcopy, and biopsy, if indicated. A 20% to 33% chance of spontaneous abortion, premature labor, or hemorrhage exists if conization is used. If further treatment is indicated, it usually is conservative with cryocautery or CO_2 laser evaporation after delivery, or with the use of newer surgical techniques.

Invasive cancers of the cervix diagnosed during the first or second trimester call for aggressive treatment. Irradiation may be necessary for the more advanced disease. Diagnosis during the third trimester may permit a delay in treatment until the fetus is viable.

Malignant melanoma may be affected by pregnancy because increased pigmentation results from stimulation of melanocytes in pregnant women. Any suspicious skin lesions should be biopsied during pregnancy.

Lymphoma and leukemia are more difficult to treat during pregnancy because the usual staging techniques of isotopic scans or laparotomy pose hazards to the fetus.

Leukemia during pregnancy is associated with spontaneous abortion, hemorrhage, and increased risk of infection. A diagnosis of acute myelogenous leukemia during the first half of pregnancy results in a healthy infant in less than half of the cases. If chemotherapy is instituted during the first trimester, the likelihood of teratogenic effects is high, and termination may be necessary. To protect the mother, chemotherapy should not be performed before exacerbation but should not be delayed once exacerbation has occurred. Chemotherapy begun during the second or third trimesters is less likely to cause teratogenic problems, and safe continuation of the pregnancy with regard to the fetus may occur.

Asthma and pregnancy

Asthma is probably the most common medical problem that exists during pregnancy. Maternal hypoxia or acidosis may necessitate the use of oxygen therapy during an acute gestational asthma attack to prevent impaired fetal oxygenation.

Presently, it appears that asthmatic women who are identified early in pregnancy, and treated appropriately, are probably at no greater risk of important perinatal complications than those without asthma. If possible, antigen immunotherapy should be avoided if systemic reactions are anticipated, because these reactions are associated with abortions. If needed, allergen immunotherapy should be continued carefully during pregnancy for those women who are already receiving it and who are unlikely to have systemic reactions. Women on maintenance therapy may have to receive a lower dose to decrease the chance of a systemic reaction. For women on an increasing antigen schedule, it may be necessary to stabilize the dose or increase the dose conservatively. Women who were not previously on immunotherapy should not start such treatment during pregnancy and should not be skin tested, because systemic reactions may occur in response to the tests (Schatz, et al, 1984, p 195).

Drugs used during pregnancy must be evaluated for the possibility of teratogenic or other effects on the fetus, as well as for effectiveness in the treatment of maternal asthma. Table 16-5 offers information about drugs used to treat asthma during pregnancy.

Seizure disorders and pregnancy

Anticonvulsant therapy is necessary for pregnant women who would suffer seizures without its use. Major seizures may precipitate hypoxia, leading to fetal damage or death. Antiepileptic drugs have teratogenic effects, with an increase in the number of microcephalic children born to the women on these drugs.

Seizure control may be lost during pregnancy, with a fall in the anticonvulsant drug level. Blood levels should be checked monthly. Women on short-acting drugs need to maintain the blood level to prevent seizures during the delivery, since seizures may result in anoxia in the neonate (Conley & Olshansky, 1987, p 326). Neural tube defects may be related to valproic acid. Other anomalies noted in the children include dysmorphic craniofacial features and hypoplasia of the distal phalanges (Robert & Guibaud, 1982, p 937; Nelson & Ellenberg, 1982, p 1247). Mental retardation and nonfebrile seizures are more common in these offspring. According to Rayburn and Lavin (1986, p 567), these women should receive phenytoin 500 mg IV during a 30-minute period in a non-glucose solution to prevent intrapartum or postpartum seizures. The infants should be observed for generalized depression or drug withdrawal. The authors also state that prophylactic oral folic acid (1 mg per day) is

Table 16-5. Drugs used for treatment of asthma during pregnancy

Drug name*	Usual dosage	Mechanism of action	Additional information
theophylline, sustained action or release	80–400 mg daily, in 2–3 divided doses: adjust dose according to serum concentrations (optimal between 10 and 20 µg/ml)	Bronchodilator	Placental transfer, but rarely affects fetus Treatment of choice for mild to moderate symptoms of asthma Monitor serum theophylline levels and clinical response; cigarette smoking decreases half-life, may require larger dose May inhibit uterine contractions, lengthening labor in multiparous women
prednisone, prednisolone	Lowest effective dose	Corticosteroid	Those who are corticosteroid dependent before pregnancy should have dose tapered to lowest possible effective level Use only when indicated for moderate to severe symptoms ineffectively controlled with a non-steroid regimen Possible hypoadrenalism is present in neonate or nursing infants
β-Adrenergic stimulant aerosols or tablets (albuterol, metaproterenol, isoetharine)	*Inhalation:* 1 or 2 inhalations every 3–4 hours *Oral tablets:* 12.5–25 mg every 4 hours (varies with manufacturer)	α- and β-receptor stimulant	
ephedrine	Lowest effective dose	Sympathomimetic	Short-term use for patients on theophylline during exacerbation of asthma

* Note: None of these drugs can be considered totally safe during pregnancy. Their use must be weighed in terms of risks of uncontrolled asthma vs. possible adverse effects of the drug on the fetus.

needed throughout pregnancy to offset any folic acid antagonism caused by the anticonvulsants, and that oral vitamin K (5–10 mg daily) should be taken during the last month of pregnancy to prevent neonatal coagulopathy.

The blood level of anticonvulsants may increase slowly after delivery and should be drawn weekly for early detection of toxicity (Conley & Olshansky, 1987, p 326).

Sexually transmitted diseases and pregnancy

Routine screening for syphilis and gonorrhea alert health care providers to the presence of these diseases so that proper treatment can be instituted to protect mother and infant. Other sexually transmitted diseases also require treatment during pregnancy to prevent complications for mother and child. Of concern to all engaged in maternal and child health programs is the increase of about 7,000 cases of syphilis from 1985 to 1990 in the U.S., a fivefold increase (Sharts-Engel, 1991). In a related finding, the Centers for Disease Control report that cases of congenital syphilis more than doubled between 1983 and 1986. In addition, the cases of penicillin-resistant gonorrhea doubled in 1986, and again in 1987.

Perhaps the greatest health fears are generated by the acquired immunodeficiency syndrome (AIDS). In 1990, more than 2,628 cases of the disease had been reported in children (with over 700 new cases in 1990)

and a mortality rate of 61%. This case load will undoubtedly increase as the number of women with AIDS expands from its present 11% of all AIDS clients, increasing the likelihood of transmission of the disease to the fetus.

Health workers should follow the procedures listed in Chapter 38 when caring for AIDS clients, with special care in labor and delivery units. The neonate should be aspirated with a bulb syringe or gentle mechanical suction, never with a mouthpiece-type suction, to prevent provider aspiration or ingestion of the newborn's secretions. Placing mother and infant in a private rooming-in unit facilitates carrying out blood and secretion precautions for both (Loveman, Colburn & Dobin, 1986, p 92). Any anti-AIDS drugs should be administered as ordered. Zidovudine triphosphate (AZT) and didanosine (DDI, also known as dideoxyinosine) are the only drugs approved by the FDA for treating AIDS. The development of a vaccine is at the point of clinical study (Segal, 1987, p 11). (See Chapter 38 for more information on sexually transmitted diseases.)

Toxoplasmosis and pregnancy

If toxoplasmosis is acquired during pregnancy, usually through contact with the feces of an infected cat or eating inadequately cooked meat, the organism causes congenital condition in the newborn, particularly cataracts. Normally, the active stage is treated with a combination of pyrimethamine and sulfadiazine or with sulfa drugs. Pyrimethamine is not used in the treatment of pregnant women because it is a known teratogen. Therefore, sulfa alone is used for treatment during the first trimester.

Differing risks of maternal medication

Medication may be needed to treat a maternal condition throughout pregnancy and during lactation. It is important to be aware of the possible differing effects of the same medication during both periods of time. Table 16-3 presents the comparisons of fetal risk during pregnancy and neonatal risk during lactation (Briggs, Freeman & Yaffe, 1986).

Intervention in fetal medical problems

Because of the fact that certain medications given to the mother pass through the placenta and reach a specific fetal organ, and other drugs introduced directly into the amniotic fluid are then swallowed by the fetus, researchers are examining ways to treat fetal medical problems that are amenable to drugs. Nurses should be aware of research in these areas so that they can help clients understand the various methods of treatment that may be suggested (Table 16-6).

The fetus, rather than the mother, may demonstrate cardiac problems. Intrauterine treatment of fetal tachycardia (over 200 beats per minute) can be accomplished by medicating the mother. Funk and Buerkle report on several cases treated with digoxin, propranolol, digoxin with propranolol, or digoxin with verapamil, and with procainamide (Funk & Buerkle, 1986, pp 298–304). Achieving and maintaining adequate fetal blood levels is imperative to prevent fetal or neonatal congestive heart failure. The daily dosage for the mother must be regulated to keep her serum level at the point at which the fetal tachycardia is controlled.

Both mother and fetus must be observed for toxicity or other side effects of the drugs. Digoxin is the drug used most frequently; it has been used successfully alone or in combination with other drugs. Propranolol may have adverse effects in the fetus or neonate (*eg*, intrauterine growth retardation, postnatal bradycardia, hypoglycemia, respiratory depression af-

ter delivery) and should therefore be used only if the expected benefits outweigh possible fetal or neonatal risk. If used, it should be withdrawn before the onset of labor. Verapamil, a calcium channel blocker, requires care in attaining and maintaining adequate maternal levels. Procainamide has the potential to cause maternal hypotension, which can lead to uteroplacental insufficiency. This drug may also cause problems to the neonate, since it is eliminated slowly, with resultant higher levels in the neonate than in the mother.

Summary of adverse effects

Teratogenicity

Because the teratogenic effects of most medications are unknown, to be safe, only those drugs that are absolutely necessary should be used and even then only with the permission of a knowledgeable practitioner. Ongoing research may prove that some abortions, miscarriages, and birth defects are unwittingly caused by maternal use of certain drugs. Some of these effects are due to one drug, others to the synergistic action of combinations of drugs. Either effect may be influenced by the genotypes of mother or fetus, which increase or decrease vulnerability.

Animal research on the safety or teratogenicity of drugs cannot be applied with certainty to humans because of the differences between species in drug reactions (Catz & Giacoia, 1972). For example, the initial laboratory studies of thalidomide on rats did not indicate the possibility of deformities in humans. Later studies on monkeys and rabbits did disclose this problem. More recent research techniques have tried to find the appropriate animal species to be used in the testing process. Again, fetal safety cannot be completely assured for humans using results extrapolated from animal studies.

The potential harm that a specific drug poses to the fetus has to be weighed against its benefits to the mother. Tables 16-4 through 16-9 contain information that can help make the decision about taking a certain drug.

Other adverse effects

Some drugs taken by the mother, although not necessarily teratogenic or carcinogenic, may cause other

---

Table 16-6. Drugs administered during pregnancy for therapeutic effect on the fetus

Fetal condition	Cause	Therapeutic drug
Heart failure	Severe anemia	digoxin
Hypothyroidism	Maternal use of propylthiouracil	sodium levothyroxine
Exposure to syphilis	Maternal syphilis	penicillin
Biotin dependency	Genetic disorder	biotin
Candidate for neonatal development of respiratory distress syndrome	Anticipation of neonatal prematurity	Glucocorticoids
Rh incompatibility, jaundice, hydrops	Rho(D)-negative mother with a Rho(D)-positive fetus	Rho(D) immune globulin

Table 16-7. Drugs used frequently for pain relief during labor

Drug name	Usual dosage	Type/desired action	Possible side-effects		Precautions
			Maternal	*Fetal*	
amobarbital (Amytal)	15–200 mg	Barbiturate/sedative	Nausea, vomiting, hypotension, vertigo, restlessness, slow labor	Apnea, CNS depression	Avoid late in labor
diazepam (Valium)	2–10 mg	Tranquilizer/antianxiety, potentiates narcotics and barbiturates	Hypotension, vertigo, drowsiness	Hypothermia, CNS depression, may remain active in fetus for 10 days	Decrease narcotics or barbiturates to ½ dose
hydroxyzine (Vistaril)	10–100 mg IM	Tranquilizer/antianxiety, potentiates narcotics and barbiturates	Hypotension, vertigo, drowsiness	CNS depression	Decrease narcotics or barbiturates to ½ dose
meperidine* (Demerol)	25–100 mg every 3 to 4 hours	Narcotic/analgesic, increased pain tolerance	Nausea, vomiting, some circulatory and respiratory depression	Respiratory depression in the neonate	Avoid within 2 hours of delivery; found in neonate's urine for 3 days
pentobarbital (Nembutal)	30 mg	Barbiturate/sedative, sleep inducer	Nausea, vomiting, hypotension, vertigo, restlessness, slow labor	Apnea, CNS depression	Avoid late in labor
phenobarbital (Luminal)	15–100 mg	Barbiturate/sedative	Nausea, vomiting, hypotension, vertigo, restlessness, slow labor	Apnea, CNS depression	Avoid late in labor
secobarbital (Seconal)	30 mg	Barbiturate/sedative	Nausea, vomiting, hypotension, vertigo, restlessness, slow labor	Apnea, CNS depression	Avoid late in labor

* Newborn respiratory depression due to narcotization can be reversed within 2 minutes by IV administration of naloxone hydrochloride (Narcan), a narcotic antagonist. Infant must be watched for subsequent episodes of apnea.

adverse effects on the embryo, fetus, or neonate. See Table 16-2 for these drug effects during pregnancy.

■ Summary

Exposure to some substances during the first 3 weeks after conception can be so destructive to the embryo that spontaneous abortion occurs. Major malformations are most likely to occur from the 3rd to the 10th week of gestation, when the organs are being formed. From the 11th week after conception through delivery, exposure mostly slows down the growth process or creates physiologic deficits, which appear in the fetus or neonate.

Nursing management

Nursing implications

Once pregnant, a woman must be aware of the effects that her lifestyle and any medications she uses have, not only on herself, but on the fetus as well. Self-deprivation is not easy for most people and is probably more difficult for the pregnant woman, who has to adjust to a radical change in body image and the thought that her actions affect an unknown being in her uterus. Why should she give up the substances that she may have previously relied on most for comfort—cigarettes, coffee, alcohol, perhaps illicit drugs—for a child who may or may not appreciate her efforts? It is important for the nurse to recognize the woman's own needs, while helping her overcome any feelings of frustration associated with placing the fetal needs on a par with (or even ahead of) her own.

Nurses who smoke while advising clients to abstain cannot be effective in their health teaching. In addition, smoking in the presence of a pregnant client exposes her to increased contamination of the air, which increases her craving for cigarettes and may be potentially harmful to the fetus.

Nursing process

Assessment   A woman who has had medical problems before pregnancy may have to modify regimens that have kept her functioning well because the medications may be contraindicated for the fetus. Other women may develop medical problems during pregnancy and may have to take medications or follow diets that make them feel uncomfortable. Some women may be reluctant to discuss feelings or anxieties, fearful of disapproval from others if they are not fully committed to doing everything that is best for the fetus. It is important for the nurse to be nonjudgmental and supportive and to be a sounding board as the client works through her feelings.

Obstetric care incorporates wellness care, as most pregnant women are in good health. It is a time for health teaching that can provide a basis for family care throughout life. Assessments should therefore include information about the lifestyle, nutrition, responses to stress, and health practices of the client.

History-taking is important, especially the taking of prescribed or OTC medications, smoking, and the use of drugs, including alcohol. For example, a history of the client's use of alcohol (quantity and frequency), the substances used (wine, whiskey, beer), as well as information about the presence of fetal alcohol syndrome in other family members may be significant. Tact must be used in obtaining the history so that the client does not become defensive and drink even more heavily to overcome her sense of guilt and inadequacy. A social history may reveal her reasons for drinking, including the possibility that she does not want the baby or lacks the proper coping mechanisms to deal with stressful situations.

Nursing diagnosis Using the data collected during the assessment, the nurse can determine the areas in which the client needs help, including the following:

> *Pain: stress that must be managed without the use of tobacco, alcohol, or other mind-altering drugs*
> *Knowledge deficit concerning maternal, fetal, or neonatal harm that may result from the medical status or medication regimen of the client*
> *Knowledge deficit concerning nutritional needs, including caloric requirements and food choices*

Planning Since most pregnant clients are well and capable of determining their own care, any desired changes should be presented as possible options by the nurse, rather than absolute demands for change. Incorporation of the client as a full partner in the planning of her care is likely to be more acceptable and therefore gain greater compliance.

If the client must carry out certain medical regimens, including medications or, as for those with diabetes, home glucose monitoring at specific times, it is wise for the nurse to help the client plan her time to accommodate whatever has to be done. The client should be helped to feel that she has a part in setting the goals for her own care.

Intervention Whatever is done must take the mother as well as the baby into consideration. If medications taken before pregnancy must be changed to protect the baby, full explanations are in order; client education is of great importance.

Client education. Pregnant women are often unaware that the drugs they are taking may affect the fetus. The general public believes that OTC preparations are safe, or that all physicians are aware of fetal reactions to drugs prescribed for maternal conditions unrelated to the pregnancy. As a result, nearly 20% of the pregnant population uses some systemic medication during the first trimester. Pregnant women should also be told to inform any health care professionals of their pregnancy before accepting any medications.

The gravida's cooperation in following medication regimens to prevent or cure fetal or neonatal disorders is necessary. For example, the pregnant syphilitic mother must take a course of penicillin not only to treat her own disease, but also to prevent congenital syphilis in her baby.

Evaluation Any intervention must be judged by its value to both mother and baby. Medications that may cause problems for the neonate at birth may have to be discontinued or modified before labor. At the same time, medications that may help the fetus but potentially harm the mother during labor may also have to be changed. Plans for stress reduction should be evaluated in light of the mother's behavior during labor and the postpartum period. Plans for eliminating or reducing drug (including alcohol) use during pregnancy can be objectively evaluated by determining intake during pregnancy (see the Example of Nursing Process and Treatment for Alcoholism during Pregnancy).

Drug use during labor

Premature labor

A normal pregnancy lasts about 280 days (40 weeks, 9 calendar months, or 10 lunar months). In the normal course of events, labor is triggered about 280 days after conception. However, the full mechanism of this phenomenon of labor remains obscure. Sometimes labor starts prematurely, posing a risk to the fetus. About 85% of infant deaths that are not related to birth defects are due to prematurity.

Before the 1970s, treatment of premature labor focused on bed rest in the Trendelenburg position, adequate nutrition, avoidance of sexual activity, and sedation. Hospitalization was used when needed. At that time, neither preventive nor adequate treatment measures existed for the most serious neonatal complication, respiratory distress syndrome, then referred to as hyaline membrane disease.

In the mid-1970s, an additional treatment modality was added, 10% alcohol (ethanol), usually given as an IV drip, as a tocolytic (contraction inhibiting) agent. Although somewhat effective in the termination of contractions, women complained of uncomfortable side effects from the alcohol (headaches, nausea, hangover).

Example of nursing process and treatment for alcoholism during pregnancy

The client is a 29-year-old advertising executive who is 4 months pregnant. Her job involves a great deal of tension, long hours, and many meals with people from her major accounts in the liquor industry. Her alcohol intake has gradually increased through the years, until she is now consuming about five cocktails a day. She denies that she is an alcoholic and is angry that her obstetrician has suggested that she stop drinking. The client acknowledges that her father has been treated for alcoholism but states she is "only a social drinker."

She expressed negative feelings about the change in her physical appearance due to the pregnancy, saying that she feels "like a blimp." she is ambivalent about having a baby, saying, "It's that biological clock that's pressuring me into it now. My husband is happy, but the loss in income and prestige have to be considered a big negative. At the same time, I really want to be a mother."

Assessment data	Nursing diagnosis	Intervention	Goals and outcome criteria
Excessive alcohol intake for past 5 years	Knowledge deficit related to harmful effects of alcohol on the fetus	**Counsel** the client regarding the risks inherent in continued use of alcohol, particularly during pregnancy.	The client's use of alcohol will decline steadily.
Paternal history of alcoholism			The client will attend AA or ACOA meetings regularly.
		Refer the client to Alcoholics Anonymous (AA) or to Adult Children of Alcoholics (ACOA).	
Denial that she is more than a "social drinker"	Ineffective coping	**Encourage** the client to face reality; offer emotional support.	The client will cope with day-to-day problems without using alcohol.
Client feels that she is "like a blimp"	Body image disturbance related to changes of pregnancy	**Provide** education about fetal growth and development in an affirmative way so that the client has a sense of pregnancy as a positive experience.	The client will become more accepting of the pregnancy; positive expressions related to self-concept will increase and negative ones decrease.

The fetus was also affected, appearing intoxicated and lethargic and showing signs of hypotonicity.

Home uterine activity monitoring systems are used to determine the presence of uterine contractions that lead to preterm labor. The monitor has a sensor that is placed against the mother's abdomen for an hour, twice a day. The information is transmitted via telephone to a perinatal nurse, usually at a perinatal center. This information permits early diagnosis of labor and the use of tocolytic drugs if needed (Freda, 1991).

Ritodrine hydrochloride

In 1981, the U.S. government approved a tocolytic drug, ritodrine hydrochloride (Yutopar). It is a potent β-sympathomimetic agent that is specifically useful as a uterine relaxant. Approval came after many clinical trials, with thorough records that documented maternal, fetal, and neonatal outcomes.

Pharmacodynamics. Ritodrine relaxes the smooth muscles of the uterus, bronchial tree, and arterioles. Its effectiveness is greatest when the fetus has reached 20 to 36 weeks of gestation, no evidence of fetal distress is found, and the membranes have not ruptured.

Pharmacokinetics. Treatment is initiated with an IV infusion of ritodrine during the acute phase of preterm labor. The dose is titrated and the drug continued until contractions have been suppressed for at least 12 hours. About 30 minutes before IV therapy is stopped, oral administration is begun. The tablets are usually taken several times a day, with reintroduction of IV therapy if labor starts again. Oral therapy is usually terminated by the 38th week of gestation, because delivery by then should produce a neonate capable of maintaining the necessary life functions.

Therapeutic uses. Ritodrine is used to inhibit labor so that parturition is delayed until the fetus is mature enough to sustain vital functions. With the use of ritodrine for even 48 hours, corticosteroids (*eg*, betamethasone) can be introduced prenatally to induce fetal pulmonary maturation. However, the combined use of these two agents is suspected of causing maternal pulmonary edema (Box 16-2).

Adverse reactions. Infusion therapy required by ritodrine induction can cause fluid volume excess and maternal pulmonary edema, especially when combined with glucocorticoid medication (Alper & Cohen, 1983). Maternal and fetal heart rate and blood pressure increase with ritodrine therapy. Both cardiac and CNS stimulation are commonly seen. In addition, hyperglycemia may develop.

Ritodrine presents a new approach to the problem of preterm labor. However, its use does present certain risks.

Precautions and contraindications. Before the initiation of ritodrine medication, the utmost consideration should be given to whether it is truly needed. If fetal lung maturity is adequate, it may be better to allow delivery to occur, since infants in this situation usually have an uncomplicated course after birth. Fetal lung maturity can be evaluated by a sonogram to determine fetal age, by the lecithin/sphingomyelin rate in the amniotic fluid, or both. Contractions should be regular, occurring at least every 10 minutes and lasting at least 30 seconds, the fetal weight less than 2,500 g, and the cervical effacement less than 80%, with dilation less than 4 cm. The use of ultrasound may help distinguish women who are in premature labor with changes in the cervix and lower uterine segments from those who are having contractions without changes.

Because ritodrine therapy poses some risks, primarily to the mother, it must be monitored carefully. Maternal fluid balance must be monitored to prevent overhydration, particularly if used in combination with corticosteroids. Multiple gestations and administration of ritodrine IV for more than 24 hours may increase the risk of pulmonary edema. Maternal serum glucose and potassium levels should be checked twice a day during IV administration. Although the many effects of ritodrine do not appear to result in clinical problems, babies should be observed for changes in their renal, electrolyte, and fluid levels (Huisjes & Touwen, 1983).

Ritodrine should never be used in the presence of maternal cardiac arrhythmia, pulmonary hypertension, bronchial asthma (treated with β-agonists, corticoste-

---

Box 16-2. Suggested protocol for ritodrine hydrochloride to inhibit labor

Establish diagnosis of labor
  Observe contractions (intervals, length, intensity)
  Ultrasonography (effacement and dilation of cervix, thinning of lower uterine segment, fetal membranes in lower cervical canal)
Data collection concerning mother
  Presence of physical complications (PIH, eclampsia, cardiac or renal disease, hemorrhage, intrauterine infection)
  Ultrasonography (multiple gestation)
  Blood studies (baseline information on maternal hematocrit, sodium, chloride, potassium, serum glucose, and carbon dioxide levels)
Data collection concerning fetus
  Fetal monitoring (fetal viability)
  Ultrasonography (establish fetal age, possible anomalies)
  Amniocentesis (L/S ratio for fetal lung maturity)
  X-rays (establish fetal demise and some anomalies)
Administration of ritodrine hydrochloride
  Preparation: 150 mg ritodrine added to 500 ml 5% dextrose in water

Microdrip and infusion pump
Mother in lateral recumbent position in bed
Continuation of ritodrine IV for 12 hours to 24 hours after contractions stop, then oral administration as ordered

Nursing actions
  Constant monitoring of contractions and fetal heart rate (maternal pulse and BP checked every 15 minutes during titration of drug, every 30 minutes during maintenance of IV administration)
  Evaluation and reporting of maternal side effects (dyspnea, chest pain, pulse over 120 beats per minute, BP below 90/60 mm Hg or decrease from original baseline)
  Careful monitoring of fluid intake (limit to 90 ml–100 ml/hr) and output (measured every hour during contractions, then every 4 hours)
  Patient education if discharged on ritodrine by mouth (report pulse rate over 120 beats/min, palpitations, agitation, tremors, nervousness)

roids, or both), hyperthyroidism, or pheochromocytoma. Fetal contraindications include chorioamnionitis, fetal death, or conditions that are incompatible with neonatal survival.

Terbutaline

Terbutaline (Bricanyl) is another β-mimetic drug with tocolytic effects. It is usually administered IV initially in the hospital, 5 mg in dextrose 5% in water, 500 ml at 10 μg/min, increased every 10 minutes until contractions stop (limit 80 μg/min). The dose is then brought down to the lowest effective level. Once stabilized, the client can be discharged on oral doses of 2.5 mg every 4 hours the first day, then every 6 hours until term (Haller, 1980).

When the client cannot be maintained on oral therapy, parenteral therapy is started in the hospital for 48 hours, and the client is then treated on an outpatient basis. A miniature portable terbutaline in-

fusion pump is used in conjunction with home uterine activity monitoring, providing a continual amount of terbutaline through a tube under the skin. The subcutaneous site is usually in the upper abdomen and changed every 3 days. The client receives instruction on the operation of the pump, care of the infusion site, and monitoring of the fetal heart rate. The infusion rate is adjusted to keep the uterine contractions less than four per hour. About 80% of the contractions are found to occur over a 6-hour period for the majority of clients, with most taking place in the evening. With this system, about 3 mg or less of terbutaline are required per day, as opposed to 40 to 60 mg per day orally or 60 mg per day IV. Treatment is continued to term or until hospitalization is required again (Lam, 1988).

The perinatal nurse may be responsible for adjusting the dose of terbutaline according to the information received over the telephone from the home uterine activity monitoring strips. Agency protocols must

---

Issues in drug therapy

Use of tocolytic drugs to inhibit preterm labor or promote fetal pulmonary maturation

Pros

Use for as few as 48 hours permits prenatal introduction of corticosteroids to induce fetal pulmonary maturation.

Provides time for prenatal transfer of pregnant woman to high-risk obstetrical facility with neonatal intensive care unit.

May end premature labor, permitting pregnancy to term or to point of viability.

Cons

Neither ritodrine hydrochloride nor terbutaline lowers prenatal mortality nor reverses severe respiratory disorder in neonates.

Maternal contraindications include: arrhythmia, pulmonary hypertension, bronchial asthma treated with β-agonists or corticosteroids, hyperthyroidism, pheochromocytoma.

Maternal adverse reactions may include increase in blood pressure and cardiac and CNS stimulation. When combined with corticosteroids, client may develop pulmonary edema (need for careful monitoring of maternal fluid balance), hyperglycemia.

Fetal contraindications include fetal death, conditions incompatible with neonatal survival, chorioamnionitis.

Fetal and neonatal adverse reactions may include increase in fetal heart rate and blood pressure, cardiac and CNS stimulation, hyperglycemia, lower insulin clearance, increased bilirubin level with neonatal icterus, increased plasma renin activity, increased weight at 6 days of age (possibly due to fluid retention from fetal exposure to drug), urine excretion of vasopressin for several days after birth.

be determined and followed for this procedure to meet client and professional safety standards.

Ritodrine has FDA approval for use as a tocolytic drug, but terbutaline does not. Although both drugs prolong gestational duration and are a factor in increased birth weights, a study released in 1988 (King, et al) noted that neither drug reduced perinatal mortality or severe respiratory disorders in neonates. Several cases of maternal deaths have been associated with β-mimetic administration, usually due to fluid overload. The positive aspect of the use of these tocolytic drugs is that they may provide sufficient time for the transfer of the client to a high-risk obstetric facility with a neonatal intensive care unit. In addition, the time can be used to administer glucocorticoids to enhance fetal lung maturation.

Induction of labor

Natural oxytocin

Although the full triggering mechanism for the beginning of labor is not known, we are aware that the posterior pituitary secretes oxytocin, a hormone with the power to stimulate uterine contractions. The myometrium of the uterus is most sensitive to this stimulation toward the end of the pregnancy. As the cervix effaces and dilates, additional oxytocin is released. This release stimulates additional contractions of the uterine fundus, resulting in greater cervical effacement and dilation. The oxytocin level seems to reach a high level during the second (expulsive) stage of delivery. Nonpharmacologic induction of labor has occurred with breast self-stimulation to ripen the cervix. Gentle massage of the nipples with a warm, moist washcloth for 1 hour, three times daily, demonstrated statistically significant changes in amount of effacement and dilation of the cervix. Tetanic contractions and other adverse contractions were not present, making this technique one to be considered when induction is necessary. Electrostimulation of the nipples has also been used, since it can be controlled more exactly than the washcloth massage. For either method of stimulation, the cervix must be inducible and the client monitored for signs of decreased fetal heart rate or prolonged uterine contractions, with intervention if either occurs (Tal, 1988).

Artificial induction of labor

In cases of fetal postmaturity, gestational diabetes, maternal diabetes mellitus, pregnancy-induced hypertension, or any other maternal or fetal condition that warrants induction of labor, the client is hospitalized and a synthetic oxytocic drug is given.

Oxytocic drugs

Pharmacodynamics. Oxytocic drugs, which are synthetic peptides, have the same properties as the naturally occurring oxytocin that appears in the posterior lobe of the pituitary gland. A selective action occurs on the smooth muscle of the uterus, stimulating contractions or increasing the forcefulness of existing contractions. Oxytocics must be administered with care to assure the proper level of contractile activity.

Pharmacokinetics. Oxytocin (Pitocin, Syntocinon) may be administered as a nasal spray, buccal tablet, intramuscular (IM) injection, or IV infusion. When administered IV, 10 units of the oxytocic drug is given in 1,000 ml of a physiologic IV electrolyte infusion. The initial dose should be limited to 1 to 2 mU/min, and may be gradually increased at a rate of no more than 1 to 2 mU/min until a contraction pattern occurs that resembles normal labor. Uterine response should start within 3 to 5 minutes, persisting for 2 to 3 hours. The infusion should be discontinued immediately if uterine hyperactivity or fetal distress occurs. Since the half-life is from 3 to 5 minutes, the effects disappear quickly after discontinuation.

Oxytocic drugs are distributed throughout the extracellular fluid and may reach the fetus as well. They are removed from the plasma by the kidney and liver.

Therapeutic uses. Oxytocic drugs can be used in controlled situations to induce or reinforce labor and to control postpartum bleeding or hemorrhage.

Adverse reactions. Oxytocic drugs have an antidiuretic effect, with the possibility of water intoxication and pulmonary edema when they are administered continuously IV and the client is taking fluids by mouth. Oxytocics are capable of causing hypertonic or tetanic contractions and therefore must be carefully monitored. For the mother, the risk of uterine rupture, hypertension, subarachnoid hemorrhage, postpartum hemorrhage, anaphylaxis, cardiac arrhythmia, afibrinogenemia, and pelvic hematoma exists. Intense uterine contractions decrease the flow of oxygenated blood to the fetus, creating the possibility of fetal damage, particularly to the brain. Arrhythmia, neonatal jaundice, low Apgar score at 5 minutes, and even fetal death may occur.

Precautions and contraindications. Oxytocics should never be used to induce labor for any reason other than medical necessity. The convenience of client or health care provider is an unacceptable reason for induction.

The cervix must be "ripe" (inducible) for the drug to be effective. Topical prostaglandin (PGE$_2$) applied to the cervix has been found to help ripen the cervix if applied the night before attempting an induction of labor with oxytocin (Sasso, 1983). These drugs should never be used if significant cephalopelvic disproportion is present, an indication that the fetal position or other problem will preclude vaginal delivery, if hypertonic uterine patterns are evident, or if hypersensitivity to the drug is indicated. Prolonged use is contraindicated in the presence of uterine inertia, severe toxemia, or fetal distress.

Throughout administration of oxytocic drugs, the flow must be accurately controlled with a constant infusion pump or similar device. Fetal monitoring is also required to determine the frequency, duration, and force of the maternal contractions, as well as the fetal heart rate. The client should be hospitalized during the procedure, with a physician available at all times.

Artificial induction of labor after fetal demise

Certain prostaglandins, which occur naturally in the body, stimulate uterine contractions. One form, PGE_2, is synthesized by the cervix and is being studied as a way to induce labor because it softens and ripens even the unfavorable cervix. The FDA has approved the use of dinoprostone (PGE_2) for expelling a fetus that dies before 28 weeks of gestation, using 20 mg suppositories inserted high in the vagina. Oxytocin is usually administered concurrently. This dose can be repeated every 2 to 4 hours until a maximum dose of 280 mg has been administered. If labor does not ensue within 24 hours, a period of 12 to 24 hours should pass before another attempt is made. The drug should not be given for more than 48 hours and should not be administered to women with active pulmonary, hepatic, cardiac, or renal disease or acute pelvic inflammatory disease.

Hypertension control during labor

During the course of pregnancy or labor, a marked elevation of blood pressure may occur. Active intervention is necessary to prevent seizures. Magnesium sulfate is the drug of choice and may be used either IM or IV to prevent or control convulsions. Severe CNS depression may occur, requiring IV administration of calcium gluconate. Oral, IM, or IV hydralazine (Apresoline) is also used as a vasodilator with antihypertensive action. Teratogenic effects have been noted when it is used in mice and rabbits, although clinical experience with the drug does not indicate any positive evidence of an adverse effect on the human fetus. Phenobarbital is another drug used as an anticonvulsant. The drawback to its use lies in its ability to cross the placental barrier, resulting in the possible depression of neonatal respiration.

Pain control during labor

Pain control during labor is a prime example of the way in which maternal and fetal needs may be in conflict. Relief of pain may be the foremost desire of the mother, whereas risk of prematurity, slow heart rate, or low level of fetal lung maturity may preclude the use of medication to relieve the mother's labor pain. For this reason, techniques such as biofeedback, hypnosis, acupuncture, therapeutic touch, and psychoprophylaxis are useful. These provide control rather than elimination of pain. The client then requires less medication than she might otherwise request.

Water immersion

Water immersion is being used in some settings to relieve pain, increase relaxation, and facilitate labor. Jet hydrotherapy (whirlpool baths) has been instituted for cases in which maternal and fetal signs are within normal limits, providing support for tense muscles and a resultant decrease in adrenaline production. This decrease leads to an increase in oxytocin and endorphin production, with an increase in contractions and cervical dilation. The immersion may also lead to a reduction in blood pressure and an increase in diuresis. The whirlpool probably increases dilation another 2 to 3 cm during a 30-minute bath. Women are helped from the bath as the second stage of labor approaches. (If an underwater birth does occur, the neonate is raised above water level immediately, and the woman helped from the bath before placental separation occurs, to prevent water embolism.)

Some women with ruptured membranes, bloody show, or less than 1% meconium staining are permitted, with physician concurrence, to use the bath. It cannot be used if continuous electronic fetal monitoring with internal scalp electrodes is ordered. The bath is also contraindicated when hyperstimulation of the uterus may occur, as with the use of an oxytocic infusion.

Maternal and fetal health are checked and documented before and after hydrotherapy, with fetal heart rate and contractions checked every 15 minutes during the 20- to 30-minute bath with the use of a hand-held Doppler. An attendant must remain with the parturient throughout hydrotherapy, offering cold fluids or ice chips to counter dehydration or overheating and to prevent chilling during longer immersion if the water cools (Aderhold, 1991, p 97–99).

Meperidine hydrochloride

Meperidine hydrochloride (Demerol) is frequently given parenterally during labor to produce analgesia and sedation. Because it readily crosses the placenta in appreciable amounts, its use in late labor is restricted because it may cause neonatal respiratory depression. It may be combined with other drugs for additional effects. Promazine hydrochloride (Sparine) reduces the excitement and anxiety that some women experience during labor, whereas scopolamine helps relax the smooth uterine muscle and reduces oral secretions. This combination of meperidine hydrochloride, promazine hydrochloride, and scopolamine results in amnesia for the labor but frequently causes the client to become excited, confused, perhaps delirious, and extremely difficult to manage, particularly during the uterine contractions.

Meperidine hydrochloride is also used in combination with hydroxyzine hydrochloride (Vistaril), which improves sedation and acts as an antiemetic during labor. (Its use is contraindicated in early pregnancy.) Propiomazine hydrochloride (Largon) and promethazine hydrochloride (Phenergan) are sometimes separately combined with meperidine for their sedative and antiemetic effects. All of these combinations must be administered with the greatest caution because they may cause neonatal respiratory depression. Pain relief during the actual delivery can be obtained through the use of a local or general anesthetic (see next section).

Table 16-11 discusses drugs that are used to control pain during labor.

■ Summary

Drugs are available to manage premature labor as well as to induce labor. In either situation, the dangers for mother, fetus, or neonate must be considered carefully, and both clients (mother and child) must be monitored closely.

Nursing management

Nursing implications

Labor and delivery usually occur in a safe manner, but they may be complicated by unexpected situations. Labor may occur before the fetus has attained sufficient maturity to sustain life, or it may be delayed beyond the time that the fetus can be nurtured properly in the uterus. Nurses must be prepared to recognize any adverse effects on the mother or child caused by drugs that are administered to delay or induce labor.

Nursing process

Assessment The client in labor may present herself in a variety of ways. She may or may not be in control and may or may not be properly prepared for the experience of labor and delivery. She may react to pain stoically, or she may want relief through medication. If an oxytocic is administered, she may need to be guided into using relaxation or other techniques for pain control, in addition to any medication that has been ordered.

The duration, forcefulness, and frequency of contractions, as well as their effect on the fetal heart rate, must be carefully observed. This observation becomes even more critical when oxytocics are used. The client needs support during her labor and delivery, whether or not she has a lay coach with her. At times, the coach may need even more support than the parturient!

Nursing diagnosis Nursing diagnoses likely to be made for clients in labor and delivery include the following:

Pain related to uterine contractions of labor
Fear of expected or unexpected situations of labor

Potential for altered tissue perfusion in the fetus secondary to labor or the medications for its control
Knowledge deficit related to expected or unexpected situations in labor

Common collaborative problems that should be differentiated from the nursing diagnoses include the following:

Potential complication: cardiac/vascular (maternal or fetal) related to labor or the medications for its control

Planning The primary goal of labor and delivery is to provide safety for mother and fetus. In addition, comfort should be considered so that the mother is able to bond with her infant more easily. (Bonding is more difficult if the mother views the baby as the cause of insufferable pain and distress.)

Intervention The mother's antepartum fantasy of labor and delivery should be examined; if it is at great variance with the actual occurrence, help should be given to facilitate her acceptance of what took place. In addition to the psychological aspects of care, the physical care throughout labor and delivery should be of the highest caliber to prevent the occurrence of iatrogenic problems. Medications must be prepared and administered accurately, with adequate follow-up as to the effects on the mother and fetus. Neonatal reactions to the medications should be observed and treated as necessary.

Evaluation Nursing care can be considered successful if both client and baby are in good health after the delivery or if complications have been met skillfully and have reversed any negative effects to the extent that is possible.

Drug use during delivery

Local anesthetics

A summary of local anesthetics used in regional anesthesia is given in Table 16-8. Anesthetics and analgesics are discussed further in Chapter 24. Clients who are otherwise reasonably comfortable may elect to have a local anesthetic if an episiotomy is needed. Lidocaine hydrochloride (Xylocaine) and procaine hydrochloride (Novocaine) are among the drugs used for pudendal or local infiltration. These two are the least toxic of all the local anesthetics. Another advantage of lidocaine is that its action is immediate and thus is helpful in an emergency episiotomy. Overdose and too rapid administration must be avoided in both because these factors may cause adverse side effects.

These same drugs are used to provide regional anesthesia, particularly for the epidural administration. Epidurals eliminate the perception of pain during uterine contractions and also maintain waist-to-toe anesthesia during cesarean sections, allowing the

Table 16-8. Local anesthetics frequently used for regional anesthesia

Drug name	Concentration or usual dosage	Onset of action	Duration of action	Nerve block	IV	Uses infiltration	Caudal	Epidural peridural	Spinal
chloroprocaine (Nesacaine)	1%–3% solution	Fast	30–60 min	✔	✔	✔	✔	✔	
lidocaine (Xylocaine)	0.5%–5% solution	Fast	1–2 hours	✔	✔	✔		✔	✔
mepivacaine (Carbocaine)	1%–2% solution	15 min	3 hours	✔	✔	✔		✔	
procaine (Novocain)	0.2%–2% solution	2–5 min	1 hour	✔		✔			✔
tetracaine (Pontocaine)	up to 15 mg	15 min	3 hours						✔

client to remain awake. They are preferable to spinal anesthesia because they do not cause postanesthetic headaches.

Epidural anesthesia does have drawbacks. Some clients develop severe hypotension, which can result in fetal bradycardia. Treatment usually consists of positioning the client on her side and administering oxygen by face mask or nasal cannula. Intravenous administration of ephedrine may also be needed to increase the blood pressure. The lack of sensation also interferes with the client's urge to push, with the possibility of ineffective pushing and the need for forceps to aid the delivery. This form of anesthesia should not be used unless the fetal descent is complete, or else the inability to push may necessitate a cesarean section.

General anesthetics

Other anesthetics used for delivery include nitrous oxide, a general inhalation anesthetic that results in moderate skeletal relaxation. In small amounts, it acts as an intoxicant. It must be combined with other anesthetic agents to be used for deeper anesthesia.

Nitrous oxide should be administered only by a trained physician or nurse. It is usually given during the last part of the first stage of labor, during delivery of the baby and the placenta, and during the postpartum internal examination immediately after the birth. According to Reeder, et al, nitrous oxide analgesia is still administered intermittently during contractions but is more effective when it is administered continuously in 30% to 50% concentration with oxygen (Reeder, Mastroianni & Martin, 1980, p 390). In a concentration of less than 50%, nitrous oxide is considered an analgesic because the client remains conscious and participates in the birth process.

Ketamine hydrochloride (Ketaject, Ketalar) is given IV and can be used alone or with nitrous oxide. It is sometimes used as an alternative to thiopental as an induction agent. However, it has a high incidence of adverse effects (particularly unpleasant dreams or hallucinations), making it less satisfactory than thiopental for induction of anesthesia for elective cesarean section.

General anesthesia that causes unconsciousness may be needed for a complicated vaginal delivery or cesarean delivery. Thiopental sodium (Pentothal sodium) and succinylcholine chloride (Anectine), administered IV, provide short-term total anesthesia. Few contraindications for their use exist, and they can be used safely in almost all cesarean deliveries.

The disadvantages of general anesthesia include a higher incidence of newborn depression, postponement of mother–infant contact, and exposure of the mother to the potentially lethal complication of pulmonary aspiration of gastric contents.

Drug use during postpartum care

Once the delivery of the placenta has been completed, oxytocin may be administered to increase uterine contraction, thereby preventing or controlling uterine hemorrhage (oxytocin is discussed earlier in this chapter and in Chapter 38).

Uterine atony can be life threatening, since it leads to severe bleeding after delivery. If the usual use of external uterine massage, oxytocin IV, or methylergonovine IM do not stop the hemorrhage, 15-methyl $PGF_2\alpha$, a synthetic prostaglandin, may prove effective. Uterine contractions should start within 45 minutes after an initial dose of 250 µg IM or by injection into the uterine wall, which can be administered through the abdomen or vagina.

The 250-µg dose can be repeated every 90 minutes as needed to a maximum dose of 15 mg. Side effects are usually limited to nausea, vomiting and diarrhea, variations in blood pressure with a possible diastolic elevation (particularly in preeclamptic women), fever, and flushing. The use of this prostaglandin may obviate the need for a blood transfusion (Few, 1987).

Ergonovine, derived from ergot, is particularly useful during the immediate postpartum period. It contracts the uterus, thus lessening the flow of blood from the placental site during the first few days after delivery. Either ergonovine maleate (Ergotrate) or methylergonovine maleate (Methergine) is usually administered three or four times daily for 2 to 7 days after delivery. If uterine relaxation recurs later in the puerperium, another course of Ergotrate or Methergine may be given.

Postpartum uterine contractions are usually painless for the primipara; however, they are increasingly painful after each successive pregnancy because the uterine fibers do not have the same ability to contract after subsequent pregnancies. Pain control may be obtained with meperidine hydrochloride, hydroxyzine hydrochloride, propoxyphene hydrochloride (Darvon), oxycodone hydrochloride, aspirin, acetaminophen (Tylenol), or various combinations.

Mothers with Rh negative blood should receive IM/Rho (D) immune globulin (RhIG) within 72 hours after delivery of an Rh positive infant. If bleeding has been severe, an additional vial of RhIG may be administered to prevent isoimmunization. If the time limit of 72 hours is exceeded, even by as much as 7 days, the American College of Obstetricians and Gynecologists (ACOG) recommends that RhIG still be given. ACOG also suggests that all Rh negative women be given RhIG after abortions, ectopic pregnancies, and second- or third-trimester amniocentesis, and possibly after antepartum hemorrhage, fetal death, sterilization, and transfusions.

While the infant is in the delivery room, its eyes are treated with drops or ointment to prevent gonorrheal infection of the eyes (ophthalmia neonatorum). The drugs of choice are erythromycin 0.5% ophthalmic ointment or tetracycline 1% ophthalmic ointment in single immediate application. Both are also effective against chlamydia trachomatis, another sexually transmitted disease that may affect the newborn's eyes and cause blindness. Silver nitrate 1% topical solution is only effective for neonatal gonococcal ophthalmia (Bryant, 1984). In addition, most newborns receive an injection of vitamin K (Aqua Mephyton) to build up their clotting capacity. The effect of drugs on the infant during lactation is discussed in the next section of this chapter.

■ Summary

Careful consideration must be given to both clients (mother and fetus) during the birthing process. The physical condition of either one may necessitate the use of a medication that has a potential for harm to the other. For this reason, any medication must be thoroughly evaluated before use to make certain that the potential for good outweighs the potential for harm to either.

Nurses should institute comfort measures to lessen the anxiety and pain that may be felt by the mother during pregnancy, labor, and delivery. Such intervention may decrease the need for drugs, which have the possibility of compromising the health of the mother, fetus, or neonate.

Nursing management

Nursing implications

The public health law in New York State was amended in 1975 to include the following section:

Drug information to be furnished to expectant mothers

The physician to be in attendance at the birth of a child shall inform the expectant mother, in advance of the birth, of the drugs that such physician expects to employ during pregnancy and of the obstetrical and other drugs that such physician expects to employ at birth and of the possible effects of such drugs on the child and mother.

A second amendment charged the nurse–midwife with the same responsibility as the physician.

Clients are increasingly aware that drugs may have negative effects on them or their fetuses and may request additional information before permitting their administration. This active consumerism requires health professionals to be knowledgeable about all medications given to the mother.

Labor and delivery call for a balance between the mother's desires and fetal safety. One mother may demand a pain-free amnesiac birth, but the health status of her infant may make that impossible. Another mother may want a drug-free experience, with herself fully in control, and that may not be possible because of a maternal or fetal emergency that requires the use of drugs or anesthesia. In either instance, the nurse can help the mother explore her disappointment, perhaps anger, at not having her wishes met. Most important, the mother may need a great deal of help so that she is not angry at the infant for what has happened, particularly if an operative scar from a cesarean section remains as a permanent reminder.

Aside from providing information to the pregnant woman about possible medications to be used during labor and delivery and discussing alternative methods, the nurse's most important responsibility in the labor and delivery room is the careful observation and monitoring of the mother and fetus. The progress of labor must be observed whether the induction of labor has been natural or artificial. The uterine contractions must be monitored carefully to prevent complications that affect the mother (*eg*, uterine rupture, cerebral hemorrhage, hypertensive crisis, cardiac arrhythmia, cervical lacerations) or the fetus (*eg*, cardiac arrhythmia, cerebral damage).

The obstetric nurse must be knowledgeable about the complications of various techniques used for pain relief, be able to recognize the signs and symptoms of adverse reactions immediately as they occur, and know what action to take until a physician or anesthesiologist is available (Reeder, Mastroianni, Martin, 1980, p 403).

Comfort measures during labor should include relaxation techniques that lessen the mother's anxiety, fear, and tension. When possible, she should be talked through contractions, lessening her need for medications to relieve pain.

Clients who receive tocolytic drugs should be observed carefully to prevent overhydration that may lead to pulmonary edema. Those who receive oxytocic drugs should be observed for any signs of uterine rupture or fetal distress.

After delivery, the mother who is not planning to breast-feed should be instructed to wear a tight bra and restrict her fluid intake to lessen breast engorgement. The use of a properly applied breast binder may be more effective than a bra. This nonpharmacologic method provides greater safety than any antilactation drug available.

Mothers of preterm or ill infants may require additions to or changes in the standard plan regularly used for guidance in breast-feeding. The modified plan may require specific information on the infant's expected abilities for its gestational age, as well as recognition of any developmental or physiologic deficits that might interfere with the feeding process. The infant should be at a gestational age of at least 34 to 35 weeks and be capable of sucking with self-regulated pauses and of maintaining its body temperature. The mother needs instruction in recognizing fatigue in the infant so that the optimal feeding time can be assured during each nursing period (Barnes, 1991).

Drug use during lactation

It has been difficult to obtain accurate information about the excretion of medications in human milk. Because of this fact, published reports include data that are based on extremely limited samples or obtained under poorly controlled circumstances. Many medications have only been studied in animals, or, if more than one report has been made about a given medication, the reports may be contradictory. Thus, care must be taken when any medication is given to the nursing mother.

In general, the administration of medications to the nursing mother is of greater concern when the infant is 1 week old than when the child is 1 year old. One of the body's principal detoxifying mechanisms is the ability to combine potentially harmful materials with glucuronic acid. This mechanism is generally not fully functioning in an infant who is 1 to 2 weeks old. This mechanism is of special importance in the case of chloramphenicol, which is almost exclusively metabolized by glucuronide conjugation. Other studies have shown that the acetylation and oxidation enzyme systems are not fully functioning either at this age. These systems are important in the metabolism of drugs, such as sulfisoxazole. Immature enzyme systems and incompletely developed kidney function make the newborn, then, susceptible to accumulations of toxic levels of drugs.

Although the immediate effects of drugs ingested in human milk have been the primary focus of the literature, an additional concern must be the long-term effects of exposure to a medication. For example, if a child nurses until the age of 2 years and has been exposed for 2 years to a drug excreted in breast milk, are there any consequences that have not yet been recognized? Is it possible that a medication that produces no immediate observable effects could have effects at a later developmental period?

It is important to realize that simply measuring the concentration of the medication in breast milk is meaningless. That is, although the drug may be present, it may be pharmacologically inactive or destroyed before absorption and therefore not pose any problem to the infant. What is meaningful is knowledge of how much of the drug is actually absorbed. On the other hand, it has been suggested that, although the amount measured at any given time may be small, the cumulative amount ingested in 24 hours may be significant for the newborn infant.

Maternal medications and the lactating woman

Principles that control passage of medications from plasma into milk

Passive diffusion is the most common mechanism by which medications pass through biologic membranes. Substances that diffuse can achieve the same concentration in milk as in plasma or different concentrations. In accord with the principles of passive diffusion, no changes in milk–plasma (M–P) ratios are noted at different plasma concentrations of the medication or at varying volumes of secreted milk (Catz & Giacoia, 1972, p 157). Back diffusion can occur when blood levels of a medication are decreasing.

Milk–plasma ratios refer to the concentrations of the protein-free fractions in milk and in plasma. Dissimilar M–P ratios reflect differences in the binding of the medications to plasma proteins. For example, the M–P ratios of different sulfonamides vary from 0.08 to 1 (Laurence, 1989, p 254). A medication with an M–P ratio of 1 has the same concentration in milk as it does in plasma. When a medication has an M–P ratio of 0.08, the level of the medication in the milk is 8% of the level of medication in the plasma. An M–P ratio of 4 means that the level of the medication in milk is four times higher than the level in plasma.

Substances may compete with medications for binding sites, a process that may result in the displacement of medication or the passage of an increased amount of medication into the breast milk.

The composition of milk goes through three phases, each with a different pH and fat content. Initially during the first 3 to 4 days postpartum, colostrum is secreted. This substance has a lower carbohydrate and fat content than whole breast milk. After several days, colostrum is replaced by transitional milk, which eventually assumes the characteristics of whole milk by the third week. Thus, the tendency for the same drug to cross the plasma into milk changes as the milk goes through these transitions.

Passive diffusion of larger molecules across membranes depends on their lipid solubility and state of ionization. The lipid solubility of a medication depends in part on the degree to which it is ionized in solution. Medications that are largely nonionized in solution are lipid soluble and, for this reason, diffuse readily through the membrane. The more lipid soluble the medication is, the greater and more rapid its absorption across a membrane. Medications with low lipid solubility diffuse rather slowly into milk. Medications like pentobarbital and secobarbital, which are more lipid soluble, tend to transfer into milk as its fat content rises. Therefore, an infant is more likely to ingest these medications under certain conditions (*ie*, when the fat content of the milk is high) than under other conditions. Catz, et al, found that the total fat excretion in human milk for a 24-hour period is relatively constant but has diurnal variations. They found that the minimal value occurs in the first morning feeding and the highest at mid morning, with progressive decline throughout the rest of the day (Catz & Giacoia, 1972, p 157).

Most medications are weak acids or weak bases. The ionization of these acids and bases depends on the *p*H of the environment and the dissociation constant of the medication (pKa). The dissociation constant is the *p*H level at which the concentrations of ionized and nonionized medication are equal. Weak bases become more ionized as the *p*H decreases. Because the *p*H of human milk (6.6–7.0) is lower than the *p*H of plasma (7.4), the ionized component of a weak base increases in milk. The opposite situation occurs with weak acids. For this reason, lincomycin, erythromycin, antihistamines, alkaloids, and isoniazid, which are all weak bases, can be expected to have concentrations in milk that are equal to or higher than those in plasma. On the other hand, barbiturates, organic acids, sulfonamides, and diuretics, which are all weak acids, should have concentrations in milk that are equal to or lower than those in plasma (Catz & Giacoia, 1972). The infant, therefore, is likely to ingest more of a medication that is a weak base than a medication that is a weak acid.

Evaluating the effects of maternal medication

Several factors should be considered when evaluating the potential effects of a medication to be taken by a mother on her nursing infant. For instance, many drugs pass more easily from plasma into colostrum during the first week after delivery than they do later into milk. Drugs administered IV reach a higher level in the maternal circulation than those given in the same dose IM, and they generally reach a higher level than those taken orally in that dose. Drugs with a molecular weight of less than 200 pass into the milk more easily than those that have higher weights. Furthermore, large molecules that are fat soluble and nonionized are more likely to enter the milk.

The amount of a drug that enters a baby through its mother's milk depends on the volume of milk ingested. What effect the drug has depends on whether it is in an active or inactive form and how it is subsequently detoxified and excreted by the infant. Drugs that are not fully excreted continue to build up in the infant's system. Toxic levels may be reached, due to accumulation, even though the maternal intake is low.

Therefore, whenever possible, perineal and other body discomfort should be relieved by nonmedication measures. Jet hydrotherapy or sitz baths help overcome soreness and promote healing. They should be offered to appropriate candidates for 10 to 15 minutes, two or three times daily. The water temperature should be at 102° to 104°F and the tubs scrupulously cleaned after each use. Local applications of compresses, ointments, and heat lamps also lessen pain, aid in healing, and decrease the need for systemic medications for perineal pain.

During the infant's first week of life, some drugs may compete with bilirubin for protein-binding sites. The resulting unbound bilirubin that remains in the infant's circulation places the infant at risk for the development of kernicterus. This risk is particularly a problem for premature babies because their livers are less capable of detoxifying drugs and because they have fewer available binding sites for the drugs or bilirubin.

As infants mature, they become more able to metabolize drugs transported in the milk. Therefore, substances that might have been harmful during the first weeks (*eg*, the sulfa drugs) may not pose a problem at a later date. One guideline in choosing maternal medications is to evaluate the safety of each medication for her infant, how it is detoxified and excreted at that particular stage in the infant's life. Another consideration is the length of time that the drug is to be taken; continuing exposure places the infant at higher risk. Long-acting drugs are also more hazardous because they are more likely to accumulate.

No drug can be considered absolutely safe during lactation. Information about the maternal need should be balanced against the drug's possible harm to the infant. The American Academy of Pediatrics and the Swedish National Board of Health have established standards to help practitioners determine the safety of drugs transferred to the infant during breastfeeding (see Box 16-3).

Drugs and their effects

Unless contrary information exists, it can be assumed that any drug absorbed by the mother is excreted to

---

Box 16-3. Standards for safety levels of drugs in human milk

American Academy of Pediatrics

1. Drug is contraindicated
2. Temporary cessation of breast-feeding suggested
3. Drug usually compatible with breast-feeding
4. Food and environmental agents that affect breast-feeding

Swedish National Board of Health

Group I. Active ingredients do not enter milk

Group II. Active ingredients present in small amounts, considered not to be a risk

Group III. Active ingredients present in sufficient quantity to present a risk

Group IV. Unknown whether active ingredients enter milk

---

some extent in the milk. Table 16-9 presents guidelines for the use of some drugs; however, it must be stressed that no drug can be considered absolutely safe.

Analgesics

Among the analgesic (nonnarcotic) drugs, acetaminophen (Tylenol) theoretically should not be given during the immediate postpartum period to lactating women because it is detoxified in the neonate's liver. However, it does not appear to harm the neonate. Although it is excreted in the milk, aspirin rarely affects the neonate unless the mother takes more than the prescribed dose.

Narcotics

Narcotics should be used cautiously, if at all. Percodan or propoxyphene (Darvon) can lead to sleepiness in the infant, poor nursing, and a subsequent loss of weight. Codeine or meperidine (Demerol) can build up in the infant, leading to neonatal depression. Morphine or heroin can be addicting to the newborn. Methadone can lead to depression and failure to thrive. Marijuana impairs DNA and RNA formation and may be inhaled by the infant if its mother or other people are smoking during the feeding. The active substance, tetrahydrocannabinol, is secreted in human breast milk and, therefore, can be absorbed by the nursing infant, resulting in drowsiness.

Antibiotics

If a mother requires an antibiotic, it is important that she be aware of its possible adverse effects on her infant. It may be appropriate for the mother to temporarily discontinue breast-feeding while being treated with antibiotics that are highly sensitizing. With the exception of cephalexin (Keflex), cephalothin (Keflin),

nystatin (Mycostatin), oxacillin (Prostaphlin), para-aminosalicylic acid (PAS), and penethamate (Leocillin), most other antibiotics are excreted in human milk. The following drugs have little, if any, effect on the neonate: colistin (Colimycin), carbenicillin (Pyopen, Geopen), cefazolin (Ancef, Kefzol), demeclocycline (Declomycin), lincomycin (Lincocin), mondelic acid, methenamine (Hexamine), penicillin G, potassium, and sodium fusidate.

The antibiotics listed in Table 16-10 may have adverse effects on the neonate.

Anticoagulants

Among the anticoagulants, heparin is not excreted in human milk, but the infant's partial thromboplastin time should be checked just to be safe. On the other hand, phenindione (Hedulin, Dindevan) is excreted in milk, causing prolonged prothrombin times in the infant; thus, it is contraindicated. Ethyl biscoumacetate (Tromexan) may cause cephalhematoma and hemorrhage around the umbilical stump and is contraindicated. The safest anticoagulants for the infant are the coumarin derivatives bishydroxycoumarin (Dicumarol) and warfarin (Panwarfin). The infant's prothrombin times should be checked regularly and the drug discontinued if the infant is scheduled for surgery or has been injured. Vitamin K should be given to the nursing infant while the mother is on a coumarin derivative.

Sedatives

If the mother requires sedation either as a sleeping aid or as an anticonvulsant, the infant receives some of the drug in the milk it ingests. Most barbiturates are excreted in milk but do not sedate the infant. Those that are contraindicated include sodium bromide (Bromo-Seltzer and OTC sleeping pills) and phenobarbital (Luminal) in hypnotic doses. However, in usual analeptic doses, phenobarbital appears safe for infants. Pentobarbital (Nembutal) should not be given until it can be detoxified by the infant's liver (normally after 1 week of age), but after that it seems safe in analeptic doses. Barbital (Veronal) and chloral hydrate (Noctec, Somnos) are considered safe for the infant.

Cardiovascular drugs

Cardiovascular drugs given to the mother also must be evaluated for their effect on the infant. Digoxin and guanethidine (Ismelin) do not affect the infant. Hydralazine (Apresoline) may cause neonatal jaundice, electrolyte disturbances, or thrombocytopenia. Methyldopa (Aldomet) may result in galactorrhea (increased milk production), whereas reserpine (Serpasil) may cause galactorrhea plus diarrhea, nasal stuffiness, and lethargy.

Diuretics

Diuretics given to the mother can cause dehydration, electrolyte imbalances, or insufficient maternal milk production. The infant's weight should be monitored

Table 16-9. Safety levels of drugs used by lactating mothers as reflected in breast milk

Drug name	Considered acceptable*	Use only with caution	Unacceptable
Nonnarcotic analgesic/sedatives			
acetaminophen (Datril, Paracetamol, Tylenol)	✔		
ibuprofen (Advil, Motrin)			✔
phenobarbitol (Nembutal)	✔ Watch for symptoms of depression, changes in sleep and feeding patterns		
primidone (Mysoline)			✔
propoxyphene (Darvon)	✔ Watch for poor nursing and sleepiness in infant		
Salicylates (aspirin, Empirin, Bufferin, Ecotrin)	✔ Acceptable for single dose; increase maternal vitamin C intake		
sodium bromide (Bromo-Seltzer)			✔
Narcotic analgesics			
codeine		✔ Build-up can lead to neonatal depression	
heroin			✔
marijuana			✔
meperidine (Demerol)		✔ Build-up can lead to neonatal depression	
methadone			✔
Antibiotics			
See Table 16-10.			
Anticoagulants			
Coumarin derivatives (Dicoumarol, warfarin)	✔ Check infant's prothrombin time, discontinue before surgery; give vitamin K to infant		
heparin	✔ PTT		
phenindione (Hedulin, Dindevan)			✔
Cardiovascular			
Digitalis (digoxin, Lanoxin)	✔		
guanethidine (Ismelin)	✔		
hydralazine (Apresoline)		✔ May cause neonatal jaundice, electrolyte imbalance, thrombocytopenia	
methyldopa (Aldomet)	✔ May cause maternal galactorrhea		
propanolol (Inderal)	✔ May cause hypoglycemia or other β-blocking effects		
quinidine	✔ May cause arrhythmia		
reserpine (Serpasil)	✔ May cause maternal galactorrhea; diarrhea, nasal stuffiness, lethargy in infant		
Diuretics†			
acetazolamide (Diamox)	✔ Watch for dehydration		
Mercurial diuretics (Dicurin, Thiomerin)			✔
spironolactone (Aldactone)		✔ Watch for sodium excretion and potassium retention	
sulfamoylanthranilic acid (Furosemide, Lasix)	✔		
Thiazides (Diuril, Enduron, Esidrix, Hydrodiuril, Oretic, Thiuretic tablets)	✔ Watch for maternal and infant dehydration		

(Continued)

Table 16-9. Safety levels of drugs used by lactating mothers as reflected in breast milk (Continued)

Drug name	Considered acceptable*	Use only with caution	Unacceptable
Central nervous system			
alcohol		✔ Drowsiness	
atropine sulfate (in prescribed and OTC drugs)		✔ May cause atropine toxicity, hyperthermia in neonate	
caffeine		✔ Excess may lead to irritability	
carisoprodol (Rela, Soma)			✔
cimetidine (Tagamet)			✔
ergotomine (Cafergot)			✔
magnesium sulfate	✔		
neostigmine (Prostigmin)	✔		
Mental problems			
chlordiazepoxide hydrochloride (Librium)		✔ May accumulate to high levels; may contribute to jaundice	
diazepam (Valium)		✔ May add to neonatal jaundice, hypoventilation, drowsiness, may accumulate to high levels	
haloperidol (Haldol)	Questionable, behavioral problems in animals		
lithium carbonate (Eskalith, Lithane, Lithonate)			✔
Phenothiazines			
chlorpromazine (Thorazine)	✔		
mesoridazine (Serentil)	✔		
thioridazine (Mellaril)	✔ Maternal galactorrhea		
trifluoperazine (Stelazine)	✔		
Tricyclic antidepressants			
amitriptyline (Elavil)	✔		
desipramine hydrochloride (Norpramin, Pertofrane)	✔		
imipramine hydrochloride (Tofranil)	✔		
Antihistamines			
brompheniramine (Dimetane)	✔		
diphenhydramine (Benadryl)	✔ Observe for decrease in milk supply, poor nursing, tachycardia		
tripelennamine (Pyribenzamine)	✔		
Hormones			
carbimazole (Neo-Mercazole)	May cause goiter, depress thyroid		
insulin	✔		
epinephrine (Adrenalin)	✔		
Cathartics			
milk of magnesia, mineral oil, saline cathartics, stool softeners, suppositories, bulkforming laxatives	✔		
aloin, cascara, rhubarb			✔
phenolphthalein			✔

*There is no "black or white" choice on drug acceptability. Before administration of a drug, careful assessment of the mother and infant must be made, considering age, physical conditions, and necessity of medication. Possibility of adverse effects must be discussed clearly with the client before drugs are administered.

†When using any diuretic, monitor infant's weight, number of wet diapers per day, and specific gravity of infant's urine.

Table 16-10. Antibiotics that may negatively affect neonates

Drug name	Additional information
amantadine (Symmetrel)	Rash, vomiting, urinary retention
ampicillin (Polycillin, Amcill, Omnipen, Penbritin)	Diarrhea, candidiasis; sensitivity if exposed repeatedly; skin rash
chloramphenicol (Chloromycetin)	Accumulative; Grey's syndrome; refusal of breast; falling asleep after feeding; vomiting after feeding
methacycline (Rondomycin)	May cause discoloration of infant teeth; inhibition of bone growth may occur; should not be given
metronidazole (Flagyl)	High milk levels; neurologic disorders; blood dyscrasia; Interrupt breast-feeding for 12–24 hr, then resume
nalidixic acid (NegGram)	Possible hemolytic anemia in infant if mother has renal failure; contraindicated in glucose-6-phosphate dehydrogenase deficiency
nitrofurantoin (Furadantin)	Contraindicated in glucose-6-phosphate dehydrogenase deficiency
penicillin G, benzathine (Bicillin)	Allergic responses
quinine sulfate	Rare thrombocytopenia
rifampin (Rimactane)	May turn secretions and milk orange
streptomycin and other aminoglycosides	Contraindicated if given for more than 2 weeks owing to ototoxicity and nephrotoxicity from extended use
sulfanilamide	Contraindicated until infant older than 1 month of age; rash; hemolytic anemia; glucose-6-phosphate dehydrogenase deficiency
sulfapyridine	Skin rash; may cause hemolysis in glucose-6-phosphate dehydrogenase deficiency
sulfathiazole	Contraindicated until infant older than 1 month of age
sulfisoxazole (Gastrisin)	Contraindicated until infant older than 1 month of age; possible hyperbilirubinemia
tetracycline (Achromycin, Panmycin, Sumycin)	May cause discoloration of teeth in infant; inhibition of bone growth may occur; not to be given repeatedly or for more than 10 days at a time
trimethoprim (Bactrim, Septra, Trimpex)	Should not be given to infants at risk for kernicterus

at intervals, the specific gravity of the urine should be checked, and the number of wet diapers over the course of a day should be noted. Furosemide (Lasix) is not excreted in milk. Acetazolamide (Diamox) may cause some dehydration, as do the thiazides (Diuril, Enduron, Esidrix, Hydrodiuril, Oretic, Thiuretic tablets). Spironolactone (Aldactone) may cause sodium excretion and potassium retention in infants. The mercurial diuretics (Dicurin, Thiomerin) are not absorbed orally, even though they are present in milk. However, they do present a risk of mercury deposits in the infant's tissue.

Autonomic nervous system drugs
Atropine sulfate deserves particular consideration because it is found in many prescribed as well as OTC drugs. Many mothers are unaware of the presence of this autonomic drug in their systems. Excreted in milk, it may cause atropine toxicity or hyperthermia in the neonate. Other autonomic drugs that can affect the newborn infant include carisoprodol (Soma, Rela), which causes drowsiness, hypotonia, and poor nursing, and ergot (Cafergot), used for migraines, which causes ergotism, vomiting, diarrhea, erratic blood pressure, and weak pulse.

Drugs used for mental health problems
Clients who require psychotropic or mood-changing drugs should be given those that exert the least possible effect on the infant, in the smallest possible dose, because all of these drugs are excreted in milk. The benzodiazepines are among the most frequently prescribed drugs in the U.S. Chlordiazepoxide (Librium) usually has little if any effect on the infant, but it may accumulate in the mother to reach high levels. Diazepam (Valium) may contribute to neonatal jaundice, possibly exerting cumulative effects. It may also lead to hypoventilation, lethargy, drowsiness, and weight loss due to poor feeding.

Other drugs used to treat mental health problems must also be monitored. Haloperidol (Haldol) has caused behavioral problems in animals. A neuroleptic drug, penfluridol, which has been responsible for learning abnormalities in animals, is particularly suspect because of its long-acting property. Lithium carbonate (Askalith, Lithane, Lithonate) has been shown to cause cyanosis, poor muscle tone, and changes in the infant's electrocardiogram.

The phenothiazines seem to be safe, creating no apparent symptoms in the infant. They include chlorpromazine (Thorazine), mesoridazine (Serentil), thioridazine (Mellaril), and trifluoperazine (Stelazine). By increasing maternal pituitary prolactin secretion, these drugs can cause maternal galactorrhea when taken in large doses.

The tricyclic antidepressants also appear to be safe for infants, although neonates should be watched for failure to feed or depression. These drugs may also cause maternal galactorrhea through an increase in maternal prolactin secretion. The frequently used medications in this group include amitriptyline (Elavil), desipramine (Norpramin, Pertofrane), and imipramine (Tofranil).

Antihistamines

Antihistamines are also excreted in milk, causing a wide variety of reactions. The infant may appear sleepy, feed poorly, or become very active and develop tachycardia. A cumulative effect may occur from those long-acting drugs. The frequently used antihistamines are brompheniramine (Dimetane), diphenhydramine (Benadryl), methdilazine (Tacaryl), and tripelennamine (Pyribenzamine).

Cathartics

For the most part, cathartics appear to have no effect on the infant. The exceptions are aloin, cascara, and fresh rhubarb, all of which may cause diarrhea and colic in the infant. The others, which are safe, include milk of magnesia, mineral oil, saline cathartics, stool softeners, suppositories, and bulk-forming laxatives. Phenolphthalein has caused increased bowel activity in some neonates.

Hormones

Hormones are sometimes required for the treatment of various maternal conditions. Those that are destroyed in the infant's intestinal tract (corticotropin, epinephrine [Adrenalin], and insulin) have no effect on the infant. Other hormones and their effects are indicated in Table 16-11.

Prednisone is considered safe if used in small doses for short periods of time. Thyroid and thyroxine are considered safe for the infant, but the antithyroid medications may cause hypothyroidism in the infant (see Table 16-11).

Oral contraceptives

Further studies are needed on the excretion of oral contraceptives or their metabolites in milk. Some effects reported are a diminished milk supply, reduced milk proteins and fats, marked decrease in all water soluble vitamins, and possible adverse long-term effects. Reports of the development of gynecomastia in male infants and the proliferation of vaginal epithelium in some females have been made.

Heavy metals

Because the heavy metals are excreted in milk, the infant and mother must be carefully observed for negative signs, particularly neurotoxicity in infants exposed to lead or mercury. Because lead may or may not cause toxicity at maternal serum levels of 40 µg or more, infants should be watched for symptoms of lead poisoning.

Radioactive agents and antineoplastic drugs

Nursing mothers should avoid certain radioactive agents (67 gallium citrate, iodine 125 and 131, and technetium 99). The analysis of data on I^{125} has shown that quite a large dose of radioactive iodine is received by the infant—about 0.1 rad (Bland, Docker, Crawford & Carr, 1969). A significant number of thyroid tumors have occurred in people who were irradiated for thymic enlargement in early infancy (Nelson, 1969). The risk of cancer due to irradiation of the thyroid has been calculated at about 100 per 10,000 rad. Based on this calculation, a dose of 0.1 rad produces a cancer incidence of 1 out of every 1,000 children irradiated.

The Committee on Drugs of the American Acad-

Table 16-11. Hormones and antithyroid medications that exert negative effects on infants

Drug name	Possible negative effects
Hormones	
chlorotrianisene (Tace)	Feminizing effects
Corticosteroids (Decadron, ACTH)	Exophthalmos, retardation of sexual development in animals
dihydrotachysterol (Hytakerol)	Hypercalcemia
estrogen	Long-term effects unknown, include possible feminization
fluoxymesterone (Halotestin, Ora-Testryl, Ultandren)	Masculinization, suppresses lactation, therefore less milk
Oral contraceptives—estrogen plus progesterone (Enovid, Ovulen, Loestrin)	Long-term effects unknown, hyperbilirubinemia; decreases milk supply; gynecomastia in males; proliferation of vaginal epithelium in females
Antithyroid medications	
carbimazole (Neo-Mercazole)	May cause goiter
methimazole (Tapazole)	May inhibit infant thyroid, requiring thyroid medication for infant
potassium iodide	May cause goiter
propylthiouracil or thioracil	May cause goiter; agranulocytosis

emy of Pediatrics notes that breast-feeding should temporarily cease for varying amounts of time, depending on the radioactive drug being used: technetium-99m for 1 to 3 days; radioactive sodium for 21 to 22 days; iodine-131 for 2 to 14 days; iodine-125 for 12 days; and gallium-69 for 14 days. The committee also notes that antineoplastic drugs, such as amethopterin and cyclophosphamide, are contraindications to breast-feeding because they may cause immune suppression, have unknown effects on growth, and are possible carcinogens.

Other substances

In addition to medications, other specific substances ingested by nursing mothers are known to cause problems in the newborn child. In 1956 in southeast Turkey, it was found that children breast-fed by mothers who ate seed wheat treated with hexachlorobenzene developed skin diseases and generalized dystrophy, and many died. It seemed that the hexachlorobenzene or one of its metabolites was excreted in the mothers' milk (Knowles, 1965). Maternal intake of caffeine (coffee, tea, cola, chocolate) may accumulate in the infant, causing the infant to remain wakeful. This effect is particularly evident if the mother also smokes cigarettes, which also produce a stimulant effect. On the other hand, the occasional use of alcohol, which reaches a level in milk equal to that in plasma, may have a calming effect but may be injurious to the infant.

Learning experience 16-2

A lactating mother states that her baby is hyperirritable. Describe how you would help her to investigate stimulants in her diet that may be responsible.

■ Summary

Some maternal conditions require the use of medications that may cause serious effects on the nursing infant, whereas other medications may have little or no effect. When considering the administration of medications to the nursing mother, the nurse should question not whether a medicated mother should be allowed to nurse but whether a nursing mother needs to be medicated.

Nursing management

Nursing implications

Nurses should remain informed about the latest research findings on how drugs given to the lactating woman affect either the mother, neonate, or older child. Updated information may necessitate discarding or replacing medications previously considered acceptable. Research studies rely on increasingly so-

phisticated techniques to evaluate medications so that infants can continue to nurse safely even though their mothers require medication.

Nursing process

Assessment Any nurse in contact with a mother who may be nursing her child should take a thorough medication history, including prescribed medications and OTC drugs. In some cases, the physician is responsible for making the decision; in some cases, the mother and nurse can decide together which is more important, the breast-feeding or the medication.

Nursing diagnosis A nursing diagnosis likely to arise is

> *Knowledge deficit related to dietary needs during lactation, the lactation process, and the effects on the infant of prescription and OTC drugs that are conveyed in breast milk*

Planning Quality care by the nurse can lessen the possibility of undesirable and unnecessary medicating of either the mother or the infant. Certainly this nursing goal is important. Another goal is the education of the mother about lactation, dietary needs during lactation, and substances conveyed in milk from mother to child.

Intervention The nurse should encourage the client to verbalize any concerns that she may have about breast-feeding. She should also encourage the client to join her in the planning process, making certain that the client's wishes are incorporated whenever possible.

It is important to plan for preventive measures to offset the need for some medications. For example, effective hand-washing and aseptic techniques by staff members are certainly preferable to reliance on antibiotics for mother or child. Mothers should also be taught these techniques. Mothers who experience painful breasts associated with nursing need assistance in managing that pain or they are unlikely to be relaxed during feedings. The resulting tension is likely to decrease milk production, as well as cause tension and poor sucking by the infant.

If the mother must take medications for a medical disorder, the nurse should evaluate the potential for harm to the mother or baby that may be caused by the medication. Some medications may have been taken through the pregnancy without harm to the fetus, but they should not be continued during lactation because of a different effect on the breast-fed baby (see Tables 16-9, 10, and 11). Another medication may have to be substituted so that the mother can continue to breast-feed.

When medications are necessary and the mother decides to continue breast-feeding, the nurse should be supportive but should not reassure the mother that no adverse consequences from taking the medication will occur. Once again, recognizing the mother's needs and openly appreciating the new mother as an individual may be major factors in helping her to accept the necessary restrictions while nursing her infant. In addition, accurate information about the effects of maternal medication on the nursing infant help protect the child from problems that can be avoided.

To provide greater safety for the child, maternal medications should be taken after the infant has been fed so that the least amount of drug is present in the milk at the next feeding. The baby should also be carefully observed for any reactions, such as development of a rash or fussiness, and any changes in responses or feeding or sleeping patterns.

When a medication that may be harmful to the baby cannot be avoided, breast-feeding may have to be discontinued temporarily. By pumping her breasts at regular intervals, a mother continues to stimulate them and should be able to resume breast-feeding after the course of medication has been completed.

Drugs that are detoxified by the liver should not be given to the lactating mother during the immediate postpartum period because the infant's liver may be too immature to detoxify them. Narcotics should also be avoided because they may build up in the infant and lead to respiratory depression.

Because caffeine taken by the mother may accumulate in her baby, lactating mothers should be discouraged from using coffee, tea, cola, or chocolate to prevent overstimulation of the infant. Even though alcohol may have a calming effect, its use is not approved because of possible long-term effects on the child, including weakness, decrease in linear growth, and abnormal weight gain and damage to the growing brain.

Client education. Breast-feeding is an ongoing activity, one in which the mother is responsible for her own food intake and use of drugs (prescribed or self-administered, including alcohol and illicit substances). Compliance will only take place if she agrees with the worth of suggestions that are made and if she is comfortable with the program that is outlined. It is important for the client to understand any changes that are made in her medication regimen if it differs from the one that had been prescribed prenatally, including any adverse effects that may occur to herself or her nursing child, with information as to what to do about them if they materialize.

Client education should include information about foods, medications, and substances that are usually used by the mother, with input as to their safety for mother and child. Dietary concerns are important. Lactation requires an adequate intake of calories and fluids, with a limitation on empty calories (*ie*, cake, cookies, candy, and other high calorie snacks that lack nutritional value). Clients who crave sweets should be encouraged to substitute fresh or dried fruits for empty calories. The food selection should be varied, with attention to the inclusion of high calcium, high protein, high vitamin foods. The cooking process should preserve nutrients but should not add calories, such as steaming, broiling, roasting, baking. Foods that contain contaminants (*eg*, chemicals, food coloring, artificial sweeteners) should be avoided, since their long-term effects on the child may not be known. The nurse should supply this information if a nutritionist is not available.

Counseling may help the mother overcome her problems, reducing their effects on her milk production and her need for particular medications. Reassurance and relief of tension through good nursing are better for mother and infant than sedation or tranquilizers.

The advantages of breast-feeding and the disadvantages of abrupt weaning should always be foremost in the nurse's mind when teaching and counseling mothers about the use of medications while nursing.

Evaluation Follow-up care should include evaluation of the mother's perception of how well breastfeeding is proceeding. The breasts and nipples should be healthy, without areas of infection, induration, or fissures. The baby's growth, feeding, sleep and waking patterns, responsiveness, and general comfort level should be within normal limits. The level of maternal–child bonding should also be examined, including the way in which the mother holds, comforts, and cares for the baby. The client may need reassurance that she is doing well in her mothering techniques.

References

Acker D, et al. (1983). Abruptio placentae associated with cocaine use. *Am J Obstet Gynecol, 146*, 220.

Aderhold K. (1991). Jet hydrotherapy for labor and postpartum pain relief. *MCN, 16*(2), 97–99.

Alper M, Cohen WR. (1983). Pulmonary edema associated with ritodrine and dexamethasone treatment of threatened premature labor. *J Reprod Med, 28*(5), 349.

Aono T, et al. (1982). Effect of sulpiride on poor puerperal lactation. *Am J Obstet Gynecol, 143*, 927.

Barnes, L. (1991a) Lactation consultation in the NICU. *MCN, 16*(3), 167.

Barnes, L. (1991b) Lactation consultants in the NICU: Staff education programs. *MCN, 16*(4), 201.

Bland EP, Docker MF, Crawford JS, Carr RF. (1969). Radioactive iodine uptake by thyroid of breast-fed infants after maternal blood-volume measurements. *Lancet, 2*, 1039.

Briggs GG, Freeman RK, Yaffe SJ. (1986). *Drugs in pregnancy and lactation*, 2nd ed. Baltimore: Williams & Wilkins.

Brooton D, Jordon CH. (1983). Caffeine and pregnancy. *J Obstet Gynecol Neonatal Nurs*, May/Jun, 190.

Bryant BG. (1984). Unit dose erythromycin ophthalmic

ointment for neonatal ocular prophylaxis. *J Obstet Gynecol Neonatal Nurs, 13*(2), 83–87.

Catz CS, Giacoia GP. (1972). Drugs and breast milk. *Pediatr Clin North Am, 19*, 157.

Clark M, Hager M. (1984, June). New warnings on smoking. *Newsweek*, p 71.

Committee on Drugs, American Academy of Pediatrics. (1983). The transfer of drugs and other chemicals into human breast milk. *Pediatrics 69*, 241.

Conley NJ, Olshansky E. (1987). Current controversies in pregnancy and epilepsy: A unique challenge to nursing. *J Obstet Gynecol Neonatal Nurs*, Sep/Oct, 321–328.

Deibel P. (1980). Effects of cigarette smoking on maternal nutrition and the fetus. *J Obstet Gynecol Neonatal Nurs, 9*(6), 333.

Donegan WL. (1983). Cancer and pregnancy. *CA*, Jul/Aug.

Edmond, S. (1990). Pre-eclampsia: Baby aspirin. *Harvard Health Letter, 16*(2), 4–6.

Eriksson UJ, et al. (1983). Diabetes in pregnancy. *Diabetes, 32*.

Fenakel K, et al. (1991). Nifedipine in the treatment of severe preeclampsia. *Obstet Gynecol, 77*(3), 331–337.

Fetal alcohol syndrome. (1990). *Mental Health, 7*(5), 1–4.

Few B. (1987). Prostaglandin F_2a for treating severe postpartum hemorrhage. *Maternal Child Nurs J, 12*, 169.

Freda M. (1991). Home care for preterm birth prevention. *MCN, 16*(1), 9–14.

Friedman JM, et al. (1990). Potential human teratogenicity of frequently prescribed drugs. *Obstet Gynecol, 75*(4), 594–599.

Funk M, Buerkle L. (1986). Intrauterine treatment of fetal tachycardia. *J Obstet Gynecol Neonatal Nurs*, Jul/Aug, 298–305.

Good-Anderson B. (1983). Home blood glucose monitoring in the pregnant diabetic. *J Obstet Gynecol Neonatal Nurs*, Mar/Apr, 89.

Greater risk of cancer is reported in children of fathers who smoke. (1991, January 24). *New York Times*, p A11.

Haire D. (1987). Drugs in labor and birth. *Childbirth Educator 30, 6*(3), 26–35.

Haller D. (1980). The use of terbutaline for premature labor. *Drug Intell Clin Pharm, 14*(80), 757–764.

Hoffmaster J. (1983). Detecting and treating pregnancy-induced hypertension. *Matern Child Nurs J, 8*, 398.

Huisjes HJ, Touwen BCL. (1983). Neonatal outcome after treatment with ritodrine: A controlled study. *Am J Obstet Gynecol*, Oct 1, 250.

Imperiale T, et al. (1991). A meta-analysis of low dose aspirin for the prevention of pregnancy induced hypertensive disease. *JAMA, 266*(2), 260–264.

Johnson G. (1981). Oxytocics for the induction of labor. In Raff B, Duxbury M, eds. *Intrapartal care*, series 3, module 2, pp 9–13. White Plains, NY: March of Dimes Birth Defects Foundation.

Jones L, et al. (1987). Occupational hazards for nurses exposed to radiation and antineoplastic agents. *Journal of the New York State Nurses Association, 18*(3), 42–60.

Knowles JA. (1965). Excretion of drugs in milk: A review. *J Pediatr, 66*, 1080.

Kritz-Silverstein D, et al. (1989). The effect of parity on the later development of non-insulin dependent diabetes mellitus on impaired glucose tolerance. *N Engl J Med*, 1214–1219.

Lam F, et al. (1988). Use of the subcutaneous terbutaline pump for long term tocolysis. *Obstet Gynecol, 72*, 810–813.

Lawrence R. (1989). *Breastfeeding: A guide for the medical profession*, 3rd ed. St. Louis: CV Mosby.

Leff E, et al. (1991). Type I diabetes and pregnancy. *MCN, 16*(2), 83–87.

Livingston I, et al. (1982). Propranolol in pregnancy: A three year prospective study. *Clin Exp Hypertens [B], 1*, 258.

Loveman A, Colburn V, Dobin A. (1986). AIDS in pregnancy. *J Obstet Gynecol Neonatal Nurs*, Mar/Apr, 91–93.

Low units of aspirin found to cut pregnancy risks. (1991). *New York Times*, p 15.

Mancino D. (1987). Overview of occupational safety and health hazards and the right to know legislation. *Journal of the New York State Nurses Association, 18*(3), 4–10.

Morris MB, Weinstein L. (1981). Caffeine and the fetus: Is trouble brewing? *Am J Obstet Gynecol, 140*(6), 607.

Moses M. (1987). Health workers and reproductive hazards. *Birth, 14*(3), 153–155.

Nelson KB, Ellenberg JH. (1982). Maternal seizure disorder: Outcome of pregnancy and neurologic abnormalities in the children. *Neurology, 32*, 1247.

Newcomb M, et al. (1979). Acute leukemia in pregnancy. *JAMA, 239*, 2691.

O'Brien TE. (1975). Excretion of drugs in human milk. *Nurs Digest, 3*, 23.

Postpartum hypertension, seizures, strokes reported with bromocriptine. (1982). *FDA Drug Bulletin, 14*(1), 3.

Rayburn WF, Lavin JP Jr. (1986). Drug prescribing for chronic medical disorders during pregnancy: An overview. *Am J Obstet Gynecol, 155*, 565–569.

Rayburn WF, Zuspan FP. (1980). Drug use during pregnancy. *Perinatal Press, 4*, 115.

Reeder SJ, Mastroianni L Jr, Martin LL. (1980). *Maternity Nursing*, 14th ed. Philadelphia: JB Lippincott.

Robert E, Guibaud P. (1982). Maternal valproic acid and congenital neural tube defects. *Lancet*, 937.

Sahni K, et al. (1981). Carcinoma of the breast associated with pregnancy and lactation. *J Surg Oncol, 16*, 167.

Sannerstedt R, et al. (1980). Medication during pregnancy and breastfeeding: A new Swedish system for classifying drugs. *Int J Clin Pharmacol Ther Toxicol, 18*, 45.

Sasso S. (1983). Prostaglandins for Ob-Gyn. *Matern Child Nurs J, 8*, 107.

Savage RL. (1977). Drugs and breast milk. *Journal of Human Nutrition, 31*, 459.

Schatz M, et al. (1984). Asthma and pregnancy. In Dawson A, Smith RA, eds. *The practical management of asthma*, pp 195–211. Orlando: Grune and Stratton.

Segal M. (1987). A progress report on AIDS research. *FDA Consumer, 21*(8), 8–12.

Sharts-Engel N. (1991). An overview of maternal-child infectious diseases (1976–1990). *MCN, 16*(1), 58.

Shortridge L. (1983). Using ritodrine hydrochloride to inhibit preterm labor. *Matern Child Nurs J, 8*, 58.

Stephens CJ. (1981). The fetal alcohol syndrome: Cause for concern. *Matern Child Nurs J, 6*, 251.

Tal Z, et al. (1988). Breast electrostimulation for the induction of labor. *Obstet Gynecol, 72*(4), 671–674.

Toxoplasmosis during pregnancy threatens fetal health. (1984). *NAACOG Newsletter, 11*(3).

Wald N. (1991). Prevention of neural tube defects: Results of the Medical Research Council's Vitamin Study. *Lancet, 338,* 131–137.

Winick M. (1981). Food and the fetus. *Natural History, 90,* 76.

Worthington-Roberts B, Weigle A. (1983). Caffeine and pregnancy outcome. *J Obstet Gynecol Neonatal Nurs,* Jan/Feb, 21.

Wright JT, et al. (1983). Alcohol consumption, pregnancy and low birthweight. *Lancet, 1,* 663.

Zacharias J. (1983). A rational approach to drug use in pregnancy. *J Obstet Gynecol Neonatal Nurs,* May/Jun, 183.

Bibliography

Pregnancy

Adverse effects with isotretinoin. (1984). *FDA Drug Bulletin, 13*(3), 1.

Andermann E, et al. (1981). Dermatoglyphic changes and minor congenital malformations associated with maternal use of anticonvulsant drugs during pregnancy. In Dam M, et al, eds. *Advances in Epileptology: XII Epilepsy International Symposium,* p 613. New York: Raven Press.

Banner W, Czajka PA. (1980). Acute caffeine overdose in the neonate. *Am J Dis Child, 134,* 495.

Binkin N, et al. (1984). Preventing neonatal herpes. *JAMA, 251*(21), 2816.

Cates W Jr. (1984). Sexually transmitted diseases: The national view. *Cutis, 33*(1), 69.

Cavanagh D, Knuppel RA. (1981). Preeclampsia and eclampsia. In *Principles and practice of obstetrics and perinatology,* p 1271. New York: John Wiley & Sons.

Centers for Disease Control (1982). *Sexually transmitted diseases treatment guidelines,* vol 3, no 25. Washington, DC: U.S. Department of Health and Human Services.

Davidson S. (1981). Smoking and alcohol consumption: Advice given by health care professionals. *J Obstet Gynecol Neonatal Nurs, 10,* 256.

DeSwiet M, et al. (1983). Prolonged heparin therapy in pregnancy causes bone demineralization. *Br J Obstet Gynaecol, 90,* 1129.

Dobbing J, ed. (1981). *Maternal nutrition in pregnancy: Eating for two?* London: Academic Press.

Dubois D, et al. (1983). Beta blocker therapy in 125 cases of hypertension during pregnancy. *Clin Exp Hypertens [B], 2,* 41.

Enkin MW. (1984). Smoking and pregnancy: A new look. *Birth, 11*(4), 225.

Gant NF, et al. (1980). *Hypertension in pregnancy: Concepts and management.* New York: Appleton-Century-Crofts.

Harvey JC, et al. (1981). The effects of pregnancy on the prognosis of carcinoma of the breast following radical mastectomy. *Surg Gynecol Obstet, 153,* 723.

Howell R, et al. (1983). The risks of antenatal subcutaneous heparin prophylaxis: A controlled trial. *Br J Obstet Gynaecol, 90,* 1124.

Janz D. (1982). *Epilepsy, pregnancy and the child.* New York: Raven Press.

Javonovic L, et al. (1981). Effect of euglycemia on the outcome of pregnancy in insulin-dependent diabetic women as compared with normal control subjects. *Am J Med, 71,* 921.

Knuppel RA. (1984). Heparin prophylaxis in pregnancy. *Perinatal Press, 8*(4).

Kretchmar RM. (1980). Smoking and health: The role of the obstetrician gynecologist. *Obstet Gynecol, 55,* 403.

Lindor E, McCarthy AM, McRae MG. (1980). Fetal alcohol syndrome. *J Obstet Gynecol Neonatal Nurs, 9,* 222.

Linn S, et al. (1982). No association between coffee consumption and adverse outcomes of pregnancy. *N Engl J Med, 306,* 141.

Luke B. (1982). Does caffeine influence reproduction? *Matern Child Nurs J, 7,* 240.

Mandell GL, et al. (1982). Sexually transmitted diseases treatment guidelines. *MMWR, 31*(2s).

Needleman HL, et al. (1984). The relationship between prenatal exposure to lead and congenital anomalies. *JAMA, 251,* 2956.

Nowicki P, et al. (1984). Effective smoking intervention during pregnancy. *Birth, 11*(4), 217.

Osborne NG, Pratson L. (1984). Sexually transmitted diseases and pregnancy. *J Obstet Gynecol Neonatal Nurs,* Jan/Feb, 9.

O'Shaughnessy R, Zuspan FP. (1981). Managing acute pregnancy hypertension. *Contemp Ob/Gyn, 18,* 85.

Parsons MT, Work BA Jr. (1984). Treatment of chronic hypertension in pregnancy. *Perinatal Press, 8*(3), 35.

Parsons WD, et al. (1981). Prolonged half-life of caffeine in healthy term newborn infants. *J Pediatr, 98,* 640.

Pear R. (1984, January 31). Food program may improve mothers' health, report says. *New York Times.*

Pedley TA, Goldensohn ES. (1982). *Epilepsy: Changing concepts and approaches,* vol 4, pp 225–240. New York: John Wiley & Sons.

Perley NZ, Bills BJ. (1983). Herpes genitalis and the childbearing cycle. *Matern Child Nurs J, 8,* 213.

Riberti C, et al. (1981). Malignant melanoma: The adverse effect of pregnancy. *Br J Plast Surg, 34,* 338.

Rosa FW. (1983). Teratogenicity of isotretinoin. *Lancet, 2,* 513.

Rubin PC, et al. (1981). Beta-blockers in pregnancy. *N Engl J Med, 305,* 1323.

Schatz M, et al. (1983). Asthma and allergic diseases during pregnancy: Management of the mother and prevention in the child. In Middleton E, et al, eds. *Allergy: Principles and practice,* 2nd ed. St Louis: CV Mosby.

Sexton M, Hebel JR. (1984). A clinical trial of change in maternal smoking and its effect on birth weight. *JAMA, 251,* 911.

Sonstegard LJ, et al, eds. (1983). *Women's health: Childbearing,* vol 2. New York: Grune & Stratton.

Streissguth AP, et al. (1980). Teratogenic effects of alcohol in humans and laboratory animals. *Science, 209,* 353.

Tovey LAD, Taverner JM. (1981). A case for the antenatal administration of anti-D immunoglobulin to primigravidae. *Lancet, 1,* 878.

Tull MW, Brown AL. (1981). Effects of caffeine on pregnancy and lactation. *Pediatr Nurse, 7*(2), 51.

Turner ES, et al. (1980). Management of the pregnant asthmatic patient. *Ann Intern Med, 6,* 905.

Tyrer JG. (1980). *The treatment of epilepsy: Current status of modern therapy*, vol 5. Philadelphia: JB Lippincott.

Weiss PAM, et al. (1984). Insulin levels in amniotic fluid of normal and abnormal pregnancies. *Obstet Gynecol, 63,* 371.

Willis S. (1982). Hypertension in pregnancy: Pathophysiology. *American Journal of Nursing, 82,* 792.

Willis SE, Sharp ES. (1982). Hypertension in pregnancy: Prenatal detection and management. *American Journal of Nursing, 82,* 798.

Zamule E. (1989). Drugs and pregnancy: Often the two don't mix. *FDA Consumer, 23*(5), 7–10.

Labor, Delivery, Postpartum

Pohodich J. (1980). Selected drugs used during labor and delivery: Effects on the fetus and neonata. In Raff B, Duxbury M, eds. *Intrapartal care*, series 3, module 1, pp 9–18. White Plains, NY: March of Dimes Birth Defects Foundation.

Stephens C. (1981). The fetal alcohol syndrome: Cause for concern. *Matern Child Nurs J, 6,* 251–256.

Lactation

Anderson P. (1977). Drugs and breast feeding: A review. *Drug Intell Clin Pharm, 11,* 208.

Davidson S. (1981). Smoking and alcohol consumption: Advice given by health care professionals. *J Obstet Gynecol Neonatal Nurs, 10,* 256.

Lawrence R. (1989). *Breast feeding: A guide for the medical profession*, 3rd ed. St Louis: CV Mosby.

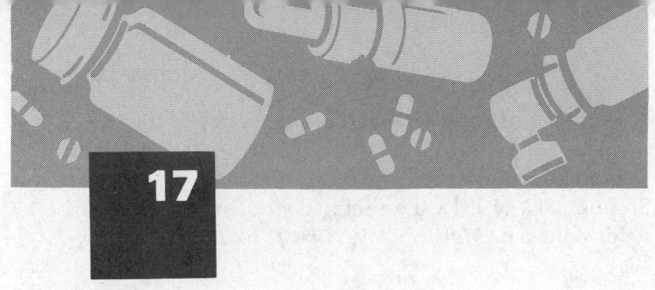

17

Drug therapy in pediatric nursing

The pediatric nurse's ability to prepare and administer children's medications is both a skill and an art. It requires not only clinical and pharmacologic expertise but also knowledge of child development and psychology, as well as a healthy dose of creativity and perseverance.

Determining the appropriate dosage

Although the physician is responsible for determining the therapeutic dosage of medication, it remains the nurse's responsibility to assess the accuracy of the dose prior to its administration. It is also the nurse's goal to determine a correct and palatable means of having the child accept the medication.

The prescribed route of administration will affect the dosage calculation. A child's water and fat mass, liver and kidney metabolism, and excretion will alter the prescribed doses (Waechter, Phillips, & Holaday, 1985, pp 197–221). Therapeutic dosage ranges are published in a variety of pharmacology texts, reference manuals, and drug inserts. These references are available to assist the nurse in the calculations process. At times, physicians use alternate criteria based on body size and organ maturity to arrive at therapeutic recommendations for medication orders. A growing subspecialty of pediatric pharmacists can assist physicians and nurses in scientifically determining therapeutic doses.

Dosages are calculated by a variety of formulae based on a child's weight or body measurements (Waechter, Phillips, & Holaday, 1985, pp 197–221) (Box 17-1).

Each formula is based on an adult model and, therefore, has some inherent limitations.

Clark's rule is computed on the child's weight and may be more accurate for determining doses. Fried's and Young's rules are calculated on a child's age and do not account for changes in body mass (*eg*, poor nutrition or obesity) (Stoklosa & Ansel, 1986, pp 88–94). Surface area guidelines use body mass as the primary criterion and provide the greatest accuracy for determining a therapeutic and safe dose. After the child's height and weight are determined, an intersecting line is drawn between these two measurements on the nomogram scale. The intersecting point represents the surface area in square meters (see Figure 17-1).

Factors influencing response
Uniqueness of the individual
Like adults, each child responds uniquely to pharmacologic interventions. Yet, because infants and children lack the medical and developmental histories of adults, their response is often unknown. Allergic manifestations and sensitivities occur quickly and without warning. For preventive health care, the nurse can educate parents about adverse signs and symptoms, necessary care measures, and access to health care.

Body system maturity and metabolism
Each child has a unique physiologic response to a medication. Research and practice have established that myriad factors influence a child's metabolism of therapeutic agents. Immature organ systems, nutritional health, genetic endowment, and physiologic variations influence drug use and effectiveness for each child.

The young infant's renal system lacks maturity and does not efficiently excrete certain substances. Fewer glomeruli and a diminished blood volume re-

Box 17-1. Formulae for determining pediatric doses

Clark's rule (based on weight)

Child's dose =

$$\frac{\text{weight of the child (pounds)}}{150 \text{ pounds}} \times \text{average adult dose}$$

Freid's rule (for infants)

Infant's dose =

$$\frac{\text{infant's age in months}}{150 \text{ months}} \times \text{average adult dose}$$

Young's rule (based on age)

Child's dose =

$$\frac{\text{child's age in years}}{\text{age of child} + 12} \times \text{average adult dose}$$

Surface area rule

Child's approximate dose =

$$\frac{\text{surface area of child (square meters)}}{1.73} \times \text{adult dose}$$

From Stoklosa MJ, Ansel HC. (1986). *Pharmaceutical calculations*, pp 88–94. Philadelphia: Lea & Febiger.

The cellular action of many pharmacologic agents is not clearly understood. Individual variations in drug metabolism affects drug use in the bodies of infants and young children. As there exists a potential for cumulative toxicity, careful observations by the nurse for adverse reactions, side effects, and alterations in laboratory values can provide vital data for adjusting dosages.

Pharmacologic toxicity

Many factors influence a child's metabolism of a given substance. Calculating drug doses according to body weight, height, or surface area provides an important, relatively safe method of standardizing dosages. Factors such as chronic illness, level of hydration, nutritional status, and heredity may influence the cumulative effects of a particular medication. Specific medications can be monitored by blood drug level concentrations. Monitoring is useful when caring for children requiring long-term medications for chronic conditions such as asthma or seizure disorders or in acute situations such as drug overdose. The limitations of using drug level concentrations include the following: 1) therapeutic levels for certain drugs vary widely;

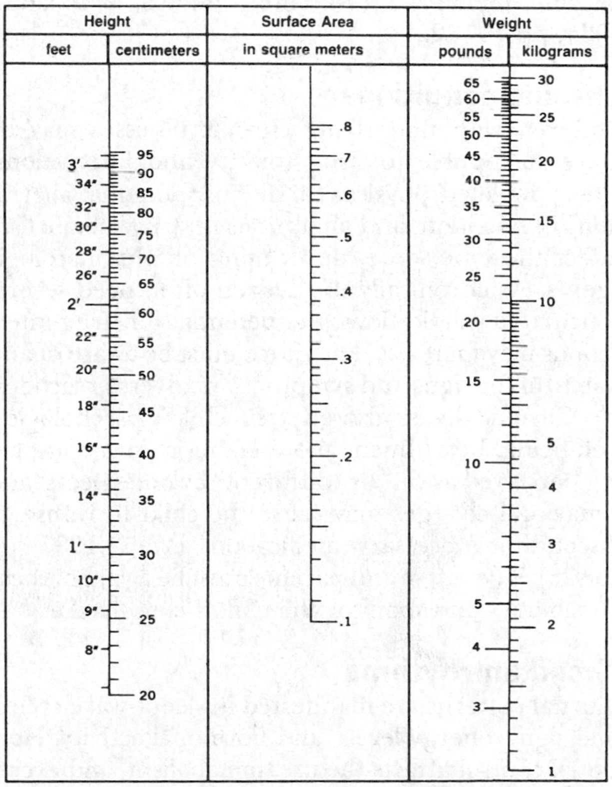

Figure 17-1. Nomogram for estimating surface area of infants and young children. To determine the surface area of the client, draw a straight line between the point representing the height on the left vertical scale to the point representing the weight on the right vertical scale. The point at which this line intersects the middle vertical scale represents the client's surface area in square meters. (Courtesy of Abbott Laboratories, North Chicago, Illinois.)

duce excretion of pharmacologic agents through the kidneys. Initial doses of medications may be given without great concern about adverse effects. However, subsequent doses may cause toxicity by increased drug retention owing to decreased glomerular filtration rates and renal tubular secretion (Waechter, Phillips, & Holaday, 1985). Despite careful, accurate drug calculations, further doses can be potentially harmful to the young infant.

During rapid physical growth and maturity of organ systems, infants are affected by many substances introduced into their environment. Neonates and breast-fed infants are affected by the mother's intake of potentially toxic substances such as alcohol, drugs, caffeine, or nicotine. Placental transfer or drug consumption through breast milk can alter growth and development. The effect of chemical substances on organ system maturity, teratogenesis, potential neonatal addiction, and congenital abnormalities are important concerns. Chemical substance intake must be considered prior to administering any additional pharmacologic substances to children.

2) concentrations of other medications may be difficult to access; 3) information may be lacking when needed; and 4) the multiple venipunctures and invasive procedures for specimen collection may cause trauma to the child. As the nurse monitors a child's response to medications, parents can be educated on signs and symptoms of drug toxicity, preventative measures, and the correct method to administer the medication.

Genetic endowment

A child's heredity may influence the metabolism and proper use of pharmacologic agents. Underlying diseases such as sickle cell anemia, disorders of vitamin metabolism, and congenital anomalies effect a child's health and ability to use certain drugs or treatments. One example of congenital defect is a hemolytic anemia associated with a deficiency of the enzyme glucose-6-phosphate dehydrogenase (G6PD). Because this anemia worsens following ingestion of chemical oxidants, these agents may be avoided or the child's closely monitored during therapy. Another example of a congenital defect is thrombocytopenia, a decreased or defective production of platelets, which may be triggered by ingestion of certain pharmacologic agents, such as quinidine, sulfisoxazole, hydrochlorothiazide, or heparin (Waechter, Phillips, & Holaday, 1985, pp 197–221).

Chronic conditions

Children with underlying chronic illnesses may be more susceptible to drug toxicity and interactions. Their depleted physical conditions, potential aberrations in nutrition, and alterations in drug metabolism affect the type, dose, and timing of pharmacologic agents. As chronically ill children often need several concurrent medications, the potential for drug interactions may increase. The nurse must be aware of and watchful for signs and symptoms of adverse reactions.

Chronic illness also effects a child's psychological well-being. Resentment about taking medications, being perceived as "ill" or "different" by one's peers, and behavioral changes may cause the child to refuse or discontinue necessary medications (Yoos, 1987, pp 25–28). The nurse and parents must be aware of these possibilities and monitor the child's compliance.

Circadian rhythms

Diurnal patterns are manifested in sleep–wake cycles, vital signs, energy levels, and hormonal activity. Hormonal control affects the use, metabolism, and excretion of pharmacologic products. Children who are ill or hospitalized are nutritionally depleted because of their altered health state. Concurrent sleep deprivation is caused by environmental stressors or lack of comfort. Their circadian rhythms are affected by illness and environment. Consequently, metabolism of pharmacologic agents may be disturbed by hormone and enzyme levels, leading to adverse reactions or toxicity.

Psychological development

The ability of children to comprehend their bodies and health status increases with age, education, and the development of abstract thinking. Young children who literally cannot visualize or perceive illness have difficulty accepting medication that is unpleasant in taste, appearance, or smell, or that is administered invasively. The cognitive ability to associate medication with relief of symptoms is an abstract and elusive concept for children (Ormond & Caulfield, 1976, pp 320–325). Paramount to the child's acceptance of medication is the nurse's knowledge of developmental theory and expertise in theory application when explaining the therapeutic value of medication to a child. Understanding and accepting medication are especially crucial for chronically ill children in need of long-term compliance (Yoos, 1987, pp 25–28).

During the initial assessment, the nurse should determine who is the primary care giver of the child. Due to changing family constellations, the primary care provider may not be the biologic parent. It may be a grandparent, sibling or nonfamily member who acts as the child's "family."

To assist the child in understanding and accepting medication, family education is essential. Prior to any drug administration by the nurse or family member, the relative should be informed of the indications, side effects, timing, and contraindications of the medication. The family may be aware of medication administration strategies that have worked in the past. Helpful ideas for administering the medication will assist the relative in supporting the treatment plan in the hospital, clinic, or at home. Family education may influence compliance with the prescribed treatment regimen. Astute relatives often report subtle changes in their children, which may actually be adverse reactions to medications. Open communication between the family, the child, and the health care provider will assist in discussion of concerns and positively influence the treatment regimen.

Before administering any medication, the nurse should collect a data base of information from the family and, if possible, the child. Developmental level, previous experiences with medications, successful interventions used in prior medication situations, and knowledge of the therapy and illness will assist the nurse in compiling a plan for administering medication. Sensitivity, creativity, and a positive approach to the child and family will assist the nurse in the process of giving medication.

The administration of analgesia to children is a complex issue. Concurrent with the aforementioned assessment, the nurse will also explore ways to anticipate and manage pain based on what are usually obvious alterations in anatomic and physiologic integrity (Broome & Slack, 1990, pp 159–162). With knowledge of the underlying pathophysiology, routine administration of analgesics to children before procedures and during selected periods following surgery would be acceptable and more widespread (Eland, 1988, pp 93–111). The issue of inadequate blood levels of analgesics due to dosage and timing of medication administration and the effect on children's pain remain an important topic in nursing research.

Factors in administering medications: a developmental perspective

Knowledge of physical, psychological, and cognitive development is, as previously mentioned, essential before administering medication to children. A therapeutic, trusting relationship between nurse and child can assist in the process. This relationship is based on frequent contact and a genuine interest in the child and family. For example, giving feedings, baths, medications, and monitoring intravenous infusions are routines that lend themselves to spending concentrated periods of time with an infant (Nugent, 1989, pp 318–321).

Creative preparation such as dissolving, crushing, or mixing the medication with a more palatable substance may be warranted. A pharmacist can assist the nurse in determining whether a change from the original medication form could alter its pharmacologic properties. Family members have information on methods that may have been successful in past situations. When gathering data, the nurse should ask specific questions about the child's concerns, behaviors, coping mechanisms, and rewards for taking medications. Older children, chronically ill children, and adolescents also have routines and preferences for the way their medication is administered (Yoos, 1987, pp 25–28).

Knowing the child's usual behavioral patterns will assist the nurse in assessing pain. Like adults, children manifest pain in different ways based on learned behaviors from previous experiences or role models and cultural variables. The nurse should interview the family to determine the child's behavior, responses to pain, and previous successful interventions.

Visual analogue and self-report scales measuring pain in children have been researched and demonstrate reliability and validity. A variety of instruments are available to the pediatric nurse. Selection of a particular instrument is dependent on the nurse's knowledge of the instrument and its interpretation, as well as the child's developmental age and health condition.

Infants manifest pain through crying, facial expressions of distress, and muscular rigidity, followed by thrashing (Johnston & Strada, 1986, pp 373–382).

However, infants have a limited repertoire of responses that serve highly differentiated sensory systems. Therefore, the absence of a response does not indicate a lack of pain (Franck, 1989, pp 65–68). Toddlers manifest pain behaviors in ways similar to infants. Because of their mobility, toddlers may show increased physical resistance to painful experiences. Normal toddlers may be perceived as restless and overactive. These behaviors may be misinterpreted in this age group and can go unrecognized as pain response.

Preschoolers react to pain with aggressive behaviors, verbal expressions, and need for comfort and support (Petrillo & Sanger, 1980). The nurse should recognize the child's need to be dependent and should provide structure to cope with the painful experience.

Increasing verbal ability, the developing interest in one's own body and health, and the desire to learn are important in helping school-aged children understand themselves and their pain. However, when expressing pain, the school-age child may regress and exhibit behaviors of younger children (Waechter, Phillips & Holaday, 1985, pp 197–221). Passive methods of dealing with pain such as holding still or bearing the pain may be coupled with aggressive outbursts. Older children sometimes describe pain in graphic detail. Despite their ability to communicate, the nurse must also be aware of the nonverbal cues used by the school-age child. When administering PRN or as needed analgesia, the nurse must be aware that requesting pain medication requires that the child be verbal, assertive, and cognizant of time, which are skills few children are consistently able to demonstrate when hospitalized and in pain (Broome & Slack, 1990, pp 159–162).

Adolescents, in their quest for identity and independence, react to pain with great self-control and might fear disclosing pain to the nurse. Seeking out verbal descriptions of pain, using pain assessment tools, and being attuned to nonverbal behaviors will assist the nurse and adolescent in collaborative planning for pain control (Waechter, Phillips, & Holaday, 1985, pp 197–221).

Infants

Infants have a natural sucking reflex that is helpful when giving them oral medications (Ormond & Caulfield, 1976, pp 320–325). Liquid medications are given with a syringe, are placed in a cheek, or are given through an empty nipple placed in the infant's mouth. The infant is held in a comfortable, upright position to aid in swallowing and to control head movements. Medications may be taken more readily if given before feeding times when the infant is still hungry. A small flexible medication cup may be used to retrieve medication that may leak from the child's mouth. Stroking the neck or cheek will facilitate swallowing. If necessary, medications are mixed in small volumes of fluids to ensure complete ingestion. Care should be taken not to force medication or inject it rapidly into the mouth since this can cause choking, aspiration, or oral trauma.

When a noxious medication is administered, infants may retain the medication more readily if they are kept in an upright position with minimal movement; regurgitation is common among young infants. A pharmacology reference or pharmacist should be consulted to determine whether a specific dose should be repeated. A second dose sometimes is administered if the infant has regurgitated the first dose. Certain medications, however, should not be repeated because they absorb rapidly through the buccal mucosa (Waechter, Phillips, & Holaday, 1985, pp 197–221).

The main criteria for repeating the medication are based on medication's potential toxicity and type of oral medication (tablet, liquid, gel capsule, and so forth). Knowledge of the relationship of the therapeutic and toxic blood levels of a particular medication is essential. If these two levels are relatively close, medications might not be repeated due to the possibility of medication toxicity. Absorption is also affected by the child's nutritional status, which varies depending upon the length of time since they have eaten or if they are NPO (nothing by mouth). A pharmacist can provide necessary information such as the rate of absorption for a particular child, which is based on the child's age, type and form of medication, nutritional status, and length of time between ingestion and regurgitation.

When administering intramuscular medication to an infant, the nurse should assess factors such as muscle mass, viscosity and volume of the medication, and frequency of injections. The suggested site for infants is the vastus lateralis muscle. The ideal location is one-third of the distance between the greater trochanter and the knee, palpating for the largest muscle mass (Evans & Hansen, 1981, pp 194–199). Following intramuscular injection, physical comforting is necessary for the child and often for the relative.

As infants grow, their feeding and tactile behaviors change. Infants aged 3–12 months may require more than one nurse to administer medications because they are more mobile and larger than younger infants. A small medication cup is helpful since older infants often retain medications in their mouth or spit them out. Palatability of medications can be improved if mixed with small amounts of soft food. However, care must be taken since infants will come to associate medications with food and possibly reject some foods. A bottle or cup of pleasant tasting liquid after medications will comfort the child, dispel the taste, and avoid oral retention of the medication. Cleansing the mouth with water or having the child brush his or her teeth after medications is encouraged to remove potentially cariogenic substances from developing teeth. Providing physical and verbal comfort after medication is also essential for the child's well-being.

Toddlers

As mobility, agility, and independence increase with age, toddlers pose a special challenge for the nurse administering medication. Independence is displayed by voluntary lip and tongue control, verbalization, and spitting. Parents should be consulted to determine prior successful medication techniques, child preferences, or routines. Simple directions, disguising medication in palatable foods, praise, and a positive, yet firm approach are strategies used with this age group. Toddlers sometimes display anxieties regarding medications through change in appetite or daily routines. Fear can also be displayed in play sessions. Careful observations by the nurse or relative will guide the nurse in opportunities for therapeutic play intervention.

Preschoolers

Preschoolers often attempt to coerce the nurse out of administering medication by bargaining and stalling. Simple, concrete directions and explanations are helpful for this age group. Fantasy thinking has begun to develop and affects the child's perception of health interventions. Preschoolers enjoy rituals and routines. The most effective medication administration method should be documented and followed by nurse and parent. Choices about medications are offered if available. Rewards, praise, and physical comfort allay the preschooler's anxiety and support cooperative behavior.

School-age children

Although developmentally able to swallow a pill or capsule, a school-aged child lacks the knowledge to associate medication with symptom relief. Since concrete thinking predominates in this age group, a child may respond as well to a warm cloth to soothe a headache as to an oral analgesic. Control and mastery of situations are sought by school-aged children. Offering choices when available, explanations using pictures and diagrams, and rewards are helpful measures.

Loss of body integrity produces fear in this age group. Invasive procedures such as surgery or parental medications cause the child great anxiety. Reassurance, information, and comfort alleviate the problem of administering medications by injection (Evans & Hansen, 1981). Of all age groups, the school-aged child most often uses play to display concerns and anxieties. The opportunity to assist the child in expressing fears is part of the nursing role with this age group.

School-aged children usually have developed adequate muscle mass to receive intramuscular injections in the gluteus maximus or ventrogluteal muscle. Older school-aged children or adolescents may have developed sufficient deltoid muscles for injections. Other considerations in the administration of injections to children include selection of correct needle size and length, volume and type of injectate, frequency of injections, as well as the child's size, muscle and skin condition, age, and medical diagnosis (Beechcroft & Redick, 1989, pp 333–336).

Immediately prior to injections, the nurse should provide a simple explanation to the child. The child may wish to choose the site or a supportive person to assist during the procedure. Adequate restraint during the procedure provides reassurance and safe administration. Praise, comfort measures, and a bandage over the injection site are also helpful.

Traumatic occurrences affect a child's behavior. Illness or hospitalization may cause regression in the school-aged or younger child. When regression occurs, the nurse should make appropriate adaptations in strategies and approaches to medication administration (Petrillo & Sanger, 1980).

Adolescents

Adolescents are developing identities and roles separate from parents and family and are more closely linked to peers. As illicit drugs continue to gain media attention, some adolescents may develop concerns about taking any type of medication. Education about prescribed or over-the-counter drugs assists the adolescent in gaining knowledge and control while encouraging pertinent questions and evaluations by this budding health care consumer.

Conversely, the adverse effects of the combination of prescribed medications and illicit drugs are assessed by the nurse. Knowledge of the adolescent's use of chemical substances often alters a therapeutic regimen. Concurrent use of alcohol and/or substances with narcotic analgesics, anticonvulsants, and other medications places the adolescent at additional risk for adverse effects and drug reactions.

Chronically ill adolescents may resist treatment regimens in their quest for identity and control (Yoos, 1987). Optimal health status can suffer during this period. A frank, honest discussion between client and nurse sometimes elicits feelings of helplessness, vulnerability, concern for addiction, a desire to be like one's peers, and a lack of knowledge. Intervention by the nurse to provide information and encourage informed decision making will enhance the client–nurse relationship.

Nursing management

Nursing implications

The child is a complex being who attempts to understand his world through the use of play and experimentation. Play is a medium for exploration, contemplation, rehearsal of life events, and gradual acceptance and integration of a given situation (Petrillo & Sanger, 1980). The value of play is extremely important when the child is in need of health care and thera-peutic interventions. It allows the child to clarify and develop some understanding of unfamiliar personnel, intrusive procedures, and unpleasant medications.

Nursing process

Assessment An assessment of the child's level of development and cognitive skills will assist the nurse in care planning. The plan of care will be geared to the child's developmental level rather than chronologic age. The child's health status will have an effect on the child's development. Some children with chronic illness have an advanced knowledge of health care procedures, while others regress due to the stress of the illness and its treatments. Assessing each child for advanced or delayed development allows for individualized care planning.

Nursing diagnosis The following statements serve as examples of nursing diagnosis that may be considered in planning care for pediatric patients and their families. Possible diagnoses are:

> *Powerlessness related to hospitalization*
> *Ineffective individual coping related to invasive procedures*
> *Knowledge deficit related to hospitalization and/or procedures*
> *Anxiety related to life-threatening, chronic or episodic disease*
> *Altered family processes concerning an ill family member*

Planning Nursing care goals are determined to assist the child and family in understanding the reasons for medical and nursing interventions. The impact of an episodic illness on the family may be extensive. Acute hospitalization may cause family dysfunction due to stress, separation, loss of parental income, as well as sibling and patient behavioral problems. Children who are chronically ill are at increased risk for these concerns and others. Peer relationships may be affected due to the child's inability to participate in activities and school. When planning for a child's care, consideration of the child's community such as family, the school, social and religious activities, and cultural background is essential.

Intervention The use of play by a nurse can assist a child in coping with a difficult procedure or hospitalization. Play allows a child to become familiar with equipment and personnel who are strange to him. Actual medical equipment can be used in conjunction with dolls, puppets, costumes, and doll houses to simulate the health care environment (Petrillo & Sanger, 1980). Children who are often in the submissive role of "patient" may choose to be the health care provider in the play scenario. Actual or replicas of health care equipment also stimulates play (Box 17-2).

Play can be guided by the nurse to recreate an

Example of nursing process and environmental factors in pediatric nursing

The client is an 18-month-old boy seen at the ambulatory pediatric center for a follow-up visit. At the last visit, his mother described pica, including ingestion of dirt and window sill paint. At the first visit, he was tested for lead poisoning and anemia.

His mother describes his appetite as poor; food preferences include large quantities of milk from a bottle and sweets. After plotting him on the growth chart, the nurse identifies his weight to be in the third percentile and his height at the 50% percentile. Throughout the visit, he sits quietly in his mother's lap and appears to lack energy. His mucous membranes and conjunctiva are pale.

His blood values show significant iron deficiency anemia and mild (class I) lead poisoning. He is placed on oral iron therapy.

Assessment data	Nursing diagnosis	Intervention	Goals and outcome criteria
Pale mucous membranes Decreased energy Poor nutrition	Altered nutrition: less than body requirements related to poor food intake	**Discuss** with the mother proper nutrition for an 18-month-old child. **Encourage** use of high caloric, iron-rich foods and snacks. **Decrease** intake of milk and sweets. **Recommend** weaning from bottle.	The child will eat proper foods and gain weight. He will exhibit increased energy and have pink mucous membranes and conjunctiva.
Order for iron supplements	Parental knowledge deficit concerning medication and iron-rich foods	**Determine** past positive medication strategies. Supply mother with written and verbal information on iron-rich foods. **Demonstrate** and have mother redemonstrate correct dose and administration of iron supplements. **Administer** water or fruit juice after medication to prevent teeth staining. Have mother keep chart of medications administered; a calendar may be helpful. **Teach** strategies for medication administration to avoid power struggle with child.	The child will receive iron supplements as ordered and have an improved hematocrit and hemoglobin in 2 months at rescreening.
Child chewing on window sills, eating dirt	High risk for injury related to ingestion of lead or other harmful substance	**Arrange** for assessment of the house for lead pollution. **Discuss** with mother lead poisoning and its effects on child. **Screen** child for blood lead levels on a regular basis and refer to lead program if necessary. **Discuss** oral behavior of child and use of substitutes or diversions.	The child will have a decreasing blood level of lead as the environment is assessed and improved. In the future, the child will demonstrate no outward effects from these ingestions.

Box 17-2. Suggested list of play materials

- Operating room cap, gown, and mask
- Stethoscope
- Toy thermometer
- Toy watch
- Sphygmomanometer
- Plastic or paper medicine cups, plastic drinking glasses
- Tongue blades
- Cotton balls, gauze, and adhesive bandages, tape
- Plastic syringes
- Plastic IV bottles and tubing
- Doll "patient"
- Other appropriate items such as wheelchairs, oxygen equipment, and respiratory or orthopedic equipment

---

event or elicit feelings about a particular procedure or intervention. Guided play involves continuous validation of the nurse's perceptions of the play situation and is useful for teaching or diminishing the child's misconceptions (Pridham, Adelson, & Hansen, 1987, pp 13–21). Experience and knowledge of the developmental process and each child's tolerance of this type of play is necessary. A given play situation may be repeated several times to incorporate it into a child's psyche or experience.

Play can also be a random event where the nurse acts as an observer. Verbal and nonverbal behaviors allow the nurse access to the child's emotions, concerns, and understanding. The opportunity exists for teaching and clarification of serial events, leading to a more formal, therapeutic intervention.

Knowledge of the child's developmental level enables the nurse to assess and intervene in a way that can facilitate understanding, coping, and growth. The nurse may also use books, dolls drawings, and concrete explanations with a school-age child. Diagrams, models, books, and explanations can assist adolescents in comprehending the need for medication or a specific interventions.

Client education. Understanding their options for treatment and providing education are important issues for children and their families. In the expanding arena of health care knowledge and pharmacology, consumers are assuming an ever-increasing role in determining their treatment plans. They require information as a necessary part of informed decision-making. Much has been written about the ethical aspects of parental consent to treating children. The nurse has a responsibility to the child and family to provide information and answer questions. Consulta-

tion with nursing experts or experts in other disciplines may also assist the nurse, child, and family. The nurse is often the advocate and liaison between children, parents, and those who prescribe medications and treatments. The nurse promotes informed consent and disseminates knowledge about pediatric health care for the benefit of the child, the family, and the community.

Evaluation   The evaluation of a child's response to a therapeutic intervention such as play involves the nurse's astute observations of verbal and nonverbal communication. The nurse's awareness of the child's developmental level, coupled with knowledge of communication, will assist in immediate interventions and future care planning. Many of the child's reactions to a well child care visit or hospitalization will develop upon discharge to home. In the child's safe home environment, the child may feel free to discuss or act out his or her concerns. Children may exhibit a change in behavior due to the stress of contact with the health care system. Family education about these behaviors and mutually planned interventions may help the child cope. Future interactions with the health care system may be improved with nursing interventions targeted at the child's behavior after discharge. (See accompanying Example of Nursing Process and Environmental Factors in Pediatric Nursing.)

Learning experience 17-1

Observe nurses administering medications to various aged pediatric clients. Note the positive approaches used by the nurses. Note the child's understanding and response to the medication administration process. What would you do differently in these situations?

References

Beechcroft PC, Redick S. (1989). Possible complications of intramuscular injections on the pediatric unit. *Pediatric Nursing, 15(4),* 333–336, 376.

Broome ME, Slack GF. (1990). Influences on nurses' management of pain in children. *American Journal of Maternal Child Nursing, 15(3),* 159–162.

Eland JM. (1988). Pharmacologic management of acute and chronic pediatric pain. *Issues in Comprehensive Pediatric Nursing, 11(2–3),* 93–111.

Evans M, Hansen B. (1981). Administering injections to different aged children. *American Journal of Maternal Child Nursing, 6(3),* 194–199.

Franck LS. (1989). Pain in the nonverbal patient: Advocating for critically ill neonates. *Pediatric Nursing, 15(1),* 65–68, 90.

Johnston CC, Strada ME. (1986). Acute pain response in infants: A multidimensional description. *Pain, 24(3),* 373–382.

Nugent, KE. (1989). Routine care: Promoting development in hospitalized infants. *American Journal of Maternal Child Nursing*, 14(5), 318–321.

Ormond E, Caulfield C. (1976). A practical guide for giving medications to young children. *American Journal of Maternal Child Nursing*, 1(3), 320–325.

Petrillo M, Sanger S. (1980). *Emotional care of hospitalized children*. Philadelphia: JB Lippincott.

Pridham D, Adelson F, Hansen M. (1987). Helping children deal with procedures in a clinic setting: A developmental approach. *Journal of Pediatric Nursing, 2(1)*, 13–21.

Stoklosa MJ, Ansel HC. (1986). *Pharmaceutical calculations*, pp 88–94. Philadelphia: Lea & Febiger.

Waechter EH, Phillips J, Holaday B, eds. (1985). Fluid and drug therapy. In *Nursing care of children*, pp 197–221. Philadelphia: JB Lippincott.

Yoos L. (1987). Chronic childhood illness: Developmental issues. *Pediatric Nursing, 13(1)*, 25–28.

Bibliography

*Bandman EL, Bandman B. (1990). *Nursing ethics throughout the life span*. Norwalk, CT: Appleton & Lange.

Broome ME, Lillis PP. (1989). A descriptive analysis of pediatric pain management research. *Applied Nursing Research, 2(2)*, 74–81.

Burokas L. (1985). Factors affecting nurses' decisions to medicate pediatric patients after surgery. *Heart Lung, 14(4)*, 373–379.

Dison N. (1988). *Simplified drugs and solutions for nurses*. St Louis: CV Mosby.

Gilman AG, Rall TW, Nies AS, Taylor P, eds. (1990) *Goodman and Gilman's the pharmacological basis of therapeutics*, 8th ed, chaps 1–4. New York: Macmillan.

*Hansen B, Evans M. (1981). Preparing a child for procedures. *American Journal of Maternal Child Nursing, 6(6)*, 392–397.

*Howry LB, Bindler RM, Tso Y. (1981). *Pediatric medicines*. Philadelphia: JB Lippincott.

*Ormond E, Caulfield C. (1976). A practical guide for giving medications to young children. *American Journal of Maternal Child Nursing, 1(5)*, 320–325.

Sallis G. (1985). Improving adherence to pediatric therapeutic regimens, *Pediatric Nursing, 11(2)*, 118–120.

Verzemnieks IL, Nash D. (1984). Ethical issues related to pediatric care. *Nurs Clin North Am, 19(2)*, 319–328.

*Recommended for further reading.

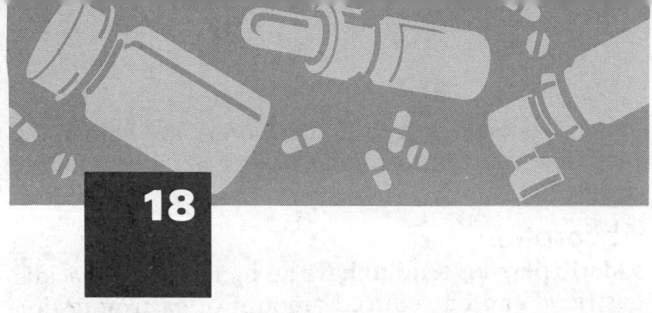

18

Drug therapy in gerontologic nursing

"Drug treatment based on ignorance—ignorance of the course of symptomatology, ignorance of the drug, the interaction of drug and drug, as well as drug and nutrition, and/or ignorance of the emotional and social environment of the patient—often leaves the older person with an exacerbation of symptoms, in the decrement of function and in the persistence of disease" (Weg, 1978, p 136).

With the progressive "graying" of our society since these words were first penned, health care providers can no longer ignore the issues of iatrogenic problems related to drug therapy in elderly clients. A continuing proliferation of new drugs, such as potent new antiarrhythmics, nonsteroidal anti-inflammatory agents, and new forms of old drugs only add to the already overwhelming medical, social, economic, and ethical dimensions of geriatric polypharmacy.*

* Polypharmacy is the use of more than one drug.

By the year 2030, 28% of the U. S. population will be over the age of 60, with more than 8 million people over the age of 85 (Fowles, 1991). It has been estimated that approximately two-thirds of physician office visits by elderly clients result in one or more new prescription drugs and that 50% of these prescriptions will not have their desired therapeutic effect due to a variety of reasons ranging from too high or too low a dosage to not getting the prescription filled (American Medical Association, 1990, pp 2459–2472).

In addition to prescription drugs, it is estimated that 40% of persons 60 years and above use over-the-counter (OTC) drugs on a daily basis and that, in general, elderly clients spend three times more on nonprescription drugs than the general population. One study found that after initiation of the prospective pricing system for hospitalized Medicare patients, the mean daily cost of prescribed drugs increased from $5.25 to $8.04 per patient (Carroll & Erwin, 1990, pp 2251–2254).

The economic impact of drug use on the individual client and on society is staggering. Whereas elderly clients currently account for only 12% of the population, they consume over 25% of all prescription drugs at a cost of more than $15 billion per year (Schmucker, 1985).

Geriatric clients are likely to have seven times more undesirable drug reactions than persons aged 20–29 (Machocki & Lamy, 1988, pp 79–81). Cardiovascular, diuretic, analgesic, psychoactive, and gastrointestinal (GI) drugs are the most frequently prescribed medications for geriatric clients. The most common OTC drugs include laxatives, analgesics, antacids, and antihistamines (Cutler & Narang, 1986). These drugs are among the most potent, have the most toxic side effects, and are interactive. In a hearing before the House Senate Aging Committee, it was revealed that 25% of health problems in nursing homes are caused by drug complications, and in 1 year, 30,000 nursing home deaths were caused by drugs (Ebersole & Hess, 1985, pp 3–22). More than 50% of drug-related deaths among elderly clients are due to bleeding associated with anticoagulant therapy (Williams & Rush, 1986, pp 109–120). These statistics demand that closer attention from health care providers be given to drug use among elderly clients.

Confounding variables of disease and the aging process interact with social, emotional, and environmental factors to impact on the pharmacokinetics and pharmacodynamics of drug therapy. Therefore, a thorough assessment by nurses of medications given to elderly clients is essential, whether in the home, the hospital, or a long-term care institution. Unfortunately, very little has been written specifically for nurses to guide them in these assessments. The study of geriatrics in nursing schools has been fragmented at best. In fact, most student clinical practice does not include experience in nursing homes, even though more than 1 million elderly persons currently reside in these institutions (Pevonka, 1988, pp 64–82).

Although aware of the general kinds of problems elderly persons have with drugs, most physicians lack formal training in using drugs with elderly clients. In recognition of this lack of preparation and the escalating medical needs of the elderly population, the American Medical Association recently released a "White Paper" on elderly health care in which they strongly recommended the following: 1) incorporation of geriatric medicine into medical school curricula; 2) emphasis on practice, research, and education on problems related to aging and health care across all specialties; 3) assessment of the knowledge of care of the aged within the certifying and recertifying procedures of specialty boards; and 4) clinical affiliation between nursing homes and resident training programs (American Medical Association, 1990, pp 2459–2472).

Consumer activist groups have helped to dispel some common myths associated with old people. Nevertheless, ageism still exists within our culture and contributes to misdiagnosed symptoms of drug-induced problems.

Factors in assessing drug use

It is beyond the scope of this chapter to present a comprehensive guide for assessing all potential drug interactions specific to elderly persons. Nonetheless, guidelines are given that can be useful when assessing the effects of drugs on elderly clients. These factors include:

- Physiologic changes and their potential effects on pharmacokinetics
- Patterns of toxicity that may not be recognized as such
- Chronic disease and polypharmacy
- Social and emotional behaviors that may affect the elderly client's perception of or compliance with medication regimens
- Diminishing financial resources and the implications on drug use
- The pharmacist as a resource in assessing drug use
- Risk–benefit ratio of drug use for each client
- Ethical considerations

Finally, the implications these factors have on nursing assessment, client advocacy, client teaching, and health-team management will be discussed.

Physiologic changes of aging

The effectiveness of drug action is subject to the pharmacokinetics of absorption, distribution, metabolism, and excretion. Although research on the effects of the aging process has been limited, there are known factors that contribute to the body's ability to handle drugs.

Absorption

Elderly persons tend to have an increased (less acidic) gastric pH and a reduced amount of gastrointestinal blood flow. There is also a tendency toward slowed or reduced gastrointestinal motility rate. All of this affects how elderly clients absorb drugs, although there is not enough evidence to identify all the implications of these changes.

Distribution

As the body ages, total body water decreases and body fat increases, resulting in a reduction of lean body mass. Weight-related drug doses, whose distribution is affected by body water or fat-free body mass may, therefore, produce higher blood or tissue concentration in elderly clients. Fat-soluble drugs also tend to accumulate in the increased body fat, producing prolonged or even toxic effects.

Serum albumin can become so decreased that, in the case of drugs that bind to albumin, less of the drug is bound. Therefore, higher concentrations of unbound drug are available to produce pharmacologic effects including increased side effects.

Metabolism

The liver is the site where many drugs become inactivated. Changes in liver function, such as decreased hepatic flow, influence the body's ability to metabolize drugs. In addition to the obvious pathologic effects of disease on the liver, there is a wide range of factors (*eg*, genetic and environmental) that can influence liver function. These effects on liver function make it difficult to establish a definitive association between drug metabolism and physiologic changes of aging.

Excretion

There is a gradual decline in renal function throughout life, which means elderly persons have a decreased glomerular filtration rate, a decreased total renal plasma flow, and an altered tubular excretory capacity. Thus, there is the potential for an accumulation of drugs normally eliminated through the kidneys.

In addition to these physiologic changes, elderly persons have a diminished homeostatic response to change. Aging autonomic nervous system reflexes, the regulation of blood pressure, temperature, vasoconstriction, and vasodilation are less stable than in younger persons. Therefore, the elderly do not rebound as rapidly from changes in sleep patterns, dietary habits, stress levels, and so forth. Because many drugs may have excitatory or depressive effects on autoregulatory mechanisms, elderly persons may be predisposed to exaggerated drug responses (Box 18-1).

Box 18-1. Physiologic changes in aging that affect drug pharmacokinetics

Diminished homeostatic responses to change

Absorption
  Increased gastric pH
  Reduced amount of gastrointestinal blood flow
  Slowed or reduced gastrointestinal motility rate

Distribution
  Decreased total body water
  Increased body fat
  Reduced lean body mass
  Decreased serum albumin

Metabolism
  Changed liver function

Excretion
  Decreased glomerular filtration rate
  Decreased total renal plasma flow
  Altered tubular excretory capacity

Patterns of drug toxicity

Pharmacokinetic data are based almost exclusively on healthy young adults. Standard dose is determined by the objective and subjective responses of young adults to drug testing with certain responses, both desirable and undesirable, to drug therapy being predictable. However, as outlined in the previous section, there are factors in the aging process that can alter these "predictable" responses among elderly persons.

Elderly persons frequently exhibit such signs of drug toxicity as behavioral changes, restlessness, confusion, irritability, anxiety, insomnia, and hallucinations suggestive of mental deterioration. Elderly clients presenting with signs of confusion secondary to drug toxicity may be diagnosed as having acute brain syndrome while the adverse drug reaction goes unrecognized. Approximately one in five elderly clients who comes to an emergency room presents with symptoms of mental deterioration or pseudodementia. Frequently, these changes are insidious and go unnoticed. Too often, health care givers dismiss such symptoms as part of the aging process without fully assessing the medication regimen of the client. Drug toxicity increases rapidly as the number of drugs taken increases. Even physical symptoms such as headache, anorexia, and visual changes are frequently attributed to the natural aging process and are overlooked as possible indicators of drug toxicity. Drug assessment should be performed initially and repeated periodically. It is essential to update the drug assessment whenever there are new symptoms.

Chronic disease and polypharmacy

Compounding the effect of physiologic aging is the presence of chronic disease among elderly clients. After age 65, a client is likely to suffer on average from one to three chronic diseases, the most common involving compromised respiratory, cardiovascular, or metabolic functions that often alter the body's ability to predictably handle drug therapy. Chronic disease often predisposes the elderly client to excessive drug use for extended periods. The rate of adverse drug reactions is directly proportional to the number of drugs taken. Nursing home residents take four to nine different drugs daily.

Ambulatory elderly clients may take as many as 11 different prescription and OTC drugs per day. In one study of noninstitutionalized clients taking an average of 11 different drugs, 91% of these clients had adverse drug reactions (Shimp, Ascione, Glazer, & Atwood, 1985, pp 766–773). Long-term management of clients with chronic disease requires much closer supervision of drug therapy than is commonly given.

The combination of an aging population and a proliferation of new drugs puts frail, elderly clients at an increased risk of polypharmacy. In a recent study, it was found that drug use in an essentially well, white, middle-class retirement community in Florida, increased by 10% over the 10-year period, 1978–1988, (Stewart, Moore, May, Marks, & Hale, 1991, pp 182–188).

The most common method for handling aches, pains, and other "complaints" of elderly people is with medication. An agitated elderly client may be given a tranquilizer, which compounds arthritic immobility problems, leading to more "complaints" to be treated with more medications. Excessive use of medications in the elderly can inadvertently create a costly (economically, psychologically, and physiologically) cycle of events from which the client may never fully recover.

A Long-Term Care Demonstration Program was set up at one hospital to deal with the increasing number of hospitalized elderly clients awaiting nursing home placement. With a multifaceted team approach, this project was successfully able to reduce the average number of prescribed medications from eight to four and to return 69% of these clients to their own homes (Mahoney, 1991, pp 45–48).

Polypharmacy is the result not only of a multidisease process, but also of multiphysician prescribing and of poorly coordinated health team management.

In one prospective study in which resident physicians were given recommendations to discontinue medications or to simplify medication regimens, the most prevalent reason for noncompliance with the recommendation was that the medicine had been prescribed by another physician (Kroenke & Pinholt, 1990, pp 31–36).

Frequently, the primary physician has minimal contact with the client and consequently takes an incomplete drug history. In the presence of an acute infectious process, new drugs may be added before a thorough assessment has been made of the effectiveness of the current regimen. Multiple drugs with varying dosages administered at different hours create confusion. Drug reactions that mimic medical–physical complaints are often treated with yet another drug. Polypharmacy increases the risk of drug interactions, increases the potential for administration error, and reduces the level of compliance. Therefore, health care providers should thoroughly evaluate all drugs their elderly clients are taking and be fully knowledgeable about potential interactions.

Social and emotional behaviors affecting drug use

One study involving elderly persons in independent living situations revealed a negative correlation between perceived physical and emotional well-being and the use of medications (Quicke, 1981). As apathy or perception of "poor health" increased, there was a significant increase in the number of pills taken. Although most clients in this study rated themselves as highly compliant about taking prescribed medications, there was significant misuse and lack of knowledge about drug regimens. Clients misnamed look-alike pills, took medication out of sequence, and stopped medication on improvement. Under such a misguided understanding of compliance, many elderly clients attempted to make up for a missed dosage by doubling the number of pills taken at the next scheduled medication hour.

Another significant behavior among aging clients is sharing medications. Many clients relate instances in which they relieved arthritic pain or other ailments by sharing medications with a relative or friend suffering from the same condition. Most elderly clients do not throw away unused prescriptions because they "might need them again." In fact, clients have inquired about taking prescription medication belonging to a deceased relative who suffered from an illness they now have. Elderly clients also hoard medications. In one study, 67% of clients had three or more hoarded drugs in their home (Shimp, Ascione, Glazer, & Atwood, 1985). Cardiovascular drugs accounted for 30% of these hoarded drugs, and almost one-third of the total drugs had not been used within the past year.

Elderly clients usually perceive the physician as the most important member of the health care team. However, most clients do not inform physicians about all the medications they are taking, including OTC drugs, nor do they tell physicians about prescriptions other health care providers have given them. In fact, elderly people frequently "do not want to bother" physicians with their complaints.

Another significant factor that predisposes the elderly to increased risk of harmful drug interaction is their use of OTC drugs and home remedies. The most common misuse of self-treatment involves laxatives. Elderly persons commonly become preoccupied with their bowel habits. Frequently, they forget to consider other changes that affect bowel function, such as decreased mobility, decreased appetite, changes in dietary patterns, or the side effects of medication. Using laxatives combined with diuretics, cardiovascular drugs, or decreased fluid intake potentiates the risk of electrolyte imbalance or drug toxicity.

Home remedies are not often thought of as drugs. It is not uncommon to find elderly clients using large amounts of sodium bicarbonate to relieve symptoms of gastric distress, yet an increased amount of sodium can be harmful in light of the decreased excretory capacity of the kidneys or the predisposition toward congestive heart failure frequently seen in this age group. The author and her students participated in a "brown-bag" exercise where they reviewed medications in a senior citizens nutrition center. The members were given large brown bags and were asked to fill the bags with all the medications found in their homes. A team of nurses, nursing students, pharmacists, and a physician reviewed the medications with the participants. Common problems included drug–drug interactions, incorrect dosages, troublesome side effects, improper storage, outdated medications, and taking different brand names of the same drug. This project was conducted among a relatively "healthy" population of elderly clients. They concluded that holistic assessment of all parameters affecting drug use must be conducted at regular intervals for all elderly clients.

Diminishing resources of elderly clients

The longer a person lives, the more diminishing physical, mental, and material resources must be taken into account. All of these factors have a direct or indirect impact on drug use.

Childproof caps become adultproof caps as the elderly person's weakened or arthritic hands are unable to open them. As a result, clients may skip medication altogether. When clients finally succeed in getting bottles opened, pills may get dumped into other containers, increasing the risk of future error, or clients may leave the tops off, exposing medication to potential rapid deterioration from air or moisture. Many people are not aware that regular (non–child-resistant) containers can be requested from their pharmacists.

In response to some of these concerns, the Consumer Product Safety Commission recently recommended changes in the test protocol for child-resistant packaging (CRP). First, they proposed that the ages of the adult panel used to test the opening and closing of child-resistant packaging be raised from the current

18–45 year age range to 60–75 years. Second, they proposed that the time limit for opening and closing these containers be reduced from the current 5-minute limit to a 1-minute limit with a 30-second familiarization period (Staff, Aging, 1991). It is hoped with the adoption of these recommendations that the elderly will properly use medication safety caps.

Most elderly persons experience a decrease in hearing. Frequently, they are too embarrassed to ask the physician or nurse to repeat instructions, thus misunderstanding their regimens. This is compounded by the fact that most prescription bottles do not contain complete instructions for use. Bottles are often labeled with "take as directed" or "take three times a day." Without adequate knowledge of peak action of drugs or the effects of drug–food and drug–drug interactions, clients and their families are left to guess at the proper drug administration.

Many elderly persons also have decreased vision. Most prescription bottles have very fine print which is difficult to read. Special instructions written on separate pieces of paper may also be difficult or impossible to read, and if elderly clients must match arrows on a childproof cap, their vision may not accommodate this.

Diet and fluid intake also become significant problems for many elderly clients. Age-related alterations in taste and smell, loss of natural teeth, and changing nutritional requirements affect food intake. The association between food and fluid intake and drugs (*eg*, the need for increased potassium with digoxin and for increased fluid intake with diuretics) is well known. A downward spiraling cycle of depressed appetite from drug effect, decreased thirst sensation, dysphagia, and difficulty in maintaining an adequate diet lead to increased side effects and decreased benefit of drug therapy.

With aging there is frequently a decrease in memory, especially for events in the immediate past. Directions for taking medications are usually given to a client when he or she is apprehensive about his or her health. Sometimes, however, when the client finally gets the medication, he or she may be unable to recall what it is for, when it is to be taken, or when it was last taken.

Diminished finances are frequently overlooked as a deterrent to taking medications. Often a large number of pills intended to last for several months is prescribed. This consumes a large portion of the client's monthly budget. It is not uncommon to find elderly clients who wait 2–3 weeks to fill their prescriptions because they must wait for their next pension or government check to arrive. If the medication is changed before all pills in a prescription are used, the client becomes reluctant to spend his or her money on another prescription (Box 18-2).

Risk–benefit ratio

The risk–benefit ratio is the weighing of adverse reactions against alleviation of symptoms. For the elderly client, the risk–benefit ratio must also include economic, physiologic, and psychological factors. Questions that need to be asked include: Will purchasing the medication drain financial resources? Do adverse reactions include compromise of an already altered respiratory, cardiovascular, or skeletal system? Will the medication alter the client's mental status, making him or her more error prone or dependent on others? Do adverse reactions of the medication or combination of medications include loss of bladder or bowel control, which might cause the loss of dignity?

Factors contributing to increased or decreased self-esteem must not be overlooked. Drug-induced dyskinesia may evoke more problems than nondrug treatment. Ethical considerations must be carefully factored into the risk–benefit ratio before starting an elderly client on medications known to have socially unacceptable side effects.

The question of drug efficacy must be asked when determining the risk–benefit ratio, particularly for drugs used routinely for chronic conditions. In one study of neuroleptic drugs used to treat demented clients in a nursing home, the behavioral problems of those taking medications were more frequent, more intense, and more problematic for the staff than for a matched group of clients not taking neuroleptics (Butler, Burgio, & Engel, 1987, pp 15–19).

These are only a few of the issues that need to be addressed in gerontologic nursing. Each client must be considered individually; it is just as important to know the client as to understand the kind of drug used. The client's unique set of circumstances must be assessed when weighing the risk–benefit ratio of a medication regimen.

Ethical considerations

It is projected that by the year 2040, life expectancy will be 83.1 years for women and 75.0 years for men; that the fastest growing group of elderly people, those

---

Box 18-2. Diminished resources of the aged

Physical resources
  Arthritic or weak hands
  Decreased hearing
  Decreased vision
  Alterations in taste and smell
  Loss of natural teeth
  Changes in nutritional requirements
Mental resources
  Decreased memory, especially of events in the immediate past
Material resources
  Diminished or limited finances

over age 85 years of age, will have increased to more than 17.8 million; and that Medicare spending for everyone 65 years and older will approach $212 billion (Schneider & Guralnik, 1990, pp 2335–2340). While many would argue vigorously against rationing health care for elderly persons, we currently have both an "unintentional" form of rationing and a formal systematic rationing of health care services. Rationing is "unintentional," for example, when an elderly person entering a busy emergency room must compete with victims of drug abuse, violence, accidents, and so forth, for scarce health services. Rationing is "unintentional" when an income-limited elderly person is unable to fill a prescription due to lack of monies, or when the physician fails to prescribe a less expensive drug which could be just as effective. The federal government initiated a prospective payment system for Medicare in 1983, a formal rationing system, which put a cap on payment for health services. By 1984, 27 states had placed a "cap" on Medicaid drug prescriptions either by limiting the number of prescriptions reimbursed per month or by requiring patient copayment. It was found in one study that there was a 30% reduction in the number of prescriptions filled in one state when this cap was put into effect. The bad news was that the Medicaid recipients predominantly affected were elderly, and the unfilled prescriptions included such "essential" drugs as insulin, thiazides, and furosemide (Soumerai, Avorn, Ross-Degnan, & Gortmaker, 1987, pp 550–556).

In addition to issues of economics, overuse and misuse of prescription drugs must be looked at from an ethical standpoint. Studies suggest that psychoactive drugs are inappropriately prescribed, overused, and may have serious complications for elderly clients (Garrard, Makris, Dunham, Heston, Cooper, Ratner, et al, 1991, pp 403–467; Beers, Avorn, Soumerai, Everitt, Sherman, & Salem, 1988, pp 3016–3020; Ray, Griffin, Schaffner, Baugh, & Melton, 1987, pp 363–369). As one writer clearly points out "pharmacokinetics in the elderly no longer is esoteric" (Riesenberg, 1988, p 3054). It is time to draw the line between unintentional misuse and the "concept of sedation as 'chemical restraint'" (Beers, Avorn, Soumerai, Everitt, Sherman, & Salem, 1988, pp 403–467).

Before any drugs are prescribed to elderly clients, nonpharmacological treatments such as behavioral modification, diet therapy, exercise training, stress management, and biofeedback must be considered. Even though these alternative therapies may not totally eliminate the need for pharmacotherapy, they may reduce the dose of medication required and probably will have other positive consequences such as additional symptom relief (McCue, 1991, pp 16–20).

As the generation of post–World War II baby boomers reaches senior citizen status, there will be continuing debates on "do not resuscitate" orders, pro-

longation of life by artificial means, living wills, and "death with dignity" issues. Adding to the complexity of these issues will be very real problems of economics, scarce resources, access to care, the proliferation of life-saving drugs, and advanced life-saving technology. These issues must be addressed within an ethically acceptable framework and must be incorporated into a more just total health care system (American Medical Association, 1990, pp 2459–2472).

■ Summary

Geriatric clients are at higher risk of adverse drug reactions than are younger clients. Factors contributing to this vulnerability include: physiologic changes that influence both the way the body handles drugs and the way it responds to them; the need for multiple prescriptions that increase the risk of drug–drug interactions; sensory-perceptual changes that may impair the client's ability to carry out the drug regimen accurately; and diminished socioeconomic resources needed for optimum adjustment to the drug regimen.

The proportion of the population that is 65 years of age or older has increased rapidly since the mid-century and will continue to do so during the foreseeable future. For this reason, health concerns of the elderly will be of increasing importance to health care professionals, including nurses.

Nursing management

Nursing implications

Physicians traditionally control the prescribing of medications. Nurses, however, administer, assess, and first note client response to drug therapy. Therefore, nurses can best serve as client advocate to physicians and other health team members. Nurses can encourage clients to take all medications to the physician's office for the next appointment. Nurses can also request that physicians label prescriptions with clear, specific instructions for use. Likewise, nurses can clearly document facts and observations pertinent to a client's drug therapy for the rest of the health team. In these ways, nurses can represent clients who are reluctant or unable to speak for themselves.

Referrals frequently come to nurses with the major problem listed as "noncompliant." Noncompliance is considered a client problem. However, there are health professionals who would argue there is no such thing as a noncompliant client; there are only unrealistic expectations or deficiencies in health teaching by health professionals. It is rare to find a client who will not take his or her heart medication knowing that by refusing he or she might die. It is not uncommon, however, to find a client who has not taken his or her heart medication because he or she was too weak to get the cap off, did not have enough money to buy a refill, or was told to take it with breakfast and never eats breakfast.

There is another view of compliance called "intelligent noncompliance," for those clients who adapt their medication therapy to their needs and who have successful clinical outcomes (Vestal, 1984). There are studies that support the notion of clients adjusting their drug therapy to obtain maximum benefit. Clients who know their own bodies are aware of undesirable side effects; clients who rationally stop their treatment (*eg*, stop digoxin when their "heart is pounding") may avoid adverse reactions by such a choice. This aspect of compliance needs to be studied by nurses as they assess drug regimen in elderly clients.

Nursing process

Assessment The nursing assessment should include a thorough drug history, asking such questions as: What do you do if you miss a dose? What reminders do you use to take your medication? Do you have any difficulty purchasing your medications?

The Appendix in this book contains a drug history guide for home use but it can be adapted for hospitals or long-term care institutions. Once this initial history is taken and placed in the chart, it should be referred to every time a new drug is prescribed. In addition, the drug assessment should be completely updated on a regular basis. Periodic assessments should include all drugs taken, including OTC drugs, because even in hospitals, family members sometimes bring in nonprescribed drugs (Box 18-3).

Nursing diagnosis Nursing diagnoses commonly found when treating older clients include the following:

Altered thought processes: confusion related to electrolyte imbalance secondary to diuretic medication
Altered comfort: nausea or vomiting related to central nervous system changes secondary to digitalis toxicity; contributing factor: potassium deficiency due to diuretic medication
Body image disturbance related to dyskinesia secondary to psychotropic medication
Altered sexual patterns: decreased libido or impotency related to CNS changes secondary to long-term medication for chronic illness
Self-esteem disturbance related to dependence on medication secondary to chronic illness
Anxiety related to life-threatening, chronic, or incurable disease
High risk for injury related to hypotension

Box 18-3. Nurse's role in drug therapy for elderly persons

Assessment of drug use

Current medication regimen
Over-the-counter drugs
Potential drug–drug, drug–food interactions
Client response

Education of client

Indication for medication
Desired effect
Potential side effects and what to do
Use of reminders to take medication
Procedure if a dose is missed

Coordination of health care team

Lowest number of drugs
Smallest possible dose
Lowest risk–benefit ratio
Client advocate

---

secondary to antihypertensive, psychotropic, antiarrhythmic, or other medication
Altered nutrition: less than body requirements related to medication regimen; contributing factor: decreased food intake related to decreased need for calories, forgetfulness, or limited financial resources

Most elderly clients will have a knowledge deficit concerning chronic illness and medication regimens used for treatment. This may be recurrent because medication regimens are often revised to meet the changing needs of the client and because managing multidrug therapy is relatively complex.

Planning Goals of nursing care include alleviating or eliminating confusion, alleviating or eliminating nausea and vomiting, enhancing self-image, optimizing sexual function, resolving fear or anxiety, maintaining tissue perfusion and good nutrition, and educating the client to properly manage drug regimens.

Intervention The nurse should note the times of drug administration, route of administration, client response, and any changes in the client since the original assessment was done. The nurse must be particularly alert to behavioral and physical changes that may signal a developing toxicity. Any time a significant change occurs in the client's condition or before a new drug is added, all drug therapy should be reviewed and evaluated against the risk–benefit ratio for that client.

Client education. Client teaching must be based on the client's drug history and assessments of the client's perception of and compliance with his or her regimen. Teaching must be carried out at a slow pace to allow time for assimilating instructions. For clients with memory impairment, aids can be used to increase compliance: calendars can be marked to show drug administration times; or nurses can use egg cartons to measure specific daily doses. As much as possible, the sequencing of drug doses should be tied in with routine events such as toileting habits, eating, or bedtime. The nurse must not "assume" routine activities are the same for every client. The client and family must be asked about routines, and teaching must be individualized. Family members can be taught to correctly administer medications to provide support. Medication schedules should be simplified as much as possible. If one single dose can be taken, it is less complicated than to give two divided doses. If the client is homebound and has an aide that comes in from 10 AM to noon, it may be easier to schedule as many medications as possible to be taken during this time when the aide can remind the client.

In the hospital, the nurse traditionally controls administration of medications. At the time of discharge, however, the client is given a variety of prescriptions to fill or a bag of medications to take home for self-administration. A more rational approach would be to provide the elderly client with all of his or her prescription medications in clearly labeled bottles a few days before discharge and use this time for supervised teaching of proper drug administration (Box 18-4). At least the nurse can spend time before discharge teaching the elderly client about his drug regimen.

Coordination of services. Finally, improved coordination of services among all health team members can reduce many of the risks of drug therapy for elderly clients. The nurse is in a unique position to facilitate this coordination and promote active participation of all health team members. This ensures that the total number of drugs prescribed is reduced to a minimum; that the risk–benefit ratio is carefully weighed before any new drug is added; that the smallest possible dosage to achieve a desired benefit is prescribed; that frequent assessments of drug therapy are made, including assessments of the effects of OTC drugs, home remedies, and drug–food interactions; that client and family teaching is instituted as early as possible; and that the client and his or her family are encouraged to ask questions and report physical or behavioral changes.

Nurses must be aware of the tendency to "medicalize" problems (*eg*, believing there is a drug cure for every condition, medical or otherwise). Nurses must be especially alert to "medicalized" social problems such

---

Box 18-4. Self-medication system used prior to discharge

1. Initiate teaching in quiet, calm environment. This is usually done during evening hours with no visitors present.
2. Start client self-administering the least toxic medication (*eg*, stool softeners, vitamins). Leave specified amount of medication at bedside, preferably in labeled container from pharmacy that client uses.
3. Each shift of nurses should check amount of medication left and reinforce proper administration. It is crucial that each health care provider be informed of the program and reinforce all teaching to the client.
4. Evaluate with client the problems, effectiveness, and progress of the medication regimen. As client is ready, add more medications for self-administration.

---

as loneliness, despair, and grief, in which a drug replaces social interaction. Interventions may involve putting the client in contact with friendly visitors, involving community resources, using staff time to listen attentively to clients, or finding appropriate social outlets to divert the elderly client from too much introspection.

Factors that predispose the elderly to increased risks from drug use point to the need for increased nursing management. Drug therapy for elderly clients must be systematically assessed at periodic intervals. Nurses must be client advocates, must be educators for the client and family, and must coordinate services for clients within a multidisciplinary environment.

Evaluation Data required for evaluation are specific to the diagnoses and goals previously established. Data collected during evaluation must be interpreted in relation to the medical regimen and to the client's physiologic state (*eg*, disease conditions and the normal changes of aging).

The effects of altered pharmacokinetics, polypharmacy, and multiple diseases on elderly clients make evaluation of drug responses extremely difficult. The desired pharmacologic effects may be associated with or even preceded by undesirable side effects. Evaluation is further complicated by "ageism" (*eg*, an 87-year-old person is "confused" on meperidine, whereas a 37-year-old person with the same symptom is having a "drug reaction"). It is important that the nurse become familiar with the "normal" status of the elderly client so that subtle departures from the norm may be recognized as possible drug reactions. (See accompanying Example of Nursing Process and Polypharmacy and Box 18-4).

Example of nursing process and polypharmacy

The client is a 71-year-old man with medical diagnoses of congestive heart failure (CHF), diabetes (recently diagnosed), end-stage cardiac failure, and hypertension with renal insufficiency. Approximately 20 years ago he underwent triple bypass surgery. His medications include: Humulin N 12U SC qA.M.; Cardizem 90 mg q8h; Isordil Tembids 40 mg bid; Captopril 25 mg q8h; Coumadin 5 mg/2.5 mg qod @ 6 P.M.; Zantac 150 mg bid; Procan SR 500 mg q6h; Colace 100 mg bid; Lasix 120 mg qA.M.; nitroglycerin SL 0.4 mg prn q5 min (maximum of 3 doses); O_2 continuous at 2 L through nasal cannula.

During a home visit, the client states he "felt too shaky to do a blood glucose (BG) chemstrip test this morning." His BG has consistently run 80–100 during the past 2 weeks. The client states he has experienced some "tightness in arms" during the past week. He appears more withdrawn this week and states he "would be better off dead," and that he wants to go to the VA hospital if he gets worse so he "will not be a burden" to his wife. He has nonpitting ankle edema and low basal lung rales. You test BG @ 80. His vital signs are: T = 36.2°C (97.2°F), P = 96, R = 24, BP = 136/86.

Assessment data	Nursing diagnosis	Intervention	Goals and outcome criteria
"Tightness" in arms	Pain related to myocardial hypoxia secondary to degenerative vascular disease	**Review** with the client and his wife the proper use of sublingual nitroglycerine. **Monitor** use of nitroglycerine.	The client will use nitroglycerine appropriately to relieve pain. The client will report a diminution of anginal pain.
Statement by client that he "would be better off dead" Stated desire to go to VA hospital so he will not be a "burden"	Fear related to seriousness of condition	**Encourage** client to express his feelings, talk with his wife about options for care, and discuss preparations for death. **Refer** to spiritual advisor as necessary.	Client and spouse will make appropriate preparations for care and for impending death; the client will express confidence about their final choices.
"Shaky" feeling Ankle edema Lung rales	High risk for altered tissue perfusion: hypervolemia related to fluid retention	**Assess** total medication regimen including over-the-counter drugs. **Teach** client: • Identity of drugs • Expected response to drugs • How/when to take drugs • Stress management techniques to minimize stress-related sodium and water retention. **Monitor** lab tests for therapeutic drug levels, prothrombin time, and electrolyte levels; report abnormal values to the physician.	Client will consistently identify the purpose and method of administration of medications. Edema will diminish. Lung rales will diminish. The client will report he feels less "shaky."
Anginal pain Edema Complex drug regimen	Knowledge deficit concerning drug regimen	**Carry** out teaching as outlined above. **Monitor** vital signs, heart/lung status, and vascular status.	Client will consistently identify the purpose and method of administration of medications. Edema and anginal pain will decrease.

(Continued)

Example of nursing process and polypharmacy (Continued)

Edema Diagnosis of end-stage cardiac failure	Knowledge deficit concerning factors leading to sodium retention and edema	**Take** measures outlined above to alleviate anxiety or fear that contributes to stress-related sodium retention. **Review** with the client and his wife techniques for reducing sodium intake.	Ankle edema and lung rales will diminish.
Coumadin therapy	High risk for ineffective management of drug regimen related to complexity of therapeutic regimen	**Analyze** the client's drug intake to verify that drug interactions will not increase the effect of coumadin and the risk of hemorrhage; if the client is using a drug such as aspirin that would have this effect, caution him about using a safer alternate drug (in the case of aspirin, substitute acetaminophen). **Advise** the client to wear a medical identification device listing specific health hazards such as coumadin medication.	Hemorrhage will not occur; if it does occur, it will be detected and treated promptly.

References

Agents in the elderly: A ten-year overview. *Age and Ageing, 20,* 182–188.

American Medical Association Council on Scientific Affairs. (1990). American Medical Association White Paper on Elderly Health: Report of the Council on Scientific Affairs. *Arch Intern Med, 150,* 2459–2472.

Beers M, Avorn J, Soumerai S, Everitt D, Sherman D, Salem S. (1988). Psychoactive medication use in intermediate-care facility residents. *JAMA, 260(20),* 3016–3020.

Butler FR, Burgio LD, Engel BT. (1987). Neuroleptics and behavior. A comparative study. *J Gerontol Nurs, 13(6),* 15–19.

Carroll N, Erwin G. (1990). Effect of the prospective-pricing system on drug use in Pennsylvania long-term-care facilities. *Am J Hosp Pharm, 47,* 2251–2254.

Cutler NR, Narang PK, eds. (1986). *Drug studies in the elderly: Methodological concerns.* NY: Plenum.

Ebersole P, Hess P. (1985). *Toward healthy aging: Human needs and nursing response,* 2nd ed. St. Louis: CV Mosby.

Fowles D. (1991). The numbers game: Pyramid power. *Aging, 362,* 58–59.

Garrard J, Makris L, Dunham T, Heston L, Cooper S, Ratner E, et al. (1991). Evaluation of neuroleptic drug use by nursing home elderly under proposed Medicare and Medicaid regulations. *JAMA, 265(4),* 463–467.

Is it really Alzheimer's? (1991). AJN, February, 52–54.

Kroenke LTC, Pinholt E. (1990). Reducing polypharmacy in the elderly: A controlled trial of physician feedback. *J Am Geriatr Soc, 38(1),* 31–36.

Machocki R, Lamy P. (1988). Adverse drug reactions. *J Am Geriatr Soc 36(1),* 79–81.

Mahoney C. (1991). Return to independence: Lessons from a hospital long-term care unit. *American Journal of Nursing, March,* 45–48.

McCue J. (1991). Elderly hypertensive patients with angina. *Geriatric Medicine Today, 10(6),* 16–20.

Pevonka M. (1988). Long-term care facilities and pharmacy services. In Delafuente J, Stewart R, eds., *Therapeutics in the elderly,* pp 64–82. Baltimore: Williams & Wilkins.

Quicke TA. An analysis of drug use and misuse by the aging in independent living: The influence of psychosocial dynamics on the dynamics of pharmacokinetics. Unpublished doctoral dissertation. Minneapolis: Walden University, 1981.

Ray W, Griffin M, Schaffner W, Baugh D, Melton L. (1987). Psychotropic drug use and the risk of hip fracture. *N Engl J Med, 316(7),* 363–369.

Riesenberg D. (1988). Drugs in the institutionalized elderly: Time to get it right? *JAMA 260(20),* 3054.

Schmucker DL. (1985). Aging and drug disposition: An update. *Pharmacol Rev, 37(2),* 133–148.

Schneider E, & Guralnik J. (1990). The aging of America: Impact on health care costs. *JAMA, 263(17),* 2335–2340.

Shimp LA, Ascione FJ, Glazer HM, Atwood BF. (1985). Potential medication-related problems in noninstitutionalized elderly. *Drug Intell Clin Pharm, 19,* 766–773.

Soumerai S, Avorn J, Ross-Degnan, & Gortmaker S. (1987). Payment restrictions for prescription drugs under Medicaid. *NEJM, 317(9),* 550–556.

Staff. (1991). Rule would make caps on medications easier to open. *Aging, 362,* 60.

Stewart R, Moore M, May F, Marks R, & Hale W. (1991). Changing patterns of therapeutic agents in the elderly: A ten-year overview. *Age and Ageing, 20,* 182–188.

Vestal RE, ed. (1984). Drug treatment in the elderly. Auckland: ADIS Health Science Press.

Weg RB. (1978). Drug interaction with the changing physiology of the aged: Practice and potential. In Kayne RC, ed., *Drugs and the elderly,* p 136. Los Angeles: University of Southern California Press.

Williams P, Rush DR. (1986). Geriatric polypharmacy. *Hosp Pract, (Feb 86),* 109–120.

Bibliography

*Beers M, Ouslander J. (1989). Risk factors in geriatric drug prescribing: A practical guide to avoiding problems. *Drugs 37,* 105–112.

Bird H. (1990). Drugs and the elderly. *Ann Rheum Dis, 49,* 1021–1024.

Burris J. (1991). Management of complicated hypertension. *Geriatric Medicine Today, 10(5),* 31–44.

Griffin M, Piper J, Daugherty J, Snowden M, Ray W. (1991). Nonsteroidal anti-inflammatory drug use and increased risk for peptic ulcer disease in elderly persons. *Ann Intern Med, 114(4),* 257–263.

Gurwitz J, Avorn J, Ross-Degnan D, Lipsitz L. (1990). Nonsteroidal anti-inflammatory drug-associated azotemia in the very old. *JAMA, 264(4),* 471–475.

Lynch R, Horowitz L. (1991). Managing geriatric arrhythmias. II: Drug selection and use. *Geriatrics, 46(4),* 41–54.

McCue J. (1991). Use of the quinolones in the elderly. *Geriatric Medicine Today, 10(1),* 40–47.

*Miller C. (1991). Driving the temperatures up and down. *Geriatric Nursing, January/February,* 44, 48.

*Miller C. (1990). Drugs and the elderly: When medication harms as well as helps. *Geriatric Nursing, Nov–Dec,* 301–302.

National Council on Patient Information and Education. (1987). Priorities and approaches for improving prescription medicine use by older Americans. Washington, DC: Report prepared under a grant from The Commonwealth Fund.

*Newbern V. (1991). Cautionary tales on using beta blockers: The side effects are perilously easy to dismiss in elders because they look like age-related problems. *Geriatric Nursing, May/June,* 119–122.

O'Neill C, Dobbs R, Dobbs S. (1991). Commentary: Measurement of compliance with medication: The 'sine qua non' of clinical trials in old age? *Age and Ageing, 20,* 77–79.

Pepper G. (1991). Monitoring the effects of anticholinergic drugs. In Chenitz C, Stone J, Salisbury S, eds., *Clinical gerontological nursing,* pp 377–389. Philadelphia: WB Saunders.

Shannon M, Lovejoy F. (1990). The influence of age vs peak serum concentration on life-threatening events after chronic theophylline intoxication. *Arch Intern Med, 150,* 2045–2048.

Stone J. (1991). Preventing physical iatrogenic problems. In Chenitz C, Stone J, Salisbury S, ed., *Clinical gerontological nursing,* 359–375. Philadelphia: WB Saunders.

Strome T, Howell T. (1991). How antipsychotics affect the elderly. *American Journal of Nursing, May,* 46–49.

*Todd B. (1990). Drugs and the elderly: Prescription for the '90's. *Geriatric Nursing, May/June,* 114–115

Weder A. (1991). The renally compromised older hypertensive: Therapeutic considerations. *Geriatrics, 46(2),* 36–47.

Yee B, Williams B, O'Hara N. (1990). Medication management and appropriate substance use for elderly persons. In Lewis CB, ed., *Aging: The health care challenge,* 2nd ed, pp 298–329. Philadelphia: FA Davis.

*Recommended for further reading.

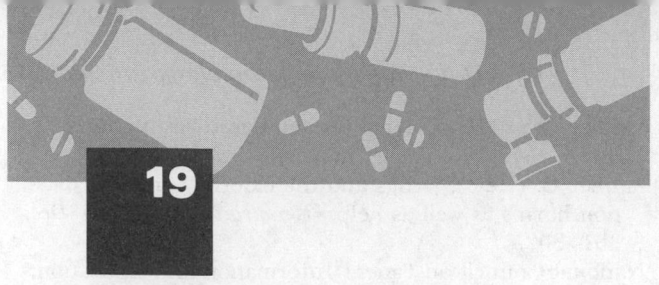

19

Drug therapy in community health nursing

Role of the nurse
  Administration of medication
  Communication and referral
  Knowledge of clients and drugs
  Knowledge of the community
    Community resources
    The community as client
Client variables
The drug history
  Nonconventional drugs
  Drug misuses
Drug effects
Storage, labeling, and disposal
Compliance/alliance
Self-care movement
  Complementary modalities
  Nursing management
    Nursing process

The expansion of the pharmaceutical industry over the last three decades, coupled with the steadily increasing trend toward home health care of acute and chronically ill populations, has presented a special challenge to both the consumer and the provider of health care. In addition to more drugs being available by prescription, a wider variety of over-the-counter (OTC) drugs are being sold.

Home drug use is a rapidly growing multibillion dollar business. Nonprescription drug retail sales (OTC products) have risen from $1.9 billion in 1964 to $11.2 billion in 1990, some 300,000 products that do not include vitamins or minerals (OTC retail sales,

1991). A new drug costs $231 million to create over a 12-year span (Tufts' study, 1990, p 20); approximately 100 new drugs appear on the market annually. Moreover, there is an increasing trend of shifting prescription drugs to OTC status, primarily due to lobbying activities by major drug manufacturers.

Health care providers must strive to increase clients' awareness of available drugs and enhance their appreciation of both the desirable and harmful effects. Moreover, many substances contained within household plants and chemicals, food, and personal care products must be considered when assessing drug use in the home. Because of the way in which these products are advertised and promoted today, there is a tendency to overlook their potentially adverse effects on the body.

The purpose of assessing drug use in the home is twofold: to promote the client's health by increasing his or her understanding of drug self-administration, and to minimize unnecessary drug reactions, incompatibilities, and harmful effects.

This chapter addresses seven factors governing drug use in the home:

- The nurse's role
- Determination of relevant client data
- Goals and method of taking a drug history
- Assessment of drug effects
- Drug storage labeling and disposal
- Compliance/alliance
- Self-care movement

This discussion of the role of the nurse emphasizes the necessary skills and approaches (including a working knowledge of the community and its resources) that can be used to encourage continuity of care within the health care delivery system. Demographic data, social attitudes, and cultural and economic factors can influence the client's safe and effective use of drugs. An approach to taking a drug history in the home is presented that should improve the client's understanding of his or her use of drugs and household products. Also discussed are methods to ensure the proper administration of drugs and ways to monitor their effects and to enhance compliance. Finally, techniques are outlined to promote the proper storage of drugs as part of the nurse's role in the ongoing assessment and monitoring of drug use in the home and community.

Enrichment experience 19-1

Search the nursing literature for a research article that investigates drug use in the home. Critique the article and compare its findings with known practice in your community.

Role of the nurse

Administration of medication

Administering medication is a skilled nursing function. In the hospital setting, it is a frequent, often complex task that requires expertise and specialized techniques. Indeed, administering medicines and monitoring their effects constitute a major part of the hospitalized client's therapeutic regimen. The hospital nurse is responsible for performing these tasks safely and effectively.

When discharged from the hospital, the client and, in some cases, the family assume responsibility for managing the therapeutic regimen. Self-administration of prescribed and nonprescribed drugs is now a recognized part of the health promotion movement in the United States. The health care consumer has begun to take greater responsibility for his or her health status and increasingly expects to be fully informed about available options. This positive, encouraging sign for our times represents a greater emphasis on health promotion and disease prevention. With medications, a potential danger lies in the lack of a natural system of checks and balances inherent in the controlled setting of the hospital. Monitoring a client's administration of medication in the home presents a challenge for the community health nurse (CHN), who must ensure compliance with the medication regimen and tailor the client's care to his or her own environment.

Communication and referral

The issue of continuity of care within the health care delivery system points to the need for faultless communication among health care providers. When making a referral to a CHN, hospital personnel must provide not only the identifying client data but also all relevant medical and nursing background data, medication information, and confirmation that the client understands his or her therapeutic drug regimen. Without this data base, it is difficult for the nurse to assess the client's home self-care reliably and systematically. One approach to alleviating this break in continuity of care would be to involve the client more in his or her discharge plans. Providing the client with medication cards that explain how to identify and administer drugs safely is one method that enhances continuity of care and aids in the nurse's home assessment of drug use.

To ascertain how the client is taking medications, the CHN needs to establish an open, trusting relationship that may take several home visits to achieve before the client is comfortable with sharing this information, especially if the client has demonstrated difficulties in complying with the recommended regimen. On the other hand, the nurse with astute interviewing skills may be able to accomplish a thorough drug use assessment successfully in one home visit.

Knowledge of clients and drugs

The value of knowing the client's health status cannot be overestimated. Obviously, if the client is a pregnant or lactating woman, any drug use must be carefully reviewed and considered. With the client taking medications for a chronic health problem such as diabetes, drug use assessment must include not only a physical assessment and a history of the disease but also the signs and symptoms of hyperglycemia and hypoglycemia; any drug side effects he or she may have experienced throughout the course of the disease; and the client's use of diet and exercise to offset the use of medication.

The CHN needs a thorough knowledge of all drugs a client is taking, including information about their method of administration (dose, route, frequency), their intended effects and the possible side effects, contraindications, and coeffects if he or she is taking two or more drugs. Substance abuse, including such things as the mixing of drugs with alcohol, must also be monitored carefully to avoid potentially harmful effects.

Because of the deinstitutionalization movement, which began in the 1960s, many chronic mentally ill and developmentally disabled persons are now being maintained at home or in group homes. These two populations are often under the care of lay personnel who are supervised by clinical nurse specialists. The complex medication regimen of these persons allows them to remain functional in a homelike community, and requires that they be monitored carefully and continuously. Nurses ministering to these populations are currently working with neuromedical specialists to bring clients toward monotherapy: the use of only one drug to control symptoms and to avoid side effects and multiple drug interactions.

Another growing home care population are hospice clients and their families, including persons with chronic debilitating conditions such as acquired immunodeficiency syndrome. The special medication needs of these persons revolves around pain control and comfort measures that frequently combine "high-tech" methods such as the use of infusion pumps for parenteral nutrition with time-tested home remedies created by families and nurses alike. With the current practice of earlier hospital discharge, clients are taking more medications at home, sometimes without sufficient supervision after beginning a new medication in the hospital. These situations demand that nurses who work with these populations be aware of the many variables that impact on the correct use of drugs in the home environment.

Supervision of the home care paraprofessional in reminding the compromised client to self-administer medication is another responsibility of the CHN. These home care personnel require regular supervision and instruction in their participation in the plan of care. When the nurse prepours the client's medications on a daily or weekly basis, it may become a function of home health aides to remind and assist a client in correctly taking drugs on their shift of care. Clients who live alone and are forgetful or confused or are too weak or incapacitated to handle drug bottles are among those for whom the nurse will involve the home health aide's help. The plan of care in the home must indicate that the aide is to remind the client to take medication. This protects the client and the aide and clarifies the aide's role to any family members involved in the home drug regimen.

Knowledge of the community

Community resources

The CHN should know about community resources available to the client, including the location of a reputable pharmacist for reference purposes, drug education classes, and the local poison control center.

A potential resource in some communities is the pharmacy department of a teaching or university-based hospital, which can provide nurses with drug information updates and new or experimental medications. It is also helpful to know how to contact companies that service drug-related equipment and supplies, such as ambulatory subcutaneous infusion pumps and portable blood glucose monitoring devices.

Nurses may also wish to call or write to the National Council on Patient Information and Education*, a coalition of constituent health-related organizations that works to improve communication about prescription drugs between patients and their health care professionals.

Computer use

Ninety percent of all American pharmacies use computers to process prescriptions (American Society for Automation in Pharmacy, 1991). The drug monitoring program includes maintaining clients' drug profiles for 2–7 years depending on state regulations. When a prescription is filled, the pharmacist enters it into the computer under the client's account. If the client informs the pharmacist of any food or drug allergies, these can be checked against each chemical ingredient in the drug. Any incompatibilities can thereby be detected, allowing the pharmacist to alert both physician and client of the situation. Furthermore, any additional prescriptions can be entered and checked against all existing data, chemical by chemical, to inform the pharmacist whether the drug combination is safe. If incompatibilities are identified, the pharmacist can choose to tell both the physician and client before dispensing the drug. This service represents an added measure of protection in ensuring the safe use of drugs in the community. To the extent that all relevant data are obtained and entered into the system, this community resource can serve as an effective, reliable, and accessible means of preventing unnecessary adverse drug interactions. The nurse should be aware of this resource to enhance the care of clients taking prescription drugs, especially in light of the increasing amount of prescription drug advertisement and use by consumers.

Other software programs available to the community-based pharmacist can provide the following:

- Cards to remind the client to refill drugs, thus encouraging compliance
- A patient education monograph that can be customized to indicate how to take and store a given drug and identify side effects
- A telephone service that allows clients to call a 900 number, key in the USP code number on their prescription label and obtain information on that drug 24 hours a day (a fee is required for use of a 900 number) (American Society for Automation in Pharmacy, 1991)

These innovative services increase the client's participation with his or her health care providers and strive to improve the effectiveness of the therapeutic regimen while reducing adverse effects.

The limitations of the computer as a community resource must be considered. As mentioned, it can only compare drugs that have been entered and these are usually only prescribed drugs. Over-the-counter preparations or drugs previously prescribed and filled at other pharmacies may be overlooked and in some cases may not even be acceptable to the particular pharmacy system. Other community resources, such as the local pharmacist or possibly a hospital-based pharmacy, should be pursued when questions arise about potential incompatibilities of a client's drugs. By combining the efforts of CHN, pharmacist, and physician, harmful drug reactions can be avoided while at the same time strengthening the lines of communication among all of the client's health care providers.

Alert system

Some communities may have an alert system for elderly clients. In these systems, a bright sticker listing the drugs the client is taking is placed in a prominent position in the household for use as reference in case of an emergency such as an overdose, a relapse of the disease process, or an adverse drug reaction. In some communities, clients who live alone may be able to subscribe to a call-in service where if the client fails to call by a particular time each day a call will be made to verify that he or she is at home. If there is no response, someone will visit immediately. Several varieties of home electronic alert systems have been developed to link clients instantly to a 24-hour emergency service. Even a bed-bound or partially paralyzed client can

---

* National Council on Patient Information and Education, 666 11th Street, N.W., Suite 810, Washington, D.C. 20001. (202) 347-6711.

enjoy the security such a system can provide. Should the client experience any difficulties or medical problems, he or she activates the device sending a signal to the emergency service operator who then calls the client to obtain further information and activate immediate assistance if necessary.

Services such as these provide the client with a level of independence while offering some protection against possible harm from unexpected drug effects.

Enrichment experience 19-2

Interview a pharmacist about his or her role in consumer education, including questions about the average cost of drug therapy (*eg*, for insulin or digoxin).

The community as client

The idea of community as client has been discussed in the nursing and public health literature and represents an aggregate approach toward identifying and solving large-scale health problems. The CHN's role will depend on how a community is defined (*eg*, a neighborhood composed of census tracts, an ethnic group within a geographic location, or a subpopulation known by their health attitudes, beliefs, or habits). Using epidemiologic methods together with the nursing process, a given community's drug-related problems may be identified, and relevant programs planned, implemented, and evaluated. Some ways to assess such problems include the following:

- Comparing the crime and death rates involving drugs in one community with a similar community to determine the magnitude of the problem;
- Determining the extent to which homeopathy is used in a given community versus the use of conventional (OTC and prescribed drugs) for home remedies; and
- Examining the effect of toxic effluents from industry on the local environment.

Examples of community as client are the ethnic populations in a given area. When health care providers consider the drug-taking practices of these clients, they must be aware of how the clients define a drug, when and how they self-administer drugs, who usually takes drugs, and generally how clients respond to drug therapy. Similarly, the nurse who cares for a client must become familiar with the client's attitudes toward drugs, as well as the common beliefs about health conditions for which drugs are used, especially the major health care problems occurring in that community. In some cases, the client may tend to use home remedies, homeopathics, and the advice of elders or nonprofessional "specialists" in the community. This background knowledge of who the client is and what resources are available to the community as a whole are important aspects of community-based nursing practice. (For further information about ethnic health care behaviors see Chapter 12.)

When drug-related problems occur in a community, specific measures can be employed by the CHN to reduce or eliminate them. These measures include educating the target population; documenting problems to local officials to enhance public awareness and participation; and working with other health care professionals to prevent misuse and abuse of drugs in the entire population or in at-risk groups only. Occupational health nurses are frequently the first to identify drug problems and harmful exposure to chemical and other environmental pollutants by carefully monitoring employees' cumulative health care complaints.

Likewise, school nurses may assess a group problem involving drugs by considering variations in students' attendance rates, grades, and excuses from school for unexplained reasons. Effective action to solve such community health problems involves a dual level approach: the community as a whole and individual members. When drug and substance abuse has been documented in a specific population (*eg*, early teenagers), parents, teachers, police, and other community leaders may institute a media campaign about the hazards of social drug and alcohol use. In addition to such collective action, individuals such as the school nurse may also provide one-to-one or small group education for students in need of a more personalized approach to their drug problems.

Based on a familiarity with the community's health patterns, the nurse can institute measures of prevention at all three levels:

1. Primary prevention aims at promoting health and well being, usually through education.
2. Secondary prevention deals with early diagnosis and screening of health care problems.
3. Tertiary prevention focuses on efforts of rehabilitation and maximizing one's abilities.

Community-based nurses should be involved with all members of the community to achieve better health and health care for the entire group.

■ Summary

The CHN assists clients to manage their drug regimens for optimum effect. Both prescription and OTC drug use must be monitored. Because clients are managing very serious health problems in the home, present day regimens may be very complex.

The CHN also participates in community programs designed to decrease the incidence of drug abuse and accidental poisoning.

Client variables

Whether clients are individuals, families, or communities, the nurse should establish a working rapport and professional relationship with the client. The nurse can then proceed to obtain an accurate data base, beginning with the collection of data for relevant client variables such as allergies, health status, length of time taking drugs, and knowledge about drug effects. (See Box 19-1 for a complete list of pertinent variables.)

Becoming acquainted with the client as a person with individual beliefs, values, and cultural background may never be fully achieved. The baseline information that is essential can, however, often be learned while assessing other aspects of the client's health care regimen. Self-care activities such as eating a well-balanced diet, regular exercise, and daily health-related habits (eg, recreation and relaxation) may suggest the client's attitude toward self-administration of drugs.

Over the course of their relationship, the astute nurse will ascertain the client's self-concept, especially as it relates to his or her attitude about drugs in general and level of motivation for following a specific drug regimen.

One of the first questions to ask clients when making a drug assessment is whether they can explain the effect of a drug on the body and on the disease process. This will provide the nurse not only with information about the client's mental state but also will give an idea of the client's *vocabulary, knowledge,* and *intellectual level.* When such information is obtained at the beginning of the drug interview, the nurse can develop a framework within which to plan further teaching and interventions.

Learning experience 19-1

Note the number and variety of drug references available in the public library. Enumerate the consumer drug literature found in a popular bookstore. Examine and compare one of these books to this text, noting how the drugs are categorized and the information presented.

The *age* of the client may also be helpful in assessing experience with drugs. The older the client, the more potential exposure he or she has had to various OTC and prescribed medications, and a greater experience with home remedies and previous advice from family, friends, and health care providers. The younger the client, the greater the chance of generally accepting drugs because of the effects of mass media, peer influence about illicit drug use, and recent proliferation of drugs from the pharmaceutical industry. Whereas older clients may be reluctant to take even prescribed medications because of their belief that drugs may be harmful, younger clients may tend to take various drugs for common ailments such as fatigue, stomachache, and feelings of depression. The reverse of this argument is also true. Because older clients have witnessed the advent and widespread successful use of drugs, they may tend to accept drug therapy without question on the advice of peers and professionals alike. On the other hand, younger clients may have observed the harmful effects of drugs on their friends or learned about adverse drug effects in health education classes and may, therefore, be hesitant to take OTC or prescription drugs for diagnosed health problems. Because this is such a complex issue, nurses must avoid stereotyping any client according to a single factor such as age.

The client's *role within the family* structure often tells the nurse the amount of responsibility he or she is assuming for administering drugs to himself or herself and to other family members. With an elderly parent, for example, a son or daughter may assume full responsibility for administering medications. On the

---

Box 19-1. Client variables that affect drug use in the home

Alliance (compliance) with drug regimen

Knowledge of drug
   Administration
   Regimen
   Action effects
   Side effects
   Contraindications

Knowledge of disease process

Mental and emotional status

Motivation

Age

Role in family

Cultural/ethnic background

Socioeconomic status

Attitudes about self-care

Health status

Lifestyle

Attitudes and beliefs about drugs

Previous experience with drugs

Length of time taking drugs

Level of education

Level of intelligence

Language barrier

Sensory and physical impairments

Allergies

other hand, the parent of teenagers may be overly cautious about their use of drugs and may not want them to assume their own self-care despite potential ability. In every case, the nurse needs to encourage the appropriate self-care and independent drug administration for the client of whatever age.

Clients' *socioeconomic status* has several different effects on compliance to the drug regimen. Such information, coupled with clients' cultural beliefs about drugs, helps the nurse to understand the level of importance that drug-taking behavior has for them. Medications may be purchased regularly and self-administered by clients regardless of the financial cost to the family. Some, however, believe that a prescribed medication such as allergy shots is nontherapeutic or a waste of money and may refuse or discontinue it prematurely even though they can afford the therapy. When drugs are not included in their insurance reimbursement plan, clients may not comply with their prescription or may replace it with a cheaper substitute or home remedy, resulting in possible embarrassment when this substitution is discovered. The nurse then has to urge correct drug compliance in the face of a situation that has external factors beyond the nurse's control. The use of less expensive generic drugs has helped to alleviate this situation somewhat, but the problem may continue for the elderly and persons on fixed incomes who have inadequate insurance coverage.

The client's *previous experience with drugs* especially during hospitalization and particularly as a result of traumatic or chronic illness must be assessed by the nurse. Experience with a previously successful cure from drug therapy is likely to enhance compliance with a current drug regimen in the home. Further, the client's understanding about the expected effect of the drug, as well as a belief that the drug therapy will promote well-being, will tend to result in accurate drug self-treatment.

The client's *health condition* at the time of the drug assessment has to be considered. Short-course drug therapy for an acute illness after either hospitalization or a visit to the physician is likely to be managed correctly by a client whose previous health status was stable and uncomplicated. The experience of living with chronic illness may also help to motivate the client's drug compliance at home.

On the other hand, clients unwilling to accept the daily responsibility for following their drug therapy accurately require additional monitoring in the home and necessitate continued teaching and assessment by the nurse. Moreover, such clients are often readmitted to the hospital owing to exacerbations of their illness that might have been prevented if a reminder or backup system had been provided for the client.

Other aspects of assessing a client's home drug use are easier to determine. If there is a language barrier, it will probably be manifested during the initial contacts with the client and may be remedied by the use of translators from the family or the community. The client's *level of education* and the related factor of *level of intelligence* can be assessed from data gathered during the rapport-building home visits. Level of education can be ascertained from the client's verbal skills; level of intelligence can be assessed through questions about drug knowledge, health status, and understanding of a medication's effect on bodily functions. A high level of education does not guarantee the desired level of compliance. Likewise, a low level of education does not necessarily mean a lack of intelligence. Mitigating factors such as fear of medication, lack of belief in their therapeutic effects, insufficient funds, illiteracy, and a poor memory can reduce drug compliance and make the assessment difficult and possibly inaccurate.

The nurse needs to be aware of cues indicating that clients understand their drug regimens. One way to obtain this information is to ask open-ended questions about the system used for taking drugs. For less articulate clients, asking them to demonstrate this system can achieve a similar outcome.

Questions about *sensory* and *physical impairments* cannot be overlooked. Asking the client to demonstrate how he or she prepares and administers drugs may be essential in this case. Partial blindness owing to glaucoma, cataracts, untreated visual disturbances, or a dyslexic condition may be detected from the client's performance of this task. Difficulty in opening a medication container or in pouring a liquid preparation or a glass of water may indicate a psychomotor disturbance, such as intentional tremors, arthritis, or Parkinsonian gestures. With any known impediment to the correct dispensing of medication by the client, the nurse should report such signs and symptoms to the physician for further medical work-up. In some cases, an alternative system of administering the medication may have to be devised in the interim; for example, soliciting the aid of a family member, friend, or neighbor, or making use of devices that aid in the correct administration of drugs. The nurse should periodically spotcheck the client in whom an impairment is suspected, preferably at different times of the day and week.

■ Summary

An open nurse–client relationship in the home setting fosters a more thorough drug use assessment. A drug assessment is best done over the course of several home visits. When time does not allow for this natural unfolding of pertinent client information, however, the nurse will need to assess these variables while taking a more formal drug history. The use of such a systematic drug history is actually a sharing of information between client and nurse, with the desired outcome being a more complete identification and proper administration of all drug forms commonly found in the home.

The drug history

If possible, the nurse should take a thorough drug history from every client and family who is visited regularly. When deciding whether a drug history should be taken, one must consider three factors: the client's degree of illness, the amount and types of medication taken, and the client's ability to comply with the drug regimen. (See goals and objectives listed in Box 19-2.)

Naturally, clients of any age with a chronic illness that requires drug therapy will need a thorough drug history. Any client taking one or more prescribed medications should also be interviewed to assess the expected action and effects of the drug.

When an acute or chronic disease that results in changes in bodily functions is newly diagnosed, the nurse must reassess the client for the need to alter the drug regimen. For a client undergoing a stressful life experience such as a job change or loss of a spouse, the nurse should be reminded to inquire about any actual or potential changes in drug use habits.

Nonconventional drugs

Another good reason to question clients about their home drug use is to increase their knowledge of the wide assortment of nonprescription drugs available to them that often are not recognizable as drugs. This process of assessment can result in teaching clients a greater awareness and appreciation of drugs and an increasing sense of responsibility for and control over self-care.

The term *drug* may be perceived by clients in various ways. Therefore, the scope of drug use in the home setting needs clarification. A drug may be defined as any substance that has a beneficial or harmful effect on the body. For purposes of an accurate and comprehensive drug history, the categorization presented below is useful.

A drug is any substance that is

- Applied: for example, deodorants, cosmetics, depilatories, soaps, detergents, hair rinses, dyes, dentifrices, lotions, ointments, transdermal patches
- Ingested: for example, tablets, pills, capsules, vitamins, minerals, syrups, house plants, leaded paints, lozenges, herbal teas, bicarbonate of soda, elixirs, alcohol
- Inhaled: for example, exhaust fumes from buses, tobacco, marijuana, spray cleaners, industrial pollutants, fumes from bleach, ammonia, and other house cleaning products
- Injected: for example, serums, insulin, vitamins, spider and insect bites, "hard" drugs, antiallergens, antileukemics, narcotics, hormones, antineoplastics
- Inserted: for example, suppositories (vaginal and rectal), contraceptives, sublingual preparations, gelatin sponges
- Instilled: for example, ear, nose, and eye drops, solutions for catheter and wound irrigations

Items prepared in the home may be seen as subcategories of applied or ingested drugs. Home remedies such as poultices and vegetable or herbal concoctions may be made from family or traditional medicinal recipes. In addition, many constituents used in the preparation of food products must also be considered drugs (*eg*, preservatives, additives, monosodium glutamate, vitamins, and herbs). Although this information may be difficult to obtain, it can be crucial for both the client and nurse when assessing the total sources of drugs in the home.

This method of categorizing drugs raises the client's awareness about the products used in daily activities. He or she may not be aware, for example, of the side effects of harsh detergents, hard water, or food additives on bodily functions. Clients taking multiple laxative preparations may be having the drug's intended effects canceled out and thus may be taking them without benefit.

Drug misuse

Apparent abuse can, in fact, be misuse owing to misinformation. Such situations arise with clients who seek medical attention from more than one source, resulting in multiple prescriptions of similar-acting drugs.

Box 19-2. Goals and objectives of completing a drug history in the home

Goals

Clarify the definition of drugs with the client and family

Assure that the drugs are having the desired effects

Prevent drug misuse

Objectives

List all drugs taken by each family member

Assess the client for understanding of the drug regimen

Observe for therapeutic and side effects

Monitor related physical signs as they are affected by drugs

Assess the client's motivation to comply with the drug regimen

Examine the household for proper storage of all products having potential pharmaceutical effects

Some clients may inadvertently take drugs that potentiate each other, especially when OTC and prescribed drugs are taken together without the physician's knowledge. The nurse must report such situations to the client's physician. In addition, the client's pharmacist should be notified so that the prescriptions can be verified and crosschecked with the client's physician. Some clients may not admit their use of illicit or recreational drugs owing to a fear of discovery by an "authority," as in the case of drug addicts both young and old.

Drug effects

Drug use in the home implies that the nurse include the routine assessment of both the intended effect and the side effects of the drugs. First, the nurse needs to ask clients general questions about whether the drug is having the desired effect. The nurse may also ask them what the physician and pharmacist, as well as family and friends, have told them about the drug. Second, questions about specific effects of the drug should be posed in an organized manner. If clients have observed any side effects, the nurse should inquire about what action they took, if any, to alleviate them. Finally, objective findings that document and measure the effects of the drug should be sought. For clients taking antihypertensive medications, for example, the nurse should take a blood pressure reading and compare it to previous data. For persons taking diuretics, the nurse should observe them for signs of dehydration, dry skin and mouth, and ankle edema; monitor their weight, urinary output and lung sounds; and assess their dietary and prescribed potassium supplements.

Side effects are best assessed by posing open-ended questions about any undesirable effects of the medications. Specific questions about the occurrence of known side effects of the client's drugs should then be asked systematically. When side effects include potential alterations in physical signs, the nurse will need to assess and record them appropriately. Any adverse or undesired drug effects should be noted, explained to the client, and promptly reported to the physician, if possible right after their discovery. Role-modeling this kind of activity in the home can teach clients self-care and enhance awareness of their responsibility for regular and safe self-medication.

Storage, labeling, and disposal

When reviewing the possible hazards involved with storing drugs, the nurse should remind the client to inspect all OTC drugs at the time of purchase for evidence of tampering. The client should suspect tampering if the package with an indicator or a barrier to entry has been breached or is missing. In addition, the appearance of all OTC drugs should be checked for

the possibility of contamination (*eg*, color and odor inconsistencies). Such an observation should be reported to the pharmacist, who could then assist the client in selecting an alternative product.

The nurse should observe how the client's medications are stored in the home. Some medications must be stored away from excessive heat, light, and moisture, whereas other preparations such as suppositories need to be refrigerated. In every case, the nurse should check to see that all drugs and chemicals are stored out of the reach of children and, except for clients who have physical handicaps such as arthritis or paralysis, that drugs are capped with childproof devices. In such extenuating circumstances, clients should request that the pharmacist use regular caps. Additionally, the nurse should check to see that each drug is stored in its own container and is labeled correctly.

When checking prescribed medications, the nurse should note whether they are all from the same physician and the same pharmacy. She should look at the number of pills, tablets, or capsules prescribed versus the number in the bottle (or quantity of liquid). The original quantity dispensed can be verified with the pharmacist by referring to the prescription number on the bottle. The quantity of pills or liquid remaining should relate to the date they were prescribed, the dose, and frequency of intended administration. Any discrepancies should be noted and discussed with the client and, if necessary, reported to the physician with the client's knowledge.

Labels on prescribed medication provide the nurse with a great amount of information. Typical information is outlined in Box 19-3. In some states, expiration dates appear only on OTC products but most liquid preparations do include them. Clients should be cautioned to check their medications regularly for expiration dates, as well as for any consistency or color changes. Some drug labels may include warnings or recommendations, such as to avoid driving, to take the drug with milk, or to refrain from the use of alcohol during a specified period after the administration of the drug. The nurse should also note if the client is taking a generic drug in addition to a similar brand name drug.

Obviously all labels should be legible and waterproof to ensure correct administration by the client. When the nurse or client has been instructed verbally by the physician to alter the administration of a drug, the label must be updated and changed to reflect the new regimen. Again, any discrepancies should be pointed out to the client and reported to the physician. Any unusual label notations or instructions should be investigated in case the physician or pharmacist has made a mistake.

A further consideration to the safe use of drugs at home includes the proper disposal of contaminated

Box 19-3. Checking the prescription label

Identifying information

- Client's name and address
- Physician's name
- Name of pharmacy, address, and telephone number
- Name of manufacturer (in most states)
- Prescription number

Medication data

- Dose
- Strength
- Route
- Directions for administration
- Warnings
- Expiration date
- Date prescription filled
- Refill information

General considerations

- Generic versus brand-name medication
- Legible
- Easy-open when necessary
- Waterproof
- Proper storage
- Appearance
- Prescriptions from multiple physicians

needles and other objects soiled with bodily wastes. Items such as used needles, syringes, drug vials, intervenous tubing, and lancets should be placed into a sturdy container—an empty thick plastic detergent bottle or preferably a metal coffee can with a tight-fitting lid. When the container is full, the contents should be covered with a solution of 1 part household bleach and 10 parts water. The container is then covered, taped tightly, and placed into two plastic bags. This parcel is then tied securely and thrown into the garbage. Naturally, it is important to wash one's hands before and after following this procedure.

The best method of disposing of leftover drugs is to burn them. If the home has a wood-burning stove, this may be done. In U.S. homes without such a stove, disposal of leftover medications involves emptying all containers and flushing the contents down a toilet. Canada has a program whereby designated community agencies such as the police or fire departments accept medications and dispose of them.

■ Summary

The nurse's interviewing and assessment skills, when employed consistently and appropriately, can create an open environment in which the client can learn about the effects of drugs on his or her health care problem. The challenge of completing a systematic drug history in the home includes increasing the client's knowledge about drugs and enhancing compliance to the drug regimen. The desired outcome of home drug assessment is the regular and safe drug self-administration by a client who is motivated, cooperative, and well informed.

Issues in drug therapy

Proper disposal of unused drugs in the home: home versus community-sponsored programs

Home disposal

Flushing into sewers is wasteful, potentially dangerous and pollutes the environment.

Control is uncertain—drugs may be diverted and misused.

This method is easy and readily available in most homes.

Disposal can be immediate and efficient.

Community program

These programs are potentially expensive.

Drug containers may be tampered with, in which case those handling the drugs may experience adverse reactions to chemical exposure, or infection from contaminated needles.

Accountable personnel must be developed.

Recycling of unused/untampered drugs may be promoted.

Can ensure destruction drugs.

Compliance/alliance

The issue of compliance is all too familiar to CHNs. Noncompliance is often the reason a referral is generated, which with a prescribed drug regimen can bear many negative connotations. The term *noncompliance* is provider-generated, and only defines the problem from the provider's perspective. Not adhering to a drug regimen may be viewed as deviant behavior by a health care provider, although the client sees this action as a cautious approach to self-administration of potentially harmful substances. A client may choose not to take a drug as prescribed for a variety of valid reasons or may not be aware of the correct doses and regimen. Whatever the reason, the nurse must avoid a one-sided judgmental approach and instead must work with the client to achieve the desired effect of the drug in a manner acceptable to both.

The term *alliance* has been suggested to replace the idea of compliance in attempting to describe client-provider interactions with drug regimes. The evolving self-care movement by health care consumers supports this less deviant and more contractual equilateral level of health care delivery in the home. A nurse researcher has presented data on a client's alliance in managing a chronic illness (Thorne, 1989). A key factor identified is clients' trust in the health care professional and trust in their own competence.

According to a survey of nurses regarding their views on drug compliance (Moree, 1985), the amount of noncompliance observed with their clients was between 10% and 75% with an average of 50%. Half of the noncompliant persons were age 65 and older. These nurses cited the causes of clients' noncompliance to include believing the drug is no longer needed, confusion about the regimen, and fear of addiction and side effects. Among suggestions to improve drug regimen compliance, the nurses cited the importance of working with physicians and pharmacists to simplify and reduce drug regimens and to clarify their instructions, and with drug companies to reduce costs and generate more once-a-day drugs. The nurse's client advocacy role assumes increasing importance in the light of the current array of drugs and drug marketing or advertising techniques in our society.

Because the CHN works with the client in the context of family and community, he or she must also view the problem of compliance from a broad perspective. Thus, the use of a thorough drug history must be emphasized to afford the nurse the greatest amount of data from which to plan interventions and evaluate outcomes of nursing care.

Self-care movement

The first decade of the diagnosis and treatment of persons with acquired immunodeficiency syndrome has led to an expanded home care population that has learned to provide complex drug treatment regimens safely at home. It is a community that continues to demand more involvement in their health care decisions.

A new technology has been developed to provide home care support to persons living with acquired immunodeficiency syndrome in the community. One nursing study demonstrated the feasibility of using home-based computer networks to provide information, communication, and decision assistance to this population (Brennan, Ripich, & Moore, 1991). The authors encourage the application of this model to other community-based populations, which could include virtually any person with access to a computer.

The self-care movement can be extended to other populations as well. Persons undergoing outpatient chemotherapy, ambulatory surgery, and ongoing blood transfusions, in addition to insulin-dependent and noninsulin-dependent diabetics, are learning to be proficient and reliable in their home care.

Consumer-oriented texts proliferate as the public seeks to become more self-directed in the treatment of their health care concerns.

In Canada, it is estimated that between 70% to 90% of all illness episodes are handled by self-treatment. The advent and use of diagnostic related groups (DRGs) in hospitals in the U.S. in the 1980s has yielded a boon to the marketing of a broad array of home care products in the 1990s. Since the regulation of for-profit home health agencies in 1985, and the change in third party reimbursement mechanisms, consumers and physicians alike have become more comfortable in adapting hospital-based drug administration policies to the home. The range of services these agencies are equipped to deliver include: management of venous access devices; stabilization therapies, that is, intravenous antibiotics parenteral and enteral feedings; pain management; chemotherapy; investigational therapies (phases 1 and 2).

The increased use of self-regulatory devices in the home is another example of the proliferation of the self-care movement. These items include: blood glucose and cholesterol monitors; self-administered sphygmomanometers; products to test for strep throat and urinary tract infection, ovulation, impotence, pulmonary function; the presence of drugs of abuse in urine; and home pregnancy tests and uterine monitors (Coons, et al, 1989). Their safe and effective use is best assessed at regular intervals by the CHN who is familiar with the client's overall health status.

Another trend in home health care is the use of complementary modalities that may enhance or mitigate the use of drugs, whether prescribed or OTC preparations. These "holistic" remedies include the use of nursing measures such as therapeutic touch to reduce pain and promote relaxation, massage to relieve sore muscles, and visualization and imagery to enhance the client's participation in the healing process. These and other contemporary nursing care interventions may be offered to clients as part of the nursing care plan with a view to involving the client, family, and home care paraprofessional in the alleviation of symptoms and the safe and optimal use of drugs in the home.

The increase in the number of home births and deaths further demonstrates the public's increasing desire to minister to a family member at these two highly charged life transition periods. For the terminally ill person in a home hospice care program, the CHN can help generate a safe, client- and family-centered plan of care that incorporates both the traditional, prescribed drug regime with the use of other measures, such as diversional and recreational therapy, music and art therapy, back rubs and warm baths, where appropriate.

■ Summary

In response to this surge in the home health self-care industry, CHNs are involved with a variety of activities at the local, state, and national levels to ensure clients' access to safe home care. Community health nurses coordinate the client's home care, which includes technical service house calls provided by contractual agencies to administer drug and other therapies, for example, oxygen, intravenous fluids, and hyperalimentation. The Intravenous Nursing Society has created home care standards in an effort to control and define their scope of practice. Clearly, nurses who work in this expanding arena require advanced clinical expertise and experience in both high-tech and home care practice (Humphrey, 1988). On the national scene, CHNs are involved in lobbying for clients' access to safe and accountable home health care. The CHN's role of client advocate is crucial at this time of transition from hospital to home-based care, and from third party reimbursement to national health care insurance mechanisms.

Nursing management

Nursing process

Assessment As in any valid assessment, the nurse first ascertains what the client knows and believes about his or her use of drugs. It is essential to listen to how the client describes or explains what he or she thinks is important to understand about the drug regimen. Corresponding to this foundational data, one nurse author cites the importance of establishing a cooperative and nonauthoritative relationship wherein the nurse is viewed as a "mutual participator" who exhibits a "no-fault" approach toward enhancing correct adherence to a drug regimen (Carey, 1984, p 161).

Assessing the client's compliance to prescribed medications begins with obtaining an accurate account of the drug regimen. For a medication that has been scheduled four times a day, the nurse may ask how the client remembers to take it, for example, with breakfast, lunch, dinner, and at bedtime. If a medication needs to be stored out of sight (away from children), the nurse would ascertain how the client is reminded to take it as prescribed. Suggestions such as a note on the refrigerator or in a familiar place, or associating a specific time or favorite snack with the medication may be offered if indicated. Employing the help of a family member has been found to be most beneficial, regardless of memory function. A home dispensing method may also be necessary (Fig. 19-1).

The nurse should check to see that the appropriate amount of medication has been left in the bottle since the last time the prescription was filled. Any discrepancy—too little or too great an amount left—should cue the nurse into further questioning about compliance. This situation may have occurred owing to memory loss, unexpressed fear of drugs, a lack of belief in the intended effects of the drug, unpleasant side effects, or a decision that the drug has achieved its effect before the prescription was exhausted. With a parent who incorrectly administers medication to a child, the possibility of child abuse or neglect should be considered. The nurse would need to document the situation thoroughly and carefully and report it to the appropriate authority.

Nursing diagnosis The most common diagnosis pertaining to medication in the home is nonalliance (noncompliance) with the prescribed drug regimen.

Planning A client's noncompliance must be addressed as openly and as clearly as possible. The nurse should strive to foster a mutually agreeable goal of

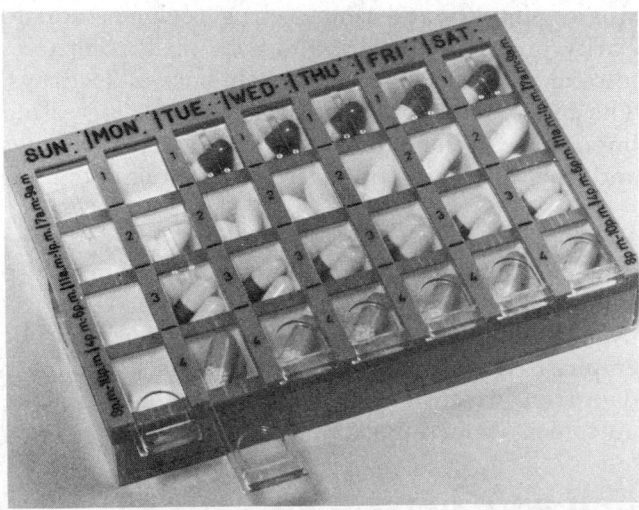

Figure 19-1. Commercial drug dispensing tray for clients to use in the home. The use of such a tray helps the client to administer the medication prescribed. (Mediset, Robbins Associates, Inc., Burnsville, MN)

compliance with the client so that a firm foundation of expected outcomes can be identified. Once this mutual contract has been established, strategies can be implemented to achieve the stated objectives. In the case of clients who are noncompliant due to a lack of knowledge about the consequences of not adhering to the prescribed regimen, the nurse verbalizes this observation and assessment. If he or she agrees with this assessment and sees the relationship between noncompliance and the signs and symptoms of exacerbations of health problems, he or she may be ready to alter drug-taking habits.

Motivation to pursue behavior change is primarily the responsibility of the client. Nonetheless, the CHN, together with the client's physician and family members, can increase motivation in several ways. First, information about the effects of the drugs on the client's condition and the risks of noncompliance must be clear, nonthreatening, and well understood by the client. Second, barriers to taking the drugs as indicated must be identified and eliminated or at the least minimized. This may include physical limitations imposed by disease or disabling conditions, or other causes that decrease access to the drug (*eg*, childproof caps). Third, the client should be approached as a partner in the drug regimen by formulating a plan in which both the nurse and client offer, implement, and evaluate solutions in the context of the same goal: a well defined concept of how the client can safely and effectively adhere to the drug regimen to foster and achieve good health.

Intervention A nurse who has identified a compliance problem owing to poor memory or an inability to open medication containers may want to initiate a home drug-dispensing system. One such system is the egg carton or ice-cube tray method for pills, tablets, and capsules (Figure 19-1). With this system, the nurse arranges the client's medications in compartments for the period of time until the next home visit. Each compartment is labeled with the time and day when that dose should be taken. A separate list of all drugs to be taken, including those prescribed on an as-needed basis, is also kept nearby, indicating what each drug is and its action, effects, and schedule. If possible, a family member or friend should be available for backup support.

Commercial products are available for this same purpose and are particularly helpful to clients who need a weekly set-up of their medication (see Figure 19-1). One system comprises a tray divided into seven sections labeled with each day of the week with four compartments per day. Each compartment has a separate cover to avoid accidental spillage. The tray is especially useful to blind persons, forgetful clients, and for those who do not want to bother with the daily dispensing of their drugs. It can be easily taken to the physician's office at the time of a check-up or on a trip when the drug regimen is likely to be disrupted because of altered time schedules. An advantage of both the homemade and the commercial product is that they promote self-monitoring by the client or client's family.

Community health nurses should become involved in community programs to increase compliance. Interventions may include public service announcements, letters to the newspaper editor, drug education classes for at-risk groups, and other methods mentioned previously. (Refer to discussion in Chapter 26 on compliance with psychoactive drugs.)

Not least among interventions is the routine practice by hospital, clinic, and CHNs of exchanging relevant information about compliance issues. Owing to the increasing number of clients of all ages with multiple chronic conditions that involve complex drug regimens, there has been a rise in the number of "revolving door" hospital admissions and emergency room visits for an apparent lapse in the client's drug regimen. Although it may be tempting to blame the client for noncompliance in these situations, the reasons for exacerbation of the disease may be caused by a host of other factors.

It is important, therefore, for health care providers to be aware of the client's situation and to be cognizant of interventions that have proved helpful in either setting. For example, when a newly diagnosed diabetic client is readmitted to the hospital for assessment and treatment of errant blood sugar levels, the CHN, with the client's knowledge, can call the hospital nurse to relate the client's drug-taking regimen at home; the occurrence of any side effects; useful practices by the client for self-administration; and possibly some background information on how the client best learns about the use and effect of drugs for this condition. When the client is ready for discharge, compliance with the new drug regimen can be fostered by the hospital nurse providing written, clear instructions for both the client and the CHN.

Furthermore, the client's subsequent visits to the clinic or physician's office should be accompanied by communication between nurses in both settings regarding the client's status and progress. These measures help to promote continuity of care, reduce noncompliance, and enhance the client's return to optimum health. In addition, they underscore the interdependence of health care providers in various settings, thus emphasizing the need for timely and pertinent communication. The nurse must remain open to trying new interventions, keeping in mind both the goals of the drug therapy and the client. This is a challenging and often rewarding nurse-client interaction that can yield a greater understanding of each other's attitudes about drugs.

Defining clients' unique sets of variables, establishing workable contracts, eliminating or reducing barriers to drug taking, and teaching about the effects of the drugs should help to increase motivation, knowledge, and compliance and thereby yield reliable self-care. Any intermittent support should be readily available from the nurse and others as necessary. Obviously, if clients are not able or do not agree to assume this responsibility, situations must be reevaluated. In some cases, perfect compliance will never be achieved. In other instances, a compromise may be sought to minimize the risks of symptom recurrence and to maximize the client's participation, especially in reporting any side effects that occur.

In any case, the client and nurse must be mutually accountable if a workable solution is to be found and incorporated into the client's drug-taking routine. The nurse must refrain from judgmental attitudes or punitive actions, remembering that ultimately the taking of any drug is the choice of the client or family (for a child or dependent adult). The client's rights must be upheld; in the broad realm of health care, this right is receiving increasing attention and discussion by consumers and professionals alike.

Evaluation Data pertaining to outcome criteria may include establishment of clear goals that are shared by the client and health care personnel; adherence of the client to the agreed-upon health care regimen; and improvements in health status of the client (as measured by changes in signs and symptoms of the client's health problems).

References

American Society for Automation in Pharmacy. (1991). Blue Bell, PA. (personal correspondence)

Brennan PF, Ripich S, Moore SM. (1991). The use of home-based computers to support persons living with AIDS/ARC. *Journal of Community Health Nursing, 8(1),* 3–14.

Caremark, Inc. (1991). New York (personal correspondence) Computers to support persons living with AIDS/ARC. *Journal of Community Health Nursing, 8(1),* 3–14.

Carey R. (1984). Compliance and related nursing actions. *Nurs Forum, 20(2),* 157–161.

Coons SJ, Fink JL. (1989). The pharmacist, the law and self testing products. *American Pharmacy, NS29 (11),* 35–38.

Fortune M. (1981). Discharge audit: A study of the adequacy and reliability of client referrals from Strong Memorial Hospital to community health nurses in Monroe County. July–August (unpublished).

Humphrey CJ. (1988). The home as a setting for care. Clarifying the boundaries of practice. *Nurs Clin North Am, 23(2),* 305–314.

OTC retail sales. (1991). Washington, DC: Nonprescription Drug Manufacturers Association.

Segall A. (1990). A community survey of self-medication activities. *Med Care, 28(4),* 301–310.

Thorne SE. (1989). Guarded alliance: Health care relationships in chronic illness. *Image—the Journal of Nursing Scholarship, 21(3),* 153–157.

Tufts' study. (1990). *Oncology, 4(7),* 20.

Bibliography

Azzarello JD. (1989). Reviewing your patient's medication regimen: A systemic approach. *Home Healthcare Nurse 7(6),* 24–26.

Beebe CA, Pastors JG, Powers MA, Wylie-Rosett J. (1991). Nutrition management for individuals with noninsulin-dependent diabetes mellitus in the 1990s: A review by the Diabetes Care and Education Dietetic Practice Group. *J Am Diet Assoc, 9(2),* 196–202.

Bennett J. (1988). Helping people with AIDS live well at home. *Nurs Clin North Am, 23(4),* 731–748.

Connelly CE. (1987). Self-care and the chronically ill patient. *Nurs Clin North Am, 22(3),* 621–629.

Gilman AG, Goodman LS, Rall TW, Murad F, eds. (1985). *Goodman and Gilman's the pharmacological basis of therapeutics,* 7th ed. New York: Macmillan.

Harden JW, Arena JM. (1974). *Human poisoning from native and cultivated plants.* Durham, NC: Duke University Press.

*Hill M. (1986). Drug compliance: Going beyond the facts. *Nursing 86, 16(10),* 50–51.

Johnson EA. (1989). Teaching the home care client. *Nurs Clin North Am, 24(3),* 687–693.

Jurgens A, Heehan TC, Wilson HL. (1987). Therapeutic touch as a nursing intervention. *Holistic Nursing Practice, 2(1),* 1–13.

Keller E, Bzdek VM. (1986). Effects of therapeutic touch on tension headache pain. *Nurs Res 35(2),* 101–106.

*Ryan SJ, et al. (1980). Symposium on community health and home care nursing. *Nurs Clin North Am, 15,* 321–322.

Schorfheide AM, Eaks GA, Hamera EK, Cassmeyer VL. (1989). Enhancing self-care in diabetes management using self-regulatory processes. *Journal of Community Health Nursing, 6(3),* 165–171.

Silvestry A, Masoorli S. (1990). PICC lines: A new dimension in home health practice. *Journal of Home Healthcare Practice 2(4),* 1–4.

*Wade B, Bowling A. (1986). Appropriate use of drugs by elderly people. *J Adv Nurs, 11(1),* 47–55.

Wickham RS. (1990). Advances in venous access devices and nursing management strategies. *Nurs Clin North Am, 25(2),* 345–364.

*Young MS. (1986). Strategies for improving compliance. *Top Clin Nurs, 7(4),* 1–8.

* Recommended for further reading.

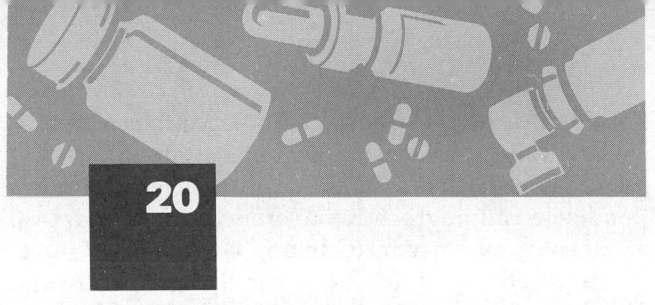

20

Drug therapy for pain relief

The pain experience

Pain may be defined as "a sensation marked by discomfort; suffering or distress of body or mind." (*The new Merriam-Webster dictionary*, 1989, p 525) Although pain is a universal experience, it is an intensely personal one. No one can actually experience the pain of another. Sympathetic observers develop psychic discomfort when signs and symptoms of pain become apparent in others but this response differs in quality and severity from that of the person who is suffering. Not even by remembering personal experiences with pain can an observer relate reliably to another's pain be-

cause pain threshold, response to pain, perception of pain, and strategies for coping with pain very greatly from individual to individual.

The point at which a stimulus is perceived as painful, called the *pain threshold*, appears to be the same for healthy people in an experimental setting. However, anyone who has had a sunburn knows that inflamed tissues become exquisitely sensitive to stimuli (touch, rubbing, slapping) that normally would cause little or no discomfort. Certain drugs such as promethazine make some people more sensitive to pain (McCaffery & Beebe, 1989, p 43). Theoretically, another factor likely to influence pain threshold is the level of endogenous analgesics such as endorphins in the brain.

Response to pain depends on many factors: the individual's past experiences of pain, learned responses to pain (which can be cultural or familial), the meaning assigned to the pain, and the success or lack of success of coping mechanisms. Most people adapt to pain to some degree. An initial response to pain may include gasping, facial grimaces, crying, moaning, muscle tension, perspiration, pallor, and alterations in vital signs. Adaptation to pain involves a reversion back to the prestimulus state, both physiologically and behaviorally. This occurs even if the pain persists. Fluctuations in pain may cause temporary loss of adaptation. For this reason, assessment of a client in pain may or may not produce objective evidence of that pain. Evidence of pain may also be masked by exhaustion or depression.

Strategies for coping with pain vary greatly from person to person. Clients may ignore the pain, use hot or cold packs, drink intoxicating beverages, exert pressure on or massage body areas, engage in diverting activities, meditate, pray, or intellectualize the experience. Coping strategies that are perceived as being helpful in the past are used repeatedly and become habitual.

Alleviation of pain

The alleviation of pain is accepted as the responsibility of health and medical care teams, especially when pathophysiology known to cause pain has been diagnosed. The traditional response of the medical profession to such pain has been the prescription of analgesic drugs. In the past, when there were few cures for painful disease, the alleviation of pain was the primary concern of the physician. Perhaps because more cures are now available, elimination of disease has become the major focus of physicians, and control of pain somewhat secondary. Whatever the reason, the health care system may not actually regard pain relief as a high priority (McCaffery & Beebe, 1989, p 1). Fortunately, many health professionals have begun to focus on pain control. Pioneers in this movement include hospice programs, which care for the terminally ill; pain clinics, some of which are multidisciplinary;

childbirth education programs; and professional organizations such as the International Association for the Study of Pain, and the International Pain Foundation. Using current theories of pain, health care professionals are beginning to apply research findings in their practice, and are conducting further research to broaden our understanding of this problem and enlarge our capability of controlling it.

Analgesic drugs

The choice of drug depends on many factors. Drugs that will eliminate the cause of pain are used when available. For example, pain due to muscle spasm can be relieved by muscle relaxants; heartburn responds to antacids or suppressants of hydrochloric acid secretion. However, when the cause of pain cannot be eliminated promptly, analgesic drugs are employed to reduce or relieve the subjective experience of pain.

Drugs used to alleviate pain range from nonnarcotic analgesics, such as salicylates and acetaminophen, to potent narcotic agents such as morphine. In choosing a drug, the type of pain to be relieved, its severity, and its expected duration must be considered. Client response will vary according to previous experience with analgesics, tolerance to drug side effects, and attitudes toward and emotional response to drugs and the pain-precipitating condition. Although the physician should consider these factors before prescribing, the initial drug order must often be adjusted to achieve the desired result.

Historically, the introduction of new analgesics or adjuncts to analgesics has been accompanied by enthusiasm for their benefits and an underestimation of their potential for causing dependence. The addictive properties of opium, morphine, heroin, cocaine, meperidine, and barbiturates were not recognized until years after their initial use. Methadone, used to treat heroin addiction, can also cause dependence. Pentazocine (Talwin) and propoxyphene (Darvon) are still generally regarded as causing few problems with dependence, although abuse, tolerance, and withdrawal syndromes can occur (Gilman, Goodman, Rall, & Murad, 1985, p 520; Brogden, Speight, & Avery, 1973). Agents that depress or stimulate the nervous system should always be regarded as potentially capable of causing dependence, whether or not physical dependence has been recognized.

The nurse's role in pain management is to devise, in collaboration with the physician and the client, a regimen of drug administration and nursing care that prevents the client's discomfort from reaching a level that interferes with the recuperative processes of the body, activities of daily living, or mental and emotional well-being. The nurse must understand the pathologic processes causing pain in each client. Knowledge of normal sensation, perception of pain, and response to stress must be combined with an understanding of the client to predict the probable course of pain and to plan interventions that prevent harmful levels of pain from developing.

There is extensive nursing literature on the pain experience and related nursing care. It is not possible in this volume to address all aspects of the problem. The following discussion will consider the use of medications to relieve acute, short-term pain, chronic pain, and pain in the terminally ill. Impediments to optimum management of pain problems will also be discussed.

Drug regimens in common use for the relief of pain

A review of the conditions discussed here and the drug regimens for them are presented in Table 20-1.

Table 20-1. Common drug regimens for various types of pain

Type of pain	Etiology	Drug regimens frequently prescribed
Acute short-term pain	Trauma, surgery, or acute medical pathology	Opioid analgesics (optimally a combination of narcotic and nonsteroidal anti-inflammatory drugs) for 3–6 days, often with tapering of doses or progressive prolongation of dosage intervals; opioids may be administered intermittently (PO or by injection), continuously (by parenteral infusion), or by the client (patient-controlled analgesia or PCA)
		Substitution of nonopioid analgesics for opioids when acute stage has resolved
Chronic pain	Chronic degenerative disease such as arthritis or neuralgia	Nonopioid analgesics or anti-inflammatory drugs (usually PO)
		Dosage intervals may be fixed (by the clock) or flexible (when necessary)
Pain of terminal illness	Life-threatening illness such as cancer or progressive neurologic disease	Nonopioid and/or opioid analgesics with progressive increases in dosage, shortening of dosage intervals, or movement from less to more potent drugs
		Drugs may be administered intermittently (PO or by injection) or continuously (by parenteral infusion)

Medication in acute short-term pain

Acute short-term pain is often the result of accidental or surgical trauma. This pain is commonly regarded as most intense in the beginning and gradually tapering off as recovery progresses. In fact, pain immediately after injury may be absent, owing to either the numbing effects of acute, sudden stress or the residual effects of anesthetics used during surgery. Pain increases when inflammation peaks (usually within 3 days of injury) and when certain activities are undertaken (ambulation, dressing changes, coughing, and so forth). Pain also fluctuates in a diurnal pattern in relation to hormonal secretion cycles, particularly that of cortisone, which blunts all sensory modalities. Clients with typical daytime patterns of cortisone production will experience more pain in the afternoon, evening, and night hours when cortisone levels are lowest.

Experienced nurses skilled in surgical care can often anticipate when medication will be most effective. They plan to administer analgesics when most needed—prior to painful procedures, rest periods, and bedtime. Medications are often ordered to be given when necessary with limitations on the frequency of dosage. With such a regimen, the need for medication should be projected tentatively over a 24-hour period. Failure to plan ahead may result in medication at an inappropriate time. For example, following surgery the nurse might anticipate the need to medicate a client with analgesics during morning care prior to a dressing change. If the medication is allowed at 4-hour intervals, the drug might be given in the afternoon to facilitate rest. A dose at bedtime also would be appropriate. If the analgesic is given at 9:00 AM and 2:00 PM with another dose planned for 10:00 PM, a question arises about medication between 2:00 PM and 10:00 PM. Will an extra dose be needed? If it will, it should be given at 6:00 PM. If it is delayed, not only will the client be unable to receive medication at bedtime but the early evening dose might cause excessive sedation during visiting hours when the client might want to be alert.

An alternative regimen for controlling acute pain is continuous parenteral infusion of analgesics. This approach facilitates uninterrupted control of pain and individual titration of dosage to the needs of the client. Continuous parenteral infusion is discussed in more detail later in this chapter.

Opioids and/or a combination of opioids and nonsteroidal anti-inflammatory drugs are the drugs most often ordered for severe, acute pain expected to be of short duration. The physician may reduce the dosage or change to a nonopioid agent as early as possible, anticipating a decrease in the client's pain and a reduced need for analgesia. Pain changes in quality and degree as convalescence progresses. Incisional pain is greatest soon after injury or surgery when the initial shock reaction or effect of anesthesia has dissipated.

Normally, this pain subsides steadily as healing takes place. When inflammatory reaction peaks, the client will experience a noticeable general discomfort. Opioid analgesics are often less effective than anti-inflammatory drugs such as salicylates in controlling this type of pain. If the physician has not prescribed a nonsteroidal anti-inflammatory drug, the nurse should request an order for one.

A given dose of an analgesic is more effective if administered before pain becomes severe. Repeated or prolonged stimulation of pain receptors causes facilitation of the nerve pathway, allowing subsequent activation of the nerves by a wider variety of stimuli and by weaker stimuli. This increased sensitivity constitutes a physiologic basis for the formation of a "habit" of pain. Early adequate control of pain will not only increase client comfort but will also reduce the overall amount of drugs required to alleviate pain. Such early control will also minimize permanent physical changes in the nervous system, which predispose a person to persistence of pain or its recurrence at a later time. Such pain habits may contribute significantly to syndromes of chronic, phantom, and intractable pain.

Although individual response to pain varies, marked deviation from the usual pattern for a given type of injury requires careful client evaluation. Unusual pain may be related to the development of complications (infection, hematoma, intestinal obstruction, and so forth); presence of pain habit developed during previous illnesses; or emotional disturbances, such as anxiety or fear, which are powerful potentiators of pain. Administering analgesics without determining the cause of inappropriate pain may mask the symptoms and prevent proper diagnosis. It is the nurse's responsibility to assess pain carefully and completely before intervening with the administration of pain medications.

Failure to control pain from trauma increases the risk of complications. Because responses to the stress of pain vary from person to person, the complications that develop are also variable. If the predominant response is sympathoadrenal activity, blood pressure and pulse tend to rise, increasing the risk of hemorrhage from injured tissue. A strong reflex vasodilation will lower blood pressure and increase the risk of shock. This response is most likely to occur in the presence of deep, visceral pain. If adrenal response is normal, cortisone levels will be high. In this state, the immune response is suppressed, the kidneys reabsorb large amounts of sodium and excrete potassium, blood volume rises, and blood pressure increases. The risks of infection, fluid and electrolyte imbalances, and hemorrhage rise proportionately. Relief of pain is, therefore, essential for the client's physical well-being.

Physical dependence on drugs is generally not considered a risk during temporary use of opioids for the relief of acute short-term pain. However, clients with a history of previous dependence will require special care to avoid a recurrence. Many of these clients will avoid or refuse narcotic analgesics. Such clients require expert and intensive nursing intervention to reduce their pain and minimize its impact on the recuperative process.

The proper use of intermittent analgesics for acute short-term pain requires conscientious application of all steps of the nursing process. The type and degree of pain perceived by the client, the physical and psychosocial responses of the client, and the orders included in the medical regimen must all be considered before a decision is made regarding drug administration. The nurse should not leave the decision of timing for analgesic administration entirely up to the client. Because the client is acutely ill and may have had little previous experience with pain, it is appropriate for the nurse to be relatively direct in the situation involving short-term pain.

Medication in chronic pain

The pain of long-term illness varies widely; it can be occasional and mild or constant and severe. Drug regimens for its treatment are equally diverse. In general, the mildest drugs adequate to control discomfort are the ones used. They may be given as necessary (PRN) with specified minimal time intervals, or regularly by the clock. When pain is persistent, using analgesics poses two problems: the risk of drug dependence and the likelihood of pain habit development.

Drug dependence

Drug dependence may be physical or psychological. *Physical dependence* is characterized by tolerance and withdrawal. *Tolerance* is the state in which a given drug dose produces a progressively weaker effect on the body over time. The client requires continually greater doses or shorter intervals between doses to achieve the same degree of pain relief. *Withdrawal* is the appearance of physical symptoms when drug dosage is interrupted. In physical drug dependence, the body has adjusted to the presence of the chemical and maintains a steady state in its presence. Removing the chemical causes disequilibrium.

Psychological dependence is a progressive need for a drug to achieve emotional well-being. The psychologically dependent person often develops some physical symptoms upon drug withdrawal. These symptoms reflect the emotional response to interruption of the habit and tend to be less specific and less severe than those of physical dependence.

Physical dependence is generally regarded as more serious than psychological dependence. No studies have been able to support this bias, however. It is relatively easy to assist dependent clients safely through physical withdrawal. In a controlled environment, they are either weaned from the drug in gradual

stages or the symptoms are controlled by other medications. Within a few weeks, the dependent person's body is usually cleared of the offending drug and physiologic stability is restored. If a psychological craving for the drug remains, however, the client may suffer a relapse. The dismally low success rate in treating narcotic addicts and alcoholics is usually due to the psychological dependence that persists after the "drying out" period.

Psychological dependence can develop whether or not the drug produces physical dependence. Susceptibility to psychological dependence varies and appears to be related to lack of self-esteem and self-confidence, as well as feelings of powerlessness. The mechanism by which psychological dependence is established may be classical conditioning, in which discomfort is the stimulus, use of drugs the response, and relief of discomfort the reward. This conditioning, initiated by the onset of physical discomfort or pain may become in a susceptible person generalized to all discomfort as the individual learns to relieve psychological and physical pain with chemical agents. However, even when very high dosages of narcotic analgesics are used, psychological dependence is very unlikely to develop in clients treated for pain unless they are predisposed to it.

The client with chronic pain is at risk for developing dependence. For this reason, drugs with the least potential for causing dependence are used, and the lowest dose adequate to control pain is prescribed. The appropriate drug or dose is, however, not always easy to determine.

The prevailing practice of underusing analgesics encourages psychological dependence by allowing the stimulus of pain to arise frequently. Minimizing or eliminating the stimulus of pain requires that ample analgesia be used to prevent pain or establish early control over it. Once the pain has been alleviated, dosage is reduced gradually until the minimal effective dose is determined.

Dependence on drugs can be minimized by carefully titrating the dosage to meet the client's individual needs, and by complementing the drug regimen with nursing interventions to minimize the perception of pain. Nursing approaches to the problems of pain and medication should not be considered alternatives but should be used in combination with drugs to provide every client with a full range of therapy to minimize the discomforts of illness. Adequate pain relief is an important factor in reducing iatrogenic drug dependence.

Whenever possible, narcotic analgesics should be avoided in treating chronic pain of indefinite duration, such as that experienced in conditions that are not life-threatening. When opioids are required, codeine or meperidine is usually prescribed. Drug regimens commonly use intermittent oral doses. The relative poten-

Table 20-2. Equipotent doses of analgesics commonly used for mild to moderate pain*

Drug name	PO dose (mg)
acetaminophen (Tylenol)	650
aspirin (ASA)	650
codeine	30
meperidine (Demerol)	50
phenacetin	650
propoxyphene hydrochloride (Darvon)	65
propoxyphene napsylate (Darvon-N)	100
sodium salicylate	1,000

*Expressed in doses approximately equivalent in total effect of ASA 650 mg. Data derived from McCaffery & Beebe, 1989, p 61.

cies of analgesics used for mild to moderate chronic pain are compared in Table 20-2.

Physiologic habit of pain

A physiologic habit of pain can develop in the client with chronic pain. This habit occurs when repeated stimulation of the neural pain pathway has altered synaptic function in the pathway, facilitating passage of impulses. Preventing this phenomenon is crucial in caring for the client over the long term. Unfortunately, the traditional approach of using the least potent drugs in the lowest dosage at the longest intervals is conducive to pain habit. If the drug regimen is advanced only in response to increasing pain, it is inevitable that the client will periodically experience significant episodes of pain. Recent experience in hospice care of the terminally ill suggests that early, aggressive treatment with large doses of analgesics given at regular intervals can achieve early control of pain. Once the client is comfortable, the drug dose is reduced gradually to determine the minimal effective amount. Such an approach, although diametrically opposed to the traditional regimen, promotes more complete relief of discomfort, reduced fear of pain, and the best overall control of pain with a minimum of drugs over the long term.

Medication in terminal illness

When life expectancy is limited because of a progressive illness, priorities for care are reordered. Cure is no longer possible. Client comfort, function, and quality of life are primary. Dependence is rarely a concern. However, the principle of adequately controlling pain with the least amount of drugs is still important if physical dependence and tolerance are to be minimized.

It is appropriate for terminally ill clients to exert control over their drug regimens because only they can determine the best quality of life for the time remaining. Generally, clients wish to remain as active and alert as possible with a tolerable level of comfort. As mentioned previously, early control of pain with gradual reduction of drug dosage to the level required by the client is the best approach.

Intermittent medication should be given regularly without waiting for pain to develop. If controlled by the health care staff, it is most effective when given at regular time intervals. Allowing the client to participate in administering drugs helps provide a sense of control and reduces anxiety. Single doses of analgesics may be left at the bedside for the client to take as desired (see Brompton's mixture discussed later in this chapter). Many institutions are, however, reluctant to adopt such permissive regimens. Nurses are uneasy with orders to leave narcotic analgesics at the bedside where they are available to anyone who might walk by. Actually, few serious problems have been reported by institutions adopting this practice. An alternative to intermittent medication is continuous parenteral infusion of analgesics. This provides a constant blood concentration of drug and good control of pain even for clients for whom regularly scheduled intermittent doses have failed to provide relief. Continuous parenteral analgesia is administered by intravenous (IV), subcutaneous, intrathecal, or epidural routes. It can be delivered by a continuous infusion using external equipment or by an implanted pump whose reservoir is refilled periodically with injections of analgesics (Pageau, Mroz, & Coombs, 1985; McGuire & Wright, 1984; Miser, Davis, Hughes, Mulne, & Miser, 1983; Waldman, Feldstein, & Allen, 1987). Equipment may be incorporated in the set-up to allow the client to infuse boluses of drug for supplemental analgesia when needed (patient-controlled analgesia).

Special techniques

Brompton's mixture

Brompton's "cocktail" or some modification of it has been used successfully as an oral form of patient controlled analgesia. This mixture is a liquid preparation containing a narcotic analgesic, a central nervous system stimulant, and one or more sedatives. Because the formula is variable, the concentration of each drug can be tailored to individual client needs.

Continuous parenteral infusion

Analgesic drugs can be administered by continuous parenteral infusion. A variety of routes are used: IV, subcutaneous, or local (at the site from which pain impulses arise, in the ganglia, or epidural). Narcotic analgesics are commonly administered by IV or subcutaneously; local infusions use local anesthetics or opioids.

Continuous parenteral infusion was first used to control the severe pain of malignant tumors refractory to usual analgesic regimens. Its use is presently being extended to acute, severe pain (*eg*, burns, multiple trauma) and to the initial control of chronic pain that has been inadequately controlled (McGuire & Wright, 1984). This therapy offers the advantages of stable serum concentrations of drug and ease in titrating dosage to individual needs. However, it requires using mechanical devices such as infusion pumps to control flow rates and prevent inadvertent overdoses.

Equipment required for administering continuous parenteral analgesia includes an IV or subcutaneous line, a volume control set, and an infusion pump with an alarm. When the drug regimen is begun, small doses of analgesic with an appropriate amount of diluent are placed in the volume control reservoir and the infusion is run at the proper rate. For example, a 1-hour dose of narcotic dissolved in 25 ml of solution will run at the rate of 25 ml/hr. The client should be assessed frequently (at least every half-hour) for therapeutic response and adverse drug reaction. Observations should be recorded on a flow sheet. During this initial period, dosage can be titrated to meet the client's needs. Once optimum dosage is established, larger doses to be infused over longer periods of time can be added, depending on the stability of the drug involved (*eg,* morphine is unstable when exposed to light and only a 4-hour supply should be added at a time). Assessment should continue on a regular basis.

Parenteral doses of analgesics may differ significantly from those administered orally (Table 20-3). Many analgesics are extensively metabolized during first pass through the liver, and only part of the oral dose reaches the circulation. Therefore, oral dosage is much higher than is parenteral dosage.

Choice of drug depends on client needs and physi-

Learning experience 20-1

Care for a client experiencing acute short-term pain who has orders for intermittent (PRN) medications for pain. Assess the adequacy of the drug regimen. Plan the administering of pain-relieving drugs during your period of care to maximize analgesia. Afterward, assess the client's response to your care. To what degree was the client pain-free? Did data relating to physiologic homeostasis (BP, pulse, and so forth) improve?

cian preference. For example, some clients may have experienced allergic reactions or other adverse effects to certain drugs. In some clients, side effects of certain drugs (*eg,* the constriction of the sphincter of Oddi by morphine) are particularly undesirable. Physicians tend to prefer and be most skilled in the use of the drugs with which they have had the most success.

When switching from intermittent to continuous medication, special care is required to achieve pain control without precipitating toxic effects. The steps for converting oral to IV doses are as follows (McGuire & Wright, 1984):

1. Determine the total oral narcotic dose the client receives in 24 hours;
2. Convert the 24-hour dose to an intramuscular dose by consulting an equianalgesic chart;
3. Divide the 24-hour intramuscular dose by two to arrive at the total daily IV dose. (Equipotent IV doses are approximately one-half the IM dose.); and
4. Divide the total IV dose by 24 to arrive at the hourly IV dose.

Table 20-3. Equianalgesic list: IM and PO doses for moderate to severe pain*

Opioid analgesic	IM (mg)	PO (mg)
buprenorphine	0.4	
butorphanol	2	
codeine	130	200
heroin	4	
hydromorphone (Dilaudid)	1.5	7.5
levorphanol (Levo-Dromoran)	2	4
meperidine (Demerol)	75	300
methadone (Dolophine)	10	20
methotrimeprazine (Levoprome, Nozinan)	20	
morphine	10	60
oxycodone (Percocet-5, oxycodone and acetaminophen; Percodan, Oxycodone and APC)	15	30
oxymorphone (Numorphan)	1	6
pentazocine (Talwin, Fortral)	60	180

*Expressed in IM and PO doses approximately equivalent in total analgesic effect of morphine 10 mg IM. Note that some doses exceed the usual recommended dosage ranges.
Data largely derived from McCaffery & Beebe, 1989, pp 61, 78, 79.

Learning experience 20-2

Care for a client receiving opioids to control chronic pain. To what degree does the medical regimen allow the client to control analgesic medication? How effective is the regimen in controlling pain? What changes in the analgesic regimen would you recommend?

The indicated dose should be increased if the oral analgesic was not controlling the pain effectively.

Continuous parenteral infusion may be supplemented by intermittent boluses when necessary. An initial bolus equivalent to 1 hour's medication may be administered when the infusion is begun. After continuous analgesia is established, bolus doses equivalent to half the usual hourly IV dose can be administered prior to painful procedures, such as moving the client or changing dressings. Should the infusion be interrupted, analgesics should be administered by an alternate route to maintain control of pain until continuous infusion can be reestablished.

Factors interfering with effective analgesia

Analgesia is a nursing goal that is often inadequately achieved. Many clients suffer needless discomfort and run high risks of complications because nursing personnel fail to manage the problem of pain effectively.

Inadequate assessment of pain

To select an appropriate approach to a pain situation, the nurse must first know the nature of the problem. Too often an analgesic is administered on the basis of inadequate information. In busy clinical settings, the medication nurse sometimes administers an analgesic automatically upon receiving a report that a client is experiencing pain. As a result, postoperative opioids have been inadvertently administered to clients suffering from toothache or arthritis rather than incisional pain. This "knee-jerk" approach to analgesia is fostered by the patterns of organization and nursing care delivery in many institutions. When medications are administered as a functional responsibility, the initial assessment of pain is unavoidably made by the staff member giving bedside care, most often an aide. To properly assess the problem, the medication nurse needs to interview the client personally. Too often, work pressures preclude this action, and it seems quicker and more efficient to administer the medication immediately.

Assumption that the client will request medication

The nurse who waits for a complaint of pain before administering medication is making several assumptions: that the client will know when discomfort becomes severe enough to qualify as pain that should be medicated; that the client knows medication is available to relieve the pain; that the client is willing to complain; and that the client regards relief of pain as desirable and beneficial. All of these assumptions may be invalid. Clients are at least as likely to believe that some pain is inevitable and must be endured and that only excruciating pain should be relieved by medication. Clients may also think that the nursing staff can detect when there is pain and will take action if warranted; that using analgesics (especially opioids) is bad and should be avoided whenever possible; that enduring pain is virtuous; and that complaining will earn dislike and disrespect from the nursing staff. Many clients assume that nothing can be done to relieve pain because they are unaware that analgesic orders have been written by the physician or because they believe they have received all the medication allowed.

Pain is a subjective phenomenon. Although its physical effects can often be measured, those effects are neither consistent nor pronounced enough to provide adequate assessment in most situations. The client should be an active participant in the process leading to effective analgesia but to do this, some preparatory teaching is required. Clients should be taught that analgesics will be ordered and available to relieve pain; that if the medications ordered do not adequately relieve the pain, the staff should be told so that adjustments in drugs or doses can be made; that adequate pain relief is essential to promote recovery and reduce the risk of complications; that pain should be reported early because at that stage it can be relieved effectively with minimum dosages; and that, although not all discomfort can be removed, most pain can be eliminated. What to emphasize to clients depends on their knowledge of and attitude toward pain and analgesia.

Inappropriate attitudes toward drug use

Attitudes toward drugs are usually colored by cultural background, moral training, and social mores. In modern American society, these attitudes tend to be polarized—some people are very permissive toward drug use and experimentation whereas others are very restrictive.

The proliferation of therapeutic drugs has contributed to the cure or control of many serious health problems. Medicines have eliminated most infectious diseases as major causes of death, reduced the mortality and morbidity rates from cancer, and reduced the populations of large residential institutions for the mentally ill. Small wonder that drugs are sometimes viewed as panaceas—ready solutions to many, if not most, of life's problems. At the same time, our society has been struggling with monumental problems of drug abuse, which have generated condemnation of drug use. Perhaps it was inevitable that antidrug biases would be generalized to include therapeutic agents, particularly analgesics, sedatives, and tranquilizers, which are also frequent substances of abuse. Unfortunately, polarization of attitudes has progressed to the point where objective, rational approaches to the proper use of chemicals are uncommon. A dispassionate appraisal by health care professionals of the need for medication is needed, particularly in relation to pain and its relief. Neither excessive reliance on drugs nor irrational fear of drug use on the part of health providers will serve clients' interests.

In health care institutions, a bias toward undermedication is often prevalent. Overmedication with analgesics can lead to oversedation and interfere with ambulation and other activities. This is rarely seen clinically. Far more frequent is a failure of analgesia—people suffering needless pain because of reluctance by health care personnel to use analgesics liberally. The paradox is that undermedication leads to refractory pain and increased client anxiety, requiring the use of greater quantities of drugs to resolve the situation.

How can the nurse develop sound judgment in managing pain problems? The first essential step is to recognize and clarify personal attitudes toward the use of analgesics. Such self-knowledge will enable the nurse to deal with the mental "sets" and emotions that could bias nursing decisions and will allow a more objective, rational approach to client care. The next step for the nurse is to develop a broad base of knowledge to support clinical judgments. In recent years, important advances have been made in understanding pain. Yet, applying this knowledge is seriously deficient because many health care practitioners have not incorporated the information into their practices. Moreover, health care personnel do not sufficiently appreciate the detrimental effects of pain. It is time to apply this knowledge clinically for the benefit of clients.

Assumption that refractory pain is psychogenic

In the health care system, there seems to be a need to assign a cause to every phenomenon and, perhaps, to place blame for failures in therapy. An infectious illness that does not respond to treatment in the usual manner may be diagnosed as a virus. This assumption is not challenged because at present we do not have specific remedies for viral infections, and there is not a conclusive diagnostic test to rule out such an illness. If demonstration of the virus by some objective test were required for such a diagnosis, it might be found that many viral illnesses were, in fact, problems of different natures. Similarly, a disease syndrome that defies diagnosis or fails to respond to treatment is often labeled *psychosomatic*. This would not be detrimental if the term were used in its true meaning (ie, involving both mind and body). In practice, the term has come to mean "arising from psychological causes." Most clients so labeled are referred to psychiatric care, and physical care is reduced to a minimal level or discontinued altogether. Health care practitioners may be very comfortable with this approach because mental or emotional causes of illness are regarded as the client's responsibility. The care provider cannot be blamed for failure of treatment because the client is at fault.

Such "scapegoating" on the part of care providers sometimes plays a part in the failure of analgesia. Lack of client response to attempts to control pain is frustrating to the nurse, particularly if several approaches have been tried unsuccessfully. When a client asks repeatedly for analgesics, watches the clock to be sure the drug is given as soon as the prescription schedule allows, and complains of discomfort despite "maxi-

mum" medication, it is very tempting to speculate that the client has a low tolerance for pain or is becoming dependent on analgesics. The tendency then is to reduce the drugs and try to manipulate the client to eliminate his or her complaints.

Placebos administered in such a situation can produce as much or more relief than drug administration. If this evidence is accepted as proof of the psychological nature of the pain, the client may be viewed as having no legitimate claim to the usual pain-relieving measures, including drugs. The fallacy of this conclusion has been exposed by recent studies indicating that effective response to placebos is characterized by production of endogenous endorphins. These autogenous analgesics interact with opioid receptors, producing effects similar to those of narcotic analgesics. These effects and the pain relief experienced are abolished when narcotic antagonists are administered. Response to placebos can no longer be regarded as good evidence that pain is mental rather than physical.

Dealing separately with the physical and psychological aspects of health problems can be harmful to the client. Such dichotomization too often leads to neglect of one aspect or the other. People cannot be divided in such an artificial way. The psychological (mental or emotional) and physical aspects of a person are inextricably interwoven. Each affects the other and anything changing one will have an impact on the other. What is needed is an integrated approach to the whole person.

In their approach to analgesia, health care personnel often fall into the trap of dealing with only part of the problem. Pain is treated by drugs or comfort measures or psychological support but rarely by all three. Instead, everyone in pain should be offered full treatment with any and all techniques needed to minimize or abolish pain.

Substitution of inappropriate drugs for analgesics

A number of drugs are useful adjuncts when used in combination with analgesics to relieve pain. Sedatives, tranquilizers, and antidepressants are most frequently used in this manner. Administering a sedative with an analgesic often provides a longer period of comfortable rest or sleep than either provides alone. Tranquilizers and antidepressants are potentiators of analgesics when the two are administered together. However, the substitution of any of these drug groups for an analgesic can fail to relieve pain and result in undesirable side effects.

Sedatives should never be substituted for analgesics for pain relief. When in pain, clients react poorly to sedation. They tend to become restless and disoriented. The pain does not seem to be reduced despite central nervous system depression, and the physiologic effects of pain persist.

Tranquilizers and antidepressants may produce

an apparent analgesia when substituted for analgesics. Perception of pain tends to decrease because the anxiety level of the client is lowered. A placebo effect may also help reduce pain. Alternating doses of analgesic and psychotropic drugs sometimes seems to provide adequate pain relief but there is no evidence that such a schedule is better than administering the drugs together. The latter is the more rational application of theoretical knowledge related to pain therapy.

Nursing management

Nursing process

Assessment When pain medication is ordered intermittently, the client should be evaluated before each dose. To help the client report the severity of pain accurately, a quantitative scale should be used. Appropriate scales may be numeric (scales of 0–10 or 0–5 with 0 representing no pain and the highest number maximum pain) or verbal (no pain, small amount of pain, moderate pain, severe pain, excruciating pain). Once chosen, the same scale should be used consistently by the individual client.

The nurse should assess factors that seem to alter the client's perception of pain. For example, the client may report increased pain at bedtime when distractors (activity, TV programs, visitors) are decreased or eliminated.

The nurse should also verify that the minimum time between analgesic doses has elapsed, that the source of pain is appropriate to the medication ordered, and that the quality and strength of the pain are appropriate to the client's condition. In addition to this minimal, immediate assessment, the pattern of pain as it is expected to recur throughout the day should be evaluated. Appropriate times for medication and maximal analgesic effect can then be projected for the next 24 hours. This approach tends to maximize control of pain and minimize the total amount of drugs required.

The daily cycle of pain should be considered within the context of the probable future course of the client's illness. Anticipating future pain patterns helps identify unusual developments that may signal complications, adjust analgesic regimens to maintain adequate pain control, and avoid inappropriate medication.

Nursing diagnosis Nursing diagnoses should be tailored to reflect the client's individual needs, which might include the following:

Pain related to nerve stimulation due to malignant tumor growth
Incisional pain related to nerve injury secondary to surgery; contributing factor: anxiety related to the outcome of treatment
Phantom pain related to irritation of nerve endings secondary to amputation
Habit of pain related to recurrent pain secondary to arthritis; contributing factors: exposure to cold and increased muscle tension
Pain related to irritability of nerve cells secondary to withdrawal syndrome during narcotic dependence
Pain related to trauma to nerve cells secondary to surgery; contributing factor: refusal of analgesia related to knowledge deficit regarding pain's adverse effects on healing

Planning Goals of nursing care are to prevent, alleviate, or eliminate pain, and educate clients concerning the physiologic effects of pain, the use of analgesia, and self-care practices to reduce the perception of pain.

Intervention Nurses often administer pain medication or teach clients to administer analgesics. They also use nursing measures to reduce pain and its percep-

Example of nursing process and palliative cancer treatment

The client is a 58-year-old factory worker who has had surgery for intestinal obstruction. An inoperable malignancy involving most of the abdominal organs was found, and no resection was attempted. The surgeon plans to refer the client to the regional medical center for palliative treatment.

The client received one dose of analgesia at 3:00 PM in the recovery room. The surgeon has ordered 75 mg meperidine IM q3h PRN for pain. At 5:00 PM the client if found lying rigidly in bed with tense facial muscles and closed eyes. Systolic and diastolic blood pressures have dropped 15 points within the last hour. When questioned, he admits to having "considerable pain" (rated as 8 on a scale of 0–10).

The client appears muscular and weighs 260 lbs. His family tells the nurses that "he never was one to complain, even when badly hurt in a shop accident a few years ago."

(Continued)

Example of nursing process and palliative cancer treatment (Continued)

Assessment data	Nursing diagnosis	Intervention	Goals and outcome criteria
Tense facial muscles	Pain: deep visceral pain related to abdominal malignancy; contributing factor: recent abdominal surgery	**Consult** with the physician to request an increase in meperidine to a dosage more appropriate to the client's size; if the physician is contacted before 6:00 PM, suggest that a dose be administered immediately.	In the morning the client will state that he had a comfortable night.
Moaning			During his hospital stay, the client will consistently rate his pain at or below 3 on a scale of 0–10 (a goal selected by the client).
Client rates his pain as 8 on a scale of 0–10			
Family states the client does not complain easily		**Administer** the maximum allowable dose of meperidine as soon as possible.	
Drop in blood pressure (Response to deep visceral pain is associated with decreases in blood pressure.)		**Refresh** the client: wash his face, hands, and back; rub his back and change his position, propping him with pillows for comfort.	During his stay at the medical center, the client will receive adequate nursing care and analgesia to control his pain.
Diagnosis of inoperable abdominal malignancy		**Give** a nursing order that analgesia is to be given at 9:00 PM after the client is settled for sleep.	On discharge, the client will be able to control his pain at home.
Order for meperidine 75 mg q3h (Usual analgesic doses of meperidine for adults range from 50–100 mg q3–4 h.)		**Advise** the night nurses to watch the client for indications of discomfort and to administer analgesia liberally to control pain.	
Weight 260 lb (muscular build)		Once the client's pain is controlled, **explore** with him his perception of pain, his usual response to it, and his wishes regarding analgesia.	
		Prepare and implement a teaching plan to educate the client to the nature of pain and its adverse effects, as well as methods for controlling it; devise a plan for pain control compatible with the client's preferences.	
		Contact the nursing service at the regional medical center and inform them of the nursing and analgesic measures that have been successful in controlling the client's pain.	

tion by the client. In addition, the nurse prepares and implements teaching plans for client education about pain and its relief.

Evaluation Data required for evaluation include (most importantly) reports from the client describing the level of comfort, discomfort, or pain in terms of the pain scale used for initial assessment. In addition, the nurse should also assess physical signs that indicate the presence or absence of pain *for the individual client.* (See accompanying Example of Nursing Process and Palliative Cancer Treatment.)

Checklist of nursing actions

- ☐ Assess pain by measuring physical changes attributable to pain and by listening to client's descriptions of pain; use a numeric or verbal scale acceptable to the client to rate pain.
- ☐ Evaluate each client's pain over the diurnal cycle; predict the likely course of pain during the client's illness.
- ☐ If the severity of pain appears inappropriate, given the client's individual reaction to discomfort and the nature of the underlying illness, evaluate the client carefully for complications.
- ☐ Consult with the physician when appropriate to request new or different orders for analgesia.
- ☐ Administer analgesics in ample amounts to control pain, reducing dosage to the minimum needed after control has been established.
- ☐ *Always* use nursing measures to decrease perception of pain.
- ☐ Educate clients to the nature of pain, its adverse effects, and the use of analgesics, and self-care measures to reduce its impact.
- ☐ Evaluate the effects of pain control measures by seeking the client's evaluation of comfort levels; monitor physiologic signs that indicate (*for the individual client*) response to pain, or its absence.

References

The new Merriam-Webster dictionary. (1989). Springfield: Merriam-Webster, Inc.

Bibliography

Baker PL. (1987). Administering a morphine drip at home. *RN, 50(3),* 72 (March).

Baquie ML. (1989). What matters most in chronic pain management. *RN 52(3),* 46–50 (March).

Bast C, Hayes P. (1986). PCA: A new way to spell pain relief. *RN, 49(8),* 18–20.

Beers L. (1988). I want to live until I die. *Nursing 88, 18(10),* 70–72 (October).

*Brown SJ. (1987). Morphine: The benefits are worth the risks. *RN, 50(3),* 20–26.

Bruera E, Brenneis C, Paterson AHG, Macdonald R. (1988). Narcotics plus methylphenidate (Ritalin) for advanced cancer pain. *Am J Nurs, 88(11),* 1555–1556.

*Burge S, et al. (1986). How painful are postop incisions? *Am J Nurs, 86,* 1262–1264.

Cancer update 90. (1990). *Nursing 90, 20(4),* 61–62 (April).

*CE: Pain. (1988). *Am J Nurs, 88(6),* 816–826.

*Clinical news: Facing pain: How much does a child hurt? (1988). *Am J Nurs, 88(2),* 155–156 (February).

Copp LA. (1990). The spectrum of suffering. *Am J Nurs, 90(8),* 35–39 (August).

Coyle N. (1990). The last four weeks of life. *Am J Nurs, 90(12),* 75–78 (December).

*Ellis JA. (1988) Managing pain in children: Using pain scales to prevent undermedication. *American Journal of Maternal/Child Nursing, 13(3),* 180–182 (May/June).

Epidural analgesics: Pain relief for children. (1990). *Nursing 90, 20(8),* 101 (August).

Fall leads to push. (1989). *RN, 52(8),* 97 (August).

*Fitzgerald JJ, Shamy PG. (1987). Let your patient control his analgesia. *Nursing 87, 17(7),* 48.

Funk SG, et al. (1989). *Key aspects of comfort: Management of pain, fatigue, and nausea.* New York: Springer Publishing Co.

Jones L, Brooks J. (1990). The ABCs of PCA. *RN, 53(5),* 54–63 (May).

Kane N, et al. (1988). Use of a patient-controlled analgesia in surgical oncology patients. *Oncology Nursing Forum, 15(1),* 29 (Jan/Feb).

*Kanner RM, Portenoy RK. (1986). Are the people who need analgesics getting them? *Am J Nurs, 868,* 589.

*Kleiman RL, et al. (1987). PCA vs regular IM injections for severe postop pain. *Am J Nurs, 87(11),* 1491–1492.

Lovasik D. (1987). An organization that helps chronic pain patients. *RN, 50(6),* 7 (June).

McCaffery M. (1985). Newer uses of NSAIDs. *Am J Nurs, 85(7),* 781 (July).

McCaffery M. (1987). Patient-controlled analgesia: More than a machine. *Nursing 87, 17(11),* 62–64 (November).

*McCaffery M, Beebe A. (1989). *Pain: Clinical manual for nursing practice.* St Louis: CV Mosby Co.

McCaffery M. (1988). When your patient is a drug abuser. *Nursing 88, 18(11),* 49 (November).

*McGrath PA, DeVeber LL. (1986). Helping children cope with painful procedures. *Am J Nurs, 86,* 1278–1279.

Mcguire L. (1990). Administering analgesics: Which drugs are right for your patient. *Nursing 90, 20(4),* 34–41 (April).

Melzack R. (1990). The tragedy of needless pain. *Sci Am, 262(2),* 27–33 (February).

O'Brien SW, Konsler GK. (1988). Alleviating children's postoperative pain. *American Journal of Maternal/Child Nursing, 13(3),* 183–186 (May/June).

O'Connor MA. (1987). The case that changed our approach to pain control. *RN, 50(9),* 44–52 (September).

Pain consult. (1987). *Am J Nurs, 87,* 64.

*Recommended for further reading.

Patt R, Subhash J. (1990). Analgesic response: Epidural sufentanil for cancer pain. *Am J Nurs, 90(5)*, 122 (May).

*Pauly-O'Neill S. (1990). Clinical news: Children demand (PCA) pain relief, too. *Am J Nurs, 90(5)*, 26 (May).

Rogers AG. What's best for this patient's pain? If the patient's on methadone maintenance. *RN, 47(10)*, 86 (October).

Schechter NL, Berren FB, Katz SM. (1988). Pain consult: PCA for adolescents in sickle cell crisis. *Am J Nurs, 88(5)*, 719–721.

Sinatra R, et al. (1989). A comparison of morphine, meperidine, and oxymorphone as utilized in patient-controlled analgesia following Cesarean delivery. *Anesthesiology, 70(4)*, 585–589 (April).

Stroud S. (1990). Drug watch: Children self-administer analgesia during fracture reduction. *Am J Nurs, 90(11)*, 53–54 (November).

*Taraglia MJ. (1987). Managing chronic cancer pain effectively. *Nursing Life, July/August*, 50–55.

Ventafridda V, et al. (1987). Antidepressants increase bio-availability of morphine in cancer patients (Letter). *Lancet, 1*, 1204 (May 23).

Waldman SD, Feldstein GS, Allen ML. (1987(. Troubleshooting intraspinal narcotic delivery systems. *Am J Nurs, 87*, 63–64.

*Recommended for further reading.

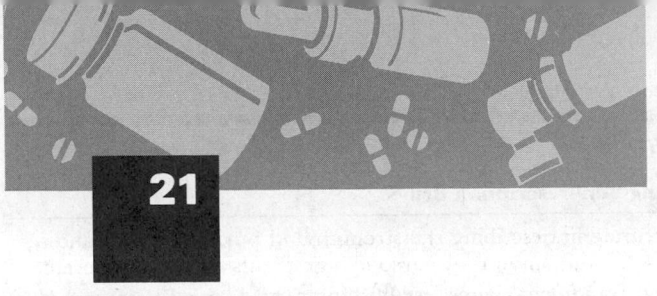

21

Self-medication with over-the-counter drugs

For centuries, people had limited access to professional medicine and relied upon herbal remedies and folk medicine to cure illnesses. With the Industrial Revolution, as people began to migrate from rural to urban areas, *patent* medicines became popular. Patent medicines were drug preparations protected by a legal document called a patent. No one other than the person who held the patent could produce or sell the preparation. Patent medicines were readily available, did not require a physician's prescription, and were advertised as cure-alls for even the most serious diseases including cancer, tuberculosis, and the plague.

Over-the-counter (OTC) drugs are drug products that can be purchased without a prescription. They are regulated by the federal Food and Drug Administration (FDA). Common properties of these drugs include low dose and a combination of ingredients. They are used as the purchaser desires and are not supervised by a physician or other health care professional who is licensed to prescribe drugs. These preparations contain active and inactive ingredients. *Active* ingredients in a drug product are those considered to have therapeutic effects (eg, reduce fever); *inactive* ingredients are those that have no therapeutic effects (eg,

preservatives, flavorings). In general, the fewer the active ingredients, the better.

As new products are developed and prescription ingredients are deemed safe for OTC use, the number of OTC preparations increases. In addition, as people become interested in maintaining health and preventing illness, the use of OTC products also increases. It is estimated that by the year 2000, consumers will save $34.1 billion in health care costs by using OTC drug products (Young, 1989). Currently, Americans spend approximately $10 billion a year on OTC drugs. Much of this cost, however, may be born by the consumer. Once a drug has been changed from prescription to OTC status, most insurance companies will not pay for the drug unless the dosage is unusual (higher than that recommended for OTC use). See Chapter 2, Standards and Controls, for more detail.

Legislative controls

By the late 1800s, many states had enacted food and drug laws to protect consumers. The first federal Food and Drug Act was not passed, however, until 1906. The initial focus of federal legislation regarding food and drugs was on dealing with adulterated products. The focus then expanded to include mislabeled products and, finally, safety and effectiveness of products (Table 21-1).

In 1906, the Food and Drug Act required that patent medicines not include harmful substances such as cocaine or morphine, which had been used in syrups for infants and small children. This law, however, did not require that new drug products be tested for safety before they were marketed. The 1938 federal Food, Drug and Cosmetic Act added the requirement that any new drug had to be safe. This did not address the problem of drugs being marketed for uses for which they actually were not effective. The 1962 Food, Drug and Cosmetic Act required that any new drug on the market had to not only be safe for humans but also effective for the purpose for which it was intended. Because the National Research Council of the National Academy of Sciences found that 75% of OTC preparations that it reviewed were not effective for at least one or more of their intended uses, the FDA established the FDA OTC Drug Review in 1972 (Federal Trade Commission, 1979). Review panels were established to determine whether OTC drugs were safe, effective, and not mislabeled. These panels continue to apply two standards in their reviews: safety and effectiveness. Safety refers to: 1) low potential for harm if the product is misused, and 2) minimal occurrence of major side effects or adverse reactions when a product is used based on clear directions and warnings about contraindications and unsafe use. Effectiveness refers to the pharmacologic effect of a product. A product is considered to be effective if it provides the type of

Table 21-1. Legislation affecting nonprescription drugs

Legislative act	Date	Provisions affecting nonprescription drugs
Federal Food and Drug Act	1906	Labels must be accurate in describing the strength and purity of drugs and must indicate the kind and amount of narcotic ingredients contained therein.
Shirley Amendment	1912	This law prohibited fraudulent claims, establishing a legal basis for control of drug efficacy.
Federal Food, Drug and Cosmetic Act	1938	New drugs must be approved as safe before they may enter interstate commerce. This act further defined labeling requirements.
Amendment to the Food, Drug and Cosmetic Act	1945	Certain drugs must be certified after batch testing at the manufacturing plant.
Durham-Humphrey Amendment	1952	This law defined prescription and nonprescription drugs and prohibited the sale of prescription drugs without medical authorization.
Kefauver-Harris Amendment	1962	Drugs of doubtful safety or efficacy can be withdrawn from the market. Adverse reactions must be reported to the government. Efficacy of new drugs must be proven before marketing. False or misleading advertising is prohibited.
Over-the-Counter Drug Review	1972	The FDA created 17 advisory panels to study ingredients in over-the-counter drugs to determine their efficacy. Ingredients are classified into Category I (safe and effective), Category II (not recognized as safe and effective), or Category III (insufficient data to classify either as Category I or II).

relief intended in a majority of the target population if used as directed. In addition, FDA regulations require that terminology used on OTC labels be clear and basic enough so that ordinary individuals have adequate directions for use and warnings about incorrect and inappropriate use.

Seventeen classes of OTC drugs were established by the OTC review. These include: antacids; antimicrobials I and II; antiperspirants; cold, cough, allergy, bronchodilator, and antiasthmatic preparations; contraceptive and other vaginal drug preparations; dentifrices and dental care drug preparations; hemorrhoidal drug preparations; internal analgesics, antipyretics, and antirheumatics; laxatives, antidiarrheals, emetics, and antiemetics; miscellaneous external drug preparations; ophthalmics; oral cavity drug preparations; sedatives, tranquilizers, and sleeping aids; and vitamins, minerals, and hemantics. Since the FDA review of OTC products began in 1972, some ingredients have been taken off the market (*eg*, phenacetin) because they are not safe. Others (*eg*, hexachlorophene) have been reclassified as prescription drugs after clinical data revealed serious side effects. The FDA review also has resulted in some prescription drug ingredients (*eg*, some hydrocortisone creams and ibuprofen) being reclassified to OTC status.

Characteristics of over-the-counter drugs

There are hundreds of over-the-counter (OTC) drug products that are available to consumers. These preparations include oral and topical drugs, cosmetics, cleansers, diagnostic agents for *in vitro* use, and contraceptives (Table 21-2). Over-the-counter products are used to prevent or treat many ailments including indigestion, the common cold, minor injuries, constipation, diarrhea, allergies, skin irritation, obesity, corns, calluses, muscle aches, and many others.

Hundreds of active ingredients can be sold without a prescription and these are marketed singly or in combination often for multiple purposes. Because federal regulations limit the dosage of OTC drugs, they tend to produce fewer adverse reactions than prescription drugs. They also may have less effect than the same ingredient in a prescription drug because of the lower dose.

The majority of OTC drugs are used to relieve symptoms rather than cure an underlying disease and the use of these products may mask serious illness (Zimmerman, 1983). It should be remembered that although OTC drugs are available to individuals of all ages, they do not necessarily have the same effect, particularly in the very young who are experiencing nonuniform biologic maturation and the very old who are experiencing nonuniform biologic deterioration. Age, therefore, influences therapeutic responses to a product in addition to its absorption and elimination.

Therapeutic uses

Over-the-counter drug preparations are used to relieve symptoms of minor, self-limiting conditions and control nonprogressive, chronic conditions. Upper respiratory infections; occasional indigestion, constipation, or diarrhea; superficial cuts and abrasions; and minor aches and pains can be treated with OTC preparations with minimal risk to the individual. Self-medication for these health problems empowers the consumer and decreases the burden on health care personnel and health care facilities.

Table 21-2. Selected nonprescription drug products

Drug category	Main active ingredient(s)	Preparation(s)	Examples of trade names
Allergy relief products	chlorpheniramine phenylpropanolamine pseudoephedrine triprolidine	Oral tablets, caplets, nasal mist, liquid	A.R.M., Actifed, Alleract, Allerest, Benadryl, Coricidin, Dristan, Drixoral, Sudafed, Teldrin, Triaminic
Analgesics	acetaminophen	Oral tablets, capsules, caplets, liquid	Anacin-3, Datril, Excedrin, Nyquil, Sine-Aid, Tylenol, Vanquish
	salicylates (including aspirin)	Oral tablets, capsules, chewing gum	Alka-Seltzer, Anacin, Arthritis Pain Formula, Aspergum, Bayer Aspirin, Bufferin, Excedrin, Ecotrin, St. Joseph's Aspirin for Adults, Vanquish
		Topical liquids, ointments	Anbesol, Ben-Gay, Heet, Icy Hot, Mobisyl, Myoflex
	ibuprofen	Oral tablets, caplets	Advil, Nuprin, Medipren, Motrin IB
Anesthetics	benzocaine	Topical liquid, gel, troches	Anbesol, Cepacol, Oracin
	dibucaine	Topical ointment	Nupercainal
	lidocaine	Topical ointment	Unguentine, Xylocaine
	phenol	Topical liquid	Chloraseptic, Phenolated Calamine Lotion
Antacids	aluminum hydroxide	Oral liquids, tablets	Aludrox, Amphojel, Di-gel Gaviscon, Maalox, Mylanta, Wingel
	calcium carbonate	Oral tablets, powder	Alka-2, Bisodol, Tums
	magnesium carbonate	Oral tablets, powder	Bisodol, Dewitt's Antacid Powder, Di-Gel, Gaviscon
	magnesium hydroxide	Oral liquid, tablets, powder	Aludrox, Bisodol, Di-Gel, Gelusil, Mylanta, Phillip's Milk of Magnesia, Wingel
	sodium	Oral tablets, effervescent tablets	Alka-Seltzer, Rolaids, Gaviscon
Antibiotics	bacitracin	Topical ointment	Baciguent, Mycitracin, Norwich Bacitracin Ointment, Septa
	neomycin	Topical ointment	N.B.P. Ointment, Myciguent, Mycitracin
	polymyxin B	Topical ointment	Polysporin, neosporin
Antidiarrheals	charcoal	Oral tablets, capsules	Requa's Charcoal Tablets, Charcocaps
	kaolin	Oral liquid	Kaopectate
	lactobacillus	Oral capsules, granules	Lactinex, Acidophilus Capsules
	bismuth subsalicylate	Oral liquid	Pepto-Bismol
Antiflatulents	charcoal	Oral tablets, capsules	Requa's Charcoal Tablets, Charcocaps
	simethicone	Oral liquid, tablets	Di-Gel, Gas-X, Gelusil, Mylanta, Mylicon, Riopan
Anti-inflammatory agents	hydrocortisone	Topical cream	Cortaid, Dermolate, Lanacort, Sensacort
Antimicrobials	povidone-iodine	Topical liquid	Betadine
	hexylresorcinol	Topical liquid	ST 37
Antiperspirants	aluminum chlorhydrate	Topical liquid, powder, cream	Ban, Mum
	zirconium-aluminum-glycine hydroxychloride	Topical liquid, cream	Secret, Sure
Antiseborrheics	selenium sulfide	Liquid shampoo	Selsun Blue
	zinc pyrithione	Liquid shampoo	Head and Shoulders
	sodium salicylate	Liquid shampoo	Phisodan, Sebulex
	sulfur	Liquid shampoo	Phisodan, Sebulex
Appetite suppressants	phenylpropanolamine	Oral tablets, capsules	Acutrim, Appedrine, Control Dexatrim
	benzocaine	Oral confections	Ayds
Bronchodilators	epinephrine	Topical liquid sprays	Bronkaid Mist, Primatene
	ephedrine	Oral tablets	Bronkaid

(Continued)

Table 21-2. Selected nonprescription drug products (Continued)

Drug category	Main active ingredient(s)	Preparation(s)	Examples of trade names
Ceruminolytics	glyceryl, carbamide peroxide	Topical liquids	Debrox, Murine Ear Wax Removal
Contact lens products	benzalkonium chloride	Liquid	Clens
	hydrogen peroxide	Liquid	Opticlens
Contraceptive spermicides	nonoxynol 9	Topical creams, foams	Emko, Koromex, Semicid, Conceptrol, Delfan, Ortho-Creme
Cough suppressants	dextromethorphan	Oral liquids, capsules	Bayer Cough Syrup for Children, Coricidin Children's Cough Syrup, Co-Tylenol Liquid Cough Formula, Dimacol, Hold, Nyquil, Robitussin DM, Triaminic-DM Cough Formula, Vick's Formula 44 Cough Mixture
Counterirritants	menthol	Topical ointments	Ben-Gay, Icy Hot, Vick's VapoRub
	phenol	Topical ointments	Unguentine
Decongestants	phenylephrine	Oral liquid, tablets	Dimetapp, Nostril
	phenylpropanolamine	Oral tablets, liquid	Congesprin, Sucrets Decongestant Lozenges
	pseudoephedrine	Oral tablets, liquid	Afrin, Co-Tylenol, Nyquil, Sine-Aid
Dental preparations anticaries	sodium fluoride	Toothpaste	Crest
	sodium mono-fluorophosphate	Toothpaste	Aim, Aquafresh, Colgate
Desensitizers	strontium chloride hexahydrate	Toothpaste	Sensodyne
Dietary supplements			
Infant formulas	soy beans, corn syrup, coconut oil	Oral liquids	Prosobee, Isomil
	predigested casein hydrolysates	Powder for suspension in water	Neutramigen
	meat, cane sugar, sesame oil	Oral liquid	MBF
Instant meals	Various combinations of soy protein, soy bean oil, vitamins, minerals, corn syrup	Oral liquids, powders for mixing in liquids	Instant Breakfast, Flexcal, Slender, Sustagen, Inosol
Digestants	pancreatic enzymes	Oral tablets	Cholagest
Diuretics	caffeine	Oral tablets	Odrinil
Electrolyte	Various combinations of salts: potassium, sodium, calcium, magnesium, citrate, sulfate, chloride, phosphate, dextrose	Oral liquid	Lytren Nursette, Pedialyte
Expectorants	guaifenesin	Oral liquid	Robitussin, Triaminic Expectorant
Karatolytics	salicylic acid	Topical liquids, ointments	Freezone, Wart-off, Compound W
Laxatives bulk	psyllium	Oral powder for mixing with liquids	Metamucil, Vegetable Powder Laxative
	vegetable hemi-cellulose	Oral granules for mixing with food	Serutan
Fecal softeners	docusate	Oral capsules	Surfak
Lubricant	mineral oil	Oral liquid	Haley's MO
Saline	milk of magnesia	Oral liquid, tablets	Phillip's Milk of Magnesia
Stimulant	bisacodyl	Oral tablets, rectal suppositories	Dulcolax
	phenolphthalein	Oral tablets	Ex-Lax, Evacugen
Pediculosides	tetrahydronaphthalene	Topical liquid	Cuprex
Scabicides	pyrethrin, piperonyl	Topical liquid	Rid
Sleep aids	diphenhydramine	Oral tablets	Nytol, Sominex, Unisom Dual Relief
	doxylamine succinate	Oral tablets	Unisom

(Continued)

Table 21-2. Selected nonprescription drug products (*Continued*)

Drug category	Main active ingredient(s)	Preparation(s)	Examples of trade names
Stimulants	caffeine	Oral tablets	NoDoz, Vivarin
Sugar substitutes	aspartame	Powdered drink mix	Crystal Light, Kool Aid (artificially sweetened)
	saccharine	Oral tablets, powder, liquid	Equal, Sucaryl, Sweeta
	sorbitol	Oral confections	Wafer Bar, Sugar-Free Hard Candy
	cyclamate		(Products available in Canada)

Adverse reactions

Over-the-counter drugs are not guaranteed to be safe even if taken as directed. Individuals who use OTC drug products should be aware not only of the therapeutic effects but also of adverse effects, including conditions that enhance: 1) toxicity, 2) interaction with prescription drugs, and 3) age-related problems. For example, if acetaminophen is taken in large doses, it can be toxic to a person who consumes more than three to four ounces of alcohol per day. In addition, there are thousands of products on the market, many of which contain the same ingredients and some products contain combinations of similar ingredients. It is important, therefore, for individuals to read labels carefully each time that they purchase a product because ingredients, directions, warnings, and indications for use of a specific drug preparation may change.

Some ingredients that are found in OTC drug products may interfere with the metabolism of specific prescription drugs (Clayman, 1988). Aluminum hydroxide, for example, may interfere with the metabolism of oral anticoagulants, corticosteroids, antibiotics such as tetracycline, digitalis preparations, and antipsychotics. It may destroy the enteric coating of tablets such as bisacodyl and cause gastric irritation.

Aspirin, a nonnarcotic analgesic and antipyretic, also helps to reduce platelet aggregation and prevent thrombus formation. This widely used drug enhances the effects of anticoagulants and increases the possibility of gastric irritation when consumed along with nonsteroidal anti-inflammatory drugs and corticosteroids. Aspirin also may decrease therapeutic effects of drugs that are prescribed for gout, especially allopurinol. Individuals who are allergic to aspirin, moreover, also are often allergic to Yellow No. 5 dye (Hecht, 1988), which is used to color both prescription and nonprescription drugs. Consumers, therefore, should avoid taking yellow-colored pills, capsules, or caplets unless the label clearly indicates that the dye used is not Yellow No. 5.

Consumers should avoid self-medication with aspirin, other salicylates, or salicylamide if they concurrently are taking prescription drugs for arthritis or gout because of the increased risk of gastric irritation and bleeding. In addition, they should avoid self-medication with salicylates if they also are taking prescription drugs for diabetes because salicylates increase their hypoglycemic effects. Major classifications of drugs that may result in adverse reactions if taken with salicylates include anticoagulants, thrombolytics, sulfonureas, corticosteroids, and antimetabolites such as methotrexate. In addition, people should avoid self-medication with salicylates if they are taking sulfa drugs and antidepressants or other mood-altering drugs. Salicylates increase the risk of bleeding due to blood dyscrasias that may occur as adverse reactions to these drugs.

Acetaminophen is widely advertised and found in many OTC preparations. It relieves pain and reduces fever but it does not relieve the redness, stiffness, or swelling of rheumatoid arthritis. Individuals should not take acetaminophen or similar drugs (*eg*, salicylates, ibuprofen) for more than 10 days for pain or 3 days for fever without checking with a health care professional. The persistence of symptoms may indicate a serious illness.

Acetaminophen may increase the blood levels of antineoplastic drugs such as methotrexate and of zidovudine (AZT or Retrovir), an antiviral drug that is used in the treatment of individuals with acquired immunodeficiency syndrome (AIDS), AIDS-related complex (ARC), or those who are human immunodeficiency virus-positive but asymptomatic (The United States Pharmacopeial Convention, Inc., 1991). Individuals who are taking zidovudine and those who are receiving antineoplastic chemotherapy should check with a health care professional before taking any OTC drug.

Several antihistamines (*eg*, brompheniramine, dimenhydrinate, diphenhydramine, and triprolidine) commonly are found in remedies for colds, allergies, and hay fever. They potentiate the effects of other drugs, prescription or OTC, that have a sedative effect on the central nervous system, including alcohol. Double-dosing of cold medications can occur if cold tablets and liquid cough preparations that contain the same ingredients are taken together. When choosing a cold remedy, therefore, a person should select a product that treats the symptoms that they have, not those that they anticipate.

Decongestants (eg, naphazoline, oxymetazoline, phenylpropanolamine, pseudoephedrine, ephedrine, triprolidine, and xylometazoline) may decrease the antihypertensive effects of drugs that include beta blockers, methyldopa, reserpine, and guanethidine. This occurs because decongestants have sympathomimetic properties that result in an increase in blood pressure due to peripheral vasoconstriction. Decongestants also may interact with a class of drugs called monoamine oxidase inhibitors to raise blood pressure. Monoamine oxidase inhibitors are psychotropic drugs that are prescribed when tricyclic antidepressants are ineffective or for certain neuroses that include depression, anxiety, or phobias. Examples of monoamine oxidase inhibitors include isocarboxazid (Marplan), phenelzine sulfate (Nardil), and tranylcypromine sulfate (Parnate).

It should be remembered that decongestants can be habit-forming when applied topically. This occurs because topical application results in a quick onset of action (ie, vasoconstriction) followed by a short duration of effect, and then vasodilation and rebound congestion, leading to overuse of the product.

Ibuprofen is a drug that had been a prescription medication but was reclassified as being safe for OTC use. It is an analgesic and anti-inflammatory drug that has fewer side effects than other nonsteroidal anti-inflammatory drugs. Ibuprofen, however, interacts with many drugs that may result in serious adverse reactions. These include potentiating the effects of oral hypoglycemics, anticoagulants, aspirin, corticosteroids, other nonsteroidal anti-inflammatory drugs, and raising blood levels of lithium.

As hundreds of OTC drugs are marketed every year, the need to examine all ingredients becomes more crucial. For example, although alcohol content in OTC preparations for children has been eliminated, the alcohol content in drug preparations made for adults varies considerably (Table 21-3). Liquid analgesics, cold and cough preparations, decongestants, mouthwashes, sleep aids, and vitamins all contain alcohol. These liquid preparations should be avoided by alcoholics because their use could result in overdosage of active ingredients (eg, diphenhydramine, phenylpropanolamine) due to a physiologic response to the alcohol content and subsequent overuse of the product. In addition, even small amounts of alcohol can cause severe adverse reactions (eg, vomiting, confusion) in individuals who are taking disulfiram (Antabuse) to maintain abstinence from alcohol. This reaction is due to markedly increased blood levels of acetaldehyde as a result of interference with alcohol metabolism.

Other OTC preparations contain sugars (eg, Beny-

Table 21-3. Alcohol content of selected nonprescription liquid drug products

Drug category	Percentage of alcohol	Examples of trade names
Analgesics	7.0	Tylenol
Cold and cough preparations	25.0	Nyquil
	23.0	Dimetapp DM
	20.0	Vicks 44M
	19.0	Medi-flu
	10.0	Vicks Day Care
Cough preparations	10.0	Vicks 44
	5.0	Benylin DM
	4.75	Robitussin CF
	3.5	Robitussin
	2.5	Sudafed cough syrup
Decongestants	10.0	Novahistine DMX, Vicks 44D
	2.3	Dimetapp elixir
Mouthwashes	26.9	Listerine
	16.6	Scope
	14.5	Signal
	12.5	Chloraseptic
Sleep aids	10.0	Benadryl plus nighttime, Excedrin PM liquid
Vitamins	12.0	Geritol
	6.6	Centrum liquid multivitamins

lin liquid preparations, Alka-Mints, Teldrin, Tums). Diabetics, therefore, need to be wary about using OTC preparations and should discuss their use with a health care professional.

Nursing management
Nursing implications

As role models, nurses should be aware of their own self-medication practices; identify the rationale for such behavior; and change habits that are inappropriate or potentially harmful. Nurses also serve as resources for information about OTC drug preparations. Even though many lay persons have access to information about OTC drug products through the mass media, they still need guidance from health care professionals. Lay persons may have little information about the meaning or severity of symptoms. Therefore, they may not be able to make informed choices about which OTC drugs can be used safely and which should not be used or used only with the guidance of a health care professional.

Nurses, therefore, should be knowledgeable about the wide variety of OTC products that are available in their geographic locations. Periodic analysis of these products should include intended therapeutic effect, directions for use, warnings and contraindications, pharmacologic properties of active ingredients, and characteristics of inactive ingredients (Box 21-1).

Cost and composition of name brand products and generic products also should be considered.

Nursing process
Assessment The use of OTC products should be included in every drug history. Many consumers do not think to mention their use of OTC products to health care providers because they do not consider OTC preparations to be medications. A nurse can elicit this information by asking direct questions such as the following: What do you do for a cold? What do you do for a headache? Do you ever take anything for indigestion? Do you take vitamins or minerals? What do you use if you have a skin rash?

Learning experience 21-1
List over-the-counter products present in the home of an acquaintance or health care consumer. Discuss with the person the purposes for which they are used, how closely instructions on the label are followed, age of the products, and age of persons who use them.

In addition to identifying the specific products used by consumers, the nurse should list reasons for use and frequency, response to the product, and any adverse reactions experienced. The same information should be obtained for prescription drugs that the consumer is taking concurrently. The interaction between OTC and prescription products can be severe.

When analyzing a client's drug history, the nurse

Box 21-1. Nurses' guide for evaluating nonprescription drugs

1. Read the label carefully for inclusion of the following:
   Description of tamper-resistant feature
   Name of product
   Active ingredients
   Inactive ingredients
   Quantity of contents
   Name and address of manufacturer, packer, or distributor
   Indications for use
   Instructions for use
   Warnings, contraindications, and interactions
   Expiration date and lot or batch code
2. Compare brand-name products with generic products, noting:
   Active and inactive ingredients
   Amount of active ingredients
   Warnings, contraindications, and interactions
   Cost
3. Compare several products recommended for the same use, noting:

Active and inactive ingredients
Instructions for use
Warnings, contraindications, and interactions
Cost
4. Using a pharmacologic data source for reference, evaluate OTC preparations:
   How does the OTC preparation compare with the recommended dosage range?
   Does the pharmacologic source recommend the active ingredient for the purpose for which it is used in the OTC preparation?
   What risks are involved in using the preparation?
   Would use of the OTC preparation be likely to result in undue delay in seeking needed care from a health care professional?
   Is the preparation safe for adults?
   Is the preparation safe for the frail elderly?
   Is the preparation safe for children?

should look for drugs that have the same effect, use of a combination of drugs for the same purpose, and potential adverse reactions to these preparations in addition to their therapeutic effects. The nurse also needs to assess the client's knowledge of the following: 1) appropriate use of prescription and OTC products, 2) therapeutic effects of preparations, 3) potential side effects, and 4) expiration date of medication.

Nursing diagnosis Many nursing diagnoses may be related to the use of OTC preparations. Examples are as follows:

> *Knowledge deficit related to unfamiliarity with information resources for use of OTC preparations*
> *Fluid volume excess related to excess sodium intake from use of antacids containing sodium*
> *Noncompliance with therapeutic regimen related to health beliefs about substitution of OTC drugs for prescription drugs*
> *Sleep pattern disturbance related to ingestion of stimulant OTC weight reduction aids and intake of beverages that contain caffeine.*

A common collaborative problem that should be differentiated from the nursing diagnoses is

> *Potential complication: GI bleeding related to interaction of anticoagulant and aspirin*

Planning The end goal of nursing care is to empower the consumer to engage in appropriate behavior in relation to the use of OTC preparations. Subgoals of nursing care, therefore, include teaching consumers to choose appropriate preparations for minor health problems and to eliminate their inappropriate use of such products, educating consumers about self-medication to reduce the risk of adverse interactions between OTC products and prescription drugs, educating consumers about health care problems for which self-medication is inappropriate, and teaching consumers to identify adverse reactions to OTC preparations and what to do if they should occur.

Intervention If OTC drug preparations are to be administered to consumers, the nurse must educate them about the use of such products. Part of this education includes directing a consumer to have a drug profile established at the pharmacy where prescription and nonprescription drugs are purchased. The nurse looks up interactions and contraindications to the use of specific products together and uses this information to give specific advice to patients about their total drug regimen. The nurse also may refer consumers to a pharmacist for additional information and guidance when appropriate.

Over-the-counter preparations should have tamperproof seals. The nurse should teach consumers to examine new packages to verify that the tamperproof seal has not been broken. The nurse should warn consumers not to use OTC products if the tamperproof seal is not intact. A broken seal could indicate that the product has been adulterated. If the seal has been broken, the package should be returned to the pharmacy or store where it was purchased and exchanged for one that is intact.

Client education. Using OTC products allows consumers to take control over some of their health care. It also decreases costs of health care to the consumer and decreases the load on an already overburdened health care system. In most instances, if recommendations on products are followed, self-medication is relatively safe and effective. Product labels are required to be accurate and to include warnings about when a preparation should not be used and when advice should be sought from a health care professional.

Even though self-medication is relatively safe, there are risks. Because most consumers are not health care professionals, they could misinterpret their symptoms and use products that are inappropriate. Self-medication also may result in the avoidance of professional health care for potentially serious problems. Over-the-counter products should be taken for minor, self-limiting conditions. Minor problems including scrapes and abrasions, occasional headaches, the common cold, occasional indigestion, or skin irritations may be treated successfully with nonprescription products. If problems or symptoms are severe, occur frequently, or are persistent, an individual should be seen by a health care professional.

Enrichment experience 21-1

Explore the sections of a supermarket or drug store that contain over-the-counter preparations, cosmetics, and soaps and other cleansers. Note the active ingredients used in various products. Identify marketing techniques used by manufacturers.

Nonprescription products (*eg*, aspirin, antacids) may be used to treat chronic medical conditions (*eg*, arthritis, coronary heart disease, peptic ulcer). The use of OTC products to treat these conditions, however, should be supervised by a health care professional.

Nurses need to advise consumers that dosages of OTC products as recommended by the manufacturer may not provide relief or may precipitate unexpected adverse reactions. This can occur because dosages are calculated for individuals who are in a specific age group and who are of average height and weight. Consumers who are of less than average weight may experience enhanced (even toxic) effects of a drug, while those who are above average weight may experi-

Table 21-4. Advantages and disadvantages of self-medication with nonprescription drugs

Advantages	Disadvantages
Over-the-counter drugs often relieve symptoms of minor or self-limiting conditions.	Relief of symptoms fosters delay in seeking professional care for potentially serious conditions.
Recommended dosages are relatively low, reducing the risk of adverse reactions.	Lack of therapeutic response may lead to use of dosages much greater than recommended.
Self-medication reduces the demand for services from health care professionals, freeing them to treat seriously ill persons.	Successful treatment may promote avoidance of professional care.
Over-the-counter drugs cost less than prescription drugs.	Fixed dosage combinations prevent tailoring of dosage to individual needs.
	Use of multiple preparations that may contain the same active ingredients increases the risk of adverse reactions.
	Over-the-counter drugs may contain inappropriate or superfluous ingredients.
	Over-the-counter drugs may increase toxicity of prescription drugs when used in combination with them.

ence little effect. The very young and the elderly, in particular, may need less than the recommended dosage.

Allergic reactions are as likely to occur with OTC preparations as with prescription products. These may be physical (*eg*, skin rash, palpitations, bronchoconstriction) or mental (*eg*, irritability, confusion). Allergic reactions may be caused by an active ingredient or an inactive ingredient such as a preservative or dye.

Consumers may be attracted to OTC products that contain multiple drug preparations. The nurse needs to caution them that more is not necessarily better. The greater the number of active ingredients, the greater are the chances of adverse reactions to the preparation and the more likely the chance of interaction with other drugs. In addition, the nurse should warn consumers that long-acting or timed-released preparations should be avoided when a new product is used for the first time. If an adverse reaction occurs, it will be prolonged and may be difficult to treat because of continued absorption of the active ingredients.

For consumers who use OTC preparations regularly, the nurse must remind them that this practice could mask symptoms of serious disease. The nurse should counsel consumers that they need to consult a health care provider periodically to avoid this problem.

When discussing OTC products with consumers, the nurse should explain not only the uses and properties of specific preparations but also the advantages and disadvantages of self-medication (Table 21-4). The nurse should teach consumers the guidelines for use of OTC products (Box 21-2).

Specifically, the nurse should instruct consumers to read labels carefully noting intended use of product, recommended dosage, potential adverse reactions, warnings, and guidelines for storage. The nurse also should instruct consumers that if an adverse reac-

tion occurs, they should stop using the OTC preparation immediately and take further action as recommended on the product label. If the adverse reaction is severe (*eg*, hives, vomiting, bleeding), the consumer should contact a health care professional immediately.

Evaluation Data required for evaluation of the efficacy of OTC preparations include a consumer's response to the preparation and evidence that the consumer is using the product appropriately. A consumer's response to

Box 21-2. Instructions to patients

1. Read the label carefully before using.
2. Check for tampering of container.
3. Use a standard measuring device for liquids.
4. If taking a capsule, caplet, or tablet with water, drink a full 8 ounces of water.
5. Check with a pharmacist or health care professional before opening capsules or crushing tablets.
6. Store preparations in their original containers.
7. Avoid using a preparation after the expiration date.
8. Use the following guidelines for storing over-the-counter preparations:
   Keep away from heat and direct light.
   Avoid storing capsules, caplets, or tablets in the bathroom medicine cabinet or near the kitchen sink (heat and moisture may cause deterioration).
   Avoid refrigerating preparations unless directed to do so.
   Keep all preparations out of the reach of children.
   Avoid freezing liquids.
   Discard outdated preparations.

Example of nursing process and over-the-counter products used in cardiovascular therapy

The consumer is a 78-year-old retired bookkeeper who comes to a walk-in clinic because of "a cold that just won't go away." He states that he has had a cold for 3 weeks and that his symptoms include a "hacking" cough that wakes him up at night, swelling in his ankles and feet, and shortness of breath with walking and doing things around the house. He has not seen a health care provider for 15 years. His drug history reveals the following over-the-counter preparations: a liquid vitamin tonic daily, over-the-counter cold medications PRN, and Rolaids PRN for "heartburn." Discharge orders include making an appointment with a family physician for a physical examination, 2,000 mg sodium diet, furosemide 40 mg daily, and digoxin 0.125 mg daily.

Assessment data	Nursing diagnosis	Intervention	Goals and outcome criteria
Use of over-the-counter vitamins, cold remedies, and antacids	Knowledge deficit related to information misinterpretation and lack of exposure to professional health care	**Explore** knowledge about symptoms and reason for over-the-counter therapy.	Consumer will state willingness to seek advice from health care professional about use of over-the-counter products.
Orders for 2,000 mg sodium diet, furosemide, and digoxin	Knowledge deficit, potential related to unfamiliarity with information resources for diet, prescription drugs and over-the-counter drugs used by the consumer	**Develop** and implement a teaching plan that will address the newly prescribed drugs and the need to take them as prescribed until seen by a family physician. Include the need to avoid taking antacids containing sodium and any other over-the-counter products until evaluated.	Consumer will have minimal edema and no episodes of nocturnal dyspnea from excessive sodium intake.

an OTC preparation includes actual effect of the product, incidence of adverse reactions, and subjective report of effectiveness. Evidence that the consumer is using the OTC product appropriately includes self-report of how closely the consumer followed the recommended dosage and instructions for use of the product and a low incidence of adverse reactions. (See Example of Nursing Process and OTC Products Used in Cardiovascular Therapy.)

Checklist of nursing actions

☐ Create a drug history including consumer's use of OTC drugs and analyze it for appropriate practices and occurrence of adverse reactions.

☐ Assess the consumer's internal and external exposure to chemicals to determine the risk of adverse reactions and advise the consumer regarding how to decrease risk.

☐ Educate consumers to use OTC products safely and effectively.

☐ Encourage consumers to use OTC drugs appropriately.

☐ Encourage clients to establish a medication profile with a pharmacist, including prescription and nonprescription drugs, and to maintain an updated profile.

☐ Counsel consumers to use OTC preparations only for minor, self-limiting health problems and to discuss their use of OTC preparations with a health care professional.

☐ Encourage consumers who use OTC products regularly, over long periods of time, or in large doses to seek advice from a health care provider for supervision of their regimens.

☐ Advise consumers to store all OTC preparations in a cool, dry, secure place that cannot be accessed by individuals who could be harmed.

☐ Refer consumers to a pharmacist if the nurse lacks knowledge or reference materials.

References

Clayman CB, ed. (1988). *The American Medical Association guide to prescription and over-the-counter drugs.* New York: Random House.

Hecht A. (1988). OTC drug labels: 'Must' reading. *FDA consumer* (DHHS Publication No. FDA 88-3157). Washington, DC: U.S. Government Printing Office.

Kaufman J, Rabinowitz-Dagi L, Levin J, McCarthy P, Wolfe S, Bargmann E, the Public Citizen Health Research Group. (1983). *Over the counter pills that don't work*. New York: Pantheon Books.

The United States Pharmacopeial Convention, Inc. (1991). *USPDI advice for the patient*, vol II. Rockville, MD: Author.

Young FE. (1989). *A doctor's advice on self-care* (U.S. Federal Document No. HE 20: 40021: Se 4). Washington, DC: The Proprietary Association in cooperation with the Food and Drug Administration.

Bibliography

*Alexander D, Spencer R. (1986). Over-the-counter analgesics, antipyretics, and anti-inflammatories: The nurse's role in selection and use. *Journal of Community Health Nursing, 3(1)*, 11–23.

*American Medical Association. (1986). *Drug evaluations*, 6th ed. Chicago: Author.

Benowicz RJ. (1983). *Nonprescription drugs and their side effects*. New York: Perigee.

*Gardner ER, Hall RC. (1983). Psychiatric symptoms produced by over-the-counter drugs. *Psychosomatics, 23*, 186.

Harkness R. (1983). *OTC handbook: What to recommend and why*, 2nd ed. Oradell, NJ: Medical Economics Books.

*Johnson JE, Moore J. (1988). The drug-taking practices of the rural elderly. *Applied Nursing Research, 1(3)*, 128–131.

*Kofoed LL. (1985). OTC drug overuse in the elderly: What to watch for. *Geriatrics, 40(10)*, 55–58, 60.

*Lehman P. (1988). Food and drug interactions. *FDA consumer* (DHHS Publication No. FDA 88-3070). Washington, DC: U.S. Government Printing Office.

McEvoy GK, ed. (1990). *American hospital formulary service drug information*. Bethesda, MD: American Society of Hospital Pharmacists.

*de Mont A. (1987). Children's medications: Sweetening the pill? *Community Outlook, August*, 28–29.

*Steil C. (1988). Over-the-counter product use. *Diabetes Educator, 14(1)*, 48–49.

*Trainor P. (1988). Over-the-counter drugs: Count them in. *Geriatric Nursing, September/October*, 298–299.

*Recommended for further reading.

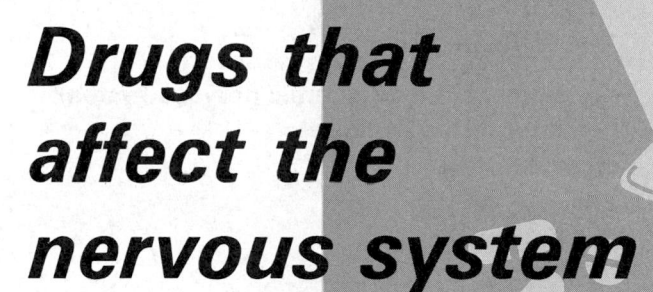

Drugs that affect the nervous system

5

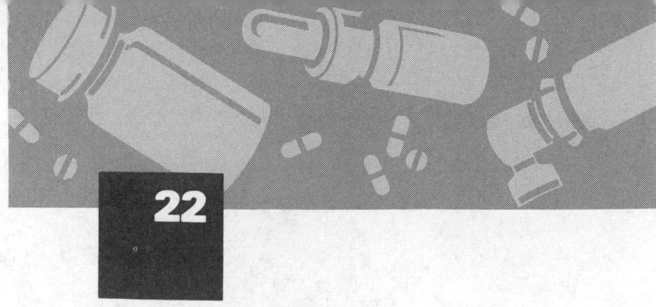

22

Autonomic drugs

The nervous system is a complex information processor and control mechanism. In conjunction with the endocrine system, it mediates the adjustments and reactions of an organism to internal and external conditions. It is responsible for physical activity, intellectual processes, and self-consciousness. Chemical substances that influence neuronal functions, therefore, have wide-ranging effects on physical functions, emotional states, and mental capacity.

The nervous system is organized into subsystems and organs (Box 22-1). Within these structures, tissues are of two types: gray matter (nerve cell bodies) and white matter (conducting fibers). Their function may be sensory or motor. Biochemical organization is complex, involving a large number of neurotransmitters, only some of which have been identified and studied to date.

Drugs may affect all or only a part of the system. The more general the action of a drug, the more side effects it causes. Selective drugs tend to generate fewer side effects and have a greater clinical usefulness.

Many nervous system drugs administered systemically affect all of the system to some degree. Local administration, as in spinal anesthesia, can restrict the action of a drug to only a portion of the system. Differences in physiologic chemistry cause the actions of certain drugs to be more pronounced in some tissues than in others. The more selective drugs affect only a small part of the system. For example, cholinergic substances mimic the effects of parasympathetic stimulation; tranquilizers profoundly depress the limbic system. In large doses, however, the effects become more widespread, causing increased side effects. Toxic symptoms tend to be similar for the major classes of drugs. Thus, excessive doses of any central nervous

Box 22-1. Categorizations of the nervous system

I. Anatomic Structures
  A. Central nervous system
    1. Brain
      a. Cortex
      b. Brain stem
        (1) diencephalon
          (a) Thalamus
          (b) Hypothalamus
        (2) Mesencephalon
        (3) Basal ganglia
        (4) Medulla
        (5) Pons
        (6) Midbrain
        (7) Cerebellum
    2. Spinal cord
  B. Peripheral nervous system
    1. Voluntary
      a. Motor
      b. Sensory
    2. Autonomic
      a. Sympathetic
      b. Parasympathetic
II. Physiologic Functions
  A. Systems
    Examples: sympathetic, parasympathetic, limbic, spinothalamic
  B. Centers
    Examples: speech, vital (respiratory, cardiac, vomiting)

  C. Circuits
    Examples: reflex arcs, reverberating circuits
  D. Subunits
    Examples: sensory cortex, motor cortex, inhibitory fibers, excitatory fibers, synapse
III. Biochemical Neurotransmitters
  A. Excitatory
    1. Known:
      a. Acetylcholine
      b. Norepinephrine
      c. Dopamine
      d. Serotonin (5-hydroxytryptamine or 5-HT)
    2. Suspected:
      a. L-glutamate
      b. L-aspartate
  B. Inhibitory
    1. Known:
      a. γ-aminobutyric acid (GABA)
      b. Glycine
    2. Suspected:
      a. Histamine
      b. Prostaglandins
      c. Polypeptide substances

---

system (CNS) depressant tend to cause hypotension, respiratory depression, and coma.

Some drugs that affect the nervous system (*eg*, opium, alcohol) are among the oldest known pharmaceutical agents. Many traditional substances (*eg*, reserpine, curare) have been purified and standardized for use in modern medicine. Other drugs are recently discovered or synthesized chemicals. As research into the nature of nervous system function continues, the potential for the development of new drugs that affect this system increases. The advent of additional drugs, however, is a double-edged sword, promising more effective treatments of nervous system disorders, while providing a greater potential for toxicity and substance abuse.

The autonomic nervous system

The autonomic nervous system (ANS) constantly controls vital functions of the body: cardiac action, temperature regulation, ionic and fluid balance, metabolism, digestion, and excretion. Through the sympathetic and parasympathetic systems, autonomic nerves influence the physiologic balance of the total organism. Somatic and visceral reflexes play a large role in coordinating this control (Fig. 22-1). Autonomic drugs are chemicals that change this balance, either by altering the function of the autonomic system or by augmenting or counteracting its effects. A thorough understanding of autonomic function, therefore, is necessary to understand the action and effects of autonomic drugs.

Physiology of the autonomic nervous system

The two main divisions of the ANS are the sympathetic (thoracolumbar) and parasympathetic (craniosacral) systems (Fig. 22-2). In each, nerves leave the CNS to synapse with other nerve fibers in ganglia (located close to the spinal cord in the case of sympathetic fibers, or near effector organs in the case of parasympathetic fibers). Postganglionic fibers extend to effector organs, where they influence and control organ function. It is in the synapses of the ganglia and the nerve–organ junction that endogenous chemicals play a role in transmitting nerve impulses. The function of the synapse is sensitive to the influence of exogenous chemicals (drugs). Therefore, drug effects on the ANS are best understood in relation to their effects on synaptic function.

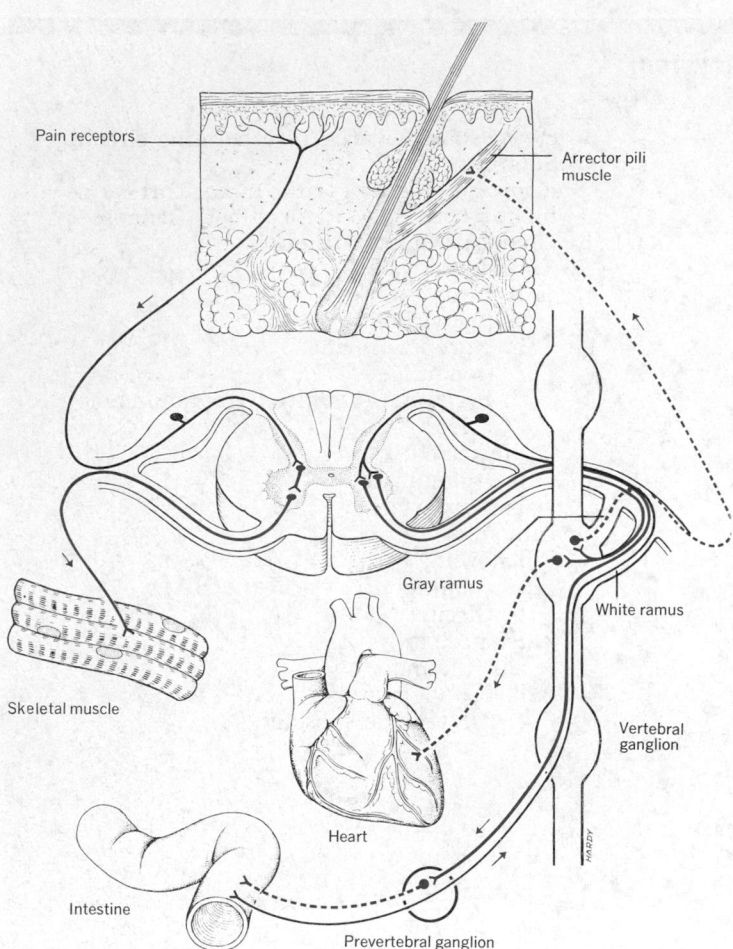

Figure 22-1. Examples of somatic and visceral reflex pathways. Arrows indicate direction of impulse transmission. Afferent neurons are shown in black; somatic central and efferent neurons are shown in color on the left. Visceral efferent neurons, shown in color on the right, are preganglionic (*solid lines*) and postganglionic (*dashed lines*); synapses occur in either vertebral or prevertebral ganglia.

Chemistry of the synapse

Synaptic transmission involves the production, storage, and release of chemical neurotransmitters, which stimulate a response in the postsynaptic cell (Fig. 22-3). Chemical substrates needed for the synthesis of neurotransmitters are transported down the axon of the nerve cell. In the nerve terminal, organelles and enzymes control the synthesis, storage, and release of the transmitter. Under normal conditions, the transmitter crosses the short distance that separates the terminal from the postsynaptic cell, where it interacts with receptors on the membrane of the cell. When sufficient receptors are activated in this fashion, an action potential is generated in the receptor cell, resulting in a second nerve impulse or effector organ response, such as muscle contraction or glandular secretion. Transmitter that has been released from the axon terminal is dissipated by at least two processes: enzymes in the extracellular space catabolize excess transmitter, and the axon terminal actively reuptakes part of the chemical. Theoretically, any step in this process could be modified by drug action. However, most drugs appear to act at the synapse by processes such as augmenting

the amount of neurotransmitter, influencing the action of catabolic enzymes in the synaptic cleft, or interacting with receptors on the postsynaptic membrane.

Because of differences in the chemical transmitters and receptors in various parts of the ANS, different drugs modify autonomic response in characteristic fashion. Acetylcholine is the neurotransmitter in ganglionic synapses, postganglionic parasympathetic synapses, and certain postganglionic sympathetic synapses (Fig. 22-4). Norepinephrine activates most postganglionic sympathetic synapses, the main exception being innervation of the sweat glands, which is mediated by acetylcholine. Cholinergic drugs that mimic or augment the effects of acetylcholine, therefore, increase parasympathetic activity, presynaptic sympathetic activity, and sympathetic stimulation of sweat glands. Sympathomimetics or adrenergic drugs produce the same general physiologic effects as sympathetic nerve stimulation. Certain drugs act only at the neuromuscular junction. The effects of others vary depending on the site of action and, in the case of receptor action, on the specific receptors affected by these chemicals (Table 22-1).

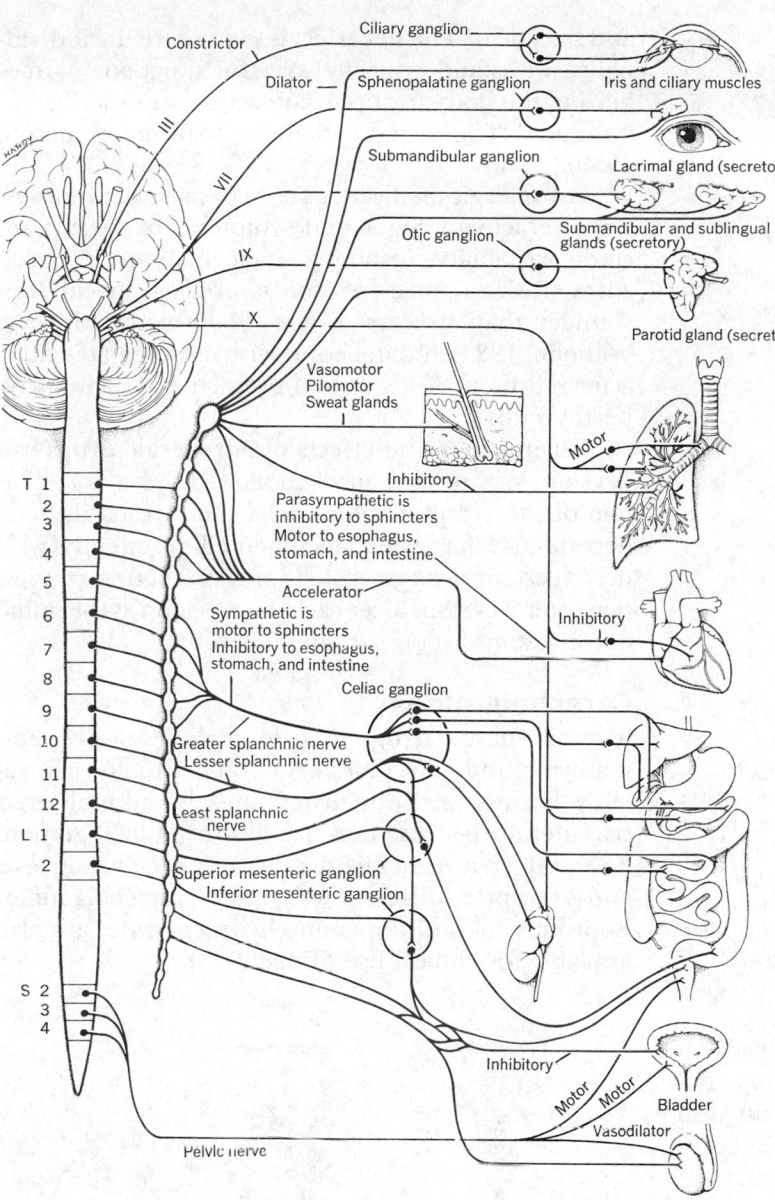

Figure 22-2. Diagram of the autonomic nervous system. Parasympathetic or craniosacral fibers are shown in black, while the sympathetic or thoracolumnar fibers are shown in color. Note that most organs have a double nerve supply. (From Chaffee EE, Lytle IM: *Basic physiology and anatomy, 4th ed.* Philadelphia: JB Lippincott Co.)

Receptors

Both the sympathetic and parasympathetic systems appear to have two distinct types of receptors (Table 22-2). In the sympathetic system, these receptors are designated by the first two letters of the Greek alphabet, alpha (α) and beta (β). The α receptors mediate responses such as vasoconstriction, contraction of the uterus, ureters, and nictitating membrane, dilation of the pupil, and inhibition of the gastrointestinal (GI) tract. The β receptor activity is characterized by vasodilation, inhibition of uterine contraction, dilation of the bronchi, and stimulation of the heart. Each type is divided further into two subclassifications according to the special tissues affected. Drugs that affect one type of receptor but not another have specific actions characteristic of the receptor involved. For example, β_1-

sympathetic blocking agents prevent sympathetic stimulation of the heart.

The parasympathetic system also has two distinct types of receptors, *nicotinic* and *muscarinic*. These names were given to the two subsystems because their specific actions were first recognized while their responses to the drug agents nicotine and muscarine were being observed. Nicotinic receptors are found in the ganglia, adrenal medulla, and striated muscle (the neuromuscular junction). Muscarinic receptors are found in the heart, smooth muscle, and glands (see Table 22-2). Many drugs affect one or the other of these receptor systems, but only a few affect both.

Autonomic drugs are best studied in relation to their specific action at the cellular level. Although agents are generally classified as adrenergic (sympathomi-

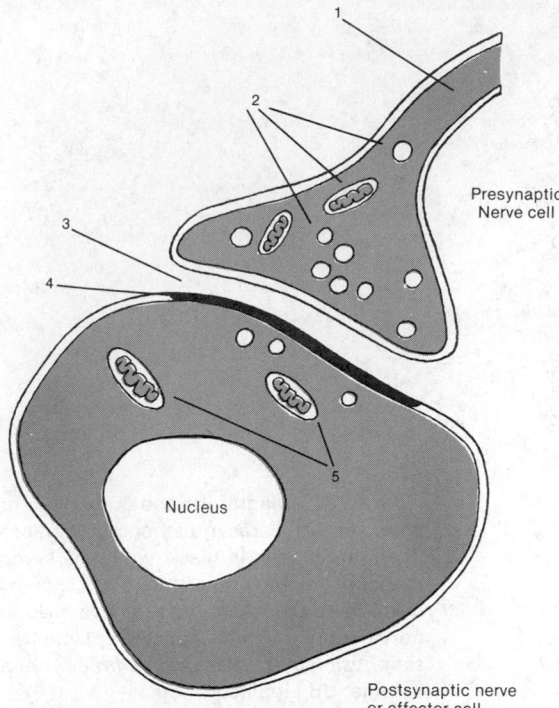

Figure 22-3. Steps in the synaptic transmission process. (*1*) Transport of substrate down the presynaptic axon; (*2*) organelles and enzymes in the nerve terminal that synthesize, store, release, and actively re-uptake the transmitter chemical; (*3*) synaptic contact zone, where extracellular enzymes catabolize the transmitter chemical; (*4*) postsynaptic receptor that triggers postsynaptic cell response to the transmitter chemical; (*5*) organelles within the postsynaptic cells that respond to receptor trigger.

metic), cholinergic (parasympathomimetic), antiadrenergic (sympatholytic), or anticholinergic (parasympatholytic), the serious student must further distinguish between muscarinic and nicotinic agents, α and β receptor drugs, and the specific site and mode of action of the particular compound.

Adrenergic compounds

Chemicals that cause an apparent increase in sympathetic nervous activity in the body are called *adrenergic*, *sympathomimetic*, or *sympathetic* drugs. The compounds in this group that contain dihydroxybenzene in their molecular structure belong to the chemical class of *catecholamines*. Other terms often applied to this group (eg, *pressor amines*, *decongestants*) reflect characteristics of their physiologic action (Box 22-2).

Although individual effects vary somewhat and these differences are highly significant in clinical practice, most adrenergic compounds share many actions. They generally stimulate the nervous system, constrict peripheral blood vessels, increase heart rate, dilate the bronchi and pupils, and cause a subjective feeling of psychological tension in the recipient. They tend to inhibit GI activity and micturition; they also mobilize energy sources in the body by increasing blood sugar

and fatty acid. The net effect is to prepare the individual to withstand critically stressful situations by mobilizing the body for necessary action, as described in Cannon's "fright–fight–flight" syndrome (Cannon, 1939).

Adrenergic medications tend to cause nervous system overactivity. Signs and symptoms of toxicity include irritability, insomnia, hallucinations, and seizures. Risk of toxic reaction is greatest in children younger than 6 years of age (Soderman, Sahlberg, Wilholm, 1984) and in people with disease states characterized by nervous system overactivity, such as hyperthyroidism.

Tolerance to the effects of adrenergic drugs can develop. Withdrawal may be followed by an exacerbation of the symptoms for which they are used. Such dependence has been documented frequently with decongestant nose drops or sprays; rebound congestion often develops after each dose as soon as the initial decongestant action subsides.

Catecholamines

Two adrenergic drugs used in clinical practice, epinephrine and norepinephrine, are actually natural body hormones. Both drugs must be administered parenterally because they are destroyed by digestion. Their effects are not identical because their action on α and β receptors differs. Two synthetic catecholamines, isoproterenol and dopamine hydrochloride, are also available for clinical use (Table 22-3).

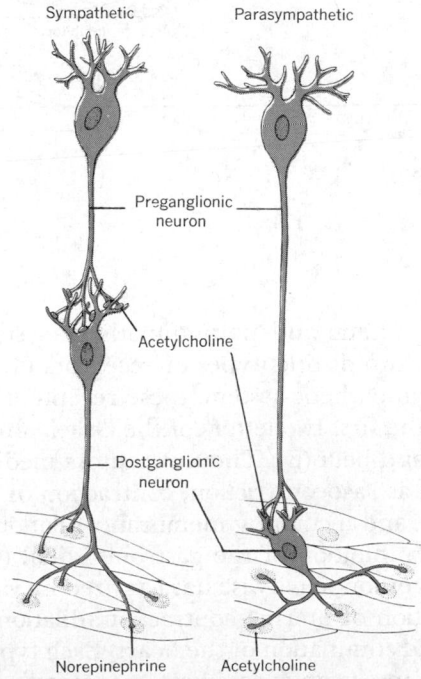

Figure 22-4. The chemical mediators. Acetylcholine is liberated by preganglionic fibers at synapses in all autonomic ganglia, and by parasympathetic postganglionic fiber endings. Norepinephrine is liberated at most sympathetic postganglionic fiber endings.

Table 22-1. General body responses to autonomic activity

Body part	Cholinergic activity	Adrenergic activity
Eye	Miosis, ciliary contraction	Mydriasis,* ciliary relaxation,† blinking*
Heart	Decreased rate and force of contraction	Increased rate and force of contraction†
	Tendency toward atrioventricular block, progressing to vagal arrest	
Blood vessels	Selective vasodilation (coronary, skin, mucosal, and cerebral arteries)	Selective vasodilation (arteries of the heart, lungs, and skeletal muscles),† generalized constriction of remainder of vasculature*
Lung	Bronchoconstriction	Bronchodilation†
	Increased secretion	
Gastrointestinal tract	Increased motility and secretion	Decreased motility and secretion*
	Relaxation of sphincters	Constriction of sphincters*
	Gallbladder contraction	Gallbladder relaxation
Ureter	Increased motility and tone	Decreased motility and tone*
Urinary bladder	Increased contractility	Decreased contractility†
	Relaxation of sphincter	Constriction of sphincter*
Uterus	Variable, depending on phase of menstrual cycle	
Nonpregnant	and hormone state	Relaxation†
Pregnant		Contraction*
Male sex organs	Erection	Ejaculation*
Skin	Generalized perspiration	Pallor
		Localized perspiration*
Adrenals	Secretion of epinephrine and norepinephrine	
Liver	Glycogen synthesis	Glycogenolysis, gluconeogenesis*†
Fat cells		Lipolysis*†

*Responses mediated by α-adrenergic receptors.
†Responses mediated by β-adrenergic receptors.

Epinephrine

The first of the catecholamines to be used widely in medicine, epinephrine (Adrenalin) has long been used in medical emergencies to stimulate cardiac function and raise blood pressure.

Table 22-2. Autonomic receptors

Receptor type	Responses mediated by receptors
Sympathetic	
α₁	Vasoconstriction, uterine contraction, blinking of the eye, ureteral contraction, mydriasis, inhibition of the GI tract
α₂	Presynaptic feedback inhibition
β₁	Increased force and rate of cardiac contractions, increased conduction velocity in the myocardium
β₂	Vasodilation, inhibition of uterine contraction, bronchodilation
Parasympathetic	
Muscarinic	Decreased rate of atrial contraction, selective (and limited) vasodilation, miosis, contraction of the ciliary muscle, increased tone and motility of the gastrointestinal tract, contraction of the gallbladder and biliary ducts, contraction of the detrusor muscle of the bladder, relaxation of the bladder sphincter
Nicotinic	Transmission in the autonomic ganglia

Pharmacodynamics. Epinephrine stimulates both α- and β-adrenergic receptors, producing the body responses described in Table 22-1 as characteristic of adrenergic activity. Stimulation of β cells activates adenylate cyclase, increasing intracellular cyclic adenosine monophosphate. Stimulation of α receptors appears to

(Text continues on p. 324)

Box 22-2. Classification of autonomic drugs

Adrenergic compounds

Catecholamines

Noncatecholamines

Antiadrenergic agents

α-adrenergic blocking agents

β-adrenergic blocking agents

Adrenergic neuron-blocking agents

Cholinergic drugs

Parasympathomimetic agents

Anticholinesterase agents

Anticholinergic drugs

Table 22-3. Adrenergic drugs

Drug names	Preparations	Usual dosage	Mode of action	Clinical uses
Catecholamines				
Dobutamine, hydrochloride (Dobutrex)	Vials that contain powder for preparing solutions for IV infusion	2.5–10 μg/kg body weight/min, adjusted according to heart rate, blood pressure, and urine flow PC: C	β$_1$-adrenergic receptor stimulation	Short-term treatment of cardiac decompensation caused by organic disease or cardiac surgery
Dopamine hydrochloride (Dopastat, Intropin)	Solution for dilution for IV infusion	Initially, 1–5 μg/kg body weight/min, increased by 1–4 μg/kg/min at 10–30-min intervals, until optimal response occurs PC: C	β$_1$, α, and dopaminergic receptor or simulation (depending on dose)	Treatment of hypotensive shock that persists after adequate fluid volume replacement, including cardiogenic shock
Epinephrine (Adrenalin, Asthma-Haler, Asthmanefrin, Broniten mist, Bronkaid Mist, EpiPen Auto-Injector, Medihaler-Epi, microNefrin, Nephron, Primatene, S-2, Vaponefrin)	Solutions for injection, oral inhalation, and topical application Ointment for topical application	Adults: 100–500 μg at intervals of 20 min–4 h (up to 5 mg/day in divided doses) Children: 10 μg/kg body weight, up to a maximum dose of 500 μg PC: C	α- and β-adrenergic receptor simulation	Treatment of acute anaphylaxis (the agent of choice) Treatment of cardiac arrest (as an adjunct) Local anesthesia (as an adjunct)
Isoproterenol hydrochloride, isoproterenol sulfate (Aerolone, Isuprel, Norisodrine)	Sublingual tablets Solutions for oral inhalation Solutions for injection	*By inhalation:* 100–200 μg, 4–6 times daily *Sublingual:* Adults: 10–20 mg q3–4 h to a maximum of 60 mg/day; children: 5–10 mg q3–4 h up to a maximum of 30 mg/day PC: C	β-adrenergic receptor stimulation	Alleviation of bronchospasm Treatment of cardiac arrest and arrhythmia (as an adjunct)
Norepinephrine bitartrate, levarterenol bitartrate (Levophed)	Solution for IV infusion	Initially: *Adults:* 8–12 μg/min *Children:* 2 μg/min Thereafter: according to blood pressure response PC: C	α- and β$_1$-adrenergic receptor stimulation	Treatment of hypotensive shock that persists after adequate fluid volume replacement
Noncatecholamines				
Albuterol, albuterol sulfate, salbutamol (Proventil, Ventolin)	Oral tablets Aerosol spray for oral inhalation	*By inhalation:* Adults and children 12 yr of age and older: 180 μg/ q4–6 h Children younger than 12 yr of age: 100–200 μg qid	β-adrenergic receptor stimulation	Alleviation of bronchospasm

320

Drug	Preparations	Dosage	Action	Uses
		Oral: Adults and children 12 yr of age and older: 2–4 mg tid-qid (with adjustments in relation to tolerance and response) PC: C		
Apraclonidine (Iodipine)	1% ophthalmic solutions	gtt ÷ to affected eye 1 h before surgery PC: C	α_2 adrenergic receptor stimulation	Prevention of high intraocular pressure associated with laser surgery
Bitoiterol mesylate (Tornalate)	Aerosol solution for oral inhalation	Adults and children older than 12 yr of age: 2 inhalations (34 µg each) q8h. Maximum dosage: 1.11 mg (3 inhalations) q6h or 740 µg (2 inhalations) q4h PC: C	β-adrenergic receptor stimulation	Prevention and treatment of bronchospasm in obstructive pulmonary disease
Ephedrine, ephedrine hydrochloride, ephedrine sulfate (Ectasule Minus, Efedron Nasal, Ephedsol-1%, Nasdro No. 3, Vatronol)	Solutions and jelly for nasal application; Capsules, syrups, and extended-release capsules for oral use; Solutions for injection	*Oral:* Adults: 25–50 mg q3–4 h PRN; children: 2–3 mg/kg body weight/day, divided in 4–6 doses. *Parenterally:* Adults: *IV:* 10–25 mg; *IM:* 25–50 mg. *Maximum daily dosage:* 150 mg (adults) PC: C	α- and β-adrenergic receptor stimulation	Alleviation of bronchospasm; Treatment of hypotensive shock that persists after adequate fluid volume replacement
Isoetharine hydrochloride, isoetharine mesylate (Beta-2, Bronkometer, Bronkosol)	Solution for oral inhalation	Adults: 0.5–1.0 ml of 0.5% solution q4h, diluted 1:3 for nebulizer administration PC: C	β-adrenergic receptor stimulation	Alleviation of bronchospasm
Mephentermine sulfate (Wyamine Sulfate)	Solutions for IM or IV injection	*Adults: IM:* 10–80 mg. *IV:* 1–5 mg/min PC: C	β- and (to a lesser degree) α-adrenergic receptor stimulation	Control and treatment of hypotension in selected situations
Metaproterenol sulfate (Alupent, Metaprel)	Tablets and solutions for oral use; Solutions for oral inhalation	Adults and children more than 9 yr of age, or more than 27.3 kg wt: 20 mg tid-qid. Children 6–9 yr of age or less than 27.3 kg wt: 10 mg tid-qid. Children less than 6 yr of age: 1.3–2.6 mg/kg body wt/day, divided in 3–4 doses. *Inhalation:* Adults and children 12 yr or older: 2–3 inhalations, q3–4 h (not to exceed 12 inhalations/24 h) PC: C	β-adrenergic receptor stimulation	Alleviation of bronchospasm

(Continued)

321

Table 22-3. Adrenergic drugs (*Continued*)

Drug names	Preparations	Usual dosage	Mode of action	Clinical uses
Noncatecholamines				
Metaraminol bitartrate (Aramine)	Solution for injection	*SC or IM:* Adults: 2–10 mg Children: 0.1 mg/kg body wt, or 3 mg/m² body surface *IV:* Adults: 0.5–5 mg as a single dose; Children: 0.01 mg/kg body weight, or 0.3 mg/m² body surface, as a single dose *IV infusion:* in accordance with blood pressure levels PC: D	α- and β₁-adrenergic receptor stimulation	Treatment of hypotensive shock that persists after adequate fluid volume replacement
Methoxamine hydrochloride (Vasoxyl)	Solution for IM or IV injection	Adults: *IM:* 5–20 mg; *IV:* 3–5 mg Children: *IM:* 0.25 mg/kg body wt, or 7.5 mg/m² body surface; *IV:* 0.08 mg/kg body weight PC: C	α-adrenergic receptor stimulation	Treatment of hypotensive shock that persists after adequate fluid volume replacement
Phenylephrine bitartrate, phenylephrine hydrochloride (Duo-Medihaler, Neo-Synephrine)	Solution for injection Solution for oral inhalation Solutions for topical application to the nose (in combination with other drugs) Cough syrups (in combination with other drugs)	*IV infusion:* Initial rate of 0.1–0.18 mg/min, thereafter, in accordance with blood pressure levels (usual maintenance dosage: 0.04–0.06 mg/min) PC: C	α-adrenergic receptor stimulation	Treatment of hypotensive shock that persists after adequate fluid volume replacement Alleviation of nasal congestion
Phenylpropanolamine hydrochloride (Anorexin, Appress, Cenadex, Control, Decongestant-P, Dex-A-Diet, Dexatrim, Dietac, Diet Gard, Nobese, Prolamine, Propagest, Resolution, Rhindecon, Westrim)	Tablets, syrup, capsules, and extended-release tablets and capsules for oral use	*Oral:* as a decongestant: Adults: 20–25 mg q4h (maximum daily dose: 150 mg); children 6–12 yr of age: 10–12.5 mg q4h (maximum daily dose: 75 mg); Children 2–6 yr of age: 6.25 mg q4h (maximum daily dose: 37.5 mg)	Indirect stimulation of α- and β-adrenergic receptors	Alleviation of nasal congestion Short-term treatment of exogenous obesity

Drug	Preparations	Mechanism	Dosage	Clinical Use
Pseudoephedrine hydrochloride (Cenafed, First Sign, Neofed, Novafed, Sinufed, Sudafed, Sudrin)	Tablets, extended-release capsules, and syrup for oral use	α- and (to a lesser degree) β-adrenergic receptor stimulation	As an anorectic: 25 mg tid or 37.5 mg bid PC: C Adults and children 12 yr of age or older: 60 mg q4–6h (maximum daily dosage: 240 mg) Children 6–11 yr of age: 30 mg q4–6h (maximum daily dosage: 120 mg) Children 2–5 yr of age: 15 mg q4–6h (maximum daily dosage: 60 mg) PC: C	Alleviation of nasal congestion
Ritodrine hydrochloride (Yutopar)	Oral tablets Solution for IV infusion	β-adrenergic receptor stimulation	IV: Initially 50–100 μg/min; thereafter in accord with response (usual maintenance dose 150–350 μg/min) Oral: 10 mg q2h or 10–20 mg q4–6h (maximum daily dosage 120 mg) PC: B	Inhibition of uterine contractions in premature labor (In practice, terbutaline is supplanting ritodrine for this purpose)
Terbutaline sulfate (Brethine, Bricanyl)	Oral tablets Solutions for subcutaneous injection	β-adrenergic receptor stimulation	Oral: Adults: 5 mg tid, administered at 6-h intervals during waking hours; children 12–15 yr of age: 2.5 mg tid Subcutaneous: Adults: 0.25 mg, repeated once after 15–30 min if necessary; children: 3.5–5 μg/kg body weight PC: B	Alleviation of bronchospasm Inhibition of uterine contraction in premature labor

KEY: PC = pregnancy category. (The validity of pregnancy categories has not been established; see Chapter 16, p 216.)

mobilize calcium ions or to increase inositol triphosphate (α_1 receptors) or to inhibit adenylate cyclase (α_2 receptors). Desired therapeutic responses depend on the clinical situation and may include mydriasis, vasoconstriction, increased heart rate and force of contraction, and bronchodilation. Epinephrine is a potent vasoconstrictor and cardiac stimulant. It also inhibits the release of histamine in allergic reactions.

Pharmacokinetics. Epinephrine must be administered parenterally or by inhalation, because its protein structure is destroyed by digestive enzymes in the GI tract. After both inhalation and injection, onset of action occurs within minutes. The drug crosses the placenta and is distributed in breast milk, but it does not cross the blood–brain barrier.

Epinephrine has a short duration of action because it is rapidly taken up and metabolized in sympathetic nerve endings. The liver and other tissues also metabolize epinephrine, in part by action of monoamine oxidase (MAO). Metabolites and a small amount of unchanged drug are excreted by the kidneys.

Therapeutic uses. Intracardiac injection of epinephrine has been a heroic measure used for decades in extreme emergencies. Although more effective means of resuscitation are now available, epinephrine is still occasionally used as an adjunct in treating cardiac arrest.

Epinephrine is the drug of choice for treating anaphylaxis and acute allergic reaction characterized by cardiovascular collapse and vasogenic shock. Injections of epinephrine reverse most of the pathology that occurs in this condition by constricting the vascular bed, stimulating heart contraction, and correcting the bronchial constriction and secretion associated with this syndrome.

Epinephrine is also a primary agent for relieving acute asthma. It brings about a rapid therapeutic effect by dilating the constricted bronchi and relieving bronchial congestion. It increases vital capacity, respiratory rate, and tidal volume. In addition, its inhibition of histamine release may add to its therapeutic action in asthma.

Historically, epinephrine has been used to treat hypoglycemic episodes in diabetics who receive insulin therapy. The rise in blood glucose that follows use of epinephrine produces a temporary remission of symptoms, restoring normal physical and mental function and allowing the victim to achieve a longer lasting correction of metabolism by consuming food that replenishes blood sugar. (Incidents are on record of spontaneous correction of such insulin reactions when a victim became angry, a state in which endogenous epinephrine is released into the circulation.) Epinephrine has been displaced for this use by glucagon, a hormone that has a more specific effect with fewer troublesome side effects.

Physicians and dentists who administer local anesthesia before performing painful procedures exploit an interaction between epinephrine and anesthetic agents. By mixing epinephrine with the anesthetic, the numbing effect of the anesthetic is prolonged without an increase of dose. Epinephrine stimulates local vasoconstriction in the area injected, reducing circulation to that site, thereby slowing the rate of absorption and dissipation of the anesthetic agent. Systemic toxicity from the anesthetic is diminished.

Epinephrine can be applied topically to control superficial bleeding. It is sometimes used to inhibit uterine contractions in premature labor and to inhibit formation of intraocular fluid in open angle glaucoma. Epinephrine has been administered intra-arterially to control severe GI or renal bleeding, to improve visualization of tumors by arteriography, and to protect kidneys from irradiation nephritis secondary to x-ray therapy.

Adverse reactions. Epinephrine increases the level of sympathetic nervous system activity and frequently causes signs and symptoms of overstimulation (*eg*, restlessness, headache, tremor, weakness, dizziness, palpitation, pallor, and subjective feelings of fearfulness, tension, and anxiety). Blood glucose levels rise, a response potentially harmful to individuals with diabetes mellitus. Blood pressure also rises, an undesirable effect in many clients. The most serious adverse reactions are increased risk of cerebral hemorrhage (one cause of stroke) and cardiac arrhythmia (including arrest).

Epinephrine interacts with many therapeutic agents. The results can sometimes be dangerous, especially for clients who are receiving general anesthetics (Table 22-4).

Precautions and contraindications. Side effects are transient but may be dangerous in clients with hypertension, angina, heart failure, hyperthyroidism, pheochromocytoma, and those forms of shock (hemorrhagic, cardiogenic) characterized by compensatory physiologic vasoconstriction. Epinephrine must be used with caution during anesthesia, because ventricular arrhythmia and cardiac arrest may occur. When local anesthetics are used to block pain in areas perfused by end-arteries (*ie*, the digits, nose, and penis), only epinephrine-free solutions can be used; local vasoconstriction can compromise circulation and cause hypoxic gangrene.

Norepinephrine

Norepinephrine (Levarterenol) differs from epinephrine in its effects in that it does not stimulate β_2-sympathetic receptors.

Pharmacodynamics. Norepinephrine stimulates α- and β_1-adrenergic receptors. It causes vasoconstriction with much less effect on other body systems than epinephrine. Although it does increase stroke volume

Table 22-4. Interactions of epinephrine with other medicinal drugs

Interacting drugs	Physiologic effect	Recommendations
Sympathomimetic drugs	Additive effects, causing toxic levels of sympathetic nervous system activity	Allow enough time between doses of sympathomimetic drugs for the effects of each to dissipate
Digitalis, mercurial diuretics, cyclopropane, halogenated hydrocarbon anesthetics	Sensitization of the myocardium to the effects of epinephrine, increasing the risk of arrhythmia	Do not use epinephrine with chloroform, trichlorethylene, and cyclopropane
		Use lidocaine or propanolol prophylactically when epinephrine is to be given with other halogenated hydrocarbon anesthetics to reduce the risk of cardiac arrhythmia
Thyroid hormone, tricyclic antidepressants	Potentiation of the cardiovascular effects of epinephrine	Reduce the dose of epinephrine and monitor clients closely during therapy
Monoamine oxidase inhibitors	Potentiation of effects of epinephrine	Do not use concurrently
Insulin	Decreased efficacy of insulin	Increase dosage of hypoglycemic drugs to meet the needs of diabetic clients when epinephrine is used
Adrenergic-blocking agents	Reduce some or all of the effects of epinephrine	Use blocking agents to ameliorate epinephrine toxicity

and coronary blood flow, norepinephrine does not effectively increase cardiac output, probably because of the increase in peripheral resistance in the vascular tree. Its metabolic effects are insignificant when compared to those of epinephrine.

Through its hypertensive action, norepinephrine increases mean arterial pressure, glomerular filtration, and urine production.

Pharmacokinetics. Norepinephrine, like epinephrine, is destroyed in the digestive tract. It is poorly absorbed from subcutaneous sites. The drug is administered by slow intravenous (IV) infusion.

Norepinephrine localizes mainly in sympathetic nervous tissue. It crosses the placenta but not the blood–brain barrier.

Norepinephrine has a short duration of action (1–2 minutes after termination of IV infusion). Like epinephrine, it is rapidly taken up and metabolized in sympathetic nerve endings. The liver and other tissues also metabolize norepinephrine, in part by MAO action. Metabolites and small amounts of unchanged drug are excreted by the kidneys.

Therapeutic uses. The principal therapeutic use of norepinephrine is the treatment of vasogenic shock, characterized by enlargement of the vascular bed disproportionate to the existing blood volume. It is administered by continuous IV drip. The pressor response is definite but disappears within minutes after drug administration is stopped. The drug produces general vasoconstriction, raising total peripheral resistance and systolic, diastolic, and pulse pressures. Compensatory vagal reflex stimulation slows the heart, and cardiac output may be decreased.

Adverse reactions. The side effects of norepinephrine are similar to those of epinephrine and include restlessness, headache, tremor, weakness, dizziness, pallor, dyspnea or apnea, and precordial pain. Blood levels of free fatty acids and cholesterol may increase. Hyperglycemia and CNS stimulation are evident when large doses are used. Like epinephrine, the drug can produce cardiac arrhythmia.

Norepinephrine can cause hypertension owing to severe peripheral vasoconstriction. Blood flow to vital organs may be reduced. The drug can also increase myocardial oxygen consumption, making the heart work harder. Toxicity is characterized by extreme hypertension, which can cause hemorrhage, including a hemorrhagic cerebral vascular accident (stroke).

Extravasation of norepinephrine solutions causes severe local vasoconstriction and reduced perfusion. Tissue necrosis can develop unless corrective measures are taken.

Precautions and contraindications. Norepinephrine therapy is not a substitute for volume replacement. Blood volume depletion should be corrected before therapy is started. Vital signs must be monitored closely during and immediately after norepinephrine infusion.

Care is required to prevent tissue infiltration of norepinephrine IV solutions. Should extravasation occur, phentolamine (5–10 mg diluted in 10–15 ml normal saline) injected directly into the affected tissues helps to prevent hypoxic necrosis.

Norepinephrine is contraindicated in hypovolemic and cardiogenic shock, during which maximal compensatory vasoconstriction is usually present. Additional vasopressin would reduce rather than increase perfusion. Instead, vasodilators are indicated to correct the circulatory problem.

Commercial preparations of norepinephrine contain sodium metabisulfite and should be used with caution for clients with known sensitivity to sulfite agents. Caution is also required when norepinephrine is administered to clients with hypertension or hyperthyroidism. Norepinephrine is contraindicated for people who are receiving cyclopropane or halogenated hydrocarbon general anesthetics, atropine, tricyclic antidepressants, MAO inhibitors, ergot alkaloids, guanethidine, and methyldopa.

Isoproterenol

Isoproterenol (Isuprel) is the most active of a group of sympathomimetic amines with alkyl substitution on the nitrogen atom of the molecule.

Pharmacodynamics. Isoproterenol acts primarily on β receptors in the sympathetic nervous system (SNS). It exerts typical β-sympathetic effects on the heart, smooth muscle of the bronchi, skeletal muscle vasculature, and GI tract. Physiologic responses include bronchodilation, cardiac stimulation, and peripheral vasodilation.

Pharmacokinetics. Isoproterenol is rapidly metabolized in the GI tract. It is readily absorbed from parenteral injection sites and the respiratory tract when inhaled. Absorption is unreliable after rectal or sublingual administration. Isoproterenol is taken up and metabolized by sympathetic nerve endings. It is also metabolized in the liver, lungs, GI tract, and other tissues. Both unchanged drug and metabolites are excreted by the kidneys.

Therapeutic uses. Isoproterenol is useful in respiratory disorders characterized by bronchoconstriction, in heart block, and in septicemic shock. It has also been used to correct circulatory abnormalities in pulmonary embolism and to aid in the diagnosis of coronary artery disease.

Adverse reactions. Serious adverse reactions to isoproterenol occur infrequently, especially when the drug is administered by inhalation. The effects of the drug tend to be short-lived but can be dangerous. The drug is a potent stimulator of the heart. Side effects are generally those of SNS stimulation: nervousness, fear, insomnia, anxiety, tremor, headache, nausea, vomiting. In addition, dizziness, tinnitus, and light-headedness may occur. Swelling of the parotid glands has been reported after prolonged use.

Disturbances in cardiac rhythm and rate can precipitate cardiac arrest. Arrhythmia is most likely to occur in people with cardiogenic shock, in those who are receiving other drugs that increase the risk of arrhythmia (*eg*, digitalis, cyclopropane or halogenated

hydrocarbon general anesthetics), and in those with hypoxia or fluid, electrolyte, or acid–base imbalances (*eg*, hypercapnia, acidosis, hyperkalemia, hypokalemia). Isoproterenol has been reported to induce Adams-Stokes seizures (a syndrome caused by heart block, characterized by sudden attacks of unconsciousness) in some individuals.

Excessive doses of isoproterenol may produce a temporary increase in blood pressure followed by hypotension. Shock may develop.

Administration of the drug by inhalation may cause bronchial irritation and edema, especially when powdered preparations are used. Isoproterenol turns pink or red on exposure to air, causing discoloration of saliva and sputum. Frequent use of sublingual tablets may damage the teeth because of the acidity of the drug.

Precautions and contraindications. Before initiation of isoproterenol therapy, hypoxia, acidosis, potassium imbalances, hypercapnia, and volume deficits should be corrected. Vital parameters of clients who receive the drug should be monitored closely, including central venous pressure, left ventricular filling pressure, and pulmonary arterial diastolic pressure. Therapy is best conducted in critical care settings.

Excessive use of isoproterenol by inhalation should be avoided. If tachyphylaxis or severe paradoxical airway resistance develops, the drug must be discontinued immediately and alternative treatment arranged. Isoproterenol should also be discontinued if precordial distress, angina, or ventricular arrhythmia occurs.

Isoproterenol should be administered with caution to elderly clients, to diabetics, and to people with renal or cardiovascular disease, hyperthyroidism, or a history of allergic sensitivity to sympathomimetic amines. It is contraindicated for individuals with a history of certain types of cardiac arrhythmia (*eg*, tachycardia). Commercial preparations of isoproterenol that contain sulfites should be used with caution in clients known to be sensitive to sulfite agents. Isoproterenol should not be administered concurrently with other sympathomimetic bronchodilators. At least 4 hours should elapse between doses if used alternately. Isoproterenol is contraindicated for clients who are receiving cyclopropane or halogenated hydrocarbon general anesthetics, as well as for clients with tachycardia caused by digitalis intoxication.

Safe use during pregnancy and lactation has not been established.

Dopamine

Dopamine is the physiologic precursor of norepinephrine.

Pharmacodynamics. Dopamine stimulates dopaminergic β$_1$-adrenergic receptors and releases norepinephrine from its storage sites. In low to moderate doses (0.5 µg/kg/min), it stimulates the heart and causes renal and mesenteric vasodilation because of an agonist action on dopaminergic receptors in these tissues. In IV doses of 2 µg/kg/min, β₁-adrenergic receptors are stimulated. In high doses (more than 10 µg/kg/min), α-adrenergic effects become more prominent, increasing vasoconstriction and peripheral resistance.

Pharmacokinetics. Because it is rapidly metabolized in the GI tract, dopamine is administered IV. The drug is widely distributed after absorption but does not cross the blood–brain barrier. Whether it crosses the placenta is not known.

About 25% of the dopamine dose is metabolized to norepinephrine in adrenergic nerve terminals. The remainder is rapidly metabolized in the liver, kidneys, and plasma, in part by MAO. Plasma half-life, normally about 2 minutes, may be as long as 1 hour in people who are receiving MAO inhibitors. Dopamine metabolites and a small fraction of the unchanged drug are excreted by the kidneys.

Therapeutic uses. The hydrochloride salt of dopamine is used as an adjunct to increase cardiac output, blood pressure, and urine flow in the treatment of severe refractory congestive heart failure. It is also used to treat shock that persists after fluid volume replacement. Somewhat less potent than isoproterenol, dopamine can be used to treat clients who experience hypotension and abnormal cardiac rhythms with isoproterenol.

Dopamine is administered by IV infusion in accordance with the client's cardiovascular response.

Adverse reactions. The toxic and side effects of dopamine are typical of adrenergic drugs. They include tachycardia, angina, palpitation, ectopic heartbeats, nausea, vomiting, and headache. Cardiac conduction abnormalities and arrhythmia may occur.

Extravasation of IV solutions may cause severe vasoconstriction and tissue damage. Prolonged use or high doses of dopamine can cause gangrene secondary to severe peripheral vasoconstriction.

Precautions and contraindications. Dopamine therapy is not a substitute for volume replacement. Adequate fluid volumes must be available to sustain adequate circulation. Because clients who receive dopamine must be closely monitored during therapy, the drug is usually used only in acute care settings, such as coronary care units.

Caution is required when dopamine is administered to clients with a history of occlusive vascular disease. Dosage should be reduced if the recipient has received tricyclic antidepressants or MAO inhibitors. In the latter case, dosage should be cut to *one-tenth* or less of the usual dosage. Phentolamine antagonizes the action of dopamine and may be administered to correct its toxic effects.

Dobutamine
Dobutamine (Dobutrex) is a synthetic sympathomimetic drug that is structurally related to dopamine.

Pharmacodynamics. Dobutamine stimulates β₁-adrenergic receptors, apparently by stimulating adenyl cyclase activity. Unlike dopamine, the drug does not cause release of endogenous norepinephrine, nor is its action dependent on this mechanism.

Pharmacokinetics. Dobutamine is administered IV. It is ineffective when administered orally because of rapid metabolism in the GI tract. The drug is also rapidly metabolized in the tissues, especially the liver, and plasma half-life is only about 2 minutes. Onset of action occurs within 2 minutes after IV administration; with cessation of the drug, therapeutic effects subside quickly. Dobutamine is excreted in urine and, to a minor extent, in feces. It is not known if dobutamine crosses the placenta or is distributed in breast milk.

Therapeutic uses. Dobutamine is used to increase cardiac output in the treatment of people with inadequate cardiac contractility from organic heart disease or cardiac surgery. Dobutamine may be preferable to dopamine for treating clients immediately after cardiopulmonary bypass, because it lowers peripheral resistance, it is relatively cardioselective, and its effects are not dependent on release of endogenous catecholamines.

Adverse reactions. The adverse effects of dobutamine are principally those of SNS stimulation of the cardiovascular system. They include cardiac arrhythmia (ectopic heartbeats and increased rate), angina, palpitation, and hypertension. Dobutamine increases the risk of cardiac arrhythmia during general anesthesia.

Precautions and contraindications. Blood volume must be restored in hypovolemic clients before dobutamine therapy is begun. Use of the drug is usually limited to critical care settings in which electrocardiographic output, vital signs, cardiac output, and pulmonary wedge pressure can be monitored. To prevent ventricular tachycardia, clients with atrial fibrillation should be digitalized before initiation of dobutamine therapy. Dobutamine should be used with extreme caution in clients with severe valvular aortic stenosis and those with recent myocardial infarction. It is contraindicated for clients with idiopathic hypertrophic subaortic stenosis.

Safe use during pregnancy and in children has not been established.

Noncatecholamines

The effects of noncatecholamine adrenergics depend on a combination of direct action on effector cells and the release of norepinephrine from stores in adrenergic nerve terminals. If the former effect predominates, β-receptor action is apparent; if the latter predominates, α activity is apparent. Many noncatecholamines are widely used in clinical conditions that require β-sympathetic stimulation. Some noncatecholamines are also incorporated in over-the-counter (OTC) drugs marketed for the treatment of respiratory conditions. The toxic and side effects of these preparations are characteristic of adrenergic drugs: tachycardia, hypertension, anorexia, nausea, and vomiting. Their use by the lay public is potentially dangerous.

Ephedrine

Ephedrine, a plant extract, was first used more than 5,000 years ago in China. Producing both α- and β-sympathetic effects, the drug acts directly on receptors and indirectly through the release of norepinephrine. The rapid reduction in effectiveness of repeated doses (tachyphylaxis) is believed to be due to depletion of norepinephrine stores. Ephedrine is effective when administered orally and has a long (2–4 hours) duration of action. Its main therapeutic uses are in bronchospasm, Adams-Stokes syndrome, narcolepsy, and allergic disorders. It acts also as a mydriatic and nasal decongestant.

Phenylephrine

Phenylephrine exerts powerful α-adrenergic stimulation, primarily by direct action on receptors. Central stimulation is minimal. The predominant actions are cardiovascular, causing a rise in blood pressure and reflex bradycardia. Phenylephrine is used therapeutically as a nasal decongestant and mydriatic. Its hypertensive effect is helpful in terminating attacks of paroxysmal atrial tachycardia, and it can be substituted for epinephrine in the administration of local anesthetics.

Terbutaline sulfate

One of a group of drugs developed for the treatment of bronchial asthma, terbutaline sulfate shares the selective activity of these drugs on β_2-receptors. This activity relaxes smooth muscle of the bronchi, the uterus, and the skeletal muscle vasculature. Cardiac stimulation is much less than with other sympathetic agents, such as isoproterenol. Terbutaline sulfate is effective when given orally. A related drug (ritodrine) is sometimes given parenterally to interrupt premature labor. Information on sympathomimetic drugs used for respiratory conditions may be found in Chapter 37.

Amphetamine

Amphetamine exerts both α and β actions common to other adrenergic agents. In addition, it is a powerful stimulant of the CNS. Amphetamines are discussed in Chapter 23.

See Table 22-3 for more information on individual noncatecholamine adrenergics. Bronchodilators are also discussed in Chapter 37.

■ Summary

Chemicals that cause responses that resemble the signs and symptoms of SNS activity are called adrenergics, sympathomimetics, or sympathic drugs. Generally, they stimulate the nervous system, constrict blood vessels, dilate the bronchi and pupils, and cause a subjective feeling of psychological tension. They tend to inhibit GI activity and micturition and to mobilize energy sources. In short, they prepare for the fright–fight–flight syndrome. Catecholamine adrenergics may appear as natural hormones or may be produced synthetically. Some noncatecholamine adrenergics are widely used in OTC drugs for respiratory conditions; their use by the lay public is potentially dangerous.

Nursing management

Nursing implications

Epinephrine therapy often requires repeated doses because the drug is metabolized quickly and may be dissipated before the desired effect is attained. Yet, repeated doses may produce side effects. Clients should be monitored carefully to detect toxicity, should it develop. Undesirable side effects can also occur during prolonged surgical procedures that involve local anesthesia in which epinephrine is used as an adjunct.

Injectable preparations of epinephrine should be routinely stocked in emergency drug supplies. Nurses who practice in situations in which acute anaphylactic reactions are likely and emergency medical care is not immediately available should obtain a supply of the drug and become familiar with its use. Standing orders for treatment in specific situations are also helpful. For example, because anaphylactic reactions to insect bites can be rapidly fatal, camp nurses should be fully prepared to initiate on-the-spot treatment.

Intravenous infusions of norepinephrine, dopamine, or dobutamine should be administered with an infusion pump or IVac regulator. The infusions must be closely monitored to maintain blood pressure within the prescribed parameters (Malcolm, Miller, 1965) and to detect infiltration promptly should it occur. An adrenergic blocking agent, such as phentolamine, should be available at the bedside during these treatments as an antidote, should the drug solution extravasate into the tissues. The α-blocking agent should be injected directly into the infiltrated tissues to prevent dangerous vasoconstriction.

If cardiovascular homeostasis is precarious, serious complications may be precipitated by the use of adrenergic agents. The potential benefits of the drug must be weighed against the risks of vasoconstriction, cardiac stimulation, and hypertension. The client who is receiving adrenergics must be carefully monitored for signs of cardiovascular problems, especially when norepinephrine or dopamine is administered IV to maintain circulation. Acute hypertension of lethal proportions may occur. In this situation, vital signs are monitored as often as every 2 minutes when dosage is being altered (Malcolm, Miller, 1965). Lethal doses vary from 10 to 30 mg.

Enrichment experience 22-1

Interview an asthmatic client to determine the subjective effects of adrenergic medication used to control acute episodes of dyspnea. What does the client do to alleviate the adverse effects of these drugs?

The use of adrenergic drugs (ritodrine or terbutaline sodium) to inhibit premature labor requires close monitoring to detect early signs and symptoms of complications, such as myocardial ischemia, cardiac arrhythmia, hypotension, and pulmonary edema. These adverse reactions can rapidly become life-threatening (Benedetti, 1981). Vital signs should be checked at least every 15 minutes. Parameters to monitor include urinary output and blood glucose levels.

Nursing process

Assessment Before adrenergic drugs are administered, the client's history should be reviewed to rule out contraindications for the prescribed drugs. The contraindications may include disease states (*eg*, thyrotoxicosis, hypertension, coronary artery disease, hemorrhagic or cardiogenic shock, occlusive vascular disease, pheochromocytoma, and allergic sensitivity to sulfite agents) or other drugs being taken (*eg*, other sympathomimetic agents, tricyclic antidepressants, and MAO inhibitors). Physical assessment should include lung and cardiac status, peripheral circulation, and blood chemistries. If hypovolemia, hypoxia, acidosis, hyperglycemia, potassium imbalance, or hypercapnia are present, the physician should be informed so that the condition can be corrected before adrenergic medication is initiated. During adrenergic therapy, clients must be assessed regularly for signs and symptoms of toxic or side effects.

Nursing diagnosis Initial diagnoses that arise from the client's illness may include the following:

> *Decreased tissue perfusion related to hypotension*
> *Impaired gas exchange related to bronchoconstriction*

A common collaborative problem that should be differentiated from the nursing diagnoses is:

> *Potential complication: hemorrhage*

Conditions that stem from the use of adrenergic drugs may include the following:

> *Anxiety related to severity of illness and to the physiologic effects of adrenergic drugs*
> *Altered comfort: perspiration, feelings of warmth related to adrenergic medication*
> *Altered nutrition: less than body requirements related to anorexia or nausea secondary to adrenergic medication*
> *Self-care deficit related to fatigue secondary to adrenergic medication*
> *Sleep pattern disturbance: insomnia related to CNS stimulation secondary to adrenergic medication*
> *High risk for altered health maintenance related to knowledge deficit concerning the prescribed drugs and the self-care measures for minimizing adverse reactions to them*

Planning Goals of treatment may include restoration of tissue perfusion, increased gas exchange, decrease in or elimination of bleeding, reduction of anxiety, alleviation of discomfort, improved nutrition, correction of care deficit by substitution of nursing care for self-care, increased rest and sleep, and teaching the client appropriate information related to the drug regimen.

Intervention Dependent nursing care involves the administration of drugs ordered by the physician. These may be given by inhalation or IV routes. Verification of the dosage and route of administration for the prescribed drugs is critical; errors in either may be life-threatening.

Interdependent interventions include consulting with the physician about the client's response to treatment and changes in orders that may be required.

Independent nursing interventions may include the following: monitoring the client for therapeutic and adverse response to the drug regiment (including close monitoring of vital signs), providing physical comfort measures (*eg*, frequent bathing, providing light clothing and bed covers, positioning for optimum

(*Text continues on p. 332*)

Example of nursing process and allergic reaction

The client is a 12-year-old girl residing in a summer camp. She has a history of allergic sensitivity to nuts and chocolate, which cause asthma attacks if she eats them when she has a "cold." She also reacts allergically to bee stings, which have caused skin rash and fever in the past.

The client brought a bee-sting kit with her to camp. The syringe in the kit contains 1 ml of 1:1000 epinephrine. Her physician has instructed her parents to administer 0.3 ml of this solution to her if she is stung by a bee. The nurse in the physician's office taught her mother how to the use the kit. The client says no one has ever told her how to avoid bee stings.

Two days before the end of the camp session, the client is stung on the ankle while hiking with a group of campers. The counselor with the group administered a dose of epinephrine immediately.

When seen in the infirmary an hour later, the client exhibited no signs or symptoms of allergic reaction, except for redness and swelling at the site of the sting. In mid-afternoon (5 hours after the client was stung) a counselor brought the client to the infirmary because she had "broken out all over with hives." The client had many large wheals on her trunk and extremities; she complained of intense itching.

The client had eaten a peanut butter sandwich, carrot sticks, milk, and an Oreo cookie for lunch.

Assessment data	Nursing diagnosis	Intervention	Goals and outcome criteria
History of asthma History of systemic reaction to bee stings	High risk for impaired gas exchange and altered tissue perfusion related to acute allergic reaction to bee stings	**Advise** the client to carry bee sting kit with her at all times and to inform a member of the camp staff immediately if stung. **Advise** the client to avoid using perfume with floral scents and areas where bees are frequently seen. **Advise** the client to report any allergic symptoms as soon as possible. **Inform** all members of the staff about the camper's allergy to bee stings; demonstrate the kit and instruct the staff in its use. **Ask** staff members to inform you as soon as possible if the camper is stung. **Verify** that the emergency supplies in the infirmary include syringes, needles, and epinephrine solutions for injection. **Review** the standing orders given by the camp physician for treating symptoms of acute allergy.	The client will not experience dyspnea or hypotension. Should an allergic reaction occur, it will be detected and treated promptly. The client will not sustain another bee sting. The client will repeat back to the nurse the information provided in teaching sessions. The client will not use floral scents; she will report to the nurse promptly if she experiences signs or symptoms of allergy. If the client is stung, she will be properly medicated by a staff member. Staff members will inform the nurse promptly if the camper is stung.
5-hour-old bee sting treated with 0.3 ml of epinephrine 1:1000 Urticaria Complaint of itching	Altered comfort: itching related to urticaria secondary to allergic reaction to a bee sting	If the standing orders indicate the use of epinephrine for urticaria, **give** the client a second dose; if necessary, consult with the physician on call regarding treatment of urticaria. If the physician concurs, give the client an antihistamine, such as Chlortrimeton.	The wheals will fade and disappear. The client will state that the itching is relieved.

(Continued)

Assessment data	Nursing diagnosis	Intervention	Goals and outcome criteria
		Apply cold packs to the affected areas.	
Urticaria Complaint of itching	High risk for infection related to scratching secondary to urticaria and itching	**Apply** phenolated calamine lotion to the wheals; advise the client to return for renewal of the calamine lotion after 4 or more hours if itching continues or returns.	The client will not scratch the inflamed skin. The client will not develop signs and symptoms of skin infection.
		Instruct the client to press on itching areas rather than to scratch them; suggest the use of cold compresses or ice packs for relief, if needed, between applications of calamine lotion.	
		Arrange with the kitchen staff for the client to obtain ice if needed.	
Allergy to chocolate and nuts Consumption of peanut butter and chocolate cookie	Knowledge deficit regarding allergy and self-care measures to control allergic reactions	**Advise** the client to avoid all substances to which she is known to be allergic (specifically nuts and chocolate) for a week or more, because reaction to them will exacerbate her reaction to the bee sting.	The client will relate to the nurse the major points of the content taught. The client will avoid contact with known allergens for the next week. The client will avoid practices that increase the risk of allergic reactions. The client will not experience a severe systemic allergic reaction.
		Prepare a teaching program for the client's parents that will cover the following: a recommendation that they secure an automatic self-injection bee sting kit (EpiPen or EpiPen Junior) for the client's use; emphasize the importance of avoiding all allergens when the client has any signs or symptoms of allergic reaction; discuss techniques for avoiding bees when outdoors; and suggest that the parents explore the possibility of desensitization treatment, to eliminate or reduce the severity of the client's reaction to bee stings.	
		The last day of camp, **meet** with the client's parents and implement the teaching plan.	
		Arrange with the staff to substitute allowable treats for the client when treats she must avoid are served to the campers.	
		Monitor the client for an increased in or recurrence of signs and symptoms of allergic reaction.	

respiration and circulation), helping to promote appetite and encouraging eating, carrying out hygienic care that the client cannot complete without undue fatigue, providing measures to promote rest and sleep (*eg*, reduction in stimuli, soothing back rubs), and developing and implementing an appropriate teaching plan.

Client education. Clients for whom adrenergic drugs are ordered are often too ill to question about knowledge of their conditions or the drugs to be used in their treatment. In this situation, the nurse gives the client clear, brief instructions and explanations during treatment. After resolution of the crisis situation, the client's knowledge should be assessed.

Clients who receive therapeutic adrenergics should be warned that they may feel fearful, anxious, tense, and restless, and that they may have difficulty sleeping. Headache, tremor, weakness, dizziness, palpitation, and pallor may occur. Clients may be reassured that feelings of apprehension and tension are direct effects of the chemicals and are not indicative of emotional breakdown or mental illness. They should be taught techniques to promote rest and sleep and to relieve muscle tension.

Adrenergic bronchodilators may be prescribed for home treatment, using an air compressor and nebulizer to generate a mist that is inhaled. The client must be taught correct use of the machine and the specifics of the drug regimen. After nebulizer treatments, the client should rinse the mouth to remove drug residues. The nebulizer should also be rinsed after each use (see Chapter 37 for more information on respiratory drugs).

Clients subject to acute anaphylaxis in response to allergens (*eg*, bee stings, foods that trigger severe allergic reactions) sometimes carry epinephrine in emergency kits. One product, EpiPen, provides a preloaded automatic syringe that can be self-administered (Lockey, 1980). Careful instruction in the use of the kit should be given to the client and to close family members or friends who may be present during an anaphylactic episode. After such an episode, medical attention should be sought promptly, because the efficacy of the epinephrine is transitory.

Nurses should caution clients against excessive use of OTC drugs that contain adrenergic compounds marketed as decongestants. Their effects are temporary and are followed by rebound congestion; therefore, they tend to cause dependence. Their short-term use (a few days) is relatively innocuous, but medical attention should be sought if they are needed for prolonged periods (more than 2 weeks).

Evaluation Data required for evaluation include information related to tissue perfusion and oxygenation, amount of bleeding, client's comfort (physical and mental), sleep patterns, and knowledge related to the drug regimen and self-care measures used to minimize adverse drug effects (see the Example of Nursing Process and Allergic Reaction).

Checklist of nursing actions

☐ Routinely stock injectable preparations of epinephrine for emergencies. Familiarize yourself with their uses.

When adrenergic drugs are prescribed

☐ Verify the dosage and route of administration for the prescribed drug.

☐ Use nursing measures to promote sleep and prevent insomnia.

☐ Bathe clients frequently.

☐ Present food when drug effects are minimal.

☐ Provide client with ample opportunities for rest.

☐ Monitor carefully for signs of cardiovascular problems and sympathetic effects on other body systems.

☐ Reassure the client that feelings of apprehension and tension are a result of the drug.

☐ Teach clients how to manage long-term medication regimens.

☐ Teach clients techniques to promote rest and sleep.

Adrenergic blocking agents

Antiadrenergic agents reduce sympathetic responses either at the receptor cell site or at the adrenergic nerve level. Sympathetic blocking agents inhibit responses by interacting with the receptor site on the effector cell in a way that prevents interaction of the receptor site with either endogenous hormones (epinephrine and norepinephrine) or other sympathomimetic amines. The inhibition is selective; some blocking agents inhibit only α-adrenergic response, while others block only β-adrenergic response. Adrenergic neuron-blocking agents interfere with the normal release of norepinephrine at nerve terminals. They reduce pulse transmission of all peripheral sympathetic fibers, whether α or β receptors are involved, but interfere with neither hormone secretion by the adrenal medulla nor response to sympathomimetic drugs.

In addition to the drugs discussed below, several antihypertensives exhibit adrenergic blocking action (see Chapter 28).

α-Adrenergic blocking agents

α-Adrenergic blocking agents include ergot alkaloids, haloalkylamines (phenoxybenzamine), and imidazole preparations (phentolamine; Table 22-5).

Ergot alkaloids

Ergot is prepared from dried parts of a fungus (*Claviceps purpurea*) that grows on grain, especially rye. The

Table 22-5. α-Adrenergic blocking agents

Drug names	Preparations	Usual dosage	Therapeutic uses
Ergot alkaloids			
Dihydroergotamine mesylate (DHE)	Solution for IM or IV injection	Adults: *IM:* Initially 1 mg, followed by 1 mg/h until relief is obtained (to a maximum dosage of 3 mg); *IV:* Up to 2 mg Maximum weekly parenteral dosage: 16 mg PC: X	Prevention or abortion of vascular headaches, including migraine and cluster headaches
Ergoloid mesylate (Deapril-ST, Hydergine, Hydro-Ergoloid, Hydro-Ergot, Hydroloid-G, Niloric, Uni-Gine)	Tablets, capsules, and solution for oral use Sublingual tablets	1–2 mg Maximum daily dosage: 12 mg PC: X	Alleviation of symptoms of senility believed to be due to cerebrovascular insufficiency
Ergotamine tartrate* (Ergomar, Ergostat, Gynergen, Medihaler Ergotamine, Wigrettes)	Sublingual tablets Solution for oral inhalation In combination with caffeine: oral tablets, extended-release oral tablets and rectal suppositories	*Oral or sublingual:* Adults: Initially 2 mg, followed by 1–2 mg q30 min up to a total of 6 mg (Maximum dosage: 6 mg/24 h or 10 mg/wk); children: 1 mg repeated once after 30 min if necessary (Safety and efficacy in children have not been established) *Inhalation:* 360 μg (one inhalation) q5min (Maximum dosage: 2.16 mg [6 inhalations]/24 hr or 5.4 mg [15 inhalations]/wk)	Prevention or abortion of vascular headaches, including migraine and cluster headaches (the agent of choice)
Methysergide maleate (Sansert)	Oral tablets	Adults: 4–8 mg/day, divided in 3 doses administered with meals. Maximum duration of treatment: 6 mo (3–4-wk intervals must separate treatment periods)	Prevention of severe refractory vascular headaches, including migraine and cluster headaches
Haloalkylamine			
Phenoxybenzamine hydrochloride (Dibenzyline)	Oral capsules	Adults: Initially 10 mg qd, thereafter increased by 10 mg daily at intervals of 4 days or more until a response occurs (Usual maintenance dose: 20–60 mg/day) Children: Initially 0.2 mg/kg body wt, or 5 mg/m², once daily (Maximum initial dose: 10 mg; usual maintenance dosage: 0.4–1.2 mg/kg body wt, or 12–36 mg/m², daily) PC: C	Control or prevention of paroxysmal hypertension and sweating in clients with pheochromocytoma Treatment of peripheral vasospastic disorders (as an adjunct)
Imidazoline			
Phentolamine mesylate (Regitine)	Vials that contain powder for preparing solutions for IM or IV injection	For diagnosis of pheochromocytoma: Adults: 5 mg IV Children: 1 mg IV or 3 mg IM	Diagnosis of pheochromocytoma Control or prevention of paroxysmal hypertension in clients with pheochromocytoma

(Continued)

Table 22-5. α-Adrenergic blocking agents (Continued)

Drug names	Preparations	Usual dosage	Therapeutic uses
Ergot alkaloids			
		To control hypertension caused by pheo-chromocytoma: Adults: 5 mg q1–2h Children: 9.1 mg/kg body weight, repeated once if necessary	Prevention of necrosis and sloughing after extravasation of IV norepinephrine
		As an antidote for infil-trated norepinephrine: 5–10 mg in 10 ml normal saline, infiltrated into the affected area	

*Also marketed in various combinations with caffeine.

KEY: PC = pregnancy category. (The validity of pregnancy categories has not been established; see Chapter 16, p 216.)

alkaloids contained in this natural material are toxic, causing abortion and peripheral vascular insufficiency (due to vasoconstriction) in poisoned mammals. Fungal contamination of grains is most likely to occur during warm moist growing seasons. The toxic potential of moldy grain has been known for centuries, but epidemics of poisoning have occurred as recently as 1953 (in France). In addition to ergot alkaloids, the mold sometimes produces lysergic acid diethylamide (LSD), causing CNS complications (perceptual disorders and hallucinations) in affected individuals.

Crude ergot is a complex substance that contains a dozen or more active alkaloids. Pure preparations are preferable for medicinal use; some drugs used today are semisynthetic.

Pharmacodynamics. The ergot alkaloids discussed below act by competitive inhibition of α-adrenergic receptors. Interaction of the blocking agent with the receptor site does not initiate effector-cell stimulation. It also prevents sympathetic hormones and sympathomimetic drugs from doing so. The drugs block pathologic effects of catecholamines, including pulmonary edema, reduced plasma volume, pericardial effusion, adrenal cortex necrosis, hyperglycemia, and cardiac arrhythmia. In addition, ergot alkaloids tend to dilate hypertonic blood vessels and constrict hypotonic blood vessels.

Pharmacokinetics. Gastrointestinal absorption of ergot alkaloids is variable. Dihydroergotamine is not well absorbed and is administered parenterally. The absorption of ergotamine tartrate varies, but the drug is administered both orally and rectally. Ergoloid and methysergide are rapidly absorbed orally. Concurrent administration of caffeine appears to enhance GI absorption of ergot alkaloids. Because all of these compounds are metabolized by the liver, a portion of each oral dose is destroyed during the first pass through the liver (in the case of ergoloid, as much as 50% of the dose is involved). Ergot alkaloids are distributed widely in the body, crossing the blood–brain barrier and probably distributing in breast milk in nursing mothers. Plasma half-lives tend to be biphasic, varying from 1.4 to 3.6 hours during the initial phase to almost 24 hours during the late phase. Excretion is by the kidneys.

Therapeutic uses. α-Adrenergic blocking ergot alkaloids are used to improve cerebral circulation. Administered early during migraine and cluster headaches, they often abort the attacks. Some ergot preparations are also used to treat senility caused by cerebrovascular insufficiency.

Adverse reactions. Common adverse reactions to ergot alkaloids include GI upset (nausea, vomiting, abdominal pain) and weakness of the legs. Withdrawal of medication may be followed by rebound headache.

Arterial spasms may cause cold painful extremities with paresthesia (numbness, tingling) and claudication. Abdominal angina or angina pectoris can occur.

Serious toxic reactions are rare but include gangrene of the extremities and myocardial or enteric infarction. In addition, methysergide can cause fibrosis in retroperitoneal, pleuropulmonary, and cardiac tissues. This condition often regresses and may disappear when the drug is discontinued.

Precautions and contraindications. The administration of ergot alkaloids should be discontinued if signs and symptoms of impaired circulation develop. The extremities should be kept warm to promote circulation, and supportive care should be given. Severe peripheral vasoconstriction may be treated by IV sodium nitroprusside or intra-arterial tolazoline.

Contraindications for ergot alkaloids include peripheral vascular disease (severe arteriosclerosis, arteritis, severe hypertension, cardiovascular disease, phlebitis) and allergic hypersensitivity to these substances. In addition, methysergide is contraindicated for clients with pulmonary disease, collagen disease, fibrotic processes, valvular heart disease, peptic ulcer, impaired hepatic or renal function, or serious infections.

Phenoxybenzamine

Pharmacodynamics. The exact mechanism of action of phenoxybenzamine is not completely understood. The compound does form stable bonds with chemical groups of α-adrenergic receptors, thereby producing a relatively long-lived blockade. Phenoxybenzamine reverses the pressor effect of epinephrine and blocks (but does not reverse) the vasoconstrictor effects of norepinephrine. The drug may also inhibit responses to some other substances, such as acetylcholine, serotonin, and histamine.

Pharmacokinetics. Phenoxybenzamine is variably absorbed from the GI tract. Onset of action is gradual, effects are cumulative for about 1 week, and biologic half-life is about 24 hours. A single oral dose produces blockade that persists from 3 to 4 days.

Because it is highly lipid soluble, phenoxybenzamine may accumulate in fat. It is not known if the drug crosses the placenta or is distributed in breast milk.

Phenoxybenzamine is metabolized by dealkylation. It is excreted by the urinary and biliary systems.

Therapeutic uses. Phenoxybenzamine is the drug of choice for the medical treatment of pheochromocytoma. It controls or prevents the paroxysmal hypertension and sweating characteristic of this disorder. It is used for clients who are awaiting surgery to remove this tumor and also for clients for whom surgery is not indicated.

Phenoxybenzamine has been used as an adjunct in the treatment of vasospastic disorders (*eg*, Raynaud's disease, frostbite sequelae).

Adverse reactions. Side effects of phenoxybenzamine stem from cardiac and GI responses to the nontherapeutic autonomic effects of the drug. Adverse reactions include postural hypotension, tachycardia, miosis, nasal stuffiness, inhibition of ejaculation, and sedation. Accommodation to postural hypotension develops with continued administration, but symptoms of dizziness and palpitations tend to recur when vasodilation is stimulated (as when eating a large meal, drinking alcohol, or exercising).

Toxic manifestations of phenoxybenzamine overdose include tachycardia, fainting, vomiting, lethargy, and shock.

Precautions and contraindications. Adverse reactions to phenoxybenzamine can be minimized by starting the drug in small doses and increasing the dose gradually until the desired therapeutic response is attained. Phenoxybenzamine should be used with caution for clients with cerebral or coronary arteriosclerosis or renal impairment. Safe use during pregnancy has not been established.

Phenoxybenzamine is contraindicated for clients for whom a decrease in blood pressure is undesirable.

Phentolamine

Phentolamine inhibits responses to adrenergic stimuli by competitively blocking α-adrenergic receptors. The action of the drug is transient, and blockade is incomplete.

Pharmacokinetics. The pharmacokinetics of phentolamine are not completely understood. To achieve similar effects, oral doses must be about five times higher than parenteral doses. About 10% of parenteral doses appears in the urine as active drug; the fate of the rest is unknown. Whether the drug crosses the placenta or is distributed in breast milk is not known.

Therapeutic uses. Phentolamine is used to diagnose pheochromocytoma in adults; the test dose temporarily reduces symptoms of norepinephrine overactivity. It is also administered before or during surgery for pheochromocytoma to prevent or control paroxysmal hypertension that may occur because of anesthesia, stress, or manipulation of the tumor.

Phentolamine is an antidote for norepinephrine and should be available at the bedside of any client who is receiving IV norepinephrine (Levophed) to maintain blood pressure. Should infiltration of extravascular tissues occur, injection of phentolamine into those tissues helps correct extreme vasoconstriction, which can compromise circulation and cause sloughing of the tissues.

Adverse reactions. The most common side effects of phentolamine are GI related (abdominal pain, nausea, vomiting, diarrhea, and exacerbation of peptic ulcer). Weakness, dizziness, flushing, orthostatic hypotension, and nasal congestion also occur.

Acute and serious reactions may follow parenteral administration. These include circulatory shock, angina, and cardiac arrhythmia. Myocardial or cerebral infarction may occur.

Precautions and contraindications. Phentolamine should be used with caution for clients with gastritis, peptic ulcer, or a history of coronary artery disease. It is contraindicated for people allergic to it or related drugs.

When phentolamine is administered, health care personnel must be prepared to treat severe circulatory shock, should it occur. Epinephrine is ineffective in this situation; norepinephrine must be readily available.

β-Adrenergic blocking agents

Pharmacodynamics. The ideal adrenergic blocking agent would selectively inhibit sympathetic response of a particular tissue, such as the heart. Four agents (atenolol, betaxolol, levobunolol, and metaprolol) exhibit differentiation, blocking β₁-adrenergic receptors without appreciably affecting β₂-adrenergic receptors. Nonselective β-adrenergic blocking agents include nadolol, pindolol, propranolol, and timolol (Table 22-6).

Pharmacokinetics. Although intestinal absorption and first pass through the liver vary among the drugs, β-adrenergic blocking agents are usually administered by mouth. Labetalol and propranolol are available in solutions for injection, and timolol is available in an ophthalmic solution. These drugs cross the placenta and are distributed in the milk of a nursing mother. Metabolism (primarily in the liver) is variable. β-Blockers are excreted by the kidneys. Half-lives tend to be biphasic, with early (distribution) half-lives shorter than later (elimination) ones.

Therapeutic uses. β-Adrenergic blocking agents are used in the management of hypertension, chronic stabilized angina pectoris, certain types of cardiac arrhythmia (mainly tachycardia), glaucoma, and thyrotoxicosis, as well as in the prevention of vascular headaches and reinfarction (in clients who have suffered a myocardial infarction). They have been used experimentally to moderate aggressive and impulsive

Table 22-6. β-Adrenergic blocking agents

Drug name	Preparations	Usual dosage	Therapeutic uses
Nonselective beta-blockers			
Labetolol (Normodyne; *Can:* Trandate)	Oral tablets Solution for IV administration	Adults: Initially 100 mg bid; maintenance, 20–400 mg bid; maximum daily dosage 2.4 g PC: C	Management of hypertension
Levobunolol (Betagan)	Ophthalmic solution (0.5%)	Gtt i qd-bid	Control of open angle glaucoma or ocular hypertension
Nadolol (Corgard)	Oral tablets	Adults: 40–320 mg/day, in single or divided doses PC: C	Management of hypertension, angina pectoris, and certain types of cardiac arrhythmia
Pindolol (Visken; *Can:* Viskazide)	Oral tablets	Adults: 100–450 mg/day, as a single dose or divided in 3 doses PC: B	Management of hypertension and angina pectoris
Propranolol (Inderal)	Tablets and sustained-release capsules for oral use Solutions for injection	Adults: initially 10–20 mg tid-qid Varies widely with indication for use PC: C	Management of hypertension, angina pectoris, cardiac arrhythmias, and thyrotoxicosis Prevention of migraine headaches and reinfarction in individuals who have suffered a myocardial infarction
Timolol (Blocadren, Timoptic)	Oral tablets Ophthalmic solution	Adults: *Oral:* Initially 10 mg bid; varies with indication for use PC: C *Ophthalmic:* Initially gtt i of 0.25% solution bid PC: C	Management of hypertension and angina pectoris Prevention of reinfarction in individuals who have suffered a myocardial infarction Control of intraocular pressure in individuals with elevated pressures
β₁-Adrenergic blockers			
Atenolol (Tenormin)	Oral tablets	Adults: 50–100 mg/day in a single dose PC: B	Management of hypertension and angina pectoris
Betaxolol (Betoptic)	Ophthalmic solution (0.5%)	Gtt i bid	Treatment of open angle glaucoma or ocular hypertension
Metoprolol (Lopressor)	Oral tablets	Adults: 100–450 mg/day in a single dose or divided in 3 doses	Management of hypertension, angina pectoris, and certain types of cardiac arrhythmia

KEY: PC = pregnancy category. (The validity of pregnancy categories has not been established; see Chapter 16, p 216.)
Can = Canadian trade name.

behavior in schizophrenia ("Betablocking" autistics' aggression, 1986), to treat stage fright (Brantigan and Joseph, 1982), and to decrease withdrawal symptoms in smokers who are trying to quit.

Adverse reactions. The most serious toxic and side effects of β-adrenergic blocking agents stem from their inhibition of sympathetic responses. The drugs tend to increase atrioventricular block, and cardiac arrest can occur in clients with preexisting partial heart block. Increased airway resistance tends to compromise respiratory function, especially in people with obstructive airway disease. Chronic "hay fever," status asthmaticus, or anaphylaxis may develop. Timolol is known to cause potassium imbalance (Steiness, 1982; Swenson, 1986) and myasthenia gravis (Coppeto, 1984).

Nervous system reactions to β-adrenergic blocking agents include unsteadiness, dizziness, weakness, confusion, sexual dysfunction (impotence and decreased libido), hearing loss, fatigue, and depression. Metabolic effects include fever, increased blood ammonia levels in cirrhosis, hyperglycemia in diabetes, and increased thyroxine (T_4) levels. Nausea, vomiting, diarrhea, or constipation also occur. Arthralgia (usually in the knee) has been reported (Sills, 1984). In combination with local anesthetics, propranolol has caused hypertensive crises (Brummett, 1984).

Clients who receive β-blockers do not exhibit a full physiologic response to stress because the action of epinephrine is inhibited. The abrupt withdrawal of these drugs may result in agitation, restlessness, tachycardia, hypertension, and exacerbation of anginal episodes. (These rebound effects reflect physiologic adaptation to the presence of the drug; the adaptation tends to compensate for the drug's effects and is given full expression when drug levels drop.)

Precautions and contraindications. β-Adrenergic blocking agents should be used with caution in clients with a history of congestive heart failure, obstructive airway disease, severe allergic reactions, diabetes mellitus, or hypoglycemia, hyperthyroidism, or myasthenia gravis. To prevent an increased risk of shock associated with general anesthesia, these drugs should be gradually withdrawn if possible before elective surgery. Reduced dosage may be necessary for clients with renal or liver impairment.

β-Adrenergic blockers are contraindicated for clients with known allergic hypersensitivity to them and for those with bronchial asthma, allergic bronchospasm, severe chronic obstructive airway disease, severe peripheral vascular disease, and certain disturbances in cardiac rhythm (bradycardia, atrioventricular block). β-Adrenergic blockers should not be used concurrently with local anesthetics. Caution should be exercised when they are used with aminophylline.

Adrenergic blocking agents should not be discontinued abruptly; after long-term use, dosages should be decreased gradually over 3 to 4 weeks (Houston and Hodge, 1988).

Adrenergic neuron-blocking agents

Two adrenergic neuron-blocking agents in present use are guanethidine and reserpine (Table 22-7). Both are used to treat hypertension. Reserpine is also used to treat certain mental illnesses; its psychotropic uses are discussed in Chapter 26.

Pharmacodynamics. Agents that block chemical mediation at postganglionic adrenergic nerve endings apparently act by several mechanisms, including depletion of neurotransmitter stores and prevention of mediator release. They tend to reduce blood pressure

Table 22-7. Adrenergic neuron-blocking agents

Drug name	Preparations	Usual adult dosage	Therapeutic uses
Guanethidine (Ismelin)	Oral tablets	*Initially:* 10 mg daily (25–50 mg daily for hospitalized patients); dosage is increased gradually at 5–7-day intervals *Maintenance:* 25–50 mg daily (up to 300 mg day may be required for some individuals) PC: B	Treatment of moderate to severe hypertension
Reserpine (Sandril, Serpalan, Serpasil, Serpate)	Powder and tablets for oral use	For hypertension: Adults: initially 0.1–0.5 mg/day; maintenance, 0.25 mg/day For psychosis: Adults: 0.1–1 mg/day PC: C	Treatment of renal hypertension secondary to pyelonephritis, renal amyloidosis, or renal artery stenosis

KEY: PC = pregnancy category. (The validity of pregnancy categories has not been established; see Chapter 16, p 216.)

and depress cardiovascular reflexes, such as those that occur in response to exercise and positional change.

Pharmacokinetics. Limited information is available about the pharmacokinetics of reserpine. It is stored in adipose tissue, crosses the placenta, and is distributed in breast milk. Reserpine is metabolized by the liver. It is excreted in both urine and feces.

Guanethidine is incompletely absorbed by the GI tract, and 50% to 97% is metabolized by the liver in the first pass. After absorption, it is rapidly taken up by the adrenergic neurons. Full effects of the drug are delayed 1 to 3 weeks after the initial therapy. It is not known whether the drug crosses the placenta, and only negligible amounts pass into breast milk. Guanethidine is metabolized by the liver and excreted by the kidneys by both glomerular filtration and tubular secretion.

Therapeutic uses. Reserpine and guanethidine are used in the treatment of hypertension. Guanethidine is used for moderate to severe disease, and reserpine is used for mild to moderate conditions. Both are used in conjunction with diuretics to achieve maximal therapeutic response at low dosages with minimal adverse reactions.

Adverse reactions. The principal side effects of adrenergic neuron-blocking agents are related to depression of the nervous system. Symptoms include drowsiness, lassitude, fatigue, dizziness, syncope, and weakness. Depression may develop. Both drugs cause postural hypotension. Reserpine may also cause extrapyramidal symptoms that resemble Parkinson's disease and an increase in dreaming (including nightmares).

Other side effects include nasal congestion and bradycardia. Congestive heart failure may develop. GI reactions include increased number of bowel movements and diarrhea. The drugs inhibit ejaculation but do not cause impotency. Hair loss may occur with prolonged use of guanethidine. Reserpine is known to be tumorigenic in animals.

Precautions and contraindications. Adrenergic neuron-blocking agents should be gradually discontinued 2 to 3 weeks before surgery. Clients who are undergoing anesthesia (as in emergencies) without this precaution are highly vulnerable to hypotensive episodes. Caution must be exercised with clients who have certain cardiac conditions (such as coronary insufficiency, heart failure not due to hypertension, recent myocardial infarction), asthma, cerebrovascular disease, ulcerative colitis, and peptic ulcer. Safe use during pregnancy has not been established. Reserpine is administered with caution to clients with epilepsy, impaired renal function, or a history of gallstones.

Both guanethidine and reserpine are contraindicated for clients with allergic sensitivity to them. Additional contraindications include pheochromocytoma for guanethidine and, for reserpine, depression (especially if the client is suicidal), lactation, and electroconvulsive therapy (see Focus on Adrenergic Neuron-Blocking Agents: Similarities and Differences).

■ **Summary**

All available antiadrenergic agents reduce sympathetic responses either at the receptor cell site or at the adrenergic nerve level. Their inhibition of responses is selective. Antiadrenergic agents include α-adrenergic blocking agents, β-adrenergic blocking agents, and adrenergic neuron-blocking agents.

Nursing management

Nursing implications

Whenever a physiologic response system is altered, homeostasis may become unbalanced. The sympathetic blocking agents interfere with the normal response to stress mediated by the SNS. This interference can inhibit adaptive compensatory mechanisms and predispose a client to circulatory shock. The nurse should eliminate unnecessary environmental stressors that may affect the client. If unusual stress develops, the client should be carefully monitored for cardiovascular malfunction, particularly hypotension.

A common and annoying side effect of β-blocking therapy is postural hypotension, which is most evident with rapid changes in posture and exercise. The normal vasoconstrictor response that maintains cerebral circulation is impaired by these drugs, and dizziness and weakness frequently occur. Supervision and assistance in ambulation by nursing personnel is prudent, especially since the clients who receive these drugs are often elderly, and the risk of serious injury from falls is high.

Fatigue and flatulence can occur during the initial stage of propranolol treatment. Ambulation promotes expulsion of flatus, but movement must be carefully regulated to provide frequent rest periods. A more serious effect of this drug is the tendency to provoke bronchospasm. Clients with obstructive airway disease who receive the drug must be monitored carefully. If respiratory impairment increases, the physician must be notified so that the drug regimen can be reevaluated.

Nursing process

Assessment Before initiation of therapy with adrenergic blocking agents, the client should be screened for factors that may increase the risk of adverse reaction to these agents. For α-blockers, these include peripheral vascular disease (severe arteriosclerosis, arteritis, severe hypertension, cardiovascular disease, Raynaud's phenomenon, Raynaud's gangrene, and phlebitis), pulmonary disease, collagen disease, fibro-

Adrenergic neuron-blocking agents: similarities and differences

Similarities

Pharmacodynamics

These agents block chemical mediation at the postganglionic adrenergic nerve endings by depleting neurotransmitter stores and preventing mediator release.

Pharmacokinetics

These agents are stored in adipose tissue, cross the placenta, and are distributed in breast milk. They are metabolized by the liver and excreted primarily in the urine with some in the feces. The maximum antihypertensive effect is achieved in 1 to 3 weeks.

Therapeutic uses

These agents are used in the treatment of hypertension.

Adverse reactions

These include: (CNS) drowsiness, lassitude, fatigue, dizziness, syncope, weakness, and depression; (CV) postural hypotension, bradycardia, and congestive heart failure; (RESP) nasal congestion; (GI) dry mouth, diarrhea; (SEXUAL) inhibition of ejaculation.

Contraindications

These agents are contraindicated for people with allergic sensitivity to them.

Precautions

These agents should be gradually discontinued 2 to 3 weeks before surgery and should be used with caution for people with coronary insufficiency, heart failure not due to hypertension, recent myocardial infarction, asthma, cerebrovascular disease, ulcerative colitis, and peptic ulcer.

Nursing considerations

Monitor the client's pulse and blood pressure frequently for changes; assess client for signs and symptoms of depression; if client is scheduled for surgery, instruct client to notify surgeon and anesthesiologist so drug can be gradually withdrawn over 2 to 3 weeks; instruct client to avoid sudden position changes; institute safety measures to prevent injury; encourage use of hard candy, ice chips, or gum to relieve dry mouth; teach client the signs and symptoms of adverse effects and the need to report them; warn client to avoid hazardous activities that require mental alertness; instruct client in drug regimen.

Differences

• **Guanethidine** depletes norepinephrine stores and prevents release of norepinephrine from adrenergic nerve endings.
• **Reserpine** depletes catecholamine and serotonin stores and reduces the uptake of catecholamines by adrenergic neurons.

• **Guanethidine** is incompletely absorbed from the GI tract. It is not known whether guanethidine crosses the placenta, and only negligible amounts are passed into breast milk. Its terminal half-life is 5 days; small amounts are excreted in the feces.
• **Reserpine** is absorbed rapidly for the GI tract. Reserpine elimination half-life occurs in two phases: in the first phase, the half-life averages 4.5 hours; during the second phase, the half-life is 11.3 days.

• **Reserpine** is also used in the treatment of agitated psychotic disorders.

• **Reserpine** may cause extrapyramidal symptoms that resemble Parkinson's disease and increased dreaming. • **Guanethidine** (prolonged use) may cause hair loss.

• **Guanethidine** is contraindicated in pheochromocytoma.
• **Reserpine** is contraindicated in depression, lactation, and electroconvulsive therapy.

• **Reserpine** should also be used with caution for people with epilepsy, impaired renal function, or a history of gallstones.

Instruct client who is taking **guanethidine** to avoid the use of over-the-counter cold and allergy medications.

tic processes, peptic ulcer, or serious infections. Clients with a history of heart blockage, congestive failure, obstructive airway disease, myasthenia gravis, cirrhosis, hyperthyroidism, or diabetes mellitus are at increased risk for adverse reaction to β-blockers. In addition, the likelihood of toxic syndromes is increased in clients with renal or hepatic impairment.

Physical assessment should include a complete evaluation of cardiovascular status, blood chemistries, urinary function, and neurologic status. A global assessment of mental and emotional status should also be carried out.

A complete drug history should be taken. Adverse drug interactions may occur if clients who receive β-blockers also take diuretics, anesthetics (both local and general), or aminophylline.

Nursing diagnosis Clients who receive adrenergic blockers usually exhibit deficits in knowledge related to their drug regimens. Other diagnoses that arise from α-adrenergic blocker therapy include the following:

Altered peripheral tissue perfusion related to vasospasm secondary to drug therapy
Impaired tissue integrity related to impaired oxygen transport secondary to drug therapy
Altered comfort: nausea or angina related to vasospasm secondary to drug therapy
Impaired physical mobility related to angina pectoris secondary to drug therapy
Activity intolerance related to angina pectoris secondary to drug therapy

A common collaborative problem that should be differentiated from the nursing diagnoses is

Potential complication: cardiovascular including decreased cardiac output

Adverse reactions to β-blockers include the following:

Sexual dysfunction related to decreased libido or impotence
High risk for noncompliance: undermedication related to sexual dysfunction or postural hypotension secondary to side effects of medication
High risk for altered nutrition: less than body requirements related to nausea and vomiting secondary to drug therapy
High risk for fluid volume deficit related to diarrhea or nausea and vomiting secondary to drug therapy
High risk for pain: arthralgia related to drug therapy

Common collaborative problems that should be differentiated from the nursing diagnoses include

Potential complication: cardiovascular including atrioventricular block, congestive heart failure, hypertensive crisis
Potential complication: respiratory including bronchospasm
Potential complication: immune including anaphylaxis
Potential complication: respiratory including tracheobronchial constriction
Potential complication: ototoxicity

Planning A major goal of treatment is teaching the client information about the drug regimen and self-care health measures that can enhance therapeutic response and reduce the risk of adverse drug reaction. In addition, alleviation of discomfort or pain, promotion of tissue perfusion, reduction of the risk of adverse drug reactions, and prompt detection and treatment of drug reactions that may occur are appropriate goals for recipients of all adrenergic blockers. For clients who receive α-blockers, other goals include increased mobility and restoration of tissue integrity. Goals for recipients of β-blockers include improved gas exchange, improved sexual function, increased compliance with the drug regimen, improved hearing, improved nutrition, and restoration of fluid volume.

Intervention Nursing interventions range from first aid treatment of acute reactions, such as severe asthma or anaphylaxis, to the preparation and implementation of a comprehensive teaching plan. An important nursing measure is the monitoring of all clients for early signs and symptoms of adverse drug reactions. A decrease in hearing acuity should be reported to the physician who may change the medication orders. Therapeutic response should also be assessed.

Clients who receive α-blockers should be monitored for impairment of peripheral circulation. They should be kept warm to promote peripheral circulation. The use of shawls, gloves, and warm socks is recommended. To protect the feet from trauma, shoes should be worn when ambulating. Special care of the feet includes daily washing and inspection for lesions; powder or lotion should be used as necessary to maintain skin integrity. Injuries or irritations should be reported to the physician and treated aggressively until they heal.

Alterations in comfort, impaired mobility, and activity intolerance are likely to remain chronic problems as long as the underlying cause, altered perfusion, remains uncorrected. The nurse collaborates with the physician to adapt the drug regimen to the client's needs. When symptoms are first noted, administration of an analgesic that contains caffeine and rest in a quiet room may abort a migraine headache and prevent the need for medication with α-blocking agents. Changes in drug orders may alleviate toxic or side effects. Comfort measures should be employed to minimize adverse reactions such as nausea. The nurse should assist clients with activities of daily living that they no longer can perform because of activity intolerance or impaired mobility.

Clients who receive β-blockers should be protected from sudden or prolonged increases in stress levels. If unusual stress develops, they should be monitored for circulatory shock, and prompt measures should be taken to combat this condition. The nurse should be prepared to take emergency measures to relieve dyspnea or asthma, anaphylaxis, or congestive heart failure, as well as nutritional and fluid deficits caused by GI upset. Sexual dysfunction may be alleviated by a change in medication. If it is not, the nurse should provide counseling to help the client develop alternative modes of sexual expression.

Client education. Teaching clients about their drug regimens corrects noncompliance when it is caused by simple errors in the administration of medicines. Noncompliance may occur for other reasons, however. The nurse should explore the client's perceptions of and emotional reactions to the prescribed treatment. If factors such as adverse drug reactions contribute to noncompliance, the physician should be consulted to see whether a change in the drug regimen could improve the client's response. When a change is not possible, it is the client's right to refuse a medication or specific doses of medicine, and the nurse must accept the noncompliance.

Clients who receive sympathetic blocking agents should avoid stressful situations and should be taught stress management techniques to moderate the impact of stress. Clients should be helped to evaluate their coping strategies and to identify the need for new approaches or improved coping skills. Clients affected by stress and those with poor stress management skills may be referred to counselors for more specialized help.

When drug therapy is initiated, clients should be reassured that physiologic side effects such as fatigue and flatulence will soon subside. Postural hypotension tends to persist, although its severity may decline. To prevent loss of balance and accidental injury, clients should be taught to move slowly, especially when rising from a bed or standing up from a sitting position. Muscular activity helps to pump blood through the venous system and reduces the pooling of blood.

Clients who receive guanethidine should be counseled to avoid the use of OTC preparations that contain adrenergic drugs. These include most cold and allergy remedies and any medicine described as a decongestant. These drugs also tend to raise the blood pressure and should not be used by clients susceptible to hypertension.

Clients should also avoid smoking, which constricts blood vessels and raises blood pressure.

Evaluation Data required for evaluation relate to the client's ability to repeat accurately the information included in the teaching plans and their ability to demonstrate self-care measures previously taught. In addition, clients who receive α-blockers should be asked about changes in comfort levels (alleviation of headache due to migraine, intermittent claudication, paresthesia in the hands and feet, and chest or abdominal pain). The extremities should be examined regularly for persistent lesions that could become gangrenous. When β-blockers are used, data is required relating to respiratory function, specifically wheezing, which indicates bronchospasm. Clients must be monitored for cardiac arrhythmia, peripheral edema, pulmonary congestion, sudden alterations in blood pressure, and nutritional status. Clients should be questioned about dizziness when suddenly changing positions, about sexual function, and about hearing. Compliance can be estimated by counting medication doses and comparing the amount consumed with the prescription.

Checklist of nursing actions

When adrenergic blocking agents are prescribed

☐ Eliminate unnecessary environmental stressors that affect the client.

☐ Control activity as recommended by the physician.

☐ Monitor for cardiovascular malfunction if unusual stress in the client develops.

☐ Supervise and assist in ambulation.

☐ Monitor carefully clients with obstructive airway disease; notify the physician if respiratory impairment increases.

☐ Teach stress management techniques to clients.

☐ Help clients evaluate coping strategies; refer to counselors those clients who need specialized help in managing stress.

☐ Reassure clients that side effects of fatigue and flatulence will subside.

☐ Teach clients to change position slowly because of postural hypotension.

☐ Warn clients who take guanethidine to avoid OTC preparations that contain adrenergic drugs.

Cholinergic drugs

Several classes of drugs act to enhance parasympathetic activity in the body (Table 22-8). Parasympathomimetic agents stimulate cells with cholinergic receptors. Their effects may be global, but the most useful therapeutic agents are selective in action. Anticholinesterase agents inhibit or inactivate cholinesterase, causing acetylcholine to accumulate at the receptor

Table 22-8. Cholinergic drugs

Drug name	Preparations	Usual dosage	Therapeutic uses
Parasympathetic agents			
Acetylcholine (Miochol)	Powder for preparing solutions for ophthalmic instillation	*Ophthalmic irrigation:* 0.5–2 ml of 1% solution	Intraocular instillation for miosis during eye surgery
Bethanechol chloride (Duvoid, Mictrol, Myetonachol, Urecholine, Urolax, Vesicholine)	Oral tablets Solution for subcutaneous injection	Adults: 40–400 mg daily, divided in 4 doses Adults: *subcutaneous:* 2.5 mg q 15–30 min (for urinary retention) or 7.5–10 mg q 4 h (for neurogenic bladder) PC: C	Treatment of acute postoperative and postpartum urinary retention Treatment of postoperative distention and postvagotomy gastric retention
Carbachol (Isopto Carbachol, Miostat)	Ophthalmic solution for topical application Ophthalmic solution for intraocular injection	*Ophthalmic irrigation:* gtt i-ii of a 0.75%–3% solution q4–8h	Treatment of glaucoma Intraocular injection for miosis during eye surgery
Muscarine	None		No medicinal uses; muscarine is the principle toxin in poisonous mushrooms, which are sometimes used for psychotropic effects
Pilocarpine (Adsorbocarpine, Akarpine, Almocarpine, E-Pilo, Isopto-Carpine, Ocusert, Pilocar, Pilomiotin, P.V. Carpine)	Ophthalmic solutions and controlled-release systems for topical application	Gtt i-ii of a 1%–4% solution q4–12h PC: C	Treatment of glaucoma
Reversible anticholinesterase agents			
Ambenonium chloride (Mytelase)	Tablets for oral use	*Initially:* Adults: 15–20 mg daily, divided in 3–4 doses; children: 300 µg/kg body weight/day, divided in 3–4 doses *Maintenance:* Adults: 45–400 mg daily, divided in 3–4 doses; children 1.5 mg/kg body weight/day divided in 3–4 doses	Treatment of myasthenia gravis
Demecarium bromide (Humorsol)	Ophthalmic solution	*Initially:* gtt i-ii of a 0.125% or 0.25% solution PC: X	Treatment of glaucoma Diagnosis and initial treatment of convergent strabismus
Echothiophate iodide (Phospholine Iodide)	Ophthalmic solution	*Initially:* gtt i-ii of a 0.125% or 0.25% solution	Treatment of glaucoma Diagnosis and initial treatment of convergent strabismus
Edrophonium chloride (Tensilon)	Solution for injection	Adults: *IV:* 1–2 mg; *IM:* 10 mg (up to 40 mg within 20 min may be required to reverse the effects of neuromuscular blocking agents used during surgery)	Diagnosis of myasthenia gravis Evaluation of response to drug regimens for myasthenia gravis Differentiation of cholinergic and myasthenic crisis Reversal of nondepolarizing neuromuscular blockade after surgery
Isoflurophate (Floropryl)	Ophthalmic ointment	0.5 cm applied q8–72h PC: X	Treatment of nondepolarizing glaucoma Diagnosis and initial treatment of convergent strabismus

(Continued)

Table 22-8. Cholinergic drugs *(Continued)*

Drug name	Preparations	Usual dosage	Therapeutic uses
Reversible anticholinesterase agents			
Neostigmine (Prostigmin)	Tablets and powder for oral use Solutions and powder for preparing solutions for injection	*Maintenance in myasthenia gravis:* Adults: 15–375 mg daily, divided in 6–12 doses; children: 0.33 mg/kg body weight or 10 mg/m² 6 times daily PC: C	Diagnosis and treatment of myasthenia gravis (neostigmine is the standard against which newer drugs are compared) Alleviation of postoperative distention and urinary retention Antidote for reversal of nondepolarizing neuromuscular blockade after surgery
Physostigmine salicylate, eserine salicylate (Antilirium, Isopto Eserine)	Solution for injection Ophthalmic solutions and ointments	Adults: *Parenteral:* 500 µg-2 mg doses repeated as indicated by response; *ophthalmic irrigation:* gtt i-ii of a 0.25% or 0.5% solution q4–8h PC: C	Treatment of atropine and tricyclic antidepressant toxicity Treatment of glaucoma Physostigmine is the active ingredient of the calabar bean used by West African natives as an ordeal poison for witchcraft trials
Pyridostigmine bromide (Mestinon)	Solution, tablets, and extended-release tablets for oral use Solution for injection	*Initially:* Adults: 180 mg daily, divided in 3 doses; children: 7 mg/kg body weight/day, divided in 5–6 doses Doses are increased gradually until maximal effective dose is determined PC: C	Treatment of myasthenia gravis Reversal of the effects of neuromuscular blocking agents

KEY: PC = pregnancy category. (The validity of pregnancy categories has not been established; see Chapter 16, p 216.)

site, thus prolonging its stimulating effect. Ganglionic stimulators such as nicotine are not used therapeutically but must be understood because of their toxic effects.

Parasympathomimetic agents

Chemicals that directly stimulate cholinergic receptors include muscarine, pilocarpine, acetylcholine, and the choline esters methacholine, carbachol, and bethanechol chloride.

Pharmacodynamics. Pilocarpine and muscarine act on muscarinic receptors in peripheral and ganglionic synapses. Acetylcholine stimulates all four classes of cholinergic nerves:

1. Cholinergic fibers within the CNS
2. Motor nerves that supply skeletal muscle fibers
3. Preganglionic autonomic fibers to ganglion cells, which stimulate sympathetic and parasympathetic response
4. Postganglionic fibers to parasympathetic effector cells

Choline esters have greater selectivity of action than acetylcholine.

When applied topically to the eye, cholinergic agents constrict the pupil, facilitating drainage of the aqueous humor through the canal of Schlemm.

Pharmacokinetics. Administered as a drug, acetylcholine penetrates poorly to the CNS, and its effects are primarily peripheral. Its action is diffuse, and it is rapidly destroyed *in vivo.* Choline esters should be administered orally or subcutaneously, never intramuscularly (IM) or IV because rapid absorption is likely to cause toxicity.

Therapeutic uses. Muscarine is not used medicinally. Other cholinergic agents are used topically to induce miosis in the treatment of glaucoma. Bethanechol is also used as a smooth-muscle stimulant to relieve postoperative distention and urine retention.

Cholinergic agents may someday be used in the emergency treatment of botulism. A substance that enhances the release of acetylcholine, 3,4-diaminopyridine, has been used experimentally to treat rats inoculated with lethal doses of botulism toxin. (Botulism: New drug buys time, 1986).

Cholinergic drugs are also being used experimentally as a treatment for Alzheimer's disease (Beller, 1988).

Adverse reactions. The side effects of cholinergic agents are typical of increased parasympathetic activity. They include increased perspiration and salivation, blurred vision, bradycardia with decreased cardiac output and hypotension, increased intestinal and ureteral peristalsis, and contraction of the bladder with urinary urgency. Incontinence of urine or stool may occur. Bronchial secretion and constriction are increased, and use of these drugs may precipitate acute asthma in susceptible clients. Cholinergic drugs can also cause atrial fibrillation in hyperthyroidism, acute angina in coronary insufficiency, and an exacerbation of symptoms in peptic ulcer. Acute toxicity is characterized by salivation, involuntary defecation and urination, sweating, tearing, hypotension, fatigability, weakness, involuntary twitchings, confusion, ataxia, slurred speech, and loss of reflexes. Generalized convulsions, paralysis, coma, and central respiratory paralysis ensue in serious poisoning.

Precautions and contraindications. Cholinergic medications are potent, and large doses should be avoided. Response to these drugs varies, and some individuals experience cholinergic toxicity from therapeutic doses. For this reason, these drugs are administered orally or subcutaneously, not IM or IV. The anticholinergic antidote, atropine, should be readily available when cholinergic drugs are administered. Cardiac monitoring, endotracheal intubation, assisted respirations, or cardiopulmonary resuscitation may also be needed.

Cholinergics exacerbate many medical conditions. They should be used with caution for clients with epilepsy, asthma, bradycardia, vagotonia, hyperthyroidism, cardiac arrhythmia, and peptic ulcer. Contraindications for their use include mechanical obstruction of or recent surgery in the GI tract or genitourinary tract, spastic or inflammatory GI conditions, parkinsonism, and obstructive pulmonary disease. They should not be used concurrently with ganglionic blocking agents (see Focus on Parasympathomimetic Agents: Similarities and Differences).

Anticholinesterase agents

Pharmacodynamics. Drugs that inhibit or inactivate cholinesterase cause acetylcholine to accumulate at the receptor site, enhancing and prolonging the nerve response to each stimulus. The effects of these agents depend on the speed with which the drug-enzyme complex can be broken down by the body to regenerate active enzyme. Under normal body conditions, cholinesterase combines with acetylcholine, forming a complex that is rapidly converted to choline, acetic acid, and regenerated cholinesterase. The reactions between cholinesterase and anticholinesterase compounds are identical in nature except that the enzyme-substrate complex is broken down less quickly, keeping the enzyme inoperative for longer periods of time.

Quantitative differences determine toxicity; those chemicals that produce "irreversible" binding of cholinesterase are more deadly. In the case of the more toxic anticholinesterase chemicals, essentially none of the enzyme is regenerated. The accumulated acetylcholine continues to induce neuron stimulation. Because cholinergic neurons are widespread, body effects are numerous and varied. They are qualitatively similar regardless of the chemical involved.

In addition to their effect on acetylcholinesterase activity, anticholinesterases also may exert either a blocking action or a cholinomimetic effect at autonomic ganglia. The importance of these "direct" actions depends on the drug involved, the dose, the site of application, and the species of the recipient organism.

The pharmacologic properties of anticholinesterases are those of physiologic release of acetylcholine by nerve impulses and the effector response to such release. These agents are capable of producing muscarine-like cholinomimetic actions at autonomic effector organs, nicotinic effects characterized by stimulation, and subsequent depression of autonomic ganglia and skeletal muscle, as well as stimulation (with subsequent depression) of cholinoreceptor sites in the CNS. Most of these effects are seen with toxic or lethal doses. With smaller doses, as in therapeutic administration, actual response depends on the balance between ganglionic and peripheral response and the distribution of drug in various body tissues.

Inhibitors of the "reversible" type that are useful drug agents include physostigmine and its derivatives (neostigmine, edrophonium chloride, pyridostigmine, and ambenonium chloride). Examples of the irreversible anticholinesterases include the insecticides parathion and Malathion and the nerve gases tabun, sarin, and soman (see Table 22-8).

Pharmacokinetics. Little information is available on the systemic distribution or metabolic fate of anticholinesterases used topically for eye conditions. Some aspects of the drugs also remain obscure when administered systemically.

Physostigmine is readily absorbed from the GI tract, mucous membranes, and subcutaneous injection sites. Ambenonium chloride, neostigmine, and pyridostigmine are administered orally but are poorly absorbed by this route. Edrophonium chloride is administered only by injection. After absorption, these drugs are all widely distributed. Physostigmine readily crosses the blood–brain barrier; edrophonium chloride does so only when large doses are used. Pyridostigmine and (in large doses) ambenonium chloride and neostigmine cross the placenta.

Duration of action varies. The action of edrophonium chloride is brief. Duration of action of ambenonium chloride, pyridostigmine, physostigmine, and neostigmine is 4 to 8 hours, 3 to 6 hours, 30 minutes to 5 hours, and 2½ to 4 hours, respectively.

Parasympathomimetic agents: similarities and differences

Similarities

Pharmacodynamics

These agents stimulate cells with cholinergic receptors to simulate the action of acetylcholine at the postganglionic neuroeffector sites.

Pharmacokinetics

The absorption, distribution, metabolism, and excretion of these agents is generally unknown. The onset of action is 10 to 30 minutes, peaking in 2 to 4 hours, and lasting 4 to 8 hours.

Therapeutic uses

These agents are used topically to induce miosis in the treatment of glaucoma. They may someday be used in the treatment of botulism and Alzheimer's disease.

Adverse reactions

These include: (CNS) dizziness, confusion, hallucinations, muscle weakness; (EENT) miosis, blurred vision, tearing; (CV) bradycardia, decreased cardiac output, hypotension; (RESP) increased bronchial secretions, bronchospasm, and bronchoconstriction; (GI/GU) nausea, vomiting, belching, incontinence, urinary urgency; (OTHER) increased perspiration and increased salivation.

Contraindications

These agents are contraindicated in mechanical obstruction or recent surgery of the GI or GU tract, spastic or inflammatory GI conditions, Parkinson's disease, obstructive pulmonary disease, and pregnancy.

Precautions

These agents should be used cautiously for people with epilepsy, asthma, bradycardia, vagotonia, hyperthyroidism, cardiac arrhythmia, and peptic ulcer.

Nursing considerations

Frequently monitor the client's cardiovascular and respiratory status for changes; institute safety measures to prevent injury; warn client that vision will be temporarily blurred and peripheral vision will be decreased; when giving topically, instruct client to apply finger pressure on the lacrimal sac for 1 to 2 minutes after instillation; instruct client in drug regimen and signs and symptoms of adverse reactions.

Differences

• **Pilocarpine** and **muscarine** act on the muscarinic receptors in the peripheral and ganglionic synapses. • **Acetylcholine** stimulates cholinergic fibers in the CNS, motor nerves that supply skeletal muscle fibers, preganglionic autonomic fibers that stimulate sympathetic and parasympathetic responses, and postganglionic fibers to parasympathetic effector cells. • **Bethanechol chloride** directly stimulates cholinergic receptors.

• **Acetylcholine** begins to act within minutes, and its duration of action is 10 to 20 minutes. • **Bethanechol chloride** is poorly absorbed from the GI tract. Its onset of action is 30 to 90 minutes (PO), 5 to 15 minutes (SC), with a duration of action that lasts 1 hour (PO) and up to 2 hours (SC).

• **Muscarine** is not used medicinally. • **Bethanechol chloride** is also used as a smooth muscle stimulant to reduce postoperative urinary retention and chap gastric retention. • **Acetylcholine** and **carbachol** are used during eye surgery to induce miosis.

• **Pilocarpine** also causes brow pain. • **Pilocarpine** and **carbachol** also cause myopia; **bethanechol chloride** also causes reflex tachycardia and decreased diastolic blood pressure.

• **Bethanechol chloride** is contraindicated for people with bradycardia, hyperthyroidism, hypotension, epilepsy, cardiac or coronary artery disease, peptic ulcer, and asthma.

• **Bethanechol chloride** should be used cautiously for people with hypertension, vasomotor instability, peritonitis, or other acute GI inflammatory conditions.

Prepare and use solutions of **acetylcholine** immediately because they are unstable; never give **bethanechol** IM or IV because of possible circulatory collapse, severe hypotension, severe abdominal cramps, shock or cardiac arrest; only give parenteral **bethanechol** subcutaneously; give oral **bethanechol** on an empty stomach to avoid nausea and vomiting associated with food; have bedpan, urinal, or commode within reach of client who is taking **bethanechol**; monitor client's urinary and bowel elimination closely.

The processes of metabolism and excretion are unknown for ambenonium chloride and edrophonium chloride. The other three drugs are hydrolized by cholinesterases; neostigmine and pyridostigmine are also metabolized by the liver. Neostigmine and pyridostigmine are excreted by tubular secretion in the kidneys. Only small amounts of physostigmine are eliminated in the urine; what happens to the remainder is unknown.

Therapeutic uses. Anticholinesterases are used to induce miosis in the therapeutic management of glaucoma, to stimulate gastric motility and secretion in clients with vagotomy, and to increase strength of skeletal muscle contraction in myasthenia gravis. The drugs also have potential value in the treatment of Alzheimer's disease (Davis and Mohs, 1982). In addition, they form the active ingredients of many insecticides and of nerve gas.

Adverse reactions. The toxic and side effects of anticholinesterases are similar to those of cholinergic agents, that is, signs and symptoms of parasympathetic activity. Exposure to insecticides, such as DDT or dioxin, can cause pronounced cholinergic effects. Skin contamination of an arm or leg may be followed by muscle spasms and paresthesia (prickling pain) that rapidly moves up the extremity. Acute systemic poisoning causes salivation, sweating, tearing, weakness, hypotension, nausea, vomiting, incontinence, ataxia, slurred speech, memory loss, agitation, hallucinations, labile mood, confusion, convulsions, and paralysis.

The effects of chronic poisoning by insecticides are not well understood. Insecticides are considered carcinogenic and may be mutagenic. Nursing mothers who have been exposed to these pollutants pass them on to their infants in breast milk. Evidence suggests that most if not all people have absorbed enough of such chemicals to be detectable in the blood (Raloff, 1985). Because concentrations in storage depots such as fatty tissue are likely to be higher than those in the blood, the threat to public health may be much greater than is generally recognized.

Precautions and contraindications. Precautions and contraindications for medicinal anticholinesterase compounds are the same as those for cholinergic agents.

When anticholinesterase compounds are used as insecticides, precautions should be taken to avoid contact with the poison. Protective gear is required. Both inhalation and skin contact can cause poisoning. The use of many insecticides has been sharply limited by law. Some agents can be used only in special circumstances when other less toxic agents are ineffective, or some agents are limited for use only by specially trained personnel (see Focus on Anticholinesterase Agents: Similarities and Differences).

■ **Summary**

Cholinergic drugs act to enhance parasympathetic activity in the body. Parasympathomimetic agents stimulate cells with cholinergic receptors, whereas anticholinesterase agents inhibit or inactivate cholinesterase. These drugs are used therapeutically to treat atony of the intestines or bladder and myasthenia gravis, as well as to maintain miosis in glaucoma. Side effects can be pronounced and may include blurred vision, hypotension or hypertension, bradycardia, bronchoconstriction, nausea, cramping, diarrhea, and excessive salivation or perspiration. Anticholinesterases are the substances used as "nerve gas" for chemical warfare.

Nursing management

Nursing implications

Muscarine has no clinical uses, but it is the principal toxin involved in mushroom poisoning. After ingestion of certain species of mushrooms, symptoms of parasympathetic overactivity begin within $1/2$ to 2 hours. These include tearing, salivation, nausea, vomiting, headache, blurred vision, colic, diarrhea, dyspnea, bradycardia, hypotension, and shock. Irritability, restlessness, ataxia, anxiety, mania, hallucinations, delirium, and convulsions are indications of CNS stimulation. Some of these effects are desired by individuals who use muscarine-containing mushrooms for psychotropic purposes, including practitioners of certain American Indian religions. Mushroom poisoning is treated by administration of atropine to reverse the peripheral manifestations and by treatment with sedatives to reduce CNS effects.

Client problems with the use of parasympathomimetic drugs depend on the condition for which the drug is given. Response to these medications in a client with myasthenia gravis is quite different from that of the postoperative "normal" client. When neostigmine is used to correct paralytic ileus or urinary retention after surgery, the client experiences the full range of side effects. In this situation, parenteral medication is often used. Response occurs within 30 minutes. The problems that result from insecticide poisoning also differ. For this reason, the nursing process for treating myasthenia gravis and insecticide poisoning is discussed separately.

Nursing process

Assessment Before any cholinergic drug is administered, the client must be carefully assessed for contraindications, such as allergic conditions (especially asthma), obstructive pulmonary disease, peptic ulcer, inflammatory conditions of the GI tract, mechanical obstructions in the intestinal or urinary tract, recent surgery that involved these two systems, cardiac ar-

Anticholinesterase agents: similarities and differences

Similarities

Pharmacodynamic

These agents block the hydrolysis of acetylcholine by cholinesterase, causing acetylcholine to accumulate at the receptor sites, enhancing and prolonging the nerve response to each stimulus.

Pharmacokinetics

These agents are poorly absorbed from the GI tract. Information about distribution, metabolism, and excretion is generally unknown.

Therapeutic uses

These agents are used to induce miosis in the treatment of glaucoma, to stimulate gastric motility and secretion in people with vagotomy, and to increase the strength of muscle contraction in people with myasthenia gravis.

Adverse reactions

These include: (CNS) headache, muscle weakness, confusion, nervousness, dizziness; (EENT) lacrimation, blurred vision, miosis; (CV) hypertension, hypotension, bradycardia, arrhythmia; (RESP) bronchial constriction, tracheobronchial secretion, bronchospasm; (GI) nausea, vomiting, diarrhea, abdominal cramps; (GU) urinary frequency and urgency, enuresis, incontinence; (OTHER) excessive salivation, sweating, pallor.

Contraindications

These agents are contraindicated for people with mechanical obstruction of the GI or GU tracts and people who are receiving ganglionic blocking agents.

Differences

• **Demecarium** and **echothiopate** inhibit the enzymatic destruction of acetylcholine.

• **Neostigmine** is metabolized by the liver and excreted in the urine. Its duration of action varies with clients, depending on the degree of physiologic and emotional stress and severity of the disease. Its elimination half-life varies from 50 to 90 minutes. • **Edrophonium** has an onset of action of 30 to 60 seconds when given IV, 2 to 10 minutes when given IM, and a duration of action of 5 to 10 minutes after IV administration and 5 to 30 minutes after IM administration. It may cross the placenta. • **Pyridostigmine** has an onset of action of 30 to 45 minutes PO, 2 to 5 minutes IV, and 15 minutes IM; its duration of action is 3 to 6 hours (PO), and 2 to 3 hours (IV). • **Pyridostigmine** is excreted in the urine. • **Physostigmine** is readily absorbed from the GI tract, mucous membranes, and subcutaneous tissues; onset of action is 3 to 8 minutes (parenterally) with a duration of action of 30 minutes to 5 hours and a terminal elimination half-life of 15 to 40 minutes; it penetrates the blood–brain barrier; it is metabolized by the liver, and small amounts are excreted in the urine.

• **Demecarium, echothiopate**, and **isoflurophate** are used in the diagnosis and initial treatment of convergent strabismus. • **Edrophonium** is also used in the diagnosis of myasthenia gravis, evaluation of response to drug regimens for myasthenia gravis, and differentiation of cholinergic and myasthenic crisis. • **Edrophonium, neostigmine**, and **pyridostigmine** are used to reverse the effects of neuromuscular blocking agents after surgery. • **Neostigmine** is also used to alleviate postoperative distention and urinary retention. • **Physostigmine** is also used in the treatment of atropine and tricyclic antidepressant toxicity.

• **Edrophonium** and **ambenonium** can cause respiratory muscle paralysis. • **Demecarium** and **echothiophate** can cause dyspnea. • **Neostigmine** can cause respiratory depression. • **Edrophonium** can also cause muscle fasiculations; **physostigmine** and **pyridostigmine** can cause convulsions. • **Pyridostigmine** can also cause thrombophlebitis when given IV.

• **Neostigmine** should not be given to people with peritonitis. • **Physostigmine** is contraindicated for people with asthma, gangrene, diabetes, cardiovascular disease, or those who are receiving choline esters or depolarizing neuromuscular blocking agents.

(continued)

Focus on

Anticholinesterase agents: similarities and differences (Continued)

Precautions

These agents should be used with caution for people with epilepsy, bronchial asthma, bradycardia, recent coronary occlusion, vagotonia, hyperthyroidism, cardiac arrhythmia, or peptic ulcer. Large doses should be avoided for people with megacolon or decreased GI motility.

• **Physostigmine** should be used with caution for people with Parkinson's disease.

Nursing considerations

Administer with food or milk to reduce the GI effects; observe the client closely for cholinergic reactions especially when using the parenteral form; have atropine available to reduce or reverse hypersensitivity reactions and to control muscarinic effects of early therapy; instruct client in disease, treatment, drug regimen, compliance, and signs and symptoms of adverse effects; monitor client's muscle strength, function, and mobility status for changes and improvements.

Use **edrophonium** to differentiate myasthenic crisis from cholinergic crisis; administer neostigmine to the client with myasthenia gravis before periods of possible fatigue.

---

rhythmia (especially bradycardia), epilepsy, parkinsonism, and hyperthyroidism.

Nursing diagnosis Clients for whom occasional doses of cholinergic drugs are ordered are likely to have nursing diagnoses such as the following:

Constipation or obstipation related to reduced cholinergic response
Urinary retention related to reduced cholinergic response
Pain related to altered patterns of elimination.

When ophthalmic solutions are prescribed, clients are likely to have:

Sensory-perceptual alteration: blurring of vision secondary to instillation of eye drops

Adverse reactions to cholinergic drugs may cause:

Altered comfort: nausea or abdominal pain related to adverse reactions to cholinergic drug therapy
High risk for injury related to blurring of vision
Functional urinary incontinence related to cholinergic drug therapy
Bowel incontinence related to cholinergic drug therapy
Decreased tissue perfusion related to bradycardia, decreased cardiac output, and hypotension

Impaired gas exchange related to bronchospasm and increased bronchial secretions or respiratory paralysis
Impaired verbal communication related to cholinergic drug therapy

All clients are likely to exhibit:

Knowledge deficit concerning cholinergic drugs

When ophthalmic solutions are prescribed, clients are likely to have sensory/perceptual alterations, with loss of vision secondary to glaucoma. All clients are likely to exhibit knowledge deficit relating to cholinergic drugs, although the magnitude of the deficit varies depending on clients' past experiences.

Planning Goals of treatment include reduction of the risk of adverse drug reaction, restoration of normal patterns of bowel and urinary elimination, elimination of discomfort or pain, conservation of vision, prompt detection and treatment of adverse drug reactions should they occur, and instruction in the necessary information or skills. Among the goals for treatment of cholinergic toxicity are improved tissue perfusion, improved gas exchange, and improved verbal communication.

Intervention Assessment of clients before administration of cholinergic medication may reveal one or more contraindications or risk factors for use of the drugs. If so, the nurse informs the physician and the drug order may be changed as a result. If not, the nurse considers the client to be at high risk for adverse drug reaction.

Atropine should be readily available as an antidote when cholinergic drugs are to be administered. Adrenalin may also be required if the client has a history of allergy. Corrective action should be taken promptly if signs or symptoms of bronchial constriction or excessive secretion (wheezing, dyspnea) develop.

When cholinergic agents are administered systemically, they must be injected subcutaneously, not IM or IV. Rapid absorption of the drug by the latter routes makes toxic reaction likely. To avoid inducing nausea, systemic doses should be administered before, rather than after, meals. When solutions are administered topically (usually as eye drops), the nurse reduces systemic absorption by exerting gentle pressure at the inner canthus of the eye to occlude the tear duct for a few seconds.

When cholinergics are administered systemically, the nurse should supply the client with a bedpan or urinal because the action of the drug is likely to cause rapid micturition or defecation. A rectal tube facilitates the passage of flatus.

Vital signs should be monitored for indications of respiratory or circulatory impairment. Acute reactions can be life-threatening and cardiorespiratory resuscitation, assisted ventilation, or treatment for shock may be necessary. The nurse should be prepared to administer injections of atropine or epinephrine to counteract the effects of the cholinergic drugs.

Client education. Before initiating cholinergic medication, the nurse should inform the client about the drugs and their effects. Clients with glaucoma require long-term therapy with miotic eye drops. Accordingly, the nurse should prepare and implement a teaching plan that covers the nature of the drugs, their therapeutic effects, common side effects, serious toxic effects, and measures the client should take if adverse reaction develops.

Evaluation Data required for evaluation include information about patterns of urinary and bowel elimination, the client's statements about comfort level, visual acuity, whether adverse reactions occurred, the time required to detect and treat such reactions, the client's response to such treatment, and the client's ability to demonstrate procedures already taught and to repeat to the nurse information included in the teaching plan.

Therapy in myasthenia gravis. The basic defect in myasthenia gravis appears to be a failure of acetylcholine to interact sufficiently with receptor sites of the neuromuscular junction to produce normal muscular contraction. Though initial muscle response may be normal, it rapidly declines, and the victim is unable to maintain voluntary muscle activity for more than brief periods. Administration of a cholinesterase inhibitor increases response to stimulation and muscle strength toward normal levels, relieving both fatigability and the respiratory depression that is life-threatening in this disease.

When cholinergic therapy is used to control and alleviate the symptoms of myasthenia gravis, nursing care focuses on the problems that stem from the disease. Tolerance to the muscarinic side effects of the drugs develops with long-term use. Until then, anticholinergic drugs such as atropine are used to control these symptoms.

Assessment Muscular function and strength of the client with myasthenia gravis should be assessed in detail. Muscle tone and strength fluctuate along with drug levels in the blood and should be tested before medication and at the peak of drug action. Orders for cholinergic medication often provide for the client to make adjustments according to symptoms; the client's schedule should be ascertained and recorded. The nurse should question the client specifically about drug effects, such as urinary urgency, abdominal cramping, dyspnea, wheezing, perspiration, or salivation. Medications or other measures taken by the client to ameliorate adverse reactions should be ascertained. Atropine may be prescribed to control these symptoms during the early period of therapy before a tolerance to the muscarinic effects of cholinergics develops. Asthmatic clients are likely to require maintenance medication to control respiratory symptoms indefinitely.

Nursing diagnosis Diagnoses related to myasthenia gravis include the following:

> *Self-care deficit*
> *Self-esteem disturbance*
> *High risk for impaired gas exchange*
> *High risk for ineffective airway clearance*
> *Sensory/perceptual alteration: diplopia*
> *High risk for urinary retention*
> *High risk for constipation*

Often there will be a

> *Knowledge deficit related to myasthenia gravis and to drugs used to treat the disease*

Diagnoses related to the use of cholinergic drugs include the following:

> *Altered comfort: excessive perspiration, excessive salivation, nausea, or abdominal cramping*
> *High risk for injury related to blurring of vision*
> *Functional urinary incontinence*
> *Bowel incontinence*

Example of nursing process and treatment of myasthenia gravis

The client is a 52-year-old male with myasthenia gravis. His wife has just died, and his daughter wants her father to live with her in a nearby city so she can care for him.

The client wishes to stay in the home he shared with his wife for "as long as possible."

The client is taking cholinergic drugs for muscle weakness.

Assessment data	Nursing diagnosis	Intervention	Goals and outcome criteria
Diagnosis of myasthenia gravis	High risk for impaired gas exchange related to muscle weakness secondary to myasthenia gravis	**Help** the client to devise a regimen that will provide maximum control of the muscle weakness and minimize risk of respiratory arrest. Suggest that the client ask his physician if a sustained release form of medication can be prescribed for the bedtime dose. Advise the client to arrange for assistance during the transition period until he ascertains whether the new medication regimen will control his muscle weakness adequately. (A relative, home-health aid, or nurse could stay with him temporarily to assist him with self-care, monitor his response to medication, and take corrective measures if necessary.) **Visit** the client regularly to ascertain whether he can safely meet his health needs and carry out activities of daily living. (Visit every day at first, gradually increasing the interval between visits in accord with his progress.)	The client will not experience respiratory depression or failure.
Recent death of wife Expressed wish to live in house he had shared with his wife "as long as possible"	Grieving (normal)	**Prepare** and implement a plan for teaching the daughter about the grieving process and identify measures she can use to support and assist her father with this process. **Encourage** the client to talk about his wife and the years he spent with her; listen and respond warmly to him if he does so.	The client will progress through the grieving process; at the end of a year, he will state that he has accepted his wife's death and is no longer experiencing acute distress because of it.

Diagnoses related to cholinergic crisis include the following:

Impaired gas exchange related to bronchospasm and increased bronchial secretion or respiratory paralysis

Impaired physical mobility

A collaborative problem that should be differentiated from the nursing diagnoses is

Potential complication: cardiovascular, including decreased cardiac output

Planning Goals of treatment include improving muscle tone to maintain adequate gas exchange, increasing tissue perfusion, maintaining mobility and self-care, and eliminating diplopia, as well as eliminating urine retention or constipation. Goals related to the drug regimen include reduction of the risk of adverse drug reaction, prompt detection and treatment of drug reaction should one occur, prevention or correction of side effects such as discomfort, blurred vision, urgency, and incontinence, and prompt correction or alleviation of impaired tissue perfusion, impaired gas exchange, and immobility and helplessness of the cholinergic crisis, should one develop. An additional goal is to teach the client information and the skills needed to manage myasthenia gravis.

Intervention When initial assessment of the client reveals risk factors or contraindications for cholinergic therapy, the nurse consults with the physician to verify that these factors were considered when the therapy regimen was determined. It is unlikely that cholinergic therapy will be cancelled because no effective alternative for control of myasthenia gravis exists. However, all health care personnel should be informed of any additional risk the client has. Atropine may be ordered to control the muscarinic effects of the cholinergic agents during the first few weeks of therapy. During long-term therapy, most clients develop a tolerance to the muscarinic action of the cholinergics, and the atropine may be slowly withdrawn. Asthmatic clients may require atropine medication indefinitely to maintain adequate respiration.

Drugs used to treat myasthenia gravis are usually administered by mouth. Medication is timed in accordance with the client's signs and symptoms of weakness: when lid lag develops, additional medication is required. Clients with severe disease must receive medication every 2 to 4 hours, during sleeping hours as well as waking hours. Sustained-release preparations are available that allow undisturbed rest for 6 to 8 hours. It is vital that medications be given at the time needed; delay may allow muscle weakness to progress to the point of respiratory arrest.

Clients should be monitored closely for response to the drug regimen. The muscle weakness should improve steadily. If a period of improvement is followed by renewed weakness, the client should be assessed for signs and symptoms of cholinergic crisis. In this toxic condition, the muscle weakness is caused by excessive cholinergic toxicity. Cholinergic crisis must be differentiated from myasthenic weakness because escalation of cholinergic drug dosage exacerbates rather than relieves the symptoms. If the client is not taking atropine, muscarinic effects (*eg*, salivation, perspiration, abdominal cramping, miosis) should allow the nurse to determine the true nature of the client's weakness. Cholinergic drugs are withheld until the crisis is resolved. The client may require mechanical assistance for respiration (Kess, 1984).

Client education. When myasthenia gravis is first diagnosed, clients require extensive teaching about the disease and its treatment. Instruction related to the drug regimen should include the action of the drugs, the expected therapeutic response, common side effects, and the phenomenon of cholinergic crisis. Clients who are beginning long-term therapy experience muscarinic effects until they develop tolerance to these actions. They may be reassured that these side effects usually decrease and disappear within a few weeks.

Clients whose illness is complicated by obstructive airway disease (especially asthma) probably require atropine indefinitely to control the pulmonary side effects of cholinergic medication. Both atropine and cholinergic drugs are quite potent, and dosage must be carefully regulated to maintain the proper physiologic balance. Clients are taught to repeat cholinergic drugs whenever they are unable to open their eyes fully. As the disease progresses, dosage intervals are likely to become shorter. If doses are scheduled for sleeping hours, the client should use a reliable alarm clock to ensure awakening. (A clock that is easy to wind should be chosen.) If an electrically powered clock is preferred, a manual one should be used as a backup, in case electrical power is interrupted. If the client is an unusually sound sleeper, a member of the family may need to awaken to verify that the client has responded to the alarm.

Clients should be taught the early signs and symptoms of urinary and intestinal obstruction and bronchial asthma. They should be urged to seek prompt medical attention should any of these symptoms develop.

Evaluation Data required for evaluation relate to muscle tone and strength, respiratory rate, skin color, peripheral circulation, mobility of the client, visual acuity, urinary and fecal elimination, and the client's statements about self-image (see the Example of Nursing Process and Treatment of Myasthenia Gravis).

Therapy in insecticide poisoning. Mild poisoning sometimes occurs in individuals who experience rapid weight loss. (Breakdown of fatty tissue releases stored insecticides into the bloodstream.) Transdermal absorption of the oily solutions applied to plants or soil may precipitate more serious toxicity. Signs and symptoms of poisoning vary with the dosage absorbed.

Assessment Whenever illness develops during or immediately after the use of insecticides, poisoning should be suspected. Signs and symptoms may range from initial transitory paresthesia and muscle cramps at the contaminated body site, to systemic parasympathetic overactivity (nausea, vomiting, abdominal cramping, wheezing, dyspnea, blurred vision, intestinal cramps, bladder spasm), or to generalized convulsions, cardiorespiratory arrest, and death.

Nursing diagnosis Nursing diagnoses may include the following:

Knowledge deficit related to procedures for safe use of insecticides
Altered comfort: nausea, vomiting, or abdominal cramping related to anticholinesterase toxicity
Impaired gas exchange related to bronchospasm and bronchial hypersecretion secondary to anticholinesterase toxicity
High risk for injury: blurring of vision secondary to anticholinesterase toxicity

A common collaborative problem that should be differentiated from the nursing diagnoses is

Potential complication: seizures

Planning Goals of treatment include termination of seizures; improved gas exchange, tissue perfusion, and clarity of vision; reduction of intestinal cramping and bladder spasm; alleviation of discomfort; and instruction to the client of procedures for safe use of insecticides.

Intervention When insecticide poisoning is suspected, contaminated clothing should be removed and residues of the solutions washed immediately from the skin at the site of the exposure. If seizures or cardiorespiratory collapse occur, an emergency medical unit should be called to treat the client and provide transportation to an acute care center. Cardiopulmonary resuscitation and continued mechanical respiratory assistance may be needed. Atropine is the antidote most likely to be ordered. Clients who experience milder systemic disturbances should also seek medical care. Administration of oral antimuscarinics (*eg*, belladonna) can accelerate recovery.

After resolution of acute symptoms, the nurse should develop and implement a teaching program to inform the client of the risks of insecticide exposure and the precautions required for their safe use.

Evaluation Data required for evaluation relate to the absence or presence of convulsive muscle movements, respiratory rate, skin color, and peripheral circulation, visual acuity, comfort level, and the client's ability to demonstrate procedures taught and to repeat the information given during the teaching sessions (see the Example of Nursing Process and Insecticide Poisoning).

Checklist of nursing actions

Before cholinergic drugs are administered

☐ Assess client for the presence of (or a history of) obstructive airway disease, peptic ulcer disease, ulcerative colitis, and urinary obstruction.

When cholinergic drugs are used

☐ Administer parasympathomimetic drugs before meals.

☐ Use a rectal tube to facilitate the passage of flatus.

☐ Provide readily available facilities for elimination (bedpan, bedside commode, or private bathroom).

☐ Watch clients for respiratory arrest and cardiovascular collapse; initiate cardiopulmonary resuscitation should they occur.

☐ Be prepared to administer atropine or epinephrine if signs or symptoms of bronchial constriction or excessive secretion develop.

☐ Monitor urinary output.

☐ Administer medications to myasthenia gravis clients every 2 to 4 hours unless sustained-release preparations are used. Repeat the drug when muscle weakness causes lid lag.

☐ Awaken myasthenia gravis clients during the night to administer their medication.

☐ Inform clients about side effects of cholinergic medication.

☐ Help myasthenia gravis clients develop dosage regimens to control the signs and symptoms of their muscular weakness.

☐ Teach clients about the early signs and symptoms of urinary and intestinal obstruction and bronchial asthma. Caution the client to seek medical attention if these signs and symptoms develop.

☐ Secure emergency care (atropine, cardiopulmonary resuscitation) for clients with systemic signs and symptoms of anticholinesterase insecticide poisoning.

☐ Teach clients exposed to cholinergic drugs or anticholinesterase agents the actions of the drugs, their toxic and side effects, and the measures required to prevent or correct them.

Anticholinergic drugs

Drugs that inhibit response to acetylcholine (anticholinergics) relax smooth muscle and reduce stimulation of postganglionic nerves. Their actions are most pro-

Example of nursing process and insecticide poisoning

The client is a 20-year-old female college student living with three schoolmates in an apartment near campus. She comes to the infirmary because of nausea, vomiting, abdominal cramping, and weakness during the last 2 hours. When questioned, she relates that she and her apartment mates had decided to spray the apartment with an insecticide in an effort to eliminate flies and silverfish. While filling the sprayer, she spilled solution on her hands, causing prickling sensations up her arms, accompanied by transitory spasms of the small muscles. She cleaned up the insecticide but felt ill and was unable to complete the spraying.

The client has come to the infirmary without changing her clothes. There is a faint odor of insecticide on her jeans.

Assessment data	Nursing diagnosis	Intervention	Goals and outcome criteria
History of insecticide spill on hands Nausea Abdominal cramping Weakness	Altered comfort: nausea, abdominal cramping, vomiting, and weakness related to adverse reaction to insecticide exposure	**Notify** the physician of the client's arrival and inform him or her of your findings. **Assist** the client in removing her clothes and showering. Provide her with a clean gown and robe or scrub gown. **Administer** anticholinergic drugs as ordered by the physician.	The client will state that she feels better, that the nausea, cramping, and weakness have decreased or ceased.
Exposure to insecticide	High risk for poisoning related to insecticide exposure	**Have** the client lie down in a quiet place until the physician arrives. Monitor her for abnormal muscle movements and be prepared to take protective measures should a convulsion occur. **Administer** atropine as noted above.	The client will not develop convulsions. If a convulsion occurs, the client will not be seriously injured.
Spillage of insecticide on hands and clothing Failure of client to change clothes and wash off all insecticide from her skin	Knowledge deficit concerning safe use of insecticides	**Prepare** a plan for teaching the client safe procedures for using insecticide sprays. Implement the plan when the client's immediate discomfort has been alleviated.	The client will repeat to the nurse the information conveyed during the teaching session. The client will develop no further signs and symptoms of insecticide poisoning.

nounced in relation to the muscarinic effects of acetylcholine. These drugs have been called *antispasmodic, spasmolytic, antiparasympathetic, cholinolytic,* and *parasympatholytic*—terms that reflect their main properties. Because most of these agents have little effect on nicotinic receptor sites, the term *antimuscarinic* is more descriptive of their true actions.

Pharmacodynamics. All drugs of the anticholinergic class resemble atropine in their action (Table 22-9). They act by competitive antagonism to acetylcholine and other muscarinic agents. Their ef-

fects are dose related, with responses occurring in orderly fashion according to a characteristic progression. Small doses of anticholinergics inhibit salivary, bronchial, and sweat secretion. Larger doses cause mydriasis, inhibition of accommodation of the eye, and increased heart rate. Still larger doses inhibit micturition and intestinal motility. At highest doses, gastric secretion is reduced.

Pharmacokinetics. Little information is available about the pharmacokinetics of most anticholinergics.
(Text continues on p. 356)

Table 22-9. Anticholinergic drugs

Drug names	Preparations	Usual dosage	Therapeutic uses
Tertiary amine compounds			
Anisotropine methylbromide (Valpin)	Oral tablets	Adults: 150 mg/day, divided in 3 doses Safety and efficacy in children have not been established	Treatment of peptic ulcer disease (as an adjunct)
Atropine, atropine sulfate	Oral tablets Solutions for injection	Adults: 400–600 μg q4–6h Children: 10 μg/kg body weight or 300 μg/m^2 (not to exceed 400 μg) q4–6h	Dilation of the pupil Inhibition of secretions preoperatively Treatment of spastic states, including biliary and ureteral colic and bronchospasm
	Solutions and ointments for ophthalmic use	gtt i of a 1% solution	Mydriasis
Belladonna, deadly nightshade (*Can:* Belladenal)	Tablet, powder, leaf, and tincture for oral use	Adults: *Extract:* 45–120 mg/day, divided in 3–4 doses; *tincture:* 0.6–1 ml tid-qid; *L-alkaloids:* 0.5–1 mg/day, divided in 7–8 doses Children: *L-alkaloids:* 0.125–0.5 mg/day, divided in 1–4 doses, *tincture:* 0.1 ml/kg body weight daily, divided in 3–4 doses Safety and efficacy of belladonna extract for children have not been established	Treatment of peptic ulcer (as an adjunct) and hypermotility problems of the gastrointestinal tract Alleviation of ureteral spasm Symptomatic treatment of parkinsonism
Dicyclomine hydrochloride (A-Spas, Antispas, Bentyl, Dibent, Dilomine, Or-Tyl, Spasmoject; *Can:* Bentylol)	Oral capsules, tablets, and solutions Solution for IM injection	Adults: *Oral:* 10–20 mg tid-qid; *IM:* 20 mg q4–6h Children 1 yr of age or older: *Oral:* 10 mg tid-qid Children younger than 12 mo: 5 mg tid-qid PC: C	Treatment of functional disturbances of GI mobility, such as irritable bowel syndrome
Homatropine, homatropine methylbromide (Homapin)	Powder and tablets for oral use	Adults: 15–40 mg/day, divided in 3–4 doses	Treatment of peptic ulcer (as an adjunct) and hypermotility problems of the GI tract
Hyoscyamine, hyoscyamine hydrobromide, hyoscyamine sulfate (Anaspaz, Cystospaz, Levsin, Levsinex; *Can:* Buscopan)	Tablets, capsules, elixir, and solutions for oral use Solution for injection	Adults: *Oral:* 0.375–1 mg/day, divided in 3–4 doses Children: 12.5–188 μg q4h (depending on weight) PC: C	Treatment of peptic ulcer (as an adjunct) and hypermotility problems of the GI tract Treatment of infant colic Treatment of hypermotility problems of the urinary tract
Methixene hydrochloride (Trest)	Oral tablets	Adults: 3–6 mg/day, divided in 1–2 doses Safety and efficacy for children have not been established	Treatment of peptic ulcer (as an adjunct) and hypermotility problems of the GI tract Management of parkinsonism
Oxyphencyclimine hydrochloride (Daricon)	Oral tablets	Adults: 10–20 mg/day, divided in 2 doses Safety and efficacy for children have not been established	Treatment of peptic ulcer (as an adjunct) and hypermotility problems of the GI tract

(Continued)

Table 22-9. Anticholinergic drugs (*Continued*)

Drug names	Preparations	Usual dosage	Therapeutic uses
Tertiary amine compounds			
Scopolamine, scopolamine hydrobromide (Transderm-Scōp, Triptone; *Can:* Transderm-V)	Tablets and capsules for oral use Solutions for injection Transdermal patches for topical use	Adults: *Oral:* 0.3–0.8 mg tid-qid PRN; *parenteral:* 0.3–0.6 mg up to qid; *topical:* one patch applied 4 h before anticipated motion (may be used up to 72 h)	Prevention of motion sickness Inhibition of secretion preoperatively
Thiphenamil hydrochloride (Trocinate)	Oral tablets	Adults: 400 mg repeated in 4 h (2–4 doses usually suffice) Safety and efficacy for children have not been established PC: C	Alleviation of smooth muscle spasm
Quaternary ammonium compounds			
Clidinium bromide (Quarzan)	Oral capsules	Adults: 7.5–20 mg/day, divided in 3–4 doses Safety and efficacy for children have been established PC: C	Treatment of peptic ulcer (as an adjunct)
Glycopyrrolate (Robinul)	Oral tablets Solution for IM or IV injection	Adults: *Oral: Initial:* 1–2 mg tid; *maintenance:* 1 mg bid (maximum daily dosage: 8 mg); *IM:* 0.1 mg tid-qid PC: C	Treatment of peptic ulcer (as an adjunct)
Hexocyclium methylsulfate (Tral)	Tablets and sustained-release tablets for oral use	Adults: 100 mg/day, divided in 4 doses PC: C	Treatment of peptic ulcer (as an adjunct)
Isopropamide iodide (Darbid)	Oral tablets	Adults: 10–20 mg/day, divided in 2 doses, administered at 12-h intervals Safety and efficacy for children have not been established PC: C	Treatment of peptic ulcer (as an adjunct) and hypermotility problems of the GI tract
Mepenzolate bromide (Cantil)	Oral tablets	Adults: 75–200 mg/day divided in 3–4 doses Safety and efficacy for children have not been established PC: C	Treatment of peptic ulcer (as an adjunct) and hypermotility problems of the GI tract
Menthantheline bromide (Banthine)	Oral tablets	Adults: 200–400 mg/day, divided in 4 doses, administered at equal intervals Children older than 12 mo: 50–200 mg/day, divided in 3–4 doses PC: C	Treatment of peptic ulcer (as an adjunct) Treatment of neurogenic bladder
Methscopolamine bromide (Pamine)	Oral tablets	Adults: 10–20 mg/day divided in 4 doses, administered ac and hs Children: 0.2 mg/kg body weight, or 6 mg/m²/day, divided in 4 doses PC: C	Treatment of peptic ulcer (as an adjunct)

(Continued)

Table 22-9. Anticholinergic drugs (Continued)

Drug names	Preparations	Usual dosage	Therapeutic uses
Quaternary ammonium compounds			
Oxyphenonium bromide (Antrenyl)	Oral tablets	Adults: 40 mg/day, divided in 4 doses Safety and efficacy for children have not been established PC: C	Treatment of peptic ulcer (as an adjunct)
Propantheline bromide (Pro-Banthine)	Oral tablets	Adults: 75 mg/day (15 mg tid ac and 30 mg qd hs) Safety and efficacy for children have not been established PC: C	Treatment of peptic ulcer (as an adjunct) and hypermotility problems of the GI tract
Tridihexethyl chloride (Pathilon)	Tablets and extended-release capsules for oral use	Adults: 75–200 mg/day, divided in 4 doses, administered ac and hs Safety and efficacy for children have not been established	Treatment of peptic ulcer (as an adjunct) and hypermotility problems of the GI tract
Antiparkinsonian agents			
Benztropine mesylate (Cogentin)	Oral tablets Solution for injection	Adults: 1–2 mg/day (Maximum daily dosage: 6 mg) PC: C	Treatment of parkinsonism (as an adjunct)
Biperiden hydrochloride, biperiden lactate (Akineton)	Oral tablets Solution for IM or IV injection	Adults: 6–8 mg/day, divided in 3–4 doses PC: C	Treatment of parkinsonism (as an adjunct)
Ethopropazine hydrochloride (Parsidol)	Oral tablets	Adults: 100–400 mg/day, divided in 1–2 doses (Maximum daily dosage: 600 mg)	Treatment of parkinsonism (as an adjunct)
Procyclidine hydrochloride (Kemadrin)	Oral tablets	Adults: 6–60 mg/day, divided in 3–4 doses PC: C	Treatment of parkinsonism (as an adjunct)
Triexyphenidyl hydrochloride	Tablets, elixir, and extended-release capsules for oral use	Adults: Initially 1 mg/day, increasing gradually to 6–10 mg/day, divided in 3–4 doses (Maximum daily dosage: 15 mg) PC: C	Treatment of parkinsonism (as an adjunct)

KEY: PC = pregnancy category. (The validity of pregnancy categories has not been established; see Chapter 16, p 216.)
Can = Canadian trade name.

Absorption is variable. Because they are completely ionized, anticholinergics that have a quaternary ammonium group are incompletely absorbed from the GI tract. Scopolamine is well absorbed percutaneously after topical application. Atropine is rapidly absorbed from IM injection sites.

Distribution of most anticholinergics has not been determined. Atropine appears to be rapidly distributed throughout the body. Quaternary ammonium anticholinergics do not readily cross the blood–brain barrier because they are poorly soluble in lipids; atropine and hyoscyamine readily enter the cerebrospinal fluid. Atropine, hyoscyamine, and scopolamine cross the placenta, but whether other anticholinergics do is not known. It is unlikely that quaternary ammonium anticholinergics enter breast milk, but atropine has been reported to do so.

Information about elimination of the anticholinergics is also incomplete. Atropine is apparently metabolized in the liver. Propantheline is hydrolyzed in the upper small intestine. Elimination of anticholinergics is mainly through the kidneys. Substantial amounts of oral doses of anticholinergics (especially quaternary ammonium compounds) may remain unabsorbed and pass from the body in feces. Atropine is apparently not removed by hemodialysis; it is not known whether the quaternary ammonium compounds are dialyzable.

Therapeutic uses. Anticholinergic drugs are used in the treatment of conditions characterized by hypersecretion (asthma, peptic ulcer, parkinsonism), smooth muscle spasm (hypermotility of the bowel, bladder spasms), abnormal parasympathetic activity (toxicity from cholinergic or anticholinesterase drugs and motion sickness), and sinus bradycardia. These drugs are often administered preoperatively to decrease respiratory secretions. Topical preparations are used to dilate the pupils before opthalmic examinations.

Adverse reactions. The side effects of anticholinergics vary depending on the purpose for which the drugs are used and the dosage involved. Thus, when atropine is administered in large doses, the client experiences a full range of side effects: dry mouth, visual disturbances, constipation, and an increased tendency for urine retention. A relatively small dose administered as an adjunct to sympathomimetic treatment of asthma may cause only a dry mouth. With drug use over a period of time, sexual dysfunction characterized by impaired tumescence may develop.

Toxic effects include rapid and weak pulse, blurred vision, hyperthermia or hypothermia, ataxia, restlessness, and excitement. The affected client appears flushed, and the iris is virtually obliterated. The skin feels hot and dry. Hallucinations, delirium, and coma occur in extreme poisoning.

The effects of atropine are heightened by many drugs that possess anticholinergic properties. Included among these are meperidine, diphenylate with atropine (Lomotil), flurazepam hydrochloride, diphenhydramine, phenothiazine tranquilizers, and tricyclic antidepressants. Combining two or three of these drugs (*eg*, atropine, meperidine, and a tranquilizer) in preoperative medication may be a major factor in the development of postoperative delirium (Tune, et al, 1981).

Precautions and contraindications. Anticholinergics must be administered with great caution to clients with benign prostatic hypertrophy, because the force of micturition is diminished and acute urinary retention may occur. Extreme caution is also required in individuals with GI infections, because the drugs inhibit the protective hypermotility that eliminates organisms and toxins. Other conditions in which the drug may be harmful include glaucoma, hyperthyroidism, hepatic or renal disease, or hypertension. Use of anticholinergics in febrile clients and those exposed to high environmental temperatures increases the risk of hyperthermia. The drugs also may cause drowsiness or blurred vision, a safety hazard in situations that require mental alertness.

Anticholinergics are contraindicated for clients with glaucoma, obstructive uropathy, myasthenia gravis (except for mitigating the initial side effects of cholinergic medications or for treating cholinergic crisis), and those with allergic hypersensitivity to them.

Atropine

The first anticholinergic substances were natural alkaloids found in the belladonna plant. Atropine is the primary agent of this ancient herb. The drug was first isolated in the early 19th century; its pharmacology is well understood. Atropine is found in many plants, including deadly nightshade, jimson weed, and thorn apple. Extracts of the deadly nightshade plant that contain atropine were often used by poisoners during the Middle Ages. The official preparation, tincture of belladonna, owes its clinical activity mainly to its atropine content.

Pharmacodynamics. Atropine stimulates the medulla and higher brain centers. It induces mydriasis, cycloplegia, and photophobia. Respiration is enhanced by bronchodilation and decreased secretions of the respiratory passages. Atropine inhibits vagal activity, thus increasing heart rate and inhibiting gastric secretion and motility. This action is most evident in healthy young adults; little or no effect may occur in infants or the elderly. Atropine also selectively inhibits CNS centers that stimulate muscle tremor and rigidity.

Pharmacokinetics. Atropine may be administered orally, topically (to mucous membranes), IM, or by inhalation. It is readily absorbed from mucous membranes and the upper small intestine. Transcutaneous absorption is limited. After absorption, atropine is widely distributed in the body. It readily crosses the blood–brain barrier and the placenta. Although evidence is limited, it is believed that the drug is not secreted in breast milk in large quantities. Binding to plasma protein (albumin) equals about 18%. Atropine is metabolized by the liver; metabolites and unchanged drug are excreted in urine. Plasma half-life is about 2 to 3 hours.

Therapeutic uses. Atropine is frequently administered preoperatively to inhibit respiratory secretion, to dilate the bronchi, to treat cardiac arrhythmias, such as bradycardia, to reduce the risk of laryngospasm, and as an adjunct in the treatment of asthma.

In the past, an atropine preparation, tincture of belladonna, was frequently prescribed to reduce gastric secretion and motility in clients with symptoms of excessive gastric acid secretion or peptic ulcer disease. In medical practice, it has now been largely supplanted by histamine-receptor inhibitors (see cimetidine and ranitidine). Belladonna's antispasmodic properties have been valued by folk herbalists, who used it as a remedy for colic and dysmenorrhea. Belladonna is useful in treating enuresis in children, urinary frequency in paraplegia, muscle tremor and rigidity in parkinsonism, and hypertonic bladder.

Atropine is a specific antidote for the treatment of cholinergic toxicity, including poisoning by mushrooms, insecticides, and nerve gas. It is used as an adjunct in the treatment of propranolol overdose and to reduce the risk of cardiovascular collapse as a result of vagus nerve stimulation by emetics, such as ipecac.

Adverse reactions. Atropine is a potent drug. Except for the treatment of cholinergic poisoning, doses for adults are measured in micrograms. Adverse effects range from dryness of the mucous membranes to delirium and death (Table 22-10). Overdoses are hazardous and can be life-threatening.

Precautions and contraindications. Atropine should be used with caution in asthmatics and in elderly men likely to have a hypertrophied prostate. It is contraindicated in acute urine retention, constipation or obstipation, diarrhea caused by enteric infections, glaucoma, and myasthenia gravis (except for the treatment of asthma or cholinergic crisis).

Scopolamine and synthetic and semisynthetic antimuscarinics

Like atropine, scopolamine is found in plant sources, including deadly nightshade. Its effects are overshadowed by the more potent atropine when the unrefined plant extract is used. Scopolamine shares many of the properties of atropine but has some distinct ones that are valuable in certain clinical situations.

The effect of scopolamine on the CNS is characterized by depression rather than excitation. Its antinauseant properties are useful in the treatment of

motion sickness and postoperative nausea. Scopolamine causes drowsiness, euphoria, and amnesia. For these reasons, it may be preferable to atropine for preoperative use. It has been used in combination with a narcotic for obstetric analgesia.

Attempts have been made to develop antimuscarinic drugs with more selectivity of action for use in specific disease conditions. While the drugs developed to date continue to exert most of the effects of the natural anticholinergics, those with a quaternary ammonium structure are not as well absorbed or widely distributed as atropine. They generally do not cause CNS effects because they pass the blood–brain barrier with difficulty. They are of little value in ophthalmology because penetration of the conjunctiva is poor. Because these drugs are more active ganglionic blockers than atropine, impotence, urinary retention, and postural hypotension are more likely to occur.

The quaternary ammonium compounds in common use include methscopolamine bromide (Pamine), methantheline (Banthine), and propantheline (Pro-Banthine). They have been used primarily to control GI activity in peptic ulcer clients. The introduction of histamine H_2-receptor antagonists has reduced reliance on these drugs for this condition.

The use of synthetic anticholinergics is contraindicated in acute urinary retention and acute glaucoma. Caution is required when they are given to people with prostatic hypertrophy or chronic glaucoma.

■ Summary
Anticholinergic drugs inhibit response to acetylcholine. They tend to relax smooth muscle and reduce postganglionic stimulation. As a class, anticholinergic drugs are potent and have a high potential for toxicity. They are used to treat asthma, peptic ulcer, parkinsonism, motion sickness, and toxicity from cholinergic substances.

Nursing management

Nursing implications

All anticholinergic drugs predispose the client to dry mouth, delayed digestion, constipation, and urinary retention. Frequent mouth care, measures to stimulate the appetite, and precautions to promote regular fecal and urinary elimination are needed by clients who receive these drugs.

Atropine is an extremely potent drug and inappropriate exposure to small amounts can cause adverse reactions. One source of toxicity is mucosal absorption of ophthalmic solutions that have drained into the nose through the tear duct. Systemic poisoning in children has resulted from conjunctival instillation of anticholinergic drugs.

Table 22-10. Systemic doses of atropine with resultant toxic effects

Dose	Effects
0.5 mg	Some dryness of the mouth, inhibition of sweating, slight cardiac slowing
1 mg	Definite dryness of the mouth, thirst, slow heart action followed by acceleration, mild dilation of the pupil
2 mg	Marked dryness of the mouth, rapid heart rate, palpitation, dilated pupils, some blurring of near vision
5 mg	All previous symptoms increased, speech disturbance, dysphagia, restlessness, fatigue, headache, dry hot skin, difficulty in micturition, reduced intestinal peristalsis
10 mg	Above symptoms pronounced, pulse rapid and weak, iris nearly obliterated, vision very blurred, skin flushed, hot, and dry, ataxia, restlessness, and excitement, hallucinations and delirium, coma

(Gilman AG, Goodman LS, Rall TW, Murad F, eds. [1985]. *Goodman and Gilman's The pharmacological basis of therapeutics*, 7th ed, p 138. New York: Macmillan.)

Exposure to atropine is an occupational hazard for nurses. Surgical nurses sometimes experience a persistent blurring of vision from accidental introduction of minute quantities of the drug into the eye while preparing preoperative injections. Nurses can avoid accidental exposure to atropine by using correct technique when drawing solutions into syringes. The dose should be adjusted exactly *before* the needle is withdrawn from the vial of medication. Accidental ejection of drug from the syringe, either while eliminating air from the syringe or while discarding excess solution, should be avoided. If such a maneuver is necessary, care should be taken to point the needle away from the eyes.

Atropine poisoning can occur in users of OTC preparations that contain scopolamine; the nurse should advise clients not to exceed the recommended dosages of such nonprescription drugs. Ingestion of berries or seeds that contain belladonna alkaloids can also cause adverse reactions. Clients should be warned against ingesting plant materials that have unknown toxic potential; children should be prevented from doing so as well.

Symptoms of belladonna poisoning include widespread paralysis of organs innervated by parasympathetic nerves, dry mucous membranes, unresponsive and widely dilated pupils, tachycardia, flushing, fever, and acute mental and neurologic symptoms. Any client with acute onset of bizarre behavior should be assessed for possible drug poisoning. Treatment involves gastric lavage and other measures to limit GI absorption. In extreme cases, physostigmine should be administered. Diazepam may help control seizures and may be useful for sedation.

Atropine as an antidote. As the specific antidote to nerve gas, atropine is a crucial substance in any military conflict in which gas chemical agents are used. Atropine must be administered at the moment of exposure to nerve gas, before the agent induces convulsions that completely incapacitate the victim and lead to respiratory arrest.

Nursing process

Assessment Before initiating atropine therapy, the nurse should assess the client for risk factors of adverse reaction to the drug. Among these are dehydration, a tendency toward hypotension, prostatic hypertrophy or other predisposition to urine retention, glaucoma, cardiac arrhythmia (especially tachycardia), infection of the GI tract, hyperthyroidism, hypertension, and fever. A complete drug history should be taken with specific queries about drugs that interact with atropine: meperidine, flurazepam, diphenhydramine, phenothiazine tranquilizers, and tricyclic antidepressants. The nurse should also ask clients if they have taken atropine in the past and, if so, how they responded to it.

Nursing diagnosis Diagnoses related to atropine therapy include the following:

Altered comfort: dry mouth, abdominal distention, and restlessness
Altered tissue perfusion: postural hypotension
Urinary retention
High risk for injury related to blurred vision
Sexual dysfunction related to impaired tumescence and impotence
Knowledge deficit related to anticholinergic drugs and self-care measures to prevent or ameliorate adverse reactions to them

Planning Goals of treatment include improved comfort (relief of dry mouth, abdominal distention, and restlessness), instruction of techniques to minimize the signs and symptoms of postural hypotension, promotion of fecal and urinary elimination, improved vision, correction of sexual dysfunction (or assistance in the adoption of alternative modes of sexual expression), and instruction about the drug regimen, adverse reactions to the drugs, and self-care practices to minimize adverse reaction to them.

Intervention When anticholinergic drugs are ordered for a short time only, the adverse reactions dissipate on withdrawal from the drugs. Clients should be informed of the cause of such symptoms as dry mouth and blurred vision and should be reassured that they are temporary. Frequent mouth care should be administered and, if allowed, oral fluids may be encouraged. Nursing measures to promote micturition are appropriate, but if acute retention cannot be relieved, catheterization may be necessary. A rectal tube may relieve abdominal distention.

Postural hypotension, constipation, and sexual dysfunction are more likely to occur with long-term therapy. Nursing measures to minimize dizziness and weakness of postural hypotension include promoting fluid intake and changing the client's position slowly. Hydration as well as fiber in the diet are important in preventing constipation. The client should also engage in physical activity and develop a habitual pattern of defecation. Moderate use of laxative foods, such as pears and prunes, may be recommended. When sexual dysfunction occurs, the physician should be consulted for a possible change in the drug regimen. If a change in drug is inadvisable, the client should be taught alternatives to intercourse. Referral to a sex therapist may be appropriate.

Client education. When long-term therapy with anticholinergic drugs is prescribed, the nurse should develop and implement a teaching program to inform the client about the drug regimen, adverse drug effects, and self-care measures that promote therapeutic response and decrease risk of adverse reactions. Cli-

Example of nursing process and reaction to anticholinergic medications

The client is an 18-year-old male college student who reports to the infirmary in the evening, complaining of blurred vision. On examination, the pupils of both eyes appear dilated and do not react to light. The client states that the blurring began in the morning and has neither increased nor decreased during the day. He denies use of drugs, stating that he has been on a field trip all day. With a tense expression on his face, the client asks, "What has happened to my eyes?"

When asked for a drug history, the client states that he uses aspirin occasionally for headache but takes no medication regularly.

Examination reveals a small round area of redness behind the left ear. When questioned, the client states that he placed a "carsickness patch" on that spot to prevent nausea during the field trip bus ride.

Assessment data	Nursing diagnosis	Intervention	Goals and outcome criteria
Tense expression on face Question: "What has happened to my eyes?" Blurred vision Use of anticholinergic medication patch Dilated pupils that do not react to light	Fear of loss of vision related to blurred vision secondary to dilation of both pupils	Explain to client the likely cause of his blurred vision. Arrange for examination of the client by a physician to verify the cause of pupil dilation. If the physician agrees that the pupil dilation is due to transfer of anticholinergic drug to the eye from the medicated disk, reassure the client that the change in vision is temporary and innocuous.	Facial muscles will relax and the client will state that he knows that no permanent damage to his eyes has occurred.
Client's exclusion of patch medication from list of drugs used Pupil dilation coinciding with use of anticholinergic patch	Knowledge deficit concerning patch medications and safe practices for their use	Instruct the client to handle medicated disks with clean hands and to wash the hand thoroughly and immediately after affixing the disk on the proper site. Warn the client not to touch the disk without washing his hands immediately.	The client will repeat back to the nurse the information conveyed during the teaching session. The client will not experience a change in vision in the future when using medicated disks.

ents should be warned about early symptoms of drug intoxication (see Table 22-10).

Male clients should report any diminution of the urinary stream to the physician, especially elderly men, who are likely to have prostatic enlargement. Clients should be taught measures to prevent constipation and to minimize the symptoms of postural hypotension. If blurred vision persists, the client should be referred to an ophthalmologist or optometrist for a change in corrective lenses.

Evaluation Data required for evaluation include measurement of abdominal girth, amount and patterns of urinary output, patterns of fecal elimination, improved visual acuity, and statements by the client describing changes in symptoms. Data pertinent to the teaching plan include the client's ability to demonstrate techniques taught and to repeat information conveyed during teaching sessions (see the Example of Nursing Process and Reaction to Anticholinergic Medications).

Checklist of nursing actions

☐ Warn clients of the toxic potential of berries and seeds that contain anticholinergic alkaloids.

☐ Warn clients who use OTC preparations that contain anticholinergics not to exceed the recommended dosages.

☐ When sudden, bizarre behavior occurs, assess the client for poisoning, including anticholinergic toxicity.

When anticholinergic drugs are prescribed

☐ Remember that atropine is extremely potent and toxic.

☐ Use correct techniques when drawing solutions into syringes so that no accidental exposure to atropine occurs.

☐ When administering eye drops, occlude the tear ducts by external pressure until solutions are completely dispersed over the conjunctival sac.

☐ Warn clients of early symptoms of drug intoxication.

☐ Tell male clients to report any diminution of their urinary stream to their physicians.

☐ When sexual dysfunction is a problem, give sexual counseling or refer to a counselor for alternatives to intercourse.

☐ Advise the client that blurring of vision may occur. If anticholinergic therapy is to be long-term, recommend refraction for corrective lenses after the drug dosage is stabilized for maintenance.

☐ Monitor clients for toxic and side effects.

☐ Alleviate mouth dryness by administering frequent mouth care.

☐ Encourage oral intake of fluids, when allowed.

☐ Promote fecal and urinary elimination.

☐ Report urine retention to the physician promptly.

☐ Catheterize as ordered to relieve retention.

☐ Instruct clients in methods to prevent or control adverse drug reactions.

Ganglionic stimulants

Impulse transmission through autonomic ganglia is more complex than was previously believed. The basic acetylcholine–cholinesterase system is modified by secondary pathways and possibly by an intermediary neuron that uses a catecholamine transmitter. Consequently, drug actions at the ganglion level do not always correspond to the effects predicted by previous theories of cholinergic mechanisms.

With the exception of a nicotine chewing gum and the nicotine patch used to reduce withdrawal symptoms in clients who attempt to quit smoking, no therapeutically useful ganglionic stimulating drugs exist. Two natural alkaloids, nicotine and lobeline, as well as a number of synthetic compounds are useful as experimental tools. Because of its nonmedicinal uses and abuses, nicotine is the drug of most interest to health care practitioners.

Nicotine

Pharmacodynamics. Nicotine has potent effects on the nervous system. Its action consists of two stages: initial stimulation followed by depression. Stimulation of the CNS is pronounced, whereas stimulation of the peripheral nervous system is more transitory. Effects vary with dosage; small amounts produce only stimulation, whereas larger doses initiate the full biphasic response. The drug acts on the brain, spinal cord, autonomic ganglia, adrenal medulla, various sensory receptors, and the neuromuscular junction. It can increase basal metabolic rate and thus inhibit weight gain or enhance weight loss (Weiss, 1989). In addition, nicotine causes release of catecholamines by a number of isolated organs. As a consequence, small doses of nicotine produce increases in respiratory and heart rates, an increase in blood pressure and mental alertness, reduced urine production, vasoconstriction, and muscle tremor. Nicotine also reduces production of bicarbonate by the pancreas.

Cigarette smoke preferentially depresses the function of immune cells that lie within the lung tissues; prolonged smoking affects immune cells elsewhere in the body (Smoking inhibits . . . 1989).

Pharmacokinetics. Nicotine is readily absorbed by the GI tract, the lungs, mucous membranes, and the skin. The drug is widely distributed, crosses the blood–brain barrier and placenta, and is secreted in milk. Nicotine absorbed from the lungs reaches the brain within 7 seconds. Nicotine is detoxified by the liver and to a lesser degree by the kidneys and lungs. Excretion is accomplished entirely by the kidneys, except in lactating women whose milk contains the drug in amounts proportional to the dose used.

Adverse effects. Nicotine is a highly toxic drug; the dose contained in two or three cigarettes, taken orally, is sufficient to kill an adult. Symptoms of poisoning include nausea, salivation, abdominal pain, dizziness, disturbed hearing and vision, mental confusion, and weakness. Respiratory arrest, cardiovascular collapse, and convulsions may occur. Death is caused by respiratory paralysis. Tolerance and dependence develop with chronic use.

Nicotine is the major active drug in tobacco. Transcutaneous poisoning is an occupational hazard of tobacco handlers. Many health problems are related to the use of tobacco, whether it is snuffed, chewed, or smoked. Even nonusers who are exposed to cigarette smoke are at increased risk for disease. Smoking is a known risk factor for cardiovascular disease, including myocardial infarction. Nicotine increases collagen levels in major blood vessels and accelerates the atherosclerotic process. It also constricts blood vessels, elevating blood pressure and reducing peripheral perfusion.

Respiratory diseases seen in smokers include flu, chronic bronchitis, emphysema, and asthma. Babies born to mothers who smoke are more likely to develop infantile apnea than are babies of nonsmokers (Toubas, 1986).

Smokers have a higher than normal incidence of cancer of the mouth, larynx, and lungs.

In the past, the carcinogenic effect of smoking was attributed to products of combustion other than nicotine. However, nicotine now appears to be a true carcinogen. Users of snuff have an increased risk of mouth cancer. Cancers of the lung, larynx, and cervix are more common in smokers than nonsmokers.

Smoking is a known risk factor for peptic ulcer. This effect may be related to nicotine's inhibition of pancreatic secretion of bicarbonate, which prevents the normal reversal of acidic pH to basic pH in the duodenum.

Although low doses of nicotine increase alertness, the drug impairs long- and short-term memory.

Nicotine has numerous effects on sexual function and fertility. In males, smoking is associated with decreases in testosterone levels, abnormal destruction of sperm, decreased sperm mobility, delayed tumescence, and impotence. Women who are smokers conceive less readily, are more likely to develop placental inadequacy, and have babies of low birth weight. Their infants have a 40% higher incidence of respiratory distress syndrome.

Drug interactions. Two types of interactions occur between nicotine and other drugs. Absorption of medications administered IM or subcutaneously is delayed because of vasoconstriction and reduced peripheral perfusion. Nicotine also induces liver enzymes, increasing metabolism and lowering blood levels of drugs such as propranolol, theophylline, insulin, propoxyphene, analgesics, nonsteroidal anti-inflammatory drugs, and tricyclic antidepressants.

■ **Summary**

Nicotine is the major toxin in tobacco. It acts biphasically on the nervous system, producing stimulation followed by depression. Nicotine is highly poisonous to both users and nonusers; users develop tolerance and dependence. The use of tobacco is associated with high risks of such diseases as respiratory disease, cancer, cardiovascular disease, impairment of sexual function, and high-risk pregnancy.

Nursing management

Nursing implications

Smoking increases the risk of many serious diseases, some of which are among the major causes of death in developed countries. All are associated with serious illness and permanent disability. Prevention is the only remedy of lasting value, and prevention requires elimination or at least a reduction in the use of tobacco products.

The elimination of smoking is considered an essential element in the medical treatment of chronic bronchitis, emphysema, and peripheral vascular in-

sufficiency. Eliminating smoking helps control peptic ulcers, asthma, and cardiovascular disease. When clients are able to abstain completely, damaged tissue tends to repair itself, and the abnormally high risks of diseases associated with smoking decline rapidly. If abstinence cannot be achieved, cutting back is beneficial. However, it has been found that switching to pipes or cigars has no advantage for the habitual cigarette smoker, because the user continues to inhale. Moreover, use of low-nicotine cigarettes does not significantly reduce consumption of nicotine.

Instruction in the dangers of smoking and nicotine is the aspect of counseling that is probably the least important for nurses, because public education campaigns have already distributed vast amounts of information about the dangers of smoking. Probably the best approach is to ascertain what the client knows and to provide only information that appears to be lacking. What is important is for the client to develop a healthier lifestyle.

Physiologic and psychological factors in tobacco use. Nicotine is an addictive substance that causes both physical and psychological dependence. Abrupt abstinence precipitates a withdrawal syndrome with physical and psychological manifestations. Physiologic disturbances include irritability, reduced pain tolerance, and sore throat (believed to be caused by regrowth of cilia on mucous membranes). Psychologically, withdrawal is accompanied by tension, anxiety, depression, a need for oral gratification, and a constant severe craving.

Nicotine dependence is one of the most difficult addictions to treat. Four out of five adult smokers say they would like to quit, but the success rate among smokers who try is less than 40%.

Box 22-3. Computation of "pack-years"

While taking a history, you are told by the client that he started smoking at the age of 14, but never smoked more than 1/2 pack of cigarettes a day until he left high school and went to work at age 18. Since then, he has smoked 1 1/2 packs of cigarettes daily. He is now 30 years old. He has never used a pipe or smoked cigars. What is his total exposure to tobacco, expressed in pack-years?

18 − 14 = 4 years of smoking		
	1/2 pack daily	
	4 × 1/2 =	2 pack-years
30 − 18 = 12 years of smoking		
	1 1/2 packs daily	
	12 × 1 1/2 =	18 pack-years
Total		20 pack-years

Nursing process

Assessment Exposure to tobacco and nicotine in cigarette smokers is measured by computing the number of pack-years accumulated by the client. The number of years smoked is multiplied by the packs used per day (Box 22-3). Use of cigars, pipe, snuff, or chewing tobacco should also be noted.

Elements in the client's lifestyle that influence tobacco use should be recorded. A client's attitude toward tobacco and perceptions of its psychological and social benefits should be explored. During the physical examination, particular attention should be given to signs and symptoms of diseases associated with tobacco use. If the client is a young nonsmoker, factors that may predispose him or her to smoke (*eg*, smoking by family members, by classmates in school, or by fellow workers as well as peer pressure to learn to smoke) should be ascertained.

Nursing diagnosis Diagnoses related to nicotine use include

For the nonuser:

Decisional conflict related to peer pressures to smoke tobacco and pressures from family and health care personnel not to smoke

For users:

High risk for infection of the respiratory tract
Sexual dysfunction

A common collaborative problem that should be differentiated from the nursing diagnoses include

Potential complication: cancer
Potential complication: cardiovascular
Potential complication: GI bleeding

For users trying to quit:

Anxiety related to anticipated tension and craving

Diagnoses related to nicotine use for smokers who are trying to quit include pain related to reduced pain tolerance, sore throat, tension, anxiety, and craving.

Planning Goals for treatment include preventing tobacco use, reducing its use, preventing respiratory inflammation and infection, improving signs and symptoms of atherosclerosis and peptic ulcer disease, confirming the absence of malignant tumors, improving self-concept, and alleviating the signs and symptoms of nicotine withdrawal.

Intervention Nurses are involved in the prevention and reduction of nicotine use in every setting—with individuals, families, and groups—and at every level of nursing. The most important measure is setting an example of nonuse. Smoking by the nurse is apt to render ineffective any attempt to influence the client's behavior toward nonsmoking.

The problem of tobacco dependence can be approached in a number of ways. Drug education in elementary and secondary schools relies heavily on providing information about the health consequences of nicotine dependence. This approach has not proved effective; curiosity about the effects of drugs is not the critical factor in susceptibility to drug use. More important are inadequacies of self-image that make children vulnerable to drug use. Enhancing self-image in children is likely to be the most effective way to prevent substance abuse, including smoking.

Methods used to assist smokers in quitting include individual counseling, group counseling (in short-term, intensive sessions, or repeated sessions over a few weeks), self-help (buddy or group) arrangements, media campaigns, and national "smokeout" days. Treatment measures include substituting innocuous behaviors for smoking behaviors (*eg*, chewing gum instead of smoking), aversion therapy (stressing offensive aspects of smoking), and hypnosis. Two medications used to ameliorate withdrawal symptoms are clonidine and nicotine. Clonidine relieves craving and blunts anxiety, irritability, and poor concentration. Nicotine gum or patches are used to provide regulated doses of nicotine for gradual weaning from the drug.

Client education. Few clients are completely ignorant about the effects of nicotine and tobacco use. It is important, however, that information be as complete as possible. Despite its apparent failure as a deterrent, education is an important element in any program to reduce tobacco use.

Clients who use nicotine gum or patches must be warned about the risks associated with these products, including nicotine poisoning. Accidental use by children could be life-threatening. The gum also tends to become sticky after a short period. It has damaged dental prostheses (crowns and bridges) and may be difficult to remove from dentures. Removing the gum and letting it stand outside the mouth decreases its stickiness. Chilling the gum causes it to become brittle, making it easier to remove from dentures. Directions for use should be followed accurately to control nicotine dosage and to achieve the desired weaning effect. Patches have proved to be more effective than nicotine gum. However, the client who continues to use tobacco while using these aids is at very high risk for nicotine poisoning.

Smokers who are attempting to quit should avoid exposure to the smoke of others because cigarette odor intensifies the craving for tobacco.

Evaluation Data required for evaluation include whether a nonuser begins to use tobacco, the amount of tobacco used during and after an attempt to withdraw, the incidence and severity of respiratory infection, clients' reports related to self-concept, whether slowing of the atherosclerotic process or improvement in the signs and symptoms of peptic ulcer disease occur, and whether incidences of malignancy associated with tobacco use or incidence and severity of withdrawal symptoms are present.

Checklist of nursing actions

☐ Set an example by not using tobacco.
☐ Provide information about the effects of tobacco and nicotine use.
☐ To reduce drug use and dependence, promote a positive self-image in people at risk.
☐ Participate in campaigns and programs to encourage discontinuation of nicotine and tobacco use.
☐ Advise smokers trying to quit to avoid smoke from other users and situations associated with previous tobacco use.
☐ Warn users of nicotine gum and patches about their toxicity; teach users of nicotine gum how to prevent damage to dentures.

Ganglionic blocking agents

A number of drugs block transmission in autonomic ganglia by occupying receptor sites and preventing response to acetylcholine. Two agents are presently available for medical use: mecamylamine (Inversine), an oral preparation, and trimethaphan camsylate (Arfonad), a parenteral preparation. These drugs are used to reduce vasoconstriction in clients with hypertensive cardiovascular disease or hypertensive crisis and to produce controlled hypotension for certain surgical procedures where hemorrhage in the operative field must be kept to a minimum (see the section on drugs that affect vascular tone in Chapter 28).

References

Botulism: New drug buys time. (1986). *Science News, 130,* 76.
Bower B. (1986). "Betablocking" autistics' aggression. *Science News, 129,* 344.
Cannon W. (1939). *The wisdom of the body.* New York: WW Norton.
Cigarettes: The low-tar irony. (1989). *Science News, 136,* 398.
"Low-Yield" cigarettes are not low risk. (1989). *American Journal of Nursing, 89,* 1118.
Miller P, et al. (1988). Association of low serum anticholinergic levels and cognitive impairment in elderly presurgical patients. *Am J Psychiatry, 145,* 342–345.
Smoking inhibits lung's immune cells. (1989). *Science News, 135,* 255.
Swenson E. (1986). Severe hyperkalemia as a complication of timolol, a topically applied beta-adrenergic antagonist. *Arch Intern Med, 146,* 1220–1221.

There is no safe way to smoke. (1986). *University of California at Berkeley Wellness Letter, 2*(8), 7.
Toubas P, et al. (1986). Effects of maternal smoking and caffeine habits on infantile apnea: A retrospective study. *Pediatrics, 78,* 159–163.
Weiss R. (1989). Nicotine boosts a busy body's metabolism. *Science News, 135,* 214.

Bibliography

Ades P, et al. (1988). Hypertension, exercise and beta-adrenergic blockade. *Ann Intern Med, 109,* 629–634.
Atenolol reduces MI mortality. (1986). *American Journal of Nursing, 86,* 244.
Bailey PL, et al. (1990). Transdermal scopolamine reduces nausea and vomiting after outpatient laparoscopy. *Anesthesiology, 72,* 977–980.
Beller S, et al. (1988). Long-term outpatient treatment of senile dementia with oral physostigmine. *J Clin Psychiatry, 49,* 404.
Berkelman R, et al. (1986). Beta-adrenergic antagonists and fatal anaphylactic reactions to oral penicillin (letter). *Ann Intern Med, 104,* 134.
Blake GJ. (1988). Pharmacist on call: Atrovent-aerosol anticholinergic for C.P.O.D. *Nursing 88, 18,* 142.
Bowen JJ. (1989). Smokeless tobacco: Safer than smoking? *Nursing 89, 19,* 82.
*Cerrato PL. (1989). Don't let weight gain keep a smoker from quitting. *American Journal of Nursing, 89,* 73–74.
*Clinical news: Even one cigarette a day increases cardiac risk. (1988). *American Journal of Nursing, 88,* 155.
*Dalgas P. (1985). Understanding drugs that affect the autonomic nervous system. *Nursing 85, 15*(10), 58–63.
Danziger Y, Garty M, Volwitz B, Ilfeld D, Varsano I, Rosenfeld JB. (1985). Reduction of serum theophylline levels by terbutaline in children with asthma. *Clin Pharmacol Ther, 37,* 469–471.
Desperately seeking smokers. (1987). *Science News, 132,* 204.
Drug news: Breaking a deadly addiction. (1989). *Nursing 89, 19,* 30.
Dyer J. (1989). Clinical news: Cure for the "salsa sniffles"? *American Journal of Nursing, 89,* 798.
*Ferguson T. (1989). *The no-nag, no-guilt, do-it-your-own-way guide to quitting smoking.* New York: Ballantine Books.
Ferree C. (1986). Apparent anaphylaxis from labetalol. *Ann Intern Med, 104,* 729–730.
*The fifteen minute, five percent solution. (1986). *American Journal of Nursing, 86,* 891.
Gengo F, et al. (1988). The effect of β-blockers on mental performance on older hypertensive patients. *Arch Intern Med, 148,* 779–784.
Gengo F, et al. (1987). Lipid-soluble and water-soluble beta-blockers: Comparison of the central nervous system depressant effect. *Arch Intern Med, 147,* 39–43.
Gilkeson G, Delaney R. (1987). Effectiveness of sublingual clonidine in patients unable to take oral medication. *Drug Intell Clin Pharm, 21,* 262–263.
Glassman AH, Jackson WK, Walsh BT, Roose ST. (1986). Cigarette craving, smoking withdrawal, and clonidine. *Science, 226,* 864.

Hiatt W, Stoll S, Nies A. (1985). Effect of beta-adrenergic blockers on the peripheral circulation in patients with peripheral vascular disease. *Circulation, 72,* 1226–1231.

Hayes L, et al. (1989). Timolol side effects and inadvertent overdosing. *J Am Geriatr Soc, 37,* 261–262.

Houston M, Hodge R. (1988). Beta-adrenergic blocker withdrawal syndromes in hypertension and other cardiovascular diseases. *Am Heart J, 116,* 515–523.

Kottke T, et al. (1988). Attributes of successful smoking cessation interventions in medical practice. *JAMA, 259,* 2883.

Lustgarten J. (1988). Topical timolol-induced arthropathy (letter). *Am J Ophthalmol, 105,* 687–688.

Martin TR, Bracken MD. (1986). Association of low birth weight with passive smoke exposure in pregnancy. *Am J Epidemiol, 124,* 633–642.

McEvoy GK, ed. (1987). *Drug information, 87,* pp 519–663. Bethesda: American Society of Hospital Pharmacists.

Metz S, et al. (1987). Rebound hypertension after discontinuation of transdermal clonidine therapy. *Am J Med, 82,* 17–19.

Miller LG. (1989). Recent developments in the study of the effects of cigarette smoking on clinical pharmacokinetics and clinical pharmacodynamics. *Clin Pharmacokinet, 17*(2), 90–108.

A new beta-blocker for blaucoma. (1986). *RN, 49*(4), 55.

Pearce KI. (1986). Clonidine and smoking (letter). *Lancet, 2,* 810.

Reyes P, et al. (1987). Mental status changes induced by eye drops in dementia of the Alzheimer type (letter). *J Neurol Neurosurg Psychiatry, 50,* 113–114.

*Samonds RJ, Cammermeyer M. (1985). Bladder dysfunction responds well to anticholinergic medication. *Nursing 85, 15*(9), 63–64.

*Scherer P. (1989). More evidence links smoking to carotid artery disease. *American Journal of Nursing, 89,* 1605.

Scherer P. (1989). "Low-yield" cigarettes are not low risk. *American Journal of Nursing, 89,* 1118.

Silberner J. (1986). Smoking, heart attack link. *Science News, 130,* 360.

*Smoking boosts death risk for diabetics. (1990). *Science News, 138,* 61.

Stricker B, et al. (1986). Fever induced by labetalol. *JAMA, 256,* 619–620.

Sudan B. (1988). Rash from nicotine gum: Nicotine as a hapten (letter). *South Med J, 81,* 287.

Talmi Y, et al. (1988). Reduction of salivary flow with Scopoderm TTS. *Ann Otol Rhinol Laryngol, 97,* 128–130.

*Teplitz L. (1989). Clinical close-up on atropine. *Nursing 89, 19,* 44–46.

Tonnesen P, et al. (1988). Effect of nicotine gum in combination with group counseling on the cessation of smoking. *N Engl J Med, 318,* 15–18.

*Recommended for further reading.

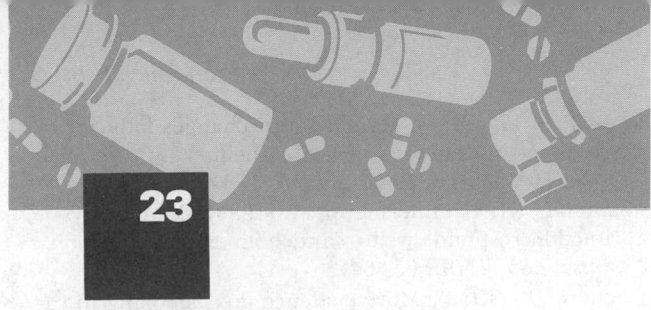

23

Central nervous system stimulants

Physiology of the central nervous system

The central nervous system (CNS) includes the organs and tissues enclosed in the cranium and in the spinal column, namely the brain and spinal cord. Its function somewhat resembles that of a computer. Information enters through sensory fibers, is processed by the system, and is then emitted as instructions through motor fibers. The process is a continuous one, providing for appropriate responses of the organism to changing conditions. In addition, the brain carries out intellectual processes and is responsible for consciousness and subjective awareness.

Many functions of the CNS are spatially distributed (Figs. 23-1 through 23-4). Others, such as memory, seem to be more pervasive. Selectivity of drug action depends on a drug's ability to affect one area or type of tissue more than others. For example, drugs that affect the cerebral cortex tend to influence sensory perceptions, motor activity, and intellectual processes. Those with pronounced effect on the limbic system change emotional status.

The distribution of chemicals to the brain is controlled by a mechanism known as the blood–brain barrier. Cells in the cerebral capillaries are tightly joined, almost fused. The spaces between these cells lack the slit-pores found in other capillary membranes. For this reason, only very small molecules pass through these openings. Normally, water, carbon dioxide, oxygen, sodium, chlorine, phosphorus, and lipid soluble substances penetrate to the brain. The efficiency of the barrier is influenced by the condition of the tissues. It may be impaired by inflammation such as meningitis, allowing entry of therapeutic drugs that are normally poorly distributed in the CNS.

Response to CNS drugs depends largely on the status of the individual. Underlying personality, physiologic function, and mental "set" reflect and influence CNS physiology, which is the milieu in which drugs must act. Response is also influenced by the client's history and situation. Previous exposure to the drug can produce tolerance or sensitization. Environmental stimuli can alter CNS activity and can promote or inhibit response to pharmacologic agents.

Central nervous system stimulants include amphetamines, xanthines, analeptics, levodopa (L-dopa), cocaine, khat, betel, and hallucinogens such as marijuana and LSD (Box 23-1).

In small doses, these drugs increase mental alertness and capacity for work, improve motor performance, and impart a feeling of well-being. They tend to stimulate the respiratory system, cardiac system, and general metabolism. In large doses, they cause tremor, restlessness, and insomnia. Motor performance deteriorates. Prolonged use can lead to hypertension and exhaustion. As toxicity increases, hallu-

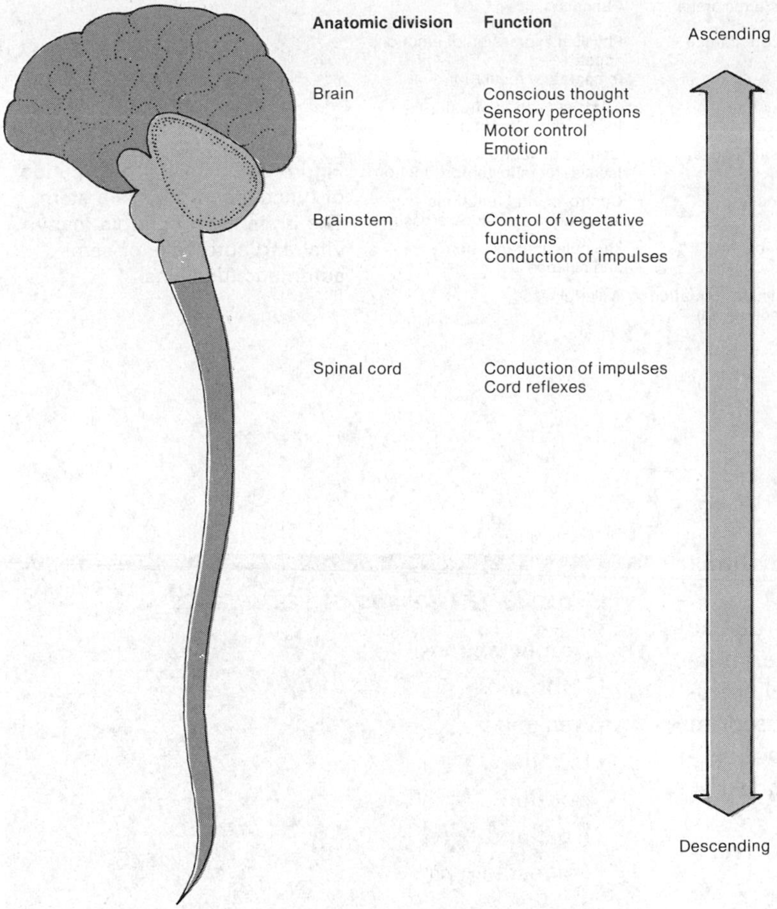

Anatomic division	Function
Brain	Conscious thought Sensory perceptions Motor control Emotion
Brainstem	Control of vegetative functions Conduction of impulses
Spinal cord	Conduction of impulses Cord reflexes

Ascending

Descending

Figure 23-1. Spatial distribution of functions of the central nervous system: divisions of the central nervous system. Functions of the brain are considered "higher" functions; those of the spinal cord "lower" functions. Drugs that exhibit an ascending pattern of activity affect first the function of the spinal cord, then successively higher functions, affecting the brain last of all. Drugs that exhibit a descending pattern of activity affect the cortex of the brain first, then successively lower functions.

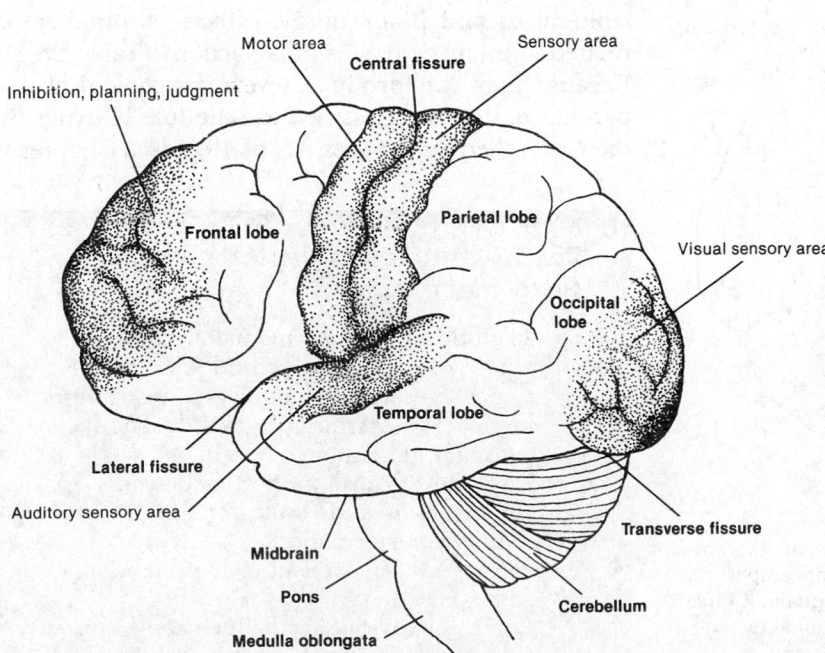

Motor area
Central fissure
Sensory area
Inhibition, planning, judgment
Frontal lobe
Parietal lobe
Visual sensory area
Occipital lobe
Temporal lobe
Lateral fissure
Transverse fissure
Auditory sensory area
Midbrain
Pons
Cerebellum
Medulla oblongata
Spinal cord

Figure 23-2. Spatial distribution of functions of the cortex of the brain.

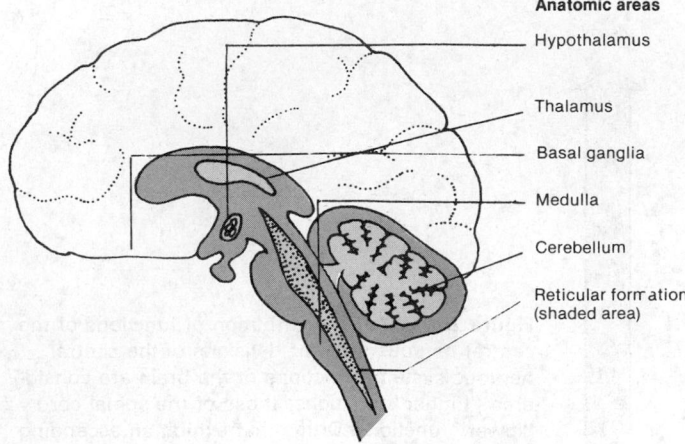

Anatomic areas	Functions
Hypothalamus	Physical expression of emotion; appetite; temperature regulation
Thalamus	Crude sensation of pain; focusing of attention
Basal ganglia	Control of habitual (semiautomatic) motor function
Medulla	Control of vital functions (respiration and blood pressure)
Cerebellum	Muscular coordination and balance
Reticular formation (shaded area)	Wakefulness

Figure 23-3. Spatial distribution of functions of the brain stem. The brain stem controls many vital and automatic or semi-automatic functions.

cinations, convulsions, and serious cardiac arrhythmia can develop (Box 23-2).

Stimulant substances have a long history of use and abuse for nonmedical purposes. Tea, coffee, chocolate, cola drinks, cocaine, yerba mate, betel, mescaline, and peyote are among the agents used in various cultures. New synthetic chemicals surface regularly in the illicit drug trade. These agents tend to be highly potent and dangerously toxic.

CNS stimulants are useful in the medical treatment of selected clinical conditions.

Box 23-1. Classes of stimulants

Amphetamines

Xanthines

Analeptics

Levodopa

Cocaine

Khat and betel

Hallucinogens

Amphetamines

Amphetamine (β-phenylisopropylamine) is a synthetic derivative of ephedrine. It exerts CNS and peripheral α- and β-adrenergic effects. A number of related substances have similar actions (Table 23-1). Because they can produce severe psychological dependence, they are classified as schedule II drugs by the Controlled Substances Act of 1970 (see Chapter 2

Figure 23-4. Spatial distribution of the limbic system. The limbic system includes the cingulate gyrus, parahippocampal gyrus, uncus, thalamus, hypothalamus, and amygdala. It functions as a storehouse for memories of past emotional experiences (pain, pleasure, sexual activities) and odors and controls emotional responses such as excitement, aggression, and sexual behavior.

Box 23-2. Action of central nervous system stimulants

- Small doses increase mental alertness and capacity for work, improve motor performance, impart a feeling of well-being, and stimulate the respiratory and cardiac systems and general metabolism.
- Large doses cause tremor, restlessness, and insomnia and result in deterioration of motor performance.
- Prolonged use can lead to hypertension and exhaustion.
- Results of toxicity are hallucination, convulsions, and serious cardiac arrhythmia.

Table 23-1. Amphetamines and related substances

Drug name	Preparations	Usual dosage	Therapeutic uses and additional information
Amphetamine (Benzedrine, "bennies")	Oral tablets and capsules	Adults: 5–30 mg daily, divided in up to 3 doses PC: C	Treatment of narcolepsy, attention deficit disorder, and obesity; abused as a stimulant
Benzphetamine (Didrex)	Oral tablets	Adults: 25–150 mg/day, divided in 1–3 doses PC: X	Treatment of obesity
Deanol (Deaner)	Oral tablets	Children: 100–300 mg daily on awakening	Treatment of learning problems, behavior problems, and hyperkinesis
Dextroamphetamine (Dexampex, Dexedrine, Oxydess, Spancap #1, "dexies")	Oral tablets, capsules, elixir, and extended-release capsules	Adults: 5–60 mg daily, divided in up to 3 doses Children: 2–15 mg daily, divided in 3 doses PC: C	Treatment of narcolepsy, attention deficit disorder, and obesity; abused as a stimulant
Diethylpropion (Depletite-25, Tenuate, Tepanil)	Oral tablets and extended-release tablets	Adults: 25–100 mg/day, divided in 3–4 doses, administered before meals PC: C	Treatment of obesity
Fenfluramine (Ponderal, Pondimin)	Oral tablets	Adults: 60–120 mg daily, divided in 3 doses, administered before meals PC: C	Treatment of obesity
Mazindol (Mazanor, Sanorex)	Oral tablets	Adults: 2–3 mg/day; 2-mg dose is administered as a single dose before lunch; a 3-mg dose is divided in 3 doses, administered before meals PC: C	Treatment of obesity
Methamphetamine (Desoxyn, Methampex, "speed")	Oral tablets and extended-release tablets	Adults: 5–30 mg daily, divided in up to 3 doses PC: C	Treatment of obesity and attention deficit disorder
Methylphenidate (Ritalin)	Oral tablets and extended-release tablets	Adults: 20–60 mg daily, divided in 2–3 doses Children 6 yr of age and older: 250 µg/kg body weight/day, divided in 2 doses, administered before breakfast and lunch PC: C	Treatment of attention deficit disorder and narcolepsy
Pemoline (Cylert)	Oral tablets and chewable tablets	Children: *Initially:* 37.5 mg/day; *maintenance:* 56.25–75 mg/day, administered as a single daily dose on awakening PC: C	Treatment of attention deficit disorder in children older than 6 yr of age
Phendimetrazine (Bontril, Dyrexan, Melfiat, Plegine, Prelu-2, SPRX, Statobex, Weh-Less)	Oral tablets, capsules, and extended-release capsules	Adults: 70–105 mg/day, divided in 2–3 doses (extended-release forms administered as a single daily dose on awakening) PC: C	Treatment of obesity
Phenmetrazine (Preludin)	Oral tablets and extended-release tablets	Adults: 25–75 mg daily, divided in 2–3 doses PC: C	Treatment of obesity
Phentermine (Adipex-P, Fastin, Ionamin, Obephen, Obermine, Parmine, Phentrol, Tora, Unifast, Wilpowr)	Oral tablets, capsules, and extended-release capsules	Adults: 24 mg/day, divided in 3 doses, administered before meals (extended-release forms administered as a single daily dose on awakening) PC: C	Treatment of obesity

KEY: PC = pregnancy category. (The validity of pregnancy categories has not been established; see Chapter 16, p 216.)

Table 23-2. Dose-related effects of amphetamine drugs

Dose	Effect on central nervous system biochemistry	Physiologic effects
Low	Release of norepinephrine from nonadrenergic neurons	Increased alertness, decreased appetite, limited locomotor stimulation
Medium	Release of dopamine from dopaminergic neurons in the neostriatum	Increased locomotor activity, stereotypic behavior
High	Release of serotonin from tryptaminergic neurons Release of dopamine in the mesolimbic system	Perceptual disturbances, overt psychotic behavior

for more information on the Controlled Substances Act).

Pharmacodynamics. The major actions of the amphetamines derive from the drugs' stimulation of neurotransmitter release in the brain. Norepinephrine, dopamine, and serotonin are involved at successively higher doses (Table 23-2). The drugs may also exert a direct agonistic action on central receptors for serotonin. The resulting effects include increased alertness, mood elevation, decreased perception of fatigue, increased ability to concentrate, a reduction in appetite, and an increased capacity for work. Psychologically, initiative and self-confidence increase. Physiologic changes include bronchial relaxation, changes in peristalsis (which can increase or decrease), and increased tone in the urinary bladder sphincters. Rapid-eye-movement (REM) sleep is suppressed.

Pharmacokinetics. Amphetamines are readily absorbed from the gastrointestinal (GI) tract. They are widely distributed throughout the body, with high concentrations occurring in the brain and cerebrospinal fluid. Varying proportions of the drugs are metabolized, but the sites and mechanisms of metabolism are not well understood. Excretion is by the kidneys and depends on urinary pH. An acidic urine enhances elimination.

Therapeutic uses. The amphetamines are recommended for treatment of narcolepsy and hyperkinetic syndrome or treatment of learning disabilities in children affected by attention deficit disorder (ADD; formerly called minimal brain dysfunction). In narcolepsy, amphetamines prevent sleep attacks and decrease catalepsy. Drug treatment of children with hyperkinesis or ADD results in improved concentration and coordination, lengthened attention span, scholastic achievement, and a paradoxical calming effect.

The use of amphetamines as anorectics in the treatment of obesity is controversial. Tolerance develops rapidly to this effect of the drug, and prolonged use is contraindicated. Drug therapy must be accompanied by a prescribed reduction in caloric intake.

The amphetamines are sometimes used as adjuncts in the treatment of epilepsy. Most stimulant drugs are contraindicated in epilepsy, but the amphetamines are capable of abolishing abnormal electroencephalogram discharges and seizures in some epileptics. They also counteract the depressant effects of sedative anticonvulsants. Other medicinal uses include the treatment of enuresis, depressive psychoneuroses such as nervous exhaustion, and Parkinson's disease when L-dopa cannot be used.

Adverse reactions. Administration of amphetamines to children can precipitate Tourette's syndrome*; uninterrupted therapy can retard growth. Muscle stiffness sometimes develops when the drugs are first used, but this subsides with continued treatment. Other undesirable effects of the drugs are largely related to toxic signs and symptoms. Their appearance with normal doses of the drug is considered idiosyncratic.

Toxic symptoms occur as dosage increases. Intermediate dosage produces elation, euphoria, talkativeness, increased motor activity, sleeplessness, and restlessness. Libido tends to increase. Both systolic and diastolic blood pressure rise, and reflexes become hyperactive. A metallic taste and dryness in the mouth can occur, as well as a tendency toward anorexia, nausea, vomiting, and abdominal cramps. Sweating and tremor are common. Hyperactivity may cause a rise in body temperature.

Incoordination, irritability, headache, palpitation, dizziness, dysphoria, apprehension, anxiety, agitation, and confusion are often seen as toxic levels are approached. Confusion, delirium, paranoid hallucinations, and overt psychotic behavior may develop. Panic states and suicidal or homicidal tendencies also sometimes occur. Cardiac signs and symptoms include arrhythmia and angina. The blood pressure may rise or fall. In extreme toxicity, circulatory collapse, convulsions, and coma precede death. Numerous cerebral hemorrhages are found on autopsy.

Chronic amphetamine toxicity is characterized by psychotic behavior, in addition to the signs and symp-

---

*This condition is characterized by motor tics (eye-blinking, throat-clearing, jaw-jerking, chin-dropping, arm-jerking, hip-turning) and abnormal phonation (snorting and snuffling, humming and panting noises, puppylike sounds, and language outbursts).

toms of acute toxicity. The client may present the classic symptoms of schizophrenia. Weight loss is common. Dermatitis is sometimes seen. Continuous long-term use by children inhibits growth and may permanently stunt it. Dermatitis is sometimes seen.

Tolerance to the drug's effects varies. Tolerance can develop rapidly in relation to appetite suppression in clients who take the drug for control of obesity. It is rarely seen in treatment regimens for narcolepsy. Chronic ingestion of high dosage, common in drug abusers, produces considerable reduction in the response to a given dose.

Severe mental depression and fatigue are experienced on withdrawal from prolonged or high doses. To what extent these conditions are due to psychological or physical dependence is uncertain.

Precautions and contraindications. Amphetamines should be used with caution in malnutrition, restlessness, and insomnia. They are contraindicated for clients with hypertension, cardiovascular disease, hyperthyroidism, anxiety states, motor tics, or a personal or family history of Tourette's syndrome.

Clients who receive amphetamines must be under continual medical supervision. During amphetamine therapy, clients should be monitored for signs and symptoms of overstimulation, such as increased blood pressure, tremor, muscle stiffness, and hyperactive reflexes. They should be questioned about nervousness, sleeplessness, and irritability. Adjustment in dosage may be required to eliminate these undesirable side effects. After extended use, amphetamine dosages should be reduced gradually to prevent withdrawal symptoms. Amphetamine medication for hyperkinesis or ADD should be discontinued at the first sign of motor or phonic tics. During long-term treatment of children, medication should be interrupted frequently to allow for resumption of growth. Growth during these drug holidays is usually rapid and sufficient to prevent permanent stunting.

The use of amphetamines to eliminate fatigue and prolong performance should be condemned as extremely dangerous. Amphetamine-induced hallucinations have been cited as a cause of motor vehicle accidents. In addition, chronic use is associated with malnutrition and reduced resistance to disease. Homicidal and suicidal behavior can occur. An increased risk of developing schizoid psychoses by susceptible individuals is suspected.

■ **Summary**

Amphetamines are CNS stimulants used in the treatment of narcolepsy, hyperkinesis, and ADD. Side effects include hypertension, irritability, and anxiety. Psychotic behavior develops in toxic states. The drugs can cause both physical and psychological dependence.

Nursing management

Nursing implications

Because amphetamines have been widely abused, they have acquired a reputation of being harmful drugs. Clients who recognize the nature of the compounds are often reluctant to take them as prescription drugs, fearing chemical dependency.

Hyperkinesis and attention deficit disorder. Fear of amphetamine use has been a particular problem in the case of children with hyperkinesis and attention deficit disorder (ADD). When the benefits of amphetamine therapy in the treatment of hyperkinesis and learning disabilities were first recognized, their use proliferated rapidly. Some school systems promoted their use. Opposition developed to this practice by individuals and groups concerned about excessive drug use by young people. Some questioned the value of medication for any children, advocating instead the use of psychotherapy, behavior modification, and other techniques for controlling ADD symptoms. A few parents feared loss of control over their children to the institutions that supervised the drug programs (see Focus on Amphetamines and Related Substances: Similarities and Differences).

More than 20 years of experience with chemotherapy for ADD provides a perspective for reevaluating the practice. People closest to the affected children—parents, teachers, and private physicians—are most supportive of this method of treatment. They report that treated children are happier, perform better in school, and are better achievers. Problems of discipline and family relationships are less severe with treatment. Fears of drug dependence have proved unfounded; dependence among drug-treated individuals is no higher than in the general population. It was found that use of the drugs could be discontinued as the children reached physical maturity. As adults, they have no apparent need for amphetamines.

Researchers theorize that ADD arises from a disruption of norepinephrine metabolism. By stimulating norepinephrine release, amphetamines may alter brain chemistry to a more normal state. Hyperkinesis may be caused by an immaturity of brain tissue that controls selective screening of stimuli and motor inhibition. Stimulation of these brain areas tends to normalize behavior.

Treatment of ADD should be established by the family's physician and should remain in the control of the parents. Drugs should be prescribed only after a complete examination and evaluation. Doses are given in the morning and, if a second dose is required, at noon. It may be necessary for second doses to be given by the nurse in the school setting. This nurse should work closely with the child's family to coordinate treatment.

Focus on

Amphetamines and related substances: similarities and differences

Similarities

Pharmacodynamics

These agents stimulate the release of nor-epinephrine in the brain, promoting nerve impulse transmission. They exert CNS and peripheral α- and β-adrenergic effects.

Pharmocokinetics

These agents are readily absorbed from the GI tract within 3 hours and last from 4 to 24 hours. They are widely distributed throughout the body, with high concentrations occurring in the brain and cerebrospinal fluid. The sites and mechanisms of metabolism are not well understood. They are excreted by the kidneys depending on the urinary *p*H.

Therapeutic uses

These agents are recommended for use in the treatment of narcolepsy, hyperkinetic syndrome, learning disabilities in children affected by attention deficit disorder, and exogenous obesity.

Adverse reactions

These include: (CNS) incoordination, nervousness, irritability, headache, dizziness, dysphoria, apprehension, agitation, insomnia, anxiety, elation, euphoria, talkativeness, increased motor activity, hyperactive reflexes, tremors that can precipitate Tourette's syndrome; (CV) increased blood pressure, palpitations, arrhythmia, angina, and tachycardia; (EENT) mydriasis; (GI) anorexia, nausea, vomiting, abdominal cramps, metallic taste, dry mouth, diarrhea, and constipation; (SEXUAL) increased libido, (OTHER) sweating.

Contraindications

These agents are contraindicated for people with hypertension, cardiovascular disease, hyperthyroidism, motor tics, personal or family history of Tourette's syndrome, concomitant use of monoamine oxidase inhibitors and history of drug abuse.

Precautions

Use these agents with caution in people with malnutrition, diabetes, restlessness, and insomnia and in geriatric, debilitated, and asthenic clients.

Differences

• **Fenfluramine** produces CNS depression more often than stimulation.

• **Dextroamphetamine** peaks in 2 to 4 hours after oral administration. • **Mazindol's** onset of action is 30 to 60 minutes. • **Fenfluramine, benzphetamine, phendimetrazine, methamphetamine,** and **methylphenidate** are metabolized by the liver. • **Methylphenidate** peaks in 1 to 2 hours. • **Pemoline** is partly metabolized by the liver into active and inactive metabolites with a half-life that ranges from 9 to 14 hours. • **Fenfluramine** is also excreted in small amounts in saliva and sweat.

• **Amphetamine** and **dextroamphetamine** are used and abused as stimulants.

• **Fenfluramine** can cause dysuria and urinary frequency.
• **Fenfluramine** and **mazindol** can cause impotence.
• **Mazindol** can also cause difficulty in initiating voiding.
• **Methamphetamine, methylphenidate,** and **phendimetrazine** can cause blurred vision. • **Pemoline** can cause increased liver enzymes and jaundice. • **Phendimetrazine** can cause glossitis and stomatitis. • **Phentermine, diethylpropion,** and **phenmetrazine** may also cause menstrual irregularities, gynecomastia, and bone marrow depression.

• **Fenfluramine** is contraindicated for people with alcoholism.
• **Pemoline** is contraindicated for people with hepatic disease.
• **Diethylpropion** and **methylphenidate** are contraindicated for clients with epilepsy.

Some formulations of **phenmetrazine, benzphetamine, methamphetamine,** and **dextroamphetamine** contain tartrazine dye and should be used with caution with people who are sensitive to it. Use • **fenfluramine** with caution in clients who are undergoing general anesthesia.

(continued)

Amphetamines and related substances: similarities and differences (Continued)

Similarities	Differences
Nursing considerations	
Instruct the client in disease, treatment, compliance, and signs and symptoms of adverse reactions; monitor cardiovascular and neurologic status frequently for signs of overstimulation; question the client about any feelings of nervousness, sleeplessness; reduce the dosage gradually to prevent withdrawal signs and symptoms; when given for clients with attention deficit disorder, assess client's growth patterns; evaluate sleep habits and institute measures to help client sleep; administer 30 to 60 minutes before meals when using for obesity; assist with meal planning, calorie counts, and calorie restriction; instruct client to avoid the intake of other stimulants such as caffeine; avoid giving amphetamines within 6 hours of bedtime; warn client to avoid activities that require alertness and coordination until the effects of the drug are known; institute safety measures to prevent injury; assess client for signs and symptoms of abuse or dependence.	When clients take **pemoline**, monitor their liver function studies, including liver enzymes; monitor blood counts for clients who receive **phentermine**, **diethylpropion**, and **phenmetrazine**; discontinue **fenfluramine** gradually because abrupt withdrawal may cause depression.

Intermittent treatment is advised to abolish tolerance of the drug and to minimize its growth-retarding effect. Suspension of therapy (drug "vacations") should coincide with school vacations. When therapy is initiated (or resumed), slight muscle stiffness may develop. With continued treatment, this symptom, which is most noticeable in the neck, tends to subside.

Narcolepsy. Narcolepsy affects older people, often beginning in late adolescence or early adult years. Diagnosis may be difficult because the affected individual may underestimate the frequency and length of sleep episodes or attribute no significance to them. The development of cataplexy (sudden collapse due to loss of muscle tone) may prompt the seeking of medical care. Narcolepsy is a safety hazard because sleep episodes are uncontrollable and occur suddenly. Amphetamine therapy can eliminate sleep episodes and lessen the severity of cataplexy. Tolerance to and dependence on the drugs are not a problem in this situation.

Amphetamine overdose. Amphetamines are frequently abused for psychotropic effect. The effect of the drugs on the user varies widely, depending on the user's physiologic and psychologic state at the time a dose is taken. Toxicity is most likely to occur in the neophyte user. Acute overdoses can occur because of the user's increased susceptibility to the drug or because an unusually potent preparation was purchased "on the street."

Treatment of amphetamine overdose is an emergency procedure. As soon as amphetamines are identified as the causative agent in drug overdose, treatment is instituted to promote excretion of the drug and counteract its most serious effects. Ammonium chloride is administered to acidify the urine and promote rapid renal elimination of the drugs. If the blood pressure is high, a rapidly acting α-adrenergic blocking agent (phentolamine) is given to reduce it toward normal range. Fever is reduced by cooling procedures. Symptoms related to CNS overstimulation are ameliorated by the administration of chlorpromazine or a short-acting barbiturate.

In addition to the physical treatment for amphetamine toxicity, these clients need supportive care and

---

**Attention deficit disorder:
treating children with amphetamines**

Pros

Children medicated with amphetamines become calmer and exhibit fewer episodes of undesirable behavior.

Schoolwork of treated children improves.

Adverse reactions to the drugs are minimal and controllable.

Drug therapy need not be constant; medication may be suspended during school holidays.

The need for medication appears to wane during adolescence; as adults these people do not develop dependence on drugs of abuse more often than others.

Cons

Children should not be medicated with stimulating drugs, especially drugs deemed to be psychotropic.

Children who receive stimulant drugs may have difficulty sleeping and may experience delays in growth, which depends in part on adequate sleep during which growth hormone secretion increases.

Children who receive stimulant drugs over long periods of time may develop dependence on them or may be at higher risk for abuse of other psychotropic drugs.

Some schools have controlled the administration of the drugs; parents fear losing control of their children.

---

counseling to reduce the risk of continued substance abuse and recurrent overdoses.

Educational programs to reduce chemical abuse should include involvement of children and adults. The facts about therapeutic drug effects and adverse reactions should be presented as a foundation for discussion. It is important that the presentation be factual and balanced. In addition, the discussion of attitudes toward drugs and the factors that shape these attitudes is essential. The potential for abuse is increased in clients with low self-esteem and low self-confidence, as well as in clients conditioned to view drugs as a primary therapy for physical and mental symptoms. Classes in parenting, in which techniques for building self-esteem and self-confidence are stressed, theoretically have a greater potential for reducing chemical abuse than other approaches.

Nursing process: therapeutic use of amphetamines

Assessment Data required for assessment before initiation of amphetamine therapy include previous use of and response to stimulant drugs, history and current status of the condition for which amphetamines have been prescribed, and history of conditions for which the drugs are contraindicated (hypertension, cardiovascular disease, hyperthyroidism, anxiety states, motor tics, and Tourette's syndrome). Any family history of Tourette's syndrome should be noted.

Physical examination should include height and weight measurements as well as an assessment of GI, cardiovascular, neuromuscular, endocrine, and emotional status. Attention span and speech patterns should be noted.

Nursing diagnosis Diagnoses related to the conditions for which amphetamines are prescribed include the following:

*Altered growth and development related to hyperkinesis and attention deficit disorder
Ineffective coping (family, individual, or both) related to shortened attention span and hyperkinesis of child
Altered nutrition: more than body requirements related to ingestion of more food than required for activity*

Amphetamine therapy increases the risk of:

*Pain related to muscle stiffness
Altered nutrition: less than body requirements, related to anorexia
Anxiety related to central nervous system stimulation
Sleep pattern disturbance: insomnia related to hyperactivity and CNS stimulation
High risk for injury related to confusion, dizziness, panic, or suicidal ideation secondary to CNS stimulation*

Most clients will exhibit:

*Knowledge deficit concerning the medical use
of amphetamines*

Some will be at risk for:

*Noncompliance related to fear of stimulant
drug use
Ineffective management of therapeutic
regimen related to knowledge deficit and/or
mistrust of regimen*

A common collaborative problem that should be differentiated from the nursing diagnoses is

Potential complication: hypertension

Planning Goals of treatment for hyperkinesis and ADD include promotion of growth and development, improved family dynamics, and improved coping (individual and family). In narcolepsy, a reduction in daytime sleep episodes, improved nighttime sleep, and reduction in cataplexy are desired. Weight reduction is the goal when the drug is used as an anorexic. Additional goals for all clients who use the drugs include prevention of drug dependence, amelioration of muscle stiffness and pain, maintenance of good nutrition, prevention of injury, promotion of rest and nighttime sleep, and teaching about the drug regimen. Prevention or prompt detection and treatment of toxic signs and symptoms such as anxiety, panic, hyperthermia, incoordination, confusion, dizziness, angina, stroke, and suicidal tendencies is also important. The goal of teaching is to help the client and family manage the drug regimen.

Intervention When the initial assessment of the client is completed, the nurse should inform the physician of any contraindications for amphetamine use, as well as any evidence of CNS and sympathetic overactivity.

Amphetamine drugs used for extended therapy should be administered with breakfast and, if a second dose is required, with lunch. Amphetamines prescribed for weight control should be taken 30 to 60 minutes before meals. If noontime medication is required for school children, the school nurse should work closely with the family to coordinate treatment. Frequent drug holidays help prevent dependence and stunting of growth. The drugs should be given on school days and at other times when a high performance level is required of the child. Drug free periods are best scheduled for school vacations or other recesses. Drug holidays for adult clients should also be scheduled for periods of relative leisure. Adults do not require as much drug-free time as do children. If signs and symptoms of withdrawal develop during drug holidays, a weaning schedule may be needed. Caffeine-

containing beverages (coffee or cola) can ameliorate withdrawal.

During the first few weeks of treatment, massage and applications of heat (particularly to the neck) help prevent or relieve muscle stiffness. Appetizing meals of foods favored by the client help maintain food intake. Both muscle stiffness and anorexia tend to dissipate with continued treatment.

Although school performance will probably improve with drug treatment, children with hyperkinesis or ADD may need special education to compensate for residual academic deficits. Psychological counseling may also be helpful to the client and family in resolving long-standing interpersonal conflicts.

All clients who receive amphetamines over a long term should be monitored regularly for early signs and symptoms of amphetamine toxicity. If these develop, the physician should be consulted for a reduction in dosage. Frank toxicity requires discontinuation of the drugs and definitive treatment (see following section on treatment of amphetamine toxicity).

Client education. The nurse should develop and implement a teaching plan to help the client and family manage the drug regimen.

Clients on long-term therapy should be advised to avoid other stimulant substances, including caffeine, except for periods when the amphetamines are temporarily withheld. The drugs should be taken with breakfast and, if a second dose is ordered, with lunch. Doses of the stimulants should be avoided for at least 6 hours before bedtime. Clients who need to lose weight should take the medications 30 to 60 minutes before meals. All clients may be taught measures to promote rest and sleep: a period of quiet activity such as reading before bedtime, retiring at about the same time every night, and adherence to a bedtime ritual. If family members are willing, they may be taught to give the client a soothing back rub at bedtime.

Clients may need assistance in planning diets to meet their nutritional needs. Calorie requirements may be increased while amphetamines are used. Unless clients are overweight, they should be advised to consume enough food to maintain weight. Clients who need to lose weight should be cautioned to limit use of the drugs to the first 2 to 4 weeks, when their use facilitates adjustment to a reduced food intake. Emphasis should be on the diet rather than the drugs as the cause of weight loss.

Clients should be warned that they may experience muscle stiffness during the first few weeks of treatment and again when treatment is resumed after drug holidays. Applications of heat and massage may be recommended, and the techniques for these treatments should be demonstrated. The nurse may recommend monitoring of blood pressure, especially in elderly clients. They or family members should be

Example of nursing process and treatment with methylphenidate

The client is an 8-year-old boy with a history of night terrors, periodic temper tantrums, and inconsistent performance in school. Teachers report that, at times, the child seems "wrapped in a coccoon and cannot be reached." His intelligence as measured by standard tests is rated "bright normal."

The family consists of the parents, a boy aged 10, the client, and a girl aged 5. The mother states that the child is usually well behaved, but sometimes he has sudden temper tantrums, often on arriving home from school.

The client has had intermittent attacks of asthma since age 3 and one episode of pneumonia at age 4. The mother recalls that, during the latter illness, the child's color was "very dark until he was put into an oxygen tent."

The child's physical development is in the upper quartile for his age and sex. He appears to be well developed and well nourished.

A diagnosis of attention deficit disorder (ADD) is made. Methylphenidate is prescribed in gradually increasing doses: 5 mg bid with meals, increased at weekly intervals to 10 mg, 20 mg, and 30 mg per dose. After optimum dosage is determined, a timed-release preparation will be given once daily.

Assessment data	Nursing diagnosis	Intervention	Goals and outcome criteria
New diagnosis of ADD Prescription of methylphenidate	Probable knowledge deficit concerning diagnosis and proposed treatment of ADD	**Explore** the client's knowledge of ADD. **Develop** and implement a plan for teaching the client and his mother about ADD and methylphenidate treatment. Content should include the therapeutic, toxic and side effects of the medication, as well as techniques for alleviation of the side effects.	The mother (and child as appropriate) will correctly demonstrate techniques and repeat information taught by the nurse.
Methylphenidate medication (CNS stimulants increase muscle tone; stiff neck is a known adverse reaction to amphetamines.)	High risk for altered comfort: pain in the neck and other muscles related to CNS stimulation by methylphenidate	**Advise** the mother to apply warm compresses to the neck and use massage to reduce muscle tension; demonstrate massage technique.	The client will report that pain from muscle stiffness is absent or minimal and is quickly relieved.
Methylphenidate medication (Amphetamines are known to slow growth, possibly by reducing time spent in sleep; growth hormone is usually secreted during sleep.)	Potential for altered growth and development: stunting of height related to inhibition of growth by methylphenidate	**Teach** the mother measures to promote rest and sleep. **Recommend** that the drug be withheld on days when a high level of performance is not required of the child. **Inform** the mother that the client's appetite is apt to be reduced during the initial period of therapy (until about 2 weeks after optimum dosage is reached). Warn about rapid or excessive weight loss and failure to gain weight during the adolescent growth spurt.	Overall increases in height will be within normal limits expected for the age, sex, and growth patterns characteristic of the family.

(Continued)

Example of nursing process and treatment with methylphenidate (Continued)

Assessment data	Nursing diagnosis	Intervention	Goals and outcome criteria
Methylphenidate medication (A known side effect of amphetamines is a decrease in appetite.)	Potential for altered nutrition: less than body requirements related to decreased food intake secondary to CNS stimulation by methylphenidate	**Explore** the mother's knowledge of nutrition. Caution the mother to serve high quality food rather than high calorie foods that are lacking in nutrients; suggest serving high quality foods that are high in calories when the client's appetite is smaller than usual.	Weight loss will be confined to the initial period of medication and will not exceed 5 lb. The client will not develop signs and symptoms of nutritional deficiency.
Methylphenidate medication ordered in gradually increasing dosages (Amphetamine toxicity causes CNS overactivity.)	High risk for altered comfort: restlessness, anorexia, and anxiety related to CNS overstimulation by methylphenidate	**Discuss** with the client and his mother the signs and symptoms of amphetamine toxicity, specifying those that should be reported to the primary health care provider.	The client will not develop signs and symptoms of advanced drug toxicity; if early signs and symptoms develop, they will be promptly detected and treated.

taught how to use a sphygmomanometer. If possible, the family should purchase an instrument for this purpose, since blood pressure should be monitored daily or several times a week.

Clients or family members should be taught the early signs of amphetamine toxicity. Instructions for consulting the physician for an adjustment in dosage should include the specific signs and symptoms the physician wishes to know about.

Clients who are reluctant to take amphetamines over a long term should be reassured that medical use does not usually lead to psychological dependence. If a mild physical dependence develops, clients can be weaned gradually from the drugs with little or no discomfort.

Evaluation Data required for evaluation of children include information related to academic achievement and behavior, physical growth compared to norms for the client's age group, and family interaction and coping. As the child matures, parents as well as health care personnel should evaluate performance during drug-free periods to determine when amphetamine therapy may be discontinued. To evaluate adult clients with narcolepsy, sleep–wake patterns should be assessed, as well as incidence of cataplexy. Body weight is monitored at regular intervals (usually weekly or biweekly) to evaluate weight reduction regimens.

The presence or absence of toxic and side effects of the drugs (tolerance and dependence, discomfort from muscle stiffness, confusion, inappropriate affect, fever, angina, stroke, and injury) should be ascertained. Food intake should be recorded and compared with appropriate intake for the client.

To evaluate client education, the nurse should ask the client and family to repeat information conveyed during teaching and to demonstrate techniques that have been taught.

Amphetamine overdose

Assessment Assessment of clients suspected of drug overdose requires evaluation of both mental and physical status. Amphetamine overdose may be characterized by elation and euphoria or anxiety, agitation and panic, restlessness and hyperactivity, fever, hypertension, hyperpnea, hyperactive reflexes, or GI upset (nausea, vomiting, diarrhea). The client may appear to be suffering from seizure disorder, stroke, or schizophrenia. Physical examination should include a complete neurologic assessment. After resolution of the immediate health crisis, the client's coping skills should be evaluated.

Nursing diagnosis Nursing diagnoses related to amphetamine overdose may include the following:

Anxiety related to nervous system overstimulation
Hyperthermia related to hyperactivity
Fatigue related to hyperactivity
Sleep pattern disturbance: insomnia and restlessness related to nervous system overstimulation
High risk for injury related to seizures
Impaired physical mobility related to coma and paralysis secondary to stroke
Impaired gas exchange related to coma and paralysis
High risk for injury related to suicidal ideation

Clients who are habitual abusers of stimulants may have ineffective coping skills.

Planning Goals for treatment include amelioration of anxiety or panic, reduction of fever and hypertension, promotion of rest, and prevention of injury or self-injury. For comatose clients, prevention of complications from immobility (*eg*, hypoxia, decubiti, thrombophlebitis) is important. A long-term goal is development of more effective coping skills.

Intervention Hyperactive clients should be removed to a quiet room and protected from unnecessary stimuli. An emotionally supportive environment should be provided. The presence of a supportive relative or friend can be helpful. Seizure and suicide precautions should be instituted. Treatment is largely symptomatic. A hypothermal blanket may be ordered to reduce body temperature. The nurse administers urinary acidifiers, antihypertensives, or sedatives as ordered
by the physician. Temperature and blood pressure should be monitored closely. Clients with anxiety or panic may benefit from reassurance and a matter-of-fact attitude.

Clients should be monitored closely for a reversal in symptoms as levels of amphetamines in the body decline. A withdrawal period of lethargy, depression, and sleep characterized by a high proportion of REM sleep is common. This may be severe if depressant drugs have been administered.

After resolution of the immediate crisis, drug-dependent clients should be encouraged to enter a drug treatment program that stresses development of coping skills.

Evaluation Data required for evaluation include assessment of skin color, body temperature, blood pressure, emotional affect, energy level, psychomotor function, incidence of injury, and level of consciousness. To evaluate the client's coping skills after lengthy treatment programs, the incidence of recurrent drug abuse should be ascertained (see the Example of Nursing Process and Treatment with Methylphenidate).

Checklist of nursing actions

☐ Assess clients who are to receive amphetamines for contraindications and for risk of adverse drug reactions.

☐ Advise clients who receive prescription amphetamines to limit drug dosage to morning and early afternoon hours.

☐ Encourage clients on amphetamine treatment to adhere to the prescribed regimen, including specified drug vacations.

☐ Monitor clients who receive amphetamines for changes in appetite, hypertension, hyperactive reflexes, muscle tremors, hyperactivity, and sleep disorders.

☐ Emphasize dietary management more than drug therapy as effective treatment of obesity.

☐ Inform concerned people about the therapeutic benefits of amphetamine use.

☐ Provide a quiet supportive environment for victims of amphetamine overdose.

☐ During emergency treatment of victims of amphetamine overdose, give priority to control of high fever, hypertension, and seizures.

☐ Teach about the problems related to overuse and abuse of amphetamines.

☐ Promote good parenting designed to increase self-confidence and self-esteem in children as an important factor in the prevention of stimulant abuse.

Xanthines

The methylated xanthines—caffeine, theophylline, and theobromine—are natural alkaloids that are structurally related to uric acid (Fig. 23-5). They are found in plant materials used for the preparations of foods and beverages, such as coffee, tea, cola, and chocolate (Table 23-3). They are descending stimulants that affect the brain before the spinal cord and lower structures.

Pharmacodynamics. The physiologic action of the xanthines are not completely understood. Xanthines are known to increase the turnover of monoamines in the CNS, augment the release of sympathoadrenal catecholamines, inhibit the degradation of cyclic adenosine monophosphate, and decrease cytosolic concentration of calcium ions. These mechanisms could explain many physiologic effects of the drug family, but cause–effect relationships remain unknown. Caffeine has been shown to block adenosine receptors in the

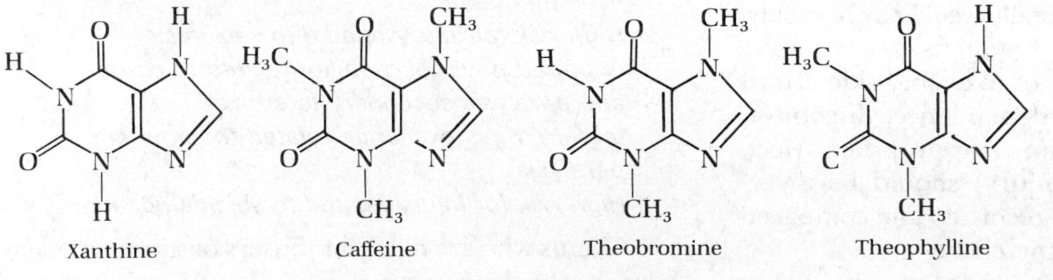

Xanthine   Caffeine   Theobromine   Theophylline

Figure 23-5. Chemical structures of xanthine and xanthine drugs. Caffeine, theobromine, and theophylline are methylated xanthines. Chemically, all are related to the nitrogenous waste product, uric acid.

Table 23-3. Xanthine stimulants

Drug name	Preparations	Additional information
caffeine		Caffeine is relatively potent as a CNS stimulant. It has little diuretic action.
Coffee	Beverage	One 5-oz cup contains 50–250 mg caffeine, depending on method of preparation.
		Drip coffee contains about 150 mg per 5-oz cup; percolated coffee about 110 mg per 5-oz; instant (regular) about 50 mg per 5 oz, and (decaffeinated) about 2 mg per 5 oz.
Tea	Beverage	Steeped brew contains about 10–50 mg per 5-oz cup.
		One-minute brew contains about 10–30 mg per 5-oz cup, 3-min brew about 20–45 mg per 5 oz; 5-min brew about 20–50 mg per 5 oz; and canned iced tea about 20–40 mg per 12-oz container.
		Strong tea, especially if boiled, can contain more caffeine than coffee.
		Tea also contains significant amounts of theophylline (see below).
Cola	Beverage	12 oz of cola drink contain 35–55 mg caffeine, about half of which is added by the manufacturer as the alkaloid.
Chocolate	Beverage and foods	Chocolate contains theobromine as well as caffeine (see below).
		Cocoa contains 5–10 mg caffeine per 6-oz cup.
		Milk chocolate contains about 5 mg caffeine per oz; bitter chocolate about 35 mg per oz.
Carbonated citrus "sodas"	Beverage	Certain brands of carbonated fruit drinks contain caffeine added as the alkaloid. The presence of this additive must be indicated on the product's label.
Over-the-counter headache remedies (Anacin, APC, others)	Oral tablets	These preparations are sometimes useful in aborting migraine headaches.
caffeine sodium benzoate	Solution for intramuscular injection	This drug is often stocked among emergency medications.
theophylline		Theophylline is a potent CNS stimulant and an effective diuretic and bronchodilator.
Tea	Beverage	One cup contains 1–6 mg theophylline. Tea also contains caffeine (see above).
theophylline anhydrous	Oral tablets, capsules, elixir, liquid, and suspension	This drug is employed in the management of chronic asthma.
theophylline ethylene diamine (aminophylline)	Oral tablets	This drug is widely used in the treatment of chronic obstructive lung disease.
	Solution for injection, rectal suppositories	
theobromine		Theobromine is a weak CNS stimulant and a diuretic of intermediate strength.
Chocolate	Beverage and other foods	Cocoa contains about 250 mg theobromine per 6-oz cup.
		Cocoa also contains caffeine (see above).

brains of rats, rendering the system hyperactive (A second cup of coffee, 1983). Adenosine is a neurotransmitter with a pronounced sedative effect. This adaptation to caffeine represents a type of tolerance and could explain the sedation and craving for caffeine that can occur when caffeine is abruptly withdrawn from a habitual user.

General effects of the xanthines in the body include CNS stimulation constriction of cerebral blood vessels, diuresis, cardiac stimulation, and relaxation of smooth muscle, including that of the bronchi. Xanthines apparently serve as natural insecticides, protecting plants such as coffee, tea, coca, and kola from insect pests.

Pharmacokinetics. The solubility of the xanthines can be increased by formulation of salts such as theophylline ethylenediamine (Aminophylline) or other complexes such as caffeine and sodium benzoate. They are absorbed rapidly from the digestive tract and parenteral sites of administration. Protein binding varies, being highest at 50% with theophylline. The methylated xanthines distribute widely to all tissues and cross the placenta. Relative concentration in the

CNS is greater for caffeine than theophylline. Xanthines are deactivated primarily by the liver microsomal enzymes. Small amounts are excreted by the kidneys.

Therapeutic uses. Beverages that contain xanthines are used socially and as part of the diet because of their stimulant properties. They decrease drowsiness and fatigue, increase mental alertness, reduce reaction time, and increase the capacity for physical and intellectual work without appreciably impairing the performance of accustomed tasks.

Caffeine is incorporated in many over-the-counter headache remedies. Its vasoconstriction action reduces blood flow to the brain. When taken at the first symptom of an attack, these preparations sometimes abort migraines, a type of headache associated with cerebral vasodilation and congestion.

Prescription use of the xanthines as CNS stimulants for maintaining vital functions has become less frequent than in the past, when adequate supportive measures to treat respiratory and cerebral depression were unavailable. Caffeine is still occasionally used as an adjunct in the treatment of toxicity from use of CNS depressants.

Xanthines are valuable as respiratory stimulants in the treatment of chronic obstructive airway disease in adults and in the treatment of apnea in premature infants. They are particularly useful in obstructive airway disease associated with bronchoconstriction. In infants, plasma levels of theophylline maintained between 2 and 10 μg/ml (11–53 μmol/liter) reduce the frequency and length of apneic episodes of undetermined origin. The drug has also been reported to be beneficial in treating sleep apnea in babies, which is suspected as one cause of sudden infant death syndrome (SIDS).

Caffeine has been suggested as a treatment for hyperkinetic behavior in children with ADD when amphetamines are poorly tolerated. Xanthines are also used therapeutically as diuretics and bronchodilators (see Chapters 37 and 40). They have been used experimentally to augment electroshock therapy for psychosis (Greenburg J, Bower B, 1987).

Caffeine is useful as an adjunct in electroconvulsive treatment of severe depression (Greenburg, Bower, 1987). Xanthines also have a potential for development as a potent insecticide that is relatively safe for people.

Adverse reactions. Side effects of the xanthines include nervousness, restlessness, insomnia, tremor, and hyperesthesia. Anxiety, nervousness, fear, nausea, restlessness, and panic disorder are increased by caffeine use (Bruce, Lader, 1989). The drugs impair the performance of motor skills that have been imperfectly or incompletely mastered. They are irritating to the gastric mucosa whether administered orally or systemically. Xanthines increase plasma free fatty acid and glycerol levels, elevate blood pressure, increase the risk of coronary artery disease, and may stimulate cardiac arrhythmia.

Evidence linking xanthines to increased severity of fibrocystic breast disease is controversial. Whereas some studies show a strong association between use of these chemicals and severity of disease, other studies refute those findings (Levinson, Dunn, 1986).

Heavy caffeine use by mothers who are smokers is associated with increased rates of infantile apnea in their offspring (Toubas, 1986). Excessive intake before and during labor increases the risk of fetal cardiac arrhythmia (Oei, et al, 1989). Xanthine toxicity can cause focal and generalized seizures. Lethal doses for humans range from 3,000 to 10,000 mg. Theophylline frequently causes toxic symptoms when plasma levels exceed 20 μg/ml. Toxicity from this drug is more difficult to treat than that caused by other xanthines.

Chronic use of caffeine produces both tolerance and dependence in some individuals. Withdrawal is characterized by severe headache.

Xanthines increase the toxicity of other CNS stimulants, including therapeutic drugs such as the amphetamines and theophylline. Xanthines may antagonize the effects of hypnotic sedatives, antidepressants, and antipsychotics (Bezchlibnyk, Jeffries, 1981). Caffeine increases renal excretion of lithium, requiring higher than normal dosages of this antipsychotic. If caffeine is suddenly withdrawn without reducing lithium dosages, serum concentrations of the latter drug may reach toxic levels (Jefferson, 1988). Caffeine also increases the risk and severity of nausea in people treated with levodopa for Parkinson's disease (Ebadi, 1985).

Precautions and contraindications. Xanthines are contraindicated in hyperthyroidism, pheochromocytoma, and cardiac conditions in which the risk of serious arrhythmia is increased. They should be avoided when other CNS stimulants (*eg*, amphetamines) are used. Seizure disorders may be worsened by use of xanthines. Xanthines should not be used by stimulant-sensitive individuals, in whom they cause restlessness, tremor, and insomnia. Women with fibrocystic breast disease should avoid using xanthines.

Regular tests for theophylline plasma levels must be performed on clients who receive long-term theophylline therapy. Diazepam should be readily available to treat seizures should a toxic reaction occur.

Xanthine drinks and oral medications should be taken with food to prevent direct irritation of the gastric mucosa.

■ Summary

Xanthines are CNS stimulants in common use as dietary components. They reduce fatigue and improve work performance. Medically, they are used to treat chronic obstructive airway disease. Xanthines can exacerbate the symptoms of psychotic states, panic disorder, sleep disorders, and fibrocystic breast disease. They also increase the effects of other CNS stimulants and antagonize the effects of CNS depressants. Chronic use can cause a toxic syndrome characterized by restlessness, irritability, and insomnia. Both tolerance and dependence can develop in long-term users.

Nursing management

Nursing implications

Dietary restriction of xanthine beverages is often ordered by physicians in the treatment of clients with thyroid toxicity, pheochromocytoma, heart disease, or peptic ulcers. Clients who receive narcotic analgesics should avoid caffeine because it diminishes the effectiveness of these drugs. Decaffeinated products may be used by most of these clients, but even decaffeinated preparations should be avoided by clients subject to gastric hypersecretion and cardiac tachyarrhythmia.

Response to caffeine varies from individual to individual. Children are generally more sensitive to it than adults. Most infants are unable to degrade caffeine until they reach the age of 7 to 9 months (Curatolo, Robertson, 1983). Some people have no difficulty sleeping after drinking coffee, whereas others must avoid even small amounts of caffeine. Chronic use of caffeine may produce tolerance to the stimulant while emphasizing the hyperglycemic and cardiovascular effects of the drug.

Xanthine-containing beverages and foods have side effects that stem from substances other than xanthines. Whether or not coffee is decaffeinated, it increases the rate of glycogenolysis (raising blood sugar), stimulates peristalsis, and induces extrasystole in the cardiac rhythm. It is a suspected carcinogen and contains a narcotic antagonist capable of interfering with the effectiveness of narcotic analgesics. Tea is an astringent and tends to cause constipation. Foods that contain chocolate are usually high in sugar and calories.

Xanthine-containing beverages and foods may help control withdrawal symptoms when amphetamines are withheld temporarily from clients on extended therapy. If xanthines are used to prevent exacerbations of symptoms during drug holidays, the physician should be informed so that evaluation of the client's responses to drug withdrawal is accurate.

Nursing process

Assessment No drug history is complete without a comprehensive evaluation of caffeine intake. In addition to the habitual use of coffee, use of tea, soft drinks, and chocolate should be explored. Clients who report high levels of caffeine intake and those who receive medicinal xanthines should be assessed for fine muscle tremors and subjective symptoms such as nervousness, headache, irritability, fatigue, and insomnia. Pulse and respirations may be elevated.

Nursing diagnosis Diagnoses that derive from either social or medicinal use of xanthines include the following:

Altered comfort: restlessness related to CNS stimulation
Disturbance in self-concept related to tremulousness, nervousness, and irritability
Ineffective individual coping related to irritability and fatigue
Sleep pattern disturbance: insomnia related to CNS stimulation
Knowledge deficit concerning the health effects of xanthine drugs
Ineffective management of therapeutic regimen related to knowledge deficit, mistrust of regimen, or powerlessness

Abrupt withdrawal of xanthines from dependent clients can cause the following:

Pain: headache possibly related to hypoglycemia
Altered thought process related to decreased alertness, depression, and lethargy
Sensory/perceptual alteration: decreased sensory acuity related to CNS depression

Planning Goals of treatment for clients who receive xanthine medication include increased rest and sleep, reduced fatigue by conservation of energy, and decreased restlessness. For clients affected by excessive use of xanthines in the diet, the goal is a reduction of xanthine intake. Improved self-concept, improved coping skills, and increased knowledge about xanthines are appropriate goals for all clients. For clients who experience withdrawal, goals include alleviation of pain (headache) and stimulation to increase wakefulness and sensory acuity.

Intervention When xanthine medications are used to treat acute illness such as exacerbations of respiratory disease, they may be administered intravenously. Because the margin of safety is relatively narrow, the rate of flow must be carefully controlled, preferably by an infusion pump. Regardless of the route of administration, blood levels of the drug should be monitored when repeated doses are required.

Three combination drugs that contain caffeine and ergotamine titrate (Cafergot, Cafetine, Cafetide) have been confused with Carafate, a drug used to treat peptic ulcers. The nurse must differentiate carefully between drugs such as these with similar trade names. Comparison of generic names (in this case caffeine, ergotamine, and sucralfate) helps clarify these differences (King, Krumlovsky, 1986).

Clients are monitored closely for early signs of toxicity, such as tremor, agitation, or irregular pulse. The aim of most theophylline regimens is to maintain plasma levels of 10 to 20 μg/ml (55–100 μmol/liter); symptoms of toxicity may appear when plasma concentrations approach 20 μg/ml (100 μmol/liter). Parenteral preparations of diazepam must be readily available for emergency use if convulsions occur.

Clients medicated with xanthines require nursing care to alleviate side effects of the drugs. Clients who receive xanthine medications require assistance with activities of daily living. They have limited energy, especially if they are affected by pulmonary disease that restricts gas exchange in the lungs. All nursing measures to promote rest and sleep should be used. The nurse should accept client irritability as a manifestation of both hypoxia and adverse drug effects. When long-term use of xanthines is necessary (as in the control of chronic asthma), clients or their families may benefit from psychological counseling to improve self-image and coping skills.

Individuals who attempt to reduce xanthine intake need considerable support and assistance during the period of withdrawal. The nurse should acknowledge that withdrawal from caffeine can be as distressing as withdrawal from nicotine and other dependence-producing substances. For the first few days, the client may need treatment for headache. Nursing measures for headaches include administrating (or recommending) nonopioid analgesics such as acetaminophen, eliminating unnecessary stimuli such as strong light and noise, encouraging rest in a quiet room with subdued light, and applying cold applications to the head. Usual patterns of social behavior ("coffee breaks" or "klatches") should be encouraged, with substitution of caffeine-free beverages and foods for regular coffee, tea, and so forth. Clients should also be encouraged to participate in activities that provide pleasure and enhance their self-image. If energy levels decline or clients feel lethargic, the nurse may recommend increased exposure to light (especially in winter or cloudy climates), stimulating activities such as dancing or other exercise, and alternating hot and cold showers.

Therapeutic communication designed to promote a positive self-concept is appropriate for all clients. Clients who receive xanthine therapy may need counseling to help them adjust to the side effects of treatment. They must learn to cope with limited energy, fatigue, irritability, and restlessness. Clients who are withdrawing from excessive use of caffeine may have used the drug to compensate for inadequate coping skills. They need help controlling environmental stressors and managing their stress responses.

Client education. All clients should understand the nature of xanthine drugs, their therapeutic uses, and toxic and side effects. Clients who receive xan-

thine medications should be reassured that the irritability, restlessness, and insomnia are effects of the drugs and subside when drug dosages are reduced. They should be taught relaxation techniques and measures to promote rest and sleep. Clients often seek counseling about the use of stimulant beverages. Moderate use in the absence of symptoms probably poses little risk. However, before reassurance is given, an assessment for fine muscle tremors and subjective symptoms should be made. Many clients do not recognize the association between difficulty in sleeping or "nervousness" and the use of beverages that contain these drugs. The nurse should identify stimulant drinks as possible causes of these problems.

Some clients should be warned not to use beverages and food that contain xanthines. The drugs are relatively contraindicated in peptic ulcer disease, poorly controlled epilepsy, heart disease characterized by irregular heart rhythm, insomnia, severe dysmenorrhea, and "coffee nerve" syndrome. They should be used with caution in gastric hyperacidity. Xanthines are not recommended for normal children. They should be used only in moderate amounts during pregnancy, in well controlled epilepsy, and in diabetes. Decaffeinated products, beverages prepared from roasted grains, and herbal teas may be recommended for clients not affected by gastric hyperacidity.

Most people recognize the toxic potential of coffee but may not realize that tea, cola, many other soft drinks, and chocolate cause similar problems (Box 23-3).

Clients who have difficulty eliminating all such beverages and foods should first omit coffee. If toxic symptoms persist, weak tea may be substituted for stronger brews. Although an infrequent offender, chocolate is not tolerated by some individuals. Light use of xanthines early in the day may be better tolerated than larger doses in the evening hours. Occasionally, sensitivity is so high that no foods that contain stimulants can be used. For such clients, all xanthine-containing beverages and foods, including chocolate desserts and candy, should be avoided.

Clients who receive xanthine medications should be taught measures to promote rest and sleep: elimina-

---

Enrichment experience 23-1

Interview a member of a Latter Day Saints or Seventh Day Adventist religious group to determine the viewpoint of the church regarding the use of substances that contain caffeine. What specific foods or beverages are forbidden by the discipline of the church? What substitutes are used in place of these items? Are any substances that contain xanthine drugs allowed?

Box 23-3. Caffeine content of selected foods

Coffee (5 oz)

Instant	40–108 mg
Percolated	64–124 mg
Drip	90–150 mg
Decaffeinated	2–5 mg

Tea (5 oz)*

1-minute brew	9–33 mg
3-minute brew	20–46 mg
5-minute brew	20–55 mg
Instant	12–28 mg
Decaffeinated	2–4 mg

Chocolate**

Cocoa (5 oz)	5–15 mg
Chocolate bar (1 oz)	6 mg

Soft drinks (12 oz)

	0–50 mg

* Tea also contains about 1 mg theophylline per serving; green and oolong tea have less than black tea.
** Cocoa contains up to 250 mg theobromine per serving.

tion of disturbing stimuli such as strong lights and noise from the environment, quiet activities for a period before bedtime, warm nonchocolate milk drinks before retiring, and warm baths or sedative massages. Blue and green colors are preferred for bedrooms, as they are less stimulating than reds and oranges. Consistency in rituals associated with preparing for sleep promotes a better sleep response.

Evaluation Data required for evaluation of xanthine medication include observations about the length of time clients slept, statements by clients that they feel rested, an increase in activity of choice by clients, and statements by clients that headache is diminished or absent. Evaluation of programs to decrease intake of dietary xanthines depends on reports from clients that indicate the amounts of xanthine-containing beverages and foods consumed, the incidence or absence of withdrawal symptoms such as headaches, and changes in self-concept. Coping skills may be observed directly

---

Learning experience 23-1

Interview several people to determine their daily caffeine consumption, their responses to the drug, and their attitudes toward its use. Are adverse reactions apparent in any of these people?

---

if the client is stressed in the presence of the nurse. Teaching is evaluated by asking the client to repeat information conveyed or to demonstrate techniques previously taught.

Checklist of nursing actions

☐ When taking drug histories, assess use of xanthine-containing beverages and foods.

☐ Assess clients who use large amounts of xanthine-containing beverages and foods for signs and symptoms of CNS and sympathetic overstimulation.

☐ Counsel clients about the nonmedicinal use of xanthines.

☐ When clients wish to decrease use of xanthines, assist and support them through the withdrawal period; teach clients measures to relieve withdrawal symptoms.

Before initiating therapy with xanthine drugs

☐ Screen clients for contraindications to stimulant drugs; assess clients for signs and symptoms of CNS and sympathetic overstimulation; consult with the physician to verify the drug order if contraindications or risk factors are found.

☐ Administer intravenous solutions of aminophylline slowly, using an infusion pump.

☐ Monitor clients for CNS and sympathetic overstimulation.

☐ Monitor clients who are receiving theophylline for excessive blood plasma levels (more than 20 μg/ml).

☐ Use nursing measures to alleviate side effects of xanthine therapy.

Levodopa

Levodopa (L-dopa) is a precursor of dopamine in normal body biochemistry. It is used in the medical treatment of idiopathic parkinsonism and parkinsonian syndrome to reduce the muscle tremors and rigidity characteristic of these conditions. The pathology of Parkinson's disease is not fully understood. The condition is characterized by akinesia, rigidity, and resting tremors that involve the skeletal muscles.

Dopamine, an intermediate product in the synthesis of norepinephrine from tyramine, is one of the stimulant neurotransmitters involved in brain function. The caudate nucleus and putamen are among the neural structures in the brain that require dopamine for proper function. These structures play a role in integrating stereotyped motor functions, such as backward extension of the head and upper trunk. An adequate level of dopamine in the caudate nucleus and putamen depends on normal function of pigmented nerve cells in the substantia nigra.

Among the physiologic abnormalities found in Parkinson's disease is a decrease of dopamine in the caudate nucleus and putamen associated with lesions in the pigmented nuclei of the substantia nigra and locus ceruleus. The disease is considered to involve a relative deficiency of dopamine in brain structures that control unconscious motor activity.

Pharmacodynamics. Levodopa is enzymatically converted to dopamine in the basal ganglia. Administration of the drug elevates the levels of this neurotransmitter in the brain, helping to correct one biochemical manifestation of parkinsonian syndrome. Muscular function and control are improved as a result.

Levodopa also stimulates the release of pituitary growth hormone. This effect may potentiate the cerebral effects of the drug.

Pharmacokinetics. The administration of dopamine does not result in improvement in parkinsonian syndrome because it is unable to cross the blood–brain barrier. Levodopa crosses the blood–brain barrier readily, however, and is converted in the brain to dopamine.

When levodopa is administered orally, it is so rapidly converted to dopamine in extracerebral tissues that only a small portion of the dose is transported to the CNS. Administered alone, the drug must be given in large amounts for therapeutic effect. In such doses, high levels of extracerebral dopamine cause distressing side effects. To reduce peripheral use of levodopa and to increase the proportion of each dose available to the CNS, a drug that inhibits decarboxylation of peripheral levodopa may be administered concurrently with levodopa. The drug used for this purpose is carbidopa, a decarboxylase inhibitor that does not cross the blood–brain barrier.

Excretion of levodopa is primarily in the urine in the form of catecholamine metabolites.

Therapeutic uses. Levodopa is used in the management of idiopathic parkinsonism and parkinsonian syndrome. In therapeutic doses, the drug produces symptomatic improvement by reducing tremor and rigidity and improving motor function. It does not alter the course of the disease.

Levodopa is available in capsule and tablet dose forms under various trade names. It is also marketed in combination with carbidopa (Sinemet). Doses must be individually titrated, starting with low doses and increasing gradually to optimal levels. The usual initial dosage for adults is 0.5 to 1 g daily, divided into two or more doses administered with food. This dose may be increased gradually in increments of 0.75 g or less every 3 to 7 days as tolerated. Total dosage should usually not exceed 8 g daily. When used with carbidopa, much smaller amounts are used. Maintenance dosage is 75 to 150 mg of carbidopa with 300 to 600 mg levodopa daily, divided in three to six doses.

Therapeutic response to levodopa includes short duration improvement that occurs after each dose and lasts about 5 hours and long duration improvement that persists for 3 to 5 days after administration of the drug is discontinued. The drug has a narrow margin of safety; slight increases of doses above optimal levels produce toxic symptoms.

A monoamine oxidase inhibitor deprenyl (seligiline, Eldepryl) is sometimes used as an adjunct in levodopa therapy. It prolongs the duration of action of levodopa by delaying the breakdown of dopamine. During the early stage of parkinsonism, deprenyl alone delays the progression of symptoms and the need for levodopa.

Adverse reactions. Adverse reactions are frequent, usually being dose dependent and reversible. The most serious reactions are choreiform, dystonic, dyskinetic, and other adventitious movements that develop when doses exceed optimal levels. Involuntary movements may occur in 50% of clients on long-term therapy.

Nausea and vomiting are common reactions, especially when levodopa is given alone without a decarboxylase inhibitor. The use of caffeine (coffee, tea, chocolate) tends to increase the severity of these responses (Ebadi, 1985). These side effects tend to subside with continued administration of the drug. Other GI effects include constipation, diarrhea, epigastric and abdominal distress, flatulence, dry mouth, dysphagia, hiccups, and changes in taste sensation. Duodenal ulcer and GI bleeding may develop.

Orthostatic hypotension occurs frequently but is usually mild and subsides with continued administration. Other cardiovascular side effects stem from peripheral sympathetic activity and include palpitation, sinus tachycardia, ventricular tachycardia or extrasystole, atrial flutter or fibrillation, and atrioventricular block. Flushing and hypertension may occur.

CNS manifestations are both intellectual and emotional in nature. These may include decreased attention span, memory loss, nervousness, anxiety, agitation, restlessness, confusion, insomnia, nightmares, daytime somnolence, euphoria, malaise and fatigue, depression, dementia, delirium, delusions, hallucinations, and inappropriate or excessive sexual behavior.

Respiratory side effects appear as episodic hyperventilation and other alterations in breathing patterns, hoarseness, and excessive nasal discharge. Ocular side effects include blurring of vision, diplopia, mydriasis or miosis, widening of the palpebral fissures, and oculogyric crisis. Phlebitis, blood dyscrasias, and convulsions have been reported. The drug may adversely affect glucose balance in diabetic clients.

Drug interactions. Levodopa interacts with many other drugs. Hypotension can occur when antihypertensives, such as methyldopa or guanethidine, are administered at the same time. Reserpine, phenytoin, and papaverine diminish client response to levodopa. The risk of cardiac arrhythmia during general anesthesia induced by cyclopropane or halogenated hydrocarbon agents is increased in clients who have received levodopa.

When levodopa is administered alone, its therapeutic effects are antagonized by the benzodiazepines chlordiazepoxide (Librium) and diazepam (Valium) and by pyridoxine (vitamin B_6). When a decarboxylase inhibitor (carbidopa) is used, pyridoxine does not reduce levodopa's therapeutic action; in this situation, pyridoxine can be administered to inhibit some of levodopa's undesirable side effects.

Precautions and contraindications. Levodopa is contraindicated in clients who are receiving monoamine oxidase inhibitors, in clients with narrow angle glaucoma, and in clients with a known hypersensitivity to the drug. It should not be used in clients with a history of melanoma or in clients with undiagnosed pigmented lesions because it may exacerbate malignant melanoma.

Extreme caution must be used when levodopa is administered to clients with a history of myocardial infarction who have residual atrial, nodal, or ventricular arrhythmia. Caution is required also with clients with bronchial asthma or emphysema who may require sympathomimetic drug therapy. The presence of peptic ulcer disease or severe cardiovascular, renal, hepatic, or endocrine disease or psychosis is also reason for caution.

During levodopa therapy, hepatic, hematopoietic, cardiovascular, and renal functions should be evaluated periodically. Safe use for pregnant women or for children younger than 12 years of age has not been established. Levodopa should not be administered to nursing mothers because the drug appears in the milk and tends to inhibit lactation.

Drug administration is best initiated in an acute care facility. Intensive coronary care facilities must be available if drug therapy is attempted for clients with cardiac arrhythmia.

■ **Summary**
Levodopa, the metabolic precursor of dopamine, is used medicinally for the palliative treatment of idiopathic parkinsonism and parkinsonian syndrome. The drug crosses the blood–brain barrier and is metabolized intracerebrally to dopamine, producing a reduction in the tremor and rigidity characteristic of these conditions.

Levodopa has a narrow margin of safety; drug therapy must be initiated cautiously and monitored carefully. Side effects, some of which are characteristic of sympathetic nervous system activity, affect many body systems.

Nursing management

Nursing implications

During the early stages of levodopa treatment, clients require considerable emotional support. The tremors characteristic of parkinsonism may increase initially, before a therapeutic response occurs. In addition, distressing side effects from the drug often develop. Clients may become quite discouraged before a therapeutic response to the drug becomes manifest.

Nursing process

Assessment Before levodopa therapy is initiated, clients must be evaluated for factors that increase risk of drug use. A careful history should be taken with particular attention to the presence of glaucoma or cardiovascular, hepatic, renal, endocrine, peptic ulcer, or chronic obstructive airway disease. The drug history should include information about previous use of levodopa and response to it. Clients should be asked specifically about recent use of monoamine oxidase inhibitors, antihypertensives, phenytoin, and papaverine.

During the physical examination, the nurse should assess for cardiac arrhythmia. If the client is a woman of childbearing age, pregnancy and lactation should be ruled out before drug dosage is begun. A complete appraisal of signs and symptoms of parkinsonian syndrome should be made as a baseline for comparison with the client's condition after response to drug therapy.

Nursing diagnosis Diagnoses related to signs and symptoms of parkinsonism may include the following:

Impaired physical mobility related to paralysis and tremor
Body image disturbance related to involuntary body movement secondary to paralysis and tremor
Self-esteem disturbance related to disability secondary to paralysis and tremor
Altered role performance related to disability secondary to paralysis and tremor
Altered nutrition: less than body requirements related to difficulties in chewing and swallowing
Sexual dysfunction related to paralysis

Among the conditions that can develop during drug treatment are the following:

Altered nutrition: less than body requirements related to nausea and vomiting, dysphagia, and altered taste sensation
Constipation
Diarrhea
High risk for injury related to dizziness secondary to postural hypotension
Anxiety
Sleep pattern disturbance
Sexual dysfunction: inappropriate or excessive sexual behavior
Sensory/perceptual alteration related to ophthalmic changes secondary to levodopa therapy

Many clients exhibit a

Knowledge deficit about Parkinson's disease and its treatment with levodopa.

Some clients may demonstrate

Ineffective management of therapeutic regimen related to knowledge deficit, powerlessness, or mistrust of regimen

Planning Goals for treatment include prevention of injury, improved physical mobility, improved body image and self-esteem, resumption of role performance, resumption of usual sexual function, improved nutrition, alleviation of constipation or diarrhea, improved sleep, improved vision, and increased knowledge about levodopa therapy.

Intervention Levodopa therapy is initiated with small doses that are gradually increased until early toxic signs and symptoms appear. At this time, the dosage is decreased slightly and continued for maintenance.

Until dosage is stabilized, clients must be monitored carefully for toxic effects and side effects. Cardiovascular status should be watched closely with particular attention to cardiac rhythm. Other significant signs and symptoms include changes in respiratory, renal, liver, and visual functions. Transient elevations in alkaline phosphatase, serum glutamic-oxaloacetic transaminase, serum glutamate pyruvate transaminase, lactic dehydrogenase, bilirubin, and blood urea nitrogen may occur. Glucose balance in diabetic clients may be unstable. All of these changes should be reported promptly to the physician to facilitate correction of the drug dosage.

Clients should be referred for physiotherapy to help them recover normal mobility as nerve function improves. To prevent falls, clients should be supervised and assisted during ambulation.

Clients should be encouraged to maintain an adequate diet, especially clients who are already malnourished owing to difficulties in eating that sometimes occur in Parkinson's syndrome. A mechanically soft diet may be required until mastication and swallowing improve. All nursing measures to stimulate the appetite and alleviate nausea should be used. Xanthine-containing foods may aggravate the nausea and should be eliminated from the diet. Laxative foods may be offered to clients who have constipation. Other nursing measures to correct alterations in bowel function should be instituted as needed (see Chapter 31 for a detailed discussion of these nursing interventions).

Clients need warm acceptance from health care personnel. They should be encouraged to talk about their feelings toward their disabilities. The etiologic role of parkinsonism in these deficits should be pointed out. Health care personnel should maintain a positive attitude toward the prospect of improvement as a result of treatment. As clients progress, their achievement should be acknowledged and praised.

Inappropriate sexual activity usually is verbal in nature. Clients may be embarrassed by unintended suggestive comments or allusions. Health care personnel should inform the client that such behavior is considered a side effect of the drug and is not unusual during the initial treatment period. The client should be encouraged to anticipate a return to usual sexual activity when the drug regimen is stabilized and the signs and symptoms of parkinsonism decrease.

Sleep pattern disturbance and visual changes may subside as the client adjusts to maintenance therapy. Until then, nursing measures to promote rest and sleep are appropriate. The client may need assistance with activities that require visual acuity. Relatives or friends may read to the client. If visual difficulties persist, clients should be referred to an ophthalmologist. A change in glasses may improve acuity.

After dosage has been established and maintenance levels prescribed, clients should continue to be monitored for adverse reactions to the drug. Clients who experience epigastric distress should be monitored for GI bleeding because the drug is ulcerogenic. Levodopa has a narrow therapeutic index and can produce toxic effects with minimal increases in serum blood levels.

Client education. Clients who are to receive levodopa should be cautioned that the drug does not cure parkinsonism. Its action is palliative. However, a positive attitude should be fostered toward the benefits of therapy.

Reassure clients that the postural hypotension and GI distress that may occur initially will subside with continued treatment. If involuntary tremors increase when the drug is first taken, inform clients that this effect is temporary. Clients should be told that optimal response to the drug requires 6 to 8 weeks of therapy.

To minimize dizziness and risk of falling, advise clients to wear elastic hose and move slowly and deliberately until this side effect disappears. Help the client adjust dietary intake to minimize nausea and vomiting to maintain nutrition.

The client is a 54-year-old man who has been hospitalized for treatment of a stroke with right-sided paralysis and expressive aphasia. In general, recovery has progressed well. He is receiving speech and physiotherapy, is ambulating well, and speech is much improved. He has developed a coarse tremor of the hand that resembles pill rolling. The neurologist has ordered L-dopa 75 mg with carbidopa 150 mg (Sinemet) tab i bid. Dosage will be increased as tolerated until optimum dosage is determined.

During the first few days of treatment, the client complained that the tremors were worse than before, but with continued therapy these movements subsided, and a noticeable improvement occurred.

The client was upset when told that he had Parkinson's syndrome. He stated that his grandmother suffered with this condition for years before her death and it was "a disease he never wanted to have." He expressed fears that he would be unable to resume employment, his responsibilities for home maintenance, or his craft hobbies of woodworking and gardening.

Assessment data	Nursing diagnosis	Intervention	Goals and outcome criteria
Comment by the client that parkinsonism "was a disease he never wanted to get" because his grandmother "suffered for years with it."	Possible knowledge deficit concerning Parkinson's disease and current modes of treatment for it	**Prepare** and implement a teaching plan that explains Parkinson's syndrome and its present-day treatment. Emphasize that new drugs and other modes of therapy have been developed since the 1940s, when his grandmother was still alive.	The client will repeat accurately information conveyed during teaching sessions. He will become more cheerful and resume active participation in therapeutic regimens and planning for the future.
Pronounced tremors Diagnosis of Parkinson's syndrome (Parkinsonism often alters the gait and causes unsteadiness and shuffling gait.)	Impaired physical mobility: resting tremor of the hands related to impaired integrity of tissue in the basal ganglia secondary to Parkinson's syndrome	**Administer** L-dopa with carbidopa as ordered. Encourage the client to continue treatment, advising that it takes a little time to establish optimum response to the drugs.	Within 2 weeks, the resting tremor will be decreased or abolished, except for times when the patient is under unusual stress.
L-dopa therapy (L-dopa can cause nausea, altered taste sensations, or altered bowel function.)	High risk for altered nutrition: less than body requirements related to nausea, altered taste sensations, or alteration in bowel elimination secondary to L-dopa therapy	**Implement** all possible nursing measures to promote adequate food intake (*eg*, serve food favored by the client, serve moderate portions of food, offer between-meal snacks, eliminate noxious stimuli at mealtime, make sure food trays are neat and inviting in appearance and that food is at the proper temperature).	The client will not lose weight during the period of dosage titration.
Fears that his lifestyle will be greatly altered Diagnosis of Parkinson's syndrome Pronounced tremors Unpleasant memories of his grandmother's condition when she had Parkinson's "disease"	Body image disturbance related to tremors and memories of his grandmother when she had Parkinson's "disease"	**Explain** to the client that muscle tremors are side effects of the medications he is receiving and that they will subside when dosages are reduced or discontinued. When appropriate, compliment the client (*eg*, about his appearance, his cooperation with the treatment regimen).	The number of negative comments made by the client relating to self-concept and body image will decrease; the client will begin to say positive things about himself.

(Continued)

Example of nursing process and treatment with levodopa (Continued)

Assessment data	Nursing diagnosis	Intervention	Goals and outcome criteria
L-dopa therapy (L-dopa can cause alteration in bowel function.)	High risk for constipation or diarrhea related to nerve stimulation secondary to L-dopa medication	**Monitor** bowel function; if constipation or diarrhea occurs, institute nursing measures to counteract them (see Chapter 31).	The client will state that he does not experience disabling or discomfiting alterations in bowel function.
Muscular tremors L-dopa therapy (L-dopa can cause weakness, dizziness, and visual changes.)	High risk for injury related to weakness, dizziness, and visual changes secondary to medication with L-dopa	**Warn** the client that he may experience visual changes as well as weakness and dizziness when changing position rapidly; teach him to change position slowly, especially when rising from a lying or sitting position. If these symptoms develop, provide assistance for ambulation.	The client will not sustain accidental injury.
L-dopa therapy (Inappropriate sexual expression tends to occur when L-dopa therapy is instituted.)	High risk for self-esteem disturbance related to inappropriate or excessive sexual expression secondary to L-dopa therapy	**Explain** to the client that unusual sexual impulses sometimes occur during the initial stages of L-dopa therapy. Assure him that overt sexuality reverts to normal with continued treatment.	The client will accept the temporary changes in sexuality as a side effect of the drug.

When emotional, intellectual, or sexual changes occur, the nurse should explain to the client that these are side effects of the drug, which can be reduced or eliminated by adjustment of drug dosage.

Caution clients that successful therapy requires continued close health care supervision, including periodic blood tests.

Evaluation Data required for evaluation include the absence or incidence of injury, measurement of activity and mobility, statements by the client indicative of self-esteem and body image, and observation of role activities or statements by the client or family about participation by the client in role activities, including sexual activity. Nutrition can be evaluated by observing foods consumed by the client and by assessing the parameters of nutrition, such as body weight and integrity of the skin and mucous membranes. Frequency and consistency of stools should be noted. Sleep time can be measured, and clients can be asked if they feel rested. Visual function is tested with wall charts and reading materials. The teaching plan is evaluated by questioning the client about information conveyed during the teaching sessions (see the Example of Nursing Process and Treatment with Levodopa).

Checklist of nursing actions

- [ ] Assess clients who are to receive levodopa therapy for factors that increase risk of adverse reactions. Inform the physician if significant factors are present.
- [ ] Monitor clients closely for side effects and toxic effects, especially during the initial 6 to 8 weeks of therapy.
- [ ] Take precautions to prevent falls and accidental injury of clients who experience postural hypotension as a side effect of therapy.
- [ ] Promote dietary intake in clients who experience anorexia, nausea, or vomiting as side effects of therapy.
- [ ] Provide emotional support to clients, especially during the initial stage of therapy before optimal response occurs.
- [ ] Inform clients that side effects are due to the medication and may be ameliorated by continued administration of the drug or adjustment of dosage.
- [ ] Be accepting of behavioral changes that may occur in response to drug therapy.
- [ ] Advise clients of measures that help minimize

side effects of the drug (*eg*, the use of elastic hose for postural hypotension, dietary modification to promote nutrition).

☐ Advise clients to avoid use of vitamin supplements that contain large doses of pyridoxine.

Analeptics

An analeptic is a substance that is restorative because of its stimulation of the CNS. This descriptive title has been applied to a group of drugs once widely used to counteract depressed physiologic functions characteristic of sudden severe illness or toxicity. Supportive care to maintain vital functions is currently regarded as much more effective, and the use of analeptics has declined considerably. Common analeptic drugs are listed in Table 23-4.

Strychnine

Strychnine is a vegetable alkaloid derived from the seed of a tree native to India. It acts as a competitive antagonist of glycine at the postsynaptic receptor that inhibits nerve cells on activation. Strychnine is an ascending stimulant that acts first on the lower centers (such as those in the spinal cord). In toxic doses, strychnine causes exaggerated motor reflexes, tetanic convulsions, which are symmetrical and coordinated, and respiratory arrest. Face and neck stiffness progress to spasms that produce characteristic facies called *risus sardonicus*.

Strychnine was formerly used in small doses as a stimulant in nonprescription tonics. Because of its bitter taste, it stimulates intestinal secretion and improves the appetite. Toxic doses are incorporated into pesticides and rodenticides. Strychnine is a major source of accidental poisoning in children. Its only recognized medicinal use is in the treatment of the rare congenital metabolic disorder nonketotic hyperglycemia.

Pentylenetetrazol

Pentylenetetrazol (Metrazol) is a synthetic compound used for its stimulant and convulsant properties. Its mechanism of action is unknown; it may act by reducing neurologic recovery time or by increasing nerve cell permeability to potassium ions. The drug is sometimes used in small doses to increase physical and mental activity in elderly clients. It is also used as a provocative agent in the diagnosis of epilepsy. Subconvulsant doses activate latent epileptogenic foci, which alter the electroencephalogram tracing in characteristic patterns. In the laboratory, pentylenetetrazol is used as a tool to screen anticonvulsant drugs.

Table 23-4. Analeptics

Drug name	Preparations	Medicinal uses	Usual dosage	Additional information
strychnine	Rat and crow poison	Nonketotic hyperglycinemia (a rare condition)	Not used medicinally	Strychnine is a frequent cause of poisoning in children.
picrotoxin ("fishberries")	None	None	Not used medicinally	Berries of the plant are used to incapacitate fish in East Indies.
pentylenetetrazol (Cardiazol, Leptazol, Metrazole, Pentrazol)	Tablets and elixir for oral use; solution for injection	Stimulant and convulsant	To diagnose epilepsy: 2 mg/kg body weight IV, followed by 1 mg/kg body weight/30 sec until EEG spike activity occurs or a maximum dose of 350 mg is reached As a stimulant for adults: 100–200 mg tid, orally	This drug is used as a laboratory tool to evaluate anticonvulsant drugs, as a provocative agent to diagnose epilepsy, and (sometimes) to enhance mental and physical activity in the elderly.
ammonia (aromatic spirits of ammonia, "smelling salts")	Mesh-covered ampules to be crushed for administration by inhalation Oral solution	Prevent or terminate fainting	*By inhalation:* whiffs of the vapors of a 4% solution until a response occurs *Orally:* (adults) 2–4 ml of a 4% solution well diluted in water	Whiffs are sufficient; excessive concentration may cause choking. In high doses it can be damaging to tissues.

Ammonia

Ammonia is an irritating chemical that stimulates vital centers in the medulla through peripheral reflexes. The drug may be inhaled or taken orally as a dilute solution. Stimulation of sensory nerves in the pharynx, esophagus, and stomach cause reflex stimulation of respiration and vasoconstriction.

Aromatic spirits of ammonia is marketed in the form of ampules enclosed in a net meshwork ("smelling salts"). The preparation is used to prevent and treat fainting. The ampule is crushed and held near the nose of the recipient. Whiffs of the vapors are sufficient to produce the desired stimulation. Excessive concentration may cause choking.

In high doses, ammonia can damage the tissues that it contacts. Exposure to ammonia is an occupational hazard in the refrigeration industry. Environmental pollution can result if a container is accidentally damaged during shipment. Tissues exposed to ammonia should be flushed with copious amounts of water. Emergency medical care should be sought without delay.

■ Summary

Analeptics are chemicals that stimulate central vital centers and thus tend to correct depressed physiology due to illness or toxicity from depressant drugs. They are infrequently used in medical practice because more effective means of maintaining vital functions are available. Analeptic drugs include strychnine, pentylenetetrazol, and ammonia.

Nursing management

Nursing implications

Because analeptics are seldom used in medical practice, the nurse does not encounter them often in the care of ill clients. These drugs are sometimes prescribed to improve function of elderly clients and as an aid in the diagnosis of epilepsy.

Analeptics are capable of stimulating convulsions; the degree of risk is related to the seizure threshold of the client.

Spirits of ammonia is a useful drug for the prevention and treatment of fainting. It is often stocked in nursing units in health care institutions. The drug may be used cautiously to restore consciousness and to strengthen the client until other supportive measures can be carried out. The cause of the fainting episode should be determined and appropriate corrective measures taken.

The use of analeptics by lay people for medical purpose should be discouraged. The drugs are believed to serve no therapeutic purpose when incorporated into nonprescription preparations.

Pesticides that contain strychnine must be carefully controlled to prevent accidental ingestion. Unused portions of such materials should be destroyed promptly, preferably by incineration.

Treatment of acute strychnine poisoning is similar to that of other CNS stimulants. Gastric lavage can reduce intestinal absorption of ingested poison. Solutions for lavage include tincture of iodine (1:250), tannic acid (2%), strong tea, potassium permanganate (1:5000), or activated charcoal slurry. A quiet environment is essential, since slight stimuli can trigger convulsions. Diazepam is administered as an anticonvulsant. The client must be watched closely for respiratory depression, and mechanical assistance should be supplied as necessary.

Nursing process

Assessment Before initiating pentylenetetrazol therapy, the nurse should question the client about previous seizures or a family history of epilepsy. Clients with a positive history are at increased risk for a toxic reaction. Muscle tone and reflexes should be assessed. Increased muscle tone, muscle spasms, and hyperactive reflexes also increase the risk of toxicity.

Nursing diagnosis Clients for whom pentylenetetrazol is prescribed are likely to have

Self-care deficits related to lethargy and fatigue

Those receiving analeptic drugs are at

High risk for injury related to seizures

Planning Goals of treatment are improved self-care, increased energy, and prevention of seizures.

Intervention Nursing actions include administering the analeptic medication and monitoring the client's response. Seizure precautions should be instituted. Diazepam or other anticonvulsants should be readily available for treating seizure, should it occur. Nursing measures to reduce the risk of seizures include alleviating acute stressors that could stimulate sympathoadrenal response or hyperventilation, encouraging regular meals to prevent hypoglycemia, and eliminating from the environment repetitive stimuli such as strobe lights, which can trigger seizures.

Client education. Clients should be cautioned against factors that increase the risk of seizures: missed meals, exposure to febrile contagious diseases, excessive sodium intake, alcoholic intoxication, and (for diabetics) insulin reactions.

Evaluation Data required for assessment include statements by clients indicating that they have more energy and tire less readily than before medication, observations that the clients participate more fully in activities of daily living, and the absence or incidence of seizures.

Checklist of nursing actions

☐ Before initiating analeptic therapy, assess clients for factors that increase the risk of seizures.

☐ Monitor clients who receive analeptics for toxic and side effects.

☐ Be prepared to institute emergency treatment for convulsions when pentylenetetrazol is administered.

☐ Administer spirits of ammonia sparingly for the treatment and prevention of fainting.

☐ Warn clients about controlling strychnine pesticides to prevent accidental poisoning.

☐ Advise clients to avoid proprietary remedies that contain analeptics.

☐ Advise clients who use analeptics without prescription about alternative measures to relieve health problems.

Cocaine

Cocaine is an active alkaloid produced by the coca shrub native to Peru and Bolivia and grown in both South America and the Far East. For centuries, Indians of the Andes Mountains have used the plant to reduce fatigue, increase endurance, and promote a feeling of well-being. They combine the leaves with lime and chew the material as a masticatory. The lime is believed to accelerate the absorption of cocaine. Although this mixture may contain other active drugs, CNS effects are attributed primarily to cocaine. The stimulant properties of cocaine resemble those of the amphetamines. Like those drugs, it is classified as a schedule II drug under the Controlled Substances Act of 1970 (see Chapter 2).

Pharmacodynamics. Cocaine blocks peripheral nerve conduction. The drug is both potent and rapid acting. Local anesthesia is apparent within 60 seconds of topical application. Cocaine potentiates the effects of catecholamines in the CNS by inhibiting their uptake by sympathetic neurons after liberation from the presynaptic fiber. Cocaine thus prolongs and enhances sympathetic nerve activity. It also inhibits vagus nerve transmission. The drug's central action is biphasic; initial stimulation is followed by depression.

General effects of systemic doses of cocaine include pronounced vasoconstriction, mydriasis, and reduction in REM sleep. Topical application causes local vasoconstriction and paralyzes sensory fibers, abolishing smell and taste when applied to the nose and tongue.

Pharmacokinetics. Cocaine is absorbed from GI and other mucosae and from sites of parenteral injection. Application to inflamed membranes results in accelerated absorption and accentuated systemic effects. The drug is degraded by plasma esterases and hepatic enzymes. Urinary excretion is normally low but becomes significant when the urine is acidified. Cocaine is deactivated rapidly by the body, having a half-life of only 1 hour.

Therapeutic uses. Medicinal uses of cocaine are limited to topical application to mucous membranes to produce local anesthesia. It is employed mainly in nose and throat procedures. Although injection is not recommended, some surgeons use this practice during procedures such as tonsillectomy. Cocaine solutions for topical use are prepared in strengths from 1% to 10%.

Abuse. See Chapter 15 for a discussion of cocaine abuse.

Adverse reactions. Side effects of cocaine include CNS and sympathetic nervous system stimulation. Temperature, pulse, respirations, and blood pressure all increase. High doses cause pronounced fever, tremor, headaches, dizziness, hyperexcitability, and cardiac arrhythmia. Seizures, cardiac failure, and cardiovascular collapse may occur.

Toxic and side effects are more likely to develop when anesthesia is prolonged and involves repeated applications of drug solution.

Chronic use of cocaine tends to cause nausea, vomiting, weight loss, and insomnia. CNS hyperexcitability can produce delirium, hallucinations, and muscle twitching or spasms. Stereotypic behavior can become pronounced. A psychopathic state characterized by paranoia, delusions of power and superiority, and homicidal tendencies may develop. Repeated doses of cocaine progressively lower the seizure threshold. Cardiovascular effects include tachycardia and hypertension. Sudden seizures, heart attack, or stroke can cause death.

The intense vasoconstrictive action of cocaine can damage tissues exposed to concentrations of the drug. The practice of snorting causes erosion of the nasal mucosa and may result in perforation of the septum. Because of tissue loss, plastic repair can be difficult and incomplete. A similar destruction of lung tissue is suspected from using crack; black sputum is sometimes expectorated by cocaine smokers.

Cocaine is both physically and psychologically addictive. Some tolerance occurs, in part from increased excretion of the drug. Chronic abusers do not eat well and tend to exhibit the characteristic ketoacidosis and ketonuria of weight loss; this acidification of the urine promotes renal excretion of cocaine. In dependent users, withdrawal is characterized by fatigue, listlessness, inability to concentrate, restlessness, depression, hyperphagia, hypersomnia, and a rebound increase in REM sleep. Craving for the drug is intense.

Mothers-to-be who use cocaine are more apt than are nonusing women to experience spontaneous abortion, abruptio placentae, premature delivery, and fetal distress. Their babies are smaller, have smaller heads, and are shorter than are normal babies. Growth impairment is directly related to duration of cocaine abuse by the mother during pregnancy (Fackelman, 1989; When cocaine use . . . , 1989). "Cocaine" babies also exhibit neurologic impairment. They test poorly on the Neonatal Behavioral Assessment Scale, have attention and orientation problems, and are less likely than are unexposed infants to respond to a human voice or face. They may be irritable or, conversely, may sleep excessively. These babies are also at increased risk of SIDS.

Precautions and contraindications. Medicinal use of cocaine is contraindicated in clients with a history of severe idiosyncratic reaction to or dependence on the drug. It should not be used by clients who suffer from epilepsy, hyperthyroidism, and anxiety states. Caution must be exercised when used in cardiovascular disease because cocaine can induce angina, cardiac arrhythmia, and elevated blood pressure.

Administration of a barbiturate before use of cocaine reduces the incidence and severity of side effects. Injection of the drug should be avoided because rapid absorption can lead to cardiac arrest.

■ **Summary**

Cocaine is a natural plant alkaloid with CNS stimulant properties similar to those of amphetamines. It is used medicinally as a topical local anesthetic. Side effects include hypertension and excitation.

Cocaine abuse is a major health problem. Use of the drug can cause sudden death from seizure, heart attack, or stroke. Cocaine dependence has devastating physiologic, psychological, and social effects. Recovery and rehabilitation are slow and difficult.

Nursing management

Nursing implications

When cocaine is applied to the throat, the gag and swallowing reflexes are abolished temporarily. After the procedure, the client should be in a prone position, with head down to promote drainage of secretions and to prevent aspiration. Close observation of respirations and cardiovascular status is required. The client should remain under close observation until vital signs are stable and reflexes are fully recovered.

Acute cocaine toxicity is characterized by hyperactivity and fever. Acute emotional disturbances such as paranoia or panic can occur. A high risk of seizure, stroke, myocarditis heart attack, cardiac arrhythmia or cardiovascular collapse is present. Treatment is directed at controlling fever and seizures and at supporting vital functions. After resolution of the crisis situation, every effort should be made to persuade the cocaine-dependent client to enter a drug treatment program.

Treatment of cocaine abuse is similar in many respects to that of alcohol abuse. (See also Chapter 15 on substance abuse.) Initial detoxification is uncomfortable and distressing. Some symptoms of cocaine withdrawal (fatigue, oversleeping, overeating) differ from those of alcohol withdrawal (tremulousness, insomnia, lack of appetite). However, with both drugs, withdrawal can cause inability to concentrate, irritability, and restlessness. Drugs used to ameliorate the CNS depression of cocaine withdrawal include tricyclic antidepressants (imipramine and desipramine), bromocriptine, and amantadine. All of these drugs influence the function of dopamine in the CNS, either as dopamine-receptor agonists or inhibitors of catecholamine reuptake. They tend to relieve CNS manifestations of withdrawal and relieve fatigue, depression, irritability, anorexia, and sleep disturbance. Some of these drugs also block the action of cocaine, preventing the "high" that users seek from the drug. It is reported that carbamazepine (Tegretol), lithium, desipramine, and bromocriptine reduce the craving for cocaine (Mrazik, Mrazik, 1991). Some investigators have prescribed large doses of amino acids (particularly tyrosine and L-tryptophan) in the hope of accelerating the regeneration of brain neurotransmitters that become depleted with extended cocaine use.

Group therapy and peer support are important components of prolonged treatment. Two national programs that have recently been established are Cocaine Anonymous, which is similar to Alcoholics Anonymous, and the toll-free National Cocaine Hotline, 1–800–COCAINE. As with alcohol, support programs stress abstinence and interruption of the pattern of drug use.

Cocaine abuse is no longer limited to the more affluent drug users. With advent of the cheap rapidly effective form of cocaine crack, abuse can be seen at all social levels. In 1987, emergency admissions for cocaine abuse out-numbered those for any other drug of abuse. Cocaine ranked third as a cause of drug-related deaths (Cocaine: High on the list, 1988). Nurses should actively participate in drug education programs for the public and for users. However, education alone is not highly effective against drug abuse. In the long run, promotion of parenting skills capable of increasing self-esteem and positive self-image could be more effective in reducing the risk of drug dependence among future generations.

Nursing process: therapeutic use of cocaine

Assessment Before application of cocaine as a topical anesthetic, the client should be questioned about

Example of nursing process and cocaine anesthesia

The client is a 39-year-old woman who has just been transferred from the operating room to the recovery room after a fiberoptic bronchoscopy and lung biopsy. Topical cocaine anesthesia was used for the procedure. The client is awake and alert.

The client is prone in Trendelenburg's position. When questioned, she states she has no pain. Acetaminophen and codeine have been ordered for pain.

The client has no gag reflex.

Assessment data	Nursing diagnosis	Intervention	Goals and outcome criteria
Cocaine anesthesia for fiberoptic bronchoscopy Absent gag reflex	High risk for impaired gas exchange related to impaired gag reflex secondary to cocaine anesthesia	**Maintain** the client in prone, Trendelenburg's position to promote drainage of respiratory secretions from the lungs. Do not allow the client to ingest food or fluids until the gag reflex returns. **Monitor** the quantity and color of secretions.	The client will not develop signs and symptoms of respiratory congestion and infection caused by aspiration.
Cocaine anesthesia for fiberoptic bronchoscopy	Altered comfort: restlessness, irritability, hyperactive reflexes related to CNS hyperactivity secondary to cocaine anesthesia	**Place** the client in an environment with minimal stimuli (away from noise and bright lights). **Use** nursing measures to promote rest. **Monitor** the client for signs and symptoms of CNS hyperactivity: restlessness, irritability, hyperactive reflexes.	The client will remain quiet and will state that she feels comfortable.

previous use of and response to the drug. Dependency on cocaine or idiosyncratic reaction to the drug should be ruled out. Nursing history should include evaluation for epilepsy, thyrotoxicity, psychological disturbance, hypertension, and angina or other cardiovascular conditions. Sensitivity to sympathomimetic drugs should be assessed. Factors that tend to increase the risk of cocaine anesthesia should be reported to the physician.

Nursing diagnosis Diagnoses that stem from use of topical cocaine include the following:

High risk for impaired gas exchange related to aspiration secondary to impaired gag reflex
High risk for altered body temperature: hyperpyrexia related to neuromuscular stimulation and vasoconstriction
High risk for injury related to seizures

Common collaborative problems that should be differentiated from the nursing diagnoses include

Potential complication: myocardial infarction
Potential complication: stroke
Potential complication: cardiac arrest
Potential complication: cardiopulmonary collapse

Planning Goals of treatment are to prevent or to promptly detect and treat adverse drug reactions, including aspiration, fever, injury, cardiovascular malfunction, and stroke.

Intervention During and after surgery that involves cocaine anesthesia, the client should be monitored closely for signs and symptoms of adverse drug reaction. Health care personnel must be prepared to treat acute reactions should they occur. Diazepam may be needed if seizure occurs. Hyperthermia may be controlled with a hypothermal blanket. Mechanical assistance for respiration and circulation may be required. After the procedure, the client should be prone, with head down, to promote drainage of secretions and prevent aspiration. The client should remain under close observation until vital signs are stable and reflexes are fully recovered. Vital signs, including temperature, should be monitored closely.

Evaluation Data required for evaluation include the absence or incidence of adverse drug reaction, the time required for detection and treatment of adverse reactions that occur, and the absence or presence of permanent sequelae (see the Example of Nursing Process and Cocaine Anesthesia).

Checklist of nursing actions

☐ Evaluate clients who receive cocaine anesthesia for sensitivity to sympathomimetic drugs and for conditions in which the drug is contraindicated.

☐ Monitor clients who receive cocaine for signs and symptoms of systemic cocaine toxicity.

☐ Position clients who are recovering from cocaine anesthesia of the throat should lie prone, with head down. Keep them under close observation until gag and swallowing reflexes are completely recovered.

☐ Warn against the abuse of cocaine for psychotropic effects.

Khat and betel

Khat and betel are plant derivatives similar to cocaine in their ability to stimulate the nervous system. They are used for their psychotropic effect by populations in areas where the plants are indigenous.

Khat is derived from the leaves of a shrub found in east Africa and east Arabia. It may be chewed as a masticatory or brewed to make a sweet, astringent, licorice-flavored tea. Khat contains active alkaloids similar to the phenylalkylamines norepinephrine and amphetamine.

The betel or Areca nut is produced by a palm tree in east India. It contains the alkaloid arecoline. In addition to increased CNS activity and euphoria, the drug stimulates parasympathetic activity, resulting in sweating, salivation, and miosis. The betel nut is mixed with lime and leaves of the pepper plant to form a mass chewed as a masticatory. As with coca, the lime is believed to accelerate absorption of the active alkaloid. Use of betel stains teeth, saliva, urine, and feces red. Betel may increase the risk of cancer. A squamous cell carcinoma is frequently seen on the inside of the cheek of betel chewers.

The active alkaloid of betel, arecoline, is used as a vermifuge in veterinary medicine.

Hallucinogens

Hallucinogens are chemical substances that stimulate sensory perceptions in the absence of environmental stimuli. Chemicals with hallucinogenic properties are found in many plant materials that are widely distributed throughout the world. They have been employed historically as poisons, magical brews, and elements of religious rituals (Table 23-5).

Physiology

Sensory perceptions normally result from a complex process that involves interaction between nerve stimuli that enter the brain from the periphery, stored memory traces, and activity in the limbic system. Stimulation of sensory receptors in the periphery of the body gives rise to nerve impulses, which travel to specific areas of the brain where they register as crude sensations (*eg*, of light, sound, odors). Perception also involves the meaning assigned to these sensations through modification of impulses in the associative areas of the brain. Factors that affect the interpretation of sensory stimuli include attention focused on them, conditioned response to previous experience with similar stimuli, emotional associations with similar stimuli, and the "mind set" (or nature of background activity in the brain) at the time the stimulus occurs. Although each stimulus can be modified to a considerable degree by these influences, the interpretation of identical stimuli nevertheless has an underlying consistency. The primary function of sensation is to inform the organism of the nature of the external world so that appropriate response behaviors may be initiated.

Pathophysiology

Sensory perceptions that are incongruous with the environment may be of two types, illusions or hallucinations. Illusions are misinterpretations of stimuli that originate from the environment. Hallucinations are sensory perceptions that occur in the absence of any external stimulus. Everyone experiences both illusions and hallucinations from time to time. For example, a fearful person may "see" the illusion of a mugger in a moving shadow, which is actually cast by a branch blowing in the wind. Hallucinations may arise from traumatic stimulation of nerves within the CNS or any time that the sensory areas of the brain receive abnormal stimulation. For example, visual hallucinations ("seeing stars") are not uncommon after a blow to the head. Tinnitus ("ringing in the ears") is an auditory hallucination that can result from a degenerative disease process or from an ototoxic drug that irritates the eighth cranial nerve. Sensory hallucinations are experienced by some clients during the aura that precedes seizure activity in epilepsy.

Certain kinds of hallucinations are associated with specific pathologies. For example, visual hallucinations are frequently experienced by alcoholics during the acute withdrawal syndrome known as delirium tremens. Although the lay stereotypic impression of these experiences is that of "seeing pink elephants," in the author's experience spiders or snakes are more commonly perceived. Tactile hallucinations (the "monkey on one's back") are characteristic of opiate

Table 23-5. Representative hallucinogenic substances

Source	Active principles	Dose	Preparations	Method of administration
Cannabis sativa, a hemp plant native to temperate areas of both hemispheres, now found in most parts of the world (marijuana)	tetrahydrocannabinols (several isomers are active)	100–230 mg/kg body weight, depending on species of subject Pure THC: 300–400 μg/kg body weight po; 200–250 μg/kg body weight when smoked	Bhand (green plant material which is dried and powdered) Ganja (pistillate tops with exuded resin, which are dried) Charas (pure resin removed from leaves and stems) Cigarettes (dried, crushed flowering tops and leaves) Hashish (the resin from recently fertilized pistillate flowers)	Oral, in drinks or candies Inhalation, when smoked with tobacco Oral, as an infusion Inhalation, by smoking Oral, mixed with spices Inhalation, by smoking Inhalation, by smoking Oral, in food or drinks
Amanita muscaria, a mushroom also known as fly agaric, native to the north temperate zone of Eurasia	ibotenic acid, muscimole, muscazone	One to four mushrooms	Dried whole mushrooms	Absorption from mucous membranes, by holding the moistened mushroom in the mouth Oral, in water, milk, or alone Oral, by drinking urine containing active drug or metabolities
Psilocybe mexicana, a mushroom mainly distributed in the temperate areas of the world	psilocybin and psilocin	4–8 mg psilocybin or about 2 g dried mushroom	Fresh or dried mushrooms	Oral, sometimes eaten with honey
Myristica fragrans, the nutmeg tree native to eastern Malaysia and east India	myristicin and other aromatic amines	400 mg pure myristicin or 20 g nutmeg	Dried, powdered seeds of the nutmeg tree	Oral, as a powder Absorption from mucous membranes, by sniffing
Lophophora williamsii, a cactus found in the deserts of Mexico and southwestern United States	mescaline and other active alkaloids	4–30 buttons	Mescal buttons, the dried crowns of the cactus	Oral, whole or as an infusion
Ipomoea violacea, a morning glory vine native to Mexico	lysergic acid amide and related alkaloids	2–5 mg lysergic acid or about 10–15 seeds	Seeds of the morning glory plant	Oral, whole or as an infusion
Chemical synthesis	D-lysergic acid diethylamide (LSD)	0.05 mg	Crystals or solution	Oral, often taken as a solution-treated sugar cube
Atropa belladonna, an herb native to Europe	scopolamine		Thought to be an ingredient in hallucinogenic witches' brew of medieval Europe	Oral, as an infusion
Mandragora officinarum (mandrake), a stemless herb indigenous to Mediterranean Europe	scopolamine		Thought to be an ingredient in hallucinogenic witches' brew of medieval Europe	Oral, as an infusion

withdrawal syndrome. Auditory hallucinations ("hearing voices") are commonly experienced by clients who suffer from psychoses, such as schizophrenia. Olfactory hallucinations are most often associated with brain tumors.

Hallucinations stimulated during use of hallucinogenic drugs may involve a greater disruption of perceptual function than those associated with alcohol or opiate withdrawal syndrome or brain tumor or psychoses. Abnormal perceptions may be multiple, involving more than one modality of sensation. Transposition of sensation has also been reported. In transposition, stimuli that normally produces a sensation in one modality may be experienced in another modality; for example, sounds may be experienced as colors, or sights as sounds.

Hallucinogenic drugs

A variety of substances have been exploited historically for their hallucinogenic properties (see Table 23-5). Fly agaric (*Amantia muscaria*) and marijuana (*Cannabis sativa*) were among the earliest hallucinogens used by humans. Fly agaric has long been employed by tribes of northern Eurasia and may have been the god-narcotic, soma, worshiped in India for a time after its introduction from the north around 1500 BC. Marijuana has been widely used in Asia, Asia Minor, and parts of Africa but is known world-wide. Both belladonna and mandrake were employed in subhallucinogenic doses by folk healers in medieval Europe. Larger amounts were added to witches' brews in that era. In the New World, a variety of hallucinogenic plants were used by American Indians, often as a part of their religious practices. Among the substances used were a cactus, tree resins, morning glory seeds, and a variety of fungi. Nutmeg is hallucinogenic only in large doses and is used primarily as a substitute for stronger hallucinogens by people such as prisoners and clients in controlled drug treatment centers who have lost access to their usual drug supplies. Synthetic hallucinogens, such as LSD, are structurally related to the active principles of natural hallucinogens. Because they are easily and economically produced, they are often sold as illegal "street" drugs.

Pharmacodynamics. The pharmacodynamics of the hallucinogens are still unknown. The active principles of these substances have chemical structures that resemble those of neurotransmitters in the CNS. Many contain indole structures that derive from tryptamine or lysergic acid that are structurally related to the neurotransmitter serotonin. Mescaline resembles the neurohormone norepinephrine. It is believed that these hallucinogens act by agonistic interaction with receptors on nerve cells that normally are stimulated only by autogenous neurotransmitters.

Physiologic effects. The physiologic effects of hallucinogens begin generally with abnormal skeletal muscle activity (twitching, tremor, slight convulsions, and ataxia). A subjective feeling of lightness and a desire to dance follow. The extremities may feel numb and cold. A dreamy state of consciousness and uncontrollable disruption of ideation develop. Euphoria or exaltation may alternate with depression or reverie. Hallucinations are usually visual, but sometimes they are auditory. Distorted perceptions, such as altered time perceptions and macropsia, may occur. Transposition of perceptions have also been reported. Altered behavior, such as a mad rushing about, violence, or sexual activity, sometimes occurs with the use of mushrooms.

In addition to these central effects, marijuana reduces intraocular pressure, dilates the bronchi, has antiemetic effects, and stimulates the appetite, especially for sweets.

Pharmacokinetics. Hallucinogenic drugs are taken by various routes. Most are ingested orally, either whole, added to foods, or infused (made into tea) and drunk as beverages. Many are inhaled by smoking. Fly agaric, nutmeg, and tree resins may be applied to mucous membranes for absorption, either whole or in powdered form. All are systemically absorbed and travel through the circulation to the brain. They appear to cross the blood–brain barrier readily. Most are widely distributed in the tissues. Marijuana tends to bind to fatty tissue and persist in fatty tissue depots.

The active principles of hallucinogens are metabolized mainly in the liver and excreted in urine. Many metabolites of the active principles of hallucinogens retain hallucinogenic activity. Although plasma concentrations decline rapidly after marijuana is smoked, tetrahydrocannabinol is detectable in the urine for up to 72 hours.

Uses. Scopolamine is employed in subhallucinogenic doses as a preanesthetic medication. Although exhibiting some depressant actions on the CNS in therapeutic doses, scopolamine can produce delirium, especially when administered to people in pain, in the absence of adequate analgesia. The amnesia produced by scopolamine is considered desirable in some clinical situations.

Two cannabinoid derivatives, dronabinol (Marinol) and nabilone (Cesamet) have been approved by the U.S. Food and Drug Administration for use as an antinausea agent in chemotherapy. These are effective antiemetics but tend to produce psychotomimetic effects characteristic of marijuana. Because they are likely to be abused, they are classified as schedule II controlled substances.

Experimentally, marijuana has been used to reduce intraocular pressure in glaucoma. As a folk medicine, it has also been used to manage asthma. LSD and other psychotomimetics have been employed in research that investigated the nature of psychotic illness, notably schizophrenia. It was hoped that the chemical effects of the drugs, which closely resemble those of the psychoses, would help explain the basic nature of these illnesses and suggest drug treatment that could reverse the processes.

Hallucinogens are widely abused for their psychotropic effects. In most areas of the world, such use is illegal. In areas where it has been sanctioned in the past, such as India, authorities are attempting to restrict the use of these substances because of the detrimental effects on people after long-term use.

Adverse reactions. Undesirable responses to a single dose of hallucinogen is termed a "bad trip." Affected individuals sometimes experience dysphoria, panic, and fear of death. During such episodes, attempts to escape the perceived threat may cause accidental injury. Suicidal behavior sometimes occurs.

Effects on the CNS sometimes appear to outlast the presence of the active drugs. Marijuana can affect memory adversely for up to 6 weeks after cessation of drug use (Marijuana mangles memory, 1989). A return of the signs and symptoms of drug effects in the absence of repeated use is termed a "flashback." Flashbacks can occur weeks or months after use of a drug has been discontinued. They tend to subside gradually over time. Some users develop permanent psychoses after use of hallucinogens. Whether the drugs trigger incipient psychosis or produce a lasting change in brain function is not known.

Marijuana smoke produces lung damage similar to that of tobacco smoke. When both marijuana and tobacco are smoked, adverse effects on the lungs are additive (Marijuana: Rough stuff, 1988).

Immature users and unstable personalities are more likely to experience adverse reactions than are stable adults. The risk of harm is greatest in clients known to have had psychotic illnesses.

While under the influence of hallucinogens, people are prone to accidents. Psychomotor performance deteriorates, and alterations of time and sensory perceptions interfere with appropriate response to environmental stimuli. Sometimes delusions lead to foolhardy action, such as stepping out of a high window while convinced that one is capable of flying.

Some hallucinogens adversely affect reproductive function. Hallucinogens are suspected to be mutagenic. Users of both marijuana and LSD sometimes exhibit increased incidence of chromosome breakdown in their cells. Whether or not the drugs increase the incidence of anomalies in children born to users is still controversial. Prolonged use of marijuana is reported to reduce potency and fertility in males and to disrupt menstrual cycles in women.

At least one hallucinogen, phencyclidine (PCP, "angel dust"), may act as an immunosuppressant. *In vitro* studies have demonstrated a reduced antibody production by B immunocytes and inhibited DNA synthesis and glucose metabolism in both B and T cells exposed to phencyclidine. PCP also inhibits production by monocytes of interleukin-1, a substance that stimulates DNA synthesis by B immunocytes.

Possibly the most damaging aspect of the use of hallucinogens is a reduced involvement in normal developmental activities. Crucial maturation periods may pass without progress toward goals. Users may be permanently handicapped by retarded or incomplete maturation.

Precautions. The risk of a bad trip is reduced by establishing an atmosphere conducive to relaxation and a feeling of security. Users of hallucinogens usually employ special religious or social settings to promote a good response and to enhance the desirable effects of the drugs. Often one or more people in the group are designated to abstain from using drugs to safeguard, monitor, and assist those who indulge.

■ Summary

Hallucinogens are substances that contain active principles that resemble neurotransmitters in the CNS. They act as agonists on receptors of brain cells responsible for sensation, producing abnormal perceptions. Most are not employed medicinally but are used and abused for their psychotropic effects.

Use of hallucinogens is hazardous. Effects sometimes persist, producing psychosis. The risk of accidental injury is high while drug effects last. Attempts at suicide may occur, especially when the subjective perceptions are unpleasant or frightening. Habitual use interferes with the completion of developmental tasks by diverting the attention and activity of the user from normal work and study.

The use of hallucinogens is restricted or prohibited in most areas of the world.

Nursing management

Nursing implications

Adverse reactions to hallucinogens are sometimes seen in clients treated in emergency departments or those who seek help from telephone "hotline" services. During a bad trip, affected individuals need support to carry them through the acute phase of the reaction. To minimize external stimuli, a quiet environment should be provided. To prevent accidental injury, clients must not be left alone until the acute reaction subsides.

It is often possible to ameliorate the symptoms

through therapeutic communication. This approach, termed "talking down" the client, involves persuading the client that some degree of voluntary control can be exerted over the mental processes, despite the effects of the drug. This type of crisis intervention helps clients alter their own mind sets so that the abnormal brain activity assumes a less threatening form of ideation and perception. The client should also be reassured that the experiences are temporary in nature and disappear as the drug is cleared from the body.

Sometimes clients under the influence of hallucinogens have experienced physical trauma as a result of an accident or attempts at self-destruction. In such situations, the physical care required to treat the injury may have to be administered at the same time as the psychological care needed to ameliorate the residual effects of the hallucinogen. Occasionally, inappropriate hyperactivity or aggression by clients must be controlled.

Withdrawal from hallucinogenic drugs appears not to produce a physical abstinence syndrome. The client may have become exhausted during the drug episode, however, and depression can develop. In habitual users, psychological dependence may produce discomfort and vague physical symptoms during withdrawal.

When the acute episode has resolved, the nurse should initiate counseling to help clients reevaluate their involvement with drugs. Referral to drug treatment programs is appropriate for receptive clients.

Nursing process

The process of nursing care in substance abuse is discussed in detail in Chapter 15.

Client education. The nurse should be actively involved in programs to educate the lay public about the hazards of abuse in using hallucinogenic drugs. Education of the young is particularly important. The facts about the risks and supposed benefits of drug use should be presented in a matter-of-fact manner so that informed decisions about drug use can be made.

The inclination to experiment with drugs is associated with a poor self-image and lack of self-confidence. It is increased by inactivity and boredom. Nurses should support programs that promote good parenting and provide ample educational and recreational opportunities. Such activities greatly enhance preventive mental health services.

People with strong egos, good self-images, and self-confidence are not likely to be attracted by the purported benefits of drug use or to be influenced by peer pressure to experiment with drugs.

Nurses should caution against indiscriminate experimentation with plant materials of unknown toxicity. Some bizarre preparations have been recommended for psychogenic effects (*eg,* baked banana

skins). Clients should be warned of the dangers of gathering wild mushrooms for food. Unless the forager is skilled in the identification of edible specimens, toxic plants may accidentally be selected. Not only do many mushrooms contain hallucinogenic drugs but some also contain deadly poisons.

Checklist of nursing actions

When clients are treated for adverse reactions to hallucinogens

☐ Provide a quiet environment to minimize external stimuli.

☐ Provide emotional support and reassurance.

☐ Employ therapeutic communication to help clients exert voluntary control over thought processes to influence them toward nonthreatening channels.

☐ Monitor clients constantly until the acute reaction subsides.

☐ Protect clients from accidental or self-imposed injury.

☐ Counsel clients about the need for referral to drug treatment programs.

To reduce the risk of abuse of hallucinogenic substances

☐ Promote good parenting practices that foster the development of strong egos, good self-images, and self-confidence in children.

☐ Provide educational programs that present the facts about the effects and risks of hallucinogens.

☐ Support programs that provide wholesome recreational and educational activities for the public.

☐ Warn against indiscriminate use of plant materials of unknown toxicity, including wild mushrooms.

References

Bruce M, Lader M. (1989). Caffeine abstention in the management of anxiety disorders. *Psychol Med, 19,* 211–214.

Curatolo PW, Robertson D. (1983). Health consequences of caffeine. *Ann Intern Med, 98,* 641–649.

Fackelmann KA. (1989). Drug slows Parkinson's progress. *Science News, 136,* 84.

Greenburg J, Bower B. (1987). Caffeine jolt for ECT. *Science News, 131,* 328.

King A, Krumlovsky F. (1986). Cafergot substitution for Carafate (letter). *N Engl J Med, 314,* 1642.

Marijuana mangles memory. (1989). *Science News, 136,* 332.

Marijuana: Rough stuff. (1988). *Harvard Medical School Health Letter, 14*(1), 5.

Mrazik MJ, Mrazik T. (1991). Drug hot line: Easing cocaine withdrawal. *Nursing 91, 21*(2), 77.

Oei. (1989). Fetal arrhythmia caused by excessive intake of caffeine by pregnant women. *Br Med J, 298,* 568.

When cocaine use is double jeopardy. (1989). *RN, 52* (8), 71.

Bibliography

*Acee AM, Smith D. (1987). Crack. *American Journal of Nursing, 87,* 614–617.

Arnaud M. (1987). The pharmacology of caffeine. *Prog Drug Res, 31,* 273.

Aro A, et al. (1987). Boiled coffee increases serum low density lipoprotein concentration. *Metabolism, 36,* 1027.

Bartels A. (1988). The effects of cocaine. *Nursing 88, 18*(2), 82.

Blake GJ. (1988). Drug news: Synthetic marijuana for chemotherapy patients. *Nursing 88, 18*(3), 21.

Bower B. (1989). Drug delays Parkinson's progression. *Science News, 136,* 365.

Bower B. (1988). Stepping out of social phobias. *Science News, 133,* 331.

Bower B. (1987). Parkinson's protection? *Science News, 131,* 359.

Bower B. (1986). Steady cocaine use linked to seizures. *Science News, 130,* 214.

Chocolate without guilt. (1986). *University of California, Berkeley, Wellness Letter 2*(5), 1–2.

Clementz G, Dailey J. (1988). Psychotropic effects of caffeine. *Am Fam Physician 37,* 167.

Complex courier delivers dopamine. (1983). *Science News, 123,* 249.

Cowen R. (1990). Cocaine and the nervous system. *Science News, 137,* 238.

Cowen R. (1990). Probing cocaine in the heart and the brain. *Science News, 137,* 406–407.

Cowen R. (1989). Receptor encounters. *Science News, 136,* 248–250.

Dubiel D. (1990). Action STAT! Cocaine overdose. *Nursing 90, 20*(3), 33–35.

FDA OKs marijuana drug. (1985). *American Journal of Nursing, 85,* 951.

Geller E, Ritvo ER, Freeman BJ, Yuwiller A. (1982). Preliminary observations on the effect of fenfluramine on blood serotonin and symptoms in three autistic boys. *N Engl J Med, 307,* 165–169.

*House MA. (1990). Cocaine. *Am J Nurs, 90*(4), 41–45.

Important brain proteins synthesized. (1983). *Science News, 123,* 236.

*In the case of ritalin, more is NOT better. (1985). *American Journal of Nursing, 85,* 526.

Isner JM, Estes NA 3d, Thompson PD, Costanzo-Nordin MR, Subramanian R, Miller G, Katsos G, Sweeney K,

Sturner WQ. (1986). Acute cardiac events temporarily related to cocaine. *N Engl J Med, 315,* 1438–1443.

Jacques J, Snyder N. (1991). Newborn victims of addiction. *RN, 54*(4k), 47–51.

Jefferson J. (1988). Lithium tremor and caffeine intake: Two cases of drinking less and shading more. *J Clin Psychiatry, 49,* 72–73.

Lacroix A, et al. (1987). Does coffee contribute to heart disease? *RN, 50*(7), 66.

Levy G, Hickey JV. (1991). Fighting the battle against drugs. *RN, 54*(4), 44–47.

Lovallo W, et al. (1989). Caffeine may potentiate adrenocortical stress responses in hyper-tension-prone men. *Hypertension, 14,* 170.

Marijuana mangles memory. (1989). *Science News, 136,* 332.

Marijuana: Rough stuff. (1988). *Harvard Medical School Health Letter 14*(1), 5.

Myers M. (1988). Effects of caffeine on blood pressure. *Arch Intern Med, 148,* 1189–1193.

National Institute of Mental Health. (1986). *Useful information on phobias and panic.* Rockville, MD: Department of Health and Human Services.

Newcombe P, et al. (1988). High-dose caffeine and cardiac rate and rhythm in normal subjects. *Chest, 94,* 900–994.

Schairer C, Brinton LA, Hoover RN. (1986). Methylxanthines and benign breast disease. *Am J Epidemiol, 124,* 603–611.

Silberner J. (1987). Cocaine cardiology: Problems, mysteries. *Science News, 131,* 69.

*Smith J. (1988). The dangers of prenatal cocaine use. *Matern Child Nurs J, 13,* 174.

Smits P, et al. (1987). Coffee and the human cardiovascular system. *Neth J Med, 31,* 36.

Suspended THA trials are on again. (1988). *Science News, 133,* 284.

Tarlotta D, Lisanti P. (1989). Countering Parkinson's assault on your patient's will. *RN, 52*(11), 34.

Tenant F, et al. (1987). Double-blind comparison of amantadine and bromocriptine for ambulatory withdrawal from cocaine dependence. *Arch Intern Med, 147,* 109–112.

Toubas PL, Duke JC, McCaffree MA, Mattice CD, Bendell D, Orr WC. (1986). Effects of maternal smoking and caffeine habits on infantile apnea: A retrospective study. *Pediatrics, 78,* 159–163.

*Vandegaer F. (1989). Cocaine: The deadliest addiction. *Nursing 89, 19*(2), 72–73.

Weiss R. (1988). Alzheimer's aging and acetylcholine. *Science News, 134,* 350.

*Recommended for further reading.

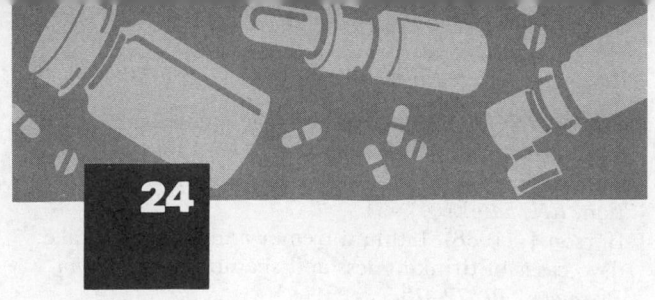

24

Central nervous system depressants

Drugs that depress the central nervous system (CNS) tend to reduce general body activities. A slowing of psychomotor functions occurs in mild sedation. Decreased alertness, apathy, lethargy, sleep, and coma occur in succession as CNS depression increases. Vital functions such as heart rate, circulation, respiration, and metabolism are slowed with deep sedation.

Some drugs affect specific functions before general depression becomes apparent. These drugs produce tranquility, analgesia, skeletal-muscle relaxation, or amnesia. Such drugs are selective at lower doses, but depression becomes more generalized as doses increase. At toxic levels, all CNS depressants tend to produce coma, cardiovascular collapse, respiratory arrest, and death.

Certain depressant drugs appear to act initially as stimulants, because they first affect the inhibitory functions of the brain. For example, alcohol initially depresses the limbic system and forebrain. This action decreases learned inhibitions, foresight, and judgment. If the recipient has impulses toward "unacceptable" behavior, the elimination of forebrain control may result in acting out that behavior. For this reason, some people become overactive, hostile, garrulous, or otherwise increasingly active when a few alcoholic drinks have been taken. As intoxication progresses, activity levels decline, and stupor may appear.

CNS depressants include drugs classified as anesthetics, analgesics, sedatives, hypnotics, anticonvulsants, and tranquilizers. Combinations of depressant drugs are often synergistic. For example, tranquilizers and analgesics in combination provide more relief from pain than either does alone. Analgesics potentiate the action of hypnotics when pain is a factor in sleeplessness. CNS depressants are indispensable agents for anesthesia during surgery, the alleviation of pain, and the control and treatment of many other clinical states (Boxes 24-1 and 24-2).

CNS depressants are major drugs of abuse. Dependency on opiates, barbiturates, and alcohol are major public health problems in many countries. The distribution and use of depressant drugs are strictly controlled in most parts of the world.

Anesthetics

Anesthesia is a state of insensibility or loss of sensation, especially the sensation of pain. Although this state can be achieved through other means (hypnosis, hypothermia, or acupuncture), anesthetic drugs are the primary agents used in modern western medicine (Box 24-3).

The pain experience provides essential protection to the organism by warning of harmful influences or processes in the environment or within the body and by motivating the individual to eliminate them. Pain sensation involves stimulation of pain receptors, transmission of impulses to the CNS, modification of these impulses by certain central structures (the substantia gelatinosa, thalamus, and frontal lobe), and interpretation of the resulting nerve tissue activity by the cortex to produce a characteristic perception (see Chapter 20 for a more detailed description of pain).

Drugs can eliminate the pain experience by interrupting the pain impulse before it reaches the CNS or by rendering the person unconscious. The pain experience may be further ameliorated by reducing the anxiety that makes the pain impulse more disturbing or by eliminating memory of past pain (amnesia). Interruption of the peripheral pain impulse prevents both physiologic and psychological effects of pain. Interference with consciousness alone does not prevent autonomic and hormonal responses to this stressor, because the pain impulse continues to influence subcortical brain processes.

The advent of anesthesia was a great impetus to the practice of surgery. Before the discovery of the first anesthetics (nitrous oxide and ether), surgery was limited to procedures that could be completed quickly. Although pain could be blunted by the use of alcohol or opium, the physical and psychic trauma of surgery could be endured for only a short time. Speed was a major criterion for successful surgery. Humanitarian concern was not the only reason for time restrictions. Clients subjected to lengthy procedures did not progress well postoperatively. We now know that acute stress, such as severe pain, induces hormonal changes in the body that disturb fluid and electrolyte balance, decrease resistance to infection, and delay healing. Most of the surgical procedures performed today would not be possible without the control of pain that modern anesthesia affords.

Anesthetic drugs are of two types: general and local (or regional). General anesthetics abolish perception of all sensations and render the client unconscious. Local anesthetics eliminate pain from a part of the body without affecting wakefulness. The affected area feels numb because sensation of heat, cold, and light pressure are also eliminated. Sensitivity to heavy pressure and motor function may or may not remain.

Whether anesthesia is local or general, the recipient needs protection from injury during this period. The degree of protection needed and the duration of the vulnerable period are directly related to the number of physiologic functions that have been interrupted by the anesthetic drug. Effects may include insensitivity to pressure, immobility, and depression of vital functions, such as respiration and circulation (Box 24-4 and 24-5).

General anesthetics

Drugs capable of producing general anesthesia include inorganic gases, hydrocarbons, ethers, and barbiturates (Table 24-1). The degree to which they

Box 24-4. Points of interest concerning pain and drugs

1. The pain experience provides protection to the organism
2. Pain sensation involves
   - Stimulation of pain receptors
   - Transmission of impulses to the CNS
   - Modification of these impulses by certain structures
   - Interpretation of resulting nerve–tissue activity by the cortex to produce pain perception
3. Drugs eliminate pain by
   - Interrupting the pain impulse before it reaches the CNS
   - Rendering the client unconscious
4. Additionally, drugs decrease response to pain by
   - Reducing anxiety
   - Eliminating memory of past pain

Box 24-5. Definitions

Anesthesia: a state of insensibility or loss of sensation, especially the sensation of pain

General anesthesia: a rapid loss of consciousness without permanent damage or immediate risk of death

Local anesthesia: elimination of sensation in a limited area of the body due to interference with impulse transmission in peripheral or spinal cord nerves

induce analgesia and relaxation vary, but all are descending CNS depressants that alter the level of consciousness. A general anesthetic should induce rapid loss of consciousness without causing permanent damage or risk of death. The ideal drug would be safe for all occupants of the surgical suite and would be effective and pleasant for the client.

Anesthetics that are chemically unstable are dangerous. They tend to be flammable, explosive, and also corrosive to structural materials used in the equipment for administration. Compatibility with catecholamines is important for two reasons: anxiety or fright elevates catecholamine levels in most surgical clients, and catecholamine medication may be needed during surgery to stimulate vital functions.

Anesthesia deep enough to produce skeletal-muscle relaxation is required for surgical access to deep organs and tissues. Rapid response to changes in dosage is desirable because it allows easy control of the depth of anesthesia.

Of particular concern for reasons of safety are an anesthetic's propensity to depress vital functions or induce cardiac arrhythmia. Some anesthetics in combination with catecholamine stress hormones pose a high risk of cardiac arrest. Agents that produce a rapid pleasant induction are desirable as they prevent pronounced emotional reactions that can disturb hormonal and nervous status.

Inhalant anesthetics should be nonirritating to the mucous membranes so as to limit stimulation of respiratory secretions, which can obstruct breathing.

Injectable drugs should not induce phlebitis or damage other tissues. Any tendency to promote capillary bleeding increases blood loss during surgery.

Anesthetic drugs vary somewhat in their properties and physiologic effects (Table 24-2). None is ideal. Agents are chosen to provide the characteristics most critical to a given situation: the status of the individual to be treated, the operative procedure, and the expected duration of surgery. Often a combination of agents is employed to achieve the best balance of efficacy and safety. The depth of anesthesia and the degree of muscle relaxation needed for different stages of surgery vary, requiring adjustments in the dosage of the drugs used for anesthesia. In addition, analgesics, sedatives, tranquilizers, and other pharmacologic agents are employed as adjuncts to promote the effectiveness of anesthetic agents or to counteract their undesired effects.

Pharmacodynamics. The mechanism of action of most anesthetics is unknown. Some drugs (ethers, al-

Table 24-1. Chemical nature of common general anesthetics

Chemical	Example(s)	State
Inorganic gases	Xenon, nitrous oxide	Gaseous
Hydrocarbons		
Straight chain	Ethylene	Gaseous
Cyclic	Cyclopropane	Gaseous
Halogenated hydrocarbons	Divinyl ether, methoxyflurane	Volatile liquid
Barbiturates	Thiopental	Solid

Table 24-2. Representative general anesthetics

Drug name	Preparations	Additional information
Inhalant anesthetics		
methoxyflurane (Penthrane)	Liquid in bottles	Nonflammable and nonexplosive in anesthetic concentrations
		Induction is slow and associated with excitement
		Recovery period is prolonged
		Light planes of anesthesia have little effect on uterine contractions
		High doses can cause liver and kidney damage
halothane (Fluothane)	Liquid in unit packages PC: C	Nonflammable and nonexplosive
		Used to maintain anesthesia after induction
		Provides moderate muscle relaxation
		Not recommended for obstetrical anesthesia except when uterine relaxation is required
		Can cause hepatotoxicity
		Is suspected of being teratogenic; increased incidence of interrupted pregnancies and birth defects among operating-suite staff members has been reported where halothane is used frequently
nitrous oxide ("laughing gas")	Liquid under pressure in steel cylinders	Produces analgesia and decreased reflexes
		Nonflammable but supports combustion
		Associated with hypoxia; oxygen given during and after anesthesia
Intravenous anesthetics		
thiopental sodium (Pentothal, "truth serum")	Powder for preparing solutions for IV injection PC: C	May precipitate acute neurologic signs and symptoms in clients with low reserves of vitamin B_{12} (Schilling, 1986)
		Used for induction or light general anesthesia
		Rapid induction
		Pleasant emergence with little nausea
propofol (Diprivan)	Ampules containing solution for IV administration PC: D	Rapid onset of action
		Short duration of action
		Relatively little nausea and vomiting during recovery
		Safety during pregnancy or parturition is not established
		Contraindicated for clients with increased intracranial pressure or decreased cerebral circulation
		Reduced dosages required for elderly, debilitated, or hypovolemic clients
		Reduced dosages required when other CNS depressants are used
Rectal anesthetics		
paraldehyde	Liquid for rectal administration PC: C	Possesses sedative and anticonvulsant properties
		Useful for alcoholics, psychotics, and extremely apprehensive candidates for surgery
		Absorption may be variable

KEY: PC = pregnancy category. (The validity of pregnancy categories has not been established; see Chapter 16, p 216.)

dehydes, halogenated hydrocarbons) are potent in proportion to their lipid solubility. They may alter the nerve cell membrane in such a way as to inhibit impulse transmission. Different classes of drugs probably act in different ways. It has been theorized that some anesthetics interfere with biochemical processes such as oxidation, phosphate uptake, and synthesis of adenosine-triphosphate and acetylcholine. Why interruptions of such fundamental cell processes fail to cause permanent harm to tissues has not been explained. Investigation continues into the molecular processes involved in anesthesia; it is hoped that an explanation of these processes will emerge in the near future. In the meantime, the drugs continue to be used on an empirical basis.

A considerable amount is known about the effects of anesthetic agents. Depression of nervous tissue progresses in a generally descending order, affecting cortical and higher brain functions before the lower functions. Vital centers in the medulla are usually spared longest. Progressive nervous system depression during anesthesia has been categorized into stages (Table 24-3). Progression through these stages is a continuous process; abrupt changes or physiologic landmarks do

Table 24-3. Characteristics of the stages of anesthesia

| Physiologic effects | Stage I | Stage II | Stage III planes | | | | Stage IV |
			1	2	3	4	
Consciousness	Present Altered perceptions Analgesia Euphoria Amnesia	Absent	Absent	Absent	Absent	Absent	Absent
Skeletal muscles	Normal tone	Increased tone	Small muscle relaxation	Large muscle relaxation	Complete relaxation	Complete relaxation	Flaccidity; diaphragmatic paralysis
Eyes							
Lacrimation	Increased with some agents			Decreased	Decreased	Absent	
Pupils	Normal reaction to light	Dilated	Constricted	Partially dilated	Partially dilated	Partially dilated	Full dilated
Movement	Normal	Increased	Increased	Absent	Absent	Absent	Absent
Reflexes							
Lid	Present	Present	Absent	Absent	Absent	Absent	Absent
Corneal	Present	Present	Present	Absent	Absent	Absent	Absent
Pharyngeal	Present	Present	Absent	Absent	Absent	Absent	Absent
Laryngeal	Present	Present	Present	Absent	Absent	Absent	Absent
Cough	Present	Present	Present	Present	Absent in large bronchi	Absent in small bronchi	Absent
Cutaneous	Present	Present	Present to absent	Absent	Absent	Absent	Absent
Respirations	Normal or somewhat increased and irregular	Rapid, irregular	Deep and regular	Regular, expirations longer than inspirations	Shallow	Depressed	Absent
Cardiovascular function							
Heart rate	Unchanged	Increased	Decreased	Decreased	Decreased	Decreased	Decreased to absent
Blood pressure	Normal	Increased	Normal	Normal	Decreased	Decreased	Decreased to absent
Venous pressure	Normal	Increased	Normal	Normal	Normal	Normal	Increased initially

not always signal transition from one stage to another. Modern techniques of induction move the client so rapidly through stages 1 and 2 that these changes may be imperceptible. Planes 2 and 3 of stage 3 are preferred for most surgical procedures. As plane 3 deepens, the risk increases of entering stage 4, life-threatening toxicity.

Pharmacokinetics. General anesthetics may be administered intravenously (IV), rectally, or by inhalation. Absorption by the IV or inhalation routes is rapid and dependable. Absorption from the rectal mucosa is less reliable. Once in the bloodstream, anesthetics rapidly affect the brain, inducing loss of consciousness. At the same time, the movement of drugs into tissue depots causes a gradual drop in plasma concentration. This redistribution lowers CNS concentration, necessitating repeated doses to maintain the proper level of anesthesia. Most drugs are stored in fatty tissues; thiopental is also bound by plasma albumin. The greater the duration of surgery, the greater the saturation of such tissue depots. When dosage is discontinued and plasma levels of free drug decline, stored drug redistributes into the blood, prolonging the duration of anesthesia.

Volatile anesthetics are eliminated mainly by the respiratory tract. About 15% is metabolized by the liver microsomal enzymes. Thiopental is largely metabolized by the liver; the remainder is excreted by the kidneys.

Therapeutic uses. Anesthetics are used principally to control pain and to promote relaxation during surgical procedures. They are also employed to alleviate pain during labor and delivery and to terminate refractory convulsive seizures.

Anesthetics are often used in combination with oxygen, muscle relaxants, analgesics, and other anesthetic agents. A typical drug regimen may include any or all of the following drugs:

A hypnotic to promote sleep the night before surgery

Premedication by administration of an opioid, anticholinergic, and/or tranquilizer

Induction by a rapid-acting general anesthetic (often IV thiopental)

A mixture of agents to maintain anesthesia

Skeletal muscle relaxants

Additional analgesia when weakly analgesic anesthetics are employed

In addition, oxygen is administered to maintain oxygenation of tissue, and a variety of agents may be employed to control vital functions and to counteract adverse reactions to drug agents or surgical trauma.

Adverse reactions. General anesthesia carries with it a small but definite risk of death or permanent disability. The margin of safety for most agents is relatively narrow; toxic doses are sometimes only two to four times those required for therapeutic effect. Acute reactions to general anesthetics include cardiac arrest, anaphylaxis, and irreversible progression through the stages of anesthesia to cardiovascular collapse and respiratory arrest.

Anesthetics tend to decrease respiratory and cardiac function. They may elevate or depress blood pressure. By irritating local tissues, agents administered by inhalation stimulate respiratory secretions and predispose to laryngospasm. Some drugs increase tissue sensitivity to catecholamines. A few stimulate excitation during induction or delirium during emergence. Muscle pains, nausea, vomiting, and inhibition of peristalsis may also occur postoperatively.

Complications of general anesthesia include atelectasis, aspiration pneumonia, urine retention, paralytic ileus, and liver or kidney damage. Hypersensitive or anaphylactic reactions can occur in allergic clients. Malignant hyperpyrexia may develop rapidly when halogenated agents are administered to genetically predisposed people. Anesthetics also interact with many other pharmacologic agents in unfavorable ways (Table 24-4).

Precautions and contraindications. A discussion of all medical conditions that require special consideration in the choice or administration of general anesthetics is beyond the scope of this book. It is the responsibility of the anesthesiologist or anesthetist to screen the client for such factors and to plan anesthesia accordingly. Before surgery, a complete evaluation is made

Table 24-4. Examples of drug interactions that involve general anesthetics

Interacting drugs	Adverse reaction
Adrenergics (with halothane and cyclopropane)	Increased risk of cardiac arrhythmia including cardiac arrest
Hormone (oxytocin)	Vasoconstriction and myocardial ischemia
Antihypertensives	Bradycardia, hypotension, and impaired circulation
Opioids, tranquilizers (and other CNS depressants)	Exaggerated CNS depression, hypotension, respiratory depression
Electrolyte (lithium)	Prolongation of muscle relaxation

to identify conditions such as infection; disease of the respiratory, cardiovascular, or renal systems; or endocrine abnormalities that increase the risk of surgery. Chest x-ray, complete blood cell count, chemical profile, urinalysis, and electrocardiogram are common tests carried out for this purpose. Together with a complete history and physical examination, including knowledge of allergies, these procedures provide a comprehensive data base for evaluating the client (Table 24-5).

General anesthetics are not administered to clients with marginal respiratory function, severe anemia, or serious cardiac conditions unless an emergency situation exists. Every effort is made to stabilize the client's condition, to eliminate infectious disease, and to promote a high level of health before surgery is attempted. Among the factors that may indicate the need to modify plans for anesthesia are prior use of drugs that interact with anesthetics, pregnancy, a morbid fear of death, or a personal or family history of malignant hyperpyrexia.

Because of the complexities of modern balanced anesthesia, the administration of general anesthetics is reserved for specially trained physicians or nurses. These highly skilled professionals have the expertise to select appropriate drug agents, operate the complicated machinery used for administration, monitor the client's condition, and intervene when necessary to prevent or terminate adverse reactions to treatment. They have primary responsibility for the client's safety and comfort during surgical procedures.

■ **Summary**

General anesthetics are systemic drugs that prevent or alleviate pain by reducing the level of consciousness. They are used to prevent pain during surgery, reduce the discomfort of labor and delivery, and terminate refractory seizures. They have a narrow margin of safety, tending

Table 24-5. Factors that increase the risk of general anesthesia

Risk factor	Nature of the increased risk
Obesity	Need for increased dosage of anesthetic due to large deposits of fat for drug storage; delayed emergence from anesthesia; decreased vital capacity; difficulty in ambulating postoperatively
Habitual use of alcohol	Cross-tolerance to anesthetic agents that increase dosage requirements for anesthetics and analgesics
Smoking	Impairment of respiration and circulation that increases risk of poor vital function during and after anesthesia; inflammation of lung tissues that increases risk of respiratory obstruction during anesthesia
Diabetes	Increased likelihood of cardiovascular deterioration and circulatory problems during anesthesia; abnormal blood sugar levels increase risk of CNS malfunction during anesthesia
Respiratory infection	Increased risk of respiratory impairment during anesthesia
Excessive fear	Increased risk of cardiac arrhythmia leading to ventricular fibrillation
Use of glucocorticoids within previous 3 months	Adrenal atrophy that reduces ability of body to withstand stress; tendency toward hypotension.

to produce hypotension, circulatory collapse, and respiratory arrest.

A combination of pharmacologic agents is commonly used to produce a balanced anesthesia characterized by adequate analgesia and muscle relaxation. Because safe administration of anesthetics requires special preparation and training, the practice of anesthesiology is reserved to physicians with specialty training and to certified nurse-anesthetists.

Nursing management

Nursing implications

Exposure to anesthetics is an occupational hazard for nurses and other health care professionals who work in operating suites. Despite the use of closed anesthetic delivery and scavenger ventilation systems, present practice does not prevent vaporous anesthetics from contaminating the ambient air in operating and recovery rooms. These gases are absorbed by health care personnel in the area. In addition, skin contact with at least one anesthetic (halothane) increases exposure because the anesthetic diffuses through the skin. Studies have shown detectable blood levels of nitrous oxide and halothane in operating room personnel that persisted for at least 2 days after exposure (Mattia, 1983).

Such occupational exposure is not innocuous. Operating room personnel experience increased incidence of spontaneous abortion, stillbirths, low-birth-weight babies, birth defects (particularly defects in the cardiovascular and musculoskeletal systems), myeloneuropathy, interference with vitamin B_{12} metabolism, cancer, and hepatic and renal diseases. In addition, halothane is linked to elevated serum bromide levels. Chronic exposure to nitrous oxide may alter hormonal cycles and impair fertility (Flam, 1989). Moreover, the immediate effects of subanesthetic

levels of anesthetic gas cause a slowing of response time and a decrease of recent memory (Mattia, 1983). Acute exposure to anesthetics may also cause lethargy, dizziness, fatigue, and nausea.

Scavenger ventilating systems are important safeguards for recovery rooms, as well as for operating suites. Nurses who care for clients who have received general anesthetics should avoid inhaling the vapors exhaled by clients. Time spent in close proximity to the client's head should be kept to a minimum. For optimum reproductive safety, acute care facilities should encourage female staff members of child-bearing age to transfer temporarily from the operating room or recovery room to other less hazardous work areas before planned pregnancies are begun or, if unplanned, as soon as pregnancy is suspected.

Nursing process for preoperative care

Assessment The client who is to undergo general anesthesia must be carefully appraised for factors that increase the risk of this procedure (see Table 24-5). The nursing history should include information about previous responses to anesthetics and information about diseases that might cause complications (*eg,* poor nutritional status, obstructive airway disease, cardiovascular conditions, diabetes, porphyria, myasthenia gravis, liver or renal disease, and allergies). The drug history should describe allergies to drugs, as well as the use of prescription, nonprescription, social, and illegal drugs. Specific inquiries should be made about the use of glucocorticoids within the preceding 3 months and tobacco or alcohol consumption. All drugs used within the preceding 2 weeks should be listed. Of particular importance are hormones (insulin, cortisone, estrogens), antibiotics, sedatives, cardiovascular drugs, sympathomimetics, and psychotropics.

Clients should be examined for signs and symptoms of infection of the skin, respiratory tract, and urinary tract. Cardiovascular assessment should rule out abnormalities; vital signs are recorded to provide a baseline for comparison with postoperative values. The client's emotional state and stress level should also be evaluated.

In addition, the nurse should determine the client's knowledge of and experience with surgery and anesthesia.

Nursing diagnosis Nursing diagnoses for the preoperative period may include the following:

> *Anxiety related to impending surgery*
> *High risk for injury related to dizziness and weakness secondary to depressant medication*
> *High risk for altered comfort: nausea or dizziness related to reaction to depressant medication*
> *Knowledge deficit concerning surgery and anesthesia*

Planning Goals of treatment include reducing anxiety, reducing the risk of cardiac arrest during surgery, preventing injury, preventing or ameliorating nausea, and educating the client about surgery and anesthesia.

Intervention Risk factors for adverse reaction to surgery and medications should be drawn to the attention of the physician. In particular, verbal expressions of premonitions about the outcome of surgery must be reported and recorded. Preoperative medications usually include a hypnotic to promote sleep the evening before surgery, as well as a combination of narcotic analgesic and anticholinergic or tranquilizer to be given about 1 hour before surgery.

Before administering the hypnotic the night before surgery, the nurse should verify that the permission for surgery has been signed. Permissions executed after medication with a CNS depressant are not considered legally valid. In addition to administering the hypnotic, the nurse should use all possible nursing measures to promote rest. Because most clients are ambulatory before surgery, routinely scheduled care may not include nursing measures to promote sleep. However, a soothing back rub given after administration of the sedative enhances response to the drug and helps induce prompt sleep. Inadequate sleep causes fatigue on the day of surgery, which could increase the risk of surgery.

To minimize risk of injury, both the bedtime hypnotic and the preoperative medication are given after all other scheduled procedures have been completed. The client is settled in bed with the side rails up.

Supportive care must be continued on the day of surgery to prevent undue apprehension. The client should not be left alone. Family members or significant others should be encouraged to sit with the client when the nursing staff is not involved in direct care.

The preoperative medication is usually ordered to be given about 1 hour before inducing anesthesia. Timing of this medication is crucial, because the drugs' actions should coincide with anesthesia induction. Premature or delayed administration increases the difficulty of induction and the need for higher doses of the initial anesthetic. Delayed administration also increases the risk of CNS depression, because drug action then occurs after anesthesia is begun. To enhance the effect of the preoperative medication, stimuli should be reduced to a minimum after administration, and the client should be instructed to relax and rest.

Client education. Preoperative teaching is a critical part of preparing the client for the surgical procedure and eliminating apprehension. Most clients who are candidates for surgery need to know what to expect of the operating experience. When general anesthesia is used, clients are aware of the environment until induction has begun. The nurse should inform clients that premedication will make them drowsy before they are transported to the operating room and that an IV line will probably be established before surgery.

Older adults often are quite fearful of surgery because of their conditioning from a time when anesthesia deaths and other complications of surgery were more common. These clients should be reassured that recent developments in surgery have produced safer anesthetic agents and procedures and that the incidence of unpleasant or dangerous reactions has been reduced.

Preoperative teaching is critical to secure clients' cooperation with treatment procedures aimed at preventing complications of general anesthesia after surgery. Clients should practice deep breathing, coughing, turning, splinting, and maneuvers that promote comfort during ambulation.

The nurse should inform the client, in terms of the subjective experience, what to expect during the surgical experience. Clients should be informed about the usual postoperative regimens, including medication for pain relief. A scale for reporting pain (one that is familiar to the nursing staff) should be introduced (*eg*, numbers 1–5, with 1 representing slight pain and 5 representing excruciating pain). The client should be instructed to ask for pain medication early, instead of waiting for pain to become severe.

Clients who are particularly fearful of surgery should be shown the operating suite and introduced to staff members before the scheduled date of surgery. It is helpful to meet the nurse who will be assisting with the surgery. A familiar face in the operating room on the day of surgery can be reassuring. Children benefit from a rehearsal of the events before surgery. This can be done through play with dolls that represent the child and the operating staff. Reassurance is important; excessive levels of catecholamine stress hormones during surgery increase the risk of cardiac arrest and death from the anesthetic.

Clients should be cautioned to remain in bed with side rails up after medication with CNS depressants. They should request assistance from the health care staff if they need to get out of bed. Lying quietly in bed minimizes the risk of falling and the likelihood of nausea in response to narcotic medications. (Head movements tend to augment the stimulation to the CNS centers for nausea and vomiting that may occur after administration of narcotic analgesics.)

Evaluation Data required for evaluation include statements by clients that they are more relaxed or less apprehensive about the impending surgery and that they are (or are not) nauseated; and the absence or incidence of accidental injury from falling or cardiac arrest during anesthesia.

Nursing process during surgery

Assessment When clients arrive in the operating suite, they should be assessed for signs and symptoms of sympathetic nervous activity that reveal anxiety. Their level of consciousness and speech patterns should also be monitored to determine their degree of sedation. The chart should be checked for previous assessments of the client and for the time of preoperative medication. Signs and symptoms of adverse reaction to the preoperative medication should also be noted.

Nursing diagnosis Nursing diagnoses may include the following:

Anxiety related to surgery
High risk for ineffective breathing pattern related to CNS depression secondary to the combined effects of preoperative sedatives and general anesthetics
High risk for impaired tissue integrity related to prolonged pressure on dependent tissues secondary to positioning for surgery

A common collaborative problem that should be differentiated from the nursing diagnoses is

Potential complication: decreased cardiac output

Planning Goals of treatment include reducing anxiety, reducing the risk of adverse reactions to anesthesia, and reducing the risk of injury related to malpositioning.

Intervention Nursing care to minimize the stress response should continue in the operating room. Stimuli should be kept to a minimum. Expression of a warm personal concern for the client and competent execution of procedures provide continued reassurance.

If the preoperative medication was administered at a time other than ordered, or if the client seems unusually apprehensive, this fact should be drawn to the attention of the anesthetist. When the client is transferred from stretcher to operating table, excessive motion that can exacerbate nausea should be avoided. Until anesthesia has been induced, clients should be protected from stimulation that could reduce the level of sedation or increase apprehension.

If the client is positioned for surgery before induction, the nurse should verify that the position is completely comfortable. After anesthesia is induced, the client will be unable to complain of discomforts or pain from improper positioning. If positioning is delayed until after the client is unconscious, particular care should be taken to ensure proper body alignment and support.

When an IV agent is used for induction, the position of the needle within the blood vessel must be carefully checked. Improper placement in the extravascular tissues delays the effect of the drug and can cause tissue necrosis. During induction, the nurse should remember that hearing is the client's last function to be lost, and therefore the nurse should avoid talk that may be disturbing.

Once the client is under the influence of a general anesthetic, consciousness is lost, and total nursing care appropriate to this state is required. The unconscious person is completely helpless and vulnerable. Vital functions must be maintained, and the client must be protected from injury. In the operating suite, the primary responsibility for monitoring the status of the client and for maintenance of vital functions belongs to the anesthetist. However, all members of the health care team share in this responsibility.

Safety precautions in the operating room should include eliminating static electricity or other sources of sparks, which can ignite flammable anesthetics and cause an explosion within the client's lungs, as well as injury to others in the immediate vicinity. The operating suite is at high risk for fires because of the flammable substances and oxygen used in the area. The area should be well ventilated to minimize the risk of fire and to protect the health care staff from exposure to anesthetic drugs exhaled by the client.

Client education. When an IV agent is used for induction, clients should be warned that they will feel a slight stinging sensation at the IV site just before they lose consciousness. If a gaseous agent is used for induction, the client breathes through a mask just before losing consciousness. Children who receive a gaseous agent for induction may be told to "blow away the smell" to promote deep breathing and rapid induction.

Evaluation Data required for evaluation include client facial or verbal expressions that show apprehension or discomfort, absence or incidence of adverse reaction to anesthesia, absence or incidence of fire or explosion during surgery, and the course of recovery of the client from the anesthetic after surgery.

Nursing process during recovery from anesthesia

Assessment When the client is transferred to the recovery room, charting for the operative period should be complete. The anesthetist, surgeon, or nurse from the operating room should give a comprehensive verbal report to the recovery room nurse, stressing the client's current status, drugs administered during surgery, and any unusual occurrences during the surgery. The nurse must assess the client's respiratory and cardiovascular status, level of sedation, responses indicative of pain, and risk factors for postoperative complication, such as hemorrhagic shock, dehiscence, pneumonia, or intravascular thrombi.

Nursing diagnosis Nursing diagnoses may include the following:

High risk for inability to sustain spontaneous ventilation related to general anesthesia
High risk for injury related to altered level of consciousness (confusion, delirium) secondary to emergence from anesthesia
Impaired tissue integrity: delay in wound healing related to increased cortisone levels secondary to stress
Pain (incisional) related to surgical trauma
Altered comfort: thirst related to decreased oral intake of fluids and preoperative administration of anticholinergic agents
Altered comfort: nausea or vomiting related to emergence from anesthesia

Common collaborative problems that should be differentiated from the nursing diagnoses include:

Potential complication: hemorrhage
Potential complication: thrombus formation
Potential complication: hypokalemia, hypernatremia

Planning Goals of treatment include improved gas exchange, reorientation of the client on emergence from anesthesia, prevention of injury, maintenance of IV therapy, reduction in stress, increased comfort, and prevention of hemorrhage and thrombophlebitis or their prompt detection and treatment, should they develop.

Intervention The client must be carefully monitored after surgery to ensure that vital functions continue uninterrupted. Oxygen is frequently administered because respirations tend to be depressed, resulting in hypoxemia. This tendency is particularly important to consider if clients have received nitrous oxide, which predisposes them to hypoxia. Clients should be stimulated verbally to breathe deep to promote elimination of gaseous anesthetics and secretions from the lungs.

Under the influence of stress hormones, clients retain sodium and fluid, thus predisposing themselves to hypervolemia, hypertension, and hemorrhage. IV infusions are administered at flow rates that replace fluid losses but do not unduly raise blood pressure. To avoid disturbance of traumatized tissue, dressings are usually left undisturbed.

The nurse should reduce noxious stimuli (especially noise) and other stressors that impinge on the client. As much as possible, the emotional tone of the recovery room should be that of quiet competence.

Restlessness that persists in the well oxygenated client is most likely due to pain, which should be controlled by regular administration of analgesics. Liberal use of drugs prevents severe pain from developing, reassures clients that they are not expected to bear severe pain, reduces their stress, and results in greater analgesic effects with minimal drug use (see Chapter 20 for management of pain).

Some anesthetics are not potent analgesics, and the client may need pain relief before fully reacted. The drugs used for anesthesia must be reviewed to determine whether the dosage of depressant analgesics should be reduced. If the client is at all hypotensive, vital signs should be monitored closely at least every 5 minutes after administration of the analgesic. Hypotension that is due to pain should respond within a half hour after administration of the drug. If the blood pressure remains low, the anesthesiologist or surgeon should be notified.

Throughout this period, the nurse should monitor the client regularly for signs and symptoms of hemorrhage, shock, and respiratory infection. If any indications are present, the physician is notified promptly.

Client education. As clients become more alert, they are oriented to time and place and told that the surgery is over. They are reminded repeatedly to breathe deeply and, if allowed, to cough. They are also reminded to begin the postoperative regimens of turning and exercising that were taught before surgery.

Evaluation Data required for evaluation include the client's vital signs, color, energy level, rate of wound healing, physical signs of pain, statements by the client indicating the absence or alleviation of discomfort, the absence or incidence of hemorrhage or thrombophlebitis, and the speed with which these are detected and treated, if they develop.

Nursing process during the postoperative period

Assessment Assessment, nursing diagnoses, planning, intervention, and client education for the client after transfer from recovery room to nursing unit is similar to that required during transfer from operating room to recovery room. A joint review of the chart by recovery room nurse and unit nurse is accompanied by a verbal report of significant data. The receiving nurse should be informed of any unusual events during surgery and recovery, treatments in progress, drains and other equipment that remain in place, and amount and timing of pain medication since surgery. The unit nurse also examines the client immediately to determine vital signs, level of consciousness, signs and symptoms of pain, and signs and symptoms of other adverse reactions. As the effects of anesthesia wear off and throughout convalescence, nurses use the comprehensive data provided by the chart as a basis for continued care. Dietary and fluid intake, as well as urinary and fecal elimination, are assessed until normal function is reestablished. Nurses should be alert to signs and symptoms of pain or other discomfort. In addition, clients must be assessed daily to monitor healing and detect complications (particularly hemorrhage, wound infection, pneumonia, and thrombophlebitis).

Nursing diagnosis   In this period, most complications of surgery become evident. Clients may develop the following:

> *Altered urinary elimination related to immobility and residual effects of anesthesia*
> *Constipation related to immobility, lack of fiber, and residual effects of anesthesia*
> *Pain related to altered tissue integrity secondary to surgery*
> *Fluid volume deficit related to inability to drink*
> *Impaired physical mobility related to surgery*
> *Altered nutrition: less than body requirements related to inability to eat*
> *Self-care deficit related to surgery*

All clients are at

> *High risk for infection related to surgical wounds and high levels of catecholamine stress hormones*

Some clients may also have a

> *Knowledge deficit concerning the normal course of convalescence and measures they may take to promote recovery; or*
> *Ineffective management of therapeutic regimen related to knowledge deficit and social support deficits*

A common collaborative problem that should be differentiated from the nursing diagnoses is

> *Potential complication: dehiscence or evisceration*

Planning   Goals of treatment are improved nutrition and hydration, rapid wound healing, control of pain, and improved mobility. Personal care should be complete, with health care personnel administering care that the client is unable to manage. Prevention of surgical complications, prompt detection and treatment of any complications that may develop, and reduction in knowledge deficit related to convalescence are additional goals.

Intervention   IV fluids are administered to prevent fluid and electrolyte imbalance. Diet should be offered according to the schedule preferred by the physician and the client's tolerance. Nursing measures to encourage eating should be instituted. The client is encouraged, with assistance from the nurse, to ambulate progressively, as rapidly as possible. Personal care procedures that the client cannot manage are performed by the staff. Pain should be controlled as necessary with both nursing measures and medication. Strict aseptic technique is used when caring for the wound. The client should continue to be protected from stressors and is encouraged to verbalize concerns and problems so that the nurse can help resolve them. The family should resolve minor matters without involving the client during the immediate postoperative period. The client should be monitored throughout convalescence for signs and symptoms of complications.

Significant data should be recorded and reported promptly so that immediate corrective measures can be taken. Nursing measures alone may alleviate difficulties in elimination. Medical intervention is needed for complications such as infection, thromboemboli, or dehiscence. The nurse should develop and implement a plan for teaching the client the usual course of convalescence and self-care measures to promote recovery.

Evaluation   Data required for evaluation include records of fluid and food intake, urinary and fecal elimination, exercise, vital signs, and ability of the client to resume self-care. The condition of the wound should be noted daily. Requests by the client for pain medication and statements related to both physical and emotional comfort indicate subjective symptoms. The ability of the client to relate information conveyed during the teaching sessions or to demonstrate a technique taught is required to evaluate client teaching. The absence of complications implies the success of preventive measures; if complications develop, the speed with which they were detected and treated should be determined (see the Examples of Nursing Process and Preoperative Opioid Medication, Recovery from Surgical Anesthesia, and Postoperative Effects of CNS Depressants).

Checklist of nursing actions

☐ Throughout the perioperative period, protect clients from stressors and assist them in managing stress levels.

☐ Before surgery, assess clients for factors that increase the risk of adverse reactions to anesthesia.

Example of nursing process and preoperative opioid medication

The client is a 36-year-old woman who was admitted yesterday for an elective cholecystectomy. She is 5'5", weighs 205 pounds, and smokes ½ pack of cigarettes a day. She admits to social drinking ("a drink or two on a weekend night out"). Preoperative care the evening before included teaching her about the postoperative regimen and administering a sedative. She appears to be slightly apprehensive this morning, but states she slept well the night before. Preoperative medication is scheduled for 7:00 A.M. Her husband and sister are waiting to see her; they plan to be at the hospital as long as necessary.

Assessment data	Nursing diagnosis	Intervention	Goals and outcome criteria
Obesity Smoker (½ pack/day) Impending surgery	High risk for ineffective breathing pattern related to general anesthesia, history of smoking, and obesity	**Reinforce** the preoperative teaching of turning, coughing, and deep breathing. **Advise** the client to discontinue smoking, at least until after surgery.	The client will cough and breathe effectively postoperatively and will not develop hypoxia or pulmonary congestion.
Impending surgery	High risk for anxiety related to impending surgery	**Use** therapeutic communication to ascertain the degree of apprehension felt by the client. **Express** interest in and concern for the client. **Perform** procedures in a competent manner. Do not leave the client alone; invite the family to sit with the client when the preoperative procedures are completed.	The client will talk openly about her feelings concerning surgery. The client will appear more relaxed by the time the preoperative procedures are completed. The client will state that she "feels better" about the surgery.
Preoperative orders include administering an opioid medication	High risk for altered comfort: dizziness or nausea related to adverse reaction to opioid medication	**Advise** the client to lie quietly in bed after receiving the preoperative medication; advise the family to sit quietly with the client and encourage her to rest. When transporting the client to the operating room, avoid sudden turns that might cause motion sickness.	The client will not complain of nausea or dizziness.
Preoperative orders include administering an opioid medication	High risk for injury related to weakness or dizziness secondary to opioid medication	**Raise** the side rails and caution the client to remain in bed after receiving the preoperative medication.	The client will not fall or sustain injury.

- [ ] Teach preoperative clients what the experience of induction will involve.
- [ ] Teach preoperative clients about measures they can take to promote uncomplicated recovery from anesthesia.
- [ ] Alleviate undue apprehension by realistic reassurance about the safety of modern anesthesia; administer personalized concerned care.
- [ ] Promote rest and relaxation before surgery.
- [ ] Administer preoperative medication at the time ordered.
- [ ] Protect the anesthetized client from injury

Example of nursing process and recovery from surgical anesthesia

Surgery for the client described in the previous Nursing Process has been completed, and she has been transferred to the recovery room. Her vital signs are stable. An airway is in place, and clear fluids are running in an IV infusion. The dressing is dry and intact.

The client is unresponsive to stimuli. The anesthetist states that the client is not expected to react immediately, because the amount of anesthetic used was more than usual for the duration of the surgery.

Assessment data	Nursing diagnosis	Intervention	Goals and outcome criteria
High doses of anesthetic	High risk for impaired gas exchange related to central nervous system depression secondary to use of high doses of anesthetic	**Administer** oxygen as ordered. **Turn** the client at least q2h. **Use** Ambu bag to inflate the lungs periodically until the client begins to respond, at which time she should be stimulated to deep breathe and cough. **Splint** the client's incision when she is about to cough.	The client's color will remain pink; she will not develop cyanosis. The client will not become restless.
High doses of anesthetic	High risk for infection: pneumonia related to immobility and impaired breathing secondary to prolonged period of anesthesia	In addition to the interventions noted above, **suction** the client's upper breathing passages as necessary to remove secretions.	The client will not develop signs and symptoms of respiratory infection (fever, hyperpnea, cyanosis, rales.)
Prolonged period of anesthesia	High risk for peripheral neurovascular dysfunction	**Turn** the client at least q2h. Passively **exercise** the legs while the client is unresponsive. When the client responds, **stimulate** her to exercise the feet and legs as instructed preoperatively. **Do not elevate** the knee gatch of the client's bed or put pillows under her knees.	The client will not develop signs and symptoms of neurovascular dysfunction

and monitor closely for impairment of vital functions.

☐ Stimulate the client who is recovering from anesthesia to breathe deeply to promote excretion of gaseous anesthetic agents.

☐ Monitor postanesthesia clients for signs and symptoms of complications related to anesthesia.

☐ Avoid personal exposure to anesthetic gases exhaled by the anesthetized client.

☐ Encourage early ambulation postoperatively to minimize complications of anesthesia.

Local anesthetics

Local anesthesia is the elimination of sensation in a limited area of the body because of interference with impulse transmission in peripheral or spinal-cord nerves. Such a state is characterized by absence of pain in a circumscribed part of the body without loss of consciousness. Local anesthesia may be produced by a variety of forces, including mechanical trauma, low temperature, anoxia, and a variety of chemical agents. Anesthesia may be temporary or relatively permanent. Usually, a return to function is desirable within a short period of time (*eg*, after completion of a surgical pro-

Example of nursing process and postoperative effects of CNS depressants

Our same client described in the previous two Nursing Processes has been transferred from the recovery room to the surgical care unit. She is responsive to verbal stimuli but sleeps intermittently. Her blood pressure and pulse were within normal limits, but her respirations are 14/min. She lies quietly in bed and offers no complaints of pain.

 The client is unable to void; the edge of her bladder is palpable three fingers below the umbilicus.

Assessment data	Nursing diagnosis	Intervention	Goals and outcome criteria
Client lies quietly in bed Respirations 14/min High dose of anesthetic	High risk for infection: pneumonia related to immobility and hypopnea secondary to prolonged effect of anesthesia	**Stimulate** the client to cough and deep breathe at least 2h. Ambulate her as soon as she is alert.	The client will not develop signs and symptoms of pneumonia (fever, cough, cyanosis).
Inability to void Bladder palpable 3 fingers below the umbilicus High dose of anesthetic	Urinary retention related to nervous system depression secondary to prolonged anesthesia	**Use** all nursing measures to promote micturition. If none is effective, consult with the physician for an order for catheterization. If necessary, **catheterize** the client to empty the bladder.	The client's bladder will be emptied.

cedure). In certain clinical states (refractory pain), permanent anesthesia may be desired and may be accompanied by some degree of nerve damage.

An ideal drug for inducing temporary local anesthesia has the following properties:

- A wide margin of safety as shown by an absence of local tissue irritation, nerve or muscle damage, or systemic toxicity
- Effectiveness when administered topically or by injection
- Appropriate duration of effect as shown by a rapid onset of action, duration of action appropriate to the clinical use, and rapid elimination from the body when anesthesia is no longer required

Chemicals with local anesthetic properties generally contain in their molecules both hydrophilic amine and lipophilic (aromatic) structures. These are usually separated by an intermediate alkyl chain. Either an ester or amide linkage may join the aromatic group to the intermediate chain. The nature of this linkage influences both the properties of the drug and the mode of its deactivation within the body. Chemicals with local anesthetic properties are listed in Table 24-6. The guanidine structures are not used medicinally.

Pharmacodynamics. Most local anesthetics inhibit nerve impulses by impeding sodium influx across the cell membrane during depolarization. The drugs appear to compete with calcium for occupation of a receptor site on the internal surface of the cell membrane, which must be unoccupied to allow sodium influx to occur. During normal impulse transmission, calcium leaves its position on the receptor, thus opening the membrane sodium channel. The anesthetic receptor interaction results in a blockade of this sodium channel, preventing depolarization.

Interruption of sensory function in a nerve in response to these agents progresses in a definite order. The sensation of pain is usually the first to disappear, followed in order by cold, warmth, touch, and response to deep pressure. Motor function is last to be obliterated.

Pharmacokinetics. To reach their site of action (the neural membrane), local anesthetics must traverse the tissues that surround the nerve and penetrate in turn the epineurium, perineurium, and endoneurium, in addition to the connective tissue or myelin sheath that surrounds individual cells. The drugs are administered either topically or by injection, using a variety of routes (Table 24-7). Because only a local effect is desired, the spatial distribution of the drugs is critical. Penetration of soft tissues may be hastened by the addition of hyaluronidase (Wydase) to the drug solution. Systemic absorption may be delayed by various strategies, including the judicious use of tour-

Table 24-6. Chemicals with local anesthetic properties

Chemical	Source
Alcohol	Fermentation processes
Phenol	Chemical derivative of benzene
Amino-esters	
Cocaine	Leaves of the coca plant
Benzocaine	Chemical synthesis
Procaine	Chemical synthesis
Dibucaine	Chemical synthesis
Tetracaine	Chemical synthesis
Amino-amides	
Lidocaine	Chemical synthesis
Chloroprocaine	Chemical synthesis
Mepivacaine	Chemical synthesis
Prilocaine	Chemical synthesis
Bupivacaine	Chemical synthesis
Etidocaine	Chemical synthesis
Guanidine structures	
Tetrodotoxin	Tissues of the Japanese puffer fish
Saxitoxin	Tissues of marine dinoflagellates that cause "red tide" and shellfish in areas affected by red tide

niquets on extremities, the administration of vaso-constrictors in conjunction with the local anesthetic, or the positioning of the client to control migration of the drug by gravity flow. Eventually, all drugs do escape into the systemic circulation and are metabolically deactivated or excreted. Amino-ester drugs are degraded largely by a plasma enzyme, pseudocholinesterase, while amino-amide compounds are metabolized by liver enzymes. Excretion of both drugs and metabolites is primarily through the kidneys.

Therapeutic uses. Local anesthesia is used to eliminate pain during surgical procedures, especially when general anesthesia is considered unnecessary or unduly risky. It is often employed during nose and throat procedures and endoscopy. The drugs are applied topically for the relief of surface pain or itching. Intractable pain is treated by local anesthetics with relatively permanent effect. Representative agents are listed in Table 24-8.

Adverse reactions. Cocaine is atypical among the local anesthetics in that it acts as a CNS stimulant rather than depressant (see Chapter 23 for a discussion of the systemic effects of cocaine on the body).

Phenol is irritating to tissues; when administered in large amounts, or frequently, tissue damage may develop.

The effects of ester-amide and amino-amide anesthetics on conduction of impulses are not limited to pain fibers or peripheral nerves. Impulse transmission is reduced in the CNS, autonomic ganglia, smooth muscle, neuromuscular junction, and muscle fibers. For this reason, these agents can produce a variety of side effects when they are absorbed systemically.

In the CNS, inhibitory fibers may be depressed before other structures are affected, producing signs of paradoxical stimulation (restlessness, tremors, and clonic convulsions). If the drug levels continue to rise, depression follows, culminating in respiratory failure. When systemic concentration of these anesthetic agents rises rapidly, the "stimulation" phase may be fleeting or absent.

Blockade of neuromuscular junctions and ganglionic synapses varies with the preparation. Some compounds reduce release of acetylcholine by the motor nerve endings as well as impair impulse conduction. These drugs tend to antagonize physostigmine and add to the effects of curare.

Local anesthetics generally decrease the conduction rate, force of contraction, and electrical excitability of the myocardium. (Lidocaine and procainamide, a derivative of procaine, are used as antiarrhythmic drugs to suppress ectopic foci in the myocardium.) Depression of cardiac conduction and response by these agents tends to reduce cardiac output and can induce arrhythmia, including ventricular fibrillation. The drugs also promote arteriolar dilation by reducing sympathetic activity. Several anesthetics (benzocaine, lidocaine, procaine, and prilocaine) have caused methemoglobinemia. The combined effects on the cardiovascular system, especially when the drugs are inadvertently administered IV, can produce cardiovascular collapse or cardiac arrest.

Although the direct effect of these drugs on smooth muscle fibers is depression, paralysis of the sympathetic nervous system may cause a net increase in the tone of the gastrointestinal (GI) mucosa.

The side effects of local anesthetics are commonly manifested as nausea, vomiting, tachycardia, talkativeness, and syncope. When administered to clients who are taking β-adrenergic blockers, these drugs can produce a brief hypertensive crisis followed by a drop in heart rate or cardiac arrest (Brummett, 1984). Respiratory difficulties, shock, and convulsions can occur in severe reactions.

Allergic hypersensitivity is most common in relation to the ester-amide compounds. Reactions may be manifested by dermatitis, bronchoconstriction, or anaphylaxis. The latter can be fatal.

In a few people, local anesthetics fail to produce the desired blockade of pain impulses. This fact may be related to genetic factors that interfere with the drug's mechanism of action or that promote rapid breakdown of the drugs in the body.

(*Text continues on p. 419*)

Table 24-7. Routes for administration of local anesthetics

Route	Clinical uses	Effective agents	Advantage	Disadvantages
Topical				
Skin	Relieve skin irritations; initial anesthesia before infiltration	cocaine tetracaine dibucaine lidocaine	Limited systemic toxicity	Application and absorption are variable
Mucous membranes	Surface anesthesia before instrumentation or infiltration anesthesia			
Infiltration				
Extravascular (intradermal, subcutaneous)	Prevention of pain during dental procedures and minor surgery	procaine lidocaine prilocaine bupivacaine propoxycaine	Rapid onset of action	Prolonged use requires the use of vasoconstrictors
Intravascular (Bier's block)	Prevention of pain during surgery on the arm	procaine chloroprocaine lidocaine mepivacaine prilocaine bupivacaine etidocaine	Reduces dose of anesthetic required; analgesia disappears rapidly with termination of procedure	Produces tissue hypoxia and ischemic pain secondary to the use of occlusive tourniquets to delay absorption of the anesthetic
Peripheral nerve blockage (field block anesthesia)				
Minor nerve block (single nerve block)	Relief of pain and relaxation of the extremities, anterior abdominal wall, or neck	procaine lidocaine mepivacaine prilocaine	Less drug required and greater area of anesthesia than infiltration anesthesia	Motor function is usually eliminated
Major nerve block (multiple nerve or nerve plexus block)	Relief of pain and relaxation of the extremities, anterior abdominal wall, or neck	bupivacaine etidocaine tetracaine	Minor nerve block; rapid onset of activity Major nerve block; long duration of analgesia	Short duration of effect of minor nerve block Slow onset of action of major nerve block
Spinal subarachnoid				
Blockade	Surgery on the lower extremities, lower abdomen, and pelvis	tetracaine procaine lidocaine	More rapid onset than epidural administration; area of anesthesia more readily controlled than with epidural administration	Shorter duration of action than with epidural administration
Central neural blockade (epidural/peridural anesthesia)				
Cervical	Rarely used medicinally	procaine chloroprocaine lidocaine mepivacaine		
Thoracic	Relief of pain after thoracic or upper abdominal surgery			
Lumbar	Adjunct in surgery of the lower abdomen, pelvis, perineum, lower extremities, and in obstetrical procedures	prilocaine tetracaine bupivacaine etidocaine	Longer duration of action than with spinal	Slower onset than spinal anesthesia; area of anesthesia less readily controlled than with spinal anesthesia
Caudal	Pelvic and perineal surgery and vaginal deliveries			

Table 24-8. Representative drugs used medicinally to produce local anesthesia

Drug name	Preparations	Therapeutic uses	Usual dosage	Additional information
Topical anesthetics				
Esters				
benzocaine (Anbesol, Americaine, Hurricaine, Ora-Jel, Rid-A-Pain)	Oral lozenges, gels, solutions, and otic solutions for topical use	Relief of pain that arises from skin or mucous membrane inflammation	Apply q1–2h as needed, for a maximum of 2 days if self-administered	Benzocaine is often added to over-the-counter preparations.
butacaine (Butyn)	Topical ointment	Temporary relief of denture pain	Apply topically as needed (effects persist for about 1 h)	Local allergic reactions may occur, requiring discontinuation of the drug.
cocaine	Topical solutions Crystals and tablets for preparing topical solutions	Surface anesthesia, before superficial surgical procedures or injection of parenteral anesthetics	Dependent on area and vascularity of tissue to be anesthetized and individual tolerance; *maximum single dose:* 1 mg/kg body weight	Cocaine is not recommended for injection or ophthalmic use.
Amides				
dibucaine (Nupercaine)	Ointment, jelly, and cream for topical (including rectal) use	Temporary relief of pain and itching of the skin Temporary relief of pain and itching caused by hemorrhoids	Adults: *Maximum dosage:* 1 oz of 1% ointment (containing 300 mg dibucaine)/day Children: ¼ oz of 1% ointment (containing 75 mg dibucaine)/day	Dibucaine is added to some over-the-counter preparations. Dibucaine is one of the most potent and toxic of local anesthetics
Miscellaneous				
cyclomethycaine (Surfacaine)	Cream, jelly, and ointment for topical or urogenital use	Relief of pain and itching of the skin Surface anesthesia of the nose, throat, urethra, rectum, or vagina	Adults: *Maximum dosage:* 30 ml of 0.75% jelly (containing 22.5 g of cyclomethycaine)/12 h	A transient stinging or burning sensation sometimes occurs before the onset of anesthesia.
dyclonine (Dyclone)	Topical solutions	Surface anesthesia before superficial surgical procedures or injection of parenteral anesthetics	Dependent on area and vascularity of tissue to be anesthetized and individual tolerance; Adults: 200 mg; *maximum dose:* 30 ml of 1% solution (300 mg) PC: C	Adverse reactions from systemic toxicity include CNS and cardiovascular malfunction.
phenol (Carbolic acid)	Solution for topical application to the skin	Relief of skin irritations	1% solution applied at intervals of at least 3 h	Phenol is added to some over-the-counter skin preparations. Repeated application may cause painless burns.
pramoxine (Perifoam, proctoFoam, tronolane, tronothane)	Cream, aerosol foam, and suppositories for rectal use Cream, jelly, and aerosol foam for topical use	Relief of pain and itching associated with inflammation of the skin or rectal mucosa	Apply q3–4h PRN	The aerosol container is never inserted into the anus.

(Continued)

Table 24-8. Representative drugs used medicinally to produce local anesthesia (*Continued*)

Drug name	Preparations	Therapeutic uses	Usual dosage	Additional information
Systemic anesthetics				
phenazo-pyridine* (Aqua-Ton, Azo-100, Azo-Standard, Ci-Azo, Phenazodine, Phenylazo, Pyridiate, Pyridium, Pyrodine, Urodine)	Oral tablets	Symptomatic relief of discomforts that result from irritation of the lower urinary tract	Adults: 200 mg tid pc Children: 12 mg/kg body weight/day, divided in 3 doses PC: B	Because it is an azo dye, phenazopyridine may interfere with urinalysis based on spectrometry or color reactions. Phenazo-pyridine colors the urine a bright orange-red.
Parenteral				
Esters				
chloroprocaine (Nesacaine)	Solutions for injection	Infiltration anesthesia Block anesthesia	Adults: (with epineph-rine) 1 g; (without epi-nephrine) 800 mg PC: C	Onset of action is more rapid and dura-tion of action longer than that of procaine.
piperocaine (Metycaine)	Solutions and powder for preparing solutions for injection	Infiltration anesthesia Block anesthesia	Adults: *Maximum single dose:* 1 g	Onset of action is more rapid and dura-tion of action longer than that of procaine.
procaine (Anduracaine, Anu-ject, Novocain)	Solutions for injection	Infiltration anesthesia Block anesthesia	Adults: *Initially:* up to 1 g PC: C	Procaine acts within 2–5 min; duration of action is about 1 h. Severe allergic reac-tions may occur. Procaine is painless when injected.
propoxycaine (Ravocaine)	Solution containing a combination of pro-poxycaine, procaine, and levonordefrin	Dental block	Adults: 9 ml of solu-tion (containing 36 mg propoxycaine and 180 mg of procaine) Children: 0.275 ml/kg body weight up to a maximum of 9 ml	Onset of action is the same as that of pro-caine; duration of ac-tion is longer (2–3 h).
tetracaine (Pontocaine)	Solutions for injection	Spinal anesthesia	Variable, depending on the site and dura-tion of anesthesia required Adults: 5–15 mg; *max-imum dosage:* 20 mg PC: C	Onset of action is delayed up to 15 min in large nerve trunks. Duration of action is about 1.5–3 h.
Amides				
bupivacaine (Marcaine, Sensorcaine)	Solutions for injection	Infiltration anesthesia Block anesthesia	Adults: Without epinephrine—175 mg q3h; with epi-nephrine—225 mg q3h; *maximum dosage:* 400 mg PC: C	Bupivacaine is not rec-ommended for use in children younger than 12 years.
dibucaine (Nupercaine)	Solutions for injection	Spinal anesthesia	Adults: 0.5–2 ml of 0.5% solution (2.5–10 mg)	Dibucaine has a longer duration of action than does procaine.

(Continued)

Table 24-8. Representative drugs used medicinally to produce local anesthesia (Continued)

Drug name	Preparations	Therapeutic uses	Usual dosage	Additional information
Parenteral				
etidocaine (Duranest)	Solutions for injection	Block anesthesia	Adults: 225–300 mg q2–3h PC: B	Safe use of etidocaine in children younger than 14 yr of age has not been established.
lidocaine (Dolocaine, L-Caine, Lidoject, Nervocaine, Nulicaine, Ultracaine, Xylocaine)	Solutions for injection	Infiltration anesthesia Block anesthesia	Adults: Without epinephrine—single doses of up to 4.5 mg/kg body weight; with epinephrine—up to 7 mg/kg body weight (or 500 mg) PC: B	Solutions for anesthesia contain no preservatives; they may or may not contain epinephrine. Solutions for anesthesia must be distinguished from those used to treat cardiac conditions. Lidocaine is the drug of choice for individuals allergic to amino-ester anesthetics.
mepivacaine (Carbocaine, Xylonest)	Solutions for injection	Infiltration, epidural, or block anesthesia	Adults: *Maximum single dose:* 400 mg; *maximum daily dose:* 1 g Children: 5–6 mg/kg body weight	Mepivacaine has a more rapid onset and longer duration of action than does lidocaine.
prilocaine (Citanest)	Solutions for injection	Infiltration, epidural, or block anesthesia	Adults: *Maximum dosage:* 600 mg q2h	Dosage must be reduced for debilitated clients and for those with liver impairment.
Miscellaneous				
alcohol	Solution for injection	Relief of intractable pain	2–4 ml injected around a nerve or ganglion	Anesthesia may last for several months.
hexylcaine (Cyclaine)	Solution for topical or urogenital use	Surface anesthesia of intact mucous membranes of the upper respiratory, upper GI, or urinary tracts	Adults: *Maximum dose:* 500 mg (in the form of 0.5%, 1%, 2%, or 5% solutions)	Low doses and concentrations should be used for geriatric or debilitated persons.
proparacaine (AK-Taine, Alcaine, Ophthetic; *Can:* Ophthaine)	Ophthalmic solutions	Prevention of pain during eye surgery Surface anesthetic before injection of parenteral anesthetics for eye or orbital surgery	gtt i-ii q 5–10 min for up to 5–7 doses	Rarely, proparacaine can cause a severe allergic keratitis, iritis, or contact dermatitis.
tetracaine (Pontocaine)	Topical solution Ophthalmic solutions and ointments	Surface anesthesia of the eye, nose, and throat	Apply as necessary; *maximum adult dosage:* 20 mg PC: C	The manufacturer recommends the addition of 0.1% epinephrine solution to tetracaine solutions used to anesthetize the larynx, trachea, or esophagus. Tetracaine is the most potent of amino-ester compounds.

*Although administered orally, this drug exerts its therapeutic effect only in the urinary tract, where it is concentrated on excretion.

KEY: PC = pregnancy category. (The validity of pregnancy categories has not been established; see Chapter 16 p 216.)

The topical spray, ethyl chloride, is highly combustible and can cause serious burns if ignited.

Prilocaine can cause methemoglobinemia in up to 15% of recipients. Viscous lidocaine, an oral topical anesthetic, has caused seizures in young children (Hess, 1988).

Precautions and contraindications. Cocaine should not be used to treat clients with a history of dependency on that drug.

The ester-amides are contraindicated for people known to be allergic to one or more of these drugs. Cross-sensitivity is fairly complete. An amino-amide drug should be used, or a sensitivity test should be carried out before anesthesia. Before the administration of anesthesia, a test dose of the drug should be given to a client who has a history of unresponsiveness to local anesthetics. Both ester-amide and amino-amide agents may be ineffective. If local anesthesia must be attempted, the client should be observed closely to determine the response to the chosen drug.

Test doses should also be administered to clients who have cardiac, thyroid, or other endocrine diseases to determine tolerance to the drug chosen for anesthesia. The physician orders small doses initially, followed by careful comprehensive assessment of client response.

Local anesthetics for use in obstetrical procedures are chosen with consideration of their effects on uterine contraction. Small doses of agents that depress uterine muscle function are acceptable if cacsarean section is planned but are contraindicated if vaginal delivery is desired.

Local anesthetics should be administered slowly, avoiding inadvertent IV administration. Appropriate techniques should be used to control the systemic rate of absorption.

Reactions can be severe and must be treated aggressively. Oxygen is required to prevent and ameliorate seizures. Diazepam is the agent of choice for terminating convulsions. An IV line should be established promptly. Fluids are given to prevent or to treat shock. Vasopressors may be required in cardiovascular collapse. Endotracheal intubation and assisted respirations may be required in respiratory collapse.

Ethyl chloride should not be used for topical anesthesia if need of a heated or electrical apparatus, such as a cautery, is anticipated.

■ **Summary**

Agents used for local anesthesia include cocaine, phenol, and a variety of ester-amide and amino-amide compounds. They act by blocking conduction of impulses along nerve fibers. Agents are administered by a number of techniques designed to limit action to an area or region of the body while preserving consciousness and minimizing systemic absorption. Systemic actions cause side effects that range from nausea and vomiting to convulsions or cardiovascular collapse. Adverse reactions are treated by controlling symptoms and maintaining vital functions during the relatively short time period required for metabolic degradation of the compounds.

Nursing management
Nursing implications

In the preparation of solutions for topical application or injection, the usual precautions to ensure accuracy of medication are observed. Additives to the anesthetic drug (vasoconstrictors or hyaluronidase) must be ordered specifically. Solution labels must be read carefully, because concentrations vary and some commercial preparations contain combinations of drugs. Most common are solutions marketed with vasoconstrictors, such as epinephrine, already added to the primary drug. Solutions that contain epinephrine are *not* used in tissues supplied by endarteries (fingers, toes, ears, nose, or penis) because the vasoconstrictor can compromise circulation, resulting in gangrene. When assisting the physician in drawing up solutions, the nurse should announce verbally the exact preparation and concentration being used. The label should also be shown to the physician for visual confirmation. Solutions that appear cloudy or that contain solid crystals should not be used.

Nursing process

Assessment   The client who is to undergo local anesthesia should be assessed for factors that increase the risks of the drugs. Reactions to previous use of local anesthetics should be explored, with particular attention paid to lack of response or adverse reactions. The client should be questioned about possible cardiac or endocrine disease (specifically thyroid or cortisone imbalance and pheochromocytoma). Drugs used currently or in the recent past should be determined.

During the history, the degree of knowledge the client has about local anesthesia can be estimated.

Nursing diagnosis   Nursing diagnoses may include the following:

Knowledge deficit concerning effects of local anesthesia
High risk for pain related to inherited refractoriness to local anesthetics

A common collaborative problem that should be differentiated from the nursing diagnoses is

Potential complication: hypovolemic shock

Planning Goals of treatment are to teach the client about the surgical procedure, including local anesthesia, to reduce the risk of adverse reaction to the anesthetic, to maintain tissue perfusion should adverse reaction occur, to limit toxic reaction to vasoconstrictors, and to prevent pain during the procedure.

Intervention If the client has a history of adverse reaction or inadequate response to local anesthetics, the physician should be notified promptly.

During surgical procedures under local anesthesia, the nurse should monitor the amount of anesthetic used and watch the client for signs of side effects, toxicity, or allergic reaction. These include restlessness, talkativeness, respiratory difficulty, rash, and changes in vital signs. These should be reported to the physician unless they are already apparent to the operating suite staff. The physician should be alerted if the client's condition indicates possible toxicity or allergic reaction. The total dose of anesthetic used and the time span elapsed since initiation of anesthesia should also be reported.

The surgical staff must be prepared to administer corrective action should a reaction occur. Oxygen, IV therapy, and assisted respirations may be required. Vasoconstrictors and diazepam should be readily accessible. Endotracheal intubation and cardiopulmonary resuscitation may be necessary.

It should be remembered that, even when sedated, the client usually remains aware of events that occur in the environment. Sights, sounds, and smells associated with surgery that are accepted as a matter of course by the staff may be disturbing to the lay person. Clients need reassurance and emotional support.

If the planned procedure interferes with verbalization by the client, a signal should be established whereby he or she can indicate to the surgical staff that pain or other adverse reaction is being experienced.

Positioning is critical to control spread of the drug when spinal or epidural anesthesia is administered. Rapid changes may be necessary. After surgery, the client should be protected from injury to the anesthetized area until numbness has disappeared.

Clients who have undergone lumbar puncture for regional anesthesia experience paralysis of the lower part of the body until the drug concentration falls. These people require special nursing care to prevent complications of immobility, especially thrombophlebitis and pressure necrosis. They should be positioned with pillows to maintain body alignment and to distribute pressure to all tissues. Because of leakage through the puncture site, the volume of cerebrospinal fluid may be reduced and spinal headache can occur. The head should be kept flat, but the client need not remain supine. Turning is required at least every 2 hours. The lower back and hips should be massaged frequently. The client should be monitored for headache, which tends to occur when fluid has been removed from the spinal canal. Nonopioid analgesics may be given for relief. Prolonged headache usually indicates that spinal fluid is leaking from the puncture site. The physician should be notified if headache persists for more than a few hours. Leakage of spinal fluid may be corrected by the creation of a small hematoma at the site. (A small amount of the client's blood is drawn from a vein and injected at the puncture site.) Ample fluid intake also hastens recovery from spinal headache by accelerating the regeneration of spinal fluid.

Client education. Inform clients about the procedure. Tell them that numbness will occur, but sensations of deep pressure may not be lost. Warn those who are undergoing spinal anesthesia that motor function will be lost temporarily. Smells of cauterization and sounds of bone sawing or chiseling are particularly distressing to lay people; if these are anticipated, clients should be informed ahead of time. Instruct the client to inform the staff if pain, nausea, restlessness, or difficulty in breathing occurs.

Many clients fear spinal anesthesia because they have heard reports of permanent paralysis after this procedure. The origin of such rumors is difficult to track down, but they may stem from instances of progressive paralysis in clients who have had lumbar punctures performed to diagnose an existing spinal cord disease process. Clients should be informed that the site of lumbar punctures is below the level of the spinal cord and is in an area that provides ample space for the needle without encroachment on nerve structures. In the rare instances when a nerve is touched by the needle, irritation is limited to one or, at most, a few fibers. Symptoms are therefore confined to one or a few dermatomes. Moreover, nerves usually recover completely from such irritation. The client may need reassurance that reports of paraplegia after this procedure are not related to the procedure but rather to an existing progressive disease process.

After spinal anesthesia, advise the client to remain flat in bed for the rest of the day and to drink plenty of fluids to promote regeneration of the cerebrospinal fluid. Explain the nursing measures (turning, coughing, and deep breathing) that will be carried out to promote respiration and circulation. Encourage the client to report headache if it develops, so that corrective action may be taken.

Caution the client to avoid injury to the anesthetized areas during the interval before numbness disappears. This warning is particularly important for the client who leaves the health care setting before the effects of anesthesia have completely dissipated.

Checklist of nursing actions

☐ Assess the client who is undergoing local anesthesia for previous response to drug agents used in such procedures.

☐ Determine whether the client has recently taken medication that may interact with local anesthesia.

☐ Assess clients for heart or endocrine disease that increase the risk of adverse reaction.

☐ Inform the client about the procedure, including the effects of the anesthesia.

☐ Instruct the client to notify the staff of pain or symptoms of adverse reaction.

☐ Reassure fearful clients that lumbar punctures do not cause permanent paralysis of the lower body.

☐ During local anesthesia, monitor the client for lack of response and signs and symptoms of adverse reaction.

☐ Provide reassurance and emotional support during the procedures.

☐ Verify the accuracy of medications used for anesthesia.

☐ Monitor the amount of drugs used for local anesthesia.

☐ Be prepared to control seizures and maintain vital functions if an acute drug reaction occurs.

☐ Caution clients to avoid injury to anesthetized parts of the body until numbness wears off.

☐ Provide appropriate care for the client who is recovering from spinal anesthesia to prevent complications of immobility and to prevent or alleviate spinal headache.

Alternative anesthetic regimens

Three alternative anesthetic regimens are available: neuroleptanesthesia, dissociative anesthesia, and twilight sleep. Their important features are listed in Table 24-9.

Neuroleptanesthesia

Neuroleptic compounds are sometimes used in conjunction with opioid analgesics to produce analgesia during diagnostic procedures or minor surgery. While under the influence of these drugs, clients appear indifferent to the environment and exhibit lack of anxiety and reduced motor function. They remain responsive to commands and can cooperate with the health care staff when necessary. Analgesia may be converted to anesthesia by the administration of nitrous oxide with oxygen by inhalation.

The most common agent for inducing neuroleptanalgesia is Innovar, a commercial mixture of droperidol and fentanyl (Sublimaze). This preparation is diluted in 5% dextrose in water, to be administered slowly by IV injection. The rate of administration must be carefully controlled to prevent adverse reactions, such as excitement, laryngospasm, and spasm of the chest wall. Should the latter develop, respirations can be restored by the administration of succinylcholine.

After neuroleptanesthesia, respirations may be depressed, especially if potent analgesics are employed. Dosage of such drugs must be reduced, and the client should be monitored carefully for respiratory function.

Dissociative anesthesia

Certain chemicals produce a state similar to neuroleptanalgesia that is characterized by marked analgesia, immobility, sedation, amnesia, and a strong feeling of disassociation from the environment. The most com-

Table 24-9. Alternative anesthetic regimens

Characteristics	Neuroleptanesthesia	Dissociative anesthesia	Twilight sleep
Effect on recipient	Indifference to surroundings	Marked analgesia	Analgesia
	Lack of anxiety	Immobility	Amnesia
	Responsiveness to commands retained	Sedation	Decreased alertness
	Residual respiratory depression	Amnesia	Ability to respond to commands retained
		Mental disassociation from surroundings	Self-control over behavior may be lost
Agents employed	Innovar (a combination of fentanyl and droperidol)	Ketamine (*Can:* Ketalor)	Various combinations of analgesics and amnesics
Precautions required (for all three regimens, clients must be protected from injury and watched closely for adverse reactions)	Carefully control rate of administration	Minimize environmental stimuli	Observe for and control inappropriate behavior
	Support respirations during and after anesthesia	Observe and treat for psychic disturbance (nightmares or hallucinations)	
	Reduce dosage of potent analgesics until anesthetic effects are completely dissipated		
Uses	Diagnostic procedures or minor surgery (with opioid analgesics)	Burn dressing changes	Historically: labor

KEY: *Can* = Canadian trade name.

Box 24-6. Actions of analgesics

- Inhibit transmission of pain impulses
- Reduce cortical response to pain stimuli
- Alter nerve activity in brain areas that control perception of pain

---

mon agent used to induce this type of anesthesia is ketamine (Ketalar). Ketamine acts on the cortex and limbic system rather than on the reticular formation. Administered intramuscularly (IM) or IV, it induces anesthesia in less than a minute. Anesthesia lasts 10 to 15 minutes and may be prolonged by succeeding doses. Analgesia persists for more than a half hour, and amnesia is evident for 1 to 2 hours.

A quiet environment is essential for smooth progress of dissociative anesthesia. Muscular movement may occur in response to extraneous stimuli. Ketamine reduces airway resistance and helps maintain an unobstructed airway. It is particularly useful for burn dressing changes that involve the face and neck.

Nightmares and hallucinations may occur when the client emerges from ketamine anesthesia and sometimes recur subsequently. Valium may be prescribed to reverse the dissociative anesthesia.

Twilight sleep

Various combinations of potent analgesics and amnesia-inducing agents have been used to alleviate pain during procedures that require some participation by the client. This procedure, termed *twilight sleep*, was used for some time in the management of labor but has fallen out of favor because the medicated client often loses control and is unable to cooperate or participate appropriately in the necessary procedures.

Analgesics

Analgesics are drugs that relieve or decrease pain without loss of consciousness. They may act by inhibiting transmission of pain impulses, by reducing cortical response to pain stimuli, or by altering nerve activity in areas of the brain (the frontal lobe and limbic systems) that moderate perception of pain. Analgesics include both natural and synthetic compounds (Box 24-6).

Analgesics are commonly described as narcotic or nonnarcotic agents. The use of these terms is unfortunate, because the word narcotic has two distinct definitions that tend to be confused. Originally, a *narcotic* was defined medically as a substance that induces sleep or stupor. A legal definition was established by the Harrison Narcotic Act in 1914. This legislation designated as narcotics various classes of drugs (opium, coca, and marijuana) believed to be habit-forming. It further forbade sale or use of these drugs or their derivatives

without a medical prescription. Legally, therefore, narcotics are dependency-producing drugs, the use of which is strictly controlled by legislation. Since 1914, prescription controls have been extended to other drugs characterized by dependency, but the term narcotic is not usually applied to them. Because of the potential for confusion, the term narcotic is not used in this discussion without qualification.

Opiates and opioids

Drugs derived from the juice of the opium poppy (*Papaver somniferum*) are termed *opiates*. Because a number of synthetic substitutes have been developed with opiumlike properties, the term *opioid* has been coined to designate both opiates and their synthetic substitutes. The active drugs contained in opium are alkaloids of two types: phenanthrene and benzylisoquinoline. Phenanthrene alkaloids, which include morphine and codeine, exhibit potent analgesic and sedative properties not characteristic of benzylisoquinolines. The major alkaloid of the latter type, papaverine, is used medicinally as a vasodilator (see Chapter 28). In addition to the natural phenanthrene derivatives, synthetic phenylpiperidine and diphenylheptane derivatives are available for use as analgesics. Meperidine and fentanyl are the major phenylpiperidine derivatives; the only diphenylheptane derivative used medicinally is methadone (Box 24-7).

Used since antiquity, opium is one of the oldest analgesics known. It was first used in Asia Minor, the geographic area where the opium poppy is indigenous. From Asia Minor, knowledge of the substance spread to Greece, Arabia, and the Orient. In China, it was originally used to treat dysentery, but habitual use became a problem after the opium trade was commercialized by European powers.

Until the 19th century, only crude opium was used. Crude opium is a brownish gum or powder pro-

---

Box 24-7. Active drugs in opium and opioids

- Phenanthrene alkaloids (morphine and codeine): exhibit potent analgesic and sedative properties
- Synthetic phenylpiperidine derivatives (meperidine, fentanyl): exhibit analgesic and sedative properties
- Diphenylheptane derivatives (methadone): relieve signs and symptoms of opioid withdrawal; they are easier to wean from than other opioids
- Benzylisoquinoline alkaloids (papaverine): dilate blood vessels (discussed in Chapter 28)

duced by drying the liquid exudate from unripe seed pods of the poppy. During the 19th century, the active alkaloids were isolated and became available for use in pure form. The invention of the hypodermic syringe and needle facilitated the use of these drugs in medical practice. Opioid drugs in current use are listed in Table 24-10.

Pharmacodynamics. Opioid analgesics act as agonists by interacting with receptors in the brain and other tissues. These stereospecific saturable binding sites are the normal sites of action of endogenous ligands (endorphins and enkephalins), which function to control the pain response and modify the psychological state of a person. Several subtypes appear to be distinguished by the functions that they mediate and the action of various chemicals that interact with them (Table 24-11). Receptors are most numerous in the limbic system, thalamus, striatum, hypothalamus, midbrain, and substantia gelatinosa of the spinal cord but are also present in nerve plexuses and exocrine glands of the stomach and intestines. Agonistic interaction with these receptors decreases adenylate cyclase activity within the cell, thereby decreasing cell activity and producing characteristic tissue responses.

Opioids may also alter the chemical environment in the brain. They inhibit release of acetylcholine and norepinephrine and modify dopamine release. Morphine decreases calcium ion concentration in the brain and prevents its uptake in brain cells.

A number of central effects occur as a consequence of these and possibly other unknown mechanisms. Activity decreases in the locus ceruleus (responsible for the alarm responses of panic, fear, and anxiety). Perception of pain is selectively inhibited more than other sensory modalities. Reaction to pain or perception of the stimulus as a stressor is reduced to a greater degree than specific pain sensation. At the same time, mood elevation and some degree of euphoria are produced.

Table 24-10. Opioid analgesics

Drug name	Preparations	Dosage	Additional information
Agonists			
alphaprodine (Nisentil)	Solutions for IV, SC, or submucosal injection	Adults: *IV:* 0.4–0.6 mg/kg body weight; *SC:* 0.4–1.2 mg/kg body weight; *maximum daily dosage:* 240 mg PC: C	Alphaprodine should not be administered IM because of erratic absorption. This drug is used to relieve moderate to severe acute pain.
codeine (*Can:* Ancasal)	Oral tablets (In combination with other ingredients) oral tablets and syrups Solutions for SC or IM injection	Adults: 15–60 mg q4h PRN Children: 3 mg/kg body weight or 100 mg/m² daily, divided in 6 doses PC: C (D for prolonged use or use of high doses at term)	Codeine is used to relieve mild pain.
fentanyl (Innovar, *Can:* Sublimaze)	Solutions for SC or IM injection	Adults: *IM:* 50–100 µg q1–2h PRN Children aged 2–12 yr: 1.7–3.3 µg/kg body weight PC: B (D for prolonged use or use of high doses at term)	Fentanyl exhibits little hypnotic activity. Histamine release rarely occurs.
heroin ("horse," "smack")	(Nonmedicinal) Powder for oral use, topical application to mucous membranes, or preparation for injection	Adults: *Oral:* 2–8 mg	Manufacture, sale, and use is illegal in the U.S.
hydrocodone (Dicodil, Hycodan)	Oral tablets	Adults: 5–10 mg q4–6h PRN	Hydrocodone is used for the relief of moderate to severe pain.
hydromorphone (Dilaudid)	Oral tablets Solutions for SC or IM injection	Adults: *Oral:* 2–4 mg q4–6h PRN; *SC or IM:* 2 mg q4–6h PRN; *rectally:* 3 mg q6–8h PRN Children older than 12 yr: 1 mg q3–4h Children 6–12 yr of age: 0.5 mg q3–4h PC: B (D for prolonged use or use of high doses at term)	Hydromorphone produces minimal hypnotic, euphoric, and GI side effects. This drug is also used in children to control cough.

(Continued)

Table 24-10. Opioid analgesics (Continued)

Drug name	Preparations	Dosage	Additional information
Agonists			
levorphanol (Levo-Dromoran)	Oral tablets Solutions for SC or slow IV injection	Adults: *Oral or SC:* 2 mg q6h PRN PC: B (D for prolonged use or use of high doses at term)	Levorphanol is used to relieve moderate to severe pain. Safe use for children or during pregnancy has not been established.
meperidine (Demerol)	Oral tablets and syrup Solutions for SC or IM injection	Adults: 50–100 mg q3–4h PRN Children: 1.1–1.8 mg/kg body weight q3–4h PRN or 175 mg/m²/day, divided in 6 doses; *maximum single pediatric dose:* 100 mg PC: B (D for prolonged use or use of high doses at term)	Meperidine has limited effects on the GI tract.
methadone (Dolophine)	Oral tablets Solutions for SC or IM injection	Adults: 2.5–10 mg q3–4h PRN; *maximum parenteral dose:* 10 mg PC: B (D for prolonged use or use of high doses at term)	Oral doses of up to 20 mg are used for severe, chronic pain (*eg,* in the terminally ill). Methadone may accumulate with repeated doses. Methadone produces weaker sedative and euphorigenic effects than does morphine.
morphine (*Can:* MOS MS Contin)	Oral tablets and capsules Solutions for SC, IM, and IV injection Rectal suppositories	Adults: *Oral:* 10–30 mg q4h PRN; *SC or IM:* 5–20 mg q4h PRN; *IV:* 2.5–15 mg over 4–5 min; *rectal:* 10–20 mg q4h PRN Children: *SC:* 0.1–0.2 mg/kg body weight q4h PRN; *maximum single pediatric dose:* 15 mg PC: B (D for prolonged use or use of high doses at term)	Morphine is a standard for comparison of strong analgesic effect of other drugs. Morphine acts as an agonist at μ and κ opioid receptors.
opium (Pantopon)	Powder Solutions for SC or IM injection Rectal suppositories	Adults: *SC or IM:* 5–20 mg q4–5h PRN; *rectal:* 30–60 mg qd-bid	The medicinal preparation, *concentrated opium alkaloids hydrochlorides,* contains the same alkaloids in about the same proportions as does crude opium.
oxycodone (Percocet, Percodan)	Oral tablets and solution	Adults: 5 mg q6h PRN Children 12 yr of age or older: 2.44 mg q6h PRN Children 6–12 yr of age: 1.22 mg q6h PRN PC: B (D for prolonged use or use of high doses at term)	Oxycodone is used to relieve moderate to severe acute pain. It is also used in combination with mild analgesics.
oxymorphone (Numorphan)	Solution for SC, IM, or IV injection Rectal suppositories	Adults: *IM (initially):* 1–1.5 mg; *IV (initially):* 0.5 mg (dosage may be increased cautiously until desired therapeutic response is attained); *rectal:* 5 mg Doses may be repeated q4–6h PRN PC: B (D for prolonged use or use of high doses at term)	Oxymorphone causes fewer GI side effects than does morphine.
sufentanil (Sufenta)	Solutions for parenteral administration	Adults (Initially): 1–8 μg/kg body weight; additional: 25–30 μg/kg body weight PC: C (D for prolonged use or use of high doses at term)	Sufentanil is used in conjunction with nitrous oxide and oxygen for anesthesia.

KEY: PC = pregnancy category. (The validity of pregnancy categories has not been established; see Chapter 16; p 216.)
Can: Canadian trade name.

Table 24-11. Hypothetical subtypes of opioid receptors

Receptor type	Functions mediated by the receptor
μ	Supraspinal analgesia, miosis, hypothermia, respiratory depression, euphoria, physical dependency
κ	Spinal analgesia, miosis, hypothermia, sedation, possible respiratory depression
o	Dysphoria, hallucinations, respiratory and vasomotor stimulation
δ	Alterations of affective behavior, possible respiratory depression

Pharmacokinetics. Opioids are readily absorbed from the GI and nasal mucosae, the surface of the lungs, and the peripheral tissues after injection. Medicinally, the drugs are administered by oral, rectal, subcutaneous, IM, IV, and epidural routes. When abused, the compounds may be applied to the nasal mucosa as snuff, inhaled by smoking, or injected.

IV injections take effect immediately. Absorption from subcutaneous and IM sites is directly related to lipid solubility. The effectiveness of oral administration is variable, because many preparations undergo significant ("first-pass") metabolism in the liver immediately after intestinal absorption. Because of this mechanism, morphine and related compounds must be given in larger doses when administered orally. Meperidine, codeine, and methadone are less affected and are relatively more effective when administered orally.

After absorption, opioids are widely distributed in body tissues. Morphine concentration is greatest in parenchymatous tissues (liver, kidney, spleen, and lungs) and intermediate in muscle tissues. About one-third binds to plasma proteins. Although relatively little morphine passes the blood–brain barrier in adults, this fraction is responsible for its central actions.

Codeine and heroin pass more readily than morphine into the CNS but exert few central effects until converted by the tissues to morphine. Heroin is rapidly metabolized to morphine, but only a small fraction of codeine follows this pathway.

Initially, most methadone binds to plasma proteins. Subsequently, it becomes firmly bound to tissue proteins. This depot is responsible for its accumulation with repeated administration and its prolonged effects in suppressing the withdrawal syndrome in morphine- or heroin-dependent people. As with morphine, only fractional parts of a methadone dose cross the blood–brain barrier.

All opioids are metabolized by the tissues. Most are deactivated by the liver microsomal enzymes. Drugs and their metabolites are excreted mainly by renal tubule filtration, but small amounts (10% or less) enter the enterohepatic circulation. Some of the latter are excreted in the feces, but a portion is reabsorbed and prolongs the duration of drug effect.

Therapeutic uses. Opioid analgesics are widely used for the symptomatic relief of pain due to acute or terminal illness. Codeine and related compounds are prescribed for moderate pain; meperidine, morphine, and morphine's relatives are reserved for severe pain. In countries outside the U.S., heroin is often preferred for the treatment of intractable pain. Methadone is used mainly in the treatment of the withdrawal syndrome in heroin- or morphine-dependent people and as an oral analgesic for the relief of severe pain, particularly in terminal cancer.

Equipotent doses of opioid analgesics are shown in Table 24-12. High doses of opioids are sometimes used as primary agents for general anesthesia. They have traditionally been administered preoperatively to facilitate the induction of anesthesia but are gradually being displaced for this purpose by antianxiety agents. Their value as antidiarrheals and antitussives is discussed in Chapters 31 and 37. In addition, opioids are used on an empirical basis in such clinical situations as left ventricular failure with pulmonary edema despite a lack of knowledge of the specific mechanisms involved.

Administration. Opioid analgesics are usually administered by the oral, subcutaneous, IM, or IV routes. They are also infused intrathecally and epidurally. Buccal administration is under investigation (New way to give morphine, 1985). Doses administered IM or subcutaneously are not absorbed unless vascular circulation is adequate. Ineffective doses should not be repeated. They remain in tissue deposits and tend to be absorbed simultaneously when circulation is restored, causing a toxic reaction because of overdose.

Increasingly, the administration of pain medication is carried out by equipment that allows clients to administer their own analgesics. This patient-

Table 24-12. Doses of opioid analgesics with effects comparable to morphine

Drug	Dose equivalent to MS 10 mg IM
codeine	130 mg IM
hydromorphone	1.5 mg IM
levorphanol	2 mg IM
meperidine	75 mg IM
methadone	10 mg IM
oxymorphone	1 mg IM

(Adapted from McEvoy GK, ed. [1991]. *Drug information 91*, p 1153. Bethesda, MD: American Society of Hospital Pharmacists.)

controlled analgesia usually employs a parenteral line with reservoirs that contain analgesic solutions and controls that allow clients to use an amount up to the maximum prescribed.

Adverse reactions. Side effects of opioid analgesics relate to both central and peripheral actions of the drugs. They appear in many tissues and systems of the body and cause a variety of physiologic responses (Table 24-13).

After the administration of opiates, respiratory rate and depth decline in direct proportion to the dose given. Irregular periodic breathing can occur. Coughing is suppressed. Asthmatic attacks may occur in susceptible individuals.

Cardiovascular effects are limited to dilation of the peripheral arterial and venous vessels. This produces some degree of postural hypotension but no obvious changes in blood pressure or cardiac rates in recumbent subjects. Because they produce fewer cardiovascular changes than other general anesthetics, opioids are sometimes used as anesthetic agents in cardiac surgery.

Skin manifestations include flushing, itching, and increased perspiration. Pruritus is most noticeable at the site of parenteral injection and in the nose. The extremities feel heavy and warm. Continuous subcutaneous infusion has produced painful plaques at the injection site (Adams, et al, 1989).

GI effects include nausea, vomiting, constipation, and biliary colic. Nausea and vomiting are most pronounced during ambulation. This response varies greatly among clients and differs with specific drugs in the same person. A number of effects combine to produce constipation: delays in stool passage that increase absorption of water from the intestinal contents, central sedation that decreases response to the impulse to defecate, relative lack of propulsive peristalsis, and increased sphincter tone.

Biliary colic is most likely to occur with the use of morphine. Meperidine causes less smooth muscle spasm and is less likely than other opioids to produce or exacerbate this condition.

Urinary retention is most apt to occur in postoperative clients who have received anesthetics or other depressant drugs along with opioids. It is particularly likely in male clients with prostatic hypertrophy, who are at increased risk for this complication.

Opioids are sometimes administered to interrupt labor in threatened abortion. When used in labor at term, they tend to prolong the process and may produce respiratory depression in the newborn.

Chronic use of opioids can suppress pituitary gonadotropins in both sexes, causing infertility. Extended use of meperidine can cause CNS excitation as a result of an accumulation of normeperidine, a metabolite that acts as a CNS stimulant (McCaffery, 1984).

Pupillary constriction is characteristic of the response to opioids. It is considered pathognomonic of opioid toxicity.

Central nervous system side effects are responsible for the opioids' appeal as drugs of abuse. The mood elevation, tranquility, and euphoria sought by the dependent person are most obvious after the administration of heroin, which rapidly enters the CNS, where it is converted almost entirely to morphine.

Toxic effects. The adverse effects of opioid drugs increase in incidence and severity as dose rises. With higher doses, subjective effects such as euphoria are accentuated, nausea and vomiting become apparent in more subjects, and respirations become slow and shallow. Muscle rigidity and catalepsy tend to develop. Behavior may become stereotypic. The T waves on electrocardiograms are depressed or inverted. Very high doses of opioids are accompanied by hypoxia secondary to respiratory impairment. Blood pressure and pulse rate decline, in part due to depression of the central vasomotor center and in part to lowered oxygen tension. Bronchoconstriction and convulsions may also develop. Death from overdose is usually due to respiratory failure.

Tolerance. Chronic administration of opioids produces tolerance in relation to many of their effects. Repeated opioid-receptor interaction leads to an adaptation of cell physiology that compensates for the presence of the drugs. Adenylate cyclase production increases, bringing cellular levels back to normal and restoring normal cell function. Tolerance is fairly complete to pain relief, sedation, mood elevation, and respiratory effects. Only partial tolerance develops to responses of the GI and male reproductive systems. Eye response does not change with repeated use of drugs, and pupillary constriction provides a reliable index of opioid exposure.

Withdrawal of opioids for the person who has developed tolerance produces signs and symptoms of abnormal physiology that stem from overactivity in cells in which adenylate cyclase levels have become abnormally heightened to compensate for the presence of the drugs. These manifestations are generally opposite to the normal effects of opioid administration. Clients in withdrawal experience dysphoria and increased sensations, particularly of pain and touch. Tactile hallucinations tend to develop (referred to as "a monkey on the back"). Nasopharyngeal secretions, GI secretions, and propulsive peristalsis increase. The pupils dilate. The affected person experiences photophobia, rhinorrhea, and diarrhea. When tolerance is highly developed and withdrawal of drugs is abrupt, this syndrome can be severe (so-called "cold turkey"). When used to treat physiologic pain, opioids rarely cause psychologic dependence. If the cause of the pain is corrected, clients respond well to weaning sched-

Table 24-13. Common side effects of opioid analgesics

Signs or symptoms	Underlying mechanism
Respiratory system	
Reduced rate and depth of respirations	Depression of response of the central respiratory center to increased carbon dioxide in the blood
Irregular or periodic breathing	Depression of the medullary and pontine centers that regulate respiratory rhythms
Decreased cough	Inhibition of cough reflex
Bronchoconstriction	Release of histamine
Cardiovascular system	
Postural hypotension	Peripheral vasodilation
Skin	
Flushing	Peripheral vasodilation and histamine release
Increased perspiration	Histamine release
Pruritus	Histamine release
Gastrointestinal system	
Nausea and vomiting	Increased vestibular sensitivity and stimulation of the vomiting center
Delayed passage of stools	Decreased secretion of hydrochloric acid, bile, and pancreatic juice
	Increased tone of valves and sphincters
	Changes in peristaltic patterns (a decrease in propulsive waves and an increase in nonpropulsive waves)
Increased pressure in the biliary system	Spasm of the sphincter of Oddi
Urinary tract	
Urgency	Increased tone of detrussor muscle
Retention	Increased sphincter tone
	Central sedation that reduces attentiveness to the need to void
Reproductive tract	
Interrupted or prolonged labor	Decrease in oxytocin-induced hyperreactivity of the uterus
Respiratory depression in the newborn	Depression of the fetal respiratory center by drug that crosses the placenta
Decreases in motility of sperm, volume of ejaculate, and testosterone levels in males	Inhibition of luteotropin hormone production by the pituitary
Endocrine system	
Reduced gluccocorticoid levels	Inhibition of pituitary production of adrenocorticotropin
Fluid retention	Enhanced antidiuretic hormone release by the pituitary
Musculoskeletal system	
Increased muscle rigidity	Stimulation of the spinal cord
Eye	
Pupillary constriction and decreased visual acuity	Excitation of autonomic fibers of the oculomotor nerve
Central nervous system	
Inability to concentrate and difficulty in mentation	Depression of the cortex
Lethargy, sedation, or sleep	Depression of the reticular formation
Mood elevation, tranquility, euphoria, and apathy	Depression of the limbic system and brain stem
Decreased temperature	Resetting of the hypothalamic temperature-regulating mechanism
Electroencephalogram changes	Increased voltage and decreased frequency of electrical activity in the brain

ules and do not abuse the drugs after weaning is completed.

Withdrawal signs and symptoms may be minimized during treatment of dependency by first substituting methadone for the drug in use and then gradually withdrawing the person from methadone. Methadone alleviates the most pronounced withdrawal symptoms of the opioids and produces less pronounced physiologic problems during its withdrawal. Physiologic function can be returned to normal and physical dependence eliminated within a few weeks or months. Psychological dependence is much more persistent, and relapses are frequent when the dependent person returns to an environment that is stressful and is offered the opportunity to resume drug use. Chapter 15 provides more information on opiate withdrawal syndrome and its treatment.

Idiosyncratic reactions. Responses to opioids vary from person to person and in the same person over time. Nausea, vomiting, dizziness, mental clouding, dysphoria, increased biliary pressure, and diarrhea do not appear invariably or uniformly in all drug users, but they do tend to emerge in characteristic patterns. Rarely, delirium may occur. Some clients experience an increased sensitivity to pain when the analgesic effect of the drugs subsides. Changes in physiology influence individual response to the drugs. For example, the presence of pain temporarily increases tolerance to these drugs, allowing the administration of sizable doses without the development of side effects. Should the pain subside before drug effect is dissipated, drowsiness and other side effects of the opioids may appear. Pathologic states also may alter toxic and side effects. Clients affected by hypothyroidism, myasthenia gravis, and multiple sclerosis are unusually sensitive to opioids, whereas hyperthyroid individuals are relatively insensitive. Liver or renal impairment interferes with elimination of the drugs and prolongs the duration of their effect. Clients with a low blood volume are prone to develop hypotension in response to opioids. Clients with chronic hypercapnia (due to obstructive airway disease, kyphoscoliosis, obesity, or cor pulmonale) are hypersensitive to the depressant effects of opioids on respirations.

Age also influences response to the drugs to some degree. Infants are prone to respiratory depression, presumably owing to increased permeability of the blood–brain barrier. People older than 60 years of age exhibit enhanced analgesic response to the drugs, perhaps because of their decreased sensitivity to pain.

Allergy. Serious allergic reaction to the opioids is uncommon. When it occurs, allergy is usually manifested by urticaria or skin rash. Contact dermatitis has been reported in people occupationally exposed to opioid compounds (nurses and pharmaceutical workers). IV administration of morphine has rarely produced anaphylaxis.

Precautions and contraindications. No absolute contraindications to the use of opioids exist, provided that equipment, supplies, and trained personnel are available to sustain vital functions and reverse acute adverse reactions. Mechanical respirators may be required to maintain oxygenation. Opioid antagonists are administered to reverse the physiologic manifestations of toxicity. Intensive therapy may be required for several hours to resolve life-threatening reactions when opioids are administered to high-risk clients.

The administration of opioids in head injury or severe obstructive lung disease is considered generally inadvisable. Brain-injured people are highly vulnerable to respiratory arrest, and the analgesic and hypnotic properties of the drugs tend to mask signs and symptoms of increasing pathology, especially rises in intracranial pressure. Great caution must be exercised when opioids are administered to people with a decreased respiratory reserve. When opioids must be used, lower doses than normal should be used, and clients must be monitored closely for reduced respiratory function. Opioids also tend to increase the degree of hypoxemia.

Opioids are also used with caution in other clients at risk for pronounced side effects. Hypovolemic people should be monitored closely to detect circulatory shock. Urinary output must be carefully assessed in clients prone to urinary retention.

When used together with other CNS drugs, the dosage of opioids is usually reduced. Alcohol, tranquilizers, hypnotics, antihistamines, and some antidepressants tend to enhance the central effects of these drugs and hence their toxicity (see Focus on Opioids/Opiates: Similarities and Differences).

■ Summary

Opiates and related compounds remain the drugs of choice for the alleviation of severe pain, especially in terminal illness. When administered orally or by injection, these drugs diminish discomfort due to pain and may reduce or abolish the sensation of pain. Mood tranquility and euphoria enhance the positive response to medication. Undesirable side effects include respiratory depression, constipation, and (in some recipients) nausea, vomiting, and dizziness. Toxicity may produce respiratory arrest and convulsions.

Opioids induce both physiologic and psychological dependency with chronic use. Tolerance develops in many people after as little as 2 weeks of regular medication. Withdrawal produces a syndrome characterized by dysphoria,

Focus on

Opioids/opiates: similarities and differences

Similarities

Pharmacodynamics

These agents act as agonists by interacting with the receptors in the brain and tissue. They act on several sites within the CNS, involving systems of neurotransmitters to produce analgesia by altering the pain perceptions at the spinal cord or higher levels in the CNS; they also alter the person's emotional response to pain.

Pharmacokinetics

These agents are readily absorbed from the GI tract, nasal mucosa, surface of the lungs and peripheral tissues after injection. They are given orally, rectally, SC, IM, or IV. They are metabolized by the liver enzymes but also by the CNS, kidneys, lungs, and placenta. They are excreted primarily in the urine, with small amounts excreted in feces.

Therapeutic uses

These agents are used for temporary analgesia in symptomatic relief of moderate to severe pain, during diagnostic and orthopedic procedures, for preoperative sedation, and as a supplement to anesthesia.

Differences

• **Morphine** decreases the calcium ion concentration in the brain cells. • **Sufentanil** has a high affinity for opiate receptors.

• **Morphine** must be given in larger doses orally; **meperidine**, **codeine** and **methadone** are more effective orally. • **Morphine** concentrations are greatest in the lungs, liver, kidney, and spleen, with half binding to plasma proteins. Most of **methadone** binds to plasma proteins. • **Codeine** has an onset of 15 to 30 minutes (PO or SC) and a duration of 4 to 6 hours with negligible amounts found in feces. • **Fentanyl** is given parenterally, onset of 7 to 15 minutes, peak of minutes, duration of 30 to 60 minutes (IV), 1 to 2 hours (IM). • **Hydromorphone** is given orally, rectally, or parenterally with an onset of 15 to 30 minutes, duration of 4 to 5 hours with no excretion in feces. • **Levorphanol** is well absorbed orally or SC; peaks in 20 minutes (IV), 60 to 90 minutes (SC), with a duration of 6 to 8 hours and no excretion in feces. • **Meperidine** peaks in 1 hour (PO), 40 to 60 minutes (SC), 30 to 50 minutes (IM), with a duration of 2 to 4 hours; 60% to 80% is bound to plasma proteins, it crosses the placenta and is found in breast milk; has a half-life of 2 to 11 minutes and then 3 to 5 hours (elimination half-life is prolonged in people with liver dysfunction) with no excretion in the feces. • **Methadone** is bound to tissue protein and has a duration of 4 to 6 hours. Morphine peaks in 60 minutes (PO), 20 to 60 minutes (R), 50 to 90 minutes (SC), 30 to 60 minutes (IM), and 20 minutes (IV); small amounts are found in breast milk. • **Oxycodone** is only given orally; its onset is 10 to 15 minutes, peaks in 30 to 60 minutes, with a duration of 3 to 6 hours with no excretion in the feces. • **Oxymorphone** can be given rectally, SC, IM, or IV; its onset is 15 to 30 minutes (R), 5 to 10 (IV), 10 to 15 minutes (SC or IM), with a duration of 3 to 6 hours and no excretion in feces. • **Sufentanil** is given IM or IV with an onset of 1 to 2 minutes (IV); rapidly eliminated from the tissues; with a duration of 40 to 80 minutes (IV), 2 to 4 hours (IM); elimination half-life is 2 to 3 hours; small amounts have been found to be metabolized in the small intestines.

• **Codeine** and **hydrocodone** are used as cough suppressants; **methadone** is used as detoxification and maintenance treatment, as oral substitute for heroin and other morphine like drugs; **opium** preparations are rarely used for analgesia; tinctures and paregoric are used as antidiarrheals; **morphine** is used to allay anxiety and cardiovascular effects in pulmonary edema and is the drug of choice in relieving the pain of acute myocardial infarction.

(continued)

Opioids/opiates: similarities and differences (Continued)

Similarities   **Differences**

Adverse reactions

These include: (CNS) mood elevation, eu-   • **Sufentanil** and **fentanyl** in high doses produce amnesia and
phoria, lethargy, sedation, dizziness, sleep,   loss of consciousness. • **Sufentanil** can also cause increased air-
coma, weakness, fainting, agitation, ner-   way resistance, apnea, tachycardia, bronchospasm, and chills.
vousness; (CV) postural hypotension, cir-
culatory depression, bradycardia; (RESP)
decreased rate and depth, irregular
breathing patterns, bronchoconstriction;
(EENT) pupil constriction, decreased visual
acuity; (GI) nausea, vomiting, constipation,
biliary colic; (GU) urinary retention, urgency, fluid retention; (SKIN) flushing,
itching, increased perspiration, pruritus
at injection site; (MS) increased muscle
rigidity; (ENDO) reduced glucocorticoid
levels, impotence, decreased libido;
(OTHER) tolerance, psychologic dependence, physical dependence (with chronic
use), painful placques with continuous
SC infusions.

Nursing considerations

Instruct in disease, drug treatment   Monitor cough type and frequency when giving **codeine**;
regimen, adverse reactions, and need for   do not use **codeine** when cough is helpful in clearing the air-
compliance; assess respiratory status and   way; keep resuscitative equipment available when giving **fen-**
do not administer if rate is less than 12   **tanyl**, **hydromorphone**, **levorphanol**, and **sufentanil**; rotate
breaths per minute; monitor skin color;   injection sites when giving **hydromorphone** parenterally, give
evaluate laboratory results for indication of IV **hydromorphone** slowly; warn that **levorphanol** has a bitter
tissue ischemia; monitor liver and renal   taste; administer IV **morphine** slowly and diluted (SC adminis-
function studies; assess pain characteristics, tration is painful); give **methadone** maintenance as an oral liq-
including onset, type, location; assess level uid—dissolve in 120 ml of orange juice or powdered citrus
of orientation and neurologic status; insti-   drink; monitor blood pressure closely when giving **morphine**
tute measures to reduce anxiety and stress;   parenterally; keep in mind that **fentanyl** and **sufentanil** reduce
help to divert attention from pain; monitor   muscle rigidity with neuromuscular blockers.
pain relief; instruct in measures to pro-
mote bowel elimination including the use
of stool softeners, laxatives as necessary,
and high fiber diet; monitor urinary elimination status, including I and O; institute
safety measures to prevent injury; raise
side rails and assist in moving and getting
in and out of bed; instruct to change position slowly; instruct to avoid driving or activities that require mental alertness until
the effects of the drug are known.

---

increased pain and other sensations, tactile hal-   ## Nursing management
lucinations, rhinorrhea, and diarrhea. Physical
dependence is treated by substitution of meth-   ### Nursing implications: substance abuse
adone for other opioids and then gradual with-
drawal from methadone. Sustained cure rates   Education of the lay public is important to resolution of
in opioid dependence are low, apparently owing   the drug-dependence problem. Young people must
to the persistence of psychological dependence.   understand the nature of these substances and the
                                                     risks inherent in their abuse. Families should be aware

of the signs and symptoms of developing drug dependence so that care can be sought early.

The problems of drug abuse are not resolved, however, by these measures alone. It is even more important to eliminate the personality problems that lead to psychological dependence on drugs. Child-rearing practices that foster the development of psychological maturity, self-reliance, and self-confidence go far to eliminate the need for chemical crutches.

Control of narcotics.
Preparation of opioids for administration is somewhat more involved than with other medications. These drugs are strictly controlled by law. They are usually stored in cabinets with double locks, the keys to which are retained by only one staff member. An accurate record must be made of the amount of the drug removed from the supply, the name of the client who is to receive the drug, the time the drug was administered, and the name of the physician and nurse involved (Fig. 24-1).

PRN medication.
The management of analgesic therapy when drugs are ordered *PRN* (as necessary) is frequently a problem for the nurse. Aware of the dependence potential of these drugs, the nurse may wish to use the least amount possible. If the client is not kept relatively pain free, however, this approach can be counterproductive. Recurring pain that is relieved by medication sets up a stimulus-response-reward sequence that conditions the client to psychological dependence on the drugs. Psychological dependence is much more difficult to resolve than physical dependence once the pain-producing pathology has been controlled. Careful nursing management of medication regimens to prevent the development of pain avoids such conditioning while keeping the client comfortable. Regular medication before events likely to increase pain (such as dressing changes or ambulation) reduces stress in the client and minimizes psychological dependence. Clients with patient-controlled analgesia should be informed of scheduled events likely to increase discomfort, so that they can plan for medication before they occur.

Research has shown that such regimens result in greater control of pain with the same or reduced drug dosages than the traditional approach of medicating only when the pain becomes unbearable to the client. Tolerance and physical dependence are also less likely to develop.

Toxicity.
Toxic reactions to opioids may occur in high-risk clients who receive drugs by prescription, but these reactions are seen more often in abusers who overdose. A major sign of toxicity is respiratory failure. Support of respirations is the first priority of care. An IV line is established for rapid administration of medications and treatment of shock should it develop. Administration of opioid antagonists may produce dramatic improvement, but this tends to be short-lived because these drugs are eliminated from the body more rapidly than opioids. Repeated doses are usually necessary. The client is kept under intensive care for at least 24 hours.

Dependency.
When pain is severe or is due to a progressive terminal condition, some degree of physical dependence is acceptable. Should the illness resolve, this type of dependence is readily amenable to treatment by a weaning regimen (provided psychological dependence has been avoided).

The treatment of chronic opioid dependence during the initial phase requires a controlled environment. Usually the client is given methadone in place of the preferred drug, and a schedule of decreasing dosage is instituted for weaning off the drug. Physical dependence can often be eliminated in a relatively short time (2 weeks to 6 months). During the weaning period, clients experience some discomfort. The intensity of this discomfort is inversely related to the speed of the weaning process. Psychological dependence is more persistent and generally requires a much longer period of treatment. It is not unusual, for example, for addicts to remain in drug treatment facilities for a year or more. Elimination of psychological dependence is crucial to long-term prognosis. The high rate of relapse after discharge from the protected environment is due to the failure to resolve psychological dependence. The success rate is sometimes improved by gradual resumption of independence. Halfway houses provide a degree of protection, along with the support of other people with similar problems. The use of self-help groups, some patterned after Alcoholics Anonymous, also improves the success rate.

Nursing process for clients who receive opioid analgesics

Assessment
The client who is to receive opioid analgesics must be assessed carefully to determine the degree of risk of such therapy. The history of previous use or abuse of these drugs and responses to them should be explored. The specific drugs involved and the nature of the reaction should be delineated if the client has experienced adverse reactions. The physician must be informed of this history; if a drug to which the client is intolerant has been prescribed, the nurse should request a change in the drug order.

Clients who are dependent on opioids may exaggerate the dosages used to establish a high tolerance and influence the physician to prescribe higher than normal dosages for relief of pain related to the condition for which they have been hospitalized (Adams, 1988).

Respiratory function must be carefully appraised. Clients with a history of multiple sclerosis, myasthenia gravis or other paralytic disorder that involves the

PHARMACY NARCOTIC CONTROL RECORD
AND 24-HOUR NURSING AUDIT RECORD

Floor 5 WEST Date 1/16/83

TIME	PATIENT	Codeine Tablet 25 mg	Codeine Tablet 30 mg	Codeine Ampule 30 mg	Demerol Tablet 50 mg	Demerol Ampule 25 mg	Demerol Ampule 50 mg	Demerol Ampule 75 mg	Demerol Ampule 100 mg	Dilaudid Ampule 2 mg	Lomotil Tablet	Morphine Ampule 10 mg	Morphine Ampule 15 mg	Pantopon Ampule	Percodan Tablet		NURSE'S SIGNATURE	PHYSICIAN'S NAME
	BROT. FORD.	21	17	14	7	9	16	12	8	—	—	5	11	—	18			
	REC'D.				10				10			10						
	TOTAL	21	17	14	17	9	16	12	18			15	11		18			
7 45 AM	R. Smith											1					Ann Smith	Raymond Jones
8 00 AM	a. Moore							1									Ann Smith	James Dudd

8-HOUR NURSING AUDIT RECORD

																	SIGNATURE ON-COMING NURSE	SIGNATURE OUT-GOING NURSE
ON HAND	AT 3:00 PM																	
ON HAND	AT 11:00 PM																	
ON HAND	AT 7:00 AM																	
	TOTAL USED IN 24 HOURS																	

Completed form inspected and approved
by _____, Nurse Date _____   Completed form inspected and approved by _____, Pharmacist Date _____
Indicate loss, waste, or a patient refusal in "Patient's Name Column" and in the appropriate drug column.

Form PH–1

Figure 24-1. Example of a narcotic control record.

respiratory muscles, obstructive airway disease, or myxedema are at high risk for acute respiratory depression when opioids are given.

Clients with liver or renal impairment are unable to metabolize opioids at a normal rate. Drug dosage for these individuals is usually reduced, or the interval at which they are administered is lengthened.

The client should be examined to assess further risk factors. Obese clients are at high risk for respiratory complications. Respiratory rate and depth and skin color should be noted. Opioids are not usually given to clients with a respiratory rate less than 12 per minute because further depression of respirations can be dangerous.

Laboratory data should be explored for indications of conditions that impair tissue perfusion (*eg*, anemia, poor cardiac function) and liver or renal dysfunction.

A careful assessment of pain should be made before each dose when opioids are ordered to relieve pain. Objective signs of distress as well as subjective symptoms should be explored. The location, severity, quality, and intensity of pain should be determined. The purpose for which the drug has been ordered should be specified by the physician; the drug should not be given to relieve pain of a different type or in a different location than that for which it was prescribed.

The nurse should determine when the last analgesic medication was administered to the client. All drugs received by the client for the previous 24 hours should be reviewed to determine if substances antagonistic to or synergistic with opioids have been given. If so, the physician should be consulted to determine if a change in dosage is appropriate. For example, if clients receive Innovar during anesthesia, dosage of opioid analgesics should generally be cut in half for a period of time until the Innovar is eliminated from the body.

Immediately before administering opioids, the nurse should count the respirations and note their depth. The degree of pupillary constriction should also be noted. If the effects of opioids that have been previously administered have worn off, the pupils are usually normal. Persistent constriction is an indication of developing tolerance, because the symptoms for which the drug is used are recurring before the drug has been eliminated by the body. (Tolerance does not develop to pupillary constriction.)

Nursing diagnosis
Diagnoses may include the following:

Pain related to trauma
High risk for impaired gas exchange related to hypopnea secondary to use of depressant drugs
Constipation related to decrease in propulsive peristalsis secondary to use of depressant drugs
Altered tissue perfusion: cerebral hypoxia related to postural hypotension secondary to use of depressant drugs
Urinary retention related to increased sphincter tone and decreased bladder contractility

Many clients exhibit a knowledge deficit related to opioid analgesics and their use to control pain. Although most people are aware of the undesirable aspects of opioid drug use, especially of physical or psychological dependence, they may not understand the therapeutic uses.

Planning
Goals of treatment are to alleviate pain, maintain respirations and gas exchange, prevent or alleviate constipation, maintain cerebral circulation, alleviate urinary retention, and decrease or eliminate knowledge deficit.

Intervention
Every client in pain should receive intensive nursing care to reduce perception of and reaction to pain and to enhance the analgesic effect of drugs. Measures to reduce anxiety and stress in the client, to promote relaxation, and to divert attention from the pain are critical.

Drug regimens in progressive conditions usually begin with the least powerful analgesics and progress to more potent preparations. Aspirin or acetaminophen may be sufficient early in the illness. Propoxyphene or pentazocine may be used next. As pain increases in severity, codeine and eventually meperidine or morphine may be required. It is the responsibility of the nurse to monitor the client's pain and response to medication so that the drug regimen may be adapted to the client's needs. It is important that acute discomfort be avoided; such episodes foster the development of psychological dependence on analgesic drugs.

Response to each dose of the analgesic to be administered should be carefully assessed. The client should be evaluated for pain control and toxic and side effects from the medication. If pain relief is inadequate or adverse reactions to the drug are apparent, the physician should be consulted for a change in the drug order.

If respirations become unduly depressed (less than 12/minute), assisted respirations or an opioid antagonist may be ordered. Administration of an opioid antagonist may temporarily abolish the analgesic effect of previous doses of opioids, precipitating acute severe pain. Intensive nursing care to decrease the perception of pain should be instituted. As effects of the opioid antagonist dissipate, the analgesic effects recur.

Nursing measures to facilitate fecal elimination are appropriate but may not be sufficient if long-term use of opioids is necessary. A stool softener should be used daily. Enemas or stimulant laxatives may also be needed. Care should be exercised to avoid obstipation or fecal impaction.

Clients subject to postural hypotension when medicated for pain should be taught to change position slowly, especially when arising from a bed or chair. Support hose may be used to minimize pooling of blood in the lower extremities.

Nursing measures to promote micturition should be used to prevent retention. As with constipation, however, these measures may be inadequate, particularly in elderly men who are prone to prostatic hypertrophy. Catheterization may be necessary.

Client education. When opioids are given for the relief of pain, the client should be informed of the purpose of the medication. The effect of the drug is usually enhanced by the placebo effect of suggestion. Moreover, clients must be aware of the nature of the drugs they are receiving if their consent to treatment is to be valid.

Occasionally, clients are reluctant to use opioid substances. Unless the person has a history of opioid dependence or religious or philosophical scruples, this fear is usually unwarranted. The client may need instruction regarding the deleterious effects of pain in the healing process to provide a rational base for the decision for or against medication. If the client wishes to avoid drug use, the nurse should provide him or her with detailed instruction in nonpharmacologic approaches to the treatment of pain.

Clients on long-term opioid treatment should be instructed in assessment techniques to evaluate their need for the drug and to assess their undesirable reactions to the drug. Respirations should be counted before each dose. The rate should be 12 or more per minute before more drug is used. Dosage schedules should be maintained, and the physician should be notified if pain relief is inadequate.

Clients or their families benefit from instruction in techniques to reduce the perception of pain and to enhance analgesic effect. Relaxation techniques, the control of other stressors, and diversion are helpful. Some people benefit from instruction in self-hypnosis.

Most clients who receive opioids develop some degree of constipation. They should be cautioned to maintain full hydration, regular exercise, and a diet that contains adequate bulk. A regular schedule of defecation should be established (daily, if possible). A stool softener such as docusate sodium (Colace) or bulk-forming laxatives such as psyllium hydrophilic mucilloid (Metamucil) may be recommended.

Clients should be warned about providing secure storage for drug supplies to prevent inadvertent ingestion, overdose, or theft. Locked containers are recommended.

While under the influence of opioids, clients tend to be less alert and less proficient than normal in psychomotor performance. They should avoid driving or operating other types of power machinery while these drug effects persist.

Learning experience 24-1

Care for a client in the hospital or nursing home who has an order for opiate medication to control pain. What special procedures are used to account for the drugs? Is the dosage ordered within the recommended range? How does the client respond to the drugs? What nursing measures are employed to enhance the analgesic effects of medication?

Evaluation Data required for evaluation include statements by clients indicating that they are comfortable or that the pain has been relieved. Respirations, color, and peripheral tissue perfusion should be monitored to determine gas exchange. Adequacy of elimination is indicated by consistency and frequency of stools and patterns of micturition. The ability of clients to repeat information conveyed during teaching sessions and their acceptance of appropriate analgesic regimens may be used as indicators of teaching effectiveness (see the Example of Nursing Process and Codeine Side Effects).

Checklist of nursing actions

☐ Assess clients who are to receive opioids for increased risk of adverse reactions, particularly history of use or abuse and risk of respiratory impairment.

☐ Assess respirations before administration of opioids; respirations should be 12 or more per minute in adults.

☐ Assess individual response to opioid medication carefully in relation to pain relief, toxic and side effects, and signs and symptoms of developing allergy or tolerance.

☐ Request a change of medication if response is undesirable or signs of allergy develop.

☐ Teach clients who manage their own opioid regimens to monitor their responses to the drugs.

☐ Teach clients who manage their own opioid regimens about self-care techniques to enhance response to the drugs and to reduce side effects.

☐ Caution clients who manage their own opioid regimens not to engage in potentially dangerous activities while under the influence of the drugs.

☐ Caution clients who manage their own opioid regimens to secure drug supplies to prevent inadvertent poisoning.

☐ Counsel parents in techniques to promote opti-

Example of nursing process and codeine side effects

The client is a 50-year-old man discharged from the hospital four weeks ago following diagnosis of adenocarcinoma of the lung, with metastases to the cervical vertebrae.

The client complains of back pain, stating that the pain pills provided relief until three days ago. Now, they "take the edge off the pain" but never make him "really comfortable." His prescription for pain medication specifies codeine 30 mg PO q3h for chest or back pain. He has taken one dose at 6 A.M. and another at noon. It is now 4 P.M. He states he is reluctant to take more of these pills because they "are not working," and he "doesn't want to become addicted."

The client's vital signs (blood pressure, pulse, and respirations) are elevated above his normal range. His pupils are equal and react to light.

The client also complains of constipation, which began in the hospital and has not improved much since his discharge.

Assessment data	Nursing diagnosis	Intervention	Goals and outcome criteria
Diagnosis of metastatic cancer Complains of back pain Client statement that the pain medication never makes him feel "really comfortable."	Knowledge deficit related to severe pain and therapeutic regimens for its relief.	**Discuss** with the client the meaning pain has for him, its impact on his quality of life, and the therapeutic use of opioid medications, stressing the adverse effects chronic pain has on health. **Advise** the client to take another dose of analgesic immediately.	The client will accept pain medication.
Client takes pain medication infrequently because he "doesn't want to become addicted." Elevated vital signs	Pain: back pain related to irritation of pain receptors by metastatic lesions in the vertebrae	**Advise** the client to take the pain medication by the clock until the pain is under control, then to gradually increase the time interval between doses until the optimum dosage schedule is determined. **Advise** the client to contact the physician for a change in medication if the pain is not controlled within 24 hours **Notify** the physician about the client's pain and the recommendations given him.	The client will state that his pain is under control and that he is comfortable. The client's vital signs will drop to levels normal for him.
Use of opioid medication	Constipation related to increased sphincter tone and decreased propulsive peristalsis secondary to use of opioid medication	**Inform** the client that constipation is a side-effect of opioid analgesics and is likely to be a continuing problem. **Recommend** that the client take an over-the-counter stool softener. **Advise** the client of hygienic measures that help to counteract constipation. **Recommend** the use of a saline or stimulant laxative of the client's choice.	The client will state that the constipation has been alleviated or eliminated

mum psychological and personality development in children to reduce the risk of drug abuse.

☐ Educate members of the lay public to the risks of nonmedicinal use of opioids.

☐ Store opioid drugs in secure places; keep an accurate record of their use and disposition.

☐ Maintain good tissue oxygenation when treating opioid toxicity.

☐ Monitor clients with opioid toxicity for at least 24 hours, administering opioid antagonists as necessary.

(For more information on medication regimens for management of pain, see Chapter 20.)

Nursing process for the hospitalized opioid abuser

Assessment   The signs and symptoms of opioid dependence depend on the time lapse since the latest dose ("fix") of the abused substance. Somnolence, indifference to pain, and contracted pupils are characteristic of the period of peak action of the drug. As these subside, the client appears normal. Later, during early withdrawal, pupils dilate (the client may experience photophobia), "sniffles" may occur, and the clients experiences discomfort and exhibits restlessness. Full-blown withdrawal may be manifested by pain, nausea, vomiting, diarrhea, and seizures. Injection sites may be visible on the arms and legs.

If clients admit to using drugs, ask specific questions to delineate the "habit"—which drugs are used, usual dosages, and usual effects. Clients may exaggerate dosages to establish that they are highly tolerant of opioid effects (Adams, 1988).

To detect opioid dependence, the physician may order naloxone drops in one eye; the test is positive if the pupil in the treated eye dilates and becomes larger than the pupil in the unmedicated eye (Creighton, Ghodse, 1989).

Nursing diagnosis   Diagnoses may include the following:

Pain related to CNS hyperactivity secondary to withdrawal from opioids
Sleep pattern disturbance: restlessness and insomnia related to CNS hypersensitivity secondary to withdrawal from opioids
Constipation related to hypertonic and hypomotile colon secondary to long-term use of opioids
Diarrhea related to hyperactive bowel secondary to withdrawal from opioids
Anxiety related to withdrawal from opioids
Fear related to hospitalization and loss of control of opioid intake

A common collaborative problem that should be differentiated from the nursing diagnoses is

Potential complication: seizures

Planning   Goals of treatment may be to minimize the signs and symptoms of withdrawal, to avoid escalation of the client's habit (if pain medications are required for the condition for which the client was hospitalized), and to inform clients of existing facilities for the treatment of drug dependence.

Intervention   The nurse collaborates with the physician in planning a medication program that meets clients' needs for pain control but at the same time does not exacerbate the client's drug dependence. Regularly decreasing doses of opioids may be ordered to "wean" the client from the drug of abuse. Nonopioid analgesics should be used for disease-related pain when possible. Nursing measures to control pain should be employed. These might include applications of heat (warm packs, hot water bottles) or cold (ice packs, cold moist packs), positioning for comfort, pleasant sensory stimuli (art, music, attractive food, flowers, back rubs), and diversion. Measures to promote sleep and rest, restore normal bowel elimination, and provide emotional support are needed by most clients. Nonopioid analgesics that may be prescribed for pain include nonsteroidal anti-inflammatories (including aspirin) or acetaminophen.

Client education.   Counseling may help prepare clients to accept referral for treatment of their drug dependence. If clients are receptive, referrals should be completed and initial contact with agencies arranged before discharge of the client.

Evaluation   Data required for evaluation include absence or presence and severity of signs and symptoms of opioid withdrawal syndrome, absence or presence of pain due to disease processes other than opioid dependence, and refusal or acceptance of referral for drug dependence treatment.

Checklist of nursing actions

☐ When one or more signs of drug dependence or withdrawal syndrome are present, assess clients for drug dependence.

☐ Collaborate with the physician to develop a regimen to maintain clients (or wean them from the drug of abuse) while meeting their needs for control of pain due to other disease conditions.

☐ Use nursing interventions to control pain and to minimize signs and symptoms of opioid withdrawal.

☐ Counsel (or obtain counseling for) clients to promote acceptance of treatment for drug dependence.

"Nonnarcotic" opioid receptor agonists

Several relatively weak opioid receptor agonists are in common use as analgesics (Table 24-14). Although they are derivatives of the more powerful opioid drugs, these compounds are not classified legally as narcotics. They are subject only to prescription controls under schedule IV of the Controlled Substances Act.

Pharmacodynamics. These drugs act as agonists or partial agonists that occupy opiate receptors, producing some of the pharmacologic effects of narcotic opioids; in general, the effects are milder, and certain effects (*eg*, antitussive, GI) may not occur. Because they compete with the stronger opioids for placement on the receptor, these drugs are capable of acting as agonist-antagonists of narcotic opioids.

Table 24-14. Nonnarcotic opioid receptor agonists*

Drug name	Preparations	Usual adult analgesic dosage	Additional information
buprenorphine (Buprenex)	Solutions for IM and IV administration	0.3–0.6 mg q4–6h PC: C (D for prolonged use or use of high doses at term)	Should respiratory depression develop, give doxapram (Dopram).
butorphanol (Stadol)	Solution for IM or IV injection	*IM:* 1–4 mg q3–4h PRN *IV:* 0.5–2 mg q3–4h PRN PC: B (D for prolonged use or use of high doses at term)	Butorphanol is used for the treatment of moderate to severe pain. Structurally, butorphanol resembles morphine; pharmacologically, it is similar to pentazocine and nalbuphine.
dezocine (Dalgan)	Vials, syringes and multiple-dose vials for IM or IV administration	(IM) 5–20 mg q3–6h (IV) 2.5–10 mg q2–4h PC: C	Dezocine's effectiveness is comparable to that of morphine sulfate. Dezocine can depress respirations but less so than morphine. Dezocine contains sodium metabisulfate; it is contraindicated for clients with allergic sensitivity to sulfites. Dezocine is too irritating to administer SC.
nalbuphine (Nubain)	Solution for SC, IM, or IV injection	10 mg q3–6h PRN In nontolerant persons, *maximum single dose:* 20 mg; *maximum daily dosage:* 160 mg PC: B (D for prolonged use or use of high doses at term)	Nalbuphine is used for the treatment of moderate to severe pain. Structurally, nalbuphine resembles naloxone and oxymorphone; pharmacologically, it is similar to pentazocine and butorphanol.
pentazocine (Talwin)	Solution for SC, IM, or IV injection Oral tablets	30 mg q3–4h PRN 50–100 mg q3–4h PRN PC: C (D for prolonged use or use of high doses at term)	Pentazocine is used for the treatment of moderate to severe pain. When given orally, a higher dose is required to achieve effects equal to parenteral administration.
propoxyphene hydrochloride (Darvon)	Oral capsules	65 mg q4h PRN PC: C (D for prolonged use or use of high doses at term)	Propoxyphene is used for the treatment of mild to moderate pain.
propoxyphene napsylate (Darvon-N)	Oral tablets and suspension	100 mg q4h PRN	Owing to its greater solubility, the hydrochloride is absorbed more rapidly than the napsylate.

* In the legal sense

KEY: PC = pregnancy category. (The validity of pregnancy categories has not been established; see Chapter 16; p 216.)

Pharmacokinetics. Nonnarcotic opioid receptor agonists are administered orally and by injection. After absorption, they are widely distributed in the body, including to the brain, into breast milk, and across the placenta. Metabolism is by the liver, and excretion is primarily by the kidneys.

Therapeutic uses. The weaker opioid receptor agonists are used to relieve pain that is not responsive to anti-inflammatory analgesics and acetaminophen. Their use allows postponement of administration of narcotic opioids considered to have a greater abuse potential and to carry greater risk of dependence. Propoxyphene has been used as a supplemental agent during methadone detoxification of opiate-dependent people.

Adverse reactions. Toxic and side effects resemble those of the stronger opioids. However, tolerance and dependence appear to develop more slowly than to most narcotic opioids. Abuse and withdrawal have been documented.

Precautions and contraindications. Precautions and contraindications are similar to those for narcotic opioids. Except for propoxyphene, these drugs are not used in the treatment of withdrawal from narcotic opioids because they do not effectively alleviate the symptoms of this syndrome.

Nonnarcotic opioid receptor agonists are not generally recommended for use in children or during pregnancy or lactation. Nonopioid analgesics are discussed in Chapter 47.

Opioid antagonists

Certain drugs that interact with opioid receptors in the CNS produce little or no agonistic effect at these sites. Because they are capable of displacing the opioid molecule from the receptor site, they tend to reduce the physiologic effects of these drugs and are termed *opioid antagonists*. Some of these substances do exert opioid effects when given to people who have neither received prior medication with opioids nor developed physical opioid dependence. However, when administered to people under the influence of opioids, they displace these more active analgesics from the receptor sites, producing a reduction in overall effect. When administered to opioid-dependent people, they displace residual drugs from the receptor and precipitate withdrawal signs and symptoms.

Pharmacodynamics. Opioid antagonists interact with opioid receptors, producing various degrees of agonistic or antagonistic effects (Table 24-15). In the absence of either opioid molecules or opioid tolerance at the site, the physiologic effects exerted by these drugs depend on the degree to which they act as agonists at the sites. Naloxone and naltrexone appear to exert little or no agonistic action and are considered to be relatively pure antagonists.

The physiologic actions of these drugs are substantially different when administered to subjects under the influence of opioid compounds. By displacing the opioid molecule from the receptor site, antagonists either abolish their physiologic effects or greatly diminish them. The person who suffers from acute opioid toxicity responds to their administration with a lessening of symptoms such as respiratory depression. If no underlying physical opioid dependence is present, physiology can be returned to near normal by the judicious use of opioid antagonists.

Response to these drugs is influenced by physical dependence on opioids in the recipient. Whether or not these clients exhibit signs and symptoms of opioid toxicity initially, administration of opioid antagonists tends to elicit the withdrawal syndrome.

Opioid antagonists have been shown to reduce analgesia induced by placebos and acupuncture. This evidence suggests that the therapeutic effectiveness of these treatments is mediated by the production of endogenous chemicals that exert agonistic effects on

Table 24-15. Opiate antagonists

Drug name	Action at opioid receptors			Usual dosage	Additional information
	μ	κ	o		
naloxone (Narcan)	Antagonist	Antagonist	Antagonist	Adults: *IV:* 400 μg q2–3 min for up to 3 doses Children: *IV:* 5–10 μg/kg body weight q2–3 min PC: B	Naloxone is a pure antagonist and is considered the drug of choice in most situations that require an opioid antagonist.
naltrexone (Trexan)	Antagonist	Antagonist	Antagonist	Adults: *Initially:* 25 mg po, repeated after 1 h if withdrawal does not occur; *maintenance:* 50–150 mg daily PC: C	Naltrexone is a pure antagonist; it is the first oral narcotic antagonist approved by the FDA to treat narcotic addiction.

KEY: PC = pregnancy category. (The validity of pregnancy categories has not been established; see Chapter 16; p 216.)

opioid receptors. These substances have been identified as endorphins and enkephalins produced by the CNS. These chemicals may also be responsible for the abolition of pain perception, which is observed in situations that involve extreme excitement or stress, and for the euphoric "high" during vigorous exercise that has been reported by many athletes. Chronic exposure to both danger and active exercise appears to have some addictive potential as shown by reports of restlessness, varying degrees of depression, and other mild withdrawal symptoms by devotees during periods of abstinence.

In summary, physiologic response to opioid antagonists depends upon a number of factors:

- The degree of agonistic action of the chosen drug
- Whether or not opioid drugs are present at the receptor site
- The presence of endogenous endorphins or enkephalins at the receptor site
- The degree of physical dependence on opioids previously developed by the recipient
- Concentration at the receptor site as determined by dosage

Pharmacokinetics. Naloxone and levallorphan are administered by injection rather than by mouth; levallorphan is poorly absorbed enterically, and both drugs are rapidly deactivated during first pass through the liver. Naltrexone is administered orally.

Serum half-lives of these drugs are shorter than are those for opioid drugs. The drugs are excreted by the kidneys.

Therapeutic uses. Narcotic antagonists are used primarily to treat acute opioid toxicity. When given to people who have taken an overdose of opioid drugs, they dramatically reduce the respiratory depression and sedation characteristic of this condition. Vital functions can be stabilized relatively quickly. Because of their short half-lives, narcotic antagonists must often be administered repeatedly when used to treat opioid overdose.

Narcotic antagonists given to the newborn or (preferably) to the mother just before birth serve to prevent or reverse the respiratory depression seen in infants whose mothers received opioid analgesics late in labor. The drugs are best given prophylactically to prevent respiratory depression.

Opioid antagonists can be used to diagnose physical opioid dependence. A dependent person, whose appearance and function appear normal because of residual opioids in the body, exhibits signs and symptoms of withdrawal when antagonists are administered. No response is apparent in nondependent people.

Because of its agonist effects, pentazocine is widely used as an analgesic. Maintenance doses of naltrexone are used to block the desirable effects of opioids during long-term treatment of opioid dependence. Because illegal drugs no longer produce euphoria, the use of naltrexone is believed to decrease drug-seeking and drug-use behavior.

Investigationally, naltrexone has had beneficial effects in autistic children (Campbell, et al, 1989). Naloxone has also been used successfully to resolve hypotension due to clonidine toxicity.

Adverse reactions. The pure antagonists, naloxone and naltrexone, exhibit few effects in the absence of opioid use or dependence. Naloxone sometimes causes nausea and vomiting and can aggravate hypertension. When administered for opiate overdose, it has caused abrupt return to consciousness accompanied by tremor and hyperventilation. Naltrexone can cause adverse GI effects (pain, cramps, nausea, and vomiting). Elevations of liver enzymes, CNS symptoms (nervousness, insomnia, anxiety, lassitude, or depression), musculoskeletal pain, rash, and upper respiratory congestion have also been reported.

Levallorphan, which possesses some agonist activity, may cause dysphoria, miosis, pseudoptosis, drowsiness, sweating, nausea, respiratory depression, and a sense of heaviness in the limbs. High doses may precipitate a pseudopsychosis characterized by disturbed sleep, bizarre dreams, visual hallucinations, disorientation, and feelings of unreality.

Precautions. Opioid antagonists should be used with caution in people suspected of opioid dependence if concurrent medical problems make an acute withdrawal syndrome dangerous (see Focus on Opioid Agonists/Antagonists: Similarities and Differences).

■ Summary

Opioid antagonists are substances that interact with opioid receptors while exerting little or no agonist effect. By displacing more powerful agonists from these receptors, they reduce the physiologic effects of these drugs. In opioid drug-dependent people, opioid antagonists elicit withdrawal syndrome. Opioid antagonists are used to treat acute opioid toxicity and opioid overdose, as well as to diagnose physical dependence on opioids.

Nursing management

Nursing implications

When opioid antagonists are administered to diagnose opioid dependency, the health care staff must be prepared to cope with the acute withdrawal syndrome that may result. The client is likely to experience nausea, rhinorrhea, and diarrhea. In addition, any "high" the user has experienced from recent drug "hits" is reversed.

Opioid agonists/antagonists: similarities and differences

Similarities

Pharmacodynamics

These agents act by displacing the opioid molecule from the receptor site, reducing or abolishing the physiologic effect of opioids. They produce varying degrees of agonistic or antagonistic effects.

Pharmacokinetics

These agents are excreted by the kidneys and metabolized by the liver. It is unknown if these agents cross into breast milk.

Therapeutic uses

These agents are used to treat opioid toxicity and overdose. They are also used prophylactically to prevent respiratory depression in infants whose mothers have received opioid analgesics during labor. They can be used to diagnose physical opioid dependence.

Adverse reactions

These agents exhibit few effects in the absence of opioid use or dependence; however, some nausea and vomiting have been reported.

Contraindications

These agents are contraindicated for people with a known hypersensitivity to the drug.

Precautions

These agents should be used with caution in people suspected of opioid dependence.

Differences

• **Naloxone** and **naltrexone** have no agonist properties. They are thought to act as competitive agonists at the opiate receptor sites. • **Levallorphan** has both agonistic and antagonistic properties.

• **Naloxone** and **levallorphan** are administered by injection; **naltrexone** is given orally. • **Naloxone** has an onset of action of 1 to 2 minutes (IV), 2 to 5 minutes (S or IM); its duration of action depends on the dose and route given; it is rapidly distributed into body tissues and fluids and crosses the placenta; its plasma half-life is 60 to 90 minutes for adults and 3 hours for neonates. • **Naltrexone** is rapidly and completely absorbed from the GI tract; its onset of action is 15 to 30 minutes, peaking in 1 hour with a terminal half-life of 95 hours; it is unknown if it crosses the placenta.

• **Naltrexone** has been used investigationally in the treatment of autistic children. • **Naloxone** is used to reduce hypertension due to clonidine toxicity.

• **Naltrexone** can cause painful cramps, elevated liver enzymes, nervousness, insomnia, anxiety, lassisitude, depression, musculoskeletal pain, rash, and upper respiratory congestion. • **Levallorphan** can cause dysphoria, miosis, pseudoptosis, drowsiness, sweating, respiratory depression, and sensation of limb heaviness.

• **Naltrexone** is contraindicated for people with acute hepatitis or liver failure, people who are receiving opiate agonists, people who are experiencing acute withdrawal, nondetoxicated people or those physically dependent on opioids, and people who experience opioid withdrawal after the **naloxone** challenge test. • **Naloxone** should be avoided after the use of opiates in surgery.

• **Naloxone** should be used with caution in people with pre-existing cardiac disease or those who are receiving potentially cardiotoxic drugs.

(continued)

Focus on

Opioid agonists/antagonists: similarities and differences (Continued)

Similarities	Differences
Nursing considerations	
Assess the person's level of consciousness and neurologic status for signs and symptoms of opioid overdose; assess cardiopulmonary status and have resuscitative equipment readily available; monitor for signs and symptoms of opioid dependence or withdrawal; institute CPR as necessary; check pupil dilation for drug effectiveness; institute measures to combat withdrawal symptoms; inform people of measures to be taken and ways they can assist in the treatment; continue monitoring until physiologic stability persists beyond the duration of activity of the last dose of opioid agonist drug; assist in coping with withdrawal signs and symptoms; provide a quiet environment; refer for treatment of drug abuse or dependence as necessary.	Make sure the person is opiate-free before starting **naltrexone**; instruct in using over-the-counter nonopiate drugs for relief of pain, diarrhea, or cough; administer the **naloxone** challenge test before giving **naltrexone**; if there are signs of opiate withdrawal do not give.

Because opioid withdrawal causes hypersensitivity to stimuli, a quiet environment should be provided for the diagnostic test. If results of the test are positive, health care personnel should avoid judgmental or punitive attitudes.

Various opioid antagonists may be stored together in the hospitals stock supplies of emergency drugs. The nurse must take care to identify the agent to be used accurately and to differentiate among several drugs with similar names.

Nursing process

Assessment

Drug overdoses are seen most commonly in emergency departments of acute care facilities. Initial assessment should focus on vital functions and on determining the drug agent involved. Clients with opioid toxicity are likely to be unconscious and to exhibit decreased pulse, blood pressure, and respirations. Clients who are responsive, or the people who accompany them, should be asked to identify the drugs taken and whether or not the client is dependent on opioids.

Nursing diagnosis The most common diagnoses are the following:

Impaired gas exchange related to respiratory depression secondary to CNS depressant toxicity
Altered tissue perfusion related to cardiovascular depression

If opioid dependence is confirmed or is likely, the client will exhibit

Altered comfort: cramping, pain, and respiratory congestion related to opioid withdrawal

Planning Goals of treatment are to maintain vital functions (respiration and circulation) until the effects of the drugs are reversed. If the client is opioid dependent, elimination of the dependence is a long-term goal.

Interventions Cardiopulmonary resuscitation is initiated as necessary. Mechanical assistance of respirations must be instituted immediately for any client with a respiratory rate of 10 per minute or less. If opioid drugs have been confirmed as the chemicals taken, injection of an opioid antagonist may be ordered. Repeated doses of the antagonist are usually required because antagonists are metabolized more rapidly than are opioids. As body levels of antagonist drop, its molecules leave the opioid receptors, which are immediately reoccupied by opioid molecules, producing a relapse to the toxic state.

Clients must be monitored closely to verify that their condition remains stable. Pupil dilation is one indicator of response to opioid antagonist medication. A rise in respiratory rate should occur within 1 to 2 minutes after injection of the opioid antagonist. A rapid but transitory improvement in general condition should occur. Repeated doses of antagonist may be required before the client's condition stabilizes.

Nursing measures should be instituted to ameliorate withdrawal symptoms, if they develop.

Client education. Clients who receive emergency treatment should be kept informed of what is to happen, even when they appear unresponsive or comatose. Instructions should be given to enable them to cooperate with treatment procedures. However, this is not the appropriate time to discuss the dangers of drug abuse or dependence. Client education should be focused on measures to assist the person in coping with the immediate situation.

After resolution of the medical crisis, clients who have experienced pronounced withdrawal should be referred for long-term treatment of drug dependence.

Evaluation Data required for evaluation include vital signs, particularly respirations, color, peripheral circulation, pupil size, and level of consciousness. The success of referral is judged by evidence of attendance at a drug treatment facility. Abstinence from drug use in the future determines whether or not the long-term goal, elimination of drug dependence, is achieved (see the Example of Nursing Process and Codeine Overdose).

Checklist of nursing actions

When treating victims of opioid toxicity

☐ Give first priority to the maintenance of vital functions, particularly respiration.

☐ Inform clients of measures to be taken and ways they can assist in the treatment.

☐ Monitor response to opioid antagonist medication closely.

☐ Continue monitoring clients until physiologic stability persists beyond the duration of activity of the last dose of opioid antagonist medication.

When opioid antagonists are administered to diagnose drug dependence

☐ Assist the client in coping with withdrawal signs and symptoms.

☐ Provide the client with a quiet environment.

☐ Refer clients for treatment of drug abuse or dependency as necessary.

Hypnotics

Hypnotics are drugs that induce sleep. Chemicals with hypnotic properties have been used for centuries to relieve insomnia and to promote rest. They have also been employed less admirably to produce stupor or coma for the purpose of victimizing the affected individual. Most hypnotic drugs are general CNS depressants that have dose-related effects. In small doses, they produce sedation, a state characterized by reduced excitation and activity and increased relaxation and lassitude. Moderate doses promote drowsiness or sleep. In large doses, many hypnotics induce general anesthesia.

Physiology of sleep

Sleep is a temporary state of altered consciousness characterized by amnesia and reduced perception of and responsiveness to the environment. Unlike unconscious states that result from disease processes or the administration of anesthetics, sleep can be interrupted by appropriate stimulation to arousal. Sensory and motor activity during sleep are virtually suspended and body processes slow down. This hiatus provides an opportunity for reparative processes to restore tissues and organs to optimum condition. During this period, the molecular and cellular biochemical changes that occur during the waking hours are reversed to prepare the body for another cycle of activity. Functionally, the brain appears to use sleeping time for sorting and storing in permanent memory the perceptions of the previous waking period. At the psychological level, the psyche similarly attends to psychological perceptions and tensions.

Stages and patterns of sleep

Sleep is not a steady state. Specific stages of sleep have been identified and described. These reflect the basic rest–activity cycles (BRACs) that characterize both waking and sleeping hours. BRACs, which last from 60 to 120 minutes, are related during the waking hours to fluctuations in efficiency and spontaneous behaviors such as food-seeking. During sleep, BRACs can be traced by monitoring brain-wave patterns, muscular activity, and vital signs. Stages in the cycles have been divided into two main classes: rapid eye movement (REM) sleep and nonrapid eye movement (NREM) sleep. REM sleep, also known as paradoxical or desynchronized sleep, is the stage during which most dreams occur. NREM sleep, or slow-wave sleep, has been further divided into four distinct stages (Table 24-16).

Sleep is one of the several body functions that exhibit rhythmic diurnal patterns. Physiologic processes characterized by such circadian rhythms include maintenance of body temperature, endocrine hormone secretion, mental alertness, and psychomotor function. Body temperatures, alertness, and activity levels are generally highest during the daylight hours and lowest during the nighttime hours. Activity patterns that vary from this norm can, however, induce changes in the chronology of other functions to conform to their rhythms. Completion of such adjustments usually requires a minimum of 2 weeks.

Each complete sleep cycle is characterized by progression from stages I through IV of NREM sleep, reversal of this sequence to return to stage I, and a subsequent period of REM sleep (Fig. 24-2). In normal people, the cycle always begins with stage I NREM

Example of nursing process and codeine overdose

The client is a 76-year-old woman admitted to the intensive care unit from the emergency department after ingesting between 20 and 30 codeine tablets containing 30 mg each. (The codeine was prescribed to control pain caused by metastatic cancer of the breast.) When she was found, she was comatose with respirations of 6/min. Respiratory resuscitation was begun by ambulance personnel, and she was placed on a demand respirator in the emergency department.

Gastric lavage and instillation of activated charcoal slurry were also performed in the emergency department. Administration of naloxone increased spontaneous respirations to 12–14/min, but these dropped to 8/min within half an hour.

The client's physician believes that chronic pain is a major factor in what was apparently a suicide attempt.

Naloxone 0.4 mg is to be administered by IV infusion every 30 minutes, until spontaneous respirations rise to 12 or more per minute. No further therapy is planned, other than maintenance of vital functions until the client becomes responsive. Consideration is being given to implantation of an infusion pump for automatic administration of morphine for pain relief once the crisis of the codeine overdose is resolved.

Assessment data	Nursing diagnosis	Intervention	Goals and outcome criteria
Coma Opioid overdose Hypopnea	Ineffective breathing pattern: hypopnea related to CNS depression secondary to opioid overdose	**Continue** assisted breathing by respirator, assessing spontaneous respirations by trial periods off the machine according to medical orders. **Administer** naloxone as ordered. **Monitor** the client for neurologic signs and symptoms indicating changes in the degree of CNS depression.	The client will not become cyanotic; arterial blood gases will remain within normal limits.
Coma	High risk for impaired tissue integrity: phlebitis or decubiti related to immobility secondary to CNS depression	**Turn** the client at least q2h. **Carry** out passive range of motion at least q4h. **Massage** the skin over pressure points at least q4h. **Place** an egg crate or alternating pressure air mattress under the client.	The client will not develop signs of phlebitis (redness and swelling of the calf) or of decubiti (persistent redness over pressure points, breaks in the skin).
Opioid overdose History of chronic pain due to metastatic malignancy	Ineffective individual coping: depression related to chronic pain and life-threatening illness	**Perform** procedures in a caring manner; handle the client gently, talk to her, and explain what will be done. **Postpone** interventions that require verbal communication until the client is alert and a good therapeutic relationship has been established.	When she is alert, the client will cooperate with the health care staff in therapeutic communication designed to improve her individual coping skills.

Table 24-16. Comparison of the characteristics of wakefulness and the stages of sleep

Characteristics	Wakefulness	Drowsiness	Non-rapid eye movement sleep				Rapid eye movement sleep
			Stage I	Stage II	Stage III	Stage IV	
Electroencephalogram tracing*	Rapid irregular waves	Alpha rhythms	Uneven low voltage waves with frequencies of 2–7 cycles per second	Larger script with spindles and K complexes	Delta waves comprise 20% to 25% of the tracing Occasional sleep spindles	Delta waves comprise more than 50% of the tracing	Wild oscillations; desynchronized beta waves similar to wakeful tracing
Subjective sensations	Alert, aware of environment	Serene, without deliberate thought, dreamlike thoughts, floating images	None—if wakened may deny sleeping	None—if wakened may report vague dreams or reveries	None—dreams not reported by wakened subjects	None—dreams not reported by wakened subjects	None—wakened subjects usually report dreaming
Peripheral muscle tone	Moderate to high	Moderate	Moderate	Fair	Fair	Fair	Atony
Muscle activity	Voluntary, varying with basic activity–rest cycles	Diminished	Minimal to absent	Minimal to absent	Minimal to absent	Minimal to absent	Rapid conjugate eye movements
Duration	6–20 h per day	Limited to a few minutes	Various	Various	Various	Various	5 to 20 min about every 90 min throughout sleep, increasing in length of each episode as sleep progresses
Persistence		Very easily disrupted	Easily wakened	Not hard to waken	Hard to waken	Hard to waken and slow to arouse	Very hard to waken
Probable chemical mobilization in the brain	Catecholamine	Serotonin	Serotonin	Serotonin	Serotonin	Serotonin	Catecholamine
Physiologic signs	Normal waking patterns	Progressive slowing of the pulse and respirations and reduction of temperature and blood pressure from non-REM stages I through IV					Variable vital signs; irregular pulse and respirations; temperature is at its nadir; bursts of autonomic activity

* See continued portion of table on facing page.

Table 24-16. Comparison of the characteristics of wakefulness and the stages of sleep (Continued)

		Electroencephalogram tracings	
Pattern	Voltage	Frequency (cycles per second)	Occurrence
Alpha waves	Low (about 50 microvolts)	8–13	Most intensive over the occiput. Characteristic of quiet resting cerebration in awake people
Beta waves	Low	14–30	Most frequent over parietal and frontal regions of the head
Theta waves	Low	4–7	Mainly in parietal and temporal regions of children and adults during frustration
Delta waves	High	1–2	Characteristic of the cortex when not subject to stimulation by the reticular activating system
Spindles	High	12–14	Intermittent bursts that last 0.5 or more sec
K complexes	High. Biphasic, with both negative and positive phases		Intermittent waves that last 0.5 or more sec

sleep and progresses through the usual sequence. Interruption of sleep, which returns a subject to wakefulness, causes the cycle to begin again at stage I NREM sleep. People who have been deprived of REM sleep by repeated awakenings before or at the initiation of this phase of the cycle, eventually adopt an abnormal sleep pattern characterized by an immediate onset of the REM phase on falling asleep. This phenomenon implies that the REM phase of sleep is necessary for important functions that cannot be performed adequately during NREM stages of sleep.

While variations in sleep patterns do exist from person to person and for a given person over time, divergence is not apparent among normal subjects. A typical sleep pattern is graphically illustrated in Figure 24-3. NREM sleep tends to predominate during the early hours of sleep, while periods of REM sleep tend to lengthen progressively during later hours.

Pathophysiology of sleep disturbances

Sleep disruptions are fairly common and are disturbing to their victims. Disruptions range in seriousness from an occasional delay in falling asleep to serious sleep deprivation that leads to psychotic manifestations. Inability to sleep may be caused by imbalance in brain neurotransmitters, environmental overstimulation, or both. Etiology may be exogenous, endogenous, or a combination of both (Box 24-8).

Adequate rest and sleep are essential if robust health is to be maintained. They are particularly important to the person who must regenerate tissue or restore physiologic or psychological equilibrium. For these reasons, promotion of adequate rest and sleep is a matter of concern to all health care professionals.

Hypnotic drugs

The ideal hypnotic would induce sleep soon after administration, promote natural sleep without disrupting normal patterns of sleep stages, allow sleep to end at the usual time of awakening, and produce no resid-

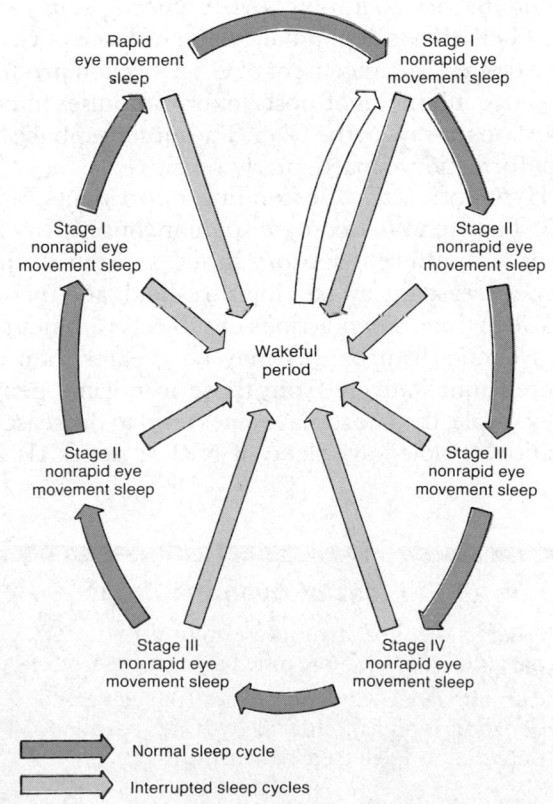

Figure 24-2. Sleep cycles.

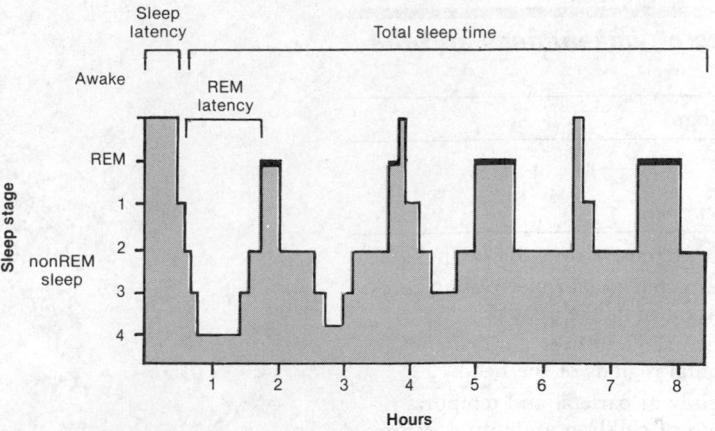

Figure 24-3. An idealized night of sleep in a normal young adult. (Mendelson WB. [1980]. *The use and misuse of sleeping pills*, p 7. New York: Plenum Medical Book Co.)

Box 24-8. Sleep disorders

Dyssomnias associated with disruptions of the diurnal sleep–wake cycle:

Phase shift in sleep cycles: a change in cycle induced by rapid travel across time zones ("jet lag") or a change in work schedule ("shift work" syndrome)

Fixed-phase sleep cycle: inconvenient or inappropriate sleep–wake cycle (the "owl" and "lark" syndromes)

Inappropriate length of sleep–wake cycle: a cycle that is shorter or longer than 24 hours. Such a cycle is "out of phase" with normal day–night patterns much of the time

Disorders of initiating and maintaining sleep:

Psychophysiologic insomnia: disturbances in sleep due to the presence of unaccustomed cues or other situational stressors

Psychiatric insomnia: sleep disturbances accompanying psychiatric illness that may be due to the psychosis, may contribute to the psychosis, or may be caused independently by the processes underlying the psychosis

Insomnia associated with medical conditions: interruption of sleep by pain, dyspnea, urinary frequency, or other discomfort

Sleep-induced ventilatory impairment: sleep apnea syndromes characterized by brief awakenings stimulated by respiratory embarrassment

Nocturnal myoclonus: brief awakenings after clonic movements of one or both legs

Childhood insomnia: early onset of insomnia usually associated with a positive family history of a similar problem

Insomnia due to drug use: chronic use of CNS stimulants or withdrawal from chronic use of CNS depressants that interfere with sleep by heightening CNS activity

ual ("hangover") or other undesirable effects on the body. No known chemical conforms to these criteria, but present-day hypnotics are equally effective as and safer than many that have been used in the past.

Drugs such as alcohol, bromides, chloral hydrate, paraldehyde, opiates, and barbiturates have historically been used for their soporific effects. Currently, prescriptions to promote sleep are largely limited to sedative-tranquilizers (particularly the benzodiazepines), chloral hydrate, paraldehyde, and selected barbiturates (Box 24-9).

Pharmacodynamics. Both the benzodiazepines and barbiturates appear to act by mimicking or enhancing the effects of τ-aminobutyric acid (GABA) in the brain. The specific effect of the barbiturates is not known; however, the benzodiazepines appear to antagonize a protein that acts to inhibit GABA binding to its receptors. Their effects depend on adequate levels of GABA in the tissues. Enhancement of GABA action produces a selective inhibition of postsynaptic impulses in polysynaptic pathways in the CNS. The mesencephalic reticular formation is particularly sensitive.

Hypnotics act as descending depressants of the CNS. They tend to decrease spontaneous activity and response to afferent sensory input, shorten sleep latency, increase the awakening threshold, and increase total sleep time. Their actions in subjects with neurotic or psychotic disturbances may be greater than and different qualitatively from those in normal people. For example, the benzodiazepines tend to decrease the duration of slow-wave sleep of NREM stages III and

Box 24-9. Types of hypnotic drugs

Historic: alcohol, bromides, chloral hydrate, paraldehyde, opiates, and barbiturates

Current: sedative-tranquilizers (particularly benzodiazepines), chloral hydrate, paraldehyde, and selected barbiturates

IV in normal people but increase the duration in people subject to neuroses or endogenous depression.

Because they affect the limbic system, the benzodiazepines exert some tranquilizing effect. Barbiturates sedate through general CNS depression.

Pharmacokinetics: dosage and administration. Most hypnotics are administered orally and are well absorbed by the GI mucosa. Chloral hydrate is irritating to mucous membranes and is administered in capsule form. It also can be administered in olive oil as a retention enema.

Paraldehyde, barbiturates, and benzodiazepines may be administered parenterally. Table 24-17 lists preparations and dosage. Paraldehyde is sometimes injected IM. Both IV and IM solutions of the benzodiazepines are available. Barbiturates may be administered IV but are never injected IM, because they cause pain and necrosis at the injection site.

After absorption, chloral hydrate, barbiturates, and benzodiazepines are bound to plasma proteins in proportion to their lipid solubility. Binding may range from minimal (as with flurazepam) to 99% (diazepam). These drugs can displace other drugs from protein-binding sites, thus increasing their physiologic action and accelerating their metabolism and excretion.

Hypnotic drugs are rapidly taken up by the gray matter of the brain. They are then redistributed to the white matter and adipose tissue and other tissues of the body. Eventually, they reach all tissues. Fetal blood levels are comparable to maternal levels, and the drugs are secreted in the breast milk.

Some hypnotics, notably phenobarbital and the benzodiazepines, circulate in the enterohepatic cycle (Goldberg, Berlinger, 1982; Gilman, et al, 1985). Metabolism of hypnotic drugs is carried out mainly by the liver microsomal enzyme system. Many metabolites are physiologically active, and an accumulation of these substances may prolong the action of a given dose. For this reason, the full effect of the drugs may not be apparent until they have been administered for several days. Persistence of active metabolites also contributes to prolonged residual effect ("hangover").

Excretion of most hypnotic drugs is performed by the kidneys. Renal filtration of unchanged drug is inversely proportional to the degree of protein binding and is insignificant for many drugs. Drug metabolites are readily eliminated in the urine, however. Renal excretion of free barbiturates may be increased by alkalinization of the urine (which increases solubility of the acid salts) and by osmotic diuresis. Small amounts of chloral hydrate and the benzodiazepines are excreted in the feces after their secretion in the bile.

Because many hypnotics persist in the body longer than 24 hours, repeated use is accompanied by accumulation and a gradual increase in physiologic effects. Toxicity is likely to develop.

Therapeutic uses. Hypnotic drugs are frequently prescribed to promote rest and sleep in ill or insomniac clients. They are also administered preoperatively to prepare clients for anesthetization. They are most useful in ameliorating temporary sleep disturbances that result from short-term illness or unavoidable environmental stimuli.

Adverse reactions. All hypnotic drugs alter sleep stages to some degree. The significance of many of the changes is unknown, but reduction in REM sleep, a common effect, is generally considered detrimental. Chronic use of hypnotics may produce pronounced REM deprivation. This condition could underlie the personality changes often seen in clients after prolonged use of these drugs. Distortion of sleep phases also can alter daytime perception; the benzodiazepines sometimes cause "daymares," phenomena analogous to nightmares that occur during sleep.

Side effects of hypnotic drugs include impairment of psychomotor and cognitive function and a decrease in inhibitions. Reaction time increases; weakness, vertigo, and confusion may occur. Behavior resembling that of alcohol intoxication is common with higher dosages.

Some individuals, particularly the elderly, react paradoxically to hypnotics. They become more wakeful and have increased difficulty in falling asleep (Johnson, 1985). Confusion and delirium have also been reported (Patterson, 1987). Hypnotic drugs may also cause sleep apnea, particularly in obese middle-aged men (Mendelson, et al, 1981). The use of phenobarbital in the treatment of epilepsy in children is associated with depression (Ferrari, Matthews, 1983).

The effects of hypnotic drugs and other CNS depressants are additive and can produce serious toxicity when multiple drugs are used. Combinations of barbiturates or tranquilizers with alcohol have been implicated in many deaths from sedative overdose.

Hypnotics share with other CNS depressants a potential for producing drug dependence. Tolerance is both pharmacokinetic and pharmacodynamic. Induction of liver microsomal enzymes by some hypnotics causes an acceleration of the rate of biotransformation in the bodies of habitual users. To maintain a constant response, an increase in dose is required. Of greater quantitative importance is the homeostatic response to the depression caused by these drugs. An excitatory feedback response compensates by increasing basal CNS activity. This phenomenon is common to all CNS depressants, and cross-tolerance is apparent among these drugs. Discontinuation of hypnotics precipitates physical withdrawal syndromes characterized by wakefulness, depression, anxiety, bizarre dreams, agitation, delirium, and psychosis. Seizures, coma, and death may occur, particularly in the case of barbiturate withdrawal. Because their addictive properties make

(Text continues on p. 451)

Table 24-17. Selected hypnotic drugs

Drug name	Preparations	Usual dosage	Additional information
Benzodiazepines			Some benzodiazepines are also employed as tranquilizers, sedatives, skeletal muscle relaxants, and anticonvulsants. Benzodiazepine may cause fetal damage when taken during pregnancy.
chlordiazepoxide (A-Poxide, Libritabs, Librium, Limbitrol, Murcil, Sereen, SK-Lygen, Tenax)	Oral tablets and capsules Solutions for deep IM or slow IV injection	*Preoperatively:* Adults: 50–100 mg IM 1 h before surgery; children 12–18 yr of age: 25–50 mg PC: D	Safe use in children younger than 12 yr of age has not been established.
flurazepam (Dalmane, Somnol)	Capsules for oral use	Adults: 15–30 mg PC: D	Safe use in children younger than 15 yr has not been established.
lorazepam (Ativan)	Oral tablets Solutions for IM or IV injection	*Preoperatively:* Adults: *IM:* 0.05 mg/kg body weight at least 2 h before surgery; *IV:* 0.44–0.5 mg/kg body weight 15 min before surgery; *maximum dosage:* 4 mg PC: D	Lorazepam causes amnesia proportional to dosage. Safe use or oral lorazepam in children younger than 12 yr of age and of parenteral lorazepam in children younger than 18 yr of age has not been established.
oxazepam (Serax)	Capsules for oral use	Adults: 10–30 mg PC: C	Although not approved for use in sleep disorders, oxazepam is preferred by some physicians for the treatment of sleep disorders in elderly people.
midazolam (Versed)	Solutions for injection	70–80 µg/kg body wt PC: D	Midazolam is used as a preoperative sedative and amnesiac. Adverse reactions to midazolam are similar to those of other benzodiazepines.
quazepam (Doral)	Tablets for oral use	Adults: 15 mg For some clients, dose may be halved after a few nights of therapy PC: X	Long duration of action may prevent withdrawal signs and symptoms when medication is discontinued. Teratogenic contraindicated during pregnancy. Concurrent use with cimetidine may prolong effects of quazepam. Safety and effectiveness in clients younger than 18 years of age are unproven.
temazepam (Restoril)	Oral capsules	Adults: 15–30 mg PC: X	Safe use in children younger than 18 yr of age has not been established.
triazolam (Halcion)	Oral tablets	Adults: 0.25–0.5 mg PC: X	For geriatric clients, the usual adult dosage should be halved. Safe use in children younger than 18 yr of age has not been established. Triazolam has been used successfully to prevent "jet-lag" upsets in workers on 12-h shift of sleep schedules.

(Continued)

Table 24-17. Selected hypnotic drugs (*Continued*)

Drug name	Preparations	Usual dosage	Additional information
Barbiturates			Barbiturates are also used to prevent cerebral edema after brain injury; to antagonize the unwanted CNS stimulation by other drugs; to reduce jaundice in kernicterus and obstructive liver conditions; and as sedatives, anesthetics, and anticonvulsants.
amobarbital (Amytal)	Powder Oral tablets, capsules, and elixir Powder for preparing solutions for deep IM or slow IV injection	*Oral or IM hypnotic dose for adults:* 65–200 mg *IV hypnotic dose for both adults and children older than 6 yr of age:* 65–500 mg; *maximum IV dose:* 1 g *IM hypnotic dose for children:* 2–3 mg/kg body weight	Amobarbital should not be used as a hypnotic for longer than 2 weeks. After long-term use, amobarbital should be withdrawn gradually.
aprobarbital (Alurate)	Oral solution	*Hypnotic dose:* Adults: 40–160 mg PC: D	Aprobarbital should not be used as a hypnotic for longer than 2 weeks. After long-term use, aprobarbital should be withdrawn gradually. Dosage for children has not been established.
butabarbital (Buticaps, Butisol)	Powder Oral tablets, capsules, and elixir	*Hypnotic dose:* Adults: 50–100 mg PC: D	Butabarbital should not be used as a hypnotic for longer than 2 weeks. After long-term use, butabarbital should be withdrawn gradually.
mephobarbital (Mebaral)	Oral tablets	*Oral sedative dose:* Adults: 32–100 mg tid or qid; children: 16–32 mg tid or qid PC: D	Mephobarbital is used primarily for sedation.
pentobarbital (Nembutal, Nova-Rectal, Novopentabarb)	Powder Oral capsules and elixir Solutions for deep IM or slow IV injection Rectal suppositories	*Oral hypnotic dose:* Adults: 100–200 mg *Rectal hypnotic doses:* Adults: 120–200 mg; children 12–14 yr of age: 60–120 mg; children 5–12 yr of age: 60 mg; children 1–4 yrs of age: 30–60 mg; children 2 mo to 1 yr of age: 30 mg *IM hypnotic doses:* Adults: 150–200 mg; children: 2–6 mg/kg body weight or 125 mg/m²; *maximum dose:* 100 mg PC: D	Pentobarbital should not be used as a hypnotic for longer than 2 weeks. After long-term use, pentobarbital should be withdrawn gradually.
secobarbital (Seconal)	Powder Oral tablets, capsules, and elixir Solutions for injection	*Oral or IM hypnotic dose:* Adults: 100–200 mg *IM hypnotic dose:* Children 3–5 mg/kg body weight or 125 mg/m²; *maximum dose:* 100 mg PC: D	Secobarbital should not be used as a hypnotic for longer than 2 weeks. After long-term use, secobarbital should be withdrawn gradually.

(Continued)

Table 24-17. Selected hypnotic drugs (*Continued*)

Drug name	Preparations	Usual dosage	Additional information
Miscellaneous hypnotics			
chloral hydrate (Aquachloral, Noctec, Oradrate, SK-Chloral Hydrate; also called "knock-out drops" or "Mickey Finn" when combined with alcohol)	Crystals Oral capsules and solution Rectal suppositories	*Hypnotic dose:* Adults: 500 mg–1 g, given 15–30 min before retiring; children: 50 mg/kg body weight or 1.5 g/m²; *maximum dose:* 1 g PC: C	Gastric irritation may be minimized by diluting oral solutions with extra water or taking other oral dosage forms with ample liquids. Chloral hydrate has been found to lose much of its effectiveness for inducing and maintaining sleep after 2 weeks of use.
ethanol ("alcohol")	Liquid for preparation of drinks (wine, beer, distilled liquors) Solutions for parenteral administration	Adults: 5–15 ml Total abstinence is recommended during pregnancy.	Alcohol has been administered in a social setting in some extended care facilities. In the past, it has been used parenterally to inhibit premature labor.
ethchlorvynol (Placidyl)	Oral capsules	*Hypnotic dose:* Adults: 500 mg hs; for awaking in the early morning hours: 100–200 mg PC: C	Ethchlorvynol should not be used as a hypnotic for longer than 1 week. Ethchlorvynol dependence resembles dependence on barbiturates.
glutethimide (Doriden)	Powder Oral capsules and tablets	*Hypnotic dose:* Adults: 250–500 mg hs; *maximum daily dosage:* 1 g PC: C	Tolerance of and dependence on glutethimide resembles that of the barbiturates. Glutethimide should be used as a hypnotic for no longer than 1 week.
hydroxyzine (Atarax, Durrax, E-Vista, Hyzine-50, Hy-Pam, Orgatrax, Quiess, Vistacon, Vistaject, Vistaril)	Oral tablets, capsules, solutions, and suspensions Solutions for IM injection	*Preoperatively:* Adults: 50–100 mg orally or 25–100 mg IM; children: 0.6 mg/kg body weight orally or 1.1 mg/kg/ body weight IM PC: C	Hydroxyzine must not be administered SC, IV, or intraarterially.
methyprylon (Noludar)	Oral capsules and tablets	*Hypnotic dose:* Adults: 200–400 mg, 15 min before retiring; *maximum daily dosage:* 400 mg *Hypnotic dose:* Children older than 12 yr of age: 50 mg; *maximum dose:* 200 mg PC: B	Safe use of methyprylon during pregnancy and lactation has not been established.
paraldehyde (Paral)	Oral, rectal, and parenteral liquids	*Hypnotic dose:* Adults: 10–30 ml orally or 10 ml IM PC: C	Paraldehyde is preferred by some physicians for hypnosis in elderly people. Do not administer if a vinegar odor is present. Mix with juice or wine and chill to administer orally. Dilute in 2 volumes of olive oil for enemata. Paraldehyde reacts to plastics and rubber; measure in glass containers; use only freshly opened containers. IV administration is hazardous; IM administration may cause sterile abscess or tissue sloughing.

KEY: PC = pregnancy category. (The validity of pregnancy categories has not been established; see Chapter 16; p 216.)

treatment difficult, abuse of hypnotic drugs is a major health problem.

Many tranquilizer drugs have exhibited significant teratogenic effects. Thalidomide, the notorious drug responsible for multiple cases of phocomelia, a severe congenital malformation of the extremities, belongs to this class. Results from retrospective studies suggest an increased risk of congenital malformations in infants of mothers who received benzodiazepines.

Allergic reactions to hypnotic agents include skin rashes (from chloral hydrate and barbiturates) and precipitation of acute allergic attacks in clients subject to asthma, urticaria, and angioedema (from barbiturates). Many tranquilizers have some degree of antihistamine action, but, paradoxically, these agents also can cause allergic reactions in some people.

Among other undesirable effects of hypnotics are nausea and vomiting (most common with chloral hydrate). The barbiturates increase porphyrin and somatotropin production and decrease adrenocorticoid secretion. Both barbiturates and chloral hydrate cause hyperalgesia. Paradoxical excitement occurs in some clients (especially the elderly) who receive barbiturates or benzodiazepines.

Toxicity from hypnotics is similar to that from other CNS depressants. Somnolence tends to progress to coma. Respiratory depression is especially severe in barbiturate toxicity. Cardiovascular collapse is a relatively late sign.

Precautions and contraindications. The barbiturates and chloral hydrate are absolutely contraindicated in the treatment of clients with a history of acute intermittent porphyria. Administration of barbiturates or chloral hydrate is likely to precipitate a severe life-threatening attack of this disease. Hypnotic drugs are usually contraindicated for people with a history of drug abuse, especially when the drugs abused are depressants.

Because of the potential for dependence, hypnotic drugs should be discontinued whenever an increased dose is needed to sustain the therapeutic effect. Limited amounts of drugs are prescribed at a given time; precautions should be taken to ensure that clients do not obtain multiple prescriptions from different physicians.

Clients with chronic obstructive pulmonary disease should take these drugs only with extreme caution (if at all), and they must be monitored closely when hypnotics are used. Dosages should be minimal, and respiratory function should be assessed at frequent intervals.

■ **Summary**
Hypnotic drugs are often useful to promote rest and sleep when illness or environmental changes temporarily disrupt normal sleep patterns. Chronic use is undesirable because sleep stages are disrupted to some degree, waking function is impaired, and dependencies tend to develop.

The benzodiazepine tranquilizers are presently considered the safest drugs to use in most situations. They are most commonly prescribed for hypnosis, although chloral hydrate, paraldehyde, selected barbiturates, and other drugs are occasionally used.

Hypnotic drugs tend to accumulate in the tissues; toxicity may develop with prolonged use. They often influence the action of other drugs by altering their storage or metabolism in the body.

Withdrawal from chronic use of hypnotics produces abstinence syndromes that can be life-threatening, particularly in barbiturate dependence.

Nursing management

Nursing implications

The promotion of rest and sleep is of major concern to nurses. Inadequate sleep is associated with many physical and psychological health problems and tends to delay recovery from illness. Inadequate sleep is an appropriate diagnosis for nurses to make because it is a health problem largely amenable to nursing treatment. The use of hypnotic drugs is an important adjunct to this treatment.

Sleep patterns. To diagnose inadequate sleep, the nurse must understand normal sleep patterns. Sleep requirements vary but tend to conform to certain normal ranges. Factors such as age and cultural conditioning affect sleep patterns. The need for sleep is highest in the early years of life, decreases gradually throughout childhood, and levels off early in the third decade of life (Fig. 24-4). Conversely, the number of awakenings after sleep onset increases with age. Cultural conditioning and personal preference influence the rest–activity pattern but do not appreciably change the overall need for sleep.

People who suffer from disease or trauma need more sleep than usual.

Toxicity. Acute hypnotic toxicity is a medical emergency. It usually results from accidental or deliberate overdose. The client exhibits signs of severe CNS depression and somnolence or coma. Respiratory depression is the major threat to life. Cardiovascular collapse and convulsions can occur, particularly in severely hypoxic individuals. Treatment is supportive. Mechanical assistance to respiration and the administration of oxygen are required to maintain tissue oxygenation. Adrenergic vasopressors are administered

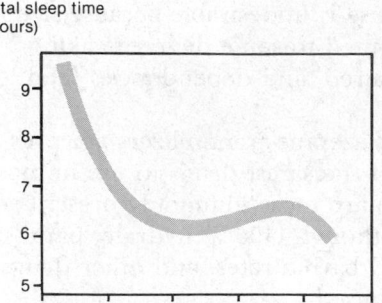
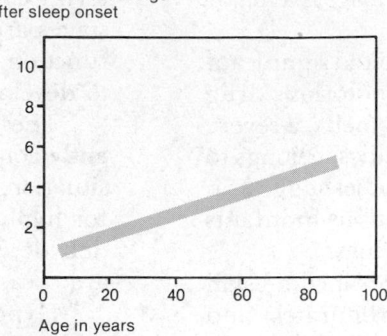

Figure 24-4. Sleep changes with age. (*A*) Total sleep time decreases steadily throughout childhood, remains low during the adult years, increases with advancing age until the late 70s and then declines toward the minimal levels of young adulthood. (*B*) Number of awakenings after sleep onset increases steadily throughout the life span. (Mendelson WB. [1980]. *The use and misuse of sleeping pills*, p 8. New York: Plenum Medical Book Co.)

IV to maintain circulation. Cardiotonics may also be required. The stomach is lavaged to remove any residual drug. In severe toxicity, hemodialysis may be instituted to remove the offending drug from the bloodstream. Until plasma drug levels subside, the client requires intensive nursing care appropriate to the comatose condition.

Storage of hypnotics. Schedule II, III, and IV hypnotic drugs such as barbiturates and benzodiazepines must be stored under secure conditions. Double locks and detailed records of the disposition of all doses may be required. All prescription hypnotics should be monitored, and careful records should be kept of their use. Automatic expiration of orders for hypnotic drugs and special records of the disposition of dispensed supplies are wise precautions for the control of all sedatives.

Drug abuse. Abuse of sedative drugs is a major health problem. Worldwide, more prescriptions are written for CNS depressants than for any other drug class. Illegal use of these compounds is also widespread. Education of the lay public to the effects of drugs and the risks of abuse is crucial, but the elimination of dependence on drugs requires consideration of underlying factors that increase the risk of dependence in some people.

Counseling and instruction designed to improve self-care and parenting techniques are basic to promoting optimal physical and emotional health. Robust health and competence in coping with minor illnesses and psychological stresses are the best insurance against the need for habitual drug use. Self-confidence and a good self-image decrease the need for chemical use as a psychological crutch. In addition to this foundation, young people need information about the physiologic and psychological effects of drugs and the detrimental effects of dependence to make intelligent decisions about drug use.

Nursing process

Assessment To assess the adequacy of sleep, current data must be compared with both baseline data from pertinent age and cultural groups and baseline data from the client's health history. A complete sleep history should be taken before drug therapy is initiated. The client's normal sleep pattern as well as the disturbed sleep pattern should be determined. Measures to promote sleep, including use of over-the-counter preparations (such as Nytol) and the client's response to them, should be explored. Risk factors that affect the individual must be assessed before administering any hypnotic. Of particular significance are habitual or chronic use of hypnotic drugs and the presence of chronic obstructive airway disease. When barbiturates or chloral hydrate are ordered, clients should be asked about any history of porphyria. The client's general attitude toward the use of chemical agents should be carefully considered as one indicator of the risk of habituation.

Nursing diagnosis The primary nursing diagnosis should be

> Sleep pattern disturbance: insomnia related to central nervous stimulating effects of therapeutic drugs or fear of impending surgery

It is useful to delineate the underlying factors for ultimate correction of the sleep disturbance. When hypnotics are used, the following diagnoses may be applicable:

> High risk for ineffective breathing pattern related to respiratory depression
> High risk for injury related to falls secondary to dizziness or sleepiness

Planning Goals for treatment include promoting sleep, maintaining effective respirations, and preventing accidental injury.

Intervention If the underlying cause for sleep disturbance is known and amenable to correction, it should be eliminated.

All appropriate nursing measures to promote sleep should be employed. General nursing measures can be taken to decrease arousal by reducing cerebral and skeletal muscle activity that interferes with sleep by maintaining arousal (Figs. 24-5 and 24-6). Such measures include the elimination or masking of environ-

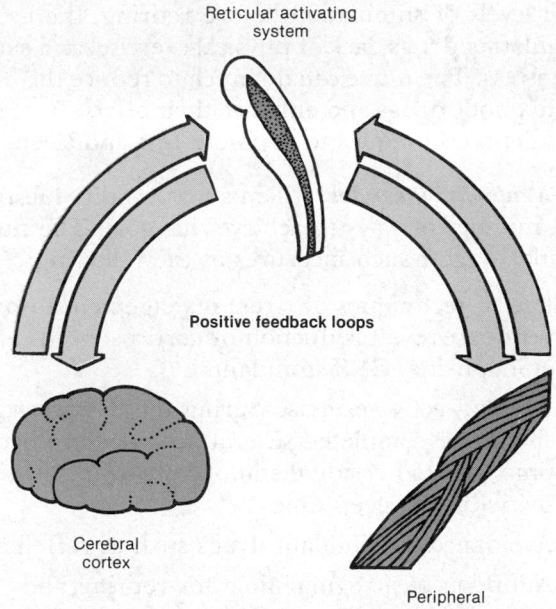

Figure 24-5. Arousal feedback cycles that affect the onset of sleep. Wakefulness is maintained by positive feedback systems that involve the reticular activating system (RAS), the cerebral cortex, and peripheral muscles. Activity in the RAS excites both the cortex and peripheral muscles; cortical and muscular activity in turn activates the RAS. Arousal levels rise until neuronal discharge rates approach saturation, at which point a steady state is established.

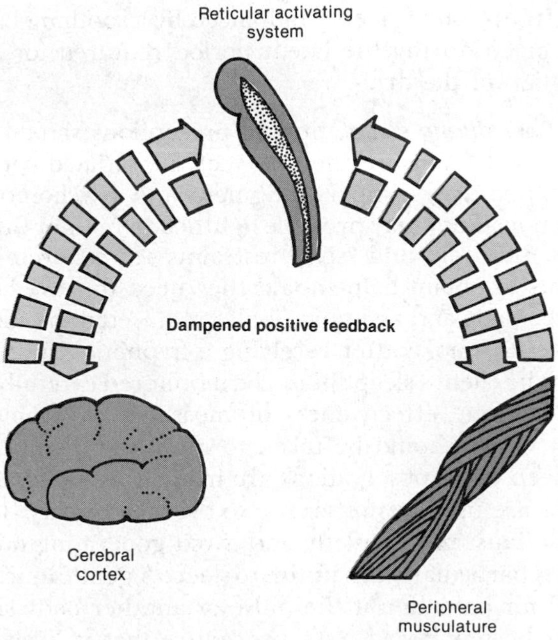

Figure 24-6. Arousal feedback cycles that affect the onset of sleep. Fatigue reduces activity levels, lowering the excitation level of all three components of the system. Interventions that promote relaxation and eliminate stimuli from the system further dampen the positive feedback mechanism. The reduction in RAS activity levels necessary for onset of sleep cannot be achieved if the cerebral cortex or peripheral musculature remains active.

mental stimuli, the promotion of muscle relaxation, the reduction of anxiety, and the promotion of physical and psychological comfort.

Before retiring, the client should engage in quiet activities in an environment that is characterized by reduced sensory stimuli. As much as possible, the client should follow a bedtime ritual (toileting, mouth care, special clothing, and so forth). Through conditioning, habitual routines become stimuli for relaxation and induction of sleep (Box 24-10).

Any critical judgments required of the client should be made before hypnotic drugs are administered. The validity of legal documents is questionable if they were signed while under the influence of CNS drugs.

The use of hypnotic drugs may be efficacious when the factors that interfere with rest cannot be controlled adequately to maintain normal sleep patterns. However, in view of the potential toxicity of such drugs and their effects on the stages of sleep, such use should be kept to a minimum. Drugs should never be used as a substitute for nursing care that is directed at promoting sleep.

The hypnotic may be administered when the client has been made comfortable. If the client tolerates milk and is not at high risk for gastric hyperacidity, warm milk given with oral hypnotics enhances their effects. Tryptophan, an amino acid in milk, is a natural sopo-

rific, while the additional heat promotes relaxation. Cocoa should not be used; the xanthines in chocolate tend to stimulate the nervous system. Malt or vanilla flavoring may be used instead.

Analgesics should usually be administered with the hypnotic if pain is a problem. While hypnotic tranquilizers sometimes relieve pain because of their antianxiety effects, other hypnotics have no analgesic properties and may cause hyperalgesia. Pain alters response to sedatives, causing an increased incidence of disorientation and paradoxical excitement. For optimum hypnotic effect, the nurse should manage the administration of analgesia through the day so that a dose is available for use at bedtime.

Box 24-10. General nursing measures to promote sleep

- Eliminate or mask environmental stimuli
- Promote muscle relaxation
- Reduce anxiety
- Promote physical and psychological comfort
- Maintain a regular bedtime ritual for retiring

Induction of sleep is enhanced by a soothing back rub given during the latent period required for absorption of the drug.

Care during sleep. Special precautions should be employed to ensure the safety of the sedated client. Hypnotic drugs impair judgment and psychomotor function. They may produce lightheadedness or dizziness. Side rails and "soft" restraints serve to remind clients to obtain help should they need to leave bed. Supervision and assistance is also required if the client wishes to smoke after receiving a hypnotic drug.

The client's sleep should be monitored carefully to evaluate the effectiveness of measures to promote sleep. Care should be taken to minimize disruption of sleep when observations are made. Shielded flashlights are used in preference to overhead lights. The nurse must move quietly and avoid generating noise that is particularly disruptive to sleep. A gentle touch is used for palpation if the pulse or another body sign must be monitored. If a procedure that is likely to interrupt sleep is required, it should be delayed until after cessation of REM to avoid depriving the client of REM sleep.

During the hours of sleep, the client's respirations should be monitored. Although serious respiratory depression is unlikely when therapeutic doses are employed, it can occur in clients who are unusually sensitive to sedatives, in the obese, and in those with respiratory diseases. Respiratory rates in adults should not drop below 12 per minute.

Postmedication care. The day after the use of hypnotic drugs, the client should be assessed for sedation or other residual effects from the drug. If significant "hangover" is evident, it may be necessary to reduce the hypnotic dose or change to another drug. The client should be questioned about subjective feelings of fatigue or dysphoria and the occurrence of "daymares."

Regular use of hypnotic drugs over long periods should be avoided. If chronic health problems make this impossible, the client must be monitored closely for personality changes that could indicate deprivation of sleep phases such as REM sleep. Such changes, or a decrease in or failure of sedative effect, indicate that the soporific should be discontinued. Hypnotic drugs must be withdrawn gradually from clients who have received them over a period of time. Abrupt withdrawal is likely to precipitate uncomfortable and dangerous abstinence syndromes. During the weaning period, the client should be assessed for wakefulness, restlessness, agitation, or depression. If pronounced symptoms develop, seizure precautions must be taken and the physician should be asked to increase temporarily the hypnotic dose or slow the weaning schedule.

Client education. Inability to sleep may arise because of erratic activity–rest patterns, daytime naps, high levels of stimulation before retiring, the use of stimulating drugs, lack of physical exercise, and excessive stress. The nurse can do much to reduce the need for hypnotic drugs and enhance their effects by teaching clients techniques to promote rest and sleep.

Modifying lifestyles. Clients may modify lifestyles in a number of ways to achieve this goal. The nurse should suggest such measures as the following:

Use of techniques of stress management to prevent excessive production of corticosteroids and epinephrine, CNS stimulants

Regular, active exercise during the day; exercise should be completed several hours before bedtime to avoid residual stimulation from the activity during sleep time

Avoidance of stimulant drugs such as caffeine

Adoption of a regular time for retiring and arising (which allows sufficient time for sleep to meet the client's needs)

Deliberate reduction in stimuli before bedtime (sedentary activity, absence of bright lights and loud noises)

Use of a comfortable warm bed and night-clothes

Adequate ventilation in the sleeping area

Taking a warm protein snack that is rich in tryptophan (such as milk) before retiring

Elimination of pain, if present, through pain-control techniques and, when necessary, the use of a bedtime dose of analgesic

Use of routine comfort measures before retiring to eliminate the need for interruption of rest in bed

Elimination of disturbing stimuli after retiring through the use of eye shades and ear plugs

Counseling about risks. Clients for whom hypnotic drugs are prescribed should be cautioned about the risks inherent in their use. Supplies of the drugs should be kept in a place other than the bedside table. A place should be chosen that is far enough away from the bedroom so that the client is roused to full alertness before repeating a dose. Clients who take hypnotics for sleep can develop amnesia about their drug use; it is believed that many cases of hypnotic overdose arise from repeated doses taken by a client during waking periods. Measures should be taken to prevent such automatism. It may be necessary to place drug supplies under the control of a second person.

The client should avoid ambulation after onset of hypnotic drug effect unless assistance is available. Impairment of psychomotor function, dizziness, and impaired judgment while under the influence of these drugs increase the risk of accidental injury. The making of critical decisions and the use of power machinery (including cars) should be avoided while drug effects persist.

Some cases of chronic overdose arise because clients receive prescriptions from more than one physician, each of whom is unaware of the orders of other doctors. Clients should be cautioned to inform each physician of all drugs being used. Over-the-counter preparations may also increase the effects of hypnotics; use of these drugs should also be disclosed to the nurse and the physician. Clients should be warned specifically of the risk of concurrent use of more than one CNS depressant. Of particular importance is the use of opioids, tranquilizers, and alcohol, all of which depress the CNS. Antihistamines also have an additive effect when taken with sedatives. Dangerous combinations of drugs are more likely to be identified if the client purchases all medicines from the same pharmacy. Most pharmacists maintain drug profiles on their clients and monitor the records for inappropriate or potentially dangerous drug combinations.

Checklist of nursing actions

To decrease the need for hypnotic drugs
☐ Use all available nursing measures to promote rest and sleep:
    ☐ Encourage the clients to maintain bedtime rituals.
    ☐ Recommend reduced activity by clients before bedtime.
    ☐ Reduce pain and promote comfort for clients at the time they retire.
    ☐ Administer a soothing back rub at the hour of sleep.
    ☐ Eliminate or mask sensory stimuli after clients retire.
    ☐ Minimize sleep interruptions, particularly during REM sleep.
    ☐ Teach clients techniques for promoting rest and sleep.

When hypnotic drugs are prescribed
☐ Assess the risk of drug use by taking a careful history. Ask specifically about previous use of hypnotics, porphyria, and chronic obstructive pulmonary disease. Note attitude toward use of sedation.
☐ Monitor client's sleep to evaluate effectiveness of the drug and to detect hypopnea or other adverse reaction to the drug.
☐ Institute safety measures to protect clients from accidental injury while sedated.
☐ Evaluate clients during waking hours for residual effects of the drug.
☐ Assess clients who use hypnotics over a long term for personality changes or other signs of sleep phase deprivation.

☐ Reevaluate the hypnotic regimen if a need for increased dosage becomes apparent.
☐ Teach clients who control their own drugs about safe management techniques.
☐ To enhance the effects of hypnotics, use nursing measures to promote rest and sleep.

When hypnotic overdose produces toxicity
☐ Administer care supportive of respiration and circulation.
☐ Assist with medical measures to remove the drug from body systems (gastric lavage, hemodialysis).
☐ Give supportive nursing care appropriate to the client's condition.

To reduce the incidence of drug abuse and dependence
☐ Teach self-care and parenting skills designed to promote robust physical and emotional health.
☐ Inform clients of the properties of sedating drugs and the risks inherent in their use.

Alcohol

Alcohols are hydroxy derivatives of aliphatic hydrocarbons formed by the fermentation of sugars by yeasts. They are produced naturally during the decomposition of carbohydrate substances and have been well known throughout history. They have long been used for a variety of purposes such as foods, medicines, and industrial chemicals. They are useful solvents, fuels, and disinfectants. As drugs taken internally, they tend to be toxic, and their pharmacologic uses have declined with the development of safer, more efficacious agents. They remain useful in limited situations, however, and are still widely employed by the lay public.

Ethyl alcohol

Ethyl alcohol (ethanol, grain alcohol, ETOH) is the least toxic of the alcohols when taken internally. This alcohol is produced by the fermentation of the carbohydrates of fruits and grains. It is the active pharmacologic component of beer, wine, and other intoxicating beverages. The concentration of alcohol in beverages is sometimes increased by fractional distillation of the ferment, as in the production of whiskey, brandy, and other "spirits" (Table 24-18). Virtually every human culture has some form of alcohol in common use as a foodstuff or drug. In the body, ethanol functions primarily as a CNS depressant, although it produces many other changes, affecting virtually every body tissue in some manner.

Pharmacodynamics. Ethanol acts primarily as a CNS depressant. It appears to reduce the resting action potential on nerve membranes by decreasing so-

Table 24-18. *Composition of common alcoholic beverages*

Beverage	Source	Method of preparation	Alcohol concentration (average range)	Additional information
Beer	Grain	Treatment with malt to produce sugar, then fermentation with hops (for flavor)	3%–5%	Beer contains carbohydrates and other nutrients. Absorption is relatively slow because of slow gastric emptying.
Wine	Fruits and berries	Fermentation	Up to 14%	Wine contains some vitamins. Dry wines have a higher alcohol content than sweeter wines. Wines made from berries are used as folk remedies for diarrhea.
Sherry wine	Fruits and berries	Fermentation, fortification, addition of brandy, refermentation	18%–20%	
Brandy	Fruits and berries	Fermentation and subsequent distillation	30%–45% (60–90 proof)	Brandy is flavored by volatile substances from the substrates that distill along with the alcohol.
Whiskey (*Spiritus frumenti*)	Grains	Treatment with malt to produce sugar, fermentation, and subsequent distillation	40%–60% (80–120 proof)	Concentration is generally reported as proof, which is equal to twice the percentage of alcohol.
Vodka	Grain or potatoes	Fermentation and subsequent distillation	40%–60%	Vodka was originally produced in Eastern Europe.
Sake (beer)	Rice	Fermentation	14%–16%	Sake was originally produced in Japan.
Sake (liquor)	Rice	Distillation of sake beer	57%–74%	

dium and potassium ion conduction across the cellular membrane. The reticular activating system and portions of the cortex are especially sensitive to the effects of ethanol.

Ethanol first affects the higher functions, particularly learned inhibitions, often producing a temporary increase in activity that has given it an undeserved reputation as a stimulant. In moderate amounts, alcohol functions as a tranquilizer, reducing anxiety and inducing euphoria. As dosage increases, hypnosis develops. Hypnosis is followed by complete anesthesia. Depression of the CNS is reflected by progressive loss of function. Inhibition of the hypothalamus reduces antidiuretic hormone production, causing a noticeable diuresis.

Ethanol enters the metabolic pool as a source of calories. Its oxidation requires enzymes and vitamins, especially the B vitamin complex. Because many alcoholic beverages contain few nutrients other than calories, they are generally considered to be "empty calories." Although each milliliter of ethanol provides about 29.4 kcal of energy, it is not an efficient source of calories because of its high specific dynamic action. The drug increases lipid anabolism and raises the ratio of high-density lipoproteins to low-density lipoproteins in the blood plasma.

Ethanol is an irritant and stimulant to local tissues. Small amounts stimulate intestinal peristalsis and gastric secretion of acid. Psychogenic stimulation of pepsin secretion also occurs in people who enjoy the use of alcohol.

Ethanol is biphasic in many of its reactions. Initially, it lowers blood pressure by vasodilation. Over time, it tends to produce or exacerbate hypertension. Alpha brain waves are slowed and convulsions suppressed immediately, but, later, nervous hyperirritability increases the risk of seizures.

Applied topically to skin or inanimate surfaces, alcohol is an effective disinfectant, provided sufficient time (30 minutes on a clean surface) is allowed for its action. It does *not* sterilize.

Pharmacokinetics. Ethanol is rapidly absorbed by both the lungs and the GI system. Skin absorption is negligible. When infused IV, alcohol is well tolerated. Absorption from subcutaneous sites varies with concentration; dilute solutions dissipate rapidly, whereas concentrated solutions are poorly absorbed because of pronounced local vasoconstriction. Necrosis and sloughing of tissues may occur with highly concentrated solutions. Ethanol distributes readily throughout the body, reaching comparable levels in most tissues of the body. It readily crosses the placenta.

Metabolism of ethanol is initiated by the liver, which oxidizes alcohol to acetaldehyde by enzymatic action. Acetaldehyde is rapidly converted to acetyl coenzyme A, which may then enter the citric acid cycle or be used for anabolic reactions that produce cholesterol, fatty acids, and other tissue components. A part of a given dose can be metabolized by the microsomal enzymes of the endoplasmic reticulum of the liver. Small percentages (2%–10%) are excreted unchanged by the lungs and kidneys. Ethanol is metabolized at a steady rate that seems not to vary appreciably with changes in the concentration of alcohol in body fluids. A normal adult is capable of metabolizing about 10 ml of alcohol per hour, roughly the amount present in a typical American "drink" (*eg*, 10 oz of beer, 3–4 oz of wine, 1 oz of whiskey).

In nontolerant people, clinical effects of ethanol vary proportionately with blood concentration (Table 24-19). Few overt signs of alcohol toxicity exist until alcohol levels reach 0.1%. The level designated by law to indicate intoxication is 0.15% in many states. Levels in excess of 0.5% are generally believed to be fatal, although these and higher levels are occasionally reported in people with a developed tolerance to the chemical.

Therapeutic uses. At one time ethanol was widely used as an analgesic, anesthetic, and tranquilizer by the medical profession. Professional use has declined with the development of safer and more selective agents for these purposes. It is still commonly used by the lay public for its psychoactive effects. Ethanol is considered a useful hypnotic tranquilizer for elderly clients who tolerate other sedative drugs poorly.

Because all alcohols are organic solvents capable of breaking down toxicodendrol, the molecule responsible for the irritant properties of poison ivy, they can be applied topically to treat this condition. Alcohols applied to the intact skin tend to disinfect, dry, toughen, and cool the skin. Alcohols are used in the prevention of decubiti in people with tender moist skin. Mixtures that contain alcohols also act as rubefacients and counterirritants when applied topically. Ethanol is widely used as a solvent and vehicle for other drugs in the form of elixirs.

Solutions that contain low concentrations of ethanol are sometimes prescribed as stomachics, medicines designed to promote appetite and digestion. Alcohol is also an effective antiseptic.

Local injections of ethanol are used medically to produce a relatively permanent nerve block to relieve intractable pain or promote peripheral vasodilation. The drug may be administered IV to boost the caloric value of IV fluids, to suppress uterine contractions in premature labor, or to suppress chronic severe pain. Table 24-20 lists medicinal preparations that contain alcohol.

Adverse reactions. Alcohols are protoplasmic poisons that precipitate and dehydrate the protein within cell membranes. Only ethanol is applied to mucous membranes or taken internally; other alcohols are toxic when absorbed systemically. Ethanol is irritating when applied to denuded skin or mucous membranes. It should not be applied to extensive or deep wounds because an eschar forms that tends to trap tissue debris beneath the surface, increasing the risk of secondary infection. Topical applications of alcohol may also cause undue drying of the skin.

When injected into the tissues, alcohol may cause degeneration of the treated nerves, even when only a temporary nerve block is desired. Concentrated solutions are astringent in nature and can compromise the local blood supply when injected subcutaneously, resulting in tissue necrosis and sloughing. Extravasation of IV solutions is also highly irritating to the tissues.

Systemic cardiovascular effects of alcohol include

Table 24-19. Clinical manifestations of alcohol toxicity in nontolerant persons

Approximate blood alcohol level	Corresponding urine levels	Usual signs and symptoms
0%–0.10%	0%–0.14%	No overt signs: slight deterioration of performance on tests of specific learned motor and mental skills, decreased feelings of fatigue
0.10%–0.20%	0.14%–0.28%	Slowing of reaction time, slight incoordination, loss of inhibitions, emotional lability, loss of discrimination
0.20%–0.30%	0.28%–0.40%	Analgesia, staggering gait, slurred speech, confusion, loss of concentration
0.30%–0.40%	0.40%–0.54%	Relative lack of response to stimuli, loss of insight, marked incoordination, stupor
0.40%–0.50%	0.54%–0.66%	Depressed reflexes, coma, anesthesia, subnormal temperature, circulatory collapse
0.50% and above	more than 0.66%	Death

Table 24-20. *Medicinal preparations of ethanol*

Name	Preparation	Administration	Therapeutic uses
Alcohol for injection	5- and 50-ml vials	Local injection	Long-term nerve block
	5% alcohol with dextrose	IV infusion	Interruption of premature labor
			Control of intractable pain
Elixirs	Aromatic sweetened solutions used as flavored vehicles for medicinal agents	Oral	Depends on medicinal agent involved (*eg*, elixir of phenobarbital, a CNS depressant used as a sedative)
Tinctures	Alcohol or hydroalcoholic solutions of drugs in 10% or 20% concentration	Oral or topical	Depends on drug involved (*eg*, tincture of iodine, used as a topical antiseptic)
Fluid extracts	Alcoholic solutions of drugs in 100% concentration	Oral	Depends on drug involved (*eg*, glycyrrhiza fluid-extract, used as a flavoring agent; cascara sagrada extract used as a cathartic)

vasodilation. When combined with other CNS depressants (barbiturates, benzodiazepines), it can cause cardiorespiratory collapse and death. Conversely, chronic use tends to increase the severity of hypertension. Alcohol's vasodilating action may underlie its aggravation of ear discomfort associated with flying or other reduction of barometric pressure. Nasopharyngeal vasodilation increases congestion in those tissues, blocking the eustacian tube.

IV administration of ethanol can produce inebriation identical to that of oral ingestion. Fluid flow rates must be carefully controlled to prevent accumulation of ethanol above the desired therapeutic level.

Except in small doses, ethanol interferes with sexual function and reproduction. Temperate use of alcohol may enhance sexual performance in people unable to function well because of learned inhibitions. Indulgence in more than 10 ml per hour tends to erode performance, however, despite increased sexual desire. Chronic alcoholism alters the balance of sexual hormones by increasing estrogen retention and promoting testosterone metabolism. Men become feminized and suffer from impotence and relative infertility. Women also experience decreased libido.

Ethanol is teratogenic and its use by pregnant women seriously endangers the fetus. Because it readily crosses the placenta, concentration in fetal tissues reflects those in maternal tissues. The drug inhibits embryonic cellular proliferation, causing congenital anomalies and growth retardation. Newborns with full-blown fetal alcohol syndrome exhibit characteristic facial deformities, joint, cardiac, and genital anomalies, and microcephaly. Virtually all such infants suffer permanent mental retardation. After birth, alcohol withdrawal syndrome may be evident in the infant.

Ethanol is also carcinogenic. Immoderate use of alcohol increases the risk of developing cancer of the mouth, larynx, esophagus, liver, and lungs.

Acute alcoholism. Acute alcoholism is accompanied by profound CNS depression. Because of the accompanying euphoria, fatigue may be ignored and exhaustion may develop. Convulsions, cardiovascular collapse, and death may occur. Hyperglycemia, acute gastritis, pylorospasm, nausea, vomiting, and dehydration often accompany the acute phase of alcohol abuse (brain glucose levels of 300–600 mg per 100 ml approach the danger level). During the subsequent withdrawal ("hangover") period, hypoglycemia develops, contributing to the subjective symptoms of headache and malaise engendered by residual dehydration and exhaustion. Both alcohol toxicity and withdrawal increase the risk of seizure in epileptics.

Chronic alcoholism. Chronic alcoholism clearly shortens one's expected lifespan. Leukocyte response to the inflammatory process declines; resistance to infectious disease is reduced. Poor nutrition often accompanies this condition, further compromising basic physiologic defenses (*eg*, ethanol antagonizes folate, predisposing a person to anemia). If food intake is reduced to compensate for the calories ingested as alcohol, a general malnutrition can develop. Deficiencies of vitamin B complex are particularly pronounced because these vitamins are required for the metabolism of ethanol. Chronic use of alcohol may also contribute to loss of bone mass and promote osteoporosis (Alcoholism in the bones, 1983).

Chronic exposure to excessive ethanol can damage any tissue of the body. These effects may stem from the drug's irritating and poisonous properties. Alcoholism increases the incidence of CNS degeneration characterized by memory loss, sleep disturbances, and psychoses. Brain damage produces encephalopathies characteristic of Wernicke's encephalopathy or Korsakoff's syndrome (Box 24-11).

Peripheral neuritis is also frequently seen, especially in malnourished people. In chronic alcohol use, the liver tends to develop fatty degeneration with eventual cirrhosis. This process stems both from the toxic effect of alcohol itself and from the nutritional deficiencies that commonly accompany alcoholism. Both acute and chronic pancreatitis have increased inci-

Box 24-11. CNS syndromes associated with chronic alcoholism

Korsakoff's syndrome: A personality disorder characterized by amnesia (loss of both long-term and short-term memory), confabulation, psychosis, disorientation, confusion, muttering, delirium, insomnia, illusions, hallucinations, and polyneuritis.

Wernicke's encephalopaphy: An inflammatory, hemorrhagic, degenerative condition of the brain caused by thiamine deficiency and manifested by double vision, involuntary and rapid movements of the eyes, lack of muscular coordination, and decreased mental function.

dence in drinkers. Ethanol stimulates pancreatic function while predisposing the pancreas to obstruction of the pancreatic duct. Effects on the normal kidney are less pronounced, but some authorities believe high concentrations of ethanol in urine can also damage these organs. Chronic alcoholism is associated with degeneration of both skeletal and cardiac muscle tissue. Ethanol use increases the risk and severity of peptic ulcer disease, hypertension, and stroke, as well as the incidence of seizures in epileptics.

Tolerance and dependence. Repeated exposure to ethanol produces tolerance and dependence similar to that characteristic of opioid addiction. It is believed that chemical reactions between biogenic amines and acetaldehyde, an intermediate metabolite of ethanol, form opioidlike alkaloids that affect the brain in similar fashion to opioids. Abrupt withdrawal produces a syndrome characterized by muscle tremors, restlessness, hyperthermia, anxiety, agitation, and visual hallucinations. Seizures and death may occur. This syndrome, termed the "shakes" by alcoholics, is known also as delirium tremens (or DTs). Although the death rate from delirium tremens has declined with improved treatment, it still ranges from 5% to 20%. People particularly prone to alcoholism may have a genetic predisposition to dependence because their metabolisms cannot break down acetaldehyde at normal rates.

Tolerance to alcohol produces cross-tolerance to most CNS depressants, including anesthetics. Because large doses of anesthetics are required for surgery, and because of the high incidence of malnutrition and poor resistance to infection, habitual users of alcohol tend to be poor surgical risks.

Drug interactions. Ethanol interacts with many other drugs. Because it induces the liver enzyme system, it enhances the metabolism of warfarin anticoagulants and propranolol, decreasing the effectiveness of a given dose. The effects of other CNS depressants are enhanced, particularly in nontolerant

individuals, causing life-threatening depression in naive users. Aspirin and alcohol taken together tend to cause severe gastric damage and can precipitate active GI hemorrhage. Disulfiram and many medicinal drugs taken concurrently with alcohol can produce a disagreeable reaction characterized by flushing, increased pulse and respirations, nausea and vomiting, headache, dyspnea, and palpitations. Chronic alcoholics are at increased risk of liver damage from acetaminophen (Fleckenstein, 1985).

Precautions and contraindications. Ethanol must be used with extreme caution (if at all) in hypertension, peptic ulcer disease, hepatic disease, extreme obesity, alcoholic myopathy, and pregnancy. People known to have been alcohol dependent also should not receive ethanol. Epilepsy, acute genitourinary infections, and kidney disease are relative contraindications. Caution should be employed by diabetics who use alcohol to avoid wide fluctuations in blood sugar.

Pain associated with alcohol ingestion may indicate Hodgkin's disease. The pain occurs at or near the tumor site within minutes of ethanol ingestion. It may be sharp and stabbing or dull and aching (Bobrove, 1983).

Alcohol intake in a social setting by normal adults usually does not produce acute intoxication if ingestion is limited to 10 ml or less per hour.

When alcohol is administered IV, flow rates must be carefully controlled to prevent inebriation. After an initial loading dose equivalent to 10 ml of ethanol, flow rates should be limited to the volume that will deliver 10 ml or less of ethanol per hour.

Exposure to alcohol fumes should be reduced to a minimum, because inhalation can deliver a toxic dose to systemic tissues. Deaths from acute toxicity after exposure to concentrated fumes have been reported.

■ Summary

Ethanol is a hydroxy derivative of ethane that is produced by fermentation of sugars by yeasts. It is the active ingredient in alcoholic beverages such as wines and beers. Ethanol is a potent CNS depressant with tranquilizing, hypnotic, and anesthetic properties. Its margin of safety is more narrow than that of many newer depressant drugs that have replaced its use for most medicinal uses. Ethanol is still used medicinally as a hypnotic tranquilizer and intravenously to interrupt premature labor and suppress severe pain.

Alcohol is generally toxic to most tissues and can produce both acute and chronic medical problems. Acute toxicity can cause death due to cardiovascular collapse and severe central depression. Chronic alcoholism predisposes the body to degeneration of the nervous system, liver, pancreas, heart, and other organs. It is an important risk factor for certain forms of cancer, hypertension, and peptic ulcers. Chronic alcoholics tend to develop either obesity from excess calorie consumption or malnutrition due to nutritional deficiencies. Alcohol use during pregnancy poses a serious risk of congenital malformations to the fetus as well as mental and growth retardation.

Nursing management

Nursing implications: acute ethanol toxicity

Acute ethanol toxicity may be life-threatening, especially in a naive drinker with no acquired tolerance to the drug. Because the ethanol molecule dialyzes readily, hemodialysis may be ordered to achieve rapid reduction of blood levels. The client needs support of vital functions similar to that required in overdoses of any CNS depressant. Neurologic vital signs must be monitored and respiration and circulation supported as necessary. In addition, the client who has been on a drinking bout may be physically exhausted, chronically malnourished, and overcome by shame and guilt.

As blood alcohol levels decline and the severe CNS depression lessens, the client may exhibit hostility or aggression. While paraldehyde or tranquilizers may be prescribed, restraints are generally considered safer than chemical measures to control the client's behavior. Ethanol blood levels may rise after discontinuation of hemodialysis (owing to movement of the drug from tissue depots into the bloodstream), adding to the depressant effects of such medication and increasing the risk of serious depression.

Clients who are treated in acute care facilities for alcohol toxicity often face legal action as a consequence of the episode. Because of this fact, and because of the guilt and shame associated with alcoholism, clients are often under considerable stress during the treatment period. The success of attempts to refer for follow-up care may depend on the quality of the nurse–client relationship developed during this crisis situation. The nurse must be nonjudgmental and accepting of clients while meeting their many needs for nursing care.

Chronic alcohol dependence. Habitual ingestion of alcohol usually results in the development of tolerance and physical dependence. If no psychological dependence is present, a period of weaning from alcohol, or abstinence combined with decreasing doses of other tranquilizers, corrects the problem. Psychological dependence is what makes recovery from alcohol dependence difficult.

Chronic alcoholics are likely to experience multiple serious health problems. The individual who maintains a nutritious diet is likely to become obese because total caloric intake is excessive. More often, food intake is reduced and the individual is chronically malnour-

ished. The combination is a deadly one, predisposing to infection (especially pneumonia), cirrhosis of the liver, and central and peripheral nervous system degeneration. Alcoholics are also at increased risk for cancer, heart disease, peptic ulcers, and pancreatitis. Sexual function and fertility in males are impaired. Women also experience a decreased libido and may bear defective children.

Habitual users of ethanol who are treated for acute toxicity are less likely than naive users to exhibit life-threatening depression but more likely to develop withdrawal symptoms as drug levels decline. During the "drying out" period, the client should be watched closely for tremors, restlessness, agitation, and fright that arises from hallucinations. Seizure precautions should be taken. Small frequent doses of mild tranquilizers or treatment with clonidine (Catapres) may be prescribed to control withdrawal symptoms. The client should be weaned gradually from these drugs after the acute phase of withdrawal has passed.

Hidden alcohol dependence. Alcohol withdrawal may occur in clients who enter the hospital for treatment unrelated to ethanol use or abuse. Individuals who are alcohol dependent are often reluctant to reveal this fact. They may delay hospitalization as long as possible, attempt to take liquor into the health care facility, or arrange for it to be brought in by visitors. The nurse should be alert to indications that hidden alcohol dependence may be a problem. These indications include restlessness and agitation that develop after several hours in a controlled setting, or a sudden insistence by the client on leaving the health care setting. The presence of alcoholic beverages in the client's possession on admission may alert the staff to potential problems. (When cut off from supplies of alcohol, the dependent person may ingest mouth wash, shaving lotion, or any other substance that contains alcohol.) Clients whose behavior changes noticeably after seeing visitors may have received alcoholic beverages during the visit.

Whenever a chronic alcohol-dependence problem seems likely, the nurse should discuss it openly with the client. It should be stressed that the use of alcohol in combination with other therapeutic drugs required for treatment can be dangerous and that withdrawal symptoms can seriously complicate the client's recovery. Only if all the facts are known can the health care team successfully manage the client's treatment. If clients are assured that their needs will be met by the health care team, they are often relieved to acknowledge the problem. In any case, the physician must be alerted to facts that point to dependency as a problem and be consulted regarding changes in the treatment regimen.

Alcohol withdrawal. Acute alcohol withdrawal is treated symptomatically and by administration of sedatives, IV fluids, and replacement nutrients (vitamins and minerals). Clonidine may be used to decrease hypertension, heart rate, and nausea and vomiting.

Clients in acute withdrawal need constant monitoring and emotional support. To minimize visual hallucinations, the client's environment should be kept lighted.

Follow-up care. The nurse who is capable of establishing a therapeutic relationship with the alcoholic client is in an excellent position to promote action toward resolution of this health problem. After treatment in a health care facility, most clients have progressed through the worst of the withdrawal period. Receptive clients should be referred to available treatment programs. These may range from the short-term residential programs to out-patient facilities. Self-help lay groups modeled after Alcoholics Anonymous are most effective in promoting long-term control.

Clients known to have an alcohol-dependence problem need a careful general health assessment. Special attention should be given to evidence of malnutrition, peptic ulcer disease, cancer, and hypertension. Such clients are at high risk for infections and delayed healing. They require excellent supportive care both physically and psychologically.

Alcohol education programs. Education of the lay public about the uses and abuses of ethanol is vital for long-term control of the dependency problem. Introduction to alcoholic beverages is considered a rite of passage to adulthood in many modern subcultures. Children should be acquainted with the facts about alcohol before they reach the age at which they are likely to be introduced to the drug. Despite the fact that the use of alcohol by minors is illegal in most states, exposure to alcoholic beverages usually occurs at a relatively early age—often well before puberty. Alcohol education programs, therefore, should be carried out in the early years of elementary education. Scare tactics should be avoided. The beneficial as well as the harmful effects of the drug should be presented. This presentation may be best done within the context of a program in which all drugs of abuse are discussed, along with their potential to produce dependency.

Education in parenting skills is of fundamental importance for the long-term control of drug dependence. People who have grown up with a healthy self-image and with self-confidence are least likely to need the chemical crutch of psychotropic drugs.

Women of childbearing age should be warned against drinking during pregnancy. The risk of fetal alcohol syndrome in offspring is directly related to the amount of alcohol used by the mother; the use of any alcohol during pregnancy is considered unsafe.

Abstinence and temperance. Clients with a family history of alcohol dependence may be at an increased risk for dependence. Their physiologic reactions to alcohol are more blunted than are those of people not related to alcoholics (Schuckit, Gold, 1988). They should be alert to indications of developing dependence. Complete abstinence may be advisable.

Diabetics may include one daily alcoholic beverage in their diet, provided it is computed at the proper exchange value (Table 24-21). Because these beverages contain few nutrients other than calories, ample vitamins and minerals should be provided by the rest of their diet.

Management of hangovers. Clients who seek advice on the management of "hangovers" can be advised to eat and drink fluids to restore hydration, raise blood

Table 24-21. Dietary exchange values for alcoholic beverages

Beverage	Approximate measure	Substitute
Beer (average)	1 12-oz bottle	1 bread exchange and 2 fat exchanges
Brandy	1 brandy glass	1½ fat exchanges
Cordials	1 cordial glass	2 fat exchanges
Highball (with water)	1 glass	4 fat exchanges
Martini	1 cocktail	3 fat exchanges
Manhattan	1 cocktail	3 fat exchanges and ½ bread exchange
Rum	1 jigger (½ oz)	2 fat exchanges
Tom Collins	1 cocktail	1 fruit exchange and 3 fat exchanges
Whiskey, rye	1 jigger (1½ oz)	3 fat exchanges
Whiskey, scotch	1 jigger (1½ oz)	2 fat exchanges
Wine, California sauterne	1 wine glass	½ fruit exchange and 1 fat exchange
Wine, California red	1 wine glass	1 fat exchange
Wine, port	1 wine glass	1 bread exchange and 2 fat exchanges
Gin, dry	1½ jigger	2 fat exchanges
Champagne	1 wine glass (½ cup)	2 fat exchanges (3 glasses equal 1 fruit and 6 fat exchanges)

sugar levels, and maintain proper nutrition. A mild analgesic such as aspirin or acetaminophen may be recommended to relieve headache. The significance of hangovers as indications of excessive drinking should be pointed out, and clients should be encouraged to evaluate their use of alcohol critically.

Medicinal alcohol. Ethanol is most often prescribed as a hypnotic tranquilizer for elderly clients. It is best given with meals to stimulate the appetite and to minimize gastric irritation through dilution of medication. Brandy, whiskey, wine, or beer may be prescribed.

Parenteral ethanol. Parenteral ethanol is sometimes used to interrupt premature labor or to assist in controlling refractory pain. During labor a 5% solution of ethanol in 5% dextrose in water is administered IV. To achieve and maintain therapeutic blood levels, 200 ml of solution that contains 10 ml ethanol are usually given rapidly as a loading dose, after which the rate of flow is reduced to 200 ml or less per hour. In clients with good kidney function, urine output rises and may exceed input due to the suppression of antidiuretic hormone by the ethanol. If this response does not occur, the client should be watched closely for signs and symptoms of overhydration, because this rate of fluid input is nearly twice that required for normal hydration. Fluid flow should be controlled closely, preferably through the use of an IVac or controlled volume pump device. The client should be monitored for signs and symptoms of inebriation. Because excessive stress is a contributing factor in both premature labor and refractory pain, supportive nursing care to reduce stress levels is an important adjunct to this therapy. β-Adrenergic agonists such as terbutaline are increasingly used instead of alcohol for premature labor.

Ethanol injections are used to interrupt pain transmission by selected peripheral nerves. These treatments may result in obliteration of specific nerve pathways.

Nursing process when alcohol is prescribed as a sedative-hypnotic

Assessment Before administering alcohol as a sedative, the nurse should assess the client for risk of adverse reaction. Previous history of alcoholism, encephalopathy, peripheral neuritis, pancreatitis, seizure disorder, or liver, heart, or peptic ulcer disease are contraindications for alcohol use. The client should also be assessed for acute infections, since alcohol decreases resistance and may delay recovery. A complete drug history should be taken. Use of other CNS depressants greatly increases the risk of toxic reaction to alcohol.

Nursing diagnosis The nursing diagnosis for which alcohol may be prescribed is

> *Sleep pattern disturbance: insomnia*

Clients who receive alcohol are at increased risk for the following diagnoses:

> *High risk for infection related to immunosuppression*
> *Altered nutrition: less than body requirements related to substitution of alcohol for a part of the diet*
> *Sexual dysfunction: decreased libido*

Common collaborative problems that should be differentiated from the nursing diagnoses include

> *Potential complication: hepatitis*
> *Potential complication: pancreatitis*
> *Potential complication: gastric acidity*

Planning The goals of treatment are to avoid adverse drug reaction and toxicity while increasing socialization and promoting sleep induction.

Intervention When increased socialization is desired, alcohol should be served as a beverage in surroundings conducive to group interaction. Alcohol is used in this way most often for elderly persons. Many extended-care facilities have regular "cocktail" hours or other social events at which alcoholic beverages are provided to clients for whom it has been medically ordered. It is most important to control the amount of alcohol each client receives. Generally, each client is given tokens or tickets which can be exchanged for one alcoholic drink. In addition. the staff must supervise the distribution of drinks to prevent swapping of tokens or tickets and to prevent unauthorized access to the alcohol supply.

When clients are properly screened for risk factors and consumption of alcohol is limited to one or two drinks over a 2-hour period, the likelihood of intoxication or other adverse effects is minimal. Clients who receive alcohol should be assessed for adverse reactions to alcohol, including intoxication, adverse alcohol–drug interactions, and signs and symptoms of withdrawal if the alcohol is withdrawn abruptly.

Evaluation Data required for evaluation include evidence of increased interaction with others, acceleration of sleep onset, maintenance of adequate food intake, and absence or incidence of signs and symptoms of other alcohol-related health problems.

Nursing process for hidden alcohol dependence in acute care settings

Assessment The problem of alcohol dependence may be discovered if a careful drug history is taken on admission to the facility. Each client should be questioned specifically about use of alcohol and other social drugs, as well as prescription drugs, nonprescription medicinals, and illegal drugs. The nurse must be non-judgmental if clients are to be open and frank when giving a history. Many clients underreport use of alcohol because they fear a judgmental reaction from health care personnel, or because they do not acknowledge, even to themselves, the magnitude of their alcohol intake.

Other data indicative of alcohol dependence include finding of bottles that contain alcoholic beverages among clients' belongings, progressive restlessness, tremulousness, and irritability after several hours in a setting where alcohol is unavailable, and restlessness and irritability before visiting hours followed by relaxation and serenity after visiting hours (indicating possible consumption of alcohol brought by visitors). Sometimes the first overt indication of alcohol withdrawal is the sight of a client cowering and crying on the floor or in a corner after the advent of terrorizing visual hallucinations. In the case of clients admitted in the late afternoon or evening, these hallucinations are likely to occur in the middle of the night. If unexpected alcohol dependence becomes manifest, a more comprehensive assessment for other alcohol-related health deficits may be in order.

Nursing diagnosis The nursing diagnoses may include the following:

> *Sensory/perceptual alteration: visual hallucinations related to CNS hyperactivity secondary to alcohol withdrawal*
> *Fear related to visual hallucinations*
> *Altered nutrition: less than body requirements related to vitamin and mineral deficiencies due to increased need for and decreased intake of nutrients such as B vitamin complex*
> *Ineffective individual coping: concealing alcohol dependence in a controlled setting in which alcohol is not available*

A common collaborative problem that should be differentiated from the nursing diagnoses is

> *Potential complication: seizures*

Planning The goals of treatment are to decrease the client's fear, prevent seizures, prevent injury should a seizure occur, improve nutrition, and provide emotional support by fostering a warm nonjudgmental nurse–client relationship.

Intervention If evidence points to an alcohol problem before acute withdrawal develops, the nurse should confront the client and attempt to determine the magnitude of dependence. The nurse must maintain an attitude of concern and helpfulness, explaining to the client the risks associated with medical treatment undertaken in ignorance of a major health problem such as alcohol dependence. The client should be reassured that the physician will take action (usually by prescribing alcohol or other tranquilizer drugs) to control withdrawal symptoms. This is not an appropriate time to broach the need for treatment of the dependence, which is likely to be perceived as threatening to the client.

Clients should be asked to allow the nurse to secure any alcoholic beverages among their belongings. These are usually locked up in the medicine room or cupboard. If visitors have supplied the client with alcohol, the nurse should explain the dangers posed by this action and enlist their help in safeguarding the client from hidden alcohol consumption. It should be explained that the health care staff can safely treat the client only if it is fully informed of the drugs the client is taking (including alcohol).

The physician should be informed of the nurse's findings regarding alcoholism (or suspicion of alcoholism, if the client continues to deny dependence). The physician usually prescribes a tranquilizing drug to prevent withdrawal symptoms. Tranquilizing medication should be administered promptly (unless the client has ingested alcohol within the past 2 or 3 hours), even if the prescription was not an immediate order. Seizure precautions should be instituted. Other orders may be altered in light of the client's dependence. In the unlikely event that the physician does not take action to prevent withdrawal, the nurse should inform the nursing supervisor of that fact, because the care facility shares the responsibility of protecting the client from injury.

If the alcoholism remains hidden until overt delirium tremens (hallucinations, fear, and tremor) develop, the nurse should attempt to reassure the client that what he or she is seeing is not real but represents the manifestations of alcohol withdrawal. The client should not be left alone. A staff member who is capable of intervening appropriately in the event of seizures should be assigned to stay with the client. A plastic airway and pillow or other material for padding should be available. The client's attendant must maintain an attitude of caring and reassurance. The physician should be informed immediately, and orders for sedative medication should be administered as soon as possible.

A high-quality diet should be offered to the client. The nurse should consult with the physician about the need for nutritional supplements. After correction of nutritional deficiencies, the client's craving for alcohol appears to decline somewhat (Cerrato, 1986).

Special care should be taken to ensure that the client is not given any food or medicine that contains alcohol. Cooked foods prepared with wine, beer, or other alcoholic liquid should be omitted even if it is cooked after preparation, as the alcohol does not always "burn off" or evaporate completely before it is

Learning experience 24-2

Review your personal experiences with alcoholic beverages. How does your use of alcohol compare with the "norm" for your peers? Have you ever become intoxicated? "Hung over"? What factors influenced your early decisions regarding acceptance or rejection of alcoholic beverages? In the light of the information on alcohol previously presented, how would you evaluate the drinking habits of yourself and your peers?

---

served. Drug preparations that contain alcohol should be avoided (see Table 24-20 for a list of medications that contain alcohol).

Evaluation Data required for evaluation include observations that the overt signs of fear have decreased and statements by clients that they feel better, that the fear has subsided, or that the hallucinations have ceased. The incidence or absence of seizures should be noted. If a seizure occurs, the incidence or absence of injury is significant. The client's willingness to rely on the staff and respond to their attempts at reassurance indicates a good client–nurse relationship (see Chapter 15 for further information).

Checklist of nursing actions

- ☐ Administer prescribed alcoholic beverages in a social setting to enhance their effects on interpersonal interaction.
- ☐ Administer alcoholic beverages with food to prevent gastric irritation and to delay intestinal absorption.
- ☐ Control the rate of flow of parenteral ethanol solutions carefully; monitor clients who receive IV ethanol for fluid imbalance and for signs and symptoms of inebriation.
- ☐ Support vital functions in clients who suffer from acute ethanol toxicity.
- ☐ When taking a drug history from clients, inquire specifically about alcohol use.
- ☐ When clients with a history of alcohol abuse are treated in a controlled setting, monitor them for withdrawal symptoms.
- ☐ Be alert to signs and symptoms of alcohol withdrawal in clients who have been in controlled health care settings for several hours; the appearance of such symptoms may indicate a hidden problem of alcohol abuse.
- ☐ Maintain an accepting nonjudgmental attitude toward clients with alcohol-related problems.
- ☐ Teach good parenting skills to reduce the potential for drug dependence in young people.
- ☐ Teach clients the facts about alcohol use and abuse.

- ☐ When diabetic clients wish to use alcohol, help them incorporate the exchange value of an alcoholic beverage into their daily diet.
- ☐ Encourage clients with alcohol-related problems to seek help in overcoming dependency. Refer them to appropriate community agencies.

Toxic alcohols

Two alcohols, isopropyl alcohol and methanol, are of interest primarily because of their toxicity when administered systemically. Illegally produced alcoholic beverages may also be toxic.

Isopropyl alcohol

Isopropyl alcohol, a constituent of some rubbing alcohols, is a useful disinfectant and topical agent but is unsuitable for internal use. When misused as a beverage, it causes initial symptoms similar to ethanol intoxication, which then progress to life-threatening coma. Isopropyl alcohol is used to "denature" (or render unfit for internal consumption) ethanol intended for uses other than as beverages or internal medicines. Ethanol so treated is exempt from federal internal revenue taxes levied on alcoholic beverages. Although the percentage of isopropyl alcohol in denatured alcohol is low, the consumption of this preparation has been the cause of serious poisoning.

Methanol

Methanol (wood alcohol) is an industrial chemical sometimes imbibed by alcoholics. Within the body, it is metabolized to formic acid, which causes severe acidosis. Abdominal pain, nausea and vomiting, headache, and blurred vision are followed by delirium, convulsions, coma, and death. The drug is highly toxic to the optic nerve, and permanent blindness frequently results from nonfatal poisoning. As little as 10 ml has been considered toxic; the lethal dose is considered to be between 60 and 240 ml (Haddad, Winchester, 1983).

Methanol toxicity is treated by administration of ethanol to saturate liver enzymes and thus slow their conversion of methanol to the toxic metabolite. Dialysis may be employed to remove the toxin from the body.

Illegal alcoholic beverages

Small amounts of alcoholic beverages may be produced privately by people for their own consumption, but the production of such beverages for sale is strictly controlled in the U.S. Beverages that are illegally produced and sold without the collection of internal revenue taxes may present health hazards owing to adulteration or faulty production practices. For example, the use of lead containers or coils in the production of "moonshine" whiskey may add toxic quantities of lead to the resulting distillate. Clients should be warned of the hazards involved in the use of such illegal products.

Disulfiram therapy

Disulfiram (Antabuse) is a chemical that reacts with ethanol in the body to produce toxic substances that engender an unpleasant physiologic reaction. Its mechanism of action is not completely understood. It is known that disulfiram blocks the conversion of acetaldehyde to acetate, but whether the systemic effects of the drug combination are due to accumulation of this or other chemicals formed from the disulfiram–alcohol combination is unknown.

Disulfiram is administered to selected people who wish to abstain from alcohol ingestion. When the chemical is present in the body, the ingestion of even small amounts of alcohol produces an unpleasant reaction characterized by vasomotor instability, respiratory changes, and nausea and vomiting. An initial flushing of the upper body is followed by hyperventilation and tachycardia. Nausea, pallor, hypotension, and vomiting follow. The affected person experiences severe headache, palpitations, and dyspnea. The reaction is usually severe enough to require medical attention and can be life-threatening because of cardiovascular collapse and respiratory depression.

Disulfiram therapy is reserved for highly motivated people under close supervision during the treatment of alcoholism. Clients must be fully aware of the therapy and understand the disulfiram–alcohol reaction. They must be warned against drinking alcohol while taking disulfiram and for a period of 2 full weeks after discontinuing its use, because residual drug in the body can produce a reaction during this period. Accidental exposure to alcohol, such as could occur from breathing fumes, shampooing with beer, or ingesting foods or medicines prepared with alcoholic ingredients, must also be avoided.

Disulfiram produces significant side effects and interactions with other drugs. Its use is not without risk, but it can prevent impulse drinking that often disrupts the process of recovery from chronic alcoholism. The act of taking the daily dose of disulfiram serves as a rededication of the client to sobriety.

Certain other drugs in combination with alcohol cause similar reactions to that produced by disulfiram. Clients who receive the drugs that are described in the literature as "causing disulfiram-like reactions" (*eg*, metronidazole, chlorpropamide) should be warned to avoid contact with alcohol in any form. Both they and clients on disulfiram therapy should carry a suitable medical identification device to warn of the potential for dangerous reaction to alcohol.

Drugs that act selectively on the CNS are discussed in Chapters 25 and 26.

References

Adams FE. (1988). Drug dependence in hospital patients. *American Journal of Nursing, 88, 18*(4), 477.

Bower B. (1991). Alcohol's fetal harm lasts a lifetime. *Science News, 139,* 144.

Campbell M, et al. (1989). Naltrexone in autistic children: An acute open dose range tolerance trial. *J Am Acad Child Adolesc Psychiatry, 28,* 200–206.

Cerrato PL. (1986). Can diet control the urge to drink? *RN, 49*(7), 63–64.

Creighton EJ, Ghodse AH. (1989). Naloxone applied to conjunctiva as a test for physical dependence. *Lancet, 1,* 748.

Flam E. (1989). She who laughs gas conceives last. *Science News, 135,* 182.

Hess G, Walson P. (1988). Seizures secondary to oral viscous lidocaine. *Ann Emerg Med, 17,* 725–727.

Lukasiewicz-Ferland P. (1987). When your ICU patient can't sleep. *Nursing 87, 17*(11), 51–53.

Patterson J. (1987). Triazolam syndrome in the elderly. *South Med J, 80,* 1425–1426.

Schilling R. (1986). Is nitrous oxide a dangerous anesthetic for vitamin B12-deficient subjects? *JAMA, 255,* 1606.

Schuckit M, Gold E. (1988). A simultaneous evaluation of multiple markers of ethanol/placebo challenges in sons of alcoholics and controls. *Arch Gen Psychiatry, 45,* 211.

Sotaniemi EA, Anttila M, Rautio A, Stengard P, Jarvensivu P. (1981). Propranolol and sotalol metabolism after a drinking party. *Clin Pharmacol Ther, 29,* 705–710.

Bibliography

*Adams FE, et al. (1989). Plaques may complicate subcutaneous opioid infusions. *American Journal of Nursing 89,* 109.

*Adams FE. (1988). Drug dependence in hospital patients. *American Journal of Nursing 88, 18*(4), 477.

Alcoholics lose some VA benefits. (1988). *Science News, 142,* 284.

Alcoholics: Where's the treatment? (1986). *Science News, 130,* 26.

Alternative for alcohol withdrawal (letter). (1991). *Nursing 91, 21*(3), 4.

*Angarola JD. (1988). World narcotic consumption. *American Journal of Nursing 88, 15,* 1021.

*Babb D, Jenkins B. (1990). Action STAT! Alcohol withdrawal syndrome. *Nursing 90, 20*(10), 33.

Baumgartner G, Rowen R. (1987). Clonidine vs chlordiazepoxide in the management of acute alcohol withdrawal syndrome. *Arch Intern Med, 147,* 1223–1226.

Beil L. (1988). Awakenings in anesthesia. *Science News, 134,* 110–111.

Blake GJ. (1988). Morphine: New routes for better pain relief. *Nursing 88, 18*(3), 111.

Blake GJ. (1989). Pharmacist on call: Versed—a powerful sedative/hypnotic. *Nursing 89, 19*(9), 95.

Bower B. (1990). Gene may be tied to "virulent" alcoholism. *Science News, 137,* 246.

Bower B. (1989a). Alcohol abuse grows among pregnant poor. *Science News, 136,* 230.

Bower B. (1989b). Drinking while pregnant risks child's IQ. *Science News, 135,* 68.

Bower B. (1989c). Early alcoholism: Crime, depression high. *Science News, 135,* 180.

Bower B. (1988). Intoxicating habits. *Science News, 134,* 88–89.

Bower B. (1986). Chemical clues to alcohol intoxication. *Science News, 129,* 21.

*Brown SJ. (1987). Morphine: The benefits are worth the risks. *RN, 50*(3), 20–28.

*Burden N. (1988). Regional anesthesia: What patients—and nurses—need to know. *RN, 51*(5), 56–61.

Butz AM, et al. (1990). Alcohol-impregnated wipes as an alternative in hand hygiene. *Am J Infect Control, 18*(2), 70–76.

Campbell M, et al. (1989). Naltrexone in autistic children: An acute open dose range tolerance trial. *J Am Acad Child Adolesc Psychiatry, 28*, 200–206.

Cerrato PL. (1988). Is alcohol always bad for your patient? *RN, 51*(12), 61–63.

Cerrato PL. (1986). Can diet control the urge to drink? *RN, 49*(7), 63–64.

Clinical news: Innocent addicts. (1990). *Nursing 90, 20*(11), 92.

*Clinical highlights. (1991). Where do you refer alcoholics who are turned off by AA? *RN, 54*(1), 113.

Cowen R. (1990). Alcoholism treatment under scrutiny. *Science News, 137*, 254.

Creighton EJ, Ghodse AH. (1989). Naloxone applied to conjunctive as a test for physical dependence. *Lancet*, 748.

*Cucchiara R, et al. (1988). Myocardial infarction in carotid endarterectomy patients anesthetized with halothane, enflurane, or isoflurane. *Anesthesiology, 69*, 783–784.

Easing alcohol withdrawal. (1989). *Nursing 89, 19*(10), 78.

Eichner E. (1985). Alcohol versus exercise for coronary protection. *Am J Med, 79*, 231.

Ericson H, Kallen A. (1985). Hospitalization for miscarriage and delivery outcome among Swedish nurses working in operating rooms. *Anesth Analg, 64*, 981.

Estes NJ, Heinemann ME. (1986). *Alcoholism: Development, consequences and interventions*, 3rd ed. St. Louis: CV Mosby.

Eye openers about sleeping pills. (1985). *Science News, 128*, 152.

Fischler RL, et al. (1988). Comparison of continuous epidural infusion of fentamyl-bupivacaine and morphine-bupivacaine in management of postoperative pain. *Anesth Analg, 67*, 559.

Fisk NB. (1986). Alcoholism: Ineffective family coping. *American Journal of Nursing, 86*, 586.

Flam E. (1989). She who laughs gas conceives last. *Science News, 135*, 182.

Fleckenstein J. (1985). Nyquil and acute hepatic necrosis (letter). *New Engl J Med, 313*, 48.

*Fraulini KE, Borchardt AC. (1988). Guide to solving post-anesthesia problems. *Nursing 88, 18*(5), 66–86.

Fuller RK, et al. (1986). Disulfiram treatment of alcoholism. *JAMA, 256*(11), 1449.

Gever LN. (1986). Buprenorphine—the newest narcotic agonist-antagonist. *Nursing 86, 16*(11), 122.

*Goodman L. (1988). Would your assessment spot a hidden alcoholic? *RN, 51*(8), 56–60.

Haddox VG, et al. (1987). Clorazepate use may prevent alcohol withdrawal convulsions. *West J Med, 146*, 695.

Hard proof about cooking with alcohol. (1990). *Tufts University Diet and Nutrition Letter, 8*, 4.

Hess G, Walson P. (1988). Seizures secondary to oral viscous lidocaine. *Ann Emerg Med, 17*, 725–727.

How to dilute morphine. (1988). *Nursing 88, 18*(5), 95.

How you eat when you drink. (1990). *Science News, 138*, 95.

*Janke RJ, Young M. (1989). More knowledge does not improve alcoholics' compliance. *American Journal of Nursing, 86*, 251.

Johnson J. (1985). Drug treatment for sleep disturbances: Does it really work? *Journal of Gerontologic Nursing, 11*, 9.

Jones AW. (1987). Elimination half-life of methanol during hangover. *Pharmacol Toxicol, 60*, 217–220.

*Joyner AJ. (1991). Sharing: Not just a drunk. *Nursing 91, 21*(7), 96.

*Kavey N, Anderson D. (1986). Why every patient needs a good night's sleep. *RN, 49*(12), 16–19.

Kelley RD. (1987). Addiction—and recovery. *American Journal of Nursing 87*, 176.

Legal questions: Informed consent—was it valid? (1986). *Nursing 89, 19*(11), 86.

Lidocaine incites morbid fears. (1987). *RN, 50*(9), 96.

Little BB, et al. (1990). Failure to recognize fetal alcohol syndrome in newborn infants. *Am J Dis Child, 144*(10), 1142.

*Litwack K. (1991). Perioperative series: Managing post-anesthetic emergencies. *Nursing 91, 21*(9), 49–51.

Lukasiewicz-Ferland P. (1987). When your ICU patient can't sleep. *Nursing 87, 17*(11), 51–53.

Lukewarm turkey: Drug firms balk at pursuing a heroin-addiction treatment. (1989). *Scientific American, 260*(3), 32.

Maany I, et al. (1987). Interaction between thioridazine and naltrexone (letter). *Am J Psychiatry, 144*, 966.

*McCaffery M. (1987). A practical "postable" chart of equianalgesic doses. *Nursing 87, 17*(8), 56.

*McCaffery M, Ferrell B. (1990). Do you know a narcotic when you see one? *Nursing 90, 20*(6), 62–63.

Methadone maintenance has a tragic price. (1988). *American Journal of Nursing, 88*(12), 1630.

Moulin DD, Coyle N. (1986). Spinal relief of cancer pain. *American Journal of Nursing 86*, 1050AA–1050BB.

*Narcotic addiction breakthrough. (1985). *American Journal of Nursing 85*, 16.

One too many narcotics. (1990). *Nursing 90, 29*(12), 30.

Patterson J. (1987). Triazolam syndrome in the elderly. *South Med J, 80*, 1425–1426.

Poliquin CM, et al. (1988). A closer look at delirium tremens. *Nursing 88, 18*(3), 79.

Pollack CV, Swindle GM. (1989). Use of diphenhydramine for local anesthesia in "caine"—sensitive patients. *J Emerg Med, 7*, 611–614.

*Powell AH, Bethbova M. (1989). How do you give continuous epidural fentanyl? *American Journal of Nursing 89*, 1197.

*Powell AH, Minick MP. (1988). Alcohol withdrawal syndrome. *American Journal of Nursing 88*, 3123–3315.

*Ramsden M. (1986). Alcohol's effects on the fetus. *Nursing 86, 16*(10), 73.

Report raises blood pressure awareness. (1988). *Science News, 133*, 284.

Rodman MJ. (1986). Naloxone alleviates clonidine toxicity. *RN, 49*(12), 80.

Schilling R. (1986). Is nitrous oxide a dangerous anesthetic for vitamin B$_{12}$-deficient subjects? *JAMA*, *255*, 1606.

Schuckit M, Gold E. (1988). A simultaneous evaluation of multiple markers of ethanol/placebo challenges in sons of alcoholics and controls. *Arch Gen Psychiatry*, *45*, 211.

Silberner J. (1986). Heavy drinking increases stroke risk. *Science News*, *130*, 276.

*Tuttle S. (1991). Letter to a nurse-addict's friend. *American Journal of Nursing 91*, 11, 48–49.

Walsh TD. (1990). . . . About oral morphine for cancer patients. *Nursing 90, 20*(8), 28.

Wickelgren I. (1989). Weakness for alcohol borne by muscles. *Science News, 135*, 117.

Young GP, et al. (1987). Intravenous phenobarbital for alcohol withdrawal and convulsions. *Ann Intern Med, 16*, 847.

*Recommended for further reading.

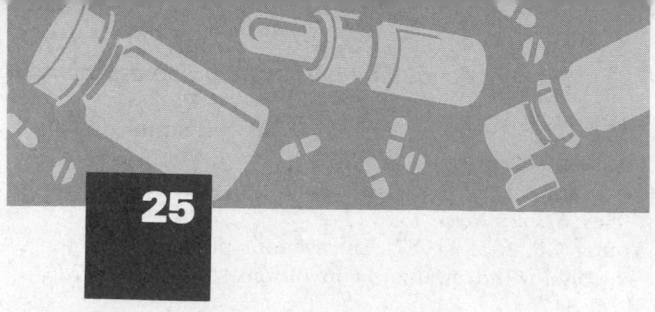

Anticonvulsants

Anticonvulsant drugs are used to eliminate or reduce seizure activity in persons subject to epilepsy.

Pathophysiology of seizures

Seizures are uncontrollable physiologic responses to abnormal electric discharges in the central nervous system (CNS). These responses are usually sporadic and self-limiting. Seizure disorders, known as *epilepsy* are indicative of neuronal hyperexcitability but do not indicate the underlying cause for the condition. The seizures are considered symptoms rather than disease entities.

The nervous system normally exhibits a basal level of excitability that increases with nervous system activity. Whenever the degree of excitability exceeds a certain critical threshold, called the *seizure threshold*, impulse transmission tends to become pronounced and generalized, stimulating abnormal discharges in nerve cells that would otherwise not be active. In seizure disorders, the seizure threshold is either lower than normal, or one or more areas in the brain spontaneously discharge, triggering generalized nerve activity. In some cases, both conditions occur. The physiologic changes that occur during seizures are unresponsive to both the usual inhibitory controls of the nervous system and to voluntary inhibition. If the entire cortex and diencephalon are involved, consciousness is lost.

Seizure activity reflects the areas of the nervous system affected by the abnormal discharges. The more common disorders are classified into types according to the presenting signs and symptoms (Table 25-1). A few types of seizures remain unclassified because of incomplete data.

Factors affecting the occurrence of seizures

Three factors affect the occurrence of seizures: the level of the basal seizure threshold, the presence of foci that initiate abnormal stimuli, and irritation of nerve cells as a result of biochemical changes in the body (Box 25-1).

Basal seizure threshold varies from person to person and is influenced by genetic inheritance and environmental factors. Because nerve function and excitability are affected by the biochemical environment, inherited metabolic patterns that influence brain chemistry play a major part in determining predominant nerve activity patterns and vulnerability to seizures. A low basal threshold predisposes a person to seizure activity and seizure disorders but it does not by itself determine whether a person will develop epilepsy.

Foci in the nervous system that are hyperirritable tend to initiate abnormal stimuli that can spread to adjacent tissue. These foci may develop because of inflammation, abnormal pressure, or other factors. Often, they represent scars from previous lesions that over time have contracted or have undergone other changes that cause irritation to adjacent tissue.

Changes in body chemistry that increase nerve irritability include hypoxia, hypoglycemia, hypocalcemia, hypomagnesemia, alkalosis, high levels of stimulant hormones such as epinephrine, and the use of stimulant drugs. A high fever increases CNS activity and the risk of seizures. Deprivation of oxygen and glucose, two substances essential for normal brain function, also can induce convulsions. Such changes lower the seizure threshold and increase the likelihood of seizure activity.

Table 25-1. International classification of epileptic seizures*

Seizure type	Symptoms
Partial seizures (focal seizures)	
Partial seizures with elementary symptoms	Motor symptoms (Jacksonian)
	Special sensory or somatosensory (Jacksonian)
	Autonomic symptoms
	Compound form
Partial seizures with complex symptoms (temporal lobe or psychomotor epilepsy)	Impairment of consciousness only
	Cognitive symptoms
	Affective symptoms
	Psychosensory symptoms
	Psychomotor symptoms
	Compound forms
Partial seizures secondarily generalized	
Generalized seizures	
	Absences (petit mal)
	Bilateral massive epileptic myoclonus
	Infantile spasms
	Clonic seizures
	Tonic seizures
	Tonic-clonic seizures (grand mal)
	Atonic seizures
	Akinetic seizures
Unilateral seizures (predominantly)	
	Involvement of one side of the body
Unclassified epileptic seizures (incomplete data)	

*This table is based on the International Classification of Epileptic Seizures.

Theoretically, any one of the just mentioned factors could precipitate seizures. However, usually more than one factor is required. In a given situation, it may not be possible to identify the factors responsible for a seizure. The family history may or may not yield a pattern of epilepsy. Although seizure patterns indicating an irritable focus imply localized brain damage at some time in the past, the initial insult may not be known. (Among the events suspected as etiologic agents are prenatal or perinatal hypoxia and head trauma.) Internal chemical changes related to emotional reactions or altered metabolism are rarely obvious as causative factors.

As symptoms, seizures may suggest some primary neurologic disease (such as brain tumor) that must be diagnosed and treated, or they may be the outward manifestation of biochemical imbalance or residual scars from past injury to the nervous system. In either

Box 25-1. Factors affecting the occurrence of seizures

- The level of the basal seizure threshold (a low threshold increases risk of seizure)
- The presence of foci that initiate abnormal stimuli
- The irritation of nerve cells as a result of biochemical changes in the body

Usually more than one factor is required for a seizure to occur.

case, abnormal nerve discharges must be controlled. Frequent seizures may cause further brain damage; if prolonged—as in status epilepticus—they are life-threatening.

Treatment with drugs

Drug treatment of seizure disorders is directed at preventing abnormal nerve activity by decreasing impulse discharge from initiating foci, thus inhibiting the spread of such impulses. This may be accomplished by inhibition of the movement of sodium, potassium, and calcium ions across the membranes, decreasing focal activity, dampening the post-tetanic potentiation of synaptic transmission, or potentiation of inhibitory pathways in the CNS. These actions stabilize nerve cell membranes and elevate the seizure threshold.

Treatment regimens rely heavily on the use of depressant drugs, although at least one stimulant drug is used to manage absence seizures (petit mal epilepsy). Among the drugs employed to control epilepsy are the hydantoins, barbiturates, benzodiazepines, succinimides, and carbamazepine. Oxazolidinediones, magnesium sulfate, and acetazolamide are also used in selected situations (Box 25-2 and Table 25-2).

(Text continues on p. 473)

Box 25-2. Drugs used to control seizures

- hydantoins
- barbiturates
- benzodiazepines
- succinimides
- carbamazepine
- valproic acid
- oxazolidinediones*
- magnesium sulfate*
- acetazolamide*

*Used in selected situations.

Table 25-2. Anticonvulsant drugs

Drug name	Preparation	Usual dosage	Additional information
Hydantoins			
phenytoin (Dilantin, Diphenylan)	Capsules, chewable tablets, and suspension for oral use Extended release forms Solution for injection	Adults: 300–600 mg/day, divided in three doses Children: 4–8 mg/kg body weight, divided in two to three doses PC: C	Therapeutic serum concentrations (10–20 μg/ml) may be achieved more rapidly by giving a loading dose (1 g to adults or 500 mg to children). Initial dosage should be reduced for the elderly, newborns, and others with impaired hepatic function. Phenytoin is frequently used with phenobarbital for the control of major motor seizures. A frequent side-effect is gingival hypertrophy. Absorption of intramuscular doses may be erratic owing to crystallization of the drug in the injection site.
ethotoin (Peganone)	Oral tablets	Adults: 2–3 g/day, divided in four to six doses, administered after food Children: 500 mg–1 g/day, divided in four to six doses, administered after food PC: C	Ethotoin does not have the antiarrhythmic properties of phenytoin. Ethotoin is both less effective and less toxic than phenytoin; it is usually used in conjunction with other anticonvulsant drugs.
mephenytoin (Mesantoin)	Oral tablets	Adults: 200–600 mg/day, divided in three equal doses Children: 100–400 mg/day, 3–15 mg/kg body weight/day, or 100–450 mg/m²/day, divided in three equal doses PC: C	Mephenytoin causes greater sedation and risk of serious blood dyscrasias than phenytoin. Mephenytoin is used for the management of grand mal, Jacksonian, and psychomotor seizures in persons who are refractory to less toxic anticonvulsants.
phenacemide (Phenurone)	Oral tablets	Adults: 2–3 g/day, divided in three equal doses Children: 0.75–1.25 g/day, divided in three equal doses PC: D	Phenacemide is extremely toxic and is used only when other less toxic anticonvulsants are ineffective in controlling seizures.
Barbiturates and derivatives			
amobarbital (Amytal)	Powder Oral tablets Powder for preparing solutions for intramuscular injection or intravenous infusion	(As an anticonvulsant used only to treat acute seizure states) Usual dosage for adults: intravenous infusion at a *maximum* rate of 100 mg/min (*ie* 1 ml of 10% solution over 1 minute) For insomnia: 60–200 mg for adults; for children: 2–3 mg/kg body weight For sedation: 60–150 mg daily, divided in two to three doses for adults; for children: 2 mg/kg body weight/day, divided in four doses PC: B	Preparation of solutions: add diluent and rotate; do not shake; use within 30 min. Intramuscular doses must be injected deeply to avoid sterile abscesses or tissue sloughing. Do not use for insomnia for more than 2 weeks. After long-term use, wean over at least 5–6 days.

(Continued)

Table 25-2. Anticonvulsant drugs (Continued)

Drug name	Preparation	Usual dosage	Additional information
Barbiturates and derivatives			
phenobarbital (Barbital, Luminol, Sulfoton)	Tablets, capsules, elixir, solution, powder, and extended-release capsules for oral use Rectal suppositories Solutions and powders for preparing solutions for injection	Adults: 100–300 mg/day, preferably in a single dose at bedtime Children: 3–5 mg/kg body weight daily, divided in one or two doses PC: D	Phenobarbital may be used for initial treatment of all forms of epilepsy except petit mal. It is often given concurrently with phenytoin or other anticonvulsants. Phenobarbital may impair intellectual ability.
mephobarbital (Mebaral, Mebroin)	Powder Oral tablets	Adults: 400–600 mg/day, taken as a single dose or in divided doses Children younger than 5 yr of age: 16–32 mg tid-qid Children older than 5 yr of age: 32–64 mg tid-qid PC: D	Mephobarbital is metabolized to phenobarbital. Mephobarbital is used in place of phenobarbital in the management of seizures in persons who exhibit undesirable reactions to phenobarbital (excessive drowsiness, hyperexcitability, irritability, or mood disturbance).
metharbital (Gemonil)	Oral tablets	Adults: 100–800 mg/day, divided in one to three doses Children: 50–100 mg qid-tid; or 5–15 mg/kg body weight/day, in divided doses	Metharbital is used in the management of seizures in persons who have adverse reactions to phenobarbital.
primidone (Myidone, Mysoline)	Chewable tablets and suspension for oral use	Adults and children 8 yr of age or older: 250 mg tid-qid Children younger than 8 yr of age: 125–250 mg tid; 10–25 mg/kg body weight/day, in divided doses; or 1.25 g/m²/day, divided in two to four doses PC: D	Primidone is considered by some physicians to be the drug of choice for the treatment of psychomotor epilepsy. Primidone is partially (15%–25%) metabolized to phenobarbital.
Oxazolidinediones			
paramethadion (Paradione)	Capsules and solution for oral use	Adults: 900–2,400 mg/day, divided in three to four equal doses Children: 300–900 mg/day and up, depending on the appearance of toxic signs and symptoms PC: D	Paramethadione is used in the management of petit mal (absence seizures) in persons who have not responded to other anticonvulsants (*eg*, ethosuximide).
trimethadione (Tridione)	Tablets, capsules, and solution for oral use	Adults: 900–2,400 mg/day, divided in three to four doses Children: 40 mg/kg body weight/day, divided in three to four doses PC: D	Trimethadione acts selectively to suppress petit mal epilepsy. Trimethadione is used only for refractory absence seizures because of its high toxic potential.
Succinimides			
ethosuximide (Zarontin)	Capsules and solution for oral use	20 mg per kg body weight/d (up to a maximum of 1.5 g for adults or 1 g for children) in divided doses PC: C	Ethosuximide is considered to be the agent of choice for petit mal seizures.
methsuximide (Celontin)	Oral capsules	10 mg/kg body weight/day, in divided doses; or 600 mg/m²/day, in divided doses PC: C	Methsuximide is used in the management of petit mal (absence seizures).

(Continued)

Table 25-2. Anticonvulsant drugs (Continued)

Drug name	Preparation	Usual dosage	Additional information
Succinimides			
			Because it does not usually precipitate grand mal (tonic-clonic seizures), it is particularly useful in managing (with other anticonvulsants) combined absence and tonic-clonic seizures.
phensuximide (Milontin)	Oral capsules	1–3g/d, divided in two to three doses PC: D	Phensuximide is the least toxic and least effective of the succinimide-derivative anticonvulsants.
			Phensuximide is used in the management of petit mal (absence seizures).
Valproate			
valproic acid (Dalpro, Depakene, Depakote, Myproic acid)	Capsules, enteric-coated tablets, and solution for oral use	15–60 mg/kg body weight/day, in one or more doses. PC: D	Valproate is used to treat absence seizures, both simple and complex.
			Valproic acid capsules must *not* be chewed (to prevent local irritation to the mouth and throat).
			Gastrointestinal side-effects can be minimized by starting with low doses and increasing gradually.
			A plasma level of 50–100 µg/mL has been suggested as the therapeutic range.
Benzodiazepines			
clonazepam (Klonopin; *Can:* Rivotril)	Oral tablets	Adults: 1.5–20 mg/day, divided in two to three doses Children: 0.01–0.2 mg per kg body weight daily, divided in two to three doses PC: C	Clonazapam is useful in the treatment of petit mal and myoclonic seizures in children.
			Also used to treat akinetic seizures.
diazepam (Valium)	Solutions for injection	Not used for maintenance In the management of status epilepticus: Adults: 5–10 mg q 10 min up to a maximal dose of 30 mg (this regimen may be repeated q2h–q4h up to a maximal dose of 100 mg/24 hr) PC: D	Diazapam is the drug of choice for initial treatment of status epilepticus (intravenous route preferred).
Miscellaneous agents			
carbamazepine (Epitol Tapazine, Tegretol; *Can:* Apo-Carbamazepine)	Oral tablets and chewable tablets	Adults and children 12 yr of age or older: 800–1.2 g/day, divided in three to four doses Children 6–12 yr of age: 400–800 mg/day, divided in three to four doses PC: C	Carbamazepine is structurally related to the tricyclic antidepressants.
			Carbamazepine is extremely toxic to a small percentage of persons and is not used unless other anticonvulsants have been ineffective in controlling seizures.

(Continued)

Table 25-2. Anticonvulsant drugs (Continued)

Drug name	Preparation	Usual dosage	Additional information
Miscellaneous agents			
magnesium sulfate	Solutions for intramuscular or intravenous injection	Not used for maintenance in the management of seizures due to toxemia of pregnancy: *Intravenous*: up to 150 mg/min *Intramuscular*: Adults: Initially: 8–10 g (as a 50% solution), divided in two doses and administered in the buttocks; thereafter; 4–5 g q4h; dosage is adjusted according to response and must be discontinued as soon as the desired therapeutic effect is obtained. PC: B	Magnesium sulfate is useful in the treatment of convulsions of eclampsia or pre-eclampsia of pregnancy.
acetazolamide (Ak-Zol, Diamox)	Tablets and sustained-release capsules for oral use Powder for preparing solutions for injection	Adults and children: 8–30 mg per kg body weight/day, divided in one to four doses PC: C	Acetazolamide is used in the management of refractory epilepsy, especially petit mal and grand mal seizures.

KEY: PC = pregnancy category. (The validity of pregnancy categories has not been established; see Chapter 16; p 216.)
Can = Canadian trade name.

Hydantoins. Hydantoin drugs are used primarily for the control of major motor and psychomotor seizures. Individual drugs are also effective in other types of epilepsy: phenytoin in autonomic seizures, as well as ethotoin and mephenytoin in focal seizures. Hydantoin drugs are not useful in petit mal epilepsy and may increase the frequency of seizures of this type. Because it is the most frequently prescribed of the hydantoins, phenytoin will be discussed in detail.

Phenytoin

Pharmacodynamics. Phenytoin is known to stabilize cell membranes and decrease the movements of sodium, calcium, and potassium ions involved in depolarization and propagation of membrane action potentials. Although these effects have not been demonstrated by therapeutic levels of the drug, they may underlie its therapeutic actions. Phenytoin decreases focal activity in the nervous system; reduces post-tetanic potentiation of synaptic transmission; decreases the spread of the seizure process from an active focus; limits the development of maximal seizure activity; and reduces abnormal hyperexcitability toward a normal level. It causes little sedative or hypnotic effect.

In the heart, phenytoin reduces the force of myocardial contraction, depresses pacemaker action, improves atrioventricular conduction (especially when depressed by digitalis), and prolongs the refractory period.

Pharmacokinetics. Phenytoin is absorbed slowly whether administered intramuscularly or orally. Because the drug precipitates in the tissues, the former route should be avoided when possible. Phenytoin is sometimes administered intravenously. Gastrointestinal (GI) absorption is variable. Bioavailability among commercial preparations is also inconsistent. When prompt release forms are used, plasma levels peak in 1.5–3 hours, whereas levels of extended-release capsules peak in 4–12 hours.

Phenytoin is highly bound to both tissue and plasma proteins; about 95% binds to plasma proteins. The drug distributes widely. Levels in the cerebrospinal fluid are equal to levels of unbound drug in the plasma.

With normal renal function, only 2% of phenytoin is excreted unchanged by the kidneys. The rest is degraded by liver microsomal enzymes, then is secreted in bile and becomes part of the enterohepatic cycle. Eventually, the metabolites are excreted by the kidneys. Metabolism in the liver is a saturable process. Thus, small increases in dosage can result in substantial increases in plasma phenytoin concentration. Plasma half-time is variable but averages 24 hours.

Therapeutic and toxic effects correlate most closely with unbound serum levels of the drug. Although these levels are not always proportionate to total serum levels, the total serum levels are used most frequently to monitor drug levels. The recommended total phenytoin serum levels for therapeutic effect range from 10 to 20 µg/ml. Drug therapy is begun with relatively low doses that are increased gradually until the optimal therapeutic response is obtained.

Therapeutic uses. Phenytoin is used in the control of seizures in most forms of epilepsy except petit mal. It is often prescribed in conjunction with phenobarbital. Phenytoin is sometimes administered intravenously (IV) as an adjunct in the treatment of status epilepticus. Other uses of the drug include the treatment of disturbed nonepileptic psychotic patients, seizures associated with head trauma and increased intracranial pressure, trigeminal and related neuralgias, and cardiac arrhythmias.

Dosage and administration. The daily dose of phenytoin is divided initially to minimize gastric irritation and toxic effects. After stabilization, the use of extended-release phenytoin capsules (one daily) may be considered. To avoid hypotension and marked CNS depression, IV solutions of phenytoin should be administered slowly; the rate must not exceed 50 mg/min and should be even slower in the elderly and those unable to metabolize the drug at a normal rate. Phenytoin must be administered with normal saline because it is incompatible (forms a precipitate) with dextrose and acidic solutions.

Adverse reactions. Side effects are generally dose-related, and dosage should be carefully regulated to minimize them. Adverse reactions to phenytoin are common and can be serious. They vary widely and may involve the GI, cardiovascular, central nervous, integumentary, lymphatic, hepatic, or hematologic systems. Nausea, vomiting, constipation, epigastric pain, difficulty in eating, and weight loss can occur. The drug depresses pacemaker activity in the heart and may cause arrhythmias. Early neurologic changes include nystagmus, ataxia, and visual changes. These may progress to nervousness, dizziness, insomnia, confusion, tremor, and chorea. Skin reactions range from rashes to serious conditions such as systemic lupus erythematosus or Stevens-Johnson syndrome, a severe form of erythema multiforme. A syndrome resembling mononucleosis may occur. Lymphadenopathy associated with phenytoin may be manifested by lymph node hyperplasia, lymphoma, or Hodgkin's disease. In addition to the liver changes seen in the mononucleosis syndrome, toxic hepatitis or other liver abnormalities may develop. Anemia usually responds to folic acid therapy but bone marrow depression is sometimes fatal.

Until recently, it was believed that phenytoin interferes with vitamin D metabolism and contributes to the development of osteomalacia. The validity of these findings has been questioned because the persons in the studies were institutionalized with little access to sunshine and may have been deficient in vitamin D.

Phenytoin does decrease intestinal absorption of folic acid and can cause anemia if folic acid intake is not increased to compensate for this effect.

Phenytoin causes cosmetic changes. A very common side effect especially in children is hyperplasia of the gums. This may become so severe that surgical removal is required. Excess hair growth and coarsening of the features may also develop.

Phenytoin is a suspected carcinogen and teratogen. In addition to lymphoma and Hodgkin's disease in persons under treatment, the drug may cause a fetal hydantoin syndrome, congenital defects such as spina bifida, or malignancies (including neuroblastoma) in children exposed *in utero*.

Toxic effects of phenytoin are associated with varying blood concentrations (Table 25-3). Although most clients tolerate blood concentrations of less than 25 µg/ml, at this point some will experience nystagmus, ataxia, and diplopia. Certain persons with inherited enzyme deficiencies metabolize phenytoin slowly and exhibit toxic effects even with reduced dosages.

Intravenous administration of phenytoin can cause cardiovascular collapse or CNS depression. The drug is irritating to blood vessels and may cause phlebitis. Rapid administration tends to cause hypotension and to damage blood vessels. Phenytoin can damage the cerebellum, causing permanent ataxia.

Drug interactions. Phenytoin interacts with numerous other drugs, usually by changing the rate of drug metabolism. It stimulates the metabolic breakdown of the hormones T_3 and T_4, of estrogens, and of corticosteroids. It can cause signs and symptoms of hypothyroidism in clients with marginal thyroid function, as well as in clients with known hypothyroidism who are taking hormone replacements. Phenytoin also decreases the effectiveness of corticosteroid medications when taken concurrently. The metabolic breakdown of phenytoin is decreased (causing blood levels to increase) by concurrent administration of ethanol (alcohol), chloramphenicol, cimetidine, dicumarol, disulfiram, isoniazid, miconazole, or certain sulfonamides. Not only do carbamazepine and theophylline decrease phenytoin levels but their own blood levels

---

Table 25-3. Plasma concentration and toxic side-effects of phenytoin

Plasma concentration	Toxic manifestations
10–20 µg/ml	Few—this is the therapeutic range
>20 µg/ml	Nystagmus, diplopia, ataxia
>30 µg/ml	Lethargy, drowsiness, asterixis
>40 µg/ml	Extreme lethargy
>50 µg/ml	Coma

are also decreased by phenytoin. Cisplatin also lowers serum phenytoin levels.

Interaction between phenytoin and phenobarbital may cause blood levels of either drug to decrease or increase. Mechanisms involved in these changes may include induction of microsomal enzymes in the liver, competition for binding sites on plasma proteins, and changes in intestinal absorption.

Phenytoin can damage the cerebellum, causing permanent ataxia.

Precautions and contraindications. Phenytoin is contraindicated in persons with allergic hypersensitivity to it and should be discontinued at the first allergic reaction such as rash or dyspnea. To prevent permanent damage to the cerebellum, the drug should be discontinued at the first sign of ataxia.

When phenytoin is administered intravenously, vital signs should be monitored. Clients with known cardiac disease, the elderly, and those with unstable vital signs should be continuously monitored via electrocardiogram. Because it is teratogenic, phenytoin should not be used during pregnancy. When its use is necessary, blood phenytoin levels should be monitored closely. Mothers taking phenytoin should not breastfeed their infants. (See Focus on Hydantoin Anticonvulsant: Similarities and Differences.)

Barbiturates

All barbiturates exhibit anticonvulsant activity but only three (phenobarbital, metharbital, and mephobarbital) are capable of suppressing seizure activity in subhypnotic doses.

Because it is effective, low in cost, and was believed to be relatively nontoxic, phenobarbital has been the barbiturate most widely used as an anticonvulsant. It will be discussed here as the prototype of this class of drugs.

Phenobarbital

Phenobarbital was the first organic agent found to be effective in the treatment of seizures. It has often been used in conjunction with other anticonvulsants particularly phenytoin.

Pharmacodynamics. The anticonvulsant activity of phenobarbital is relatively nonselective. It elevates the seizure threshold and limits the spread of seizure activity. These effects appear to stem from the potentiation of inhibitory pathways in the CNS. Phenobarbital does stimulate gamma-aminobutyric acid (GABA) receptors, thus, inhibiting microsomal activity. However, its action on GABA is less than that of barbiturates with more pronounced sedative properties. (Activation of GABA receptors causes inhibition of neuronal activity.)

Pharmacokinetics. Oral doses of phenobarbital are absorbed slowly but relatively completely (in amounts of 70%–90%). The development of peak blood levels requires 8–12 hours; peak levels in the brain occur 2–3 hours later. Delayed onset of action is also apparent with IV administration, which requires about 5 minutes for effects to appear. Up to half of a given dose binds to plasma proteins. Tissue binding, including that in the brain, occurs to a similar degree. Because phenobarbital is relatively nonlipophilic, it penetrates and leaves the brain slowly, resulting in both slow onset and long duration of effect.

Phenobarbital crosses the placenta and appears in the milk of nursing mothers.

Approximately three-fourths of phenobarbital is degraded by the hepatic microsomal enzymes. The remainder is eliminated unchanged by the kidneys. Renal excretion is pH dependent—it is most rapid when urine is mostly alkaline. Plasma half-life in adults is about 90 hours; in children it tends to be shorter and more variable. To maintain anticonvulsant activity without toxic effects, a serum level of 10–25 μg/ml is recommended. For the control of febrile convulsions, at least 15 μg/ml are needed. The daily maintenance doses may be divided to minimize toxicity.

Therapeutic uses. Phenobarbital has been a primary agent for treating grand mal and cortical focal seizures, particularly in children. It is ineffective in petit mal epilepsy. Phenobarbital is frequently administered concurrently with phenytoin and may be part of a mixed medication regimen in the treatment of epilepsy characterized by several forms of seizures. It is used to prevent recurrent seizures in children who have experienced one or more febrile seizures and who are judged to be at high risk for repeated episodes. Because of its slow onset of action, phenobarbital is seldom used in treating status epilepticus.

Dosage and administration. The usual oral daily anticonvulsant dose of phenobarbital is 1 mg to 3 kg body weight (60—250 mg for adults). Several weeks are required to attain a steady plasma level. Loading doses (double dosage for the first 4 days of treatment) can shorten the latency period but these dosages produce marked sedation. Recommended dosages for initiating treatment of children are 3–5 mg/kg body weight. Only one dose is required daily because phenobarbital has a long half-life. Dosages are adjusted in accord with individual response to the regimen until the minimal effective dosage for maintenance is determined.

Plasma levels of phenobarbital may be used to monitor drug therapy. Although these do not correspond exactly with therapeutic response, concentrations of 10–25 ug/ml are recommended as the therapeutic range. To prevent febrile convulsions, a level of at least 15 ug/ml is required. In most individuals, levels between 30 ug/ml and 60 ug/ml produce signs and symptoms of toxicity.

Hydantoin: anticonvulsants

Similarities	Differences

Similarities

Pharmacodynamics

These agents are thought to stabilize the neuron cell membrane at the cell body, axon, and synapse to limit the spread of seizure activity. They are thought to decrease focal activity, reduce post-tetanic potentiation of synaptic transmission, reduce spread of seizure progress from active focus, limit development of maximal seizure activity, and reduce abnormal hyperexcitability.

Pharmacokinetics

These agents are rapidly absorbed from the GI tract. They are primarily metabolized by the liver and excreted in the urine as metabolities; some are excreted in feces and breast milk, and small quantities are excreted in saliva.

Therapeutic uses

These agents are used as anticonvulsants in all forms of epilepsy except petit mal seizures.

Adverse reactions

These include: (CNS) ataxia, slurred speech, dizziness, insomnia, nervousness, nystagmus, behavioral changes, hand trembling; (CV) diminished pacemaker activity; (GI) nausea, vomiting, constipation, epigastric pain, difficulty eating, weight loss, gingival hyperplasia; (HEMA) anemia, bone marrow depression; (OTHER) rash, erythema multiforme, Stevens-Johnson syndrome, exfoliative dermatitis, lymphadenopathy, excessive hair growth.

Contraindications

These agents are contraindicated in persons with hypersensitivity to hydantoins.

Precautions

Use these agents cautiously in persons taking other hydantoins.

Differences

• **Phenytoin** decreases sodium, potassium, and calcium ion influx into the cell involved in depolarization and propagation of membrane action potentials; it also decreases the force of heart muscle contraction, depresses pacemaker activity, improves atrioventricular conduction and prolongs refractory period.

• **Phenytoin** is slowly absorbed orally or IM; IM route is not recommended because of erratic absorption; it may be given IV. • **Phenytoin** excretion is enhanced by an alkaline urine. • **Phenytoin** has a half-life averaging 22 hours, an onset of 1½–3 hours (4–12 hours with extended release preparations). • **Ethotoin** has a half-life of 3–9 hours. • **Mephenytoin** has a half-life of 7 hours, peaks in 45 minutes to 4 hours with a duration of 24–48 hours. • **Phenacemide** has a duration of 5 hours.

• **Phenytoin** is used in the treatment of status epilepticus, disturbed nonepileptic psychosis, trigeminal neuralgia, and cardiac arrhythmias. • **Phenacemide** is extremely toxic and used only when other less toxic anticonvulsants are ineffective.

• **Phenytoin**, given intramuscularly can cause pain, necrosis, and inflammation at the injection site; intravenous administration may cause cardiovascular collapse and central nervous system depression. • **Phenacemide** may cause hepatitis, jaundice, acute psychosis, paresthesias, muscle pain, and nephritis.

• **Ethotoin** is contraindicated in persons with hepatic or hematologic disorders. • **Phenytoin** IV is contraindicated in persons with sinus bradycardia, sinoatrial block, second or third degree atrioventricular block, or Stokes/Adams syndrome. • **Phenacemide** is contraindicated in persons with jaundice or liver dysfunction.

Use **phenacemide** with caution in persons with history of drug allergy, personality disorders, or those taking other anticonvulsants. Use **phenytoin** cautiously in persons with acute intermittent porphyria, hepatic or renal dysfunction, myocardial insufficiency, respiratory depression, and in elderly or debilitated clients.

(continued)

Hydantoin: anticonvulsants (Continued)

Similarities	Differences
Nursing considerations	

Similarities

Nursing considerations

Instruct in disease, treatment, drug therapy, adverse effects, and compliance; assess seizure disorder, including characteristics of seizures; never withdraw drug suddenly; warn person to avoid activities requiring mental alertness; monitor complete blood count and platelets initially and at frequent intervals; give drugs with meals to avoid gastric upset; warn that alcohol use may decrease the benefit of drug; evaluate for signs and symptoms of neurologic abnormalities including effects of drug; assist in eliminating or controlling factor that might precipitate seizure activity; begin drug therapy with a low dose, gradually increasing until adequate control is achieved; monitor behavior and neurologic function closely; administer regularly at consistent intervals; assess response to drug therapy; assist in maintaining an acceptable appearance; instruct in measures to diminish the side effects of the drug; and institute safety and privacy measures.

Differences

When giving **phenacemide**, monitor liver function studies and urinalysis; instruct to watch for personality changes; increase dosage slowly while other anticonvulsants are being discontinued; and assess for signs and symptoms of jaundice or hepatitis. When giving **phenytoin**, mix only with saline; give within 1 hour of preparation; and administer infusion over 30–60 minutes or as intravenous bolus at 50 mg/min. Instruct that **phenytoin** may change urine to pink, red, or reddish brown. Administer **phenytoin** into a large vein; avoid using hand veins because of tissue irritation; advise not to change brands or dosage forms of **phenytoin** once regimen is stabilized.

Adverse reactions. Anticonvulsant dosages of phenobarbital may cause CNS depression, GI upset, pain, and allergic hypersensitivity. Side effects include respiratory depression, lethargy, vertigo, headache, nausea, vomiting, diarrhea, myalgia, neuralgia, and arthralgia. Phenobarbital is suspected of being teratogenic. Doses administered during pregnancy affect the fetus, and barbiturates given to nursing mothers may cause toxicity in the infant.

A recent study (Farwell et al, 1990) found that children treated with phenobarbital scored lower on the Stanford-Binet IQ test while taking the drug and for as long as 6 months after the drug was discontinued. An adverse psychologic effect is depression associated with low self-esteem, high levels of anxiety, self-destructive behavior, and complaints of persecution. Some epileptic children taking barbiturates have attempted suicide. It is known that the barbiturates interfere with rapid eye movement sleep, and rapid eye movement sleep deprivation sometimes leads to psychotic episodes. However, whether this is the mechanism by which phenobarbital causes depression is not known. When phenobarbital is withdrawn, the psychologic depression lifts.

Allergic hypersensitivity to phenobarbital often produces skin reactions, some of which progress to life-threatening conditions such as Stevens-Johnson syndrome. Early symptoms of hypersensitivity include headache, fever, stomatitis, conjunctivitis, rhinitis, and urethritis (or balanitis). Phenobarbital also enhances porphyrin synthesis. Rarely, blood dyscrasias develop during its use.

Some degree of tolerance develops with continued administration of phenobarbital. The seizure threshold is lowered when the drug is withdrawn; abrupt discontinuation may precipitate status epilepticus.

Excitement or confusion can occur when phenobarbital is administered to the elderly. Children also may exhibit paradoxic excitement and hyperactivity. These effects are attributed to a disproportionate depression of CNS inhibition by the drug. Subtle personality changes (distortions of mood and impairment of judgment) also develop in some clients, especially with prolonged therapy.

Drug interactions. Phenobarbital is known to stimulate liver microsomal enzymes that inactivate many drugs and change them to metabolites, which are easily eliminated by the body. Although there is little evidence that the drug stimulates the rate of its own breakdown, it does alter the rate of metabolism of many other drugs. In addition, phenobarbital interferes with absorption or secretion of some chemicals. Drugs whose effects are decreased because of more rapid metabolism by liver enzymes include coumarin, digitalis, corticosteroids, tricyclic antidepressants, and doxycycline. Phenobarbital interferes with pituitary secretion of corticotropin.

A few drugs affect serum levels of phenobarbital. For example, disulfiram and monoamine oxidase inhibitors restrict the metabolism of phenobarbital, prolonging its half-life in the body. Phenobarbital competes with other weak acids for binding to plasma albumin. Displacement of thyroxine from these sites may produce clinically significant increases in free thyroxine levels. This could be a factor in the excitation seen in some clients.

Precautions and contraindications. Phenobarbital is contraindicated in clients with bronchopneumonia and in clients with known allergic hypersensitivity to the drug. It is not given to persons with a history of porphyria. Caution should be used when phenobarbital is used to treat clients with pulmonary insufficiency and children with hyperactivity. The drug should be withdrawn if depression develops.

To prevent serious allergic syndromes, the drug should be promptly discontinued if a skin rash develops.

When phenobarbital is prescribed concurrently with drugs known to interact with it, the dosage of each drug must be carefully regulated to achieve optimal effects. If the dosage of one drug is altered, the dosage of the other may need adjustment.

Following prolonged therapy, phenobarbital should be withdrawn gradually. (See Focus on Barbiturates: Similarities and Differences.)

Oxazolidinediones

The oxazolidinediones are a class of drugs that act to control petit mal (absence) seizures. They are not effective in major motor seizures but rather tend to precipitate or exacerbate grand mal epilepsy.

One of the oxazolidinediones, trimethadione, was the first truly selective anticonvulsant discovered. It will be discussed here as a prototype of the class.

Trimethadione

Pharmacodynamics. In addition to suppressing petit mal seizures, trimethadione has some sedative activity. It acts to raise the seizure threshold of the thalamocortical system, which appears to be particularly important in the genesis of absence seizures. The drug depresses projection of seizure activity from cortical foci to the thalamus. It does not affect cortical spread of activity or post-tetanic potentiation in the spinal cord or stellate ganglia.

Pharmacokinetics. Trimethadione is rapidly absorbed from the GI tract. It is uniformly distributed in the tissues but does not bind to plasma proteins. Trimethadione is readily metabolized by liver enzymes to an active metabolite, dimethadione, which is responsible for its therapeutic effects. Eventually, dimethadione is excreted by the kidneys. It has a half-life of 6–13 days.

Dimethadione serum levels are more indicative of therapeutic levels than are trimethadione levels. Therapeutic serum levels of dimethadione range from 700 to 800 μg/ml. Therapy is initiated with low doses that are increased gradually until a therapeutic effect is achieved, a process requiring several weeks.

Therapeutic uses. Trimethadione is used to control petit mal epilepsy that is refractory to ethosuximide. If dosage is adequate, up to 80% of clients achieve control of absence seizures. It can be used in combination with most other anticonvulsants to treat epilepsy with mixed types of seizures.

Adverse reactions. Trimethadione is a relatively toxic drug. Drowsiness is the most frequent side effect. This tends to subside with continued administration. Visual disturbances are fairly common and include hemeralopia (blurred vision in bright or glaring light), diplopia, and photophobia. Allergic reactions include neutropenia, skin rashes, hepatitis, nephrotic syndrome, and a syndrome resembling myasthenia gravis. Other side effects are alopecia, paresthesias, vaginal bleeding, and changes in blood pressure. Trimethadione may be teratogenic; congenital malformations have occurred in children born to women taking the drug.

Precautions and contraindications. Trimethadione is used only for petit mal seizures that fails to respond to other less toxic drugs. It is not recommended for use by women who are or may become pregnant. The drug is contraindicated in persons known to be allergic to it.

Extreme caution is required when trimethadione is prescribed for patients with retinal or optic nerve disease.

Therapy must be closely monitored, especially during the first year of treatment. Regular white blood cell counts are taken and the drug discontinued if the neutrophil count falls to 2,500/mm^3. If symptoms of nephrosis, hepatitis, or myasthenia gravis occur, the drug is also discontinued.

To reduce the risk of precipitating seizures, trimethadione is best withdrawn slowly.

Succinimides

The frequency and severity of toxic reactions to the oxazolidinedione anticonvulsants have limited their

Focus on

Barbiturates: similarities and differences

Similarities

Pharmacodynamics

These agents act as nonselective CNS depressants. They depress the sensory cortex, decrease motor activity, alter cerebral function, and produce sedation and hypnosis. They enhance or mimic the inhibitory synaptic action of gamma-aminobutyric acid. They also decrease the rapid eye movement phase of sleep.

Pharmacokinetics

These agents are absorbed in varying degrees after oral, parenteral, or rectal administration. They are rapidly distributed to all tissues and fluids. They are primarily metabolized by the liver and excreted in the urine. Their onset occurs in 20–60 minutes for oral administration, slightly faster for intramuscular, and seconds to 5 minutes for IV administration. The average half-life ranges from 24 to 34 hours.

Therapeutic uses

These agents are used for sedation, hypnosis, insomnia, and preanesthetic sedation.

Adverse reactions

These include: (CNS) confusion, depression, paradoxical excitement, drowsiness, lethargy, vertigo, headache, central nervous system depression, hangover effect, impaired judgment and motor skills; (CV) hypotension, bradycardia, circulatory collapse; (RESP) respiratory depression, apnea, laryngospasm, bronchospasm: (GI) gastric upset, nausea, vomiting, diarrhea; (HEMA) megaloblastic anemia, agranulocytosis, thrombocytopenia; (OTHER) exfoliative dermatitis, Stevens-Johnson syndrome, dependence, rash, fever, myalgia, neuralgia.

Contraindications

These agents are contraindicated in those with known hypersensitivity to barbiturates and in those with bronchopneumonia, status asthmaticus, severe respiratory distress, depression or suicidal ideas, uncontrolled or chronic pain, or porphyria.

Differences

• **Phenobarbital**, **mephobarbital**, and **metharbital** depress the monosynaptic and polysynaptic transmission in the CNS; they increase the threshold for electrical stimulation of the motor cortex.

• **Mephobarbital**, **metharbital**, and **phenobarbital** have an average duration of 10–12 hours (PO). • **Amobarbital**, **butabarbital**, and **aprobarbital** have an average duration of 6–8 hours. • **Pentobarbital** and **secobarbital** have an onset of action of 10–15 minutes (PO) and average duration of 3–4 hours (PO).

• **Phenobarbital**, **mephobarbital**, and **metharbital** are also used as anticonvulsants in treating tonic-clonic or absence seizures. • **Metharbital** is also used for treating myoclonic and mixed seizures. • **Phenobarbital** and **secobarbital** are used to treat status epilepticus. • **Primidone** is used for generalized tonic clonic and complex partial seizures. • **Mesoridazine** is used as an adjunctive treatment for alcohol depression.

• **Phenobarbital**, **secobarbital**, and **amobarbital** can cause thrombophlebitis, pain, and tissue damage at the injection site; **primidone** can cause alopecia, impotence, polyuria, edema, and thirst.

• **Mephobarbital**, **metharbital**, and **primidone** are contraindicated in suspected pregnancy or near-term pregnancy.

(continued)

Barbiturates: similarities and differences (Continued)

Similarities	Differences

Similarities

Precautions

These agents should be used cautiously in persons requiring mental alertness to work, and those with renal or hepatic dysfunction.

Nursing considerations

Assess neurologic status and level of consciousness frequently; check vital signs frequently for changes; assess sleeping patterns before and during therapy to determine drug's effectiveness; institute nonpharmacologic measures to assist with sleep; institute safety measures to prevent falls and injury; anticipate possible rebound excitement; assess bowel and bladder elimination for changes; assist with measures to promote urinary elimination; instruct in measures to promote bowel elimination, including high fiber diet; monitor blood studies frequently for changes; discontinue slowly to avoid withdrawal symptoms; instruct in diseases, drug therapy, treatment, adverse effects and need for compliance; and monitor for signs and symptoms of overdose.

Differences

• **Parenteral amobarbital**, **pentobarbital**, and **phenobarbital** should be given cautiously to those with hypotension, severe pulmonary or cardiovascular disease, shock, and uremia.
• **Primidone**, **metharbital**, and **mephobarbital** should be used cautiously in those persons using alcohol, CNS depressants, monoamine oxidase inhibitors, narcotic analgesics, or anticoagulants.

Administer IM deep into a large muscle to prevent tissue damage; have resuscitative equipment available when giving IV; do not mix **pentobarbital** with other medications; **secobarbital sodium** injection is not compatible with Ringer's lactate solution; do not mix **secobarbital** with acidic solutions; rotate ampul of **secobarbital**, and do not shake.

---

usefulness in treating epilepsy. Continued research led to the development of the succinimides: ethosuximide, methsuximide, and phensuximide. Ethosuximide is the primary agent in this group.

Ethosuximide

Pharmacodynamics. Ethosuximide exhibits frequency-dependent effects on cortical response to stimuli. Response to stimuli occurring at intervals greater than 200 milliseconds is markedly decreased. Ethosuximide reduces focal activity responsible for spike and wave electroencephalogram patterns even more effectively than does phenytoin. Reduction of thalamocortical excitation is similar to that of phenytoin.

Pharmacokinetics. Ethosuximide is administered orally; however, the extent of GI absorption is unknown. Peak plasma concentrations occur within 4–7 hours after administration. The drug does not bind significantly to plasma proteins. It distributes widely and evenly in the tissues, producing concentrations in the cerebrospinal fluid comparable to that in plasma.

Plasma half-life averages 30 hours in children and 60 hours in adults. Four to seven days of treatment are required to achieve steady-state concentrations.

Ethosuximide is largely metabolized by the liver. About 80% is degraded by the microsomal enzymes and is subsequently eliminated by the kidneys. Most of the remainder is excreted unchanged by the kidneys. Small amounts appear in bile and feces.

Therapeutic uses. Ethosuximide is considered by many to be the agent of choice in treating absence seizures. It is sometimes used to control myoclonic or psychomotor seizures.

Adverse reactions. The most common side effects of ethosuximide are GI. These include anorexia (with weight loss), nausea, vomiting, and epigastric distress. Central nervous system manifestations include drowsiness, headache, fatigue, dizziness, euphoria, ataxia, irritability, and hiccups. Parkinsonism and photophobia sometimes occur. Myopia, vaginal bleeding, and swollen tongue have also been reported.

The most serious complications of therapy are allergic reactions to the drug, blood dyscrasias, and syndromes resembling systemic lupus erythematosus and Stevens-Johnson syndrome. Leukopenia, eosinophilia, agranulocytosis, pancytopenia, and aplastic anemia may occur.

Recent reports indicate that ethosuximide, like other anticonvulsants, may be teratogenic.

Precautions and contraindications. If ethosuximide is used to treat mixed epilepsy, concurrent medication with adequate doses of anticonvulsants must be given to control major motor seizures. Dosage of ethosuximide must be adjusted carefully and slowly. Abrupt withdrawal should be avoided because it may precipitate frequent seizures or petit mal status (prolonged absence seizure).

Blood counts must be monitored regularly to detect changes indicative of bone marrow malfunction. The skin is inspected frequently for lesions and rashes. Ethosuximide must be discontinued if either of these conditions occurs. Fatalities have resulted when such side effects have been allowed to progress.

Carbamazepine

Carbamazepine is structurally related to the tricyclic antidepressants.

Pharmacodynamics. Like phenytoin, carbamazepine limits seizure propagation by reducing post-tetanic potentiation of synaptic transmission. The drug exhibits sedative, anticholinergic, antidepressant, muscle relaxant, antiarrhythmic, antidiuretic, and neuromuscular transmission-inhibitory actions. It has only slight analgesic properties.

Pharmacokinetics. Following oral administration, carbamazepine is slowly absorbed from the GI tract. Two to four days may be required to achieve steady-state plasma concentrations. Therapeutic ranges of plasma concentrations are reported to be 3–11 µg/ml (8–34 µmol/liter). Signs and symptoms of abnormal CNS function may occur when concentrations exceed 4 µg/ml and are common when concentrations are 10 µg or greater per milliliter.

Following absorption, carbamazepine is widely distributed to body tissues and fluids, including the brain, cerebrospinal fluid, bile, and saliva. The drug crosses the placenta and accumulates in fetal tissues. It is distributed in breast milk in concentrations 60% of maternal plasma levels. Carbamazepine is 75% to 90% bound to plasma proteins.

Only 1% of carbamazepine is excreted unchanged by the kidneys. The metabolism of the drug is poorly understood, although it is known that some is metabolized by microsomal enzymes in the liver, and that the drug is a liver enzyme inducer. The plasma half-life of the drug is relatively long and has been reported to range anywhere between 8 and 72 hours.

Therapeutic uses. Carbamazepine is used in the management of seizures (with the exception of absence [petit mal], myoclonic, and akinetic seizures). It is sometimes used in conjunction with phenytoin, phenobarbital, or primidone. Carbamazepine has also been used for treating schizophrenia manic-depressive illness that does not respond to lithium, and pain associated with true trigeminal neuralgia.

Adverse reactions. Carbamazepine shares the toxic potential of the hydantoin-derivative anticonvulsants (see Phenytoin). The most frequent side effects are nausea, vomiting, dizziness, drowsiness and unsteady gait. In addition, carbamazepine can cause renal and liver impairment. Genitourinary changes include frequency, retention, oliguria with hypertension, impotence, albuminuria, glycosuria, elevated blood urea nitrogen, and microscopic deposits in the urine. Acute renal failure has been reported. Inflammation can develop in both the liver and biliary system. Liver failure has caused at least one death in a child (Scheffner, 1986). Exposure to carbamazepine *in utero* increases to 1% the incidence of spina bifida in the newborn (Rosa, 1991). Rarely, a manic reaction may develop (Drake & Peruzzi, 1986).

Carbamazepine is known to interact with several drugs. It increases metabolism (decreasing blood levels) of phenytoin and valproate. In turn, phenytoin may increase carbamazepine degradation, lowering its blood levels. Propoxyphene, erythromycin, and two calcium blockers, verapamil and diltiazem, inhibit carbamazepine metabolism. Isoniazid increases serum levels of carbamazepine. Carbamazepine accelerates the conversion of primidone to phenobarbital.

Precautions and contraindications. Carbamazepine may be extremely toxic to a small percentage of recipients and should be used only when other less toxic anticonvulsants are ineffective or contraindicated. Clients should be informed of the potential toxicity of the drug. Blood cell levels, liver function tests, and ophthalmic status should be assessed before carbamazepine therapy is begun and continued regularly thereafter. Treatment must be discontinued if evidence of bone marrow depression, hepatotoxicity, or eye changes is found. The drug is best withdrawn gradually to prevent abrupt declines in blood levels, which can precipitate seizures.

Clients who perform work requiring mental alertness or physical coordination should be warned about the possible neurologic effects of the drug.

Safe use of carbamazepine in children and during pregnancy and lactation has not been established.

Carbamazepine is contraindicated for persons with a history of bone marrow depression or hypersensitivity to the drug or to any of the tricyclic antidepressants. The drug should be administered with extreme caution, if at all, with other drugs that may increase the possibility of adverse reactions.

To maintain its efficacy, carbamazepine should be stored in a dry location in tightly closed containers.

Valproate (valproic acid)

Valproic acid's anticonvulsant properties were discovered when it was used as a vehicle for other compounds tested for anticonvulsant activity.

Pharmacodynamics. The specific mechanism of action of valproic acid is unknown. It appears to affect GABA function at the synapse by inhibiting enzyme degradation of this neurotransmitter or by inhibiting its reuptake by glial cells and nerve endings. This selective increase in synaptic concentration of GABA, which is an inhibitory neurotransmitter, decreases impulse transmission.

Pharmacokinetics. Valproate is rapidly and almost completely absorbed by the GI tract. Peak plasma concentration occurs 1–4 hours after administration of oral doses. Protein binding varies between 80% and 95%. Tissue concentrations appear highest in the extracellular fluid. The drug is metabolized by the liver; little of the unchanged drug is excreted in the urine. Some drug appears in the feces. Plasma half-life is about 10 hours.

Valproic acid treatment is initiated with low doses that are gradually increased to achieve a therapeutic effect. Therapeutic plasma levels do not correlate well with efficacy but are considered to be 50–100 µg/ml.

Therapeutic uses. Valproic acid is particularly effective in the treatment of both simple and complex absence seizures. Although this is the only approved use for the drug in the United States, it has exhibited some therapeutic effect in intractable hiccups and in myoclonic and grand mal seizures. It is less effective in partial seizures.

Adverse reactions. Valproic acid has a low incidence of side effects. The most common side effects are GI: anorexia, nausea, and vomiting. The drug has caused hepatotoxicity and liver failure. It decreases hepatic conversion of ammonia to urea, causing blood ammonia levels to rise. Valproic acid is irritating to the tissues and can cause stomatitis if dosage forms are chewed. Central nervous system manifestations—sedation, ataxia, and incoordination—occur infrequently. The drug causes thrombocytopenia in some clients. It may also be teratogenic.

Drug interactions. Valproic acid and phenobarbital used together in therapy may result in plasma concentrations of phenobarbital greater than those occurring from phenobarbital when used alone (valproic acid may inhibit the liver enzymes that degrade phenobarbital). When the two drugs are used concurrently, valproic acid may produce either increased or decreased plasma levels of phenytoin. When used with clonazepam, absence seizure status may occur.

Precautions and contraindications. Hepatic function should be tested before valproic acid therapy is begun and for every 2 months thereafter as long as the drug is used. The drug should not be used by clients who have decreased liver function. If possible, valproic acid should be discontinued if ammonemia or a change in liver function tests develops. Alternatively, ammonemia may be moderated either by decreasing protein in the diet or by adding arginine or carnitine to it.

Gastrointestinal complaints may be minimized by beginning with very low doses and slowly increasing the dose.

When valproic acid is used concurrently with phenobarbital or phenytoin, dosage levels must be carefully adjusted for therapeutic effect; if the dosage of one agent is altered, then that of the other may also require adjustment.

Benzodiazepines

A detailed discussion of benzodiazepine drugs is given in Chapter 26. Two agents from this group are used in the treatment of epilepsy. Clonazepam is employed for the chronic treatment of certain seizures in children, whereas IV diazepam is the agent of choice for the treatment of status epilepticus (see Focus on Benzodiazepines: Similarities and Differences).

Clonazepam

Clonazepam is administered orally for prolonged management of absence or myoclonic seizures in children. It acts by facilitating GABA action at the synapses, apparently by increasing the affinity of this neurotransmitter for binding sites. (GABA acts to inhibit nerve impulse transmission.) About half of the clients who take clonazepam develop drowsiness, somnolence, fatigue, and lethargy. These symptoms usually subside with continued treatment. Muscular incoordination and ataxia are fairly common. Other side effects include hypotonia, dysarthrias, dizziness, anorexia (or hyperphagia), and increased salivation and bronchial secretion. Behavioral problems such as aggression, hyperactivity, irritability, or inability to concentrate may necessitate discontinuation of the drug.

Diazepam

Diazepam is administered parenterally in the treatment of status epilepticus. When treating adults or older children, 5–10 mg are administered slowly by IV to initiate treatment. This may be repeated at 10–15-minute intervals to a maximal total dose of 30 mg. If necessary, the regimen may be repeated every 2–4 hours. No more than 100 mg should be administered in any single 24-hour period. Because diazepam is

Benzodiazepines: similarities and differences

Similarities

Pharmacodynamics

These drugs act on presynaptic neuronal pathways in various areas of the CNS to enhance the action of GABA, an inhibitory neurotransmitter. Most have anxiolytic and sedative action by depressing the CNS at the limbic and subcortical levels, affecting the reticular activating system and decreasing arousal.

Pharmacokinetics

These drugs are well absorbed from the GI tract. Onset of action is generally 30 to 60 minutes. They are highly bound to plasma proteins. They are metabolized by the liver to several active and inactive metabolites and are excreted in the urine. Elimination half-lives are relatively long.

Therapeutic uses

These drugs are used for anxiety and tension as well as to control seizures.

Adverse reactions

These agents may cause: (CNS) drowsiness, lethargy, dizziness, confusion, tremor, depression, impaired motor function; (GI) constipation, diarrhea, nausea and vomiting, change in appetite, abdominal discomfort, taste alterations; (CV) bradycardia, hypotension, palpitations; (OTHER) visual disturbances, urinary incontinence or retention, physical dependency, withdrawal syndrome, paradoxical reactions, change in libido, hepatic dysfunction and rash.

Contraindications

These drugs are contraindicated in clients who have known hypersensitivity, acute narrow angle or untreated open-angle glaucoma, clients in shock and coma, and clients in acute alcohol intoxication.

Precautions

Use cautiously in patients with psychosis, myasthenia gravis or Parkinson's disease, impaired renal function, in elderly or debilitated, and those prone to addiction or abuse.

Differences

• **Clonazepam, clorazepate dipotassium**, and **diazepam** have anticonvulsant action by enhancing presynaptic inhibition, suppressing the spread of seizure activity produced by epileptogenic foci in the cortex, thalamus, and limbic structures.
• **Diazepam, lorazepam**, and **midazolam** have amnesic action by unknown mechanism. • **Diazepam** has skeletal muscle relaxant action by inhibiting polysynaptic frequent pathways.

• **Chlordiazepoxide, diazepam**, and **midazolam** can be given IM or IV. A small amount of **diazepam** is excreted in the feces. • **Midazolam** and **triazolam** have the shortest half-lives, under 6 hours. • **Clorazepate dipotassium** is hydrolyzed in the stomach and **diazepam, halazepam**, and **prazepam** are metabolized in the liver to the active metabolite **desmethyldiazepam**, whose half-life is 30–200 hours.

• **Diazepam, midazolam**, and **lorazepam** are used as surgical adjuncts for conscious sedation and amnesia. • **Diazepam** and **chlordiazepoxide** are used for skeletal muscle spasm and tremor.

Agents administered IV may cause pain, phlebitis, and desquamation at the injection site. • **Clonazepam, diazepam**, and **flurazepam** may cause blood dyscrasias. • **Clonazepam** and **diazepam** may cause dysrrhythmias. • **Diazepam** IV may decrease gag reflex.

• **Chlordiazepoxide, clorazepate dipotassium**, and **diazepam** are contraindicated in infants less than 30 days old. • **Clonazepam** is contraindicated in significant hepatic or chronic respiratory disease. • **Lorazepam** is contraindicated in tartrazine or ASA hypersensitivity. • **Temazepam** and **triazolam** are contraindicated in pregnant patients.

Use **lorazepam** and **midazolam** cautiously in impaired respiratory function such as COPD.

(continued)

Focus on

Benzodiazepines: similarities and differences (Continued)

Similarities

Nursing considerations

Assess level of consciousness, vital signs, and neurologic status before administration. Assess sleep pattern routinely. Institute safety precautions such as use of side rails. Warn patients to avoid activities that require alertness and good psychomotor skills until CNS response is determined. Warn patients to avoid other CNS depressants such as alcohol and over-the-counter cold preparations.

Differences

Use IV agents slowly and have resuscitation equipment on hand. Tell clients that **flurazepam** is most effective after 3 or 4 nights, and not to increase dosage without doctor's advice.

---

absorbed by plastic tubing, therapeutic response to infusions will increase gradually until the tubing is saturated by the drug. Tolerance increases with long-term use of diazepam and physical dependence may develop.

Miscellaneous agents

Other agents used to control seizures in selected situations are magnesium sulfate and acetazolamide.

Magnesium sulfate

The seizures of magnesium deficiency and acute eclampsia are best treated with magnesium solutions. The mechanism by which magnesium depresses the CNS is unknown, although the drug is known to decrease the amount of acetylcholine liberated by the motor nerve impulse. Magnesium solutions also act osmotically to reduce brain edema—a factor contributing to irritability and lowered seizure threshold.

Magnesium sulfate is the drug of choice for managing convulsive toxemia in pregnancy. It is also used as an anticonvulsant in preventing and controlling severe eclamptic seizures. Magnesium sulfate is usually administered by slow IV infusion. Serum magnesium levels are monitored as a guide to dosages. Maximum recommended dosage is 150 mg/min. (Consult stat: Use caution when administering magnesium sulfate, 1990.) Excessive use may result in hypermagnesemia (manifested by severe CNS depression).

Acetazolamide

Acetazolamide is sometimes useful as an adjunct to other anticonvulsants in the prophylactic management of certain types of epilepsy, particularly petit mal. It resembles carbon dioxide in its anticonvulsant properties; acetazolamide's inhibition of carbonic anhydrase activity may act by reducing carbon dioxide elimination from glial cells. Elevation of the seizure threshold

and selective depression of spinal cord monosynaptic pathways result. Because tolerance to the action of acetazolamide develops rapidly, the drug has limited therapeutic value.

Calcium channel blockers

Calcium channel blockers, although used primarily to control hypertension and angina pectoris, are now occasionally used as adjuncts in treating seizure disorders. They are discussed in Chapter 28.

■ Summary

Anticonvulsants are drugs that control seizures by raising the seizure threshold and limiting the spread of nerve activity from initiating foci. Most anticonvulsants are CNS depressants. Many are relatively toxic, causing CNS symptoms, GI upset, and various allergic reactions. Most are also teratogenic. Despite the risks of therapy, anticonvulsant drugs enable the majority of epileptic clients to control their seizures and lead relatively normal lives.

Learning experience 25-1

Compare and contrast the adverse reactions commonly associated with anticonvulsant medications. What precautions are necessary during treatment with each agent?

Nursing management

Nursing implications

Seizures and seizure disorders pose many risks to the affected person. The occurrence of an unexpected seizure can result in serious accidental injury: drowning or near drowning if it occurs while the person is in water; fractures or head trauma from falling; collision with objects in the environment; or injury by powered machinery that the person may have been near at the time of the attack. Status epilepticus is a threat to life and can cause brain injury. In addition, frequent seizures interfere with the normal activities of life (school, work, recreation, socializing).

Consciousness is frequently lost during seizure episodes and may be clouded for some time afterward, especially following major motor seizures. Moreover, psychomotor seizures can mimic unacceptable behavior, alienating people who are unaware of the true nature of the episode. In addition, failure to control seizure activity may result in legal constraints, specifically, loss of a license to drive a car. Inability to control the symptoms of the condition also reinforces the stigma attached to the disease, leading to rejection of the affected person. The uncontrolled epileptic, therefore, is at a disadvantage in accomplishing critical developmental tasks. Optimal control of seizures is vital for the client's normal development and enjoyment of life.

With current drug therapy, seizures can be virtually eliminated in the majority of clients. Depending on the criteria used for determining "control," up to 85% of persons subject to seizures are reported to be adequately controlled with proper drug regimens. The nurse can do much to enhance the therapeutic effects of drugs and to reduce the incidence of seizures for those few clients whose response to drugs is less than complete.

Anticonvulsant drugs cause many side effects, especially when a new drug regimen is instituted. Most are CNS depressants and affect levels of consciousness, motor coordination, and behavior. Sedation is common but may lessen with continued drug therapy. Nystagmus, ataxia, tremor, dizziness, hyperactivity, or behavioral changes may occur, especially in cases of drug toxicity. Long-term phenobarbital therapy, multidrug therapy, or use of high dosages may impair intellectual function. The nurse should appraise mental and neurologic function and behavior carefully.

Gastrointestinal symptoms also affect the person receiving anticonvulsants. Nausea, vomiting, and diarrhea are most common. If pronounced, they may interfere with retention or absorption of the medications, thereby lowering serum levels and allowing seizures to occur.

Many anticonvulsant drugs also have individual side effects not shared by other agents of this class (Table 25-4).

Many anticonvulsants appear to increase the risk of birth defects when given to pregnant women. However, most mothers treated with these drugs do give birth to normal children; seizures during pregnancy pose a significant risk to the embryo, and it is usually inadvisable to discontinue medication during preg-

nancy. When possible, dosage is reduced to a minimum before conception is attempted.

A failure to control seizures, or frequent or severe side effects may indicate inappropriate dosages. Initial dosages may need to be revised before optimum control is established. Changes in the client's health status may alter response to dosages that previously had been adequate. In addition, clients may not comply with the prescription owing to a misunderstanding of the dosage regimen, or to an attempt to decrease undesirable side effects.

Most adverse reactions are dose-dependent and are minimized by careful regulation of dosages to the least amount required for therapeutic effect. The objective of treatment is the best control of seizures with the least amount of drug.

Pronounced or persistent side effects may require a change in the drug agent.

Nursing process

Assessment Because of the stigma still attached to the diagnosis of epilepsy, clients will sometimes seek to conceal seizure disorders. The presence of gingival hypertrophy, a side effect of phenytoin, is suggestive of seizure disorder. Depression may be a clue to prolonged barbiturate therapy. If these signs are apparent, the nurse should ask specifically about seizure disorders when taking an initial history.

Some affected clients may be unaware of seizure episodes; their only clues may be an unexplained lapse of time. Only when incontinence or mental clouding occur are many clients able to detect episodes. A family member may be able to give more accurate information regarding the frequency of seizures. The nurse should determine what clients know about their seizures.

Data required for assessment include a history of the seizure disorder: the type of seizures experienced by the client, including behavior before, during, and after the seizures; pattern of progression of the seizure; precipitating circumstances; the presence and type of aura; whether any (and how many) have occurred recently; usual anticonvulsant treatment regimen; and the client's acceptance of and adaptation to therapy.

During physical examination, the nurse should evaluate the client for signs and symptoms of neurologic abnormality, as well as for toxic and side effects of anticonvulsant drugs. Skin integrity, level of consciousness, and signs and symptoms of allergy should be assessed.

Laboratory blood tests should be evaluated for abnormalities related to the drug regimen.

The reproductive status of women of childbearing age (*ie*, plans to have children in the near future, pregnancy, or lactation) should be determined.

Table 25-4. Adverse effects of commonly prescribed anticonvulsants

Drug name	Side-effects	Adverse effects on children	Toxic effects
phenytoin (Dilantin,* Diphenylan, Mebroin)	Gingival hypertrophy Gastric irritation Hyperglycemia Hirsutism, facial coarsening Increased risk of birth defects when used during pregnancy Inappropriate antidiuretic hormone secretion* Allergy:* fever, rash, exfoliative dermatitis, bone marrow depression, systemic lupus erythematosis	Unsteady gait, involuntary movements, fatigue, altered emotions Impaired problem-solving and visuomotor skills Short attention span	Nausea and constipation Nystagmus, ataxia, drowsiness, tremor, increased frequency of seizures Hyperactivity, behavioral change, confusion, or dullness Hallucinations After rapid intravenous administration: cardiovascular collapse, hypotension, and central nervous system depression Lymphadenopathy
phenobarbital (Barbital, Luminal, Sulfoton)	Stevens-Johnson syndrome* Excitation in the elderly and very young* Pain in muscles, nerves, or joints Physical dependence Personality changes Depression and suicidal tendencies* Increased risk of birth defects when used during pregnancy Porphyria in susceptible persons* Inflammation of the mouth, conjunctiva, nose, urethra, and glans penis Allergy:* fever, rash, bone marrow depression, systemic lupus erythematosus	Lethargy, depressive symptoms Irritability, hyperactivity, sleep disturbance Stubbornness, disobedience Impaired memory Impaired concentration	Sedation Gastrointestinal disturbances Vertigo, headache, depression Nystagmus, ataxia Respiratory depression
trimethadione (Tridione, Trimedone)	Stevens-Johnson syndrome* Hemeralopia, diplopia, photophobia Alopecia, paresthesias, vaginal bleeding Changes in blood pressure Increased risk of birth defects when used during pregnancy Neutropenia, hepatitis, nephrotic syndrome Myasthenia syndrome (muscle weakness) Allergy:* rash	Drowsiness	Sedation Major motor seizures
valproic acid (Dalpro, Myproic acid; Depakene)	Transient hair loss Drowsiness, ataxia, incoordination Gastrointestinal disturbances Inhibition of platelet aggregation Increased risk of birth defects when used during pregnancy Hepatotoxicity and thrombocytopenia	Drowsiness, lethargy	Coma

(Continued)

Table 25-4. Adverse effects of commonly prescribed anticonvulsants (Continued)

Drug name	Side-effects	Adverse effects on children	Toxic effects
ethosuximide (Zarontin)	Headache Epigastric distress Hiccups Myopia Vaginal bleeding Increased risk of birth defects when used during pregnancy Allergy:* urticaria, erythema multiforme, pancytopenia, rash, bone marrow depression, systemic lupus erythematosis	Drowsiness Minimal deficits on psychosocial function	Anorexia, nausea, and vomiting Dizziness, drowsiness, fatigue, euphoria, ataxia, irritability, photophobia Parkinsonism
clonazepam (Clonopin, Klonopin, *Can:* Rivotril)	Stevens-Johnson syndrome* Drowsiness, fatigue, lethargy Muscular incoordination, ataxia Anorexia or hyperphagia Increased risk of birth defects when used during pregnancy Allergy:* rash, bone marrow depression	Irritability, hyperactivity Antisocial behavior, aggression, disobedience	Thick speech, hypersalivation Excessive bronchial secretions Hypotonia Aggression, hyperactivity, irritability, inability to concentrate
carbamazepine (Epitol Tapazine, *Can:* Apo-Carbamazepine)	Bone marrow depression* Aggravation of cardiovascular disease Hepatotoxicity Nephrotoxicity Urinary frequency, retention Impotence Nausea, vomiting, abdominal pain, diarrhea, constipation, glossitis Rash, Stevens-Johnson syndrome*, aggravation of systemic lupus erythematosis, alopecia Chills and fever Arthritis	Emotional lability Irritability, agitation Insomnia Impaired task performance	Ataxia, dizziness, stupor opisthotonus, agitation, disorientation, tremor, adiadochokinesis, abnormal reflexes Mydriasis, nystagmus Cyanosis Urinary retention Glycosuria, acetonuria Coma

* Indications for discontinuation of the offending drug.
KEY: *Can* = Canadian trade name.

Nursing diagnosis Diagnoses may include:

High risk for injury related to lapses in consciousness and uncontrollable muscle activity secondary to seizures
High risk for impaired gas exchange related to apnea during grand mal seizures
Body image disturbance related to seizure disorder and to cosmetic effects of medication
High risk for impaired skin integrity related to side effects of anticonvulsant drugs
Impaired social interaction related to the stigma of epilepsy, the client's negative self-image, and cosmetic side effects of anticonvulsant drugs
High risk for altered growth and development in nursing infants of female clients related to CNS depression secondary to exposure to anticonvulsant drugs in maternal milk
Knowledge deficit concerning seizure conditions and treatment regimens
High risk for injury related to seizures secondary to inappropriate drug dosages or to noncompliance with the drug regimen.

A common collaborative problem that should be differentiated from the nursing diagnoses is:

Potential complication: congential defects

Planning Goals of treatment are to achieve the best control of seizures with the lowest possible dosages of anticonvulsant drugs; to improve clients' self-image; to increase their social interaction; to reduce intrauterine or neonatal exposure of female clients' children to anticonvulsant drugs; to increase clients' knowledge about the disease and its treatment; and to prevent or promptly detect and treat toxic and side effects of anticonvulsant drugs.

Intervention Nursing measures may help reduce the number of seizure episodes. Many factors increase the risk of seizures by changing the biochemical environment in the CNS (Table 25-5). The nurse should strive to eliminate or control these factors in the acutely ill client and to teach clients who manage their own regimens about techniques for reducing their impact. Acute intercurrent illnesses must be vigorously treated; fever and hypoxia must be controlled or eliminated. Maintaining fluid and electrolyte balance is critical. Reducing stress and promoting good mental health help minimize the impact of endogenous biochemicals conducive to seizures. Good habits contribute not only to vigorous physical health but also to a feeling of general well-being. These benefits can enhance seizure control. Good nutrition, including ample intake of vitamin D and folic acid, is needed to maintain optimal health.

If the nurse finds that the client is pregnant or is planning to have children in the near future, the physician should be consulted. For the protection of the fetus, drug dosages should be reduced as much as possible before and during pregnancy. The client should inform the physician promptly if seizures occur because episodes during pregnancy can be harmful to the fetus. Breast-feeding is generally contraindicated for mothers on anticonvulsant drugs. Health measures to reduce the risk of seizure and the need for high drug doses are particularly beneficial to women of childbearing age.

Managing the drug regimen. Clients must be monitored closely for therapeutic, toxic, and side effects of the drugs, especially when drug therapy is initiated, when dosages or drug agents are changed, or when intercurrent illness complicates the clients' response to treatment. When anticonvulsant therapy is initiated, side effects are common. To limit their severity, drug dosages are begun at a low level and are gradually increased until adequate control is achieved. Seizures should decrease as serum levels approach the therapeutic range.

Many anticonvulsants share common side effects. Most are CNS depressants and affect the level of consciousness, motor coordination, and behavior. Sedation is common but may lessen as the client adapts to the drug. Nystagmus, ataxia, and tremors are signs of toxicity. Hyperactivity or behavioral changes may occur. The nurse should appraise mental and neurologic function and behavior carefully. Common GI symptoms include nausea, vomiting, and diarrhea. If pronounced, they may interfere with retention or absorption of the medications, thereby lowering serum levels and allowing seizures to occur. Nursing measures to

Table 25-5. Nursing management of factors predisposing to recurrent seizure activity

Factors	Intervention
Fever	Prompt and vigorous treatment of febrile illness
	Control of high temperatures with tepid baths, hypothermia blankets, cold applications, or antipyretic drugs
Hypoxia	Prevention of chronic respiratory disease by avoidance of smoking and air pollution
	Prompt and vigorous treatment of respiratory infections
	Careful attention to oxygen needs in sports such as scuba diving
Hypoglycemia	Regular, nutritious meals
	Avoidance of concentrated carbohydrates by clients subject to reactive hypoglycemia
	Avoidance of insulin reactions by diabetics
Calcium ion deficiency	Prevention of hyperventilation by good emotional hygiene and bag rebreathing at the beginning of an episode
	Regular, moderate exercise to induce mild physiologic acidosis
Sodium imbalance	Avoidance of excessive sodium intake, especially by female clients during the premenstrual period and by those on oral contraceptives
	Avoidance of water intoxication and hyponatremia by adequate salt intake in environments conducive to excessive perspiration
Sympathoadrenal response	Stress management techniques and good emotional hygiene
	Avoidance of exhaustion
Alcohol	Avoidance of intoxication of any degree (mild intoxication depresses central nervous inhibition and severe intoxication is often complicated by dehydration and hypoglycemia)
Repetitive stimuli of specific frequencies (strobe lights, repetitive bells)	Avoidance of discotheques or other environments where such stimuli are pervasive
	Avoidance of looking at emergency strobes on ambulances and police vehicles

improve GI function are important in maintaining effective control. Administering the medications with meals reduces the incidence of gastric symptoms. The client needs considerable support during this period. Nursing measures to ameliorate side effects may encourage compliance by increasing comfort.

Many anticonvulsant drugs also have individual side effects not shared by other agents of this class (Table 25-4). The nurse must be aware of these effects and monitor the client carefully for them. Preventive measures should be taken when possible. For example, gingival hypertrophy from phenytoin is less common and less pronounced when meticulous oral hygiene and gum massage are practiced.

Once an optimal regimen is established, doses should be administered regularly, at consistent intervals in relation to diurnal patterns of rest or activity and in relation to meals. The drug regimen may change from time to time because of allergy, side effects, toxicity, or loss of seizure control. Most adverse reactions are dose-dependent and are alleviated by careful reduction of dosage.

Whenever drugs are added to or deleted from the treatment regimen, client response to all drugs is likely to be altered. Assessment of client response and side effects from medication is critical to proper evaluation of the new drug regimen. When available, serum drug levels provide pertinent data but they should never be the sole basis for this evaluation.

Allergic reactions to anticonvulsants include liver impairment, blood dyscrasias, and skin eruptions. Allergic hypersensitivity may progress to life-threatening pathology and should be reported immediately to the physician. In most cases, the drug will be discontinued, and loading doses (higher than normal doses) of a different anticonvulsant drug may be ordered to prevent seizures during the transition period. Initially, side effects from loading doses are likely to be pronounced. Omitting doses may cause seizure activity to occur. Abrupt, complete withdrawal of anticonvulsants may precipitate status epilepticus.

Emergency treatment of status epilepticus. The treatment of status epilepticus requires intensive medical and nursing care. For rapid effect, medications are commonly administered intravenously. Diazepam is the agent of choice. If response is inadequate, other drugs may be added. A general anesthetic may be administered in refractory cases. Treatment is best carried out in an intensive care unit where skilled nursing care is available. Vital signs must be closely watched.

Because medications are administered by IV, the rate of infusion must be controlled carefully; use of infusion pumps is recommended. If IV phenytoin is ordered, saline solution must be used as the vehicle, and no other drugs may be added to it. The rate of infusion should not exceed 50 mg/min. Phenytoin precipitates out of solution easily; it is incompatible with glucose or acid solutions and most other drugs. Infusions should be monitored closely for particle formation, phlebitis and infiltration. Because phenytoin can cause cardiac dysrhythmias, clients receiving it intravenously (especially the elderly, those with heart disease, and those with unstable vital signs) should be monitored for cardiac arrhythmias.

Phenytoin solutions are very irritating to the tissues. Should discoloration or edema develop distally to the IV site, the IV should be *removed immediately* and the physician notified. Continued infusion can lead to ischemia and tissue necrosis manifested by purple discoloration of the hand (or foot), skin blisters, and sloughing of tissues (so-called "purple glove syndrome"). The limb should be elevated above the chest and warm compresses applied to the hand or foot. The nurse should monitor peripheral pulses, skin color and temperature, and capillary refill. Purple glove syndrome can lead to extensive tissue damage and subsequent amputation.

Status epilepticus is very disturbing to clients' families or friends who are present during such episodes. These significant others should be offered emotional support and sufficient explanation of what is occurring in order to allay anxiety. Care should be taken to protect the privacy of clients brought to the medical facility by strangers or casual acquaintances. The nurse should ascertain the status of those persons accompanying clients and use judgment in discussing the client's condition with them.

Following resolution of the acute episode, clients are commonly lethargic and mentally confused. The duration of this postictal state is proportional to the duration of the seizure. As mental alertness returns, clients will need an explanation of what has happened and will need to be oriented to their surroundings. They may be disturbed by the recurrence of seizures. In addition to the usual emotional impact of sudden illness and institutionalization, disruption of seizure control may arouse feelings of embarrassment or shame. There may also be practical consequences, such as the loss of a driver's license. In many states, the right to drive is suspended until the person has again been free of seizures for at least 1 year. Clients will need considerable emotional support and assistance in coping with such stressors.

Maintaining self-image. Control of seizures with a stable drug regimen is an important factor in enhancing the client's self-image and social interaction. In addition, health care personnel should treat the client with respect and warm acceptance. The client should be encouraged to maintain existing social relationships and develop new ones. This can be facilitated if the client is taught techniques for countering drug-related cosmetic changes and for enhancing physical appearance.

Client education. In the past, epilepsy has been regarded as an indication of genetic inferiority, mental incapacity, and personal deficiency. The traditional stigma attached to this condition has not entirely disappeared. The emotional reaction to the diagnosis of this condition may be so severe that neither clients nor their families are receptive to teaching until they are able to cope with their emotional response to the illness.

Clients and their families need reassurance that seizure disorders have a physical cause and are not a form of mental illness. The nurse's own attitude toward epilepsy will have a pronounced effect. If the nurse regards the client with respect and warm acceptance and discusses the disease matter-of-factly, client and family acceptance of the diagnosis will be facilitated.

The nurse should provide a careful explanation of the client's condition and a plan of treatment. A discussion of general health measures that will decrease the risk of seizures should be included. Because there is a large amount of material to be covered, several teaching sessions may be required; written materials should be given to the clients for perusal.

If clients are unaware of seizure occurrences, someone close to them should monitor the frequency of those seizures. This should be discussed openly with clients, and permission should be obtained before a family member is recruited for this responsibility. The designated monitor should receive an explanation of the different types of seizure manifestations. This will help detect episodes that may differ from the client's usual pattern.

Many clients need help in maintaining an acceptable appearance. Facial coarsening and hirsutism from phenytoin are particularly disturbing to the female client. Excessive hair loss is a transient effect of valproic acid. Phenytoin causes unsightly gingival hypertrophy in many recipients. Some anticonvulsants cause acne.

For women, bleaching of undesirable facial hair is usually preferable to shaving since the stubble that appears after shaving is more noticeable than light-colored hair. Electrolysis may effectively destroy hair follicles; however, treatment by this process is prolonged, uncomfortable, and expensive. Moreover, the elimination of all hair follicles will result in an unattractive shiny appearance to the skin because the fine hairs that impart a downy appearance have been eliminated. When alopecia is a problem, a wig or hair piece may be used to disguise hair loss.

Meticulous skin care will minimize acne, which develops with some anticonvulsants. Facial features can be defined and enhanced with makeup. Careful oral hygiene, which includes flossing, helps to minimize gingival hypertrophy.

Clients may inquire how long medication must be continued. In some cases of childhood and post-traumatic epilepsy, medication can eventually be discontinued after a suitable weaning period. However, this is usually not attempted until after 2–4 years of treatment. Most clients with idiopathic epilepsy will need anticonvulsant therapy indefinitely. The nurse should prepare clients for the prolonged drug therapy and should never promise that the therapy will be temporary. Clients should be cautioned to avoid abruptly discontinuing drug therapy and to consult with their physician if conditions occur that interfere with medication. Women of child-bearing age should be cautioned to consult their physicians prior to conceiving. Because anticonvulsant drugs tend to be teratogenic, it is advisable to use the minimum dosages required for control during pregnancy. Dosages must not be decreased or discontinued without medical advice, however, because seizures are also detrimental to the fetus (Fackelmann, 1991).

Clients for whom phenytoin is prescribed should be cautioned to buy the same trade name preparation each time the prescription is filled to avoid variation in blood levels of the drug that stem from differing bioavailability among different brands.

Clients should be taught to take anticonvulsant drugs with food to minimize GI side effects. They should be cautioned about missing doses, which can precipitate seizures.

Evaluation Data required for evaluation include absence or incidence of seizures; changes (reductions) in drug dosages; statements by the client relating to self-image, self-confidence, and social interactions; absence or incidence of congenital anomalies or anticonvulsant drug effects in female clients' children; absence or incidence of toxic or side effects in clients; and ability of the client to repeat to the nurse information conveyed during teaching sessions. (See the accompanying Example of Nursing Process and Change in Anticonvulsant Drug Regimen.)

Checklist of nursing actions

When maintenance anticonvulsant therapy is ordered

☐ Teach the client to avoid strobe lights and conditions that may cause hypoxia, hypoglycemia, exhaustion, and sodium and water retention. (These may increase the frequency of seizures.)

☐ Assist the client to develop effective stress management techniques to prevent sympathoadrenal reactions.

☐ Caution clients to avoid alcohol intoxication.

☐ Stress the importance of good seizure control, especially when absence seizures are the only evidence of epilepsy.

☐ Urge clients to take the drugs as ordered. Warn

Example of nursing process and change in anticonvulsant drug regimen

The client is a 19-year-old secretarial school student who is on anticonvulsant drugs for control of psychomotor epilepsy, diagnosed 3 years ago. Her seizures take the form of inappropriate behavior, such as irrelevant answers to questions and apparent failure to pay attention to verbal communication.

During the first week of school after Christmas recess, the client was counseled by her faculty advisor that instructors had reported that her academic performance had deteriorated, that she was not applying herself, and that she was not paying attention to directions. In view of her medical history, the counselor advised the client to consult with her physician to rule out seizure disorder as a factor in the change in performance.

In the physician's office, the client appears anxious and defensive. She states that she is "afraid the school is going to dismiss her because she is an epileptic." The client was last seen by the physician during the holiday recess, at which time the drug regimen was changed. A low dose of phenobarbital was added to the regimen, and the dosage of phenytoin was increased.

Assessment data	Nursing diagnosis	Intervention	Goals and outcome criteria
Anxious appearance Defensive demeanor Perception of academic counseling as preliminary to dismissal from school	Fear of dismissal from school related to unusual behavior, possibly secondary to exacerbation of psychomotor seizures	**Remind** the client of her 3-year record of excellent seizure control; reassure her that it is likely that control can be regained; inform her that there are several drugs that can be used if necessary to develop a successful drug regimen for her. **Point** out that the school advisor has recommended medical attention; the client should view this as a positive sign that the school administration regards epilepsy as a medical problem amenable to medical treatment.	Signs and symptoms of anxiety will decrease and the client will appear more relaxed.
Behavior suggestive of exacerbation of psychomotor epilepsy Recent change in medication regimen	High risk for noncompliance related to knowledge deficit regarding the new drug regimen	**Examine** the client's medication bottles; count the remaining doses and compare the number taken with the number required for compliance with the new drug regimen. Ask the client how and when she is taking the drugs. If noncompliance is confirmed, explore with the client the reasons for the noncompliance. Intervene as necessary to promote improved compliance. Schedule a return visit by the client for reevaluation of the new regimen.	The client will take the drugs accurately, in accord with the prescribed regimen. An accurate evaluation of the new drug regimen will be made.

(Continued)

Example of nursing process and change in anticonvulsant drug regimen (Continued)

Assessment data	Nursing diagnosis	Intervention	Goals and outcome criteria
		(In this case, as a result of this approach it was determined that the client had taken the correct number of drug doses, but had taken the total day's dosage at one time instead of taking phenytoin tid. With correction of the timing of doses, the signs and symptoms of seizures ceased.)	

against abrupt discontinuation of medication.
☐ Teach clients to take anticonvulsant drugs with food.
☐ Teach clients the toxic and side effects of their anticonvulsant drugs that indicate the need for medical reappraisal.
☐ Teach clients how to minimize side effects of medication.
☐ Monitor clients carefully for therapeutic response, toxic effects, and side effects, especially when combinations of drugs are ordered.
☐ Refer clients to the physician for adjustment of dosage if response to drugs is inadequate or if toxic effects occur.
☐ Teach clients receiving phenytoin the techniques of good oral hygiene and gum massage.
☐ Warn clients that anticonvulsant drugs can cause drowsiness and incoordination that make operation of a car or other powered machinery dangerous.
☐ Advise clients to verify that the pharmacist consistently refills prescriptions for phenytoin with the same trade name drug.

When anticonvulsants are given
for status epilepticus
☐ Monitor clients closely for toxic signs of drugs given intravenously.
☐ Be prepared for treatment if cardiovascular shock or cardiac arrest occurs.
☐ Support family members or friends who accompany the client to the health care facility.
☐ Protect the privacy of the client.

References

Consult stat: Use caution when administering magnesium sulfate. (1990). *RN, 53(11)*, 100–101 (November).

Drake M, Peruzzi W. (1986). Manic state with carbamazepine therapy of seizures. *J Natl Med Assoc, 78*, 1105–1107 (November).

Fackelmann KA. (1991). Epilepsy and pregnancy: A drug dilemma. *Science News 140*, 11 (July 6).

Farwell Jr, et al. (1990). Phenobarbital for febrile seizure—effects on intelligence and on seizure recurrence. *N Engl J Med 322(6)*, 364 (February 8).

Rosa FW. (1991). Spina bifida in infants of women treated with carbamazepine during pregnancy. *N Engl J Med 324(10)*, 674.

Scheffner D. (1986). Letter: Fatal liver failure in children on valproate. *Lancet, 2*, 511.

Survey finds physicians not always aware of phenytoin release forms. (1990). *FDA Drug Bulletin (10)*, 11 (October).

Bibliography

Allen M. (1988). Don't switch anti-seizure medications. *Am J Nurs 99(2)*, 166–168 (February).

Barker E. (1990). Brain tumor: Frightening diagnosis, nursing challenge. *RN 53(9)*, 50–52 (September).

Blake GJ. (1991). Carbamazepine for trigeminal neuralgia and pain. *Nursing 91, 21(3)*, 102 (March).

Brodie M, MacPhee G. (1986). Carbamazepine neurotoxicity precipitated by diltiazem. *Br Med J, 292*, 1170–1171.

Callaghan N, et al. (1988). Withdrawal of anticonvulsant drug in patients free of seizures for two years. *N Engl J Med 318*, 942–946 (April 14).

Callanan M. (1988). Epilepsy: Putting the patient back in control. *RN, 51(2)*, 48–55 (February).

Cohen MR, Wieland K. (1988). Drug hot line: Gingival hyperplasia and Dilantin. *Nursing 88, 18(10)*, 14 (October).

Dreifuss F, et al. (1989). Valproic acid hepatic fatalities: II US experience since 1984d. *Neurology 39*, 201–207 (February).

Drug news: Dampness warning. (1990). *Nursing 90, 20(9)*, 95 (September).

Fishel, et al. (1990). When you give phenytoin IV. *RN, 53(9)*, 58–59 (September).

Friedman D. (1989). Nursing consult: Controlling the seizures. *Nursing 89, 19(4)*, 98 (April).

Friedman D. (1988). Taking the scare out of caring for seizure patients. *Nursing 88, 18(2)*, 52–59 (February).

Gever LN. (1986). Dilantin: Questions of compatibility. *Nursing 86, 16(1)*, 30.

Grossman SA, et al. Decreased phenytoin levels in patients receiving chemotherapy. *Am J Med, 87*, 505–510 (November).

*Guyton A. (1986). *Textbook of medical physiology*, 7th ed. pp 674–675. Philadelphia: WB Saunders.

Herrera JJ, et al. (1987). Efficacy of adjunctive carbamazepine in the treatment of chronic schizophrenia. *Drug Intell Clin Pharm 21*, 355 (April).

Jaster P, Abbas D. (1986). Erthromycin-carbamazepine interaction (letter). *Neurology 36*, 594–595 (April).

Kutcher J. (1987). How to administer IV Dilantin. *RN, 50(1)*, 68.

MacPhee G, et al. Verapamil potentiates carabamazepine neurotoxicity: A clinically important inhibitory interaction. *Lancet 1*, 700–703d (March).

Obeso JA, et al. (1989). The treatment of severe action myoclonus. *Brain 112*, 765.

Pedley T. (1988). Discontinuing antiepileptic drugs. *N Engl J Med 318*, 982–984 (April).

Raebel M. (1983). Nonequivalence of phenytoin capsules and tablets. *N Engl J Med, 309*, 925.

*Recommended for further reading.

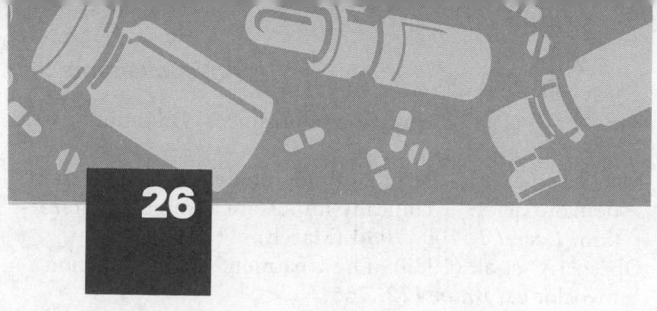

26

The psychoactive drugs

Historic treatment of the mentally ill

Before the advent of modern psychotropic drugs, the mentally ill were treated with psychoanalysis, insulin or electroshock, hydrotherapy, drugs, and psycho-surgery. All of these therapeutic measures had severe limitations, which offset their beneficial effects. Psychoanalysis, which requires private sessions with a psychiatrist for a number of years and, as a result, costs a great deal of money, was within the means of only a privileged few. Early insulin shock and electroconvulsive therapy (ECT), costly both in time and number of personnel involved, often proved hazardous. Hydrotherapy, the forcible restraint of a client in a water bath, yielded short-term benefits and was really only a relaxation technique used in conjunction with drugs. Psychosurgery meant, in most instances, prefrontal lobotomy. This procedure, which severed associative fibers between the frontal lobes and the thalamus, left the client in a vegetative state. The drugs administered ranged from opiates and alcohol (both in use for many centuries) to chloral hydrate, given in doses large enough to keep the client in a constant drowsy state.

Chemotherapy has been used for centuries to produce or intensify moods and emotions or to alleviate distressing mental symptoms. There is evidence that herbs, roots, mushrooms, hashish, opium, and alcohol have been used as psychoactive drugs throughout the history of mankind. Whether they were used to drive out "evil spirits," to elevate the user's mood, or to relieve disturbing symptoms, drugs have always had a place in society and in the treatment of the mentally ill.

The role of drugs in treating mental illness was minimal until the 1950s, however, when the development of two drugs, reserpine and chlorpromazine, revolutionized the use of chemotherapy in mental illness. Reserpine, the alkaloid rauwolfia serpentina, had been widely used in India for many years. Chlorpromazine was synthesized in France, the result of investigations into antihistamines. Since then, the development of psychoactive drugs has been rapid. Today, there are approximately 1,800 compounds classified as psychoactive agents. As a result of this wide range of drugs to choose from, fewer adverse reactions, and more rapid effect, chemotherapy is often the first treatment of choice for the disturbed client. In fact, antianxiety agents are the most widely prescribed drugs in the United States.

The increased, widespread use of drugs, as well as the extensive research on hallucinogens and drug-induced behavioral changes, strongly support the possibility that emotional and mental disturbances may have a chemical basis. There is also evidence that a relationship exists between behavior and the amine level in the brain. Researchers suspect that schizophrenia and major depression are linked to abnormalities in neurotransmission of chemical transmitters such as dopamine. Moreover, evidence increasingly supports the existence of a genetic link in mental and emotional disturbances. As yet, research trying to locate genes responsible for mental illness has not been successful.

Recent research on addiction suggests that drugs developed to treat addiction may be useful in treating mental illness. Antidepressant drugs, acting to inhibit dopamine uptake, seem effective in treating addiction (Holloway, 1991).

Physiology of the nervous systems

The physiology of the autonomic nervous system (ANS) and the central nervous system (CNS) is discussed in Chapters 22 and 23. When reference is given in this chapter to those systems, it is suggested that the reader refer to those chapters. Some of the physiologic actions of psychoactive drugs are discussed in the next section of this chapter.

The use of psychoactive drugs

Chemotherapy is not a cure for mental illness, but when used in conjunction with other therapies, it is a valuable part of the total therapy. The psychoactive drugs, which are used in the treatment of both psychoses and neuroses, affect behavior indirectly. The chemical composition of the drug interacts with chemicals and enzymes in body cells. The resulting interaction affects behavior—the way a person interacts with others and with the environment. The violence of mental illness, manifested either inwardly or outwardly, is thereby reduced. These drugs help to normalize behavior, to alleviate the psychotic process, to enable the client to participate in other therapies and yet remain at home while undergoing treatment, or to return to the community after only a shortened stay in a mental health facility, and to maintain a minimal daily level of functioning.

Although the full action of the psychoactive drugs remains unknown, these agents depress the CNS. Generally, they inhibit the function of the subcortical areas of the brain: the hypothalamus, the limbic system, and the reticular activating systems (Fig. 26-1), thereby lessening the effect of anxiety on the ANS. As a result, the client's emotional response to both external and internal stimuli is lessened. It is thought that this occurs due to changes in the functions of the following:

1. The *hypothalamus*, which controls and integrates the ANS and aids in regulating basic life functions;
2. The *limbic system*, which assumes a major role in controlling patterns of behavior and emotional set; and
3. The *reticular activating system*, which monitors sensory input.

The antipsychotic drugs prevent nerve cells from responding to dopamine by blocking specific receptors on cell surfaces that bind it. Dopamine, a neurotransmitter, carries signals between nerve cells. Acetylcholine, norepinephrine, and serotonin are other neurotransmitting substances that influence behavioral responses. It has been found that phenothiazines affect these cholinergic receptors. When an antipsychotic drug is administered, dopamine activity is inhibited through blockage of dopamine receptors in the brain. Because these drugs also block the dopamine receptors of the pituitary cells, excessive amounts of prolactin are secreted by these cells, leading to menstrual abnormalities and gynecomastia. In addition, because metabolism of the antipsychotic drugs takes place in the liver and the drugs are excreted by the

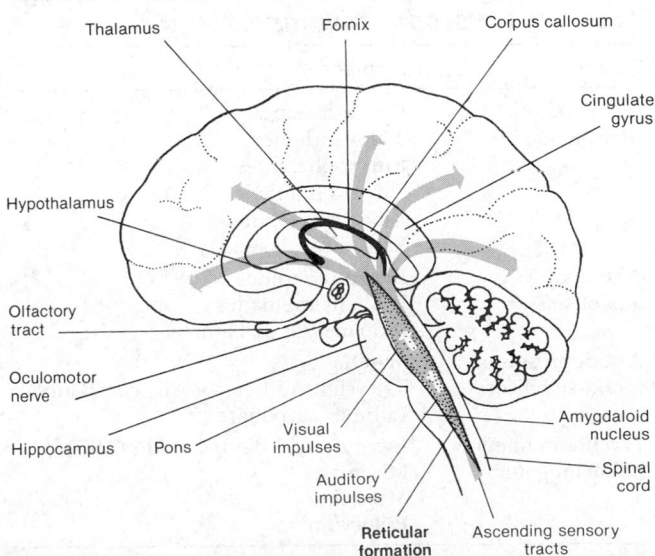

Figure 26-1. Subcortical areas of the brain: the hypothalamus, limbic system, and reticular activating systems.

kidney, these agents must be used cautiously in clients with renal or hepatic dysfunction. Since these agents interfere with transmission of nerve impulses in many areas, a broad range of drug interactions and adverse responses may result.

Categories of psychoactive drugs

The psychoactive drugs are classified as antipsychotic agents, antianxiety agents, and antidepressant agents/ mood stabilizers. They are classified according to the major use of the drug class. Another class of psychoactive drugs is the psychotomimetics or hallucinogenics. Although they are being administered experimentally, their use is illegal. (The abuse of these drugs is discussed in Chapter 15.) Table 26-1 lists the members of the various categories of psychoactive drugs. Another group of drugs used in conjunction with psychoactive drugs are anticholinergic or antiparkinsonism agents, which are effective in treating drug-induced extrapyramidal symptoms.

Indications for these drugs are given in Table 26-2. Psychoses are treated with antipsychotic agents and antidepressants; these drugs affect the psychotic processes of schizophrenia, organic brain syndrome, depression, mania, and severe anxiety. Psychosis distorts clients' perceptions of reality, impairing their ability to function on a daily basis. Classes of drugs used to alleviate psychotic symptoms include phenothiazines, rauwolfia alkaloids, butyrophenones, thioxanthenes, dihydroindolones, and dibenzoxazepines. Neuroses are usually treated with antianxiety agents, which provide symptomatic relief of anxiety and neuromuscular tension. Tolerance, however, develops after prolonged use of antianxiety drugs.

Table 26-1. Psychoactive drugs

Category	Member
Antipsychotic/ neuroleptic	Phenothiazines Thioxanthenes Butyrophenones Dihydroindolones Dibenzoxazepines Rauwolfia alkaloids
Antianxiety/ anxiolytics	Benzodiazepines Diphenylmethanes Propanediol carbamate
Antidepressants/ mood stabilizers	MAOIs Tricyclic and heterocyclic compounds Lithium carbonate
Psychotomimetic/ hallucinogenics*	Lysergic acid diethylamide (LSD) Marijuana Mescaline Psilocybin

*These agents currently are illegal except for some accepted experimental uses and the use of a marijuana derivative to treat nausea and anorexia associated with cancer chemotherapy.

Disadvantages of psychoactive drugs

Adverse reactions

Along with the benefits of psychoactive drugs, there are also drawbacks. Pharmacologically, these drugs initially produce sedation, depending on the drug and dosage. The client often shows minimal response to the environment, frequently sitting in a state of drowsiness, unable to focus on conversation. Fortunately, tolerance to these sedative effects develops rapidly.

Other responses are a fall in blood pressure, restlessness, tachycardia, decreased salivation, decreased motor activity, and a reduced ability to carry out complex intellectual tasks. Common adverse reactions, most notably extrapyramidal syndromes (parkinsonism, akathisia, dystonia), necessitate the use of anticholinergic drugs such as benztropine (Cogentin) and trihexyphenidyl (Artane). These reactions are usually associated with antipsychotic agents.

Other problems occur with food and alcohol interactions, drug–drug interactions, idiosyncratic responses, changes in sleep patterns, changes in sexual activity, compliance with the drug regimen, attitudes of the client and the health professional toward drug therapy, variations in effective doses for each client, and physical illnesses.

Antipsychotic drugs can affect sleep through their sedative effect or by enhancing or inhibiting rapid eye movement (REM) sleep. The antianxiety agents affect sleep patterns by decreasing the time it takes to fall asleep, prolonging the stage of nonrapid eye movement, and decreasing the duration of REM sleep. Although antipsychotic drugs tend to normalize sleep disturbances, some clients experience fatigue or a "hangover" the following morning. Similarly, an increase or decrease in libido or impotence may occur, characterized by a desire for sexual activity but an inability to achieve orgasm or continue intercourse. The phenothiazines and monoamine oxidase (MAO) inhibitors inhibit ejaculation without interfering with erection. Added to this is the possibility of feminization in some men. Any of these adverse reactions can cause extreme distress in clients already experiencing disturbances in sexual relationships and difficulties with their own sexuality. Other adverse effects are discussed in more detail in this chapter.

Usage during pregnancy is not usually recommended for many of the psychoactive drugs. However, the necessity of moderating severe symptomalogy must be weighed against the potential for harmful side effects. In all clients, the benefits gained in alleviating distressful symptoms must be measured against the accompanying problems. The continuing search for drugs that block the dopamine receptors yet create fewer adverse reactions will lead to a greater understanding of drug actions and to safer drugs. Currently,

Table 26-2. Psychoactive drugs: major indications for use

Drug name	Major indication
Antipsychotics	
Phenothiazines	
chlorpromazine (Thorazine, Largastel)	Thought disorder, psychomotor agitation in acute and chronic psychoses, agitation in alcohol withdrawal, mania
	Antiemetic
thioridazine (Mellaril)	Similar to chlorpromazine with little antiemetic action
trifluoperazine (Stelazine)	Withdrawal, apathetic schizophrenia with psychomotor retardation, delusions, hallucinations
	Chronic psychosis
fluphenazine (Moditen, Modecate, Prolixin)	Similar to chlorpromazine
acetophenazine (Tindal)	Psychotic disorders
carphenazine (Prodetazine)	Psychotic disorders
mesoridazine (Serentil)	Schizophrenia, organic brain disorders, psychoneurosis
perphenazine (Trilafon)	Moderate to severe anxiety and agitation, schizophrenic depression
piperacetazine (Quide)	Psychotic disorders
prochlorperazine (Compazine)	Psychotic disorders, psychoneurosis with moderate to severe anxiety and tension, nausea and vomiting
promazine (Sparine)	Psychotic disorders
triflupromazine (Vesprin)	Psychotic disorders and severe nausea and vomiting
Thioxanthenes	
chlorprothixine thiothixine (Taractan)	Similar to phenothiazines with both stimulating and relaxing actions
Butyrophenones	
haloperidol (Haldol, Peridol)	Thought disorders
	Psychosis with moderate and severe agitation, anxiety, overt aggressiveness, hostility
	Delusions, hallucinations, hyperactivity manifested in schizophrenia, manic phase of manic-depressive syndrome, organic brain syndrome (OBS), mental retardation, Gilles de la Tourette's syndrome
	Torticollis
	Withdrawal from opiate addiction
droperidol (Inapsine)	Tranquilization and sedation, as well as preoperative reduction of nausea and vomiting
Dihydroindolone	
molindone (Lidone, Moban)	Management of schizophrenia
Dibenzoxazepine	
loxapine (Loxapac, Loritane)	Psychotic disorders
Rauwolfia alkaloids	
reserpine (Serpasil)	Acute and chronic schizophrenia
Antianxiety agents	
Benzodiazepines	
diazepam (Valium, Vivol)	Tension and anxiety
	Emotional tension leading to somatic complaints
flurazepam	Psychoneurotic tension, depression, agitation
	Skeletal muscle spasm
halazepam	Convulsive disorder, status epilepticus
prazepam	Reverse effects of LSD and mescaline, anxiety disorders
triazolam	Enuresis
	Anxiety with phobias
oxazepam (Serax)	Anxiety disorders or anxiety associated with depression
chlordiazepoxide (Librium)	Anxiety, tension, apprehension
	Adjunct for agitation in chronic alcoholism
	Alcohol withdrawal

(Continued)

Table 26-2. Psychoactive drugs: major indications for use (Continued)

Drug name	Major indication
Antianxiety agents	
chlorazepate (Tranxene)	Anxiety, anxiety disorders, adjunct therapy in management of partial seizures
lorazepam (Ativan, Novolorazem)	Anxiety, anxiety with depression
alprazolam (Xanax)	Anxiety disorders
temazepam	Insomnia
Diphenylmethane	
hydroxyzine (Atarax, Vistaril)	Apprehension stemming from organic problems
Propanediol	
meprobamate (Equanil, Miltown)	Anxiety, tension, phobias, psychosomatic disorders
Antidepressants/mood stabilizers	
MAO inhibitors	
phenelzine (most toxic) (Nardil)	Phobias
	Moderate to severe depressive states
	Endogenous depression, exogenous depression
	Psychomotor retardation
trancyclopromine (Parnate)	Severely depressed clients who have not responded to other treatment and cannot undergo ECT
isocarboxazid (Marplan)	Depression unresponsive to ECT and other antidepressants
Tricyclic heterocyclic compounds	
imipramine (Tofranil)	Retarded depression, periodic endogenous depression, reactive depression
	Depressive phase of manic-depressive state
	Senile and organic brain depression
	Cocaine addiction
clomipramine (Anafranil)	Obsessive-compulsive behaviors
desipramine (Norpramin)	Depressive syndromes, especially endogenous depression
amitriptyline (Elavil, Etrafon, Triavil)	Depression with anxiety and agitation
	Endogenous depression
doxepin (Sinequan, Triadepin)	Psychoneurotic anxiety
	Depressive reaction
	Mixed anxiety and depression
	Psychotic depression
	Alcoholism-anxiety with or without depression
nortriptyline (Apo-Trimip, Aventyl)	Acute panic states in phobias
protriptyline (Triptil)	Depression with withdrawal
trimipramine (Rhotriamine)	Endogenous depression
maprotiline (Ludiomil)	Depressive neurosis, manic depression, major depressive disorders
trazodone (Desyrel)	Major depressive episodes
amoxapine (Asendin)	Depression in neurotic or reactive depressive disorders, endogenous and psychotic depression, depression with anxiety
lithium carbonate	Manic episodes of manic-depressive psychosis
	Maintenance to prevent recurrent manic episodes
fluoxetine (Prozac)	
Antiparkinsonian agents	
diphenhydramine (Benadryl)	Extrapyramidal symptoms of antipsychotic agents
benztropine (Cogentin)	
trihexyphenidyl (Artane)	
procyclidine (Kemadrin)	
biperiden (Akineton)	

it takes about 10 years for each new drug that is synthesized to reach the market.

Accumulation

Psychoactive drugs, when administered over a period of time, accumulate in body tissue; they tend to have large volumes of distribution. When administration of a drug is discontinued, the tissues slowly release the accumulated supply. Traces of a drug can be found in the urine for several weeks after drug therapy is discontinued. This factor must be considered when contemplating the following:

- Instituting other drug regimens
- Calculating necessary time intervals between noncompatible drugs
- Discontinuing drugs that require gradual withdrawal
- Alleviating behavioral symptoms while waiting to initiate drug therapy

■ Summary

Psychoactive drug therapy is not a cure for mental illness; instead, it is a valuable part of total therapy and is used in conjunction with other therapies. Although the full action of psychoactive drugs is unknown, they depress the CNS and alleviate the effect of anxiety on the ANS. This occurs possibly by changing the amounts of neurotransmitters available at receptor sites. As a result, they help to normalize behavior, alleviate the psychoactive process, and help the client function on a daily basis. The categories of psychoactive drugs are antipsychotic, antianxiety, and antidepressant/mood-stabilizing agents. Psychotomimetics or hallucinogens are psychoactive but are illegal; their only legal use is in experiments. Anticholinergic and antiparkinsonism agents are used in conjunction with antipsychotic drugs for the treatment of drug-induced parkinsonism.

Antipsychotic agents

Antipsychotic agents are effective in modifying psychotic symptoms, yet do not affect the underlying pathology. Their usefulness lies in relieving symptoms, not in effecting cures. Antipsychotic drugs decrease aggressive, highly active behavior; produce little or no psychic or physical dependence; produce extrapyramidal symptoms; lower the seizure threshold; and do not produce coma when large doses are given (Box 26-1).

Antipsychotic drugs modify the most disabling symptoms of the client's behavior and modify the client's affective state without diminishing the intellectual processes to any great extent. Selection of the appropriate drug for the individual client depends on the psychopathology, the target behavior, and the client's medical status. Metabolic differences and receptor site structure could cause the client to be unresponsive to a drug in one class, yet responsive to another in that same class. Choosing the proper drug, therefore, necessitates a full understanding of the pharmacology of each drug used and its possible range of effects on a client. Physicians should be experienced in using one or two agents in each class, rather than randomly selecting an agent from the many available. Administering more than one agent in a class often is of no therapeutic value, making it difficult to evaluate the benefits of each drug. The trend has moved away from using the low-potency agents such as chlorpromazine toward using high-potency drugs such as haloperidol. Cross-sensitivity between classes exists. It is important for the nurse to know the criteria used by the physician when selecting a drug for the client. This leads to more accurate evaluation of behavioral and physiologic changes. The major indications for antipsychotic drugs are thought disorders and severe agitation in acute and chronic psychoses. The diagnostic classifications include schizophrenia, organic psychoses, and manic–depressive illnesses (Box 26-2).

The classes of antipsychotic drugs are phenothiazines, butyrophenones, thioxanthenes, dihydroindolones, dibenzoxazepines, and rauwolfia alkaloids. Psychotic behaviors resulting from hostility and withdrawal and perceptual disturbances, such as delusions and hallucinations, can be modified by using these agents.

Box 26-1. Advantages of antipsychotic agents

- Decrease aggressive, highly active behavior
- Produce little or no psychic or physical dependence
- Do not produce coma when given in large doses

Box 26-2. Major indications for the use of antipsychotics

- Thought disorder and severe agitation in acute and chronic psychoses
- Diagnostic classifications for which they are used—schizophrenia, organic psychoses, manic-depressive illnesses
- Psychotic behaviors due to hostility, withdrawal, and perceptual disturbances, such as delusions and hallucinations.

Phenothiazines

The widespread use of phenothiazines (the major group of antipsychotic drugs) resulted from a French surgeon's (Laborit) search in 1951 for a drug to calm preoperative clients. Chlorpromazine had already been synthesized when antihistamines were developed but its sedative effects were too powerful for use as an antihistamine. Laborit gave chlorpromazine to clients before surgery, found it worked well, and suggested that it be given to psychiatric clients to make them more manageable. It became widely accepted as the drug therapy of choice for the mentally disturbed client (Kolata, 1979). Many derivatives of phenothiazine now exist.

Phenothiazines usually add to or potentiate the effects of other CNS depressants. There is some cross-sensitivity between phenothiazines. Initially, the ability to tolerate phenothiazines and to respond to them, is usually greater in the actively psychotic client. Generally, all phenothiazines have similar actions; their usefulness lies primarily in their antipsychotic and antiemetic actions. Differences are determined by the potency of a particular drug and the severity of the adverse effects it causes; the piperazine group is the most potent. It usually takes weeks for the antipsychotic effects of these drugs to be felt fully; however, their sedative effects are rapid. Phenothiazines are divided into three groups: aliphatic, piperazine, and piperidine. Thioxanthenes are structurally similar to phenothiazines but are less likely to produce serious adverse reactions.

Pharmacodynamics

Sedative action. The drug depresses the lower levels of the CNS without depressing the vital centers. The depression of the lower levels of the CNS (the vomiting center and the temperature-regulating center) has an antiemetic effect, results in minor drops in body temperature, and suppresses shivering. Vasodilation occurs in the extremities, salivary and gastric secretions are decreased, and smooth muscles relax.

Antipsychotic action. Antipsychotic action is characterized by the alleviation or elimination of psychotic activity. This results when the response of the receptors to dopamine is blocked. There is a reduction in behavioral activity while neurophysiologic stimulation occurs. The suppression of the nervous center's sympathetic activity leads to reduced psychomotor agitation.

Therapeutic uses

Phenothiazines potentiate CNS depressants, thereby enhancing the sedative effects of alcohol, analgesics, hypnotics, and anesthetics. In animal studies, the drug has reduced conditioned avoidance responses without affecting escape responses (Gilman, Goodman, & Gilman, 1980). The sedative effect reduces activity and produces a calming effect. Sedation occurs rapidly, making phenothiazines useful for agitated, anxious clients. Sleep disturbances are alleviated, leading to increased sleeping time and a normalization of sleep patterns. The sedative actions of aliphatic phenothiazines make them useful in acute schizophrenic and manic states. Phenothiazines reduce hallucinations, delusions, aggression, panic, fear, and agitation, making them useful in treating acute and chronic psychoses. On the other hand, some members of the piperazine group and thioxanthenes stimulate the withdrawn, apathetic client.

Dosage and administration

Because there are so many preparations of phenothiazines and because they can be administered both orally and by injection, the reader is referred to a current reference for specific doses. However, the basic daily doses are given in Table 26-3.

Adverse reactions

Because clients vary in their ability to tolerate phenothiazines and because there is a wide range of adverse reactions, the effectiveness of phenothiazines often depends on the clients' responses to these side effects. Effects from these drugs result from action on the CNS, the ANS, the cardiovascular system, and the endocrine system. The cholinergic blocking activity of phenothiazines results in parkinsonism. Aliphatic phenothiazines are responsible for a high incidence of parkinsonism and high sedation, whereas piperidine compounds create fewer symptoms of parkinsonism and less sedation. Piperazine compounds are the most likely to produce extrapyramidal symptoms and to cause the least sedation. As with many of the psychoactive drugs, safety of usage during pregnancy has not been established and prescribing phenothiazines is left to the judgment of the physician.

Behavioral effects. Feelings of tension and restlessness usually occur early in phenothiazine therapy. This is often unpleasant for the client receiving antipsychotic drug therapy. A prolonged sense of fatigue decreases the client's ability or desire to participate in activities of any kind. A somnolent stage, varying from drowsiness to deep sleep, usually occurs shortly after administration (most obvious with chlorpromazine). Depressing effects may lead to attempts at suicide or to the client's reluctance to take the drug.

Eye and skin reactions. Eye and skin reactions include blurred vision, photosensitivity, and pigmentary changes in the conjunctiva. In addition, allergic skin reactions, contact dermatitis, and jaundice may occur. Exposure to the sun can cause pigmentation changes (blue-gray spots) in a client receiving high doses over an extended time. If jaundice occurs within the first several weeks, the drug should be discontinued.

Orthostatic hypotension. Phenothiazines exert direct depressant action on the heart. Orthostatic hypotension occurs, especially with chlorpromazine and

Table 26-3. Antipsychotic drugs: phenothiazines

Drug and name	Usual daily dosage (mg)	Additional information
Aliphatic phenothiazines		
chlorpromazine (Thorazine)	30–1000 PC: C	Strong sedative effects, orthostatic hypotension, fewer extrapyramidal side effects
promazine (Sparine)	60–1000 PC: C	
triflupromazine (Vesprin)	30–150	
Piperazine phenothiazines		
acetophenazine (Tindal)	40–120 PC: C	High potency, antiemetic, high incidence of extrapyramidal side effects, minimal sedation, lesser orthostatic hypotension
carphenazine (Proketazine)	25–400	
fluphenazine (Prolixin)	1.25–10 PC: C	
perphenazine (Trilafon)	4–16 PC: C	
prochlorperazine (Compazine)	15–100 PC: C	
trifluoperazine (Stelazine)	2–40 PC: C	
Piperadine phenothiazines		
piperacetazine (Quide)	20–160	Moderate sedation, fewer extrapyramidal side effects, orthostatic hypotension
thioridazine (Mellaril)	150–800 PC: C	
mesoridazine (Serentil)	100–400 PC: C	

KEY: PC = pregnancy category risk. (The validity of pregnancy risk categories has not been established. See Chapter 16, p 216.)

thioridazine, although tolerance may develop after several weeks of administration. Hypotension, leading to complaints of dizziness or faintness, is most likely to occur when the client arises in the morning. This occurs most frequently with the initial doses, particularly with parenteral administration, or when higher doses are given. Usually the client adjusts to this. If severe hypotension occurs, intravenous fluids or norepinephrine are given. It may be necessary to discontinue the drug or to lower the dosage.

Extrapyramidal effects. Extrapyramidal effects can appear after one or many doses and are common responses to this drug therapy. It is thought that this results from the blockade of postsynaptic dopamine receptors in the caudate nucleus.

Parkinsonism is characterized by a masklike facial expression, muscular rigidity, drooling, and restlessness. This syndrome is also indicated by the less distressing signs of akinesia—the slowing of voluntary movement with complaints of weakness in the arms and legs. Tremors and pill-rolling movements are observed. The flat facial expression and retarded move-

ments are similar to depression. Drug-induced parkinsonism is reversible through the administration of the antiparkinsonian agents benztropine (Cogentin), trihexyphenidyl (Artane), or procyclidine (Kemadrin). These cholinergic blocking agents are thought to reverse symptoms of parkinsonism by balancing the cholinergic and dopaminergic activity as the action of acetylcholine on neurons is blocked. Anticholinergics are used for rapid control of early extrapyramidal symptoms.

Akathisia—an extreme restlessness in which the client feels compelled to move (stand up and walk around)—occurs early in phenothiazine therapy. Unable to control this restlessness, the client will sit for only a few moments before getting up, possibly walking around or pacing, then sitting again, only to repeat these actions minutes later. Clients continually move their hands, body, and mouth. Although these symptoms are similar to those of agitation in the psychotic client, treatment differs. Antiparkinsonian agents relieve these symptoms.

Dystonia—facial grimacing, muscle rigidity, abnormal posturing, and difficulty in swallowing or in opening the mouth—can occur within 2–8 weeks of treatment. It is necessary to differentiate between an hysterical reaction and these symptoms, which the prompt administration of antiparkinsonian agents can alleviate. *Tardive dyskinesia* is a syndrome that occurs late and more frequently in the elderly. It is thought to be due to heightened sensitivity of dopamine receptors after prolonged use of antipsychotic drugs. It is characterized by rhythmic, stereotyped involuntary motions, such as sucking and smacking the lips, repetitive protrusion of the tongue, tongue tremor, chewing movements, and facial spasms. All of these actions subside during sleep. The sudden onset of these symptoms can be disconcerting to clients and staff alike. Autopsies on clients with dyskinesia have revealed lesions in the substantia nigra. Early symptoms of facial tics, oral motions, or rocking call for reduction of the drug dosage and discontinuation of the drug. At this stage, the condition may be reversible, or it may be kept from progressing further. However, symptoms may persist indefinitely.

Agranulocytosis. Depression of leukocyte production occurs within 3–6 weeks after the initiation of phenothiazine therapy. This condition occurs very infrequently, its onset is sudden, and it can result in death during the acute phase. Symptoms of sore throat, elevated temperature, and lesions in the mouth should be reported immediately. Treatment consists of discontinuing the drug and administering broad-spectrum antibiotics. Corticotropin may also be used. White blood cell levels should be monitored.

Other side effects. Other side effects include changes in the activity of the hypothalamus with resulting effects on the endocrine system, and changes in the concentrations of adrenocorticotropic hormone, prolactin, gonadotropin, estrogen, and progestin. As a result, growth may be diminished and inappropriate lactation can occur, as well as amenorrhea, infertility, feminization in men, and hypoglycemia. Inhibition of ejaculation in men and ventricular arrhythmias are adverse reactions to thioridazine therapy. The seizure threshold can be lowered; this necessitates concurrent anticonvulsive drug therapy in epileptics. Use of chlorpromazine may also result in decreased motility and constipation. Other adverse reactions to phenothiazines are hypoglycemia that develops into diabetes and autonomic disturbances, such as nasal congestion, dry mouth, headache, leg pains, menstrual dysfunction, inappropriate lactation, and weight gain.

Drug interactions
Phenothiazines have a potentiating or additive effect when given with either CNS depressants or anticholinergic agents. Because phenothiazines increase the sedative effect of narcotics, lower doses can be given to relieve pain. There also appears to be an antagonistic action to stimulants, such as amphetamines. Susceptibility to the effects of alcohol may also increase. Cross-sensitivity between phenothiazines exists. Interaction with CNS depressants may lead to deepened sedation and severe hypotension.

Phenothiazines used in conjunction with narcotic analgesics increase respiratory depression. The phenothiazine chlorpromazine may counteract the antihypertensive effect of guanethidine; this can lead to difficulties because the onset of guanethidine's antihypertensive action is slow. Giving such phenothiazines to clients receiving guanethidine or witholding them necessitates close monitoring of their blood pressure. There are indications that antacids may interfere with the absorption of phenothiazines. For this reason it is suggested that the administration of these two agents be separated by approximately 2 hours.

Because phenothiazines block the effect of levodopa (L-dopa), they should not be given to a client on L-dopa therapy. Furthermore, L-dopa is ineffective in alleviating phenothiazine-induced extrapyramidal symptoms.

Interaction between phenothiazines and tricyclic antidepressants or antiparkinsonian drugs may produce cumulative anticholinergic effects. Symptoms include constipation, urinary retention, dry mouth, orthostatic hypotension, and fuzziness of vision. (See Focus on Phenothiazines: Similarities and Differences.)

Other classes of antipsychotic agents
Thioxanthenes, butyrophenones, dihydroindolones, dibenzoxazepines, and rauwolfia have actions similar to phenothiazines but with a few variations. These drugs are used in the treatment of acute and chronic psychoses, especially states of excessive psychomotor activity, panic, severe agitation, hostility, and aggression. The depressant effect of antipsychotic drugs on the vomiting center makes them useful as antiemetics. See Table 26-4 for more information on these drugs.

Butyrophenones
In comparison to phenothiazines (chlorpromazine is used as the model), butyrophenones have a more rapid effect on acute schizophrenia, acute manic attacks, and paranoid excitement. These drugs are particularly effective in multiple tic syndromes.

Dibenzoxazepines
Dibenzoxazepines are similar in action to phenothiazines. Loxapine (Loxitane), a fairly inexpensive drug, has been used with some effect in treating tardive dyskinesia.

Thioxanthenes
Thiothixene (Navane) is one of the most potent of the thioxanthenes, frequently producing extrapyramidal

Phenothiazines: similarities and differences

Similarities

Pharmacodynamics

These agents act at the subcortical levels of reticular formation, limbic system, and hypothalamus. They are believed to antagonize dopamine transmission at the synapses or block postsynaptic dopamine receptor sites. They also have antagonistic activity at the alpha adrenergic, serotonergic, histamine (H-1 receptors) and muscarinic receptors.

Pharmacokinetics

These agents are primarily metabolized by the liver. They generally have a gradual onset, peaking in 4–7 days. They are absorbed well from the GI tract and parenterally; are distributed in most body tissues; readily cross the placenta; and are excreted in urine and feces. The average onset of action is 30–60 minutes with a duration of 4–6 hours when given orally.

Therapeutic uses

These agents are used to treat acute or chronic psychoses and for sedation.

Adverse reactions

These include: (CNS) lethargy, restlessness, hyperactivity, bizarre dreams, depression, headache, dizziness, insomnia, nocturnal confusion, pseudoparkinsonism, motor restlessness, dystonias, tardive dyskinesias, euphoria, catatonic-like state, paranoid reactions, increase in psychotic symptoms; (EENT) photophobia, worsening of glaucoma, blurred vision, mydriasis, ocular lesions; (CV) tachycardia, syncope, cardiac arrest, postural hypotension, hypertension; (RESP) nasal congestion, laryngospasm; dyspnea, bronchospasm; (GI) dry mouth, nausea, vomiting, anorexia, constipation, diarrhea, weight gain, increased appetite, cholestatic jaundice; (GU) urinary retention, glycosuria; incontinence; (HEMA) agranulocytosis, eosinophilia, leukopenia, anemia, aplastic anemia, hemolytic anemia, thrombocytopenia, pancytopenia; (ENDO) breast enlargement, amenorrhea, blood sugar changes, impotence; (DERM) urticaria, pigment depositions, photosensitivity, eczema, erythema; (OTHER) hypothermia or hyperthermia.

Differences

• **Triethylperazine**, **triflupromazine**, **perphenazine**, **prochlorperazine**, and **chlorpromazine** are believed to directly block the chemotrigger zone (CTZ).

• **Fluphenazine** has an onset of 1 hour (PO or IM), and peaks in 2 hours with a duration of 6–8 hours. • **Promethazine** has an onset of 20 minutes (PO or IM), 3–5 minutes (IV), with a duration of 6–12 hours. • **Acetophenazine** has a duration of 4–6 hours. • **Prochlorperazine** peaks in 2–4 hours.

• **Triflupromazine**, **prochlorperazine**, and **chlorpromazine** are used as antiemetics. • **Promethazine** is also used as an antihistamine. • **Chlorpromazine** and **thioridazine** can be used to control combativeness and hyperexcitability in children with behavior problems. • **Chlorpromazine** is also used to treat intractable hiccups and acute intermittent prophyria.

• **Fluphenazine** can also cause polyuria, fecal impaction, peripheral edema, and mental depression. • **Promazine**, when given IM, can cause severe orthostatic hypotension.
• **Prochlorperazine**, when given IM, can cause necrosis at the injection site.

(continued)

Phenothiazines: similarities and differences (Continued)

Similarities

Contraindications

These agents are contraindicated in hypersensitivity, severe toxic CNS depression, persons in a coma, or those with subcortical brain damage, bone marrow depression or those receiving L-dopa therapy.

Precautions

These agents should be used cautiously in persons with seizure disorders or those receiving anticonvulsants; those with cardiovascular disorders; those exposed to high environmental temperatures; the elderly or debilitated; those with hepatic or renal disorders, glaucoma, prostatic hypertrophy, chronic respiratory conditions, or hypocalcemia; and those persons who have a severe reaction to insulin or electroconvulsive therapy.

Nursing considerations

Instruct client in disease, treatment regimen, compliance, and signs and symptoms of adverse reactions; avoid direct contact of drug with skin; obtain baseline information about the overt signs of emotional disturbance, anxiety level, depression, suicidal ideation; obtain baseline information about vital signs and usual patterns of elimination; monitor vital signs frequently during therapy for changes; assess intake and output for signs of urinary retention; obtain blood studies, including CBC, platelet counts, and liver function studies; evaluate emotional status for changes and institute safety and suicide precautions as necessary; assess neuromuscular status for involuntary movements; instruct not to withdraw or stop taking the drug suddenly; instruct client to avoid beverages and over the counter drugs containing alcohol; warn client to avoid activities requiring mental alertness and coordination until effects of drug are known; administer with milk or foods to minimize GI upset; instruct client that excessive exposure to sunlight may cause photosensitivity reactions; teach client to avoid extreme heat or cold temperatures because of risk of hypothermia and hyperthermia; suggest measures to relieve dry mouth such as ice chips, gum, hard candy; warn client that urine may become discolored; dilute concentrate with 2–4 ounces of liquid such as water, carbonated drinks, fruit juice, tomato juice, milk or puddings; avoid using apple juice or caffeine-containing products.

Differences

• **Triflupromazine** is contraindicated in children and adolescents with suspected Reye's syndrome.

Some preparations of **trifluperazine, promazine, perphenazine,** and **chlorpromazine** contain sulfites and should be used cautiously in persons with sulfite sensitivity to prevent a possible allergic reaction. Some preparations of **mesoridazine** and **promazine** contain tartrazine and should be used cautiously in persons who have a sensitivity to tartrazine.

Administer IM **chlorpromazine, fluphenazine, mesoridazine, perphenazine** and **promazine** deep into the upper outer quadrant of the buttocks and massage afterwards to prevent abscess formation; protect liquid concentration from light. When giving **promethazine** by IV drip, wrap solution container in foil to protect from light. Monitor the client's blood pressure closely, sitting, standing and lying, when giving promazine IV.

Table 26-4. Other antipsychotic agents

Class	Drug name	Usual daily dosage (mg)	Additional information
Butyrophenones	droperidol (Inapsine) haloperidol (Haldol)	2.5–10 1–100	High potency, antiemetic, high incidence of extrapyramidal side effects, minimal sedation, minimal orthostatic hypotension
Dihydroindolones	molindone (Lidone, Moban)	15–225	Extrapyramidal side effects
Dibenzoxazepines	loxapine (Loxitane)	50–250	Extrapyramidal side effects
Thioxanthenes	chlorprothixene (Taractan) thiothixene (Navane)	30–600 5–60	
Rauwolfia alkaloids	reserpine (Serpasil)	0.5–1.0	Extrapyramidal side effects, depressive reactions, nightmares, nasal congestion, edema, excessive gastric secretion

symptoms and insomnia. Chlorprothixene (Taractan) is less likely to produce these symptoms.

Rauwolfia alkaloids

Rauwolfia alkaloids are rarely prescribed today because they have been superseded by phenothiazines. The adverse reactions caused by large, single doses limit their usefulness. As a result, it is necessary to use small daily doses, which delays the therapeutic effectiveness of these drugs as antipsychotic agents. They are used primarily as antihypertensive agents.

■ Summary

Antipsychotic agents modify psychotic symptoms without affecting underlying pathology. They relieve symptoms but do not effect cures. Antipsychotics are used in schizophrenia, organic psychoses, and manic-depressive illness. The derivatives of phenothiazine have been widely accepted as the drug therapies of choice for the mentally disturbed client. Other classes of antipsychotics have actions similar to phenothiazines and are used especially in states of excessive psychomotor activity, panic, severe agitation, hostility, and aggression.

Nursing management of clients using antipsychotic agents

Because many of the implications for nursing management and client education are similar for all psychoactive drugs, they are discussed at the end of this chapter. They should be studied carefully. However, implications for client education that are specific for antipsychotic agents are given here.

Nursing implications

Concentrations of antipsychotic drugs, particularly chlorpromazine, may cause dermatitis. The nurse should avoid direct contact with these chemicals. Antiparkinson drugs may be prescribed concurrently to reduce extrapyramidal symptoms.

Nursing process

Assessment Before drug therapy is initiated, baseline data should be recorded in relation to overt signs of emotional disturbance, anxiety level, depression, and suicidal ideation; vital signs, particularly blood pressure; and usual patterns of elimination. Clients should be screened for possible adverse reactions to antipsychotic drugs, including a history of allergic dermatitis, predisposition to constipation or urinary retention, and a history of hypotension or postural hypotension.

Nursing diagnosis Possible nursing diagnoses include the following:

Anxiety related to mental changes
Altered comfort: dizziness related to postural hypotension secondary to antipsychotic drugs
High risk for injury related to postural hypotension secondary to antipsychotic drugs
Altered comfort: abdominal distention and/or painful defecation related to decreased peristalsis secondary to antipsychotic drug regimen
Altered comfort: bladder distention related to urinary retention secondary to anticholinergic effects of drug regimen
Sexual dysfunction related to antipsychotic drug regimen
Noncompliance: omitted drug doses related to increased anxiety secondary to discomforting drug side effects
Knowledge deficit secondary to antipsychotic medications and drug regimens

Planning Goals of nursing care relate specifically to the nursing diagnoses and may include reduction of anxiety, increased comfort, reduction in the risk of falls, maintenance of normal elimination, maintenance of normal sexual function, maintenance of optimal blood levels of antipsychotic drugs, and education of the client regarding antipsychotic medications and drug regimens.

Intervention   When administering oral medications, concentrates are mixed with at least 2 ounces of juice for drinking. Parenteral solutions should not be mixed with other drugs in the same syringe. Directions for administration should be followed carefully.

Clients must be monitored carefully for reactions to the drug regimen. To determine therapeutic response, emotional status (anxiety, depression, suicidal ideation) should be assessed at regular intervals. Among the parameters that should be monitored for adverse drug reaction are blood pressure, cardiac action, dizziness, steadiness of gait, urinary and fecal elimination, vision (for brownish discoloration), blood cell counts, and skin color (for jaundice).

Antipsychotic drugs should be discontinued if signs and symptoms of agranulocytosis (sore throat, fever, weakness) develop. Increased irritability or agitation, urinary retention, jaundice, and laboratory reports indicating abnormally low levels of blood cells should be reported promptly to the physician. Drug doses should not be given if, in the nurse's judgment, they are:

- Prescribed in unsafe dosages
- Contraindicated with another drug or a medical condition
- Creating serious adverse reactions

In such a case, the decision not to give a drug and the reasons for the decision should be reported to the nursing superior and to the physician. An accurate record of observations, nursing actions, and the client's response must be kept in the client's chart.

Agranulocytosis is a rare but potentially fatal adverse reaction to antipsychotic drugs. If signs and symptoms of infection develop, the drug should be discontinued and blood counts should be monitored.

Nursing measures to reduce the risk of constipation and urinary retention should be instituted. If necessary, the physician should be consulted for laxative prescriptions or orders for catheterization.

Dry mouth, a usual side effect, can be alleviated by encouraging the client to suck on ice chips or hard candies, chew gum, sip small amounts of fluid frequently, or rinse the mouth frequently.

Administration of an antiparkinsonian agent prescribed by the physician will reduce pronounced or persistent extrapyramidal symptoms. If symptoms are severe, encourage the client to lie down in a quiet, darkened room; someone should remain with the client until symptoms subside.

Clients affected by postural hypotension should be encouraged to remain in a recumbent position from 45 minutes to 1 hour after the drug is administered. If symptoms persist, the dosage may need to be reduced or the medication changed. Side rails or assisted ambulation may be necessary.

Client education.   Educating the client early in the treatment helps to reduce anxiety about adverse reactions and promotes compliance. Advise clients and their families that it will take 3–6 weeks for a therapeutic response. Also advise clients and their families that drugs must be taken exactly as prescribed; tell them whether a missed dose can be taken with the next one. Caution them not to discontinue their medication before consulting the doctor because sudden discontinuance can cause relapse or deterioration. If adverse drug reactions (including sexual dysfunction) are severe or persistent, advise the client to consult with the physician for a change in the drug regimen.

Lightheadedness and dizziness may be reduced by doing the following:

- Advise clients to rise or to change position gradually.
- Advise clients to sit on the edge of the bed for a few minutes before standing.
- Offer clients reassurance that they will adjust to the drug within a few days.

Clients taking antipsychotic drugs should be cautioned about taking care when driving an automobile, operating machinery, or performing tasks requiring fine motor coordination. Advise the client that alcohol, barbiturates, and analgesics, which interact with antipsychotic agents, cause further CNS depression. Advise clients that if photosensitivity occurs, they should wear protective clothing, sunglasses, and sun screens and avoid direct sunlight.

Clients may be reassured that extrapyramidal and hypotensive reactions tend to diminish with continued therapy. Pronounced or severe reactions should be reported to the primary health care provider because dosages may need to be adjusted.

Evaluation   Data required for evaluation relate to specific goals and predetermined criteria. They may include serial assessment of emotional status, serial vital signs (including postural blood pressures), absence or occurrence of falls, absence or occurrence of constipation or urinary retention, serum drug levels, reports by the client of comfort levels, and ability of the client to manage the drug regimen and maintain accurate medication.

Checklist of nursing actions

☐   Do not give any drug that you think is prescribed in unsafe doses, that is contraindicated with another drug or medical condition, or that you observe creating serious adverse reactions.

☐   Report and accurately record your observations, the steps taken, and the outcome.

Table 26-5. Usefulness of antianxiety agents in various conditions

Useful	Questionable	Not effective
Moderate anxiety and muscle tension associated with psychoneurotic and psychosomatic conditions	Anxiety associated with phobias and neurasthenia	Psychoses Long-term treatment of psychotic states
Conjunction with chemotherapy		

☐ Advise the client and family that therapeutic responses take 3–6 weeks.

☐ Advise the client and family that the drug must be taken exactly as prescribed.

☐ Caution clients not to discontinue medication without consulting the physician.

☐ Caution against driving an automobile, operating machinery, or performing tasks that require fine motor coordination when taking antipsychotic drugs until the drug response is known.

☐ Advise clients about the interaction between their drug and alcohol, barbiturates, and analgesics.

☐ Advise the client to wear protective clothing, sunglasses, and sun screens and to avoid direct sunlight if photosensitivity occurs.

☐ Encourage clients to suck on ice chips or hard candies, chew gum, sip small amounts of fluid frequently, or rinse their mouths frequently if they develop dry mouths.

☐ Follow directions for administering the drug carefully.

☐ Avoid contact with drug concentrates.

☐ Promptly report complaints of brownish discoloration of vision because this is a sign of pigmentary retinopathy.

☐ Discontinue antipsychotics 48 hours before surgery upon the physician's order.

☐ Remain with the client until medication is swallowed.

☐ Monitor blood pressure for hypotension and observe for CNS depression.

☐ Encourage the client to remain in a recumbent position for 1 hour after initial doses.

☐ Advise the client to rise or change positions gradually and to sit on the edge of the bed for a few minutes before standing.

☐ Use side rails and supervise ambulation if necessary.

☐ Carefully observe the elderly client.

☐ Observe for signs of depression and possible suicidal ideation. Be alert to increased irritability or agitation.

☐ Check bowel movements and abdominal distention, as well as change in the color of urine and stools.

☐ Observe for signs of sore throat, fever, or weakness.

☐ Allow the client with extrapyramidal symptoms to lie down in a quiet, darkened room if symptoms are severe. Remain with the client until symptoms subside.

(See accompanying Example of Nursing Process and Haloperidol Treatment.)

Antianxiety agents

Antianxiety agents or anxiolytics, commonly referred to as *minor tranquilizers*, are used to alleviate moderate anxiety and muscle tension associated with psychoneurotic and psychosomatic conditions (Table 26-5). Symptoms of anxiety include muscle tension, restlessness, fatigue, insomnia, sexual dysfunction, excessive perspiration, and gastrointestinal (GI) upsets (Box 26-3). Antianxiety agents are not effective for psychoses and are not recommended for long-term treatment of psychotic states. When these drugs are taken over an extended period of time, tolerance develops, as well as the possibility of withdrawal reactions. The use of these drugs for decreasing anxiety associated with phobias and neurasthenia is questionable.

Antianxiety agents are highly useful in conjunction with psychotherapy. Unfortunately, in a health care system geared to the remedial treatment of conditions with an acute onset, all too often the antianxiety drugs are prescribed without considering the preventive or long-range effects of an adjunct psychotherapy.

Box 26-3. Symptoms of anxiety

Muscle tension

Restlessness

Fatigue

Insomnia

Sexual dysfunction

Excessive perspiration

Gastrointestinal upset

Example of nursing process and haloperidol treatment

John Johnson, a 41-year-old man, has been on the unit suffering from psychotic behavior manifested by hallucinations, delusional thinking, with the possibility of doing harm to his wife and children. John was started on Haldol yesterday and complains of feeling dizzy and lightheaded. The symptoms are most severe when rising from bed or a chair.

Assessment data	Nursing diagnosis	Interventions	Goals and outcome criteria
Baseline blood pressure	High risk for injury (falling) related to postural hypotension secondary to Haldol therapy	**Monitor** and record blood pressure.	Blood pressure stabilizes to usual level.
Drug history: especially antihypertensives and diuretics		**Ensure** adequate fluid intake.	John makes positional changes slowly.
Age		**Have** John rise or change positions slowly and sit on the side of the bed or chair until dizziness passes.	John ambulates without falling.
Physiologic status: Cardiovascular Neurological		**Remain** with client during early ambulation.	Complaints of lightheadedness decrease or cease.
Knowledge level of Haldol		**Reassure** John that the symptoms will disappear as his body adjusts to the drug.	John continues to take medication.
		Educate John about drug actions and effects.	
		Administer medication, remain with John to be sure he takes the medication.	
		Observe for signs of change or continued orthostatic hypotension.	

Emphasis should be placed on other approaches, as well as on drug therapy to help clients develop more positive methods of coping with stressful experiences. Pharmacotherapy would then be a secondary support therapy, alleviating anxiety so that the clients could cope with their problems.

Drugs used in the treatment of anxiety include barbiturates, antihistamines, antidepressants, benzodiazepines, and propanediol carbamates. Because barbiturates and antihistamines are covered in other chapters, this chapter focuses on benzodiazepines, propanediol carbamate, and diphenylmethane.

Pharmacodynamics. Antianxiety agents depress the polysynaptic reflexes of the spinal cord and the limbic structures, reducing skeletal muscle tension and inhibiting behavioral responses. The depressant action appears to affect the brain stem reticular activating systems along with the limbic system (see Fig. 26-1). The depressant effect of anxiolytics reduces a client's reaction to stressful stimuli.

Precautions. Caution should be taken to prevent dependence on these drugs by closely monitoring clients taking them over extended periods of time, as well as clients with a history of alcohol or drug addiction, and the elderly. Common adverse reactions by the elderly are confusion, drowsiness, and ataxia. Clients with histories of impaired renal or hepatic function, allergies, and blood dyscrasias, and pregnant women should be carefully assessed and monitored. Every client taking one of these agents should be cautioned about driving an automobile, operating dangerous machinery, drinking alcoholic beverages, and taking phenothiazine at the same time.

Benzodiazepines

Because of their effectiveness in alleviating symptoms of anxiety, benzodiazepines are the most widely prescribed drugs on the market today; they are readily prescribed by practitioners in every branch of medicine. Unlike barbiturates, they may not reduce mental alertness and do not suppress REM sleep. The various drugs and their doses are given in Table 26-6. The benzodiazepine derivatives, temazepam (Restoril) and flurazepam (Dalmane), are used only as hypnotics.

Pharmacodynamics. The pharmacologic action of these agents is not fully understood. Antianxiety agents have little effect on neurotransmitters but they depress the polysynaptic reflexes of the spinal cord. Anxiolytic action appears to take place in the limbic system, suppressing anxiety for extended periods. Paradoxically, hostility, rage, and physical violence can occur, especially in the severely disturbed or psychotic client. Benzodiazepines also may raise the seizure threshold.

Pharmacokinetics. These agents are well absorbed from the GI tract, becoming effective within 30 minutes to 1 hour and exerting an effect for 12–24 hours after a single dose has been ingested. Excretion varies with the drug being used, with a half-life of 24 hours for chlordiazepoxide and 2–8 days for diazepam.

Therapeutic uses. Benzodiazepines are most effective for short-term drug therapy. They are not intended for long-term therapy or for the minor stresses of daily living. The muscle relaxant and anticonvulsant potentials of benzodiazepines make them useful in controlling the psychomotor excitability of acute psychotic episodes. Chlordiazepoxide is used in alleviating symptoms of alcohol withdrawal. The conditions under which these agents can be effective are listed in Box 26-4.

Dosage and administration. These agents are generally given in one to three doses daily. Administering the larger doses at bedtime ensures full use of the sedative effect for sleep and the anxiety-reducing effect for daytime. Combining benzodiazepines with

other CNS depressants is not recommended because the CNS will be even further depressed.

Adverse reactions. Drowsiness, ataxia, and lethargy are the most common adverse reactions. Headaches, vertigo, rash, nausea, increased or decreased libido, and jaundice occur less frequently; they are apparently dose-related and are seen more often in the elderly. Decreasing the dose usually alleviates these symptoms. Slurred speech is another indication that dose should be decreased.

Reactions of rage, excitement, hostility, physical violence, and depersonalization can occur when benzodiazepines are administered to severely disturbed clients. Hyperexcitability and hyperactivity may occur after the first dose. Benzodiazepines can cause sleep disturbances, nightmares, and vivid dreams.

Dependence and tolerance may occur if these drugs are taken over an extended period of time; some clients report as withdrawal symptoms the inability to sleep, restlessness, extreme irritability, and nervousness.

Less common adverse reactions are mild hypotension, dry mouth, constipation, retarded ejaculation, and sexual impotence. Amenorrhea often occurs but can be alleviated by reducing the dose. The combination of diazepam and alcohol may prove fatal.

The possibility of congenital deformities exists from usage during the first trimester. Although this has not been conclusively proven, use of antianxiety agents during pregnancy is not recommended.

Precautions. If benzodiazepines are given intramuscularly (IM) or intravenously, extreme caution must be taken to use the proper dilutant. Intramuscular administration is not recommended because absorption by this route is slow and erratic. Cumulative effects occur over a period of repeated administration. As metabolism occurs in the liver, accumulation may prove hazardous for clients with impaired liver functions, necessitating reduced doses. (Oxazepam and lorazepam, which do not have this cumulative effect, may be substituted for another benzodiazepine.) Traces of benzodiazepine can be found in the urine long after the drug has been discontinued.

Drug interactions. Chlordiazepoxide, frequently used in doses of 50–100 mg IM for controlling acute withdrawal symptoms (delirium tremens and agitation) of alcoholism, ironically has resulted in narcosis when given to alcoholics in doses of 25–50 mg (Hartshorn, 1976, p 104). Additive effects of CNS depression can occur when chlordiazepoxide is given concurrently with other drugs having CNS depression activity. This necessitates close monitoring of these clients. In such instances, drug dosages may be lowered or discontinued to decrease the possibility of further CNS depression.

Box 26-4. Conditions for which benzodiazepines are effective

Neurotic anxiety

Neurotic or reactive depression

Spasticity of cerebral palsy, multiple sclerosis, cerebrovascular accident

Adjunct therapy to analgesia during labor and delivery

Preoperative sedation

Nonepileptic convulsions

Status epilepticus (diazepam)

Acute alcohol intoxication (chlordiazepoxide)

Cigarette smoking may decrease the sedative effects of selected benzodiazepines. Cimetidine may impair the hepatic metabolism of benzodiazepines, such as diazepam, resulting in enhanced effects.

Propanediol compounds

Meprobamate, a synthetic drug sold as Equanil or Miltown, acts as an antianxiety agent, a muscle relaxant, and an anticonvulsant.

Pharmacodynamics. Meprobamate selectively synchronizes interneuronal electric activity and relaxes skeletal muscle. A centrally acting muscle relaxant, meprobamate is believed to have no effect on the ANS.

Pharmacokinetics. Meprobamate is readily absorbed from the GI tract, reaching a peak concentration within 1–2 hours. Meprobamate has a half-life of 10 hours.

Dosage and administration. See Table 26-6 for information about doses and administration.

Therapeutic uses. Meprobamate is used to alleviate symptoms associated with anxiety and tension. Relief of tension leads to decreased irritability and a greater sense of well-being. Propanediol compounds have proven effective in treating psychosomatic disorders, abnormal fears (or phobias), and behavior disorders. Meprobamate is effective in relieving symptoms of premenstrual tension. Although it is not a potent hypnotic, meprobamate promotes sleep by relieving tension. Propanediol also relieves tension headaches and headaches resulting from constant contractions of the posterior neck muscles (Box 26-5).

Adverse reactions. Common reactions are drowsiness, skin sensitivity (skin rash, itching), and bronchial spasm. The allergic reactions can be relieved with antihistamines. Large doses of meprobamate may lead to respiratory and vasomotor collapse.

Precautions and contraindications. Tolerance and both psychological and physical dependency can develop from continued use of meprobamate over a long period of time. Addiction to meprobamate is similar to that caused by chronic use of barbiturates or alcohol. Gradual withdrawal is essential if dependence develops. Abrupt withdrawal results in anxiety, insomnia, delirium, and convulsions.

Drug interactions. It has been suggested that meprobamate decreases the effectiveness of anticoagulants. This, however, has not been proven clinically. Of particular interest is meprobamate's interaction with alcohol and other CNS depressants. The combination of alcohol and meprobamate enhances the depressant action of meprobamate, further impairing the client's performance.

Diphenylmethanes

Diphenhydramine (Benadryl) and hydroxyzine (Vistaril, Atarax) are antihistamines and antianxiety agents with strong sedative action. Diphenhydramine is effective in controlling drug-induced extrapyramidal symptoms, whereas hydroxyzine is useful in treating clients with high levels of anxiety resulting from organic problems or psychoneuroses. These antihistaminic and anticholinergic agents are used for sedative–hypnotic effect. Diphenhydramine, used for its antihistaminic and anticholinergic effect, is discussed in Chapter 41.

Pharmacodynamics. Little is known about the action of these antianxiety agents on the CNS. However, it is thought that a central antimuscarinic action exists for diphenylmethanes. Central nervous system depression decreases tension and produces sedation and muscle relaxation. Tolerance occurs with chronic use.

Therapeutic uses. Diphenylmethanes are used to alleviate anxiety, reduce muscular tension, control drug-induced extrapyramidal reactions, relieve urticaria and pruritus, and promote sedation.

Dosage and administration. Hydroxyzine is given orally or IM in doses ranging from 200 mg to 400 mg daily. Diphenhydramine is given orally in doses of 25–200 mg and IM in doses of 10–50 mg (Table 26-6).

Adverse reactions. Sedation and dry mouth are common side effects; others include drowsiness, ataxia, and thickening of bronchial secretions.

Contraindications. The use of hydroxyzine is contraindicated in early pregnancy.

■ **Summary**

Antianxiety agents (anxiolytics), commonly referred to as *minor tranquilizers*, are used to alleviate moderate anxiety and muscle tension associated with psychoneurotic and psychosomatic conditions. They are not effective for

---

Box 26-5. Conditions for which propanediol compounds are effective

Anxiety and tension states

Psychosomatic disorders

Abnormal fears or phobias

Behavior disorders

Insomnia

Premenstrual tension

Tension headaches

Table 26-6. Antianxiety agents

Drug name	Route of administration	Usual daily dosage (mg)
Benzodiazepines		
alprazolam (Xanax)	Oral	0.75–4 PC: D
chlorazepate (Tranxene)	Oral	15–60 PC: C
chlordiazepoxide (Librium, Libritabs)	Oral, IM, IV	10–100 PC: D
diazepam (Valium)	Oral, IV	5–40 PC: D
halazepam (Paxipam)	Oral	60–160 PC: D
lorazepam (Ativan)	Oral, IM, IV	1–10 PC: D
oxazepam (Serax)	Oral	30–120 PC: C
prazepam (Centrax)	Oral	20–60 PC: C
Propanediol compounds		
meprobamate (Equanil, Miltown)	Oral	1200–2400
Diphenylmethane		
hydroxyzine (vistaril, Atarax)	Oral, IM / Oral	200–400 / 200–400

KEY: PC = pregnancy category risk. (The validity of pregnancy risk categories has not been established. See Chapter 16, p 216.)

psychoses and not recommended for long-term treatment of psychotic states. Tolerance may develop with the use of these drugs, and the possibility exists that withdrawal reactions can occur. Antianxiety drugs are highly effective in conjunction with psychotherapy, although, unfortunately, they are not often used in this way. Drugs used in anxiety treatment include barbiturates, antihistamines, tricyclic depressants, benzodiazepines, and propanediol carbamates. Benzodiazepines are the most widely prescribed drugs on the market today. They are most effective for short-term therapy. Unlike barbiturates, they do not produce as much loss of mental alertness (although this is dose-related) and do not suppress REM sleep. Propanediol compounds have proven effective in alleviating a variety of anxiety and tension states.

Nursing management of clients using antianxiety agents

General nursing management for all psychoactive drugs is discussed at the end of this chapter. Implications specific to antianxiety agents follow.

Nursing process

Assessment Care must be taken in identifying the types and dosages of drugs the client is taking because there is increased sedative effect when antianxiety agents are given with other CNS depressants or antidepressants (MAO inhibitors, tricyclics). It is important to know the client's age because the elderly client may become confused or ataxic when taking the usual or lowered dosages. Other areas of assessment include drug sensitivity or possible dependence. It is also necessary to identify the degree of anxiety.

Nursing diagnosis Possible diagnoses include:

*Altered thought processes: oversedation or confusion related to overmedication or increased sensitivity to drugs secondary to changes of aging
Impaired social interaction related to overmedication and drug dependence*

Planning Goals of nursing care may include decreasing sedation, decreasing dependence, and reducing the severity of adverse drug reactions.

Intervention Close observation in monitoring the sedative effects is maintained. Discuss with the physician the possibility of decreasing the drug dosage if the client is overly drowsy. Observe elderly clients for drowsiness, ataxia, and confusion. Side rails and supervised ambulation may be necessary.

Continue to monitor the client for hypersensitivity and drug dependence. Hypersensitivity is signified by rash, fever, chills, nausea, and vomiting. Signs of dependence are requests for steadily increasing doses of drugs, administration of medication before the prescribed time, and irritability if administration is delayed.

When administering medication, it is important to give parenteral doses exactly as the manufacturer instructs. Despite medication, the highly anxious client may at first remain tense. It is helpful to stay with such clients and encourage them to verbalize their concerns.

Client education. Clients need to be advised about drug regimen and activities while under medication. Clients should be advised to take the medication exactly as prescribed and not to change their drug regimen without consulting the physician. Clients must be warned not to abruptly discontinue medication because that may induce withdrawal symptoms. The nurse should advise clients that antianxiety agents and alcohol taken together seriously impair alertness and may increase the effects of the alcohol. Clients should be advised to take care when operating dangerous machinery, driving a car, or performing tasks requiring fine motor coordination while taking these drugs.

Evaluation Effects of sedation should decrease with fewer complaints of drowsiness noted. Symptoms of anxiety and tension lessen as the drug regimen is followed. There should be no symptoms of dependency or hypersensitivity.

Checklist of nursing actions

☐ Advise clients to take medication as prescribed.

☐ Caution clients about changing their drug regimen without consulting the physician.

☐ Advise clients not to discontinue drugs abruptly.

☐ Advise clients that antianxiety agents and alcohol taken together seriously impair functioning and alertness.

☐ Advise clients to maintain precautions when operating dangerous machinery, driving a car, or performing tasks requiring fine motor coordination while taking these drugs.

☐ Give parenteral doses exactly as instructed by the manufacturer.

☐ Remain with the highly anxious client.

☐ Observe carefully for sedative effects. Excessive drowsiness may necessitate lower doses.

☐ Observe the elderly client for drowsiness, ataxia, and confusion.

☐ Observe for signs of dependency.

☐ Be alert for hypersensitivity.

Antidepressants/mood stabilizers

Depression

Depression, a condition that has plagued people throughout history, is a commonly diagnosed illness, as well as a major health problem. Dissatisfaction resulting from disruptions in daily living and from the negative effects of interpersonal relationships cause many persons to seek medical treatment for depression. Yet, many more individuals with severe symptoms of depression do not seek help. Depression and mania, classified as affective disorders, are characterized by changes in mood and are often accompanied by anxiety. Psychosis, with symptoms of thought disorder and delusions, may also be present. Depression can be classified as endogenous, reactive, or neurotic, also known as a *depressed personality* (Table 26-7). It can be manifested in depressive episodes only or marked by shifts between manic and depressive episodes. Manic–depressive episodes are evidenced by mood swings of a cyclic nature. During the manic phase, speech and body movements accelerate to the point where the person is unable to stop voluntarily. There is an accompanying flight of ideas, grandiosity, and euphoria. Lithium is the preferred drug for treating the manic states, whereas the tricyclic compounds

Table 26-7. Types of depression

Classification	Factors	Symptoms
Endogenous	Internal (psychopathological)	Loss of pleasure
		Loss of appetite
		Suicidal ideation
		Handwringing
		Inability to make decisions
		Pacing
		Psychomotor retardation
		Drooping facial expression
Reactive	External (situational)	Loss of appetite
		Withdrawal—social isolation
		Loss of pleasure
		Psychomotor retardation
		Weeping
		Thoughts focus on the event
		Feelings of loss, grief
Neurotic	Chronic (personality)	Unhappiness
		Dissatisfaction
		Irritability
		Anger
		Negative outlook
		Overreaction to disappointment
		Helplessness
		Low self-esteem

and psychomotor stimulants are prescribed for the depressive states.

Classifications

Endogenous depressions apparently of psychopathologic origin have no clear precipitating factors. These depressions involve an inability to function with occasional hallucinations or delusions. The person in this state usually exhibits readily identifiable symptoms, such as loss of pleasure, loss of appetite, suicidal ideation, hand wringing, inability to make decisions, sleep disturbance, pacing, or psychomotor retardation.

Reactive depressions usually are abnormal depressive responses in a normally functioning person. A clearly defined external cause precipitates the depressive response. Situational stressors, such as loss of a loved one, loss of a job or possessions, or loss of health, give rise to a variety of symptoms associated with depression. Reactive depressions are usually self-limiting.

Neurotic depressions are chronic disorders characterized by low self-esteem, unhappiness, and dissatisfaction with much of life; irritability or anger; a negative outlook; overreaction to disappointments; and feelings of helplessness. Psychotherapy is a necessary adjunct to antidepressant or antianxiety drug therapy in treating attitude and behavior changes.

People suffering from neurotic depressions may exhibit further symptoms of depression—delusions of a self-accusatory nature, apathy, or drooping facial expression. Other symptoms are given in Box 26-6.

Treatment

A variety of methods have been used to alleviate the distress of depression, notably ECT and drugs. Electroconvulsive therapy is still being given to those who do not respond to drug therapy and to those with strong suicidal impulses. Antidepressant agents are referred to by a variety of names: mood elevators, psychomotor stimulants, and psychic energizers. They all exert preferred effects on mood and behavior. Tricyclic and heterocyclic compounds, MAO inhibitors, psychomotor stimulants, and antimanic drugs are the pharmacologic agents used in treating depression. The decision to use an antidepressant depends on the symptoms. Psychomotor stimulants are used for mild depression but have a high potential for abuse.

The first modern antidepressant drug, the hydrazine, iproniazid (Marsilid), was used in 1951. This drug, which had been used previously in the treatment of tuberculosis, induced euphoria in some recipients. By 1957, it was used in treating the mentally ill, producing the added benefits of improved appetite and increased vitality. Since that time, several other related drugs have been synthesized. Prozac, one of the newest drugs on the market, has gained widespread use due to its effectiveness in alleviating depression.

Iproniazid, an MAO inhibitor, prevents serotonin and epinephrine breakdown in the brain by inhibiting the enzyme MAO. As with other psychoactive drugs, the exact action is not understood. However, serious adverse reactions limit its use. In 1957, the first tricyclic drug (Tofranil) was used clinically to treat depression. Continued research into drug action in depression indicates that this syndrome is genetically based. Manic depression is thought to be caused by a gene located on the X-chromosome (This month in mental health, 1987).

Before these drugs were used clinically, convulsive therapy was the usual treatment for depression, using aleptic drugs, insulin, and ECT. Although their exact action is not known, it is thought that these agents disrupt brain patterns, thereby allowing neuronal activity to return to normal. It is believed that a disturbance in the regulation of brain receptors occurs in depression. The antidepressant agents work to change the sensitivity of these receptors.

Tricyclic and heterocyclic antidepressants

Tricyclic antidepressants are similar in structure to phenothiazines. Currently, the drugs of choice for depression, the tricyclic drugs, are effective in endogenous depression. They cause an elevation in mood, an increase in activity and appetite, and improved sleep patterns. During clinical investigation in 1958, imipramine, the prototype tricyclic, was found to be ineffective in quieting agitated psychotic clients. Surprisingly, imipramine was beneficial for some depressed clients. The tricyclics have not been effective in treating agitated depressions. Changes in mood do not occur within the first week of administration; usually 2–4 weeks are required for maximum benefit. Indications point to the fact that 80% or more of depressed clients will eventually recover without treatment.

As the drug becomes effective, the client becomes less self-deprecatory and has fewer psychosomatic complaints; this is followed by increased socialization.

Pharmacodynamics. The tricyclic drugs stimulate the limbic structure. Pharmacologically, they affect the biogenic amines, norepinephrine and serotonin, making them more available yet preventing their resorption into the activating nerve endings. In this way, they increase the action of the neurotransmitters and their resulting excitatory behavior. These agents have anticholinergic effects, creating adverse reactions similar to those of atropine (dry mouth, blurred vision, urinary retention). This antidepressant action on the aminergic systems has led to a strong belief that depression has a biochemical basis. Heterocyclic antidepressants (unicyclic, bicyclic, and tetracyclic compounds) are similar to tricyclic compounds. They block amine absorption and are categorized by the drug's ability to bind to neurotransmitter receptors.

Pharmacokinetics. Because it is rapidly absorbed from the GI tract, oral administration of tricyclics and heterocyclics is preferred. For maximum benefit, the initial dose should be minimal, allowing for a gradual increase. Excretion of these agents is rapid: 70% within the first 72 hours with wide variations depending on the individual metabolism.

Box 26-6. Other manifestations of depression

Loss of interest

Fatigue

Constipation

Guilt

Feelings of inadequacy

Sleep disturbances (insomnia or the desire to sleep most of the time)

Dependence

Sexual disturbances (lower or absent sex drive or impotence)

Amenorrhea

Psychomotor agitation

Therapeutic uses. Tricyclic and heterocyclic drugs have been found effective in the depressive phase of manic-depressive states and in endogenous depressions. They are not effective for agitated depressions and are only somewhat effective for depressive reactions with organic brain syndromes. However, the effectiveness of tricyclic drugs on neurotic depression is limited. They have also been useful for some clients with chronic pain and for some phobic states.

A newer drug, Anafranil, has been proven useful in the management of obsessive-compulsive behaviors. It is questionable whether any of these drugs are useful for the treatment of enuresis in children. Although they act as sedatives, increasing length of sleep periods and decreasing REM time, the use of tricyclic drugs as hypnotics is not recommended. The effectiveness of tricyclics lies in their ability to dull depressive ideation rather than to produce stimulation. Imipramine is effective in relieving the craving for cocaine and in blocking its euphoric effect (Wilbur, 1986, p 42).

Dosage and administration. Various tricyclic antidepressants and doses are given in Table 26-8. Single doses at bedtime have been found effective, although divided doses may be more beneficial for elderly persons, who are more inclined to suffer hypotensive effects. If insomnia occurs due to the mild stimulative effect, the drug should be administered early in the day. The client should remain on this drug regimen for several months because symptoms recur with withdrawal. After 3–6 months of satisfactory behavioral change, the drug should be discontinued. It should be withdrawn gradually to prevent headache, nausea, and vomiting. If an improvement in behavioral responses is not observed within 4 weeks, another tricyclic agent may be tried. If drug therapy does not appear to be alleviating the symptoms of deep depression, some physicians initiate a series of ECT.

Adverse reactions. Although a variety of adverse reactions are common, most are considered minor. The most noticeable are the anticholinergic effects; almost everyone who takes these drugs experiences dry mouth and, paradoxically, excessive perspiration around the head and neck. Blurred vision, constipation, headaches, and urinary retention are commonly observed.

Such cardiovascular effects as postural hypotension, tachycardia, dizziness, and palpitations occur frequently, especially in the elderly and hypersensitive clients. Arrhythmias and heart blocks have occurred in some clients using these drugs. Tricyclics lower the blood pressure and increase the incidence of arrhythmias, possibly due to the high concentrations of norepinephrine in cardiac tissue. The resulting orthostatic hypotension is common.

The tricyclics exert a slight depressant effect on the CNS. Serious reactions, such as confusion, disorientation, delirium, nightmares, numbness, and tremor occur from larger doses, again more frequently in elderly clients. Insomnia sometimes occurs when drug therapy is initiated.

Allergic reactions such as skin rash may occur, making it necessary to discontinue the drug. Petechiae, photosensitivity, and edema have also been observed in some clients. An allergic type of obstructive jaundice may be produced.

Fever and sore throat, indicating possible blood dyscrasias, may occur. Eosinophilia is fairly common, although leukopenia and agranulocytosis occur much less frequently. Gastrointestinal effects, such as nausea, vomiting, anorexia, diarrhea, and epigastric distress, are seen.

Responses of the endocrine system include swelling of the testicles, enlarged breasts, and impotence in men, as well as enlarged breasts and galactorrhea in women. Both men and women may experience changes in libido and in blood sugar levels. Some clients may go from a depressive to a hypomanic state.

Usage during pregnancy is not recommended because the possibility exists for congenital malformation.

Precautions. Because tricyclic antidepressants have significant effects on the cardiovascular system, caution is imperative when prescribing for a client with cardiac disease. There is less concern when using heterocyclics for clients with cardiac disease. As with all antidepressant drugs, the health caregiver should be

Table 26-8. Tricyclic, heterocyclic, and other antidepressants for mood elevation and sedation

Drug name	Routes of administration	Usual daily dosage (mg)
amitriptyline (Elavil, Endep)	Oral, IM	50–300
amoxapine (Asendin)	Oral	150–300
clomipramine (Anafranil)	Oral	25–250
desipramine (Norpramin, Pertofrane)	Oral	50–300
doxepin (Adapin, Sinequan)	Oral	50–300
fluoxetine (Prozac)	Oral	20–60
imipramine (Tofranil, Imavate)	Oral, IM	50–300
maprotiline (Ludiomil)	Oral	75–300
nortriptyline (Aventyl)	Oral	25–100
protriptyline (Vivactil)	Oral	10–60
trazodone (Desyrel)	Oral	150–600
trimipramine (Surmontil)	Oral	75–300

Although administered daily, antidepressant effects may not be observed for 1–3 weeks.

alert for increased risk of suicide as the depressive state alleviates.

Drug interactions. Tricyclic antidepressants are incompatible with some drugs due to their stimulation or inhibition of the liver's metabolic processes. Individual genetic differences may be responsible for these interactions. Other agents enhance or diminish the effectiveness of tricyclic compounds. Drug interactions occur between tricyclic compounds and the following drugs: guanethidine, MAO inhibitors, CNS depressants, thyroid preparations, methylphenidate, phenothiazines, barbiturates, alcohol, and anticholinergics.

Administration of MAO inhibitors and a tricyclic agent concurrently or close together may result in severe reactions, such as convulsions, coma, and hyperpyrexia. Two-week intervals should be allowed between discontinuing an MAO inhibitor and initiating a tricyclic agent. Barbiturates increase the metabolic breakdown, thereby diminishing the therapeutic potential of a tricyclic drug. The antihypertensive effects of guanethidine are blocked. Serious adverse reactions, such as coma, delirium, tachycardia, urinary retention, and hyperpyrexia, have occurred in children receiving a tricyclic agent for enuresis. (See Focus on Tricyclic Antidepressants: Similarities and Differences.)

Monoamine oxidase inhibitors

The MAO inhibitors are second-line agents used in treating depression. The severity of adverse, and sometimes fatal, reactions to them has resulted in some MAO inhibitors being withdrawn from use. However, others have been introduced and remain in use.

Pharmacodynamics. Monoamine oxidase is an enzyme responsible for destroying body chemicals, such as epinephrine, norepinephrine, and serotonin. The MAO inhibitors block oxidative deamination of these naturally occurring monoamines. The resulting central stimulation occurs from this inactivation of the MAO enzyme, thereby increasing psychomotor activity. Anticholinergic effects result in dry mouth and blurred vision. These inhibitors cause the enzyme to become irreversibly inactivated, leading to long-term effects that last until the enzyme regenerates, a process which takes weeks.

Therapeutic uses. Countering depression or causing an elevation in mood, increasing psychomotor activity, and stimulating appetite are the major therapeutic actions of the MAO inhibitors. The MAO inhibitors are most effective in elevating mood, in treating some phobic-anxiety states, and possibly in treating narcolepsy (in other words, in clients with atypical depression).

However, hypomanic or manic reactions may result from the use of an MAO inhibitor. These drugs also suppress REM. Their capacity to prevent the breakdown of serotonin and epinephrine in the brain through inhibition of the MAO enzyme leads to a rise in the cerebral levels of these enzymes.

Because these drugs are potentially toxic, the choice of an MAO inhibitor rather than a tricyclic agent depends on how potential clients have responded previously to these drugs and how reliably they would adhere to a strict drug regimen. Furthermore, it takes weeks before a therapeutic response is noticed. Tricyclic compounds are considered safer for depressive disorders than MAO inhibitors. Tricyclics are often more successful with persons exhibiting vegetative characteristics. The therapeutic response is characterized by latent periods of days or weeks (usually 1–4 weeks) before relief of symptoms is noticed.

Dosage and administration. Monoamine oxidase inhibitors are readily absorbed when given orally. The initial doses should be minimal; gradually, they may be increased to obtain maximum effectiveness. Once this is achieved, the doses may be gradually reduced. It is recommended that the drug regimen be continued for several months after remission of symptoms before gradually discontinuing the drug. These agents may be given in a single dose or in divided dosages. Use of these agents should be limited to a supervised setting to prevent serious adverse reactions. Table 26-9 lists the prominent MAO inhibitors and their daily doses.

Adverse reactions. A number of adverse reactions to MAO inhibitors can occur. Paradoxically, the most dangerous toxic reaction is hypertensive crisis, which is caused by interactions with other drugs, overdosage, and foods containing tyramine. Tyramine is a pressor amine, and the drug-induced lack of MAO in the body prevents destruction of tyramine or other norepinephrine-releasing amines. (See Precautions and contraindications.)

An adverse reaction common to all MAO inhibitors is orthostatic hypotension, indicative of interference with sympathetic venoconstriction. The dizziness and feelings of faintness can be reduced by encouraging the client to remain prone and then to shift position gradually. If this condition persists, it

Table 26-9. Monoamine oxidase inhibitors for delayed action

Drug name	Usual daily dosage (mg)
isocarboxazid (Marplan)	10–30
phenelzine (Nardil)	15–90
trancyclopromine (Parnate)	10–30

Although administered daily, antidepressant effects may not be observed for 1–3 weeks.

Tricyclic antidepressants: similarities and differences

Similarities

Pharmacodynamics

These agents stimulate the limbic structure affecting the biogenic amines, norepinephrine and serotonin, making them more available yet preventing their reabsorption into the activating nerve endings. They are thought to act by inhibiting the reuptake or norepinephrine and serotonin in the CNS nerve endings, resulting in increased concentration and enhanced activity of the neurotransmitters at the synaptic cleft. They also have anticholinergic effects.

Pharmacokinetics

These agents are rapidly and well-absorbed from the GI tract. They are widely distributed to the lung, heart, brain, and liver and breast milk; they are primarily metabolized by the liver and extensively bound to protein. Onset of action is approximately 2–3 weeks. There are wide variations in half-life. They are excreted as metabolites in the urine.

Therapeutic uses

These agents are used to treat major depressive affective (mood) disorders, depression in manic depressive disorders, and endogenous depression.

Adverse reactions

These include: (CNS) dizziness, confusion, drowsiness, disorientation, delirium, nightmares, sedation, insomnia, numbness, tremors; (CV) postural hypotension, tachycardia, palpitations, arrhythmias, heart block, and ECG changes; (EENT) blurred vision, photosensitivity, tinnitus, increased intraocular pressure; (GI) dry mouth, constipation, nausea, vomiting, anorexia, paralytic ileus, epigastric distress, obstructive jaundice; (GU) urinary retention; (ENDO) testicular swelling, breast enlargement, impotence, libido changes, galactorrhea, blood sugar fluctuations; (SKIN) rash, petechiae; (HEMA) blood dyscrasias; (OTHER) edema, fever, sore throat.

Differences

• **Amoxapine, desipramine, trimipramine, nortriptyline, protriptyline** inhibit the reuptake of norepinephrine.
• **Amitriptyline** blocks serotonin. • **Doxepine** is a moderate inhibitor of norepinephrine and a weak inhibitor of serotonin.
• **Maprotiline** does not appear to influence the reuptake of serotonin.

• **Amoxapine** has an onset of 1–2 weeks, peaks in 90 minutes, a plasma half-life of 8 hours with small amounts excreted in feces. • **Nortriptyline** crosses the placenta. • **Amitriptyline** is rapidly absorbed parenterally, peaks in 2–12 hours (PO or IM), with a plasma half-life of 10–50 hours; small amounts are excreted in feces. • **Desipramine** peaks in 4–6 hours, is distributed in breast milk, and has a plasma half-life of 7–60 hours. • **Doxepine** peaks in 2 hours and has a plasma half-life of 6–8 hours. Imipramine peaks in 1–2 hours (PO), 30 minutes (IM), has a plasma half-life of 8–16 hours and is excreted in small amounts in feces. • **Maprotiline** is slowly absorbed from the GI tract, peaks in 8–24 hours (PO), has a plasma half-life averaging 51 hours and is one-third excreted in feces. • **Nortriptyline** peaks in 7–8½ hours, has a plasma half-life of 16–90 hours and excreted in small amounts in feces. • **Protriptyline** peaks in 24–30 hours with very little excreted in feces. • **Trimipramine** peaks in 2 hours (PO) with a plasma half-life of 9 hours.

• **Anafranil** is used in the treatment of obsessive compulsive disorders. • **Imipramine** is used to treat childhood enuresis. • **Amitriptyline, desipramine, doxepine,** and **nortriptyline** are used to treat chronic severe neurogenic pain. • **Amitriptyline** and **desipramine** are used to treat bulimia. • **Doxepine, amitriptyline, trimipramine** are used to treat peptic ulcer disease. • **Desipramine** is used to decrease the cravings and severe depression for cocaine withdrawal. • **Maprotiline** is used to treat depression mixed with anxiety.

• **Protriptyline** has the least sedative effect but the most pronounced effect on the blood pressure and heart. • **Maprotiline** and **amoxapine** can cause seizures.

(continued)

Focus on

Tricyclic antidepressants: similarities and differences (Continued)

Similarities	Differences

Contraindications

These agents are contraindicated in known hypersensitivity, acute recovery of myocardial infarction, persons with coma or severe respiratory depression, or within 14 days of drug therapy with MAO inhibitors.

• **Doxepine** is contraindicated in breast-feeding women and persons with tardive dyskinesias.

Precautions

These agents should be used cautiously in persons with benign prostatic hypertrophy, glaucoma, history of urinary retention, hyperthyroidism, history of seizures, history of cardiac disease, respiratory disorders, scheduled ECT therapy, diabetes, paralytic ileus, hepatic or renal dysfunction, Parkinson's disease, and in those undergoing surgery with general anesthesia.

Some **desipramine** and **imipramine** preparations may contain tartrazine, causing a possible allergic reaction to susceptible individuals.

Nursing considerations

Instruct in disease, treatment regimen, compliance, and signs and symptoms of adverse reactions; assess cardiovascular status, including blood pressure, frequently; instruct clients to avoid activities requiring mental alertness until CNS effects of drug are known; assess neurologic status frequently for changes; institute safety measures and suicide precautions as necessary. Assess for mood changes to monitor drug's effectiveness; gradually withdraw drug to avoid rebound effect; instruct to avoid foods and fluids containing alcohol and to check with physician before taking any over-the-counter drugs; instruct to change positions slowly and dangle before getting out of bed; assist with ambulation as necessary; administer drug with food to minimize GI upset; advise client to avoid excessive exposure to sunlight; offer ice chips, gum, hard candy to alleviate dry mouth; stay with the client and make sure the client has swallowed the drug to prevent hoarding; monitor urinary and bowel elimination; institute measures to alleviate constipation, such as high fiber diet, increased fluids; monitor intake and output; instruct in measures to facilitate voiding; instruct to take full dose at bedtime and warn about the possibility of morning hypotension.

Be aware that **trimipramine's** effectiveness for enuresis may decrease over time. When giving **desipramine**, **doxepine**, **nortriptyline**, or **amitriptyline** for pain, evaluate the effectiveness of pain relief.

---

may be necessary to reduce doses or to discontinue the drug.

Effects on the cardiovascular system result in lower blood pressure. Furthermore, while MAO inhibitors provide relief for angina pectoris by suppressing the warning signal of pain, it is for this same reason that their use is contraindicated for clients with cardiovascular conditions.

Just as many of the psychoactive agents do, MAO inhibitors also cause dry mouth, constipation, difficulty in urination, and confusion. Some men experience delayed ejaculation.

Another adverse reaction is the possible increased risk of suicide. This occurs initially due to the drug's delayed action and later as the depressive state lessens.

Jaundice and leukopenia have occurred in a few clients receiving MAO inhibitors. Because of this possible adverse reaction, extreme care should be taken in prescribing an MAO inhibitor to clients with impaired liver or kidney function.

Toxic reactions due to the cumulative action of MAO inhibitors include agitation, tremor, hallucinations, convulsions, and insomnia. There may be a transition from a depressed to a hypomanic state. Toxic reactions can occur within hours after the drug is ingested.

Precautions and contraindications. Monoamine oxidase inhibitors should be given with caution to clients with kidney dysfunction, cardiovascular disease, pheochromocytoma, and epilepsy; clients who are agitated and overstimulated; and pregnant women.

Monoamine oxidase inhibitors act to store abnormal amounts of norepinephrine in neuronal storage sites, to potentiate the effects of many other drugs, and to lower blood pressure. They also interact with foods or beverages rich in amines, which can lead to hypertensive crises (Table 26-10). Through MAO inhibition, the actions of these amines are potentiated. Tyramine releases the stored catecholamines in nerve endings and, with the already raised level of amines, the pressor responses are effected. There are marked cardiovascular changes with a rise in blood pressure caused by the action of the tyramine.

The most commonly implicated foods and beverages are aged cheeses, red wines, and chicken liver. The interaction between MAO inhibitors and tyramine increases the norepinephrine (a vasoconstrictor) level in the blood. Such foods and beverages should not be ingested for 2–3 weeks after the drug is discontinued. The onset of severe occipital headaches is usually the first indication that a client may be going into a

hypertensive crisis. These headaches may be accompanied by nausea, vomiting, fever, pallor, sweating, pain and rigidity in the neck, elevated blood pressure, photophobia, dilated pupils, and tachycardia or brachycardia. Subsequent intracranial bleeding followed by death can occur. The occurrence of any of these symptoms requires discontinuing the drug immediately and administering intravenously an α-adrenergic blocking agent (Regitine). Such drugs as tricyclic antidepressants, amphetamines, meperidine, methyldopa, and other MAO inhibitors combine with MAO inhibitors to produce a hypertensive crisis.

Drug interactions. Interactions between MAO inhibitors and other drugs may occur through the release of norepinephrine, through altered metabolism of a drug by an MAO inhibitor, or through inhibition of the enzymes that metabolize a drug. Although there are many drugs that interact with MAO inhibitors, few cause severe adverse reactions.

The interaction of MAO inhibitors and tricyclic antidepressants can lead to a hypertensive crisis. Serious adverse reactions resulting in death can occur when these drugs are given concurrently. Two-week intervals should be allowed to elapse between the end of one drug therapy and the initiation of another. However, some researchers report successful combined use of these drugs and believe that the adverse reactions have been overemphasized. The severe atropine-like reactions, convulsions, and hyperpyrexia that have occurred in some clients do justify extreme caution.

Administering combinations of MAO inhibitors can also lead to hypertensive crises or convulsions because each MAO inhibitor potentiates the other. Again, a 2-week interval should elapse between discontinuing one MAO inhibitor and initiating another.

Concurrent use of an MAO inhibitor and methyldopa can result in hallucinations and hypertensive crises. Monoamine oxidase inhibitors potentiate the effects of alcohol, ingesting red wines may lead to a hypertensive crisis; antianxiety agents, enhancing sedative effect; antihistamines, increasing sedative and anticholinergic effects; CNS depressants, causing severe hypotension, coma, muscle twitching, hyperpyrexia; antihypertensives, enhancing hypotension; insulin, potentiating and prolonging hypoglycemia; and amphetamines and sympathomimetic amines, creating a rapid rise in blood pressure, hypertensive response. Concurrent use of an MAO inhibitor and L-dopa may cause transitory elevation of blood pressure.

Administration of an MAO inhibitor with any other agent should be done with extreme care. It should not be given with tricyclic antidepressants, other MAO inhibitors, and certain tyramine-rich foods. (See the accompanying Example of Nursing Process and Imipramine Treatment and Focus on MAO Inhibitors: Similarities and Differences.)

Table 26-10. Common interactions with monoamine oxidase inhibitors

Foods and beverages	Medications
Cheese—aged, especially Cheddar, Gruyere	Diet pills
Wine—especially Chianti	Cold and cough remedies
Beer	Hay fever preparations
Chicken livers	Decongestants
Avocados	Central nervous system depressants
Bananas	Anesthetics
Broad beans	
Pickled herring	
Yogurt	

Example of nursing process and imipramine treatment

Mrs. S., a 52-year-old widow, has been on the nursing unit for 6 days. She expresses a wish to die, saying she "has nothing to live for." She frequently becomes teary but does not cry. Mrs. S. has been observed sitting alone most of the time, staring at the floor. She refuses to participate in unit activities. During mealtimes, Mrs. S. either picks at her food or remains in her room, stating that she is not hungry. Since admission, Mrs. S. has been in imipramine; however, she does not think the medication is helping and would like to stop taking it.

Assessment data	Nursing diagnosis	Interventions	Goals and outcome criteria
Drug history	High risk for self-mutilation related to feelings of depression	**Assess** for suicidal ideation.	Absence of suicide ideation or attempts
Nursing psychosocial history to include family history, mood patterns, suicide assessment, sleep patterns, and nutritional habits	Altered nutrition: less than body requirements related to lack of appetite secondary to depression	**Maintain** suicide precautions.	Outlook brighter, interested in unit activities and participates at least once daily
Physiologic status	High risk for noncompliance related to knowledge deficit concerning imipramine and its slow therapeutic effect	**Administer** imipramine as ordered.	Maintains compliance with drug regimen
Knowledge level of drug actions, effects, and precautionary measures		**Remain** with Mrs. S. to ensure she has swallowed the drug.	Nutritional intake increases
		Monitor BP and pulse.	Verbalizes drug knowledge
		Observe for mood changes.	
		Encourage adequate nutritional intake.	
		Have someone eat with her.	
		Monitor sleep patterns.	
		Discuss with Mrs. S. that it takes several weeks for drug's effectiveness to be felt.	
		Remain supportive and positive about expected mood changes.	
		Educate Mrs. S. about drug actions, effects, precautions, and need for compliance.	

Mood stabilizers

Lithium carbonate

Lithium was first used to treat gout in the mid 1800s, then as a hypnotic in the 1920s, and finally as a salt substitute in 1940. Hazardous results prevented its widespread use until the 1960s when it was introduced as an experimental drug in the United States. During the 1940s, John Code of Australia used it experimentally on laboratory animals; results of this research led him to try it in 1949 on manic persons. By 1970, lithium was widely used to modify the manic and hypomanic behaviors of clients suffering from manic-depressive psychoses.

By controlling the acute symptoms of hyperactivity—flights of ideas, aggressiveness, and decreased sleep time—lithium produces an observable calming effect. In contrast to the antipsychotic agents, lithium does not impair intellectual activity, consciousness, or the quality of emotional life because it does not produce the sedative or euphoric effects of the other psychoactive drugs. Clients who experience frequent alternations between manic and depressive episodes benefit less from this drug than clients who suffer predominantly manic or hypomanic states. About 70%–80% of the latter group are effectively helped.

Currently, lithium is most often the treatment of

MAO inhibitors: similarities and differences

Similarities

Pharmacodynamics

These agents block the oxidative deamination of the enzyme, monoamine oxidase, resulting in increased concentration of neurotransmitters in the storage sites in the CNS. They prevent the inactivation of tyramine resulting in increased release of norepinephrine from sympathetic nerve endings.

Pharmacokinetics

These agents are well absorbed from the GI tract. They are metabolized by the liver. Their onset is from 7 to 10 days but may take 3–4 weeks to achieve a therapeutic effect. Their duration is 10 days. They have a half-life of $2^{1}/_{2}$ hours. Their distribution is unknown and they are excreted in the urine as metabolities.

Therapeutic uses

These agents are used in the symptomatic management of neurotic or atypical depression, in the treatment of phobic and anxiety states, and to elevate mood.

Adverse reactions

These include: (CNS) dizziness, faintness, confusion, increased risk of suicide, headache, agitation, tremors, hallucinations, convulsions and insomnia; (EENT) blurred vision; (CV) hypertensive crisis with tyramine food, orthostatic hypotension; (GI) dry mouth, nausea, vomiting, constipation, anorexia, jaundice; (GU) difficulty urinating; discolored urine, dysuria; (SKIN) rash, purpura, flushing, increased perspiration; (HEMA) leukopenia, agranulocytosis; (ENDO) transient impotence; (OTHER) arthralgia, peripheral edema.

Contraindications

These agents are contraindicated in persons with hypertension, seizure disorders, and known hypersensitivity.

Precautions

These agents should be used cautiously in persons with kidney dysfunction, angina, cardiovascular disease, diabetes, pheochromocytoma, epilepsy, Parkinson's disease, agitated or overstimulated clients, and pregnant women.

Differences

• **Pargyline** inhibits the vasomotor centers, resulting in hypotension. • **Tranylcypromine** produces greater CNS stimulation.

• **Isocarboxazid** peaks in 3–5 hours with some excretion in feces. • **Tranylcypromine** peaks in $1–3^{1}/_{2}$ hours. • **Phenelzine** peaks in 2–4 hours with some excretion in feces.

• **Pargyline** is used to treat moderate to severe hypertension. • **Isocarboxazid** is used to treat severe depression not responsive to ECT therapy.

• **Pargyline** may also cause fluid retention and increased appetite.

• **Pargyline** is contraindicated in pheochromocytoma, cerebrovascular and cardiovascular disease, paranoid schizophrenia, hyperthyroidism, advanced renal failure, persons taking centrally-acting or peripherally-acting sympathomimetic agents, and in persons with labile or malignant hypertension.

• **Pargyline** is contraindicated in persons with seizures, and in persons taking alcohol, barbiturates, sedatives, tranquilizers, narcotics, and dextromethorphan.

(continued)

Focus on

MAO inhibitors: similarities and differences (Continued)

Similarities	Differences
Nursing considerations	

Similarities

Nursing considerations

Instruct client in disease, treatment, regimen, compliance, and signs and symptoms of adverse reactions; assess level of consciousness and neurologic status frequently; monitor vital signs, especially blood pressure and cardiovascular status for changes; advise client to avoid activities requiring alertness until effects of drug are known; stay with the client when giving the drug and make sure he or she swallows it to prevent hoarding; institute suicide precautions as necessary; instruct to avoid beverages containing alcohol and not to take any over-the-counter drugs without the physician's approval; institute safety precautions; encourage client to change positions slowly and to dangle prior to getting out of bed; gradually withdraw the drug and continue precautions for 10–14 days after therapy has stopped; encourage use of identification bracelet stating use of MAO inhibitor therapy; instruct client in foods containing tyramine and explain why avoidance is necessary; supervise diet to restrict tyramine-containing foods; instruct in signs and symptoms of hypertensive crisis and need for immediate medical intervention; monitor urinary and bowel elimination status; monitor intake and output; institute measures to facilitate voiding; instruct client in measures to prevent and relieve constipation; have phentolamine (Regitine) available to counteract severe hypertension if it occurs; assess extremities for signs of peripheral edema; obtain complete blood count and liver functions studies frequently to monitor for changes; do not administer tricyclic and MAO inhibitors together; Separate by at least 2–3 weeks.

Differences

When giving **pargyline**, monitor client's weight for signs of fluid retention; monitor blood pressure while standing; discontinue 2 weeks before any elective surgery; be aware that psychotic symptoms may unmask in persons with preexisting emotional problems; keep in mind that antihypertensive effects may be potentiated by fever and stress. Store **phenelzine** in a tight container away from heat and light.

---

choice for the manic and hypomanic phases of manic-depressive states. When thought disorders are also present, lithium is given in combination with phenothiazine. However, some physicians prefer to try haloperidol initially; if this drug is ineffective, then lithium becomes the drug of choice. Lithium therapy can be carried out over a number of years to maintain a stable behavior state. Differences of opinion, however, do exist about whether it is preferable to use lithium alone as the drug of choice or in conjunction with other agents, such as antipsychotic or antidepressant drugs. In some instances, using lithium with a course of anti-depressants induces a more rapid therapeutic effect. It is believed this occurs because manic behaviors develop from an underlying depression. Some physicians believe that antipsychotics are more effective because they reduce acute symptoms more rapidly. Others prefer to rely solely on lithium or to use it after trying a phenothiazine initially.

Appearance of adverse reactions, fear of toxicity, denial of illness, and enjoyment of feelings of exhilaration during manic episodes have led some clients to refuse lithium therapy or to abandon treatment once they are removed from the treatment setting.

Pharmacodynamics. The specific mechanism of lithium's action in manic-depressive states is not clear, even though definite changes in biochemical, electrolyte, and endocrine functions can be observed. Lithium increases norepinephrine turnover rates in the brain, increases the synthesis of serotonin in the brain, and can replace sodium in the isolated nerve. There is an interference with the action of vasopressin on the nephron, which leads to a diabetes insipidus-like syndrome. Initially, lithium administration leads to diuresis, saluresis, and kaluresis; however, this reverses after 3 days of treatment, and sodium retention reappears. Sodium restriction and diuretics enhance lithium toxicity.

Pharmacokinetics. A peak serum lithium level is reached within 1–4 hours, although a therapeutic behavioral effect does not occur for 7–10 days. Lithium is excreted almost exclusively through the kidneys. A direct relationship exists between sodium intake and lithium excretion. Because a lowered sodium intake slows the excretion of lithium, the resulting accumulation leads to drug toxicity.

Therapeutic uses. Lithium is administered to persons experiencing acute manic and hypomanic attacks. It calms the sufferer and controls acute symptoms of motor hyperactivity, elation, talkativeness, flight of ideas, restlessness, poor judgment, aggressiveness, hostility, and lack of sleep, all of which are characteristic of hypomanic and manic states. Lithium may be administered concurrently with antidepressants to alleviate symptoms of endogenous depression.

Dosage and administration. High solubility in water and rapid absorption make lithium suitable for oral administration. Doses are individualized (higher doses given during acute states) and administered two to three times daily, based on the client's serum level and clinical response (Table 26-11).

Because a narrow margin exists between therapeutic and toxic levels, the serum lithium level must be routinely monitored. Levels between 1.0 mEq and 1.5 mEq/liter are the most effective. Generally, levels are on the higher end during the acute phase and on the lower end during the maintenance phase. When serum lithium levels exceed 1.5 mEq/liter, toxicity usually occurs, making it necessary to discontinue the drug and to resume drug therapy at a lower dose.

Table 26-11. Lithium as an antimanic and mood-stabilizing drug

Drug name	Usual daily dosage (mg)
lithium carbonate (Lithane, Lithonate, Eskalith)	600–1800

Table 26-12. Adverse reactions to lithium therapy

Minor	Moderate	Major
Nausea	Blurred vision	Weight loss
Vomiting	Slurred speech	Marked lethargy
Diarrhea	Tinnitus	Coarse tremors
Fine hand tremors	Abdominal cramps	Muscular twitching
Polyuria	Dizziness	Ataxia
Muscle weakness	Sluggishness	Confusion
Headache		Toxic psychosis
		Convulsions
		Circulatory failure
		Coma

Blood samples should be obtained initially twice weekly, then once weekly during the stabilization phase of therapy, then monthly during maintenance therapy.

Adverse reactions. The severity of adverse reactions depends on the lithium level in the blood. Minor toxic effects occur during the first weeks of lithium therapy, then usually subside. To some clients, the continued fine tremor of the hands can be disconcerting; if they need steady hands, clients may require a muscle relaxant. If the symptom persists, the drug should be discontinued or the dose decreased. A generalized slowing of the electroencephalogram and a tendency toward normalized sleep occurs during lithium administration, usually within 24 hours. Lithium suppresses REM, increases cortisol excretion, modifies aldosterone excretion, and lowers protein-bound iodine.

Thyroid disorders (goiter and hypothyroidism) have been reported in some clients, prompting treatment with small doses of thyroid. This may be a result of the lithium ion blocking active transport of iodine. It has been suggested that this occurs only in those clients with a family history of thyroid disease (Vogel, 1986, p 9).

Weight gain may occur but can be controlled with a low-calorie diet containing sodium (2 + g daily). However, too much sodium interferes with treatment and has been observed to increase manic activity.

Toxic effects of lithium therapy are listed in Table 26-12. Toxic symptoms in the early stages can be reversed by lowering the dose of lithium or by promptly discontinuing the drug and by restoring the fluid and electrolyte balance.

Early symptoms of toxicity include nausea, vomiting, diarrhea, abdominal cramps, muscle weakness, polyuria, and thirst. If the drug dose is not lowered at this time, toxicity increases, causing blurred vision, slurred speech, tinnitus, coarse tremor, and muscle twitching. Convulsions, coma, and death can occur from the severe electrolyte imbalance.

Major toxic effects necessitate immediately discontinuing the drug. Because the onset of toxicity is gradual, and a small margin exists between therapeutic and toxic doses, close monitoring for symptoms is necessary. Maintaining a proper fluid and electrolyte balance helps to reverse toxic symptoms. Measures to increase lithium excretion are necessary. However, there is no specific antidote for severe toxicity.

Precautions and contraindications. As with other psychoactive drugs, lithium is not recommended for use during pregnancy. Again, the risk of usage must be weighed against the severity of the symptomatology. Lithium administration is contraindicated or used with extreme caution in clients with impaired renal function, congestive heart failure, sodium-restricted diets, organic brain disease, and impaired CNS functioning and in pregnant women. Close evaluation is indicated for clients with thyroid disorders, cardiovascular disease, and diabetes mellitus.

During pregnancy renal clearance tends to rise. This may show up later in the lithium level of breast-fed babies. There have also been reported cases of congenital malformation of infants born to lithium-treated mothers.

A diabetes insipidus-like syndrome of thirst and polyuria may persist throughout the course of lithium therapy.

Drug interactions. Diuretics should not be given in conjunction with lithium therapy because the fluid and sodium depletion greatly increases the possibility of lithium toxicity.

Phenothiazines are used in conjunction with lithium when there is impairment of thought processes with delusions or hallucinations. However, some of these antipsychotic agents block the nausea that indicates the onset of toxicity.

One study demonstrated that lithium enhanced the effect of tricyclic antidepressants in endogenous depressions.

Iodine and lithium given concurrently may act synergistically to produce a hypothyroid effect. Steroids may produce electrolyte imbalance.

Learning experience 26-1

While caring for a depressed client, determine which of the three classes of depression the client is experiencing. Identify drugs used in the treatment of this type of depression. What drugs have been prescribed for this client? What therapeutic effects are expected? For what adverse reactions should you watch?

■ **Summary**

Depression is a major health problem; it is the most commonly diagnosed illness today. Depression and mania, classified as affective disorders, are characterized by changes in a person's mood. Depression can be classified as endogenous, reactive, or neurotic. It can manifest itself by depressive episodes only or by shifts between manic and depressive episodes. Antidepressant drugs do not treat the underlying causes of depression but merely provide relief from its symptoms.

Nursing management of clients using antidepressants

General nursing management for all psychoactive drugs is discussed at the end of this chapter. The information here pertains to antidepressant agents.

Nursing process

Assessment Before antidepressant drug therapy is initiated, the client should be evaluated for emotional status, particularly suicidal ideation and depth of depression. Fluid and electrolyte status and vital signs, particularly blood pressure should also be assessed. Clients should be screened for risk factors for adverse reaction to antidepressant drugs, including hypotension or hypertension, impaired glucose metabolism (diabetes mellitus or reactive hypoglycemia), habitual use of alcohol, predisposition to thyroid disease, constipation or urinary retention, and predisposition to conditions such as asthma or congestive heart failure that normally require treatment with drugs that increase the risk of adverse reaction to antidepressants. A complete drug history should be taken.

Baseline data to be recorded include weight, blood pressure, and diet (particularly fluid, sodium, and fiber intake).

Nursing diagnosis Nursing diagnoses might include the following:

High risk for self-mutilation related to depression and to increased energy levels secondary to antidepressant medication
High risk for fluid volume excess related to sodium and fluid retention secondary to lithium therapy
High risk for infection related to bone marrow depression secondary to antidepressant medication
High risk for injury related to postural hypotension secondary to antidepressant therapy
Knowledge deficit concerning antidepressant drugs and their use

A common collaborative problem that should be differentiated from the nursing diagnoses is

Potential complication: hypertensive crisis

Planning Goals of nursing care are specific to the nursing diagnoses and the individual client. They may include reduction in the risk of accidental or self-injury, maintenance of normal tissue perfusion, reduction in the risk of adverse drug reaction such as agranulocytosis or hypertensive crisis, and education of the client regarding the therapeutic regimen.

Intervention Tricyclics and MAO inhibitors should generally not be administered together; they must be given 2–3 weeks apart. Some clients may require doses of medication earlier in the day to decrease the possibility of insomnia. Others benefit from the sedative effect by taking the entire dose at bedtime to assist in sleeping. If dry mouth is a problem, ice chips, hard candies, gum, frequent sips of liquids, and frequent mouth rinsing will reduce the discomfort. One of the important tasks for a nurse of depressed persons is to be alert for suicide attempts. The nurse should watch for risk of suicide throughout therapy because symptoms of potential suicide may be masked. The danger of suicide increases as clients' depressive states lift and their energy increases.

Other assessments and observations must be made while clients are taking antidepressant medications. Clients should be monitored for signs and symptoms of adverse reaction specific to the drug used for treatment. Weight, fluid intake and output, and fecal elimination should be assessed regularly. Signs and symptoms of intercurrent illness should be carefully evaluated in relation to the drug regimen; blood counts should be ordered if infection develops. If skin rashes occur, the drug may have to be discontinued. Elderly clients, who are especially prone to orthostatic hypotension, may experience this adverse effect. If so, they may require side rails and assistance with ambulation. Monitoring of blood pressure and pulse for hypotension or hypertension, tachycardia, or possible arrhythmias is necessary.

Care with MAO inhibitors. Headaches and elevated blood pressure must be promptly reported because these may signify a hypertensive crisis. Regitine should be kept available in case this occurs. The diabetic client must be observed for hypoglycemia when on MAO inhibitor therapy.

Care with lithium administration. Lithium levels should be monitored carefully. Transient symptoms of nausea, tremor, diarrhea, thirst, and polyuria may appear when lithium therapy is initiated but usually rapidly diminish or disappear. At this point, the client should be monitored closely to determine whether the symptoms are early signs of toxicity or merely transient.

Because of lithium's action, which alters sodium transport in nerve and muscle cells, a client taking lithium must maintain a normal intake of salt and water and should not take diuretics concurrently with lithium. The client must be observed for signs of restlessness and insomnia. When these occur, the dose may need to be increased. Dosage is also adjusted on the basis of normalization in sleep patterns.

Client education. It is very important that clients taking antidepressant medication and their families receive instruction about these drugs and their use. First, the client should be advised to take the medication as prescribed. Withdrawal symptoms of headache and nausea can occur if the drug is stopped abruptly. Clients and their families should be advised that it takes 2–4 weeks for a therapeutic response. Alcohol is not to be used with antidepressant drugs because antidepressants potentiate the effects of alcohol. The client should also be cautioned not to drive a car or operate dangerous machinery if drowsiness occurs. Advise clients that orthostatic hypotension can be reduced if they rise slowly and change positions gradually, sitting on the edge of the bed for a few minutes before standing. Tell them that elderly persons are especially prone to this reaction when taking antidepressants.

Education about MAO inhibitors. Because MAO inhibitors are toxic, the advice you give clients and their families is important. Diet should be carefully supervised. Tyramine-rich foods, such as aged cheeses and chicken livers, and alcohol, such as Chianti wines, must be restricted. Write out a list of foods and beverages to be avoided and instruct the client to tape it to the refrigerator at home. Be sure that the family understands the serious consequences of giving the client tyramine-rich foods; family members must refrain from bringing such foods into the hospital if the client is hospitalized. Two to three weeks should elapse between discontinuing the drug and ingesting these foods. The client must be cautioned not to take cough medicine and cold preparations while on MAO inhibitors. Keep an accurate drug profile of prescribed medication and over-the-counter drugs that the client may use.

Education about lithium medication. The client's diet must be supervised to ensure adequate salt and fluid intake. Advise clients and their families that they must include an adequate amount of salt in the diet. Crash diets and fasting lead to sodium depletion and must be avoided. The nurse should discuss with the client and family the symptoms of lithium toxicity (drowsiness, diarrhea, confusion, vomiting, muscle weakness, ataxia) and the need to discontinue the drug and notify the physician immediately if these symptoms occur. The need for regular testing of serum levels should be stressed.

Any physical illness should be reported to the physician promptly. Caution clients not to change their drug therapy, and discuss the need with clients for maintaining the lithium level in the blood even after they feel better. Doses should not be increased by the client because the margin between the toxicity level and therapeutic level is very small. Increased sodium loss through increased sweating or any condition where sodium depletion occurs entails an adjustment of dosage.

Taking lithium with meals controls nausea. Pregnant women should not breast-feed because toxicity develops in the infant through ingesting the milk.

Evaluation Data required for evaluation relate to specific goals and include affect (a lessening of depression should occur within 2–4 weeks of therapy); behavior (manic behavior should decrease); absence or occurrence of adverse drug reaction; the ability of the client to manage the drug regimen; and client compliance with the treatment regimen (drug dosages, dietary restrictions, and laboratory tests).

Checklist of nursing actions

☐ Monitor for suicidal risk throughout the therapy, particularly on emergence from depression.
☐ Advise the client to rise slowly and change positions gradually, sitting on the edge of the bed for a few minutes before standing.
☐ Check for urinary retention or constipation and take necessary action.
☐ Check for fever and sore throat. If these are present, order blood counts.
☐ Observe for skin rashes.
☐ Check weight for gain or loss.
☐ Use ice chips, hard candies, gum, frequent sips of liquids, and frequent mouth rinsing to alleviate dry mouth.
☐ Do not administer tricyclics and MAO inhibitors together. They must be given 2–3 weeks apart.
☐ Give doses earlier in the day if insomnia is a problem.
☐ Advise the client to take the medication as prescribed.
☐ Advise the client and family that a therapeutic response takes 2–4 weeks.
☐ Caution client not to use alcohol with antidepressant drugs.
☐ Caution client not to drive a car or to operate dangerous machinery if drowsiness occurs.
☐ Monitor and accurately record normalization of sleep patterns.

With MAO inhibitors

☐ Supervise the client's diet. Restrict tyramine-rich foods and alcohol.

☐ Be sure the family understands the consequences of the diet.
☐ Caution the client not to take cough and cold preparations with MAO inhibitors.
☐ Keep an accurate drug profile of prescribed and over-the-counter drugs.
☐ Promptly report headaches and elevated blood pressure. Regitine should be kept available for hypertensive crises.
☐ Observe the diabetic client for hypoglycemia.

With lithium therapy

☐ Supervise the client's diet to ensure adequate salt and fluid intake.
☐ Advise clients and their families that it is necessary to provide adequate salt intake in the diet.
☐ Do not give diuretics concurrently with lithium.
☐ Discuss the symptoms of lithium toxicity, and advise clients to discontinue the drug and notify their physician immediately if they occur.
☐ Discuss with clients the need for regular testing of serum levels.
☐ Notify the physician of any physical illness.
☐ Observe for signs of restlessness and insomnia.
☐ Caution clients not to make any changes in drug therapy.
☐ Discuss the need to maintain the lithium level in the blood even after the client feels better.
☐ Caution the client not to increase doses.
☐ Advise pregnant women not to breast-feed.
☐ Advise the client to take lithium with meals to control nausea.

Anticholinergics/ antiparkinsonian agents

Although there are many drugs available for treating parkinsonism, only those synthetic anticholinergic agents that are used to alleviate the drug-induced extrapyramidal reactions to antipsychotic drugs will be considered here. The other anticholinergic agents are effective in treating parkinsonism but ineffective in relieving drug-induced extrapyramidal reactions.

Symptoms of drug-induced parkinsonism

Clinically, the symptoms of drug-induced parkinsonism are similar to the symptoms of Parkinson's disease. They include muscle rigidity, slow movement, a shuffling gait, pill-rolling tremor, and drooling. These reactions are reversible when treated with antiparkinsonian agents. Other extrapyramidal reactions of akathisia, akinesia, and dyskinesia are also controlled by the antiparkinsonian agents. However, persistent tardive dyskinesia, usually appearing late in drug therapy and more often in the elderly, may become irreversible even after the antipsychotic agent is discontinued. Tardive dyskinesias are not controlled by antiparkinsonian agents. Early signs of tardive dyskinesia (facial tics, chewing, rocking, swaying, and oral or ocular movements) indicate a necessity to discontinue antipsychotic drug therapy while it is still possible to reverse these symptoms.

Development of antiparkinsonian agents

Antiparkinsonian agents were developed in response to a need for a drug that would produce fewer disturbing side effects than those drugs currently in use—the belladonna alkaloids (atropine and scopolamine) and related agents. Research led to the development of L-dopa. However, L-dopa is not effective in treating the extrapyramidal reactions produced by antipsychotic agents. Further research led to the development of the synthetic anticholinergics in current use. Benadryl, an antihistamine, is also an effective antiparkinsonian agent, especially in elderly persons, because it is less likely to produce mental confusion.

The antiparkinsonian agents are not intended for prolonged use. They are sometimes prescribed prophylactically with antipsychotic drugs or only after extrapyramidal symptoms appear. Difficulty arises when antipsychotic and antiparkinsonian agents are given concurrently before extrapyramidal symptoms occur because the more disturbing symptoms may be masked. Antiparkinsonian agents alleviate these disturbing extrapyramidal symptoms, and as the symptoms decrease or disappear, the drugs can be withdrawn. Once these agents have been withdrawn, the symptoms usually do not recur. Only a small percentage of the clients taking an antiparkinsonian agent requires continued treatment with the drug after the initial symptoms disappear.

Pharmacodynamics. The anticholinergic action results from partial blockade of the cholinergic receptors, lowering the excitation of the cholinergic pathways, which arises when the inhibitory control of the dopaminergic pathways is blocked. Depression of the synaptic transmission occurs in the CNS. These agents, which also make more of the dopamine transmitter available to receptors, are anticholinergics, smooth muscle relaxants, and antihistamines. They relieve the spasticity of voluntary muscles by acting on the cerebral motor center.

Pharmacokinetics. Antiparkinsonian agents are well absorbed from the GI tract, making them suitable for oral administration.

Therapeutic uses. Antiparkinsonian agents, which are short-term muscle relaxants, reduce rigidity and tremors. These agents are used to control extrapyramidal effects caused by antipsychotic agents and to treat parkinsonism by relieving spasms, tremors, rigidity, akinesia, and akathisia. Their effectiveness in

dyskinesia is increased if the symptoms are treated early.

Dosage and administration. Drug therapy consists of small doses divided throughout the day. Some clients may tolerate one drug better than another (Table 26-13). Depending on the drug, the dosage, and the client, relief from the extrapyramidal symptoms may occur within a few hours.

Adverse reactions. All of these drugs provoke similar adverse reactions: dry mouth, blurred vision, urinary disturbances, and dizziness. In addition, there is the probability of constipation, fecal impaction, increased ocular tension, tachycardia, dilated pupils, nausea, suppression of perspiration, and nervousness. The antiparkinsonian agent benztropine, given in small doses, may cause or aggravate glaucoma due to its ability to produce mydriasis. Overdoses of trihexyphenidyl, biperiden, and procyclidine cause cerebral excitement, hallucinations, and delirium. Large doses may produce CNS symptoms of mental confusion, delirium, hallucinations, and ataxia.

Contraindications. These drugs should not be given to clients with glaucoma or prostatic hypertrophy.

Drug interactions. Concurrent administration of antiparkinsonian agents, tricyclic antidepressants, and antipsychotic agents can lead to additive effects and increased extrapyramidal symptoms. MAO inhibitors potentiate the antiparkinsonian drugs, intensifying tremors.

■ Summary

The symptoms of drug-induced parkinsonism are similar to the symptoms of Parkinson's disease. Research for an antiparkinsonian agent led to the development of L-dopa. However, L-dopa is not effective in treating the extrapyramidal reactions produced by antipsychotic agents. Further research led to the synthetic anticholinergics now in use. Antiparkinsonian agents are muscle relaxants not intended for long-term use. They may be prescribed along with antipsychotic drugs or only after extrapyramidal symptoms appear.

Table 26-13. Antiparkinsonian agents

Drug name	Routes of administration	Usual daily dosage (mg)
benztropine (Cogentin)	Oral, IM, IV	0.5–6
biperiden (Akineton)	Oral, IM, IV	2–8
procyclidine (Kemadrin)	Oral	6–15
trihexyphenidyl (Artane)	Oral	5–15

Nursing management of clients using antiparkinsonian agents

General information pertaining to all psychoactive drugs follows this section. The information given here concerns nursing care of clients receiving antiparkinsonian agents.

Nursing process

Assessment A nursing history should include past responses to drug therapy, blood pressure reading, elimination patterns, diagnosis of glaucoma or prostate problems, or visual disturbances.

Nursing diagnosis Possible diagnoses would be

> Constipation, colonic, related to side effects of drug therapy
> Altered comfort: thirst, decreased secretions secondary to anticholinergic medication
> High risk for injury related to falls due to dizziness and blurred vision secondary to anticholinergic medication
> Knowledge deficit concerning the drug regimen

Planning Goals for nursing care would include alleviation of constipation and thirst, prevention of injury, and an increase in the client's knowledge about the drug regimen.

Intervention The client must be monitored for blood pressure and urinary and bowel habits. Because hypotension may occur, monitoring blood pressure is important. Record fluid intake and output. Urinary hesitancy or retention may occur; constipation and fecal impaction commonly occur. High-residue diet, increased fluid intake, and laxatives may be necessary. Dry mouth can be alleviated with ice chips, hard candies, gum, frequent sips of fluid, and frequent rinsing of the mouth. If dizziness or blurred vision occur, side rails may be necessary, and the client may require supervised ambulation. Visual changes should be reported because the drug can increase intraocular pressure.

Client education. Caution the client to exercise care when driving a car or operating dangerous machinery while on antiparkinsonian medication.

A teaching plan to prevent further problems with elimination would include dietary changes and an increase in fluid intake.

Evaluation Extrapyramidal symptoms should decrease or disappear. Elimination patterns should return to normal and dietary changes should be maintained.

Checklist of nursing actions

- ☐ Monitor blood pressure for hypotension.
- ☐ Monitor fluid intake and output.
- ☐ Monitor bowel habits for constipation and fecal impaction. A high-residue diet, laxatives, and increased fluid intake may be necessary.
- ☐ If dizziness or blurred vision occur, use side rails and supervise ambulation.
- ☐ Alleviate dry mouth with ice chips, hard candies, gum, frequent sips of fluid, and frequent rinsing of the mouth.
- ☐ Caution client about driving a car or operating dangerous machinery.

Nursing management related to all psychoactive drugs

Nursing implications

Successful drug therapy for the mentally ill calls for accurate diagnosis, knowledge of the drug's effects and drug interactions, sensitivity in interpersonal relations, and an understanding of underlying psychodynamics. Psychiatric diagnoses are often arbitrary in spite of efforts toward accurate diagnostic classification. As a result, a neurosis can be as incapacitating as a psychosis or more so. Drug therapy, therefore, usually is based on the drug's effect on presenting symptoms. After the psychotic responses are alleviated with drug therapy, a client is more likely to benefit from various psychotherapies.

Although there has been some controversy about whether time, itself, is the significant healing factor, occasionally it is not feasible to initiate psychotherapy with acutely psychotic clients until their symptoms have been alleviated by drug therapy. It is important for you as a nurse to understand a drug's action, interaction, adverse reactions, doses, contraindications, and desired effects before administering any psychoactive agent. If it is an unfamiliar or infrequently used drug, take the short time that it requires to familiarize yourself with the drug; this caution may well prevent hazardous consequences. Because you initiate and maintain drug therapy, it is necessary for you to understand the rationale for the drug regimen, as well as to obtain an accurate nursing history.

As with any drug therapy, you must be knowledgeable and accurate about drug doses, routes of administration, drug actions, and drug effects. This, however, is only a small part of drug therapy. Quite often the administration of drugs is carried out by health care personnel other than professional nurses. Where this occurs, you will function in a supervisory or coordinating capacity while maintaining responsibility for proper administration. Beyond the administration of the drug and observation of effect, you will provide client education, an ongoing evaluation of the drug regimen, and clear communication (orally and written) of significant information. These functions remain the same whether you serve the public in the community or in a private facility.

Nursing process

Assessment Evaluation of drug therapy begins with your initial contact with the clients and continues through their discharge from an inpatient facility or their supervision in the community. Since the effects of drug therapy are often individualized, it is important for you as the nurse to know not only the drug actions but the client. This enables you to compare correctly the client's past and present behavior with the possible expected effects of the drug on current and future behavior.

Drug profile and nursing history. Client needs in drug therapy are varied and individualized. You can gain an understanding of these needs through the compilation of a drug profile and a nursing history. This information would include data from the identified client, the client's family and friends, health team members, old records, and community agencies.

When gathering information for a drug profile, ask about drugs taken in the past, as well as those being taken currently (both over-the-counter and prescription drugs). Furthermore, it is necessary to know what effect such drugs have had, the client's reasons for taking them, how long they have been taken, and when (if at all) they were discontinued. Information should be elicited from the client or the family about their knowledge of the drug's desired effects and possible adverse reactions; the client's medication schedule (times taken during the day and regularity of schedule); doses or number of pills taken; the client's activity level; and ways of coping with alterations in the drug schedule (forgetting a pill, increasing the number taken). Organizing all of this data on one form helps you to identify readily any potential or actual problems with cross-medication (some of the psychoactive drugs take several weeks to leave the system) or with hypersensitivity.

Drug interactions. Initiating a new drug regimen before the old drug has left the system could precipitate a hazardous reaction, such as convulsions or circulatory collapse. There is always the possibility that one drug could counteract the effects of another, creating cross-tolerance or potentiating the effects of another with fatal consequences. Extreme caution should be taken with the client who uses alcohol, barbiturates, or antihypertensives, or who has a history of seizures.

Alcohol. There is a wide variation in the amount of alcohol that must be ingested before adverse reactions occur. It has been found that drug interactions occur not only in the heavy drinker but also in the recovering or dry alcoholic. The client with a history of past or present alcohol abuse must be closely monitored for CNS depression, profound vasodilation (tachycardia, palpitations, facial flushing, dysphoria), hypotension, anticoagulation effects, convulsions, and toxic manifestations of impaired liver function. With the parallel increase in the use of alcohol and drugs, the number of accidental and suicidal deaths related to combining alcohol and drugs is approximately 20% (US Dept HEW Public Health Service, 1979). Information on the drinking habits of a client should include the type of alcohol consumed because Chianti and beer, which contain tyramine, interact with MAO inhibitors to produce a hypertensive crisis.

Diet. Another influence on drug therapy is the client's dietary habits. The chemical components of particular foods, such as cheeses containing tyramine (Gouda, Stilton, Cheddar, & Limburger), interact with the psychoactive drugs with hazardous effects (hypertensive crises). It has been found that tyramine releases norepinephrine, which, in turn, raises blood pressure and increases peripheral vascular resistance.

Further assessments. In assessing the client's mental and emotional state, the nurse gains insight into the client's ability to comprehend what is being communicated, the client's ability to communicate directly and accurately, the client's attitude toward drug therapy, the family's involvement, and the client's capacity for self-medication. Further data required for assessing the client's needs include sleep patterns, sexual habits, and mental and emotional status.

Nursing diagnosis Because of the highly individualized responses to the drug therapy, diagnoses can be varied. Possible nursing diagnoses would include the following:

> *High risk for injury related to sedation,*
> *postural hypotension, or weakness secondary*
> *to medication*
> *High risk for altered thought process:*
> *confusion related to interactions between*
> *medications*
> *Noncompliance related to knowledge deficit*
> *concerning medication regimen*
> *Ineffective management of therapeutic*
> *regimen related to knowledge deficit, mistrust*
> *of regimen and/or health care personnel, and*
> *lack of perceived benefits*

Planning A plan of action would include the goals of minimizing adverse effects and maximizing drug effectiveness and client education.

Intervention Although it may take weeks to effect a therapeutic response, other segments of the CNS are more quickly affected, producing common adverse reactions before the alleviation of behavioral symptoms. There are serious adverse reactions and contraindications for all of the psychoactive drugs but this does not mean that with careful monitoring some drug regimens should not be initiated and effectively maintained.

Consequently, it is important to monitor the type of drug given to the client, the doses, the mode of administration, and the client's need for antiparkinsonian agents. Especially close monitoring is necessary for clients with diabetes, cardiac problems, liver impairment, epilepsy, respiratory problems, and suicidal impulses, and for pregnant women. Consideration must be given when treating elderly persons, debilitated persons, and children. The recommended lower doses for elderly persons and the doses computed by body weight for children should be strictly followed.

Accurate recording. Finally, it is necessary to record accurately drug administration, refused or missed dosages (with the reason), and specific observed behaviors. This should be done as soon after drug administration as possible.

Attitude of the care giver. Promoting a supportive environment that enhances drug therapy and allows for growth of a working nurse-client relationship is necessary. Until more definitive evidence is found about psychiatric treatment, we must continue to treat the mentally ill client holistically, that is, we must be cognizant of environmental, interpersonal, sociocultural, and physiologic differences.

Moreover, the influence of the care giver cannot be overemphasized. It has been found that the way the client perceives the care giver can either promote or detract from the total therapy. This makes it necessary for nurses to understand their own attitudes toward the drug regimen and toward the client. A positive attitude enhances the effectiveness of the drug regimen. Are we as accepting of every client for whom we care, whether child molester, drug or alcohol abuser, or client who attempted suicide? Do we view drug therapy as the last resort or the initial step? In administering a medication, do we give it as a punishment, a bribe, or to make our job easier? Do we view the client as an active participant in drug therapy? Through a positive attitude and knowledge of the drug therapy, the client, and ourselves, the effectiveness of drug therapy can be increased. Medications are no substitute for excellent nursing care.

Client education. A major part of psychiatric drug therapy is client education, which adds to the effectiveness of the drug regimen. Education of the client begins with the administration of the initial drug dose and continues throughout the course of the therapy. More than one session is necessary to ensure that the client understands. The instruction can be given formally or informally, in groups or individually. Some agencies have found it beneficial to hold regular drug information classes for clients. Additional help can be given in the form of clearly written, easily understood instructions. The more knowledgeable clients are about the drug therapy, the more apt they are to comply with a drug regimen. In many instances, drug education will include family members, who often supervise drug administration in the home (Boxes 26-7 and 26-8).

Diet planning. Through knowledge of the client's customary diet, the nurse and the client together can compile a list of foods to be avoided and a list of permissible foods to avoid some of the adverse reactions of psychoactive drugs. With a knowledge of the client's dietary habits and an understanding of the drug action, it is easier to plan a diet that will relieve other distressing reactions, such as constipation, hyperglycemia, hypoglycemia, or headaches. We are only beginning to understand the effect of diet on drug therapy and behavior.

Compliance. Noncompliance is a major problem with the psychiatric client. There are many reasons behind noncompliance (Box 26-9). The client may be refusing to take a drug for secondary gains, or as a means of getting attention or even displacing other issues onto the drug therapy, such as difficulty in relating to authority figures. Noncompliance may be related to the size, odor, or lasting taste of drugs or to a fear of injections.

Whatever the reason for a client's noncompliance, you must remain supportive, encouraging the client to talk about concerns. Listening to the client's concerns and educating the client about drug therapy enhances drug effectiveness. Every client should know the name of the drug being taken, the dose, a desirable time schedule; the desired effects and possible adverse reactions; the length of time required for the drug's action to take effect; the impact of the drug on daily activities; how to adjust for missed doses; the necessity of monitoring vital signs and blood levels; contraindi-

---

Box 26-7. Information every client should know about a prescribed drug

- Name of the drug being taken
- Dose
- Desirable time schedule
- Desired effects and possible adverse reactions
- Length of time required for the action to take effect
- Impact on daily activities
- How to adjust for missed doses
- Necessity of monitoring vital signs and blood levels
- Drugs and foods that are contraindicated
- Measures to take if adverse reactions or toxicity occur

Box 26-8. Points to remember in drug therapy with the mentally or emotionally distressed client

- Heavy use of psychoactive drugs is of recent origin, although use of behavior-modifying drugs is centuries old.
- The complex actions of these drugs on the human system are not fully understood.
- Drug therapy is most useful in conjunction with other therapies when treating psychiatric disorders.
- Difficulties arising from drug therapy include distressing adverse reactions, contraindications, adjusting doses to the individual client, cross-medication, interactions with food and alcohol, noncompliance, and differences in the attitudes and values of the client, family, and health care providers.
- Clients should actively participate in their drug therapy.
- Whether administering or supervising the administration of medications, the nurse is responsible for the implementation of the drug regimen. This means that the nurse must continually assess and evaluate the behavioral and physical responses of the client, including the resulting decision either to administer or to withhold the drug.
- Complete nursing histories and drug profiles should be maintained for every client receiving drug therapy.
- Knowledge of the pharmacologic properties and actions of every drug given by the nurse is essential.
- A major function of the nurse in drug therapy is client education.
- The nurse is responsible for conveying accurate, clear information orally and in writing to other health team members.

Box 26-9. Reasons for noncompliance

- Lack of understanding and motivation
- Denial of illness and the limitations it imposes
- Fear of the unknown
- Values
- Disorientation or impaired intellectual ability
- Means to an end
- Dislike or fear of medication in general

cated drugs and foods; and measures to take should adverse reactions or toxicity occur.

It is unrealistic to keep such information from the client under the rationale that it might be harmful, when it could prevent overdoses, discontinuance, and hazards due to cross-medication. The knowledgeable client is more likely to adhere to the drug regimen.

Noncompliance occurs within the treatment facility, as well as within the community. Within the facility, the client may refuse a medication (every client has this right), exchange medications with other clients, hide the medication in the cheek or under the tongue only to spit the medication out when the nurse leaves, or acquire a supply of pills for future use.

Direct administration of psychoactive drugs enables you, the nurse to verify if clients have swallowed their pills. This may be the only way to ensure greater compliance within the confines of the facility but this does not prepare the clients for their return to the community. There are many more people living in the community who are on psychoactive drugs than who remain in the hospital.

Early drug education and client involvement in the drug therapy has far broader consequences for effective drug therapy. Preparing the client for self-medication and all of its ramifications early in the treatment can decrease the rate of noncompliance and can enable you to determine if the client and the family will possibly sabotage the drug therapy. Changing to long-range injectables can alleviate this problem. Being alert to toxicity, adverse reactions, and contraindications encourages the client to seek out health team members for possible changes in doses, other drugs, or discontinuance of drug therapy for a period of time.

Evaluation Data required for evaluation relate to the goals of nursing care and include physical and behavioral reactions and signs and symptoms of adverse drug reactions.

References

Vogel P. (1986). Lithium and the thyroid. *J Psychosoc Nurs Ment Health Serv*, 24(2), 9.

Wilbur R. (1986). A drug to fight cocaine. *Science*, 86(March), 42.

Drugs affecting the cardiovascular system

6

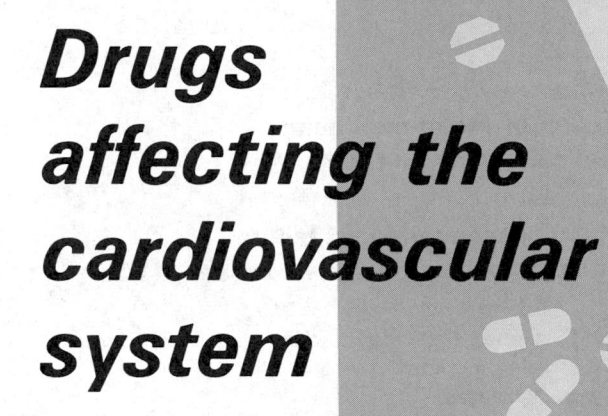

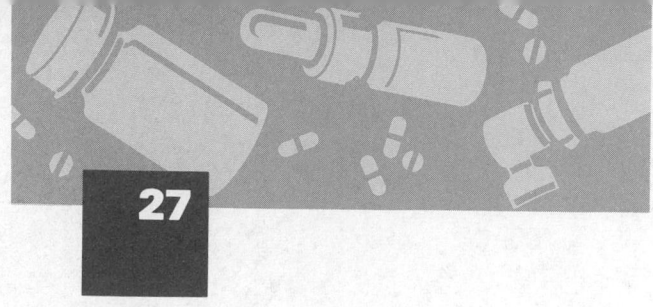

27

Cardiac drugs

Physiology of the heart

The heart is a muscular pump whose function is to move blood through the vascular system. Circulating blood provides the cells of the body with oxygen, nutrients, and other chemicals essential to their continued life and function. The blood also carries away the waste products of cell metabolism. As the moving force behind circulation, the heart is vital to life.

Although subject to the influence of autonomic nerves, hormones, and other control systems of the body, the heart is designed to perform its function consistently, efficiently, and independently, if necessary, for years without respite. This is fortunate; cessation of circulation for even a few minutes causes immediate and widespread cell death. Absence of cardiac function has long been a criterion for death. It is only in recent years, with the development of heart-lung machines capable of maintaining tissue perfusion, that we have been able to sustain life temporarily while the heart is nonfunctioning. These machines enable surgeons to perform open heart surgery and heart transplants. Extracorporeal perfusion is required for the performance of these and other procedures.

Function of the normal heart

The heart is really two pumps in one that function side-by-side (Fig. 27-1). The right side receives blood from the peripheral body and pumps it into the lungs where its carbon dioxide is exchanged for fresh supplies of oxygen. This blood then enters the left side of the heart, which propels it through the peripheral vascular system to nourish the cells of the body.

Each side of the heart is, itself, two pumping chambers: an atrium and a ventricle. To move blood most effectively, these chambers must function out of phase with each other. Both atria contract while the ventricles are relaxed, allowing blood to flow freely and rapidly from the upper chambers to the lower. When the ventricles contract, the atria are relaxed and filling with blood. The maintenance of this complex, rhythmic pumping pattern without cessation, weakening, or desynchronization depends upon a unique system for periodic stimulation of muscle contraction.

Cardiac tissue differs from other muscles in its automaticity or ability to generate spontaneous impulses. Because the cell membranes are more permeable to sodium than are other muscle cells, sodium leaks gradually across the membrane, triggering impulses at periodic intervals. The rate at which this occurs differs from one area to another in the heart and is most rapid in the specialized conduction tissues. Because all cardiac muscle fibers respond to each stimulus, and each impulse is followed by a refractory period (during which the muscle fibers are unable to respond to stimuli), heart rate is controlled by the tissue with the most rapid rate of spontaneous impulse

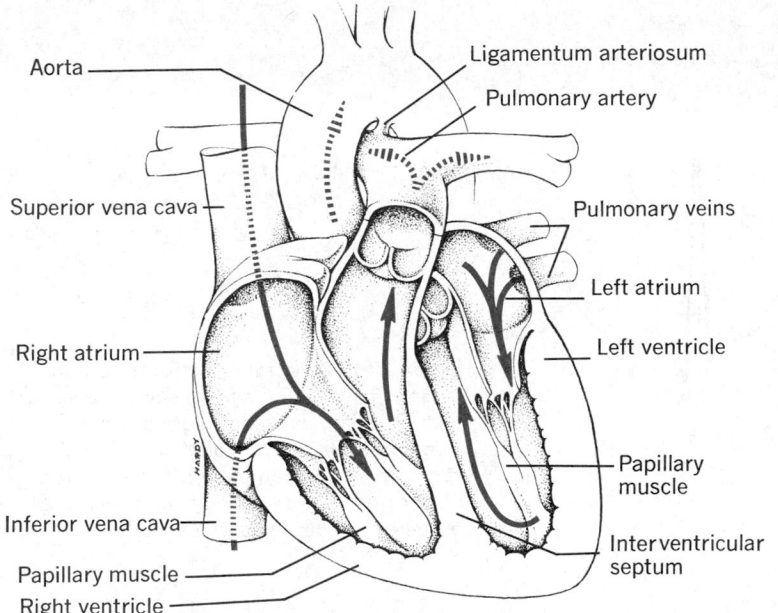

Figure 27-1. The heart, and the direction of pumped blood.

Labels on figure:
- Aorta
- Ligamentum arteriosum
- Pulmonary artery
- Superior vena cava
- Pulmonary veins
- Left atrium
- Left ventricle
- Right atrium
- Papillary muscle
- Inferior vena cava
- Interventricular septum
- Papillary muscle
- Right ventricle

formation. This normally is the sinoatrial (SA) node with a rate of 50 or more per minute. Each impulse from this pacemaker spreads throughout the atria and to the atrioventricular (AV) node. Atrial contraction occurs almost immediately.

At the AV node, the impulse is first delayed briefly and then transmitted down the bundle of His and Purkinje fibers to the muscles of the ventricle. Ventricular contraction follows. This sequence allows for alternating atrial and ventricular contraction, the most effective pattern for pumping. The electric changes occurring during impulse transmission can be recorded graphically by electrocardiogram (ECG) tracings (Fig. 27-2).

Should initiation and conduction of the impulse fail to occur in the expected pattern, the automaticity of the rest of the conduction system provides a measure of safety. If a stimulus is not received by the AV node, spontaneous impulses will develop in this tissue with subsequent ventricular contraction. The new (nodal) rate will be slower than normal sinus rhythm. Cardiac function will be sustained but at the slower rate (30–40 per minute), which is characteristic of ventricular automaticity. Should the AV node not function properly, bundle fibers can initiate impulses. Even cardiac cells outside the specialized conduction tissue can initiate stimuli, especially when they are injured or otherwise irritated.

Chemical effects on the heart

Cardiac muscle contraction is influenced by the nature of the chemical changes that occur upon impulse transmission. At the time of stimulation, sodium ions flow across the cell membrane into the cell. They are accompanied by an influx of calcium ions, which increase the force and duration of contraction of the myofibril. A rise in calcium levels in the body favors this mechanism and is accompanied by more forceful and prolonged contraction during systole. Very high levels of the electrolyte can cause *calcium rigor*, a sustained cardiac contraction. The effect of calcium is opposed by that of potassium whose concentration is directly related to the degree and duration of relaxation during diastole. A balance of the two electrolytes is required for normal alternations in contraction and relaxation. Other chemicals affecting cardiac action include central nervous system (CNS) depressants and cholinergic drugs, which slow the heart, and stimulants, sympathomimetic agents, and anticholinergics, which accelerate it.

Direct effects upon the heart are of three general types: 1) inotropic, affecting the strength of contraction of cardiac muscle; 2) chronotropic, affecting the rate of contraction; and 3) dromotropic, affecting conductivity of cardiac tissue. Each can be influenced positively or negatively. Thus, a positive inotropic agent increases the strength of cardiac contraction, whereas a negative dromotropic would reduce conductivity (Box 27-1).

Cardiotonics

A number of natural glycosides share a specific and powerful action on the myocardium that increases the force of contractility. The chemicals are found in plants such as foxglove, sea onion, and lily of the valley. They are also present in the tissues of certain toads. Crude preparations that contain cardiac glycosides have a long history of use as poisons and medicines by populations familiar with their properties. They were used as arrow and ordeal poisons by natives in various parts of the world. For centuries, the Chinese have

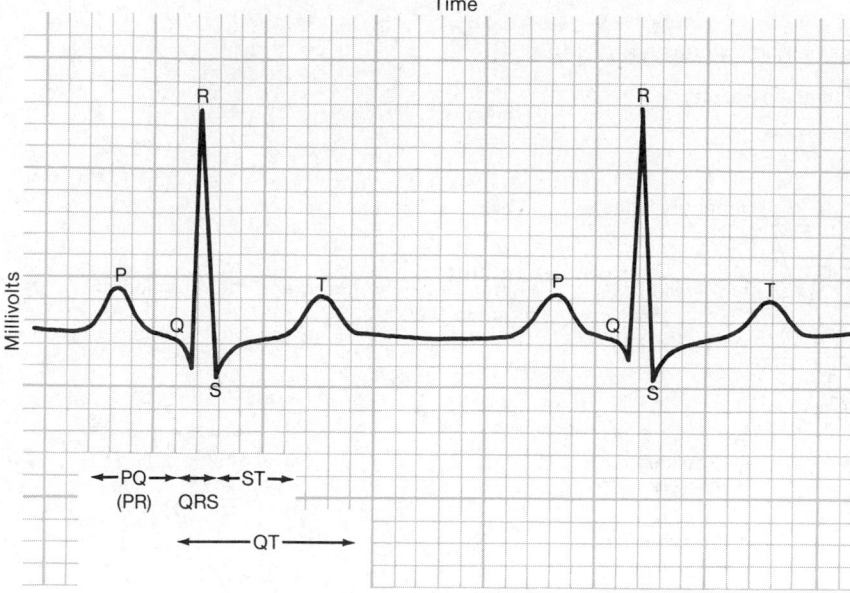

Time

Millivolts

Figure 27-2. A normal electrocardiogram tracing. The electric changes associated with atrial repolarization normally coincide with the QRS complex and are obscured by it. The amplitude and direction of tracings vary depending on placement of the electrodes for various leads.

Key:

Each vertical square represents one tenth of a millivolt of electrical charge

Each horizontal square equals 0.04 seconds of time.

Approximate values for normal intervals:

PQ(PR) interval—0.16 sec.
QT interval—0.3 sec.
QRS interval—0.08 sec.
P wave—0.08 sec.
ST interval—0.1 sec.

P wave = Electrical changes associated with atrial depolarization
QRS Complex = Electrical changes associated with ventricular depolarization
T wave = Electrical changes associated with ventricular repolarization
The electrical changes associated with atrial repolarization normally coincide with the QRS complex and are obscured by it.

used diced toad skin as a drug. Squill, a derivative of sea onion, was used as a medicine by both the Egyptians and the Romans.

More recently, the active principle in foxglove, digitalis, has been widely used for the treatment of cardiac problems by physicians practicing Western medicine. In 1783, the properties of foxglove and its uses in edema were described in the book *An Account of the Foxglove and Some of Its Uses: With Practical Remarks on Dropsy and Other Diseases.* Its author, William Withering (1977), recognized the cardiac effects of digitalis but considered these to be secondary in importance to its diuretic action. Although the primary nature of its cardiac actions was soon recognized, digitalis was not

employed rationally for many decades. Rather, it was administered indiscriminately, often in toxic doses, to treat many disorders. In the present century, the efficacy of digitalis for the treatment of congestive heart failure has been established as its main therapeutic value. Because of the high incidence of cardiac disease in the aging populations of developed countries, derivatives of digitalis are among the most frequently prescribed drugs.

Pathophysiology of heart failure

Failure of the heart to pump sufficient volumes of blood to meet the body's needs triggers a series of events that produce the characteristic symptoms of congestive heart failure. A loss of functioning myocardial tissue, disruptions of rhythmic patterns, or fatigue from long periods of excessive workloads can impair the heart's ability to pump blood. Weak, ineffective cardiac contractions fail to empty the chambers completely. During subsequent cycles, the chambers overfill, causing dilation. This stretches the myofibril, causing stronger contractions in accordance with Starling's law. The effect is temporary, and the cycle tends to be repetitive, resulting in progressive dilation. When heart muscle becomes unduly stretched, contraction becomes weaker, and cardiac output drops markedly. Circulatory stasis develops with congestion

Box 27-1. Types of chemical effects on the heart

Inotropic: affect the strength of contraction of cardiac muscle

Chronotropic: affect the rate of contraction of cardiac muscle

Dromotropic: affect the conductivity of cardiac tissue

in both peripheral and pulmonary circulation. Because of an increase in stress and a tendency toward hypotension, body mechanisms that increase blood volume through sodium and water retention are activated. This increases circulatory congestion. The affected person develops symptoms of peripheral and pulmonary edema (swelling of dependent tissues, moist respirations, cough productive of frothy sputum, and dyspnea).

Cardiac glycosides in the treatment of heart failure

The administration of cardiac glycosides strengthens the force and prolongs the duration of cardiac contraction. Cardiac output increases and tissue perfusion improves. In addition, the effects of the drugs promote recovery of the ailing heart by various secondary mechanisms. Improved blood supply to the kidneys increases their ability to excrete water and salts. This diuretic effect is enhanced by a reduction of the compensatory mechanisms that favor sodium and water retention. By reducing blood volume, diuresis reduces peripheral resistance, further improving cardiac output. In addition, the drugs improve coronary circulation, inhibit responsivity to ectopic stimuli within the heart, and tend to eliminate premature contractions. Enhancement of perfusion reduces the general level of stress by improving the function of other body organs impaired by congestion.

Each of the cardiac glycosides has a chemical structure consisting of a sugar, a steroid, and a five- or six-member lactone ring (Fig. 27-1).

Variations in the sugar, lactone, or side groups attached to various carbon atoms in the steroid structure alter the drug's chemical and physical properties. Although a large number of compounds with cardiotonic properties have been produced, only a few are customarily used in clinical practice (Table 27-1).

Pharmacodynamics. The exact mode of action of cardiac glycosides is not known. At the molecular level, these drugs are believed to increase the influx of calcium ions across the membrane of the stimulated myocardial cell. They also inhibit adenosine triphosphate, a chemical involved in the active transport of sodium and potassium ions during repolarization of nerve and muscle cell membranes. These effects alter the electrochemical properties of myocardium, influencing contractility, conduction, and automaticity.

The main therapeutic effect of the cardiac glycosides is the increase in the force and velocity of myocardial systolic contraction (positive inotropic effect). In persons with failing hearts, this improves the pumping efficiency of the heart, resulting in increased cardiac output, more complete emptying of the cardiac chambers, and a reduction in elevated ventricular end-diastolic pressure and venous pressures. As peripheral (including kidney) perfusion improves, diuresis occurs. Thus, the cardiac glycosides tend to correct the basic cause of congestive failure and ameliorate the signs and symptoms of this condition.

The cardiac glycosides have a negative chronotropic action. The reduction in heart rate derives largely from vagal reflexes initiated by the carotid baroreceptors in response to increased systolic pressure. This effect is enhanced by direct actions of the drugs—a reduction in the positive chronotropic action of catecholamines and an enhancement of the SA response to acetylcholine.

Other cardiac effects of the glycosides include a decrease in conduction velocity (a negative dromotropic effect) and an increase in automaticity. Refractory periods may be increased or decreased, depending on the area of myocardium involved.

Pharmacokinetics. Gastrointestinal (GI) absorption of cardiac glycosides varies with the polarity* of the drugs. Relatively nonpolar compounds (*eg*, digitoxin) are completely absorbed. Digoxin, which is more polar than digitoxin, is less completely absorbed. The extent of absorption varies greatly from one manufacturer's preparation to another. Deslanoside, even more polar than digoxin, is poorly absorbed after oral administration and is administered only parenterally. Binding by plasma proteins also varies with polarity with more polar compounds being less bound than nonpolar drugs. At therapeutic plasma concentration, digitoxin is 97% protein bound, and digoxin is 20%–30% protein bound.

Cardiac glycosides are widely distributed in body tissues. Concentrations are highest in the heart, kidneys, intestine, stomach, liver, and skeletal muscle; lowest concentrations are in the plasma and brain. The drugs cross the placenta and are distributed in breast milk.

Metabolism varies with polarity. Highly polar glycosides (*eg*, digoxin and deslanoside) are not metabolized appreciably; less polar compounds such as digitoxin are extensively metabolized by the liver. Excretion is primarily by the kidneys but some glycosides

---

* Polar drugs are those having electrical charges on the molecule. Although the molecule as a whole is electrically neutral (because the number of negative and positive charges are equal), one or more sites on it will exhibit a negative charge while one or more others are positively charged.

Table 27-1. Comparison of cardiac glycosides

Drug name	Preparations	Loading dose*	Maintenance dose	Onset of action	Maximal effect	Elimination	Therapeutic plasma concentration
deslanoside (Cedilanid-D)	Solution for IM and IV injection	Adults: 1.6 mg, divided in 1–2 doses (maximum digitalizing dose: 2 mg)	Not used for maintenance	*IV:* 10 min *IM:* 30 min	*IV:* 20 min–4 hr	20%/d (renal) $t_{1/2}$ = 33–36 hr	Unknown
digoxin (Lanoxin, Lanoxicaps)	Tablets, capsules, and elixir for oral use; Solution for IM and IV injection	*Oral tablets and elixir:* Premature neonates: 20–30 µg/kg body weight; Full-term neonates: 25–35 µg/kg body weight; Infants, 1–24 mo of age: 35–60 µg/kg body weight; Children, 2–5 yr of age: 30–40 µg/kg body weight; Children, 5–10 yr of age: 20–35 µg/kg body weight; Adults and children older than 10 yr of age: 10–15 µg/kg body weight. *Liquid-filled oral capsules:* Children, 2–5 yr of age: 25–35 µg/kg body weight; Children, 5–10 yr of age: 15–30 µg/kg body weight; Adults and children older than 10 yr of age: 8–12 µg/kg body weight	*Oral tablets and elixir:* Premature neonates: 20–30% of oral loading dose. All others: 25–35% of oral loading dose	0.5–2 hr	6–8 hr	30%/d (renal) $t_{1/2}$ = 34–44 hr	0.5 ng–2.0 ng/ml (>2 ng/ml are usually considered toxic)

Drug	Preparations	Dosage	Onset	Peak	Maintenance	Excretion	Serum levels
digitoxin	IV solutions	Premature neonates: 15–25 μg/kg body weight					
		Full-term neonates: 20–30 μg/kg body weight					
		Infants, 1–24 mo of age: 30–50 μg/kg body weight					
		Children, 2–5 yr of age: 25–35 μg/kg body weight					
		Children, 5–10 yr of age: 15–30 μg/kg body weight					
		Adults and children older than 10 yr of age: 8–12 μg/kg body weight					
	Oral tablets						
	Solutions for IM or IV injection	Premature and full-term neonates: 22 μg/kg body weight, or 300–350 μg/m², infants, 2 wk–1 yr of age: 45 μg/kg body weight	30 min–2 hr	4–12 hr	10% of total digitalizing dose	10%/day (hepatorenal) $t_{1/2}$ = 5–7 days	20 ng–35 ng/ml (>40–45 ng/ml are usually considered toxic)
		Children, 1–2 yr of age: 40 μg/kg body weight					
		Children, 2–12 yr of age: 30 μg/kg body weight, or 750 μg/m²					
		Adults and children, 12 yr of age and older: 1.2–1.6 mg					
ouabain (G-Strophanthin)	Solution for IV injection	Adults: 0.25–1 mg	3–10 min	½–2 hr	Not used for maintenance	50%/d (renal) $t_{1/2}$ = 1 day	
gitalin (Gitaligin)	Oral tablets	Adults: 5–6 mg			0.25–1.25 mg		
digitalis (Digifortis, Digiglusin)	Powder Oral tablets and capsules	Adults: 1.2–1.8 g	30 min–2 hr	12–20 hr	100 mg (1 USP digitalis unit)	Therapeutic effects persist 2–3 wk after withdrawal of the drug	

*Total loading doses are divided and fractional doses administered q4h–q12h during the first 24 hour of treatment.

and their metabolites are excreted in the feces. Cardiac glycosides are not removed by dialysis.

Plasma concentrations of cardiac glycosides are helpful but not absolute indicators of therapeutic and toxic effects of the drugs. Individual response to a given concentration is influenced by serum electrolytes (particularly potassium, calcium, and magnesium), acid-base balance, nature of the cardiac disorder, thyroid status, autonomic nervous system activity, and other drugs administered concurrently. For example, both quinidine and verapamil increase serum digoxin concentration and may precipitate toxic reactions; hypokalemia increases the toxic potential of a given drug level; clients with supraventricular tachycardias (atrial fibrillation or atrial flutter) may require higher plasma concentrations than do clients with heart failure; infants appear to require higher plasma concentrations than do adults.

Dosage and administration

Loading doses. If a prompt response to cardiac glycosides is desired, the initial doses must usually be several times the magnitude of those required for maintenance. Tissue depots (plasma proteins and other body tissues) must be saturated before therapeutic serum concentrations of the drugs are stabilized. Such accelerated dosage regimens are termed *digitalization.*

Loading doses in a given situation vary depending on the age, body size, and medical condition of the recipient, and the particular glycoside and route of administration chosen (Table 27-1). The dose is usually divided and administered over a period of about 24 hours (usually every 6 hours). Clients who are not acutely ill may receive intermediate doses (more than maintenance doses but below the usual digitalizing doses) over 1 or 2 weeks to gradually establish therapeutic plasma levels.

Rapid digitalization is best accomplished in a controlled environment with facilities for continuous assessment of cardiac function and prompt treatment of serious cardiac arrhythmias. Intravenous (IV) administration, which may be required in serious failure, is particularly hazardous. These clients are usually admitted to special coronary care hospital units and placed on cardiac monitors.

Maintenance doses. Maintenance doses are proportional to the daily losses from metabolism or excretion. They are relatively high for the glycosides that are eliminated by the kidneys (if the client has normal renal function) because approximately one-third of the drug is excreted in the urine daily. Digitoxin is metabolized more slowly in the liver; its maintenance dose is only about one-tenth of the loading dose. Renal or liver impairment will slow elimination of certain drugs and requires reduction of the maintenance dose. Because it is not eliminated by the kidneys, digitoxin may be the drug of choice for clients with renal disease; agents excreted through the kidneys are preferable for persons with hepatic impairment. Most children require proportionately higher doses of the cardiac glycosides—up to 50% more than adults according to weight. Premature and immature infants are very sensitive and require reduced dosages.

Digitalis has been said to be a cumulative drug (*ie,* one with a tendency to increase in concentration and cause toxicity). The drug is probably no more likely to accumulate in body tissues than many other substances with long half-lives (*eg,* digoxin $t_{1/2} = 36$ hours; digitoxin $t_{1/2} = 136$ hours) that are bound by the tissues. Thus, it can take 1 week or longer to reach steady-state conditions with digoxin and 4 weeks or longer with digitoxin. Whether the concentration of a chemical increases or decreases is determined by the relation of the maintenance dose to the rate of elimination from the body. Because of its narrow safety margin, however, digitalis causes toxic symptoms with only slight excesses above the therapeutic range. Drifts toward higher concentrations are poorly tolerated and hence are potentially dangerous.

Therapeutic uses. Cardiac glycosides are the drugs of choice for the treatment and prevention of heart failure.

They are also used with clients with certain atrial arrhythmias, such as atrial fibrillation and atrial flutter. Atrial arrhythmias, characterized by rapid or chaotic transmission of impulses, subject the ventricles to excessive stimulation. Ventricular rates increase and filling time is markedly reduced. Only small amounts of blood are ejected with each ventricular contraction; cardiac output drops despite the great number of contractions. Clients with these arrhythmias are at risk for heart failure because of the reduced efficiency of cardiac function. By inhibiting the conductivity of the heart, the cardiac glycosides reduce the number of impulses that reach the ventricles and slow the rate of ventricular contraction. This prolongs diastole, improves ventricular filling, and increases cardiac output.

Adverse reactions. Cardiac glycosides are toxic. The minute size of harmful doses makes them some of the most poisonous substances known. Moreover, the therapeutic margin of safety is narrow. Therapeutic doses are fully 50%–60% of toxic doses. So close are toxic to therapeutic doses that, historically, loading (digitalization) was accomplished by giving large doses until toxic symptoms appeared, whereupon doses were reduced to a maintenance level. More careful control of initial doses and frequent monitoring of plasma concentrations have reduced, but not eliminated, the frequency of toxicity.

There are few nontoxic side effects of cardiac glycosides. The drugs are irritating to tissue and cause nausea when administered orally. They are rarely injected intramuscularly because pain, muscle fasciculation, and necrosis can occur at the injection site.

Most adverse reactions to cardiac glycosides are symptoms of toxicity (Box 27-2). Their appearance indicates the need for a careful appraisal for overdose and possible reduction of dose. Toxic symptoms include bradycardia (apical rate of less than 60/min in adults); tachycardia, which is rare (apical rate greater than 100/mm in adults); and symptoms of CNS dysfunction: nausea, anorexia, vomiting, headache, fatigue, malaise, disorientation, confusion, aphasia, delirium, and seizures. Changes in the level of consciousness may produce drowsiness or restlessness and nervous irritability. Changes in vision include some effects that are unique to these drugs. Yellow and green color perception may be abnormal; white halos or outlines might be seen around objects. Diplopia and scotomata also occur. If toxicity is allowed to progress,

various arrhythmias could develop including premature ventricular contractions, bundle branch block, complete heart block, and tachycardia. Ventricular fibrillation can also occur. Toxicity is most likely in elderly persons and in persons with a tendency toward hypokalemia, hypomagnesemia, hypercalcemia, hypoxia, and acid-base imbalances.

The symptoms of toxicity of the cardiac glycosides resemble those of the heart conditions for which they are prescribed. Differentiation of the two requires careful assessment. A comparison of serum glycoside with the usual therapeutic range is sometimes helpful but can be misleading because physiologic response to the drugs can be excessive when serum levels are not. The best diagnostic tool is the ECG, which graphically reveals the electric changes in the myocardium throughout the cardiac cycle. Therapeutic levels of digitalis tend to alter certain segments of the ECG; they narrow the QRS complex, depress or invert the T waves, and slow the heart rate (Fig. 27-3). With increasing drug effects, the P-R interval is prolonged and the Q-T interval is shortened. Large doses produce altered P waves.

Drug interactions. Digoxin interacts with many drugs (Table 27-2). Drugs that decrease absorption of digoxin when they are given concurrently include antacids, antidiarrheals, and ion-exchange resins. By decreasing absorption, the effectiveness of the digoxin is decreased. In a study with antacids, magnesium trisilicate, magnesium hydroxide, and aluminum hydroxide all reduced digoxin bioavailability. One small study showed a decrease in bioavailability of digoxin tablets but not digoxin capsules. It is felt that spacing the doses to minimize mixing in the GI tract (about 2 hours

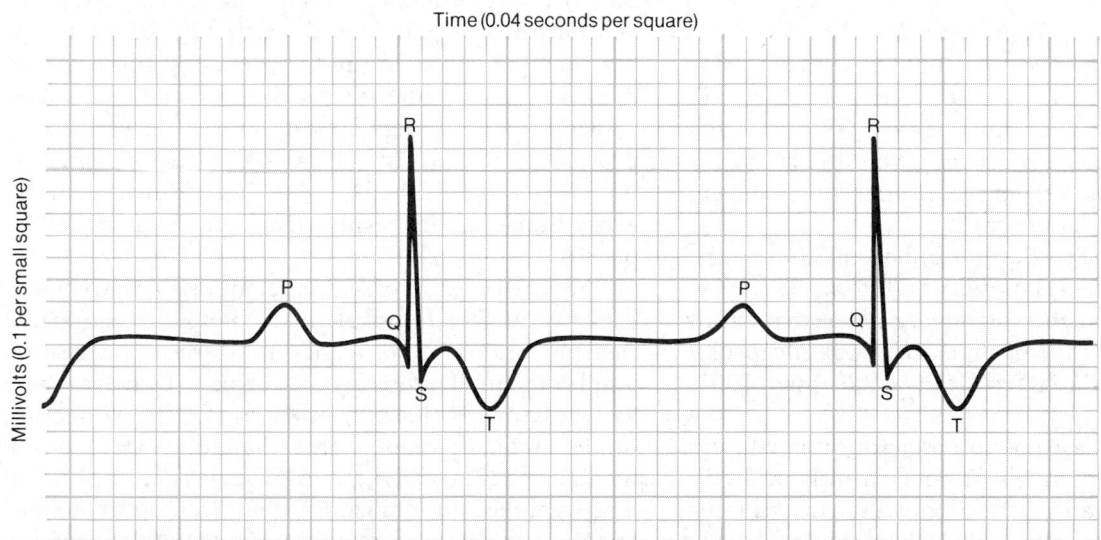

Figure 27-3. A typical electrocardiogram in therapeutic digitalization. In comparison with the normal electrocardiogram (Fig. 27-2), the tracing in digitalized patients is likely to show a prolonged P–R interval, a shortened Q–T interval, and T wave inversion.

Table 27-2. Selected drug interactions involving digoxin

Agent	Mechanism of action	Result
antacids	Decrease GI absorption	Decreased digoxin effect
kaolin-pectin	Decrease GI absorption	Decreased digoxin effect
cholestyramine	Decrease GI absorption	Decreased digoxin effect
metoclopramide	Decrease GI absorption	Decreased digoxin effect
propantheline	Increase GI absorption	Increased digoxin effect
calcium	Calcium action on myocardium	Increased digoxin effect
thiazide and loop diuretics	Cause hypokalemia	Increased digoxin effect
amphotercin B, corticosteroids	Cause hypokalemia	Increased O_2 effect
quinidine	Displacement of digoxin from tissue-binding sites, decrease renal clearance	Increased digoxin effect
barbiturates	Enzyme induction, enhanced metabolism	Decreased digoxin effect
erythromycin	Enzyme inhibition	Increased digoxin effect
spironolactone	Decrease renal clearance	Altered digoxin effect
amiloride	Increase renal clearance	Altered digoxin effect
thyroid preparations	Change renal clearance of digoxin	Increased or decreased digoxin effect
verapamil	Decrease renal clearance	Increased digoxin effect

apart) may reduce the inhibitory effect of antacids on digoxin absorption. The use of digoxin capsules may also be indicated.

Kaolin-pectin (Kaopectate) appears to produce a reduction in the bioavailability of digoxin tablets by inhibiting absorption but digoxin capsules do not appear to be affected. If kaolin-pectin must be used, it should be given 2 hours after the digoxin tablets.

Cholestyramine, and possibly colestipol, appears to reduce the serum concentrations of digitoxin by binding digitoxin in the gut, thus interrupting the enterohepatic circulation of the digitoxin and shortening its half-life. Giving the digitalis product 1–2 hours before the cholestyramine may lessen the magnitude of the interaction.

Metoclopramide, which increases GI motility, has been shown to reduce serum digoxin concentration when it is coadministered with slowly dissolving digoxin tablets. Absorption may be decreased. It is felt that this interaction can probably be minimized by the use of rapidly dissolving digoxin preparations, such as Lanoxin tablets or Lanoxicaps.

Propantheline (Pro-Banthine) has anticholinergic activity and decreases GI motility and stomach-emptying rate. It has been shown to increase absorption of slowly dissolving brands of digoxin. Digoxin capsules do not appear to be affected (Hansten & Horn, 1991, p 288).

Drugs that increase the potential for dysrhythmias and bradycardia when given concurrently with digoxin include beta-adrenergic blockers, calcium salts, thyroid preparations, and succinylcholine.

Parenteral calcium generally should be avoided in clients receiving digitalis glycosides, because it may precipitate cardiac arrhythmias in such clients. The calcium ion and digitalis have some similar effects on the myocardium. The positive inotropic effect of digitalis is probably mediated via an effect on calcium.

In the hypothyroid client, the half-life of digoxin is prolonged, while in the hyperthyroid client, it is shortened. These changes appear to be due to an enhancement of renal clearance in the hyperthyroid individual and a diminished clearance in the hypothyroid individual (Craig & Stitzel, 1990, p 318).

Cardiac arrhythmias have occurred following the administration of succinylcholine to fully digitalized clients. One manufacturer of succinylcholine states it should not be used in digitalized clients unless absolutely necessary. Succinylcholine appears to potentiate the cardiac conduction effects of digitalis preparations and may produce increased ventricular irritability. It has been proposed, but not proven, that this is due to the effect on cholinergic receptors that release catecholamines. Also, depolarizing muscle relaxants may produce a sudden shift of potassium from inside the muscle cell to outside. In the digitalized myocardium, arrhythmias could result (Hansten & Horn, 1991, p 289).

Some drugs increase the potential for digoxin toxicity by causing hypokalemia. These drugs include thiazide and loop diuretics that waste potassium, amphotericin B, and corticosteroids. Diuretics such as furosemide (Lasix), ethacrynic acid (Edecrin), bumetanide (Bumex), chlorthalidone (Hygroton), metolazone (Zaroxolyn), and thiazides are implicated. The magnesium deficiency that can occur following diuretic therapy may also contribute to digoxin toxicity.

Other drugs that increase the potential for digoxin toxicity include quinidine and erythromycin. The quinidine–digoxin interaction may be the single most important interaction involving digoxin. If the client with atrial fibrillation does not respond satisfactorily to digoxin, quinidine has often been added. Unfortunately, this combination can result in a marked increase in toxicity to digoxin because quinidine administration raises serum digoxin levels in about 90% of clients using the combination. The extent of the rise in serum digoxin is related to the dose of quinidine. Two different mechanisms seem to be involved in this interaction. Quinidine apparently displaces digoxin from peripheral tissue-binding sites in striated muscle, without affecting binding to cardiac receptors, and competes with digoxin for carrier-mediated excretion mechanisms in the proximal tubule. By these mechanisms, digoxin levels may be elevated to twice the normal level, thus bringing it into the toxic range. The client may manifest toxicity with arrhythmias and the other usual symptoms of digitalis toxicity (McInnes & Brodie, 1988, p 95).

A significant amount of oral digoxin is normally inactivated by intestinal bacteria. Administering erythromycin to the client on digoxin has increased serum concentration of active digoxin by up to 100%. Apparently, the erythromycin reduces the population of bacteria that inactivate the digoxin. With the rise in serum levels of digoxin, there is the increased likelihood for digoxin toxicity.

Drugs that decrease activity of digitalis preparations by hepatic enzyme induction include the barbiturates, phenytoin, rifampin, and possibly phenylbutazone. Thus, the effectiveness of the digitalis preparation is decreased and the dose of the preparation may need to be increased. Decreased plasma digitoxin concentrations and a shortened digitoxin half-life have been demonstrated when phenobarbital is given to clients receiving digitoxin. The increased conversion of digitoxin to digoxin and other metabolites could decrease the therapeutic effect since digoxin has a much shorter half-life than digitoxin. Digoxin would seem less likely to be affected by enzyme induction and may be preferable to digitoxin if this interaction becomes a problem (Hansten & Horn, 1991, p 283).

The renal clearance of digoxin may be affected by verapamil, spironolactone, and amiloride. When verapamil and digoxin are used together, the renal clearance of digoxin is reduced. The negative inotropic effect of verapamil could negate some of the benefits of the positive inotropic effect of digoxin.

Spironolactone may reduce the renal excretion of digoxin, produce false elevations in plasma digoxin as determined by certain serum digoxin assays, and possibly inhibit the positive inotropic effect of digitalis glycosides. Spironolactone also appears to enhance the metabolism of digitoxin. It appears that digoxin assays using sheep antibody may be less likely to be affected by spironolactone than digoxin assays using rabbit antibody. To manage the assay problem, clients receiving the two drugs should have the monitoring of digoxin response done by means other than serum digoxin concentration unless the laboratory has proven that the digoxin assay method used is not affected by spironolactone therapy (Hansten & Horn, 1991, p 288).

Amiloride administration has been associated with an increase in renal digoxin clearance and a decrease in nonrenal digoxin clearance. The net effect was to decrease the total body digoxin clearance and to increase serum digoxin concentrations slightly. Thus, in a client with impaired renal excretion of digoxin, amiloride might be expected to cause substantial increases in serum digoxin concentrations. On the other hand, a client with impaired nonrenal digoxin excretion might develop a decreased serum digoxin concentration due to amiloride-induced increase in renal digoxin clearance. Clients receiving both drugs should be watched for altered responses to digoxin (Hansten & Horn, 1991, pp 282–283).

Precautions and contraindications. Adequate levels of potassium must be maintained in clients receiving cardiac glycosides. General nutrition should be supported to ensure optimal levels of other electrolytes such as magnesium and calcium.

When initial signs or symptoms of toxicity develop, one or more daily doses of the glycosides are omitted. Medication is not resumed until these indicators disappear.

Cardiac glycosides are contraindicated in heart block, hypertrophic subaortic stenosis, and some cases of ventricular tachycardia. Caution is advised in acute or toxic myocarditis, such as that which follows myocardial infarction.

■ Summary

Cardiotonic glycosides exert positive inotropic, negative chronotropic, and negative dromotropic effects on the heart. They are widely used to treat and prevent congestive heart failure in clients whose cardiac function is marginal.

These drugs have a narrow margin of safety, and clients should be assessed for toxicity before each dose. Anorexia, nausea or vomiting, disturbances in vision, and very slow or very rapid cardiac rate are indications of toxicity.

Nursing management of clients with heart failure

Clients with heart failure usually can be identified as being in acute left-sided heart failure (acute pulmonary edema), in chronic left-sided heart failure, or in chronic right-sided heart failure. Nursing manage-

Cardiac glycosides: similarities and differences

| Similarities | Differences |

Similarities

Pharmacodynamics

These agents increase the force and velocity of myocardial systemic contractions (positive inotropic action). They increase the influx of calcium ions across the myocardial cell membrane and inhibit the transport of sodium and potassium across the cell membrane. These agents decrease the rate of conduction and refractory period in the AV node. They exert a negative chronotropic action resulting in a decrease heart rate.

Pharmacokinetics

These agents are absorbed and metabolized in varying degrees depending on their polarity. They are widely distributed in body tissues, with highest concentrations in the heart, kidney, intestines, stomach liver, and skeletal muscle. They are primarily excreted by the kidneys, cross the placenta, and are found in breast milk.

Therapeutic uses

These agents are used in the prophylactic management and treatment of heart failure, and the treatment of arrhythmias such as atrial fibrillation and atrial flutter, paroxysmal atrial tachycardia or AV junctional rhythms, and myocardial infarction.

Adverse reactions

These include: (CNS) headache, fatigue, malaise, drowsiness, disorientation, vertigo, generalized muscle weakness, restlessness, irritability; (CV) bradycardia, tachycardia, heart block, hypotension; (GI) anorexia, nausea, vomiting, abdominal pain, diarrhea; (GU/REPRO) gynecomastia, electrolyte imbalance such as hypokalemia, hypomagnesemia, and hypercalcemia; (EENT) abnormal yellow/green perception, halos around visual images, diplopia, scotomata, photophobia; (SKIN) hypersensitivity; (OTHER) acid base imbalances.

Differences

• **Digitoxin** and **digitalis** (relatively nonpolar) are completely absorbed; **digoxin** (more polar than digitoxin) is less completely absorbed; **deslanoside** (more polar than digoxin) is poorly absorbed. IV **deslanoside** and **digoxin** are rapid acting; oral **digoxin** is intermediate acting; **digitoxin** and **digitalis** are long-acting. • **Deslanoside** is only minimally metabolized and is only given IV; it has an onset of 10–30 minutes, peaks in 1–3 hours, has a duration of 2–5 days and an elimination half-life of 33–36 hours. • **Digitoxin** is rapidly and completely absorbed by the GI tract; it has an onset of action 1–4 hours (PO), $\frac{1}{2}$–2 hours (IV), peaks in 8–14 hours (PO), 4–12 hours (IV), has a duration of action of 14 days and an elimination half-life of 5–7 days with metabolism by the liver to active and inactive metabolites. • **Digoxin** has an onset of action of 5–30 minutes (IV), $\frac{1}{2}$–3 hours (PO), 30 minutes (IM), peaking in 1–4 hours (IV), 2–6 hours (PO), 4–6 hours (IM), a duration of 6 days and an elimination half-life of 32–48 hours, undergoing slight metabolism by the liver.

When **digoxin** is given IM, it may cause pain, muscle fasciculation and necrosis at the injection site.

(continued)

Cardiac glycosides: similarities and differences (Continued)

Similarities	Differences

Contraindications

These agents are contraindicated in persons with ventricular fibrillation, digoxin toxicity and hypersensitivity.

Precautions

These agents should be used with caution in persons with idiopathic hypertrophic subaortic stenosis, incomplete AV block without artificial pacemaker, hypertensive carotid sinus syndrome, Wolff-Parkinson-White syndrome, sinus node disease, acute glomerulonephritis and congestive heart failure, severe pulmonary disease, hypoxia, myxedema, acute MI, severe heart failure, acute myocarditis, chronic constrictive pericarditis, those having frequent premature ventricular contractions or ventricular tachycardia, and those persons with low cardiac output, conditions that increase cardiac sensitivity, such as hypokalemia, chronic obstructive pulmonary disease, and acute hypoxemia.

IV **deslanoside** and **digoxin** should be used cautiously in persons with hypertension.

Nursing considerations

Instruct client in disease, treatment, drug therapy regimen, adverse effects and compliance; assess cardiopulmonary status as a baseline and ongoing, especially, heart rate, rhythm, and blood pressure; obtain serum electrolyte levels prior to initiating therapy and frequently thereafter, monitoring for changes indicative of electrolyte imbalance; monitor apical-radial pulse for 1 full minute and note any discrepancies—obtain 12 lead ECG and blood pressure if any discrepancies are noted; hold the drug if client's pulse rate is below 60 beats/min; notify MD of any significant changes in pulse rate or blood pressure; assess I and O and nutritional status, paying particular attention to fluid, electrolyte and acid-base balance; monitor bowel elimination status for signs of constipation or diarrhea; assist with hygiene as necessary; elevate the head of the bed if client is experiencing shortness of breath; administer after meals and avoid giving with high fiber foods; institute measures to correct electrolyte imbalances; monitor client's response to drug therapy watching for signs of toxicity; institute any dietary measures such as low sodium and calorie restriction; instruct client and family in technique for monitoring pulse rate and in dietary measures; teach client to take the medication at the same time each day and not to switch brands.

Administer **digoxin** IM only when other routes (PO or IV) are not available; administer deep into a large muscle and massage the injection site afterwards; watch for possible cumulative effects when giving **digitalis leaf** and **digitoxin** since they are long-acting drugs.

ment varies somewhat depending on the acuity of the condition, the origin of the condition, and the signs and symptoms manifested.

Nursing implications

Clients in acute heart failure are usually hospitalized in coronary care units where equipment for direct cardiac monitoring is available. Medical care is intensive and focuses on maintaining vital functions and tissue perfusion. Drugs are the major mode of therapy and include cardiotonics and diuretics. Clients' nursing care needs are intense. They must cope with the stress of sudden, life-threatening illness, a strange environment, and acute discomfort.

Clients who continue to experience some degree of congestive failure following an acute episode, and those who experience repeated exacerbations of this condition, are often placed on complex medication regimens, including cardiac glycosides. Dosages of all drugs must be carefully adjusted for optimal effect. All clients require assistance in managing their medications for optimal therapeutic effect.

Nursing process

Assessment A detailed history should be secured. The client is interviewed, if possible, depending on mental and emotional status. A family member or another significant other may need to be the primary source of data. The client's consciousness may be impaired owing to poor oxygenation of the brain. Most clients in acute failure will be fearful and anxious because they are aware of the life-threatening nature of the illness; anxiety is heightened if admission is to the coronary care unit. Significant others also are prone to fear, anxiety, and feelings of helplessness. If these feelings are evident in significant others, they may exacerbate those of the client.

A drug history has to be secured. Clients with more chronic failure often require several drugs, some of which may interact in a nonbeneficial manner. All drugs used by the client should be documented, including prescription, over-the-counter, and social drugs such as caffeine, nicotine, and alcohol. Risk factors predisposing to drug toxicity should be identified. These include hepatic or renal impairment, use of potassium-wasting diuretics, and hormonal use. Hepatic or renal impairment causes accumulation of drugs; unusual stress contributes to depletion of potassium. Immobility may be accompanied by hypercalcemia associated with bone demineralization.

Assessment should also involve physical assessment including vital signs, apical-radial pulse, cardiac rhythm and sounds, color, tissue turgor, edema, peripheral perfusion, level of consciousness, level of energy, and some measure of central venous pressure. Cyanosis, dyspnea, increased venous pressure, edema,

---

delayed capillary refill, lack of energy, and altered level of consciousness are signs and symptoms of cardiac decompensation.

The nutritional status should be appraised with particular attention to fluid, electrolyte, and acid-base balance. Hypokalemia, hypercalcemia, hypomagnesemia, and alkalosis predispose to digitalis toxicity. Bowel status is also important. Constipation causes vagal stimulation, which tends to slow the heart; diarrhea can cause rapid potassium depletion.

The nurse should appraise the client's current health practice. Compliance with the current medical regimen should be determined. Evaluation of the client's ability to incorporate self-care measures appropriate to the level of disability into his or her lifestyle is necessary. Chronic dependence on medication or other special treatment may be difficult to accept and integrate into living patterns. The success of treatment is measured by quality of life, as well as by compliance with the medical regimen.

These data are supplemented by information from cardiac monitors and laboratory tests. Monitors provide a sophisticated measure of heart function (see Fig. 27-3 for ECG changes characteristic of therapeutic digitalization). Laboratory data include arterial blood gases and electrolyte levels.

Nursing diagnosis Diagnoses most likely to be made are the following:

Altered tissue perfusion related to weak heart action, hypervolemia, and edema
Fluid volume excess related to sodium and fluid retention and altered renal perfusion
Impaired gas exchange related to pulmonary edema
High risk for impaired skin integrity related to tissue hypoxia, malnutrition, and immobility
Self-care deficit related to exhaustion secondary to tissue hypoxia
Anxiety related to deprivation of familiar stimuli and overload of unfamiliar stimuli

In addition, some clients will experience:

Fear of dying related to the life-threatening nature of the illness

*Body image disturbance related to visible
edema and cyanosis
Self-esteem disturbance related to feelings of
helplessness, exhaustion, and immobility*

Both client and family may have knowledge deficit related to heart failure and its treatment. Either the client or family may respond with:

*Ineffective individual coping with the stressors
of the illness
Altered family processes concerning the
incapacity of the hospitalized member*

Diagnoses related to the drug regimen include potential toxic effects such as the following:

*Altered nutrition: less than body requirements
related to anorexia, nausea, or diarrhea
Decreased cardiac output related to
arrhythmias, impairment of cardiac
conductivity, and shortening of diastole
Visual sensory/perceptual alterations:
disturbance in yellow and green color vision*

A nursing diagnosis of noncompliance with the treatment regimen may also apply.

*Ineffective management of therapeutic
regimen related to complexity of therapeutic
regimen and knowledge deficit*

A common collaborative problem that should be differentiated from the nursing diagnoses is

*Potential complication: hypokalemia related to
digitalis toxicity and diuretic therapy*

Planning Goals of treatment are to increase cardiac output and tissue perfusion, decrease interstitial and blood fluid volumes, improve gas exchange in the lungs, alleviate or eliminate dyspnea, decrease the risk of skin breakdown, provide physical care needed by the client, alleviate or eliminate anxiety, provide clients with the information needed to cope with the illness, promptly detect and treat digitalis toxicity, improve intake of potassium, and increase compliance with the treatment regimen. For some clients, additional goals should be to reduce their fear and help them to adjust to a new body image and more effectively cope. Appropriate goals for the family are to more effectively cope and to develop new patterns of effective family process.

Intervention Nursing care administered to the client may involve provision of all personal care. Exertion is contraindicated. The client should be positioned to facilitate breathing; the upper torso should be elevated. The lower extremities may be lowered to facilitate movement of edematous fluid out of the lungs. Much of the physical care administered to the client depends on the medical plan of care. The nurse ad-

ministers medications (including oxygen), monitors the client's response to treatment, and adjusts treatment in accord with this response, following standard protocols when appropriate. Administering digitalis preparations requires special care. Because of the drug's potency and narrow safety margin, medication errors of small magnitude may have serious consequences. An overdose of only one-eighth of a milligram could represent a doubling of the therapeutic maintenance dose. The nurse must clearly differentiate between maintenance and loading doses, which may differ by a magnitude of tenfold.

Errors in dosage are particularly likely to occur in medication areas where many different digitalis preparations are stored. The names of digitalis preparations are similar enough to make differentiation difficult. For example, the generic names digitoxin and digoxin are very easy to confuse, yet the drugs differ significantly in their maintenance dose, onset of action, half-life, and routes for metabolism and elimination. Drug errors may be reduced by stocking only those preparations in common use and those needed in emergencies. The unit dose system using individual rather than stock drug supplies is preferred.

Oral preparations of cardiac glycosides should not be administered with meals that have a high fiber content. Studies have shown it binds with the fiber, reducing the amount of medication available for absorption. In addition, they may be irritating to the gastric mucosa and are best given following a meal. Because they are usually administered only once a day, they are customarily given after breakfast.

Cardiac glycosides may be ordered intramuscularly if the client cannot tolerate oral administration. These injections are uncomfortable because the solutions contain two tissue irritants: the glycoside and alcohol. They must be injected deep into a large muscle mass; sites should be rotated on a regular basis. As soon as possible, cardiac glycosides should be administered orally because digoxin is erratically and unpredictibly absorbed from intramuscular (IM) sites

---

Learning experience 27-1

Identify the cardiac glycoside preparations available on a medical nursing unit for both routine and emergency use. Examine medication records to determine which are used most frequently. Which preparations contain doses within the usual ranges for daily maintenance doses? Do any contain digitalizing doses? What precautions are taken to prevent the erroneous administration of digitalizing doses for maintenance doses?

owing to the nature of its vehicles: alcohol and other organic solvents.

The nurse must monitor clients' responses to cardiac glycosides carefully. A normal therapeutic response is characterized by a stronger, slower pulse, diuresis, and a decrease in dyspnea. Because these drugs have a narrow margin of safety, therapeutic response may be followed by signs and symptoms of toxicity.

Toxicity of cardiac glycosides. Clients most likely to develop toxicity are those who have difficulty maintaining adequate potassium levels. Because the source of potassium is normally dietary, clients who have difficulty eating are at high risk. Potassium is present in large amounts in the contents of the lower GI tract, and abnormal losses due to diarrhea or fistula drainage place the client in danger of hypokalemia. A common cause of potassium loss in clients with cardiac disease is urinary loss due to the administration of potassium-wasting diuretics.

In addition, all clients subject to high stress levels will lose potassium through the kidneys in response to high levels of the adrenocortical hormones, aldosterone and cortisone. Toxicity can also develop in clients who are unable to detoxify and eliminate the drug at the normal rate (people with marginal liver or kidney function). Infants may be unable to handle the drug efficiently because their organs are immature; elderly persons are likely to have some degree of damage to these organs. If the client has adequate kidney function, the nurse should encourage consumption of foods rich in potassium to reduce the risk of digitalis toxicity.

Because cardiac glycosides have such narrow safety margins, monitoring of the client must include careful attention to indications of therapeutic response and early signs of toxicity. Laboratory tests for drug concentrations must be considered carefully but they are relative rather than absolute indicators of the potential for toxicity. Individual response to specific drug concentrations is altered by many factors, including electrolyte and hormone levels, acid-base balance, and degree of cardiac pathology. Laboratory data must be interpreted in view of the total clinical picture.

Because many of the signs and symptoms of toxicity from the glycosides are identical to those of congestive failure, they cannot be relied on for the diagnosis of drug toxicity. The client with congestive failure is likely to experience malaise, anorexia, nausea, vomiting, or alterations in levels of consciousness. Changes in vision are good evidence of toxicity but they do not occur consistently. The timing and sequence of symptoms may be helpful. Early nausea is more likely to be due to poor perfusion of the intestinal tract than to drug overdose. If a period of improvement (indicating therapeutic response to medication) is followed by renewed GI problems, toxicity is much

---

Box 27-3. Characteristic ECG changes in digitalis toxicity

Bradycardia

Prolongation of the P–R interval

Shortening of the Q–T interval

Alterations in P waves are danger signs.

---

more likely to be the cause. An apical pulse slower than 60 or greater than 100 in adults is suggestive of toxicity as is an increase in pulse deficit.* Judgment in interpreting such data is developed with experience.

When heart action is assessed continuously by cardiac monitor, the ECG can be used to diagnose digitalis toxicity. The interpretation of ECGs is a specialized skill of the coronary care personnel. However, any hospital nurse should be able to identify the characteristic changes of cardiac glycoside toxicity. These changes include bradycardia, prolongation of the P-R interval, and shortening of the Q-T interval. Alterations in P waves are danger signs (Box 27-3).

Nursing measures designed to eliminate stressors and help the client minimize stress response allay toxicity by conserving body potassium stores. Both the family and the client need emotional support and teaching. The client is given information required to allay apprehension, to gain informed consent for treatment, and to enlist cooperation with the treatment regimen. The next of kin must be fully informed of the client's condition and the plan of medical care. In addition, family members should be encouraged to maintain adequate self-care, particularly rest, sleep, and nutrition.

Assessment for toxicity should be performed before each scheduled dose of medication. It is particularly important to be alert to early signs and symptoms of toxicity. Diagnosis at this stage allows early correction of the problem. For example, assessment of the client's appetite for breakfast (before the drug is administered) will be helpful. Anorexia or nausea at this time cannot be attributed to the local GI effect of the drug, therefore, such complaints are good indicators of possible drug toxicity. By the time late symptoms develop, when the diagnosis is obvious, the client is likely to be in serious difficulty. Advanced toxicity is signalled by tachycardia faster than 100 beats a minute, accompanied by nausea, vomiting, diarrhea, and abnormal color vision. At this level, ventricular fibrillation and cardiac arrest can occur.

---

*The number of cardiac contractions per minute that fail to produce a palpable pulse wave, as measured by the difference between apical and radial pulse rates per minute.

If a diagnosis of toxicity seems likely, cardiac glycosides should be withheld and the physician notified of the client's condition. If tolerated, orange or tomato juice may be offered to supply potassium, which will tend to ameliorate the symptoms. Juice is usually tolerated better by the anorexic client than are other sources of potassium. Alleviation of stress (which favors potassium excretion) will also increase tolerance to the drug. The physician may order potassium supplements if the client's levels are low. Usually omission of one or more doses of the glycosides will suffice to lower serum concentrations below the toxic level. Nursing measures to support general physiologic function and maintain fluid and electrolyte balance are helpful not only to correct toxicity but also to delay or prevent its occurrence.

The use of cardiac glycosides in treating acute heart failure will often alleviate the symptoms of congestive failure and restore homeostasis. Unless the underlying cause of cardiac impairment can be corrected, however, failure can recur. Although cardiac glycosides may be withdrawn following resolution of an acute episode, they are sometimes required for prolonged periods of time. Many clients treated for congestive failure continue to take maintenance doses of cardiac glycosides for years, often for life, to maintain the required level of cardiac function.

Client education. Clients in acute heart failure cannot absorb large amounts of information at one time, nor can their families or significant others. The nurse should develop and implement a teaching plan appropriate to their status. Comprehensive teaching should be postponed until the client's physical condition appears to be stabilized.

Clients who live at home and manage their own care need teaching that is designed to help them manage their drug regimen. Instructions should include the importance and ways of maintaining adequate potassium intake, techniques for self-monitoring for early signs and symptoms of digitalis toxicity, and actions to be taken when those signs appear.

When compliance is a problem, the nurse should ascertain and try to eliminate the underlying reasons. Sometimes clients omit drug dosages when they are feeling well, believing that medicines can be taken on an "as needed" basis. Sometimes the client has too little money to cover both medication and essential living expenses. If during cold weather the client must choose, for example, between medicine and heat, it should not be surprising if compliance with the drug regimen suffers.

If clients have difficulty remembering to take all their drugs, a system can be developed to ensure regular dosage. Preparing all medications needed for the day, sorted according to the time of administration, is usually helpful. Poured drugs may be stored temporarily in the individual compartments of an egg carton.

To maintain therapeutic blood concentrations, cardiac glycoside preparations should be given at approximately the same time each day. This is particularly important if digoxin is used because more than one-third of the drug is excreted normally in 24 hours, and blood levels can drop by half if the daily dose is delayed, for example, from morning to evening.

Clients should be taught to monitor their own pulses. The daily dose of cardiac glycoside should be omitted if the pulse drops below 60 per minute, especially if the appetite has declined. The physician should be consulted if GI upset (anorexia, nausea, vomiting, or diarrhea) has developed.

Because digitalis preparations are potent poisons, they must be stored in secure places that are not accessible to children.

Evaluation Data required for evaluation include vital signs (especially blood pressure, pulse, and respirations); descriptions of color perception, tissue turgor, and peripheral circulation; absence or presence of rales and rhonchi; absence or presence of skin breakdown; evidence of good grooming and hygienic care; serum potassium levels; serum digoxin levels; and statements by the client relating to difficulty or ease in respirations and level of fear and anxiety. The client's ability to repeat to the nurse information conveyed during teaching sessions also provides data for evaluation. Additional data include statements by the client and family concerning their perceptions of stress and interpersonal relationships. (See the accompanying Example of Nursing Process.)

Checklist of nursing actions

When acute heart failure is the diagnosis

☐ Assess clients directly for cardiorespiratory status; supplement observations with ECG and blood pressure monitoring and laboratory data.

☐ Assess emotional reaction of clients and families to the life-threatening illness.

☐ Protect the client from exertion by providing complete physical care.

☐ Differentiate carefully between digitalizing and maintenance doses of cardiotonic glycosides.

☐ Rotate sites used for IM injections of cardiotonic glycosides.

☐ Monitor client for therapeutic and toxic reactions to cardiotonic medication; evaluate clients carefully each time before administering these drugs.

☐ Withhold cardiotonic drugs when clients exhibit early signs and symptoms of toxicity.

☐ Unless otherwise contraindicated, encourage ingestion of foods and fluids rich in potassium.

☐ Eliminate unnecessary stressors and assist the client in reducing stress levels.

☐ Teach the client essential information for un-

Example of nursing process and digoxin therapy

The client is a 67-year-old male machinist who has been admitted to an acute-care facility with complaints of increasing dyspnea in the last 24 hours. The client sustained an anterior wall myocardial infarction due to occlusion of the left anterior descending coronary artery 3 weeks ago. The client appears weak and fatigued, as well as tense and anxious. He reports he has felt anorexic and has eaten less than usual in the last 2 days.

Examination revealed a 13″ ankle circumference bilaterally with apparent edema (but with no pitting), prolonged capillary refill, a purple-blue discoloration of the lips, and labored respirations at 26 per minute. His temperature was 56.5°C (97.8°F) and blood pressure was 98/70. On auscultation, moist rales/crackles were heard in the lungs. Heart sound assessment identified the presence of an S_3 and S_4.

According to the bedside scale, the client weighed 210 pounds. On hearing this, the client exclaimed, "I have never weighed more than 195 pounds in my life!"

The physician's orders included an immediate chemical profile, complete blood count, arterial blood gases, urinalysis, and electrocardiogram. The chest x-ray done in the emergency room shows an enlarged heart. Oxygen by nasal cannula at 3–4 L/min was ordered, telemetry monitoring was instituted, and a saline lock was inserted. An IV of D5W with 20 mEq of potassium added was started at a "keep open" rate. Digoxin and furosemide were started.

Assessment data	Nursing diagnosis	Intervention	Outcomes
Dyspnea Moist rales/crackles on auscultation Slow capillary refill Cyanosis Hyperpnea Gallop rhythm Enlarged heart	Decreased cardiac output related to an inability of heart to pump effectively, secondary to myocardial damage and cardiac hypertrophy	**Perform** interventions to improve respiratory status. **Perform** interventions to treat fluid volume excess. **Instruct** client to avoid activities that create a Valsalva response. **Provide** frequent, small meals rather than three large ones. **Discourage** intake of foods/fluids high in caffeine. **Monitor** for therapeutic and nontherapeutic effects of digoxin and any other cardiovascular drugs ordered.	Client will have improved cardiac output as evidenced by: blood pressure within normal range for client; apical pulse audible, regular, and between 60-100 beats/minute; resolution of gallop rhythm; less labored respirations; improved breath sounds and fewer rales/crackles; usual mental status; palpable peripheral pulses; improved skin color and temperature; capillary refill time less than 3 seconds; urine output at least 30 cc/hr; and resolution of peripheral edema.
Unusual weight gain Swelling of ankles	Fluid volume excess related to high levels of aldosterone and antidiuretic hormone secondary to impaired renal perfusion secondary to heart failure	**Administer** furosemide as ordered; monitor for therapeutic and nontherapeutic effects. **Maintain** fluid restrictions as ordered; limit IV intake as ordered. **Restrict** sodium intake as ordered (usually to about 2 gm/d). **Monitor** intake and output; keep accurate records.	Client will experience resolution of fluid imbalance as evidenced by: decline in weight toward client's normal; Blood pressure and P within normal range for client and stable with position change; resolution of gallop rhythm; balanced I and O; resolution of peripheral edema;

(Continued)

Example of nursing process and digoxin therapy (Continued)

Assessment data	Nursing diagnosis	Intervention	Outcomes
		Monitor laboratory values for electrolytes, especially potassium and sodium. **Monitor** circumference of ankles. **Monitor** and record relative amount of edema in extremities (degree of pitting, 0–4†). **Monitor** weight daily; same time of day, same amount of clothing. **Teach** good nutritional habits and use of seasonings to make lower sodium diet more palatable.	less labored respirations; improved breath sounds and fewer rales/crackles; usual mental status; and BUN and serum creatinine levels within normal range.
Dyspnea Moist rales/crackles on auscultation Anxiety	Impaired gas exchange related to thickened alveolar-capillary membrane secondary to pulmonary edema and decreased systemic tissue perfusion	**Perform** interventions to improve cardiac output. **Place** client in semi-to-high Fowler's position; position overbed table so client can lean forward on it if desired. **Assist** client as needed to reposition self at least every 2 hours. **Instruct** client to deep breathe or use inspiratory exerciser at least every 2 hours. **Maintain** O_2 therapy as ordered. **Perform** actions to facilitate removal of pulmonary secretions as needed. **Instruct** client to avoid gas-forming foods.	Client will experience adequate respiratory function as evidenced by: normal rate, rhythm, and depth of respirations; decreased dyspnea; improved breath sounds; usual mental status; client report that breathing is easier; and blood gases within normal range.
Weakness Fatigue	Activity intolerance related to tissue hypoxia secondary to impaired alveolar gas exchange and decreased tissue perfusion	**Perform** interventions to promote sleep. **Perform** interventions to improve respiratory status. **Perform** interventions to increase cardiac output. **Maintain** activity restrictions as ordered. **Increase** client's activity gradually as allowed and tolerated (ie, set an increased ambulation distance goal for each shift). **Assist** client with measures to conserve strength, such as resting before and after activities like meals, bath, and ambulation.	Client will demonstrate an increased tolerance for activity as evidenced by: verbalization of feeling less fatigued and weak; and ability to perform activities of daily living without dyspnea, chest pain, diaphoresis, dizziness, or significant change in vital signs.

(Continued)

Example of nursing process and digoxin therapy (Continued)

Assessment data	Nursing diagnosis	Intervention	Outcomes
Digoxin therapy Anorexia	Altered nutrition: potential for less than body requirements related to stimulation of vomiting center secondary to vagal and/or sympathetic stimulation	**Instruct** client on how to monitor physiological response to activities. **Instruct** client to stop any activity if fatigue or other signs of hypoxia occur. **Perform** activities to improve cardiac output. **Be alert** to factors in client's situation that may cause an increased sensitivity to digitalis preparations (*eg*, MI, potassium depletion, kidney dysfunction, liver dysfunction, diuretic therapy, any diarrhea, advancing age). **Take** apical pulse before administering each dose of digoxin and report any deviations from established parameters. **Monitor** serum digoxin levels. **Monitor** serum potassium levels. **Provide** opportunity for oral hygiene before meals. **Provide** attractive, small servings of easily digested meals. **Offer** foods rich in potassium. **Eliminate** noxious sights and smells from environment. **Instruct** client to eat dry foods and avoid drinking liquids with meals if nausea does occur. **Instruct** client to rest after eating with head of bed elevated. **Encourage** client to change positions slowly.	Client will not exhibit signs and symptoms of digoxin toxicity as evidenced by: serum digoxin level 0.8–1.6 ng/mL; serum potassium level between 3.5 and 5.0 mEq/L; absence of nausea and vomiting; absence of changes in color vision; apical pulse audible, regular, and between 60–100 beats/min; and adequate intake of meals.

Adapted from Ulrich SP, Canale SW, Wendell SA. (1990). *Nursing care planning guides, A nursing diagnosis approach*, 2nd ed. Philadelphia: W. B. Saunders Co.

derstanding and cooperating with the treatment regimen; postpone detailed and comprehensive teaching until the client's condition has stabilized.

When congestive heart failure has become chronic
☐ Periodically perform a general health assessment with emphasis on cardiovascular function.

☐ Before each dose of cardiac glycosides, evaluate client for abnormal pulse and anorexia.
☐ Administer cardiac glycosides daily at about the same time.
☐ Analyze the client's drug regimen for risk of adverse drug reactions and interactions.
☐ Monitor the client for signs and symptoms of adverse drug reactions and interactions.

☐ Encourage digitalized clients with good renal function to increase their intake of dietary potassium, especially when potassium-wasting diuretics are used concurrently.

☐ Advise against constipation; teach hygienic measures to promote fecal elimination.

☐ Inform clients about signs and symptoms of adverse drug reactions or interactions; teach them (or their family members) how to monitor the pulse.

☐ When clients need financial aid, refer them to social agencies for assistance.

☐ Assist the client in devising a system that promotes accurate administration of all drugs.

☐ To prevent accidental poisoning, warn clients to store medicines in secure areas.

Nursing management of acute toxicity from cardiac glycosides

Nursing implications

Acute digitalis toxicity carries a definite risk of cardiac arrest and death. Immediate medical attention is required. Clients are usually hospitalized because cardiac monitoring greatly facilitates treatment, and because IV medication is usually required. A parenteral antidote for digoxin toxicity, digitalis immune Fab, is now available to treat severe toxicity.

Digitalis immune Fab. Digoxin immune antibody fraction (Digibind) is the first biologic preparation to be approved as a specific antidote to a drug. The antigen-binding fragments (Fab) are made from anti-digoxin antibodies produced by sheep.

Pharmocodynamics. Digoxin immune Fab removes digoxin molecules from receptor sites and binds with them to reverse digoxin toxicity. It can reverse cardiac arrhythmias of digoxin toxicity within 30 minutes. All signs and symptoms of toxicity can be abolished in a few hours.

Pharmacokinetics. Digoxin immune Fab is administered IV, either by bolus or by infusion over a 30-minute period. The onset of action is in less than 1 minute and its half-life is 15–20 hours. While antigen-binding fragments are circulating in the blood, laboratory assays for digoxin may indicate an increase in serum levels. This is because the drug that is bound to the antigen-binding fragments will be measured along with the free digoxin. Elimination from the body of the fragments and the digoxin they bind depends on kidney function and may require several days. During this interval, digoxin immune Fab remaining in the blood is likely to render further doses of digoxin ineffective.

Therapeutic uses. Use of digoxin immune Fab is limited to life-threatening overdoses in clients who have severe cardiovascular disruption (shock, cardiac arrest, severe ventricular dysrhythmias, progressive bradycardia) or serum potassium exceeding 5 mEq/liter.

Dosage and administration. The dose of digoxin immune Fab is computed according to the amount of digoxin taken by the client or drug serum levels. Usually a 40-mg dose of digoxin immune Fab will bind approximately 0.6 mg of digoxin or digitoxin. Average doses used in clinical testing were in the range of 120–400 mg. The drug is marketed in vials containing 40 mg each and is expensive, costing a hospital pharmacy about $245.00 per vial.

Digoxin immune Fab is administered IV over 30 minutes, and it is recommended that it be infused through a 0.22 μm membrane filter.

Adverse reactions. Experience with this antidote is limited and few adverse reactions have been reported. Because it is an animal product, it has the potential to cause allergic reactions in persons allergic to sheep or products made from them. Allergic hypersensitivity to wool is relatively common, and should be considered a risk factor for adverse reaction to digoxin immune Fab.

The use of this antidote is likely to withdraw all digoxin from the client's system and precipitate the cardiac malfunctions for which the cardiotonic glycoside was originally prescribed. For this reason, its use is likely to be followed by low cardiac output, congestive failure, and atrial tachycardia. Hypokalemia could also develop.

Precautions and contraindications. Clients at risk for allergic reaction to this drug (those with allergy to sheep protein and those who have previously received digoxin immune Fab) should be skin tested before the drug is administered. Skin testing is not recommended as a routine procedure for all clients, however, because it delays the initiation of treatment.

If possible, serum digoxin concentrations should be obtained before the antidote is given. Potassium levels should be monitored carefully for several hours after giving the drug.

Nursing process

Assessment Data required for assessment include signs and symptoms of digitalis toxicity, a complete drug history, and laboratory data defining electrolyte values. Serum drug levels can also be helpful. Plasma concentrations of 0.5–2.0 ng/ml for digoxin and 10–35 ng/ml for digitoxin are considered to be "therapeutic." A definitive diagnosis can be made from an ECG exhibiting a prolonged P-R interval, a short Q-T interval, and abnormal P waves.

Nursing diagnosis Nursing diagnoses related to toxicity from glycosides include the following:

Altered comfort: anorexia, nausea, vomiting, or diarrhea
Fluid volume deficit related to decreased intake and increased loss secondary to nausea, vomiting, and diarrhea
Visual sensory/perceptual alterations: changes in yellow and green color vision

Common collaborative problems that should be differentiated from the nursing diagnoses include

Potential complication: hypokalemia related to cardiac glycoside toxicity
Potential complication: cardiac arrest related to cardiac glycoside toxicity

Planning Goals of treatment are to increase the client's comfort, correct fluid volume deficits, increase blood potassium level, prevent cardiac arrest by controlling arrhythmias, and promptly detect and treat cardiac arrest should it occur. For clients with life-threatening digoxin toxicity, the physiologic effect of the drug may be reduced or abolished by administering the antidote, digoxin immune Fab.

Intervention The medical treatment of frank glycoside toxicity requires immediate suspension of drug dosages and general supportive measures to promote metabolism or excretion of the drug, or both. Medical treatment usually involves the administration of IV solutions and medication, including potassium. Antiarrhythmic drugs may be required to correct disruptions of cardiac rhythm. Therapy carries a risk of serious complications because overmedication with antiarrhythmics and parenteral potassium may further disrupt heart function and cause cardiac arrest. Digoxin immune Fab may be used in severe cases.

Clients are usually cared for in coronary care units where cardiac monitoring is available. Nurses may be responsible for IV bolus medication (in accordance with established protocols), as well as infusions. The rate of medication must be carefully controlled, preferably by infusion control devices.

The staff must be prepared to initiate cardiopulmonary resuscitation should cardiac arrest occur. Clients receiving digoxin immune Fab should be monitored very closely for allergic reactions to the antidote, hypokalemia, and recurring symptoms of cardiac failure.

Nursing measures to alleviate discomfort from GI disturbances (nausea, vomiting, and diarrhea) should be instituted. As the client improves, juices and foods rich in potassium should be offered. Intravenous potassium is relatively dangerous because it can rapidly raise blood potassium levels to toxic levels. However, it cannot be discontinued until the client is able to ingest adequate potassium, either as a food or in the form of supplemental medication.

Nursing measures that limit stressors impinging on the client and help the client to manage stress levels may be crucial. The stress response, which includes loss of potassium through the kidneys, is detrimental to clients receiving cardiac glycosides.

If the client is disturbed by visual changes, abnormal perceptions may be diminished or masked by manipulating environmental stimuli. If the client's color vision is disturbed, visual stimuli should be minimized and pleasant stimuli provided to the other senses. A radio with pillow speaker is helpful if local programming is enjoyed by the client. Back rubs provide tactile stimulation. When the client resumes oral intake, food from home may be appreciated.

Nursing care to ameliorate GI symptoms should be instituted. Food and fluids should be withheld if active nausea is apparent. When tolerated, warm tea or ginger ale helps relieve nausea. Medications may be ordered to control nausea or diarrhea.

Recovery is relatively rapid when the glycoside involved has a short half-life, provided renal function is adequate. Digitoxin, which is metabolized by the liver, is more slowly eliminated from the body. Its metabolism may be accelerated by the administration of a liver enzyme inducer such as phenobarbital.

When clients have recovered from the acute phase of illness, it is imperative that the reason for the imbalance be identified. The nurse should explore with clients their self-medication practices. Examination of drug containers from the client's home will ensure that the proper drugs and doses are available. If a change in prescription has occurred, the client may have confused the physician's instructions and taken both old and new medications. A complete assessment of drug use—prescription and nonprescription—is necessary to identify drug interactions that may have contributed to the toxic reaction.

Factors that affect electrolyte balance must also be investigated. A diet poor in potassium, a temporary digestive upset, unusual stress, or acid-base imbalance may deplete body potassium. Hypercalcemia and hypomagnesemia potentiate the effects of digitalis and may precipitate toxicity (the softening of drinking water reduces magnesium intake). Changes in electrolyte levels can cause toxicity to develop despite a constant serum concentration of drug.

Client education. Once the factors contributing to the development of toxicity are identified and the medical emergency resolved, the client should be taught to avoid recurrence. Preventive measures include careful attention to diet, correction of medication errors, and control or better management of stress. The client should be cautioned to seek early medical attention for changes in health status that are likely to predispose to toxicity. These include impairment in kidney or liver function, acute digestive upsets, and a recurrence of frank congestive failure (which increases myocardial sensitivity to cardiac glycosides).

Evaluation Data required for evaluation include the absence of incidence of cardiac arrest; the correction of cardiac arrhythmias, should they occur; laboratory data indicating normal potassium levels and drug serum levels below the toxic range; alleviation or elimination of signs of toxicity; and statements by clients that they feel better and that any visual disturbance has subsided. (See the accompanying Example of Nursing Process.)

Example of nursing process and treatment for digoxin toxicity

The client is a 62-year-old retired waitress who has been under treatment for chronic congestive heart failure for a year and a half. She has been admitted to an acute-care facility, with complaints of nausea, vomiting, and diarrhea since the previous day. She thinks she may have "picked up a stomach bug" but is concerned because her pulse is irregular and she has occasional periods of palpitations.

On admission, her vital signs are: temperature 37.5°C (98°F), radial pulse 60/min, apical pulse 104min, respirations 22/min, and BP 112/86. Tissue turgor is poor as evidenced by tenting when skin fold is pinched; mucous membranes appear dry. The client is being maintained at home with digoxin, and hydrochlorothiazide 50 mg/day.

The client is transferred to the coronary care unit, where a printout from her cardiac monitor shows a short Q–T interval and prolonged P wave. A diagnosis of digoxin toxicity is made.

Results of blood tests show a potassium level of 3.4 mEq/liter and a plasma digoxin level of 2.4 ng/ml. An IV infusion of 1,000 ml of D5W with 40 mEq potassium is ordered to run at a rate of 125 ml/hr.

Assessment data	Nursing diagnosis	Intervention	Goals and outcome criteria
Nausea, vomiting, and diarrhea Blood pressure 112/86 Tenting of skin	Fluid volume deficit related to increased loss from the intestinal tract due to vomiting and diarrhea secondary to digoxin toxicity	**Administer** IV fluids as ordered; control the rate of flow with an infusion control device. **Keep** an accurate record of fluid intake and output.	Within 24 hours, tissue turgor will improve as shown by decreased or absent tenting on pinching of the skin. Systolic blood pressure will rise above 120 mm Hg.
Vomiting and diarrhea Serum potassium 3.4 mEq/liter Plasma digoxin level 2.4 ng/ml	High risk for for decreased cardiac output related to cardiac arrhythmias secondary to digoxin toxicity	**Monitor** client for ECG changes characteristic of digitalis toxicity. **Initiate** cardiopulmonary resuscitation if client develops a potentially lethal ventricular arrhythmia. **Offer** client clear fluids that help correct nausea such as ginger ale or tea. When nausea subsides, **offer** the client foods rich in potassium.	Ventricular flutter or fibrillation will not occur; if one does occur, circulation will be promptly restored by cardiopulmonary resuscitation. Serum potassium level will increase to normal range. The client will report that she no longer feels nauseated.
Client's lack of awareness of the nature of her illness	High risk for knowledge deficit concerning the drug regimen used to treat congestive failure	**"Coach"** client through procedures necessary for immediate care. **Prepare** a plan for teaching client about cardiac failure and the drug regimen used to treat it; postpone teaching until current crisis is resolved.	The client will actively collaborate in the treatment regimen. The client will not experience a recurrence of serious digitalis toxicity

Checklist of nursing actions

When cardiac glycosides are prescribed

☐ Before administering the drug, assess clients for evidence of drug toxicity. Withhold the dose if bradycardia or anorexia and tachycardia are present.

☐ Administer oral preparations after a meal at the same time each day.

☐ Administer parenteral preparations by deep IM injection; rotate sites regularly.

☐ If renal function is adequate, encourage the client to use ample amounts of potassium-rich foods.

☐ Assist clients in developing stress management skills.

☐ Carefully assess self-care practices of clients who experience episodes of toxicity.

Other drugs used in congestive heart failure

The ideal drug for the treatment of congestive heart failure should increase ventricular performance, decrease filling pressure, and augment cardiac output by decreasing afterload (Craig & Stitzel, 1990, p 319). Cardiac glycosides can accomplish the first two objectives but not the last.

Vasodilators

There are agents whose primary effect is the ability to dilate systemic blood vessels, which can be used if clients have not responded to the glycoside and diuretic therapy. Agents that dilate venules sufficiently decrease preload and decrease left ventricular filling pressure. These effects tend to improve cardiac output and decrease pulmonary congestion in congestive heart failure clients. Agents that dilate arterioles tend to decrease left ventricular afterload and increase stroke volume and left ventricular ejection fraction. In advanced heart failure, symptomatic benefits may only be realized by improving peripheral circulation.

Nitrates (like isosorbide dinitrate) are venodilators and in high doses they dilate arterioles. They are especially helpful in clients with heart failure related to ischemic heart disease. Angiotensin converting enzyme inhibitors (such as captopril/Capoten and enalapril/Vasotec) are smooth muscle vasodilators that improve peripheral circulation, decrease afterload, and, therefore, left ventricular filling pressure, thereby increasing cardiac output and exercise tolerance. Combining hydralazine hydrochloride/Apresoline (vasodilator) with isosorbide dinitrate, cardiac glycoside, and diuretic therapy has been demonstrated as beneficial at times. The action of calcium channel blockers results in peripheral vasodilation which may lead to reduced afterload, increased cardiac output, and increased exercise tolerance. Afterload may be decreased and cardiac function augmented by the actions of dopamine.

Phosphodiesterase III inhibitors

Phosphodiesterase III inhibitors act by preventing the breakdown of cyclic adenosine monophosphate through their inhibition of phosphodiesterase. The subsequent increase in cyclic adenosine monophosphate leads to an increase in myocardial contractility. This action is similar to the action of methylxanthines (*eg*, theophylline) but the drugs being studied in relation to congestive heart failure are more cardioselective. Two groups of drugs are being studied: bipyridine derivatives (amrinone and milrinone) and imidazole derivatives (enoximone and piroximone).

Amrinone has both inotropic and vasodilatory properties. It has been used with clients with severe congestive heart failure, which has been shown to be refractory to glycoside and diuretic therapy. Its full mechanism of action is unknown but it reduces preload and afterload, increases myocardial contractility, and increases resting cardiac output.

Amrinone therapy usually involves a dosage of 0.75 mg/kg body weight given by slow IV injection over 2–3 minutes. The 5 mg/ml solution is diluted to 1–3 mg/ml with normal sterile saline for use. Amrinone cannot be diluted in any solution containing glucose and cannot be infused into lines containing furosemide.

Monitoring of cardiac output, pulmonary capillary wedge pressure, and central venous pressure helps evaluate response. The initial dose is followed by maintenance infusion of 0.005–0.01 mg/kg/min with additional bolus injections (0.75 mg/kg) after 30 minutes, if needed.

Amrinone's half-life is about 3.6 hours after rapid IV injection and 5.8 hours after IV infusion. It is metabolized by the liver and excreted by the kidneys (approximately 63%) and feces (about 18%). Amrinone does improve cardiac function but it appears to have a high incidence of adverse effects (such as GI symptoms, myalgias, arrhythmias, dose-dependent thrombocytopenia, and hypersensitivity reactions). It must not be administered concurrently with disopyramide because severe hypotension has occurred.

Milrinone is approximately 20 times as potent as amrinone and does not cause thrombocytopenia. Adverse reactions include arrhythmias, lightheadedness, hypotension, nervousness, and headache (DiBianco et al, 1989, p 677).

Client survival does not appear significantly improved with either amrinone or milrinone (Craig & Stitzel, 1990, p 320).

Enoximone and piroximone are also phosphodiesterase III inhibitors shown to have short-term favorable effects on left ventricular function. Further studies are necessary to determine their role in the treatment of congestive heart failure.

Antiarrhythmics

Antiarrhythmic drugs are substances that alter the automaticity and conductivity of the heart in ways that help correct abnormal patterns of contraction or marked increases or decreases in the heart rate. Such abnormalities of heart function decrease cardiac output and predispose to congestive heart failure. Certain arrhythmias are immediately life-threatening.

Pathophysiology of abnormal cardiac rhythms

Arrhythmias are, as the name implies, disturbances in the normal rhythm of the heart beat. These disturbances in impulse generation or conduction cause abnormalities not only of heart rate and rhythm but of site of origin as well. They may be manifested by unusually rapid heart rate (tachycardia), unusually slow heart rate (bradycardia), or irregular heart beats (See Table 27-3).

Tachycardias may affect the atria or the ventricles, be constant or paroxysmal, and range from 100 beats a minute to flutter or fibrillation that is too rapid to count. Moderate tachycardia can occur naturally as the result of fever or sympathetic nerve stimulation. Other causes include the use of stimulant drugs, such as caffeine, nicotine, or amphetamines; myocardial inflammation (*eg*, following infarction); or myocardial irritability (*eg*, during ischemia). Flutter and fibrillation are conditions characterized by very rapid, incoordinated contractions of the myocardium. The frequency of contraction in flutter is lower than in fibrillation, and there is sufficient coordination to pump small quantities of blood. Atrial flutter or fibrillation reduces cardiac output but is generally not a serious emergency. Ventricular fibrillation is incompatible with life and requires immediate intervention to sustain perfusion of body tissues.

When the AV node is bombarded by rapid impulses from the atria, it is unable to respond to all of them. If the atrial impulses are regular as they may be in atrial tachycardia or flutter, ventricular response also may be regular but at a fractional rate. If the ventricles respond to half of the stimuli, it is said that the heart is in a two-to-one rhythm. Three-to-one and (rarely) four-to-one rhythms also occur. The ventricular rate is apt to be very irregular in atrial fibrillation.

Bradycardias also may affect the atria or the ventricles. Except in athletes (whose stroke volume output is large), rates lower than 60 beats per minute are considered abnormal. Stimulation of either the carotid sinus reflex or the vagus nerve temporarily slows the heart. Disease conditions that characterize bradycardia include carotid sinus syndrome, in which the carotid sinus is unusually sensitive to pressure due to arteriosclerosis, and Stokes-Adams syndrome in which the atrial impulse does not reach the ventricles, which then beat at their own, slower, intrinsic rhythm.

Irregular heart beats may arise from irritable (ectopic) foci in the myocardium or blocks in impulse transmission. These foci produce extrasystoles, or premature atrial or ventricular beats. Sometimes ectopic foci generate impulses fast enough to capture control from the SA node and dictate the rhythm of cardiac contraction. At other times, they generate extra beats out of synchrony with the basic rhythm of the heart.

Blocks in impulse transmission also cause rhythm irregularities. They may occur when part of the cardiac muscle is depressed by biochemical abnormalities or nonfunctioning because of necrosis or scarring. Blocks tend to deflect impulses, causing them to follow abnormal pathways. This may produce circuitous impulses that reverberate indefinitely, the characteristic pattern of fibrillation. Circuitous impulses are more likely to develop in enlarged hearts in which the conduction of impulses through the myocardium is prolonged.

Cardiac arrest is the cessation of all contraction of the heart. The underlying cause is usually hypoxia. Although the term as strictly defined does not apply to other cardiac arrhythmias, it is often used to indicate any arrhythmia that reduces cardiac output to a level incompatible with life. These states, chiefly ventricular fibrillation, will rapidly cause severe hypoxia and progress inexorably to true cardiac arrest if not treated.

Treatment of cardiac arrhythmias

Many arrhythmias respond well to mechanical or physical treatment methods. Cardiac massage is sometimes effective in maintaining circulation when heart function is inadequate to sustain life. Electric shock is used to abolish the chaotic impulses of fibrillation. Following defibrillation (or *cardioversion* as the procedure is termed when used to correct atrial fibrillation), the heart is temporarily refractory to all stimuli. Upon recovery, normal impulse conduction is usually resumed by the heart. Conduction deficiencies (heart block, cardiac arrest) are controlled by the use of pacemakers, which deliver periodic electrical stimuli to the ventricles. Drug therapy is limited mainly to normalizing as much as possible heart rhythm, suppressing

---

Table 27-3. Cardiac arrhythmias

Arrhythmia	Contributing factors
Tachycardias (atrial or ventricular, constant or paroxysmal, including flutter and fibrillation)	Increased body temperature
	Sympathetic nerve activity
	Stimulating drugs (caffeine, nicotine, amphetamine, epinephrine, thyroxine, marked digitalis toxicity)
Bradycardias	Vagal stimulation
	High cardiac output characterized by large stroke volume, as in athletes
	Carotid sinus syndrome

Irregular rhythms
  Sinoatrial block
  Atrioventricular block
	AV ischemia, compression, inflammation, or extreme vagal stimulation

Intraventricular block	Tachycardia
Premature atrial contractions	Ectopic atrial foci, excessive smoking, lack of sleep, excessive caffeine, alcoholism
Premature AV nodal or AV bundle contraction	Excessive smoking, lack of sleep, excessive caffeine, alcoholism
Premature ventricular contractions	Excessive smoking, excessive caffeine, lack of sleep, milk toxic states, emotional irritability

ectopic impulses, and restoring cardiac control to the normal pacemaker.

Although positive chronotropic agents such as atropine, epinephrine, and isoproterenol are occasionally administered to correct bradycardia, drugs commonly used as antiarrhythmics are all myocardial depressants. They may be grouped into four classes according to their mechanism of action (see Table 27-4). Within each class, individual drugs differ as do their therapeutic effectiveness in any individual. If a therapeutic response is not achieved with one drug, the client may respond to another within the same class.

Class I drugs: Sodium channel blocking agents

Drugs of this class include several local anesthetic-type antiarrhythmic drugs (lidocaine, procainamide, tocainide, encainide, flecainide); an isomer of quinine (quinidine); and an anticonvulsant (phenytoin).

Class I. A drugs

Drugs in this subgrouping include quinidine, procainamide, and disopyramide (See Table 27-5).

Quinidine

Pharmacodynamics. Quinidine was among the first drugs observed to possess antiarrhythmic activity and is an isomer of quinine. It blocks the fast sodium channel in the myocardial membrane, therefore, slowing the rate of the rise of the action potential. It also prolongs both repolarization and the refractory period of isolated cardiac tissue.

Pharmacokinetics. Quinidine is almost completely absorbed (70%–80%) from the GI tract after oral administration. Peak plasma concentrations are achieved for quinidine gluconate in 3–4 hours and in 1–1.5 hours for quinidine sulfate. It is extensively bound to plasma protein with 10%–20% of adminis-

tered dose free in the circulation. It is metabolized extensively in the body, primarily by the liver, with some active metabolites. The elimination phase half-life is approximately 5–8 hours. Renal disease may require a reduction in dosage or an increase in the dosing interval. Liver disease also requires reduction of quinidine dosage. Urinary excretion of metabolites of quinidine accounts for 75%–90% of the administered dose with the rest excreted as unchanged drug (Antonaccio, 1990, pp 396–397). The proportion of quinidine eliminated in urine could be increased by acidifying the urine.

Therapeutic uses. Quinidine is used to treat atrial flutter, established atrial fibrillation, after cardioversion of atrial flutter/fibrillation; paroxysmal atrial fibrillation, atrial tachycardia, AV junction rhythm, ventricular tachycardia not associated with complete heart block; and premature atrial/ventricular contractions.

Dosage and administration. The quinidine content varies among the three forms of quinidine available: quinidine sulfate/Cin-Quin (83%), quinidine gluconate/Duraquin, Quinaglute (62%), and quinidine polygalacturonate/Cardioquin (60%). Therefore, dosage adjustment may be needed if one form is substituted for another.

The usual dosage every 6 hours does depend partly on the form selected. The typical oral dose for quinidine gluconate would be 324–648 mg every 8–12 hours.

The effective dosage varies widely due to several factors, including the specific arrhythmia being treated. Clients with rapid elimination, often due to concomitant administration of metabolic inducers, may require a higher dosage. If the drugs that induce hepatic metabolism are discontinued, the quinidine dosage may need to be reduced.

Table 27-4. Classification of antiarrhythmic drugs

Class	Mechanism of action	Examples
I	Sodium channel blockade	quinidine, procainamide, disopyramide
	A. Moderate depression of sodium influx during depolarization; prolonged repolarization	
	B. Minimal depression of sodium influx during depolarization; shortened repolarization	lidocaine, mexiletine, phenytoin, tocainide
	C. Marked depression of sodium influx during depolarization; little effect on repolarization	encainide, flecainide, lorcainide, propafenone
II	Beta-adrenergic blockade	acebutol, esmolol, propranolol
III	Prolonged repolarization	amiodarone, bretylium, N-acetylprocainamide, sotalol
IV	Calcium channel blockade	verapamil

Table 27-5. Antiarrhythmic drugs, class I. A

Drug names	Preparations	Usual dosage	Adverse reactions
disopyramide (Norpace)	Oral capsules Oral controlled-release capsules	Adults: conventional tablets: 150 mg q6h; controlled-release capsules: 300 mg q12h PC: C	Urinary hesitancy and retention, constipation, blurred vision, dry mouth, nose, and eyes, esophageal reflux
procainamide (Procan SR, Pronestyl)	Oral capsules Oral tablets Oral extended-release tablets IM IV	Adults; initially: 500 mg–1 g followed by 750 mg 1 hr later if needed; maintenance: 500 mg–1 g q4h–q6h PC: C	Lupuslike syndrome, agranulocytosis
quinidine gluconate (Duraquin, Quinaglute)	IM IV Oral tablets Oral capsules Oral extended-release tablets	Adults: 324–648 mg q8h–q12h; Children: 30 mg/kg body weight divided in 5 doses PC: C	Hypotension, conduction block with pre-existing conduction system disease, widening of QRS complex, cardiac asystole, ventricular ectopic beats, paradoxical tachycardia, atrial embolism, serious blood dyscrasias

KEY: PC = pregnancy risk category. (The validity of pregnancy risk categories has not been established. See chapter 16, p 216.)

Adverse reactions. Serious hematologic reactions such as acute hemolytic anemia, hypothrombinemia, thrombocytopenic purpura, and agranulocytosis are rare but do occur.

Cardiovascular reactions that may occur include hypotension, conduction block in clients with preexisting conduction system disease, widening of QRS complex, cardiac asystole, ventricular ectopic beats, paradoxical tachycardia, and atrial embolism. Prior to the initiation of therapy to alleviate atrial flutter or fibrillation, anticoagulants might be administered to reduce the risk of thrombotic complications.

Quinidine should not be used in clients with a long QT syndrome or hypokalemia due to the possibility of arrhythmia aggravation. Metabolic problems that may be contributing to the arrhythmia, such as hypokalemia or other electrolyte imbalances, hypoxia, and acid–base imbalances should be corrected before drug therapy is initiated.

Drug interactions. Quinidine raises serum digoxin levels in about 90% of clients using the combination of digoxin and quinidine. The extent of the rise in serum digoxin is related to the dose of quinidine. The client may manifest toxicity to the combination with cardiac arrhythmias and the other usual symptoms of digitalis toxicity (McInnes & Brodie, 1988, p 95).

Quinidine metabolism is inhibited by cimetidine and induced by phenytoin, phenobarbital, and rifampin with the latter agents leading to subtherapeutic quinidine concentrations. Quinidine inhibits the liver cytochrome P450 specific for debrisoquine metabolism and may, therefore, interfere with the biotransformation of pharmacologic agents dependent on cytochrome P450 for their metabolism (Woosley & Funck-Brentano, 1988, p 62A).

Procainamide
Pharmacodynamics. Procainamide is a class I. A drug and the mechanism of action of these drugs is described under quinidine.

Pharmacokinetics. After oral administration, 75%–95% of the administered dose is absorbed rapidly. Only 15%–20% of the drug is bound to plasma proteins. Peak plasma concentrations are achieved 60–90 minutes after oral administration. Procainamide is metabolized extensively in the liver by the enzyme N-acetyltransferase to N-acetylprocainamide. The rate of metabolism of procainamide varies widely among individuals and is under genetic control. Rapid acetylators have higher plasma concentrations of N-acetylprocainamide and excrete larger amounts of N-acetylprocainamide in urine than slow acetylators.

Acetylation of procainamide may occur predominantly as a first pass effect after oral administration. N-acetylprocainamide has actions similar to those of procainamide although it is less potent. The elimination half-life is approximately 2.5–4.5 hours for procainamide and 6 hours for N-acetylprocainamide. Renal elimination is the primary route for removal of procainamide with 50%–60% eliminated unchanged. N-acetylprocainamide has a slower rate of renal elimination and accumulates rapidly in the presence of renal failure, whereas the concentration of procainamide under those circumstances may be within the therapeutic range (Antonaccio, 1990, pp 402–403).

Therapeutic uses. Procainamide is often prescribed to prevent recurrence of arrhythmias following cardioversion of atrial fibrillation. It is also used to treat atrial flutter, paroxysmal atrial tachycardia, and premature ventricular tachycardia.

Dosage and administration. Tablets and capsules come in 250-mg, 375-mg, and 500-mg strengths. The sustained-release preparations (250 mg – 1 g) allow dosing every 6–8 hours. A typical maintenance dose would be 500 mg every 6 hours.

Adverse reactions. Procainamide should not be used in clients with a long QT syndrome or hypokalemia due to the possibility of arrhythmia aggravation.

The incidence of adverse effects associated with long-term procainamide therapy limits its usefulness. Fifteen percent develop a lupuslike syndrome, characterized by arthralgia, myalgia, and skin rash. If this syndrome is recognized, treatment with procainamide is discontinued. Continuing procainamide after the development of the syndrome is dangerous because of the possibility of pleural effusion and potentially lethal pericardial tamponade (Woosley & Funck-Brentano, 1988, p 63A).

Antinuclear antibodies develop in clients during chronic therapy but are not, by themselves, reason for discontinuing procainamide. Procainamide is associated with the development of agranulocytosis and some feel the sustained-release form of the drug may be especially responsible for this toxicity.

Drug interactions. Procainamide interacts with cimetidine, which blocks its tubular secretion.

Disopyramide
Pharmacodynamics. Disopyramide is a class I. A drug and the mechanism of action of these drugs is described under quinidine.

Pharmacokinetics. Disopyramide is rapidly and almost completely absorbed from the GI tract (83%) after oral administration. Peak plasma concentrations occur in 30 minutes to 3 hours after an oral dose. It is moderately bound to plasma proteins (about 50%) but this may range from 35% to 95%, depending on plasma concentration. An increase in the administered dose may produce a disproportionately large increase in the unbound plasma drug concentration and a more pronounced pharmacologic effect.

As a result of this and the ability of disopyramide to produce cardiovascular depression, the dosage of the drug must be increased slowly. Dosage reduction is necessary for clients with hypotension, possible cardiac decompensation, reduced left ventricular function, or cardiomyopathy. The hepatic metabolism of disopyramide is not well understood but one metabolite is active as an antiarrhythmic agent. With normal renal function, the half-life is 7 hours; with renal impairment the half-life may range from 8 to 18 hours. Approximately 80% of the drug is eliminated in the urine with 50% being unchanged and the remainder is metabolites. Excretion into the bile, hence fecal excretion, accounts for 15% of the administered dose (Antonaccio, 1990, pp 480–409).

Therapeutic uses. Disopyramide is used in the treatment of cardiac arrhythmias, including unifocal and multifocal premature ventricular contractions, paired ventricular contractions, and episodes of ventricular tachycardia. In contrast to procainamide, it is well suited for long-term therapy.

Dosage and administration. The usual dosage is 150 mg three to four times a day with a maximal dose of 800 mg/d.

Adverse reactions. Disopyramide should not be used with clients with long QT syndrome or hypokalemia due to the possibility of arrhythmia aggravation.

Anticholinergic side effects are dose-related and include urinary hesitancy and retention, constipation, blurred vision, dry mouth, nose, and eyes, and esophageal reflux. Because of the anticholinergic effects, the drug is contraindicated in clients with glaucoma or obstruction uropathy. However, recent studies indicate the anticholinergic effects can be prevented by concomitant use of acetylcholinesterase inhibitors such as physostigmine and neostigmine (Woosley & Funck-Brentano, 1988, p 63A).

The controlled-release form of disopyramide may reduce adverse effects because it reduces the fluctuations of free disopyramide in plasma.

Clients with compensated congestive heart failure can be treated with disopyramide if the dosage is carefully adjusted but disopyramide is contraindicated in uncompensated heart failure.

Drug interactions. Phenytoin, rifampin, and phenobarbital induce liver metabolism of disopyramide, thus increasing its elimination and perhaps lowering its therapeutic effect.

Class I. B drugs
Drugs in this subgrouping include lidocaine, mexiletine, phenytoin, and tocainide (Table 27-6).

Lidocaine
Pharmacodynamics. Drugs in class I. B have less effect on sodium influx than those of class I. A and they shorten rather than prolong repolarization. They depress ventricular automaticity. Both the duration of the action potential and the effective refractory period are shortened.

Pharmacokinetics. Lidocaine is the drug of choice for the short-term management of serious ventricular arrhythmias (*eg*, following myocardial infarction and during heart surgery or cardiac catheterization). Unlike class I. A drugs, it can be used with clients with long QT syndrome.

Dosage and administration. Initial bolus dose is often 50–100 mg IV and it may be repeated in 5 minutes. Dosage should not exceed 200–300 mg in 1

Table 27-6. Antiarrhythmic drugs, class I. B

Drug names	Preparations	Usual dosage	Adverse reactions
lidocaine (Xylocaine)	IM solutions IV solutions N. B.: these must be marked "for cardiac arrhythmias"; preparations for local anesthesia that contain preservatives or vasopressors should not be used	IV: *initially*: 1–1.5 mg/kg body weight, repeated after 5 min if needed (no more than 200–300 mg should be administered within a 1-hr period); *maintenance*: 20–50 mcg/kg/min PC: B	Seizure activity, drowsiness, dizziness, disorientation, hypotension, bradycardia
mexiletine (Mexitil)	Oral	Adults: *initially*: 400 mg loading dose, then 200 mg 8 hr later; maintenance: 200–400 mg q8h (not to exceed 1,200 mg/d) PC: C	Tremor, dizziness, or lightheadedness, nervousness, difficulties with coordination, nausea, vomiting, heartburn
phenytoin (Dilantin)	Oral tablets Oral capsules Oral suspension IV solutions	Adults: oral: 200–400 mg qd, divided in up to 4 doses; IV: 100 mg q 5 min up to a *maximum* of 1 g PC: D	Hypotension and respiratory arrest with rapid IV administration, giddiness, ataxia, tremors, nystagmus, diplopia, blurred vision, slurred speech, sedation, ptosis, anemia
tocainide (Tonocard)	Oral film-coated tablets	Adults: *initially*: 200–400 mg q8h, increase dosage only every 3–4 days PC: C	Tremor, nausea, vomiting, paresthesia, rash, dizziness, confusion, pneumonitis and pulmonary fibrosis, agranulocytosis

KEY: PC = pregnancy risk category. (The validity of pregnancy risk categories has not been established. See chapter 16, p 216.)

hour. The usual maintenance infusion rate is 1–4 mg/min. Due to extensive first-pass hepatic metabolism, it is not given orally.

Adverse reactions. Central nervous system changes (*eg*, seizure activity, drowsiness, dizziness, disorientation) are early signs of lidocaine toxicity. Hypotension and bradycardia may occur.

Drug interactions. Use of lidocaine with beta-blockers or with cimetidine increases lidocaine serum levels.

Mexiletine
Pharmacodynamics. Mexiletine is an analogue of lidocaine and is structurally similar to tocainide. It is a class I. B drug and the mechanism of action of these drugs is described under lidocaine.

Pharmacokinetics. Its half-life of elimination ranges from 8 to 20 days with the time to reach steady state as 1–3 days. It is considered to be twice as potent as tocainide. The most important difference between tocainide and mexiletine is the mexiletine is extensively metabolized by the liver prior to elimination.

Therapeutic uses. Mexiletine is used for treatment of symptomatic ventricular arrhythmias, including premature ventricular contractions, tachycardia, and unifocal and multifocal couplets.

Dosage and administration. Dosage should be 150 mg every 8 hours and it should be given with food.

Mexiletine doses should be increased only every 2–3 days. The daily dose should not exceed 1,200 mg.

Adverse reactions. Common adverse effects include dizziness, tremor, nervousness, difficulty in coordination, nausea, vomiting, and heartburn.

Drug interactions. Phenytoin, rifampicin, and phenobarbital induce liver metabolism of mexiletine, thus increasing its elimination and perhaps lowering its therapeutic effect.

Phenytoin
Pharmacodynamics. Phenytoin (diphenylhydantoin) is structurally related to barbiturates and was introduced in 1938 for use in convulsive disorders. It was first used in 1950 for treatment of cardiac arrhythmias.

Phenytoin's electrophysiologic actions differ from those of quinidine and procainamide and somewhat resemble the actions of lidocaine. It produces less alterations in SA node function than do other antiarrhythmics. It decreases automaticity of the atria, AV node, and His-Purkinje system.

Pharmacokinetics. Phenytoin is absorbed almost completely after oral administration. It is poorly and erratically absorbed after IM administration and is not recommended for administration by this route.

It is metabolized by hepatic microsomal enzymes and one metabolite is conjugated with glucuronic acid and excreted in the urine. Other metabolites have also been found in the urine. About 93% of phenytoin is bound to plasma proteins.

Therapeutic uses. Phenytoin's most effective use is in the treatment of supraventricular and ventricular arrhythmias associated with digitalis toxicity. An important use is for prophylactic action to prevent post-cardioversion arrhythmias, especially in the digitalized client. It has been used with ventricular arrhythmias that have followed myocardial infarction, open-heart surgery, anesthesia, cardiac catheterization, cardioversion, and angiographic studies. It is not effective with atrial flutter or atrial fibrillation.

Dosage and administration. Intravenous doses of 100 mg can be given every 5 minutes until the arrhythmia is abolished or until 1,000 mg have been given. Oral maintenance therapy can then be started.

Adverse reactions. Rapid IV administration of doses in excess of 50 mg/min has been associated with serious toxicity, such as hypotension and respiratory arrest.

It is important to note that the diluent supplied with phenytoin is not pharmacologically inert and certain of the adverse effects attributed to phenytoin may indeed be due to the diluent. The diluent has a high *p*H of 11 and contains propylene glycol and ethyl alcohol. Because of the high *p*H, IV administration may cause local irritation of the vein and each dose should be followed by normal saline to flush the vein.

The CNS manifestations of toxicity include giddiness, ataxia, tremors, nystagmus on far lateral gaze, diplopia, blurring of vision, slurring of speech, sedation, and ptosis.

Hematologic evidence of toxicity includes anemia, pancytopenia, and reticuloendothelial disorders that decrease when the drug is discontinued. It may produce a megaloblastic anemia, which responds to folate therapy.

Phenytoin does not produce the anticholinergic effects seen with quinidine, procainamide, and disopyramide.

Drug interactions. Caution should be exercised when phenytoin is used in conjunction with other drugs that alter the metabolism of phenytoin (salicylates, sulfonamides, phenylbutazone—all displace phenytoin from plasma proteins) (Antonaccio, 1990, pp 416–422).

Tocainide

Pharmacodynamics. Tocainide is a class I. B drug, a primary amine analogue of lidocaine, and the mechanism of action of these drugs is described under lidocaine. It was first marketed in 1984.

Pharmacokinetics. Tocainide's pharmacokinetics are not known to be altered by concurrent administration of other drugs. It does not appear to have pharmacologically active metabolites. It is not extensively bound by plasma proteins. About 90% of tocainide is absorbed after oral administration. Half of it is eliminated via the kidneys unchanged while the rest of it undergoes glucuronidation before renal excretion.

Therapeutic uses. Tocainide is used for suppression of symptomatic ventricular arrhythmias. It has no appreciable effect on atrial arrhythmias.

Dosage and administration. Because of the variation in individual responsiveness to tocainide, the initial doses should be around 200–400 mg every 8 hours. The elimination half-life determines the time required to achieve steady-state plasma concentrations and the time to achieve the steady state is 3–4 elimination half-lives. Therefore, tocainide doses should be increased only every 3 or 4 days (Roden & Woosley, 1986a, p 42). More frequent increases in dose might suppress the arrhythmias but this approach increases the risk of accumulation of high plasma concentrations of tocainide that will produce adverse reactions.

Tocainide is often most effective when used in combination with a Class I. A action drug (*eg*, quinidine).

Adverse reactions. About 30% of clients have significant side effects, depending on the dose. Tremor, nausea, and vomiting are common; the effects can be decreased or eliminated by giving the drug with a meal or snack to slow absorption. Paresthesia may occur. Rash occurs, as well as dizziness and confusion. A serious problem is the incidence of severe reactions like pneumonitis and pulmonary fibrosis and agranulocytosis. The neutropenia can be reversed if detected early (*eg*, white blood cell counts can be done frequently on clients receiving tocainide and they can be advised to promptly report fever or sore throat to the doctor).

Drug interactions. To date, no drug interactions have been identified.

Class I. C Drugs

Encainide

Pharmacodynamics. Encainide is a class I. C drug (See Table 27-7). Structurally it resembles procainamide but it has different actions. It prolongs normal intracardiac conduction with minimal effects on repolarization. It has no effect on the SA node and, thus, does not alter the heart rate.

Pharmacokinetics. Its absorption is nearly complete. Absorption is prolonged in the presence of food but its bioavailability is not altered. It is highly bound to plasma proteins (75%–80%). It is metabolized in the liver rapidly and extensively, forming two active metabolites. In fast metabolizers, it is metabolized in 1–2 hours, while in slow metabolizers, it is metabolized in

Table 27-7. Antiarrhythmic drugs, class I. C

Drug names	Preparations	Usual dosage	Adverse reactions
encainide (Enkaid)	Oral capsules	Adults: initially: 25 mg q8h, increase dosage every 3–5 days; maintenance: 100–200 mg qd in 2–4 divided doses PC: B	Arrhythmias, dizziness, blurred vision
flecainide (Tambocor)	Oral tablets	Adults: 50–100 mg q12h PC: C	Dizziness, headache, tremor, difficulty in visual accommodation, arrhythmias, thrombocytopenia, exfoliative dermatitis
lorcainide	Oral IV	Adults: oral: 100 mg q12h, increased to maximum of 800 mg qd; IV: 1–2 mg/kg over 15–60 min, then 200 mg per 24 hr PC:	Feeling of warmth and/or lightheadedness with IV administration, sleep disturbances, gastrointestinal disturbances, metallic taste in mouth, dizziness, headaches, impotence
propafenone (Rythmol)	Oral	Adults: 150 mg q8h; increase q 3–4 days as necessary, up to maximum of 900 mg/d PC: C	Constipation, nausea, vomiting, dizziness, fatigue, metallic taste in mouth, arrhythmias, exacerbation of CHF, agranulocytosis

KEY: PC = pregnancy risk category. (The validity of pregnancy risk categories has not been established. See chapter 16, p 216.)

6–12 hours. Its peak plasma concentration is reached in 30–90 minutes. Monitoring plasma levels of encainide has not been a useful guide in adjusting its dose due to the differences among clients in blood concentration of the drug and due to the active metabolites. The kidneys are the predominant route of elimination although some drug is also eliminated via the feces.

Therapeutic uses. It has been used in the treatment of clients with symptomatic ventricular arrhythmias and in the management of clients with supraventricular tachyarrhythmias. It is not used with sick sinus syndrome or with a conduction block unless a pacemaker is present.

Dosage and administration. A dosage of 100–200 mg per day given in two to four divided doses is effective in suppressing 75%–100% of chronic nonsustained ventricular arrhythmias in 88% of clients. This is a better performance than observed with quinidine (Antonaccio, 1990, p 435). The initial oral dosage in clients with normal renal function would be 25 mg given every 8 hours and the dose may be increased to 35 mg and then 50 mg. Dose increases should be made only every 3–5 days.

Adverse reactions. Side effects are relatively few when the daily dosage is less than 150 mg/d. There is a potential proarrhythmic effect with an increase in dose. The proarrhythmic effect is a tendency for a drug to worsen certain arrhythmias or cause new arrhythmias. Side effects include transient dizziness and blurred vision. A reduced level of dosage should be used in clients with renal impairment.

Drug interactions. The only reported drug interaction is with cimetidine, which increases the plasma level of encainide (Woosley & Funck-Brentano, 1988, p 65A).

Flecainide

Pharmacodynamics. Drugs in class I. C have the greatest effect on sodium influx and do not effect repolarization appreciably. They depress cardiac conductivity, especially in the His-Purkinje system. Structurally a portion of the flecainide molecule is similar to that of procainamide, except it lacks the section that is probably responsible for the lupuslike syndrome seen frequently with procainamide.

Pharmacokinetics. Flecainide is well-absorbed after oral administration. Ten to fifty percent of a dose is excreted unchanged in urine and the remainder of the drug is biotransformed to two major metabolites, which are conjugated and undergo renal excretion. The fact that the metabolites are not active makes blood level monitoring of flecainide potentially useful. The half-life ranges from 12 to 30 hours. Flecainide is not extensively bound by plasma proteins (32%–47%).

Therapeutic uses. Flecainide is used for treatment of frequent premature ventricular contractions and sustained or symptomatic nonsustained ventricular tachycardia. It has no appreciable effect on atrial arrhythmias. Studies indicate flecainide appears to provide better antiarrhythmic therapy than quinidine or disopyramide (Roden & Woosley, 1986b, p 38).

Dosage and administration. To reduce incidence of adverse reactions, flecainide therapy should start with low dosage and this dosage should be maintained until steady state is reached (4 days). A typical dosage would be 50–100 mg every 12 hours.

Adverse reactions. The occurrence of transient CNS symptoms, such as dizziness, headache, tremor, and difficulty in visual accommodation, is fairly common. Unlike procainamide, quinidine, and disopyramide, flecainide less commonly produces GI or urinary tract disorders. Exacerbations of arrhythmias may be seen in clients with severe heart disease. Sinus node dysfunction and second- or third-degree AV block may occur.

Flecainide increases the pacing threshold so that pacemaker-dependent clients may need reprogramming of their pacemaker. New or worsening congestive heart failure occurs in a small but significant percentage of those receiving flecainide. Thrombocytopenia and exfoliative dermatitis occur.

Drug interactions. Evidence suggests that cimetidine, digoxin, and propranolol all have the potential to cause a clinically important drug interaction with flecainide, however, definitive data are not available (Roden & Woosley, 1986b, p 38). Use with disopyramide or verapamil requires extreme caution.

Lorcainide
Pharmacodynamics. Lorcainide exhibits class I. C properties. It is an acetanilid derivative with local anesthetic properties.

Pharmacokinetics. Absorption is essentially complete and bioavailability approaches 100%. There is extensive hepatic metabolism and one metabolite has antiarrhythmic activity. The half-life is 8 hours.

Therapeutic uses. It appears to be effective against both ventricular and supraventricular arrhythmias.

Dosage and administration. The IV dose is 1–2 mg/kg over 15–60 minutes, then 200 mg per 24 hours. The usual oral dose is 100 mg every 12 hours initially, increasing to a maximum of 800 mg per day.

Adverse reactions. Intravenous infusion of lorcainide has been associated with a feeling of warmth or transient lightheadedness. Oral therapy is frequently associated with sleep disturbances, which may lessen with further therapy. The sleep disturbances have been characterized by frequent awakening, vivid dreams, feelings of warmth, chilliness, or diaphoresis, and anxiety. Other adverse reactions include GI disturbances, metallic taste in the mouth, dizziness, headaches, and possibly impotence.

Drug interactions. Long-term studies of this drug are limited. Drug interactions have not been studied systematically (Michelson & Dreifus, 1988, pp 293–294).

Propafenone
Pharmacodynamics. Propafenone exhibits class I. C properties (reduces upstroke velocity of the action potential and decreases conduction velocity in the atria, ventricles, and Purkinje fibers). It also exhibits local anesthetic, beta-adrenergic-blocking, and weak calcium channel-blocking actions.

Pharmacokinetics. Its absorption after oral administration is 100% but its bioavailability is usually less than 20% due to extensive first-pass metabolism. More than 95% of the drug is bound to plasma proteins. The drug undergoes oxidative metabolism and one metabolite is known to possess antiarrhythmic properties. It reaches its peak plasma concentration after 2–3 hours. Elimination is primarily hepatic with a mean elimination half-life after oral administration of 5.5 hours in extensive metabolizers and 17.2 hours in poor metabolizers. Therefore, plasma concentrations have limited usefulness in adjusting doses.

Therapeutic uses. It is used for suppression of sustained ventricular tachycardia and has been tried with certain supraventricular arrhythmias. The drug should not be used with the less serious ventricular arrhythmias because of its proarrhythmic effect.

Dosage and administration. The initial dose is 150 mg every 8 hours and it may be increased at intervals of 3–4 days up to 900 mg per day. It is recommended that it be administered with food. Clients with impaired hepatic function should receive only 20%–30% of the recommended dose.

Adverse reactions. Side effects include constipation, nausea, vomiting, dizziness, fatigue, metallic taste in the mouth, and conduction abnormalities. Exacerbation of congestive heart failure is a potential problem and the potential proarrhythmic effect must be considered also. Agranulocytosis has occurred, but rarely.

Drug interactions. Propafenone increases serum digoxin levels modestly. It should be used cautiously with warfarin; plasma warfarin levels may rise. It should be used cautiously with propranolol and metoprolol because plasma levels of these beta-blockers may rise. Propafenone may have additive beta-blocking effects so it is contraindicated for clients with bronchospastic disorders. Quinidine can inhibit metabolism of propafenone (Hussar, 1990, p 43).

■ Summary
Class I antiarrhythmic drugs depress cardiac action by blocking the sodium channel in the myocardial membrane, generally exerting negative inotropic, chronotropic, and dromotropic effects. They are used to treat or prevent the recurrence of tachyarrhythmias. They can cause a variety of adverse reactions, including arrhythmias and decreased cardiac output.

Although maintenance therapy to prevent recurring arrhythmias is prescribed for nonhospitalized clients, therapy is usually initiated in critical care facilities in which cardiovascular function can be monitored closely and cardiopulmonary resuscitation can be initiated without delay, if necessary.

Class II drugs: Beta-adrenergic blocking agents

Beta-adrenergic blocking agents used as antiarrhythmics include acebutolol, esmolol, and propranolol (See Table 27-8). The drug with the longest history of use, propranolol, will be discussed as the prototype of this group. Until 1978, this was the only FDA-approved drug in this class in the United States.

Propranolol

Pharmacodynamics. Propranolol and other members of class II will prevent the effects of the adrenergic nervous system or adrenergic drugs (norepinephrine, epinephrine, isoproterenol, dopamine) on the heart.

Several of the physiologic responses mediated by activation of beta-adrenergic receptors include: 1) increases in heart rate and cardiac contractile force in response to exercise, stress, excitation, and other factors; 2) an increase in AV conduction velocity; 3) relaxation of bronchial smooth muscle and a decrease in airway resistance; and 4) release of insulin from beta cells in the islets of Langerhans.

With the administration of propranolol, the adrenergic system can no longer initiate these responses (Antonaccio, 1990, p 444). The blockade's consequences on the overall regulation of the cardiovascular system must be considered when a beta-adrenergic blocking agent is used. Clients with normally functioning cardiovascular systems may be able to tolerate a blockade of adrenergic transmission to the heart, however, those with compensated heart failure are dependent on adrenergic tone to maintain adequate cardiac output. Removal of such tone may precipitate acute congestive heart failure or pulmonary edema (Antonaccio, 1990, p 444).

Propranolol also has a membrane-stabilizing property that can contribute to its antiarrhythmic action.

This property resembles a property that quinidine has and can account for propranolol's antiarrhythmic effect against arrhythmias in which beta receptor stimulation does not play a role.

As a result of the two properties, heart rate decreases and the cardiovascular system's potential for response to stressors is diminished. Impulse conduction through the SA and AV nodes is delayed and myocardial automaticity is reduced. Blood pressure also declines.

At low plasma concentrations of propranolol, less than 100 ng/ml, the antiarrhythmic action is a result of beta-adrenergic blockade. However, plasma concentrations of above 100 ng/ml are often needed to reduce ventricular rate in certain situations. At this plasma concentration, in addition to beta-adrenergic blockade, the direct depressant action of propranolol on AV transmission occurs.

Pharmacokinetics. Propranolol is almost completely absorbed from the GI tract after oral administration. Peak plasma concentrations are observed 2 hours after administration. First-pass metabolism does result in significant decrease in bioavailability. Ninety-three percent of the drug is bound to plasma proteins. It is metabolized in the liver by four different pathways. Certain of its metabolites are known to be capable of beta-adrenergic blockade. Clients with hepatic disease have a decreased rate of metabolism of propranolol and possibly experience increased bioavailability. Hepatic disease also decreases the plasma-protein-bound fraction and increases free propranolol. Hyperthyroidism may increase propranolol clearance by the liver. The half-life for propranolol is 3–5 hours and its route of elimination is the kidney (fecal elimination also occurs). Following absorption, propranolol is widely distributed across the blood–

Table 27-8. Antiarrhythmic drugs, class II

Drug names	Preparations	Usual dosage	Adverse reactions
acebutolol (Sectral)	Oral	Adults: initially: 200 mg bid; maintenance: 600–1200 mg in single or divided doses PC: B	Fatigue, weakness, bradycardia, hypotension, CHF, impotence
esmolol (Brevibloc)	IV	Adults: initially: 500 mcg/kg/min for 1 min, then 50 mcg/kg for 4 min, continued until effect reached; maintenance: 25–50 mcg/kg/min, used for 24 hr or less PC: C	Hypotension, diaphoresis, dizziness, headache, nausea, inflammation at injection site
propranolol (Inderal)	Oral tablets Oral extended-release capsules IV	Adults: oral: 10–30 mg qid, up to 160–480 mg/d; IV: 1–3 mg, 1 mg/min PC: C	Bradycardia, hypotension, peripheral vascular insufficiency, heart block, CHF, disorientation to time and place, short-term memory loss, emotional liability, clouded sensorium, nausea, vomiting, diarrhea or constipation, epigastric discomfort, flatulence, hypersensitivity

KEY: PC = pregnancy risk category. (The validity of pregnancy risk categories has not been established. See chapter 16, p 216.)

brain barrier and the placenta. It is also secreted into breast milk.

Therapeutic uses. Propranolol is usually used with another agent in the treatment of arrhythmias. Propranolol in conjunction with a cardiac glycoside is of value in managing the ventricular rate in clients with atrial flutter or fibrillation. It is also used in managing clients with recurrent supraventricular tachyarrhythmias associated with the Wolff-Parkinson-White syndrome. Propranolol is highly effective in the treatment of digitalis-induced arrhythmias but it is not the drug of choice in digitalis toxicity because of its additional effects on the cardiovascular system.

Propranolol has not proved effective in preventing the recurrence of atrial fibrillation after cardioversion but combining propranolol with quinidine in that situation may be more effective than quinidine alone. Combining propranolol and procainamide has been helpful in managing clients with persistent ventricular fibrillation. Orally administered propranolol has not improved the survival rate nor decreased the incidence of arrhythmia in clients with acute myocardial infarction (Antonaccio, 1990, p 454).

The arrhythmias associated with halothane or cyclopropane anesthesias have been attributed to the interaction of the anesthetic with catecholamines and have been shown to be suppressed by IV administration of propranolol.

It has been used to relieve ventricular outflow obstruction in hypertrophic obstructive cardiomyopathy and hypertrophic subaortic stenosis. It is used in prophylactic management of clients who experience migraine headaches (it apparently inhibits cerebral vasodilation and arteriolar spasms). It has been used to relieve acute panic symptoms (*eg*, stagefright) and a variety of other uses may be encountered.

Dosage and administration. Propranolol may be administered orally or IV. Ten to 30 mg three or four times a day is a typical dose for supraventricular arrhythmias but the treatment of ventricular arrhythmias may require over 300 mg/d. When given IV for arrhythmias occurring under anesthesia, the usual dose is 1–3 mg and the rate of administration should not exceed 1 mg (1 ml/min).

Adverse reactions. Many adverse effects relate to the comments made under the section on pharmacodynamics. Adverse effects include bradycardia, hypotension, peripheral vascular insufficiency, heart block, congestive heart failure, or cardiac arrest. Any degree of AV block prior to the onset of a tachyarrhythmia is a contraindication to the use of propranolol because propranolol can further depress AV transmission.

Central nervous system reactions include disorientation to time and place, short-term memory loss, emotional lability, and clouded sensorium. They are usually reversible once the drug is withdrawn. Gastrointestinal reactions include nausea, vomiting, diarrhea or constipation, epigastric discomfort, and flatulence. Other adverse reactions include allergic signs and symptoms.

The presence of chronic obstructive pulmonary disease is a contraindication to the use of propranolol because the resulting blockade would intensify the degree of airway obstruction.

Hypoglycemia has been reported in diabetes mellitus clients on insulin, in children during recovery from anesthesia, and in clients following partial gastrectomy. The mechanism may be related to the fact that the beta receptor blockade prevents adrenergic stimulation of glycogenolysis in skeletal muscle, which would normally result in an increase in plasma lactate. Lactate is subsequently converted by the liver to glucose. At the same time, insulin reactions are more difficult to detect in the client receiving propranolol because signs and symptoms relating to sympathoadrenal hyperactivity, which normally assist the nurse in identifying the occurrence of hypoglycemia, will be absent. On the other hand, hyperglycemia may be seen and this seems to be related to the blocking of insulin release from the pancreas.

Abrupt withdrawal of beta-adrenergic blocking agents may be followed by rebound sympathetic overactivity. A withdrawal syndrome of tremulousness, sweating, severe headache, malaise, palpitation, rebound hypertension, myocardial infarction, and arrhythmias has been identified. It should always be decreased gradually when it is being discontinued, over a period of 1–2 weeks. The manufacturer recommends that it be withdrawn gradually 48 hours prior to major surgery in most cases but some physicians prefer to continue propranolol at lower doses. Many other side effects have been reported.

Drug interactions. Interactions have been reported with cardiac glycosides, quinidine, phenothiazines, cimetidine, lidocaine, and verapamil. Enzyme inducers increase hepatic elimination of propranolol and, thus, reduce its serum concentration.

■ **Summary**
Propranolol is a nonselective beta-adrenergic blocking agent (blocks both beta 1 and beta 2 adrenoreceptors). In addition, it has membrane-stabilizing properties. It is administered for the control of hypertension and certain arrhythmias, and in a variety of other situations. There are many potential adverse reactions, including bradycardia, hypotension, congestive heart failure, bronchospasm, and hyperglycemia or hypoglycemia.

Other beta-adrenergic blocking agents

Acebutolol (Sectral) is a cardioselective beta-adrenergic blocking agent with partial agonist activity (intrinsic sympathomimetic activity). It is approved for use in the management of clients with premature ventricular complexes and in treating essential hypertension.

Atenolol (Tenormin) is a cardioselective beta-adrenergic blocking agent. Cardioselectivity is not absolute and beta 2-adrenoreceptors are blocked at higher doses.

Metoprolol (Lopressor) is a selective beta 1-adrenergic blocking agent. Its cardioselectivity is not absolute. It is used primarily in the management of clients with essential hypertension and angina pectoris.

Nadolol (Corgard) is a nonselective beta-adrenergic blocking agent which is used primarily for the management of clients with angina pectoris.

Pindolol (Visken) is a nonselective beta-adrenergic blocking agent which is used primarily for the management of clients with hypertension.

Timolol (Blocadren) is a nonselective beta-adrenergic blocking agent which is used for the management of clients with essential hypertension. A special ophthalmic preparation of this beta-blocker has found use in the treatment of chronic open-angle glaucoma.

Esmolol (Brevibloc) is an ultrashort-acting, cardioselective beta-adrenergic blocking agent, which is used for short-term management of clients with supraventricular tachyarrhythmias (Antonaccio, 1990, p 446).

Other, newer, beta-adrenergic blocking agents being used at this writing include labetalol (Normodyne), betaxolol (Kerlone, Betoptic), penbutolol (Levatol), and carteolol (Cartrol).

Class III drugs: Drugs that prolong repolarization

The Class III drugs include amiodarone, bretylium, N-acetylprocainamide (NAPA), and sotalol (See Table 27-9).

Amiodarone

Amiodarone was approved for use in December 1985. It is a benzofuran derivative and much of the drug is iodine.

Pharmacodynamics. Amiodarone does have potent sodium-channel blockade ability. It is unusual among sodium-channel blockers in that its blockade occurs almost totally when sodium channels are inactivated (during phase 2 and part of phase 3 of the cardiac action potential). It prolongs repolarization in myocardial tissue, reduces sinus node automaticity, increases conduction time and refractoriness of the atrioventricular node, and reduces conduction velocity in the myocardium and the Purkinje tissue.

The effects that give it value in the management of angina pectoris include relaxation of smooth muscle, increases in systemic and coronary vasodilation, increases in coronary blood flow, and reduction of myocardial oxygen consumption. It is also a weak noncompetitive alpha- and beta-adrenergic blocking agent.

Pharmacokinetics. Absorption after oral administration is slow and variable with 20%–55% being absorbed. Its bioavailability is low and varies among individuals. It concentrates in the body in adipose tissue, liver, spleen, and lungs. A high percentage (96%) is bound to plasma proteins. It is metabolized in the liver, producing one active metabolite. The low availability is thought to be due to intestinal mucosal cell dealkyla-

Table 27-9. Antiarrhythmic drugs, class III

Drug names	Preparations	Usual dosage	Adverse reactions
amiodarone (Cordarone)	Oral tablets	Adults: 800–1600 mg qd for 1–3 wks, then 600–800 mg qd for 4 wks, then 200–600 mg qd in single or divided doses PC: C	Arrhythmias, CHF, pulmonary fibrosis and pneumonitis, elevations in liver enzymes, blurred vision or smokey hue or halos, photosensitivity, blue-gray skin discoloration, hypothermia or hyperthyroidism, tremors of hands, sleep disturbances, ataxia, peripheral neuropathy, myopathy
bretylium (Bretylol)	IV IM	Adults: initially: 5–10 mg/kg body weight, q15–30 min, up to 30 mg/kg body wt/24 hr PC: C	Transient hypertension, hypotension, vertigo, dizziness, lightheadedness, bradycardia, nausea, vomiting, diarrhea, swelling, and tenderness of parotid gland
N-acetylprocainamide (NAPA)			Arrhythmias, gastrointestinal symptoms, visual symptoms
sotalol	Oral IV	Adults: 160–480 mg qd in divided doses	Transient hypotension, bradycardia, arrhythmias, bronchospasm, peripheral ischemia

KEY: PC = pregnancy risk category. (The validity of pregnancy risk categories has not been established. See chapter 16, p 216.)

Focus on

Beta adrenergic blocking agents: similarities and differences

Similarities	Differences

Similarities

Pharmacodynamics

These agents block the agonistic effect of the sympathetic neurotransmitter by competing with receptor binding sites. They block β1 receptors in cardiac muscle and β2 receptors in bronchial and vascular smooth muscle.

Pharmacokinetics

These agents are adequately absorbed by the GI tract, minimally metabolized by the liver, removed by hemodialysis and most are excreted by the kidneys; they peak in 1–4 hours after oral administration, with an average half-life of 3–5 hours.

Therapeutic uses

These agents are used in the treatment of hypertension.

Adverse reactions

These include: (CNS) disorientation, short-term memory loss, emotional ability, clouded sensorium, fatigue, dizziness, nightmares, depression; (CV) bradycardia, hypotension, congestive heart failure, cardiac arrest; (RESP) bronchospasm; (GI) nausea, vomiting, diarrhea, constipation, epigastric distress, flatulence; (ENDO) impotence; (OTHER) hypersensitivity, cold extremities.

Contraindications

These agents are contraindicated in people with known hypersensitivity, and those with overt cardiac failure, cardiogenic shock, 2nd or 3rd degree AV block, sinus bradycardia, and bronchial asthma.

Differences

• **Labetalol** is also an alpha-adrenergic blocking agent. • **Propranolol** and **nadolol** also decrease the myocardial oxygen demand by blocking catecholamines. • **Propranolol, acebutol**, and **esmolol** also prolong the refractory period of the AV node and slow AV conduction. • **Acebutolol, atenolol, betaxolol, esmolol**, and **metoprolol** are cardioselective and block only B1 receptors. • **Pindolol** also has partial beta-agonist activity, decreasing cardiac output less than other beta blocking agents.

• **Nadolol** is poorly absorbed from the GI tract. • **Penbutolol, timolol, propranolol, metoprolol**, and **labetalol** are not removed by hemodialysis; it is unknown if **carteolol** and **pindolol** are removed by hemodialysis. • **Nadolol** is not metabolized. • **Acebutolol, labetalol** and **timolol** are also excreted in feces. • **Atenolol** has an elimination half-life of 6–7 hours; **carteolol** has an elimination half-life of 6 hours; **labetalol** has an elimination half-life of 6–8 hours (PO), 5.5 hours (IV); **metoprolol** has an elimination half-life of 3–7 hours; **nadolol** has an elimination half-life of 20–24 hours.

• **Propranolol, metoprolol**, and **nadolol** are used to treat angina pectoris. • **Propranolol, acebutol**, and **esmolol** are used to treat arrhythmias. • **Betaxolol, levobunolol**, and **timolol** are used to treat open-angle glaucoma. • **Timolol, propranolol**, and **metoprolol** are used as prophylaxis for myocardial infarction in susceptible persons. • **Propranolol** is used in the treatment of recurrent migraine headache attacks. Parenteral **labetalol** is used to produce controlled hypotension during surgery to decrease bleeding in the surgical field.

• **Pindolol** may also cause bone pain. • **Propranolol** may cause mental depression and paresthesias. • **Betaxolol** may cause eye discomfort, tearing, erythema, photophobia, and keratitis. • **Esmolol** may cause induration, inflammation at the infusion site, pallor, flushing, diaphoresis, and breathing difficulties. • **Labetalol** may cause vivid dreams, urinary retention, increased airway resistance, nasal stuffiness, orthostatic hypotension. • **Levobunolol** may cause cerebral ischemia, arrhythmias, urticaria, transient burning or stinging, decreased visual acuity, and blepharoconjunctivitis. • **Metoprolol** may cause agranulocytosis, shortness of breath, fever, and arthralgias. • **Nadolol** may cause dry mouth, tinnitus, and reversible alopecia. • **Penbutolol** may cause laryngospasm, cerebrovascular accident, and edema.

• **Penbutolol** is contraindicated in persons with congestive heart failure.

(continued)

Beta adrenergic blocking agents: similarities and differences (Continued)

Similarities

Precautions

These agents should be used cautiously in persons with impaired hepatic or renal function, coronary insufficiency, diabetes, hyperthyroidism, and bronchospastic chronic airway disease.

Nursing considerations

Instruct client in disease, treatment, drug therapy, regimen, adverse effects and compliance; assess cardiopulmonary status for baseline and ongoing for changes; assess blood pressure sitting, lying and standing for changes; check pulse rate prior to administering—if any extreme changes are noted or if rate is below 60 beats/min, hold the dose and notify the physician; assess client's heart rhythm continuously; follow weaning schedule when discontinuing the drug; institute safety precautions to prevent injury; monitor urinary and bowel elimination status for problems; instruct client in measure to reduce stress and manage diet.

Differences

• **Levobunolol** and **betaxolol** should be used cautiously in persons with closed-angle glaucoma and those with myasthenic-like symptoms, history of heart failure, or restricted pulmonary dysfunction. • **Carteolol** should be used with caution in persons with congestive heart failure who are controlled with digitalis and diuretics. • **Esmolol** should be used cautiously in atopic clients. • **Labetalol** and **penbutolol** should be used cautiously in persons with pheochromocytoma. • **Metoprolol** should be used cautiously in persons with sinus node dysfunction.

Use **esmolol** for short-term therapy only (48 hours); do not give by direct IV injection—dilute and administer as an infusion; change IV site if local reaction occurs. When giving **propranolol** IV, continuously monitor client's heart rate, rhythm, blood pressure, and ECG; administer a vasopressor if ordered for severe hypotension; administer orally with meals to enhance absorption; always double check route of administration since IV doses are much smaller than PO doses; administer glucagon to treat **propranolol** overdose. Instruct clients taking **labetalol** to change positions slowly and dangle prior to getting out of bed; tell client to remain supine for 3 hours after IV infusion for hypertension. Administer **metoprolol** with meals. Notify anesthesiologist that client is taking **propranolol** or **acebutol** if surgery is scheduled. Be aware that **labetalol**, **nadolol**, **propranolol**, **acebutolol**, **atenolol**, **metoprolol**, **pindolol**, and **timolol** may mask the symptoms of shock and hypoglycemia. Instruct clients taking **timolol eye drops** not to touch the dropper to the eye or surrounding tissue; instruct client in proper technique for instilling eye drops, teaching them to lightly press the lacrimal sac with the finger after administration to decrease systemic absorption.

---

tion of amiodarone before it reaches the liver (Mason, 1987, p 455). Half-life of elimination is biphasic with a mean of 53 days. It may be detected in the plasma for up to 9 months after drug discontinuation. It reaches peak plasma concentration after 3–7 hours. Less than 1% of the dose is excreted in the urine unchanged. Twenty-five percent of an administered dose is excreted in breast milk.

Some of these pharmacokinetic characteristics are unusual and mean that loading doses need to be used, there is a delay in the achievement of full effects, and there is a prolonged period of elimination of the drug.

Therapeutic uses. Amiodarone is only approved for use for treatment of life-threatening recurrent ventricular tachyarrhythmias that are resistant to control by other means. It is effective in maintaining sinus rhythm in most clients with paroxysmal atrial fibrillation and in many other clients with persistent atrial fibrillation. The drug is effective in preventing atrial fibrillation in clients with Wolff-Parkinson-White syndrome. It is contraindicated in clients with sick sinus syndrome.

Dosage and administration. Loading doses are needed to achieve a therapeutic effect within a reasonable period and a typical loading dose is 800–1,600 mg/d for 1–3 weeks until a therapeutic response is achieved. The dose is reduced to 600–800 mg/d after 1 month with a maintenance dose after that of around 400 mg/d. The IV form is not approved for use in the United States. Blood level monitoring may prove useful in avoiding adverse reactions and a concentration of 1–2 µg/ml is probably appropriate.

Adverse reactions. Its use is limited, as described above, due to the potential for significant toxicity. The adverse reactions of greatest concern are exacerbations of arrhythmias, worsening of congestive heart failure, and pulmonary fibrosis and pneumonitis. If pulmonary toxicity is suspected, the drug must be discontinued because about 10% of clients who show evidence of pulmonary toxicity die.

Hepatic toxicity is manifested by elevations in liver enzyme levels and the drug should be discontinued if they exceed three times the normal values.

Many clients experience blurred vision, smokey hue, or halos caused by corneal microdeposits of the drug. The deposits are reversible on stopping the drug. Photosensitization occurs and blue-gray skin discoloration occurs.

Alterations in thyroid function occur and manifestations of both hypothyroidism and hyperthyroidism have been reported. Hypothyroidism manifestations may require thyroid replacement therapy.

Neuromuscular side effects that have been reported include tremors of hands, sleep disturbances such as vivid dreams and nightmares, ataxia, peripheral neuropathy, and myopathy.

Drug interactions. Amiodarone binds covalently to cytochrome P450, thus blocking metabolism of many other drugs. Because of its slow elimination, its potential for interaction with other drugs persists for months after it is discontinued. It has been shown to interact with digoxin, flecainide, phenytoin, procainamide, quinidine, and warfarin, increasing the concentration of these drugs in each instance. Amiodarone may also have interactive effects with drugs such as beta-blockers and calcium channel blockers.

Bretylium

Bretylium was introduced in 1959 as an antihypertensive agent but it is not now used for that purpose.

Pharmacodynamics. At therapeutic concentrations, to control arrhythmias, bretylium prolongs the action-potential duration. This results in prolongation of the effective refractory period in atrial tissue. It increases the effective refractory period in Purkinje cells and ventricular muscle; this action is greater than that observed with other antiarrhythmic agents, which is the property that distinguishes it as a class III drug.

Bretylium's actions on the sympathetic nervous system include: 1) an initial release of neuronal stores of norepinephrine; and 2) an inhibition of norepinephrine release resulting from sympathetic nerve stimulation. The initial phase of catecholamine release may be associated with transient hypertension (Antonaccio, 1990, p 457).

A unique property of bretylium as an antiarrhythmic agent is its positive inotropic action; this action is related to the initial release of norepinephrine.

Pharmacokinetics. Bretylium is administered by IV or IM injection; oral absorption is poor. The drug accumulates in sympathetic ganglia and post-adrenergic neurons and protein binding is negligible. Its half-life is 5–10 hours with a range of 4–17 hours. More than 90% of the administered dose is excreted in the urine as the unchanged drug. Thus, the dose should be reduced in clients with impaired renal function (Antonaccio, 1990, p 459).

Therapeutic uses. Bretylium is not a first-line antiarrhythmic agent but it has been found useful in the treatment of life-threatening ventricular arrhythmias, principally recurrent ventricular tachycardia and/or fibrillation, especially when conventional agents have proven to be ineffective. It should not be used in circulatory shock and its associated release of catecholamines could increase myocardial oxygen consumption in a client with ischemic heart disease. This could precipitate difficulties with angina in the client.

Dosage and administration. Undiluted bretylium is administered at a dose of 5 mg/kg body weight by rapid IV injection. If ventricular fibrillation persists, the dose may be increased to 10 mg/kg and be repeated at 15–30-minute intervals until a total dose of not more than 30 mg/kg body weight has been given. To prevent recurrent ventricular tachycardia and/or fibrillation, a dosage of 5–10 mg/kg body weight is given by IV infusion over an 8-minute period. More rapid infusion may cause nausea and vomiting. A second dose may be given in 1–2 hours if tachyarrhythmia recurs. Present indications limit bretylium's use to a 5-day period.

Adverse reactions. The most important adverse reaction is hypotension as a result of peripheral vasodilation caused by adrenergic blockade. Hypotension is most commonly postural but marked hypotension in the supine position has been reported. Hypotension with a systolic blood pressure of 75 mm Hg or below needs to be treated and may be reversed by IV fluid to increase circulating blood volume and by cautious administration of IV norepinephrine.

Bradycardia, nausea, vomiting, diarrhea, swelling and tenderness of parotid gland (especially at mealtime), and vertigo have all been reported.

Drug interactions. If used with antihypertensive agents and certain arrhythmics, the hypotensive effects may be additive. It may worsen digitalis-induced arrhythmias and concurrent use is not recommended.

N-acetylprocainamide (NAPA)

Pharmacodynamics. The main action of this metabolite of procainamide is prolongation of action potential duration.

Pharmacokinetics. NAPA has a bioavailability of 85%. Ten to fifteen percent of it is bound to plasma proteins. Eighty percent of it is eliminated unchanged via the kidneys; the half-life of elimination is 6–10 hours (Jaillon & Drici, 1989, 67J).

Therapeutic uses. NAPA is mainly effective in ventricular arrhythmias.

Adverse reactions. Potentially significant arrhythmias can occur in the presence of low potassium. Digestive and visual symptoms do occur.

Sotalol
Pharmacodynamics. Sotalol is a nonselective beta-adrenergic blocking agent without significant membrane stabilizing activity. It does prolong repolarization at therapeutic plasma levels. This property is its major distinguishing feature and is the reason it is classified as a class III agent (Michelson & Dreifus, 1988, p 301). It reduces heart rate, cardiac contractility, and blood pressure.

Pharmacokinetics. It is absorbed rapidly after oral administration. Bioavailability varies from about 75% to 100%. Eighty percent of it is excreted unchanged in the urine and apparently there are no active metabolites. The elimination half-life varies from 7 to 10 hours. Fifty percent of it is bound to plasma proteins (Jaillon & Drici, 1989, 67J).

Therapeutic uses. It has been used as an effective antiarrhythmic agent for the suppression of both ventricular and supraventricular arrhythmias, including some clients with sustained ventricular tachyarrhythmias and some clients with Wolff-Parkinson-White syndrome.

Dosage and administration. The usual dosage is 160–480 mg per day in divided doses but larger doses have also been used as once-daily dosing. Intravenous doses of 0.2–1.0 mg/kg have been used in acute arrhythmia situations.

Adverse reactions. Transient hypotension, bradycardia, proarrhythmic effects, bronchospasm, and peripheral ischemia have been reported. Side effects are related to beta-blockade, prolongation of repolarization, and myocardial depression.

Drug interactions. Potentially malignant arrhythmias can occur in the presence of low potassium. It should be used with caution with drugs that have cardiac depressant properties.

■ Summary
Class III drugs alter cardiac dysrrhythmias by slowing down heart action. They act by prolonging the action potential duration or prolonging repolarization in the myocardium. Individual effects of these drugs that supplement the antiarrhythmic action include sodium channel blockade, increase in conduction time, reduction in sinus node automaticity, adrenergic blockade, and increased refractory period in the heart. Adverse effects include impairment of cardiovascular, pulmonary, hepatic, and GI function, and exacerbation of cardiac arrhythmias. When drug therapy using these drugs is initiated, clients are usually under close observation in acute care facilities.

Class IV drugs: Calcium channel blockers
Class IV antiarrhythmics are calcium channel blockers. Within this class, verapamil is the drug most frequently used to treat arrhythmias (See Table 27-10).

Pharmacodynamics. Calcium ions, like the sodium ions affected by class I antiarrhythmics, contribute to depolarization and repolarization by moving back and forth across cardiac cell membranes. Verapamil alters the action potential by inhibiting the influx of calcium ions through slow channels across the cell membrane of cardiac smooth muscle cells. It decreases AV conduction and prolongs the refractory period.

Verapamil produces peripheral vasodilation also by a relaxant effect on vascular smooth muscle cells, which reduces systemic peripheral resistance and myocardial afterload. It, thus, reduces myocardial oxygen consumption, which probably explains its ability to improve exercise tolerance in clients with angina pectoris.

Pharmacokinetics. Verapamil may be administered orally or IV. Oral doses are well absorbed but bioavailability is 20%–35% because of extensive first-pass hepatic metabolism. Approximately 90% of it is

Table 27-10. Antiarrhythmic drugs: class IV

Drug names	Preparations	Usual dosage	Adverse reactions
verapamil (Calan)	Oral film-coated tablets Oral extended-release tablets IV	Adults: initially: 40–80 mg q8h, increase dose q2d–3d; maintenance: 240–480 mg qd in 3–4 divided doses PC: C	Constipation, nausea, gastric discomfort, hypotension, bradycardia, fatigue, vertigo, ankle edema, headache, nervousness, pruritus, abnormal liver enzyme tests

KEY: PC = pregnancy risk category. (The validity of pregnancy risk categories has not been established. See chapter 16, p 216.)

bound to plasma proteins. After oral administration peak plasma concentration is achieved in 1–2 hours but it does show wide individual variation. Half-life ranges from 4.5 to 12 hours; half-life increases with repetitive dosing due to saturation of hepatic enzyme system. Steady-state plasma concentration is usually achieved within 48 hours. Fifty percent of it is eliminated via the kidney within the first 24 hours. The therapeutic plasma concentration is 125–400 ng/ml (Antonaccio, 1990, p 471).

Therapeutic uses. Verapamil is used in managing supraventricular tachyarrhythmias, angina pectoris (Prinzmetal's angina, effort-induced angina), and hypertension.

Dosage and administration. Oral doses of 240–480 mg/d in three to four divided doses are typical. The usual starting dose is 40–80 mg every 8 hours. The dose can be increased every 2 or 3 days. Use of a sustained release preparation may allow less frequent dosing. The IV dose has been 10 mg over 10–15 minutes, with a second dose in 30 minutes if necessary. It has been given as a continuous infusion at the rate of 0.1 mg/min.

Adverse reactions. The administration of verapamil is well tolerated by the majority of clients. Most complaints are about constipation, and perhaps nausea and gastric discomfort. Other adverse reactions include hypotension, bradycardia, fatigue, vertigo, ankle edema, headache, nervousness, and pruritus. If abnormal liver transaminase tests occur and are persistent, the drug may need to be discontinued. It should not be given to clients with sick sinus syndrome, severe congestive heart failure, or beta-adrenergic receptor blocking agents, except with great caution.

Drug interactions. The major interaction has been with digoxin; clearance of digoxin is reduced. The negative inotropic effect of verapamil could negate some of the benefits from the positive inotropic action of digoxin. Digoxin dosing adjustments will be necessary. Other interactions have been verapamil and quinidine (hypotension) and beta-adrenergic receptor blocking agents (hypotension, decreased cardiac output). Highly protein bound drugs could displace or be displaced by calcium channel blockers.

■ **Summary**

Verapamil is the calcium channel blocker used most frequently as an antiarrhythmic drug. It can be administered IV or orally in treating supraventricular tachycardias, angina pectoris, and hypertension. Adverse reactions include constipation, hypotension, bradycardia, and others.

Nursing management of all clients using antiarrhythmic agents

Nursing implications

Any agent capable of correcting cardiac arrhythmias is also capable of inducing other arrhythmias. The lack of fundamental knowledge of both the mechanism of arrhythmias and the mode of action of antiarrhythmic drugs makes accurate predictions of clinical response impossible. The use of these drugs should be considered hazardous, particularly during the initial stages of therapy.

Nursing process

Assessment Data required for assessment include a history of health problems related to cardiovascular disease, a complete drug history, and appraisal of current cardiovascular status, an assessment of the client's attitudes and feelings toward the life-threatening illness, and evidence of the client's and family's knowledge about cardiac arrhythmias and their treatment. Clients should be asked about specific risk factors for adverse reaction to the drugs to be used. Finally, the degree of stress and specific stressors affecting the client should be determined.

Nursing diagnosis Nursing diagnoses for clients affected by cardiac arrhythmias include the following:

Activity intolerance related to decreased energy secondary to imbalance between oxygen supply and demand
Fear of death related to risk of cardiac malfunction secondary to arrhythmia
Self-care deficit related to fatigability secondary to impaired tissue perfusion

Diagnoses stemming from the use of antiarrhythmic drugs include

Altered tissue perfusion related to hypotension secondary to inadequate sympathetic stress response
Fluid volume excess: edema related to decreased cardiac output and increased sodium and water retention
Impaired gas exchange related to bronchoconstriction or pulmonary edema
Constipation related to depression of intestinal nerve function
Diarrhea related to GI irritation
High risk for injury related to dizziness, weakness, and syncope due to postural hypotension

Other diagnoses include

Pain related to inflammation at sites of parenteral injections

Sexual dysfunction: gynecomastia, impotence, and decreased fertility
Body image disturbance related to hirsutism, gynecomastia, and impotence
High risk for infection related to impairment of immune response secondary to bone marrow depression

Many clients are at risk for

Noncompliance
Knowledge deficit concerning drug treatment of arrhythmias

Common collaborative problems that should be differentiated from the nursing diagnoses include the following:

Potential complication: iatrogenic ventricular fibrillation or bradycardia related to heart block
Potential complication: thromboembolism formation related to movement of clots formed in nonfunctioning atria
Potential complication: systemic lupus-like syndrome
Potential complication: gingival hypertrophy
Potential complication: osteomalacia

Many clients are at risk for noncompliance and knowledge deficit related to drug treatment of arrhythmias.

Planning Goals of care include increased activity tolerance; efficient use of the limited energy available to maximize the client's quality of life; maintenance of hope and, at the same time, acceptance of the reality of eventual death; and provision of personal care that the client is no longer able to carry out.

Goals related to the drug regimen are to prevent or promptly detect and treat cardiac arrest, thromboembolus, acute bronchospasm, or congestive failure if they occur; reduce the client's stress levels; maintain adequate blood pressure; decrease risk of accidental injury; alleviate or eliminate constipation or diarrhea; and promptly detect and treat other adverse reactions specific to the prescribed drugs.

Goals for the noncompliant client include correcting possible misinformation about the drug regimen, ameliorating adverse reactions to prescribed drugs, and altering the drug regimen in response to client decisions about treatment.

The major goals for clients and families with knowledge deficits are to help them understand and participate in the treatment regimen, and to provide information and teach skills necessary to effectively manage the client's home care after discharge.

Intervention For the acutely ill hospitalized client, the nurse will intervene directly to achieve treatment goals. At the same time, a teaching program is initiated

to prepare the client and family to assume care once the client returns home.

When antiarrhythmic medication is begun, the client should be under close observation, preferably in a special-care unit equipped with cardiac monitors. Under these conditions, many clients have or develop life-threatening cardiac arrhythmias that require cardiopulmonary resuscitation, cardioversion, or pacemaking. Allergic hypersensitivity and idiosyncratic drug reactions are also likely to surface during this period. Nursing assessment requires close attention to signs and symptoms of the adverse reactions that are characteristic of the specific agent being used. Small doses may be ordered to precede administration of the first full doses. The response to these test doses should be carefully evaluated before the first full dose is given.

Special care should be taken to prevent errors in the use of parenteral antiarrhythmics. The rate of flow of IV solutions containing antiarrhythmic drugs should be controlled by infusion controller to prevent inadvertent overdose, which could cause cardiac arrest.

Quinidine solutions that appear brownish in color must be discarded. Lidocaine solutions should be clearly marked "for cardiac arrhythmias." Preparations of this drug for local anesthesia contain preservatives and vasopressors that are contraindicated for the cardiac client. Some drugs are incompatible with emergency drugs that may be needed by the client. The IV equipment must provide for separation of the incompatible substances. The antiarrhythmic may be "piggy-backed" into an IV line that can be flushed of the drug if needed for administration of other drugs.

Cumulation of antiarrhythmic drugs can occur in clients with liver or renal impairment. Recipients of the drugs should be observed carefully for evidence of increasing toxicity. Although the margin of safety of antiarrhythmic drugs is wider than for digitalis, toxicity can induce sudden catastrophic cardiac malfunction.

When antiarrhythmic treatment is initiated, clients are usually kept in bed and continuously monitored for ECG and blood pressure. Signs and symptoms of hypotensive shock, heart block, congestive heart failure, or bradycardia may develop. Clients with atrial flutter or fibrillation should be watched for signs and symptoms of thromboemboli (pulmonary or peripheral). Color, respirations, and peripheral pulses should be monitored. Any of these complications may require emergency measures to maintain adequate cardiopulmonary function.

During this acute period, the client and family are aware of the life-threatening nature of the illness. Nursing staff should discuss the illness and its treatment realistically, acknowledging the gravity of the situation. They should support the client's and family's hope of the condition stabilizing, at the same time helping them to accept the guarded prognosis. Clients with poor prognoses may need assistance in completing tasks related to impending death (eg, making a will, arranging a visit with long-absent relatives). Both clients and families also may be involved in anticipatory grieving.

If the staff providing the client's physical care cannot assist with this emotional work, a psychiatric nurse, religious counselor (rabbi, pastor, priest), or other counselor should be consulted. Severe stress among everyone concerned should be minimized by controlling all possible stressors (eg, noise, glaring lights, missed meals, lack of sleep). Some of these—lack of food and sleep, debilitation, and anxiety—increase myocardial excitability and will increase the client's risk of arrhythmias.

The client's physical care should be performed initially by the nursing staff; when circulation improves and energy levels increase, the client may begin to participate in self-care. The choice of activity to be undertaken should be a joint decision shared by client and nursing staff.

A diet low in sodium and saturated fat that provides ample vitamins, potassium, trace minerals (especially magnesium, a lack of which promotes arrhythmias), and fluids should be encouraged. Small, frequent feedings are preferable to large meals.

Eliminate factors favoring vagal stimulation, including the ingestion of very hot or icy cold food or fluids, ingestion of large quantities of food or fluids at one time, and pressure in the rectum from fecal mass or instrumentation.

When clients are ambulated, they may be weak, dizzy, and prone to fainting from their prolonged immobility and postural hypotension as a result of antiarrhythmic medication. All possible safety precautions to prevent accidental falls should be taken.

When long-term antiarrhythmic medication is prescribed, a cardiovascular assessment should be performed during each nursing visit. The client should also be assessed for adverse reactions to the prescribed drugs. The nurse should encourage clients to report adverse drug reactions, so that measures can be taken to minimize their effects. Drug-related problems that cannot be corrected to the client's satisfaction should be reported to the physician so that the therapeutic regimen may be altered to better meet the client's needs.

Client education. Although antiarrhythmic therapy is more risky than some drug regimens, it can significantly improve cardiac function in many clients. Maintenance doses can be administered for long periods of time. These clients or their families should be aware that cardiac emergencies may arise. They should be taught the signs and symptoms of cardiac arrest, congestive failure, and pulmonary and peripheral embolism. Training in cardiopulmonary resuscitation techniques should be provided for the family. Knowing what emergency help to summon (rescue units, ambulances, police) requires investigation of available services and ready availability of such information as telephone numbers.

Education of the client receiving long-term antiarrhythmic therapy should include instructions regarding accuracy of dosage, proper drug storage, and monitoring of response. The side effects of the prescribed drug and measures to be taken when side effects occur must be described. Clients should be taught to monitor their pulses and to recognize bradycardia and signs and symptoms of congestive failure. Specific instructions should be given regarding normal parameters and the action required when abnormalities develop.

Clients may be receiving several other drugs (such as anticoagulants, digitalis, and diuretics) along with the antiarrhythmic agent. Such multiple drug regimens require careful attention to the risks attendant, not only with the use of individual agents, but also with interactions among the drugs that alter client response and increase the risk of adverse reactions. (See Chapter 9 for a discussion of drug interactions that can develop from multidrug therapy.)

The teaching plan should also include instruction in stress, diet, and fluid management (with diet, usually cholesterol, calorie, and sodium restriction but ample hydration to maintain blood volume); techniques for minimizing the effects of postural hypotension (maintaining ample hydration and gradually or slowly rising from a prone or seated position); and measures to promote optimal elimination (intermittent catheterization for clients who experience urinary retention, and hygienic measures for normalizing bowel function for those who develop diarrhea or constipation. (See Chapter 31 for a discussion on hygienic measures for alleviating disturbances in bowel elimination.)

Evaluation Data required for evaluation relate to activity tolerance, adaptation of lifestyle, incidence or absence of complications (cardiac arrest, thromboembolus, bronchospasm, congestive failure), serial blood pressures, fecal elimination, incidence or absence of injury, congruence between the medical regimen and the client's self-care, client acceptance of care by others, and client reports regarding quality of life and perceived prognosis.

Checklist of nursing actions

When antiarrhythmic drugs are ordered

☐ Screen clients for risk factors for adverse drug reactions; verify that the physician is aware of all such factors.

☐ Monitor ECG and blood pressure continuously; assess respirations and peripheral circulation frequently.

☐ Evaluate client status and laboratory data for response to treatment.

☐ Control the rate of infusion carefully if the drug is administered IV.

☐ Prevent errors in the use of antiarrhythmics, especially IV solutions of lidocaine.

☐ Be prepared to administer emergency care for cardiac arrest, thromboemboli, or heartblock when necessary.

☐ Watch for signs and symptoms of thromboemboli in clients who have had atrial flutter or fibrillation.

☐ Carefully observe clients with liver or renal impairment for signs of toxicity.

☐ Help client and family to accept a guarded prognosis while maintaining hope of stabilization.

☐ Support the client and family in maintaining hope of improvement.

☐ With a guarded prognosis, help client and family in anticipatory grieving; obtain counseling for them when needed.

☐ Minimize stressors on client and family, and teach them stress management techniques.

☐ During the medical crisis, conserve clients' energy by administering personal care; as clients improve, encourage them to take over personal care tasks of their choice.

☐ Provide assistance when clients ambulate; take safety measures to protect them from falling.

☐ Institute nursing measures to reduce the risk of adverse reactions specific to the antiarrhythmic drugs used; monitor clients for their signs and symptoms; when necessary, institute corrective nursing measures and consult with the physician for medical treatment.

☐ Prior to discharge, help families prepare for managing medical emergencies for which the client is at high risk.

☐ Teach clients and families how to manage the drug regimen at home.

☐ Teach clients and families to avoid stressors that increase the risk of arrhythmia.

References

Antonaccio M. (ed.) (1990). *Cardiovascular pharmacology*, 3rd ed. New York: Raven Press.

Craig CR, Stitzel RE. (1990). *Modern pharmacology*, 3rd ed. Boston: Little, Brown and Co.

DiBianco R, Shabetai R, Kostuk W, Moran J, Schlant R, Wright R. (1989). A comparison of oral milrinone, digoxin, and their combination in the treatment of patients with chronic heart failure. *N Engl J Med, 320*, 677–683.

Hansten P, Horn J. (1991). *Drug interactions and updates*, 7th ed. Philadelphia: Lea and Febiger.

Hussar DA. (1990). New drugs. *Nursing 90, 20(12)*, 41–51.

Jaillon P, Drici M. (1989). Recent antiarrhythmic drugs. *Am J Cardiol, 64*, 65J–69J.

Mason J. (1987). Amiodarone. *N Engl J Med, 316*, 455–465.

McInnes GT, Brodie MJ. (1988). Drug interactions that matter: A critical reappraisal. *Drugs, 36*, 83–110.

Michelson E, Dreifus L. (1988). Newer antiarrhythmic drugs. *Med Clin North Am, 72(2)*, 275–319.

Roden D, Woosley R. (1986a). Tocainide. *N Engl J Med, 315*, 41–45.

Roden D, Woosley R. (1986b). Flecainide. *N Engl J Med, 315*, 36–41.

Withering W. (1977). *An account of the foxglove and some of its uses: With practical remarks on dropsy and other diseases.* (Reprint of 1785 edition.) Wakefield, NH: Longwood Publishing Group.

Woosley RL, Funck-Brentano C. (1988). Overview of the clinical pharmacology of antiarrhythmic drugs. *Am J Cardiol, 61*, 61A–69A.

Bibliography

Brozena S, Jessup M. (1990). Pathophysiologic strategies in the management of congestive heart failure. *Annu Rev Med, 41*, 65–74.

Cardiac therapy: Digitalis glycosides, diuretics, antianginals, and antiarrhythmics. *Nursing 86, 16(11)*, 92–93.

Colucci W, Wright R, Braunwald E. (1986). New positive inotropic agents in the treatment of congestive heart failure. *N Engl J Med, 314*, 290–297.

Farah A. (1986). Historical perspectives on inotropic agents. *Circulation, 73 (suppl III)*, III-4–III-9.

Gandy W. (1989). Severe epinephrine-propanolol interaction. *Ann Emerg Med, 18(1)*, 98–99.

Gever LN. (1984). Giving procainamide safely. *Nursing 84, 14(5)*, 116.

Knobler H, Levy IS, Gavish D, Chajek-Shaul T. (1986). Quinidine-induced hepatitis: A common and reversible hypersensitivity reaction. *Arch Intern Med, 146*, 526–528.

Mahler R, Sissons W, Watters K. (1986). Pigmentation induced by quinidine therapy. *Arch Dermatol, 122*, 1062–1064.

Ordog GJ, Benaron S, Bhasin V, Wasserberger J, Balasubramanium S. (1987). Serum digoxin levels and mortality in 5,100 patients. *Ann Emerg Med, 16*, 32.

Rehnqvist N. (1989). Arrhythmias and their treatment in patients with heart failure. *Am J Cardiol, 64*, 61J–64J.

Scherer P. (1987). New drugs: Hands-on experience, part I. *Am J Nurs, 87*, 448–484.

Smith T. (1988). Digitalis: Mechanisms of action and clinical use. *N Engl J Med, 318*, 358–364.

Surawicz B. (1989). Ventricular arrhythmias: Why is it so difficult to find a pharmacologic cure? *J Am Coll Cardiol, 14(6)*, 1401–1416.

Wellens H, Brugada P, Smeets J. (1988). Antiarrhythmic drugs for supraventricular tachycardia. *Am J Cardiol, 62*, 69L–73L.

Yacone L. (1988). The nurse's guide to cardiovascular drugs, part I. *RN*, 36–44.

Yacone L. (1988). The nurse's guide to cardiovascular drugs. part II, *RN*, 40–47.

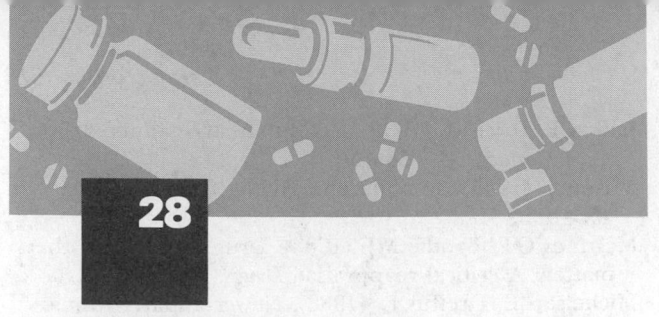

28

Vascular drugs

Drugs that affect the blood vessels are used to enhance circulation. They may be administered to correct temporary, acute conditions such as shock or hypertensive crisis, or to combat the slow degenerative process of atherosclerosis. However, drug therapy is not the best approach to these problems, which usually occur secondary to trauma and disease resulting from unhealthy lifestyles.

Physiology of the vascular system

The circulatory system is a continuous, closed circuit of tubes that carry the blood pumped by the heart through the lungs and periphery of the body. The flow of fluid through this system depends on the patency of the vessels and pressure gradients, which propel liquids from the arteries to the veins and back to the heart. Maintenance of the pressure gradients requires adequate pumping action by the heart to establish high pressure in the vessels opening from the ventricles; elasticity of the arteries to moderate and prolong this pressure; and a degree of peripheral resistance sustained by partial constriction of the smaller vessels. The volume of the vascular bed must be appropriate for the blood volume.

In a healthy person's circulation, the heart pumps a bolus of blood into the arteries during systole (Fig. 28-1). This fluid volume distends the blood vessel, stretching the muscle fibers and raising the intraluminal pressure above that of the distal arterioles, capillaries, and venules. The pressure gradient established in this way causes blood to flow rapidly toward the capillary bed.

As the heart relaxes, the elastic walls of the arteries contract, exerting continuing pressure, which subsides gradually until it is equal to the peripheral resistance. Because pressure in the venous system remains much lower than pressure in the arterioles and capillaries, a pressure gradient and blood flow are maintained throughout the cycle, although the flow is most rapid

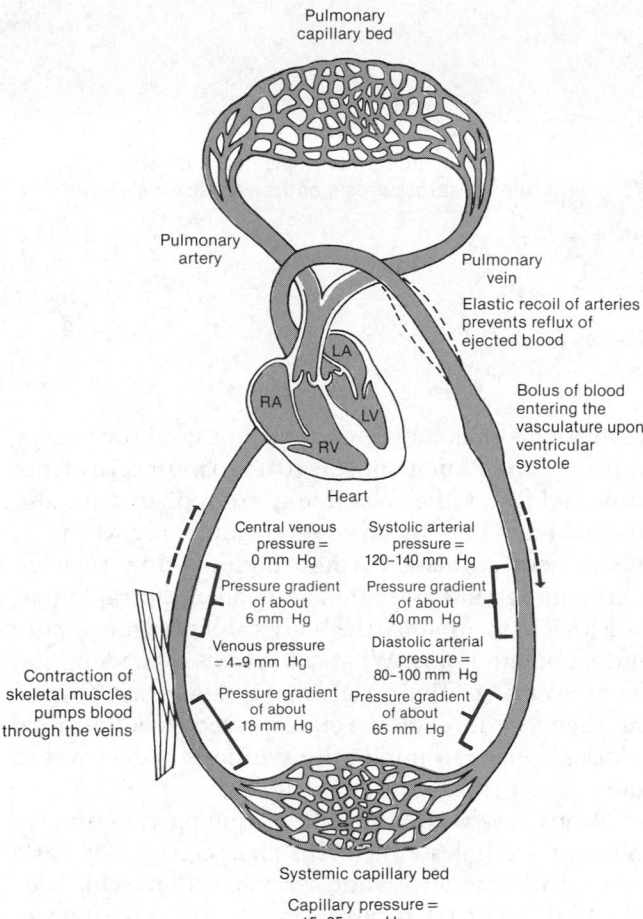

Figure 28-1. Forces moving blood through the systemic circulation.

when the heart contracts. The flow of venous blood is promoted by skeletal muscle contraction. Valves in the veins allow the blood to flow only toward the heart.

Vascular pathology

In addition to cardiac malfunction and changes in the volume of circulating blood, changes in the blood vessels can decrease blood flow. Circulation is reduced by processes that decrease the patency of the blood vessels, impair their elasticity, cause inappropriate vasoconstriction or vasodilation, or interfere with the venous return. Patency may be reduced by external pressure (the cause of decubitus), internal obstructions (thrombi, emboli, tumors), and atherosclerosis. Elasticity is reduced in arteriosclerosis, a degenerative process involving progressive fibrosis and calcification of the vascular wall. Inappropriate vasodilation is seen in neurogenic shock and postural hypotension, whereas excessive vasoconstriction is characteristic of hypertension. Venous pooling occurs in varicosities owing to the destruction of the valves and increased volume capacity in the tortuous vessels.

The best approach to circulatory problems is cor-

rection of the underlying cause whenever feasible. Treatment ranges from surgery to correction of health practices detrimental to the vascular system (such as a high-fat diet). When such approaches are not sufficient to correct the problem, drug therapy may be helpful. Research to improve the treatment of vascular disorders, including drug therapy, is continuing at an active pace, spurred on by the high mortality and morbidity rates associated with vascular disorders. Drugs presently available that affect the blood vessels include antilipemics, vasoconstrictors, vasodilators, and sclerosing agents.

Drugs used to combat atherosclerosis

Pathophysiology of atherosclerosis

Atherosclerosis is a disease of the large- and medium-sized arteries. It is characterized by the formation of plaques, which narrow the vessel lumen. It is associated with *arteriosclerosis*, a word that means hardening of the arteries (Fig. 28-2). Risk factors for atherosclerosis have been identified but there are still unanswered questions about how the risk factors contribute to the development of atherosclerosis. Two theories about atherosclerosis that have received much attention in recent years are: 1) the vessel injury hypothesis, and 2) the lipid infiltration hypothesis.

The vascular endothelial layer acts as a selective barrier that protects the subendothelial layers. Some feel that repeated injury may impair the ability of the endothelium to regenerate. Injurious agents would include products associated with smoking and mechanical stress associated with hypertension. With injury to the endothelium and pulling apart of endothelial cells, the opportunity may be provided for platelet adherence, aggregation, and thrombosis (Porth, 1990, pp 269–271).

Types of lipids

Considerable evidence links hypercholesterolemia to atherosclerosis. Lipids are insoluble in plasma and are carried in lipoproteins. There are five classes of lipoproteins: 1) chylomicrons, 2) very low-density lipoproteins (VLDLs), 3) intermediate-density lipoproteins, 4) low-density lipoproteins (LDLs), and 5) high-den-

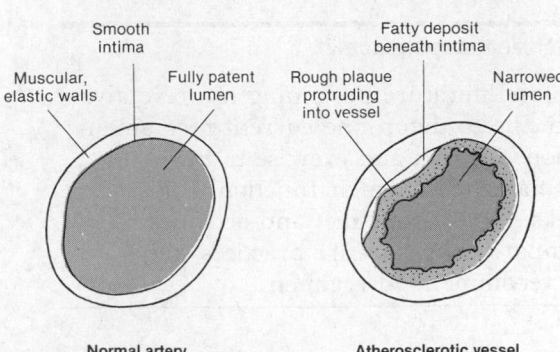
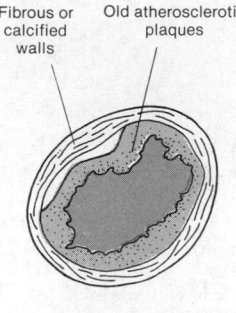

Figure 28-2. Typical lesions of atherosclerosis and arteriosclerosis.

sity lipoproteins (HDL) (Table 28-1). The higher the density of the compounds, the smaller the particles.

Although general increases in plasma lipids and lipoproteins were implicated in atherosclerosis and coronary artery disease in early studies, later research has indicated that the type of lipids present may also be significant (Porth, 1990, p 273). High concentrations of all lipids except the HDLs are associated with an increased risk of atherosclerosis. High serum levels of triglycerides and LDL lipoproteins are associated with coronary heart disease. Triglycerides form a high percentage of the chemical composition of both chylomicrons and VLDLs. Low-density lipoproteins contain a high proportion of cholesterol. High-density lipoproteins may exert a protective effect against atherosclerosis and may promote the mobilization and metabolism of cholesterol, thereby reducing deposition of it in blood vessel walls.

Associated factors

Among the factors believed to affect the level and composition of blood lipids are diet, genetic predisposition, hormone status, and level of activity (Box 28-1).

Diets high in calories, saturated fats, and cholesterol create a predisposition toward hyperlipidemia. The body is capable of synthesizing cholesterol from all nutrients that contain calories not used for energy or tissue repair but it appears to do so most easily from saturated fats. Other blood lipid components are also derived from both dietary sources and body synthesis. Metabolism of fats is further moderated by such dietary components as lecithin and polyunsaturated fats, which seem to enhance the body's ability to metabolize and eliminate lipids. What constitutes a prudent diet for preventing atherosclerosis remains controversial but diets low in cholesterol, saturated fats, and total calories appear to inhibit the synthesis of fats and to lower blood concentration of lipids.

Many *genetic influences* affect lipid metabolism. Familial hypercholesterolemia is characterized by early onset of atherosclerosis and serious cardiovascular disease. Inherited traits also create a predisposition to diabetes mellitus, hypothyroidism, obesity, and other conditions associated with hyperlipidemias.

The hormones estrogen and thyroxine, tend to reduce atherosclerosis. Thyroxine lowers cholesterol and triglyceride levels. Part of this effect stems from thyroxine's diversion of calories for energy, which reduces the substrate available for the body's synthesis of cholesterol and fats. Estrogens increase the proportion of HDL in the serum. It is known that women of childbearing age, whose estrogen levels are high, do not develop vascular degeneration as often or as early

Table 28-1. Properties of the plasma lipoproteins

Lipoprotein class	Density	Electrophoretic mobility (paper)	Chemical composition (% by weight)				
			Free cholesterol	*Cholesterol esters*	*Phospholipids*	*Triglycerides*	*Protein*
Chylomicrons*	0.95	origin	3.1	6.0	7.1	81.3	2.5
Very low density (VLDL)†	0.95–1.006	pre-β	6.0	16.2	17.9	51.8	7.1
Low-density (LDL)‡	1.006–1.063	β	7.5	39.4	23.1	9.3	20.7
High-density (HDL)§	1.063–1.21	α	2.0	17.4	26.1	8.1	46.4

*These lipids derive from intestinal absorption and provide fat for storage in adipose tissue.
†Produced by liver synthesis, in part from carbohydrates, these lipids are also stored in adipose tissue.
‡These lipids contain the major portion of the plasma cholesterol.
§These protective lipids are increased by exercise and estrogens.
Data from Gilman AG, Goodman LS, Rall TW, Murad F. (1985). *Goodman and Gilman's the pharmacological basis of therapeutics*, 7th ed, pp 827–832. New York: Macmillian; and Katcher BS, Young LY, Koda-Kimble MA. (1983). *Applied therapeutics*, 3rd ed, p 651–655. Spokane: Applied Therapeutics, Inc.

Box 28-1. Factors that influence the progress of atherosclerosis*

Genetic predisposition

Smoking

Diet rich in fats and calories

Obesity

Blood cholesterol levels

Stress

Hormone status

Disease (*eg*, diabetes mellitus)

Hypertension

Aging

*Accelerated in developed countries with advanced technology

as their male counterparts. After menopause, when estrogen levels drop, the incidence of disease in women soon rises to equal that of men. Other hormones also may play a role in fat metabolism, especially the glucocorticoids, which affect body metabolism of all three energy nutrients: fats, carbohydrates, and proteins.

Exercise has long been valued for its protective effect on the vascular system. It uses up calories, reducing the substrate available for lipid synthesis and storage in adipose tissue. Exercise also tends to blunt the appetite and increases the proportion of protective HDL in the blood.

Classification of hyperlipemias

Hyperlipidemia is defined in various ways. According to the National Cholesterol Education Panel, cholesterol concentrations of less than 200 mg/dl are desirable; 200–239 mg/dl are borderline high risk of coronary heart disease; and values of 240 mg/dl or higher are elevated and of high risk (Gilman, Rall, Nies, & Taylor, 1990, p 879).

With the aim of tailoring treatment to the particular type of hyperlipoproteinemia, a system of classifying clients with hyperlipemia has been developed (Table 28-2). The hyperlipoproteinemias can be designated as primary or secondary. Primary hyperlipoproteinemias can be divided into two groups: those that are caused by an inherited, single-gene defect and those that appear to be caused by a combination of several genetic factors that act together with various environmental insults (such as diets high in saturated fats and cholesterol).

Secondary hyperlipoproteinemias are complications of a more generalized metabolic disturbance, such as diabetes mellitus, hypothyroidism, or excessive alcohol intake.

Table 28-2. Classification of primary hyperlipoproteinemias

Disorder (naming varies)	Possible phenotype	Predominant lipid abnormalities	Incidence	Age of detection	Commonly used drugs
Primary hyperchylomicronemia, exogenous hyperlipemia	I	Increased chylomicrons,* increased triglycerides	Very rare	Early childhood	—
Familial hypercholesterolemia	IIa	Increased total cholesterol, increased LDLC*	Common	Early childhood, in severe cases over age 20	lovastatin resin probucol niacin
(Familial) combined hyperlipidemia	IIb	Increased total cholesterol, increased VLDLC,* increased LDLC,* increased triglycerides	Common —		gemfibrozil niacin resin
Familial dysbetalipoproteinemia	III	Increased total cholesterol, increased VLDLC, increased IDLC,* increased LDLC, increased triglycerides	Relatively uncommon	Over age 20	gemfibrozil niacin clofibrate
Familial hypertriglyceridemia, endogenous hyperlipemia	IV	Increased VLDLC,* decreased HDLC, increased triglycerides	Common	Adulthood	niacin gemfibrozil clofibrate
Mixed hypertriglyceridemia	V	Increased total cholesterol, increased chylomicrons, increased VLDLC,* increased IDLC, increased triglycerides	Uncommon	Early adulthood	gemfibrozil niacin clofibrate

*Primary abnormality.
KEY: VLDLC = very low-density lipoprotein cholesterol; IDLC = intermediate-density lipoprotein cholesterol; LDLC = low-density lipoprotein cholesterol; HDLC = high-density lipoprotein cholesterol.

The LDL cholesterol should be the indicator for management decisions, together with any other coronary artery disease risk factors that are present. A minimal goal is to reduce LDL cholesterol to 160 mg/dl or less (serum cholesterol 240 mg/dl or less) in the client who has no coronary disease and fewer than two risk factors. Levels of serum triglycerides in excess of 250 mg/dl are excessive.

In many clients, diet alone can bring lipoprotein levels within the desired range and several months of effort may be made for this purpose. If hypercholesterolemia is severe, however, drug therapy might have to be initiated earlier. A saturated fat intake of less than 8%–10% of total calories and a restriction of daily cholesterol intake to 200 mg or less is recommended (Kane & Malloy, 1990, p 477).

The drugs discussed below should only be used in conjunction with a low saturated fat and low cholesterol diet.

Antilipemic drugs

An active search for agents that can safely control blood lipid levels is in progress. A number of useful drugs are presently prescribed (Table 28-3).

HMG CoA reductase inhibitors

The introduction of a new class of drugs derived from fungi has been important in the therapy for the hyperlipoproteinemias. The first such drug was mevasatin, isolated in Japan in 1976. The drugs undergoing trials at the present time include mevasatin, lovastatin, simvastatin, and provastatin.

Lovastatin

Lovastatin (Mevacor) has been the most extensively studied HMG Coenzyme A (CoA) reductase inhibitor and is the only one currently approved for use in the United States. It was isolated from cultures of *Aspergillus terreus.*

Pharmacodynamics. This newest antilipemic agent reduces cholesterol synthesis by competitively inhibiting HMG CoA reductase, an enzyme that is necessary to convert HMG CoA to mevalonate (an early step in the biosynthesis of cholesterol). Additional mechanisms contribute to a reduction in VLDL and LDL production and/or rate of production. The serum levels of VLDL, LDL, cholesterol, and plasma triglycerides are reduced while the plasma concentration of HDL cholesterol is increased. Since the enzyme is not completely inhibited, mevalonate is available in amounts necessary to maintain homeostasis.

Pharmacokinetics. Lovastatin is absorbed after oral administration. Peak plasma concentrations are obtained in 2–4 hours. It crosses the blood–brain and placental barriers. The drug is metabolized in the liver to active metabolites. About 80% of a dose is excreted in the feces via the bile, and approximately 10% is excreted in the urine.

Therapeutic uses. Lovastatin is indicated as an adjunct to diet in the treatment of primary hypercholesterolemia (types IIa and IIb). It is used with clients with a significant risk of coronary artery disease or clients with coronary artery disease who have not responded to other cholesterol-lowering measures.

Dosage and administration. Lovastatin is available in 20-mg or 40-mg tablets and doses of 20–80 mg per day are used with the total dose divided into two smaller doses. Dosage adjustments may be made as

Table 28-3. Drugs employed to reduce blood lipid levels

Drug names	Preparations	Usual dosage	Therapeutic effect
HMG CoA reductase inhibitor: lovastatin (Mevacor)	Oral tablets	Adults: 20–80 mg per day, divided into two doses with meals	Reduction of cholesterol and LDL serum levels
Bile acid-sequestering resins: cholestyramine (Questran, Questran Light, Cholybar)	Powder in packets or cans Chewable bars	Adults: 4 g, tid–qid ac Children: 80 mg/kg body weight, tid	Reduction of cholesterol and LDL serum levels
colestipol (Colestid)	Powder in bottles	Adults: 15–30 g/d, divided in 2–4 doses	Reduction of cholesterol and LDL serum levels
nicotinic acid of niacin (Nicolar)	Oral tablets Oral extended-release tablets	Adults: 1.5–6 g/d, divided in 2–4 doses, with meals	Reduction of LDL and LVDL serum levels
Fibric acid derivatives clofibrate (Atromid S)	Oral capsules	Adults: 500 mg, qid	Reduction of triglyceride and VLDL (and in some recipients, LDL) serum level
gemfibrozil (Lopid)	Oral capsules, tablets	Adults: 600 mg, bid, before morning and evening meals	Reduction of triglyceride and VLDL serum level
probucol (Lorelco)	Oral tablets	Adults: 500 mg, bid, with morning and evening meals	Reduction of cholesterol serum levels

necessary every 4 weeks. Peak effect of the drug will be achieved in 6–8 weeks.

If a single daily dose is used, it is recommended that it be administered with the evening meal. The reasons for this recommendation are that the highest rate of cholesterol production occurs during the night and that a larger percentage of the drug is absorbed when it is taken with food.

As with other antilipemic drugs, the client should also be on a cholesterol-lowering diet and an appropriate exercise regimen. The treatment will probably be ongoing for several years or for the rest of the individual's life.

Adverse reactions. Side effects include various gastrointestinal (GI) symptoms (constipation or diarrhea, dyspepsia, flatus, abdominal pain or cramps, heartburn, nausea), dizziness, headache, rash, and insomnia. In a small percentage of clients, it causes marked elevation of hepatic transaminases. The drug is contraindicated in clients with known hepatic dysfunction. In a small percentage of clients, it causes a myopathy, which can lead to myolysis with risk of renal failure. This type of problem has been seen particularly with clients on other drugs such as immunosuppressants (cyclosporin) as might be used with cardiac transplant surgery.

In the laboratory, this drug inhibits cholesterol synthesis in the lens and this might cause cataracts (this has happened in dogs). To date, it has not been found to produce cataracts in humans although less than 2% of clients did report blurred vision.

Bile acid-sequestering resins

Cholestyramine (Questran) and colestipol (Colestid) are anion-exchange resins used as antilipemics. These resins, since they are not absorbed from the GI tract, appear to be the safest antilipemics available.

Pharmacodynamics. Cholestyramine and colestipol are called *bile acid sequestrants*. Cholesterol is the major precursor of bile acids that are normally secreted from the gallbladder and liver into the small intestine. After bile acids perform their physiologic functions, they are normally returned to the liver.

Cholestyramine absorbs and combines with bile salts in the intestine in exchange for chloride. An insoluble complex is formed and is excreted in the feces. In an attempt to compensate for the loss of bile salts, the body increases the rate of metabolism of cholesterol to bile acids. Over time, the use of cholestyramine causes a reduction in serum cholesterol and LDL. The agent has either no effect on or increases triglycerides, VLDL, and HDL.

Colestipol binds bile acids in the intestine, forming an insoluble complex that is excreted in the feces. To compensate for the loss of bile acids removed by the drugs, the liver increases the rate of oxidation of cho-

lesterol by converting more sterol to bile acids. Thus, over time, the long-term fecal loss of bile acids causes a reduction of serum cholesterol and LDL. This agent has either no effect on or may increase triglycerides, VLDL, and HDL.

Pharmacokinetics. Anion-exchange resins are poorly absorbed systemically. They act locally within the GI tract and are excreted in the feces.

Therapeutic uses. Both resins may be used to treat familial hypercholesterolemia (type IIa) or familial combined hyperlipidemia (type IIb). In clients with elevated concentrations of VLDL and HDL, they are not helpful; they should not be used in types III, IV, or V.

Cholestyramine may be used to relieve pruritus associated with biliary disease. In individuals with partial biliary obstruction, excess bile acids may be deposited in the dermal tissues, resulting in pruritus.

Dosage and administration. These resins come in packets, cans, or bottles of powder. These resins must not be given in dry form. To avoid esophageal irritation or obstruction and intestinal obstruction, these resins must be well diluted in fluids prior to administration. These preparations have a sandy or gritty quality and may be mixed in pulpy fruits or pureed foods. Cholestyramine is also available in chewable bars containing 4 g of anhydrous resins (Cholybar).

The usual daily dosage is 12–16 g (cholestyramine) or 15–30 g (colestipol) divided into two or four doses and taken before or during meals and at bedtime (Gilman, Rall, Nies, & Taylor, 1990, p 891).

Adverse reactions. Anion-exchange resins are nondiscriminatory in their actions; they bind drugs and nutrients as well as bile acids, leading to decreased intestinal absorption of them (Box 28-2). Parenteral supplements of fat-soluble vitamins may be required in long-term therapy.

The most common adverse reactions to cholestyramine and colestipol involve the GI tract. These drugs should be used with caution in clients with preexisting bowel disease or intractable constipation. Constipation occurs in 10%–20% of recipients of these drugs: fecal impaction may occur and hemorrhoids

Box 28-2. Drugs binding with bile acid-sequestering resins

Antibiotics, including penicillin, tetracyclines, cephalexin, clindamycin, trimethoprim

Anticoagulants

Chenodiol

Corticosteroids

Digitalis preparations

Fat-soluble vitamins (A, D, E, K)

Folic acid

Iron preparations

Mefenamic acid

Phenobarbital

Phenylbutazone

Thiazide diuretics

Thyroxine, thyroid hormones

may be aggravated. Measures should be taken to prevent constipation, especially in persons with coronary artery disease. Other GI problems include abdominal or rectal discomfort, distention or "bloating," flatulence, anorexia, nausea, vomiting, diarrhea, heartburn, steatorrhea. Dysphagia, sour taste, hiccups, ulcer attack, melena, pancreatitis, and diverticulitis have been reported.

Because it liberates chlorides in the GI tract, cholestyramine can cause hyperchloremic acidosis. This condition accelerates urinary calcium excretion and increases the risk of osteoporosis.

Cholestyramine contains tartrazine and is contraindicated for asthmatics with aspirin allergy because these persons also tend to be allergic to tartrazine.

Colestipol may also affect other body systems. Symptoms of central nervous system involvement include headache, dizziness, anxiety, vertigo, drowsiness, fatigue, and weakness. Skin rash, urticaria, elevated liver enzymes, musculoskeletal pain, and arthritis may occur.

Drug interactions. The resins may bind other compounds in the intestine, including drugs administered concurrently. This has been noted with thyroxine, anticoagulants, and various digitalis preparations (among others). Therefore, it is recommended that other drugs be taken 1 hour before or 4 hours after the resin.

Nicotinic acid

When administered in very large doses, nicotinic acid (niacin) is capable of lowering plasma cholesterol and triglyceride concentrations. Cholesterol is decreased by about 10% but triglycerides may be reduced by

20%–80%. Niacin decreases the hepatic secretion of VLDL, which, in turn, results in decreased plasma levels of LDL.

Pharmacodynamics. It is believed that the antilipemic effect of niacin derives, in part, from a lowering of plasma concentration of free fatty acid. Circulating free fatty acid is derived mostly from adipose tissue and niacin is an inhibitor of lipolysis in adipose tissue. Circulating free fatty acid is a main source for synthesis of triglycerides in the liver. Thus, a reduction in free fatty acid can decrease triglyceride synthesis (Craig & Stitzel, 1990, p 242).

Niacin may also accelerate the activity of lipoprotein lipase, which transports triglyceride to adipose tissue, thereby facilitating the removal of this from the blood.

Pharmacokinetics. Niacin is a water-soluble vitamin readily absorbed following oral administration on an empty stomach. It is metabolized to niacinamide, which is widely distributed in the body, including breast milk. The liver further metabolizes niacinamide; both unchanged niacin and its metabolites are excreted by the kidneys. In the doses used to treat hyperlipidemia, large amounts of unchanged drug are excreted in the urine.

Therapeutic uses. Niacin is considered effective in all types of hyperlipoproteinemia except type I. It is especially useful in type V with those clients who do not respond to gemfibrozil (discussed in next section). Because of niacin's adverse reactions, in type IV, gemfibrozil may be more suitable and lovastatin may be more suitable in type IIa.

In one study, men with previous myocardial disease were given 3 g per day of niacin for 6 years. At the end of the study, the drug on the average had lowered serum cholesterol by 10% and reduced nonfatal myocardial infarctions (MIs) by 70%. The clients also had a significant reduction in mortality 9 years after discontinuing the drug, compared to a placebo group (Dujovne & Harris, 1989, pp 277–278).

Dosage and administration. Niacin (Nicolar) is available as 100-mg tablets, 500-mg tablets, and extended-release tablets in amounts of 25–500 mg. Niacin is a vitamin of the B group and the recommended dietary allowance is 20 mg per day. However, the usual daily dose for antilipemic effect is 1.5–6 g in three doses, taken orally with meals or just after meals. Therapy with niacin is started with three 100–200-mg tablets per day and over a 1–3-week period additional tablets are added. This slow increase in dosage seems to help decrease difficulties with certain adverse reactions.

Adverse reactions. In the high doses required for treatment of hyperlipemias, niacin initially produces an intense cutaneous flush and pruritus over the face and upper body. After continued treatment, these reactions subside. Hyperglycemia and hyperuricemia occur. Diabetes mellitus is more difficult to control, and gouty arthritis may develop in clients receiving the drug. Gastrointestinal reactions include vomiting, diarrhea, dyspepsia, and altered hepatic function accompanied by jaundice. Niacin causes histamine release, which increases hydrochloric acid secretion in the stomach; peptic ulcers have been reported.

Other adverse reactions to niacin include skin problems (rash, dry skin, increased sebaceous gland activity, hyperpigmentation, pruritus); visual changes (amblyopia, blurred vision, loss of central vision); and central nervous system changes (headache, nervousness, panic). Vasodilation induced by the drug may cause hypotension, dizziness, tachycardia, and syncope. Vasovagal attacks may occur. Some niacin preparations contain tartrazine and may cause acute asthmatic attacks in persons with aspirin allergy.

Niacin in large doses should not be used during pregnancy or lactation unless the possible benefits outweigh the potential risk. Safety and efficacy for children have not been established; the drug is not recommended for prepubertal children.

Drug interactions. Niacin may interact with some antihypertensive drugs to increase postural hypotension.

Fibric acid derivatives

Fibric acid derivatives used to decrease plasma concentrations of triglycerides and cholesterol are gemfibrozil (Lopid) and clofibrate (Atromid S). A related compound, fenofibrate, is available in Europe.

Pharmacodynamics. Clofibrate's primary effect is to increase the activity of lipoprotein lipase, which, in turn, promotes the catabolism of the triglyceride-rich lipoproteins, VLDL and intermediate-density lipoproteins. Hepatic synthesis and secretion of VLDL may also be decreased. High-density lipoprotein is raised indirectly as a result of the decrease in the concentration of VLDL. The effect on LDL plasma levels is variable; it may increase or decrease. Lowering of LDL may be related to enhanced hepatic clearance of VLDL and intermediate-density liproproteins, which would reduce the production of LDL. Gemfibrozil is less effective in lowering LDL.

Pharmacokinetics. Clofibrate and gemfibrozil are readily absorbed from the GI tract. Following absorption, clofibrate is hydrolyzed to an active metabolite. This metabolite and unchanged gemfibrozil are highly protein bound. Both drugs cross the placenta. Both are metabolized by the liver and excreted by the kidneys. In healthy adults, clofibrate has an elimination half-life of 12–25 hours; in persons with low serum albumin or renal impairment, half-life is prolonged.

Gemfibrozil has an elimination half-life of 1.3–1.5 hours.

Therapeutic uses. Clofibrate appears to be helpful in clients with familial dysbetalipoproteinemia, type III.

The Helsinki Heart Study in 1987 has demonstrated gemfibrozil's efficacy in reducing the manifestations of coronary artery disease. The clients in the study had hypercholesterolemia with or without hypertriglyceridemia and were treated for 5 years. Gemfibrozil reduced total cholesterol by 11%, LDL by 10%, and triglycerides by 43%. It increased HDL by 10%. Fatal and nonfatal MIs were reduced by 34% (Gilman, Rall, Nies, & Taylor, 1990, pp 887–888).

Dosage and administration. Clofibrate is available as 500-mg capsules and is administered in two or four doses daily for a total dose of 2 g. Gemfibrozil is available as 300-mg capsules and 600-mg tablets. The usual dose is 600 mg twice daily, taken 30 minutes before meals.

Adverse reactions. Fibric acid derivatives cause numerous adverse reactions, some of which are potentially serious. The most frequent effects are GI effects (anorexia, nausea, diarrhea, vomiting, abdominal discomfort, gastritis, and stomatitis). Hypogeusia, or blunting of the sense of taste, is an additional effect. These effects tend to decrease with continued therapy.

The fibric acids increase the lithogenicity of bile, and they have been associated with an increased incidence of cholelithiasis and cholecystitis. The drugs promote gallstone formation by increasing the hepatic secretion of cholesterol into the bile and by decreasing the conversion of cholesterol into bile acids in the liver. Both of these changes increase the saturation, or lithogenicity, of bile (Gilman, Rall, Nies, & Taylor, 1990, p 889).

The fibric acids infrequently cause a myopathy (severe muscle cramps, tenderness, stiffness, and weakness). The syndrome is associated with elevated creatine phosphokinase.

Sexual changes in men (impotence, decreased libido, and gynecomastia) do occur. Fibric acid derivatives are contraindicated in clients with impaired renal or hepatic function. They should not be prescribed for pregnant or lactating women. Long-term use of clofibrate may be associated with a slightly increased incidence of various tumors.

Drug interactions. Clofibrate has been demonstrated to potentiate the effect of oral anticoagulants and to displace these drugs from their binding sites on albumin. In addition, the clofibrate may induce alteration in the synthesis of clotting factors, disposition of vitamin K, or characteristics of the warfarin receptor (Gilman, Rall, Nies, & Taylor, 1990, p 888).

Probucol

Probucol (Lorelco) is a synthetic lipophilic antioxidant.

Pharmacodynamics. Probucol appears to increase excretion of bile acids, increase the clearance of LDL, and, to some degree, inhibit cholesterol biosynthesis. It is a potent inhibitor of LDL oxidation, which results in decreased uptake of LDL by macrophages.

Enthusiasm for the drug has been limited because it reduces HDL even more then LDL-cholesterol. The reduction in LDL is usually less than 10% but the reduction in HDL is around 30% (Gilman, Rall, Nies, & Taylor, 1990, p 891).

Pharmacokinetics. It is administered orally but less than 10% of a dose is absorbed. Peak concentrations are higher and less variable when the drug is taken with food. It accumulates in adipose tissue and persists for 6 months or longer after the last dose is taken. It is eliminated primarily via the bile and feces.

Therapeutic uses. It has been used with familial hypercholesterolemia, type IIa. In studies with clients with this hyperlipoproteinemia, there was a modest lowering of cholesterol but a marked reduction in cutaneous and tendon xanthomas. In these clients, it did not lower HDL-cholesterol.

It has not yet been clearly determined whether probucol can prevent or control atherosclerosis or its sequelae in man.

Dosage and administration. Probucol is available as 250-mg and 500-mg tablets and the recommended dosage is 250–500 mg twice daily with morning and evening meals.

Adverse reactions. The most common adverse reactions are diarrhea, flatulence, abdominal pain, and nausea. Occasional effects include eosinophilia, paresthesia, hyperhidrosis, fetid sweat, and hypersensitivity reactions.

Probucol should not be given to clients with evidence of recent myocardial damage or with ventricular arrhythmias. Clients with a prolonged Q-T interval or taking a drug known to produce this effect should also not take probucol.

Combined drug therapy

Single drug therapy may fail to achieve the desired plasma concentrations of the lipids of concern. Several regimens combine more than one antilipemic.

Miscellaneous drugs

Other drugs known to affect lipid metabolism include neomycin, estrogens, dextrothyroxine, beta-sitosterol, and omega-3 fish oils.

Neomycin

This aminoglycoside antibiotic is largely unabsorbed when taken orally. At a dose of 1–3 g per day, it lowers serum cholesterol by precipating bile acids and preventing their resorption in the ileum. Its mechanism of action seems, thus, to be similar to that of the bile acid-sequestering resins. It can reduce total serum cholesterol levels 10%–20% (LDL cholesterol is reduced).

However, in clients with impaired renal function, the potential for nephrotoxicity and ototoxicity exists. Diarrhea and malabsorption of nutrients are other possible side effects (Dujovne & Harris, 1989, pp 279–280).

Estrogens

The decrease in natural estrogens with menopause frequently leads to increased levels of LDL cholesterol and a rise in cardiovascular risks for the client. Estrogen replacement therapy lowers elevated LDL and raises HDL in these clients and appears to reduce the risk of coronary artery disease. Effects are variable with different estrogen preparations (Dujovne & Harris, 1989, pp 280–281).

Dextrothyroxine

The optical isomer of L-thyroxine (dextrothyroxine [Choloxin]) has documented hypocholesterolemic activity and lowers plasma concentrations of LDL modestly. For a time, this drug was tried for the treatment of hypercholesterolemia, especially type II. However, when it was used in a large clinical trial as an alternative to niacin, it was found to be associated with an increased incidence of cardiac mortality and morbidity. This seemed related to arrhythmias and its general hypermetabolic effects. Therefore, it is no longer recommended for treatment of hypercholesterolemia (Dujovne & Harris, 1989, p 281).

Beta-sitosterol

Beta-sitosterol is a plant sterol with a structure similar to that of cholesterol. It is not absorbed and its mechanism of action is unknown but it may relate to an inhibition of the absorption of dietary cholesterol. It is used only for those with excessive LDL who appear extremely sensitive to dietary cholesterol. Adverse reactions include a mild laxative effect, nausea, and vomiting. The dose is 6 g (mixed with coffee, tea, fruit juice, or milk to increase palatability) and it is taken 30 minutes before meals and at bedtime (Gilman, Rall, Nies, & Taylor, 1990, p 894).

Omega-3 fish oils

Health food stores and pharmacies currently advertise omega-3 fish oils to lower serum cholesterol and decrease triglyceride levels. The clearest indication for their use is hyperlipoproteinemias types IV and V and possibly III. The basis for their use is epidemiologic studies and observation (such as with Greenland Eskimos), rather than well controlled clinical trials.

Oily fish such as salmon, mackerel, herring, and sardines are rich sources of these fish oils. The products currently available commercially that contain these oils are Max EPA, Super MaxEPA, Promega, and

Proto-Chol. All contain two major n-3 fatty acids (eicosapentaenoic, EPA, and docosahexaenoic acid, DHA). Doses of 2–3 g (6–9 1-g capsules) per day have been effective in lowering triglyceride levels. A dose of 3 g is equivalent to 8 ounces of salmon.

These oils also competitively inhibit synthesis of thromboxane A2, a vasoconstrictor that promotes platelet aggregation. Although they have the ability to inhibit platelet function, clinically significant bleeding has not been reported.

■ Summary

Treatment for hyperlipemia is considered necessary when both cholesterol and triglyceride levels are elevated. Initial treatment involves diet and exercise. Drugs are used only when these approaches are ineffective and are used in conjunction with diet. The antilipemics that are used medically include HMG CoA reductase inhibitors, bile acid-sequestering resins, nicotinic acid, fibric acid derivatives, probucol, and selected miscellaneous drugs.

Nursing management

Nursing implications

For most clients, the prevention and treatment of hyperlipemia depends on maintaining a healthy lifestyle, in particular, a sound diet and regular exercise (Box 28-3). The most effective approach is a "prudent" diet of a variety of foods rich in essential nutrients (vitamins, minerals, fiber); adequate in protein; low in cholesterol and saturated fats; and containing calories sufficient to maintain ideal body weight. Fish is recommended over red meats. Exercise should involve all body muscles without stressing joints or bones; swimming and walking are considered ideal. Exercise should last 20–30 minutes at least three times weekly and be vigorous enough to stimulate the heart and lungs.

It is vital that the general public understands the palliative nature and risks of hypolipemic drugs. Although these drugs are helpful to clients at high risk due to genetic factors, they are not panaceas that can be relied on to correct the detrimental effects of poor health practices. Many adverse reactions have been documented with only limited use of hypolipemics: their long-range effects are not fully established. Given the present pace of pharmaceutical research, it is likely that more antilipemic drugs will appear in the near future. However, their use will be limited to those persons with hereditary hyperlipemia and those at high risk of atherosclerosis and early death from heart disease.

Drug treatment for hyperlipemia may involve the use of more than one agent. If clients have contribut-

---

Box 28-3. Self-care measures recommended to decrease the risk of cardiovascular disease

Diet

Decrease overall fat intake, substituting poly-unsaturated (liquid or soft) fats for saturated (hard) fats. Avoid animal fats and saturated vegetable fats such as solid baking shortening and coconut oil. Use skim milk and evaporated skim milk in preference to whole milk or cream. Decrease the use of foods rich in cholesterol and the use of alcoholic beverages. Serve fish entrees frequently and decrease the use of red meats. Increase fiber intake by using more legumes, whole grains, fruits, and vegetables. Use recipes low in fat and cholesterol; decrease fat by one-third to one-half. Trim visible fat from meats; boil, broil, or bake foods rather than fry them. Decrease use of salt; season foods with herbs and spices. Adjust calories to a level that maintains a lean body weight.

Activity

Participate in active exercise for at least 20 minutes three times each week. Choose activities that are recreational (*ie*, ones that reduce stress levels and promote relaxation). Provide for adequate rest and sleep.

Drug use

Eliminate (or decrease) use of tobacco and alcohol.

Medical care

Take measures to prevent or control diabetes mellitus, hypertension, and hormone imbalances.

---

ing illnesses, such as hormone imbalances, they are likely to be taking several drugs concurrently, some of which may interact. This could make management of the drug regimen more difficult.

Nursing process

Assessment The assessment of clients who are candidates for antilipemic therapy would identify specific cardiovascular risk factors such as lack of exercise, undue stress, obesity, a diet high in cholesterol-rich foods and saturated fat, and such diseases as hypertension, diabetes mellitus, and hypothyroidism. The drug history should include specific data on use of estrogens, alcohol, tobacco, and such drugs as anticoagulants, nitroglycerin, or antilipemics. Significant laboratory data include cholesterol and triglyceride levels. If endocrine disease is present, serum glucose and thyroid function tests may be pertinent. Blood lipid electrophoresis would be required when a primary familial hyperlipidemia is suspected.

A complete examination of current cardiovascular status is in order. The reproductive status of women of childbearing age should be determined.

By the time treatment with antilipemic drugs is considered, clients have experienced failure to reduce blood lipid levels through dietary manipulation and exercise. They may have become discouraged by their "failure." The prescription of drugs may be seen by some as the only remaining hope for control of a life-threatening condition. Conversely, other clients may erroneously view drugs as an alternative to diet and exercise. The nurse must assess the client's attitude toward the use of antilipemics and determine the impact that a drug prescription has had on the client's emotions and motivation for compliance.

The client's knowledge (and that of significant others) about atherosclerosis and regimens to delay its onset should be assessed.

Nursing diagnosis Clients for whom antilipemics are prescribed are likely to be affected by the following:

> *Anxiety related to perception of a (long-term) poor prognosis secondary to high risk of atherosclerosis*
> *Altered nutrition: more than body requirements related to excessive amounts of fat, cholesterol, and calories*
> *Powerlessness related to failure of diet and exercise to control blood lipid levels*
> *Self-esteem disturbance related to increased risk of life-threatening disease secondary to genetic predisposition toward hyperlipemia, and supposed "failure" to correct lipemia with lifestyle changes*

Nursing diagnoses will vary, depending on the medications prescribed. Most of the drugs place clients at risk for

> *Constipation (diarrhea) related to prescribed medication.*

Clients using bile acid-binding resins may also have:

> *Altered nutrition: less than body requirement of fat-soluble vitamins related to fat malabsorption*

Common collaborative problems that should be differentiated from the nursing diagnoses when clients are using bile acid-binding resins include

> *Potential complication: calcium loss from bones*
> *Potential complication: liver impairment*

Clients taking large doses of niacin may develop the following:

> *Altered comfort: cutaneous flush and pruritus related to vasodilation*

A common collaborative problem that should be differentiated from the nursing diagnoses when clients are using niacin is

> *Potential complication: metabolic imbalance*

When fibric acid derivatives are prescribed, clients may have the following diagnoses:

> *Altered comfort: nausea, abdominal discomfort, or muscle discomfort*
> *Impaired tissue integrity: inflammation of the mouth or stomach*
> *Sexual dysfunction: impotence and decreased libido in men*

Common collaborative problems that should be differentiated from the nursing diagnoses when clients are using fibric acid derivatives include

> *Potential complication: impaired liver function*
> *Potential complication: impaired renal function*

Probucol also can cause the following:

> *Altered comfort: nausea (abdominal pain, itching eyes, chest pain), dizziness, syncope, or palpitation*
> *Body image disturbance related to hyperhidrosis and fetid sweat*

Most clients will have a

> *Knowledge deficit concerning antilipemic drugs and the self-care regimen required for management of atherosclerosis*

Planning The goals of nursing care are to lower serum cholesterol, alleviate or eliminate anxiety, maintain the prescribed diet, replace feelings of powerlessness with self-confidence, improve self-image, reduce knowledge deficits, and alleviate or eliminate adverse reactions to antilipemic drugs.

Intervention Nursing interventions to reduce anxiety include assisting the client in delineating its cause, usually a vaguely perceived threat. When the long-term prognosis is "poor," the specific fears may relate to losses, such as separation from loved ones or inability to fulfill role functions (*eg*, providing financially for the family). Once these are defined, the client may be assisted to take steps to use available time more efficiently in realizing life goals. At the same time, hope must be fostered for the client. The fact that there are medical interventions (*ie*, antilipemic drugs) that improve the prognosis, and the fact that research continues to find new treatment modalities, should encourage the client.

Many clients receiving prophylactic drug treatment are relatively young. Dietary limitations and drug therapy may be poorly accepted if clients still have a great need to conform to their peers. On the other hand, because food preferences are less well entrenched in the young, they may adapt to dietary changes somewhat more easily than older people. The nurse must assist clients in integrating their regimen into daily activities to minimize its impact on their lifestyle. Both the client and the dietary "gatekeeper" (whoever does the shopping and cooking) should be involved in this process.

Nursing interventions to improve self-image and decrease feelings of powerlessness include acceptance of the client's feelings; positive reinforcement for appropriate action by the client; and counseling of close family members to help them understand the client's reaction to the illness and to provide the support needed. Clients for whom probucol is prescribed should be advised to bathe frequently and use antiperspirant deodorants to control body odor.

After the drug regimen begins, the nurse should monitor clients for adverse reactions characteristic of the drugs prescribed. Clients receiving clofibrate or niacin should be monitored for hyperglycemia. Clients receiving niacin should be monitored for hyperuricemia. Those receiving clofibrate or cholestyramine must be watched for abnormal bleeding.

Client education. The nurse should prepare and implement a teaching plan designed to provide the facts and skills needed by the client to achieve maximum effect from the diet, exercise, and drug regimens. The teaching plan should stress measures the client can take to delay vascular degeneration. Clients should be assisted in correcting any factors that may have produced limited success in the past with the dietary and exercise regimens. Clients should be referred to sources of additional help, for example, to a dietitian for planning satisfying, nutritional meals, or to the American Heart Association for literature, including a cookbook on foods low in cholesterol and saturated fats. Exercise should be convenient, accessible in all seasons, and enjoyable. Brisk walking or swimming are generally suitable. Clients for whom bile acid-sequestering resins are prescribed should rely on weight-bearing exercise rather than swimming to stimulate calcium deposition in bone and reduce the risk of osteoporosis.

Adverse reactions to the drugs may affect compliance. The client should be informed of the side effects most likely to occur and those with serious implications that require medical attention. It should be stressed that many adverse reactions are temporary and tend to subside as treatment is continued. In addition, because antilipemic drugs have a short history of use, health care personnel should be informed of any unusual signs and symptoms that may be due to a previously unrecognized adverse drug reaction.

When niacin is used, to deal with the cutaneous flush, warm sensation, or pruritus that occurs when the drug is started or the dose increased, an aspirin tablet may be taken 20–30 minutes before the niacin. The aspirin will decrease the sensation, which seems to be mediated by a prostaglandin. Niacin must be taken with meals and antacids may be used to minimize nausea and abdominal discomfort.

Anion-exchange resins must never be ingested dry. Care should be taken while measuring the powder to avoid inhalation, which can cause serious lung reactions. These powders should be mixed with at least 90 ml of fluids (fruit juices, soup, milk, pureed fruit). If carbonated beverages are used, the powder should be stirred slowly into the liquid to prevent excess effervescence. Anion-exchange resins should be taken before meals and at least 1 hour before or 4 hours after ingestion of other oral drugs. The resins can interfere with absorption of drugs such as thyroxine, anticoagulants, and various digitalis preparations (among others). Clients should increase intake of fat-soluble vitamins to promote adequate absorption of these nutrients. To prevent or decrease constipation that may occur with use of the resins, bran may be added to the diet or a psyllium seed preparation may be mixed with the resin.

Antilipemic drugs do not correct the faulty metabolism that causes abnormal blood lipid levels. The aim of treatment is control. In this respect, the use of antilipemic drugs is similar to the use of insulin by the diabetic. Therapy is required for a long period, perhaps for life. The client must adjust to living with a chronic condition and incorporate the treatment regimen into a new lifestyle that can be maintained indefinitely.

Evaluation Data required for evaluation include statements made by the client indicating a reduction in anxiety or fear, increased self-esteem, incidence or absence of adverse drug reactions, and the ability of the client and significant others to implement the self-care measures recommended during the teaching sessions. (See accompanying Example of Nursing Process and Clofibrate Therapy.)

Checklist of nursing actions

☐ For each client, assess risk factors for cardiovascular disease.

☐ Encourage lifestyles that promote cardiovascu-

Example of nursing process and clofibrate therapy

The client is a 28-year-old male psychology professor with a family history of early and severe cardiovascular disease. His father died of a coronary thrombosis at age 39. An older brother is under treatment for hypercholesterolemia.

Two years ago, the client was warned that his plasma cholesterol was high. He was treated with niacin and cholestyramine but these regimens did not lower plasma cholesterol below 260 mg/dl.

The client is 6' 1" and weighs 170 lbs. He tells the nurse that he always has been aware that men in his family tend to die early, and that he has tried to live life to the fullest because his time may be limited. He has completed requirements for his doctorate in psychology and he dotes on his family (wife and two children).

The physician is now prescribing clofibrate 500 mg qid.

Assessment data	Nursing diagnosis	Intervention	Goals and outcome criteria
Family history of early and severe cardiovascular disease Hypercholesterolemia refractory to niacin and cholestyramine therapy Clofibrate therapy	Knowledge deficit concerning hypercholesterolemia and its treatment	**Assist** the client in managing diet and drug regimen for optimum therapeutic effect. Review the diet and exercise prescriptions. Assess the client's attitude toward and emotional reaction to the treatment regimen. Assist the client in identifying problems he may have with the regimen. If the diet is difficult for him to manage, refer him to a nutritionist for further assistance.	The client's plasma cholesterol will decline slowly but consistently.
		Inform the client of signs and symptoms of adverse drug reactions and urge him to report these promptly, should they occur.	Adverse drug reactions will be promptly detected and treated while still in the early stages.
Altered comfort: abdominal discomfort and diarrhea related to irritation secondary to clofibrate medication		**Advise** the client to avoid irritating and laxative foods while taking clofibrate.	The client will report that abdominal discomfort is absent or mild; stools will be solid or semisolid.
Sensory-perceptual alteration: hypogeusia related to clofibrate therapy		**Advise** the client to increase the quantity of herbs and nonirritating spices to flavor foods.	The client will report that interest and pleasure in food have not noticeably declined.
Sexual dysfunction: impotence, decreased libido, and gynecomastia related to antiandrogenic effects of clofibrate		**Inform** the client of the potential for antiandrogenic effects of clofibrate therapy. Inform him or her of alternatives available to him, should the drug cause sexual dysfunction. Advise him to contact his primary health care provider for assistance and referral if a sexual problem develops.	The client will report no sexual problems *or* he will request assistance and referral for sexual dysfunction.

lar health by teaching clients to choose a "prudent" diet, exercise regularly, avoid smoking and excessive alcohol, and learn to manage stress.

☐ Give emotional support to clients for whom antilipemic drugs are prescribed, and reassure them that the therapeutic regimen is capable of lowering plasma levels of harmful cholesterol.

☐ Refer clients to nutritionists or to the American Heart Association for helpful literature and other assistance in adopting more healthful lifestyles.

☐ Foster a positive self-image in clients at high risk for early cardiovascular disease.

☐ Teach clients to manage the therapeutic regimen for maximum effect.

☐ Teach clients receiving antilipemic drugs self-care measures that assist them in integrating the therapeutic regimen into a new lifestyle.

☐ Teach clients the therapeutic and adverse responses to antilipemic drugs, and when to con-

sult with the physician for modification of the regimen.

☐ Avoid inhalation of bile acid-binding resins when preparing them for administration.

Drugs that affect vascular tone
Physiology

Vascular tone is influenced by the nervous and endocrine systems. The vasomotor center in the medulla sends both stimulating and inhibiting impulses to the smooth muscle of the blood vessels. Stimulating impulses normally predominate, maintaining sufficient tone in the vasculature to keep blood pressure at optimal levels. These stimuli pass down the spinal cord through the sympathetic ganglia and postganglionic fibers to the vessel walls. Their effects are augmented by catecholamines, angiotensin, vasopressin, and (possibly) prostaglandins (Fig. 28-3).

Many factors can alter vascular tone by affecting the control system. Impulses from the carotid and

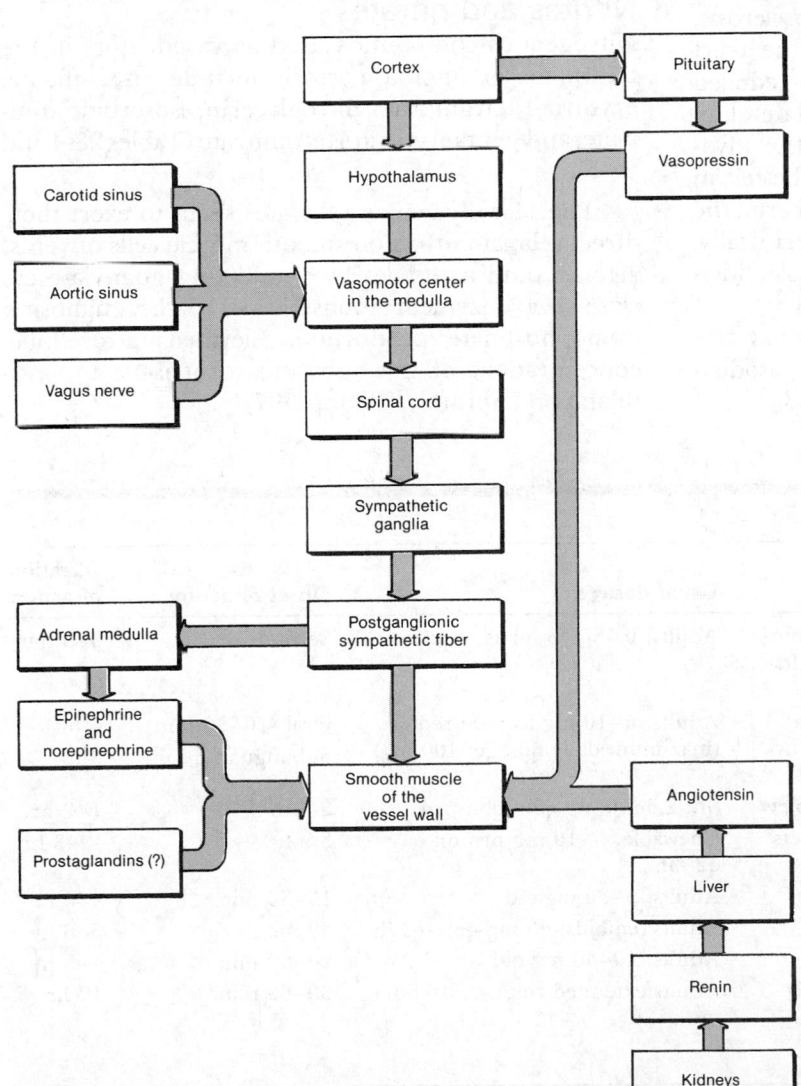

Figure 28-3. Nervous and hormonal influences contributing to vasoconstriction.

aortic sinuses adjust vasomotor center activity in accordance with changes in pressures and blood gases in these sinuses. Stress moderates the activity of the center by way of the cerebral cortex. Alterations in hormone balance can influence the control system at many points in the chain. Drugs also affect the system. Depending on their particular actions, they can cause constriction or dilation of the vasculature.

Pathophysiology of angina pectoris

Inappropriate constriction or dilation of the blood vessels is associated with several disease conditions. Excessive vasodilation is the cause of neurogenic shock. Conversely, compensatory vasoconstriction in response to hypovolemic or cardiogenic shock seriously impairs peripheral circulation while preserving the perfusion of vital organs. Local vasospasm contributes to hypoxia in such conditions as transient ischemic attacks and angina pectoris.

Angina pectoris is a condition characterized by intermittent myocardial ischemia. When the coronary vessels become narrowed by progressive atherosclerosis, less blood and oxygen can be transported to the heart tissues. If the workload of the heart is not reduced proportionately, some degree of hypoxia will develop. Acidosis and other chemical changes in the myocardium initiate impulses of pain that may be felt in the chest, or referred to the left shoulder and arm, the throat and chin, or the epigastrium. Characteristically, this pain is precipitated by exertion or stress and is relieved by rest.

The pain of persistent angina pectoris may frequently be relieved by the administration of a vasodilator, such as nitroglycerin.

Vasodilators

Drugs that relax the smooth muscle of blood vessel walls may exert their effects on smooth muscle cells of vessels directly, on the brain, the vasomotor center, the sympathetic nervous system, or the hormones that influence vascular tone.

Vasodilation increases the lumen of blood vessels, allowing greater fluid flow through them. As long as pressure gradients from the arterial to the venous circulation are maintained, circulation improves. The work of the heart is made easier as peripheral resistance diminishes. If vasodilation is widespread, however, blood pressure decreases, and the pressure gradients are reduced. Blood flow drops. The heart will be reflexly stimulated to increase its rate of contraction.

Vasodilators are important agents for the treatment of angina pectoris and hypertension. They are sometimes helpful in peripheral vascular disease or as adjuncts in the treatment of some kinds of circulatory shock.

Nitrites and nitrates

Nitrogenous compounds used as vasodilators in the treatment of angina pectoris include amyl nitrite, erythrityl tetranitrate, nitroglycerin, isosorbide dinitrate, and pentaerythritol tetranitrate (Tables 28-4 and 28-5).

Pharmacodynamics. Nitrates seem to exert their direct relaxant effect on smooth muscle cells of veins, arteries, and arterioles by stimulating guanylate cyclase, the enzyme responsible for cyclic guanosine monophosphate production. Elevated intracellular concentrations of this substance contribute to vasodilatation (Abrams, 1988, p 397).

Table 28-4. Nitrites and nitrates

Drug names	Preparations	Usual dosage	Onset of action	Duration of action
amyl nitrite (Amyl Nitrate Aspirols, Amyl Nitrate Vaparole)	Perles for administration by inhalation	Adults: 0.18–0.3 ml as required	Seconds	3–5 min
erythrityl tetranitrate (Cardilate, Carvasin, Cedocard-SR, Coradur, Coronex, Dilatrate)	Oral/sublingual tablets (taken by either route)	Adults: 5–10 mg as required (maximum daily dosage: 100 mg)	Oral: 15–30 min Sublingual: 5 min	6 hr 3 hr
isosorbide dinitrate (Iso-Bid, Isordil, Isoket, Isordil, Isoket, Isosorb, Isosorbide, Isotrate, Novosorbide, Onset, Risordan, Sorate, Sorbitrate)	Sublingual tablets	SL: 2.5–10 mg q2h–q3h prn	2–5 min	1–2 hr
	Chewable tablets Oral tablets	Chewable: 5–10 mg prn or q2–3h	3 min	1/2–3 hr
	Oral extended-release tablets	Adults: 5–30 mg qid Adults/tembids: 40 mg q8h–q12h	15–30 min 30 min	4–6 hr 6–8 hr
pentaerythritol tetranitrate (Desatrate, Duotrate, Mycardol, Naptrate, Neo-Corvas, Nitrin, Pentraspan, Pentritol, Pentylan, Peritrate, Vasolate)	Oral tablets	Adults: 10–40 mg qid	20–60 min	4–5 hr
	Oral extended-release tablets, capsules	Adults/extended release: 30–80 mg q12h	30–60 min	12 hr

Table 28-5. Nitroglycerin: preparations and dosage

Preparations	Usual dosage
Extended-release capsules (*eg*, Nitroglyn Extended-Release Capsules)	Initially 2.5 mg tid or qid, titrated to response
Controlled-release capsules (*eg*, Nitro-Bid Plateau Caps, Nitrocine, Nitroglyn)	
Extended-release tablets (*eg*, Nitrong)	
Ointment (*eg*, Nitrol Ointment, Nitrong Ointment)	1–2 inch ribbon q8h but some require 2 inch q4h or 5 inch q8h
Buccal tablets (*eg*, Nitrogard (transmucosal extended release nitroglycerin tablets))	1–3 mg in buccal pouch q3–5h during waking hours
Transdermal (*eg*, Deponit, Mintran, Nitrodisc, Nitro-Dur II, Transderm-Nitro, NTS)	5 mg/24 hrs, titrated to response
To relieve acute attack or prophylaxis before stressful activity	
Sublingual tablets (*eg*, Nitrostat (nitroglycerin tablets))	gr $^1/_{400}$ (0.15 mg)–gr $^1/_{150}$ (0.4 mg); may repeat q5 min 3 times
Translingual spray (*eg*, Nitrolingual Spray)	1–2 doses sprayed onto or under the tongue, may repeat q3–5 min to maximum of 3 doses within a 15-minute period
Emergency relief of acute attack	
IV infusion (*eg*, Tridil [nitroglycerin], 5–50 mg/ampul, 50–100 mg/vial)	5–20 mcg/min or more, titrate to client situation, need to use special infusion set specific to trade name preparation and an infusion pump, no fixed optimum dose
Nitrostat IV, 8–100 mg/ampoule, or vial	
Nitro-Bid IV, 5 mg/ml	

A reduction in myocardial work and requirement for oxygen is the major action of the nitrites and nitrates. They relax vascular smooth muscle, resulting in reduction of blood pressure by generalized vasodilation. This lowers peripheral resistance against which the heart must pump.

The workload of the heart is diminished, and the oxygen need of the myocardium drops. When the need for oxygen is reduced below the level supplied by coronary circulation, ischemia is relieved and chest pain subsides. The vasodilating effects on arteriolar resistance are not as great as the action on the venous side. This decreases the pressure gradients between the veins and the right side of the heart, causing pooling of blood in the venous system.

Stress on the ventricular wall is affected by a number of factors, which together constitute preload. The venous pooling related to nitrate use reduces venous return and contributes to a diminished preload.

Nitrite and nitrate action favors subendocardial perfusion. This is important because the subendocardium is particularly vulnerable to ischemia during angina attacks. Distended ventricles, without nitrate use, mechanically interfere with blood flow through the arteries supplying the subendocardial areas. Diminished preload with nitrate use decreases left ventricular volume. A reduction in volume relieves mechanical pressure and allows more blood flow through the subendocardium.

At higher concentrations nitrites and nitrates also decrease afterload.

Pharmacokinetics. Nitrites and nitrates are available for sublingual, buccal, oral, dermal, inhalant, and intravenous (IV) use (Tables 28-4 and 28-5). Amyl nitrite is administered by inhalation and is readily absorbed by the respiratory tract. Other nitrites or nitrates are absorbed from the oral mucosa or GI tract. When given orally, the drugs undergo first-pass metabolism by the liver. Nitroglycerin is readily absorbed through intact skin when applied topically.

The onset and duration of action of the nitroglycerin preparations are influenced by the route of administration. Intravenous nitroglycerin begins in 1–2 minutes and lasts 3–5 minutes; sublingual and translingual nitroglycerin begins in 1–3 minutes and lasts 30–60 minutes; buccal nitroglycerin begins in 1–3 minutes and lasts 3–5 hours; extended or controlled release preparations begin in 20–45 minutes and last 3–8 hours; and transdermal preparations begin in 30–60 minutes and last 12–24 hours or more.

Preparations other than nitroglycerin, including erythrityl tetranitrate, isosorbide dinitrate, and pentaerythritol tetranitrate, are reviewed in Table 28-4.

These drugs are rapidly and efficiently metabolized in the liver by the enzyme glutathione-organic nitrate reductase. Excretion is through the kidney.

Therapeutic uses. Nitrites and nitrates are used to control the pain of angina pectoris. For medicinal use, organic nitrates are generally preferred to nitrites. They act as rapidly and are much more potent.

Intravenous nitroglycerin can be used to lower blood pressure during cardiovascular procedures when perioperative hypertension occurs; to produce controlled hypotension during surgical procedures; and to treat acute congestive heart failure (Antonaccio, 1990, p 318).

In addition to their use in the treatment of angina pectoris, nitrites and nitrates are also prescribed for the relief of paroxysmal nocturnal dyspnea, diffuse esophageal spasm, and biliary colic. They may be helpful in ureteral colic and bronchial asthma. Amyl nitrate is used as an adjunct in the treatment of cyanide poisoning.

Topical application of nitroglycerin ointment is sometimes prescribed to provide local vasodilation in the treatment of trophic ulcers and Raynaud's disease. It has also been used to dilate peripheral veins to facilitate insertion of needles or intracatheters.

When administered IV concurrently with packed red blood cells, nitroglycerin reduces the risk of excessive preload and pulmonary edema secondary to the increased blood volume. Using this technique, it is possible to transfuse clients with congestive heart failure.

Adverse reactions. Common adverse reactions to vasodilators reflect the general effects of the drugs. Dilation of cutaneous vessels causes flushing. Vascular congestion in cerebral vessels produces throbbing headaches. Hypotension reduces perfusion in some areas of the body, causing nausea, vomiting, faintness, and dizziness. Reduced pressure in the aortic and carotid sinuses triggers reflex tachycardia. A moderate, but persistent, vasodilation may produce none of these effects but may still interfere with the normal compensatory vasoconstriction that maintains cerebral circulation in the upright position. This produces orthostatic or postural hypotension, which is characterized by weakness, dizziness, and fainting with sudden changes in position. Venous pooling can cause ankle edema.

Other adverse reactions include drug rash (seen more frequently with pentaerythritol tetranitrate and topical nitroglycerin) and methemoglobinemia. The latter is most common and dangerous in infants, who can be poisoned by relatively small amounts of nitrates. Such poisoning can be caused by accidental ingestion of nitrate medications, by explosive powders, or by the use of well water with a high nitrate content. Older children and adults are relatively unaffected by ingested nitrates but the use of water high in nitrates for dialysis carried out in the home can cause toxic methemoglobinemia.

Intravenous nitroglycerin contains substantial amounts of ethanol as a diluent. When high doses are used, ethanol intoxication may develop.

Tolerance. Tolerance can develop in persons under medical treatment with these chemicals and in persons with occupational exposure to these chemicals.

Considerable evidence has accumulated that the development of tolerance is common in the client treated with nitrates. The mechanisms responsible for nitrate tolerance are not completely clear. The appearance of tolerance is somewhat variable and unpredictable and does not occur in all clients or to the same degree in each client. Variables responsible for diverse findings relative to tolerance may include size of dose, dosing interval, and duration of action of specific preparation. To avoid tolerance, it is now felt shorter-acting nitrates, smallest effective doses, fewer daily doses, and a nitrate-free interval (usually at night and of 8–12 hours) are principles that must be applied in nitrate therapy (Abrams, 1988, pp 399–400).

Industrial exposure to organic nitrates induces both tolerance and physical dependence. Workers involved in the manufacture or detonation of explosives are in frequent contact with nitroglycerin or nitroglycol. With first exposure, these substances produce typical adverse reactions but the reactions soon subside. This tolerance dissipates after a few days' interruption of exposure to nitrates, causing renewed symptoms when contact with the chemicals resumes, typically on a Monday after a weekend off. Workers may wear work clothes impregnated with the chemicals or rub the chemicals on their skin during their time off to maintain tolerance and prevent a recurrence of discomfort when they return to work.

Chronic exposure can produce dependence. Withdrawal from contact with the substance has been reported to produce severe myocardial ischemia and pain, MI, or sudden death. (See Focus on Nitrites/Nitrates: Similarities and Differences.)

Miscellaneous agents

Vasodilator drugs have been promoted for use in peripheral and cerebrovascular diseases but currently are felt to be of little value. They have been advocated for disorders of the chronic occlusive type such as arteriosclerosis obliterans, and Buerger's disease (thromboangiitis obliterans), and for disorders of the vasospastic type such as Raynaud's disease. They have also been advocated for night leg cramps, frostbite, and disturbances from labyrinth artery spasm or obstruction.

Drugs used in these disorders have included adrenergic blocking agents and agents that have a direct relaxing effect on smooth muscles of peripheral arterial walls (Table 28-6). The rationale for use was to increase peripheral blood flow to areas where perfusion is compromised, however, these agents primarily

Focus on

Nitrites/nitrates: similarities and differences

Similarities

Pharmacodynamics

These agents directly relax the vascular smooth muscle and all smooth muscles. They produce vasodilation and reduce the myocardial oxygen demand. They also reduce preload and afterload.

Pharmacokinetics

These agents are rapidly absorbed through the skin, oral mucous membranes, and GI tract. They are rapidly and efficiently metabolized by the liver and excreted by the kidneys

Therapeutic uses

These agents are used as prophylaxis and treatment of angina pectoris. They also provide relief of paroxysmal nocturnal dyspnea and are used in the treatment of diffuse esophageal spasms, biliary colic, and ureteral colic

Adverse reactions

These include: (CNS) throbbing headache, faintness, dizziness, weakness, restlessness; (CV) reflex tachycardia, orthostatic hypotension, syncope, cardiovascular collapse; (EENT) blurred vision; (GI) nausea, vomiting, dry mouth, and sublingual burning; (SKIN) flushing, cold sweats; (OTHER) ankle edema

Differences

• **Amyl nitrate** converts hemoglobin to methemoglobin which reacts with cyanide to form cyanmethemoglobin

• **Amyl nitrate** is readily absorbed by the respiratory tract. It has an onset of action of 30 seconds, and duration of 3–5 minutes. • **Erythritol tetranitrate**, when administered SL has an onset of action of 5 minutes, and duration of 3 hours; when given PO, it has an onset of action of 15–30 minutes, peaking in 60 minutes and a duration of 6 hours. • **Isosorbide dinitrate**, when given SL, has an onset of 2–5 minutes, a duration of 1–2 hours and a half-life of 60 minutes; when given PO, it has an onset of 15–40 minutes, a duration of 4–6 hours and a half-life of 4–6 hours; when given PO, as extended release form, it has an onset of 30 minutes and a duration of 12 hours. • **Pentaerythritol tetranitrate**, when given PO, has an onset of 30 minutes, a duration of 4–5 hours and a half-life of 10 minutes; when given PO, as extended release form, it has a slow onset with a duration of 12 hours; this agent is also excreted in small amounts in feces as inactive metabolites. • **Nitroglycerin (NTG)** when given by the buccal route, has an onset of 3 minutes, a duration of 5 hours and a half-life of 1–4 minutes; when given SL, it has an onset of 1–3 minutes, duration of 30–60 minutes; when given by IV infusion, it has an immediate onset, and a duration of several minutes; when given as an ointment, it has an onset within 30 minutes, and a duration of 4–8 hours; when given as a transdermal patch, it has an onset within 30 minutes and a duration of 8–24 hours.

• **Topical NTG** is used to provide vasodilation in the treatment of trophic ulcers and Raynaud's disease; it is used to dilate peripheral veins for IV therapy. • **IV NTG** is used to control blood pressure during surgery and as an adjunctive treatment for congestive heart failure associated with a myocardial infarction. • **Amyl nitrate** is used to treat cyanide poisoning; it is seldom used for angina.

• **IV NTG** can cause ethanol intoxication in high doses. • **Amyl nitrate** can cause methemoglobinemia, palpatation, and muscle twitching.

(continued)

Focus on

Nitrites/nitrates: similarities and differences (Continued)

Similarities

Contraindications

These agents are contraindicated in persons with open-angle glaucoma, head trauma, or cerebral hemorrhage, severe anemia or hypersensitivity to the drug

Precautions

These agents should be used cautiously in persons with diuretic-induced fluid depletion, systolic blood pressure less than 90, increased intracranial pressure or impaired hepatic or renal function

Nursing considerations

Instruct client in disease, treatment, drug therapy regimen, adverse effects and compliance; assess cardiopulmonary status for baseline and ongoing for changes; assess client's complaints of chest pain, and any factors associated with it, such as activity, stress; assess measures client uses to relieve pain and their effectiveness; administer oral forms on an empty stomach with a full glass of water; institute safety precautions and warn client to change positions slowly; instruct client not to discontinue drug abruptly; monitor vital signs, frequently for changes; instruct client in technique for proper administration and storage of drug; institute measures to relieve headache, such as cool compresses, rest, and mild analgesics; warn client to avoid alcohol when taking drug

Differences

Extended release preparations of **isosorbide**, **NTG**, and **pentaerythritol** are contraindicated in persons with functional organic GI hypermotility or malabsorption syndrome. • **IV NTG** is contraindicated in persons with hypotension, uncontrolled hypovolemia, or normal or low pulmonary capillary wedge pressure. • **NTG** injectable is contraindicated in persons with cerebral hemorrhage, head trauma, pericardial tamponade, or constrictive pericarditis.

• **NTG**, **isosorbide**, and **erythritol** should be used cautiously in persons who are in the initial days after an acute myocardial infarction. • **Pentaerythritol** should be used cautiously in persons with hypotension.

Dilute **NTG** for IV use in 5% dextrose and water or normal saline; avoid skin contact with topical preparations and wash hands thoroughly after administering; store **NTG** in a cool dry place; instruct client to take SL form immediately after the onset of chest pain and to repeat dose in 5 minutes if no relief up to a maximum of 3 tablets—if still no relief, instruct client to seek medical attention; apply topical preparations to non-hairy, nonfatty areas of the torso or upper extremities; remove previous topical applications before applying a new dose; avoid giving buccal **NTG** at bedtime to prevent the risk of aspiration; instruct client to avoid hot liquids when taking buccal forms; when administering **NTG** as IV infusion, use special nonabsorbing tubing supplied by manufacturer; instruct client not to chew buccal form; wrap **amyl nitrate** ampule in cloth and crush holding it near the client's nose and mouth so vapor is inhaled; keep **amyl nitrate** away from flame, it may ignite.

---

increase blood flow to nonischemic areas rather than to the ischemic areas.

■ **Summary**

Nitrites and nitrates are vasodilators used for the treatment of angina pectoris. They reduce blood pressure by generalized vasodilation, thus decreasing the preload and afterload on the heart. For therapeutic use, organic nitrates are generally preferred to nitrites; they act just as rapidly and are more potent.

Side effects of nitrites and nitrates include headache, hypotension, and some degree of tolerance with continued use.

Nursing management

Nursing implications

Clients under treatment for angina pectoris suffer from coronary artery disease, which has reduced the blood flow to the myocardium below the level required for optimal function. Ischemia and chest pain develop when the myocardium's need for oxygen exceeds the capacity of the coronary circulation to deliver it. Pain occurs at first only with extreme exertion but as vascular degeneration progresses, less strenuous activity precipitates discomfort. In the final stages of coronary artery disease, oxygen supplies to the myocardium are

Table 28-6. Vasodilators for peripheral vasodilation

Drug names	Preparations	Usual dosage	Adverse reactions
cyclandelate (Cyclospasmol)	Oral capsules and tablets	100–200 mg qid	Flushing, tachycardia, headache, weakness, GI symptoms
isoxsuprine (Duradilan, Vasodilan)	Oral tablets IM	10–20 mg tid or qid	Hypotension, tachycardia, nausea, vomiting, abdominal distress, dizziness, rash
nylidrin (Arlidin Dilatol, Peridilatal, PMS Nylidrin)	Oral tablets	3–12 mg tid or qid	Orthostatic hypotension, dizziness, anxiety, nausea, vomiting, flushing
papaverine (Genabid, Pavabid, Pavagen, Pavaspan, Pavasule, Pavatym, Paverolan, Vasospan)	Oral tablets Oral extended-release capsules Elixir IM IV	100–30 mg, 3–5 times daily	Flushing, tachycardia, drowsiness, GI symptoms, elevation of hepatic enzymes

so low that even minimal work by the heart exhausts them, and pain is constant even during rest.

Judicious use of nitrate vasodilators can improve the client's quality of life by alleviating pain and increasing tolerance to exercise. Therapy is usually initiated by the prescription of sublingual nitroglycerin tablets to be taken "as necessary" to terminate a pain episode. Use of these tablets before exertion may prevent the occurrence of pain. Because excessive use may cause severe adverse reactions and some degree of tolerance, clients need considerable assistance in managing their medication regimens for optimal benefit.

When using topical nitroglycerin preparations, the nurse should avoid cutaneous contact with the drug and wash the hands thoroughly after administering the dose.

Storage of nitroglycerin. Nitroglycerin is sensitive to air, light, heat, and moisture. It requires special handling and storage to preserve its therapeutic efficacy. Sublingual tablets are dispensed in small, brown, tightly stoppered, glass bottles. They should not be transferred to pill boxes or other containers. Because the drug is somewhat volatile, no cotton, paper, or other material that could absorb the vapors should be allowed to remain in the bottle with the tablets. The drug must be kept secure from small children, who are

highly susceptible to nitrate poisoning. To protect it from body heat, nitroglycerin should not be carried in pockets of close-fitting garments. Despite these precautions, the drug will deteriorate over time. Tablets should be discarded 3 months after the seal has been broken. Nitroglycerin should not be stored in the bathroom or refrigerator but should be stored in a dark, dry place.

Nursing process

Assessment Data required for initial assessment of clients for whom nitrates are prescribed include complete assessment of cardiovascular status. Specific information should be included regarding activities that cause anginal pain and whether or not rest relieves the pain. The nurse should determine the client's knowledge of coronary artery disease, attitude toward drug use, and the client's goals for therapy.

Nursing diagnosis Most clients for whom nitrates are prescribed are affected by

Activity intolerance: chest pain upon exertion related to myocardial ischemia secondary to coronary artery disease

As coronary artery disease advances, clients have

Pain at rest related to severe myocardial ischemia secondary to coronary artery occlusion

Nitrate drugs pose the following:

Pain: headache related to vasodilation Altered tissue perfusion: impaired cerebral perfusion related to postural hypotension secondary to use of vasodilators

Many clients will have a

Knowledge deficit related to vasodilators and their use to control angina pectoris

---

Learning experience 28-1

Ascertain the policies and practices in local health care institutions regarding use of nitroglycerin by clients subject to angina pectoris. What drug preparations are used most frequently? Are any self-administered? If so, how does the nursing staff monitor use of the drugs?

Planning The goals of treatment are to alleviate or eliminate chest pain, increase activity tolerance, prevent or alleviate adverse drug reactions such as headache and postural hypotension, and increase knowledge on the client's part of the prescribed drug regimen.

Intervention The dosage and timing of nitroglycerin medication varies considerably, depending on the route of administration and the drug in use. Relatively small doses are required for sublingual administration. When administered by this route, nitroglycerin has an onset of action within 3 minutes and duration up to 60 minutes. If a single dose is not effective, it may be repeated after 5 minutes. No more than three doses should be taken for any one episode because additional doses are not likely to be effective. If pain is not relieved, the client should immediately seek medical attention. Because such pain may be due to MI rather than simple ischemia, prompt treatment is vital.

Nitroglycerin is most effective in controlling angina when it is administered immediately after the onset of pain. For this reason, even in acute-care settings, nitroglycerin is usually kept in the client's possession and is self-administered. Proper assessment of the client requires that the amount of drug used be monitored and recorded. A record may be kept by the client, or the nursing staff may place a limited supply of the drug at the bedside, noting the number of tablets used and replacing them periodically.

Transdermal preparations include ointment and skin patches. Nitroglycerin absorbed transdermally exerts its effects over a period of several hours.

Before applying ointment, take the client's baseline blood pressure and heart rate after the client has been at rest for 10 minutes. Repeat the vital signs 1 hour after drug administration. An appropriate dosage produces a 10 mm Hg fall in blood pressure with the client in a resting position.

Both ointment and patches should be applied to clean, dry, hairless skin area of chest or upper extremities. Before a new dose is applied, the site of the previous dose should be washed to remove drug residues. Rotate sites to prevent inflammation. Doses should be placed where they will not interfere with auscultation of the heart. Avoid skin folds, areas distal to knee or elbow, and irritated or scarred areas. Do not rub in ointment because rapid absorption will interfere with drug's desired action. Avoid any contact between nurse's fingers and ointment.

Three transdermal nitroglycerin systems (patches) are currently available (*eg*, Transderm-Nitro, Nitro-Dur II, and Nitrodisc). Each system has a different mechanism of drug delivery. For example, Nitrodisc contains nitroglycerin mixed in a solid polymer similar to silicone. The drug is absorbed through the skin from the polymer, which also contains a cosolvent to enhance skin penetration. On the other hand, Transderm-Nitro contains a semipermeable membrane between the drug and the skin that is the controlling factor for drug delivery. Drug absorption in all systems is by passive diffusion.

The three systems are not interchangeable because nitroglycerin content and average amount of nitroglycerin delivered in 24 hours can differ.

Some practitioners feel that maintaining stable nitroglycerin serum levels over 24 hours is not always desirable because tolerance to the drug and the need to increase dosage would occur. Thus, some prescribe application for 12–16 hours and, then, removal for the night. Research is ongoing in this area.

Drug discontinuation should be gradual, not abrupt. Weaning the client off the drug is recommended to prevent rebound symptoms or sudden changes in pressures.

Intravenous nitroglycerin may be used to treat acute congestive heart failure in the critical care setting. It is diluted in 5% dextrose in water or in normal saline. Glass bottles are used. Special infusion sets may be used. Polyvinyl chloride tubing of IV administration sets in general use absorb nitroglycerin. Some filters absorb nitroglycerin. Some infusion controllers may not work well with the special infusion set (*ie*, the special tubing tends to be less pliable than conventional polyvinyl chloride tubing). Infusion pumps should be pretested with the infusion set when a special set is used. No other drug should be administered in the same solution or via the same tubing. During IV administration, the blood pressure and heart rate will be monitored constantly, and other measurements such as pulmonary capillary wedge pressure will often be made. As response is observed, the dose will be reduced and the interval between increments lengthened. Clients may be very sensitive to the effects of nitroglycerin.

Nursing care for adverse reactions. The throbbing headache induced by nitrates tends to disappear if the drug is used on a regular basis. Cold compresses to the head and rest in a quiet environment help relieve discomfort. Mild analgesics (*eg*, acetaminophen) may be necessary to reduce the pain. The client should be encouraged to continue using the drug for an adequate trial period to see if tolerance develops. Regular use helps maintain tolerance.

Nitrates reduce blood pressure and can cause dizziness, fainting, and weakness. If these symptoms are troublesome, rest in a recumbent position will relieve them. Vital signs should be monitored. If the client is susceptible to shock from some other medical condition, an alternative treatment for the angina (oxygen and rest) may be used in preference to the drug. Clients who experience these symptoms or postural hypotension should avoid alcohol, which tends to intensify the reactions.

Slow movement when changing position helps to reduce these symptoms. To reduce the risk of falls, clients may need assistance when ambulating. A reduction in dosage is sometimes necessary to relieve side effects.

Client education. The nurse should prepare and implement a teaching plan to inform clients about nitrate drugs and to assist them in managing the drug regimen effectively. Because clients usually control and manage nitroglycerin therapy themselves, it is important that they receive complete information about the drug. Proper storage and administration techniques should be explained. The mouth must be moist to dissolve sublingual tablets for rapid absorption. The client should be advised to drink fluids before using sublingual tablets if the mouth tends to be dry.

Management of the drug regimen should allow for maintenance of those activities perceived by clients as important to their quality of life. Nitroglycerin may be taken prophylactically before undertaking activities known to precipitate anginal episodes. Planning for such activity on a regular basis may be highly desirable. Not only will it keep the client relatively active, a factor in developing collateral circulation in the myocardium, but daily use of the drug will maintain resistance to nitrate-induced headaches. Of course, the kinds and frequency of activities must be appropriate to the severity of coronary artery disease. The client who cannot walk without chest pain will not be able to undertake strenuous activities simply by using the drug.

Although clients often express a preference that the ointment or patches be applied to their chest, the drug's effect is exerted systemically through the circulation, and other sites may be used just as effectively. The distal portions of the extremities should not be used. Application of the ointment to the chest probably enhances the psychologic effect and is as convenient and comfortable as any other site. Because drug, papers, and patches are somewhat irritating, the client should be taught to rotate the sites of application.

Accidental exposure to topical nitrates can be a problem. The tubes of ointment have been mistaken for toothpaste or dentifrice fixatives. Rapid absorption of this form of the drug from the oral mucosa causes acute hypotension. To reduce the risk of such an accident, the medication should not be stored in the same area as dental preparations. A strip of tape on the tube may be used to alert clients with poor vision to the nature of the tube's contents. Skin patches or ointment sometimes become displaced from the client to the skin of another person. Signs and symptoms caused by this type of exposure are usually less severe but can be discomforting.

Because they contain metal foil or paste, skin patch medications can cause accidental burns. When subjected to microwaves, ultrasound, or electrical currents, metal becomes hot. Microwave ovens in good repair do not pose a significant hazard but second degree burns have resulted from exposure to units with microwave leaks. Burns have been reported also if patches remain in place when electrical shock is delivered for defibrillation during cardiopulmonary resuscitation.

Evaluation Data required for evaluation include statements by the client indicating that the anginal pain has subsided or disappeared, that the client's physical activity has increased, and that headache and postural hypotension have decreased or disappeared; and evidence that the client is correctly managing the drug regimen (including a decrease in blood pressure, and correct pill counts indicating that all the prescribed medicine is taken). (See the accompanying Example of Nursing Process and Nitro-Dur Therapy.)

Checklist of nursing actions

When nitroglycerin is prescribed
for angina pectoris

☐ Instruct clients to allow sublingual tablets to dissolve under the tongue.

☐ Monitor the amount of drug used and the client's response to it.

☐ Instruct clients in proper storage of the medication.

☐ Instruct clients to replace their supply of tablets every 3 months or whenever the drugs no longer sting when placed under the tongue.

☐ Apply transdermal patches to clean, dry, hairless skin of the upper body.

☐ Instruct clients to rotate the site used for transdermal preparations.

☐ Apply cold compresses to the head and administer analgesics to relieve headache when it occurs.

☐ Instruct the client to rest quietly when headache or faintness occurs following medication.

☐ Encourage clients to continue the therapeutic regimen until tolerance to the drug's side effects develops.

☐ Assist the client in managing the drug regimen for optimal therapeutic effect, including maintenance of normal lifestyle.

Example of nursing process and Nitro-Dur therapy

The client is a 58-year-old man with a 3-year history of angina pectoris, which has been fairly well controlled until recently with sublingual nitroglycerin medication. He does not wish to undergo cardiac catheterization or other invasive procedures "unless it cannot be avoided." Lately, because he has needed medication more often, he has returned to the physician for further assistance. The physician has prescribed Nitro-Dur, one patch worn for 12 hours daily.

Assessment data	Nursing diagnosis	Intervention	Goals and outcome criteria
Nitro-Dur therapy	High risk for impaired tissue integrity: burns related to exposure to electrical current	**Advise** the family that should the client experience a heart attack and require cardiopulmonary resuscitation (CPR), the emergency personnel should be informed by them about the patch so it can be removed before defibrillation.	The client will not sustain burn injury related to the medicated patch.
Nitro-Dur therapy (patch medications can be dislodged and after normal use there is enough residual nitroglycerin in patch that patch may be potential hazard to children and pets)	High risk for accidental poisoning of others related to contact with the patch	**Teach** the client to apply the patch to a flat, smooth, hairless area of skin not subject to any friction, which could dislodge the patch. Teach client to discard patch safely and thoroughly. Advise client to check periodically to verify patch is in place.	Others will not become medicated by the client's patch.
Nitro-Dur therapy	High risk for impaired tissue integrity: skin inflammation related to irritation secondary to patch	**Advise** client to rotate the application site for the patch, to remove the old patch, and to clean skin thoroughly before applying new patch.	The client will not develop skin irritation or inflammation.

Drugs used to treat hypertension

Pathophysiology of hypertension

Blood pressure is considered excessive when systolic pressure is consistently above 140 mm Hg or diastolic pressure is consistently above 90 mm Hg (Wollam & Hall, 1988, p 365). Hypertension places an increased workload on the heart and increases the risk of degenerative changes in the blood vessels, themselves, as well as in other body organs such as the kidneys, brain, heart, and eyes.

The primary factor in hypertension is an increase in peripheral resistance resulting from vasoconstriction or narrowing of the internal lumen of blood vessels. Hypervolemia is a contributing factor. In a small number of clients, a specific, correctable cause (endocrine imbalance, cardiovascular abnormality, certain forms of kidney disease) can be determined. In these cases, definitive treatment can eliminate the cause.

In the majority of affected persons, however, the disease, termed *idiopathic*, is nonspecific. Such hypertension appears to be related to lifestyles and is associated with factors such as obesity, excessive dietary intake of sodium, high levels of stress, and progressive atherosclerosis and arteriosclerosis.

Management of hypertension requires elimination or modification of as many risk factors as possible. Sometimes weight reduction, better stress management, or a reduced salt intake is sufficient to return blood pressure to normal levels. However, drug regimens are frequently instituted to reduce excessive pressures and maintain them at the desired level. Diuretics may be prescribed alone initially but common drug regimens include both diuretics and other antihypertensive agents. (See Chapter 40 for information on diuretics.)

Antihypertensives

A number of different types of agents are available for use as antihypertensives. These include diuretics, sympathetic inhibitors, direct-acting vasodilators, inhibitors of the renin-angiotensin system, and calcium-channel blocking agents (Table 28-7.)

Sympathetic inhibitors

The sympathetic inhibitors as a group include five subgroupings: adrenergic blocking agents, central action inhibitors, blockers of neuroeffector transmission, ganglionic blocking agents, and an undefined grouping.

Adrenergic blocking agents

The adrenergic blocking agents can further be divided into five subcategories: combined alpha-1 and alpha-2 adrenoreceptor blockade; selective alpha-1 adrenoreceptor blockade; nonselective, combined beta-1 and beta-2 adrenergic blockade; cardioselective, predominantly beta-1 adrenergic blockade; and combined alpha and beta adrenergic blockade.

The combined alpha-1 and alpha-2 adrenergic blocking agents reduce systemic and pulmonary resistance and, thus, lower blood pressure. They prevent catecholamines from activating smooth muscle alpha-receptors, which normally cause vasoconstriction. With these drugs, there will be reflex increases in heart rate, contractile force, and plasma renin activity. These drugs prevent vasoconstriction in both arterial and venous beds. Because of the venous dilation, orthostatic hypotension is common.

The selective alpha-1 adrenoreceptor blockers differ from combined alpha-1 and alpha-2 blockers in that venous smooth muscle is little affected by the selective blockers. Consequently, orthostatic hypotension is less of a problem, and increases in heart rate, contractile force, and plasma renin activity are less prominent.

The nonselective, combined beta-1 and beta-2 adrenergic blockers depress cardiac output and reduce arterial pressure with long-term use. It is not completely understood how these drugs produce a persistent reduction in blood pressure. Some feel that with chronic treatment there is an adaptation of peripheral resistance as a consequence of reduced blood flow. This would result in persistently reduced peripheral vascular resistance, regardless of the cardiac output (Craig & Stitzel, 1990, p 286).

The cardioselective, predominantly beta-1 adrenergic blockers, exhibit greater antagonism of cardiac beta (beta-1) receptors and cause less blockade of vascular and pulmonary beta (beta-2) receptors. The cardioselective blockers are 50–100 times more potent in inhibiting beta-1 receptors but the cardioselectivity is not an absolute quality. As the dose of these blockers is increased, more inhibition of vascular and pulmonary receptors does occur.

Labetalol is the first of a new category of drugs that is a nonselective combined beta-1 and beta-2 adrenergic blocking agent and is a selective alpha-1 adrenergic blocker. It is more potent as the former than the latter. In addition, it has a direct vasodilator effect. Cardiac output is not always changed, although it may be decreased during exercise. Volume expansion occurs and may be more common than with agents that are in the combined beta-1 and beta-2 category. Renal blood flow and glomerular filtration rate are unchanged.

Agents with central antihypertensive action

The second major subgrouping of sympathetic inhibitors includes the agents that have a central antihypertensive action (Table 28-7). This subgrouping includes clonidine, guanabenz, guanfacine, and methyldopa. Methyldopa was introduced over 15 years ago; methyldopa and clonidine have comparable antihypertensive potency. The mechanism by which methyldopa lowers arterial pressure is not completely understood. Several mechanisms have been proposed.

However, it is felt the major site of action is in the central nervous system and involves the cardiovascular regulatory centers of the lower brain stem, particularly the region of the nucleus tractus solitarius of the medulla oblongata. One of its metabolites, alpha-methylnorepinephrine, stimulates postsynaptic alpha-2 receptors in the cardiovascular regulatory centers, leading to decreased sympathetic outflow from the central nervous system and lowered arterial pressure (Wollam & Hall, 1988, p 322). Cardiac output is usually unchanged or somewhat reduced. Renal blood flow and glomerular filtration rate are maintained and myocardial and cerebral blood flow are reported to be increased. It does cause plasma volume expansion and may produce fluid retention.

The major difference between clonidine and methyldopa is that clonidine acts directly but methyldopa had to be first be converted to alpha-methylnorepinephrine.

Agents causing blockade of neuroeffector transmission

The agents which cause a blockade of neuroeffector transmission include guanethidine, guanadrel, and reserpine (Table 28-7). The first two work differently from the third. The accumulation of guanethidine in adrenergic neurons leads to a disruption of the process by which action potentials trigger the release of stored norepinephrine (Craig & Stitzel, 1990, p 288).

However, the exact mode of action is unknown. Parasympathetic function is not altered, which distin-

(Text continues on p. 601)

Table 28-7. Antihypertensive agents

Drug names	Preparations	Usual dosage	Adverse reactions
Combined alpha-1 and alpha-2 adrenergic blocking agents			
phenoxybenzamine (Dibenzyline)	Oral tablets IV	Adult: 10 mg qd, increase by 10 mg/d at 4-day intervals; maintenance dosage 20–40 mg bid or tid	Miosis, nasal congestion, vomiting, hypotension
phentolamine (Regitin, Regitine)	Oral tablets IM, IV	Adult: 5 mg 1–2 hr preoperatively, repeat as needed Child: 1 mg 1–2 hr preoperatively, repeat as needed	Hypotension, tachycardia, arrhythmias, angina, abdominal pain, nausea, vomiting, diarrhea
tolazoline (Priscoline)	IV	Newborn: 1–2 mg/kg over 5–10 min through scalp vein or directly into pulmonary artery initially; then, 1–2 mg/kg/hr via IV infusion	Hypotension, GI bleeding, acute, renal failure, hypochloremic alkalosis, thrombocytopenia
Selective alpha-1 adrenergic blocking agents			
doxazosin mesylate (Cardura)		Adult: 1–4 mg daily	
prazosin (Hypovase, Minipress)	Oral capsules	Adult: Initially 1 mg at bedtime; maintenance: 2–20 mg/d, divided in 2–3 doses	Dizziness, drowsiness, headache, weakness, orthostatic hypotension, palpitations, nausea, "first-dose effect" (syncope 30–90 min after initial dose, more common in those also receiving beta-blockers and/or diuretics; minimize this by low first dose)
terazosin (Hytrin)	Oral	Adult: Initially 1 mg, then slowly increase up to 5 mg/d; may be given as single dose or in two divided doses, not to exceed 20 mg/d	Dizziness, weakness, headache, nasal congestion, nausea
Nonselective, combined beta-1 and beta-2 adrenergic blocking agents			
carteolol (Cartrol)	Oral filmtab tablets	Adult: 2.5–5 mg/d, up to 10 mg/d	Bradycardia, weakness, lethargy, GI disturbances, insomnia, nightmares, hallucinations, depression, hyperlipidemia, hyperglycemia and hypoglycemia (extra care needed with diabetics), CHF (in clients with diminished cardiac reserve), bronchospasm (in clients with asthmatic tendency), aggravation of arterial insufficiency, sexual dysfunction
nadolol (Corgard, Syn-Nadolol)	Oral tablets	Adult: Initially 40 mg/d; maintenance: 80 mg/d; maximum dosage: 320 mg/d; taken once daily	See above
penbutolol (Levatol)	Oral tablets	Adult: 20 mg/d; maximum dosage: 80 mg/d	See above
pindolol (Apo-Pindol, Syn-Pindolol, Viskazide, Visken)	Oral tablets	Adult: Initially 10 mg/d, divided in two doses; maintenance: 10–30 mg/d, divided into three doses; maximum dosage: 60 mg/d	See above
propranolol (Inderal, Inderal LA, Inderide, Novopranol, PMS Propranolol)	Oral tablets Oral extended-release capsules IV	Adult: Initially 40 mg bid (prompt preparation), 80 mg qa (extended-release preparation); maintenance: 160–480 mg/d (prompt preparation), 120–480 mg/d (extended-release preparation)	See above
timolol (Apo-Timol, Apo-Timop, Betim, Blocadren, Temsorin, Timacor Timoptic, Temoptol)	Oral tablets Ophth	Adult: 10–60 mg/d in divided doses Adult/Child: Ophth: 1 drop of 0.25 or 0.5 solution bid	See above With ophthalmic use, systemic reactions may occur.

(Continued)

Table 28-7. Antihypertensive agents (*Continued*)

Drug names	Preparations	Usual dosage	Adverse reactions
Cardioselective, predominantly beta-1 adrenergic blocking agents			
acebutolol (Monitan, Sectral)	Oral capsules	Adult: Initially 400 mg/d in 1 or 2 doses; maintenance: 200–800 mg/d	Fatigue, weakness, dizziness, headache
atenolol (Apo-Atenol, Atenol, Premormine, Tenormin)	Oral tablets IV	Adult: Initially: 50 mg/d in one dose; maximum: 100 mg daily	Fatigue, weakness, dizziness, nausea
betaxolol (Kerlone, Betoptic)	Oral tablets Ophth solution	Adult: 5–10 mg daily Adult: Ophth: 1 drop bid	Ophthalmic use has caused ocular stinging
esmolol (Brevibloc)	IV	50–200 µg/kg/min; maintenance: 25–50 micrograms/kg/min; used for 24 hr or less	Hypotension, nausea, dizziness, infusion site reactions, diaphoresis
metoprolol (Betalor, Lopressor, Novametoprolol, Seloken)	Oral film-coated tablets	Adult: Initially: 100 mg/d, in single or divided doses	Dizziness, diarrhea, depression, fatigue, weakness
Combined alpha and beta adrenergic blocking agents			
labetalol (Normodyne, Trandate)	Oral tablets IV	Adult: Initially: orally, 100 mg bid; maintenance: 200–400 mg bid; IV, 2 mg/min or 20 mg initially, 20–80 mg every 10 min, maximum cumulative dose 300 mg	Fatigue, weakness, orthostatic hypotension
Centrally acting adrenergic inhibitors			
clonidine (Catapres, Catapres TTS, Dixarit)	Oral tablets Pouched transdermal system	Adult: Initially 0.1 mg bid, increase to 0.2–0.8 mg daily in divided doses; maximum dosage 2.4 mg; transdermal dosage is one pouch once every 7 days	Dry mouth, drowsiness, fatigue, weakness, sedation, dizziness, constipation, GI disturbances (nausea, vomiting), impotence, agitation
guanabenz (Wytensin)	Oral tablets	Adult: Initially 8 mg/d, divided in two doses; maximum dosage: 64 mg daily	Dry mouth, drowsiness, dizziness, weakness, headache
guanfacine (Tenex)	Oral tablets	Adult: 1 mg at hs; maximum dosage: 3 mg daily	Dry mouth, drowsiness, dizziness, weakness, headache, insomnia, constipation
methyldopa (Aldomet, Dopamet, Novomedopa, Presinol, Sembrina)	Oral tablets Oral suspension IV	Adult: 250 mg bid, may be increased to 2 g/d	Somnolence, dry mouth, nasal congestion, orthostatic hypotension, impotence, positive direct Coombs test, hepatitis, drug fever
Blockade of neuroeffector transmission			
guanadrel (Hylorel)	Oral tablets	Adult: Initially: 10 mg/d, divided in two doses; maintenance: 25–75 mg/d, divided in two doses	SOB/DOE, palpitations, chest pain, cough, orthostatic hypotension, faintness, nocturia, urinary dysfunction, ejaculation disturbance, anorexia, indigestion, flatus, diarrhea, drowsiness, fatigue, leg cramps, myalgia, paresthesias, headache, confusion, visual disturbances
guanethidine (Ismelin)	Oral tablets	Adult: Initially: 10 mg/d, increased at 3–5 day intervals; maintenance: 25–150 mg/d	Orthostatic hypotension, dyspnea, chest pain, nocturia, ejaculation disturbance, myalgia, weight gain, fluid retention, diarrhea, bradycardia
reserpine (Novoserpine, Reserpoid, Sandril, Serfin, Serpalen, Serpasil)	Oral tablets	Adult: 0.05–0.25 mg/d in 1–2 doses	Bradycardia, lethargy, drowsiness, impotence, diarrhea, abdominal cramps, depression, activation of peptic ulcer, nasal congestion, weight gain, Parkinsonian state
Ganglionic blocking agents			
mecamylamine (Inversine)	Oral tablets	Adult: Initially: 2.5 mg bid; maintenance: 25 mg, divided in 2–4 doses	Orthostatic hypotension, mydriasis, dry mouth, urinary retention, paralytic ileus

(Continued)

Table 28-7. Antihypertensive agents (Continued)

Drug names	Preparations	Usual dosage	Adverse reactions
Combined alpha-1 and alpha-2 adrenergic blocking agents			
trimethaphan (Arfonad)	IV	Adult: Initially: 500 mg put into 500 ml D5W, 0.5–1 mg/min, increased gradually to 1–5 mg/min; adjusted in accordance with client's blood pressure	See above
Undefined			
pargyline (Eudatin, Eutonyl, Eutron)	Oral tablets	Adult: Initially, 25 mg qd, increased at weekly intervals by 10 mg until desired response attained; maintenance: 25–50 mg qd; maximum dosage: 200 mg daily; maintenance for those over 65 years and those who have undergone sympathectomy: 10–25 mg daily	Orthostatic hypotension, drowsiness, dizziness, sedation, dry mouth
Direct-acting vasodilators			
Arterial			
diazoxide (Hyperstat, Proglycem)	IV Oral capsules Oral suspension	Adult: 1–3 mg/kg over 30 sec or less, may repeat in 5–15 min; do not use longer than 10 days Child: 5 mg/kg as bolus over 30 sec or less	Dizziness, weakness, hypotension, sodium and water retention, tachycardia, nausea and vomiting, hyperglycemia
hydralazine (Apresoline)	Oral tablets IM IV	Adult: Orally: initially, 10 mg qid; maintenance 50–200 mg daily in divided doses; rarely up to 400 mg/d; IV: 10–40 mg q4h–q6h prn Child: 0.75–3 mg/kg q6h–q12h with maximum dosage of 7.5 mg/kg/24 hr	GI disturbances, reactions resembling SLE or rheumatoid arthritis, headache, palpitations, dry mouth, tachycardia, flushing, nasal congestion, blood dyscrasias, drug fever, rash, depression, precipitation of CHF in clients with myocardial disease
minoxidil (Loniten)	Oral tablets	Adult: Initially, 5 mg qd; increased gradually to 2.5–20 mg qd, in 1–2 doses; maximum dosage: 100 mg daily Child under 12: Initially, 0.2 mg/kg body weight once daily, increased gradually to 1 mg/kg/d in 1–2 doses; maximum dosage: 50 mg/d	Hypertrichosis, edema and severe cardiac complications (*eg*, CHF, pericardial effusion with tamponade, aggravation of coronary insufficiency)
Arterial and venous			
nitroprusside (Nipride, Nitropress)	IV	May be prepared as 50 mg/1000 ml, which equals 50 μg/ml; up to 200 mg/1000 ml; need infusion pump	Headache, dizziness, nausea, abdominal pain
Inhibitors of renin-angiotensin system			
Angiotensin converting enzyme inhibitors			
captopril (Capoten)	Oral tablets	Adult: Initially: up to 25 mg tid (increased only after 1 wk–2 wk of therapy); maintenance: 25 mg–150 mg tid; maximum dosage: 450 mg daily	Rash, fever, cough, hypotension, proteinuria, hypogeusia
enalapril (Vasotec)	Oral tablets IV	Adult: Oral, initially: 2.5–5 mg/d, increasing as tolerated; maintenance: 10–40 mg/d in one or 2 doses; IV, hypertension, 1.25 mg over 5-min period, repeat q6h; in client taking diuretic, 0.625 mg over 5 min, repeat in 1 hour, then 1.25 mg q6h	Headache, dizziness, fatigue, hypotension
lisinopril (Prinivil, Zestril)	Oral tablets	Adult: 5 mg/d if on diuretics or 10 mg/d, may be increased up to 20–40 mg daily	Headache, dizziness, fatigue
Angiotensin II analogues			
saralasin (Sarenin)	IV		Hypotension, rebound hypertension

(Continued)

Table 28-7. Antihypertensive agents (*Continued*)

Drug names	Preparations	Usual dosage	Adverse reactions
Calcium-channel blocking agents			
diltiazem (Cardizem, Cardizem SR, Tilazem)	Oral tablets Oral sustained release capsules	Adults: Initially 30 mg, increased gradually until desired response; maximum dosage 360 mg/d; SR 60–120 mg bid initially; may be increased to 240–360 mg/d	Dizziness, headache, fatigue, hypotension, conduction abnormalities, edema, nausea
nicardipine (Cardene)	Oral capsules	Adults: 20 mg tid	Dizziness, headache, tachycardia, palpitations, edema, flushing
nifedipine (Adalat, Apo-Nifed, Novonifedin, Procardia)	oral capsules	Adults: Initially 10 mg tid, maintenance 30–60 mg/d, divided in three doses; maximum dosage 180 mg/d	Dizziness, headache, fatigue, hypotension, conduction abnormalities, edema, nausea, GI symptoms, hepatic dysfunction
nimodipine (Nimotop)	Oral capsules	60 mg q4h for 21 consecutive days after SAH	
verapamil (Apo-Verap, Calan, Calan SR, Cordilox, Dilacoran, Isoptin, Manidon, Novoveramil, Verelan)	Oral tablets Oral sustained release preparations IV	Adults: Initially 80 mg q8h, maximum dosage 360 mg/d; SR from 180 mg given in morning to 240 mg q12h IV: adults: Initially 5–10 mg, given over 2 min, followed by second dose of 10 mg in 30 min if needed	Dizziness, headache, fatigue, hypotension, conduction abnormalities, edema, nausea

guishes this class from the ganglionic blocking agents. There is little or no change in peripheral vascular resistance. With chronic treatment with guanethidine, catecholamine stores are slowly depleted. With the prevention of release of norepinephrine, the contraction of vascular smooth muscle due to sympathetic nerve stimulation is reduced and blood pressure decreases.

Guanethidine is an example of a drug that demonstrates the concept that initial physiologic changes during the early treatment period may change with chronic use of the agent. During early treatment period, there is a reduction in cardiac output and a proportional decrease in renal, splanchnic, and cerebral blood flow. With long-term therapy, hemodynamic adjustments occur and cardiac output gradually increases to pretreatment levels. A reduction in renal blood flow and glomerular filtration rate occurs in the early treatment period but there do not seem to be significant changes in renal function with long-term therapy.

Guanadrel acts similarly to guanethidine and is as effective but its antihypertensive effect is of short duration.

Rauwolfia serpentina (snakeroot), found in India, Sri Lanka, Burma, and Java, contains 20 antihypertensive alkaloids; one of them is reserpine. Although the net result is similar, reserpine does not interfere with norepinephrine in the same way that guanethidine does. Under the normal physiologic situation, when an action potential invades the sympathetic nerve terminal, a portion of released norepinephrine is recycled.

First, norepinephrine is transferred across the neuronal membrane into the cytosol by an energy-dependent, carrier-mediated active process. Secondly, the recaptured amine is transported from cytosol into noradrenergic storage vesicles. Reserpine inhibits the second uptake process and as a consequence of this inhibition norepinephrine cannot be stored intraneuronally (Craig & Stitzel, 1990, p 291).

In addition, reserpine also impairs vesicular uptake of dopamine, the immediate precursor of norepinephrine. Since dopamine must be taken up into the vesicles to go through the process of being made into norepinephrine, reserpine also indirectly impairs norepinephrine synthesis. The occurrence of reserpine-induced extrapyramidal symptoms (Parkinsonian syndrome) is believed to be a result of the impaired uptake of dopamine.

Ganglionic blocking agents

The ganglionic blocking agents (Table 28-7) act by preventing the attachment of acetylcholine to the receptor sites of the autonomic ganglia. They prevent the interaction of acetylcholine with the nicotinic receptors on postsynaptic neuronal membranes of both the sympathetic and parasympathetic nervous systems. Their blockage of impulse transmission decreases vascular tone, cardiac output, and blood pressure.

Undefined group

The undefined grouping of sympathetic inhibitors includes one drug: pargyline. Pargyline is known to be a monoamine oxidase inhibitor and it is the only inhibitor used for treatment of hypertension. It lowers blood pressure by blocking the release of norepinephrine at the sympathetic neuroeffector junctions, thereby interfering with vasoconstriction (see Table 28-7).

Direct acting vasodilators

Hydralazine is an example of a direct-acting vasodilator, which produces vasodilation of precapillary resistance vessels by direct relaxation of arteriolar smooth muscle. It has little or no effect on postcapillary venous capacitance vessels. The cellular mechanism is not completely understood. Minoxidil is a piperidinopyrimidine derivative and is not related chemically to hydralazine but its action is similar. Sodium nitroprusside's mechanism of action is similar to that described under the discussion of nitrites and nitrates earlier in this chapter.

Postural hypotension is not a problem with hydralazine because cardiovascular reflexes and postcapillary venous capacitance vessels are not affected. However, hydralazine does result in an increase in cardiac output, which reduces its antihypertensive effect and causes certain side effects. There is a reflex increase in sympathetic stimulation of the heart, an increase in plasma renin, and an increase in salt and water retention.

Captopril is an example of an angiotensin converting enzyme inhibitor. Enalapril and lisinopril are other examples (Table 28-7). They suppress the renin-angiotensin-aldosterone system by inhibiting angiotensin-converting enzyme and thereby preventing the conversion of angiotensin I to angiotensin II. Angiotensin II is a vasoconstrictor that stimulates the production of aldosterone. With less angiotensin and aldosterone, vasodilation and decreased blood pressure occur (see Focus on ACE Inhibitors: Similarities and Differences.)

Calcium-channel blocking agents

The calcium-channel blocking agents are a very important group of drugs (see Table 28-7). Intracellular free Ca^{2+} plays an important role in the excitation-contraction coupling process. Vascular contraction is directly related to the rise of intracellular calcium. Calcium-channel blocking agents lower intracellular calcium concentration through a reduction of the transmembraneous slow calcium influx, which occurs during membrane depolarization. The inhibition of calcium influx into cells prevents the rise in calcium levels and results in diminished vascular tone, vascular smooth muscle relaxation, and, consequently, vasodilation and lowering of blood pressure. Vasodilation is more pronounced in smaller arteries and arterioles. The cerebral, coronary, and skeletal muscle beds or arteries and arterioles are the most sensitive to the action of these agents (see Focus on Calcium-Channel Blocking Agents: Similarities and Differences).

Therapeutic uses of antihypertensives

It is evident that there are many individual antihypertensive agents from which to choose. In addition, there are even more combination drugs, often including a diuretic (Table 28-8). The combined alpha-1 and alpha-2 adrenergic blocking agents, specifically phenoxybenzamine and phentolamine, are used to manage the hypertension and sweating of pheochromocytoma (tumor of adrenal medulla). Phentolamine is used to control the blood pressure during the surgical removal of the pheochromocytoma. They are used to treat hypertension associated with adrenergic excess, such as that produced by tyramine-containing foods when clients are on monoamine oxidase inhibitor therapy. Phentolamine is also used to prevent and treat dermal necrosis and sloughing following extravasation of norepinephrine, phenylephrine, or dopamine. To manage extravasation, it can be injected directly into the affected area (5–10 mg in 10 ml of 0.9% sodium chloride).

Tolazoline is used in treatment of persistent pulmonary hypertension or "persistent fetal circulation" of the newborn when oxygenation cannot be satisfactorily provided by other means.

Prazosin is an example of the selective alpha-1 adrenergic blocking agents. Its potency is comparable to that of propranolol, methyldopa, and clonidine. It should be used with a diuretic because this will enhance its therapeutic action. In clients requiring multidrug therapy, a beta blocker and hydralazine might also be used with prazosin and the diuretic.

Prazosin may also be useful in managing clients

Table 28-8. Examples of drug combinations used as antihypertensive agents

Drug name	Active ingredients
Aldoclor	methyldopa and chlorothiazide
Apresazide	hydrochlorothiazide and hydralazine
Capozide	hydrochlorothiazide and captopril
Combipres	chlorthalidone and clonidine
Corzide	bendroflumethiazide and nadolol
Esimil	hydrochlorothiazide and guanethidine monosulfate
Hydrotensin	hydrochlorothiazide and reserpine
Inderide	hydrochlorothiazide and propranolol
Minizide	polythiazide and prazosin
Regroton	reserpine and chlorthalidone
Salutensin	reserpine and hydroflumethiazide
Ser-Ap-ES	hydrochlorothiazide, hydralazine, reserpine
Tenoretic	chlorthalidone and atenolol
Timolide	hydrochlorothiazide and timolol
Vaseretic	enalapril and hydrochlorothiazide
Zestoretic	lisinopril and hydrochlorothiazide

Focus on

ACE inhibitors: similarities and differences

Similarities	Differences

Similarities

Pharmacodynamics

These agents inhibit the action of angiotensin converting enzyme. They prevent the conversion of angiotensin I to angiotensin II resulting in a suppression of the renin-angiotensin-aldosterone system. They decrease vasoconstriction, reducing peripheral vascular resistance and decrease sodium and water retention and extracellular fluid volume

Pharmacokinetics

These agents are adequately absorbed by the GI tract and are not affected by food intake. They are metabolized by the liver and eliminated unchanged by the kidneys

Therapeutic uses

These agents are used to treat hypertension

Adverse reactions

These include: (CNS) headache, fatigue; (CV) tachycardia, hypotension, orthostasis; (GI) loss of taste perception, nausea, diarrhea; (GU): proteinuria, nephrotic syndrome; (Heme) neutropenia, agranulocytosis, anemia, thrombocytopenia; (Skin) rash; (Other) hyperkalemia, angioedema of hands and face, fever, joint pain

Contraindications

These agents are contraindicated in persons with hypersensitivity to the drug

Precautions

These agents should be used with caution in persons with impaired renal function

Differences

• **Captopril** decreases systemic vascular resistance and preload.

• **Captopril** is rapidly absorbed from the GI tract but the absorption is diminished with food intake; it has an onset of action of 15–60 minutes, peaking in 60–90 minutes, a duration of 2–12 hours and a half-life of less than 3 hours. Small amounts (1%) are excreted in breast milk. • **Lisinopril** is poorly absorbed and not metabolized. It has an onset of 1 hour, peaking in 6 hours, with a half-life of 12 hours. • **Enalapril** is well absorbed and metabolized to the active metabolite—**enalaprilate**. It has an onset of 1 hour, peaking in 4–6 hours, a duration of 24 hours and a half-life of 11 hours; one-third is excreted in feces.

• **Captopril** and **enalapril** are also used to treat congestive heart failure in conjunction with cardiac glycosides and diuretics.

• **Lisinopril** may also cause depression, paresthesia, impotence, decreased libido, dyspepsia, nasal congestion and muscle cramps; **captopril** may also cause angina, congestive heart failure, pericarditis, renal failure and urinary frequency; **enalapril** may cause insomnia; **enalapril** and **captopril** may cause a cough.

• **Enalapril** and **captopril** should be used with caution in persons with hepatic impairment and in those persons with sodium depletion, those receiving diuretics and hemodialysis. • **Enalapril** should be used with caution in persons with collagen vascular diseases. • **Captopril** should be used with caution in persons with serious autoimmune disease or those exposed to other drugs affecting the white blood cell counts or immune response.

(continued)

ACE inhibitors: similarities and differences (Continued)

Similarities	Differences

Nursing considerations

Instruct client in disease, treatment, drug therapy, regimen, adverse effects and compliance; monitor vital signs especially blood pressure for changes; assess cardiopulmonary status for changes; check blood counts, renal function studies and urinalysis frequently; instruct client in signs and symptom of infection and need to notify physician; institute safety measures to prevent injury; instruct client to change position slowly; monitor serum potassium levels for changes; instruct client to limit the use of caffeine-containing products; instruct client in technique for self-monitoring of blood pressure; institute dietary restrictions, such as low sodium and instruct client in dietary restrictions; advise client to continue to take drug even if he or she feels better

Administer captopril 1 hour before meals and separate doses of drug and antacids by 1–2 hours; Administer **IV enalaprilate** slowly over 5 minutes; stop **thiazide diuretic** therapy 2–3 days before giving **lisinopril**.

---

with hypertension with hyperlipidemia because it tends to decrease serum cholesterol and triglycerides.

The nonselective, combined beta-1 and beta-2 adrenergic blockers include carteolol, nadolol, penbutolol, pindolol, propranolol, and timolol. They are widely used to treat angina pectoris and hypertension (alone or with other agents) and certain tachyarrhythmias. They have also been used to decrease certain manifestations of hyperthyroidism, such as tachycardia and muscle tremors. They cannot be used alone because the underlying pathology must be treated; they might come into use during the management of hyperthyroid crisis or during initial use of antithyroid drugs.

They are used for the prophylactic treatment of migraine headaches. The headache's pain is felt to be related to vasodilation and the blockage of craniovascular beta-receptors may result in decreased vasodilation.

Timolol can be used topically to reduce intraocular pressure in clients with chronic open-angle glaucoma and ocular hypertension. The decrease in ocular pressure seems to relate to decreased production of aqueous humor.

The cardioselective, predominantly beta-1 adrenergic blocking agents include acebutolol, atenolol, betaxolol, and metoprolol and are used for the treatment of angina pectoris and hypertension (alone or with other agents). Esmolol is used for short-term management of supraventricular tachyarrhythmias. A nonapproved use is the lowering of blood pressure during surgical procedures.

Labetalol's antihypertensive effect is comparable to that of the nonselective, combined beta-1 and beta-2 adrenergic blockers. Therapy should include the use of a diuretic to counteract the volume expansion that occurs.

Methyldopa is used for mild to moderate primary hypertension. Because it lowers blood pressure without compromising renal blood flow or glomerular filtration rate, it is particularly helpful in hypertension complicated by renal disease. However, it is often not effective with end-stage renal disease and the accompanying severe hypertension.

Clonidine is used for mild to moderate hypertension. It may be used in combination with a diuretic, vasodilator, and beta-blocker. It also is especially useful in clients with renal disease. Nonapproved uses include management of narcotic withdrawal, prophylaxis of vascular headaches, treatment of dysmenorrhea, and treatment of menopausal syndromes.

Guanethidine is an extremely potent antihypertensive agent. However, due to a number of side effects related to the imbalance between sympathetic and parasympathetic functions that it produces, its use is declining. It should always be used with a diuretic and a vasodilator is also sometimes added. A number of drug interactions have been identified (including tricyclic antidepressants and phenothiazines).

Reserpine and related compounds were once widely used in the treatment of mild to moderate hypertension. Their use has decreased with the advent of newer agents. A diuretic should be administered concurrently when reserpine is used. The orthostatic hy-

Focus on

Calcium channel blockers: similarities and differences

| Similarities | Differences |

Similarities

Differences

Pharmacodynamics

These drugs inhibit calcium influx across the slow channels of myocardial and smooth muscle cells, lowering intracellular calcium and ultimately dilating coronary arteries, peripheral arterioles and arteries, and slowing cardiac conduction.

• **Verapamil** has the most pronounced affect on specialized cells of the sinoatrial and atrioventricular nodes of the heart, slowing cardiac conduction.

Pharmacokinetics

All are well absorbed from the GI tract but undergo significant first-pass metabolism. Onset of action within 30 minutes. Most are bound to plasma proteins, metabolized by the liver, and excreted in the urine.

Onset of action is quickest with sublingual **nifedipine** (5 min) and **verapamil IV** (1–5 min). • **Diltiazem** and **nifedipine** are also excreted in the feces. Elimination half-life for **diltiazem** is 3–9 hours, for **nifedipine** is 2–5 hours, for **verapamil** is 6–12 hours.

Therapeutic use

All are used as antianginal and antihypertensive agents. Also used in Raynaud's disease and migraine headaches.

• **Verapamil** is used as an antiarrhythmic.

Adverse reactions

All may cause dizziness, headache, fatigue, hypotension, conduction abnormalities, edema, and nausea.

• **Verapamil** also causes bradycardia, constipation, and elevated liver enzymes. • **Nifedipine** also causes flushing, weakness, syncope, lightheadedness, headache, dyspnea, palpatations, worsening of angina, MI, edema, heartburn, diarrhea, and muscle cramps. • **Diltiazem** also causes drowsiness, nervousness, depression, insomnia, confusion, bradycardia, vomiting, diarrhea, elevated liver enzymes, rash, photosensitivity.

Contraindications

All are contraindicated in history of hypersensitivity.

• **Diltiazem** and **verapamil** are contraindicated in severe hypotension, second and third degree heart block, and sick sinus syndrome. • **Verapamil** also contraindicated in severe left ventricular dysfunction.

Precautions

All must be used cautiously in clients with congestive heart failure or impaired left ventricular function.

• **Nifedipine** must be used cautiously in aortic stenosis. • **Verapamil** must be used cautiously in hypertropic cardiomyopathy, sick sinus syndrome, Wolff-Parkinson-White syndrome, wide complex ventricular tachycardia, and impaired liver or kidney function. • **Diltiazem** must be used cautiously in conduction abnormalities, clients on beta blockers or digoxin, and impaired liver or kidney function.

Nursing considerations

Monitor heart rate and rhythm and blood pressure when starting therapy and increasing dose. Warn client not to stop drug or change dose without doctor's advice. If client on **digoxin**, monitor **digoxin** level and observe for signs of toxicity.

Reduced dosage of **carbamazepine** needed when patient is also on **verapamil**, observe for signs of **carbamazepine** toxicity. • **Nifedipine** may exacerbate angina briefly; reassure patient and adjust dosage slowly. Monitor EKG continuously for patients on IV **verapamil**.

potension seen with reserpine is usually less severe than that seen with guanethidine.

The ganglionic blocking agents are extremely potent antihypertensive agents but with the availability of sodium nitroprusside, they are no longer widely used. One use might be the IV preparation in hypertensive emergencies or in surgical procedures in which hypotension is desirable to decrease the possibility of hemorrhage. Blockage of impulse transmission in both the sympathetic and parasympathetic nervous systems produces marked side effects, such as orthostatic hypotension, visual changes, urinary retention, and paralytic ileus.

The sympathetic inhibitor, pargyline, is not widely used. It is only used when hypertension is refractory to safer drugs.

The direct-acting vasodilators include diazoxide, hydralazine, and minoxidil. Diazoxide is used intravenously for hypertensive emergencies, particularly malignant hypertension, hypertensive encephalopathy, and eclampsia. It is frequently administered with a diuretic.

Hydralazine is used in the treatment of clients with primary hypertension of moderate severity. It is rarely used alone and is likely to be combined with a diuretic and a beta-blocker. This combination affects three of the chief determinants of blood pressure: cardiac output (beta-blocker), plasma volume (diuretic), and peripheral vascular resistance (hydralazine). It was used intravenously in the past for hypertensive emergencies but it is not now so used, largely due to its slow onset of action after IV injection and its somewhat unpredictable actions.

Minoxidil can produce a greater reduction in blood pressure than hydralazine and is used for hypertension resistant to other forms of therapy and severe hypertension that may be life-threatening. It is especially used for hypertension in clients with renal failure because it produces no significant changes in renal blood flow or glomerular filtration rate. It is often used in combination with a beta-blocker and a diuretic.

Sodium nitroprusside is used in the management of hypertensive emergencies, especially hypertension with acute MI or left ventricular failure. Due to venodilation, it reduces preload and due to arteriolar dilation it reduces afterload. Thus, it improves ventricular performance and may be used with congestive heart failure in the absence of hypertension.

Captopril and enalapril are used alone or in combination with other antihypertensives. Captopril is often used with a diuretic and enalapril is 10 times more potent than captopril. Their effects on preload and afterload also make them useful in the treatment of congestive heart failure.

The calcium-channel blocking agents as a group are used in the management of angina pectoris and when ischemic disease accompanies hypertension. Ve-

rapamil, a class IV antiarrhythmic, is discussed as such in Chapter 27.

Clinical studies have proved the efficacy and safety of calcium-channel blocking agents in the treatment of hypertension, alone or in combination with other drugs. One reason they can be used alone is that they are not accompanied by the reflex tachycardia or volume retention that occur with some other antihypertensives and that mandate combination therapy. However, they are helpful in combination with captopril in severe hypertension accompanied by renal complications. They seem particularly effective in older individuals who tend to have low plasma renin activity and possibly also in black clients (who tend to respond less well to beta-blockers or inhibitors of the renin-angiotensin system) (Buhler & Kiowski, 1988, p 594). However, the most reliable predictors of their effectiveness are the dose employed and the pretreatment level of hypertension.

Peripheral vasospasm (Raynaud's disease) may respond to therapy with nifedipine.

Many new members of this class of drugs are in clinical trial. Slight structural changes in the first calcium-channel blocking agents have yielded second-generation drugs with improved selectivity of action. Some have greater cerebrovascular selectivity, such as nimodipine. Cerebral ischemia can be produced by acute occlusion of brain vessels, cardiac arrest, and subarachnoid hemorrhage. The ischemia elicits an alteration of normal Ca^{2+}, K^+, and Na^+ gradients across cell membranes, due to depletion of adenosine triphosphatase stores, and there is a move toward intracellular Ca^{2+} overload and vasospasm.

Vasospasm, which appears at two points after rupture of an intracranial aneurysm in subarachnoid hemorrhage (1–3 hours after the bleeding and then several days after the bleeding) has been considered the main cause of mortality in these clients. Nimodipine may prevent vasospasm by blocking the intracellular Ca^{2+} overload, thus, increasing cerebral blood flow. The calcium-channel blocking agents have been administered intracisternally and by other routes (Marin, 1988, pp 301–303).

Calcium-channel blocking agents have also been studied to use in prophylaxis of migraine headaches. Nimodipine has demonstrated reduction in the frequency, severity, and duration of migraine attacks and may do so by decreasing vasoconstriction. (See accompanying Example of Nursing Process and Nifedipine Therapy.)

■ Summary

Hypertension is an all-too-common cardiovascular health problem. Some individuals may have their hypertension managed nonpharmacologically but many will require a drug regimen. There are many types of antihypertensives, in-

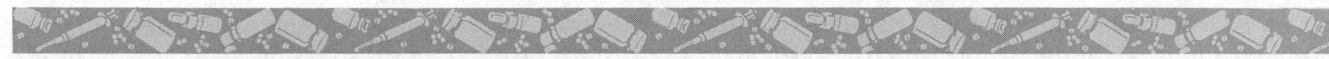

Example of nursing process and nifedipine therapy

The client is a 40-year-old black male with a 6-month history of moderate hypertension. He has been treated with hydrochlorothiazide and methyldopa with good response. He is now requesting a change in the drug regimen because he has experienced sexual dysfunction. The physician is planning to phase out the methyldopa according to a weaning schedule, replacing it with gradually increased doses of nifedipine (beginning with 10 mg tid).

Assessment data	Nursing diagnosis	Intervention	Goals and outcome criteria
Complaint of sexual dysfunction associated with methyldopa therapy Change in antihypertensive medication	Sexual dysfunction related to antihypertensive medication	**Assist** the client in integrating methyldopa weaning schedule and nifedipine medication into his drug regimen.	The client will report that sexual function is improved.
Nifedipine therapy	Altered comfort: intestinal disturbances related to irritation and decreased smooth muscle tone secondary to nifedipine therapy	**Advise** the client to avoid foods that can cause intestinal disturbance. Recommend a high quality, easily digested diet with adequate fiber. Advise him to avoid fatty foods and concentrated carbohydrates. **Urge** the client to consult with his primary health care provider if discomforting signs and symptoms of intestinal disturbance develop.	The client will not experience intestinal disturbance; if intestinal disturbance develops, it will be detected and treated in an early stage.
Nifedipine therapy	Pain: headache related to nifedipine medication	**Teach** the client the side effects of nifedipine therapy that are likely to occur; advise the client on measures to relieve pain.	If headache develops, the client will be knowledgable about methods to relieve the pain.
Nifedipine therapy	Knowledge deficit concerning the adverse effects of nifedipine medication on liver function	**Advise** the client of the importance of regular medical supervision and periodic laboratory tests to detect adverse reactions to medication. Monitor liver function tests and alert the physician if these indicate liver impairment.	The client will report regularly for office appointments and laboratory tests. If liver impairment develops, it will be detected and treated during an early stage.

cluding sympathetic inhibitors (adrenergic blocking agents of several types, agents with central antihypertensive action, agents causing blockade of neuroeffector transmission, and ganglionic blocking agents); direct-acting vasodilators; the inhibitors of the renin-angiotensin system; and calcium-channel blocking agents. Clients will often experience adverse reactions related to the medications because the agents influence various body processes.

Nursing management of chronic hypertension

Nursing implications

The importance of early and vigorous treatment of hypertension has been recognized only recently. Adequate control of blood pressure reduces the risk of death from cardiovascular disease.

It is estimated that about 20% of adults in the United States has blood pressures above the "normal" range. At least half of this number are unaware of the problem. Only half of the people who have been diagnosed are treated, and of these only half are under adequate control. These figures imply that only one person in eight who is at risk is receiving adequate treatment. Casefinding and referral are important nursing responsibilities.

Medical regimens for the treatment of hypertension generally follow a well defined progression, according to a "stepped care" model. Within the guidelines of this concept, drug therapy begins with one drug (usually a diuretic or a beta adrenergic-blocking agent) at minimal dosage. Dosage is increased until a therapeutic response is attained.

If the client does not respond adequately, a second drug is added (a beta-blocker or diuretic, depending on which was used at step one). Clients with moderate to severe disease may require a third drug (usually a vasodilator) or a fourth drug (usually an additional beta-blocker). Within each step, there are alternative drugs that may be substituted for agents to which the client does not respond adequately. Thus, captopril or enalapril may be substituted for an ineffective beta-blocker at step two, or be used as the additional drug at step four. If hydralazine is inadequate at step 3, minoxidil may be substituted. Certain drugs require others to control adverse effects: a beta-blocker is usually given whenever hydralazine is prescribed; captopril and enalapril (which stimulate sodium and water retention) should be given only in conjunction with diuretics; a potent loop diuretic is often required when minoxidil is prescribed.

Response to therapy for hypertension can be greatly enhanced by nursing measures to reduce contributing factors such as obesity, excessive intake of sodium, lack of exercise, and stress. A reduction of excess weight often lowers blood pressure, sometimes to normal. Sodium intake must be limited to prevent hypervolemia. Moderate exercise is helpful, not only to accelerate weight loss but also to promote sleep and reduce emotional stress. The client may need to learn new techniques for managing stress to minimize psychologic and physiologic reactions. Some people benefit from biofeedback training or hypnosis to promote vasodilation. Such measures can be used prophylactically in persons at risk for hypertension and for those in the early, mild stages of the disease. Once signs and symptoms have advanced, nursing management must be coordinated with the medical plan of care.

The fact that half of the people under treatment for hypertension are not adequately controlled implies that compliance with prescribed regimens is difficult. Many factors are involved. It is difficult to appreciate the importance of therapy when the condition is asymptomatic (as is usual with hypertension). Treatment is long-term and may be necessary for the duration of the client's life. Buying drugs is a financial drain. Adverse reactions to the drug can be uncomfortable or otherwise distressing. The nurse can improve compliance by assisting the client in following the prescribed regimen. It is important to explore the factors associated with noncompliance and work with the client to reduce their impact. Treatment must be incorporated into the client's lifestyle and integrated into the daily routine. Consistent dosage may be difficult, especially for clients with memory deficits. The nurse should assist clients in devising a system for taking medication that will help prevent dose omissions.

Nursing process

Assessment   Nurses are in a position to refer many clients with previously undetected hypertension for definitive diagnosis. Screening clinics for cardiovascular disease are often initiated and managed by nurses. Individuals with high blood pressures above 140 systolic or 90 diastolic should be referred to a physician for evaluation.

Initial assessment of clients with chronic hypertension should include a complete health evaluation with emphasis on risk factors for cardiovascular disease and current cardiovascular function. A complete drug history should be included. (See Chapter 3, Nursing Process in the Management of Drug-Related Problems, for a discussion of drug histories.) The nurse should take a family history pertinent to cardiovascular disease. The client's knowledge of hypertension and cardiovascular disease and their treatment should be assessed.

The client should be screened for contraindications for given antihypertensive agents and for risk factors for adverse reactions to antihypertensive agents.

Nursing diagnosis   Nursing diagnoses for clients with hypertension may include the following:

> *(If the client is obese) altered nutrition: more than body requirements*
> *Fluid volume excess: edema related to excessive sodium intake secondary to hypertension*

Many clients receiving antihypertensive agents have a

> *High risk for injury related to dizziness, lightheadedness, and syncope secondary to orthostatic hypotension*

Most clients for whom drugs are prescribed have been under nonpharmacologic treatment for hypertension. Therefore, they should have knowledge about the disease and its treatment. However, most will have a knowledge deficit concerning the prescribed drugs (*eg*, signs and symptoms of side effects to report to the health care provider).

Common collaborative problems that should be differentiated from the nursing diagnoses include

Potential complication: stroke
Potential complication: renal failure

Planning Goals of nursing care include reduction in blood pressure; for the obese client, weight loss; reduction in risk of hypervolemia and edema; for tobacco users, reduction or elimination of tobacco use; for clients using alcohol, reduction of alcohol use; improved management of stress; reduction in the incidence and severity of postural hypotension; reduction in knowledge deficit; and compliance with the treatment regimen. Another goal should be reduction in risk of, amelioration, or elimination of adverse reactions.

Intervention Nursing care of clients with chronic hypertension includes assisting the client in adopting a lifestyle conducive to cardiovascular health and assisting the client in managing the drug regimen for maximum benefit.

A client experiencing dizziness, lightheadedness, or syncope while on an antihypertensive should be assisted in actions to take to compensate for these difficulties. The client should rise from a lying to standing position by sitting up slowly, sitting quietly for a few minutes, and then standing slowly. To decrease peripheral venous pooling, the client should avoid prolonged standing and possibly wear support stockings. To decrease further vasodilation, hot baths or showers should be avoided.

A client may experience GI symptoms while on an antihypertensive, including anorexia, nausea, vomiting, abdominal discomfort, diarrhea, and constipation, among others. These symptoms, in some cases, may be minimized by taking the drugs at fixed times in relation to meals, with food, or with antacids. On the other hand, some of these drugs cannot be taken with antacids because drug interactions will occur.

Likewise, certain other drugs commonly taken for GI problems can negatively *interact with* certain antihypertensives (*eg*, cimetidine with nonselective, combined beta-1 and beta-2 adrenergic blockers or with calcium-channel blockers). Thus, it should be evident that nursing interventions depend upon the nurse securing information about the specific antihypertensive being used.

To adapt to the drowsiness and fatigue characteristic of some agents, clients should be advised that these effects may make driving dangerous. Alcohol or any other depressants can increase these side effects.

Client education. Public education and case finding are vitally important to identify those adults with undiagnosed hypertension. Many lay people are unaware of the importance of early and continuing treatment of this condition. Information campaigns through the media are beginning to convey this message to the public. Screening clinics held at fairs, shopping malls, hospitals, and many other community sites are proliferating. Nurses play an active role in informing people of the risks of hypertension and in identifying persons with the disease.

Regular medical supervision is as important for clients under long-term therapy for hypertension as it is for clients with other chronic conditions. The number of visits to health care providers can be reduced, however, if clients learn to monitor their own progress. Most clients or a family member can be taught to use a sphygmomanometer to measure blood pressure. They will need assistance in choosing a reliable instrument and in developing skill in the procedure. Readings should be taken regularly, at the same time of day and under similar conditions. Morning pressures are apt to be lower than those taken in the afternoon.

Activity, emotional stress, eating, and sleep all affect readings. The client should select a time when monitoring is convenient and take daily readings for comparison. For example, pressures taken each morning before breakfast but after bathing and dressing would provide a good baseline. A log should be kept of the results and be taken to each follow-up visit with the health care provider. The log can provide data that will help a provider assess the effects of the drug regimen and adjust a treatment regimen if necessary.

The nurse should prepare and implement a teaching program to inform the client about their specific antihypertensive drug regimen. Printed materials should accompany verbal instruction. Clients should be advised that medication should not be stopped abruptly due to the potential for adverse reactions to this action (*eg*, rebound hypertension).

The client needs to be told to continue taking the medication, even if feeling better. The client needs to be advised that some adverse reactions that are experienced early in therapy will subside with continued therapy. If the client forgets to take the antihypertensive, the client should not take the forgotten dose and should not try to catch up by taking two doses next time. The client should generally be advised to limit coffee, tea, and cola drinks because caffeine has been shown to raise blood pressure and increase abnormal heart rhythm.

Clients will need assistance in carrying out recommendations for health measures designed to enhance the medical treatment of hypertension. Counseling and instruction are required in the areas of diet, exercise, emotional hygiene (*eg*, techniques for minimizing stressors and managing stress), discontinuation of smoking, and moderation or elimination of alcohol consumption.

Example of nursing process and hydralazine therapy

The client is a 76-year-old man with a history of non-insulin-dependent diabetes mellitus, mild hypertension, and one episode of congestive heart failure. His diabetes is controlled by diet (1,800 calories/d). Antihypertensive medication has been limited to hydrochlorothiazide 50 mg/d. Until recently, his blood pressure has ranged between 130–160/70–86. However, for the last 2 months, it has risen to 170–180/90–100.

The physician is adding hydralazine to the drug regimen. The initial dosage of 10 mg qid will be increased gradually, until optimal response is obtained.

Assessment data	Nursing diagnosis	Intervention	Goals and outcome criteria
New drug added (hydralazine) to regimen for control of hypertension	Knowledge deficit related to new drug regimen	**Assist** the client in developing a system for drug administration that will ensure that drugs will be taken as prescribed. Advise the client to take doses of hydralazine at fixed times in relation to meals (either always before meals or always after meals).	The client's blood pressure will decline gradually and consistently in response to the proper implementation of new drug regimen.
Therapy involving a smooth muscle relaxant (smooth muscle relaxants decrease peristalsis)	Potential for constipation related to decreased peristalsis due to decreased tone of intestinal smooth muscles caused by antihypertensive medication	**Recommend** self-care measures to prevent constipation: increased intake of fiber and fluids; use of laxative foods such as prune juice, pears, bran, and coffee; establishment of a routine of defecation and active exercise. Recommend the use of a bulk laxative such as psyllium hydrophilic mucilloid.	The client will report that defecation is not difficult or uncomfortable; stools will be of a soft consistency.
Hydralazine therapy	High risk for injury, falls related to postural hypotension secondary to hydralazine	**Inform** client of potential for injury. **Teach** measures to prevent: change to sitting and standing positions slowly. Allow time to adjust to change of position before walking.	The client will report that he has not fallen.

Evaluation The client should be monitored carefully for both therapeutic and adverse reactions to the antihypertensive agents. Because doses are tailored to individual needs and minimally effective dosages are desirable, evaluation of response is critical for proper adjustment of dosage by the health care provider. Data required for evaluation include serial measures of weight and vital signs, and absence or incidence of signs and symptoms of vascular complications such as stroke, coronary heart disease, and chronic renal failure. Additional data from the client include reports about use of tobacco and alcohol, food consumption in relation to the recommended diet, serial measure-ments of blood pressure taken at home, subjective assessment of stress levels, and incidence or absence of adverse reactions. (See accompanying Example of Nursing Process and Hydralazine Therapy.)

Checklist of nursing actions

☐ Play an active part in identifying persons with hypertension. Assist clients in improving self-care practices designed to enhance the medical regimen (*eg*, stress reduction, increased exercise, diet modification).

☐ Assess clients for risk factors for adverse reactions to prescribed drugs.

☐ Assist clients in following their prescribed regimens. Help integrate treatment into the clients' lifestyles.

☐ Monitor at regular intervals the status of clients on therapy for hypertension (*eg*, vital signs, weight, specified laboratory tests) for therapeutic reactions to therapy.

☐ Monitor at regular intervals for known adverse reactions to the drugs and for changes in health status that may indicate previously unrecognized, individualized adverse reactions to the drugs.

☐ Reassure clients that some adverse reactions are transient and are likely to subside with continued therapy.

☐ Teach appropriate coping strategies for use with adverse reactions experienced in response to drugs (*eg*, orthostatic hypotension).

☐ Advise clients of signs and symptoms that should be reported promptly to the health care provider that may require adjustment of the therapeutic regimen.

Nursing management of hypertensive crisis

Pathophysiology of hypertensive crises

Acute hypertensive crises are infrequent but life-threatening when they occur. The blood pressure rises rapidly to very high levels. There is a risk of cerebrovascular hemorrhage or convulsions. Vigorous treatment to lower the blood pressure rapidly is essential.

The etiology of hypertensive crisis is variable. It may be a complication of pregnancy, hormone toxicity, or antidepressant drug therapy. Treatment is influenced by the nature of the underlying condition. Thus, magnesium sulfate is the drug of choice to reduce cerebral edema in preeclampsia or eclampsia of pregnancy. Episodes due to excessive catecholamine secretion in pheochromocytoma respond well to an alpha-adrenergic blocking agent. Intravenous administration of vasodilators is frequently an important part of treatment for this medical emergency.

Certain agents, including nitroprusside, diazoxide, trimethaphan, labetalol, and hydralazine have been used intravenously in hypertensive crisis.

Nursing implications

Intravenous antihypertensives act very quickly. Constant and close supervision is required to prevent dangerous complications. Although rapid reduction of blood pressure is desired, abrupt or excessive drops can compromise circulation to vital organs. Use of these drugs can be dangerous.

Treatment of hypertensive crisis is best carried out in special care units where the client can be closely monitored, and emergency measures can be instituted quickly and easily should the need arise. Cardiac monitoring is recommended. Drugs administered by infusion should be controlled by an IV infusion controller. Drastic changes in blood pressure can occur within 2–5 minutes. Vital signs must be watched closely.

Nursing process

Assessment The client treated for hypertensive crisis is acutely ill and likely to be anxious and fearful. Evaluation should include assessment of emotional reaction to the life-threatening situation, vital signs, and signs and symptoms of complications, such as hemorrhage, stroke, or MI.

Nursing diagnosis Diagnoses for these clients include the following:

Anxiety related to perception of threat to life

Administration of antihypertensive drugs may cause the following:

Altered tissue perfusion related to hypotension secondary to vasodilation
High risk for fluid volume excess related to IV administration of medication

A common collaborative problem that should be differentiated from the nursing diagnoses is

Potential complication: stroke

Planning Goals of treatment include reduction of anxiety and fear; reduction of the risk of stroke, MI, or hemorrhage; reduction of blood pressure to more normal levels; and prevention of, or prompt detection and correction of, hypotension or excess fluid volume.

Intervention To protect the anxious or fearful client, the nurse should establish a therapeutic relationship as soon as possible, characterized by the nurse's warm concern for the client's welfare and the client's trust in the nurse. Once the client's trust is won, the nurse will be effective when offering reassurance. Clients should not be told "everything will be all right." Instead, the nurse should remind clients that the health care staff is skilled, and that they will use every means possible to improve the medical condition and resolve the crisis.

The administration of IV infusions is a nursing responsibility. The nurse should maintain infusions at the proper rate (using an automatic control device such as an infusion pump). The nurse should also monitor the client for complications, such as abrupt drops in blood pressure or infiltration, and protect sensitive drugs from conditions conducive to deterioration. The client should be observed closely for response to treatment. Blood pressure should decline steadily but gradually. The client should rest in bed until the blood pressure has stabilized at a safe level. A strict accounting of fluid intake and output is required. Fluid intake should err on the low side rather than excess because hypervolemia further increases blood pressure. Clients should be monitored closely for peripheral edema or respiratory difficulty signifying pulmonary edema.

Client education. The client treated for hypertensive crisis is acutely ill. Teaching is confined to explanations of the treatment regimen designed to allay apprehension and to secure the cooperation of the client. Health teaching should be deferred until the acute phase of illness has been resolved.

Evaluation Data required for evaluation include serial measurements of vital signs, especially blood pressure, incidence or absence of stroke, MI, hemorrhage, peripheral edema, or pulmonary impairment, and reports from clients concerning their physical and emotional comfort.

Checklist of nursing actions

When IV antihypertensives are administered for hypertensive crisis

☐ Establish a nurse/client relationship characterized by concern (nurse) and trust (client).
☐ Offer the client reassurance and emotional support.
☐ Use an infusion control device to maintain a steady infusion rate.
☐ Monitor the client closely for response to treatment; take frequent vital signs, especially blood pressure.
☐ Monitor the client closely for adverse drug reactions, including abrupt drops in blood pressure, infiltration, respiratory impairment, and hypervolemia.
☐ Promote rest in bed for the client.
☐ Maintain a strict accounting of fluid intake and output; maintain a minimal intake to avoid hypervolemia.

Vasoconstrictors

Vasoconstrictor drugs include vasopressin and a number of sympathomimetic agents (Table 28-9). They are discussed in detail in Chapter 37 and Chapter 22, respectively.

Therapeutic uses

Vasoconstrictor (vasopressor) drugs are effective in reversing shock due to inappropriate dilation of the peripheral blood vessels. They are the treatment of choice in anaphylactic and neurogenic shock. They are sometimes used in the treatment of orthostatic hypotension and when the drop in blood pressure is induced by spinal anesthesia.

Vasoconstrictors are no longer used for the treatment of other types of shock as frequently as in the past. Although their administration does raise blood pressure, it may not improve blood flow. In cardiogenic and hypovolemic shock, significant reflex vasoconstriction is usually present. Intensification of this response by drugs may seriously compromise circulation. Only when these types of shock are associated with a failure of the normal compensatory vasoconstriction are vasopressor agents helpful.

Vasopressors are customarily mixed with local anesthetics to produce constriction of nearby blood vessels. This slows systemic absorption and prolongs the local effect of the anesthetic, allowing adequate anesthesia with minimal doses.

Vasopressors are also active ingredients in nose drops and eye drops, designed to reduce local congestion. A rebound hyperemia often occurs when the effect of a dose wears off. If the drug is repeated, physical dependency may develop. Psychological dependency does not usually develop. Excessive use of such topical agents may cause systemic toxicity due to repeated absorption of the drug.

Drugs used to treat varicose veins
Pathophysiology of varicose veins

Normal blood flow through the veins of the lower extremities and abdomen is often impaired by varicose veins. Tortuous, distended veins with incompetent valves develop most often in persons subject to increased hydrostatic pressure in the veins or obstruction of venous flow. Familial predisposition (apparently due to relatively weak vein structures) increases the risk. Factors associated with early onset of varicosities include obesity, pregnancy, abdominal tumors, long periods of sitting or standing in one place, and constricting clothing. When venous pressure rises for prolonged periods of time, the veins become overdistended. This weakens the wall and prevents the valves from closing completely, further reducing venous return and increasing congestion. Venous distention tends to progress with eventual destruction of the valves and development of enlarged, tortuous vessels. Increased venous pressure is reflected by increased capillary pressure, and peripheral perfusion is reduced. Painful, weak muscles and edema ensue. Stasis ulcers or gangrene can develop.

Conservative treatment of varicose veins includes frequent elevation of the legs to promote drainage and the use of elastic hose to reduce distension. When these measures prove inadequate, venous pooling can be reduced by the elimination of some of the incompe-

Table 28-9. Selected vasoconstrictors

Drug name	Route(s) of administration	Usual dosage	Common therapeutic uses	Mechanism of action
ephedrine (Efedron, Vick's Vatronol)	Oral Topical	Adults: 25–100 mg, daily, divided in 1–4 doses Children: 3 mg/kg body weight/d, divided in 4–6 doses	Allergy (hay fever/asthma)	Sympathomimetic (stimulates α- and β-adrenergic receptors)
	SC/IM/IV	*SC or IM*: Adults: 25–50 mg for 1–2 doses *IV*: Adults: 10–25 mg q 5–10 min to a maximum of 150 mg/d; children: 3 mg/kg body weight/day divided in 4–6 doses	Orthostatic hypotension Hypotension induced by spinal anesthetic	
	Topical	Solution strength of 0.5%–3%	Nasal congestion	
epinephrine (Adrenalin, Epi-Pen)	SC IV	Adults: 0.1–0.5 mg Children: 0.01 mg/kg body weight Adults: 0.1–0.25 mg, well diluted and slowly administered	Anaphylaxis	Sympathomimetic (stimulates α- and β-adrenergic receptors)
norepinephrine (levarterenol/ Levophed)	IV infusion	Adults: *Initially*: 8–12 μg/min Children: *Initially*: 2 μg/min Subsequent dosage is adjusted in accordance with blood pressure.	Hypotension induced by drug overdose, shock, or anesthesia	Sympathomimetic (stimulates α- and β-adrenergic receptors)
metaraminol (Aramine, Pressonex)	SC/IM/IV infusion	*SC or IM*: Adults: 2–10 mg, at intervals of at least 10 min; children: 100 μg/kg body weight, at intervals of at least 10 min *IV*: Adjusted in accordance with blood pressure	Hypotension associated with vasodilation	Sympathomimetic (stimulates α- and β-adrenergic receptors)
dopamine (Intropin, Revimine)	IV infusion	*Initially*: 1–5 μg/kg body weight/min Subsequent dosage is adjusted in accordance with blood pressure.		Sympathomimetic (stimulates dopaminergic and α- and β-adrenergic receptors)
vasopressin (Pitressin, Pressyn)	IV	Adults: 20 units over 5–30 min	(Rarely used as a pressor agent to raise blood pressure) Control of bleeding from esophageal varices Reduction of portal hypertension during abdominal surgery	Direct stimulation of smooth muscle Antidiuretic effects

tent, overdistended vessels. Surgical removal of the varicosities is often preferred. When this is contraindicated or less than optimal, veins can be obliterated by the injection of irritating sclerosing drugs, which induce fibrosis of the vessels (Box 28-4).

Sclerosing agents

Drugs used presently as sclerosing agents include sodium morrhuate (Scleromate) and sodium tetradecyl (Sotradecol).

Pharmacodynamics. Sclerosing agents irritate the vein, producing inflammation and stimulating fibrous scarring that obliterates the vessel.

Pharmacokinetics. Sclerosing agents are injected directly into the affected veins. They are not absorbed systemically but act locally at the injection site.

Therapeutic uses. Morrhuate and sodium tetradecyl are used to treat superficial varicosities of the lower extremities.

Box 28-4. Varicose veins

Factors associated with early onset

- Obesity
- Pregnancy
- Abdominal tumors
- Long periods of sitting or standing in one place
- Constricting clothing on lower extremities
- Genetic predisposition

Treatment of varicose veins

- Frequent elevation of the legs to promote drainage
- Use of elastic hose to reduce distention
- Surgical removal of varicosities
- Injection of irritating sclerosing drugs

These substances are administered by the physician, usually in an outpatient or office procedure. Sclerosing agents also can be used to treat other conditions benefited by the production of fibrous tissue, such as the closure of hernial rings and the removal of condylomata acuminata.

Adverse reactions

With sodium morrhuate, burning or cramping sensations indicate local reactions and urticaria may result. With sodium tetradecyl, a permanent discoloration of skin along the path of the sclerosed vein segment may result. Tissue sloughing results if the drug is allowed to extravasate. Hypersensitivity reactions and anaphylaxis occasionally occur. Injection therapy is contraindicated for clients with acute thrombophlebitis or for those in whom there is significant valvular or deep venous incompetence. Only a limited number of vessels can be treated at one time, and the total number so obliterated must be controlled to prevent permanent venous insufficiency.

Nursing management

Nursing implications

Excessive obliteration of venous vessels can compromise circulation and, in extreme cases, require amputation of a lower limb. The physician will consider past history in determining the number of injections the client can tolerate.

Nursing process

Assessment   Initial assessment of the client seeking sclerotherapy should include a complete history of venous disease, including episodes of phlebitis, vein

surgery, and previous sclerotherapy. The client should be examined to determine the extent of superficial vein involvement. A phlebogram is usually performed to evaluate venous circulation. The client should be questioned to determine the potential for allergic reaction to the sclerosing drugs. A client with multiple allergies or a family history of allergy, particularly of reactions to sclerosing agents, is at increased risk for allergic reaction during treatment, especially if the client has been treated with these drugs in the past.

Nursing diagnosis   A nursing diagnosis arising from sclerotherapy is:

> *Pain related to phlebitis secondary to sclerotherapy*

A common collaborative problem that should be differentiated from the nursing diagnosis is

> *Potential complication: anaphylaxis*

Planning   Goals of treatment are to alleviate or eliminate pain and to prevent or promptly detect and treat allergic reaction to the prescribed drugs.

Intervention   The nurse supports and assists the client as necessary during the treatment procedure. Equipment and supplies for the treatment of anaphylaxis should be at hand before the procedure is started. The health care staff must be prepared to treat anaphylaxis should it occur. The nurse also prepares and implements a teaching plan to assist the client in managing self-care at home following the procedure.

Client education.   The client should be instructed that severe pain or local tissue sloughing, which indicate adverse reactions to the drugs, must be reported promptly for follow-up care. Warm compresses and a mild analgesic such as aspirin, ibuprofen, or acetaminophen may be recommended to relieve discomfort at the injection sites. Injection therapy is an adjunct to, rather than a substitute for, other methods of treating varicose veins. Delay in the progression of venous degeneration depends on such health measures as the reduction of excess weight, periodic elevation of the extremities, avoidance of long periods of standing, elimination of restricting clothing, and the use of elastic support hose. The client should avoid the use of round garters, panty girdles, or other clothing that constricts circulation in the legs. Encouragement is needed for clients to continue such practices even when injection therapy is used.

Evaluation   Data required for evaluation include the following: absence or incidence of allergic reaction to sclerosing drugs; absence or incidence of edema; decreased sensation; temperature or color change or skin breakdown in treated extremities; and the client's reports of absence or incidence of pain.

Checklist of nursing actions

☐ Assess candidates for injection therapy as to previous treatment of varicosities.

☐ Screen candidates for allergic sensitivity to sclerosing agents.

☐ Be prepared to treat sensitivity reactions, including anaphylaxis, when sclerosing agents are used.

☐ Instruct clients to report to the physician severe pain or tissue sloughing at the sites of injection.

☐ Teach clients health measures that will delay the progression of venous degeneration (reduction of excess weight, intermittent exercise, and avoidance of restrictive clothing and long periods of standing or sitting).

References

Abrams J. (1988). A reappraisal of nitrate therapy. *JAMA, 259*, 396–401.

Antonaccio M. (ed.) (1990). *Cardiovascular pharmacology*, 3rd ed. New York: Raven Press.

Buhler FR, Kiowski W. (1988). Calcium antagonists and their potential for antihypertensive therapy. *Ann N Y Acad Sci, 522*, 594.

Craig CR, Stitzel RE. (1990). *Modern pharmacology*, 3rd ed. Boston: Little, Brown and Co.

Dujovne CA, Harris WS. (1989). The pharmacological treatment of dyslipidemia. *Annu Rev Pharmacol Toxicol, 291*, 265–288.

Gilman AG, Rall TW, Nies AS, Taylor P. (eds.) (1990). Goodman and Gilman's *The pharmacological basis of therapeutics*, 8th ed. New York: Pergamon Press.

Kane JP, Malloy MJ. (1990). Treatment of hyperlipidemia. *Annu Rev Med, 41*, 471–482.

Marin J. (1988). Vascular effects of calcium antagonists. Uses in some cerebrovascular disorders. *Gen Pharmacol, 19(3)*, 301–303.

Porth CM. (1990). *Pathophysiology: Concepts of altered health states*, 3rd ed. Philadelphia: J.B. Lippincott Co.

Wollam GL, Hall WD. (1988). *Hypertension management: Clinical practice and therapeutic dilemmas.* Chicago: Year Book Medical Publishers, Inc.

Bibliography

Brown L, Langer R. (1988). Transdermal delivery of drugs. *Annu Rev Med, 39*, 221–229.

Chan L, Schrier RW. (1990). Effects of calcium channel blockers on renal function. *Annu Rev Med, 41*, 289–302.

Cherner R. (1987). Antihypertensive agents and diabetes: Side effects that demand careful consideration. *Consultant, 27(2)*, 22.

Delabays A, et al. (1989). Hemodynamic and humoral effects of the new renin inhibitor enalkiren in normal humans. *Hypertension, 13*, 941.

Detection, evaluation, and treatment of high blood pressure, NIH Publication No. 88–1088. (1988). U.S. Department of Health and Human Services: Public Health Service National Institutes of Health.

Gleeson B. (1991). Loosening the grip of anginal pain. *Nursing 91, 21*, 33–39.

Gleeson B. (1991). Teaching your patient about his antianginal drugs. *Nursing 91, 21*, 65–72.

Gotto AM. (1988). Lipoprotein metabolism and etiology of hyperlipidemia. *Hosp Pract, 23(Suppl 1)*, 4.

Illingworth DR, Bacon S. (1989). Treatment of heterozygous familial hypercholesterolemia with lipid lowering drugs. *Atherosclerosis, 9(Suppl)*, 1-121–1-134.

Manninen V, et al. (1988). Lipid alteration and decline in the incidence of coronary heart disease in the Helsinki Heart Study. *JAMA, 260*, 641–651.

Mulinari R, et al. (1989). Bradykinin antagonism and prostaglandins in blood pressure regulation. *Hypertension, 13*, 960.

Report of the expert panel on detection, evaluation and treatment of high blood cholesterol in adults, NIH Publication No. 88–2925. (1988). U.S. Department of Health and Human Services: Public Health Service National Institutes of Health.

Report of the national cholesterol education program's expert panel on detection, evaluation, and treatment of high blood cholesterol in adults. (1988). *Arch Intern Med, 148*, 36–69.

Rodman MJ. (1991). Hypertension: Step-care management. *RN, 54*, 24–31.

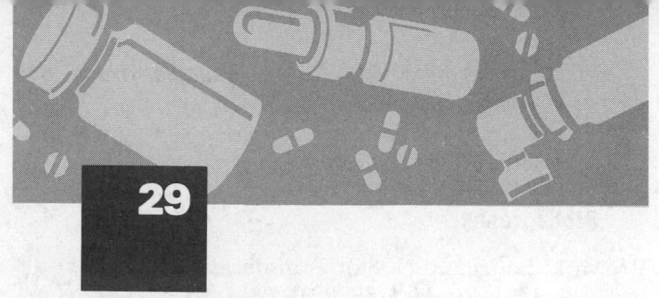

29

Drugs affecting coagulation

Blood is a delicately balanced chemical mixture that remains fluid while circulating in an undamaged vascular system, becomes solid to seal off leaks in the system, and dissolves old clots to reopen healed vessels. The blood's ability to coagulate is influenced by heredity, nutrition, hormone levels, and the function of such body organs and systems as the bone marrow, liver, and kidneys. The complex mechanism of coagulation is not completely understood at present. Enough is known, however, to correct some coagulation deficiencies and to manipulate coagulation to arrest or ameliorate certain disease conditions.

Physiology of coagulation

Blood coagulation involves an enzymatic chain reaction that culminates in the formation of fibrin, the structural matrix of a clot. Coagulation is initiated when damaged platelets release a chemical that activates thromboplastin. Thromboplastin catalyzes the conversion of prothrombin to thrombin, which then mediates the formation of fibrin out of fibrinogen. At least 12 clotting factors have been identified. Once formed, blood clots are dissolved by another series of chemical interactions. To date, only a few natural anticoagulants have been identified (see Boxes 29-1 and 29-2).

Clotting may be triggered by tissue damage or by exposure of blood to subendothelial collagen (Fig. 29-1). Clots differ in their characteristics depending on the rate of blood flow at the site of formation. In the arteries, where blood flow is rapid, clots characteristically have a large platelet head and a small fibrin tail. In the venous system, where blood flow is slower, clots form with a large fibrin head and a small platelet tail. These differences, depending on the specific action of the drug involved, will influence a client's response to therapeutic agents administered to alter the blood's coagulability.

Pathology

Diseases characterized by inappropriate coagulation are of two general types: deficient coagulation, resulting in excessive bleeding, and inappropriate coagulation, which obstructs blood flow within the vasculature. These disorders are serious, life-threatening conditions. Drug agents used to treat clients with coagulation problems include substances to restore coagulation, anticoagulants, and agents to dissolve clots.

Clotting disorders

Clotting disorders characterized by excessive or prolonged bleeding are often associated with deficiencies of one or more clotting factors. For example, significant decreases in blood levels of calcium or prolonged

vitamin K deprivation can delay clotting. An inherited inability to maintain levels of clotting factors IX and XIII underlies two congenital "bleeding" diseases: the hemophilias. Other clients lose the ability to produce certain clotting factors owing to liver, bone marrow, or other diseases. Whenever possible, the underlying problem is eliminated but often replacement of the deficient clotting factors is necessary. Of increasing importance are iatrogenic conditions that cause defects in clotting; they result from massive blood transfusions, drug therapy, or radiation (see Table 29-1 for hemostatic agents).

Hemostatics

Systemic hemostatics

Blood and blood products

Fresh, whole, uncitrated blood contains all the factors necessary to sustain clotting. Direct transfusions, therefore, are effective in correcting most episodes of abnormal bleeding. However, because this procedure is difficult, inconvenient, and poses serious health risks, it is generally reserved for emergencies. Banked citrated blood will correct most emergencies, provided only one or two units are needed. Administration of massive amounts of citrated blood produces an iatrogenic clotting problem caused by lowered blood levels of ionic calcium. Normally, the quantity of a transfusion is limited to that required to replace a portion of the blood loss.

Fractional components of blood are also useful in treating deficiencies in clotting factors. Blood plasma

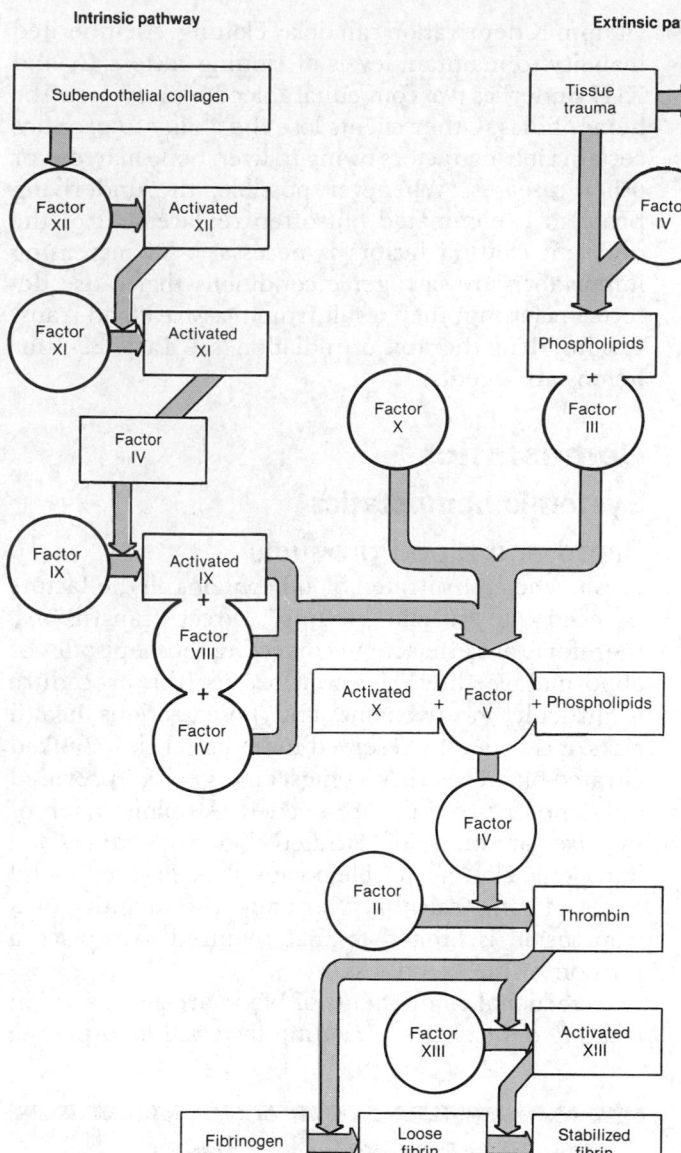

Intrinsic pathway

Extrinsic pathway

Figure 29-1. The mechanism of coagulation.

contains most of the clotting factors but cannot be administered in large amounts due to the danger of fluid overload. The fractional parts of plasma, which contain high concentrations of specific clotting factors, are of greater value in the treatment of bleeding problems. Two such products are presently available, antihemophilic factor (coagulation factor VIII) and human factor IX complex (coagulation factors II, VII, IX, and X).

Whole blood

See Chapter 51 for a detailed discussion of blood therapy.

Pharmacodynamics. Fresh whole blood provides all the factors necessary for clotting; citrated blood supplies all factors except for calcium.

Pharmacokinetics. Whole blood is administered intravenously and is absorbed immediately into the general circulation. It is metabolized by the body in essentially the same way as endogenous blood.

Therapeutic uses. Whole blood is effective in hemorrhage associated with deficiencies of clotting factors whether they are iatrogenic or result from disease.

Adverse reactions. Whole blood can cause serious antigen-antibody reactions and can cause infection by introducing pathogens harbored by the donor. A particular risk is the transmission of hepatitis B or of acquired immunodeficiency syndrome (AIDS). In addition, administering the volumes of blood necessary to arrest hemorrhage may cause hypervolemia and circulatory overload.

Precautions and contraindications. Blood used for transfusion is tested for the presence of infectious organisms or for antibodies indicative of probable infec-

Table 29-1. Drugs used to control hemorrhage

Drug name	Preparations	Usual dosage	Additional information
Systemic agents			
Blood and blood products			
whole blood	Citrated or fresh blood in sterile containers for IV administration	1–2 pints	Direct transfusion of uncitrated blood provides all clotting factors.
			Only 1–2 units of citrated blood can be used before calcium binding will cause further clotting impairment.
plasma	Fluid fraction of blood in sterile containers for IV administration	1 or more pints	Doses required for correction of bleeding problems pose high risk of fluid overload.
antihemophilic factor: factor VIII (Factorate, Hemofil, Koāte, Profilate)	Powder for preparing solution for IV administration	8–25 U/kg body weight q8h–q24h PC: C	Dosage must be calculated in relation to the degree of deficiency of factor VIII as shown by coagulation studies, the clinical situation, and the level of coagulants desired.
factor IX complex (Alpha Nine, Konyne, Profilnine, Proplex T)	Powder for preparing solutions for IV administration	*Initially:* 75 U/kg body weight PC: C	Dosage must be calculated in relation to the degree of deficiency of clotting factors as shown by coagulation studies, the clinical situation, and the level the coagulants desired.
Vitamin K preparations			
menadione (Hykinone, vitamin K3)	Oral tablets	Adults: 2–10 mg/day Children: 50–100 µg/day PC: C except near term when it is X	Menadione is contraindicated for neonates and women during the last weeks of pregnancy; it is ineffective in the treatment of oral anticoagulant-induced hypoprothrombinemia.
menadiol sodium diphosphate (Kappadione, Synkavite, Synkayvite, vitamin K4)	Oral tablets and solutions for parenteral injection	Adults: 5–15 mg qd–bid Children: 5–10 mg, qd–bid PC: C except near term, when it is X	Menadiol sodium diphosphate is contraindicated for neonates and women during the last weeks of pregnancy; it is ineffective in the treatment of oral anticoagulant-induced hypoprothrombinemia.
phytonadione (Aqua-MEPHYTON, Konakion, Mephyton)	Oral tablets Solution for IM administration Solution for IV, IM, and SC administration	Adults: 2.5–10 mg, q12h–q48h PRN Infants: 0.5–1 mg, q6h–q8h PRN PC: C	Phytonadione reverses the inhibitory effect of coumarin and indanedione derivative anticoagulants.
Heparin antagonist			
protamine sulfate	Powder for preparing solutions for IV administration	0.25–1.75 mg/100 U of heparin administered, depending on the time elapsed since the heparin dose PC: C	One milligram of protamine sulfate will neutralize 90–115 units of heparin, depending on the specific preparation of heparin involved.
Enzyme inhibitor			
aminocaproic acid (Amicar)	Tablets and solution for oral use Solution for IV administration	Adults: *Oral or IV:* Initially 4–5 g over the first hour; thereafter: 1–1.25 g/hr (maximum daily dosage: 30 g) Children: *IV:* Initially: 100 mg/kg body weight or 3 g/m² body surface over the first	Aminocaproic acid inhibits action of proteolytic enzymes including SK and UK

(Continued)

Table 29-1. Drugs used to control hemorrhage (Continued)

Drug name	Preparations	Usual dosage	Additional information
Systemic agents			
		hour; thereafter: 33.3 mg/kg body weight/hr or 1 g/m^2 body surface/hr (maximum daily dosage: 18 g/m^2 body surface) PC: C	
tranexamic acid (Cyclokapron)	Capsules for oral use Powder for preparing parenteral solutions	Adults: *Oral:* Initially: 25 mg/kg body weight tid or qid for 24 hrs prior to tooth extraction and for 2–8 days after *IV* 10 mg/kg body weight PC: B	Tranexamic acid should not be mixed with blood or penicillin solutions. If visual changes develop, tranexamic acid should be discontinued.
Local and topical agents			
epinephrine (Adrenalin, Epifrin)	Solution for injection or topical application	Solution strength of 1:20,000–1:100,000 PC: C	Large doses are readily absorbed and cause systemic toxicity.
oxidized cellulose	Treated gauze for topical application	Quantity depends on area of tissue involved in bleeding	Used internally, the material is eventually absorbed.
absorbable gelatin	Powder, sponge, or film for topical application	Quantity depends on area of tissue involved in bleeding	Material is eventually absorbed. Allergic hypersensitivity may occur.
thrombin (Thrombostat, Thrombinar, Thrombogen)	Powder, solution, or spray for topical application	Solution strength of 1000–2000 U/ml	Solutions must never be administered by IV since they cause fatal clotting.
thromboplastin	Powder for topical application	Quantity depends on area of tissue involved in bleeding	Produced from human blood, this product is available in limited quantities.
human fibrin foam	Powder for topical application	Quantity depends on area of tissue involved in bleeding	

KEY: PC = pregnancy risk category. (The validity of pregnancy categories has not been established. See chapter 16, p 216).

tion in the donor. Immediately before administration, the blood must be typed and crossmatched to ensure compatibility with the blood. Special precautions are taken to prevent errors that could result in administration to the wrong client. (See Chapter 51 for a detailed discussion of blood transfusion.) Blood is administered through tubing in which filters prevent the movement of solid particles such as clots into the bloodstream.

Plasma

Blood plasma is the liquid remaining after removal of the cellular components of the blood.

Pharmacodynamics. Plasma provides most of the clotting factors needed to sustain coagulation. It tends to correct deficiencies of all coagulation factors except for platelets.

Pharmacokinetics. Plasma is administered intravenously. It is incorporated into the blood, and its components are metabolized like those of endogenous plasma.

Therapeutic uses. Plasma is not used extensively to treat hemorrhage. One or more units may be ad-

ministered in the treatment of hemorrhagic conditions in which blood volume is depleted and whole blood is either contraindicated or unavailable.

Plasma is processed to produce blood fractions containing clotting factors (see sections on antihemophilic factor and factor IX complex in this chapter).

Adverse reactions. Plasma can transmit blood-borne disease such as hepatitis B and AIDS. In the amount required to arrest hemorrhage, it tends to cause hypervolemia and circulatory overload.

Precautions and contraindications. Blood used for the preparation of plasma is tested to detect the presence of infectious organisms. Most pathogens can be screened out but the tests for hepatitis B and AIDS are not completely effective.

Antihemophilic factor

Antihemophilic factor is a product of plasma derived from whole blood.

Pharmacodynamics. Antihemophilic factor provides coagulation factor VIII, which is deficient in persons with hemophilia A (classic hemophilia).

Pharmacokinetics. After reconstitution with sterile water, antihemophilic factor is administered intravenously (IV). It moves rapidly into the extravascular compartment in both normal and hemophilic subjects.

Therapeutic uses. Antihemophilic factor is used to arrest bleeding in clients with hemophilia A or acquired factor VIII inhibitors when replacement of blood volume or red blood cells (RBCs) is not required.

Adverse reactions. Rapid administration of antihemophilic factor tends to cause headache, flushing, tachycardia, paresthesia, nausea, vomiting, back pain, hypotension, decreases in the level of consciousness, changes in vision, chest tightness, and rigor. Mild allergic reactions and jaundice may occur. Like other blood products, this preparation can convey the causative organisms of hepatitis B and AIDS. When large doses are administered, trace amounts of blood groups A and B isohemagglutinin may reach levels high enough to cause intravascular hemolysis. Safe use during pregnancy has not been established.

Precautions and contraindications. During processing, blood factors are heat-treated in an attempt to attenuate any viruses.

Antihemophilic factor VIII should be administered slowly. It should be filtered before injection or infusion. Pulse rate should be monitored during treatment, and the infusion should be slowed if there is a substantial increase in pulse.

Clients who may receive antihemophilic factor repeatedly should be actively immunized against hepatitis B. Clients who have received this or other human blood products should be advised to report to the physician any signs or symptoms of AIDS, should they develop.

Factor IX complex

Factor IX complex is a fractional part of plasma produced from donated whole human blood.

Pharmacodynamics. Factor IX complex provides coagulation factors II, VII, IX, and X, temporarily correcting deficiencies of these factors.

Pharmacokinetics. Factor IX complex is administered IV. It appears to be distributed to both intravascular and extravascular compartments. Reported half-lives range from 12 to 40 hours depending on the commercial product.

Therapeutic uses. This blood fraction is used to treat hemorrhage caused by hemophilia B (Christmas disease) when the level of factor IX required cannot be achieved with plasma infusions without the danger of hypervolemia and proteinemia. It may be used to treat hemorrhagic disease in newborns (who do not produce vitamin K due to a lack of microscopic flora in the gastrointestinal tract.) It is also used to treat hemorrhage caused by coumarin anticoagulants when prompt reversal is required.

Adverse reactions. Rapid injection of factor IX complex can cause tingling sensations, fever, chills, headache, flushing, and changes in pulse rate and blood pressure. Because this drug is derived from human plasma, there is a small (but real) chance that it may contain the hepatitis B virus or the causative factor of AIDS. Persons with blood groups A, B, or AB who receive large doses may experience intravascular hemolysis, owing to the presence of blood groups A and B isohemagglutinins. Postoperative thrombosis in clients treated with factor IX complex has been reported.

Safe use during pregnancy has not been established.

Precautions and contraindications. Factor IX complex should be administered slowly; vital signs should be monitored throughout therapy. When treated with factor IX complex, clients who have had surgery must be closely observed for signs and symptoms of thrombosis. Should these develop, the drug should be discontinued.

To prevent the development of disseminated intravascular coagulation (DIC), the blood level of factor IX should usually not be raised above 50% of normal. When large doses of the drug are required, prophylactic anticoagulation should be considered. Persons who may receive factor IX complex repeatedly should be actively immunized against hepatitis B. Clients who have received blood or blood products such as this preparation should be monitored for signs and symptoms of AIDS.

Factor IX complex is contraindicated for persons in whom DIC or fibrinolysis is suspected, including those with liver disease.

Vitamin K preparations

Vitamin K is a nutrient necessary for the production of prothrombin. Although its mechanism of action is unknown, vitamin K is believed to be involved in activating an enzyme required for the synthesis of this clotting factor by the liver. Deficiencies of vitamin K are rare in healthy persons because it is found in many foods, and additional amounts are manufactured by microorganisms in the intestinal tract. Deficiencies of clinical significance can arise in infants who have not yet acquired microscopic flora in the gastrointestinal (GI) tract when GI absorption is inadequate due to prolonged inflammation (colitis, sprue) in obstructive biliary tract disease, or when intestinal flora are reduced by antibiotic medication.

Vitamin K is widespread in nature. It was first isolated from hog liver and alfalfa. Green leafy vegetables and vegetable oils are good dietary sources. The natural substance exists in two forms: K_1 and K_2 (Fig. 29-2). Three medicinal preparations—menadione,

Chemical Structure Common to All K Vitamins

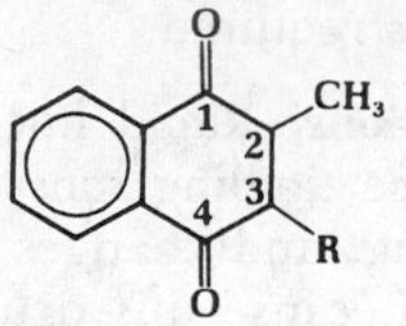

Structural Variations in Specific Forms of Vitamin K

Vitamin Form	Structure of R
K_1	$CH_2—CH=C—CH_2—CH_2—CH_2—CH—CH_3$ (with CH_3 groups)
K_2	$CH_2—CH=C—CH_2—CH_2—CH=C—CH_3$ (with CH_3 groups)
K_3	H

Figure 29-2. Chemical structure of the K vitamins.

menadiol sodium diphosphate, and phytonadione—are currently available.

Menadione and menadiol sodium diphosphate

Menadione is a fat-soluble, synthetic analogue of vitamin K; menadiol sodium diphosphate is a water-soluble preparation that is similar in activity.

Pharmacodynamics. Menadione and menadiol act similarly to naturally occurring vitamin K in the production by the liver of blood coagulation factors II (prothrombin), VII (proconvertin), IX (plasma thromboplastin component), and X (Stuart-Prower factor).

Pharmacokinetics. Menadione is administered orally and requires bile salts for absorption. Menadiol does not require bile salts for absorption and may be given either orally or by injection. Information is not available on the onset of action of oral doses. Following intramuscular or subcutaneous administration, bleeding may be controlled within 1–2 hours. Response to IV administration tends to be more prompt but of shorter duration.

Menadione crosses the placenta. Little is known about the excretion of vitamin K preparations.

Therapeutic uses. Menadione and menadiol are used in the prevention and treatment of coagulation deficits caused by limited absorption of vitamin K due to malabsorption syndromes or the use of drugs that interfere with vitamin K production or absorption by the GI tract. They are not effective in treating inadequate coagulation stemming from hereditary hypoprothrombinemia, severe liver disease, or anticoagulant therapy.

Adverse reactions. Oral doses of menadione or menadiol can cause nausea, vomiting, gastric upset, and headache. Allergic hypersensitivity may also oc-

cur. High doses may prolong the prothrombin time (PT), paradoxically impairing coagulation.

When menadione or menadiol is administered to persons with glucose-6-phosphate dehydrogenase deficiency, hemolysis can occur. Safe use during pregnancy has not been established.

When administered to neonates, menadione and menadiol can cause severe hemolytic anemia, hyperbilirubinemia, hemoglobinuria, kernicterus, brain damage, and death (Gilman, Goodman, Rall, & Murad, 1985). Risk is inversely related to maturity of the infant; premature infants are particularly vulnerable.

Precautions and contraindications. Menadione in concentrated form is irritating to the tissues. The powder can cause inflammation of the skin or respiratory tract; alcoholic solutions act as vesicants. Care should be taken by health care personnel to avoid exposure to menadione, whether in powder or solution form.

Menadione and menadiol are contraindicated for neonates, women during the last few weeks of pregnancy, and persons with hypersensitivity to the drugs.

Phytonadione

Phytonadione is a fat-soluble synthetic compound that is identical to naturally occurring vitamin K_1.

Pharmacodynamics. Phytonadione acts in the body as does naturally occurring vitamin K_1, which is required for liver synthesis of blood coagulation factors II (prothrombin), VII (proconvertin), IX (plasma thromboplastin component), and X (Stuart-Prower factor). In adequate doses, phytonadione reverses the inhibitory effect of coumarin and indanedione-derivative anticoagulants.

Pharmacokinetics. Phytonadione may be administered either orally or by injection. The drug requires the presence of bile salts in the GI tract for oral absorption. Onset of action, as shown by increased levels of coagulation factors, occurs 1–2 hours after injection and 6–12 hours following oral doses.

Only small amounts of phytonadione are stored in the tissues. The drug does cross the placenta. Little is known about the excretion of vitamin K preparations.

Therapeutic uses. Phytonadione is used in the prevention and treatment of hypoprothrombinemia caused by vitamin K deficiency secondary to malabsorption or use of drugs that inhibit vitamin production or absorption in the GI tract. It is also used to prevent and treat hemorrhagic disease in newborns, including that arising from the mother's use of anticonvulsants during pregnancy. It may be useful in the treatment of coumarin or indanedione-derivative anticoagulants overdose.

Phytonadione is not effective in the treatment of hereditary hypoprothrombinemia, hypoprothrombinemia caused by severe liver disease, or bleeding from heparin anticoagulation.

Adverse reactions. Phytonadione is relatively non-toxic. However, reactions resembling allergy or anaphylaxis can occur following injection. Signs and symptoms include abnormal contractions of skeletal and smooth muscle, chest pain, cyanosis, flushing, a sense of chest tightness, circulatory collapse, bronchospasm, dyspnea, altered level of consciousness, and cardiac or respiratory arrest. The reactions may occur in persons receiving the drug for the first time; they tend to be most severe when the drug is administered intravenously. Local inflammation at the injection site may develop. Safe use during pregnancy has not been established.

Precautions and contraindications. When phytonadione is administered parenterally, equipment and trained personnel should be available for immediate treatment of adverse reactions, including anaphylaxis.

Although adverse reactions in infants occur less frequently than with other vitamin K preparations, large doses of phytonadione in neonates should be avoided. The drug is contraindicated for persons with hypersensitivity to it.

Heparin antagonist: protamine

Protamine is a low molecular weight, cationic protein derived from the sperm or mature testes of fish.

Pharmacodynamics. When administered to normal persons, protamine acts as a weak anticoagulant. However, when administered to clients who have been treated with heparin, protamine combines chemically with the acidic heparin to form a stable compound that has no anticoagulant properties.

Pharmacokinetics. Protamine is administered IV. It acts to neutralize heparin within 30–60 seconds. The compound is subsequently degraded, thus freeing heparin.

Therapeutic uses. Protamine is used intravenously in the treatment of severe heparin overdosage. It is also used to terminate heparin anticoagulation following extracorporeal circulation or dialysis procedures.

Adverse reactions. Allergic reactions to protamine have been reported. They are most likely in persons who are allergic to fish. Rapid injection of protamine has caused anaphylactoid reactions.

Although there is a theoretic risk of protamine anticoagulation when excess protamine is administered, effects seem to be mild and transient.

Precautions and contraindications. No more than 50 mg of protamine should be administered in any 10-minute period. Dosage is calculated in relation to the dose of heparin, its route of administration, and the time elapsed since it was given.

Coagulation tests should be performed 5–15 minutes after protamine is administered. Recipients of the drug should be watched for 12 hours following administration for signs and symptoms of anticoagulation due to heparin rebound.

Protamine should be used only with extreme caution in clients with a history of fish allergy.

Enzyme inhibitors

Aminocaproic acid

Aminocaproic acid is a synthetic monoaminocarboxylic acid that inhibits fibrinolysis.

Pharmacodynamics. Aminocaproic acid inhibits the activation of proteolytic enzymes including profibrinolysin (plasminogen), fibrinolysin (plasmin), and trypsin. It also inhibits the action of streptokinase (SK) and urokinase (UK), enzymes administered medicinally to promote the resolution of intravascular clots in selected clinical situations.

Pharmacokinetics. Aminocaproic acid is administered orally and intravenously. It is rapidly and completely absorbed from the GI tract. It is distributed in both intravascular and extravascular compartments and penetrates body cells, including RBCs. It does not appear to bind to plasma proteins.

Aminocaproic acid is excreted in the urine as unchanged drug. Renal clearance is approximately 75% that of the creatinine clearance.

Therapeutic uses. Aminocaproic acid is used to treat excessive bleeding resulting from overactivity of the fibrinolytic system. It has been used following surgery, especially urinary tract procedures, and for clients with cirrhosis of the liver, carcinomas of the lung, stomach, prostate, and cervix, abruptio placentae, and aplastic anemia. It has been used investigationally as an adjunct in the treatment of hemorrhage in persons with hemophilia. The drug is considered promising as an antidote for thrombolytic agents such as SK and UK.

Adverse reactions. Reactions to aminocaproic acid are usually mild and disappear when the drug is discontinued. Signs and symptoms include nausea, cramps, diarrhea, dizziness, tinnitus, malaise, headache, nasal stuffiness, conjunctival suffusion, and skin rash. Myopathy and renal failure have been reported. Hypotension and bradycardia may occur when the drug is administered by IV.

If aminocaproic acid is administered to persons with intravascular clots, the clots may not undergo lysis as they do normally. Safe use during pregnancy has not been established.

Precautions and contraindications. Use of aminocaproic acid is limited to acute, life-threatening hemorrhage, which has been demonstrated to be caused by overactivity of the fibrinolytic system. Dosage should be reduced in persons with renal impairment. Caution is required if the drug is administered to clients with cardiac, renal, or hepatic disease.

Aminocaproic acid is contraindicated for women in the first or second trimester of pregnancy and for clients with active intravascular clotting with possible active fibrinolysis and bleeding.

Tranexamic acid

Tranexamic acid is an antifibrinolytic that inhibits plasminogen activation and opposes the effects of plasmin by competitive inhibition. It is administered orally and IV. Tranexamic acid is used to control bleeding in hemophiliacs, especially when teeth are extracted. Adverse reactions to tranexamic acid include nausea, vomiting, and diarrhea, as well as changes in color vision, visual acuity, visual fields, and eye grounds. When this drug is used, clients should be monitored for visual changes. Tranexamic acid is contraindicated for clients with subarachnoid hemorrhage. It is unsafe for people with defective color vision because they would not detect color changes that indicate degradation of the drug.

Topical hemostatics

A number of substances are available that can be applied topically to bleeding tissue to retard blood loss or promote coagulation.

Epinephrine

Solutions of epinephrine stimulate vasoconstriction, slowing blood flow and allowing normal clotting to occur. It is particularly useful in controlling bleeding from tissues to which pressure cannot be applied. Some of the drug may be absorbed systemically, especially if it is applied to large areas (see Chapter 22).

Oxidized cellulose

A specially treated surgical gauze, oxidized cellulose, reacts with blood to form an artificial clot. It can be left in place and will be absorbed gradually. Because the material will interfere with formation of new skin, it is not used on exterior wounds. Oxidized cellulose is not suitable for use as permanent packing since it also interferes with bone regeneration.

Absorbable gelatin

Available as a powder, sponge, or film, gelatin absorbs blood and water. It is most effective when moistened with thrombin solution. It is absorbed systemically and need not be removed. Because gelatin is an animal protein, allergic hypersensitivity may develop.

Clotting intermediaries

Three products helpful in controlling bleeding are chemicals involved in the normal process of clotting: thrombin, thromboplastin, and human fibrin foam. Thrombin is available as a powder, solution, or spray. It is often applied to absorbable gelatin. The solution must not be administered IV because if it is, fatal intravascular clotting will ensue. Thromboplastin is applied as a powder. Human fibrin foam is a solid. Because both thrombin and thromboplastin are animal derivatives, they can induce allergic hypersensitivity. All three substances promote coagulation chemically by inducing the latter steps in the coagulation process, thereby bypassing the earlier reactions usually necessary for clotting.

■ Summary

There are various clotting disorders characterized by excessive or prolonged bleeding. Some are associated with hereditary deficiencies of one or more clotting factors. Other clients lose their ability to produce certain factors due to disease. Of increasing importance are iatrogenic conditions arising from massive blood transfusions, drug therapy, or radiation. The underlying problem is eliminated whenever possible but replacement of the deficient clotting factors often is necessary.

Hemostatics include whole blood, blood plasma, fractional parts of plasma, vitamin K, enzyme inhibitors, and topical hemostatics. Fractional parts of plasma contain high concentrations of specific clotting factors but carry some risk of serious infection. Protamine corrects abnormal bleeding caused by heparin, whereas vitamin K corrects that caused by a low concentration of prothrombin. Enzyme inhibitors interfere with the normal processes for clot dissolution. Topical hemostatics include epinephrine, oxidized cellulose, absorbable gelatin, and clotting intermediaries.

Nursing management

Nursing implications

Whenever systemic hemostatics are administered, there is a chance of overcorrecting the clotting deficiency and producing a state of hypercoagulation. Such a condition is actually more dangerous than bleeding; lost blood can be replaced but intravascular clots are difficult to remove or to dissolve. The stressed client is particularly vulnerable to this complication because stress hormones induce an underlying hypercoagulability that is manifested once the coagulation defect is remedied. For this reason, treatment for most clients is aimed at restoring clotting factors to a minimally effective level. A gradual correction of the coagulation defect is desirable. Clients, who often feel desperate, may become impatient if treatment does not produce prompt improvement. They must be reassured that their blood loss can be replaced if necessary, and that a conservative approach is preferable in these situations.

Blood and blood products. The single clotting factor presently available for medicinal use is human antihemophilic factor. Several preparations of this drug are produced. The processes used to manufacture them, their concentrations, and their impurities vary. This medication is the drug of choice to treat classic hemophilia (hemophilia A).

Antihemophilic factor is presently used only to treat acute problems associated with hemophilia, such as frank hemorrhage, hemarthrosis, or the risk of hemorrhage during surgery. Although daily dosage as replacement therapy is thought to have potential in controlling the disease, at present, such a regimen is seldom prescribed for the following reasons:

1. As a product of human blood, antihemophilic factor is in limited supply.
2. At present, antihemophilic factor must be administered IV.
3. The drug requires careful handling to maintain its efficacy.

Human factor IX complex contains coagulation factors II, VII, IX, and X. It is useful in treating Christmas disease (hemophilia B), which is characterized by a deficiency of clotting factor IX. It is sometimes used to treat life-threatening hemorrhagic disease in newborns.

Incompatibility reactions. When blood or blood products are administered, there is always a danger of incompatibility reactions. These are most frequent and most serious with whole blood but they occasionally occur with fractional components such as antihemophilic factor. The student is referred to Chapter 51 for precautions required during the administration of blood. Specific recommendations for blood products are available in the accompanying literature.

The client must be observed closely for adverse reactions, which may be manifested by headaches, flushing, tachycardia, back pains, hypotension, fever, chills, and neurologic changes. To minimize reactions, avoid the rapid administration of IV preparations. Jaundice may develop within hours or days following a reaction. The sclerae and skin of all clients who have recently received blood or blood derivatives should be observed regularly for yellow discoloration. Jaundice is not apparent under fluorescent lights because there is little yellow in its spectrum. For this reason, normal sunlight is preferred when examining a client for jaundice.

Infections can also be transmitted by these medications. During the course of processing, blood and blood products are screened for most infections but the tests for hepatitis B and AIDS are not entirely reliable. Clients who have received human blood products should be monitored for signs and symptoms of hepatitis B (jaundice, malaise) and AIDS (frequent infections that do not resolve with the usual treatment).

Storage and handling of blood. Blood and its derivatives are easily damaged by temperature extremes and rough handling. The nurse must understand the particular requirements of the preparation being used and adjust procedures for its preparation and administration accordingly. For example, solutions (blood, plasma, reconstituted antihemophilic factor) are refrigerated until they are administered but they must be protected from freezing. Both RBCs and protein molecules are damaged by vigorous agitation or rough handling.

Vitamin K preparations. Vitamin K is administered either orally or parenterally. Fat-soluble preparations require bile salts for intestinal absorption but water-soluble preparations do not. An emulsion of fat-soluble vitamin K can be administered intramuscularly; water-soluble injectable solutions are administered by all parenteral routes.

Two major uses of phytonadione (vitamin D_1) are the prevention and treatment of hemorrhage in the newborn and the treatment of coumarin anticoagulant overdose. Administering large doses of vitamin K_1 will restore the liver's production of prothrombin even in the presence of warfarin. However, because the effect is not immediate, cases of severe bleeding may require transfusion. Vitamin K_3 is not effective in treating coumarin toxicity.

When used medicinally, vitamin K has a wide margin of safety and in normal doses appears nontoxic. However, when it is administered to animals in large doses, it has produced anemia, polycythemia, splenomegaly, renal and hepatic damage, and death (Gilman, Goodman, Rall, & Murad, 1985). Infants appear to have a limited tolerance for menadione and menadiol; these drugs have been implicated in hemolytic anemia, hyperbilirubinemia, and kernicterus in newborns, especially in premature infants. In clients with severe hepatic disease, large doses of vitamin K can further depress liver function.

When preparing doses of menadione, care should be taken to avoid personal contact with the drug. Inhalation of the powder can cause irritation of the lungs, and both powder and alcoholic solutions can damage the skin.

Nursing process

Assessment Data required for assessment include history of bleeding disorders (onset, duration, and severity of bleeding), evaluation of current rate of blood loss, vital signs, color, warmth of and circulation return to peripheral tissues, and results of laboratory tests for RBCs, hemoglobin, platelets, PT, partial thromboplastin time (PTT), and blood type. Previous exposure and reaction to hemostatic agents should be determined. If protamine is to be used, clients should be screened for allergy to fish, a risk factor for allergic reaction to protamine.

Nursing diagnosis Clients with prolonged or excessive bleeding will experience the following:

Fear of dying
High risk for altered tissue perfusion related to neurogenic vasodilation secondary to stress response
Pain related to altered tissue perfusion due to hypotension and to multiple venipunctures, injections, and mechanical devices used to control bleeding

A common collaborative problem that should be differentiated from the nursing diagnoses is

Potential complication: hypovolemia related to hemorrhage

When hemostatic drugs are employed, adverse reactions may cause the following:

Altered comfort: nausea, vomiting, diarrhea, cramping, headaches, back pain, chills and fever, and back pains related to tissue irritation
Altered tissue perfusion related to vasodilation and bradycardia
High risk for infection related to possible exposure to the hepatitis B or AIDS viruses
Body image disturbance related to jaundice or skin rash

Common collaborative problems that should be differentiated from the nursing diagnoses include

Potential complication: visual impairment
Potential complication: tinnitus
Potential complication: hypotension related to anaphylaxis

Clients and families may also have

Knowledge deficits related to coagulation deficiencies and their treatment

Planning Goals of treatment are to increase coagulability of the client's blood to a minimally effective level, to improve tissue perfusion and circulation, to alleviate the client's discomfort and fear, to reduce the risk of adverse drug reactions, to promptly detect and treat any adverse reactions that develop, and to teach clients and their families about coagulation problems and treatment.

Intervention Nursing interventions to alleviate fear include promoting the client's trust in health care personnel by demonstrating competence in nursing skills and a warm concern for the client's welfare. Both clients and family should be encouraged to express their concerns, and the gravity of the client's situation should be acknowledged. The nurse may realistically reassure the client that modern medicine has various treatments effective in controlling abnormal bleeding.

Nursing measures should be taken to reduce the client's stress levels. Often the clinical situation is characterized by an atmosphere of worry and hurry. This should be minimized as much as possible. Unnecessary stressors such as prolonged fasting, pain, noise, and glaring lights should be eliminated. The family should be advised to maintain as healthful a routine as possible, taking regular meals, sleep, and rest. For both client and family, the nurse should emphasize stress management techniques such as regular participation in activities that provide diversion and recreation.

Nursing measures to minimize pain include preventing multiple needle sticks when possible. Blood samples can sometimes be taken from existing IV lines if fluid equal to the dead space between port and catheter or needle end is aspirated and discarded. This technique also prevents additional bleeding sites, which may develop at new needle stick sites.

To promote tissue perfusion, the hypotensive client should be maintained at bed rest, in shock position (flat with legs raised on pillows). Antishock leggings that exert pressure on blood vessels in the lower limbs to prevent excessive dilation may be ordered. Fluid replacement to reverse hypovolemia and medication to restore coagulation are important factors in treatment.

Administration of hemostatics. If hemostatic drugs are administered IV, an infusion pump or other device is required to control the rate of flow. Rapid infusion is usually contraindicated. Safe administration of blood requires special precautions to prevent administration of mismatched blood. The student is directed to Chapter 51 for a detailed discussion of the use of blood.

Topical hemostatics are often left in place to be absorbed by the body. When materials applied to bleeding sites must be removed, it is important to moisten them thoroughly with a sterile liquid such as normal saline. Removal of dry, adherent substances can traumatize blood vessels, causing further bleeding. This principle also applies to the removal of nasal, vaginal, or other packings. Normally such packs are not moistened before removal but when a bleeding disorder is present, moistening is vital to prevent further tissue trauma.

Clients should be monitored for adverse reactions specific to the prescribed hemostatic drugs. Clients to whom protamine or topical hemostatics of animal origin have been administered should be assessed regularly for allergic reaction to these substances. Health care staff should be prepared to give emergency treatment for anaphylaxis should it occur. Clients receiving blood require close observation, especially during the infusion of the first 50 ml. The signs and symptoms of early blood reactions include headaches, flushing, tachycardia, back pain, hypotension, fever, chills, and neurologic changes. If these develop, the transfusion must be stopped immediately, and the tubing should be disconnected from the IV catheter or needle and flushed before resuming infusion of clear IV fluids. The amount of incompatible blood to which the client is exposed can be further decreased if a small amount of blood is aspirated from the catheter or needle while the tubing is disconnected.

Both jaundice as a result of transfusion and uncontrolled bleeding alter body image. Clients may feel that they are ugly and that their bodies have betrayed them by failing to seal off bleeding sites. The nurse may reassure clients with jaundice not caused by active liver disease or an ongoing hemolytic process that the discoloration is temporary and will subside with time. Nursing measures to promote a positive self-image are appropriate. Judicious use of cosmetics by women can conceal yellow facial discoloration. The nurse should point out improvement in the client's condition when it occurs.

Client education. Clotting deficiencies are often chronic health problems and most clients and their families eventually learn a great deal about the specific disorder. However, it cannot be assumed that they do not need further education. There may be deficits in their knowledge, and, under the stress of an acute bleeding episode, they may be unable to recall facts or think rationally. The nurse should offer clients information necessary for coping with the treatment procedures without conveying an assumption that this knowledge is new. If time allows, the nurse should question clients to determine how sophisticated they are about their condition. However, even clients who are very knowledgeable should continue to receive the "coaching" instructions that help them to participate in treatment procedures.

During convalescence, clients who have received blood products should be instructed to seek medical attention if signs of hepatitis or AIDS develop. The onset of these conditions is usually delayed until the client is discharged from the hospital.

When signs and symptoms of serious adverse drug reactions appear, such as sensory perceptual changes, the physician should be notified immediately and medication withheld until the client is reevaluated. Intestinal upsets may be amenable to nursing intervention. (See Chapter 31 for a discussion of nursing measures for diarrhea.)

Clients deficient in vitamin K due to alterations in intestinal flora may benefit from foods containing lactobacillus cultures, such as buttermilk or yogurt. These kinds of foods help restore normal flora, thereby increasing the production of vitamin K in the GI tract.

Clients on long-term warfarin therapy may be advised by their physicians to carry vitamin K preparations and to ingest a dose in the event of trauma or spontaneous bleeding. Only vitamin K_1 preparations are recommended for this purpose. Other preparations of the vitamin are not effective. Clients should seek medical attention as soon as possible after such an episode. These clients must also maintain a steady intake of vitamin K because fluctuations in this nutrient interfere with a constant anticoagulant effect. Foods rich in the nutrient (green leafy vegetables and vegetable oils) should not be eliminated from the diet but rather included each day in normal, controlled amounts.

Evaluation Data required for evaluation include statements by the client indicating that fear and stress have decreased and that symptoms such as pain, dizziness, and weakness have decreased or disappeared. The presence or absence of bleeding and the results of laboratory tests for RBCs, hemoglobin, platelets, partial thromboplastin time (PTT), or PT will indicate changes in coagulability, replacement of blood losses, and contained blood loss. Color, tests for peripheral circulation, and vital signs indicate changes in tissue perfusion. The presence or absence of adverse drug reactions and their severity are required to evaluate their prevention, detection, and treatment. Teaching is evaluated by the client's ability to cooperate with treatment procedures and to repeat information conveyed during teaching sessions. (See Example of Nursing Process and Dysfunctional Uterine Bleeding.)

Checklist of nursing actions

When clients are treated for abnormal bleeding

☐ Eliminate or ameliorate stressors where possible.

☐ Assist the client in coping with stress.

☐ Reassure the client that blood loss can be replaced and that a conservative approach is desirable.

☐ Take measures to keep the number of needle sticks to a minimum.

☐ Implement nursing measures to reduce circulatory shock in hypotensive clients.

☐ Use the proper procedures in handling, storing, and preparing blood and its derivatives.

☐ Avoid rapid administration of IV preparations.

☐ Moisten topical hemostatic materials thoroughly with a sterile liquid before removing them.

☐ Take measures to reduce the risk of adverse drug reactions.

☐ Observe clients closely for adverse drug reactions. Where possible, use nursing measures to

Example of nursing process and dysfunctional uterine bleeding

The client is a 45-year-old secretary with a history of prolonged vaginal bleeding who has been admitted to an acute-care institution. For the last 4 months, the client's menstrual flow has been heavy and prolonged. This month the flow has been uninterrupted for 3 weeks.

Upon examination, the client appears pale and anxious. She states that her father "bled to death" as a result of injuries sustained in a motor vehicle accident.

The client lives alone in an apartment in a suburban residential complex. She has never married and is childless.

Laboratory tests show RBCs 2.9 million mm^2 and Hgb 8.7 g/dl. Vital signs are temperature 35.4°C (97.6°F), pulse 104/min, respirations 24/min, blood pressure 102/80.

The physician has ordered typing and cross-matching for three units of blood; one unit is to be administered as soon as possible, with repeat CBC and Hgb 1 hour after completion.

Assessment data	Nursing diagnosis	Interventions	Goals and outcome criteria
Low RBC count and Hgb levels	Impaired peripheral gas exchange related to low levels of RBCs and hemoglobin due to loss of blood, possibly secondary to menopausal menorrhagia and coagulation deficiency	**Administer** the blood as ordered. Monitor blood loss by counting the number of perineal pads used by the client, the color of the vaginal discharge, and the degree of saturation of used pads.	The client's color will become pinker, hemoglobin and red blood cell levels will rise; bleeding will decrease gradually and then cease.
Prolonged bleeding Client's statement that her father "bled to death"	Fear of dying related to severe blood loss and memory of her father's death	**Encourage** the client to express her feelings about her illness and about her father's death. Establish a relationship characterized by competence and personal concern for the client (by the nurse) and trust of the nurse (by the client). Offer realistic reassurance; tell the client that today modern medicine has more and better ways of controlling abnormal bleeding than a few years ago.	The client will appear more relaxed; she will make statements that indicate that she is less anxious and fearful.
Age: 45 year Childless	Possible anticipatory grieving related to beginning menopause and state of childlessness	**Encourage** the client to explore her feelings about menopause and childlessness. Listen to her and provide emotional support.	If the client is grieving, she will be able to express her feelings and begin to work through the stages of grief.

reduce the severity of these reactions; report reactions requiring medical attention to the physician.

☐ Instruct clients receiving blood or blood products about the signs and symptoms of hepatitis and AIDS and warn them to seek immediate medical attention if such reactions develop.

☐ Advise clients about including foods rich in vitamin K in their diet.

☐ When preparing doses of menadione, avoid personal exposure to the drug.

Anticoagulants

Drugs that inhibit clotting may be used either for the prevention or treatment of thromboembolic disorders. Anticoagulant therapy is used in the treatment of such conditions as venous thrombosis, pulmonary embolism, coronary thrombosis, and disseminated intravascular coagulation (DIC). These drugs will not dissolve existing clots but do interrupt the extension of these clots, which tend to increase in size due to the autocatalytic nature of the coagulation process. Long-term oral anticoagulant therapy is used to prevent thromboembolic disorders in clients considered at high risk, including persons with rheumatic heart disease (especially if atria are enlarged or fibrillating), clients with prosthetic heart valves, or clients with a history of myocardial infarction (MI) due to coronary thrombosis. Subanticoagulant doses of heparin (low-dose heparin) have been used to prevent thrombi in hospitalized clients at high risk: postpartum mothers, older clients undergoing surgery, and victims of long bone fractures.

Heparin

Heparin is a mucopolysaccharide found in most tissue cells, notably in the liver and lungs. It is a strong organic acid whose anionic groups appear to react with clotting factors.

Pharmacodynamics. Heparin inhibits activated factors IX, X, XI, and XII, which are involved in the conversion of prothrombin to thrombin, thereby reducing thrombin formation. Heparin inhibits clotting both *in vivo* and *in vitro*. It prolongs whole blood clotting time and thrombin time.

Pharmacokinetics. Heparin must be administered parenterally because it is broken down by the digestive process. It is readily absorbed when administered intramuscularly, subcutaneously, or intravenously. However, when injected into vascular tissue, large ecchymotic areas develop. For this reason, injection of heparin into a muscle or thin layers of subcutaneous tissue is avoided. In acute situations requiring full anticoagulation, the drug is usually given intravenously, by continuous drip, or as a bolus in an existing IV line or heparin lock. Low doses are commonly administered by subcutaneous injection.

Following administration, heparin is widely distributed in the body; much of it is trapped in the interstitial fluid and reticuloendothelial cells. It does not cross the placenta and is not distributed into breast milk. Although heparin is eliminated through the kidneys, it is not removed by hemodialysis. When administered IV, heparin becomes effective immediately. The duration of its action is 3–4 hours. Doses are determined by biologic assay and measured in units. An initial dose of 10,000 units is given to adult clients, followed by 5,000–10,000 units every 4–6 hours. The drug is also administered by continuous IV infusion.

Therapeutic uses. Heparin is approved for use in the prevention and treatment of venous thrombosis, pulmonary embolism, and embolism caused by atrial fibrillation. It is also used in the diagnosis and treatment of DIC; the prevention of cerebral thrombosis in evolving stroke; the prevention and treatment of peripheral arterial embolism; the control of angina pectoris; and as an adjunct in the treatment of coronary occlusion.

Heparin is the anticoagulant of choice when an immediate effect is required. Heparin is also used to prevent clotting in equipment used for extracorporeal circulation (artificial kidney, heart-lung machine), intermittent IV infusions (indwelling IV catheters, implanted central venous lines), and for laboratory test specimens requiring unclotted blood.

Adverse reactions. Heparin is well tolerated by most clients. High-dose heparin therapy is used only in institutional settings where the recipient is under close medical supervision. The greatest risk is that of excessive bleeding. When this occurs, discontinuing the medication is usually sufficient to eliminate the symptoms. In severe cases, protamine is administered as an antidote. Low-dose heparin increases the incidence of postoperative wound hematoma in clients undergoing surgery (van Ooijen, 1986).

Heparin can cause clotting in some individuals by inducing platelet aggregation, causing the formation of a "white clot." Kappa (1987) describes a syndrome (heparin-induced platelet aggregation; HIPA) that develops 4–10 days after heparin is started, and is characterized by new thrombi, a falling platelet count, and laboratory evidence of irreversible platelet aggregation. Chong (1982) reported a similar "delayed allergic reaction," characterized by heparin-dependent antiplatelet antibody and thrombocytopenia that develops 9–25 days after initiation of heparin. These disorders have a high morbidity and mortality rate, with some survivors losing limbs due to impairment of peripheral circulation.

Heparin therapy may increase loss of blood during menstruation. Prolonged heparin therapy increases the risk of osteoporosis and pathologic fracture because it inhibits renal production of calcitriol, the most active form of vitamin D. Allergic and local reactions at injection sites are also frequently seen.

Precautions and contraindications. Response to full dose heparin must be carefully assessed by monitoring thrombocytes and PTT. Anticoagulation is considered therapeutic if PTT is $1\frac{1}{2}$–$2\frac{1}{2}$ times normal levels. Thrombocytopenia is undesirable and may indicate dangerous allergic hypersensitivity. If thrombocytes drop 30%–35%, heparin therapy should be discontinued.

When intermittent doses of heparin are given, monitoring tests should be performed 1 hour or less before heparin medication is administered. Heparin may also prolong the PT. Caution is required when evaluating this test in cases where clients are receiving oral anticoagulants and heparin together.

Low-dose heparin therapy is usually not monitored by blood tests.

Due to the risk of uncontrolled bleeding, heparin is contraindicated for clients suffering from active bleeding or bleeding tendencies, threatened abortion, subacute bacterial endocarditis, GI ulcers, severe hypertension, visceral malignancies, or suspected intracranial hemorrhage. It is also not given to clients undergoing regional or lumbar block anesthesia, eye surgery, central nervous system (CNS) surgery, or tube drainage. Hematuria in a client on anticoagulants is not always caused by the anticoagulant. Blood in the urine should be investigated by a diagnostic workup, especially if it persists after withdrawal of the anticoagulant (Schuster & Lewis, 1987).

Heparin treatment must be discontinued and not resumed after HIPA or delayed allergic reactions. Resumption of heparin in these clients can cause rapid development of massive thromboemboli. If the use of heparin is unavoidable, dosage should be kept to a minimum and aspirin administered in antiplatelet dosages (Laster et al, 1989).

Warfarin

Warfarin (coumarin) was first discovered when it was identified as the cause of an animal disease characterized by abnormal bleeding. Improperly cured clover hay was found to contain a substance causing this syndrome. The affected animals recovered when the fodder was discontinued.

Pharmacodynamics. Coumarin drugs have a chemical structure that resembles vitamin K (Fig. 29-3). It is believed that they act mainly by competitively inhibiting this nutrient. The drug molecule is accepted by the liver in place of vitamin K, thereby decreasing the production of clotting factors II, VII, IX, and X.

Chemical Structure Common to All K Vitamins

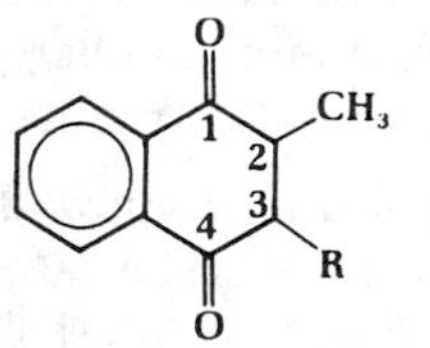

Chemical Structure Common to Coumarin Anticoagulants

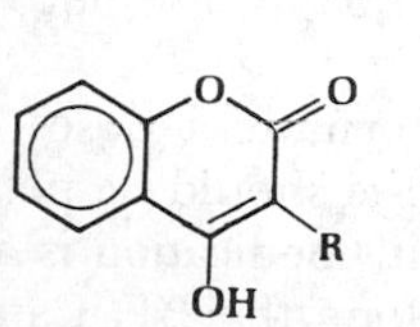

Figure 29-3. Comparison of the chemical structures of coumarin and vitamin K.

Pharmacokinetics. Coumarin anticoagulants may be given orally. The various preparations available vary in the degree to which they are absorbed in the GI tract. Dicumarol is poorly absorbed, whereas warfarin is rapidly absorbed. Dosages are listed in Table 29-2. Large amounts of the drug are bound to plasma albumin; it also accumulates in the lungs, liver, spleen, and kidneys. A period of 12–24 hours is required for the development of peak levels in the blood. A further lag of 24–72 hours occurs before a therapeutic response is evident due to existing clotting factors in the system, which are not affected by coumarin and are eliminated gradually.

Warfarin is usually administered once a day. While the client is in the hospital, doses are adjusted daily in accordance with prothrombin tests. Because blood is customarily drawn in the early morning for such tests and the results are not available for several hours, warfarin is administered to the client in the afternoon or evening.

Warfarin has a half-life of approximately 48 hours. It is metabolized by the hepatic microsomal enzyme system and excreted by the kidneys. Coumarin, which can cross the placental barrier, is secreted in the breast milk of lactating mothers.

Therapeutic uses. Coumarin and indanedione derivatives are approved for the prevention and treatment of venous thrombosis and pulmonary embolism; the treatment of embolism caused by atrial fibrillation; and as an adjunct in the treatment of coronary occlusion. Because serious toxic reactions have occurred with the indanedione derivative phenindione, coumarin is usually used for oral anticoagulation. It is generally prescribed for follow-up therapy after the effects of full-dose heparin therapy have been established and when long-term anticoagulant therapy is indicated. Warfarin has been reported to be effective in the treatment of aggression associated with chronic dementia. (Walsh, 1989)

Because the effects of coumadin are delayed, it must be administered for several days before heparin is discontinued.

Adverse reactions. As with heparin, the most serious risk with warfarin therapy is abnormal bleeding.

Toxicity is often manifested first by hematuria. Although alarming, this sign does not necessarily indicate kidney damage.

Rarely, warfarin may cause necrosis of fatty soft tissue (breast, buttocks, thighs, abdomen, and penis). This can happen after a single dose. Obese, middle-aged women and clients undergoing open heart surgery are at increased risk. This reaction can be severe and refractory to treatment. Extensive debridement, skin grafting, or amputation may be required (Weinberg, Lieskovsky, McGehee, & Skinner, 1983). Warfarin-induced hepatic injury associated with choles-

Table 29-2. Coumarin and indanedione derivative anticoagulants

Drug name	Preparations	Usual dosage	Additional information
Coumarin derivatives			
anisindione (Miradon)	Oral tablets	Adults: *Initially:* 300 mg the first day, 200 mg the second day, 100 mg the third day; *thereafter:* 25–30 mg daily	Dosage is individualized in accordance with prolongation of PT as shown by laboratory tests.
dicumarol	Oral tablets and capsules	Adults: *Initially:* 200–300 mg; *maintenance:* 25–200 mg/day PC: D	Dosage is individualized in accordance with prolongation of PT as shown by laboratory tests.
phenprocoumon (Liquamar)	Oral tablets	Adults: *Initially:* 24 mg; *maintenance:* 0.75–6 mg/d	Dosage is individualized in accordance with prolongation of PT as shown by laboratory tests.
warfarin (Athrombin-K, Coufarin, Coumadin, Panwarfin)	Oral tablets Solution for IM or IV injection	Adults: *Initially:* 10–15 mg/d for 2–5 days until desired prothrombin time is reached; *maintenance:* 2–10 mg/d PC: D	Panwarfin contains tartrazine (FD&C yellow dye #5) which can cause allergic reactions in susceptible persons. Dosage is individualized in accordance with prolongation of PT as shown by laboratory tests.
Indanedione derivative			
nicoumalone (Sintrom)	Oral tablets	Adults: *Initially:* 8–12 mg; *maintenance:* In accordance with Quick value of blood	
phenindione (Hedulin)	Oral tablets	Adults: *Initially:* 300 mg; *second day:* 200 mg; *thereafter:* 100 mg/d	Phenindione is rarely used because it has caused serious, sometimes fatal, toxic reactions involving the hematologic, renal, and hepatic systems.

KEY: PC = pregnancy risk category. (The validity of pregnancy risk categories has not been established. See Chapter 16, p 216.)

tasis has also been reported (Adler, Benjamin, & Zimmerman, 1986).

So many drugs affect the body's response to these anticoagulants that the interactions are considered a prototype for the study of drug interactions. Drugs that reduce therapeutic response to coumarin include griseofulvin, cholestyramine, barbiturates, ethchlorvinyl, glutethimide, rifampin, vitamin K, and chlorthalidine.

Precautions and contraindications. Warfarin is administered in milligram doses. However, because individual responses vary widely, laboratory monitoring of the drug's effect is required. Hospitalized clients receive daily doses adjusted to the results of one-stage PT (Quick Time). Anticoagulation is considered therapeutic when the PT reaches 1.2–2.0 times the control (a normal established by the laboratory for each test).

Coumarin anticoagulants may be administered over long periods of time on an outpatient basis. The client must first be stabilized with a maintenance dose. Periodic (usually monthly) PT tests are necessary to monitor the client's response to the drug. The physiologic effect of the drugs is altered by many factors, including diet, intestinal absorption, function of the liver and kidneys, and concurrent medications.

When abnormal bleeding occurs, anticoagulation should be partially or completely reversed. In addition, all possible causes other than anticoagulant toxicity should be ruled out, especially if the bleeding is not affected by restoration of normal coagulation.

Long-term warfarin therapy is contraindicated for clients suffering from alcoholism, malignant hypertension, active tuberculosis, or conditions that require the administration of salicylates. Coumarin anticoagulants are not recommended during pregnancy because the drugs cross the placenta and increase the risk of hemorrhage for the fetus. In addition, there is some evidence that prenatal therapy may induce other pathologic conditions in the fetus. Except for heparin sensitivity, the contraindications previously listed for heparin apply also to warfarin therapy.

Indanedione anticoagulants

Indanedione anticoagulants, such as anisindione and phenindione, are similar to coumarin compounds in their action and adverse reactions. They are somewhat more toxic and are used primarily to treat clients who do not tolerate coumarin drugs.

Drugs that affect platelet aggregation

A number of drugs interfere with the aggregation of platelets and prolong bleeding time. These include aspirin, dextran (both 40 and 70), sulfinpyrazone (Anturane), dipyridamole (Persantine), beta-adrenergic agents, and calcium channel blocking agents. Aspirin is the most widely used.

Aspirin

Aspirin appears to affect platelets by acetylating them and by blocking ADP-mediated secondary aggregation. Small doses (50–75 mg q12h–q24h for adults) appear to be more effective than dosages at the levels required for anti-inflammatory or analgesic effect. This is fortunate because it allows use of aspirin by clients who cannot tolerate larger doses. (See Chapter 47 for a detailed discussion of aspirin.)

Aspirin is recommended as an antiplatelet agent by many physicians for clients suffering from arteriosclerosis or other conditions believed to increase the risk of thrombotic disease such as coronary thrombosis. Doses ordered twice a day should be spaced 12 hours apart. If only one dose per day is required, it should be taken at the same time each day.

Aspirin is recommended for reducing the risk of a second MI in men who have a first MI. One study found that in men age 50 and older one 325 mg aspirin tablet every other day decreases the risk of MI, although it does not appear to reduce the total cardiovascular mortality. Subjects in this study who received aspirin did exhibit increased risk of hemorrhagic stroke and peptic ulcer (Steering Committee of the Physicians' Health Study Research Group, 1989).

Dipyridamole

Dipyridamole (Persantine) is an inhibitor of platelet aggregation that acts also as a vasodilator.

Pharmacodynamics. Dipyridamole inhibits adenosine deaminase, an enzyme involved in the metabolism of adenosine. It thereby leads to an accumulation of adenosine, which acts as an inhibitor of platelet phosphodiesterase, and also as a potent vasodilator. Its effects include prolonged survival of platelets, delayed coagulation, and dilation of small resistance blood vessels, particularly in the coronary vascular bed.

Dosage and administration. Dipyridamole is marketed as oral tablets ranging in dosage from 25 to 75 mg. The usual adult dosage is 150–400 mg daily (given in divided doses). When used for long-term for treatment of chronic angina pectoris, usual dosage is 50 mg three times daily (a daily total of 150 mg).

Pharmacokinetics. When administered orally, dipyridamole is absorbed incompletely from the GI tract. Peak plasma concentrations from a single dose occur in 45–150 minutes. The drug is widely distributed and is highly bound to plasma albumin. Animal studies indicate that small amounts cross the placenta; it is known to be excreted in human milk. Serum half-life during the distribution phase is 40–80 minutes; during elimination phase, half-life is 10–12 hours. Dipyridamole is metabolized by the liver. The drug and its metabolites enter the entero-hepatic cycle via secretion in bile, and eventually are eliminated in the feces.

Therapeutic uses. Dipyridamole is used as an adjunct with coumarin for anticoagulation therapy, particularly after cardiac valve replacement and bypass surgery. It is used in chronic (but not acute) angina pectoris, and to prevent strokes caused by thrombi. Combined therapy with dipyridamole and aspirin prolongs the survival of platelets in clients with thrombotic diseases.

Adverse reactions. Adverse reactions are generally transient, dose-related, and reversible with withdrawal of the drug. They affect the CNS (headache, dizziness, syncope), the GI tract (nausea, vomiting, diarrhea), and the peripheral vascular system (vasodilation, flushing). Weakness, rash with pruritus, and worsening of angina have occurred. Rarely, acute MI has occurred in recipients with coronary artery disease.

Precautions and contraindications. The manufacturer claims that there are no contraindications for dipyridamole. Caution should be exercised when the drug is prescribed for individuals who tend to be hypotensive and for nursing mothers (who pass some drug on to the infant). Safety and efficacy remain unproven for children less than age 12.

See Table 29-3 for a comparison of aspirin and dipyridamole antiplatelet therapy.

Dextran

Dextran coats the platelets and forms a complex with some clotting factors. It may be given concurrently with either heparin or warfarin. The drug can be used only in selected clients because it increases blood volume markedly.

■ Summary

Anticoagulants may be used either for preventing or treating such conditions as venous thrombosis, pulmonary embolism, coronary thrombosis, and DIC. These drugs will not dissolve existing clots but they interrupt the extension of these clots. The most serious risk with heparin and warfarin therapy is excessive bleeding. Many drugs affect responses to the oral anticoagulants.

Nursing management
Nursing implications

Anticoagulant therapy is often used to treat acute, life-threatening conditions such as pulmonary or arterial embolism and cerebral or coronary thrombosis. Hep-

Table 29-3. Comparison of dipyridamole and aspirin

	Aspirin	Dipyridamole
Route of administration	Oral	Oral
Dosage	50–400 mg daily, divided in 1–2 doses	100–150 mg daily, in divided doses
Effect on blood vessels	None	Dilation
Uses	Chronic angina pectoris	Prevention of recurrent myocardial infarctions
	Prevention of recurrent strokes due to thrombi	(With warfarin) treatment of thrombotic disease
	(With warfarin) treatment after cardiac valve replacement and by-pass surgery	
Pregnancy risk category*	(D in the third trimester)	C

*The validity of pregnancy risk categories has not been established. See Chapter 16, p 216.

arin therapy is usually used at first. If the thrombus is in a vein, warfarin may also be administered immediately so that heparin may be discontinued in 2–3 days when the PT is sufficiently delayed. Because arterial thrombi do not respond as well to oral anticoagulants, heparin alone is used for treating this condition. (See Table 29-4 for a comparison of heparin and warfarin therapy.)

Accuracy in heparin medication. Special care must be taken when measuring doses of heparin because overdoses can be disastrous. The drug is available in solutions of various concentrations: 10, 100, 1,000, 5,000, 7,500, 10,000, 15,000, 20,000, or 40,000 units per milliliter. Care must be exercised when reading the label and computing doses. Many hospitals require that every heparin dose be verified by a second nurse. This is always a wise precaution.

Continuous IV drip administration is accomplished by adding a specified amount of heparin to a standard bottle of IV solution. Either 5% dextrose in water or normal saline may be used. Regular flow is critical to establish a stable therapeutic state. An infusion regulator or IV pump is recommended for all IV

lines containing heparin. Special care is taken to minimize movement of the needle or catheter to prevent infiltration or irritation of the vein. The client receiving anticoagulants is particularly vulnerable to trauma.

Nursing process

Assessment Data required for initial assessment of the client who is to receive anticoagulants include signs and symptoms of thrombi or emboli; previous exposure to anticoagulants; level of knowledge about thromboembolic disease and its treatment; emotional response to the life-threatening condition; and general stress level. Baseline data should include color, vital signs, peripheral pulses, warmth of peripheral tissues, and results of laboratory tests such as thrombocytes, bleeding time, coagulation time, PT, and arterial blood gases. A complete drug history should be taken.

Before any anticoagulant is administered, it must be determined if the client is at risk for adverse reactions to the drugs. A careful history must be taken to rule out contraindications to anticoagulants. A history of peptic ulcers or abnormal bleeding tendencies

Table 29-4. Comparison of heparin and warfarin

	Heparin	Warfarin
Dosage measures	Units	Milligrams
Route of administration	Parenteral	Oral
Onset of action	Immediate (IV)	Delayed
Crosses the placenta	No	Yes
Laboratory tests	PTT	PT
Antidote	Protamine sulfate	Vitamin K
Indications for treatment	Venous and arterial thrombi	Venous thrombi
Source	Animal	Plant
Setting for care	Acute care agency	Home or community after dosage is stabilized
Cost	Expensive	Inexpensive
Pregnancy risk category*	C	D

*The validity of pregnancy risk categories has not been established. See Chapter 16, p 216.

is particularly important. If heparin is to be used, the client should be questioned about any previous heparin therapy. Because heparin is an extract from animal tissues, initial exposure may induce allergic hypersensitivity. If warfarin therapy is planned, pregnancy should be ruled out in women of childbearing age. Although anticoagulation poses risks during pregnancy, heparin is sometimes used during gestation to prevent venous thrombi and systemic embolism associated with heart disease or prosthetic heart valves (Ginsberg & Hirsh, 1989, p 29). A careful drug history is crucial to identify risks of complications from drug interactions.

Nursing diagnosis Diagnoses stemming from thromboembolic disorders may include the following:

> *Altered tissue perfusion related to increased blood coagulability and thrombus or embolus*
> *Pain related to vascular inflammation secondary to clot formation*
> *Impaired physical mobility related to bed rest therapy to prevent emboli*
> *Fear of death related to sudden disruption of circulation due to thromboemboli*

Diagnoses stemming from anticoagulant therapy include the following:

> *Body image disturbance related to ecchymoses and petechiae*
> *Pain related to multiple needle sticks*
> *Fear of death related to uncontrollable bleeding*

Most clients will have

> *Knowledge deficit concerning thromboembolic disorders and their treatment*

Common collaborative problems that should be differentiated from the nursing diagnoses include

> *Potential complication: hemorrhage*
> *Potential complication: anaphylaxis*
> *Potential complication: hypovolemic shock related to hemorrhage*

Planning Goals of treatment include improved tissue perfusion, elimination of pain and discomfort, reduction in fear, improved self-image, reduction in the risk of adverse drug reaction, prompt detection and treatment of adverse drug reactions that may occur, increase in the client's knowledge related to thromboembolism and its treatment, and the client's return to normal mobility.

Intervention: altered tissue perfusion Extremities affected by thrombi or emboli usually become edematous due to impaired venous return. Elevation of the part promotes drainage and reduces swelling.

Applications of either heat or cold may be ordered to promote vasodilation.

Fear. The client's anxiety and fear must be dealt with during the initial stages of treatment. Most clients experience fear of sudden death from embolism, heart failure, stroke, or other catastrophic complications of the disease process. Also, clients may equate anticoagulation with bleeding disorders, such as hemophilia, and believe that they can "bleed to death from a scratch." Nurses must listen to and acknowledge such concerns.

Demonstration of technical competence and a warm personal concern for the client promotes trust in the nursing staff. The nurse should provide the client with adequate information to understand the regimen and cooperate with the treatment. The client must be informed that there is risk involved with both the disease and its treatment but detailed description of complications and disastrous outcomes is inappropriate.

Controlling client fear is particularly important because the normal hormone response to this emotion (increased adrenaline and cortisone secretion) increases the blood coagulation, thereby requiring larger doses of medication. Fluctuations of emotional status contribute to an uneven response to anticoagulant drugs. For these reasons, the nurse should be particularly diligent in reducing all factors that contribute to stress. Prompt attention to call bells makes the client feel confident that treatment will be immediate should complications develop. A calm, confident demeanor on the nurse's part that conveys a concern for the well-being of the client is reassuring. Correcting misconceptions about anticoagulant therapy reduces fear. The nurse should reassure clients that the drugs do not eliminate clotting but only delay it.

Nursing measures to enhance the client's self-image, especially body image, are appropriate. The use of attractive bedclothing and grooming aids should be encouraged. Men should be shaved daily (using an electric shaver rather than razor blades). Women should be encouraged to continue normal use of cosmetics. Clothing should cover ecchymoses. Accidental injury likely to produce further ecchymoses should be avoided. Hazards in the environment that increase the risk of falls, cuts, abrasions, or other injury must be eliminated.

Multiple needle sticks contribute to both pain and the development of ecchymoses. If an IV line is established, it should be used whenever possible for the collection of blood specimens for the daily laboratory tests. The smallest gauge needle possible should be used for specimen collection. The client with a history of previous heparin therapy should be given a test dose of 1,000 units to rule out allergy. Hypersensitivity is usually manifested by asthma, urticaria, lacrimation, rhinitis, or fever. Clients exhibiting allergic symptoms after the test dose may undergo rapid desensitization to develop tolerance to the drug. The first dose must be small enough to be tolerated by the client; succeeding doses are escalated as rapidly as possible without inducing an allergic response.

Hypersensitivity can develop during the course of treatment, especially in clients with a history of allergic disorders. Any respiratory distress, skin rash, symptoms of a "head cold," or fever should receive prompt attention. The physician may order antihistamines or other palliative medications. Cold compresses are soothing to the client with "hives." If antipyretics are required, acetaminophen is preferable to aspirin, which enhances the response to anticoagulants.

Administration of heparin. When large volumes of IV fluids are contraindicated, intermittent IV therapy may be ordered. Drugs so ordered are usually administered by means of a "heparin" lock, an IV needle with a small "well" covered by a rubber diaphragm (Fig. 29-4). The presence of heparin in the needle inhibits clot formation in the lumen, thereby maintaining patency despite the absence of fluid flow for long periods of time. To administer drugs through the lock, clean the rubber diaphragm and insert the needle into the well. Inject the medication and withdraw the needle. Flush with saline or (when ordered) heparin. To prevent damage to the diaphragm and subsequent leakage, use a small-gauge (25 or 26) needle. Injection should be slow, as with all IV push medications.

Subcutaneous administration is commonly ordered for small doses of heparin. Whenever a needle is inserted into tissue, small blood vessels may be penetrated and damaged. If an anticoagulant is then injected into the tissue or if the client has already been medicated, these blood vessels may not close off but continue to bleed slowly, causing large ecchymoses to form. For this reason, special care must be taken to minimize vascular damage while injecting heparin. The abdominal subcutaneous fat tissue is preferred as a site for injection because it contains fewer blood vessels than other injection sites. Injections should be positioned at least 2 inches from any scar and from the umbilicus. The nursing care plan should specify a schedule of site rotation to minimize trauma. When administering heparin subcutaneously, omit aspiration and postinjection massage to minimize blood vessel damage. Subcutaneous injection is not appropriate for very thin or cachexic clients because their fat deposits are inadequate to protect them from inadvertent intramuscular injection.

Administration of warfarin. When warfarin is prescribed, the coagulability of blood is more stable when doses are given regularly; a specific hour should be established for medication. The diet should be monitored to ensure that there are no sudden large fluctuations in vitamin K content. Most clients are on a regular diet.

The timing of doses for the outpatient is continued on the same basis. The periodic blood tests are likely to be scheduled for the morning hours, and the usual afternoon administration of the drug is continued. This provides stability and continuity in the client's medication regimen.

Monitoring. While therapy is in progress, the recipient must be monitored carefully for toxic effects or side effects. Heparin therapy is normally given for periods of 7–10 days. Warfarin, however, may be used over periods of months or years. The degree of anticoagulation is monitored by bleeding time or PTT (for heparin) and PT for warfarin. Thrombocytes are monitored also when heparin is used because a decrease may warn of impending platelet aggregation.

Careful attention must be paid to signs of hemorrhage, such as red or smoky urine, bloody or tarry stools, petechiae, and excessive bruising. Hemarthrosis may cause painful, enlarged joints. Chemical tests of stools and urine for occult blood should be performed at regular intervals. Any frank bleeding, such as epistaxis, hemoptysis, or wound hemorrhage should be reported immediately. Equipment and appropriate personnel must be readily available for IV treatment, including transfusion. Whole blood, plasma, or vitamin K are required for the treatment of warfarin toxicity; protamine is the antidote for heparin.

Adverse reactions. Surgical or obstetric clients receiving subanticoagulant doses of heparin are at increased risk for hemorrhage. Heparin also retards healing. Nurses should be alert to any indications of dehiscence in surgical wounds. Removal of stitches may need to be delayed.

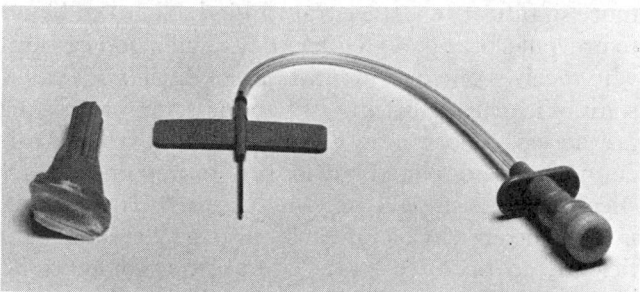

Figure 29-4. One type of heparin lock (with the needle sheath removed). The flaps on either side of the needle are flexible and make the needle easy to handle and anchor. There is a sterile plug at the end of the tubing. Medication is administered by inserting the needle of the syringe or IV tubing through the rubber tip.

Because the risk of GI hemorrhage is serious in clients receiving anticoagulants, measures to reduce the risk of peptic ulcer and prevent gastric irritation should be taken. Aspirin is contraindicated for clients receiving heparin or warfarin. Aspirin is sometimes used as an antiplatelet agent in the treatment of thromboembolic disorders.

Acetaminophen is well tolerated by most people and can be recommended as a substitute for aspirin used for analgesia or antipyresis; it does not have the anti-inflammatory effects of aspirin. Most anti-inflammatory drugs that might be used in place of aspirin are themselves ulcerogenic. For this reason, victims of severe arthritis have particular problems with heparin or warfarin anticoagulant therapy. Not only are many of their usual arthritis medications contraindicated but should they develop hemorrhages in the joints, their arthritic symptoms will increase. Nursing measures to ameliorate the arthritic symptoms include reduction of stress, prevention of chilling (which increases muscle tone), applications of heat, and promotion of adequate sleep.

Hospitalized clients receiving anticoagulants are subject to daily venipunctures to collect blood for the necessary blood tests. Bleeding does not stop readily from these sites. The nurse should verify that a pressure dressing has been applied to the site to minimize leakage of blood. Despite all precautions, large ecchymoses are common. The usual site is the antecubital space. Discomfort in the area may be diminished by the intermittent application of warm packs. Clients may be distressed by the appearance of their arms. They may be encouraged to wear gowns or bed jackets with long sleeves to enhance appearance. Reassurance is needed that the change is temporary and that the ecchymoses are not dangerous. Clients may require much emotional support due to these ecchymoses and because successive venipunctures become increasingly painful.

Food/warfarin interactions. Body levels of vitamin K depend not only on diet but on the maintenance of normal intestinal flora. Intestinal organisms, which synthesize vitamin K, play an important role in maintaining adequate levels. Adding an antibiotic to the regimen of a client receiving warfarin may reduce the intestinal flora and deplete body levels of vitamin K. This will increase the effect of warfarin and may lead to spontaneous bleeding. Neomycin, which acts only within the lumen of the intestine, and broad-spectrum drugs are especially harmful to intestinal organisms. If antibiotics are necessary, close medical supervision is required. The ingestion of buttermilk, yogurt, or other dairy product containing live lactobacilli helps restore normal intestinal flora and may ameliorate these effects.

Diet can affect the body's response to warfarin. Vitamin K inhibits the effect of the anticoagulant. Some of the literature advises that clients receiving warfarin avoid foods rich in vitamin K. This advice is potentially dangerous because long-term avoidance of whole groups of foods increases the risk of malnutrition. The goal is consistency and regularity of intake. Clients should be advised to eat a diet consistent in this nutrient. They may choose to eat one or two servings of a food rich in vitamin K daily. This level of intake should be maintained as long as the anticoagulant is used. A low to moderate fat intake is also recommended because a high fat intake may increase the tendency toward thrombosis.

Throughout anticoagulant therapy, response to warfarin and other drugs used concurrently should be monitored carefully for adverse reactions caused by drug interactions. Dosages of both warfarin and other drugs may need to be manipulated to compensate for these effects. When warfarin or other drugs are discontinued, further dosage adjustments may be needed. The physician may need to be reminded of the client's total drug regimen so that appropriate adjustments can be made.

Heparinized blood. When heparin is used to control clotting in extracorporeal circulation (hemodialysis, heart-lung machines), it is introduced into the blood as it leaves the client to enter the machine; protamine is added to the blood as it reenters the client. If the doses of the two drugs are carefully controlled, clients will not experience a significant change of coagulation within the body. Such clients should be watched carefully for tendencies to bleed, however, because any imbalance in the proportions of heparin and protamine can cause clotting problems.

Transfused blood occasionally can cause bleeding problems in recipients. Aspirin is not considered a factor in these reactions. The concentration of aspirin in donated blood is generally not high enough to affect the client who receives one or two units of blood. Of more significance is the citrate added to banked blood to prevent clotting. A client with normal blood calcium who receives one or two units of blood will not exhibit signs of impaired clotting. When massive transfusions are necessary, commonly in severe hemorrhage, calcium may be depleted sufficiently to impair clotting. Bleeding persists and may increase if further blood is administered. Calcium may also be depleted sufficiently to produce tetany. The physician must be informed of such situations. Calcium rather than additional blood may be required.

Client education. Initial education is directed at assisting the client to cope with the impact of institutionalization, dependence, and anxiety.

Clients on heparin. The nurse should inform the client about procedures to be performed, the effects of the drugs, and safety precautions. Large ecchymotic areas usually develop at the site of the daily venipunctures required for laboratory tests. The nurse should offer reassurance that no permanent damage will result from this phenomenon. Another source of concern to the client receiving heparin is injection into the subcutaneous tissue of the abdomen. This site is seldom used for parenteral medication but it is the preferred location for subcutaneous injections of heparin. The client should be informed that the needle does not penetrate any abdominal organ; the medication is deposited into the "pocket" below the subcutaneous tissue. The medication is actually safer and more comfortable in this area since there are fewer blood vessels, and bleeding at the site is minimal.

Before discharge from the hospital, the client should be informed of two complications that can occur. A transient alopecia is experienced by some clients 4–12 weeks after heparin therapy. This condition is self-limiting, and no permanent effects occur. Allergic hypersensitivity to heparin can also develop, especially in clients with a personal or family history of allergic conditions.

Clients who have experienced allergic reactions to heparin should be advised to secure a medical identification device that warns of this allergy.

Clients on warfarin. Clients being discharged on maintenance doses of warfarin need extensive instruction to enable them to manage their regimen successfully. Continued medical supervision is necessary, including regular visits to the physician and periodic blood tests. The client must be cautioned to maintain the regimen as prescribed without alterations. The physician must be consulted if the client wishes to discontinue or to add any medications. The anticoagulant dose to be prescribed is established under a set of controlled circumstances in the hospital. If these conditions are altered, serious complications may develop. Addition of medications may increase or decrease the effect of the anticoagulant. Changes often require adjustment of warfarin dosage. Over-the-counter and illegal drugs can alter the client's response to warfarin. Nonprescription preparations often contain aspirin, phenobarbital, or vitamins, which change the therapeutic effect of the anticoagulant. "Downers," which contain phenobarbital, reduce the efficacy of warfarin by increasing its rate of metabolism.

All outpatient clients on warfarin should carry identification information that lists the drug dosage, as well as the names, addresses, and telephone numbers of both client and physician. Clients are cautioned to avoid injury. Electric razors should be used instead of blades. Clients should be reassured that clotting is not abolished, only delayed. Although bleeding will be more persistent than usual and can be troublesome, the client will not exsanguinate rapidly if minor injury occurs. Should the client experience serious injury, bleeding will be persistent. If emergency care personnel are aware of the drug regimen, corrective measures to control the bleeding can be instituted.

Some authorities believe that abrupt cessation of warfarin therapy is followed by a rebound hypercoagulability and a temporary increase in the risk of serious clotting problems. The physician may want to wean the client off warfarin to avoid such an occurrence. Clients should be warned not to discontinue the drug without consulting their physician and to follow the recommended schedule for reducing doses.

The onset of congestive failure increases clients' sensitivity to warfarin. Cardiac clients should be taught to identify early signs and symptoms of this condition and to consult their physicians immediately. The dose of anticoagulant may need to be reduced. All clients should recognize the signs and symptoms indicating toxicity, which must be reported to the physician. These include blood in urine or stools, large "bruises," unusual bleeding from any organ, and back pain, which may indicate retroperitoneal hemorrhage.

Clients on aspirin. Clients receiving aspirin as an antiplatelet agent may not regard this drug as "real" medicine. They may have taken aspirin for years on their own for minor symptoms. Because clients may be conditioned to taking aspirin on an intermittent basis, as needed, they may need to be reminded that it is necessary to take prescription doses regularly. The nurse should emphasize that because aspirin does alter coagulability, it deserves the respect given to any effective medicine. The client may need to be taught about the potential risks and adverse reactions associated with aspirin. The nurse should determine whether the client normally takes aspirin for other symptoms, such as pain or fever. If so, the client should be advised to substitute acetaminophen for aspirin because additional aspirin may decrease the antiplatelet effect. If heartburn or gastric discomfort develops, a buffered or enteric-coated form of aspirin may be recommended.

Evaluation Data required for evaluation include vital signs, color and warmth of extremities, peripheral pulses, a more relaxed appearance on the client's part, and statements by the client indicating that fear and pain have decreased. Improvement in self-image may be evaluated by counting the number of positive and negative comments about self. The success of the teaching plan is judged by client comments indicating that information has been helpful in adapting to the treatment regimen, by the client's increased compliance to the regimen, and by the client's ability to repeat information conveyed during teaching sessions.

Checklist of nursing actions

Before anticoagulant therapy is initiated

☐ Screen clients for risk factors for adverse drug reaction, including excessive bleeding.

☐ Assess client for stress level, anxiety and fear, and knowledge about thromboembolic illness and its treatment.

During anticoagulant therapy

☐ Monitor clients carefully for adverse drug reactions.

☐ Elevate extremities affected by thrombi or emboli to promote venous return and to decrease edema.

☐ Apply heat or cold to affected extremities as ordered.

☐ Administer prescribed analgesics as needed to control pain due to inflammatory reaction to thrombi.

☐ Provide emotional support for fearful clients.

☐ Eliminate unnecessary stressors and assist the client in reducing stress levels through stress management techniques.

When anticoagulant therapy using heparin is prescribed

☐ Before administering the first dose of heparin, ascertain whether clients have been previously exposed to the drug; assess their reaction to it and whether the client is allergic to fish.

☐ Ensure accuracy of heparin dosage; when possible, have another nurse verify the prepared dose.

☐ When heparin is administered by continuous IV infusion, control the dosage by using an IV pump or infusion control device.

☐ Administer subcutaneous injections of heparin in the subcutaneous space of the abdomen; do not aspirate prior to injection or massage the site afterward.

☐ Monitor the client for signs and symptoms of abnormal or excessive bleeding.

☐ Monitor bleeding time or PTT, and thrombocyte levels.

☐ Promote a positive self-image in clients affected by large or numerous ecchymoses.

☐ Protect clients from trauma.

Learning experience 29-1

Examine preparations of heparin available in medication rooms of a local hospital. How many different solution strengths did you find? What is the policy of this institution regarding verification of doses when heparin is administered?

When warfarin is prescribed

☐ Analyze the total drug regimen to identify possible drug interactions with warfarin.

☐ Administer daily doses of warfarin at the same time each day, preferably in the afternoon.

☐ Monitor prothrombin levels reported from blood tests.

Thrombolytic agents

Physiology of clot resolution

Clots within the body are normally dissolved by the following process. Plasminogen and tissue plasminogen activator (tPA) are attracted to the fibrin of existing clots. They react to produce *plasmin*, a fibrinolytic enzyme. Fresh fibrin is degraded by plasmin, resulting in dissolution of a portion of the clot and the release of fibrin-split products and other tissue debris. In large clots, some of the fibrin remains unaffected; this clot residue produces a fibrotic scar. Excess plasmin not used for clot lysis is neutralized in blood by alpha 2-antiplasmin. If plasmin is abundant, this enzyme may be exhausted, allowing blood levels of plasmin to rise. Free blood plasmin then degrades systemic fibrinogen and other coagulation factors (*eg*, V and VIII), producing a systemic anticoagulation (See Fig. 29-5).

Pathology of internal coagulation and clot resolution

The presence of tissue debris, old blood, and purulent exudate stimulates inflammation, promotes infection, and retards healing. Clots that form in the circulatory system obstruct blood flow causing serious damage to tissue deprived of blood. Natural resorption proceeds slowly and tends to produce scars. Acceleration of this process restores circulation, prevents ischemia and tissue necrosis, and reduces fibrous scarring. This, in turn, reduces the permanent damage caused by such conditions as coronary thrombosis, cerebral thrombi, and peripheral arterial emboli.

Three fibrinolytic drugs will be discussed. Streptokinase and UK have been used in the treatment of thromboembolic disease for several years. Tissue plasminogen activator is a relatively new agent (see Table 29-5).

Streptokinase

Streptokinase is an enzyme produced by hemolytic streptococci.

Pharmacodynamics. Streptokinase activates plasminogen, causing an increase in plasmin levels throughout the body. Excessive plasmin reacts with alpha$_2$-antiplasmin (a natural substance that neutralizes plasmin) and degrades fibrinogen, producing a systemic anticoagulant action. Streptokinase also de-

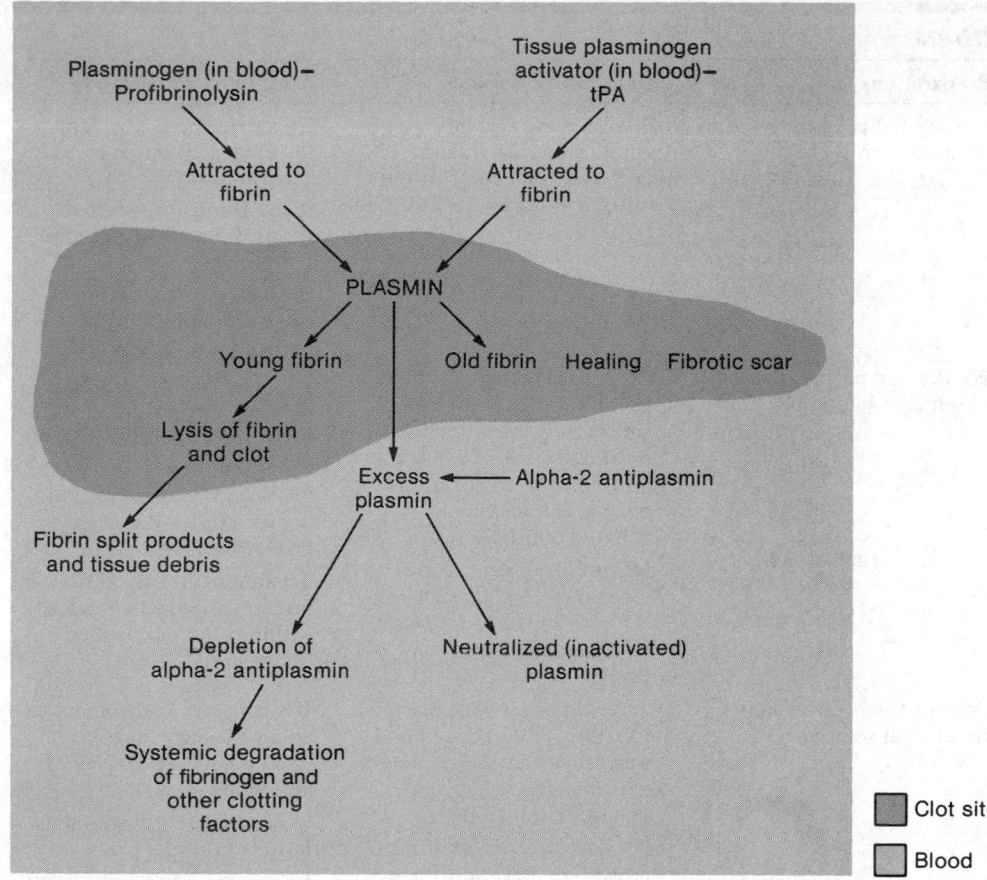

Figure 29-5. Physiologic mechanism of clot dissolution.

creases blood viscosity, decreases erythrocyte aggregation tendency, and alters platelet function.

Pharmacokinetics. Streptokinase may be administered by intracoronary infusion, intra-arterial infusion, or intravenously. Following injection, it has a circulating time of approximately 90 minutes and a duration of action of 24–36 hours. In individuals with prior exposure to the drug, it is rapidly inactivated by antibodies.

Therapeutic uses. Streptokinase is used in the treatment of massive pulmonary emboli, deep vein thrombosis, arterial thrombosis, coronary artery embolus, and arteriovenous cannula occlusion. When administered by intracoronary infusion, the treatment is reported to produce reperfusion of the affected coronary tissue in 60%–75% of cases. Intravenous administration appears to be somewhat less successful (20%–60%) (Rodriguez & Lombardo, 1987).

Adverse reactions. Febrile reactions occur in approximately 30% of clients treated with SK. In most recipients, temperature elevation is less than 40°C (104°F) (McEvoy, 1991, p 818).

Streptokinase is highly antigenic. It may produce allergic reactions characterized by redness, swelling, itching, flushing, nausea, and headache. When antibodies are produced, the recipient is rendered refractory to the drug for several months. Rarely, anaphylaxis occurs when large doses of SK are used in the treatment of thrombi in refractory clients.

The systemic anticoagulant action of SK increases the risk of hemorrhage. Premature resolution of clots allows damaged blood vessels to reopen and to resume bleeding. The client is at high risk for wound hematoma and bleeding. Bleeding during SK therapy is difficult to control.

When ischemic cardiac tissue is reperfused, arrhythmias are likely to develop. The most common reperfusion arrhythmias are accelerated idioventricular rhythm and ventricular extrasystoles, tachycardia, or fibrillation.

Safe use in children and in women during pregnancy or during lactation has not been demonstrated.

Precautions and contraindications. Caution is required if SK therapy is continued after the appearance of allergic reaction or is attempted in refractory clients. Steroids and antihistamines control some, but not all, allergic reactions.

Clients receiving SK must be closely monitored for hemorrhage. Fibrinolytic treatment is contraindicated

Table 29-5. Thrombolytic drugs

Drug names	Preparations	Usual adult dosage	Additional information
alteplase (Activase, tPA, recombinant tissue plasminogen activator)	Powder for preparing parenteral solutions	0.5–0.75 mg/kg body weight, administered as follows: 10% over 1–2 min, the rest (90%) infused over the next 60 min PC: C	This drug does not deplete fibrinogen as much as SK. Treatment for myocardial infarction must be started within 6 hours of onset of symptoms. Coronary reperfusion success rates appear to be higher than those of SK.
streptokinase (SK, Kabikinase)	Powder for preparation of parenteral solutions	*For pulmonary emboli:* 250,000 IU, infused over 30 min *For coronary artery thrombosis: Initially:* 15,000–20,000 IU, infused over 15 sec to 2 min; *maintenance:* 2,000–4,000 IU/min Maximum dosage: Intracoronary: 150,000–500,000 IU; IV: 500,000–1,500,000 IU over 30–60 min PC: B	Fever is the most frequent adverse reaction. SK is less expensive than urokinase. SK is highly antigenic; antibodies render the client refractory to the drug. Treatment for myocardial infarction should be started within 6 hrs of onset of symptoms.
urokinase (UK, Abbokinase)	Powder for preparation of parenteral solutions	For pulmonary embolism: Initially: 4,400 IU/kg body weight over 10 min; maintenance: 4,400 IU/kg body weight/hr for 12 hr For coronary artery thrombosis: 6,000 IU/min for up to 2 hr PC: C	UK is useful for treating clients with high titers (>1,000,000 IU) of SK antibodies. Occasional febrile reactions have been reported. UK is costly to produce and expensive to use in therapeutic amounts. Treatment for myocardial infarction should be started within 6 hrs of onset of symptoms.

KEY: PC = Pregnancy risk category. (The validity of pregnancy categories has not been established. See Chapter 16, p 216.)

for clients at high risk for hemorrhage, such as those with clotting defects, low serum protein, serious liver impairment, active bleeding, recent surgery, peptic ulcer, or recent cerebral vascular accident. Other contraindications include acute cellulitis without suppuration, tuberculosis, bronchopleural fistulas, and SK resistance levels exceeding 1 million international units.

Prophylactic lidocaine infusions may be used to reduce the risk of reperfusion arrhythmias; if arrhythmias occur, they should be aggressively treated with drugs or cardioversion.

Following fibrinolytic therapy, adequate anticoagulation should be instituted to reduce the risk of new clot formation and reocclusion.

Aminocaproic acid is the specific antidote for an overdose of a fibrinolytic agent. (See previous discussion of this drug.)

Urokinase

Urokinase is a trypsinlike serine protease extracted from human urine. It is costly to produce and expensive to use in therapeutic amounts.

Pharmacodynamics. Like SK, UK activates plasminogen, causing an increase in plasmin levels throughout the body. Excessive plasmin reacts with alpha$_2$-antiplasmin (a natural substance that neutralizes plasmin) and degrades fibrinogen, producing a systemic anticoagulant action.

UK does not change erythrocyte aggregation or platelet function.

Pharmacokinetics. Urokinase is administered by intracoronary infusion, intravenously, or by injection into occluded IV catheters. Following absorption, the drug concentrates in the liver and bladder. It has a circulating half-life of about 20 minutes and a duration of action of 12–24 hours. It is excreted in small amounts in bile and urine.

Therapeutic uses. Urokinase is used in the treatment of massive pulmonary emboli, deep vein thrombosis, arterial thrombosis, coronary arterial emboli, and arteriovenous cannula occlusion. It is particularly useful in the treatment of clients who are refractory to SK due to previous exposure and antibody formation.

Adverse reactions. The systemic anticoagulant action of UK increases the risk of hemorrhage. Premature resolution of clots allows damaged blood vessels to reopen and to resume bleeding.

The most frequent adverse reaction to UK is hemorrhage. Hematoma at injection sites and severe spontaneous bleeding may occur. The client is at high risk for wound hematoma and bleeding. Bleeding during UK therapy is difficult to control. Urokinase appears to be nonantigenic.

When ischemic cardiac tissue is reperfused, arrhythmias are likely to develop. The most common reperfusion arrhythmias are accelerated idioventricular rhythm and ventricular extrasystoles, tachycardia, or fibrillation.

Precautions and contraindications. Fibrinolytic treatment is contraindicated for clients at high risk for hemorrhage, such as those with clotting defects, low serum protein, serious liver impairment, active bleeding, recent surgery, peptic ulcer, or recent cerebral vascular accident. Other contraindications include acute cellulitis without suppuration, tuberculosis, and bronchopleural fistulas.

Prophylactic lidocaine infusions may be used to reduce the risk of reperfusion arrhythmias. If arrhythmias occur, they should be aggressively treated with drugs or cardioversion.

Following fibrinolytic therapy, adequate anticoagulation should be instituted to reduce the risk of new clot formation and reocclusion.

Aminocaproic acid is the specific antidote for an overdose of a fibrinolytic agent. (See previous discussion of this drug.)

Tissue plasminogen activator

Tissue plasminogen activator is a naturally occurring trypsinlike serine protease that is now produced in quantity by recombinant DNA techniques.

Pharmacodynamics. When administered within 6 hours of the occurrence of a clot, tPA acts in the presence of thrombin in formed clots. The drug activates plasminogen, increasing local concentrations of plasmin at the clot site. It does not produce systemic anticoagulation or fibrinolysis.

Pharmacokinetics. Tissue plasminogen activator is administered by intracoronary infusion and intravenously. It has a circulating half-life of 5–10 minutes and a duration of action of 25–50 minutes.

Therapeutic uses. Tissue plasminogen activator is used to resolve coronary thromboses and prevent infarction of heart muscle. When infused into the coronary artery, reperfusion success rates (66%–70%) (Rodriguez & Lombardo, 1987) are slightly higher than with SK.

Adverse reactions. The most common complication of tPA therapy is bleeding. However, because it is most active at the site of a clot, tPA does not increase the risk of bleeding as much as SK and UK. It appears to be nonantigenic.

When used alone, the withdrawal of tPA is followed by reocclusion (reformation of clots) in 20%–45% of recipients; this effect appears to be associated with elevated levels of an inhibitor of plasminogen activator.

Precautions and contraindications. The client must be monitored for signs and symptoms of abnormal bleeding. External bleeding may be controlled with dressings soaked in aminocaproic acid, the antidote for tPA. (See previous discussion of aminocaproic acid in this chapter).

Contraindications for the use of tPA include myocardial necrosis, and a history of recent surgery, organ biopsy, cardiopulmonary resuscitation, cerebrovascular accident, aneurysm, pregnancy or childbirth, or bleeding abnormalities. Candidates for tPA treatment must receive treatment as soon as possible after onset of acute chest pain. Quality of therapeutic response is inversely related to delay in treatment. Clots 3 hours or younger respond more readily to fibrinolytics than do older ones. Thrombolytic should be given within 6 hours of onset of signs and symptoms of MI (Olson, 1987), although one study (Deuce of hearts, 1989) indicated that treatment within 24 hours of onset will be beneficial to some degree. Once infarction necrosis is established, use of fibrinolytics is contraindicated.

Anistreplase

Anistreplase (Eminase) is a complex derived from lysplasminogen and SK. It activates anisolated plasminogen SK with effects on the body very similar to those of SK. However, the action of anistreplase is exerted primarily on the thrombus; it has much less systemic effect than does SK.

Anistreplase is a relatively new drug and is very expensive. Its adverse effects are relatively unknown as yet, except for those it has in common with SK. Because this drug is derived from human tissue, it may be less antigenic than is SK.

One study (Altman, 1991) has shown that the three drugs—SK, tPA, and anistreplase—are equally effective in the treatment of people who have had one MI. There was no difference in mortality rates among the three treatment groups, and those treated with SK were less likely to experience a cerebral hemorrhage than were those in the other two groups.

■ Summary
Four proteinaceous enzymes capable of stimulating or accelerating the natural fibrinolytic process are SK, UK, tPA, and anistreplase. They are useful as treatment agents to dissolve dangerous intervascular clots (*eg*, coronary thrombosis and pulmonary emboli) and to clear occlusions from arteriovenous cannulas or IV

infusion lines. They are administered intravenously, intra-arterially, into the coronary artery by way of cardiac catheterization, or into occluded cannulas or intracatheters. Adverse reactions to these drugs include systemic anticoagulation (SK and UK), allergic hypersensitivity with refractoriness to treatment (SK), and hemorrhage.

Nursing management

Nursing implications

Enzyme substances are protein in structure and require careful storage and handling. Drugs should be stored in a cool area. Although it is not usually necessary to refrigerate them, drugs should be refrigerated if room temperatures are above 70° F. When preparing solutions, add the diluent slowly and gently swirl the container (never shake it).

Most drugs dissolve readily in water. Preparations should be dated and used before the recommended period expires. Manufacturers' instructions for reconstitution and storage should be followed carefully.

Proteolytic enzymes may irritate or damage delicate tissues. They should not be allowed to enter the eyes. If accidental contamination occurs, the eyes should be irrigated with copious amounts of tepid water. To ensure that damage has not occurred, the affected individual should be examined promptly by an ophthalmologist.

Nursing process

Assessment Clients who are candidates for thrombolytic therapy are victims of sudden vascular accidents and come to the acute care facility as emergency admissions. The nurse must assess cardiovascular status, pain, and fear.

As much information as possible should be obtained from the client's family or significant other. It is helpful if prescription drugs taken by the client are brought to the health care facility in their original containers. A complete drug history will be needed. The nurse should ask specifically whether the client was taking the drugs as ordered (full dosage at the indicated times and with proper timing in relation to meals). The nurse should also ask about rest/activity cycles and the client's daily routine.

An important fact to establish is the onset time of the client's symptoms. The time elapsed between onset of symptoms and initiation of fibrinolytic therapy crucially affects prognosis. The sooner treatment is begun, the less permanent damage occurs to the tissue.

Determining risk factors for thrombolytic therapy is primarily the physician's responsibility. However, the nurse may be able to gather important information from the family while the physician is examining the client. Contraindications for thrombolytic therapy in-

clude bleeding problems (*eg*, clotting deficiencies and GI bleeding), severe liver disease, recent head trauma, recent sustained cardiopulmonary resuscitation (which may have caused internal injury), pregnancy, hypertension, and recent use of anticoagulants and antiplatelet drugs, including aspirin.

Numerous laboratory tests will be ordered. Baseline values will be needed for plasma fibrinogen, fibrin degradation products, thrombin time, PT, bleeding time, activated partial thromboplastin time, creatine phosphokinase, creatine phosphokinase isoenzymes, complete blood count, and hemoglobin (See Table 29-6).

An assessment should be made of the client's and family's knowledge about the client's condition and especially about the treatment. Fibrinolytic therapy is relatively new and the general public is not as well versed in the use of these drugs as it is about older therapies.

Nursing diagnosis Nursing diagnoses arising from the medical emergency include the following:

> *Pain related to tissue ischemia secondary to thrombi or emboli*
> *High risk for impaired tissue integrity related to ischemia secondary to vascular occlusion*
> *Fear of dying or of amputation*

Diagnoses stemming from the use of fibrinolytic drugs for SK may include:

> *High risk for altered body temperature: fever related to inflammation*
> *High risk for infection related to decreased resistance secondary to surgical wounds and immunosuppression*

Most clients and their families will exhibit

> *Knowledge deficits related to thrombolic disease and its treatment*

Common collaborative problems that should be differentiated from nursing diagnoses include

> *Potential complication: hemorrhage*
> *Potential complication: cardiac arrhythmias*

Planning Goals for treatment include elimination of pain and prevention of tissue damage by restoration of circulation, alleviation or elimination of anxiety and fear, control of fever should it occur, prevention or control of hemorrhage, prevention or control of circulatory shock, correction of reperfusion arrhythmias, reduction in the risk of infection, and alleviation of stress.

Intervention: acute care The nurse should foster the client's trust in the health care facility and its staff. Competent and rapid response to the client's needs and an attitude of warm, personal concern for the client and family promote this therapeutic relation-

Table 29-6. Laboratory tests useful during fibrinolytic treatment

Drugs	Test	Normal range	Effects of drugs	Additional information
streptokinase (SK)	SK antibody level	—	Exposure to SK stimulates production.	If level is <1,000,000 IU, SK treatment is contraindicated.
	Thrombin time (TT)	Control 5 sec (10–15 sec)	Increase (Therapeutic level = 2–5 × premedication baseline)	When drug is discontinued, level should drop to 2× the preinfarction baseline within 3 hr.
	Prothrombin time (PT)	Control 2 sec (13.5–15 sec)	Increase (Therapeutic level = 2–5 × premedication baseline)	When drug is discontinued, level should drop to 2× the preinfarction baseline within 3 hr.
streptokinase and urokinase (UK)	Plasma fibrinogen	0.2–0.4 g/100 ml	Marked decrease	Excess systemic plasmin degrades fibrinogen. Change in fibrinogen is roughly indicative of degree of anticoagulation.
	Fibrin degradation products (fibrin split products)	5 µg/ml	Marked increase	Increase in values reflects the amount of fibrinolysis.
tissue plasminogen activator	Plasma fibrinogen	0.2–0.4 g/100 ml	Decrease	Tissue plasminogen activator has no effect on TT or PT.
	Fibrin degradation products (fibrin split products)	5 µg/ml	Increase	

ship. Until the emergency situation is resolved, it is not possible to counsel the client at length. The client may be assured that the facilities of the institution and skill of the staff will be used to provide the best possible care. Crisis intervention techniques may be useful in assisting the family to cope with the emergency situation. The client's family should be kept informed about the progress of treatment.

For comfort and to facilitate respirations, the client should be placed in a reclining chair or Fowler's position. Oxygen may be ordered to increase delivery of oxygen to the ischemic tissues.

The nurse assesses the client as previously noted and assists in the administration of drugs, such as analgesics, as ordered. Clients with coronary occlusion will need continuous cardiac monitoring.

At least two intravascular infusion lines will be needed: an intracoronary, intra-arterial, or IV line for administering fibrinolytic drugs, and a separate IV line for the collection of blood specimens and administration of other drugs, such as lidocaine. Each line should include an infusion control device, such as an IV pump, to maintain a steady rate of flow at the prescribed dosages. The nurse administers fibrinolytic, antiarrhythmic, anticoagulant, and (nonaspirin) analgesic drugs as ordered.

The nursing staff should be prepared to assist with emergency surgical procedures (embolectomy, cardiac catheterization, coronary artery bypass grafts) if required.

Clients with coronary thrombosis must be closely monitored for changes in cardiac rhythm; arrhythmias are likely to develop when the clot is dissolved and perfusion restored. Cardiac antiarrhythmic drugs, such as lidocaine, should be administered in accordance with established protocols for the treatment of arrhythmias. Fibrinolytics are sometimes used to resolve purulent exudates in body cavities, such as the pleural space. Systemic reactions are minimized if the cavity is drained or aspirated repeatedly. Clients should be observed closely for signs or symptoms of fistula formation, which would require discontinuation of the fibrinolytic therapy. Clients receiving fibrinolytics, especially SK and UK should be watched closely for hemorrhage. Pertinent laboratory tests should be monitored (see Table 29-5). If IV catheters are removed from vascular puncture sites, pressure should be exerted on the sites until a clot forms. This may require 30 minutes or more. To prevent bleeding, the client should be handled gently, and bruising or other trauma should be avoided.

Fever must be controlled in clients with thromboembolic disorders. Oxygen requirements in peripheral tissue are related to temperature, and fever increases ischemia by stimulating tissue metabolism. Antipyretics (acetaminophen rather than aspirin) may be ordered. If fever is high or difficult to control, other methods of cooling the client, such as a hypothermia blanket, may be required.

Convalescence. Following resolution of the clot, fibrinolytic medication is continued briefly to reduce the risk of reocclusion. It is then discontinued and heparin is administered for anticoagulation over 2–3 days. As heparin is withdrawn gradually, the client may receive oral anticoagulants (warfarin, coumadin) or antiplatelet medication (aspirin, dipyridamole). These oral drugs are often continued indefinitely to reduce the risk of reocclusion.

Throughout the period of hospitalization, the nurse intervenes to decrease the risk of infection. Strict aseptic technique is employed with all surgical procedures. Venipuncture or arterial puncture sites should be protected from contamination by surgical dressings. Anti-infective solutions or ointments may be applied to the wound. To support general resistance to infection, the client should be provided with a nourishing diet, adequate fluids, and ample rest and sleep. High stress levels suppress the immune response; the nurse should eliminate unnecessary stressors and assist the client in controlling stress levels.

Client education. Until clients are stabilized and their clots dissolved, clients can cope only with essential information. The staff should explain to the client what is about to happen in terms relating to the client's perceptions of the experience (*ie*, what the client is likely to feel). Information about invasive procedures such as arterial or venous punctures should be given immediately before the procedure occurs. The longer the client anticipates such procedures, the higher the level of fear and stress.

During this period, the family should be kept informed in detail about the treatment and its progress. When the client is incapacitated, permission for treatment may be obtained from the next of kin.

During convalescence, both client and family should be taught (or retaught) about the disease, the treatment provided in the hospital, and the home treatment likely to be prescribed. Self-care measures to ameliorate the underlying condition (exercise, diet, stress management) should be emphasized. If long-term anticoagulant or antiplatelet medication is prescribed, clients need instruction in proper administration of the drug, signs and symptoms of adverse reaction to it, and, in specific terms, what signs and symptoms warrant a report to the physician or nurse.

Evaluation Data required for evaluation include statements by the client related to reduction in pain and anxiety or fear, reduction in general stress levels, angiograms demonstrating dissolution of the obstructive clot, vital signs (including temperature), reports or printouts of electrocardiogram monitoring, and incidence or absence of hemorrhage and infection. The teaching plan is best evaluated by observing self-care after discharge. In the interim, clients may be questioned to determine whether they can repeat to the nurse information conveyed during teaching sessions. (See Example of Nursing Process and Streptokinase Therapy.)

Checklist of nursing actions

☐ Establish a therapeutic relationship characterized by trust in the nursing staff by the client.

☐ Explain to the client procedures to be done in terms of what will be experienced.

☐ Assess clients for pain, decreased tissue perfusion, and anxiety and fear.

☐ Keep the family informed of the client's condition and the progress of treatment.

☐ Position the client to facilitate respirations. Administer oxygen to ameliorate tissue ischemia.

☐ Assist with emergency procedures, including parenteral administration of drugs.

☐ Handle enzymes gently to prevent denaturation.

☐ Store drugs in a cool area (refrigerate if room is excessively warm).

☐ Add diluent slowly and swirl container gently (do not shake).

☐ Date preparations and use before expiration period.

☐ Monitor clients with coronary artery thrombosis for cardiac arrhythmias, especially when coronary circulation is restored.

☐ Observe clients frequently for bleeding.

☐ Check wounds for bloody drainage.

☐ Control fever in clients with tissue ischemia to prevent an increase in tissue metabolism.

☐ Do not allow enzymes to come into contact with the eyes (flush eyes with copious amounts of tepid water if contact occurs).

☐ Observe for the formation of fistulas in clients receiving intercavitary injections.

☐ Observe and record reactions to administration of enzymes.

☐ Teach the client and family self-care measures to promote cardiovascular function and to delay the progress of cardiovascular disease.

To reduce the risk of infection

☐ Maintain strict aseptic techniques for surgical procedures.

☐ Promote rest and good nutrition.

☐ Take measures to limit client stress.

Drugs that enhance peripheral perfusion

Research is in progress on at least three types of pharmacotherapy using drugs with unique mechanisms of action for the treatment of ischemic conditions. One treatment involves using blood treated by two drugs to enhance oxygen release in the capillary; a second employs a stable acellular hemoglobin molecule with enhanced oxygen release; the third uses a drug that increases flexibility of RBCs, making them flow more freely through narrow lumen blood vessels. At this

Example of nursing process and streptokinase therapy

The client is a 54-year-old man admitted to the emergency room with a tentative diagnosis of right femoral artery thromboembolus.

The client has been treated with antiarrhythmics for atrial fibrillation for the past 5 months. One hour prior to admission, he experienced a sharp pain in the right leg. Subsequently, the leg became cold and mottled in appearance.

The right pedal pulse cannot be palpated.

The physician has ordered hypothermia to the right leg and an immediate right femoral arteriogram, with probable fibrinolysis of femoral thromboembolus.

The client appears tense and anxious. He asks the physician, "I'm not going to lose my leg, am I?"

The client states that he has not, to his knowledge, ever been treated with SK.

Assessment data	Nursing diagnosis	Intervention	Goals and outcome criteria
Appearance of tension and anxiety Client's question, "I won't lose my leg, will I?"	Anxiety concerning loss of leg	**Establish** client trust by demonstrating competence and efficiency in the administration of physical care and by expressing a warm concern for the client. **Offer** realistic reassurance by pointing out that the client reached medical care very quickly, that the institution is equipped and staffed to give comprehensive care for problems such as his, and that new drugs are available that are capable of dissolving intravascular clots. Give "coaching" instructions throughout the surgical procedure.	The client will relax and make statements indicating that he is more comfortable and less fearful.
Impending femoral artery arteriogram with fibrinolysis	High risk for altered tissue perfusion related to hemorrhagic shock from blood loss secondary to surgical trauma to the femoral artery and administration of a fibrinolytic drug	During the surgical procedure, **monitor** the client for hemorrhage. At the end of the procedure, **apply** digital pressure to the site of the arterial puncture until bleeding stops; apply a pressure dressing.	Visible loss of blood will be trivial. Vital signs will remain within normal limits.

writing, not all of these drugs have been approved for therapeutic use but they offer exciting indications of possible future developments in the field of cardiovascular pharmacotherapy.

Dimethylsulfoxide and phytic acid

Phytic acid is a natural analog of 2,3-diphosphoglycerate (DPG), which normally occupies a site on the hemoglobin molecule that can either weaken or tighten the bond with oxygen. When phytic acid supplants natural DPG from its binding site, oxygen binds more loosely to hemoglobin and is released more rapidly in the capillary beds. Under normal circumstances, phytic acid is unable to penetrate the cell membrane of the red blood cell. However, when RBCs are exposed simultaneously to phytic acid and dimethyl sulfoxide (DMSO), phytic acid not only crosses the cell membrane, but becomes trapped inside. DMSO readily penetrates cellular membranes and subsequently causes the cells to swell. This increases membrane permeability, allowing penetration by chemicals to which the cell is normally impervious. When phytic acid follows DMSO into the red blood cell, it displaces DMSO, forcing it out of the cell. When the cell is free of DMSO, it shrinks to normal size, trapping the phytic acid inside. Transfusion of blood treated in this way could be very helpful in dealing with such ischemic diseases as acute sickle cell anemia.

Vitamin B₆ analog

A second blood treatment designed to increase oxygen release involves stripping hemoglobin from RBCs and subsequently treating it with an analog of vitamin B_6, causing a permanent linking of the two pairs of subunits in the hemoglobin molecule. This change appears to increase available oxygen tenfold. Such a blood extract could be added to the blood of trauma victims or persons with ischemic emergencies. It also might improve oxygenation of transplant organs during transport.

Pentoxifylline

Pentoxifylline (Trental) is a xanthine derivative used to improve peripheral circulation in clients with vascular insufficiency.

Pharmacodynamics. The mechanism of action of petoxifylline is not well understood. The drug appears to modulate the phosphorylation/dephosphorylation interactions of RBC membrane proteins involved in maintaining the shape of the cell. Effects of the drug include increased flexibility of RBCs, decreased viscosity of whole blood, decreased systemic vascular resistance, improved blood flow, especially in microcirculation, and increased oxygenation of tissues. The magnitude of effect is directly related to the degree of vascular insufficiency, with greatest effect in tissue having impaired circulation and poor oxygenation. Pentoxifylline also inhibits platelet aggregation, and increases fibrinolytic activity.

Pentoxifylline has been reported to increase the duration of activity of ejaculated sperm.

Pharmacokinetics. Pentoxifylline is well absorbed from the GI tract. It undergoes extensive metabolism on first-pass through the liver; only about 10%–40% of oral doses reach the circulation unchanged. Food delays but does not decrease absorption. Distribution of pentoxifylline has not been fully characterized. The drug is secreted in breast milk. Whether or not it crosses the placenta is unknown. Approximately 45% is bound to RBC membranes where it is metabolized (McEvoy, 1991, p 805). The drug is also metabolized by the liver. Elimination is primarily renal; only a small fraction (about 4%) is excreted in feces (McEvoy, 1991, p 806).

Preparations and dosage. Pentoxifylline is available as extended-release, film-coated oral tablets. Usual adult dosage is 400 mg bid to tid, administered with meals.

Therapeutic uses. Pentoxifylline is used as an adjunct in the treatment of intermittent claudication as-

sociated with peripheral vascular disease. Investigationally, it is used in the treatment of sickle cell anemia, cerebrovascular insufficiency, vascular problems secondary to diabetes mellitus, Bell's palsy, and male fertility problems.

Adverse reactions. Pentoxifylline is generally well tolerated. The most frequent adverse reaction is GI upset (incidence 1%–3%), the majority of which is mild (McEvoy, 1991, p 806). Signs and symptoms include dyspepsia, anorexia, nausea, vomiting, bloating, eructation, flatus, dry mouth, thirst, and constipation.

Central nervous system changes also affect a few recipients. Dizziness, headache, tremor, agitation, nervousness, drowsiness, or insomnia may occur.

Incidence of cardiovascular changes is less than 1% (McEvoy, 1991, p 807). Chest pain, angina, arrhythmias (tachycardia), palpitation, flushing, edema, and hypotension have been reported.

Mutagenicity and carcinogenicity of pentoxifylline in humans is unknown. The drug is known to increase the incidence of embryo resorption in pregnant rats. Safety and efficacy in children and in pregnant women is unknown.

Precautions and contraindications. The only contraindication for pentoxifylline is a history of intolerance to the drug or to xanthine derivatives such as caffeine or theophylline. Recipients should be monitored for cardiovascular changes similar to those caused by xanthine compounds.

■ Summary

Pentoxifylline is a hemorrheologic agent used to improve peripheral circulation by increasing the flexibility of the RBC and decreasing blood viscosity. Because it is a relatively new drug, pentoxifylline's toxic and side effects are largely unknown. It does cause (mostly mild) GI upset and CNS changes in a small number of clients.

Nursing management

Nursing implications

When a relatively new drug is prescribed, an important nursing responsibility is the detection and reporting of unusual changes in the client, which may indicate previously unidentified reactions to the chemical. Such reactions are more likely to be recognized when the drug is used (as is pentoxifylline) over a long time. Drug reaction reports are filed with the federal Food and Drug Administration (see Chapter 2).

Pentoxifylline is not marketed in a prompt dosage form; at this writing, the only preparation is a sustained-release oral tablet. Adverse reactions to prompt preparations are more frequent and more severe than to sustained-action forms. Taking the drug with food favors gradual absorption and stable blood levels that further protect the client from adverse reactions.

Nursing process

Assessment Before initiating pentoxifylline treatment, a thorough evaluation of health status is needed to provide a baseline for identification of all drug-induced changes. Of particular importance are the cardiovascular, gastrointestinal, and central nervous systems, which are known to be affected by pentoxifylline. The client should be asked specifically about responses to xanthines, such as caffeine and theophylline.

Nursing diagnosis The client with intermittent claudication will be affected by the following:

> *Impaired physical mobility: limited tolerance of walking related to tissue ischemia secondary to arteriolar vascular disease*
> *Pain: leg pain related to tissue ischemia secondary to arteriolar vascular disease*

When pentoxifylline is prescribed, possible diagnoses include:

> *High risk for altered comfort: dyspepsia, nausea, bloating, dizziness, headache, nervousness, or agitation related to drug side effects*
> *High risk for constipation related to drug side effects*
> *Sleep pattern disturbance: insomnia related to CNS stimulation secondary to xanthine medication*

Clients will have a knowledge deficit about the new drug pentoxifylline. They may also have a

> *Knowledge deficit concerning cardiovascular disease and the regimen for its treatment*
> *High risk for ineffective management of therapeutic regimen related to knowledge deficits, lack of perceived benefits, and economic difficulties*

Planning Goals for treatment include increased tolerance for walking, decreased pain when walking, prevention or prompt detection and treatment of undesirable GI and CNS changes, improved sleep and rest, and elimination of knowledge deficits.

Intervention The nurse should evaluate the client regularly for changes in status, especially those resembling toxic or side effects to xanthine drugs, indicating possible reactions to pentoxifylline. Unusual reactions should be reported to the Food and Drug Administration.

The client should be encouraged to increase gradually the distance walked each day. A route should be chosen that allows periodic sitting. The client should be advised to rest until pain disappears, if leg pain occurs. The client may choose to carry a portable seat; some canes have built-in fold down seats. Alternatively, exercise may be taken in a local shopping mall; some malls are promoting such use during nonbusiness hours. Improved tolerance to walking may be anticipated as a result of the hemorrheologic actions of pentoxifylline.

A comprehensive plan for teaching the client about pentoxifylline should be prepared and implemented. The nurse should assess the client's knowledge of arteriolar vascular disease and hygienic measures for its treatment (diet, exercise). The teaching plan should provide for reinforcement of previous teaching about arteriolar vascular disease and its treatment regimen (diet, exercise, elimination of smoking).

Client education. The client should be informed about known reactions to pentoxifylline and advised of the likelihood that effects remain as yet undetected. Any unusual changes in health status should be reported to health care personnel.

To minimize the risk of adverse GI changes, the nurse should advise the client to eliminate xanthines from the diet, increase fiber and fluid intake, avoid foods known to produce intestinal gas, promote a regular habit for defecation, and avoid foods known to cause GI discomfort. If bloating and flatulence develop, the nurse may suggest the use of activated charcoal or an over-the-counter preparation containing simethicone, both of which substances absorb gas. The client should be taught measures to promote sleep. These may include quiet activity and a relaxing, warm bath. The bedroom should be free of stimuli such as noise and bright light. Soothing music may also be helpful. A regular routine for preparing for sleep will reinforce a sleep response.

If discomfiting GI or CNS side effects persist, the nurse may suggest omitting the midday dose of pentoxifylline and consult with the physician for changes in the regimen.

If abstinence from smoking is a problem, the client may be referred to a smoker's clinic for help.

Evaluation Data required for evaluation include the distance walked before onset of leg pain; client reports concerning level of comfort; incidence and severity of adverse drug effects; dietary and smoking habits; and the ability of the client to repeat to the nurse information conveyed during teaching sessions.

Checklist of nursing actions

When pentoxifylline is prescribed
- [ ] Evaluate the client regularly for therapeutic and adverse reactions to pentoxifylline.
- [ ] Advise the client to increase duration of walking gradually.
- [ ] Provide the client with facts about pentoxifylline, its therapeutic effects, and the recommended regimen for its use.
- [ ] Teach clients signs and symptoms of adverse GI

and CNS drug reactions, as well as self-care measures to prevent them or reduce their severity.

☐ Report to the federal Food and Drug Administration unusual changes in clients that could indicate previously unrecognized effects of pentoxifylline.

☐ If adverse drug reactions persist despite hygienic measures to alleviate them, advise the client to omit the midday dose of pentoxifylline and consult with the physician.

References

Adler E, Benjamin SB, Zimmerman HJ. (1986). Cholestatic hepatic injury related to warfarin exposure. *Arch Intern Med, 146,* 1837–1839.

Altman LK. (1991). Cheapest heart attack drug found to be safest. *The New York Times,* March 4, 1991.

Deuce of hearts. (1989). *Nursing 89, 19(2),* 81.

Ginsberg JS, Hirsh J. (1989). Anticoagulants during pregnancy. *Annu Rev Med 40,* 79–86.

Kappa J, et al. (1987). Heparin-induced platelet activation in sixteen surgical patients: Diagnosis and management. *J Vasc Surg 5,* 101–109 (January).

Laster J, et al. (1989). Reexposure to heparin of patients with heparin-associated antibodies. *J Vasc Surg, 9,* 677–682 (May).

McEvoy GK. (1991). *Drug information 1991,* pp 779–824. Bethesda: American Society of Hospital Pharmacists.

Olson AR. (1987). What you should know about thrombolytic therapy. *Nursing 87, 17(12),* 52–55 (December).

Rodriguez SW, Lombardo RR. (1987). Thrombolytic therapy for MI; for CE credit. *American Journal of Nursing, 87,* 631.

Rodriguez SW, Reed RL. (1987). Thrombolytic therapy for MI. *American Journal of Nursing, 87,* 632–640.

Schuster G, Lewis G. (1987). Clinical significance of hematuria in patients on anticoagulant therapy. *J Urol, 137,* 923–925 (May).

Steering Committee of the Physicians' Health Study Research Group. (1989). Final report on the aspirin component of the ongoing Physicians' Health Study. *N Engl J Med, 321,* 129–135 (July 20).

A two-pronged attack on intermittent claudication. (1984). *Nursing 84, 84(12),* 22.

Walsh A. (1989). Anticoagulant therapy for aggressive dementia patients (letter). *Am J Psychiatr 146,* 278–279 (February).

Warfarin therapy revised. (1986). *Nursing 86, 16(5),* 24.

Weinberg AC, Lieskovsky G, McGehee WG, Skinner DG. (1983). Warfarin necrosis of the skin and subcutaneous tissue of the male external genitalia. *J Urol, 130,* 352–354.

Bibliography

Adler E, Benjamin SB, Zimmerman HJ. (1986). Cholestatic hepatic injury related to warfarin exposure. *Arch Intern Med, 146,* 1837–1839.

Anderson J. (1991). *A double-blind randomized comparison of anistreplase and alteplase in acute myocardial infarction: Coronary patency results from the TEAM-3 study.* Paper presented at the 40th Annual Scientific Session of the American College of Cardiology, Atlanta, GA.

Aspirin and the second heart attack. (1986). *University of California, Berkeley Wellness Letter, 2(6),* 1.

Bangs NU, et al. (1989). Thrombolytic therapy in acute myocardial infarction. *Annu Rev Pharmacol Toxicol 29,* 323–341.

Blanck Z, et al. (1990). Thrombolysis with recombinant tissue plasminogen activator in late saphenous vein graft thrombosis. *Am Heart J 119(4),* 952–953 (April).

Braun A. (1991). Drugs that dissolve clots. *RN 54(6),* 56 (June).

Collen D, et al. (1988). Thrombolytic therapy. *Annu Rev Med, 39,* 405–423.

Cowan R. (1989). Fortifying a protein through family ties. *Science News, 136,* 23 (July 8)

*Cyganski JM, Donahue JA, Heaton JS. (1987). The case for the heparin flush. *American Journal of Nursing, 87,* 796–797.

Davidson J, et al. (1988). Immunology of a serum sickness/vasculitis secondary to streptokinase used for acute myocardial infarction. *Clin Exp Rheumatol, 6,* 381–384 (October–December).

Edwards DD. (1988). Searching for the better clot-buster. *Science News, 133,* 230 (April 9).

Fackelmann K. (1991). Prime-time clot-busting. *Science News, 140,* 334 (November 23).

Gilman AG, Goodman LS, Rall TW, Murad F. (1990). Goodman and Gilman's *The pharmacological basis of therapeutics.* New York: Pergamon Press.

Guyton A. (1991). *Textbook of medical physiology,* 7th ed. Philadelphia: WB Saunders.

Hennekens CH, Buring JE. (1988). Aspirin and risk of cardiovascular disease. *Rational Drug Therapy, 22(11),* 1–7 (November).

Hirsch J, et al. (1986). A therapeutic range for oral anticoagulant. *Chest, 89(2),* 11S–14S (Suppl, February).

Hyers TM, et al. (1986). Antithrombotic therapy for venous thromboembolic disease. *Chest 89(2),* 26S–35S (Suppl, February).

Killing the cure: The problem of t-PA inhibitors. (1988). *American Journal of Nursing, 88(8),* 1061 (August).

*Krokosky NJ, Vanscoy GJ. (1989). Running an anticoagulation clinic. *American Journal of Nursing, 89(10),* 1304–1306 (October).

Marder VJ, Sherry S. (1988). Thrombolytic therapy: Current Status. *N Engl J Med, 318(23),* 1512–1520.

Meyer J, et al. (1989). Randomized clinical trial of daily aspirin therapy in multi-infarct dementia: A pilot study. *J Am Geriatr Soc, 37,* 549–555 (June).

*Passannante A, Macik G. (1988). Case report: The heparin flush syndrome: A cause of iatrogenic hemorrhage. *Am J Med Sci, 296,* 71–73 (July).

Pauker SG, et al. (1986). A decision analytic view of anticoagulant prophylaxis for thromboembolism in heart disease. *Chest 89(2),* 99S–106S (Suppl, February).

Peritoneal catheter: Patency issue. (1990). *Nursing 90, 20(7),* 30 (July).

Peterson P, et al. (1989). Dysrhythmia stroke risk warrants warfarin. *RN, 52(4),* 139 (April).

*Piercy S. (1987). Urokinase for pediatrics. *Nursing 87, 17(3),* 5.

Raskob GE, et al. (1988). Heparin therapy for venous thrombosis and pulmonary embolism. *Blood Rev, 2,* 251–258.

Resnekov L. (1986). Antithrombotic agents in coronary artery disease. *Chest, 89(2),* 54S–67S (Suppl, February).

Resnekov L. (1987). Antiplatelet effects of aspirin and dipyridamole. *JAMA, 258,* 842 (August 14).

Rizzoni W, et al. (1988). Heparin-induced thrombocytopenia and thromboembolism in the postoperative period. *Surgery, 103,* 470–476 (April).

*Rodriguez SW, Lombardo RR. (1987). Thrombolytic therapy for MI: For CE credit. *American Journal of Nursing, 87,* 631.

Rodriguez SW, Reed RL. (1987). Thrombolytic therapy for MI. *American Journal of Nursing, 87,* 632–640.

Simmons ML. (1989). Thrombolytic therapy in acute myocardial infarction. *Annu Rev Med, 40,* 181–200.

Smith P, et al. (1990). The effect of warfarin on mortality and reinfarction after myocardial infarction. *N Engl J Med, 323,* 147 (July 19).

Soff G, Kadin M. (1987). Tocainide-induced reversible agranulocytosis and anemia. *Arch Intern Med, 147,* 598–599.

Solomon J. (1987). An enzyme that fights blood clots. *RN, 50(1),* 68.

*Swithers CM. (1988). Tools for teaching about anticoagulants. *RN, 51(1),* 57–58 (January).

Topol E, et al. (1987). Community hospital administration of intravenous tissue plasminogen activator in acute myocardial infarction: Improved timing, thrombolytic efficacy and ventricular function. *J Am Coll Cardiol, 10,* 1173–1177 (December).

Vanscoy G, Gyi F. (1988). A new era in warfarin therapy. *US Pharmacist, 13,* H24–H30 (April).

Walker MG. (1987). Subcutaneous calcium heparin in treatment of established acute deep vein thrombosis of the legs: A multicenter prospective randomized trial. *Br Med J, 294,* 1189.

*Warfarin therapy revised. (1986). *Nursing 86, 16(5),* 24.

Warkentin TE, Kelton JG. (1989). Heparin-induced thrombocytopenia. *Annu Rev Med 40,* 31–44.

Weiss R. (1989). New therapies brighten stroke horizon. *Science News 136,* 292 (November 4).

Wessler S, Gitel SN. (1986). Pharmacology of heparin and warfarin. *J Am Coll Cardiol, 8(6),* 10B–20B (December).

*Wilson V. (1991). Action STAT! Complications of thrombolytic therapy. *Nursing 91, 21(1),* 41 (January).

* Recommended for further reading.

Drugs affecting the gastrointestinal system

7

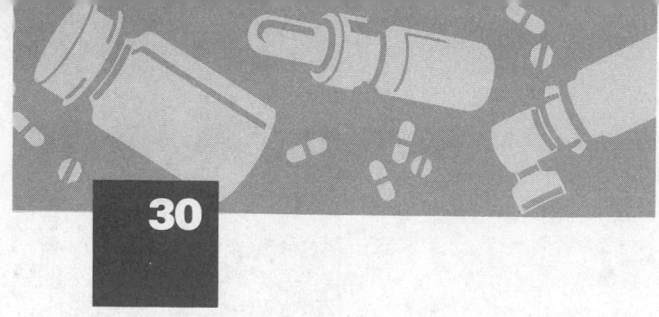

30

Agents affecting the upper gastrointestinal tract

Although healthy persons have little need for most gastrointestinal (GI) drugs, large quantities of non-prescription drugs are purchased over-the-counter for self-medication. Some of these products are harmless but others cause more health problems than they cure. With no other group of over-the-counter drugs is consumer education more needed than with GI preparations.

Drugs affecting the upper GI tract (including the stomach and proximal portion of the duodenum) are discussed in this chapter. (Drugs affecting the lower GI tract are discussed in Chapter 31.)

Most drugs affecting the upper GI tract promote digestion, prevent damage to susceptible tissues, and alleviate symptoms. Some of these agents are valuable in treating primary pathology (notably, peptic ulcers).

Agents used for the mouth

The American public is besieged by the media with advertisements implying that failure to use special cleansers in the mouth will lead to social ostracism and sexual unattractiveness. This may sell a lot of toothpaste and mouthwash but the products endorsed do not necessarily eliminate undesirable odors.

Physiology of the upper GI tract

The GI tract is designed to be self-cleaning, under "natural" (*ie*, primitive) circumstances. The flow of saliva, amounting to about a liter a day, and the washing action of ingested fluids tend to wash food particles, as well as other materials down the tract into the stomach. The consumption of raw fruits and vegetables enhances this function by mechanically cleaning tooth surfaces and stimulating the flow of secretions. (Saliva also exerts a mild antibacterial action.) Under these conditions, breath odors are not likely to come from the mouth or nasopharynx. However, certain foods (onions, garlic, leeks) can cause odors because aromatic flavors are absorbed from the intestines and subsequently excreted by the lungs.

Pathology of the upper GI tract

Diets in modern, developed societies rarely follow primitive patterns. Cooking and other food processing tend to decrease fiber content and make foods less abrasive. Teeth are not subjected to as much scouring action and are not effectively cleaned by the mechanical process of chewing. In addition, cooked foods tend to have a pasty consistency and adhere to teeth and other oral tissues. Removal of food particles requires brushing and rinsing after eating. Modern diets also promote the growth of plaque-producing microorganisms in the mouth.

Plaque and periodontitis

Plaque is a stony, adherent deposit on teeth composed of colonies of bacteria. More than 1,000 strains of microorganisms have been identified as plaque components. These bacteria develop in an organized sequence, producing a complex bacterial ecosystem.

Generally, gram-positive organisms colonize the surface of the teeth first; gram-negative organisms appear later. The various organisms coaggregate, binding together and cementing the whole mass to the tooth surface. This dense matrix, in turn, produces a low oxygen environment that favors the growth of anaerobic organisms (Miller, 1986).

Progressing toward the root of the tooth, plaque extends under the soft tissues of the gums, which become irritated. Stomatitis and periodontitis follow. This process is a major cause of tooth loss, due to suppurative infection of the soft tissues anchoring the teeth to the jawbone. Certain bacteria in plaque (*eg*, *Streptococcus mutagens*) also create dental caries, another cause of tooth loss.

The process of plaque formation is enhanced by sugars that provide food for bacterial growth and that are involved in the process of coaggregation. The presence of calcium ions tends to favor plaque formation, whereas the presence of magnesium tends to inhibit it.

Halitosis

Although some breath odors stem from retained secretions, crusts, and exudates in the mouth, these are temporary and can be controlled by simple hygienic measures. Other odors denote excretion by the lungs of alcohol, tobacco smoke, or substances ingested with foods (as noted previously). Diseases that cause breath odors include periodontitis, infections of the respiratory tract (*eg*, pharyngitis, tonsillitis, peritonsillar abscess, diphtheria, and bronchitis), ketoacidosis (in uncontrolled diabetes and in rapid weight loss), liver failure, and uremia.

Dentifrices

Toothpastes contain a variety of ingredients designed to help clean the teeth, to provide a certain consistency in the product, and to please the senses. Pumice, precipitated calcium carbonate, and milk of magnesia are among the abrasives used. Soap and alcohol aid in cleansing. Glycerin, propylene glycol, and abrasive compounds combine to produce the pasty consistency desired. Sweeteners and flavoring agents enhance the taste, whereas dyes add color and eye appeal.

Fluoride toothpastes and solutions

Some commercial dentifrices contain a fluorine compound, such as stannous fluoride or sodium monofluorophosphate. Fluoride solutions are also applied topically to teeth by rinsing. In some communities, fluorine is added to drinking water to reduce the incidence of dental caries.

Pharmacodynamics. The mechanisms of action of fluorides in reducing tooth decay are not fully understood. Fluorine ions are incorporated into the apatite crystal of teeth and bone. They stabilize the crystal, forming fluoroapatite, which is less soluble in an acid medium than hydroxyapatite, and thereby increases resistance of tooth enamel to acid and to the development of caries. Fluorides also act to desensitize exposed root surfaces of teeth.

Pharmacokinetics. Little information is available concerning the pharmacokinetics of topically applied fluoride. Because these preparations have demonstrated effectiveness in reducing tooth decay, they probably react with the exposed tooth enamel to which they are applied. Fluorides that are ingested are absorbed systemically and are incorporated into the crystalline structure of bone and growing teeth.

Dosage. Studies have shown that at levels of 1–2 mg/l of drinking water, fluoride helps fight tooth decay. Presently, the Environmental Protection Agency recommends a ceiling on fluoride concentrations in drinking water of 1.4–2.4 mg/l. Clients using fluoridated water for drinking should not take fluoride tablets as a dietary supplement.

Therapeutic uses. Preparations containing fluorides (rinsing solutions, toothpastes) are used to decrease the incidence of tooth decay in children and to desensitize exposed root surfaces.

Adverse reactions. When ingested in excessive amounts, fluorides can cause mottling of tooth enamel. Discoloration ranges from faint white flecks to brown spots; the enamel becomes roughened with advanced fluorosis. Bone is also affected; prolonged fluorosis may cause osteosclerosis.

Allergic reactions have been reported. Signs and symptoms include skin rash, stomatitis, and GI or respiratory dysfunction.

Moderate to severe fluorosis has been shown in as many as 40% of children exposed to drinking water fluoridated at the level of 4.0 mg/l (Fluoride proposal draws criticism, 1985). People at high risk of fluorosis include those who must maintain a high fluid intake (diabetics, kidney stone formers, women with recurring cystitis).

Precautions and contraindications. Oral rinsing solutions are not generally used in children younger than 6 years of age because very young children usually cannot perform the proper rinsing procedure. The solutions are contraindicated for persons with allergic sensitivity to them.

■ Summary

Dentifrices are substances used to facilitate cleaning of teeth and other oral surfaces. Preventing plaque formation is the most important goal of oral hygiene. Toothpaste containing fluorides also increase the resistance of tooth enamel to caries and decay. Excessive fluoride intake causes mottling and roughening of teeth, and osteosclerosis.

Nursing management

Nursing implications

The purpose of oral hygiene is to remove crusts, food residues, and bacteria from teeth and other oral surfaces. Secretions may form crusts during the night when saliva flow is decreased and bacterial growth is accelerated, especially in mouth breathers. Food, especially sugars and starches, promotes the growth of microorganisms and the formation of plaque. Bacteria produce acids that dissolve tooth enamel, causing cavi-

ties and promoting decay. A program of careful and frequent oral hygiene can significantly decrease the incidence and severity of dental caries and periodontitis, as well as freshen the mouth and breath.

Fluoridated toothpastes and topical rinses are valuable adjuncts in preventing tooth decay. The Council on Dental Therapeutics of the American Dental Association has stated that certain toothpastes containing fluorides are effective in reducing the incidence of dental caries. However, if fluoride intake (from drinking water or dietary supplements in tablet form) is adequate, these toothpastes may be superfluous. How and when oral hygiene is performed may be more important than the substance used for the procedure.

Brushing technique should be designed to loosen material from the surface of the teeth, gums, and tongue. The free debris is then rinsed from the mouth. A pulsating stream of water (such as that produced by *WaterPik* oral hygiene appliances) removes particles that may remain behind when oral "swishes" are the only rinsing measure. Oral hygiene should be performed after each meal or snack and before retiring for sleep. At times, when this is impossible or inconvenient the snack or meal should end with an apple or other crisp chewable food, and the mouth rinsed thoroughly.

An inexpensive and effective toothpowder can be made by mixing equal parts of salt and sodium bicarbonate. This preparation is very economic, cleans well, neutralizes mouth acids, and stimulates salivation. Although it lacks the pleasant flavor and appearance of commercial toothpaste, the taste is not offensive.

Although oral hygiene will retard the development of plaque, it cannot remove already developed plaque from teeth. This requires scraping and scaling by a dentist or dental hygienist, a procedure that should be performed at least every 6 months. Clients in whom plaque formation is rapid should have teeth professionally cleaned more frequently. Plaque formation is accelerated by carbohydrates, especially sugars, and the calcium ion. It is inhibited by the presence of magnesium.

For clients with active disease (periodontitis or caries), antiseptic mouthwashes (those containing sodium benzoate or benzoic acid) help reduce the oral microscopic flora. Hydrogen peroxide mouthwash solution is also antibacterial but prolonged use can foster the development of "hairy tongue," an unsightly fungus growth. (See Chapter 27 for more information on hydrogen peroxide.)

Oral hygiene will not affect halitosis caused by ingestion or inhalation of substances that are excreted via the lungs. These include tobacco smoke, alcohol, onions, and garlic. Halitosis that does not resolve with avoidance of offending substances and conscientious hygienic measures may indicate a medical problem.

Vincent's angina, stomatitis, oropharyngeal and lung abscess cause bad breath of relatively short duration.

Long-term symptoms may arise from catabolic metabolism (*eg*, in weight reduction regimens that produce ketosis) or from carcinoma in the mouth or respiratory tract. Intermittent halitosis can be caused by gingivitis, oropharyngeal diverticulum (which traps food particles that then decompose), nasal discharge, rhinitis, foreign body in the nose, sinusitis with postnasal drip, infection (in the throat, tonsils, adenoids, and lungs), or lung cancer.

Nursing process

Assessment Risk factors for dental plaque and caries include inadequate fluoride intake, impaired manual dexterity which interferes with good oral hygiene, high intake of carbohydrates (especially sugars), and high calcium intake (either dietary or medicinal). Clients should be questioned specifically about use of fluoridated water, fluoride tablets, fluoridated toothpastes, and calcium supplements. Examination of the mouth may reveal cavities in the teeth and crusts or discolored plaque. Colorless plaque may be revealed by chewing a tablet that stains plaque a bright color.

Nursing diagnosis Nursing diagnoses related to dental disease may include the following:

> *Impaired tissue integrity: inflammation of the gums related to plaque formation secondary to inadequate oral hygiene*
> *Body image disturbance: impaired self-image related to halitosis, dental decay, or multiple fillings secondary to inadequate oral hygiene*
> *Self-care deficit: inability to perform effective oral hygiene related to impaired manual dexterity secondary to arthritis, paralysis, or paresis*

Clients using fluoride supplements may be affected by the following:

> *Impaired tissue integrity: roughened and discolored tooth enamel related to fluorosis secondary to excessive ingestion of toothpaste, rinsing solutions, or dietary supplements containing fluorine*
> *Impaired tissue integrity: skin rash related to allergic reaction secondary to exposure to fluorine*

Many clients will have a knowledge deficit about oral hygiene and prevention of dental caries and periodontitis.

Planning Goals of treatment include improving oral hygiene, preventing dental caries and periodontitis, increasing or decreasing fluorine intake, and educating the client about good oral hygiene.

Intervention The nurse may refer the client to a dentist or dental hygienist for instruction in proper techniques for oral hygiene, or the nurse may demonstrate these techniques and instruct the client directly. Clients who are unable to perform oral hygiene because of impaired manual dexterity may employ aids such as a jet spray (WaterPik) appliance, an interdigital stimulator (StimUdent), or a dental floss holder. When clients are unable to perform oral care, the nursing staff carries out this care.

Client education. An optimum regimen for oral hygiene should include thorough brushing after each meal or snack (using salt and soda powder or a fluoride toothpaste), flossing twice a day to remove particles from between teeth, and regular professional cleaning by a dentist or dental hygienist. Clients with conditions requiring sodium-restricted diets (*eg*, hypertension, congestive heart failure) should not use salt and soda toothpowder because some of it may be swallowed during use. Dietary fluoride supplements may be recommended for clients in areas where water is low in fluoride. These supplements should not be used by people whose drinking water is fluoridated. Clients receiving calcium supplements for the control of osteoporosis should be warned that plaque will probably form more rapidly because of increased concentrations of calcium ions in the saliva.

Clients using fluoridated drinking water and dietary supplements containing fluorine should be warned that such combinations can result in excessive fluorine intake, with subsequent damage to teeth and bones.

Evaluation Data required for evaluation include cleanliness of the mouth after oral hygiene and the incidence or absence of dental caries, plaque, gingivitis, and periodontitis.

Checklist of nursing actions

- [ ] To reduce the incidence of tooth decay, recommend regular, thorough cleaning of the teeth, using either fluoride toothpaste or salt and soda toothpowder.
- [ ] Recommend regular professional cleaning by a dentist or dental hygienist.
- [ ] Recommend the use of a jet spray appliance, interdigital stimulator, or a dental floss holder to assist in oral hygiene when the client's manual dexterity is impaired.
- [ ] When clients are unable to perform oral care, clean their mouths as part of regular nursing care.

Mouthwashes and gargles

Most solutions used in the mouth and throat exert a mechanical washing action on, or apply heat to, the tissues. A few are chemically active. Their effects depend on the presence or absence of foreign material in the oropharynx, the turbulence of the fluid flow with which they are applied, and the length of time they are in contact with the tissues.

Oxidizing agents

Among the oxidizing antiseptics used to clean or treat the mouth are sodium perborate, hydrogen peroxide, and potassium permanganate.

Pharmacodynamics. Oxidizing agents aid in cleansing by stimulating secretion of saliva and by breaking down foreign material. In addition, hydrogen peroxide exerts an effervescent action that mechanically removes debris.

Therapeutic uses. Mouthwashes and gargles are often prescribed to aid in cleansing, to reduce the microscopic flora of the mouth and oropharynx, and to soothe and relieve discomfort. Prior to the development of antibiotics, potassium permanganate was used to treat oral infections.

Adverse reactions. Prolonged use of hydrogen peroxide mouthwash can produce "hairy tongue," a fungus growth that disappears spontaneously when use of the disinfectant is discontinued. Potassium permanganate coats the membranes, and can cause a persistent purple discoloration.

Ingestion of these solutions may cause toxicity. The release of concentrated oxygen can damage tissues; if fresh wounds are present in the tissues, oxidizing agents may break down the clot, causing fresh bleeding.

Precautions and contraindications. Only fresh hydrogen peroxide solutions should be used because in the presence of air and light, this compound breaks down, releasing its oxygen and leaving a residue of plain water. Mouthwashes and gargles should be expectorated; ingestion should be avoided.

Surfactants

Proprietary preparations marketed as mouth cleansers include Cepacol, Chloraseptic, and Listerine. All are available as solutions; Cepacol and Chloraseptic are also marketed as lozenges. These agents usually contain a surfactant, aromatic oils, and antiseptics.

Pharmacodynamics. Surfactants aid in cleansing by reducing the surface tension of fluid in the mouth. Aromatic oils stimulate the salivary glands and act as flavoring agents that mask odors. Antiseptics are capable of inhibiting or killing pathogenic microorganisms but may not effectively reduce plaque formation because the minimum time required for chemical antisepsis exceeds the normal period of contact between the agents and the tissues.

Mouthwashes mask odors for only a limited time, usually 15–30 minutes.

Pharmacokinetics. Mouthwashes and gargles are intended to be applied topically. There is probably little or no systemic absorption through the mucous membranes. Lozenges dissolve in the mouth and are gradually swallowed. Information regarding their absorption or metabolic fate is not readily available.

Therapeutic uses. Mouthwashes, gargles, and surfactant lozenges are used to aid in cleaning the mouth, in reducing the microscopic flora of the mouth, and in soothing and relieving local discomfort. The public employs these agents to freshen the mouth and to reduce offensive breath odors.

Antiseptic and antifungal mouthwashes may relieve candida stomatitis sometimes seen in denture wearers (DaPaola, 1987). Mouthwash has also been used as a perineal deodorant.

Adverse reactions. Some ingredients in mouthwashes and gargles (*eg*, alcohol and antiseptics) can cause toxicity when ingested. Any of the ingredients may cause adverse reactions when ingested. Some aromatic oils are pharmacologically active. Surfactants may act as stool softeners or laxatives. The toxic potential of ingesting small amounts of these substances is unknown. Solutions containing high concentrations of alcohol tend to dry the mouth and inhibit secretion of saliva.

Use of these agents to reduce breath odors may cause the client to delay seeking medical attention to determine the cause of persistent odors, which may be symptomatic of serious systemic disease.

Phenol, an ingredient in Chloraseptic, can cause painless ulcerations with excessive use.

Precautions and contraindications. Mouthwashes and gargles should be expectorated: ingestion should be avoided. Use of lozenges should not exceed the recommendations specified on the product label. Medicated preparations and those containing alcohol should be tightly secured to prevent accidental ingestion, which can cause serious toxicity, especially in small children.

Antiplaque mouthwash: chlorhexidine gluconate

Chlorhexidine gluconate (Peridex) is an antibacterial mouthwash available only by prescription.

Pharmacodynamics. Chlorhexidine gluconate is microbicidal in action, and affects both aerobic and anaerobic bacteria. Its use decreases oral bacteria count.

Pharmacokinetics. Chlorhexidine gluconate is intended as a washing agent. Following use, it is expectorated. About 30% of its active ingredient is retained in the oral cavity where it is slowly released into the oral fluids. When ingested, less than 1% of chlorhexidine gluconate is absorbed from the GI tract and subsequently excreted in urine. The rest passes unabsorbed into the feces.

Therapeutic uses. Chlorhexidine gluconate is used in the treatment of gingivitis. Following professional removal of plaque (prophylaxis), one-half ounce of a 0.12% solution is prescribed for use twice daily, following tooth brushing.

Adverse reactions. Local reaction to chlorhexidine gluconate is characterized by irritation and superficial desquamation. The solution does stain teeth and other oral surfaces but the discoloration can be removed by dental prophylaxis. Discoloration of dentures or other oral prostheses is difficult to correct. Using this mouthwash may increase the formation of supragingival calculus formation. Systemic allergic reactions have been reported.

Precautions and contraindications. Chlorhexidine gluconate is contraindicated for individuals with allergic hypersensitivity to it. Clinical efficacy and safety during pregnancy and safety for pediatric use have not been established.

Clients for whom this antimicrobial mouthwash has been prescribed should be cautioned not to swallow the solution.

Proteolytic enzyme

A useful agent for removing debris from the mouths of ill clients is papaya juice, which contains a proteolytic enzyme. It may be applied with a sponge or Toothette and is nontoxic, even if ingested. Papaya juice is available from health food stores.

Artificial saliva

Some clients are unable to secrete enough saliva to keep the mouth comfortable. Risk factors for dry mouth include dentures, mouth breathing, radiation therapy or surgery involving the parotid glands, use of anticholinergic medications, and Sjogren's syndrome. Solutions designed to replace saliva should be moderately viscous and contain electrolyte concentrations similar to natural saliva. Commercial saliva substitutes include Orex, Moi-Stir, and Xerolube.

Cetylpyridinium chloride

Active research is underway to find substances that will be effective inhibitors of plaque formation when used as mouthwashes. One promising compound, cetylpyridinium chloride, is a quarternary ammonia compound. When used twice daily as a rinse, it reduces plaque and decreases the severity of gingivitis in adults. However, the solution has an unpleasant taste and is not well tolerated. Its use has not been approved by the Food and Drug Administration.

■ **Summary**
Mouthwashes and gargles exert a mechanical washing action and apply heat to tissues. Their

Learning experience 30-1

Examine the dentifrices and vitamin preparations offered for sale in a local drug store. Which preparations contain fluorides? Ask the pharmacist what recommendations are made to customers seeking advise on supplementing their children's diets with fluorine compounds.

effect depends on the foreign material present, the turbulence that accompanies their application, and the length of time they are in contact with the tissues. The anti-infective properties of some solutions inhibit the growth of microorganisms that play a role in the formation of plaque and dental caries.

Styptics

Certain strong astringents are applied to the tissues of the mouth or lips by the lay public to treat "cold sores" or "cankers." Powdered alum and styptic "pencils" are two forms of such agents. The latter is a slender cylinder of solid aluminum sulfate, which is marketed for application to small cuts (*eg*, razor cuts) to arrest hemorrhage. Both preparations cause slight pain when applied to open lesions. They do appear to hasten healing but should be used in moderation. If the sores do not heal readily, or if repeated lesions occur, the client should seek medical care. These ulcerations often are manifestations of viral infections. Persistent problems indicate either lowered resistance or a virulent viral strain that requires professional treatment. Because styptics are poisons, they must be stored properly to prevent accidental ingestion by children.

Nursing management

Nursing implications

Recommended solution strengths for oxidizing agents used as mouthwashes vary. Sodium perborate, a white, odorless powder, is prepared as a 2% solution ($\frac{1}{2}$ tsp per 100 ml solution). Hydrogen peroxide should be prepared as a 1.5% solution. A solution is marketed in this strength specifically for use as mouthwash. The more usual hydrogen peroxide preparation, 3%, should be diluted 1:1 with water for oral use.

Because they are medicinal agents, these substances must be regarded with the respect accorded any drug substance. Medicated solutions and those containing alcohol should be stored in secure places to prevent accidental ingestion and poisoning.

Commercial mouthwashes often contain considerable alcohol; preparations with low concentrations (less than 27%) are preferred over those with higher alcoholic content.

Nursing process

Assessment Data required for evaluation include the kinds of preparations used by the client, the frequency of application, and the purposes for which they are used. If the client experiences persistent breath odors, the nurse should inquire about smoking, use of alcohol, and weight reduction regimens. Assessment for signs and symptoms indicative of disease conditions likely to produce such odors should be comprehensive. The nurse should also determine where substances used for oral hygiene are stored.

Nursing diagnosis The most likely diagnoses for clients using oral cleansers and deodorants are as follows:

> *Body image disturbance related to breath odors secondary to ineffective oral hygiene, smoking, alcohol consumption, ketoacidosis, or metabolic or respiratory disease*
> *Knowledge deficit related to oral hygiene*

Accidental ingestion of mouthwash may result in diagnoses such as:

> *Impaired tissue integrity: pharyngitis, esophagitis or gastritis related to irritation due to ingestion of oxidizing compounds*

A common collaborative problem that should be differentiated from the nursing diagnoses is

> *Potential complication: CNS depression related to alcohol intoxication secondary to ingestion of mouthwash*

Planning Nursing goals may include the detection of disease conditions contributing to breath odors and referral of affected clients for definitive medical diagnosis and treatment. Goals also include reducing or eliminating smoking and alcohol consumption; reducing the risk of poisoning by accidental ingestion of mouthwashes and gargles; reducing breath odors through improvement of oral hygiene; and educating the client about oral hygiene.

Intervention A variety of aids for oral hygiene are available for use by the nurse caring for clients unable to perform their own hygiene. Regular, routine care is conveniently performed with the aid of Toothettes, sponge-tipped applicators impregnated with a pleasantly flavored dentifrice. The removal of crusts and other debris requires other approaches. Papaya juice, which contains a proteolytic enzyme, is effective in breaking down crusts. Debris may be removed mechanically by irrigation with water, normal saline, normal saline with sodium bicarbonate, or a 1:6 solution of hydrogen peroxide and water. WaterPiks also facilitate irrigation.

Client education. There is little need for the healthy person to use special agents for cleansing the mouth or throat. Commercial solutions are formulated to enhance flavor and eye appeal. Except when prescribed by a physician, they should be regarded as cosmetics rather than medicine and used sparingly because of their potential for adverse reaction. When ordered as part of a medical regimen, the client should be encouraged to use them as prescribed.

For normal hygiene, the nurse should emphasize regular use of simple, inexpensive cleansers. A 1% solution of sodium bicarbonate ($1/2$ tsp in 6–7 ounces of water) helps remove mucus and is an excellent mouthwash. As a gargle, normal saline is nonirritating and an excellent medium for applying heat to an inflamed membrane. It can be prepared by adding $1/2$ tsp of salt to 7 ounces of warm water. A temperature of 120°F is recommended for liquids that come in contact with membranes of the upper GI tract, which are accustomed to warm fluids. These home preparations are easily flavored by the addition of a drop or two of essences, such as peppermint, wintergreen, or cinnamon. Food coloring may also be added.

In the past, some manufacturers of mouthwashes and gargles have heavily advertised their antiseptic properties. This is no longer legally permissible unless the antiseptic efficacy of the product has been proven.

Clients using oral lozenges should be cautioned not to exceed the maximum dosage specified on the product label.

Evaluation Data required for evaluation include client reports of alcohol and cigarette use and reduction of breath odors, the incidence or absence of accidental poisoning involving mouthwashes, and frequency of referral for medical care of conditions underlying halitosis.

Checklist of nursing actions

☐ When caring for clients unable to perform oral hygiene, use Toothettes for routine mouth care; avoid the use of lemon and glycerin swabs.

☐ To remove crusts and debris from the mouth, apply papaya juice to break down the material chemically, then remove by irrigating with a nonirritating electrolyte solution or diluted hydrogen peroxide.

☐ Recommend 1% sodium bicarbonate solution or normal saline for use as mouthwashes or gargles.

☐ Warn clients using antiseptic lozenges not to exceed the recommended dosage.

☐ Encourage clients using antiseptic mouthwashes or gargles prescribed by a physician to use the agents conscientiously, as with any medication.

Denture adhesive

Adhesives are applied to artificial teeth to prevent denture displacement during ordinary activities such

---

Enrichment experience 30-1

Prepare a quart or more of 1% sodium bicarbonate solution. Divide it into several portions. Using flavoring essences, flavor each portion differently. Further divide each portion in two. Add color to one half, leaving the other half uncolored. Ask several of your classmates to test the preparations, rating them for asthetic appeal and effectiveness in cleansing. Which flavoring was preferred? Did the addition of color enhance the asthetic appeal of the preparations? Compare the cost of 1 quart of this preparation with 1 quart of three different commercial mouthwashes. Would you recommend such a preparation to your clients?

---

as chewing, laughing, and sneezing. Adhesives are marketed in powder and paste forms.

Adverse reactions to denture adhesives include allergic reactions, fungal infections in the mouth, and deterioration of remaining natural teeth. The latter is caused by both retained food particles and by the action of karaya gum, a common ingredient of adhesives. Karaya gum is an acidic compound that directly attacks tooth enamel.

Clients in the habit of using denture adhesives are likely to have poor fitting dentures. Retention of dentures depends on a close fit between the artificial material and the mouth surfaces. This fit can be lost due to atrophy of tissues or weight changes that alter the amount and contour of the mouth tissues. When dentures do not remain in place, a dentist should be consulted. Relining of existing dentures may improve the fit. Clients should be encouraged to regard dentures as they do eyeglasses, that is, as prostheses requiring periodic adjustment or replacement. Denture adhesive should be used only as a temporary measure until a dentist can be consulted.

Digestants
Physiology

Digestants are endogenous chemicals that promote the breakdown of food into absorbable particles. They include hydrochloric acid, enzymes (proteases, saccharases, lipases), and bile. In normal individuals, digestants are secreted by the pancreas and liver and by the cells in the mucous membranes of the intestinal tract. Hydrochloric acid and pepsin are produced in the stomach; amylase, trypsin, and lipase by the pancreas; and bile by the liver. Hydrochloric acid promotes the activation and chemical activity of pepsin and accelerates protein hydrolysis. Pepsin and other enzymes catalyze the breakdown of calorie nutrients in chyme. Bile acts as a surfactant to emulsify fat.

Pathology

Several conditions can interfere with the production of endogenous digestants. For example, stomach cancer destroys secretory gastric cells. Pancreatitis interferes with pancreatic secretion, either temporarily by cell inhibition, or permanently by cell destruction. Liver disease or biliary obstruction may decrease the secretion of bile into the duodenum. Cystic fibrosis is characterized by production of thick secretions that obstruct ducts and inhibit secretion of several digestants. Surgical removal of secretory tissue (*eg*, gastrectomy) also reduces endogenous production of digestants.

Gastric acidifiers

Hydrochloric acid and glutamic acid hydrochloride are used to lower gastric *p*H (see Table 30-1).

Pharmacodynamics. Hydrochloric acid and glutamic acid hydrochloride restore the normal acidic environment of the stomach, thereby increasing the precipitation of caseinogen, converting pepsinogen into pepsin, and stimulating secretion by the duodenum. They also inhibit the multiplication of bacteria and stop the action of ptyalin.

Pharmacokinetics. Administered orally, gastric acidifiers enter the stomach, which is their site of action. They are handled by the body in the same way as endogenous hydrochloric acid. When the food mass containing these acids reaches the duodenum, pancreatic juice (which has a basic *p*H) neutralizes the acid. In the small intestine, the salts produced by this reaction are absorbed into the bloodstream and used as are any other salts in food.

Therapeutic uses. Gastric acidifiers are administered orally for the purpose of replacing stomach acid for clients with a deficiency of hydrochloric acid (achlorhydria or hypochlorhydria).

Adverse reactions. In the mouth, hydrochloric acid reacts with tooth enamel, breaking down the enamel and causing erosion and cavity formation. In the esophagus, it can irritate tissue and promote ulcer formation. Acid that is handled carelessly may contact the skin, producing chemical burns. In large doses, gastric acidifiers can cause metabolic acidosis.

Precautions and contraindications. Hydrochloric acid should be diluted and administered through a glass straw placed near the back of the mouth.

Gastric acidifiers are contraindicated for persons with peptic ulcers or gastric hyperacidity. These agents should be stored in a secure place to prevent accidental ingestion.

Table 30-1. Digestants

Drug name	Preparations	Usual adult dosage	Therapeutic uses
Gastric acidifiers			
hydrochloric acid	10% diluted solution for oral use	4–8 ml, tid, with meals.	Dyspeptic symptoms
glutamic acid hydrochloride	Capsules	340–680 mg with meals	Absence of free hydrochloric acid in stomach Achlorhydria Hypochlorhydria
Enzymes			
Gastric			
pepsin	Elixir of lactated pepsins	8 ml, tid, with meals	Gastric achylia in pernicious anemia
	Tablets	500–1000 mg with meals	
Pancreatic			
pancreatin (Creon, Vitalin: *Can:* Pancrex)	Enteric-coated tablets Plain tablets Powder	8,000–24,000 U of lipase activity with each meal and snack PC: C	Replacement therapy for pancreatic insufficiency
pancrelipase (Cotazym, Pancrease, Ilozyme; *Can:* Viokase)	Capsules Tablets Powders Packets	8,000 U to 24,000 U of lipase activity/17 g of dietary fat with each meal and snack PC: C	Replacement therapy for pancreatic insufficiency; treats conditions of cystic fibrosis, pancreatitis, malabsorption syndrome
Bile constituents			
Bile salts			
ox bile extract	Enteric-coated tablets	300 mg, tid, after meals.	Replacement therapy for a variety of conditions
ox bile extract with iron (Bilron)	Capsules	150–500 mg, during or after meals	Same as above
Bile Acids			
dehydrocholic acid (Atrocholin, Cholan-DH, Decholin, Hepahydrin)	Tablets	250–500 mg, tid, with meals or immediately following meals	Replacement therapy with deficiency or biliary stasis Following surgery of the biliary system Cholangitis Cholecystitis
chenodiol (Chenix)	Oral tablets	250 mg AM and HS, or 500 mg HS PC: X	Dissolution of gallstones in people at high risk for surgery

KEY: PC = Pregnancy risk category. (The validity of pregnancy risk categories has not been established. See Chapter 16, p 216.)
Can: Canadian trade name.

Digestive enzymes

Pepsin

Pharmacodynamics. Pepsin acts as a protease in the stomach. It is most active in the presence of acid (*p*H of 1.5–2).

Pharmacokinetics. Pepsin is administered orally. It acts locally in the stomach and is broken down and absorbed in the digestive tract, along with food components and other GI secretions.

Therapeutic uses. Pepsin is administered in combination with hydrochloric acid as replacement therapy for clients lacking secretory gastric mucosa. It is available in granular and elixir forms. Usual dosage is 8 ml, administered with meals.

Adverse reactions. Pepsin prepared from animal tissues has the potential to stimulate allergic hypersensitivity. Allergy to pepsin is not usually seen clinically.

Precautions and contraindications. The only contraindication for pepsin is allergic hypersensitivity to the specific preparation prescribed.

Pancreatic enzymes

Pancreatic enzymes contain lipases, proteases (trypsin and chymotrypsin) and saccharases (amylases). Pancreatin is a powder prepared from the pancreases of hogs. For medicinal use, it is formulated as an enteric-coated tablet to prevent the active ingredients from disintegrating in the stomach.

Pharmacodynamics. In the duodenum, pancreatic enzymes perform the chemical functions of digestion normally performed by endogenous enzymes.

Pharmacokinetics. Following the breakdown of nutrients in the small intestine, pancreatic enzymes are digested and absorbed along with components of food and other digestant substances.

Therapeutic uses. Pancreatic enzymes are used for replacement therapy in the treatment of malabsorption caused by exocrine pancreatic insufficiency. Conditions causing this deficiency include cystic fibrosis, chronic pancreatitis, and pancreatectomy. Pancreatin is available as plain or enteric-coated oral tablets. Pancrelipase (Cotazyme, Festal II, Ilozyme, Pancrease), a more concentrated preparation, is marketed as capsules (prompt or delayed-release), powder, and tablets (prompt or delayed-release). Dosages range from 8,000 to 36,000 units of lipase activity and should be administered with food.

Adverse reactions. Excessive doses of pancreatic enzymes can cause nausea, vomiting, or diarrhea. Extremely high doses are associated with hyperuricemia and uricosuria. Allergic reactions (most likely in persons allergic to pork) are characterized by sneezing, lacrimation, or rash.

Inhalation of powdered pancreatic enzymes causes irritation of the mucosa and can precipitate bronchospasm in persons with allergic sensitivity to the substance.

Precautions and contraindications. Initial doses of pancreatic enzymes are relatively low and are increased as necessary until steatorrhea abates. The preparation is contraindicated for persons with allergic hypersensitivity to it or to hog protein.

Bile

Pharmacodynamics. Bile acts as an emulsifier, reducing surface tension and breaking down fat globules into small particles. Small fat particles are more easily broken down into absorbable fatty acids by pancreatic lipases. Because fat-soluble vitamins are absorbed in conjunction with fats, bile is essential for the absorption of vitamins A, D, E, and K.

Bile also acts as a choleretic, stimulating the liver to secrete whole bile in larger quantities. It also stimulates the smooth muscle lining of the GI tract.

Pharmacokinetics. Bile extracts are administered orally and are treated by the body as endogenous bile. Almost all of a dose enters the enterohepatic circulation; a small fraction is excreted in feces.

Therapeutic uses. Bile is used in the treatment of clients deficient in natural bile. Pharmaceutical bile is an extract of ox bile. It is administered orally, in dosages of 300 mg tid with meals. The efficacy of bile in promoting digestion in clients with bile deficiency remains unproven.

Adverse reactions. Administration of ox bile extract stimulates endogenous production of bile and can result in toxicity. High doses act as a laxative and can cause diarrhea. Some components of bile are capable of impairing liver function. Bile is also believed to impair resistance of the upper GI tract to the corrosive action of hydrochloric acid, predisposing clients to peptic ulcers.

Precautions and contraindications. Clients receiving ox bile extract should be monitored for diarrhea, liver impairment, and signs and symptoms of peptic ulcer disease.

Bile acids

Chenodiol (Chenix), ursodiol (Actigall) and dehydrocholic acid (Decholin) are three bile salts available in drug formulations.

Pharmacodynamics. Bile acids dissolve cholesterol in bile and facilitate drainage of bile. In the intestines, bile acids emulsify fat, facilitating its enzymatic breakdown into absorbable fatty acids. Bile acids also act as choleretics (*ie*, stimulate the production of a dilute bile by the liver.)

Pharmacokinetics. Bile acids are administered orally and traverse the intestinal tract. They are subsequently digested like natural bile acids, with most entering the enterohepatic circulation and with a small fraction excreted in feces.

Therapeutic uses. Chenodiol is used to promote the dissolution of gallstones in persons who cannot be treated surgically. Ursodiol is indicated for the treatment of small noncalcified gallstones. Dehydrocholic acid is employed as a laxative and is sometimes administered after gallbladder surgery to promote T-tube drainage.

Adverse reactions. Bile acids may cause diarrhea and liver impairment. Both are reversible upon withdrawal of the drugs.

Precautions and contraindications. Caution should be used when bile acids are administered to clients with impaired liver function.

■ Summary

Digestants are pharmaceutical preparations of chemicals essential for digestion. They include hydrochloric acid, pepsin, pancreatic enzymes, bile, and bile acids. They are used in replacement therapy for clients with deficiencies of autogenous digestant compounds. In addition, bile acids are used for their laxative and choleretic effects. Digestants are well tolerated by most clients but can cause adverse reactions, including damage to the teeth, allergic hypersensitivity, diarrhea, and liver impairment.

Nursing management

Nursing process

Assessment   Before digestant therapy is instituted, clients should be evaluated for risk of adverse reaction. Individuals with a history of peptic ulcer disease are likely to experience renewed ulcer pathology if they are given hydrochloric acid or bile. Clients with jaundice should not receive bile or bile acids. When pepsin and pancreatic enzymes are prescribed, clients should be asked specifically about allergy to pork.

A complete nutritional assessment should be done, with emphasis on signs and symptoms of malabsorption.

Nursing diagnosis   Clients who are candidates for digestant therapy are likely to have

> *Altered nutrition: less than body requirements related to malabsorption*

Clients receiving digestant medication may experience the following:

> *Impaired tissue integrity: erosion of tooth enamel related to hydrochloride ingestion secondary to achlorhydria*
> *Altered comfort: sneezing, lacrimation, and dyspnea related to inflammation due to allergic hypersensitivity to pork protein in digestive enzymes*
> *Joint pain related to hyperuricemia secondary to pancreatic enzyme medication*
> *Diarrhea related to stimulation of peristalsis by bile or bile acids*

Common collaborative problems that should be differentiated from the nursing diagnoses include

> *Potential complication: peptic ulcer*
> *Potential complication: hepatotoxicity*

Many clients will also have a knowledge deficit related to digestant deficiencies and their treatment.

Planning   Goals of treatment include prevention of tooth damage by hydrochloric acid medication; prevention or prompt detection and treatment of hyperacidity in clients receiving hydrochloric acid medication; prevention or prompt detection and treatment of allergic reactions to digestant enzymes by clients allergic to pork protein; maintenance of normal fecal elimination; prompt detection and treatment of other

adverse reaction to digestant medications; and client education about digestant deficiencies and their treatment.

Intervention   Digestants are administered with food or after a meal to increase their efficacy in promoting digestion and (in the case of pancreatic enzymes) to protect them from degradation by stomach acid. They should be administered with ample fluids to propel them into the stomach. Hydrochloric acid solutions, usually 10% strength, must be further diluted 15–20 times for administration. Even at these dilutions, the acid is strong enough to injure tooth enamel and should not be allowed to contact the teeth. The solutions are administered through a glass straw placed in the back of the mouth; the solution should be swallowed without allowing contact with the teeth. Each dose should be followed by water or other liquid to ensure that it is washed from the esophagus into the stomach.

When digestant therapy is underway, clients should be assessed to determine therapeutic response to the medications. They should also be monitored for adverse reactions to these drugs. The teeth of clients receiving hydrochloric acid should be examined regularly for erosion and cavities. Clients receiving digestive enzymes may develop signs and symptoms of allergic reaction (sneezing, lacrimation, rash, wheezing) that require treatment with antihistamines or decongestants. When bile or bile acids are prescribed, clients should be monitored for hepatotoxicity and diarrhea. Clients being treated with acids (hydrochloric or bile) should be watched for signs and symptoms of peptic ulcer disease.

Client education.   Clients taking hydrochloric acid should be taught preventive measures to protect their teeth. After taking medication, they should neutralize any residual acid in their mouths by rinsing with a dilute sodium bicarbonate solution. Other digestants should be taken with 8–12 ounces of water to ensure delivery into the stomach. All digestants except pancreatic enzymes should be taken with food. Pancreatic enzymes are taken immediately after a meal to protect them from degradation by stomach acid. Fluids taken with pancreatic enzymes must not be hot because enzymes may degrade in high temperatures.

Clients taking bile or bile acids should be taught the signs and symptoms of toxicity. They should receive specific instruction regarding signs and symptoms that warrant consulting the physician regarding adjustment of the drug regimen.

There are over-the-counter preparations that contain digestants and claim to provide relief from digestive symptoms. These medicines are provided in low doses that are inadequate to correct medical conditions for which digestants are prescribed. Clients should not substitute these drugs for those prescribed by the physician but should follow the prescribed regimen. (See

Example of nursing process and hydrochloric acid therapy

The client is a 53-year-old teacher who has had a partial gastrectomy to remove a small malignancy. Her prognosis is considered good but sequelae after surgery include achlorhydria and pernicious anemia. She has been placed on maintenance doses of hydrochloric acid (4 ml of 10% solution tid with meals) and cyanocobalamine (100 μg/week). The client has never taken long-term medication, nor has she ever self-administered parenteral medication.

Assessment data	Nursing diagnosis	Intervention	Goals and outcome criteria
Medications prescribed as replacement therapy: hydrochloric acid and cyanocobalamine	Knowledge deficit relating to long-term use of hydrochloric acid and cyanocobalamine and to injection technique	**Explain** to the client the function of hydrochloric acid in digestion and that of cyanocobalamine in the production of red blood cells. Teach the client to dilute the hydrochloric acid and take it through a glass straw, avoiding any contact with teeth.	The client will be able to repeat to the nurse facts conveyed during teaching sessions. She will be able to demonstrate correct injection technique.
Lack of client experience with long-term medication and injection technique		**Instruct** the client in injection technique, using sterile asepsis.	The client will carry out the medication regimen accurately.
		Warn the client to purchase the correct concentration of cyanocobalamine; the drug is marketed in 100 μg/ml and 1,000 μg/ml strengths, and the weaker preparation is appropriate for maintenance doses.	
Hydrochloric acid prescription; this acid can damage inert materials and living tissue.	Knowledge deficit concerning adverse effects of hydrochloric acid	**Explain** to the client the corrosive properties of hydrochloric acid and warn her not to allow it to contact sensitive tissues or inert materials that can be damaged by it; urge her to keep the drug in a secure place where it will not be available to unauthorized people or children.	Neither the client nor other persons in her home will be injured by the acid solution.
			When asked, the client will report that the acid solution has not damaged objects or materials in the home.
		Instruct the client to perform oral hygiene and a sodium bicarbonate rinse after acid medications.	Dental caries will not develop.

Example of Nursing Process and Hydrochloric Acid Therapy.)

Checklist of nursing actions

☐ Before initiating digestant medication, assess clients for factors that increase risk of adverse reaction to these drugs.

☐ Administer digestants with or following meals so that they mix with the food mass in the digestive tract.

☐ Follow digestant medications with ample fluids to deliver them to the stomach.

☐ Dilute hydrochloric acid solutions 15–20 times before administration.

☐ Administer hydrochloric acid with a glass straw placed in the back of the mouth.

☐ Have clients rinse their mouths with dilute sodium bicarbonate solution after administration of hydrochloric acid.

☐ Monitor clients receiving digestants for adverse drug reactions.

☐ Teach clients receiving digestants how to administer their drugs and how to monitor themselves for adverse reactions.

☐ Caution clients for whom digestants are prescribed not to substitute over-the-counter preparations for the prescription drugs recommended by the physician.

Drug therapy for disorders associated with hyperacidity

Physiology

The hydrochloric acid produced by the stomach plays an essential role in the digestion of food. Protein digestion is initiated in the stomach by pepsin and a low pH, which promote the hydrolysis of proteins to amino acids. Not only is acidity favorable to proteolysis, it is essential for the formation of its partner, pepsin.

The conversion of pepsinogen to active pepsin proceeds most rapidly in a medium with a pH of two or less, which is highly acidic; it virtually ceases when pH rises to five or more. The hydrochloric acid produced by parietal cells in the gastric mucosa normally maintains a pH between two and five, depending on the presence of food and other chemicals taken orally. While this degree of acidity is optimal for digestion, it is highly corrosive and potentially traumatic to tissue. Any cells damaged by the acid are also vulnerable to the action of pepsin. It is no wonder that the damaging

effects of gastric secretions frequently contribute to both minor and major health problems. However, the normal GI tract has defenses against this threat (Fig. 30-1).

Gastric mucosa secretes two kinds of mucus. One type is a thin lubricant similar to that produced by other parts of the tract to promote digestion and to propel the food mass. The second is a thick, viscid substance that forms a barrier between the gastric mucosa and its corrosive secretions. This type of mucus is unique to the stomach and serves to protect the gastric mucosa from chemical damage by its own secretions. Normal gastric mucosa appears to resist penetration by acid to a degree not shared by the mucosa of persons susceptible to peptic ulcer disease.

Mechanical barriers prevent the spread of undue amounts of acid to unprotected tissues outside the stomach. The cardiac sphincter prevents reflux of acid upward into the esophagus; the pyloric sphincter prevents leakage of acid into the duodenum.

Stomach contents do enter the duodenum periodically during digestion. Under normal conditions, by the time this material leaves the stomach, some of the acid has been neutralized by buffer substances in the food. Moreover, only small volumes enter the duodenum at any one time, and they are quickly mixed with pancreatic secretions, which raise the pH to an alkaline level.

Pathology

Discomfort and tissue damage can develop whenever the delicately balanced processes of digestion are disrupted. Excess acid production, inadequate mucus se-

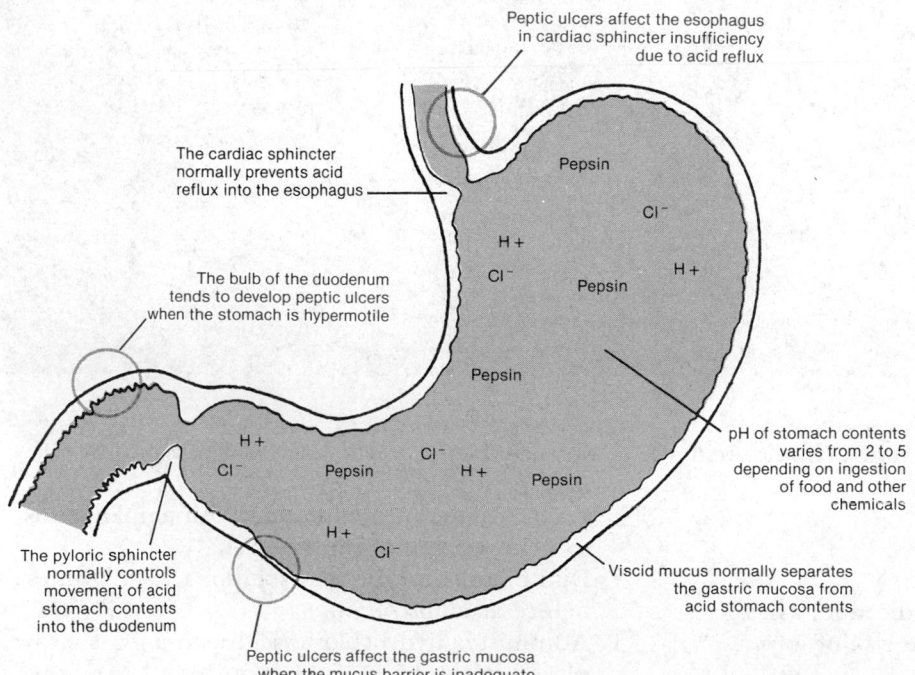

Figure 30-1. Factors influencing the development of peptic ulcers.

cretion, an impairment of mucosal resistance to acid penetration, inadequacy of the cardiac sphincter, hypermotility of the stomach, and inadequate pancreatic secretion are among the factors predisposing to problems attributed to "hyperacidity."

These are secondary to both genetic and environmental influences. The mechanisms by which the genetic predisposition is expressed are not completely understood but may include an excess number of acid-secreting parietal cells; inadequate mucus production; a mucosa susceptible to acid penetration; a metabolism favoring high levels of histamine or other substances that stimulate acid secretion; a diaphragmatic structure susceptible to the development of hiatal hernia; stress response patterns with a predominance of parasympathetic activity; and an undue sensitivity to external stimuli that normally trigger acid secretion.

Environmental factors are multiple. Smoking and the ingestion of gastric irritants are known risks. Undue stress triggers nervous system and endocrine responses, such as increased corticosteroid production and intestinal hypermotility, which are conducive to pathology. Recent evidence indicates that an infectious microorganism may play a role in the development of peptic ulcers.

Displacement of acid from the stomach to areas normally not exposed to a low pH can cause pain and irritation, as well as tissue inflammation. Excessive abdominal pressure due to pregnancy, tight clothing, overeating, or obesity can force open the cardiac sphincter and propel acid upward into the esophagus. Deficiency of the cardiac sphincter and intermittent pressure on the stomach by the diaphragm contribute to acid reflux in hiatal hernia. Abnormal passages in the tract, often surgically produced (as in gastrojejunostomy), may bypass the normal barriers and allow acid to come into contact with extragastric tissues. Peptic ulcers can result (Box 30-1).

No matter what the cause of the complaint, reducing acidity tends to alleviate symptoms and to promote healing. This is the major objective of drug therapy in these conditions, and it can be achieved by inhibiting acid production or by subsequent neutralization.

Factors influencing gastric acid production

Gastric secretion of hydrochloric acid is mediated by several stimuli: vagus nerve signals, the hormone, gastrin, and the amino acid derivative, histamine.

Vagus nerve activity is responsible for the cephalic phase of secretion, which is stimulated by the sight, sound, odor, and even thought of food. The parasympathetic system, of which the vagus is a part, is one pathway by which emotional stress stimulates the production of acid.

Gastrin is produced by the antrum of the stomach in response to such stimuli as mechanical distention,

---

Box 30-1. Factors predisposing to problems related to gastric acid

Disruption of the process of digestion

Excess acid production

Inadequate mucus secretion

Impairment of mucosal resistance to acid penetration

Inadequacy of the cardiac sphincter

Hypermotility of the stomach

Inadequate pancreatic insufficiency

Genetic factors*

Excess number of acid-secreting parietal cells

Inadequate mucus production

Mucosa susceptible to acid penetration

Metabolism that favors high levels of substances such as histamine

Diaphragm susceptible to hiatal hernia formation

Stress response patterns of parasympathetic activity

Undue sensitivity to external stimuli to acid production

Environmental factors

Smoking

Overeating

Ingestion of gastric irritants

Undue stress

Excessive abdominal pressure (pregnancy, tight clothing, obesity)

Deficiency of the cardiac sphincter

Intermittent pressure on the stomach by the diaphragm

Abnormal passages in the tract

*Genetic factors are not completely understood but may include those listed here.

---

extremes of temperatures, and chemical irritants. The specific elements of the diet that act as irritants vary from person to person, but "rich" foods containing high levels of sugar and fat, caffeine, alcohol, and strong flavoring agents, such as spices, are frequent offenders. Smoking is also believed to stimulate the parietal cells.

A negative feedback mechanism helps to control activity of the parietal cells. As pH in the stomach drops, secretion declines, becoming totally blocked at a pH of two. When food is ingested, it reacts with the acid

> ### Box 30-2. Therapeutic approaches to reduce gastric acid production
>
> Reduce sensory stimuli related to food
>
> Modify the diet to include small, bland meals at moderate temperatures
>
> Avoid ingesting highly alkaline compounds
>
> Institute drug therapy with agents that reduce vagal nerve activity; suppress production of gastrin or histamine; inactivate gastrin or histamine; and block the stimulating effects of gastrin and histamine on the parietal cell

secretions, raising the pH and stimulating further acid production.

Histamine stimulates acid secretion in much the same way as gastrin. Body levels of this chemical are increased in allergic reactions and any condition characterized by extensive tissue damage. Histamine stimulation of parietal cells may be the primary mechanism by which peptic ulcers develop. Stimuli that increase acid production also tend to relax the cardiac sphincter.

The mechanisms outlined already offer potential points of intervention for reducing acid production. Therapeutic approaches include reducing sensory stimuli related to food; changing the diet to small bland meals at moderate temperatures; avoiding ingestion of highly alkaline compounds; and drug therapy with agents that reduce vagal nerve activity, suppress production of gastrin or histamine, inactivate gastrin or histamine, or block the stimulating effects of gastrin and histamine on the parietal cell (Box 30-2). Dietary regimens and drug therapy have been the classic cornerstones of treatment. Anti-infectives may be given to eliminate the infectious organism suspected of causing ulcers. No drug agents are yet available that directly suppress gastric secretion of acid or inactivate either gastrin or histamine.

Drugs used to suppress acid production

Medications to reduce acid production include anticholinergics, tranquilizers, and histamine$_2$ receptor blockers (Table 30-2).

Tranquilizers and anticholinergics

Tranquilizers are CNS depressants that selectively inhibit brain structures involved in stress responses. They may decrease acid production by reducing vagal activity that results from a response to stress. Chlordiazepoxide (Librium) and diazepam (Valium) are common choices for treating persons with peptic ulcer disease, "nervous stomach," and other problems associated with hyperacidity.

Anticholinergics prescribed to inhibit vagal stimu-

lation of the stomach include belladonna (as a tincture) and propantheline. The use of these agents appears to be declining since the introduction of histamine-2 blockers. Both tranquilizers and anticholinergics are administered before meals. They may be combined in one preparation, as in the product Librax, which contains chlordiazepoxide hydrochloride and clidinium bromide (Quarzan). Tranquilizers and anticholinergics are discussed in detail in Chapters 24 and 26 and in Chapter 22, respectively.

Histamine$_2$ receptor antagonists

In recent decades, drugs capable of inhibiting histamine$_2$ (H$_2$) receptors have been developed. Three of these—cimetidine, famotidine, and ranitidine—have been approved by the Food and Drug Administration for use in the treatment of duodenal ulcers and conditions such as Zollinger-Ellison syndrome that are characterized by pathologic hypersecretion of gastric hydrochloric acid. Cimetidine is also approved for the short-term treatment of active benign gastric ulcers. A fourth drug of this class, nyzatidine, is available in Canada (Table 30-3).

Pharmacodynamics. Histamine$_2$ receptor antagonists competitively inhibit the action of histamine on the H$_2$ receptors that triggers parietal cell response to chemical stimulation. These receptors differ from the histamine$_1$ (H$_1$) receptors, which mediate the local tissue effects of histamine in allergic and anaphylactic reactions. The latter are blocked by the classic antihistamines, which have no effect on secretory functions stimulated by H$_2$ receptors. The fact that they reduce acid secretion attributable not only to histamine but also to gastrin and vagal activity indicates that all three mechanisms may share, to some degree, a common pathway, possibly the H$_2$ receptor, itself.

Reduction in H$_2$ receptor activity results in reduced gastric acid output and concentration, with basal secretion affected to a greater degree than secretion in response to stimuli (food, insulin, histamine, pentagastrin, and caffeine). Pepsin levels are reduced indirectly as a result of the rise in gastric pH.

Cimetidine appears to retard gastric tumors (cancers) either by attacking them directly or by stimulating the immune system. (Tonneson, 1988)

Pharmacokinetics. Cimetidine, nyzatidine, and ranitidine are rapidly absorbed from the GI tract. Cimetidine and ranitidine undergo extensive first-pass metabolism with bioavailability averaging 50% for ranitidine and 70% for cimetidine. Famotidine is incompletely absorbed and undergoes minimal first-pass metabolism; its oral bioavailability is 40%–50%. All three drugs are widely distributed to most body tissues and fluids, except in liver disease, they do not cross the blood–brain barrier readily. Protein binding is relatively low, 10%–19% for ranitidine, 15%–20% for cimetidine and famotidine, and 35% for nyzati-

Table 30-2. Antimuscarinics and tranquilizers used to treat hyperacidity

Drug name	Preparations	Usual adult dosage
Antimuscarinics		
methantheline bromide (Banthine)	Oral tablets	50–100 mg, q6h around the clock
		50–100 mg, q6h
		PC: C
methscopolamine bromide (Pamine)	Oral tablets	2.5–5 mg, ac and hs
		0.25–1 mg, q6h–q8h
		PC: C
oxyphencyclimine (Daricon)	Oral tablets	5–10 mg bid
		PC: C
propantheline bromide (Norpanth, Pro-Banthine, Prothine)	Oral tablets	15 mg ac and 30 mg hs
		30 mg, q6h
		PC: C
tincture of belladonna	Oral solution	gtt x ac and hs
		PC: C
tridihexathyl (Pathilon, Pathibamate)	Oral tablets	25–50 mg tid
Tranquilizers		
chlordiazepoxide (Librium)	Oral tablets	5–10 mg, ac and hs
	Powder for preparing solutions for injection	5–20 mg, q6h
		PC: D
diazepam (Valium)	Oral tablets	2–5 mg, ac and hs
	Solution for injection	2–5 mg, q6h
		PC: D

KEY: PC = Pregnancy risk category. (The validity of pregnancy risk categories has not been established. See Chapter 16, p 216.)

dine. These drugs are distributed in breast milk; animal studies indicate that cimetidine crosses the placenta.

Histamine$_2$ receptor antagonists are metabolized by the liver and excreted by the kidneys, with small amounts eliminated in feces. Cimetidine and ranitidine are removed by hemodialysis but famotidine is not. Elimination half-lives are approximately 2 hours and are prolonged in persons with impaired renal function.

Therapeutic uses. Histamine$_2$ receptor antagonists are used for the treatment of peptic ulcers and pathologic GI hypersecretory conditions such as Zollinger-Ellison syndrome, systemic mastocytosis, and multiple endocrine adenomatosis. Cimetidine is also approved for prophylaxis of duodenal ulcers. Although not approved by the Food and Drug Administration for these purposes, H$_2$ receptor antagonists have also been used for the treatment of other acid-related problems, such as hiatal hernia, esophagitis, acute GI bleeding, and gastritis, as well as in prevention of the development of stress ulcers.

Ranitidine has been used successfully as an adjunct in the treatment of theophylline toxicity. It is used to decrease nausea so that charcoal, administered to absorb the toxin, is not vomited (Amitai, Yeung, Moye, & Lovejoy, 1986).

Adverse reactions. Histamine$_2$ receptor antagonists are generally well tolerated. The reported incidence of any single adverse reaction is 4% or less (McEvoy, 1991). The CNS, cardiovascular system, and musculoskeletal system are affected most often. Signs and symptoms of CNS reactions include stupor, depression, headaches, dizziness, confusion, fatigue, and somnolence. Cimetidine sometimes causes feminization of male recipients (gynecomastia, impaired sexual function).

Intravenous administration of cimetidine has resulted in disorientation, hallucinations, psychosis and agitation, especially in clients over age 70 (Porter, Beard, Walker, Lawson, Jick, & Kellaway, 1986). Bradycardia, hypotension, and cardiac arrest have been reported. Musculoskeletal pain (arthralgia, myalgia) also occur.

In addition, H$_2$ receptor antagonists have been associated with rash, liver and kidney impairment, antiandrogen effects, and bone marrow depression. Ranitidine can cause chronic headaches. The most frequent adverse reactions to nyzatidine are diaphoresis and urticaria. The use of cimetidine to treat clients who have had a gastrectomy or vagotomy or to treat those who have difficulty chewing has been associated with the development of phytobezoars (masses of undigested vegetable in the stomach). Other adverse reactions include leukocytosis, blurred vision,

Table 30-3. Histamine₂ receptor antagonists

Drug names	Preparations	Usual adult dosage	Specific adverse reactions	Drug interactions
cimetidine (Tagamet)	Tablets and liquid for oral administration Solution for IM or IV injection	300 mg q6–8h or 400 mg q12h Maximum daily dosage 2.4 g PC: B	Nephrotoxicity greater than that of ranitidine Diarrhea Mania Inhibition of parathormone production Fever	Cimetidine inhibits the degradation and elimination of benzodiazepines, coumarin, lidocaine, phenytoin, beta-adrenergic blockers, triamterene, and theophylline. Antacids inhibits the absorption of cimetidine.
famotidine (Pepcid)	Oral Solution for IV injection	40 mg/d, given as a single dose; maintenance dose: 20 mg/d Maximum daily dosage (for pathologic hypersecretion states): 640 mg PC: B	Diarrhea Reversible alopecia Diarrhea Transient irritation at injection site	No significant drug interactions have been reported to date.
ranitidine (Zantac)	Oral tablets Solution for IM or IV injection	150 mg q12h Maximum daily dosage: 400 mg PC: B	Nausea and vomiting, constipation, abdominal pain Hepatotoxicity greater than that of cimetidine Increased intraocular pressure Anaphylaxis	Ranitidine inhibits the metabolism of theophylline.
Nyzatidine (Axid)	Pulvules for oral administration	300 mg hs PC: C	Diaphoresis Urticaria Somnolence	Nyzatidine increases serum levels of aspirin.

KEY: PC = pregnancy risk category. (The validity of pregnancy risk categories has not been established. See Chapter 16, p 216.)

bone marrow depression, liver abnormalities and allergic reactions.

Cimetidine is known to inhibit liver metabolism of many drugs that are administered concurrently. Drugs whose serum levels are increased when cimetidine is added to the treatment regimen include coumarin anticoagulants, tricyclic antidepressants, benzodiazepines, phenytoin, beta-adrenergic blocking agents, lidocaine, triamterene, and theophylline. Ranitidine appears to be less likely to raise levels of benzodiazepines. When administered with morphine, cimetidine has caused apnea. Cimetidine may mask the signs and symptoms of pheochromocytoma, which then recur in exaggerated form when the histamine₂ blocker is discontinued (Faryna, 1982).

Adverse reactions to famotidine resemble those caused by ranitidine.

Precautions and contraindications. Histamine₂ receptor antagonists should be used with caution for persons with renal or hepatic impairment; dosages must be reduced in renal failure. Cimetidine is contra-indicated in liver disease because liver impairment increases the permeability of the blood–brain barrier, increasing the risk of cimetidine-induced mental confusion. Symptomatic response to the drugs should not be interpreted as precluding the presence of gastric malignancy; it has been suggested (but not established) that cimetidine therapy may predispose clients to the development of gastric carcinoma.

Safe use during pregnancy has not been established. The drugs are not recommended for use in children or lactating mothers. They are contraindicated for persons with allergic hypersensitivity to them.

Ranitidine appears to decrease (minimally) the secretion of gastric intrinsic factor; clients receiving the drug over long periods of time should be monitored for vitamin B₁₂ deficiency. This drug also causes false-positive results in urine protein determinations using Multistix; a sulfosalicylic acid reagent should be used for determining urinary protein during ranitidine therapy (see Focus on Histamine₂ Receptor Antagonists: Similarities and Differences).

Focus on

Histamine₂ receptor antagonists: similarities and differences

Similarities

Pharmacodynamics

These agents inhibit the action of histamine or H_2 receptors of the parietal cells, decreasing gastric acid output and concentration regardless of the stimulating agent or basal condition.

Pharmacokinetics

These agents are rapidly absorbed from the GI tract and are metabolized by the liver. They are primarily excreted by the kidneys. Their elimination half-life ranges from 1 to 2.5 hours, peaking in 1 to 3 hours. They are widely distributed.

Therapeutic uses

These agents are used to treat acute duodenal ulcers. They are also used to treat GI hypersecretory conditions such as Zollinger-Ellison syndrome, systemic mastocytosis, and postoperative hypersecretion. They are also used in the treatment of short-term gastric ulcers and other acid-related problems such as hiatal hernia, gastritis, acute GI bleeding, and prevention of stress ulcers.

Adverse reactions

These include: (CNS) depression, stupor, headache, dizziness, confusion, fatigue, somnolence; (CV) bradycardia, hypotension, cardiac arrest; (EENT) blurred vision; (GI) kidney impairment; (MS) musculoskeletal pain, arthralgia, myalgia; (SKIN) rash, allergic reaction; (HEMA) bone marrow depression, leukocytosis; (REPRO) bilateral gynecomastia, breast soreness.

Contraindications

These agents are contraindicated for people with hypersensitivity to H_2 receptor antagonists.

Precautions

These agents should be used cautiously in people with cirrhosis and impaired renal and hepatic function.

Differences

• **Cimetidine** indirectly decreases pepsin secretion by decreasing the volume of gastric juice; it has a weak antiandrogenic effect.
• **Famotidine** and **ranitidine** produce a dose-related reduction in pepsin secretion.

• **Ranitidine** and **cimetidine** are distributed into breast milk, removed by hemodialysis, and undergo extensive first pass metabolism. The half-life of parenteral **cimetidine** is 1.6 to 2.1 hours; parenteral **ranitidine** has a half-life of 2 to 2.5 hours; parenteral and oral **famotidine** has a half-life of 2.5 to 3.5 hours. The distribution of **famotidine** is unknown. The duration of **famotidine** is 10 to 12 hours; **cimetidine** is 6 to 8 hours; **nizatidine** is up to 12 hours; and **ranitidine** is 6 to 10 hours. • **Cimetidine** is also excreted in breast milk. **Nizatidine** and **ranitidine** are also excreted in feces.

• **Cimetidine** is used in the prophylactic treatment of duodenal ulcers. • **Ranitidine** is used in the treatment of theophylline toxicity.

IV **cimetidine** may also cause disorientation, hallucinations, agitation, psychosis, and cardiac arrhythmia. • **Ranitidine** and **cimetidine** may cause itching, burning, and pain at the injection site. • **Famotidine** may cause transient irritation at the IV site. • **Famotidine** and **ranitidine** may cause constipation and diarrhea. • **Famotidine** may cause flushing, palpitations, hypertension, and tinnitus. • **Ranitidine** may cause vomiting and abdominal discomfort. • **Nizatidine** may cause hyperuricemia.

• **Cimetidine** is contraindicated for people with liver disease.

• **Cimetidine,** in large doses, should be used cautiously for people with asthma.

(continued)

Focus on

Histamine₂ receptor antagonists: similarities and differences *(Continued)*

Similarities	Differences
Nursing considerations	
Instruct client in disease, treatment, drug therapy, regimen, adverse effects, and compliance; administer as a daily dose, preferably at bedtime; instruct client to take with food if necessary; separate doses of antacids by 1 to 2 hours; encourage client to avoid cigarette smoking; monitor blood studies for changes.	Administer IV **ranitidine** over 5 minutes or as an infusion over 15 to 20 minutes; do not dilute for IM injection; administer **famotidine** IV push over 2 minutes or more and as an IV infusion over 15 to 30 minutes; infuse IV **cimetidine** slowly over 30 minutes and warn client that IM injection of **cimetidine** may be painful; do not dilute **cimetidine** with sterile water for injection; administer **famotidine** for best results at bedtime; instruct client that it may be taken with a snack and it may be taken concomitantly with antacids.

Miscellaneous inhibitors of acid secretions

Omeprazole

Omeprazole (Losec, Prilosec) is an enzyme inhibitor that blocks a step in the formation of hydrochloric acid in the stomach.

Pharmacodynamics. Omeprazole acts by inhibiting the gastric enzyme H+, K+ ATPase, which catalyzes the final step in the production of acid at the secretory surface of the gastric parietal cell. It, therefore, blocks the final common pathway by which multiple stimuli act to stimulate gastric acid secretion.

Pharmacokinetics. Omeprazole is administered orally as a capsule taken once or twice daily. It is absorbed rapidly but undergoes extensive first-pass metabolism. About 95% of the drug present in the blood is bound to plasma proteins. Peak plasma levels occur within 4 hours. Terminal half-life is about 40 minutes. Omeprazole is excreted via urine (80%) and feces (20%).

Therapeutic indications. Omeprazole is used in the treatment of conditions requiring a reduction in stomach acid concentration (peptic ulcer, reflux esophagitis, and Zollinger-Ellis syndrome).

Dosage and administration. Adult dosages of omeprazole range from 20 to 40 mg daily, given in one or two doses. Up to 120 mg daily have been used in the treatment of Zollinger-Ellis syndrome. The drug is administered orally.

Adverse reactions. To date, only mild adverse effects have been reported, and the incidence of these is low. They include headache, nausea and vomiting, abdominal pain, dyspepsia, flatulence, and diarrhea or constipation. Skin rash has been reported in a few recipients.

Precautions and contraindications. Dosage for geriatric clients and those with impaired liver function should be limited to 20 mg daily. Omeprazole is contraindicated for clients who are hypersensitive to it or any other components of its preparations.

Drug interactions. Omeprazole inhibits the metabolism of warfarin, diazepam, and phenytoin, thereby increasing blood levels of these drugs. Dosage of these drugs may need to be reduced if omeprazole is added to the drug regimen.

Misoprostol

Pharmacodynamics. Misoprostol is a synthetic analog of prostaglandin E₁ (alprostadil). It acts as a gastric antisecretory agent that reduces gastric acid secretion and protects the mucosa from the irritant effects of drugs such as nonsteroidal anti-inflammatory antirheumatics. It is believed that misoprostol exerts the same protective effects as does alprostadil, a prostaglandin that is antagonized by the nonsteroidal anti-inflammatory drugs. The effects of misoprostol appear to be local rather than systemic.

Pharmacokinetics. Misoprostol is rapidly and completely absorbed from the GI tract, and is rapidly metabolized to an active metabolite, misoprostol acid, and two inactive metabolites. Food and antacids decrease the extent and delay the rate of systemic absorption. Although its action is local, the effects of misoprostol may be prolonged due to secretion of its active metabolite into the GI tract from the blood. Misoprostol is widely distributed in animal subjects.

Onset of action occurs within minutes; action peaks at 60–90 minutes and lasts about 3 hours. Misoprostol acid (the active metabolite of misoprostol) is 80%–90% protein bound. Distribution across the placenta or into milk is unknown.

Misoprostol and its metabolites are excreted primarily by the kidneys. Small amounts appear in the feces, probably via biliary elimination. Accumulation does not appear to occur following chronic administration. Serum half-life of the misoprostol acid is biphasic; 1.5 hours during the distribution phase and 20–40 minutes during the elimination phase. The drug is not removed by hemodialysis.

Therapeutic uses. Misoprostol is used for the prevention and treatment of nonsteroidal anti-inflammatory drug-induced gastric ulcers in persons at high risk of developing complications from these ulcers, and for treatment of duodenal ulcer.

Administration and dosage. Misoprostol is marketed as tablets containing 100 μg or 200 μg each. It is administered four times a day (after meals and at bedtime) in doses of 100–200 μg for up to 8 weeks. Dosage may be reduced for recipients with renal impairment.

Adverse reactions. Adverse reactions involving the GI tract (diarrhea, nausea, abdominal pain) may occur in up to 40% of recipients. Diarrhea is dose-related and usually, but not always, self-limiting, lasting approximately a week.

Other adverse reactions appear less frequently. Reported CNS effects include headache, fatigue, dizziness, and anxiety. Other reactions involve the following systems: genitourinary and renal (menstrual irregularities, polyuria, dysuria, hematuria, urinary tract infection); hematologic (anemia, thrombocytopenia, increased sedimentation rate); sensory (visual abnormalities, conjunctivitis, earache, tinnitus, deafness); dermatologic (rash, dermatitis, alopecia, purpura); cardiovascular (blood pressure changes, cardiac arrhythmias, phlebitis, angina, chest pain, edema); hepatic (altered liver function tests); and respiratory (infection, bronchospasm, epistaxis). Misoprostol can also cause abortion, fever, thirst, breast pain, impotence, arthralgia, myalgia, stiffness, back pain, and weight changes.

Precautions and contraindications. As a new drug, misoprostol is likely to produce other adverse reactions not seen or reported to date. Package inserts should be read each time a new supply is obtained because the information in the inserts may change frequently.

Misoprostol is contraindicated during pregnancy, and for individuals with allergic hypersensitivity to prostaglandins. It is not recommended during lactation.

Caution should be used when the drug is prescribed for clients with inflammatory bowel disease, or those prone to dehydration. It should not be used concurrently with magnesium antacids or other laxative preparations. Safety and efficacy in children younger than 18 years of age have not been established.

To date, misoprostol appears to interact with few drugs. It has been effective in reversing cyclosporine toxicity in animals.

■ **Summary**

A number of drugs act to inhibit acid production by the gastric mucosa. They are effective agents for the treatment of peptic ulcers and are often used to prevent the development of stress ulcers. Adverse reactions to this group of drugs occur infrequently but are variable and affect many body systems. All of these drugs are fairly new. As of this writing, cimetidine has been in use for less than 20 years; the newest, omeprazole was approved for use in the United States less than 4 years ago. For this reason, it is important to monitor clients for signs and symptoms of long-term adverse effects that may not yet have been documented.

Antacids

Antacids are alkaline chemicals administered orally to neutralize hydrochloric acid secreted by the stomach mucosa. They are used to relieve discomfort and reduce trauma caused by the corrosive effect of acid on exposed GI tissues. Unlike the inhibitors of acid secretion, antacids can be purchased without a prescription and are widely used for self-medication without supervision by health professionals. Although generally safe, these drugs are not without side effects and toxicity.

When prescribing antacids, the physician must consider their therapeutic efficacy, their acceptability to the client, adverse reactions, and cost. Although the prescription may require adjustment to achieve optimal results, neither client nor nurse should substitute one antacid for another without consulting the physician.

Pharmacodynamics. Most antacids are alkaline salts or hydroxides of sodium, calcium, magnesium, or aluminum. They react chemically with hydrochloric acid to form neutral or weak acid salts, thereby increasing gastric pH.

Among antacid preparations, acid-neutralizing capacity varies considerably. A specific preparation may also vary over time because drug manufacturers continuously reformulate antacid preparations. Liquid formulations are generally more effective than tablets (Table 30-4).

Pharmacokinetics. The salts resulting from the chemical neutralization occurring in the stomach mix with other materials in the GI tract and are subjected to the normal digestive process. If the chemical complex is broken down and absorbed, the body gains base reserve. If it is not, acidic material is carried out of the body in the feces.

Table 30-4. Properties of selected antacids

Drug name	Preparations	Usual adult dosage	Ingredients	Acid-neutralizing capacity/dose	Sodium content/ dose
Alka-Seltzer Effervescent Antacid	Tablets	2 tablets	Sodium bicarbonate, citric acid, potassium bicarbonate	21.2 mEq/2 tablets	592 mg/2 tablets
Alka-2 Antacid	Chewable tablets	2 tablets	Calcium carbonate	21 mEq/2 tablets	4 mg/2 tablets
Alka-Seltzer Effervescent Pain Reliever and Antacid	Tablets	2 tablets in 6 oz water	Sodium bicarbonate, citric acid, aspirin	34.4 mEq/2 tablets	1102 mg/2 tablets
AlternaGEL	Liquid	2 tsp	Aluminum hydroxide	32 mEq/2 tsp	<4 mg/2 tsp
Amphojel	Liquid	2 tsp	Aluminum hydroxide	13 mEq/2 tsp	14 mg/2 tsp
	Tablets	2 tablets	Aluminum hydroxide	4 mEq/2 tablets	14 mg/2 tablets
Basaljel Extra-Strength	Liquid	2 tsp	Aluminum carbonate	29 mEq/2 tsp	46 mg/2 tsp
Basaljel	Tablets	2 tablets	Aluminum carbonate	30.8 mEq/2 tablets	4 mg/2 tablets
Camalox	Liquid	2–4 tsp	Magnesium hydroxide	32 mEq/2 tsp	5 mg/2 tsp
	Tablets	2 tablets	Magnesium hydroxide	33.4 mEq/2 tablets	3 mg/2 tablets
Delcid	Liquid	2 tsp	Aluminum hydroxide, magnesium hydroxide	41 mEq/2 tsp	3 mg/2 tsp
Maalox TC	Liquid	2–4 tsp	Aluminum hydroxide, magnesium hydroxide	42 mEq/2 tsp	2.4 mg/2 tsp
Maalox Plus	Liquid	2–4 tsp	Aluminum hydroxide, magnesium hydroxide, simethicone	23 mEq/2 tsp	5 mg/2 tsp
	Tablets	1–2 tablets	Aluminum hydroxide, magnesium hydroxide, simethicone	11.4 mEq/2 tablets	2.8 mg/2 tablets
Mylanta II	Liquid	1–2 tsp	Aluminum hydroxide, magnesium hydroxide, simethicone	36 mEq/2 tsp	2.2 mg/2 tsp
	Tablets	2 tablets	Aluminum hydroxide, magnesium hydroxide, simethicone	22 mEq/2 tablets	2.6 mg/2 tablets
Di-Gel	Liquid	2 tsp	Aluminum hydroxide, magnesium carbonate, magnesium hydroxide, simethicone	24 mEq/2 tsp	17 mg/2 tsp
	Tablets	2 tablets	Aluminum hydroxide, magnesium carbonate, magnesium hydroxide, simethicone	9.4 mEq/2 tablets	10 mg/2 tablets
Gelusil	Liquid	2 tsp	Aluminum hydroxide, magnesium hydroxide, simethicone	22 mEq/2 tsp	1.4 mg/2 tsp
Gelusil II	Tablets	2 tablets	Aluminum hydroxide, magnesium hydroxide, simethicone	16.4 mEq/2 tablets	4.2 mg/2 tablets
Milk of Magnesia	Liquid	2 tsp	Magnesium hydroxide	27 mEq/2 tsp	0
	Tablets	2 tablets	Magnesium hydroxide	21.4 mEq/2 tablets	0
Phillips' Lo-Sal	Tablets	1 tablet– 2 tablets	Calcium carbonate, magnesium hydroxide	31.2 mEq/2 tablets	Less than 0.4 mg/2 tablets
Riopan	Liquid	5–20 ml	Magaldrate*	8.8 mEq/5 ml	0.7 mg/5 ml
Riopan Plus	Liquid	1–2 tsp	Magaldrate,* simethicone	18 mEq/2 tsp	1.4 mg/2 tsp
	Tablets	1–2 tablets	Magaldrate,* simethicone	20 mEq/2 tablets	0.6 mg/2 tablets
Titralac	Liquid	1 tsp	Calcium carbonate, glycine	21 mEq/1 tsp	11 mg/1 tsp
	Tablets	2 tablets	Calcium carbonate, glycine	19 mEq/2 tablets	0.6 mg/2 tablets
Tums	Tablets (regular)	1–2 tablets	Calcium carbonate	21 mEq/2 tablets	5.4 mg/2 tablets

The above data cannot be applied to current products marketed under the designated names because commercial preparations are frequently reformulated.

*A complex hydroxy-magnesium aluminate.

Therapeutic uses. Antacids are used for the treatment of peptic ulcers and other hydrochloric acid-related conditions. They are often used in conjunction with antimuscarinics or histamine₂ receptor antagonists.

Adverse reactions. Antacids tend to increase body fluid pH and can cause metabolic alkalosis (milk-alkali syndrome). The increase in gastric pH stimulates renewed secretion of acid, causing acid rebound, which may be severe. When antacids are the sole treatment agent, they must be administered repeatedly to maintain the lowered acidity. When administration is interrupted during the night, a very low pH may develop in the stomach, reversing the beneficial effects of daytime treatment.

Some adverse reactions are specific to the metallic cations present in antacids (Table 30-5). Sodium increases the risk of overhydration and hypervolemia. Aluminum binds with dietary phosphate, forming an undigestable precipitate that is excreted in feces.

Hypermagnesemia reduces impulse transmission, causing sedation and weakness. Myocardial rhythm is affected by both magnesium and calcium. Aluminum

and magnesium, which are both neurotoxic, are associated with encephalopathies. High serum levels of metallic ions during pregnancy can affect the fetus because they cross the placenta freely, and elevations in the maternal circulation are reflected in the fetus.

The heavier metals (calcium, magnesium, and aluminum) form compounds that characteristically are not very soluble. They predispose to the formation of concretions (calculi) in both the GI tract and the renal system.

Aluminum and calcium compounds cause constipation, whereas sodium and magnesium are laxative in effect. Both disturbances are frequent problems in antacid therapy. Drug manufacturers produce multiple preparations with varying combinations of antacids to try to balance the effects on bowel function and to minimize these problems. Individual responses to the formulas vary. It is often necessary to make successive trials of several products to determine the best one.

Although antacids have the potential for causing serious physiologic problems, they have a fairly wide safety margin. Clinical problems occur mainly when large doses are prescribed or over-the-counter preparations are seriously abused. An appreciation of the risks of antacid therapy has been slow to develop; it is possible that adverse reactions are still underdiagnosed.

Some antacid preparations contain sugar, which could cause hyperglycemia in diabetic clients.

Precautions and contraindications. A certain percentage of most antacids is absorbed, altering blood chemistry and elevating the serum levels of individual metals. Sodium is contraindicated for many persons for whom water retention is harmful. Even healthy persons should avoid excessive sodium intake, which is believed to contribute to the development of hypertension.

Magnesium and aluminum compounds should be used with caution by individuals with impaired kidney function.

Antacid regimens should be tailored to the individual needs of clients. For example, combinations of both laxative and constipating agents are often needed to maintain normal fecal elimination.

Drug interactions. Antacids interact with many other drug agents. Within the GI tract, they combine chemically with some drugs, notably tetracycline antibiotics, forming complexes that resist digestion and pass unchanged out of the system. When administered with enteric-coated drugs, they may disintegrate the coating, releasing these drugs prematurely in the stomach. Elevations of pH also alter membrane transport of alkaline and acidic compounds, promoting passive diffusion of acidic chemicals and lipid membrane transport of alkaline chemicals. Passive diffusion of alkaline substances and lipid membrane trans-

Table 30-5. Adverse reactions to the metallic elements of antacids

Ion	Adverse reactions
Sodium	Water retention (increased risk of edema, ascites, effusion, hypertension, premenstrual tension, heart failure)
	Reduced iron absorption
Calcium	Constipation
	Milk—alkali syndrome (including pronounced alkalosis)
	Rebound hyperacidity
	Potentiation of digitalis
	Renal calculi
	Impaired absorption of such drugs as tetracycline and iron
Magnesium	Diarrhea (increased risk of hypokalemia)
	Iron deficiency owing to complexation of iron
	Hypermagnesemia (causing sedation, weakness, cardiac arrhythmias, and encephalopathy), especially in persons with renal impairment
	Impaired absorption of such drugs as tetracycline and iron
Aluminum	Constipation
	Phosphate depletion and osteomalacia
	Delayed gastric emptying
	Intestinal concretions (increased risk of colonic perforation and peritonitis)
	Encephalopathy
	Impairment of absorption of such drugs as tetracycline, digitalis, and isoniazid

port of acidic substances are inhibited. These effects can alter both absorption and excretion of many systemic drugs.

Digitalis is potentiated by hypercalcemia; calcium directly augments the ionic stimulation of cardiac contractility, thereby mimicking the action of digitalis. Magnesium may also potentiate digitalis by depleting potassium stores (causing hypokalemia) secondary to diarrhea.

■ **Summary**

Antacids are basic compounds that act locally in the stomach to neutralize hydrochloric acid. They are comparable to H_2 receptor antagonists in cost and in effectiveness as antiulcer drugs. However, they must be administered more often than do H_2 receptor antagonists. Antacids may alter the absorption of other drugs administered at the same time. They can also cause adverse reactions because of local and systemic actions of the cation portion of the molecules.

Sucralfate

Sucralfate is an anionic sulfated disaccharide structurally related to heparin.

Pharmacodynamics. Sucralfate's therapeutic effects appear to be local (*ie*, at ulcer sites in the upper GI tract), rather than systemic. Sucralfate reacts with hydrochloric acid in the stomach to form a pastelike substance that is highly viscous and adhesive. This material binds to the surface of the GI mucosa, exhibiting a pronounced affinity for ulcer sites. Sucralfate does not reduce gastric acid output or concentration. The combination of mechanical barrier and local acid neutralization may be important for protection of the ulcer site from the actions of pepsin, acid, and bile.

Pharmacokinetics. Following oral administration, sucralfate is only minimally absorbed from the GI tract. Only 3%–5% of an oral dose reaches the systemic circulation as sucrose sulfate. Distribution has not been determined, and it is unknown whether sucrose sulfate crosses the placenta or is distributed in breast milk. Most of the drug administered orally remains in the GI tract and is eliminated in feces. The small amount absorbed is excreted unchanged by the kidneys.

Therapeutic uses. Sucralfate is approved for use in the short-term treatment of duodenal ulcers. It has also been used for the treatment of oral ulcers (Solomon, 1986) and gastric ulcers, as well as for the prevention of aspirin-induced gastric erosions. Usual adult dosage is one 1 g tablet po qid for a course of 4–8 weeks.

Adverse reactions. Sucralfate is generally well tolerated. Constipation affects about 2% of recipients;

nausea, diarrhea, gastric discomfort, indigestion, dry mouth, rash, pruritus, back pain, dizziness, sleepiness, and vertigo have also been reported.

Sucralfate may bind to other oral drugs (cimetidine, phenytoin, tetracycline), reducing their bioavailability.

Precautions and contraindications. Safety and efficacy in children have not been established. Evidence concerning mutagenicity, carcinogenicity, and teratogenicity of the drug is incomplete. Safe use during pregnancy and lactation has not been established.

■ **Summary**

Sucralfate is an antiulcer drug that acts mechanically by forming a protective coating over the ulcer site. It appears to be comparable in efficacy to antacids and H_2 receptor antagonists. Adverse reactions are relatively minor, affecting mainly the GI tract.

Nursing management

Nursing implications

Treatment for acid-related problems is required in a variety of conditions. Prescription of the drugs discussed above is an indication that the recipient is at risk; therefore, nursing measures to minimize acid secretion are appropriate.

Stress is believed to contribute to gastric acid production by a number of mechanisms, including parasympathetic activity and the secretion of adrenergic and glucocorticoid hormones. For this reason, nursing measures to reduce stress are therapeutic for the client suffering from hyperacidity. The nurse should reduce clients' stress and assist them in managing unavoidable stress. Periodic diversion is helpful when situational stress cannot be eliminated.

Smoking and the consumption of alcohol should be discouraged. The so-called ulcer diets are no longer in common use but adaptation of food intake is important. Any food that the client recognizes as contributing to symptoms of hyperacidity should be omitted. Coffee, chocolate, and foods rich in carbohydrates, fats, and spices may increase symptoms. It is wise for the client to eliminate these items temporarily from the diet, then to test them individually for tolerance before resuming consumption.

Treatment of peptic ulcers. Peptic ulcer disease is characterized by remissions and exacerbations. Multiple drug therapy, a modified diet, and rest are usually prescribed. Compliance with the medical regimen is likely to fluctuate with the severity of symptoms. Adherence to the regimen is vital to recovery. In the case of cimetidine, at least, continuous therapy is recommended for long periods of time (Wade, 1988).

Treatment of hiatal hernias. Clients with hiatal hernias often have antacids prescribed to prevent the effects of regurgitated acid on the lower esophagus. This is not solely a comfort measure but a preventative measure to reduce the risk of esophagitis, esophageal rupture, or atresia. Repeated exposure of the mucosa to gastric acid can cause esophagitis. Peptic ulcerations of the esophagus can result in perforation, just as happens in the stomach or duodenum. Such perforation allows the escape of GI contents (food, acid, bile) into the chest cavity. This complication is apt to occur during an episode of vomiting when perforation is followed immediately by rapid propulsion of the stomach contents into the chest. Chemical damage to lung tissue and tension pneumothorax follow. This is a life-threatening emergency requiring immediate surgical intervention to drain the chest. This circumstance also calls for life-support measures in an intensive care situation.

Chronic acid regurgitation that is inadequately controlled with antacid therapy causes repeated episodes of inflammation followed by healing. Fibrotic scars develop, which tend to contract as they age. Over time, the esophagus becomes constricted, and swallowing is impaired. Esophageal atresia predisposes to acute obstruction of the esophagus, requiring surgical removal of the impacted food. Surgical correction of the esophageal deformity is often necessary.

Compliance. The critical nature of complications makes it very important that clients carry out their medical regimens accurately. Assessing clients' compliance and intervening to encourage it are important nursing functions. Many clients omit doses of medications because the preparation is unpalatable, expensive, or inconvenient to carry (especially the liquid antacids).

Although the overall cost of histamine₂ receptor inhibitors and antacids is comparable,* only drugs requiring prescriptions are covered by most prescription insurance coverage. Hence, the client usually must bear all of the cost of antiacid treatment.

Clients may be reluctant to carry large bottles of liquid to school, work, or social events because the bottles are difficult to conceal and their presence identifies the nature of the health problem. Rather than risk omitting doses, it might be preferable for the client to carry a dry (tablet) form of antacid to use in such situations. Distressing adverse reactions can also reduce clients' motivation to adhere to their dosage schedule. Identifying and eliminating specific impediments to individual acceptance of the drug regimen are critical in improving compliance.

---

* Per dose cost is higher for histamine₂ receptor antagonists than for antacid medications; however, antacid medication must be administered more frequently than are the prescription drugs.

Nursing process

Assessment Clients under treatment for hyperacidity should be evaluated to determine their general health and nutritional status. If peptic ulcer disease has been diagnosed, the nurse should look for signs and symptoms of anemia, which can develop when ulcers bleed. The nature, severity, and chronology of pain associated with hyperacidity should be delineated. In addition, the client's stress levels and stress-reduction skills should be evaluated. A complete drug history should be taken, with particular attention given to nonsteroidal anti-inflammatory drugs and other medications likely to stimulate acid production.

Nursing diagnosis Clients with hyperacidity are likely to experience the following:

Pain (burning epigastric pain, heartburn) related to hyperacidity secondary to peptic ulceration, hiatal hernia, or use of ulcerogenic drugs

Clients for whom H₂ receptor antagonists are prescribed may develop the following:

Pain: headache, muscle pains, bone and joint pain related to use of histamine receptor antagonists
Sexual dysfunction: decreased libido and potency secondary to cimetidine therapy

Common collaborative problems that should be differentiated from the nursing diagnoses include

Potential complication: hypovolemic shock related to hemorrhage
Potential complication: CNS effects
Potential complication: hepatotoxicity
Potential complication: renal toxicity

Clients receiving misoprostol or omeprazole may develop

Altered comfort: intestinal upset, nausea, vomiting, abdominal pain
Diarrhea

Additional diagnoses may be made if the client shows inadequate therapeutic response, or if toxic reactions appear to medications administered with inhibitors of hydrochloric acid secretion because of the latter's influence on the absorption or metabolism of other drugs.

Clients receiving antacids are likely to develop:

Constipation (diarrhea) related to use of aluminum, calcium (or magnesium) antacids
Altered nutrition: more than body requirements related to ingestion of sugars in antacid formulations
Pain: abdominal discomfort related to adverse reaction to sucralfate medication

Clients receiving sucralfate may develop

Altered bowel function: constipation (diarrhea) related to adverse reaction to medication

A common collaborative problem that should be differentiated from the nursing diagnosis is

Potential complication: phosphate deficiency

Many clients will have a knowledge deficit related to hyperacidity and drugs used for its treatment.

Planning Goals for treatment include increased gastric pH; decreased pain; prompt detection and treatment of upper GI bleeding (if it develops); maintenance of normal fecal elimination; prompt detection and treatment of other adverse reactions to antihyperacidity medications; prevention of adverse drug interactions; prevention of iatrogenic hyperglycemia in diabetic clients; and client education about hyperacidity and its treatment.

Intervention The nurse should regularly assess clients receiving antihyperacidity drugs for therapeutic response, gastric bleeding, known adverse reactions to prescribed drugs, changes indicative of previously unidentified adverse reactions, and compliance to the drug regimen. Reports of epigastric discomfort and tenderness, or "heartburn," are significant indicators of continued tissue damage from excess acid. Symptoms attributable to hyperacidity should decline with treatment. Gastric bleeding may be detected by testing stools for occult blood, or by the presence of tarry stools or coffee ground emesis.

Particular attention should be paid to signs and symptoms of alkalosis, changes in bowel function, and specific effects of the metallic ions contained in some of the drugs. Fecal elimination should be monitored; nursing measures may be employed to alleviate mild constipation or diarrhea.

Clients receiving sucralfate, misoprostol, omeprazole, or H_2 receptor antagonists must be carefully evaluated for side effects of and adverse reactions to these drugs. Although they appear to have wide margins of safety, they are relatively new drugs and may have unrecognized potential for toxic effects.

The physician should be informed of therapeutic response to the drug regimen and any complications such as gastric bleeding. The nurse should also consult with the physician (for possible changes in the drug regimen) if the client develops adverse drug reactions, such as persistent or severe constipation or diarrhea, impaired kidney or liver function, discomfiting nervous system changes, susceptibility to infection, or pain.

Administration. When oral antacids are administered, tablets should be chewed or sucked to dissolve the medication before being swallowed. The drugs will not combine efficiently with acid unless they reach the stomach in a solution or a finely divided form. When liquid antacids are administered, each dose should have sufficient volume and neutralizing capacity to reach the stomach. Small amounts of water may be given with antacids but large amounts (more than 4 ounces) stimulate gastric emptying and may propel the medication promptly into the small bowel.

Antacids are administered in frequent doses. Acutely ill ulcer clients may receive the drug by continuous intragastric drip. This is particularly helpful in controlling acid rebound and in reducing gastric pH during the night. Oral doses may be ordered at hourly intervals, then every 2 hours as recovery progresses. The use of anticholinergics or histamine (H_2) receptor antagonists allows less frequent dosing with antacids, which may then be given after meals and at bedtime. Palatability is an important consideration. Plain compounds tend to taste "chalky." Flavored preparations are available for many formulations.

Antacid medication is often left at the hospital bedside for self-medication by the client. Most institutions require a specific physician's order for this practice. The nurse should supervise use of the drug carefully to ensure that the regimen is carried out accurately. This situation is ideal for teaching the client, who is likely to receive continued antacid therapy after discharge.

Client education. Whereas clients requiring antacid prescriptions tend to take inadequate amounts, the lay public generally overuses them when self-prescribed. The general public has been conditioned to regard antacids as convenient home remedies for the relief of minor symptoms, rather than as prescription drugs for the treatment of illness. Family traditions of dosing with antacids, media advertisements extolling the virtues of "fast relief for overindulgence," and the reluctance of medical reimbursement plans to pay for antacid therapy are some of the reasons antacids have been traditionally accepted as casual remedies. Their value as an efficacious medical treatment, with risks of adverse reactions and toxicity, is not appreciated.

Nurses who educate the public about self-medication should discourage the use of antacids except in isolated incidents clearly related to unusual circumstances. Occasional self-medication to relieve distressing symptoms of overindulgence will probably cause no serious problems. More frequent use or the need for unusual doses are warning signals. Medical attention should be sought to determine the underlying problem. A peptic ulcer, hiatal hernia, or other disease may be found. Treatment of the underlying pathology may well include continued use of antacids, but in a more definitive fashion, with careful selection of the proper agent, a regular schedule of specific doses, and medical supervision of the client's progress. Other treatment measures are usually also added to the antacid regimen.

Clients should be cautioned particularly against using sodium bicarbonate (baking soda) as an antacid. Although temporarily effective in relieving hyperacidity, sodium bicarbonate reacts with acid to generate a considerable amount of carbon dioxide gas, causing dangerous stomach distention. If a portion of the organ's wall is weakened, as in gastric ulcer disease, perforation can occur. This is a potentially fatal condition requiring immediate medical attention. Other problems related to use of sodium bicarbonate are pronounced acid rebound and significant alkalosis (the chemical is easily and completely absorbed). Sodium bicarbonate's high sodium content can seriously disturb electrolyte balance and is particularly detrimental to persons who should restrict their sodium intake.

Abdominal pain or heartburn is sometimes experienced during cardiac ischemia or infarction. Self-treatment with sodium bicarbonate can be very detrimental if it causes a delay in seeking proper medical attention. Moreover, large doses of sodium in such situations predisposes the client to congestive heart failure.

Clients with peptic ulcer disease experience remissions and exacerbations. During acute episodes, the regimen is likely to be followed meticulously but when symptoms subside, compliance is apt to be poor. Both H₂ receptor antagonists and antacids are of proven value in the treatment of peptic ulcers. Adherence to the prescribed regimen is critical to enhance healing and to prevent complications.

Education about the serious nature of peptic ulcer disease and the critical need for compliance with the regimen should be initiated as soon as the diagnosis is made. Clients may remain inpatients in acute care facilities until response to treatment is evident and their physiologic status stabilizes. This period is ideal for teaching clients how to manage their therapeutic regimen after discharge.

Clients receiving cimetidine, ranitidine, or sucralfate should report unusual signs and symptoms that could indicate previously undetected side effects of, or adverse reactions to, these drugs.

Evaluation Data needed for evaluation include gastric *p*H, clients' reports that they are comfortable, the consistency and frequency of stools, the duration and severity of adverse drug reactions, and the blood sugar levels of diabetic clients.

The *p*H of gastric fluid may be monitored to determine the effects of antacid medication when a nasogastric tube is in place. Specimens of gastric secretions are taken before medication, 15 or 30 minutes after medi-

cation, and every 30 minutes thereafter. Testing materials for *p*H include Combistix R, Nitrozine R paper, and Phydrion paper. (See Example of Nursing Process and Therapy with Ranitidine and Antacids.)

Checklist of nursing actions

☐ Urge clients who frequently self-administer antacids to seek medical care to determine the cause of their symptoms.

☐ When drugs are prescribed to combat hyperacidity, help the client to reduce stress levels and to manage unavoidable stress effectively.

☐ Discourage smoking and the consumption of alcohol by clients experiencing hyperacidity.

☐ Assist clients in identifying and eliminating from their diets foods that stimulate acid secretions.

☐ Monitor clients receiving drugs to combat hyperacidity for therapeutic and adverse reactions to the drugs.

☐ Instruct clients to chew antacid tablets thoroughly before swallowing.

☐ Supervise clients' use of antacids when these drugs are left at the bedside in institutional settings.

☐ Stress the importance of compliance to the medication regimen for preventing the progression of the disease.

☐ Warn clients not to use baking soda as an antacid.

☐ Urge clients receiving new drugs such as misoprostol or omeprazole to report promptly unusual signs and symptoms.

Antiemetics

Nausea and vomiting are common problems that require skilled nursing care. They herald the onset of many acute illnesses and accompany chronic illnesses, drug reactions, emotional disturbances, and pregnancy. Few symptoms are more distressing.

Pathophysiology

The vomiting reflex is complex and not well understood (Fig. 30-2). Impulses from the cerebral cortex, the aural vestibular apparatus, and all parts of the GI tract stimulate the medullary centers that mediate the reflex. Many impulses are transmitted to the chemoreceptor trigger zone (CTZ) before acting on the vomiting center. Impulses from the vomiting center stimulate a sequence of motor acts in the upper GI tract, which result in rapid emptying of the stomach. Closely associated with the vomiting center is an area whose excitation produces the sensation of nausea. Nausea is often accompanied by symptoms of autonomic (mainly

Example of nursing process and therapy with ranitidine and antacids

The client is a 65-year-old machinist with a long-standing history of peptic ulcer disease. He has been treated with antacids (Mylanta II, 15 ml q2h PRN), which he takes regularly after meals and at bedtime and at other times when heartburn occurs. Until recently, he has had no pronounced signs or symptoms of recurrent ulcers for over 5 years. Six months ago, he retired from his job. He has been consulting the physician because he has had increased heartburn and epigastric pain for several days, which the antacids do not control. An upper GI x-ray series reveals a small duodenal ulcer. The physician has prescribed ranitidine 150 mg bid and continued use of antacids PRN.

Assessment data	Nursing diagnosis	Intervention	Goals and outcome criteria
The client complains of heartburn and epigastric pain, which persists despite antacid medication	Pain: epigastric pain and heartburn related to inflammation and irritation secondary to hyperacidity and peptic ulcer; possible contributing factor, the stress of retirement.	**Recommend** that the client continue to take a dose of antacid after meals and at bedtime until he is pain free.	Within a week the client will report that he is having little or no heartburn or epigastric pain.
Medical diagnosis of duodenal peptic ulcers		**Instruct** the client to take ranitidine at 12-hour intervals, to maximize its inhibitory effect on stomach secretion of HCl.	
Recent retirement		**Explore** with the client stressors affecting him since his retirement; assist him in planning to decrease them. Review with the client stress management techniques he has used in the past; teach new techniques as appropriate.	
New prescription for ranitidine	Probable knowledge deficit relating to ranitidine and histamine$_2$ receptor antagonists	**Inform** the client that a few people who take ranitidine experience adverse reactions. Instruct him to report to his primary health care provider if he develops persistent, severe headaches, muscle or joint pains, or signs and symptoms of CNS disturbance. Inform the client that ranitidine is a fairly new drug and that it may have some adverse effects that remained unreported; advise the client to inform his primary health care provider of any unusual changes that coincide with the use of ranitidine.	The client will report significant signs and symptoms to the nurse or physician.

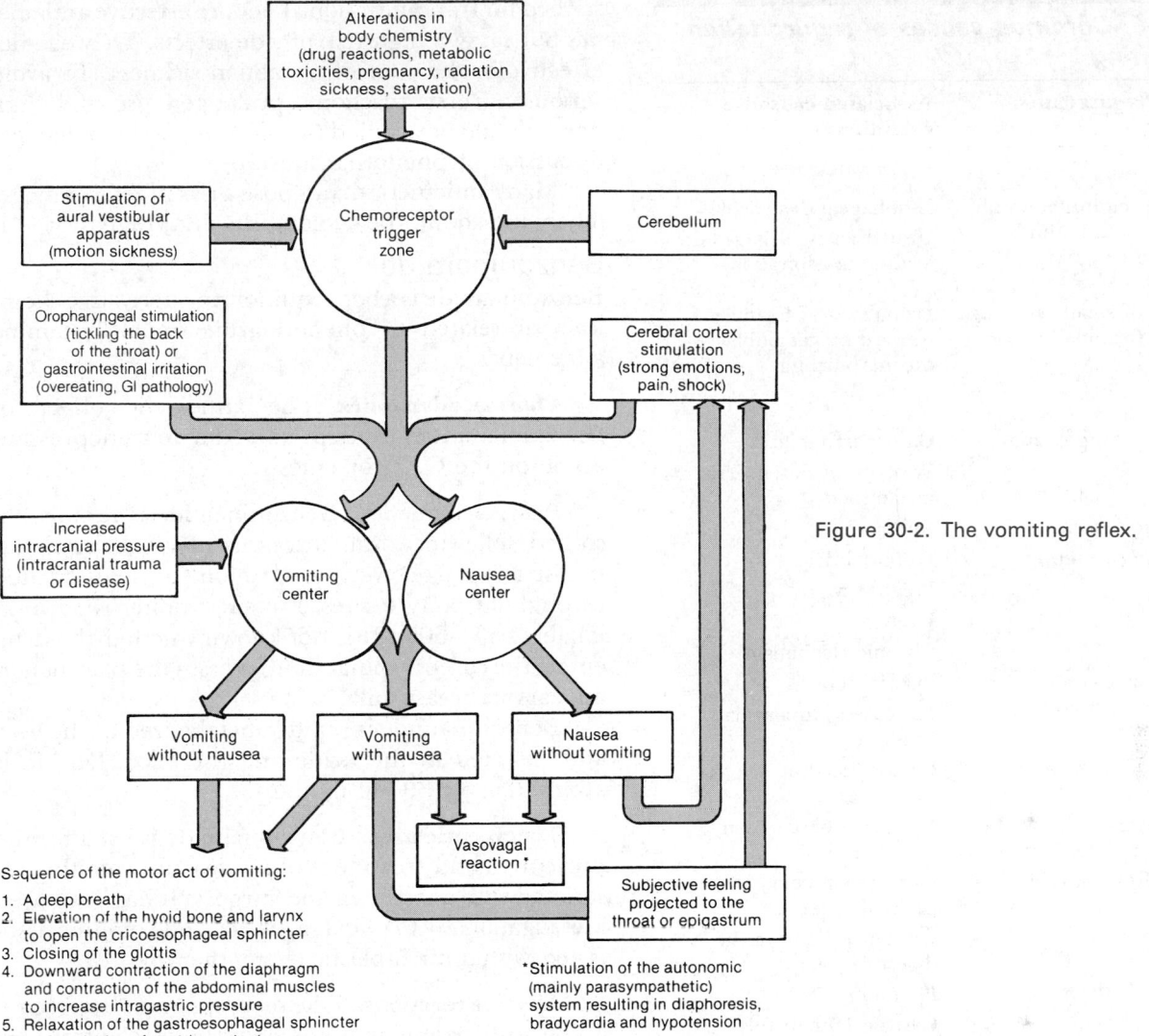

Figure 30-2. The vomiting reflex.

Sequence of the motor act of vomiting:

1. A deep breath
2. Elevation of the hyoid bone and larynx to open the cricoesophageal sphincter
3. Closing of the glottis
4. Downward contraction of the diaphragm and contraction of the abdominal muscles to increase intragastric pressure
5. Relaxation of the gastroesophageal sphincter and explusion of gastric contents through the esophagus

*Stimulation of the autonomic (mainly parasympathetic) system resulting in diaphoresis, bradycardia and hypotension

parasympathetic) stimulation: increased perspiration, salivation, pallor, bradycardia, and hypotension.

Some reports of vomiting by clients describe regurgitation rather than true vomiting. The nurse must be able to assess the phenomenon described to determine the appropriate nursing response (Table 30-6). Regurgitation is a relatively passive emission of material from the upper GI tract owing to various mechanical factors, such as incomplete swallowing, eructation, or aspiration. Vomiting is characterized by reverse peristalsis, which forcibly empties the stomach.

Causes of vomiting are many; they range from the physiologic state of pregnancy to serious pathology. It is essential that a complete assessment be carried out to determine the reason for the problem. Whenever possible, the best approach is to eliminate the cause. For many reasons, it may be impossible to correct the underlying pathology. At that point, measures are required to control nausea and to reduce vomiting.

Classification of antiemetics

Antiemetic drugs are helpful adjuncts in controlling nausea and reducing vomiting. Selected antiemetics are listed in Table 30-7.

The vomiting reflex can be interrupted at any point on its pathway. If vomiting is due to GI irritation or pain, drugs given to reduce these problems may exert an antiemetic effect. Some general CNS depressants, such as phenobarbital, also suppress vomiting. The drugs generally classified as antiemetics act on the vomiting center, the CTZ, or the aural vestibular apparatus (Fig. 30-3). Most of these drugs are anticholinergics, antihistamines, or phenothiazines (discussed in detail in Chapters 22, 35, and 26 respectively).

The *anticholinergics* depress excitatory labyrinthine impulses in the vestibular nuclei. Their GI effects (decreased motility, secretion, and spasm) also tend to reduce enteric stimulation of the vomiting center. Of this group of drugs, scopolamine is most commonly

Table 30-6. Common causes of regurgitation and vomiting

Patterns of regurgitation or vomiting	Associated causative conditions
Regurgitation	
Nonforcible regurgitation of undigested food or fluids, often during coughing episodes	Esophageal diverticula
	Insufficiency of gag reflex leading to aspiration
Spitting up of small amounts of formula by infants	Propulsion of formula upward by gas bubbles during burping
Vomiting	
Vomiting following eating	Gastric irritability
	Presence of potent irritants in the food
Deliberate or self-induced	Bulimia
Early morning vomiting	Postnasal drip
	Pregnancy
	Uremia
	Chronic alcoholism
Forceful (projectile) vomiting often without nausea	Pyloric stenosis
	Increased intracranial pressure
Bloody or coffee-ground emesis	Gastric bleeding
Vomitus of digested food 12 or more hours after eating	Duodenal obstruction
Vomitus of food with bile	Obstruction below the ampulla of Vater
Fecal vomiting	Obstruction low in the digestive tract
	Peritonitis
	Gastrocolonic fistula

employed for antiemetic effect. It carries a high incidence of anticholinergic side effects, such as tachycardia, palpitations, dry mouth, constipation, urinary hesitancy, urinary retention, impotence, dizziness, nervousness, and blurred vision. Because of its mydriatic effect, scopolamine is contraindicated in glaucoma.

The *antihistamines* depress selected portions of the CNS system, but their antiemetic effects appear to be due, in large part, to their anticholinergic properties. Hydroxyzine (Vistaril) and dimenhydrinate (Dramamine) are common antihistamine antiemetics. Dimenhydrinate has been quite popular as a preventative of motion sickness. In addition to anticholinergic side effects, antihistamines frequently cause drowsiness. (See Chapter 35 for a detailed discussion of antihistamines.)

Like antihistamines, *phenothiazines* are CNS depressants. Major antipsychotics, they are often pre-scribed for tranquilization. They are effective antiemetics but carry a high risk of side effects. They are not effective in the control of motion sickness. To avoid serious adverse reactions, prolonged use and high doses should be avoided (see Chapter 26 for a detailed discussion of phenothiazines).

Many antiemetic drugs pose a risk of fetal damage. Their use should be avoided during pregnancy.

Benzquinamide

Benzquinamide is a benzoquinolizine derivative chemically unrelated to phenothiazine or antihistamine antiemetics.

Pharmacodynamics. The antiemetic effect of benzquinamide is thought to be due to its depressant action on the CTZ for emesis.

Pharmacokinetics. Benzquinamide is rapidly absorbed following oral, intramuscular, or rectal administration. Following absorption, it is distributed throughout body tissues. Protein binding is approximately 55%–60%. It is not known whether the drug enters the cerebrospinal fluid, crosses the placenta, or appears in breast milk.

Benzquinamide is rapidly metabolized by the liver and excreted in the urine and the bile. Half-life is approximately 30–40 minutes.

Therapeutic uses. Benzquinamide is used for the prevention and treatment of nausea and vomiting associated with anesthesia and surgery. It has been used investigationally to manage nausea and vomiting associated with antineoplastic chemotherapy.

Adverse reactions. The most common adverse reaction to benzquinamide is drowsiness. Central nervous system stimulation can also occur, as manifested by tremor, insomnia, restlessness, headache, excitement, and nervousness. Gastrointestinal side effects include dry mouth, hiccups, anorexia, nausea, vomiting, abdominal cramps, and salivation. Shivering, sweating, flushing, weakness, and fatigue have been reported. Cardiovascular effects, which include alterations in blood pressure, atrial fibrillation, and premature atrial and ventricular contractions are associated with intravenous administration.

Precautions and contraindications. Intravenous administration of benzquinamide should be avoided whenever possible. This route is contraindicated for persons with cardiovascular disease or for clients who have received drugs that alter blood pressure or cause arrhythmias. Benzquinamide is also contraindicated for persons allergic to it.

Use of benzquinamide may mask the signs and symptoms of conditions such as intestinal obstruction, brain tumor, or drug overdose. These conditions should be ruled out before the drug is administered.

Table 30-7. Antiemetics

Drug name	Preparations	Mode of action	Usual dosage	Additional information
Anticholinergics				
scopolamine (Transderm, Scōp; *Can:* Transderm V)	Transdermal patch for topical application	Depression of labyrinthine impulses in the vestibular nucleus	Adults: one system programmed to deliver 0.5 mg of scopolamine over 72 hr PC: C	Scopolamine is considered one of the most effective drugs for the treatment of motion sickness but it causes a high incidence of anticholinergic side effects.
Antihistamines				Antihistamines possess CNS depressant, anticholinergic, antispasmodic, and local anesthetic activity. Antihistamines are used to control motion sickness.
buclizine (Bucladin-S)	Oral tablets	Depression of labyrinth excitability, and conduction in vestibular-cerebellar pathways	Adults: 50 mg 30 min before exposure to motion, repeated in 4–6 hr if required PC: C	
cyclizine (Marezine)	Oral tablets Solution for IM injection	Depression of labyrinth excitability and conduction in vestibular-cerebellar pathways	Adults: 50 mg 30 min before exposure to motion, repeated in 4–6 hr if required Children: 25 mg 30 min before exposure to motion, repeated in 4–6 hr if required PC: C	
dimenhydrinate (Dramamine, *Can:* Gravol)	Oral tablets and solution Solution for IM or IV injection	Inhibition of vestibular stimulation, probably by inhibition of acetylcholine in the otolith system and the semicircular canals	Adults: 50 mg–100 mg, q4h, PRN Children 2–5 yr of age: 12.5–25 mg, PO, up to tid; Children 6–12 yr of age: 25–50 mg, PO, up to tid PC: B	
hydroxyzine (Atarax, Atozine, Durrax, Hydroxacen, Hyzine, Orgatrex, Vistacon, Vistajet, Vistaquel, Visteril, Vistazine)	Oral tablets, capsules, solution and suspension Solution for IM injection	Possibly CNS inhibition of acetylcholine	Adults: *Oral:* 25–100 mg, tid–qid PRN; *IM:* 50–100 mg, q4h–q6h PRN Children: 1.1 mg/kg body weight PC: C	Hydroxyzine is used to control nausea caused by radiation therapy, drug reactions, and surgery, as well as motion sickness.
meclizine (Antivert, Antrizene, Bonine, Dizmiss, Motion Cure, RuVert-M)	Oral tablets, chewable tablets, and chewable capsules	Depression of labyrinth excitability and conduction in vestibular-cerebellar pathways	Adults: *For prevention of motion sickness:* 25–50 mg, 1 hr before exposure to motion, repeated q24h PRN; *for control of vertigo:* 25–100 mg/day, in divided doses PC: B	Safety and efficacy of meclizine in children younger than 12 yr of age have not been established.
Phenothiazines				
chlorpromazine (Somazine, Promapar, Thorazine, Thor-Prim)	Oral tablets, solution, and extended-release capsules Rectal suppositories	Possibly depression of the medullary CTZ by blockade of dopamine receptors	Adults: *Oral:* 10–25 mg, q4h–q6h PRN; *rectal:* 100 mg, q6h–q8h PRN; *IM:* initially 25 mg, then	Phenothiazines are not effective in the control of motion sickness; they are used to control nausea caused by

(Continued)

Table 30-7. Antiemetics (Continued)

Drug name	Preparations	Mode of action	Usual dosage	Additional information
Phenothiazines				
	Solutions for IV or deep IM injection		25–50 mg, q3h–q4h PRN as tolerated Children 6 mo of age or older: *Oral:* 0.55 mg/kg body weight, q4h–q6h PRN; *rectal:* 1.1 mg/kg body weight, q6h–q8h PRN; *IM:* initially 0.55 mg/kg body weight, q6h–q8h PRN PC: C	uremia, gastroenteritis, radiation sickness, carcinoma, and drug reactions.
prochlorperazine (Compazine)	Oral tablets, solution, and extended-release capsules Rectal suppositories Solutions for IV or deep IM injection	Possibly depression of the medullary CTZ by blockade of dopamine receptors	Adults: *Oral:* (prompt) 5–10 mg, tid–qid PRN; (extended-release) 15 mg once daily on arising PRN, or 10 mg q12h PRN; *rectal:* 25 mg, bid PRN; *IM:* 5–10 mg, q3h–q4h PRN (maximum daily IM dosage: 40 mg) Children: *Oral:* (depending on weight) 2.5–10 mg/d, in divided doses; *IM:* 130 µg/kg body weight/day, divided in 3–4 equal doses. PC: C	
promethazine (Anergan, Pentazine, Phenazine, Phencen, Phenergan, Prorex, Prothazine, Provigan, V-Gan)	Oral tablets and solutions Rectal suppositories Solutions for IM or IV injection	Depression of the CNS and inhibition of acetylcholine	Adults: 12.5–25 mg, q4h PRN Children: 0.25–0.5 mg/kg body weight, 4–6 times daily PRN Maximum rate of IV administration: 25 mg/min; maximum solution concentration for IV administration: 25 mg/ml PC: C	
thiethylperazine (Torecan)	Oral tablets Rectal suppositories Solution for IM injection	Depression of the vomiting center and medullary CTZ	Adults: 10 mg, 1–3 times daily PRN	
Benzoquinolizine				
benzquinamide (Emete-Con)	Solution for IM or IV injection	Depression of the medullary CTZ	Adults: 0.5 mg–1.0 mg/kg body weight, administered 15 min before emergence from anesthesia and repeated in 1 hr if required; subsequent doses q3h–q4h PRN	Benzquinamide is used for the prevention of postoperative nausea and vomiting when vomiting endangers the client or the results of surgery. Claims of freedom

(Continued)

Table 30-7. Antiemetics (Continued)

Drug name	Preparations	Mode of action	Usual dosage	Additional information
Benzoquinolizine				
				from hypotensive or autonomic effects are unproven. IV injection may cause sudden increase in blood pressure and cardiac arrhythmias; IV doses must be administered slowly.
Cannabis derivative				
dronabinol (Marinol)	Liquid filled oral capsules	Unknown	5 mg/m^2 1–3 hr before antineoplastic chemother-therapy treatment PC: B	CNS phenomena associated with marijuana use (hallucinations) may occur.
Unclassified				
metoclopramide (Clopra, Mexalon, Reglan)	Oral tablets and solution Solution for IM or IV injection	Blockade of dopamine receptors in the medullary CTZ	Adults: *Oral:* 10 mg qid, ac and hs *IV:* (In antineoplastic therapy) 1–2 mg/kg body weight, 30 min before administration of an emetogenic drug, repeated q2h–q3h PRN PC: B	Metoclopramide is used to control emesis caused by antineoplastic chemotherapy. Metoclopramide is contraindicated in persons with pheochromocytoma or in whom increased GI motility might be dangerous.
trimethobenzamide (T-Gen, Tebamide, Ticon, Tigan)	Oral capsules Rectal suppositories Solution for IM injection	Possibly inhibition of stimuli at the medullary CTZ	Adults: *Oral:* 250 mg, tid–qid PRN; *IM or rectal:* 200 mg, tid–qid Children: *Oral and rectal:* 15–20 mg/kg body weight/d, divided in 3–4 doses PC: C	Trimethobenzamide exhibits a weak antihistaminic activity.

KEY: PC = Pregnancy risk category. (The validity of pregnancy risk categories has not been established. See Chapter 16, p 216.)
Can: Canadian trade name.

Diphenidol

Pharmacodynamics. The mode of action of diphenidol has not been explained but it is believed to inhibit the medullary CTZ and conduction in vestibular-cerebellar pathways.

Pharmacokinetics. Diphenidol is well absorbed when administered orally or intramuscularly. Distribution in humans is not known. The drug is metabolized to inactive compounds; excretion is mainly in urine, with small amounts eliminated in feces. Biologic half-life has been reported as approximately 4 hours.

Therapeutic uses. Diphenidol is used in the control of nausea and vomiting associated with surgery, malignant tumors, antineoplastic chemotherapy, radiation sickness, infectious disease, and labyrinthine disturbances, including those associated with Meniere's disease (hearing loss, tinnitus, vertigo) and surgery of the middle and inner ear.

Adverse reactions. Adverse reactions to diphenidol frequently involve CNS effects, including drowsiness, mental depression, sleep disturbances, blurred vision, dizziness, headache, visual and auditory hallucinations, disorientation, and confusion. Although they affect less than 1% of clients receiving the drug, acute reactions can be disturbing.

Other signs and symptoms of adverse reactions to diphenidol include dry mouth, nausea, indigestion, rash, malaise, palpitation, and heartburn. Injection may cause transient decreases in blood pressure. Jaundice has also been reported.

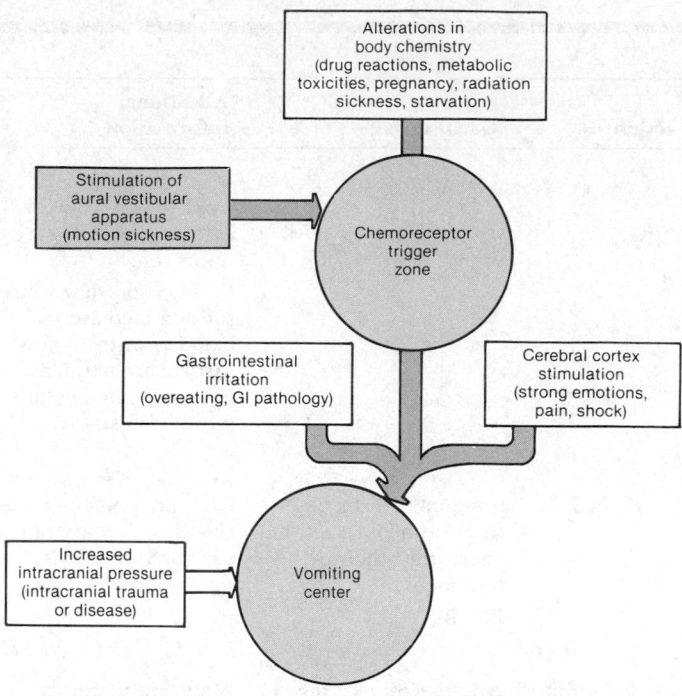

Figure 30-3. The vomiting reflex can be interrupted along its pathway. Impulses come in but are stopped at one of three locations (shown in color). Compare with Fig. 30-2.

Precautions and contraindications. The use of diphenidol is limited to settings in which the recipient is under close, continuous supervision by health care professionals. If hallucinations, disorientation, or confusion occur, the drug should be discontinued immediately.

Diphenidol should be used with caution in persons with glaucoma and in those with obstructive lesions of the GI or genitourinary tract. This drug is not recommended for treating persons with a history of sinus tachycardia.

Diphenidol is contraindicated for clients with anuria or those with a known allergic hypersensitivity to the drug. The oral tablets are contraindicated for persons with a known allergy to tartrazine, a coloring agent used in this formulation.

Metoclopramide

Metoclopramide hydrochloride is a synthetic substituted benzamide.

Pharmacodynamics. Metoclopramide acts as a dopamine receptor antagonist, an antiemetic, and a stimulant of upper GI motility. It increases GI motility in a coordinated manner that accelerates gastric emptying and intestinal transit from the duodenum to the ileocecal valve. Metoclopramide also increases the tone of the cardiac sphincter (Fink, Lange, & McCallum, 1983). The exact mechanism of action is unclear but it may be mediated by enhancement of cholinergic excitatory processes at the postganglionic neuromuscular junction, antagonism of nonadrenergic, noncholinergic inhibitory motor nerves, or a direct effect on intestinal smooth muscle.

In the CNS, metoclopramide blocks dopamine receptors in the CTZ. It increases the CTZ threshold and decreases the sensitivity of visceral nerves that transmit afferent impulses from the GI tract to the vomiting center.

Pharmacokinetics. Metoclopramide is administered orally, intramuscularly, or intravenously. It is well absorbed by all routes. Onset of action is rapid, within minutes following injection and within 1 hour following oral administration.

Distribution is not fully understood. In animals, the drug crosses the blood–brain barrier and is found in high concentrations in the area of the brain where the CTZ is located. Metoclopramide binds weakly to plasma proteins, principally to albumin. The drug crosses the placenta and is distributed in breast milk.

Metoclopramide is not extensively metabolized. Both metabolites and unchanged drug are excreted in the urine and bile. The drug is only minimally removed by dialysis.

Therapeutic uses. Metoclopramide is used in the management of GI motility disorders (*eg*, gastric stasis) and for the prevention of cancer chemotherapy-induced emesis. The drug is also used to facilitate intubation of the small intestine to reduce gastroesophageal reflux and as an adjunct during radiographic examination of the upper GI tract.

Adverse reactions. Adverse reactions to metoclopramide are usually mild, transient, and reversible with discontinuation of the drug. Central nervous system effects occur most frequently. Signs and symptoms include lassitude, drowsiness, fatigue, restlessness, insomnia, headache, and dizziness. When the drug is administered by rapid intravenous injection, feelings of anxiety or agitation may occur. Depression has also been reported. Metoclopramide tends to stimulate prolactin secretion and can cause sexual dysfunction in men.

Extrapyramidal reactions to metoclopramide are sometimes seen during the first 2–3 days of treatment. Akathisia occurs most frequently but acute dystonia, parkinsonism, and chronic tardive dyskinesia resembling the syndromes caused by antipsychotic drugs can develop. Acute dystonia occurs most frequently in young adults (incidence approximately 25%) receiving high doses (*eg*, 2 mg/kg body weight) during cancer chemotherapy. Parkinsonism and tardive dyskinesia, which may not be reversible when the drug is discontinued, are most apt to develop in elderly clients who have received the drug for years.

Gastrointestinal reactions to metoclopramide are characterized by alterations in bowel function (constipation or diarrhea). Other adverse reactions include hypertension, bronchospasm, skin rash, xerostomia, glossal or periorbital edema, methemoglobinemia, acute porphyria, galactorrhea, gynecomastia, and menstrual disorders. The drug may cause hypertensive crisis in persons with pheochromocytoma. Cardiac arrhythmias have been reported following injection of metoclopramide.

Precautions and contraindications. Clients receiving metoclopramide should be advised that the drug may impair their ability to perform activities requiring mental alertness or physical coordination. It may enhance responses to CNS depressants (alcohol, barbiturates, narcotic analgesics, and tranquilizers).

Metoclopramide should be used with caution in persons with impaired renal function and in those at risk of developing fluid retention or hypokalemia. Because of the high risk of extrapyramidal reactions, the drug should not be prescribed for children.

Metoclopramide is contraindicated for persons with a history of seizures and for those in whom stimulation of GI motility might be dangerous (*eg*, in the presence of mechanical obstruction or perforation). It is also contraindicated for clients with a history of sensitivity or intolerance to the drug. Caution should be exercised when the drug is administered to persons allergic to procainamide because the two drugs are structurally similar.

Trimethobenzamide

Trimethobenzamide is structurally related to the substituted ethanolamine antihistamines but exhibits only weak antihistaminic activity.

Pharmacodynamics. Although the precise mode of action of trimethobenzamide is not known, the drug appears to inhibit stimuli at the medullary CTZ.

Pharmacokinetics. Trimethobenzamide is well absorbed when administered orally or intramuscularly. Distribution into human body tissues and fluids is not known. In animals, the drug is distributed mainly into the liver, kidneys, and lungs.

In animals, trimethobenzamide is metabolized by the liver; its metabolism in humans has not been determined. The drug is excreted in urine of both animals and humans and is found in the feces of animals.

Therapeutic uses. Trimethobenzamide is used for the control of nausea and vomiting, especially when long-term therapy is anticipated. It is less effective than phenothiazines for the control of severe and potentially hazardous vomiting but causes fewer adverse reactions than those drugs.

Adverse reactions. Adverse effects of trimethobenzamide may involve the CNS (blurred vision, seizures, coma, depression, disorientation, vertigo, dizziness, drowsiness, and headache), the GI tract (diarrhea, jaundice, and exaggeration of preexisting nausea), and bone marrow (blood dyscrasias). Following IM injection, hypotension has been reported. Pain, stinging, burning, and inflammation may also occur at injection sites.

Adverse reactions occur infrequently in persons receiving usual dosages of trimethobenzamide and very rarely require discontinuation of the drug.

Precautions and contraindications. Trimethobenzamide should be administered with caution to persons with acute febrile illness, encephalitis, gastroenteritis, dehydration, and electrolyte imbalance. Children and the elderly or debilitated persons are especially at risk for adverse reactions to trimethobenzamide. The drug should be discontinued if signs and symptoms of allergic hypersensitivity develop.

Trimethobenzamide is contraindicated for persons who are allergic to the drug. Trimethobenzamide suppositories are contraindicated for those who are allergic to benzocaine or similar local anesthetics.

Safety during pregnancy and lactation has not been established.

Marijuana derivative: dronabinol

Dronabinol (Marinol) is a derivative of the hallucinogen marijuana, which is used medicinally to control nausea and vomiting caused by chemotherapy. (The following data are taken from Kastrup & Olin, 1987.)

Pharmacodynamics. The active ingredient of dronabinol is delta-9-tetrahydrocannabinol (delta-9-THC, or THC), the principle psychoactive substance in *Cannabis sativa*. Its mechanism of action as an antiemetic is unknown. Tetrahydrocannibinol acts primarily on the CNS, and its antiemetic effect is probably central in nature also.

Pharmacokinetics. Reliable information regarding the distribution of dronabinol is not available. Due to first-pass through metabolism in the liver, only about 10%–20% of an oral dose is available systemically. Plasma levels peak about 2–3 hours after ingestion. Tetrahydrocannabinol is known to have a predilection for fatty tissues and is believed to be stored in fatty tissues for long periods of time. The drug crosses the placenta and is concentrated and secreted in breast milk.

Therapeutic uses. Dronabinol's medicinal use is limited to the prevention or treatment of nausea and vomiting caused by chemotherapy. Dronabinol is supplied as liquid capsules. Initial dosage for adults is 5 mg/m² of body surface, 1–3 hours before administration of antineoplastic drugs. Subsequent doses are administered 2–4 hours apart for a total of 4–6 doses per day. If necessary, dosage may be increased by 2.5 mg/m² body surface increments: no dose should exceed 15 mg/m² body surface.

Adverse reactions. Dronabinol exerts all the effects of marijuana and other centrally active cannabinols, including impairment of cognitive performance and memory, loss of inhibitions, and altered perceptions of reality (hallucinations, altered time perception). It can cause psychosis. Systemic physical effects include dry mouth, conjunctival injection, increased blood pressure, diarrhea, and musculoskeletal pain. Tetrahydrocannibinol also produces sexual changes: a decreased rate of pregnancy in women and sexual impairment in men.

Precautions and contraindications. The use of dronabinol, especially for clients who have not used tetrahydrocannabinol previously, is limited to institutional settings where the recipient can be closely observed, and where adverse reactions can be treated promptly. Prescriptions are limited to a few days' supply. Clients should avoid using alcohol or barbiturates when using the drug. They should also avoid hazardous tasks, such as operating power machinery.

Dronabinol is contraindicated for clients with allergic hypersensitivity to either tetrahydrocannabinol or sesame oil.

Glucocorticoids

Glucocorticoids also act as antiemetics and are sometimes used to prevent nausea and vomiting during antineoplastic chemotherapy. These drugs are discussed in detail in Chapter 32.

■ Summary

Drugs from several chemical groups are effective in reducing nausea and vomiting. Because they may mask the symptoms of underlying disease, care should be taken to evaluate the client's condition thoroughly so that effective treatment may be prescribed for the causative condition. Pregnancy should be ruled out because many antiemetics are teratogenic. Nausea and vomiting can be reduced by the judicious use of anticholinergics, antihistamines, or phenothiazine tranquilizers, as well as individual drugs developed for their antiemetic effects.

Nursing management

Nursing implications

If allowed to persist, vomiting can undermine nutritional integrity and impair recuperative powers. Control of these symptoms is essential to the client's well-being. Pathologic conditions contributing to the problem must be treated to minimize their impact. Until a definitive diagnosis is made, the use of antiemetics may be avoided to prevent the masking of symptoms. The client must depend on nursing measures to ameliorate the symptoms.

Nausea and vomiting decrease when stimuli affecting the vomiting reflex are reduced. A decrease of all types of stimuli can be helpful. Noxious stimuli to all sensory modalities should be eliminated. Noise, offensive odors, distressing sights, emotional tension, pain, and similar stressors augment nausea. Even usually pleasant stimuli can add to reflex excitation. Body motion, which disturbs the vestibular apparatus in the inner ear, is particularly distressing. When nausea is acute, a quiet environment with subdued lighting is required; the client should be protected from the sights, sounds, and odors associated with food.

To minimize gastric irritation, it is helpful to have the client eat frequent, small, bland meals. Foods that increase nausea should be eliminated. After episodes of vomiting, warm tea, ginger ale, or cola drinks may help reduce nausea. Effervescent beverages should be exposed to air until the gas bubbles dissipate and the liquid approaches room temperature because carbonation contributes to gastric distention and increases discomfort. Large amounts of water, which stimulate nausea, should be avoided. Allow clients to choose the foods and beverages they prefer. Conditioning greatly influences response. A dish associated with a loving parent's care during childhood illness may be far better tolerated than foods believed to act pharmacologically to control nausea.

After a proper medical diagnosis is made, antiemetic drugs may be prescribed. In acute conditions, they are usually required for limited periods of time, the need declining as the underlying condition subsides. Clients with chronic conditions associated with nausea and vomiting will receive antiemetics for longer periods of time.

Nursing care during pregnancy. Antiemetics are not recommended during pregnancy. The safety of these drugs in pregnancy is not established. Some related compounds, such as thalidomide, are highly teratogenic. Vomiting in pregnancy often responds to the general measures outlined previously. Eating dry crackers before rising helps to prevent or to ameliorate morning sickness. It is believed that extra carbohydrates reduce hypoglycemia caused by the rapidly growing fetus' demands for energy. (Hypoglycemia is often associated with nausea.) In most cases, nausea and vomiting subside before the second trimester and do not seriously interfere with maternal nutrition.

Nursing process

Assessment Determining and correcting the cause of nausea and vomiting are of primary importance. Complete assessment is vital to diagnosis and treatment. Exactly what the client means by nausea or vomiting must be determined. Vomiting should be clearly differentiated from regurgitation and retching. The amount and character of emesis should be determined. Timing of the symptoms (onset, frequency, duration, and associated circumstances) provides important clues to etiology. Factors that either increase or alleviate the symptoms must be identified.

Physical assessment should include general appearance, vital signs, and an examination of the abdomen. When vomiting persists, nutritional status must be evaluated, with special attention to signs of fluid and electrolyte disturbances. Women of childbearing age should be questioned closely about the possibility of pregnancy.

A drug history should also be taken before antiemetic therapy is begun. Particular attention should be paid to previous responses of the client to anticholinergics, antihistamines, and phenothiazines. Drugs in present use and those taken recently (2 weeks for most but longer for clients with liver or renal impairment) should be listed. This information must be evaluated to determine how likely it is that the nausea and vomiting might be an adverse reaction to a drug; how great a risk there is of interactions with antiemetic agents; and what the indications are of concomitant medical conditions. The client should be questioned specifically about glaucoma. Antiemetics with anticholinergic properties are contraindicated in this condition. A family history of glaucoma indicates an increased risk of this problem in middle-aged or elderly clients.

Nursing diagnosis Clients who are given antiemetics will all have increased potential for alteration in comfort: nausea. Some clients will also have alteration in nutrition: less than body requirements related to vomiting. The contributing factors will vary, depending on the underlying health problem causing the nausea and vomiting.

Most antiemetic drugs are CNS depressants and clients receiving them are likely to develop the following:

> High risk for injury related to drowsiness secondary to CNS depression
> Altered comfort: fatigue, weakness, dizziness, disorientation, hallucinations, confusion, or depression related to CNS changes secondary to antiemetic medication
> Altered tissue perfusion: hypotension related to vasodilation secondary to antiemetic medication
> Altered comfort: headache, sweating, shivering, restlessness, nervousness related to adverse reaction to antiemetic medication
> Sensory-perceptual alterations: blurred vision or hallucinations related to antiemetic medication
> Constipation (or diarrhea) related to metoclopramide medication
> Impaired tissue integrity: skin rash related to inflammation secondary to metoclopramide medication

Many clients or their families will have knowledge deficits related to nausea and vomiting and their treatment.

Planning Goals of treatment include alleviation or elimination of nausea and vomiting, improved nutrition, improved comfort, maintenance of adequate blood pressure, restoration of normal sensory-perception, maintenance of normal fecal elimination, alleviation and elimination of skin rash, and education of the client or family about self-care measures to prevent or minimize nausea and vomiting.

Intervention The nurse's responsibilities in antiemetic therapy include administration of medications, evaluation of therapeutic response, identification of adverse reactions, and client education. Careful management of drug administration enhances the beneficial effects while it minimizes adverse effects. To achieve optimal results, nursing measures to control the symptoms are continued when drugs are employed.

Antiemetics are usually administered as needed (PRN). In active nausea, parenteral or rectal routes are used because oral doses may not be retained. Preventive doses may be given by mouth. The client must be monitored carefully for adverse reactions. Safety precautions to prevent injury are important because the client may experience postural hypotension and drowsiness. If phenothiazines are used, the drug must be discontinued at the earliest sign of akathisia. Paradoxically, nausea and vomiting can be increased by antiemetic drugs. If the client either fails to respond with improvement or develops other adverse reactions, a change in prescription or discontinuation of treatment may be required.

Chronically or terminally ill clients. Chronically or terminally ill clients often experience nausea over long periods of time. Antiemetic medication should be timed to precede events known to precipitate symptoms. If nutrition is inadequate, medication may be needed before meals. Preventive use of the drugs allows for the oral administration of medication and controls nausea more effectively than treatment after the vomiting reflex activity is well established. Establishing a medication schedule designed to meet individual needs usually increases the client's response. A PRN order does not imply that the medication is restricted to use only after full-blown symptoms develop. The client may need preventive medication.

Nausea and vomiting can persist despite vigorous treatment by conventional means. Such refractory problems often develop in clients suffering from malignant neoplasms. Whether the underlying disease, itself, or the radiation and antineoplastic drugs used for treatment cause this problem is unknown. Perhaps both contribute. Cancer clients are poorly nourished at best, and an inability to eat further erodes their nutritional status. The problem is a serious one.

Client education. Clients subject to motion sickness should be advised to take antiemetic medication at least 30 minutes before beginning a trip or activity that normally causes nausea and vomiting. If traveling in an automobile or bus, clients should sit near the front of the vehicle because they will be subject to fewer stimuli that result from the sway or bouncing of the vehicle. Such a position also will facilitate focusing on objects directly ahead, a strategy that decreases the nausea-causing impact of peripheral visual stimuli.

Clients seeking advice about the treatment of nausea and vomiting should be referred for medical assessment of the underlying condition. Habitual use of antiemetics is not advisable as a substitute for definitive medical care.

Clients with chronic or terminal conditions accompanied by nausea and vomiting should be taught how to decrease the stimuli accentuating these symptoms. Antiemetics should be taken regularly in such situations for their preventive effect. Whenever antiemetic medication is required, clients should be warned not to operate power machinery, including automobiles, because the drugs can cause drowsiness.

Evaluation Data required for evaluation include the absence or presence and severity of vomiting, clients' reports about the absence or presence and severity of nausea, absence of signs and symptoms of undernutrition (including changes in weight), clients' reports about sensory-perception, frequency and consistency of stools, absence or presence and severity of skin rash, and ability of the client or family to perform self-care

measures conveyed in teaching sessions. (See Example of Nursing Process and Dronabinol Therapy.)

Checklist of nursing actions

☐ Assess clients subject to nausea and vomiting to determine carefully the true nature of their symptoms.

☐ Refer clients for definitive diagnosis and treatment.

☐ Decrease stimuli, especially noxious stimuli, to reduce the level of nausea and vomiting.

☐ Give careful mouth care following emesis.

☐ Recommend small, frequent bland feedings to minimize gastric irritation; use warm tea or "flat" ginger ale or cola drinks instead of water.

☐ Rule out pregnancy before administering antiemetic drugs.

☐ Administer preventive doses of antiemetics orally; medication during active nausea should be given rectally or parenterally.

☐ Monitor clients receiving antiemetics for drowsiness, postural hypotension and (when phenothiazines are used) for extrapyramidal effects.

☐ Teach clients subject to motion sickness to take antiemetic medication 30 minutes before undertaking the activity that causes nausea.

☐ Teach clients subject to chronic nausea techniques to reduce the symptoms.

Emetics

Emetics are substances that induce vomiting. Theoretically, stimulation of the vomiting reflex at any point could initiate the act but most emetics act either by irritation of the GI mucosa or stimulation of the medullary vomiting center. These drugs are useful in cases of poisoning when it is desirable to remove ingested substances quickly from the stomach.

Apomorphine

Apomorphine is a morphine derivative that lacks the analgesic properties of morphine.

Pharmacodynamics. Apomorphine stimulates the CTZ directly. It may also excite the vestibular centers, producing secondary stimulation of the CTZ. The drug produces secondary depression of the CNS. When the medullary centers are capable of responding, the drug produces emesis of the contents of the stomach and upper intestines.

Pharmacokinetics. Because oral administration of apomorphine does not produce reliable results, the drug is injected. Following subcutaneous administration, emesis usually occurs within 1–15 minutes. Apomorphine is metabolized by the liver and excreted by the kidneys.

Example of nursing process and dronabinol therapy

The client is a 22-year-old college student undergoing cancer chemotherapy for acute leukemia. He is experiencing severe nausea and is seldom able to eat more than a fraction of the nourishment offered him. Compazine and related antiemetic drugs have been ineffective in controlling the nausea. The physician has decided to try dronabinol. A dose is to be administered before each chemotherapy treatment.

Assessment data	Nursing diagnosis	Intervention	Goals and outcome criteria
Prescription of a hallucinogenic agent for its antiemetic effect	High risk for sensory/perceptual alterations: hallucinations related to CNS stimulation secondary to dronabinol medication	**Inform** the client of the new medication order. Question the client to determine if he has ever been exposed to marijuana, and is so, what kind of reaction he had to it.	After chemotherapy sessions involving the use of dronabinol, the client will report that the experience was predominantly pleasant; the client will not report a "bad trip."
		Assess the client's reaction to the prospect of using dronabinol; if he is apprehensive, explain that hallucinations in response to this drug may be influenced by mental set and controlled in part by conscious thoughts.	
		While the client is under the influence of dronabinol, **monitor** him for signs and symptoms of unpleasant sensations (a "bad trip"); if necessary "talk him down" by repeating to him that he can control the hallucinations by thinking of pleasant things.	
Severe nausea Inability to eat a normal amount of food	High risk for altered nutrition: less than body requirements related to decreased food intake secondary to nausea caused by antineoplastic chemotherapy	**Administer** dronabinol before each chemotherapy treatment as ordered. **Offer** foods preferred by the client. **Ensure** that trays containing meals are attractive and that the food is at the proper temperature. **Eliminate** noxious stimuli, particularly around mealtime. **Offer** between meal snacks. **Monitor** body weight daily.	The client will not lose weight.

Therapeutic uses. Apomorphine is used to induce vomiting in the management of poisoning and drug overdosage when vomiting is not contraindicated. It has also been employed to arrest supraventricular paroxysmal tachycardia by inducing Valsalva's maneuver in children too young to "strain" voluntarily, and as an adjunct to levodopa in the treatment of parkinsonism (Stilbe et al, 1988).

Adverse reactions. Respiratory depression and circulatory depression are the chief hazards of apomorphine therapy. Sedation, weakness, perspiration, and pallor also occur. In some clients, CNS stimulation develops. Excessive doses can produce violent and protracted vomiting and acute circulatory failure associated with bradycardia. In persons with parkinsonian syndrome, apomorphine can cause mild myoclonic jerks, head bobbing, and dyskinesia.

Precautions and contraindications. Apomorphine is used only in institutional settings by trained medical personnel. Effects of the drug can be reversed by the administration of morphine antagonists, such as naloxone.

Apomorphine should be used with caution in children, geriatric or debilitated clients, and in clients with cardiac decompensation, cardiac impairment, pathologic changes of the blood vessels, or a predisposition to nausea and vomiting. It is contraindicated for clients who are unconscious, semicomatose, in shock, having seizures, or who lack a gag reflex. It is not used when the poison involved is a convulsant, CNS depressant, or corrosive or volatile oil. Its use for petroleum distillate poisoning (gasoline, kerosene, fuel oil, paint thinner, cleaning fluid) is controversial.

Safe use of apomorphine during pregnancy has not been established. The drug is distributed into breast milk, and it should be used with caution in nursing women.

Apomorphine is also contraindicated for persons with a known hypersensitivity to it or allergy to morphine or related opiates.

Ipecac

Syrup of ipecac is a sweetened solution of active compounds from the root of a plant indigenous to Central and South America. Its active ingredients are emetine and cephaeline.

Pharmacodynamics. Ipecac alkaloids act both centrally and locally, producing stimulation of the CTZ and irritation of the gastric mucosa. When medullary centers are capable of responding, contents of both the stomach and upper intestine are regurgitated.

Pharmacokinetics. There is no information on the GI absorption of small doses of ipecac. Following oral administration, vomiting occurs within 30 minutes in 90% of recipients, and it is likely that most of the drug is eliminated in the emesis.

Therapeutic uses. Ipecac syrup is used to induce vomiting in the early management of acute drug overdosage and poisoning. Ipecac is preferable to apomorphine in some situations because it can be administered orally and it does not produce CNS or respiratory depression. Ipecac has also been used to stimulate a Valsalva maneuver to treat paroxysmal supraventricular tachycardia in very young children.

Adverse reactions. In the doses (30 ml or less) usually employed, ipecac syrup produces few adverse reactions. However, if vomiting does not occur, emetine may be absorbed. Ipecac toxicity has caused serious myopathy affecting the GI tract, skeletal muscles, and myocardium.

Precautions and contraindications. Ipecac syrup should not be confused with ipecac fluidextract, which is 14 times more potent. Fatalities have occurred when the fluidextract was administered inadvertently. Safe use during pregnancy and lactation has not been established.

Ipecac syrup is contraindicated for clients who are unconscious, semicomatose, severely inebriated, in shock, having seizures, or who lack the gag reflex. It should be used with caution in persons for whom vomiting is hazardous, such as those with impaired cardiac function and pathologic changes in blood vessels.

If vomiting fails to occur after two doses, the drug should be recovered by gastric lavage.

Nursing management

Nursing implications

Before vomiting is induced for the treatment of poisoning, it is vital to determine the nature of the poison. Vomiting is generally considered to be contraindicated if either a corrosive substance or a petroleum product has been ingested. Emesis containing corrosives, such as alkalis, causes additional injury to the mucosa it contacts, virtually doubling tissue damage. Petroleum substances may injure tissue but they are also apt to be aspirated into the lungs during vomiting, causing a serious lipid pneumonia. Both types of poisons must be removed from the stomach by gastric intubation, suctioning, and lavage. Vomiting should not be induced in clients who do not have active gag or swallowing reflexes; lavage is required for them also.

When it is determined that inducing vomiting is a safe procedure, a simple approach is to touch the back of the throat with a finger. This measure is often very effective, especially in children. If the emesis produced is small in quantity, administer a glass of water and repeat the maneuver.

Ipecac has been promoted for the emergency treatment of poisoning by noncorrosive, nonpetroleum substances. The drug is marketed in 1-oz (two dose) containers for home medicine stocks. It may be used if pharyngeal stimulation does not cause vomiting or if emptying seems incomplete. One-half ounce of syrup of ipecac is given orally, followed by water. When treating children, water (or other fluid such as soft drink) may be given first, followed by the syrup of ipecac. Vomiting should occur in 15–20 minutes. If 30 minutes elapse without results, the ipecac dose is repeated. If the victim still fails to respond, the stomach must be emptied by gastric suctioning and lavage to prevent systemic absorption of the toxic ipecac.

When substances of unknown toxicity are the cause of poisoning, a poison control center may be able to identify the ingredients of a mixture, and provide treatment recommendations. Such centers have been established in most medical regions, often at the emergency department of a major teaching hospital. The telephone number of the poison control center should be available at all health care institutions. It also should be posted near home telephones, along with the numbers for police, ambulance, and other emergency assistance.

Nursing process

Assessment When poisoning by ingestion is suspected, it is important to determine what substance was taken. If the client is unable to give this information, witnesses should be questioned. Empty or partially empty containers of medicine or other toxic materials may identify the substance taken. If the client is admitted to an acute-care facility, such containers should be taken along to facilitate identification of the toxin.

The client should be examined for life-threatening toxic effects on vital functions, such as impaired respirations or circulation and CNS malfunction. Vital signs, neurologic signs, and level of consciousness should be assessed.

Nursing diagnosis The nursing diagnoses appropriate for poisoning victims vary with the toxic substances to which the client has been exposed. Priority must be given to life-threatening changes, especially impaired respirations and circulation.

If emetics are used to empty the stomach, the client may develop problems such as the following:

Impaired gas exchange related to respiratory depression secondary to adverse reaction to apomorphine
Altered tissue perfusion: hypotension related to circulatory depression and bradycardia secondary to apomorphine administration
Altered comfort: protracted vomiting and weakness related to adverse reaction to apomorphine

Some clients or families will have a

Knowledge deficit related to poison control and emergency treatment for poisoning

Common collaborative problems that should be differentiated from the nursing diagnoses include

Potential complication: seizures
Potential complication: cardiotoxicity

Planning Primary goals of treatment are to support vital functions and to remove as much of the toxin from the GI tract as possible before it is absorbed. Other goals include prompt detection and treatment of adverse reactions to emetic drugs, amelioration of toxic effects of the poison taken, and education of the client or family about poison prevention.

Intervention When poisoning occurs, the toxin involved should be identified as soon as possible. If the substance is one which can safely be removed by emesis, vomiting should be induced. Syrup of ipecac is the method of choice. If ipecac is not available, tickling the throat to gag the client should be attempted. If, in response to this treatment, the emesis is small in volume, the client may be given a drink and the maneuver may be repeated. First-aid should be given and emergency assistance summoned if vital functions are affected; these clients should be transported to an acute-care facility without delay. Gastric lavage, the most effective procedure for removing drugs from the stomach, is often carried out.

After they receive first-aid treatment, poisoning victims should always be evaluated by a physician. If possible, the package containing the ingested substance should be taken with the victim to the emergency facility to help in identifying the poisons involved. Because some substances produce delayed effects, it may be necessary to admit the victim for a period of observation.

When apomorphine is used in the treatment of poisoning, the nurse should have available its antidote, naloxone. Before injecting the apomorphine, 200–300 ml of water are administered orally. An emesis basin should be given to the client because the drug's effect is quite prompt—within 1–2 minutes in children. Only one dose of apomorphine is given. If the first dose is not effective, subsequent doses are even less likely to produce vomiting.

Client education. Following an episode of poisoning, it is important to teach the victim and family safety measures to prevent repeated episodes. The home environment should be assessed for poison hazards and the family should be assisted in improving storage arrangements and in securing hazardous chemicals. Appropriate recommendations for other poison preventive measures should be reviewed. The family should add the telephone numbers of the nearest emergency care and poison control centers to their emergency list.

If clients have stocked ipecac syrup for emergency use, the nurse should verify that they understand the types of poisons for which it is appropriate and those

Example of nursing process and accidental poisoning

The mother of a 3-year-old girl has called the poison control center for advice. Her daughter has been found with an open prescription container with five tablets remaining. The prescription is for propranolol, an antiangina adrenergic blocker. The child was out of the mother's sight less than 5 minutes. It is believed that 6–8 tablets are missing from the bottle. The mother has a bottle of syrup of ipecac in the medicine chest.

Assessment data	Nursing diagnosis	Intervention	Goals and outcome criteria
A quantity of adrenergic blocker sufficient to constitute a toxic dose is missing under circumstances suggesting that a child has ingested it.	High risk for altered tissue perfusion: bradycardia and hypotension related to absorption of a toxic dose of anti-adrenergic medication	If consistent with the protocols in effect at the poison center, **advise** the mother to administer to the child 4 ounces of water followed by ½ ounce (1 standard measuring tablespoon) of ipecac. The child should be taken promptly to the nearest emergency medical facility. To receive emesis should the child vomit enroute, the mother may **prepare** a "burp" bag by lining a paper bag with a plastic bag (like those for bagging groceries), then gathering the tops of the bags to form a funnel. Advise the mother to bring the bag and its contents to the emergency department. **Advise** the mother to keep the child comfortably warm.	The child will not develop signs and symptoms of circulatory shock: ashen color, cold extremities, weak and slow pulse, hypotension, and lethargy. If the child does develop circulatory shock, it will be detected and treated promptly.

for which it is contraindicated. Clients should be cautioned not to administer ipecac to children under 1 year of age.

Evaluation Data required for evaluation relate to vital signs; speed of recovery from signs and symptoms of poisoning; absence or presence of adverse reactions to emetic drugs; speed of treatment of and recovery from adverse reactions; ability of counseled individuals to repeat to the nurse points covered in the teaching program; and absence or incidence of recurrent problems of poisoning in individuals or families previously counseled. (See Example of Nursing Process and Accidental Poisoning.)

Checklist of nursing actions

When poisoning is suspected
☐ Determine the nature of the poison taken.
☐ Do not induce vomiting if the poison involved is corrosive or petroleum in nature.
☐ Do not induce vomiting in clients who do not have active gag or swallowing reflexes.

When emesis is indicated for treatment of poisoning by ingestion
☐ Administer water orally before administering an emetic.
☐ Do not administer ipecac to infants under 1 year of age.
☐ Monitor the client for adverse reaction to emetics.
☐ Provide the client with an emesis basin before administering the emetic.

References

Amitai Y, Yeung AC, Moye J, Lovejoy FH Jr. (1986). Repetitive oral activated charcoal and control of emesis in severe theophylline toxicity (letter). *Ann Intern Med, 105,* 386.

Attia EL, Marshall KG. (1983). Halitosis. *Can Med Assoc J, 126,* 1281.

DaPaola L. (1987). Mouthwash for denture wearers. *Privileged Information, 3(10),* 7.

Faryna A. (1982). Onset of pheochromocytoma syndrome following cessation of cimetidine administration. *Heart and Lung, 11(3),* 213–214 (May–June).

Fink S, Lange R, McCallum R. (1983). Effect of metoclopramide on normal and delayed gastric emptying in gastroesophageal reflux patients. *Dig Dis Sci, 28,* 1057–1061.

Kastrup EK, Olin BR. (1987). *Facts and comparisons,* p 259h. Philadelphia: JB Lippincott.

McEvoy GK. (1991). *AHFS Drug information 91,* 1752–1761 and 1777–1782. Bethesda, MD: American Society of Hospital Pharmacists.

Miller JA. (1986). Oral ecology. *Science News, 129* 396–397.

Porter JB, Beard K, Walker AM, Lawson DH, Jick H, Kellaway GS. (1986). Intensive hospital monitoring study of intravenous cimetidine. *Arch Intern Med, 146,* 2237–2239.

Stilbe CMH, et al. (1988). Subcutaneous apomorphine in parkinsonian on-off oscillations. *Lancet 1,* 403 (February 20).

Tonnesen H, et al. (1988). Effect of cimetidine on survival after gastric cancer. *Lancet 2,* 990 (October 29).

Wade A, Rowley-Jones D. (1988). Long term management of duodenal ulcer in general practice: How best to use cimetidine? *Br Med J, 296,* 971–974 (April 2).

Bibliography

Aasebo U, et al. (1987). High-dose metoclopramide and chlorpromazine in the treatment of cisplatin-induced emesis. *Pharmacol Toxicol, 60,* 337–339.

Auerbach PS, Osterloh J, Braun O, Hu P, Geehr EC, Kizer KW, McKinney H. (1986). Gastric lavage versus emesis induced by ipecac. *Ann Emerg Med, 15,* 692.

Ballesteros JA, et al. (1990). Bolus or intravenous infusion of ranitidine: Effects on gastric pH and acid secretion. *Ann Intern Med, 112,* 334–339 (March).

Berkowitz J, et al. (1987). Ranitidine protects against gastroduodenal mucosal damage associated with chronic aspirin therapy. *Arch Intern Med, 147,* 2137–2139 (December).

Berlin R. (1986). Metoclopramide-induced reversible impotence. *West J Med, 144,* 359–361.

Billings R, Stein M. (1986). Depression associated with ranitidine. *Am J Psychiatry, 143,* 915–916.

Brenner L. (1986). Agranulocytosis and ranitidine (letter). *Ann Intern Med, 104,* 896–897.

Bruera E, et al. (1988). Managing chemotherapy-induced emesis. *American Journal of Nursing, 88,* 367–368 (March).

Drug update 90. (1990). *Nursing 90, 20(5),* 61 (May).

Epstein C, Klopper J. (1985). Ranitidine headache. *Headache, 25,* 392–393 (October).

Few BJ. (1988). Nabilone as an antiemetic for children undergoing chemotherapy. *Matern Child Nurs J, 13,* 209 (May/June).

Gelwan JS, Schmitz RL, Pelecchia C. (1986). Ranitidine and leukocytosis. *Am J Gastroenterol, 81,* 685–687.

Gilman AG, Goodman L, Rall TW, Murad F. (1985). Goodman and Gilman's *The pharmacological basis of therapeutics,* 7th ed, pp 980–993. New York: Macmillan.

Guyton A. (1985). *Textbook of medical physiology,* 7th ed, pp 754–800. Philadelphia: WB Saunders.

Hussar DA. (1987). New drugs. *Nursing 87, 17(6),* 55.

Hussar DA. (1989). Drug update: A naturally occurring bile acid that most patients tolerate well. *Nursing 89, 19(5),* 47 (May).

Hussar DA. (1989). New drugs update: Masoprostol. *Nursing 89, 19(12),* 60 (December).

Injectable zantac. (1985). *American Journal of Nursing, 85,* 242.

Katzin L. (1988). New drugs: Hands-on experience, Gallstone dissolver. *American Journal of Nursing, 88,* 838 (June).

Kelley FM. (1990). Nursing consult: Stomatitis: Preventing oral infection. *Nursing 90, 20,* 88 (August).

Lazzara RR, Stoudemire A, Manning D, Prewitt KC. (1986). Metoclopramide-induced tardive dyskinesia: A case report. *Gen Hosp Psychiatry, 8,* 107–109.

Levy S, et al. (1988). Use of medications with dental significance by a noninstitutionalized elderly population. *Gerodontics 4,* 119–125 (June).

Malloy M, Rhoads G. (1988). Syrup of ipecac. *Am J Dis Child, 142,* 640–642 (June).

Manzo M. (1988). Pharmacist on call: Dronabinol and nabilone ease cancer chemotherapy. *Nursing 88, 18,* 81 (August).

Marks J, et al. (1984). Low-dose chenodiol to prevent gallstone recurrence after dissolution therapy. *Ann Intern Med, 100,* 376–381.

Omeprazole for duodenal ulcers: Preemptive strike. (1988). *Nursing 88, 18(10),* 102–103 (October).

O'Neil-Cutting M, Crosby W. (1986). The effect of antacids on the absorption of simultaneously ingested iron. *JAMA, 255,* 1468–1470.

Pain clinic. (1989). *RN 52(11),* 119 (November).

Plaque: Current approaches to prevention and control. (1984). *J Am Dent Assoc, 109,* 690–702.

Rodman MJ. (1985). Metoclopramide aids stomach acid backup. *RN, 48(8),* 71–72.

Rodman MJ. (1987). A new medication for duodenal ulcers (in What's new in drugs). *RN, 50(3),* 97.

Rodman MJ. (1990). A new drug controls overflow of stomach acid. *RN, 53(1),* 121 (January).

Rodman MJ. (1990). New drugs you're giving now: A preventative against drug-induced ulcers. *RN, 57(3),* 71 (March).

*Tarail J. (1987). Sjögren's syndrome: A dry-eyed diary. *American Journal of Nursing, 87,* 324–326.

Teutsch E, Hill M. (1987). Adding moisture to your life. *Am J Nurs, 87,* 327–329.

What causes bad breath? (1986). *University of California, Berkeley Wellness Letter, 2(5),* 8.

*Zantac: New adverse reactions listed. (1988). *American Journal of Nursing, 88(8),* 1101 (August).

*Recommended for further reading.

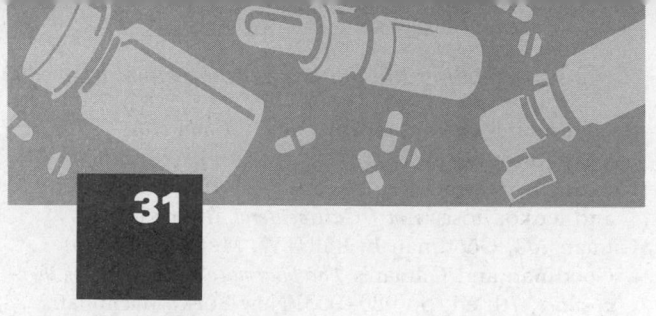

31

Agents affecting the lower gastrointestinal tract

The lower gastrointestinal (GI) tract is that portion of the gut that extends from the papilla of Vater to the anus. Drugs affecting this portion of the GI tract include antiflatulents, laxatives, and antidiarrheals.

Antiflatulents

Gases are a normal component of GI contents. Some gas is merely swallowed air. Other gases are products of fermentation in the bowel. Usually these gases are expelled from the stomach and colon promptly and cause no problems. Distention, discomfort, and pain can develop when unusual amounts of gas are present or when they cannot be expelled.

Pathophysiology

Excessive gas can be caused by compulsive air swallowing, by the use of antacids producing carbon dioxide as a by-product of the neutralization reaction, or by increased fermentation of the GI tract. Conditions promoting fermentation include the presence of large amounts of sugar, infection caused by organisms capable of fermentation, and prolonged passage time due to hypomotility or entrapment of material in diverticuli. Certain foods, such as dried beans, notorious for causing flatulence, contain undigestible sugars that remain in the tract, promoting the growth of fermenting bacteria.

    The ability of the tract to expel gas can be impaired by immaturity (as in colicky babies), immobility, inadequate dietary fiber, depression, or neuropathy, all of which reduce intestinal motility. When flatulence develops, it is important to treat the underlying causes whenever possible. Until this is accomplished and as long as chronic problems persist, antiflatulents can provide a measure of symptomatic relief.

    Antiflatulents promote the expulsion of gases by two mechanisms: mild irritation of the mucosa, which stimulates peristalsis, and defoaming, which causes small bubbles to coalesce into larger ones, which are more easily eliminated. Antiflatulents also cause an increase in eructation and passage of gas from the rectum, which can be socially embarrassing.

Carminatives

Most irritant antiflatulents (carminatives) are aromatic oils, which stimulate intestinal motility by mild irritation. They are rarely prescribed as medical treatment but are frequently used as home remedies. Alcohol (in the form of whiskey or brandy) and peppermint (oil of peppermint or peppermint water) are popular. Small amounts of an alcoholic beverage or a few drops of peppermint are mixed with hot water for oral ingestion.

Simethicone

Simethicone (Mylicon, Silain) is a greasy, translucent liquid containing a mixture of liquid dimethylpolysiloxanes. Its antifoaming and water-repellent properties derive from its capability to reduce surface tension. Simethicone decreases flatulence by causing gas bubbles in the GI tract to coalesce, forming larger masses, which are more easily expelled. Believed to be physiologically inactive, it is considered nontoxic. Simethicone is not recommended for the treatment of infant colic because safety in infants and children is unproven. The drug is frequently combined with antacids, antispasmodics, and digestants in proprietary remedies.

Dicyclomine

Dicyclomine is a synthetic antispasmodic with a tertiary amine structure.

Pharmacodynamics. The drug acts as an anticholinergic to relax smooth muscle.

Pharmacokinetics. Dicyclomine may be administered orally or intramuscularly. The relative bioavailability of oral doses is about 67% of parenteral doses. The drug acts systemically. It is eliminated in both urine and feces in approximately equal amounts. Elimination half-time is 9–10 hours.

Therapeutic uses. Dicyclomine is used to treat functional disturbances of GI hypermotility, including colic, that do not respond to other measures. Adult dosage (oral) is 20–40 mg qid.

Adverse reactions. Toxic levels of dicyclomine produce drowsiness, weakness, irritability, seizures, stridor, irregular heart rate, respiratory depression or arrest, and coma.

Precautions and contraindications. Toxic syndromes have been seen following errors in dosage, in which the recipient received twice the prescribed amount. Care is required to ensure accuracy of dosage, particularly with oral preparations used for treating infants.

Nursing management

Nursing process

Assessment When flatulence is a problem, the nurse should attempt to determine the cause. During the client history, the nurse should ask specifically about exercise and physical activity; diet (foods that worsen flatulence, amount of fiber normally consumed); events occurring when flatulence first became a problem; and general health status. If a stroke or serious glucose imbalance preceded the onset of symptoms, neuropathy may be a contributing factor. A history of diabetes mellitus, multiple sclerosis, or other disease associated with nerve damage also may signify neuropathy. A long intestinal transit time and diverticulosis favor GI fermentation and increased production of gas. During the drug history, the nurse should ask specifically about use of narcotic analgesics (*eg,* morphine, codeine) that tend to reduce propulsive peristalsis.

A complete physical examination of the abdomen should be carried out to determine the degree of distention, tympany indicative of gas accumulations, and tenderness. The client should be observed to determine if air swallowing is occurring.

Nursing diagnosis Diagnoses appropriate for the client complaining of flatulence may include the following:

> Altered comfort related to abdominal
> distention secondary to immobility (or
> neuropathy)
> Impaired social interaction related to
> embarrassment secondary to frequent (or
> uncontrolled) eructation (or rectal expulsion
> of gas)

Planning Goals of treatment are to reduce the production of intestinal gas, to reduce the volume of gas in the GI tract, or to promote the expulsion of gas.

Intervention In hospitalized clients, flatus often develops because of temporary immobility, lingering effects of general anesthetics, or the use of narcotic analgesics. The nurse should encourage ambulation as one means of stimulating peristalsis. If possible, nonnarcotic analgesics should be used to control pain. Warmth (*eg,* a hot water bottle) applied to the abdomen is often helpful. If a rectal tube is used, it should be left in place for only 15–20 minutes at a time. As soon as tolerated, a normal diet with adequate fiber should be resumed.

Nursing home residents are likely to develop flatus due to neuropathy and limited mobility. Inadequate innervation of the intestinal tract is usually irreversible. These clients are usually affected by constipation and need a bowel regimen to promote normal fecal elimination. Stimulant laxatives may be prescribed as a part of the regimen. If the regimen does not control flatus adequately, the physician should be consulted for prescription of an antiflatulent (*eg,* simethicone). Foods that cause increased flatus should be eliminated from the diet.

Client education. The nurse should assist the client in determining the cause of flatulence. The client should be informed about foods such as beans, cabbage, and concentrated carbohydrates that increase gas production in the GI tract. Beans may be tolerated if the client parboils and drains them before adding them to other ingredients. Exercise and ingestion of dietary fiber should be encouraged.

Clients affected by neuropathy or diverticulosis will have a chronic problem. For them and for colicky babies, peppermint may be recommended. It is inexpensive and readily available. Moreover, whereas medicinal preparations may not be stocked in the home, peppermint flavoring and candy often are. A drop of peppermint extract or a small piece of hard candy can be dissolved in hot water and swallowed. Adult clients may prefer to use a preparation containing simethicone. Over-the-counter medications containing simethicone include Gas-X, Tempo, Di-Gel, Riopan Plus, Gelusil II, Gelusil M, and Mylanta II. Both peppermint and simethicone are relatively innocuous; alcohol should be discouraged because of its potential for toxicity.

Evaluation Data required for evaluation are reports by clients that they are more comfortable and that flatus has diminished. For clients whose social interaction had been impaired, an increase in social contacts and interaction would be significant. (See Example of Nursing Process and Treatment of Flatulence.)

Checklist of nursing actions

☐ Assess clients affected by excessive flatus to identify causes and contributing factors.

☐ Recommend dietary measures to decrease production of gas in the GI tract.

☐ To relieve distention, recommend increased measures to stimulate peristalsis and promote the expulsion of flatus.

☐ If possible, decrease use of narcotic analgesics in clients experiencing flatus or distention.

☐ Recommend warm applications to the abdomen to stimulate peristalsis and promote expulsion of gas.

☐ If antiflatulent drugs are required, recommend essence of peppermint or preparations containing simethicone.

Drugs affecting fecal elimination

Laxatives and antidiarrheals were among the earliest drugs used. Every culture and society has had its agents for adjusting the elimination function of the intestine. Because this function has often been regarded as a mysterious, significant, and even magical process, laxatives and antidiarrheals have sometimes acquired psychological or religious overtones. Before the development of modern medicine, laxatives were among the few truly effective remedies available to the medical practitioner. As a consequence, physicians tended to overuse them, a practice that fostered undue reliance on them by the lay public. Laxatives and antidiarrheals are valuable agents for treating many conditions but their rational use requires a careful assessment of the factors associated with abnormal function and considered judgment in determining their appropriate use.

Physiology

After leaving the stomach, chyme enters the small intestine and is mixed with digestive enzymes, bile, and other secretions (Fig. 31-1). Nutrients are absorbed in this section of the GI tract, leaving a residue with the consistency of watery gruel made up of undigestible fiber, water, electrolytes, bile pigments, digestive enzymes, mucus, and microorganisms. Several times a day, most notably after a meal, the ileocecal valve opens, and peristalsis propels part of this mass into the colon.

The colon's function is to reabsorb fluids, electrolytes, and other substances (concentrating the residue into a smaller volume of soft to solid feces), to store this material for a time, and to expel it from the body during defecation. Normal feces contain about three times more water than solids. In the moist, warm environment of the colon, microorganisms proliferate rapidly. About half of the solid material in normal feces is composed of bacteria and other one-cell organisms.

Intestinal motility is regulated by local innervation, autonomic controls, nervous reflexes, and central nervous system (CNS) activity. Peristaltic waves are mediated by Auerbach's plexus, which lies between the

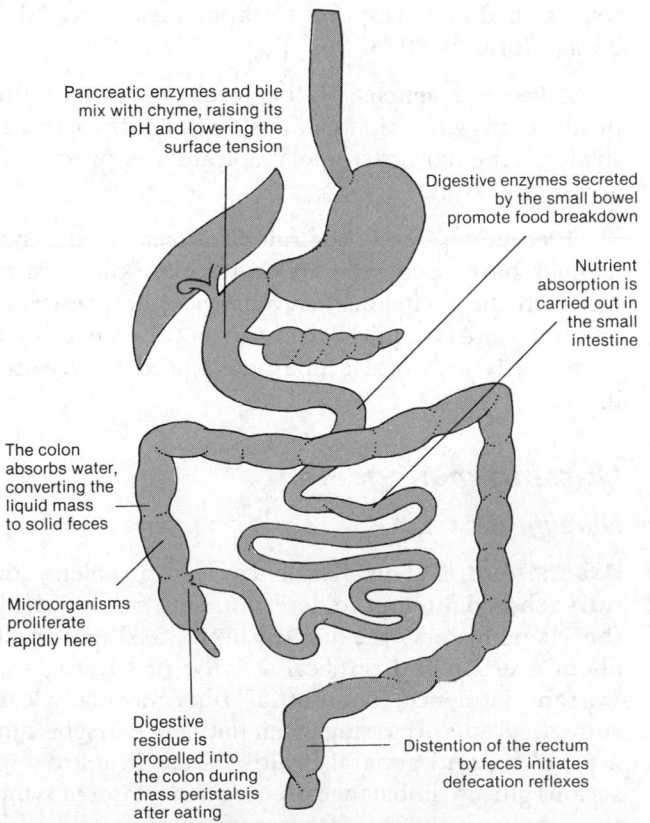

Pancreatic enzymes and bile mix with chyme, raising its pH and lowering the surface tension

Digestive enzymes secreted by the small bowel promote food breakdown

Nutrient absorption is carried out in the small intestine

The colon absorbs water, converting the liquid mass to solid feces

Microorganisms proliferate rapidly here

Digestive residue is propelled into the colon during mass peristalsis after eating

Distention of the rectum by feces initiates defecation reflexes

Figure 31-1. Lower part of the digestive tract.

Example of nursing process and treatment of flatulence

The client is a 70-year-old woman living in a skilled nursing facility. She has a history of stroke, with right-sided paresis, and hiatal hernia. She is complaining of discomfort from "gas," which she has difficulty "bringing up or passing." She states that her discomfort is relieved by eructation, or passing of flatus from the rectum, but she is embarrassed when this is audible. The client also experiences heartburn and a tendency toward constipation; the physician has ordered an antacid (magnesium salt) to control these problems. Nurses have observed that the client frequently exhibits abdominal distention.

Assessment data	Nursing diagnosis	Intervention	Goals and outcome criteria
Complaints of discomfort from "gas" and difficulty in "passing" gas	Altered comfort: abdominal distention related to inability to eliminate gas secondary to intestinal atony secondary to stroke and malfunction of the cardiac sphincter	**Monitor** food intake to assess consumption of fiber and foods such as cabbage, known to cause increased gas production in the GI tract.	Abdominal distention will decrease in severity and become less frequent.
History of stroke, paresis, and hiatal hernia		**Arrange** with the dietary service to increase fiber content in the client's diet and to eliminate foods known to increase gas production in the GI tract.	The client will report that she is more comfortable and that she is able to "pass" gas more easily.
Intermittent abdominal distention		**Take nursing measures** to promote exercise, such as walking.	
		Consult with the doctor and request an order for an antiflatulent such as simethicone, or a change in the antacid order to a preparation containing simethicone.	
Complaints of embarrassment because of audible elimination of gas	Potential for impaired social interaction related to embarrassment due to uncontrolled and audible elimination of gas	**Advise** the client to reduce her consumption of foods known to increase production of gas in the GI tract.	The client will report that she experiences fewer episodes of uncontrolled elimination of gas.
		Recommend that the client consume ample fiber in her diet.	Time spent by the client interacting with other residents will increase.
		Inform the client that the nursing staff will arrange with the dietary service for necessary dietary changes.	
		Advise the client that physical activity promotes more rapid intestinal transit of food and reduces the production of gas.	
		Encourage the client to become involved in activities and to interact with other residents of the facility.	

circular and longitudinal muscular coats of the gut. Sensory receptors in the mucous membrane transmit impulses to this myenteric plexus, which, in turn, stimulates smooth muscle contraction, producing pendulum and segmentation movements. These activities and the tone of the gut may be influenced by acetylcholine, which is present in the intestinal wall.

Both the sympathetic and parasympathetic nervous system (PNS) alter intestinal function. Sympathetic innervation is inhibitory in nature, decreasing peristalsis and relaxing the smooth muscle. Sphincters constrict and secretion decreases. Parasympathetic activity stimulates secretion and motility and relaxes sphincters. Strong stimulation of the PNS can cause colic by inducing simultaneous contraction of large segments of intestines.

Reflexes serve to coordinate functions of the GI tract. Gastrocolo-reflexes and duodenocolo-reflexes stimulate mass movements and propulsion of intestinal contents toward the anus. When feces enter the rectum, distention of the wall stimulates the myenteric plexus to initiate defecation. This weak reflex is fortified by spinal cord reflexes that increase PNS activity, augmenting peristaltic waves and initiating the Valsalva maneuver. This behavior (also called straining) involves taking a deep breath, closing the glottis, and contracting the abdominal muscles to increase intraabdominal pressure. Straining, which facilitates defecation, also has pronounced effects on the cardiovascular system and can stress the heart.

The CNS influences the colon's function through both voluntary and involuntary mechanisms. The external anal sphincter is subject to voluntary control. Defecation normally does not occur until this sphincter is consciously relaxed. The CNS also affects intestinal motility through a person's characteristic, individualized autonomic activity. The GI tract response will vary, depending on the relative proportions of sympathetic nervous system and PNS stimulation.

Pathology

Minor disturbances in fecal elimination often occur in everyday life. Changes in diet, exercise, hydration, body rhythms, and emotions alter colonic function. Disease and medical regimens, such as bed rest and drug therapy, also disrupt normal patterns. A slowing of intestinal passage fosters excessive reabsorption of water and the formation of a hard, dry stool. Rapid passage allows too little time for reabsorption; stools tend to be watery and fluid, and electrolyte loss can be great. The passage of infrequent, hard stools is termed *constipation*, whereas that of frequent, semi-liquid, or liquid stools is termed *diarrhea*. These are relative terms with no precise meanings; the norms for fecal elimination vary from culture to culture, family to family, and individual to individual.

Laxatives

Drug agents that stimulate defecation are called *laxatives*. A cathartic is a strong laxative that produces watery stools. Purgatives are even stronger agents that empty the bowel. When classified according to their mode of action, laxatives fall into five classes: irritant, hyperosmotic, bulk-forming, lubricant, and stool-softener (see Table 31-1).

Irritant laxatives

Irritant laxatives stimulate the intestinal mucosa, increasing motility and secretion. They may affect the small intestine and the colon. Stools tend to be watery and profuse, and griping (intestinal pain and cramps) may occur. Ideally, irritant laxatives should not affect the stomach or cause vomiting. They should be mild to prevent undue discomfort, and they should not induce systemic effects if absorbed.

Vegetable laxatives

Certain foods contain organic acids that act as mild laxatives. Figs, prunes, pears, raisins, and rhubarb are known for their laxative effect.

Pharmacodynamics. The organic acids contained in laxative foods irritate the intestinal mucosa, stimulating reflex peristalsis. This action is supplemented by the food's cellulose content, which adds bulk to the stool, a further colonic stimulant.

Pharmacokinetics. Laxative foods pass through the GI tract fairly rapidly, a factor that decreases the absorption of the active ingredients. However, the potential for absorption of toxic amounts of the laxative compounds is present. The active ingredient of rhubarb, oxalic acid, is sufficiently concentrated in the plant's leaves to pose a serious threat of poisoning if the leaves are eaten.

Therapeutic uses. Laxative foods should be incorporated in the diet in moderate amounts as part of a varied, balanced diet. Rhubarb is often used by the elderly as a home remedy for constipation. Prunes are frequently included in the diet to prevent constipation in such institutions as summer camps and nursing homes.

Adverse reactions. Excessive use of laxative foods will cause abdominal cramps, frequent stools, and fluid and electrolyte loss. Evacuation may be followed by a period of apparent or actual constipation. If the colon has been completely emptied, a period of time must elapse before feces accumulate sufficiently to produce another evacuation. Some foods (notably rhubarb) contain tannin, an astringent that produces constipation as an after-effect.

Irritant laxatives, including those found in foods, are contraindicated for persons with a tendency toward colonic spasticity or for those with chronic in-

(Text continues on p. 702)

Table 31-1. Drugs used to promote fecal elimination

Drug name	Preparations	Usual dosage	Additional information
Irritant (stimulant) laxatives			
Vegetable laxatives:	Foods (figs, prunes, pears, raisins, rhubarb)	One serving	Foods should be those preferred by the client.
Grain and fruit fibers (*Can:* Fibyrax)	Oral tablets	Adults: 4–8 tablets with water	Follow tablets with ample fluid (8 oz for adults).
castor oil (Alphamul, Emulsoil, Neoloid)	Oral capsules, suspension, and oil	Adults: 15–60 ml Children 2–12 yr of age: 5–15 ml Children younger than 2 yr: 1–5 ml A single dose is administered about 16 hr before surgery or procedure PC: X	Castor oil is ineffective in the absence of bile or pancreatic enzymes. Unless the taste is disguised, the oil may cause nausea and vomiting.
Dehydrocholic acid (Atrocholin, Cholan-DH, Decholin, Hepahydrin, Neocholan)	Oral tablets	Adults and children older than 12 yr of age: 750–900 mg/d, in divided doses	Dehydrocholic acid increases the volume and water content of bile.
Anthraquinones:			
Aloe	Material from the aloe vera plant	Adults: 150–250 mg (herbal remedy)	Aloe is favored as a "natural" laxative by some folk herbalists.
Aloin	Powder	Adults: 15 mg (herbal remedy)	Aloin is incorporated into the proprietary preparations Carter's Little Pills and Nature's Remedy. Although unreliable abortifacients, aloe and aloin are contraindicated for pregnant women.
cascara sagrada	Oral powder, suspension, tablets, fluidextract	Adults: 300–1000 mg Children 2–12 yr of age: 50% of adult dose; children younger than 2 yr of age: 25% of adult dose PC: C	Cascara sagrada is considered the mildest of the anthraquinone laxatives. A mixture of liquid cascara and milk of magnesia sometimes ordered for hospitalized persons is commonly termed (because of the color contrast between the two drugs) a "black and white."
senna (Black Draught, Casafru, Dr. Caldwell's Senna Laxative, Fletcher's Castoria, *Can:* Glysennid, Senokot)	Oral tablets, powder, capsules, and solution Rectal suppositories	Varies with the preparation PC: C	Senna is obtained from dried leaflets of cassia.
Diphenylmethane cathartics:			
bisacodyl (Bisco-Lax, Carter's Liver Pills, Cenalax, Codylax, Deficol, Dulcolax, Fleet Bisacodyl, Nuvac, Theralax)	Enteric-coated oral tablets Rectal suppositories and suspension	*Oral:* Adults: 5–15 mg; children older than 3 yr of age: 5–10 mg or 0.3 mg/kg body weight *Rectal:* Adults and children older than 2 yr of age: 10 mg; children 2 yr of age or younger: 5 mg PC: C	Repeated use of bisacodyl suppositories can cause inflammation of the rectal mucosa.
phenolphthalein (Alophen, Evac-U-Gen, Evac-U-Lax, Feen-A-Mint, Phenolax, Prulet)	Oral tablets, chewable tablets, and chewing gum	Adults: 30–270 mg Children older than 6 yr of age: 30–60 mg; children 2–5 yr of age: 15–20 mg PC: C	Phenolphthalein can discolor urine; alkaline urine will appear pink. Stools containing phenolphthalein turn pink if SSE are employed.

(Continued)

Table 31-1. Drugs used to promote fecal elimination (*Continued*)

Drug name	Preparations	Usual dosage	Additional information
Hyperosmotic laxatives			
glycerin, glycerol (Fleet Babylax)	Solution for enemas Rectal suppositories	Adults and children 6 yr of age or older: 5–15 ml Children younger than 6 yr of age: 2–5 ml *Rectal:* Adults and children 6 yr of age or older: 3 g Children younger than 6 yr of age: 1–1.5 g PC: C	Glycerin suppositories should be refrigerated for storage.
lactulose (Rhodiolax, Rhodialose; Can: Lactulax)	Oral syrup containing 10 g/15 ml	Adults: 15–60 ml daily as required PC: B	
Sorbitol, D-glucitol	Oral solution Rectal solution	*Oral:* Adults: 15 ml of a 70% solution *Rectal:* Adults: 120 ml of a 25%–30% solution; children 2 yr of age or younger: 30–60 ml of a 25%–30% solution	Sorbitol is sometimes used as an adjunct in therapeutic regimens employing sodium polystyrene sulfonate.
Saline laxatives			
magnesium citrate (Citromag, Evac-Q-Mag)	Oral solution	Adults: 100–200 ml Children 6–12 yr of age: 50–100 ml; children 2–5 yr of age: 4–12 ml PC: B	Compounds containing magnesium are relatively contraindicated for persons with impaired renal function.
magnesium hydroxide (Milk of Magnesia)	Oral tablets Oral suspension	Adults: 2.4–4.8 g Children 6–12 yr of age: 1.2–2.4 g; children 2–5 yr of age: 0.4–1.2 g PC: B Adults: 30–60 ml Children 6–12 yr of age: 15–30 ml; children 2–5 yr of age: 5–15 ml PC: B	
magnesium sulfate (Epsom salt)	Oral crystals and powder	Adults: 10–30 g Children 6–12 yr of age: 5–10 g; children 2–5 yr of age: 2.5–5 g PC: B	
polyethylene glycol (Klean-Prep)	Oral solution	Adults: 250 ml q10 min for up to 4 L PC: C	Solution is isotonic. No flavoring or other ingredients should be added to the solution.
potassium phosphate	Oral crystals and powder	Dosage depends on the preparation and combination of drugs used	
sodium phosphate	Oral powder	Dosage depends on the preparation and combination of drugs used PC: C	
Bulk-forming laxatives			
Bran	Food supplement, cereals	Adults: 1–4 oz	Bran is the outer husk of grain seeds, which is normally separated from the starch and germ during refinement of cereal products.

Table 31-1. Drugs used to promote fecal elimination (*Continued*)

Drug name	Preparations	Usual dosage	Additional information
Bulk-forming laxatives (continued)			
			Whole bran is somewhat irritating to the intestine and can aggravate spasticity of the bowel: it is contraindicated in intestinal obstruction, ulceration, stenosis, or adhesions.
			Bulk-forming laxatives must be given with ample fluids, and recipients must be kept well hydrated to produce a laxative effect.
calcium polycarbophil (Fibercon, mitrolan)	Oral tablets and chewable tablets	Varies with the preparation PC: C	
karaya	Oral powder	Adults: 5–10 g	
Malt soup extract (Maltsupex)	Oral tablets, powder, and solutions	Adults: 12–64 g Infants 1 mo to 2 yr of age: 6–32 g	
methylccllulose (Collothyl, Citrucel, Cologel Fiberall, Hydrocil)	Oral tablets and solution	Adults: 4–6 g Children 6–12 yr of age: 1–1.5 g PC: C	
psyllium hydrophilic mucilloid (Effersyllium, Konsyl, L.A. Formula, Laxamead, Metamucil, Modane Bulk, Mucillium, Mucilose, Naturacil, Reguloid, Serutan, Siblin, Syllact, V-Lax)	Oral powder and chewable pieces	Adults: 2.5–30 g Children 6–12 yr of age: 1.25–15 g PC: C	
Sterculia gum (Normacol)	Granules in satchet	Adults: 1–2 pkts daily	Sterculia gum interferes with absorption of other drugs; do not take 4 within 2 hrs of any other medication.
Lubricant laxatives			
mineral oil (Agoral, Kondremul, Neo-Cultol, Milkinol, Neo-Cultol, Nujol, Zymenol)	Oral liquid Oil enema	*Oral:* Adults: 15–45 ml; children older than 6 yr of age: 10–15 ml *Rectal:* Adults: 60–150 ml; children older than 6 yr of age: 60 ml PC: C	Plain mineral oil administered orally should be given only on an empty stomach to reduce the loss of fatsoluble vitamins; administer at least 2 hr before bedtime to reduce risk of regurgitation and aspiration.
Stool softeners			
docusate (Bu-Lax, Colace, Comfolax, Dioctocal, Doxidan, Doxate-C, Doxate-S, Diocto, Diosuccin, Disonate, Doxinate, Duosol, Kasof, Laxinate, Modane, Pro-Cal Sof, Regul-Aid, Regulex, Regutol, Stulex, Surfak)	Oral capsules and solution	Adults and children older than 12 yr of age: 50–360 mg/d Children 2–12 yr of age: 50–150 mg/d; children younger than 2 yr of age: 25 mg PC: C	Docusate may be administered as a single bedtime dose or in divided doses.
poloxamer 188 (Alaxin)	Oral capsules	Adults: 240 mg, 1–3 times daily	

KEY: PC = pregnancy risk category. (The validity of pregnancy risk categories has not been established. See chapter 16, p 216.)
Can: Canadian trade name.

flammatory bowel diseases such as ulcerative colitis or Crohn's disease.

Castor oil

A product of the castor bean, castor oil, is a bland, nonirritant oil used as a high-grade industrial lubricant and topical emollient.

Pharmacodynamics. Administered orally, castor oil has no effect on the stomach. During digestion, bile and pancreatic enzymes in the small intestine convert part of the oil to ricinoleic acid, a powerful irritant. Both the small and large intestines respond with increased motility and rapid passage of their contents; soft to watery stools are produced within 2–3 hours.

Pharmacokinetics. The extent of absorption of castor oil is unknown. Its active principle, ricinoleic acid, is absorbed to a small extent and subsequently metabolized like other fatty acids.

Therapeutic uses. Castor oil is used medically to empty the bowel in preparation for abdominal procedures such as x-ray studies.

Adverse reactions. Castor oil has a wide margin of safety. Large doses have little more effect than standard doses because the drug is rapidly eliminated by the purgative action it induces. Some people find the taste of castor oil very disagreeable.

Precautions and contraindications. Castor oil is contraindicated for persons in whom increased intestinal motility is hazardous (*eg*, those with obstructive disease of the GI tract) and for persons with obstructive jaundice and pancreatic disease who lack the bile and pancreatic enzymes required for activation of the drug.

Anthraquinones

Anthraquinone (anthracene, emodin) cathartics include senna, aloes, and cascara sagrada. Danthron, another drug of this class, has been recalled by the federal Food and Drug Administration because it causes cancer in mice and rats (Drug recalls, 1987).

Pharmacodynamics. Anthraquinones act by irritating the intestinal mucosa and stimulating reflex peristalsis. Evacuation usually occurs within 6–12 hours but may be delayed for up to 24 hours.

Pharmacokinetics. With the exception of danthron, anthraquinone laxatives are only slightly absorbed from the small intestine. In the colon, enzymatic hydrolysis of glycosides in the drugs free the pharmacologically active anthraquinones.

Absorbed anthraquinones are metabolized in the liver. The drugs and their metabolites are eliminated in feces by bile and in urine. Unabsorbed drug is eliminated directly in feces.

Therapeutic uses. Proprietary preparations of anthraquinone laxatives are widely used and sometimes abused by the lay public.

When laxatives are required medically, anthraquinones (senna or cascara derivatives are preferred over other stimulant drugs by many practitioners. They are prescribed for the relief of simple constipation and to prepare the bowel for diagnostic procedures, such as x-ray examination of the GI tract with contrast media. Aloe is not used medically.

Adverse reactions. Stimulant (irritant) laxatives are habit-forming. Prolonged use may result in dependency and loss of normal bowel function.

Stimulant laxatives may produce abdominal discomfort, nausea, cramping, griping, and faintness. Among the anthraquinones, cascara sagrada is relatively mild, whereas aloe (aloin) is the most irritating. Irritant laxatives can also cause electrolyte disturbances (hypokalemia, hypocalcemia, acid-base imbalance), malabsorption, weight loss, and protein-losing enteropathy. Pathologic changes include structural damage to the myenteric plexus, severe and permanent loss of colon motility, and hypertrophy of the muscularis mucosae. Atony and dilatation of the colon sometimes resemble that seen in ulcerative colitis.

Anthraquinones may discolor the urine (from pink to red or brown to black). These drugs also discolor colonic mucosa (melanosis), an effect that appears to be innocuous.

Precautions and contraindications. Anthraquinones are contraindicated for persons with symptoms suggestive of abdominal pathology (nausea, vomiting, acute abdominal pain) and for those with intestinal obstruction.

Diphenylmethane cathartics

Diphenylmethane cathartics include phenolphthalein and bisacodyl.

Pharmacodynamics. Diphenylmethane cathartics have their greatest effect on the colon. They act as irritants that stimulate reflex peristalsis.

Diphenylmethane cathartics require 6 or more hours to act. They can be given at bedtime for results in the early morning.

Pharmacokinetics. Bisacodyl is not significantly absorbed from the GI tract. Up to 15% of orally administered phenolphthalein may be absorbed; some of the absorbed drug enters the enterohepatic circulation. Following absorption into the bloodstream, diphenylmethanes are metabolized in the liver and excreted in the urine. They are distributed into breast milk.

Therapeutic uses. Proprietary preparations containing diphenylmethanes are popular laxatives used by the lay public. They have also been used medically to relieve constipation occurring secondary to neurologic disease, idiopathic slowing of transit time, or constipating drugs, as well as to cleanse the bowel prior to surgery or diagnostic procedures involving examination of the GI tract.

Adverse reactions. Side effects of diphenylmethanes include nausea, cramping, griping, and faintness. Prolonged use may lead to laxative dependency, loss of normal bowel function, fluid and electrolyte imbalance, impaired nutrition, and weight loss. Rectal suppositories containing bisacodyl may cause irritation, inflammation, and a burning sensation of the rectal mucosa.

Allergic reactions to diphenylmethane laxatives include skin manifestations, renal irritation, encephalitis, respiratory disturbances, cardiac arrest, and (rarely) death. Skin problems include polychromatic skin eruptions, which may last several months. These drugs have been associated with the development of Stevens-Johnson syndrome and systemic lupus erythematosus.

Precautions and contraindications. Stimulant laxatives, including diphenylmethanes, are contraindicated for persons exhibiting signs and symptoms of abdominal pathology (nausea, vomiting, acute abdominal pain). They are not recommended for persons with abdominal cramps, anal or rectal fissures, or ulcerated hemorrhoids. Stimulant laxatives should not be prescribed for children younger than 6 years of age. Safe use of bisacodyl during pregnancy has not been established.

Diphenylmethane laxatives are contraindicated for persons with a known allergic sensitivity to them.

Dehydrocholic acid

Dehydrocholic acid is an unconjugated, oxidized bile acid derived from cholic acid.

Pharmacodynamics. Dehydrocholic acid increases the volume and water content of bile. In the intestine, it acts as a stimulant laxative.

Pharmacokinetics. Dehydrocholic acid is readily absorbed from the GI tract. It is concentrated in the liver and is excreted in feces in the form of bile.

Therapeutic uses. Dehydrocholic acid is used to relieve temporary constipation. It has also been used to increase bile flow in persons with biliary tract dysfunction. Even though the drug produces a larger volume of bile with lower concentrations of solutes, benefits under those conditions remain unproved.

Adverse reactions. Prolonged use of dehydrocholic acid may lead to laxative dependency, loss of normal bowel function, fluid and electrolyte imbalance, impaired nutrition, and weight loss.

Precautions and contraindications. Dehydrocholic acid should not be used when signs and symptoms of acute abdominal pathology (nausea, vomiting, acute abdominal pain) are present.

Hyperosmotic laxatives

Hyperosmotic laxatives include glycerin, sorbitol, lactulose, and saline laxatives (magnesium cations and phosphate anions).

Pharmacodynamics. Hyperosmotic laxatives appear to act by increasing colonic fluid retention. The increased osmotic pressure in the lumen of the bowel may also promote movement of fluid across the intestinal mucosa from the extracellular fluid compartment. As a result, feces become more liquid, and the increased volume in the bowel stimulates stretch receptors, increasing peristalsis.

Magnesium salts may also stimulate cholecystokinin release or reduce transit time.

Hyperosmotic laxatives tend to dehydrate the client and may be preferable to other laxatives in persons for whom a negative fluid balance is desirable.

Lactulose promotes reduction of blood ammonia levels in portal-system encephalopathy. It acidifies the contents of the bowel, promotes the outward diffusion and elimination of ammonia in the GI tract, and inhibits absorption of amines.

Pharmacokinetics. Rectally administered hyperosmotic laxatives are poorly absorbed. Preparations administered orally may be absorbed systemically, particularly magnesium-containing agents. The absorbed drugs are subsequently eliminated by the kidneys, whereas unabsorbed drugs are eliminated in feces.

Therapeutic uses. Hyperosmotic laxatives, especially saline laxatives, are used to correct temporary constipation and to empty the bowel prior to surgery or procedures involving bowel examination. Saline laxatives are also used as adjuncts in the treatment of poisoning to hasten removal of some poisons from the GI tract.

In the past, hyperosmotic laxatives have been used as adjuncts with anthelmintics in the treatment of parasites. However, newer drugs used for treating helminth infestations do not require laxatives, so that this practice of using laxatives is becoming obsolete. Sorbitol is frequently used in conjunction with sodium polystyrene sulfonate to prevent constipation caused by that resin. In addition to its functions as a laxative, lactulose is used to treat portal-system encephalopathy associated with high blood ammonia levels.

Adverse reactions. Unless administered with sufficient fluid to produce an isotonic solution, saline cathartics tend to dehydrate the body and may cause electrolyte disturbances. Hypertonic preparations draw fluid into the lumen from the tissues. This fluid is excreted when the stool is evacuated. Dehydration is enhanced by the diuretic effect of these salts when the absorbed portion of the drugs is excreted in urine.

Glycerin may produce rectal discomfort, irritation, burning or griping, cramping, and tenesmus. The bitter taste of magnesium sulfate may cause nausea.

Saline laxatives are absorbed to some degree, increasing body levels of the particular metallic ion involved. These electrolyte changes are transient in clients with good renal function, who promptly excrete the salts in urine. If renal function is impaired, however, plasma content rises, and symptoms of excess may occur. Hypermagnesemia causes weakness, confusion, and sedation (about 20% of magnesium salts may be absorbed). Phosphates tend to reduce plasma levels of ionic calcium. Potassium toxicity arising from renal failure is heightened by the administration of a potassium-containing laxative. Sodium salts increase water retention and are contraindicated in congestive states, such as heart failure.

Lactulose may cause flatulence and abdominal cramping, especially when treatment is initiated. High dosages can cause diarrhea. Nausea and vomiting have also been reported. The fermentation of lactulose in the bowel may produce large accumulations of hydrogen gas.

Precautions and contraindications. Hyperosmotic laxatives are contraindicated for persons with signs and symptoms of acute abdominal pathology (nausea, vomiting, acute abdominal pain).

Magnesium compounds are contraindicated for persons with renal impairment, and sodium compounds should not be used by persons advised to restrict sodium intake.

If lactulose is used regularly, clients should be monitored for electrolyte disturbances (particularly hypokalemia) secondary to excessive loss of intestinal contents. This drug can cause high concentrations of hydrogen gas in the bowel. Cauterization of the bowel poses a theoretic risk of explosion unless hydrogen gas accumulations have been removed from the bowel by thorough cleansing prior to any endoscopic procedures.

Bulk-forming laxatives

Bulk-forming laxatives are composed of polysaccharides and cellulose derivatives that are both hydrophilic and nondigestible.

Pharmacodynamics. Within the digestive tract, bulk-forming laxatives swell in water to form gels or viscous solutions that soften the stool and increase its bulk. Peristalsis is stimulated, and transit time is reduced. Because the stool is soft, it is passed easily without trauma to rectal or anal tissues. Bulk-forming laxatives are the most physiologic of the laxatives; they mimic the action of dietary fiber in the digestive tract.

Pharmacokinetics. Bulk-forming laxatives are not absorbed and are carried out of the body in feces.

Therapeutic uses. Bulk-forming laxatives are often considered the treatment of choice in chronic constipation or laxative dependency not complicated by impairment of intestinal motility due to neural impairment.

Adverse reactions. Powdery formulations of bulk laxatives can cause suffocation or serious lung pathology if inhaled. When the drugs are taken with insufficient amounts of fluid, they may lodge in the esophagus, causing impaction and obstruction. This is most likely to occur in persons who experience difficulty in swallowing.

Precautions and contraindications. Bulk-forming laxatives should never be administered in dry form; they must be given with ample fluids (at least 8 ounces for adults) to ensure propulsion of the dose beyond the cardiac sphincter into the stomach. In addition, without sufficient fluid, no bulk can be formed in the colon. Bulk-forming laxatives are contraindicated for persons with marked dysphagia.

Lubricant laxatives

Lubricant laxatives include various oils, such as digestible vegetable oils and nondigestible liquid petrolatum (mineral oil). Because lubricant laxatives must be used in quantity to ensure that a portion reaches the colon undigested, vegetable oils are not recommended for their laxative effect.

Pharmacodynamics. Oils retard the reabsorption of water from the fecal mass in the colon, preventing hardening of the stools. Oils also act as lubricants, facilitating stool passage.

Therapeutic uses. Mineral oil is used by the lay public, and in selected cases by physicians, to control chronic constipation. Oils are used medically as retention enemas to soften stools in the treatment of constipation or obstipation.

Adverse reactions. Digestible oils are not used orally to treat constipation because they retard gastric motility and secretion and increase caloric intake.

Mineral oil is nondigestible and poorly absorbed. However, the small amounts that are absorbed can cause a foreign body reaction in the mesenteric lymph nodes, intestinal mucosa, liver, and spleen. Although these reactions seem benign, the long range safety of the drug is questionable. Mineral oil can leak past the anal sphincter, soiling undergarments, causing itching, and interfering with the healing of rectal lesions. As a lipid solvent, the drug interferes with the absorption of fat-soluble nutrients. Vitamins A, D, and K dissolved in the unabsorbed portion of the oil are carried through the tract and excreted in feces. Because mineral oil taken at bedtime may be aspirated during sleep, causing a lipid pneumonitis, there is no truly safe time for the drug to be given.

Precautions and contraindications. Mineral oil is usually administered between the last meal of the day and bedtime to minimize the risk of aspiration and the loss of fat-soluble vitamins. Persons receiving the drug over a long time should be monitored for signs and symptoms of fat-soluble vitamin deficiencies. Supplemental vitamins may be needed.

Stool softeners
Stool softeners are moistening agents. They include poloxamer 188 and sodium salts of docusate.

Pharmacodynamics. Stool softeners act by reducing surface tension in the bowel, promoting emulsification of the stool. They facilitate the incorporation of water into the fecal mass, thereby softening the stool. They may also affect motor and secretory functions of the digestive tract. The pharmacology of these compounds is not completely understood.

Pharmacokinetics. Stool softeners appear to be minimally absorbed; the portion that is absorbed is excreted in bile.

Adverse reactions. Docusate compounds are toxic to human hepatic tissue cell cultures and, theoretically, could cause adverse reactions in the liver. However, in more than two decades of clinical practice, these drugs have been well tolerated, even when prescribed over long periods. Occasionally, GI pain, cramping, and skin rash may occur.

Precautions and contraindications. Stool softeners should be administered with ample fluids to promote softening action in the bowel.

■ Summary
Laxatives are drugs that stimulate fecal elimination. They are classified as irritant, hyperosmotic, bulk-forming, lubricant, and stool-softening. Irritant laxatives stimulate intestinal motility and secretion. Hyperosmotic laxatives draw water into the intestinal lumen, preventing dehydration and hardening of the stool. Bulk-forming laxatives stimulate the bowel by distention and also soften the stool. Lubricants and stool softeners promote the production of a soft stool.

In normal persons, constipation is best prevented by dietary management, hydration, exercise, and the promotion of habit. Laxatives may be needed to relieve temporary dysfunction or to compensate for permanent impairment of fecal elimination.

Except for lubricants, laxatives should be taken with ample amounts of fluid. Excessive use of laxatives may cause dehydration, potassium loss, or toxicity from absorption of chemical components.

Nursing management
Nursing implications
The great number and variety of laxative agents available for over-the-counter purchase and the volume of their sales indicate that the lay public frequently, even habitually, uses these agents. Is constipation such a widespread problem, or are laxatives used when they are not needed? The answer to both questions is probably yes. The historic roots of the problem are multiple.

Historic roots of laxative use. Among the few truly effective treatment agents, laxatives were highly regarded by both the medical profession and the lay public for centuries. Psychological attitudes toward fecal excretion, which commonly associate excrement with evil and its elimination with the expiation of guilt, strengthened this view. Purging was considered helpful in virtually all illnesses, and there was little regard for its dangers. Some people still consider periodic use of a laxative to "clean out" the body a healthy practice.

Somewhat ironically, a number of modernizing trends in the 20th century have contributed to the increase of constipation in developed countries. Diets containing highly processed foods often are seriously deficient in fiber. Moreover, increasing use of machines to perform strenuous work has promoted a sedentary lifestyle. Increases in life expectancy have also caused a particular problem among the rising number of elderly, who tend to suffer from decreased intestinal secretion and motility. In addition, the accelerated pace of modern life allows little time for maintaining regular defecation habits. It is small wonder that many people have become preoccupied with bowel function and depend on intermittent or regular use of laxatives.

Causes of constipation. Changes in bowel habits can indicate serious, underlying conditions ranging from depression to malignant neoplasms. Clients with constipation that does not respond to hygienic measures should be referred for a diagnostic evaluation to determine the cause of the condition.

Clients who are inpatients in health care institutions frequently develop constipation due to their relative inactivity, changes in diet, use of depressant drugs, inability to assume a normal posture for defecation, a lack of privacy, and lack of opportunity to defecate at the normal time. Fasting required for diagnostic tests, anorexia, fluid and electrolyte imbalances, and increased stress levels tend to increase the risk of constipation. Many medical treatments also disrupt normal function: some reduce fluid and food intake; some cause intestinal atony, leading to constipation. Laxatives are often helpful in ameliorating or controlling such conditions.

Pathology could also cause constipation, especially when nerve function in the gut is impaired. Neurologic diseases, such as stroke, multiple sclerosis, diabetic gastroparesis, and cord injuries damage the nerves involved in stimulating motility and, thus, reduce peristalsis. Complete atony is not amendable to laxative therapy but reduced motility often is.

Fecal impaction. Fecal impaction is a complication too often seen in institutionalized clients. In this severe form of constipation, fecal mass cannot be propelled through the tract, and partial or complete obstruction develops. Because the mass irritates the colon, secretion of mucus increases, and liquid stool may be excreted around the impaction, simulating diarrhea.

Impaction can be a life-threatening condition in clients with cardiovascular problems. Pressure in the rectum stimulates vagal activity, which slows the heart and increases the risk of heart block. Use of the Valsalva maneuver while attempting to defecate subjects the heart to rapid changes in intrathoracic pressures, first reducing venous return to the heart and then flooding the heart with excessive amounts of blood. The Valsalva maneuver also increases blood pressure in the eyes and CNS. Strokes and heart attacks are not uncommon occurrences during straining.

Careful attention to the prevention of constipation will eliminate the risk of impaction for most clients. However, monitoring bowel function is critical for proper evaluation. Progression of disease in clients with secondary constipation can result in problems, even when the preventive regimen is meticulously observed. It is not enough to ask the clients every day if they have passed stools. (Even this rudimentary measure is too often neglected in busy nursing units.) The frequency, amount, and consistency of stools should be ascertained and recorded. Analysis of these data enables nurses to determine the efficacy of preventive regimens and the need for further intervention.

Indications for laxative use. Medical uses of laxatives include eliminating toxins from the GI tract in cases of food poisoning and drug poisoning, expelling parasites and toxic anthelmintics, cleansing the colon before x-rays or surgery, preventing irritation by hardened stool in rectal and colon disorders, preventing straining when it is contraindicated, and treating certain kinds of constipation (Box 31-1). Laxatives and cathartics are not appropriate in treating functional constipation stemming from dehydration, lack of exercise, or dietary deficiency of fiber. In this situation, it is necessary to correct the faulty practices.

Some substances used as laxatives are also used for different purposes. Methyl cellulose and carboxymethylcellulose, for example, have been incorporated in combination preparations designed to aid in weight

---

Box 31-1. Medical uses of laxatives

Eliminating from GI tract toxins in food poisoning and drug poisoning

Expelling parasites and toxic anthelmintics

Cleansing the colon before x-rays or surgery

Eliminating irritation by hardened stool in rectal and colon disorders

Preventing straining when contraindicated

Treating certain kinds of constipation

---

reduction. The sensation of bulk in the stomach temporarily allays hunger, and the drugs help prevent the constipation that often accompanies reduction in dietary intake.

Psyllium appears to inhibit the reabsorption of bile acids; long-term use tends to reduce plasma cholesterol levels. Agar, a dried colloid substance rich in undigestible hemicellulose is a substance related to bulk-forming laxatives. Although agar is not a very effective laxative, it is employed as an emulsifier in some combination laxative preparations containing mineral oil. It is also added to foods or prepared as a gel for culture media. Bran, aloe, and mineral oil are sometimes used as cosmetics: bran as a mild abrasive in cleansing soaps and aloe and mineral oil as skin lubricants.

Laxative abuse. The use of laxatives tends to be habit-forming. Undue reliance on these agents in preference to hygienic measures fosters psychological dependence. Cathartics and purgatives, which tend to empty the tract, cause a hiatus in stool production, which is often interpreted as continued constipation. Repetition of the laxative dose establishes a physiologic dependency. Some clients develop a cyclic pattern of alternate laxative and antidiarrheal use, failing to recognize the need to allow the tract time to reestablish normal patterns. The habitual use of laxatives by persons with normally functioning intestinal tracts is not a healthy practice.

Laxatives are sometimes abused by persons seeking to lose weight or by persons suffering from eating disorders such as bulimia. Excessive dosages may be consumed in these situations. Frequent or excessive laxative treatment also has been identified as one form of child abuse.

Nursing process

Assessment When clients complain of constipation, it is necessary to ascertain exactly what they mean. Some clients consider constipation as failure to have a bowel movement every day. Depending on food and fiber intake, a person may or may not have a stool that frequently. Constipation applies only to conditions in which the stools are hard and difficult or painful to pass. A person who has soft stools at intervals greater than 24 hours may have a prolonged intestinal transit time but does not have true constipation.

Data required for assessment include frequency and consistency of stools, the ease or difficulty of passage, and prolonged, subjective sensations of fullness and distention in the distal bowel. When stools are dry and hard, are passed with difficulty or pain, and the client feels distended, a diagnosis of constipation can be made. The nurse must then assess the client's diet, hydration, activity level, and bowel habits to determine if faulty hygiene is the cause of, or a contributing factor in, the development of the problem.

Nursing diagnosis Clients for whom laxatives are prescribed usually have a diagnosis of

Constipation, colonic related to immobility (dehydration, fiber deficiency, inadequate stimulation of peristalsis, or habitual postponement of defecation)

There are many contributing factors, including permanent nervous system or musculoskeletal disability, inability to eat, fever, and dietary deficiency. When laxatives are administered, they may cause the following:

Diarrhea related to overstimulation of peristalsis secondary to laxative use
Fluid volume deficit related to excessive loss of water from the lower intestinal tract secondary to diarrhea
Pain: abdominal cramping related to overstimulation of the lower bowel secondary to laxative use
Altered comfort: nausea (flatulence) related to laxative use
High risk for recurrent constipation related to dehydration and hypokalemia secondary to laxative use
Fear caused by coloration of the urine related to use of anthraquinone laxatives
Impaired tissue integrity: loss of normal bowel function related to repeated use of laxatives
Impaired tissue integrity: skin rash related to inflammation secondary to laxative allergy

Many clients will have a

Knowledge deficit related to normal fecal elimination, constipation, and its treatment

Common collaborative problems that should be differentiated from the nursing diagnoses include

Potential complication: hypokalemia
Potential complication: metabolic acidosis

Planning Goals of treatment are to restore normal fecal elimination, and to prevent or promptly detect and treat nausea, abdominal cramps and discomfort, dehydration, hypokalemia, acidosis, skin rash, or other adverse reaction to laxatives. Preventing fear is another goal for clients receiving anthraquinone laxatives. When client teaching is needed, increased knowledge about constipation, its prevention, and its treatment is a major goal.

Intervention When clients are identified as being at high risk for constipation, measures should be taken to prevent the condition. Emphasis should be on increasing the intake of fluids, fiber, and potassium, on increasing physical activity, and on establishing a regular pattern of defecation.

Laxative foods may be offered, if allowed, in the diet. Choice of food should be dictated by client preference. Children often refuse cooked prunes but accept dry prunes as snack foods. Pears and raisins exert laxative effects and are well liked by most people. Clients who refuse these foods may enjoy prune juice popsicles.

Constipation secondary to medical treatment regimens or illnesses can usually be prevented by regular use of a bulk laxative or stool softener. These types of laxatives must be given before the stool becomes hard and dry, 2–3 days before constipation is expected to develop.

Single episodes of temporary constipation are amenable to saline or irritant cathartics, or enemas. Temporary use of these agents is also appropriate when bulk laxatives or stool softeners are first administered, if the client has already become constipated. The choice of agent is determined by the client's general condition, associated pathology, and the preference of the client, nurse, or physician.

Enemas or rectal suppositories are required for clients unable to take oral preparations. They are preferred when immediate evacuation is desired. Traditional enema solutions include tap water, soap suds solution, and normal saline. Tap water is hypotonic and can be absorbed in large amounts. Soap suds solutions, which are very irritating, are seldom prescribed today. Normal saline, which is isotonic, disturbs fluid and electrolyte balance the least, and is essentially nonirritating. It is the solution of choice in most situations. Small hypertonic enemas, such as Fleet's Phospho-Soda, may be prescribed when fluid loss is considered beneficial.

Repeated enemas are sometimes ordered to cleanse the colon completely. These can remove excess amounts of nutrients from the intestine, however. Colonic hypermotility is reflected by increased motility of the small intestine. Chyme is propelled into the colon prematurely and removed by succeeding enemas. Clients may become very weak and exhibit signs of stress, such as diaphoresis. They should be allowed to rest. Administration of electrolyte-containing fluids (*eg,* coffee or tea) helps to correct fluid and potassium depletion and often reverses the symptoms. The physician should be informed of the client's reaction before enemas are resumed.

Oral laxatives should be administered in the most palatable form possible. Some clients prefer milk of magnesia diluted with milk. The flavor of magnesium sulfate can be disguised in chilled grape juice. Laxatives marketed in enteric-coated form are virtually tasteless but should not be chewed, crushed, or administered concurrently with antacids. Not only could the taste of the drug be evident, but premature release of the agent in the stomach could also cause irritation. Castor oil is more palatable if emulsified. Some people prefer the plain oil mixed with orange juice. This mixture can be emulsified and effervesced by the addition of a small quantity (1/2 tsp) of soda bicarbonate immediately before ingestion. Caution should be exercised when disguising drug flavors with foods. Unless the taste of the drug is well masked, the client could become conditioned to dislike the food.

An alternative to using food is chilling the tongue before the medicine is to be ingested. Chilling anesthetizes taste buds and prevents bitter sensations. The client should suck on an ice cube or a popsicle just before taking the drug. Bulk laxatives must be mixed with fluid immediately before ingestion. (They form a gel quickly after mixing.) Ample fluids (for adults, one or two glasses) should be administered with all laxatives.

When preparing doses of dry bulk laxatives, care should be taken to minimize their dispersion into the environment. Inhalation of their dusts can cause respiratory distress. These compounds can stimulate allergic sensitivity; once reexposed, symptoms in the sensitized person tend to be minor (rhinitis, itching of the eyes) but more serious reactions are possible. Powders are more frequent offenders than granular preparations because of their higher dust content. Drug allergy is an important cause of occupational illness among nurses.

Mineral oil should be administered on an empty stomach, a minimum of 2 hours before bedtime. Clients receiving mineral oil over an extended period should be monitored for deficiencies of fat-soluble vitamins.

Until appendicitis is ruled out, laxatives must not be given when abdominal pain or other symptoms of this condition are present. The risk of perforation is sharply increased in victims of appendicitis who have been given a laxative. These drugs are also contraindicated in intestinal pathology, such as obstruction, inflammations (typhoid fever, ulcerative colitis), hemorrhage, and intussusception. Pregnant women or debilitated clients should also avoid using laxatives. Because laxatives increase fluid and electrolyte loss from the lower intestine, their excessive use predisposes to dehydration, hypokalemia, nutritional depletion, and malnutrition. Repeated passage of watery stools, which sometimes contain digestive enzymes, can cause anal excoriation.

Clients who are still in possession of laxatives containing danthron should be advised to return these preparations to a pharmacy. Danthron preparations (Dorbane & Mobane) have been recalled by the Food and Drug Administration.

Client education. The client afflicted with simple, primary constipation requires considerable teaching to acquire a healthy attitude toward bowel function and to reform faulty hygienic practices.

The client's usual bowel functions in the absence of laxatives should be determined. Contrary to the prevailing opinion, infrequent defecation should not be accepted as "normal for the individual." It is more likely to be an example of abnormal bowel function resulting from modern lifestyles. Prolonged transit time for material in the bowel is associated with such diseases as constipation, obesity, diabetes, diverticulosis, hemorrhoids, and colonic cancer. These diseases are much less common in more primitive societies in which transit times are shorter. Although a cause-and-effect relationship has yet to be established, prevailing evidence is persuasive: a reduction in transit time would seem highly desirable.

Hygienic measures to correct constipation include changes in diet, physical activity, and bowel habits. Clients also should be advised of the impact of stress on bowel function, as well as the importance of proper use of over-the-counter and herbal laxatives.

Diet. Foods high in fiber should be substituted for refined carbohydrates and concentrated fats. Whole grain cereals and breads, fruits, and vegetables are recommended. Some fruits and vegetables should be eaten raw because cooking tends to break down cellulose, the main source of dietary fiber. Foods containing natural laxatives, such as prunes and rhubarb, are not necessarily helpful because dependence may be merely shifted from commercial to "natural" laxatives. Astringent foods (tea, blackberries, blueberries, elderberries) are best avoided.

Ample hydration is important to prevent excessive reabsorption of water from the stools. At least 8 glasses of fluid per day (1,500 ml) are needed by adults. Most clients must learn new cooking practices. There are numerous cookbooks on the market containing recipes for vegetarian and "natural" dishes, such as granola, whole grain breads, and vegetable casseroles. Clients may need to be cautioned against using large quantities of honey. Although a natural food, honey is a concentrated carbohydrate high in calories and low in fiber.

Since hypokalemia reduces smooth muscle motility and can cause intestinal atony, dietary potassium must also be adequate if constipation is to be avoided.

Physical activity. A graduated program for increasing physical activity and exercise helps tone all the body's muscles, including the smooth muscle of the intestine. Immobility and lack of exercise are recognized causes of constipation. Regular exercise is preferable; 20-minute workouts at least three times weekly are suggested. Activities should be chosen that reflect the client's interests, that are feasible during bad weather, and that are suitable for one or two participants. If exercise is fun and available no matter what the season or number of people available to "form a team," it is more likely to become a permanent habit. Walking, cycling, swimming, dancing, golf, and tennis may be recommended, depending on the client's age, physical condition, and lifestyle.

Defecation habits. Establishing a routine for defecation is important. If the initial defecation reflex is ignored, it will die out within 1 or 2 minutes. Habitual suppression weakens the reflex. The client should choose a time of day when leisurely attention can be paid to bowel function. Because gastrocolic reflex appears strongest after the first meal of the day, the period following breakfast may be most suitable. Clients may need to adjust their sleeping habits to allow 15–20 minutes of extra time between breakfast and the daily schedule. Sipping warm liquids while relaxing on the toilet helps promote the defecation reflex.

Stress. In some clients, constipation is brought on or increased by unusual stress. These persons appear to respond to stress with autonomic stimulation, characterized by a predominance of sympathetic over parasympathetic activity. (Other people, in whom parasympathetic activity predominates, may have a tendency toward frequent, loose stools when under stress.) For these people, learning to reduce or better manage the stress in their lives may help significantly to reduce constipation.

Glucocorticoid stress hormones increase potassium excretion by the kidneys and can deplete body stores of the electrolyte, contributing to intestinal atony.

Use and abuse of laxatives. Instruction about the use and abuse of laxatives is important. Adding prunes or pears to the diet may correct occasional problems. The rare use of saline or irritant laxatives to treat temporary constipation is probably not harmful if the cause of the disruption is minor and not likely to recur. Milk of magnesia or bisacodyl is relatively benign for such use.

Recurrent problems must be investigated to identify the underlying cause and determine the corrective measures needed. Excessive use of laxatives can cause fluid and electrolyte depletion. Some clients, who are unable or unwilling to change their lifestyles, continue to experience problems. For them, regular use of a bulk-forming laxative may be necessary. Bulk-forming laxatives must be taken prophylactically because they are not immediately effective. Peristalsis may be stimulated within 12–24 hours but the appearance of soft stools requires 2–3 days. Chronic use of other laxatives should be discouraged unless prescribed by a physician for a chronic medical condition.

When prolonged use of laxatives is necessary, clients should be taught the proper techniques for administering the drugs, the adverse reactions that can occur, and precautions necessary to prevent complications. Clients taking phenolphthalein preparations should be reassured that the pink color imparted to alkaline urine and feces is harmless.

Specific parameters should be established for bowel function and signs and symptoms of adverse reactions. This gives the client a clear understanding of the circumstances requiring renewed evaluation by a health care professional.

Herbal preparations. Clients who are advocates of herbal medicines should be cautioned about certain laxative preparations. Aloin is not recommended for laxative use or any other purpose requiring internal consumption. This drug is considered too toxic for systemic use. Although it is contraindicated during pregnancy, aloin is not a reliable or safe abortifacient.

Psyllium preparations containing the whole seed are not suitable for ingestion. The outer seed coat acts as a harsh irritant. In addition, when digested, a pigment is released that is absorbed and subsequently deposited as small granules in the renal tubules. The significance of these deposits is not known. It is claimed that refined psyllium preparations from which the seed coat has been eliminated do not cause renal pigmentation.

Mineral waters have a reputation for enhancing health. Although they do contain salts, such as magnesium or sodium sulfates, they are not reliable laxatives. Commercial mineral waters are artificially prepared, factory-made solutions which are not formulated for medicinal purposes and should not be used for the treatment of constipation.

Evaluation Evaluation depends on accurate and comprehensive monitoring of fecal elimination. The

---

Learning experience 31-1

Prepare a teaching plan for good bowel habits.

Learning experience 31-2

With a classmate, role-play a nurse's discussion with a client about constipation.

Example of nursing process and treatment to prevent constipation

The client is a 39-year-old telephone operator with a 10-year history of varicose veins. She has just been admitted to the hospital for treatment of acute phlebitis (left leg). The physician has ordered anticoagulants (heparin and dicumarol) and strict bed rest. During the drug history, the client states that she does not use laxatives, and she is not bothered with constipation unless she neglects to eat fibrous foods.

Assessment data	Nursing diagnosis	Intervention	Goals and outcome criteria
Order for bed rest Client statement implying that ample fiber is required if she is to avoid constipation	High risk for constipation related to decreased exercise secondary to enforced inactivity required for treatment of phlebitis	**Discuss** with the client her usual diet; ascertain what fibrous foods she is accustomed to eating. **Inform** the client that a diet ample in fiber will be ordered for her; advise her to specify fibrous foods when marking her menu. **Advise** the client to consume ample fluids to avoid dehydration that can contribute to constipation. **Contact** the physician and request an order for a bulk laxative. **Ascertain** from the client her usual routine for defecation; ensure that she has time and privacy to defecate at the usual time in order to maintain this pattern.	The client will produce at least one stool daily. Stools will be soft in consistency. The client will state that defecation is not uncomfortable.
Diagnosis of phlebitis (involving a clot in a vein in the leg) Risk of constipation (Movement of a clot in the leg may be caused by the pronounced negative intra-abdominal pressure that develops at the end of a Valsalva maneuver.)	High risk for altered tissue perfusion: pulmonary embolism related to thrombosis secondary to phlebitis; contributing factor, Valsalva maneuver during attempt to defecate	**Take measures** to prevent constipation as outlined previously. **Warn** the client not to strain during defecation (or for any other reasons). **Advise** the client to notify the nursing staff immediately if chest pain, respiratory difficulty, or rusty sputum develops.	Pulmonary embolism will not occur; should it occur, it will be detected and treated promptly.

amount, consistency, and frequency of stool should be recorded. Clients should report that defecation is comfortable and that there is no cramping, distention, or pain. (See Example of Nursing Process and Treatment to Prevent Constipation.)

Checklist of nursing actions

☐ Promote fecal elimination by teaching clients to exercise regularly, to include ample fluids, po-

tassium, and bulk in the diet, and to develop a regular routine for defecation.

☐ Identify clients at risk for constipation from pathology or medical regimens; recommend regular use of bulk laxatives or stool softeners to prevent alteration in fecal elimination.

☐ Monitor clients at risk for constipation; recommend a saline or stimulant laxative for temporary relief should constipation develop.

☐ Monitor clients receiving laxatives for adverse reaction to these drugs.

☐ Discourage repeated use of stimulant, saline, or lubricant laxatives.

☐ Avoid inhaling dry bulk laxatives by minimizing their dispersion in the environment.

☐ Monitor clients using mineral oil for deficiency of fat-soluble vitamins.

☐ Warn clients against using aloe as an herbal laxative.

☐ Warn clients not to use laxatives when abdominal pain or other signs and symptoms of appendicitis, intestinal obstruction, or peritonitis are present.

Antidiarrheals

Palliative treatment of diarrhea is sometimes ineffective and unwise. Acute episodes are often self-limiting because the rapid passage of stools eliminates offending irritants from the intestinal tract. In recurrent or chronic conditions, identifying and treating the underlying cause corrects the symptoms. When diarrhea is severe or refractory, restoring and maintaining fluid and electrolyte balance are of primary importance. Antidiarrheals are used primarily as a palliative measure to reduce discomfort.

Pathophysiology

Rapid passage of intestinal contents, which results in frequent, watery stools, may result from parasympathetic overactivity or local irritation of the mucosa of the bowel. These stimuli cause increased secretion and hypermotility of the bowel. The fecal mass, moistened and lubricated by large amounts of mucus, is rapidly propelled from the tract through the anus. Increased peristalsis in the large bowel is reflected in the small intestine, and chyme is carried prematurely into the colon, shortly to be eliminated by succeeding waves of peristalsis. Because absorption of nutrients, bile, and digestive enzymes is not allowed to proceed to completion, dehydration, electrolyte depletion, and nutritional deficits may develop. The stool may be green in color due to the presence of undigested bile; its odor is abnormal and may be foul. The stool, which may contain active digestive enzymes, is irritating to perianal tissues, and can cause maceration. The affected client experiences weakness, griping, abdominal pain, and anal soreness. Weight loss with diarrhea is primarily caused by dehydration, although some lean body mass and fat may be broken down if caloric intake is inadequate.

In severe diarrhea, the primary objective of treatment is to restore and maintain fluid and electrolyte balance. Imbalances can be severe and life-threatening. Fluids are given by mouth when possible but parenteral administration may be necessary. If diarrhea is caused by a chemical irritant or minor infection, these measures may be all the treatment that is needed. The rapid expulsion of intestinal contents tends to eliminate the offending substances from the tract, and the natural defenses of the body complete the recuperative process. In other instances, the underlying cause must be identified and corrected.

Causes of diarrhea

Many factors are associated with diarrhea (Table 31-2). Excessive PNS activity can occur when cholinergic drugs are used, in hyperthyroidism, during withdrawal in narcotic addiction, and as a response to stress in susceptible persons. Parasympathetic nervous system stimulation is probably the mechanism whereby emotions contribute to the incidence and severity of diarrhea. Some people respond to stress by autonomic stimulation characterized by a preponderance of PNS over sympathetic nervous system activity.

Colonic irritation may be caused by mechanical or chemical factors. Mechanical irritants are mainly poorly masticated foods containing fibers and seeds. These are particularly troublesome in diverticulosis. Impacted feces and bowel tumors can also stimulate hypersecretion or hypermotility of the bowel.

Chemical irritants include bacterial toxins, drugs, poisons, stimulant laxatives, and toxic components of foods. Salmonellosis, cholera, and amoebic dysentery are some infectious causes of diarrhea. These illnesses may be transmitted by personal contact, in food, or in water. They are associated with substandard sanitation.

Diarrhea is an adverse reaction to many drugs. Antibiotics alter the microbial flora and environment and predispose to intestinal superinfections. Broad-spectrum antibiotics are particular offenders. Barbiturates, especially in large doses, also stimulate peristalsis. In some cases, suicide attempts with barbiturates have failed because the large doses ingested precipitated prompt evacuation of the drug in diarrheal stools. The body reacts to many drugs and poisons with a similar protective catharsis.

Agents used in the treatment of diarrhea

Fluid and electrolyte solutions

As previously mentioned, correcting fluid and electrolyte imbalances is important in treating diarrhea. Solutions are administered orally when possible. Diet is limited to clear fluids to rest the bowel. If the client is unable to ingest a sufficient quantity of fluid to replace losses, or if the imbalance is pronounced, parenteral solutions are administered. Dextrose in water is usually given first to establish optimal renal function. Mixtures of electrolytes in succeeding bottles replace body deficits; excess are excreted by the kidney. Additional potassium may be ordered because losses of this elec-

Table 31-2. Common causative factors in diarrhea

Mechanism involved	Examples	Corrective measures
Excessive parasympathetic activity	Use of cholinergic drugs Narcotic withdrawal Stress-induced diarrhea Hyperthyroidism	Anticholinergic agents may be used for treatment.
Mechanical irritation	Poorly masticated foods containing fiber and seeds Bowel tumors Fecal impactions	Removal of the source of irritation is necessary for definitive treatment.
Chemical irritation	Bacterial toxins (echovirus, coxsackievirus, *Escherichia coli,* salmonella species, shigella species, *E. histolytica, Giardia lamblia,* and so on)	Some conditions are self-limiting and will resolve with supportive treatment designed to maintain fluid and electrolyte balance.
	Superinfection secondary to use of broad-spectrum antibiotics	An antimycotic or other anti-infective may be needed to treat the superinfection, or the antibiotic prescription may need to be changed.
	Reaction to drugs (iron supplements, antacids, colchicine)	A change in the drug order may resolve the problem.
Increased osmotic pressure in the intestinal lumen	Malabsorption syndrome Excessive intake of salt or sugar	Definitive treatment of the underlying syndrome or a change in diet is needed.
Inflammation of the bowel	Ulcerative colitis Crohn's disease	Definitive treatment of the underlying condition is required.
Laxative abuse	Regular use of laxatives with inability to defecate without laxatives	Reeducation and assistance in establishing regular bowel habits are needed.

trolyte tend to be severe. (Parenteral fluids are discussed in Chapter 51.) Bicarbonate is often required to correct acidosis. Common antidiarrheal medications are reviewed in Table 31-3.

Lactobacillus acidophilus

Lactobacillus acidophilus (Bacid) is an acid-producing bacterium prepared in a concentrated, dried, and viable culture for oral administration.

Pharmacodynamics. *Lactobacillus acidophilus* helps to restore the normal flora of the GI tract by inoculating the tract with a fresh culture of viable organisms. The acid produced by this bacterial growth creates an environment favorable to beneficial flora and unfavorable to potentially pathogenic fungi and bacteria that can cause diarrhea.

Therapeutic uses. *Lactobacillus acidophilus* is used to treat diarrhea arising from the modification of intestinal flora by antibiotics. It has also been used to treat infectious diarrhea, ulcerative colitis, irritable colon, diverticulitis, colostomies, functional constipation, mucous or spastic diarrhea, and diarrhea following amebiasis.

Adverse reactions. When treatment is initiated, intestinal flatus may increase temporarily.

Precautions and contraindications. *Lactobacillus acidophilus* is not recommended for infants and children under 3 years of age, unless treatment is ordered and supervised by a physician. It is contraindicated for those who are sensitive to, or intolerant of, milk products (*ie,* lactose-deficient persons).

Anticholinergics

Drugs that reduce PNS activity alleviate intestinal hypermotility and hypersecretion. They are rarely used alone in treating diarrhea but may be used as adjuncts in combination with adsorbents. Anticholinergics are particularly effective in relieving griping and tenesmus because they inhibit smooth muscle spasm. The anticholinergic effects are not confined to the bowel but affect all body systems, producing the side effects characteristic of these drugs. Overuse of anticholinergics causes subsequent constipation, which can be severe. For a detailed discussion of anticholinergics see Chapter 22.

Demulcents and protectives

Certain salts of polyvalent metals are believed to soothe and coat the intestine, thereby reducing irritation and overstimulation. Their effects seem to be limited and their efficacy has not yet been proven. Salts of bismuth, calcium carbonate, and magnesium oxide are commonly employed for this purpose. They are included as ingredients in over-the-counter remedies such as Pepto-Bismol.

Table 31-3. Antidiarrheal medications

Drug name	Preparations	Usual dosage	Additional information
Demulcents and Protectives			
Salts of bismuth, calcium, or magnesium oxide (Pepto-Bismol)	Over-the-counter remedies that "coat" the intestines	As recommended on package labels PC: C (D in the third trimester)	Efficacy of these preparations is unproven. Avoid taking aspirin with bismuth subsalicylate.
Adsorbents			
Charcoal	Tablets for oral use	600 mg–5 g PRN PC: C	Burned toast remains a traditional preparation used for "indigestion."
Kaolin } ingredients in over-the-counter preparation Pectin } (Donnagel-MB, Kaodene, K-C, Kaopectate, Kaopectolin, K-P)	Liquid for oral use	15–30 ml of kaolin with pectin (an official mixture) after each unformed stool PC: C	Kaopectate is contraindicated in the presence of fever.
Astringents			
Tea Berries Berry wines	Foods	Dosage is adjusted in accordance with response	Astringent foods are commonly used as folk remedies to treat diarrhea.
Opiates			
Diphenoxin (Motofen)	With atropine, oral tablets	Adults: 2 tablets initially; then 1 tablet q3–4h as needed up to 8 tablets in 24 hrs PC: C	Avoid giving diphenoxin with MAO inhibitors to avoid serious hypertension. Use with caution in hepatic disease.
Diphenoxylate (Lofene, Logen, Lomenate, Lomotil, Lonox, Lo-trol)	With atropine, oral tablets, and solution	Adults: 2 tablets (containing 5 mg of diphenoxylate tid–qid Children: 2–5 yr of age: 2 mg, tid; 5–8 yr of age: 2 mg, qid; 8–12 yr of age: 2 mg, up to 5 times daily PC: C	Diphenoxylate is frequently used to treat "traveler's diarrhea." This drug can trigger pancreatitis owing to spasm of the sphincter of Oddi.
Loperamide hydrochloride (Imodium)	Oral capsules	Adults: *Initially:* 4 mg; *thereafter:* 2 mg after each unformed stool (maximum daily dosage: 16 mg) Children: 0.08–0.24 mg/kg body weight/day, divided in 2–3 doses PC: B	Loperamide acts directly on the nerve endings or intramural ganglia of the intestinal wall; it may also increase segmentation and retard forward motion through the intestine by enhancing contractions of intestinal circular musculature.
Opium			
Camphorated tincture of opium (Paregoric)	Oral liquid	Adults: 5–19 ml 1–4 times daily Children: 0.25–9.5 ml/kg body weight 1–4 times daily B (D for prolonged use or use of high doses at term)	Camphorated tincture of opium is subject to Schedule III controls under the Federal Controlled Substance Act of 1970.
Tincture of opium (Laudanum, Deodorized Opium Tincture)	Oral liquid	Adults: 0.3–1 ml 1–4 times daily Children: Dilute tincture of opium 1:25 and give 0.2–0.7 ml, depending on weight B (D for prolonged use or use of high doses at term)	Tincture of opium is subject to Schedule II controls under the Federal Controlled Substance Act of 1970.
Inoculants			
Lactobacillus acidophilus (Bacid, Intestinex, Lactinex)	Oral capsules, granules, and tablets	Adults: 2 capsules, 4 tablets, or 1 pkt of granules, tid–qid	*Lactobacillus acidophilus* may be administered with food or fluids. Fermented milk products and buttermilk also contain *L. acidophilus.*

KEY: PC = pregnancy risk category. (The validity of pregnancy risk categories has not been established. See Chapter 16, p 216.)

Adsorbents

Adsorbent antidiarrheals include charcoal, chalk, kaolin, and pectin.

Pharmacodynamics. Adsorbents attract and hold other chemicals on the surface of their molecules. Their value in diarrhea is attributed to the immobilization and removal of toxins and irritants. Their actions are general rather than specific.

Pharmacokinetics. Adsorbent antidiarrheals appear not to be absorbed systemically in significant amounts.

Therapeutic uses. They are used to alleviate the symptoms of acute, short-term episodes of diarrhea.

Adverse reactions. Adsorbents affect beneficial substances, as well as harmful ones. They inhibit intestinal absorption of water, electrolytes, nutrients, and drugs (preventing even local action by the latter). Kaolin and pectin may cause constipation, especially if fever, which can cause dehydration, is present.

Precautions and contraindications. Kaolin and pectin preparations should not be used when fever is present. They should not be used in young children (under the age of 3 years) and debilitated, geriatric clients without the supervision of health care professionals. When self-administered, adsorbents should not be used for longer than 48 hours before seeking the advice of a health care professional.

Astringents

Astringents used for the control of diarrhea include many folk remedies and some beverages recommended by physicians.

Pharmacodynamics. Astringents are believed to reduce diarrhea by inhibiting secretion and forming a protective layer on the mucous membrane surface through the precipitation of protein in the tissues. The latter mechanism is not yet scientifically substantiated.

Pharmacokinetics. Astringent foods include tea, blueberries, blackberries, and elderberries. They are absorbed by the GI tract and metabolized as nutrients. The potassium they provide helps replace the losses that occur with excessive depletion of lower digestive tract contents. Elderberry wine and blackberry cordial, prized as diarrhea remedies, also provide alcohol, whose tranquilizing properties may help relieve the subjective distress caused by the ailment. The alcohol is absorbed in the upper digestive tract and does not reach the colon.

Therapeutic uses. Preparations made from berries are longstanding folk remedies used to treat diarrhea. Tea is also a traditional remedy. It is sometimes prescribed by physicians for use in self-limiting acute diarrhea, even in children.

Adverse reactions. Excessive use of astringents can cause constipation. Xanthines in tea can provoke restlessness or insomnia in inexperienced users, such as children. The alcoholic content of wines and cordials can also cause toxicity if consumed in appreciable quantities. (See Chapter 24 for adverse reactions to alcohol.)

Precautions and contraindications. Astringent preparations should be sipped or taken in small amounts at frequent intervals. As diarrhea subsides, the amount taken should be reduced gradually until the medication can be discontinued.

Opiates

Opium is a well known antidiarrheal. Constipation is a side effect of all narcotic analgesics.

Pharmacodynamics. Opium depresses the nervous system, thereby slowing the propulsive movement of the small and large intestines.

Pharmacokinetics. Opium preparations taken for the relief of diarrhea are absorbed, metabolized, and excreted, as are all opioid drugs (see Chapter 24).

Therapeutic uses. Opiates are used for the relief and prevention of acute diarrhea caused by chronic conditions such as diverticulosis or diverticulitis.

Adverse reactions. In addition to the usual adverse reactions caused by opioid drugs, antidiarrheal preparations can slow the passage and excretion of toxins from the digestive tract.

Precautions and contraindications. Opiates should not be used in infectious diarrhea or other conditions associated with the presence of toxins in the digestive tract because they slow the excretion of these irritants and prolong the pathologic condition.

The usual precautions and contraindications for opioid drugs apply to the preparations used to treat diarrhea. As narcotics, all are subject to the Controlled Substances Act.

■ **Summary**

A limited number of drug agents are available to treat diarrhea. Whenever possible, the underlying cause of the symptom should be eliminated. During acute nonfebrile episodes, an absorbent, such as Kaopectate (a combination of kaolin and pectin), is often effective. Lomotil, which combines an anticholinergic and opioid, is frequently prescribed for traveler's diarrhea and chronic diarrhea in the elderly. Overuse of astringent foods, which are common folk remedies for diarrhea, can cause subsequent constipation.

Nursing management

Nursing implications

It may be unwise to suppress diarrhea until the cause is identified because purging is a physiologic defense mechanism of the body. Once the underlying problem is identified, it can be decided how safe it is to suppress the diarrhea by palliative agents. For this reason, the cause of the bowel disorder should be determined as soon as possible and definitive treatment begun to correct it.

Treatment often involves the use of drugs. Antibiotics are corrective in many enteric infections. The judicious use of cathartics to remove impactions or to purge the gut of chemical toxins may eliminate the sources of irritation. These drugs are discussed elsewhere in this chapter and text.

Nursing process

Assessment   Assessment of the client who presents with diarrhea requires a careful history and physical examination. The nature and timing of symptoms must be thoroughly explored. Data to be collected include the time of onset, duration, frequency, periodicity, quality, severity, location, and radiation of symptoms. The nature, volume, and frequency of stools must be delineated and the presence of blood, mucus, and fiber noted.

Associated symptoms, such as fever, chills, cramping, pain, nausea, vomiting, and malaise, are clues to the nature of the underlying problem. Associated events (dietary changes, travel, wilderness outings) and exposure to animals, inadequate sanitation, or people with similar symptoms help to clarify the etiology.

During the physical examination, a careful evaluation of the client's fluid, electrolyte, and nutritional status must be made. Although fever develops in dehydration, it often suggests infection as well. Hyperpnea suggests acidosis; tachycardia suggests hypovolemia. A complete examination of the abdomen is particularly important. Excessive bowel sounds, tenderness, and hypermotility may be readily apparent. A palpable mass in the transverse or descending colon suggests a high fecal impaction or intestinal tumor.

Clients receiving broad-spectrum antibiotics are at risk for developing diarrhea secondary to overgrowth of opportunistic organisms such as fungi.

Nursing diagnosis   Diagnoses related to diarrhea include the following:

> *Diarrhea related to intestinal irritation or inflammation secondary to intestinal infection or to ingestion of laxative foods (food allergens, laxative medicines)*
> *High risk for fluid volume deficit related to increased fluid loss in stools secondary to diarrhea*
> *Altered comfort: cramping, abdominal pain, fatigue, and weakness related to intestinal irritation and diarrhea*
> *High risk for altered body temperature: fever related to dehydration secondary to diarrhea*

Common collaborative problems that should be differentiated from the nursing diagnoses include

> *Potential complication: hypokalemia*
> *Potential complication: metabolic acidosis*

Treatment by antidiarrheal medications can lead to diagnoses such as the following:

> *Constipation related to parasympathetic inhibition secondary to anticholinergic antidiarrheal medication*
> *Altered comfort: flatulence related to increased intestinal fermentation secondary to administration of* Lactobacillus acidophilus
> *Impaired tissue integrity: excoriation of perianal tissues related to irritation by diarrheal stool*
> *High risk for injury related to CNS depression secondary to ingestion of antidiarrheal medication containing alcohol*

Planning   The first priority in treating diarrhea is to prevent or promptly correct fluid and electrolyte imbalances. Such complications are the most serious threat to the client's life and well-being. Achieving this goal allows the body's recuperative power to eliminate the cause of diarrhea in many instances. The underlying cause must be treated if it is not a self-limiting condition.

Other goals include increased client comfort by reducing cramping and preventing anal excoriation. Stools must be reduced in number and in fluid content. If the condition is severe or chronic, it is important to promote nutrition and to conserve the client's strength.

Adverse reactions to antidiarrheal medication should be promptly detected and treated.

Intervention   Fluids and electrolytes administered orally can be life-saving. These may be prepared by dissolving Gastrolyte (a commercial preparation containing salts) as directed. Ready to use oral electrolyte maintenance solutions include Pedialyte, Rapolyte, and Rehydralyte. Parenteral fluids are administered when oral fluids are not tolerated, or when rapid correction of fluid and electrolyte imbalance is required. (Parenteral fluids are discussed in Chapter 51.)

Diet should be limited to clear liquids. Tea, Jell-O water, cola drinks, and Gatorade help replenish fluids and electrolytes without further irritating the GI tract.

A glucose and electrolyte solution (prepared by dissolving 3.5 g of sodium chloride, 2.5 g of sodium bicarbonate, 1.5 g of potassium chloride, and 20 g of glucose in sufficient water to make 1 liter of solution) may be offered in unlimited quantities. Artificial sweeteners, some of which are irritating to the colon, should be avoided.

Clients at risk for diarrhea caused by overgrowth of microorganisms may be given foods containing *Lactobacillus acidophilus* (buttermilk, yogurt, cottage cheese). To maintain a relatively normal intestinal flora, these foods should be taken tid to qid at times at least 1 hour after and 2 hours before oral antibiotic medication. The client with acute diarrhea should be encouraged to rest. Narcotic analgesics may be ordered for sedation and for their antidiarrheal effect.

As the client responds to treatment, the diet may be advanced to solids with the omission of milk products. Because diarrhea temporarily depletes the GI disaccharidases required for the digestion of lactose, milk should be avoided for a few days. When it is again tolerated, yogurt or buttermilk helps restore normal intestinal flora.

Progression of ambulation depends on the client's strength and the degree to which activity stimulates intestinal motility. Activity may be allowed in the absence of fatigue, dizziness, or increased diarrhea. Antidiarrheal drugs are usually given orally. Lomotil may be administered at specific hours but adsorbents and paregoric are often ordered after each stool. A maximum dose per day should be established to avoid overmedication, a frequent cause of subsequent constipation.

To avoid excoriation, the perianal area should be cleansed carefully after each evacuation. An emollient barrier such as white petrolatum or A and D Ointment may be applied. Prevention of skin breakdown is especially important in clients who are debilitated, immobile, or incontinent.

Antidiarrheal medications should be decreased in accordance with the client's improvement. They should be discontinued altogether when stools become soft and the daily frequency of stools drops to two.

Client education. Mild or temporary diarrhea is not uncommon. It is often amenable to simple home treatment. Rest and a clear liquid diet are usually effective. A physician should be consulted, however, if severe fluid losses develop or the client cannot take fluids orally. Dizziness and weakness are danger signs. If the loose stools persist beyond 24–48 hours (depending on severity), medical attention is also required. These recommendations apply to adults only. Infants and small children can quickly become seriously ill, developing fluid and electrolyte imbalances, and should always be seen by a physician very early in the illness.

A tendency toward chronic diarrhea can be reduced by eliminating gas-forming foods, such as cabbage and beans, from the diet. Milk products should be eliminated for a trial period if lactase deficiency (common in blacks) is suspected. Artificial sweeteners, laxative foods, and laxative drugs should be avoided. Assistance in reducing or managing stress is helpful to some clients. If the condition fails to respond, a diagnostic workup to determine the cause is indicated.

Clients planning trips abroad to countries where diarrhea is endemic may be advised to take with them bismuth subsalicylate (Pepto-Bismol). This may be taken in dosages of 60 ml (or four tablets) qid to control diarrhea. Prolonged use (longer than 3 weeks) can cause CNS toxicity.

Evaluation Fluid balance must be closely monitored. An accurate record of intake should be kept. The volume of liquid stools must be measured and included in output totals. The client should be carefully observed for signs and symptoms of dehydration, hyponatremia, hypokalemia, and acidosis. A careful record of number, frequency, and characteristics of stools is essential. If progress is normal, stools will decrease in frequency and become less liquid. Other data required for evaluation include client reports regarding comfort and energy levels, signs and symptoms of nutritional deficiency, and presence or absence of anal excoriation.

Checklist of nursing actions

☐ Carefully assess the client presenting with diarrhea to determine the nature of the underlying condition. Evaluate the presence of weakness, pain, or discomfort, fluid and electrolyte imbalance, malnutrition, perianal skin breakdown, and emotional effect.

☐ Administer solutions to correct fluid and electrolyte imbalances.

☐ Promote rest in the client affected by diarrhea.

☐ During the acute phase of illness, limit diet to clear fluids, progressing to a milk-free full diet as tolerated. Delay the use of milk until the normal intestinal flora are restored.

☐ Clean the perianal area carefully after each defecation; apply emollients to prevent irritation.

☐ Monitor fluid balance, electrolyte balance, and number, frequency, and characteristics of stools in clients affected by diarrhea.

☐ Use antidiarrheal medications in moderation to avoid the development of subsequent constipation.

☐ Advise clients to seek medical attention early in the course of an illness characterized by diarrhea; this is critical in children, who become dehydrated very quickly.

☐ Advise clients about measures to prevent food-related diarrhea.

References

Drug recalls. (1987). *American Journal of Nursing, 87,* 768.

Bibliography

Anderson J, et al. (1988). Cholesterol-lowering effects of psyllium hydrophilic mucilloid for hypercholesterolemic men. *Arch Intern Med, 148,* 292–296 (February).

Clinical practice: A series question. (1990). *Nursing 90, 20(5),* 18 (May).

Dupont HL, Ericsson CD, Johnson PC, Bitsura JA, Dupont MW, Cabada de la FJ. (1987). Prevention of travelers' diarrhea by the tablet formulation of bismuth subsalicylate. *JAMA, 257,* 1347.

Gever LN. (1987). Laxative options. *Nursing 87, 17(12),* 21 (December).

Hussar DA. (1989). Drug update: Difenoxin hydrochloride. *Nursing 89, 19(5),* 47 (May).

Martin R. (1987). Fatal poisoning from sodium phosphate enema. *JAMA, 257,* 2190.

McCormick PA, O'Donoghue D, Brennan N. (1985). Diphenoxylate and pancreatitis (letter). *Lancet, 1,* 752.

Saltzstein R, et al. (1988). Anorectal injuries incident to enema administration: A recurring avoidable problem. *Am J Phys Med Rehabil, 67,* 186–188 (August).

Sommer J. (1986). Suggestions for using mini-enemas. *American Journal of Nursing, 86,* 900.

Drugs affecting the endocrine system

8

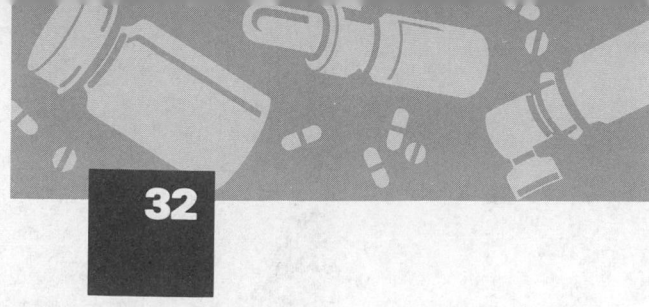

32

Steroid hormones and their antagonists

Nature of hormones

Hormones are glandular secretions produced by organs and tissues that are transported through the bloodstream to other tissues, on which they act (Fig. 32-1). Hormones are chemicals, synthesized within an organism, that alter the rate of cellular processes. Effective in minute amounts, these substances are extremely potent; few body processes are unaffected by them. They profoundly influence such functions as the following:

Digestion

Metabolism

Energy production

Mental processes

Emotions

Sexuality

Reproduction

Growth

Antihormones are substances that reduce the effects of a hormone on an organism. Some hormones themselves act as antihormones, opposing the action of other hormones.

Exactly what constitutes a hormone is subject to considerable interpretation. Chemicals produced by the endocrine glands (*eg*, pituitary, thyroid) are uni-

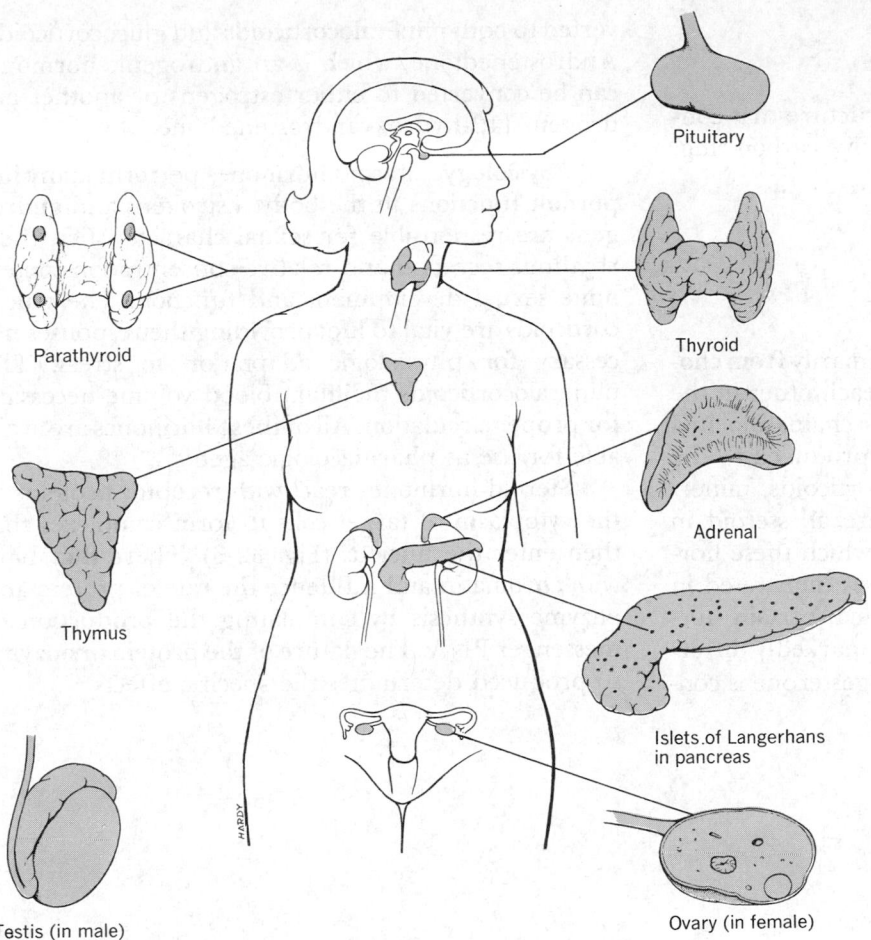

Figure 32-1. General location of the major endocrine glands.

Pituitary

Parathyroid

Thyroid

Thymus

Adrenal

Islets of Langerhans in pancreas

Testis (in male)

Ovary (in female)

versally recognized as hormones. Chemical messengers that control digestion (*eg*, gastrin, cholecystokinin) are gaining recognition as true hormones. Some authorities also include biochemicals such as histamine and serotonin in this category. The following discussion focuses on the hormones secreted by the endocrine glands.

As with most drugs, the effects of hormones depend on molecular structure. Certain subunits or molecular structures of these chemicals are associated with specific actions. Each hormone or family of hormones exerts multiple effects on the body. They act on a number of sites, affecting organized structures such as organs, tissues, or organelles. These actions are related, converging to produce an overall effect that enables the organism to carry out a physiologic function or adapt to a particular environmental or biochemical circumstance.

Hormones used as drugs are produced from animal extracts, plant materials, or fermentation processes. They are simple extracts or semisynthetic chemicals derived from substances that are chemically related to the hormone. Because most animal hormones differ chemically somewhat from their human counterparts, they often function as antigens. In gene replication processes that have been developed, microorganisms are induced to manufacture hormones identical to those produced in the human body, with reduced antigenic potential. Such techniques should also increase the production of scarce hormones.

The chemical nature of hormones is variable, but most are either steroids or glycoproteins. Molecules vary in size, ranging from the small double tyrosine molecule of triiodothyronine to macromolecules such as growth hormone, which has a molecular weight of 21,500. Some hormones are effective when taken orally (most steroids and thyroid hormone), but others (proteins) are destroyed by the digestive enzymes and must be administered parenterally.

Hormone drugs are administered to people with endocrine deficiency diseases to replace missing or insufficient biochemicals. They are also employed as drugs to manipulate the metabolism in a way that is beneficial to the recipient. For replacement therapy, the full range of action is required, and true hormones are often used. When used as drugs, a single effect is often desired, with other actions undesirable. Dissociation of multiple effects and the development of modified chemicals with single actions are goals of much pharmacologic research that involves hormones.

Steroid hormones

The steroid nucleus

Steroid hormones share a central structure that contains three six-carbon rings and one five-carbon ring.

Steroid hormones are derived primarily from cholesterol in the body, differing from each other in the number and nature of side-groups or chains attached to the various rings. The hormones produced by the adrenal cortex and gonads—glucocorticoids, mineralocorticoids, and sex hormones—are all steroid in nature. The metabolic pathways by which these hormones are synthesized in the body are illustrated in Figure 32-2. As shown in this schema, certain hormones are precursors of others with markedly differing characteristics. For example, progesterone is con-

verted to both mineralocorticoids and glucocorticoids. Androstenedione, which is an androgenic hormone, can be converted to either estrogens or another androgen, 11β-hydroxyandrostenedione.

Physiology. Steroid hormones perform many important functions in the body. Estrogens and androgens are responsible for sexual characteristics; their rhythmic secretion and relative concentrations determine sexual development and function. The glucocorticoids are vital to life, providing the responses necessary for physiologic adaptation to stress. The mineralocorticoids maintain blood volume necessary for proper circulation. All of these hormones are available for use as pharmacologic agents.

Steroid hormones react with receptor proteins in the cytoplasm of target cells to form complexes that then enter the nucleus (Fig. 32-3). There they bind with chromatin and influence the rate of protein and enzyme synthesis by stimulating the production of messenger RNA. The nature of the protein or enzyme so produced determines the specific effects.

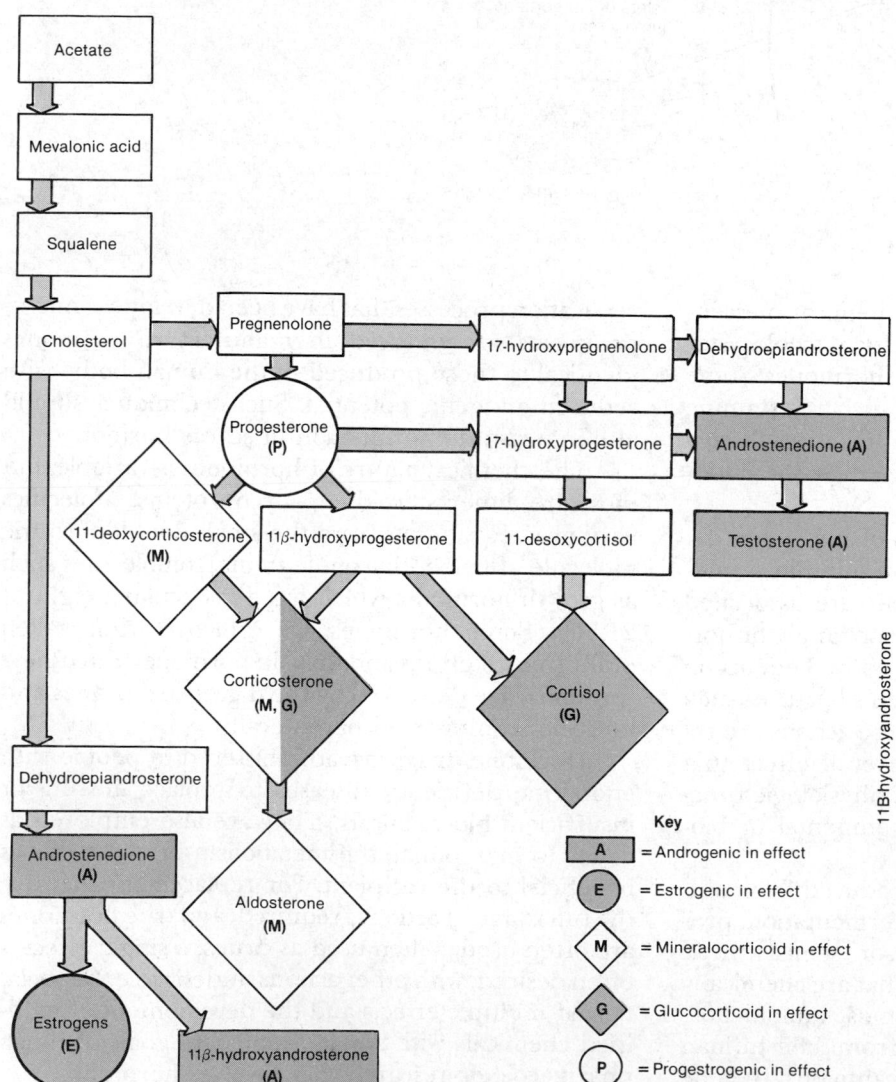

Figure 32-2. Metabolic pathways for steroid hormone synthesis.

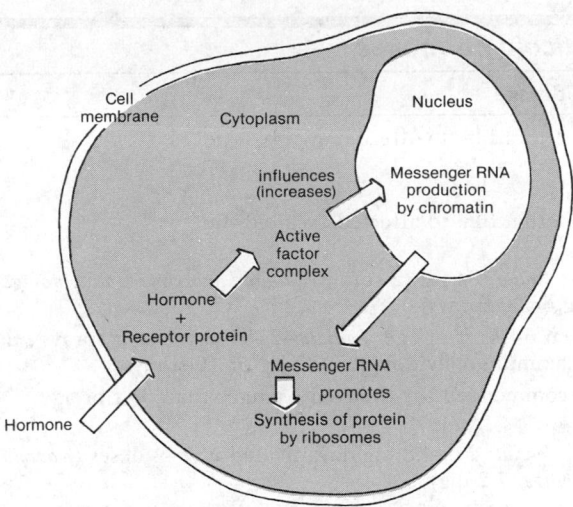

Figure 32-3. The mechanism of action of steroid hormones involves effects in cell nuclei.

For the most part, steroids are degraded by the liver and are subsequently excreted in urine. Body levels may be measured by either blood or urinary assay.

Corticosteroids

The cortex of the adrenal glands produces several steroid hormones: mineralocorticoids, glucocorticoids, and sex hormones. The term *corticosteroid* is employed to designate mineralocorticoids and glucocorticoids. Although people of both sexes produce both male and female sex hormones in the adrenals, the amounts are usually insignificant compared to the hormones secreted by the gonads. Mineralocorticoids and glucocorticoids share many functions, but the former exert greater effects on fluid and electrolyte balance, whereas the latter are characterized by widespread effects on body metabolism and immune response with less pronounced effects on fluids and electrolytes.

The two main naturally occurring mineralocorticoids, desoxycorticosterone and aldosterone, act on the renal tubule to promote sodium reabsorption and potassium and hydrogen excretion. Water reabsorption increases secondary to sodium retention. As a result, blood volume and blood pressure are maintained at levels adequate for circulatory perfusion.

Production of the mineralocorticoid hormones by the zona glomerulosa of the adrenals is independent of that of the other cortical steroids. Factors that affect mineralocorticoid secretion include potassium ion concentration in the extracellular fluid, volume of extracellular fluid, and sodium concentration in the extracellular fluid. Hormone secretion is stimulated by high potassium concentration, low blood volumes, and low sodium concentration.

Glucocorticoids significantly alter energy nutrient metabolism so as to maintain or increase the blood sugar level. This action is believed to maintain brain and other vital functions during periods of stress when increased energy is required by the organism. Other effects of these chemicals contribute to resistance to stress by stimulating the central nervous system (CNS) and skeletal muscles, inhibiting inflammation, and increasing coagulability of the blood. Their enhancement of sodium and water retention provides additional blood volume. The glucocorticoids also suppress immune responses and inhibit growth.

Pathology. Primary deficiency of adrenal corticosteroids (Addison's disease) involves inadequate production of both glucocorticoids and mineralocorticoids. This disease is caused by progressive destruction of the adrenal cortex due to infection or hemorrhage. Diagnosis during the early stages of the disease is difficult because hormone levels are maintained at levels close to normal until more than 90% of the gland is involved.

Addison's disease is characterized by general debility, hypovolemia, a weak heart action, gastrointestinal irritability, and a bronzing discoloration of the skin. All of these signs and symptoms except the skin pigmentation are caused by depletion of sodium and water and potassium excess. The skin changes are due to excesses of pituitary corticotropin that stimulate melanin deposition in the tissues.

Salt-losing adrenogenital syndrome is a congenital condition characterized by an inherited enzymatic interference with the synthesis of glucocorticoids and mineralocorticoids. When body levels of these corticosteroids are low, the pituitary is stimulated to produce large amounts of corticotropin. Although the adrenals are incapable of increasing glucocorticoid or mineralocorticoid production, they do respond to corticotropin by increasing production of adrenal androgens, causing abnormally high testosterone levels and masculinization.

Inability to produce adequate glucocorticoids in response to stress is life-threatening. Inadequate secretion of these stress hormones makes an organism vulnerable to cardiovascular collapse when exposed to sudden or severe stress. Deficient adrenal function is a characteristic of the exhaustion stage of stress response.

Glucocorticoids

Drug preparations. A large number of synthetic glucocorticoids are available for therapeutic use (Table 32-1). Some of these exhibit a degree of differentiation of effect. For example, equivalent doses of hydrocortisone and dexamethasone differ markedly in their sodium-retaining potency (Table 32-2). Glucocorti-

(Text continues on p. 727)

Table 32-1. Drug preparations that contain glucocorticoid hormones

Drug name	Preparations	Usual dosage
alclometasone dipropionate (Aclovate, Glaxo)	Topical cream and ointment (0.05%)	Apply a thin film to affected area bid–tid. PC: C
amcinonide (Cyclocort; *Can:* Mycoderm)	Topical cream and ointment	Apply a thin film to affected area bid–tid. PC: C
beclomethasone dipropionate (Beclovent, Propaderm, Vanceril; *Can:* Beclavert, Beconese)	Oral aerosol inhaler	Adults: *Initial:* 84 µg (2 sprays) tid–qid (*maximum daily dosage:* 840 µg or 20 sprays)
		Children 6–12 yr of age: *Initial:* 42–84 µg (1 or 2 sprays), tid–qid (maximum daily dosage: 420 µg or 10 sprays)
		Not recommended for children younger than 6 yr of age PC: C
betamethasone (Celestone)	Oral tablets and solution (0.6 mg/5 ml)	Adults: *Initial:* 2.4–4.8 mg/day, divided in 2–4 doses (*maximum daily dosage:* 7.2 mg)
	Solutions and suspension for injection	Children: 0.0175–0.25 mg/kg body weight or 0.5–7.5 mg/m^2 body surface, divided in 3–4 doses
		IM: 0.5–9 mg or more/day (varying with the condition being treated) PC: C
betamethasone benzoate (Baben, Uticort)	Topical cream, gel, lotion, and ointment (0.025%)	Apply sparingly and rub gently into affected area once daily to qid. PC: C
betamethasone dipropionate (Alphatrex, Diprolene, Diprosone; *Can:* Diprosalic)	Topical cream, lotion, and ointment (0.05%)	Apply sparingly and rub gently into affected area once daily to qid.
	Topical aerosol spray	Maximum weekly dosage: 45 g; *maximum course of treatment:* 14 days
		Spray an area the size of the client's hand not more than 3 sec from a distance of 15 cm tid–qid. PC: C
betamethasone valerate (Betatrex, Beta-Val, Betacort, Valisone; *Can:* Celstoderm)	Topical lotion, cream, and ointment (0.1%)	Apply sparingly and rub gently into affected area once daily to qid. PC: C
(Valisone Reduced Strength)	Topical lotion (0.01%)	Apply sparingly and rub gently into affected area once daily to qid.
clobetasol (Temovate; *Can:* Dermovate)	Topical cream and ointment (0.05%)	Apply sparingly and rub gently into affected area bid. PC: C
clocortolone (Cloderm)	Topical cream (0.1%)	Apply sparingly and rub gently into affected area once daily–qid. PC: C
cortisone (Cortelan, Cortistab, Cortoderm, Cortogen; *Can:* Cortone)	Powder and solution Oral tablets Suspension for IM injection	Dosage varies with the condition being treated and the response of the client; high doses are given initially, then decreased to the lowest effective maintenance dose. Daily dosage may be divided in 1–2 doses.
		Adults: *Initial:* Oral: 25–300 mg/day; *IM:* 20–300 mg/day
		Children: *Initial:* Oral: 0.7–10 mg/kg body weight/day or 20–300 mg/m^2 body surface/day; *IM:* 0.2–1.25 mg/kg body weight/day or 7–37.5 mg/m^2 body surface/day PC: D
desonide (DesOwen, Tridesilon)	Topical cream and ointment (0.05%–0.25%)	Apply sparingly and rub gently into affected area bid–qid. PC: C
desoximetasone (Esperson, Ibaril, Topicort-LP, Topicort, Topisolon)	Topical cream, gel and ointment (0.05%–0.25%)	Apply sparingly and rub gently into affected area bid PC: C
dexamethasone (Ak-Dex, Decadron, Deronil, Gammacorten, Hexadrol, Maxidex, Mymethasone, Oradexon)	Oral elixir, tablets, solution and solution concentrate	Adults: 0.75–9 mg daily, divided in 2–4 doses
		Children: 0.024–0.34 mg/kg body weight or 0.66–10 mg/m^2/day, divided in 4 doses PC: C
(Aeroseb-Dex, Decaderm, Decaspray)	Topical aerosol spray (0.01%–0.1%)	Apply sparingly and rub gently into affected area tid–qid

(Continued)

Table 32-1. Drug preparations that contain glucocorticoid hormones (Continued)

Drug name	Preparations	Usual dosage
dexamethasone acetate (Dalalone L.A., Decadron-LA, Decaject-L.A., Decameth L.A., Dexacen LA, Dexasone L.A., Dexon L.A., Dexone L.A., Solurex, L.A.)	Suspension for injection	Adults: *Initial:* 8–16 mg, q1–3 wk Children younger than 12 yr of age: dosage has not been established PC: C
dexamethasone sodium phosphate (Decadron Phosphate Respihaler, Dalalone, Decadrol,	Oral inhaler	Adults: 300 μg (3 inhalations), tid–qid (*maximum daily dosage: 1200 μg or 12 inhalations*) Children: 200 μg (2 inhalations), tid–qid (*maximum daily dosage: 800 μg or 8 inhalations*)
Decadron, Decaject, Decameth, Delladec, Demasone, Dexacen-4, Dexameth, Dexasone,	Solutions for injection	*IM or IV:* Adults: 0.5 mg–24 mg/day; children 6 μg–40 μg/kg body weight or 0.235 mg–1.25 mg/m² body surface, 1–2 times daily
Dexon, Dexone, Dezone, Gammacorten, Hexadrol, Savacort D, Solurex)	Topical cream (0.1%)	Apply sparingly and rub gently into affected area tid–qid PC: C
diflorasone diacetate (Florone, Flutone, Maxiflor)	Topical cream and ointment (0.05%)	Apply sparingly and rub gently into the affected area bid–qid PC: C
fluprednisolone (Alphadrol)	Oral tablets	Adults: *Initial:* 2.5–30 mg/day, divided in 3–4 doses Children: *Replacement:* 0.07 mg/kg body weight or 2 mg/m² body surface/day, divided in 3 doses
flunisolide (Aero-bid, Bromelide, Nasalide, Syntaric; *Can:* Rhinalar)	Aerosol inhalent	Use only twice a day PC: C
fluocinolone (Fluronid, Flurosyn, Synemol, Synalar)	Topical cream, ointment, and solution (0.01%, 0.025%)	Apply sparingly and rub gently into the affected area bid–qid PC: C
fluocinonide (Lidemol, Lyderm, Lidex, Metosyn, Topsyn Gel)	Topical cream, gel, ointment and solution (0.05%)	Apply sparingly and rub gently into the affected area bid–qid PC: C
flurandrenolide (Cordran, Drenison, Drocort, Sermaka)	Topical cream, lotion, and ointment (0.025%–0.05%)	Apply sparingly and rub gently into the affected area bid–tid
	Dressing (4 μg/cm²)	Apply to clean, dry affected area q12h. PC: C
halcinonide (Halog)	Topical cream, ointment, and solution (0.025%–0.1%)	Apply sparingly and rub gently into the affected area bid–tid PC: C
Hydrocortisone (Cortisol)		
hydrocortisone (Bactine, Cetacort, Cortate, Cortef, Cortenema, Cortiment, Cortril, Dermacort, Dermicort, Emo-Cort, Hi-Cort, Hydrotex, Hytone,	Powder, oral tablets, suspension for injection	*Oral:* Adults: *Initial:* 10–320 mg/day, divided in 3–4 doses; children: 0.56–8 mg/kg body weight or 16–240 mg/m² body surface/day, divided in 3–4 doses *IM:* Adults: *Initial:* 15–240 mg/day, divided in 2 doses
	Topical cream, solution, ointment, powder, and lotion	Apply sparingly and rub gently into affected area once daily–qid
Prevex, Proctocort, Synacort, Texacort, Unidort)	Topical aerosol spray	Spray each 10 cm² of affected area for 1–2 sec from a distance of about 15 cm bid–tid
	Rectal suspension (100 mg/60 ml)	Adults: 100 mg nightly administered as a retention enema
	Rectal cream, ointment (0.5%–1.0%)	Apply creams and ointments externally to the anal area
	Powder for suspension	Adults: 40 mg dissolved in 30–180 ml water, administered as a retention enema PC: C
hydrocortisone cypionate (Cortef Fluid)	Oral suspension	Adults: *Initial:* 10–320 mg/day divided in 3–4 doses Children: 0.56–8 mg/kg body weight or 16–240 mg/m² body surface/day, divided in 3–4 doses PC: C

(Continued)

Table 32-1. Drug preparations that contain glucocorticoid hormones (*Continued*)

Drug name	Preparations	Usual dosage
Hydrocortisone acetate (Alocort, Biosone, Cort-Dome, Cortocet, Cortamed, Corticreme, Cortoderm, Fernisone, Hyderm, Lanacort, Orobase, PharmCort, Rectocort, Rhulicort; *Can:* Novohydrocort)	Suspension for injection	For intrasynovial, intrabursal, or intra-articular injection, 5–50 mg, q3–5d (for bursae) or q1–4wk (for joints); dosage varies with degree of inflammation and size and location of affected area PC: C
(Cortifoam)	Rectal aerosol foam suspension (10%)	Adults: 90 mg (1 full applicator) 1–2 times daily PC: C
(Cort-Dome, Corticaine)	Rectal suppositories (10 mg, 25 mg)	Adults: 10–50 mg bid–tid PC: C
(CaldeCORT, Cortaid, Cortef, Gynecort, Lanacort, Orabase, Pharm-Cort, Rhulicort)	Topical cream, lotion, ointment, and paste (0.5%–1%)	Apply sparingly and rub gently into affected area once daily–qid PC: C
(CaldeCORT)	Topical aerosol spray (0.5%)	Spray each 10 cm² of affected area for 1–2 sec from a distance of 15 cm bid–tid PC: C
hydrocortisone sodium phosphate (Hydrocortone Phosphate)	Solution for injection	Adults: *Initial:* 15–240 mg/day, divided in 2 doses Children: 0.16–1 mg/kg body weight or 6–30 mg/m² body surface, 1–2 times daily PC: C
hydrocortisone sodium succinate (A-hydro-Cort, SoluCortef)	Solutions for injection	Adults: 100–500 mg, q2–10h Children: 0.16–1 mg/kg body weight or 6–30 mg/m² body surface, 1–2 times daily PC: C
Methylprednisolone		
methylprednisolone (Metastab, Urbason; *Can:* Medrate)	Oral tablets	Adults: *Initial:* 2–60 mg/day, divided in 4 doses Children: 0.117–1.66 mg/kg body weight or 3.3–50 mg/m² body surface/day, divided in 3–4 doses PC: C
methylprednisolone acetate (Depo-Medrol, Depo-Pred, Duralone, Medrone, Mepred, Pre-Dep, Rep-Pred)	Suspension for IM, intra-articular, intralesional, or soft tissue injection	Adults: 10–80 mg PC: C
(Medrol)	Powder for rectal suspension	40 mg dissolved in 30–180 ml water administered as a retention enema PC: C
(Medrol)	Topical ointment	Apply sparingly and rub gently into affected area once daily–qid PC: C
methylprednisolone sodium succinate (A-methaPred, Solu-Medrol)	Solutions for IM or IV injection	Adults: 10–250 mg (may be repeated up to 6 times daily) Children: 0.03–0.2 mg/kg body weight or 1–6.25 mg/m² body surface, 1–2 times daily PC: C
mometasone furoate (Elocan)	Topical cream and ointment	Apply only once a day.
paramethasone acetate (Alondra, Dilar, Haldrate, Haldrone, Monocortin, Stemex)	Oral tablets	Adults: *Initial:* 2–24 mg/day, divided in 3–4 doses Children: 0.058–0.8 mg/kg body weight or 1.67–25 mg/m² body surface/day, divided in 3–4 doses PC: C
Prednisolone		
prednisolone (Ak-Tate, Balpred, Cortalone, Delta-Cortef, Fernisolone-P, Hydeltra, Inflamase,	Powder Oral tablets	Adults: *Initial:* 5–60 mg/day, divided in 2–4 doses Children: 0.14–2 mg/kg body weight or 4–60 mg/m² body surface/day, divided in 4 doses PC: B

(*Continued*)

Table 32-1. Drug preparations that contain glucocorticoid hormones (Continued)

Drug name	Preparations	Usual dosage
Nova-Pred, Nonoprednisolone, Ophtho-Tate, Paracortol, Predoxine-5, tracortenol)		
prednisolone acetate (Fernisolone, Key-Pred, Meticortelone Acetate, Predcor, Savacort; *Can:* Pred Forte, Pred Mild)	Suspensions for IM, intra-articular, or soft tissue injection	Adults: *Initial:* 4–60 mg/day, divided in 2 doses, administered at 12-hr intervals Children: 0.04–0.25 mg/kg body weight or 1.5–7.5 mg/m^2 body surface/day, 1–2 times daily PC: B
prednisolone sodium phosphate (Hydeltrasol, Key-Pred, Pediapred, Predote, SP, P.S.P. IV, solu-Predalone)	Solution for injection	Adults: *Initial:* 4–60 mg/dose Children: 0.04–0.25 mg/kg body weight or 1.5–7.5 mg/m^2 body surface, 1–2 times daily PC: B
prednisolone tebutate (Hydeltra-T.B.A., Metalone T.B.A., Predcor T.B.A.)	Suspension for intra-articular, intralesional, or soft tissue injection	Adults: 4–40 mg, q2–3wk; dosage varies with the degree of inflammation and the size and location of the affected area PC: B
prednisone (Deltasone, Fernisone, Liquid Pred, Meticorten, Novoprednisone, Orasone, Panasol, Prednicen-M, SK-Prednisone, Sterapred)	Powder Oral tablets and solution	Adults: *Initial:* 5–60 mg/day, divided in 2–4 doses Children: 0.14–2 mg/kg body weight or 4–60 mg/m^2 body surface/day, divided in 4 doses PC: B
Triamcinolone		
triamcinolone (Apo-Triazo, Aristo-Pak, Traderm, Triamacort)	Oral tablets	Adults: *Initial:* 4–48 mg/day, divided in 1–4 doses Children: 0.117–1.66 mg/kg body weight or 3.3–50 mg/m^2 body surface/day, divided in 4 doses PC: C
triamcinolone acetonide (Acetospan, Aristocort, Cenocort, Cinomide, Flutex, Kenaject, Kenalog, Triacet, Triam-A, Triamonike, Trilog, Trymex)	Suspension for IM, intra-articular, intrasynovial, intralesional, sublesional, and soft tissue injection Oral aerosol inhaler Topical aerosol spray Topical cream, lotion, ointment, and paste (0.025%–0.1%)	*IM:* Adults and children older than 12 yr of age: 60 mg q6wk children; 6–12 yr of age: 0.03–0.2 mg/kg body weight or 1–6.25 mg/m^2 body surface q1–7days 200 µg (2 sprays) tid–qid Apply sparingly and rub gently into affected area once daily–qid Apply sparingly and rub gently into affected area once daily–qid PC: C
Triamcinolone diacetate (Amcort, Aristocort, Articulose, Cenocort, cinalone, Cino, Kenacort, Tracilon, Triacort, Triam-Forte, Triamolone, Trilone, Trisoject)	Oral solution Suspension for IM, intra-articular, intrasynovial, intralesional, sublesional, and soft tissue injection	Adults: *Initial:* 4–48 mg/day, divided in 1–4 doses Children: 0.117–1.66 mg/kg body weight or 3.3–50 mg/m^2 body surface/day, divided in 4 doses PC: C
Triamcinolone hexacetonide (Aristospan)	Suspension for intra-articular, intralesional, or sublesional injection	*Intralesional:* up to 0.5 mg/square inch of affected skin *Intra-articular:* 2–20 mg/q3–4wk; dosage varies with size of affected area PC: C

KEY: PC = pregnancy category. (The validity of pregnancy risk categories has not been established; see Chapter 16, p 216.)
Can = Canadian trade name.

coid drugs are available for oral, parenteral, or topical administration. The drugs are absorbed by all routes. Aerosol and parenteral administration can produce rapid increases in blood levels. The oral route is preferred for systemic effect when it can be used. Topical use always results in some systemic absorption and may produce systemic side effects. Whereas most gluco-corticoid medications are limited to prescription use, some ointments and creams that contain these drugs are presently available for over-the-counter purchase.

Pharmacodynamics. Glucocorticoids function within the cell to influence protein production as described earlier (see Physiology). They have the poten-

Table 32-2. Comparison of relative effects of selected glucocorticoids

Drug name	Relative anti-inflammatory potency	Relative sodium retaining potency
Cortisol (hydrocortisone)	1	1
Cortisone	0.8	0.8
Betamethasone	25	0
Dexamethason	25	0
Prednisone	4	0.8
Prednisolone	4	<1
Triamcinolone	5	0

(Gilman AG, Goodman LS, Rall TW, Murad F. [1985]. *Goodman and Gilman's The pharmacological basis of therapeutics*, 7th ed, p 1466. New York: Macmillan.)

tial to produce the full range of hormone effects, including a rise in blood sugar, sodium and water retention, increased potassium excretion, immunosuppression, CNS stimulation, mood elevation, inhibition of cell division, increased coagulability of blood, suppression of inflammation, and inhibition of corticotropin secretion. A few drug preparations are more specific in that they produce minimal sodium and water retention.

Pharmacokinetics. Glucocorticoids are effective when administered by all routes. They are absorbed through the skin and mucous membranes as well as from the gastrointestinal (GI) tract. After absorption, they are distributed to all tissues through the bloodstream.

Glucocorticoids are degraded by the liver and excreted by the kidneys.

Therapeutic uses

Replacement therapy. The glucocorticoids are used as replacement therapy to maintain appropriate physiologic stress responses in clients with deficient adrenal function. Inability to produce adequate glucocorticoids may stem from destruction of the adrenal cortex, suppression of hormone secretion (often due to a period of therapeutic administration of these hormones), adrenal exhaustion, or a lack of pituitary corticotropin. The amount of hormone needed in any given situation depends on the degree of adrenal hypofunction and the severity of stress to which the client is subject. Relatively large doses are needed to support a victim of acute addisonian crisis. (This form of circulatory shock arises as a result of a sudden inadequacy of the adrenal stress response.) Much lower doses suffice to maintain a deficient client during normal life circumstances, but need to be increased twofold or more on the advent of stress.

If the adrenal cortex malfunction is permanent in nature, drug therapy must be continued indefinitely. Temporary hyposecretion may respond to a course of glucocorticoid therapy to provide a period of rest, followed by gradual reduction of dose to zero. If pituitary corticotropin production has been suppressed by therapeutic use of the glucocorticoids, serious deficiency states can be avoided by gradual withdrawal of the drugs.

Treatment of disease. Because of their broad effects on basic physiologic processes (Table 32-3), the glucocorticoids have been exploited for the treatment of many diseases. Glucocorticoids are capable of alleviating the symptoms of painful, disabling, and potentially lethal illnesses. They are used to treat inflammatory, allergic, and malignant conditions and are adjuncts in the care of clients with recent brain injuries or organ transplants.

Inflammatory diseases that respond to the administration of glucocorticoids include rheumatic conditions, nephrotic syndromes, collagen diseases, vascular and ocular inflammations, toxic shock syndrome, chronic ulcerative colitis, and hepatitis, including acute alcoholic hepatitis. The drugs can be life-saving in acute fulminating and chronic progressive inflammations. They may also prevent or delay serious disability that stems from such conditions (*eg*, meningitis). Although palliative rather than curative in effect for most of these diseases, the glucocorticoids are often the drugs of choice in the absence of better therapeutic approaches. In a few situations, the drugs appear to produce permanent effects. For example, sympathetic ophthalmia, an inflammation of the uveal tract that is triggered by injury to the eye, can be prevented completely by a promptly initiated short course of steroid therapy.

Allergic conditions that respond to the glucocorticoids include contact dermatitis, asthma, serum sickness, drug reactions, and anaphylaxis. The drugs are most valuable for the control of acute severe allergic responses that do not respond to other treatment agents such as epinephrine or the antihistamines. Some of the inflammatory diseases cited in the preceding paragraph may eventually be classified as allergic manifestations because they are suspected of being autoimmune in nature.

Glucocorticoid therapy is used in the treatment of several types of malignant tumors. With certain other antineoplastics, these steroids are considered drugs of choice for the treatment of lymphomas. Their inhibition of cell division is most marked on lymphocytes, and long-lasting remissions may be induced through combination chemotherapy that includes these agents. In an increasing number of clients, remissions appear permanent and are considered by some to be permanent cures. Glucocorticoids are also administered to people with brain metastases to inhibit brain inflammation and edema. Although they are helpful in cer-

Table 32-3. Major physiologic effects of glucocorticoids

Organ system/mechanism of action	End result of prolonged excessive hormone action*
Nutrient metabolism	
Favors the formation of glucose from nutrients that contain calories (increases gluconeogenesis)	Increased blood sugar, diabetes mellitus in susceptible people, increased severity of pre-existing diabetes mellitus
Favors glycogenolysis	
Antagonizes the action of insulin	
Favors the breakdown of protein	Muscle wasting, osteoporosis
Inhibits protein synthesis	
Promotes lipolysis of triglycerides of adipose tissue	Abnormal fat distribution ("buffalo hump," "moon face")
Fluid and electrolytes	
Promotes sodium and water retention	Edema, hypertension, increased intraocular pressure
Favors potassium excretion	Weakness, fatigability
Tissue response to injury and infection	
Suppresses the immune response	Serious infections with few signs and symptoms, post-transplant lymphoma
Suppresses inflammation	
Gastrointestinal tract	
(Mechanisms obscure)	Peptic ulcerations, pancreatitis
Central nervous system	
Stimulates the brain	Insomnia, euphoria, manic psychosis
(Mechanisms obscure)	Blunting of the senses (pain, taste, smell, hearing)
	Dementia that resembles Alzheimer's disease (rare)
Musculature	
Protein depletion	Progressive weakness of the shoulder and pelvic girdles and the muscles of the extremities
Endocrine glands	
Inhibits adrenocorticotropin secretion by the pituitary	Adrenal atrophy (when administered as a drug)
Blood	
Increases red blood cell production	Polycythemia
Increases coagulability	Increased incidence of thrombi and emboli
Cell reproduction	
Inhibits cell division	Growth retardation, dwarfism, poor healing

*Most likely with systemic treatment, but some are seen after topical use (*eg*, eye drops, skin preparations.)

tain other malignancies, their mechanisms of action remain obscure. Glucocorticoids are effective in the treatment of nausea and vomiting secondary to antineoplastic chemotherapy.

Aggressive treatment with methylprednisolone shows promise of limiting nerve damage in spinal cord injuries if it is initiated soon (within 8 hours, or preferably 4 hours) after injury. The steroid is administered in large dosages. It is believed to act by inhibiting the damaging effects of free radicals released by injured cells. These highly reactive oxygen molecules are toxic to membranes of neighboring cells (Bracken, et al, 1990).

People with brain injury (whether traumatic or surgical) often develop serious brain edema. Because of their anti-inflammatory action, glucocorticoids suppress this complication. The drugs are administered routinely during the postoperative or post-trauma period to prevent the symptoms and permanent tissue damage that accompany cerebral edema.

Box 32-1. Therapeutic principles in determining glucocorticoid therapy

- Glucocorticoids should never be used unless the client's condition cannot be controlled by safer standard therapy.
- Each drug preparation has distinctive effects; the proper steroid should be carefully selected by the physician for each client. The appropriate dosage must be titrated for each client.
- The administration of glucocorticoid is palliative therapy, not curative.
- The physician should determine the smallest daily dose that will keep the client comfortable.
- The administration of massive doses of glucocorticoid for brief periods is virtually without harmful effects.
- When glucocorticoids are administered by a step-down dosage regimen (initial large dose and then reduction of dose each day for a week or two), there are rarely harmful effects.
- An individually tailored program may include alternate day therapy or intermittent dosage schedules.
- When therapy is prolonged or the dosage is high, the incidence of potential disabling or lethal effects increases.
- Systemic glucocorticoid toxicity may be lessened by the use of locally acting drugs.
- Abrupt withdrawal of high dosage levels of glucocorticoids can result in acute adrenal insufficiency and may be life-threatening.

Glucocorticoids are employed to suppress the immune response in recipients of organ transplants. Immunosuppression can delay or prevent rejection of these foreign tissues. The drugs are used in combination with other immunosuppressants.

Corticosteroids have also been used to prevent interruption of pregnancy in habitual abortion secondary to lupus erythematosus.

Benefits vs. harmful effects. Whenever glucocorticoid therapy is used for therapeutic purposes other than replacement of deficient hormones, the potential benefits must be weighed against the risk of harmful effects and toxicity. Box 32-1 lists principles that influence the choice for or against chemotherapy in current practice.

Treatment regimens. Choice of drug, route, dosage, and schedule of administration varies with the nature of the condition being treated. Replacement therapy requires a chemical such as hydrocortisone, which exerts all the physiologic effects of the endogenous hormone. The drug is administered so as to mimic the normal diurnal pattern of hormone secretion (Fig. 32-4). Doses are given once or twice a day: on arising and, if needed, about 6 hours later. The basal dose, which is designed to meet the client's needs under normal conditions of stress, must be increased according to the degree of additional stress that is expected. Usually, double doses are taken for mild increases in stress such as a cold or a visit to the dentist. Three or more times the basal dose may be needed to compensate for severe stress. The goal of therapy is to achieve hormone balance without symptoms of either deficiency or excess of the hormones. Drug therapy is continued for life.

Dexamethasone is the preparation of choice for the prevention of cerebral edema. This chemical has a marked anti-inflammatory effect with minimal sodium and water retention. The drug is administered orally several times a day at equally spaced intervals, for example, every 6 hours. A relatively stable blood level is desired to maintain a constant effect. The drug is withdrawn gradually when the danger of cerebral edema is considered to have passed.

Prednisone, an oral glucocorticoid, is commonly used for other conditions that require a systemic drug effect. If a short term of therapy is anticipated, the drug is administered regularly, at frequent intervals, to maintain a constant blood level. When long-term therapy is necessary, large doses are given every other day; this timing significantly reduces the incidence of side effects without seriously impairing therapeutic response. Every-other-day doses should be administered as soon as possible after waking in the morning.

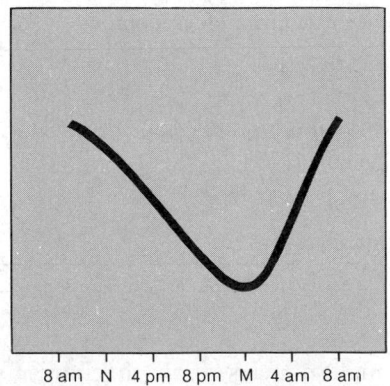

8 am   N   4 pm   8 pm   M   4 am   8 am

Figure 32-4. Spontaneous diurnal variation in 17-hydroxycorticoids in people with daytime activity schedule. In the absence of stress, adrenal production of glucocorticoids reaches a maximum at about 6 AM, after which time there is a gradual decline to the lowest level from early evening to midnight. The difference between maximal and minimal levels of active 17-hydroxycorticoids in the blood is twofold to fourfold in most subjects. The actual curve is not smooth; corticotropin is secreted intermittently by the pituitary in short bursts or boluses.

Topical preparations are normally restricted to short-term use. Therefore, they tend to be administered regularly, several times a day. Topically administered steroids are absorbed and may produce systemic effects, including toxicity.

Adverse reactions. The glucocorticoids are potent medicines. When used in high doses, or over a period of time, toxic effects are virtually universal. In extreme cases, full-blown Cushing's syndrome develops. In this condition, many if not all of the toxic effects listed in Table 32-3 are manifested. Other symptoms include leukocytosis, hiccups, abnormal hirsutism, menstrual disturbances, infertility, muscle weakening, thinning of the skin, ruddiness of complexion and striae ("stretch marks") on the torso and extremities. One report (Messer, et al, 1983) stressed that the incidence of peptic ulcer in people who were receiving glucocorticoids is low (2%). However, this represents a doubling of the 1% incidence characteristic of the general population. Clients who receive glucocorticoids must be monitored carefully for signs and symptoms of complications.

In addition to the physiologic and behavioral changes, clients on long-term therapy develop atrophied adrenal glands because of the suppression of pituitary corticotropin production, and the normal diurnal fluctuation of glucocorticoids is obliterated. The recipient is thereby rendered physically dependent on the hormones. (With prolonged treatment, the adrenals may be irreversibly damaged, resulting in permanent Addison's disease.) Psychologic dependence on the euphorigenic properties of the hormones has also occurred.

Anaphylactoid reactions to glucocorticosteroids have been reported. Allergic hypersensitivity may develop to the corticosteroid base or to the particular ester form of preparation.

Drug interactions. When used in combination with other drugs, glucocorticoids may interfere with the therapeutic effects of these drugs. Other drugs also may affect the action of the hormones. Some combinations produce increased risk of adverse reactions (Table 32-4).

Precautions and contraindications. Before initiation of long-term glucocorticoid therapy, a baseline electrocardiogram, blood pressure evaluation, chest and spinal radiographs, glucose tolerance tests, and evaluations of hypothalamic-pituitary-adrenal axis function should be performed. Parameters that require monitoring during therapy include height, weight, blood pressure, growth rate in children, serum levels of glucose, and signs and symptoms of infection. Periodically, chest and spinal radiographs, complete blood cell counts, blood chemistries (especially glucose and electrolytes), and ocular pressure should be assessed.

Table 32-4. Interactions between glucocorticoids and other drugs

Interacting drug	Effects
Hepatic enzyme inducers (*eg*, barbiturates, phenytoin, rifampin)	Enhanced glucocorticoid metabolism (need to increase glucocorticoid dosages)
Estrogens	Potentiation of effects of glucocorticoids (need to decrease glucocorticoid dosages)
	Potentiation of electrolyte imbalances and hypercoagulation effects
Ulcerogenic drugs (*eg*, indomethacin, aspirin and other nonsteroidal anti-inflammatory agents)	Increased risk of GI ulceration
Salicylates	Decreased serum concentration of salicylates
Potassium-depleting diuretics (*eg*, thiazides, furosemide, ethacrynic acid)	Pronounced hypokalemia
Anticholinesterase agents (*eg*, ambenonium, neostigmine, pyridostigmine)	Severe weakness
Vaccines and toxoids	Diminished response to toxoids or vaccines
	Potentiation of replication of attenuated vaccines
	Increased risk of neurologic reactions to vaccines
Oral anticoagulants	Increased blood coagulability and need for increased dosages of anticoagulant

When glucocorticoid therapy is initiated for people with a history of active tuberculosis, chemoprophylaxis with isoniazid may be added to the regimen. Antituberculosis drugs are sometimes ordered also for clients with a positive skin tests for tuberculosis, because glucocorticoids may reactivate dormant organisms in the body.

After prolonged use of pharmacologic doses of glucocorticoids, the drugs must be withdrawn gradually. Abrupt withdrawal can cause cardiovascular collapse and death in adrenal crisis. The route of administration does not affect the need for weaning. Dosage of topical as well as systemic preparations should be tapered off gradually. The rate at which dosages should be decreased and the length of time required for weaning vary with the dosages of drugs used and the duration of hormone therapy. Some clients who have received large doses for prolonged periods may require a weaning period of up to a year. A few clients become permanently dependent on exogenous hormones owing to irreversible adrenal damage.

Pharmacologic doses of glucocorticoid drugs are not generally recommended for use during pregnancy, lactation, or in children. (An exception is glucocorticoid therapy to prevent abortion in expectant mothers with lupus erythematosus.) When they are required for the treatment of a life-threatening condition, the risk of fetal damage or growth retardation in children must be considered. Lactating women should not nurse their infants while taking pharmacologic dosages of these drugs.

Glucocorticoids should be used with caution in people with seizure disorders, renal insufficiency, osteoporosis, or viral infections (especially those that affect the eye). Caution is also required when the drugs are ordered for those who are receiving anticholinesterase or ulcerogenic anti-inflammatory drugs. The drugs are contraindicated for clients with known allergic hypersensitivity to any of the other corticosteroids. Because of the adverse reactions that so often accompany the use of glucocorticoids, such therapy is controversial in many conditions. Unless a serious threat of death or permanent disability is obvious, many physicians avoid their prescription. The decision for or against therapy requires consideration of the expected progress of the condition, the severity of complications likely to develop with the use of drugs, the availability of alternative modes of treatment, and the life goals of the client.

■ Summary

Glucocorticoids are adrenal cortex steroid hormones that play a major role in the body's physical response to stress. They are used as replacement hormone therapy for Addison's disease and as pharmacologic agents for the treatment of dangerous inflammatory conditions, acute allergy, serious autoimmune diseases, and certain malignant neoplasms. Toxic and side effects are similar to the signs and symptoms of Cushing's disease and may be debilitating and life-threatening. Multiple preparations of both natural and modified hormones are available for drug use. Because their toxic potential is high, glucocorticoids are not prescribed unless the expected benefits clearly outweigh the risks.

Nursing management

Nursing implications

The needs of the client who receives glucocorticoid therapy vary depending on the particular situation. The underlying illness or illnesses, stage of disease, and therapeutic goal influence nursing care. The nurse must assess the client's therapeutic response carefully, provide for accurate and consistent administration of the drugs, minimize the incidence and severity of complications, and monitor the client for adverse reactions and toxic side effects. Education of the clients and their families is vital.

Nursing process: care of clients with hormone deficiency

Assessment   Clients for whom replacement therapy is prescribed should be assessed to determine the effects of the hormone deficiency. In most cases, clients complain of fatigue, depression, weakness, and increased perception of pain. They may be prone to inflammatory or allergic conditions, such as arthritis or dermatitis. A history of circulatory shock or heat exhaustion is not unusual; tissue turgor is apt to be reduced. Clients or their relatives may have noticed a marked change in personality. If pituitary function is normal, bronzing of the skin may be apparent. This abnormal pigmentation is evidence of excessive corticotropin production.

The nurse should ascertain what the client was like before the onset of symptoms. Reestablishment of this premorbid personality and level of function is a major goal of hormone therapy.

Nursing diagnosis   Nursing diagnoses before initiation of hormone replacement may include the following:

> *Activity intolerance: fatigue related to depression secondary to glucocorticoid deficiency*
> *Anxiety related to dysphoria secondary to glucocorticoid deficiency*
> *Pain: abdominal pain and cramping related to hyperkalemia secondary to glucocorticoid deficiency*
> *Diarrhea related to hyperkalemia secondary to glucocorticoid deficiency*
> *Fluid volume deficit related to increased renal excretion by the kidneys secondary to glucocorticoid deficiency*
> *Altered comfort: increased perception of pain related to sharpening of the senses secondary to glucocorticoid deficiency*

After hormone replacement is prescribed, the client is at risk for toxic reaction to the drug until optimal dosage is established. These reactions are usually minimal and easily controlled by adjusting the dosage. Diagnoses related to excessive medication may include the following:

> *Constipation related to hypokalemia secondary to glucocorticoid excess*
> *Fluid volume excess related to sodium retention secondary to glucocorticoid excess*

The client may also notice an increased tolerance of pain. Newly diagnosed clients also probably have a

Knowledge deficit related to glucocorticoid deficiency and its treatment by hormone replacement

Planning The long-range goal for treatment is to educate the client and family in managing the drug regimen to maintain proper hormone balance. Clients must learn how to administer the hormones for optimum effect, detect the signs and symptoms of both deficiency and excesses of hormones, and adjust hormone dosages to meet the increased requirements of unusual stress. Short-range goals include reducing anxiety and pain, alleviating abdominal discomfort, maintaining blood volume, restoring normal tissue turgor, conserving limited energy, and reducing the number of stools.

Intervention At the time of diagnosis, clients need emotional support and assistance in accepting a chronic health condition that requires life-long medication. The nurse assists in the grieving that precedes acceptance. Until the client has resolved the conflicts inherent in this situation, compliance may be poor. The nurse should stress the importance of maintaining the drug regimen. Failure to maintain medication can have serious life-threatening consequences. The client who has a history of an acute episode of shock may have no trouble understanding the importance of medication, but a client who was diagnosed before such an occurrence may experience a prolongation of the normal denial reaction.

Some form of identification that indicates the hormone deficiency should be carried by the client. If stricken by sudden acute illness or trauma, the client needs additional hormone doses to provide adequate protection from the stress. A meditag or wallet card alerts health care personnel to these needs even though the person may be unable to explain his or her condition.

Client education. For the short period of time until medication restores hormonal equilibrium, the client should take temporary measures to compensate for the residual deficiency. Foods rich in potassium should be avoided so that blood levels of this electrolyte begin to decline. Foods taken should be nonirritating; any food known to cause abdominal cramping or diarrhea should be excluded from the diet. The client should continue to take extra salt and fluids to maintain blood volume. Extra rest and reduction in stressors help conserve the client's energy. Higher than normal doses of analgesics may be needed for common causes of pain such as headache. These precautions need be observed for only a few days until the medication regimen is well established.

When sufficient hormone has been absorbed to meet physiologic needs, the client must be alert to beginning signs and symptoms of both deficiency and excess. The full-blown syndrome of both imbalances should be described to clarify the differences between each extreme. The client should be advised to watch for mood changes (euphoria from excess glucocorticoids, dysphoria characterized by anxiety and depression from deficiency). A tendency toward hypotension occurs in deficiency, whereas the blood pressure rises with excesses; the client or a family member should be taught to monitor blood pressure as one indicator of hormone balance.

When hormone replacement is the goal of corticosteroid treatment, the drug should be taken regularly according to a dosage regimen that produces blood levels as close as possible to those of the normal diurnal cycle (see Fig. 32-4). Usually, a morning dose and an afternoon dose are ordered. The highest level of serum corticosteroids normally occurs during the hour before awakening; therefore, the morning dose should be taken immediately on arising for the day. The client feels "below par" until blood levels of the drug are restored. The second dose should not be delayed beyond early afternoon, because high blood levels of the hormone stimulate the brain and may prevent sleep at the normal bedtime if a dose is taken late in the day. The time of dosages are not set arbitrarily to certain clock hours but should be adapted to correspond with the client's normal activity patterns. Changes in routine, such as moving from day-shift work to night-shift work, require similar changes in drug schedules. The physician's directions for increasing doses in accordance with stress must be clearly delineated. Usually, doses are doubled for moderate stress, such as a common cold or a visit to the dentist, and tripled for severe stress, such as serious illness or surgery.

Control of hormone balance is more easily achieved if the client maintains a degree of regularity in lifestyle. Consistent routines for sleep and activity are particularly helpful. Techniques for controlling and managing stress can significantly improve the client's general condition; his or her physiologic response to stress is impaired, and events such as emotional upsets, extreme exertion, dehydration, and fasting are poorly tolerated because exogenous replacement therapy cannot be adjusted as finely to physiologic requirements as can hormone secretion by a normal gland.

Evaluation The success of short-term measures to alleviate the signs and symptoms of residual deficiency are evaluated by the client and reported to the health care professional. Anxiety, dysphoria, pain, and feelings of weakness and fatigue should subside. Diarrhea should decrease. Within a few days after initiation of the drug regimen, the signs and symptoms of corticosteroid deficiency should resolve completely. The nurse should assess blood pressure and tissue turgor as indicators of fluid volume.

The success of the teaching program can be evaluated on a short-term basis by asking the client to repeat facts learned (or demonstrate procedures taught) during the teaching sessions. Over the long term, the absence of signs and symptoms of hormone imbalance (either excess or deficiency) signify successful management of the drug regimen and imply adequate teaching (see the Example of Nursing Process and Hormone Replacement Therapy).

Nursing process: care of clients who receive pharmacologic doses of corticosteroids

Assessment Initial assessment of clients for whom pharmacologic doses of glucocorticoids are prescribed vary according to the disease condition for which the hormones are ordered. Clients also should be evaluated for indications of the degree to which adrenal secretion has compensated for the stress of the illness or injury. An adequate response will have maintained homeostasis, whereas a marginal or inadequate response may have caused a tendency toward hypotension, potassium retention, hypoglycemia, emotional depression, anxiety, and increased perception of pain. Baseline data should include any history of allergy, infection, autoimmune disorder, hyperacidity or peptic ulcer disease, and usual sleep pattern. The physical examination should include evaluation of vital signs, blood chemistries (electrolytes and glucose), weight, fluid balance, and predominant mood and affect. The nurse should also note general appearance, body contours, and pattern of fat deposition and muscle mass.

Nursing diagnosis Most clients who receive pharmacologic doses of these drugs for more than a few days exhibit some degree of Cushing's syndrome. Nursing diagnoses are likely to include the following:

> *High risk for constipation related to hypokalemia secondary to glucocorticoid excess*
> *High risk for fluid volume excess related to sodium and water retention secondary to glucocorticoid excess*
> *High risk for infection related to inhibition of immune processes secondary to glucocorticoid excess*
> *High risk for injury related to muscle atrophy and decreased bone density secondary to glucocorticoid excess*
> *Potential for sensory/perceptual alterations: blunting of the senses secondary to excess glucocorticoids*
> *Sleep pattern disturbance: insomnia related to CNS stimulation secondary to glucocorticoid excess*
> *Body image disturbance related to elation, mania, and Cushingoid appearance secondary to glucocorticoid excess*

> *High risk for delayed healing secondary to glucocorticoid excess*

Most clients will also have a

> *Knowledge deficit related to treatment with pharmacologic doses of glucocorticoids*
> *High risk for ineffective management of therapeutic regimen related to knowledge deficit*

Common collaborative problems that should be differentiated from the nursing diagnoses include

> *Potential complication: hypertension*
> *Potential complication: hypokalemia*

Planning Goals should include prevention or prompt detection and treatment of constipation, hypertension, infection, injury, malnutrition, sensory deprivation, and insomnia. In addition, a positive self-image and healing of wounds that may be sustained should be promoted. With prolonged treatment, a major goal of nursing care is to educate the client in the management of the drug regimen and optimum adjustment to the changes caused by glucocorticoid excess.

Intervention Glucocorticoid treatment of medical conditions is likely to begin while a client is hospitalized. The nurse must monitor the client for therapeutic response to the regimen. Poor response is indicated by such signs and symptoms as a tendency toward shock, undiminished inflammation, or signs and symptoms of allergy. The neurologic client may develop increased intracranial pressure. The nurse must report to the physician data that indicate inadequate response, so that hormone dosage may be increased as necessary.

Once treatment begins, nursing measures become important to protect the client from adverse drug reactions. Clients should be monitored for signs and symptoms of glucocorticoid toxicity. Toxic and side effects are multiple and varied.

Diet for most clients should be low in sodium, high in potassium and fiber, moderate in calories, and free of irritating components. The physician may prescribe the diet for people with diseases that alter fluid and electrolyte balance (ileostomy, renal impairment, fistula drainage). If the physician does not so prescribe, he or she should be consulted for assistance in planning the diet. Low-sodium diets are harmful to some clients and should not be indiscriminately imposed.

Clients who receive glucocorticoids require protection from exposure to infection. Asepsis, both medical and surgical, should be meticulous. Occasionally, reverse isolation is necessary.

Clients who are to undergo surgery may need an increase in cortisone dosage because their adrenocor-

Example of nursing process and hormone replacement therapy

The client is a 35-year-old housewife and mother with a history of hypophysectomy a year ago to remove a pituitary adenoma. Since the surgery, she has taken maintenance doses of cortisone, thyroid hormone, and estrogen for replacement therapy. Her husband spent 10 years in the army as a noncommissioned officer. Since leaving the service recently, he has had difficulty in securing steady work as a civilian.

The family is also being followed by a public health nurse since the 14-year-old daughter was hospitalized 6 months ago for acute asthma.

During today's visit, the nurse finds the daughter at home recovering from a "cold" accompanied by acute asthma. She has treated the asthma with bronchodilators and a glucocorticoid inhalant medication. She is much improved and states she plans to attend school the next day. The mother, however, appears listless and depressed. She complains of "feeling like a dishrag." The house is untidy—the breakfast dishes remain on the dining table at 11:45 AM.

On examination, the mother's vital signs are T 37°C (PO), P 105 and somewhat weak, R 18, and BP 96/48. The mother feels that she might have caught her daughter's cold. When the nurse suggests that she take an extra dose of cortisone as prescribed for mild infections, the mother explains that she "ran out of that medicine 3 days ago" and that they have not had the money to renew the prescription.

The father is out interviewing for a job.

Assessment data	Nursing diagnosis	Intervention	Goals and outcome criteria
Iatrogenic Addison's disease after hypophysectomy	Altered tissue perfusion: hypotension related to fluid volume deficit secondary to hypocortism	**Advise** the mother to take salty fluids immediately; prepare and administer a cup of hypertonic salt water (1 t salt in 6–8 oz water), bouillon, or commercially prepared soup. (If the soup is "low salt," add extra salt.) Encourage the mother to take fluids (both salted and unsalted) at frequent intervals.	The mother's blood pressure will be maintained at or above the level found when first measured.
Last dose of cortisone 72 hours ago			
Blood pressure below normal limits, pulse rapid and weakened			
Lack of energy			
Emotional depression		**Monitor** the mother's vital signs. If the mother's blood pressure declines, contact the physician.	
Lack of glucocorticoid medication for lack of money			
Absence of concern regarding omission of hormone medication		If the mother develops serious shock, **call** for emergency medical assistance; inform them that the daughter has a glucocorticoid medication for asthma, should the physician wish to approve administering a dose to the mother.	
		Remain with the family until the mother's cortisone prescription is refilled and she has taken a double dose as prescribed for moderate stress.	
		When the mother's condition is stabilized, **inform** her of the life-threatening	In the future the mother will give a high priority to maintaining hormone

(Continued)

Example of nursing process and hormone replacement therapy (Continued)

Assessment data	Nursing diagnosis	Intervention	Goals and outcome criteria
		nature of glucocorticoid deficiency. Stress the importance of taking this medication without interruption. **Prepare** and implement a teaching plan to reinforce and supplement teaching carried out when the hormone replacement drug regimen was initiated. **Encourage** the family to accept public assistance, at least Medicaid, so that health-care and drug regimens are not interrupted.	therapy, with the highest priority given to glucocorticoid medication.
	Ineffective management of therapeutic regimen related to economic difficulties	**Contact** the local office of social services to obtain financial help for the family. Arrange an emergency grant so that the mother's prescription for cortisone can be filled immediately.	In the future, drug therapy will be maintained without interruption.

tical response to stress has been inhibited as a result of pharmacologic dosages of corticoids.

When clients with wounds receive glucocorticoids, wound healing is delayed. Undue stress on surgical areas should be avoided. The removal of stitches may have to be delayed to prevent dehiscence.

Ambulatory clients require protection from hazards that increase the risk of falls. The weak muscles and fatigability characteristic of glucocorticoid excess predispose to accidents, and bone fractures are more likely because of the weakening of skeletal structures.

Clients may require stronger sensory stimuli than normal. Foods should be well flavored with essences, herbs, and spices; bright colors are appropriate for decor and clothing. The client is likely to use a high-volume setting for television, radio, or stereo.

Because clients may have difficulty sleeping at night, frequent rest periods should be provided. All possible nursing measures to promote sleep at night are needed.

Clients may be prone to peptic ulcer, the early signs and symptoms of which include heartburn, epigastric pain, and bloody or coffee-ground emesis. The stools should be tested for occult blood, another indication of gastric bleeding.

Infections can develop insidiously in the client who receives pharmacologic doses of glucocorticoids. Many normal responses to such conditions (fever, increases in white blood cell counts, and changes in the differential count) are suppressed by these drugs. The skin and mucous membranes should be inspected closely and regularly for visible changes. Complaints of pain and nausea, which may be the first symptoms of serious infection, must be reported and investigated. Because the client's immune and inflammatory responses are impaired by the drugs, the risk of invasion by pathogens is increased. If a history of tuberculosis is discovered and antimycobacterial drugs are not ordered, the physician should be informed of the history. Prophylactic antituberculosis drug therapy is often required, because tuberculosis is likely to reactivate when glucocorticoid levels are high. Cough and hemoptysis may signal the development of active pulmonary infection.

Clients should be monitored for the development of diabetes mellitus. The physician usually orders periodic fasting blood sugars. Finger-prick glucose tests or urine tests for sugar and acetone are useful for more frequent testing.

Clients should be monitored for excess fluid volume. Visible edema or a general rise in blood pressure should be reported to the physician. The client should also be monitored for signs and symptoms of potassium deficiency (weakness, constipation, and increased tendency toward digitalis toxicity in clients who receive the cardiotonic drugs).

If the client has a surgical or traumatic wound, healing proceeds more slowly when glucocorticoid levels are high. Dehiscence is more likely, and the wound should be monitored closely.

Mental and emotional changes may occur when glucocorticoids are administered in high dosages or over long periods of time. Clients should be monitored for changes in affect (euphoria, excitement) and for sleep disorders (insomnia).

Clients who receive glucocorticoids over long periods of time should also be monitored for undesirable skeletal effects. The growth and development of children should be assessed and compared with normal values for their ages. Adults should be monitored for pathologic bone fractures and reduction in height (often indicative of compression of the vertebrae).

Other abnormal changes in body structure include pronounced changes in weight, rounding of the face, development of a fat pad between the upper shoulders, and atrophy of muscle of the extremities. Striae and acneiform skin eruptions may also occur.

Client education. Clients who receive prolonged glucocorticoid therapy for a chronic medical condition are likely to manage their own treatment at home. The nurse's primary objective is to assist in this task. As with the hormone-deficient person, this client must learn to monitor his or her own condition, administer the drugs, and consult with the physician when necessary. The content to be taught differs somewhat, however. In this client, a degree of toxicity from the drugs may be acceptable in return for the benefits of therapy. The client should understand in specific terms what symptoms are to be reported to the physician for adjustment of the drug regimen. Because some side effects do occur, the client also needs assistance in minimizing their severity and impact. Appropriate assessment techniques and control measures should be taught.

In addition, clients and families should be informed of the changes in appearance and emotional affect that commonly develop with use of glucocorticoids. In some conditions, dosages are high enough to produce a frank cushingoid appearance. The face becomes round and somewhat puffy. The torso thickens, and extremities become thinner. Abnormal fat deposits may appear high on the back. The client is likely to feel jittery or somewhat "high" or, conversely, may feel depressed. The family or significant other should be asked to monitor psychologic status, because the client may be unable to assess this objectively. The client should be reassured that these changes are temporary; appearance and affect revert to normal once the drugs are withdrawn.

Because the client who receives hormones for their drug effects develop adrenal atrophy secondary to suppression of pituitary corticotropin secretion, the normal response to stress may not take place. Although hormone levels are generally above normal, they are inadequate for extreme stress. The client needs help controlling stressors and managing stress response similar to clients on replacement therapy. A meditag or wallet card that states the drug and dosage should be recommended to the client.

Because glucocorticoid hormones are frequently used for medicinal purposes, education regarding their use is needed by the lay public. The importance of weighing risks against benefits in the consideration of this type of drug therapy should be stressed. Glucocorticoids have been lauded as "miracle drugs" and are requested inappropriately by some clients out of ignorance of their dangers. The ruling of the federal Food and Drug Administration (FDA) that skin ointments and creams that contain glucocorticoids may be purchased without a prescription poses a risk of abuse. The drugs are absorbed by the skin, and systemic effects may occur. The public should be cautioned against using these preparations too frequently or for prolonged periods. Recommended dosage should be adhered to, and a physician should be consulted if the condition for which it is used fails to respond within a few days.

Evaluation Data required for evaluation include the frequency and consistency of stools; serial blood pressures; presence or absence of pus formation, loss of function, or pain indicative of infection; absence or occurrence of injury; blood levels of glucose, sodium, and potassium; and presence or absence of wound complications such as dehiscence or evisceration. Reports from the client or family should indicate the quality and amount of sleep. The client should be questioned about sensory perception to determine whether increased intensity of stimuli has compensated adequately for decreased acuity. Self-image should be evaluated by comparing the number of negative and positive statements related to self-concept uttered by the client.

The client's success in managing the treatment regimen while avoiding complications implies effectiveness of the teaching plan. Questioning the client about facts conveyed during teaching sessions provides short-term evaluation.

Learning experience 32-1

Care for a client who is receiving therapeutic glucocorticoids for their anti-inflammatory or antineoplastic effects. Assess the client carefully for responses to the drug. Plan and carry out appropriate nursing care to enhance therapeutic effects of and minimize adverse reactions to the drug.

Checklist of nursing actions

When glucocorticoids are prescribed

☐ Recommend the use of a medical identification device that identifies the drug regimen.

☐ Teach the client techniques for stress management to minimize fluctuations in hormone status.

☐ Monitor clients for evidence of glucocorticoid imbalance and for response to therapy.

☐ Teach clients to manage their drug regimens.

When hormones are prescribed
for replacement therapy

☐ Protect client from stress until hormone balance is restored.

☐ Administer hormones on arising from sleep and about 6 hours later.

☐ Assist the client in the process of grieving over altered body function.

☐ Emphasize the importance of compliance with the drug regimen.

When glucocorticoids are prescribed
for drug effects

☐ Determine if the client has been exposed to tuberculosis in the past.

☐ Monitor the client carefully for signs and symptoms of hyperadrenocorticism and complications that arise from toxicity.

☐ Consult with the physician for definitive treatment to prevent or control complications of therapy when indicated.

☐ Protect the client from exposure to infection.

☐ Protect the client from undue stress.

☐ Promote rest and sleep.

☐ Recommend a low-sodium high-potassium diet with controlled levels of carbohydrates and calories, unless contraindicated by complicating conditions.

☐ If the client is receiving digitalis, monitor closely for toxicity.

☐ Inform the client of side effects of the drug, identifying signs and symptoms that should be reported to the health care provider.

☐ Emphasize the need for continued health supervision during the course of drug treatment.

☐ Warn the client not to discontinue the drug abruptly.

Mineralocorticoids

The mineralocorticoids are adrenal cortex steroid hormones that exert their most pronounced physiologic effects on fluid and electrolyte balance.

Drug preparations. Several drug preparations are available to replace the natural mineralocorticoids in deficient clients (Table 32-5).

Pharmacodynamics. The mechanisms of action of the mineralocorticoids are still poorly understood. Because a time lag (of about an hour) exists between administration of the drugs and renal response, the hormones are believed to act by altering the concentration of enzymes that affect renal tubule reabsorption. Two theories have been proposed regarding these enzyme effects: mineralocorticoids initiate transcription of RNA, which serves as a template for the synthesis of a protein that facilitates the transport of sodium ions across the renal tubule; and mineralocorticoids activate enzymes involved in the sodium pump at the tubular serosal surface. The hormones increase sodium reabsorption and increase potassium excretion by the kidneys. Secondarily, reabsorption of water and anions increases, extracellular fluid volume increases, potassium levels decrease, hydrogen ion concentration drops, and body pH tends to rise.

Table 32-5. Mineralocorticoid drug preparations

Drug name	Preparation	Usual dosage
Desoxycorticosterone		
desoxycorticosterone acetate	Powder	Adults: 1–5 mg/day (maximum daily dose 10 mg)
		Children: 1.5–2 mg/m² body surface/day
(Doca Acetate)	Solution for IM injection	Adults: 1–5 mg/day (maximum daily dose: 10 mg)
		Children: 1.5–1 mg/m² body surface/day
(Percorten Acetate, Syncortyl)	Pellets for subcutaneous implantation	250 mg for each mg desoxycorticosterone required daily; the mineralocorticoid effects usually last 8–12 months after implantation
desoxycorticosterone pivalate (Percorten Pivalate)	Suspension for IM injection	25 mg for each mg of desoxycorticosterone required daily, administered q4wk
fludrocortisone acetate (Alflorone, F-Cortef, fludrocortone; *Can:* Florinef)	Oral tablets	Adults: 50–200 µg/day PC: C

KEY: PC = pregnancy category. (The validity of pregnancy risk categories has not been established; see Chapter 16, p 216.)

When administered to clients with salt-losing adrenogenital syndrome, mineralocorticoids correct the abnormal levels of pituitary corticotropin by replacing one of the natural hormones that stimulates the pituitary when deficient. In conjunction with glucocorticoids that are given concurrently, they inhibit corticotropin production just as natural hormones do. As body levels of corticotropin decrease, adrenal production of androgens and the signs and symptoms of the disease subside.

Pharmacokinetics. The synthetic hormone fludrocortisone acetate is not inactivated by digestion and can be administered orally. Desoxycorticosterone is not effective when given orally. It is administered by intramuscular (IM) injection or surgical implantation in the tissues (see Table 32-5).

All mineralocorticoids are distributed to the tissues by the blood. They are metabolized to inactive forms by most body tissues to some degree, but the liver is the primary site for their degradation or conjugation. They are excreted in the urine.

Therapeutic uses. The mineralocorticoids are employed for partial replacement of hormones required by people with deficient adrenal cortex function due to Addison's disease or salt-losing adrenogenital syndrome. Additional glucocorticoid hormones are also needed for adequate treatment of most clients affected by these syndromes.

Adverse reactions. Overdose of mineralocorticoids produces signs and symptoms of hormone excess: edema, hypervolemia, hypertension, and cardiac enlargement and arrhythmia. Headache, arthralgia, and tendon contractures can occur. Congestive heart failure or cerebral vascular accident may develop. As potassium depletion progresses, weakness and intestinal atony are succeeded by ascending paralysis and paralytic ileus. Laboratory data usually indicate hypernatremia, hypokalemia, and alkalosis.

Allergic hypersensitivity to mineralocorticoid drugs sometimes develops. The first sign of allergy may be increasing irritation or inflammation at the site of injection.

Precautions and contraindications. Clients with Addison's disease are more sensitive to mineralocorticoids than are people with adequate adrenocortical function. Dosage must be established cautiously during initial stages of the treatment regimen. Blood tests for electrolyte levels are taken frequently. Clients must be watched for sudden gain in weight or rise in blood pressure, the appearance of edema, and cardiac enlargement. If toxic manifestations appear, sodium intake must be restricted and potassium supplements administered.

If mineralocorticoid therapy is necessary during pregnancy, the newborn must be assessed for signs and symptoms of hypoadrenalism.

Mineralocorticoids are contraindicated for clients with high levels of these hormones. They are not administered to clients who exhibit hypertension or edema. People who develop allergic sensitivity to the drugs should be treated with a preparation to which they do not react, or they must undergo desensitization.

Glucose tolerance tests are contraindicated for clients who receive mineralocorticoids unless absolutely necessary, because their marginal hormone levels make them vulnerable to severe hypoglycemia.

■ Summary
Mineralocorticoids are drugs that exert physiologic effects similar to those of the adrenal cortex steroid hormones aldosterone and desoxycorticosterone. They act to increase renal reabsorption of sodium, water, and anions and to increase renal excretion of potassium and hydrogen ions. They are used as replacement therapy for clients who suffer from Addison's disease and salt-losing adrenogenital syndrome.

Mineralocorticoid toxicity is characterized by hypervolemia, hypertension, edema, and hyperkalemia. Allergic hypersensitivity to the mineralocorticoids sometimes occurs.

Nursing management

Nursing implications

Case-finding is an important nursing function in treating adrenal corticosterone deficiencies. The earlier the hormone inadequacy is diagnosed, the easier it is to treat. Clients with signs and symptoms suggestive of adrenal cortex insufficiency should be referred to a physician, preferably an endocrinologist, for definitive diagnosis and treatment. When mineralocorticoid deficiency is found, hormone therapy is needed indefinitely. Clients must adjust to the presence of a chronic medical condition that requires regular health supervision and uninterrupted drug therapy.

Nursing process

Assessment Early manifestations of mineralocorticoid deficiency are subtle, and it may be difficult to detect at this stage. When taking the history, the nurse should inquire specifically about episodes of fainting, shock, or heat exhaustion. Baseline physical data include vital signs, weight, fluid balance, electrolytes, and blood glucose levels. The nurse should be alert to signs and symptoms characteristic of the syndrome, such as weakness, fatigue, tendency toward hypotension, hypoglycemia, and abdominal discomfort. Affected clients may crave salt; they usually maintain a high sodium intake. Ambiguous genitalia in female newborns or virilization of female children or young adults are additional manifestations of adrenogenital syndrome. Laboratory data may reveal tendencies toward hyperkalemia, hyponatremia, and acidosis. A weak cardiac action, excessive intestinal peristalsis, poor tissue turgor, hypotension, and flaccid muscles may be found on physical examination.

After medical diagnosis, clients should be assessed for emotional reaction to diagnosis of a chronic disease and for knowledge about the disease and its treatment.

Nursing diagnosis Nursing diagnoses may include the following:

Anxiety related to uncertainty about prognosis of a chronic debilitating deficiency disease
Activity intolerance related to metabolic changes secondary to mineralocorticoid deficiency
Decreased cardiac output related to hypovolemia secondary to mineralocorticoid deficiency
Fluid volume deficit related to hypovolemia secondary to mineralocorticoid deficiency
Knowledge deficit related to mineralocorticoid deficiency and its treatment

Once hormone therapy begins, a potential for hormone toxicity exists, particularly during the initial phase of treatment when dosages have not been established. Diagnoses related to mineralocorticoid excess include the following:

Activity intolerance related to metabolic changes secondary to mineralocorticoid excess
Fluid volume excess related to hypernatremia secondary to mineralocorticoid excess

Planning Initial nursing goals are to alleviate or eliminate anxiety, conserve the client's energy, and increase blood volume and cardiac output. Other goals are to prevent or promptly detect and treat hypertension and hypokalemia due to hormone excess.

Intervention Clients need emotional support and assistance in accepting the diagnosis of a chronic incurable disease. They should be encouraged to express their feelings openly. Clients should be told that their condition can be controlled with medication and that, if treated, it should not become life-threatening. However, detailed teaching should be delayed until the initial shock and disbelief have been resolved.

During the initial stages of treatment, the nurse should promote rest and relaxation to conserve the client's energy. Physical activity should be resumed gradually, as blood pressure rises and muscle strength improves.

Until hormone therapy is established, the client should be given ample sodium and water with the diet. Sodium intake should be tapered off gradually as the client responds to medication. If the client has hyperkalemia, potassium intake should be restricted.

When treatment is initiated, daily doses of desoxycorticosterone are administered until optimum dosage is established. During this period, the client must be closely monitored for manifestations of drug toxicity. To avoid hypertensive crisis, the dose is initiated at low levels and increased gradually. Fluid and electrolyte balance are assessed carefully by means of body weights and blood electrolyte levels. The nurse should assess emotional affect, tissue hydration, muscle strength, and cardiovascular and intestinal function.

Desoxycorticosterone must be administered, at first daily, by IM injection. When dosage requirements have been established, a (surgically implanted) depot preparation that provides medication for a longer period of time may be employed.

Desoxycorticosterone acetate or pivalate in oil is administered about once every 4 weeks. Because relatively large volumes of the preparation are required, the drug should be injected into the upper outer quadrant of the buttocks. The liquid is viscous, and a 20-gauge or larger needle should be used.

Implantation or IM injection sites should be monitored for irritation or inflammation indicative of allergic hypersensitivity. Development of this complication must be reported to the physician; it may be necessary to change the form of medication prescribed.

Fludrocortisone acetate, which can be administered orally, can sometimes be used for the treatment of adrenal corticosterone deficiency states. Because this preparation has glucocorticoid as well as mineralocorticoid activity, management of hormone dosages is somewhat complex when it is employed.

The client should be evaluated for hormone imbalance (either excess or deficiency) at each nursing visit. The nurse should take vital signs and assess emotional affect, muscle strength, and GI motility.

The nurse should plan and implement a teaching program that helps clients manage the drug regimen and maintain hormone balance.

Client education. Clients should take an active part in the management of their disease. To do so, they need to be fully informed of the signs and symptoms of hormone deficiency and excess and must be able to monitor themselves for signs of imbalance. Clients must be taught the skills needed to assess blood pressure, pulse, tissue turgor, and body weight. If IM drugs are prescribed, clients should learn injection technique and should administer their own medications. When clients are incapable of self-care because of age or disability, a family member may perform these functions.

Response to hormone therapy is reduced somewhat by stress, particularly exposure to hot or humid environments that increase salt loss through perspiration. Clients should be warned to avoid sauna baths and similar situations that stimulate sweating.

Adverse reactions to hormone therapy can be ameliorated through dietary adjustment of electrolyte intake. The effects of mineralocorticoids are enhanced by increased sodium intake and decreased potassium intake. Clients should be instructed to increase sodium in the diet when signs and symptoms of hormone deficiency appear. Potassium-rich foods should be avoided at these times. When signs and symptoms of excess hormone levels are noted, sodium restriction and potassium increases are appropriate. Clients must be taught techniques for altering dietary intake of these electrolytes, such as the preparation of attractive and tasty low-salt dishes, methods for reducing potassium intake, and selection of foods that are rich in each mineral.

Clients should be cautioned to maintain regular health supervision by qualified professionals. They should notify the physician when signs and symptoms of persistent or progressive hormone imbalance occur; dosage regimens may need to be altered.

Evaluation Data required for evaluation include the absence or presence of restlessness, irritability, or other signs of anxiety, statements by the client indicative of emotional tension or relaxation, duration of sleep and rest periods, serial blood pressure readings, and tissue turgor, muscle strength, and activity tolerance evaluations. The success of the teaching plan is inferred by the ability of the client to maintain hormone balance over the long term. The client should also be tested to determine retention of facts and ability to carry out procedures taught during the teaching program.

Checklist of nursing actions

☐ Assess clients for signs and symptoms of adrenocorticosterone deficiency or adrenogenital syndrome; refer clients who exhibit these signs and symptoms for definitive diagnosis and treatment.

☐ Monitor clients who receive mineralocorticoid therapy for signs and symptoms of fluid, sodium, potassium, and acid-base imbalances that indicate hormone imbalance.

☐ Administer mineralocorticoids in oily suspensions by deep IM injection in the upper outer quadrant of the buttocks, using a 20-gauge or larger needle.

☐ Provide complete perioperative nursing care for clients scheduled for surgical implantation of desoxycorticosterone pellets.

☐ Help clients to adjust emotionally to the reality of chronic endocrine illness that requires lifelong treatment.

☐ Teach clients who require injectable drug preparations to administer their own drugs.

☐ Teach clients how to monitor hormone balance and response to medication.

☐ Teach clients how to adjust sodium and potassium intake to ameliorate fluctuations in response to mineralocorticoid therapy.

☐ Caution clients to maintain regular care by qualified health professionals.

(See Example of Nursing Process and Prednisone Treatment. A detailed care plan is presented in Chapter 3.)

Male sex hormones

Male sex hormones are responsible for the differentiation, growth, and development of the male reproductive system, as well as the induction and maintenance of male secondary sex characteristics. They also influence metabolism and sex drive in both sexes.

Androgens

Physiology. Androgens are produced by both the male and female, but in significantly differing amounts. Normal adult males secrete 7 to 9 mg a day, maintaining a serum level of 0.2 to 1 μg per 100 ml. Adult females secrete about 3 mg a day; their serum levels are half or less than half those of men.

Androgens are produced in large amounts by the testes (in males) and in smaller quantities by the adrenal cortex. Some also arise from the metabolism of other steroid hormones such as estrogens and progestogens.

The differentiation of genital tissues in fetuses of both sexes is affected by male sex hormones. In the male, high levels of androgens stimulate the growth of the penis, the descent of the testicles, and the formation of normal male genitalia. Although the proportion of androgens to estrogens is much smaller in the female embryo, some male hormone appears necessary to her proper reproductive development also. However, excessively high levels of androgens *in utero* can masculinize the female fetus, producing an appearance of male gender in an otherwise normally functioning potentially fertile female.

Shortly after birth, the production of androgens in males declines sharply and remains low until puberty. At this time, the increase of male hormones to adult levels triggers a spurt in growth, rapid development of the genitalia, and the appearance of male secondary sex characteristics. The voice deepens, muscles increase in size, the skin thickens and becomes more oily, and male patterns of hair growth develop (triangular genital hair, chest hair, beard, and baldness in men who have that hereditary trait). The epiphyses close, and growth declines. Male hormone levels peak at about 20 years of age and then decline gradually; in

Example of nursing process and prednisone treatment

The client is a 59-year-old carpenter who retired on disability a year ago because of lung impairment caused by sarcoidosis. Since diagnosis, he has been treated with prednisone 20 mg every other day and followed by the public health nursing service. One month ago his prednisone dosage was increased to 30 mg every day to treat an acute attack of shingles.

On the current visit, the nurse notes that the client's appearance has changed. His face seems fuller and the shoulders more bulky. He is complaining of tenderness in the left calf. Homan's sign is positive on the left side.

The client's wife comments, "I'm glad you came today. He missed his last doctor's appointment." The client chides her, "Now, you know I've been feeling good up to now—no need to run to the doctor all the time."

Assessment data	Nursing diagnosis	Intervention	Goals and outcome criteria
High dosage prednisone therapy Tenderness in left calf Positive Homan's sign, "moon face" and "buffalo hump"	Altered peripheral tissue perfusion: pulmonary artery obstruction related to embolism secondary to phlebitis with venous clot formation	**Instruct** the client to sit down in a chair that will not cause pressure to be exerted against the calf of the leg or the back of the knees. **Caution** the client not to walk around until the physician's advice is obtained. **Contact** the physician and report the client's signs and symptoms. **Assist** the client and his wife in implementing the physician's recommendations.	The client's complication will be diagnosed and properly treated. The client will not develop pulmonary embolism.
Client's absence of concern over signs and symptoms of abnormal clotting Missed doctor's appointment while on high-dose prednisone therapy Client's statement that he has been "feeling good"	Knowledge deficit concerning adverse reactions to glucocorticoid therapy; contributing factor: iatrogenic euphoria	**Inform** the client that his signs and symptoms may indicate a serious adverse reaction to prednisone **Take initial action** to prevent embolism (see above). **Prepare** and implement a teaching plan to inform the client and his wife about prednisone therapy, including the following content; signs and symptoms of glucocorticoid toxicity, specific signs and symptoms that should be reported immediately to the primary-care provider, precautions to reduce the risk of serious adverse reactions, and the importance of maintaining dosage until a weaning schedule has been implemented.	The client will maintain medical supervision as scheduled; he will contact the physician or nurse if he is unable to appear for a scheduled appointment. The client will contact the physician or nurse should he develop signs or symptoms of serious complication; he will not contact the health care provider inappropriately for minor changes. The client will not discontinue prednisone medication without contacting the physician or nurse. The client will implement recommended precautions to decrease the risk of serious adverse reactions to prednisone.

old age they may be reduced to one-fifth of the maximum levels.

Androgens exert an anabolic effect on metabolism. They produce increases in protein synthesis, bone density, bone marrow function (especially erythropoiesis), sodium retention, and low-density and very-low-density lipoproteins in the blood. A tendency toward gain in lean body weight is accompanied by a decrease in subcutaneous fat deposits.

Male sex hormones affect emotions and behavior also. They increase libido in both sexes. Rises in androgen levels are accompanied by a subjective feeling of well-being. In animals these hormones are known to influence mating behavior and to stimulate aggressiveness; indications suggest that similar though less potent influences affect humans. In the pituitary, metabolites of these compounds inhibit gonadotropin secretion.

Drug preparations. Among the natural androgens are several distinct compounds (Table 32-6). Testosterone is the most abundant and most potent. Both natural hormones and modified drug preparations are used pharmaceutically.

Combinations of androgens and estrogens, sometimes including nutrient minerals and vitamins, are also marketed.

Pharmacodynamics. Androgenic drugs influence basic cell physiology in ways similar to endogenous male hormones. They exert antiestrogenic, anabolic, and masculinizing actions on the body. Synthetic preparations have been modified chemically in ways that enhance anabolic and minimize androgenic properties, but complete separation of these functions has not been achieved.

Pharmacokinetics. Androgenic drugs are most often administered orally, buccally, sublingually, and intramuscularly.

Natural hormone preparations are not very effective when administered orally, owing to metabolism of the drugs in the GI mucosa and on first pass through the liver. The synthetic androgens and anabolics are less extensively metabolized after oral administration.

After absorption, most androgens are highly (98%–99%) bound to plasma proteins. This inactive tissue depot prevents rapid fluctuations in the serum level of free androgen; as the level of free hormone in the serum declines, hormone is released from the protein-binding sites and becomes physiologically active.

As with most steroids, male sex hormones are deactivated by the liver and excreted in urine.

Therapeutic uses. Androgens are most valuable for the treatment of sex-hormone deficiencies in males. They restore normal sexual appearance and potency in males affected by castration or pan-

hypopituitarism. They are sometimes helpful in delayed puberty, postpubertal cryptorchidism, oligospermia, and impotence. Cases for drug therapy must be carefully selected, because these disorders do not always stem from hormone deficiency and the administration of androgens may permanently impair fertility, especially in young recipients.

Androgenic drugs are rarely used for long-term therapy in females because of their masculinizing effects. The drugs have been used for the palliation of breast cancer in women when the malignancy is considered to be hormone dependent and the less toxic anabolic derivatives are not effective. On a short-term basis, androgens have been used to prevent postpartum breast pain and engorgement by suppressing lactation.

The anabolic hormones are used in the treatment of refractory or aplastic anemias and osteoporosis in both sexes. They promote a positive nitrogen balance, bone healing in fracture clients, and tissue regeneration and weight gain in debilitated or cachexic people. They are preferred to the more masculinizing preparations for the treatment of advanced breast cancer in women.

The anabolic hormones produce some growth in pituitary dwarves but also initiate bone maturation and closure of the epiphyses, thereby terminating growth. For this reason, they are used only after somatotropin therapy has been exhausted, or when this hormone is not available.

Adverse reactions. Both male sex hormones and their anabolic derivatives exert similar adverse and toxic effects. Although the masculinizing properties are less pronounced in the anabolic compounds, they are not absent. Findings indicate that masculinizing and anabolic actions of this class of drugs are not completely separable.

Masculinization is the most obvious and troublesome adverse reaction in clients for which this is not the desired therapeutic result. The type and degree of sexual change varies with the sex and age of the recipient. Because fetuses of both sexes become masculinized, the use of male sex hormones is contraindicated in pregnancy. Women who receive these drugs experience menstrual irregularities, excess hirsutism, a deepening and weakening of the voice, clitoral enlargement, an increased incidence of acne, and male pattern baldness if they possess this genetic trait. Structural changes of the larynx are irreversible, and early withdrawal of the drugs is required to reverse voice changes. Prepubertal males exhibit enlargement of the phallus, increased frequency of erection, precocious sexuality, and permanent closure of the epiphyses, which limits stature. In postpubertal males the effects of androgens are masked if male sexual development

Table 32-6. *Male hormones and related drugs*

Drug name	Preparations	Usual adult dosage	Pattern of effects
Natural hormones			
testosterone (Andro 100, Android-T, Histerone, Malogen, Testaqua, Testoject, T Pellets)	Powder Pellets for subcutaneous implantation Suspensions for IM injection	For replacement of endogenous testicular hormone: *IM:* 10–25 mg, 2–3 times weekly; *subcutaneous (pellets):* 150–450 mg q3–6 mo For palliative treatment of carcinoma of the breast in women: *IM:* 100 mg, 3 times weekly For prevention of postpartum breast pain and engorgement: *IM:* 25–50 mg/day, for 3–4 days For treatment of impotence and male climacteric: *IM:* 25–50 mg, 2–3 times a week PC: X	Full range of androgenic and anabolic properties
testosterone cypionate (Andro-Cyp, Andronate, dep Andro, Depotest, Depo-Testosterone, Duratest, T-lonate-P.A., Testoject LA, Vigorex)	Solution in oil for IM injection	For replacement of endogenous testicular hormone: 50–400 mg, q2–4wk For the development and maintenance of testicular function in oligospermia: 100–200 mg, q2–4wk For palliative treatment of carcinoma of the breast in women: 200–400 mg, q2–4wk For treatment of impotence and male climacteric: 200–400 mg, q3–4wk PC: X	Full range of androgenic and anabolic properties
testosterone enanthate (Andro L.A., Android-T, Andryl, Anthatest, Delatestryl, Everone, Malogex, Testate, Testostroval)	Powder Solution in oil for IM injection	For replacement of endogenous testicular hormone: 50–400 mg, q2–4wk For the treatment of impotence, full range of androgenic and male climacteric: 200–400 mg, q4wk For treatment of oligospermia: to develop and maintain testicular function: 100–200 mg, q2–4wk; to suppress and produce rebound stimulation: 200 mg weekly for 6–12wk For palliative treatment of carcinoma of the breast in women: 200–400 mg, q2–4wk For adjunctive treatment of postmenopausal women or senile osteoporosis: 200–400 mg, q4wk PC: X	Full range of androgenic and anabolic properties
testosterone propionate (Androlan, Malogen in Oil, Oreton, Perandren, Testex)	Powder Solution in oil for IM injection	For replacement of endogenous testicular hormone: 10–25 mg, 2–3 times weekly For the palliative treatment of carcinoma of the breast in women: 50–100 mg, 3 times a week For the prevention of postpartum breast pain and engorgement: 25–50 mg/day for 3–4 days For treatment of impotence and male climacteric: *IM:* 10–25 mg, 2–3 times a week PC: X	Full range of androgenic and anabolic properties
Synthetic androgens			
danazol (Danocrine, Ladogal)	Oral capsules	*Initial:* For endometriosis: 200–800 mg/day, divided in 2 doses (depending on the severity of the condition); for fibrocystic disease: 100–400 mg/day, divided in 2 doses; for hereditary angioedema: 400–600 mg/day, divided in 2–3 doses *Maintenance:* Dosage is gradually reduced until individual requirements are determined PC: X	Inhibition of pituitary secretion of gonadotropins Weak androgenic and anabolic properties

(Continued)

Table 32-6. Male hormones and related drugs (Continued)

Drug name	Preparations	Usual adult dosage	Pattern of effects
Synthetic androgens			
fluoxymesterone (Halotestin, Ora Testryl, Ultandren)	Oral tablets	For replacement of endogenous testicular hormone: 2–10 mg/day, divided in 1–4 doses For palliative treatment of carcinoma of the breast in women: 15–30 mg/day, divided in several doses For prevention of postpartum breast pain and engorgement: 2.5 mg administered when active labor begins, then 5–10 mg/day, in divided doses, for 4–5 days PC: X	Androgenic activity equal to that of testosterone Anabolic properties Promotion of recalcification of osseous metastases and decrease in urinary concentration of calcium in malignant neoplasms
methyltestosterone (Android, Metandren, Neo-Hombreol, Oreton-M, Orchisterone, Testred, Vigorex, Virilon)	Powder Buccal tablets Oral tablets and capsules	For replacement of endogenous testicular hormone: *Oral preparations:* 10–50 mg/day, in divided doses; *buccal tablets:* 5–25 mg/day, in divided doses For delayed puberty in males: *Oral:* 10 mg/day; *buccal:* 5 mg/day For the treatment of carcinoma of the breast in women: *Oral:* 50–200 mg/day; *buccal:* 25–100 mg/day For the prevention of postpartum breast pain and engorgement: *Oral:* 80 mg/day; *buccal:* 40 mg/day (duration of treatment: 3–5 days after parturition) For treatment of impotence and male climacteric: *Oral:* 10–50 mg/day; *buccal:* 5–25 mg/day PC: X	Androgenic and anabolic properties comparable to those of endogenous hormones
nandrolone decanoate (Deca-Durabolin, Kabolin)	Solution in oil for IM injection	For the treatment of anemia of renal disease: 50–100 mg, q3–4wk; children aged 2–13 yr: 25–50 mg, q3–4wk PC: X	Enhanced anabolic properties Reduced androgenic and antiestrogenic properties
nandrolone phenpropionate (Durabolin)	Solution in oil for IM injection	For the treatment of metastatic cancer of the breast: 25–50 mg/wk PC: X	Enhanced anabolic properties Reduced androgenic and antiestrogenic properties
stanozolol (Winstrol)	Oral tablets	For the treatment of aplastic anemia: 2 mg, tid; children aged 6–12 yr of age: 2 mg, tid; children younger than 6 yr: 1 mg, tid PC: X	Enhanced anabolic properties Reduced androgenic and antiestrogenic properties

KEY: PC = pregnancy category. (The validity of pregnancy risk categories has not been established; see Chapter 16, p 216.)

has been completed. The drugs do produce inhibition of testicular function and oligospermia, resulting in fertility problems. Gynecomastia may also develop. The administration of androgens to hormone-deficient males may result in prostatic hypertrophy; acute urinary retention may ensue. Priapism (pronounced and persistent penile erections) may occur early in the treatment period but tends to subside with reduced dosages of the drug.

General effects in all recipients include nausea, fever, inhibition of pituitary gonadotropins, and in-

creased tendency toward acne, edema, and cholestatic jaundice. Problems in sexual function include changes in libido (increases or decreases), infertility, impotency, and orgasmic dysfunction.

Because of the metabolic effects of the hormones, changes in the results of certain laboratory tests occur. Thyroid function test results tend to decline, and the glucose tolerance test curve changes. Serum levels of sodium, potassium, phosphorus, calcium, and cholesterol increase. Hypercalcemia, which occurs in 3% to 5% of recipients, can reach dangerous levels. Clotting factors II, V, VII, and X decline. The accompanying decrease in coagulability can cause episodes of bleeding in clients who receive both anticoagulants and androgenic hormones.

Danazol, a synthetic androgen, may elevate intracranial pressure, which can cause blindness. This adverse reaction is manifested by headaches and visual disturbances such as double vision (Shag, et al, 1987). Danazol can also cause thrombocytopenia (Arrowsmith & Dreis, 1986).

Toxic effects of androgens are seen most often in athletes who abuse these drugs to promote muscle growth and to improve performance and strength. Short-term effects include sodium and water retention, tachycardia, hypertension, vertigo, headache, acne, nausea, vomiting, and diarrhea, insomnia, chills, muscle cramps, changes in libido, and elevated blood levels of sodium, cholesterol, triglycerides, and glucose; (in men) gynecomastia, decreased sperm production, and difficulty in urinating; and (in women) hirsutism, breast shrinkage, and clitoral enlargement. Long-term effects include liver damage (including cancer); (in men) atrophy of the testicles, prostate enlargement, and hair loss; and (in women) impaired fertility and permanent voice changes (deepening and weakening).

Precautions and contraindications. Male hormones must be administered with caution to people with cardiac, renal, or hepatic disease and seizure disorders. They are contraindicated during pregnancy, nephrosis, or nephrotic phase of nephritis, and for males who suffer from cancer of the prostate or breast. The drugs are not used in the treatment of non-hormone-dependent cancer of the breast in women. They should be discontinued if serum calcium concentration rises above normal in recipients with bone metastases (see Focus on Androgens: Similarities and Differences).

■ **Summary**

Male sex hormones are steroids produced by the testes and the adrenal cortex that stimulate development of the reproductive system and secondary sex characteristics in the male and promote normal sexual function. Natural hormones are prescribed for replacement therapy and the treatment of cryptorchidism. The anabolic properties of modified hormones are useful in the palliative treatment of tissue-wasting conditions and anemia. Male hormones are rarely used for prolonged treatment of females because of their masculinizing effects. Side effects of the drugs include nausea, fever, acne, and changes in sexual function. They are contraindicated in pregnancy, cancer of the prostate, and nephrosis.

Nursing management

Nursing implications

Androgen deficiencies. Adolescent males or their families who are concerned about late maturation may consult the nurse for advice regarding hormone therapy to correct the perceived condition. The nurse should advise younger clients to have patience, since the age of maturation is quite individual and ranges from the early to late teens. When anxiety persists, referral to a physician for evaluation and reassurance is appropriate. When the late teens have been reached without normal sexual development, the client must be referred for an endocrine evaluation. The nurse should caution that hormone therapy is not always helpful and may cause serious side effects; therefore, even when failure of maturation is a recognized problem, drugs may not be the appropriate treatment.

Nursing process: care of sexually immature male clients

Assessment Nurses should be alert to evidence of lack of sexual maturity in males in their late teens. Data indicative of male hormone deficiency include absence of secondary sex characteristics (body build, beard, pitch of voice) and age of the client. These data are not significant in the early teens, because many males do not experience puberty until their midteens.

When approached by clients or families who are concerned about delayed maturation, the nurse should determine the degree of concern felt and reasons for it. The usual pattern of development among family members should be considered in evaluating the significance of immaturity. If males on both sides of the family normally achieve sexual maturity in the early teens, lack of maturity in the midteens is of greater significance than it would be if a familial pattern of later maturation exists.

Nursing diagnosis Nursing diagnoses may include the following:

Altered growth and development: delay in male sexual maturation inconsistent with familial pattern
Fear of infertility and sexual impotence related to delayed development of sexual maturity
Body image disturbance related to sexual immaturity
Knowledge deficit concerning normal growth and development

Planning Nursing goals for the client whose development is within normal limits include providing information for the client and family, reducing their fear, and gaining their acceptance of the client's status as normal. When development is unusually delayed, the

Androgens: similarities and differences

Similarities

Pharmacodynamics

These agents stimulate RNA polymerase activity and RNA synthesis, resulting in increased protein production and tissue building. They suppress gonadotropin-releasing hormone, luteinizing hormone, and follicle-stimulating hormone through a negative feedback system. They promote maturation of male sex organs and male secondary sex characteristics. They stimulate production of red blood cells by enhancing the production of erythropoietic-stimulating factors.

Pharmacokinetics

These agents are administered orally, buccally, sublingually, and IM. Solutions for injection are slowly absorbed. The natural hormones undergo first pass metabolism after oral administration; the synthetic hormones undergo less metabolism after oral administration. These agents are metabolized by the liver and excreted by the kidneys.

Therapeutic uses

These agents are used for the treatment of sex hormone deficiency in males. They are also used for the palliative treatment of breast cancer and for the treatment of refractory or aplastic anemia and osteoporosis in both sexes.

Adverse reactions

These include: (CNS) headache, anxiety, mental depression, vertigo, insomnia; (CV) tachycardia; (GI) nausea, vomiting, constipation, change in appetite, weight gain, gastritis, cholestatic jaundice, hepatic dysfunction, and elevated liver enzymes; (GU) bladder irritability, frequency; (REPRO) masculinization, change in libido, priapism, clitoral enlargement, increased frequency of erection, fertility problems, diminished sperm production, gynecomastia, impotency, orgasmic dysfunction, prostate enlargement; (SKIN) acne, male pattern baldness; (ENDO) decreased thyroid function test, fluid imbalance; (HEMA) bleeding tendencies, polycythemia; (OTHER) fever, elevated sodium, potassium, phosphorus, calcium and cholesterol, deepening of voice.

Differences

• **Testosterone** and **fluoxymesterone** cause growth spurts in adolescents and terminate long bone growth. They promote the retention of calcium, nitrogen, phosphorus, sodium, and potassium. • **Danazol** suppresses the pituitary ovarian axis and inhibits the output of pituitary gonadotropins.

The half-life of **fluoxymesterone** is 9 hours; the half-life of **methyltestosterone** is 2.5 to 3.5 hours; the half-life of **testosterone** is 10 to 100 minutes; the half-life of **testosterone cypionate** is 8 days; **methyltestosterone** peaks in 1 hour after buccal administration and in 2 hours after oral administration. Some **testosterone** is excreted in feces.

• **Danazol** is used as palliative treatment of endometriosis and fibrocystic breast disease.

• **Danazol** may cause increased intracranial pressure, blindness, hypertension, visual disturbances, thrombocytopenia, muscle cramps, and sweating. • **Fluoxymesterone** may cause testicular enlargement, oligospermia, epididymitis. • **Methyltestosterone** may cause irritation of the oral mucosa with buccal administration. • **Testosterone** may cause pain at the injection site and generalized paresthesia and induration and irritation with pellet administration.

(continued)

Focus on

Androgens: similarities and differences (Continued)

Similarities	Differences

Contraindications

These agents are contraindicated in males with breast or prostatic cancer or symptomatic prostatic hypertrophy. They are also contraindicated in people with known hypersensitivity, severe cardiac, renal, or hepatic dysfunction, abnormal genital bleeding, and in women who are pregnant or breast-feeding.

• **Testosterone** and **methyltestosterone** are contraindicated in people with hyperuricemia and those who are easily sexually stimulated.

Precautions

These agents should be used cautiously in children.

Some preparations of **methyltestosterone** and **fluoxymesterone** contain tartrazine dye and should be used cautiously in people with tartrazine hypersensitivity. • **Danazol** should be used cautiously in people with seizures and migraine headaches.

Nursing considerations

Instruct client in disease, treatment, drug therapy, regimen, adverse effects, and compliance; provide emotional support; monitor serum lab studies, including electrolytes and liver enzymes; assess fluid balance and intake and output frequently for changes; institute sodium restriction if necessary; assess for edema, especially in the lower extremities; check daily weights; encourage diet high in calories and protein if not contraindicated; instruct male clients to report signs of priapism, decreased ejaculation; instruct females to report signs of virilization.

Administer **testosterone** IM deeply into a large muscle; store IM preparations at room temperature. • Encourage clients who take **danazol** for fibrocystic disease to examine breasts regularly. Instruct clients who take **danazol** to wash after intercourse and wear cotton-lined underwear to prevent possible vaginitis.

---

goal is medical evaluation and definitive diagnosis. Goals for all clients include enhancing self-concept and fulfilling appropriate role function.

When hormone replacement is prescribed, the goal of teaching is to provide the client with the knowledge and skills needed to manage the drug regimen. Goals of the medical regimen include initiation of puberty and stimulation of autogenous hormone production.

Intervention The immature client whose development is within normal limits and his family should be taught about growth and development and reassured that his progress is within normal limits. Emotional counseling may be needed to reduce fear and promote acceptance of the client's individual growth patterns. Family and client concerns should be accepted as legitimate, and they should be encouraged to seek referral for medical evaluation should puberty not begin by the late teens. If the family desires referral, the nurse should arrange for them to see a physician skilled in the area of endocrinology. These young men require a

great deal of emotional support. Everything possible should be done to enhance their perceptions of themselves as normal males. The goals of treatment and the reasons for changes in the therapeutic regimen should be carefully explained.

Client education. Clients who are diagnosed as hormone deficient receive replacement medication. They and their families need information about therapeutic and adverse reactions to the drugs and the medical tests required for monitoring drug treatment (see following section for care of clients who receive hormone therapy). They should be informed that hormone therapy is likely to be intermittent to maximize the potential for resumption of autogenous hormone production. They should be fully informed by the physician of the probable course of treatment and the prognosis.

Evaluation Success of care for clients with development within normal limits is determined by data that indicate improved body image, and a decrease in fear, such as statements by client or family that they are less concerned, or decreases in muscle tension. The teaching plan may be evaluated for the ability of client and family to relate back to the nurse facts conveyed during the teaching sessions.

Nursing process: care of clients who receive male sex hormone replacement therapy

Assessment Male hormone deficiency in adults may be secondary to trauma or disease that affects the testes or to pituitary deficiency. A history of gradual decline in sexual potency, gonadal injury, or orchiectomy may exist. Blood levels of male hormones that are below normal suggest a physiologic rather than psychologic etiology for impotence.

Nursing diagnosis Nursing diagnosis may include the following:

> *Sexual dysfunction: impotence related to deficiency of male hormone secondary to orchiectomy (testicular atrophy, pituitary gonadotropin deficiency)*
> *Body image disturbance related to sexual malfunction*
> *Knowledge deficit concerning male hormone deficiency and its treatment*
> *High risk for altered tissue integrity: inflammation of oral tissues secondary to irritation by buccal or sublingual administration of hormone drugs*
> *High risk for sexual dysfunction related to tissue damage secondary to excess male hormone levels*
> *High risk for altered urinary elimination: retention related to prostatic hypertrophy secondary to excess male hormone levels*

Planning Goals of nursing care include increased sexual potency, improved self-image, elimination of knowledge deficit, and prevention or prompt detection and treatment of adverse reactions to the prescribed drugs.

Intervention All recipients of male hormone drugs are subject to their general metabolic effects. They should be monitored for adverse reaction to the drugs.

When drugs are administered sublingually or buccally, the nurse should examine the mouth to detect oral lesions. A change to injection administration may be necessary. However, parenteral preparations are also irritating and sites for injection or implantation should be monitored for inflammation.

The client should also be assessed for nausea, fever, acneiform skin lesions, and jaundice. The nurse must monitor laboratory reports for abnormalities in thyroid function, glucose tolerance, creatinine and electrolyte levels, cholesterol levels, and clotting fac-

tors. The physician must be informed of abnormal changes. Marked deviations from normal do not usually occur when drugs are used for replacement, since tissue hormone levels seldom exceed those found with normal autogenous production.

Client education. When hormone therapy is initiated, clients should be instructed to report priapism promptly. If it occurs, drug doses are temporarily discontinued and reinstituted later at a reduced dose. Persistent priapism is associated with subsequent, sometimes permanent, impotency and must be avoided.

A reduction in urinary stream, hesitancy, or other difficulty in voiding must also be reported, since prostatic hypertrophy sufficient to interfere with patency of the urethra is likely to occur when male hormones are administered to deficient people.

Clients should be taught how to administer the prescribed drugs. If IM doses are required, injection technique must be learned. Clients must also be taught the signs and symptoms indicative of therapeutic response and of hormone excesses, with specific instructions regarding data that must be reported to the health care team.

Evaluation Data required for evaluation include development of secondary sex characteristics (beard, muscle size and strength, deepening of the voice) and the absence or incidence of adverse drug reactions and their severity. Reports from the client of improved sexual function indicate therapeutic response to the drugs. Improved self-concept may be manifested by an increase in positive comments about self, a decrease in negative comments about self, improved personal grooming and dress, or a more erect posture and striding gait. The client's knowledge about his condition and treatment is reflected by his ability to discuss these knowledgeably and his compliance with the drug regimen.

Nursing process: care of clients who receive anabolic steroids

Assessment Clients who are to receive anabolic steroids usually have chronic or severe debilitating diseases such as cancer. The nurse must assess the client's status in relation to this condition, particularly tissue wasting and other evidence of malnutrition.

Although the physician retains the primary responsibility for screening clients before prescribing male hormone therapy, the nurse must be alert to and report signs and symptoms of contraindications of which the physician may not be informed.

Nursing diagnosis Diagnoses likely to be made for clients who take anabolic steroids include the following:

Altered tissue integrity: muscle wasting (emaciation, cachexia) related to increased catabolism secondary to a chronic debilitating disease condition
Altered comfort: nausea or fever related to adverse drug reaction
Pain related to calcium renal stones due to hypercalcemia secondary to anabolic steroid therapy
High risk for sexual dysfunction related to persistent priapism secondary to male hormone excesses
Altered urinary elimination: retention related to prostatic hypertrophy secondary to male hormone therapy

A common collaborative problem that should be differentiated from the nursing diagnoses is

Potential complication: hemorrhage

Planning   The goals of treatment are increased muscle mass and prevention or prompt detection and treatment of adverse drug reactions.

Intervention   If anabolic therapy is to be successful in rebuilding tissue, the client must have adequate nutritional intake. The diet should be high in protein, minerals (except calcium), and vitamins. Calories should be adequate to prevent metabolism of protein nutrients for energy.

Stress should be reduced to a minimum, because stress hormones are generally catabolic and reduce anabolic response to the androgenic hormones. Unnecessary environmental stressors should be eliminated and measures taken to promote rest and relaxation.

To monitor therapeutic response to the drugs, the client should be regularly weighed and tested for muscle strength.

Clients should be monitored for signs and symptoms of adverse drug reaction. Significant laboratory data include decreased thyroid function, abnormal fasting blood sugars, increased creatinine level, electrolyte imbalances (especially hypercalcemia), and reduced levels of clotting factors. Nurses must watch the client for signs of abnormal bleeding: petechiae, occult blood in stool or urine, pink-tinged sputum after oral care, or nosebleeds. Urinary retention or priapism should also be reported. Some degree of masculinization is expected in females; if these are distressing to the client, the physician should be consulted and alternative therapy considered. A glucocorticoid is sometimes ordered to control fever.

Client education.   Many clients with chronic debilitating diseases are often cared for at home with the support of home nursing services. This fact increases the need for teaching of the client and family. They must be taught the information and skills necessary to effectively manage the drug regimen. Anabolic drugs are usually administered orally. The teaching program must address toxic and side effects of anabolic steroids.

Abundant fluids are needed by clients with increased serum calcium to aid in excretion of the mineral and to decrease the risk of obstipation and calcium stone formation in the urinary tract. Blood levels of calcium should be monitored at regular intervals. Marked hypercalcemia must be reported immediately, since this can lead to cardiac arrest in systole that responds poorly to resuscitation attempts.

Other adverse reactions that must be reported to the health care team include fever and jaundice.

Diabetics who receive male hormone drugs tend to be unstable and should be cautioned against loss of control during anabolic therapy.

Athletes and aspiring athletes should be warned of the dangers of male hormone abuse. The nurse should stress the value of regular intense training for body building.

Evaluation   Data required for evaluation include the absence or incidence of adverse drug reaction and its severity. Therapeutic response is indicated by increases in body weight, muscle mass, and muscle strength. Successful teaching is inferred by the ability of the client and family to manage and comply with the drug regimen. On a short-term basis, teaching can be evaluated by the ability of the client or family to repeat back to the nurse information conveyed during teaching sessions and to demonstrate proper technique in performing procedures taught by the nurse.

Checklist of nursing actions

☐ Warn clients of the risks of inappropriate use of male hormones as "body builders" or aphrodisiacs.

When male hormones are used as replacement therapy

☐ Monitor clients who receive male hormones for response to treatment and evidence of toxicity.
☐ Monitor clients for tissue irritation at administration sites.
☐ When hormones are administered buccally or sublingually, promote good oral hygiene.
☐ Teach clients and their families about anabolic male hormone therapy, including expected therapeutic response (specific to the individual client's situation), administration of the drugs, and signs and symptoms of adverse drug reactions.
☐ Reinforce a masculine self-image in clients.
☐ Warn the client to report priapism promptly.

When anabolic hormones are prescribed

☐ Assess client for contraindications for treatment (pregnancy, and heart, liver, or kidney disease).

☐ Recommend a diet high in protein, minerals, and vitamins, adequate in calories, and ample in fluids.

☐ Protect clients from undue stress.

☐ Monitor serum calcium levels and report excesses promptly to the physician.

☐ Monitor diabetics for increased severity of the disease.

Male hormone antagonists

With the exception of the female sex hormones and spironolactone, no male hormone antagonists are approved for medicinal use. However, substances that would inhibit or reverse the effects of male hormones could be useful in treating such conditions as virilization in women, precocious puberty, and cancer of the prostate. They may also function as male contraceptives. Such drugs could act by a number of mechanisms: inhibition of endogenous male hormone production, inhibition of pituitary gonadotropin, inactivation of free serum testosterone, or inhibition of tissue use of androgens. A number of experimental drugs are discussed briefly (Table 32-7).

Estrogens and progestogens

Both estrogens and progestogens (and their analogues and derivatives) are natural antagonists of the male hormones. The estrogens appear to antagonize testosterone at the tissue level and also inhibit pituitary gonadotropin secretion. Their feminizing effects limit their clinical usefulness in males. One estrogen, chlorotrianisene, has been widely used for the treatment of cancer of the prostate, a disease that affects males in late maturity. The seriousness of the disease and the effectiveness of the drug in controlling tumor growth

justify the use of this drug despite its effects on sexuality.

Spironolactone

Spironolactone, a potassium-sparing diuretic, has anti-androgenic properties and has been used to treat female hirsutism caused by idiopathic hyperandrogenism. The drug can disrupt menstruation (causing metrorrhagia) and is best given only on days 4 through 24 of the woman's cycle (Helfer, et al, 1988).

Leuprolide

Leuprolide (Lupron, Euflex) is a gonadotropin-releasing hormone analog that inhibits the production of ovarian and testicular hormones. It is used with flutamide for the treatment of cancer of the prostate. When leuprolide treatment is initiated, a brief "disease flare" occurs before a therapeutic effect begins. This exacerbation of symptoms is reduced by concurrent administration of flutamide (see below).

Investigational drugs

Flutamide

Flutamide (Enlexin) is a testosterone antagonist thought to act by competitive inhibition at the level of testosterone receptors on cell membranes. It is used in conjunction with leuprolide in the treatment of cancer of the prostate. In clinical trials, survival times were better among subjects who took both drugs than among those who took leuprolide alone. Flutamide can cause hepatitis (Drug update, 1989).

Cyproterone acetate

Investigation continues with the goal of developing other androgen antagonists, but none are presently approved for wide clinical use. One substance, cyproterone acetate, appears to be effective in several conditions and is being tested for safety. It has been used in combination with estrogens as a female con-

Table 32-7. Male hormone antagonists

Drug name	Therapeutic uses	Adverse reactions
Estrogens:		
chlortrianisene	Treatment of cancer of the prostate	Feminization and inhibition of sexual function
spironolactone	Control of female hirsutism	Metrorrhagia
cyproterone acetate	Treatment of precocious puberty (in children of both sexes)	Stunting of growth
	Control of hirsutism and virilization in women	Acne, thinning of hair
	Control of severe sexual deviance in males	Acne, baldness
flutamide (Enlexin)	Used in conjunction with treatment of cancer of the prostate	Feminization and inhibition of sexual function
ketaconazol (Nizoral)	Treatment of cancer of the prostate	Feminization and inhibition of sexual function

traceptive. Cyproterone has also been used to treat precocious puberty in both sexes, hirsutism and virilization in females, and severe sexual deviance in males. In the latter, sexuality virtually disappears after 10 to 14 days of treatment. This effect reverses 2 weeks after discontinuation of the drug. Cyproterone has some progestational action and causes inhibition of pituitary gonadotropin secretion. It can stunt growth when administered to immature individuals. Acne and baldness in both sexes have also been caused by this drug.

Although this type of therapy has obvious drawbacks, research continues, and it is likely that effective, and/or relatively safe androgen antagonists will appear on the market in the near future.

Female sex hormones

Estrogens and progestogens are the hormones responsible for the normal development and function of the female reproductive system. Like androgens, these chemicals are produced by both men and women, but they are present in much greater amounts in the female, the ovaries and placenta being their primary natural sources. The amounts secreted vary widely with the rhythms of the menstrual cycle, pregnancy, and lactation, with relative proportions of and interplay between these two kinds of chemicals controlling the progressive changes in the body necessary to promote and sustain pregnancy.

Estrogens

Physiology. Estrogens are produced by the ovary, placenta, testes, adrenal cortex, and through peripheral conversion of testosterone and androstenedione. Production in the female fluctuates during the menstrual cycle with daily secretion varying from 60 to 400 μg. During pregnancy, estrogen levels increase steadily, and near term daily production may reach 50 mg.

Estrogens are responsible for the normal maturation of the female genital tract and the development and maintenance of feminine secondary sex characteristics. Under the influence of these compounds, the uterus, fallopian tubes, vagina, and external genitalia rapidly increase in size during puberty. Fat is deposited in the mons pubis and labia majora, the vaginal epithelium becomes more stratified, and the endometrium proliferates. The girl's general appearance changes as the breasts enlarge, the pelvis widens, the skin thickens (while remaining soft and smooth), pigmentation increases, and hair develops in the axillae and pubic region. Like androgens in the male, estrogens stimulate pronounced skeletal growth, while at the same time promoting closure of the epiphyses.

Estrogens affect several metabolic processes in the body. They promote retention of calcium and phosphate and their use in the formation of bone. Protein synthesis is stimulated—especially in the uterus, breasts, bone, and fatty tissues—but the anabolic effect of estrogens is less pronounced than those of androgens. The metabolic rate rises slightly and the kidneys retain more sodium. In large amounts, estrogens inhibit glucose metabolism and favor the development of diabetes mellitus. The hormones also increase blood levels of high-density lipoproteins (HDL) and decrease those of low-density (LDL) and very low density proteins (VLDL), probably by enhancing the excretion of cholesterol in the bile.

During childbearing years, estrogen levels fluctuate regularly in response to pituitary gonadotropins, which control the menstrual cycle. As the ovarian follicle develops and matures, the ovary secretes estrogen in increasing amounts. After ovulation, secretion drops slightly but is maintained at a relatively high level until the last week of the cycle, when it drops precipitously. The sequence of endometrial stimulation followed by withdrawal of estrogen induces menstrual flow in females.

Estrogens are produced in large quantities by the placenta during pregnancy. Many of the metabolic effects of these hormones favor the nurturing of the fetus. Estrogens increase serum levels of prothrombin and clotting factors VII, VIII, IX, and X, enhancing the coagulability of the blood. This effect is progressive, with the tendency toward clotting rising steadily during continuous or repeated exposure to high levels of the hormones. By the end of a normal-term pregnancy, considerable protection against severe hemorrhage is enjoyed by the expectant mother. This helps limit blood loss at the time of parturition.

Some estrogens function in part as antiestrogens. For example, by occupying receptor sites and blocking the action of the more potent hormone estradiol, estriol can reduce total estrogen response in the body.

Drug preparations. The natural forms of estrogens—estrone, estradiol and estriol—are mostly converted to estriol by the body. Estradiol, the most potent of these compounds, is secreted in large amounts by the ovary. It is available for drug use both in its natural form and as modified by esterification (Table 32-8). Several orally active nonsteroidal estrogens are also available, the most widely used of which is diethylstilbestrol. Though not a steroid, this chemical resembles the steroid nucleus topographically, and on radiographic analysis the molecular structure appears similar to estradiol.

Estrogens that are used as drugs are marketed as tablets and capsules for oral use, injectable solutions, transdermal patches, vaginal creams and suppositories, and pellets for subcutaneous implantation.

Pharmacodynamics. Estrogenic drug preparations elicit all of the physiologic changes produced by endogenous hormones. They stimulate or maintain the development of female sex characteristics (*eg*, well

Table 32-8. Estrogenic and antiestrogenic drugs

Drug name	Preparations	Usual adult dosage
Natural hormones		
estradiol (Brevicon, Demulen, Diane, Estinyl, Loestrin, Microgynon, Minestrin, Min-Ovral, Neo-Mens, Norlestrin, Ortho, Ovral, Synphasic, Triphasil, Triquilar)	Oral tablets	For replacement therapy in female hormone deficiency: 0.05 mg, 1–3 times daily for 2 wk followed by progesterone for 2 wk to complete an arbitrary theoretical menstrual cycle For the management of menopausal symptoms: 0.02–0.05 mg/day in a cyclic regimen (21 consecutive days followed by 7 drug-free days) For palliative treatment of metastatic carcinoma of the breast in selected postmenopausal women: 1 mg, tid For the palliative treatment of carcinoma of the prostate: 0.15–2 mg/day PC: X
estradiol (Estrace)	Oral tablets	For replacement therapy in female hormone deficiency and for management of menopausal symptoms: 1–2 mg/day For palliative treatment of carcinoma of the breast in selected men and postmenopausal women: 10 mg, tid For palliative treatment of carcinoma of the prostate: 1–2 mg, tid
(Estraderm)	Skin patch	For management of menopausal symptoms: 0.05 mg twice weekly PC: X
estradiol cypionate (Depanate, Depestro, depGynogen, Depo-Estradiol Cypionate, Depogen, Dura-Estrin, E-Ionate PA, Estra-D, Estro-Cyp, Estroject-LA)	Solution in oil for IM injection	For replacement therapy in female hormone deficiency: 1.5–2 mg q1mo For the management of menopausal symptoms: 1–5 mg, q3–4wk PC: X
estradiol valerate (Delestrogen, Dioval, Duragen, Dura-Estradiol, Estradiol L.A., Estra-L, Estate, Estraval, Feminate, Femogex, Gynogen L.A., Progynova, Valergen)	Solution in oil for IM injection	For replacement therapy in female hormone deficiency and for management of menopausal symptoms: 10–20 mg, q4wk For prevention of postpartum breast engorgement: 10–25 mg at the end of the first stage of labor For the palliative treatment of carcinoma of the prostate: 30 mg or more q1–2wk PC: X
polyestradiol phosphate (Estradurin)	Solution for IM injection	For the palliative treatment of carcinoma of the prostate: 40 mg, q2–4wk PC: X
conjugated estrogens (C.E.S. Congest, Premarin)	Oral tablets Solution for IM or IV injection Vaginal cream	*Oral:* For replacement therapy in female hormone deficiency: 2.5–7.5 mg/day for 20 consecutive days, followed by 10 days without the drug (an oral progestogen is added to the regimen the last 5 days of drug treatment); alternatively: 1.25 mg/day for 21 days, followed by 7 days without the drug For the management of menopausal symptoms: 0.3–1.25 mg/day for 21 days, followed by 7 days without the drug For the prevention of postpartum breast engorgement: 3.75 mg, q4h for 5 doses, or 1.25 mg, q4h for 5 days For the palliative treatment of carcinoma of the breast in selected men and postmenopausal women: 10 mg, tid For the palliative treatment of carcinoma of the prostate 1.25–2.5 mg, tid *IM or IV:* For the emergency treatment of abnormal uterine bleeding caused by hormone imbalance: 25 mg, q6–12h *Vaginally:* For treatment of atrophic vaginitis or kraurosis vulvae: 2–4 g of vaginal cream daily for 21 days, followed by 7 days without the drug PC: X
Estrone		
estrone (Bestrone, Estronol, Femogen, Kestrone, Oestrilin, Theelin Aqueous)	Suspensions for IM injection	For replacement therapy in female hormone deficiency: 0.1–1 mg, q1wk For the management of menopausal symptoms: 0.1–0.5 mg, 2–3 times weekly For the palliative treatment of carcinoma of the prostate: 2–4 mg, 2–3 times weekly PC: X

(Continued)

Table 32-8. Estrogenic and antiestrogenic drugs (Continued)

Drug name	Preparations	Usual adult dosage
Estrone		
esterified estrogens (Estratab, Evex, Menest, Menrium)	Oral tablets	For replacement therapy in female hormone deficiency: 2.75–7.5 mg/day for 21 days, followed by 7 days without the drug or 20 days followed by 10 days without the drug PC: X
		For the management of menopausal symptoms: 0.3–3.75 mg/day for 21 days, followed by 7 days without the drug
		For the palliative treatment of carcinoma of the breast in selected men and postmenopausal women: 10 mg, tid
		For the palliative treatment of carcinoma of the prostate: 1.25–2.5 mg, 1–3 times daily PC: X
estropipate (Ogen)	Oral tablets Vaginal cream	*Oral:* For replacement therapy in female hormone deficiency: 1.5–9 mg/day for 21 days, followed by 8–10 days without the drug; for management of menopausal symptoms: 0.75–6 mg/day for 21 days, followed by 7 days without the drug
		Vaginally: For treatment of atrophic vaginitis or kraurosis vulvae: 2–4 g of 0.15% vaginal cream daily for 21 days, followed by 7 days without the drug PC: X
Synthetic nonsteroidal estrogens		
chlorotrianisene (Tace, TACE)	Oral capsules	For replacement therapy in female hormone deficiency: 12–25 mg/day for 21 days, followed by several days without the drug (dosage is resumed on the fifth day of induced uterine bleeding)
		For management of menopausal symptoms: 12–25 mg/day for 21 days, followed by 7 days without the drug
		For prevention of postpartum breast engorgement: 12 mg, qid for 7 days, or 50 mg, q6h for 6 doses, or 72 mg, tid for 2 days
		For inoperable advanced cancer of the prostate: 12–25 mg daily PC: X
dienestrol (DV, Estraguard, Ortho Dienestrol, Synestrol)	Vaginal cream and suppositories	For treatment of atrophic vaginitis or kraurosis vulvae: *Initial:* 6–12 g of 0.01% cream daily or 1–2 suppositories (0.7 mg–1.4 mg)/day, for 1–2 wk, followed by one-half the initial dosage for 1–2 additional weeks, *maintenance:* 6 g of 0.01% cream or 1 suppository (0.7 mg), 1–3 times weekly PC: X
diethylstilbestrol (Honvol)	Oral tablets and enteric-coated tablets	For replacement therapy in female hormone deficiency or the management of menopausal symptoms: 0.2–0.5 mg/day for 21 consecutive days, followed by 7 drug-free days
	Vaginal suppositories	For palliative treatment of carcinoma of the breast in selected men and postmenopausal women: 15 mg/day
		For palliative treatment of carcinoma of the prostate: *Initial:* 1–3 mg/day; *maintenance:* 1 mg/day PC: X
diethylstilbestrol diphosphate (Stilphostrol, Dymeric, Omifin, Serophene)	Oral tablets Solution for IV infusion	For palliative treatment of carcinoma of the prostate: *Initial (oral):* 50 mg, tid; *(IV):* 0.5 g, followed by 1 g/day for 5 or more days; *maintenance (oral):* 200 mg or more, tid; *(IV):* 0.25–0.5 g, 1–2 times weekly PC: X
Antiestrogenic drugs		
clomiphene (Clomid)	Oral tablets	For the treatment of infertility associated with inadequate production of pituitary gonadotropins: 50 mg/day for 5 days PC: X
tamoxifen (Alpha-Tamoxifen, Apo-Tamox, Nolvadex, Tamofen, Tamone)	Oral tablets	For palliative treatment of advanced carcinoma of the breast in postmenopausal women: 20–40 mg/day, divided in 2 doses PC: D

KEY: PC = pregnancy category. (The validity of pregnancy risk categories has not been established; see Chapter 16, p 216.)

developed genitalia, enlarged breasts, feminine fat deposition, hair distribution) and exert a weak anabolic effect. Metabolic effects include increased sodium and water retention, lowering of elevated serum concentrations of cholesterol and phospholipids, a moderate increase in anabolism, and increased coagulability of the blood. Estrogens also affect pituitary gonadotropins, inhibiting their secretion by a negative feedback system.

Pharmacokinetics. Natural unconjugated estrogens are inactivated in the GI tract and liver and are not effective when administered orally. Drug preparations with altered chemistry (synthetic conjugated and nonsteroidal compounds) may be administered orally. Most estrogens are metabolized promptly and must be administered one or more times a day. Chlorotrianisene, however, has a prolonged duration of action, owing to its storage in fatty tissue. Pellet implantations provide long-term treatment with a single dose, but absorption is gradual and slow and may be erratic. Withdrawal of the drug before the life of the pellet expires is rarely feasible because it requires removal of the pellet remnants. Topical applications are used when local (usually vaginal) effect is desired. Estrogens are readily absorbed from the skin and mucous membranes, and systemic effects from such use or exposure are not uncommon. The choice of drug preparation depends on convenience, cost, and reliability of the client as much as it depends on the therapeutic goal.

In the blood, estrogens are bound by sex hormone–binding globulin and albumin. They are metabolized by the liver, primarily by conjugation as sulfates and glucuronates. Some enter the enterohepatic circulation and thus are handled repeatedly by the liver. The end products of estrogen metabolism are excreted mainly by the kidneys.

Therapeutic uses

Hormone replacement. Deficiency of estrogens in adult women can produce such symptoms as "hot flashes" (subjective feelings of hyperthermia), flushing, inappropriate sweating, chilling sensations, and paresthesia that often takes the form of formication (sensations of ants crawling on the skin). Although the exact causes of these phenomena are not known, they are believed to be associated with hypersecretion of pituitary gonadotropins or gonadotropin–sex-hormone imbalances. The more severe and abrupt the withdrawal of estrogens, the more pronounced the symptoms. Young women of childbearing years who are surgically castrated exhibit the most pronounced symptoms. About 15% to 25% of women who experience natural menopause experience discomfort severe enough to prompt a request for medical help or advice. Administration of estrogens relieves the symptoms promptly. Hormone therapy also prevents the loss of femininity experienced with extended estrogen deficiency.

Estrogens have been administered to prevent the postmenopausal changes of aging that are associated with deficiency of these hormones. With increasing knowledge of the dangers of long-term estrogen therapy, this practice has become highly controversial. Some authorities argue that the aging skin, osteoporosis, vaginal atrophy, hirsutism, general decrease in femininity, and depression that develop in some postmenopausal women represent a true deficiency disease that warrants treatment. Others point out that many women suffer few if any severe problems at the climacteric and do not develop marked physiologic deficits as they grow older. Complicating the situation is the fact that some physiologic changes respond little or not at all to later hormone therapy once they are allowed to develop. Loss in height and "dowager's hump" due to collapse of osteoporotic bone are permanent, and vaginal atrophy and skin changes tend to persist. At present, most physicians apply the principle that the least amount of estrogens for the shortest time possible to relieve frank symptoms is the safest course. In the absence of definitive studies of hormone-deficient women, it is impossible to determine the true risks of complications for replacement therapy. Most toxicity studies to date have involved younger women who receive estrogens for contraceptive purposes and who experience abnormally high hormone levels as a result.

Estrogens are also administered to promote sexual maturation in girls who suffer from primary gonadal failure. In some of these girls, the estrogen deficiency is part of a more complex condition such as Turner's syndrome, which also involves dwarfism. Long-lasting injected forms of estrogen are often used in this type of treatment. The drugs induce full development of the reproductive tract and feminization. Unfortunately, significant growth may not occur before the epiphyses close and linear bone growth ceases.

Contraception. Estrogen and estrogen–progestogen preparations are extremely popular forms of contraception. Contraceptive uses of estrogens are discussed in detail in Chapter 38.

Treatment of disease. Estrogens have been used clinically to relieve dysmenorrhea, endometriosis, dysfunctional uterine bleeding, and acne. For most conditions, the same preparations and schedules of administration can be used as for contraception. The drugs serve to regularize and control endometrial changes through the cycle, relieving discomfort and preventing excessive blood loss. Their benefits in acne appear to stem from their antiandrogenic effects. Given the undesirable risks of estrogens, some physicians are reluctant to use them in such conditions until other therapeutic approaches have been exhausted. When oral contra-

Estrogen replacement therapy (ERT) for postmenopausal women

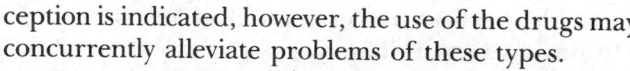

Pros

The postmenopausal condition is a true hormone deficiency.

ERT relieves most signs and symptoms of menopause (*eg*, hot flashes, paresthesia, depression).

ERT helps prevent the development of osteoporosis, muscle atrophy, and atherosclerosis in older women.

ERT maintains secondary sex characteristics in women, preserving a more youthful appearance.

Cons

Menopause is a natural event in the female life cycle.

Estrogens tend to increase the frequency and severity of migraine headaches, seizures, asthma, and renal and heart disease.

ERT increases the risk of cancer of the body of the uterus, thromboembolic disease, and diabetes mellitus.

ERT may stimulate the growth of malignant tumors of the female genital tract (ovarian, cervical, and breast cancer).

---

ception is indicated, however, the use of the drugs may concurrently alleviate problems of these types.

Excessive hirsutism in females may also respond to estrogen therapy. Treatment with cortisol is usually tried first, but if this approach is not effective, a year's course of estrogen treatment is initiated. Termination of treatment too early limits therapeutic response.

Hormone-dependent malignancies that respond to estrogens include breast cancer in postmenopausal women and cancer of the prostate in men. The presence of cytoplasmic estrogen receptors in the tumor cells increases the likelihood of response to this hormone treatment. Estrogen therapy is palliative rather than curative and may not significantly prolong life span. Combined hormone and antineoplastic regimens may be more effective than hormones alone.

Estrogens are used to suppress lactation in postpartum women and in those in whom lactation persists during weaning. Only a short term of treatment is required to interrupt breast function and prevent the discomforts associated with nonpharmacologic methods to terminate milk production.

Adverse reactions. Estrogens are considered among the most toxic of hormone drugs. This fact may be a consequence of widespread use of the compounds for fertility control, which has provided many client-years of exposure for observation of toxic and side effects. Because some effects of the drugs are life-threatening, their use even for therapeutic purposes tends to be much more cautious today than before the development of oral contraceptives. A review of adverse reactions helps to elucidate the guidelines and precautions exercised in present day practice.

Effects on females. When used for contraception in women, exogenous estrogens are superimposed onto endogenous supplies, producing body levels above those normally present in the nongravid woman. In these concentrations, the chemicals produce many of the changes characteristic of pregnancy. Nausea and occasional vomiting, dizziness, headache, breast discomfort, weight gain, and sodium and water retention are most prominent during the first few weeks of therapy. These effects tend to subside with continued administration. Changes in pigmentation may produce chloasma (the "mask of pregnancy") and darkening of the linea alba. Glucose tolerance decreases, and diabetes mellitus tends to develop in susceptible women. Corneal sensitivity increases and may preclude the use of contact lenses. The hormones inhibit pituitary secretion of gonadotropins and ovulation, causing, in this case of course, the desired therapeutic effect.

One of the most dangerous effects of estrogen excesses is the increased risk of thromboembolic phenomena. The tendency toward hypercoagulability rises steadily with continuing therapy, increasing the risk of phlebitis, thromboembolism, and cerebral and coronary thrombosis. The death rate from these disorders is significantly greater in women who receive contraceptive hormones than in normal nongravid women, but it remains considerably lower than that of pregnancy. The risk is greatest in older women and those who smoke, two factors that appear to enhance the detrimental effects of estrogens.

Estrogens also exert a carcinogenic and teratogenic effect. A history of prolonged or high levels of the hormones is associated with increased incidence of endometrial cancer in postmenopausal women. Although not yet implicated in the etiology of other human malignancies, the hormones are known to cause cancer in animals. They also stimulate the growth of most preexisting tumors that affect the female genital tract, including ovarian, cervical, and breast cancer. Congenital limb deformities, cryptorchidism, and masculinization of the fetus have been attributed to use of estrogens by expectant mothers. (Excess estrogens can be converted to androgens by metabolic processes in the body.) Among people whose mothers were given diethylstilbestrol to prevent abortion during their gestation, the incidence of vaginal cancer in females and genital malformations in males is significantly greater than in the nonexposed population.

Estrogens predispose to gallbladder disease. The hormone appears to increase the concentration of cholesterol in bile, favoring the formation of stones. Administration of the hormones increases the incidence of cholelithiasis and cholecystitis in both men and women. A similar risk affects women who experience several pregnancies in rapid succession. Liver function tests are altered by the drugs, and the risk of cholestatic jaundice is increased.

Because they increase levels of renin and angiotensin, estrogens favor sodium and water retention and induce tissue edema. They tend to increase the frequency and severity of migraine headaches, epilepsy, asthma, and renal and heart disease. When estrogen levels are high, the body's need for several nutrients (vitamin C, folate, and pyridoxine) rises. Folate absorption declines; the physiologic mechanisms that cause vitamin C and pyridoxine deficits are poorly understood.

Although estrogens induce a feeling of well-being when administered to deficient women, high levels tend to produce depression. In susceptible people, this may progress to psychotic dimensions.

When estrogens are used alone in cyclical therapy to mimic the normal menstrual cycle, mid-cycle ("breakthrough") bleeding can occur. This has been attributed to excessive endometrial proliferation in response to the stimulus of the estrogens. The addition of progesterone to the regimen often corrects this problem (see Chapter 38).

Effects on males. Males who are treated with estrogens experience reversal of secondary sex characteristics and impotence. The testes and phallus atrophy, the beard thins, and the breasts enlarge. Scalp hair may regrow in areas affected by male pattern baldness (the expression of this genetic trait depends on the influence of androgens, which are inhibited by estrogens). The body assumes feminine contours as deposition of fats conforms to female patterns.

Precautions and contraindications. Estrogen therapy is contraindicated during pregnancy and in women with a history of genital tract cancer. Because they are secreted in breast milk and tend to suppress lactation, they are not prescribed while breast-feeding is in progress. They must be used with caution when a history of cardiovascular disease (especially thromboemboli), liver or renal disease, migraine, epilepsy, or depression exists. Care must be exercised when treating immature females to minimize undesirable stunting of growth.

■ Summary
Estrogens are female sex hormones produced by the ovary, placenta, and adrenal cortex. They are necessary for normal female development and sexual function. Their metabolic effects include sodium and fluid retention, increased coagulability of the blood, and a moderate increase in anabolism. Numerous hormone preparations are on the market. They are prescribed for hormone-replacement therapy, for contraception, and to treat hormone-sensitive malignancies. Estrogen therapy increases the risk of gallbladder and thromboembolic disease, hypertension, cancer, and congenital defects in fetuses. Males who receive these drugs become feminized. Contraindications for their use include pregnancy, lactation, and cancer of the female genital tract.

Nursing management
Nursing implications: therapy in postmenopausal women

The controversy among medical practitioners over the advisability of prescribing estrogens for postmenopausal women has been disturbing to the public. Many women are aware that some physicians are reluctant to use these drugs, whereas other physicians are not. Some women who wish to receive supplemental hormones "shop" until they find a physician who is willing to prescribe them.

Certainly, the adverse effects caused by the drugs make caution advisable. Eventually, perhaps, optimum hormone levels will be established, and women will be monitored by serum assay to determine their need for therapy. At present, the decision to give estrogen therapy requires careful assessment for evidence of hormone depletion and consideration of personal risk factors for adverse reaction. The decision whether or not to use the drugs should be made jointly by the woman and her doctor.

Estrogens were the first drugs for which the FDA ruled that information must be provided to the recipient concerning the risks of use. By law, brochures that contain this information are required to be packaged with the drugs. The principle that the consumer should be informed of potential risk appears to be gaining recognition, since similar regulations are now in effect for other drugs.

Nursing process

Assessment When hormone therapy is under consideration, clients should be carefully assessed for the need for therapy and risk for adverse reaction. Both the client and the physician should weigh expected benefits against possible risks before deciding in favor of or against treatment.

Not all postmenopausal women need hormones. Most women experience no noticeable distress from menopause. A minority are plagued by frequent hot flashes or dyspareunia. Clients sometimes attribute emotional problems to menopause, but the degree to which hormonal imbalance is a factor is not known. At this stage of life, women may experience many stressors that hormone therapy is unlikely to influence.

Hormone levels in postmenopausal women vary considerably. Evidence suggests that fat tissue plays a role in estrogen metabolism; women with ample fat deposits appear to retain higher levels of these hormones than thinner women. This relative protection from estrogen deficiency is associated with an increased incidence of uterine cancer, hypertension, and diabetes.

Women with a family history of postmenopausal problems, such as dowager's hump or brittle bones, are at high risk for osteoporosis, especially if body build is slight and lifestyle does not include active weight-bearing exercise. Other factors believed to contribute to the risk of osteoporosis are an inadequate calcium intake throughout life and repeated use of weight-reduction diets. The development of strong bone structure during childhood and its maintenance during the childbearing years is believed to reduce the risk of osteoporosis. Rapid weight loss is accompanied by acidosis and aciduria, which increases calcium loss in urine. Women at high risk for osteoporosis should not be allowed to become hormone deficient, because this condition is difficult to arrest once it has begun.

Women at high risk for early cardiovascular disease include those with a family history of such disease occurring in females soon after menopause. Other risk factors are diabetes mellitus, hypothyroidism, high serum cholesterol, and obesity. Hormone replacement therapy is believed to delay the onset of cardiovascular disease, owing to its effect on HDL, which it increases.

Pregnancy must be ruled out before estrogens are prescribed. Other contraindications include a history of intravascular thrombosis ("phlebitis," coronary thrombosis, cerebral thrombosis) and malignancies of the female reproductive organs.

Surgical castration before menopause, premature menopause, and evidence of rapid or severe hormone depletion are indications for treatment. These clients are at lower risk for adverse drug reactions. The lowest effective dose is given to maintain femininity and prevent deficiency symptoms. For these women, the need for hormones is undisputed, and therapy should be continued without interruption at least until the normal age of menopause.

Nursing diagnosis Nursing diagnoses of postmenopausal women who are candidates for sex-hormone therapy include the following:

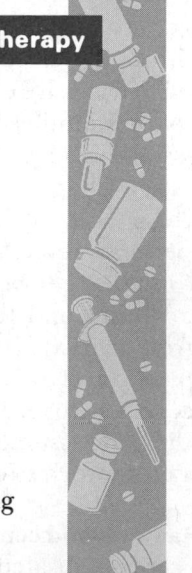

Issues in drug therapy

Factors that influence osteoporosis in postmenopausal women

Increased risk factors	Decreased risk factors
Short stature	Tall stature
Slender body type	Muscular body type
Small bone structure	Large bone structure
Dark complexion	Fair complexion
Smoking	Nonsmoking
Excessive alcohol intake	Abstinence or moderate alcohol use
Low calcium intake (throughout the life span)	High calcium intake (throughout the life span)
Sedentary lifestyle *or* a history of strenuous exercise associated with amenorrhea	Active lifestyle, including weight-bearing exercise

High risk for injury related to osteoporosis secondary to sex-hormone deficiency
Potential for sexual dysfunction: dyspareunia related to vaginal atrophy secondary to sex-hormone deficiency
Altered comfort: hot flashes related to vasomotor instability secondary to sex hormone deficiency

A common collaborative problem that should be differentiated from the nursing diagnoses is

Potential complication: cardiovascular degeneration

Collaborative problems that arise from hormone therapy are most likely in young women with normal endogenous hormone production, but they can arise in other recipients, even in men who receive the drugs for antineoplastic chemotherapy. Potential complications include the following:

Potential complication: thrombi or thromboemboli
Potential complication: cholecystitis

Many clients are likely to have a

Knowledge deficit regarding female reproduction, sex hormones, and drug therapy that involves female sex hormones

Planning Goals of nursing care are to avoid pregnancy, prevent osteoporosis and cardiovascular degeneration, preserve sexual function, and prevent or promptly detect adverse reactions to hormone therapy, such as malignant tumor growth, cholecystitis, or intravascular clotting. An additional goal is to eliminate the knowledge deficit by teaching clients about female reproduction and use of sex hormones.

Intervention During therapy, clients should be monitored for both therapeutic response and adverse reaction to the prescribed hormones. Most physicians prescribe only a 6-month supply of hormones at a time, ensuring that the client return for examination before the drug supply is renewed. (The nursing care of clients who use oral contraceptives is discussed in detail in Chapter 38.) When vaginal atrophy is the only manifestation of estrogen deficiency, the use of an estrogenic vaginal cream often is effective. The drug exerts its greatest effect on the local tissues, and systemic effect is minimized. Absorption does occur, however, and systemic effects may be evident. Such creams cannot be used when estrogens are contraindicated, as in women with a history of genital cancer. When estrogens are to be applied topically, they should be administered at regular intervals.

Any woman who receives estrogenic drugs on a regular basis should be closely monitored for signs and symptoms of adverse reactions, including the develop-ment of breast or uterine malignancy, cholecystitis, and phlebitis. Because uterine (especially endometrial) cancer can occur late in life, pap smears for cytologic examination should be continued regularly for life.

Emotional support. Regardless of the degree to which hormone depletion adds to emotional lability at this stage in life, the menopausal woman often needs help in maintaining emotional health. At this time, many women become acutely conscious of the effects that age has had on their physical appearance, energy levels, and life goals. Most children either have left home or soon will. The energy previously invested in nurturing the family must be diverted to other pursuits. In many families, menopause in the mother coincides not only with the "emptying of the nest" but with a similar midlife crisis in the father. The influences of hormone depletion on emotional balance simply add to the normally high stress level at this time. The nurse can help the family adapt to changed circumstances and promote healthy coping mechanisms and interpersonal relationships. When appropriate, further family or individual counseling with a specialist in this field should be recommended.

Client education. For women considering the use of sex hormones, the nurse should provide the facts about the potential benefits and risks of therapy. Often, the use of estrogens is elective, and the client needs facts that will enable her to make an informed decision regarding consent to treatment.

Prepubertal girls should be told that estrogens induce maturation of the reproductive tract and feminization, but—depending on the underlying condition—fertility may not be attained. If dwarfism is part of the clinical picture, estrogens do not ensure growth to normal adult stature; rather, they tend to terminate growth after an initial growth spurt because of closure of the epiphyses.

Postpubertal women who receive cyclic estrogen therapy also require a careful orientation to the effects of the drugs. The risk of adverse reactions is greatest in these clients, because the addition of estrogens used as drugs to normal endogenous hormones raises the overall levels in the body. Alternatives to hormone therapy should be thoroughly explored, including other methods of contraception and the use of antibiotics and retinoic acid for acne.

Some women who desire hormone therapy may find that their physicians oppose such treatment. The nurse should inform the client of her right to seek medical care from another physician. If no absolute contraindication to hormone therapy exists, the client may desire referral to a physician with a more compatible viewpoint.

Menopausal women for whom replacement is contraindicated, or who wish to avoid the use of drugs, should be taught health practices that minimize the effects of hormone deficiency. A diet ample in calcium, combined with active exercise, helps prevent osteoporosis. Exercise also helps maintain serum levels of HDL and helps prolong the protective effects of these substances on the cardiovascular system. Limitation of cholesterol and saturated fats in the diet remains controversial. It should be recommended to people with a history of familial hypercholesterolemia, but it may be harmful to others.

Dressing in layers allows removal of some clothing when hot flashes occur. The client may also be told that such episodes tend to subside over time as the body adjusts to lower estrogen levels and as pituitary hyperactivity declines.

Excessive facial hair may be distressing. Simple solutions include shaving or the application of bleaching solutions to make the hair less noticeable. Electrolysis provides a more permanent solution, though the treatments are expensive, tedious, and uncomfortable. It is difficult to obliterate the hair follicle completely; only about half of the hairs treated at any one session are permanently eliminated.

Skin care may need to be revised. The skin tends to become drier in postmenopausal women than in women in their childbearing years. Women who had excessively oily skin in younger years are helped by this phenomenon. These women need to reduce their use of drying cosmetics and evaluate their skin carefully to determine its current needs. Those whose skin has previously been dry need to increase their protective measures. Exposure to the sun and low-humidity environments should be avoided. These women also probably have a greater need for lotions or ointments that help prevent the loss of natural skin oils. In most cases, soap should be used less frequently.

Education during therapy. Clients who receive estrogens need considerable education to understand the risks that such treatment entails, as well as the benefits that can realistically be expected. They must remain under close medical supervision and should be taught the signs and symptoms of adverse reactions and the need to report these promptly.

Clients should watch for and report any sudden weight gain, bloating, calf tenderness, pain on dorsiflexion, or unusual vaginal bleeding. Diabetic women should be told that glucose tolerance may decline while estrogens are in use. Smokers should be warned of the high risks of cardiovascular disease posed by concurrent use of estrogens and tobacco. This risk is compounded in older women. Cessation (or at least a reduction) of smoking should be urged. If the client is receptive, referral to a smokers' clinic is appropriate.

Women for whom topical therapy is prescribed should be cautioned against its use for lubrication before intercourse. The hormones are absorbed by the skin of the penis and may cause symptoms of reduced potency and some degree of feminization in the male partner. Application of the hormone after rather than before intercourse minimizes this effect. A water soluble lubricant can be recommended if vaginal secretion is not restored by hormone replacement. The use of condoms prevents absorption of hormones by the male partner if intercourse is desired after application of the medication.

When estrogens are given to men, they are usually prescribed to treat cancer of the prostate. Because the purpose of hormone manipulation is to eliminate androgenic stimulation, some degree of impotency and feminization is expected. In fact, if this does not occur, or if it abates, further treatment to eliminate androgens (orchidectomy or adrenalectomy) may be required. The client and his partner may need help coping with this disruption of sexual function. Alternatives to genital intercourse are acceptable to some couples. For others, referral to a surgeon for implantation of a penile prosthesis may be helpful. Such a device provides an artificial erection, which allows normal intercourse that is satisfying to both partners.

Checklist of nursing actions

☐ Evaluate women who are to receive estrogens for contraindications and factors that increase the risk of complications (pregnancy, lactation, history of genital cancer, phlebitis, hypertension, diabetes mellitus, and depression).

☐ Inform the client about the medication, the benefits to be expected, and the risks of the treatment.

☐ Assist the client who declines hormone replacement therapy to develop health practices that alleviate discomforts and minimize risk of complications due to hormone depletion.

☐ When estrogen vaginal cream is prescribed, instruct the client in techniques to prevent exposure of sexual partners to the drug.

☐ When estrogens are prescribed for males, counsel the client and his partner about ways to preserve their sexual relationship.

Diethylstilbestrol

Diethylstilbestrol (DES) is a synthetic estrogen that was used widely in the mid-20th century to treat threatened abortion (spontaneous premature termination of pregnancy) and cancer of the prostate in men. The drug later was found to be carcinogenic and teratogenic. Fetuses exposed to DES *in utero* were found, later in life, to have increased risk of genital malignancies (particularly cancer of the vagina in females) and congenital abnormalities. These progeny, now middle-aged, should be monitored throughout life for cancer of the genital tract.

Antiestrogens

In addition to the antiestrogenic effects of the weaker estrogens themselves, progestogens and androgens exhibit mild antiestrogenic properties. By binding to cytoplasmic estrogenic receptors, they prevent the more potent estrogens from occupying these sites.

Two potent antiestrogens available for clinical use in the U.S. are tamoxifen and clomiphene (Clomid; see Table 32-8).

Tamoxifen

Pharmacodynamics. Tamoxifen (Nolvadex) competes with estrogen for binding to cytoplasmic estrogen receptors and translocation into cell nuclei. Within the nucleus, the tamoxifen-receptor complex does not produce the characteristic effects of the estrogen-receptor complex. Only a weak estrogenic effect occurs, and that only with large doses. By blocking the formation of the more active estrogen-receptor complexes, tamoxifen greatly reduces estrogen responses.

Pharmacokinetics. Tamoxifen is administered orally. It is well absorbed from the GI tract and is subsequently concentrated in tissues rich in estrogen receptors, such as the uterus. The drug enters the enterohepatic circulation. It is metabolized, mainly by hydrolysis and conjugation. Metabolites are excreted in both feces and urine. Elimination half-life is more than 7 days. It is not known if tomaxifen is secreted in breast milk.

Therapeutic uses. Tamoxifen is used to treat advanced cancer (especially breast cancer) that involves tissues with high levels of estrogen receptors. Early use alone may induce a remission; it is also used after mastectomy and for palliation in metastatic breast cancer (Forrest, 1989). It is most effective in the treatment of postmenopausal clients, especially if metastases involve soft tissues.

Adverse reactions. The most frequent adverse reactions to tamoxifen are nausea, vomiting, and hot flashes. Use of the drug can stimulate pituitary gonadotropin production, causing ovulation. Vaginal bleeding or discharge, menstrual irregularities, pruritus vulvae, rash, leukopenia, and thrombocytopenia have occurred. Blood calcium levels may rise, especially in clients with bone metastases. Although tamoxifen is carcinogenic in animals, it has not been identified as a human carcinogen.

The most serious adverse reaction to tamoxifen is optic neuritis, which can permanently impair vision. Eye lesions associated with tamoxifen include papilledema, atrophy of the optic disc, white deposits on the cornea, and retinal vascular lesions. Although nonmutagenic, the use of tamoxifen during pregnancy may impair growth and development of the skeleton of the embryo.

Precautions and contraindications. Reduction in dosage alleviates most adverse reactions to tamoxifen. The drug should be discontinued in favor of other antineoplastic treatment when signs and symptoms of eye damage develop. Cortisone may be required to reduce inflammation in such cases.

The manufacturer recommends caution when tamoxifen is used to treat individuals with leukopenia and thrombocytopenia. Complete blood cell counts, including platelet counts, should be monitored regularly during tamoxifen therapy.

Tamoxifen is contraindicated during pregnancy and lactation.

Nursing management

Nursing implications

Most women who receive tamoxifen as antineoplastic therapy are postmenopausal. However, younger women may retain the ability to reproduce. If they do not have a dependable method of contraception, one should be instituted before drug therapy is initiated.

Nursing process

Assessment   Clients for whom tamoxifen therapy is considered should be evaluated for risk factors for adverse drug reactions. These include leukopenia, thrombocytopenia, and impaired vision. Pregnancy and lactation should be ruled out before drug therapy is initiated.

Nursing diagnosis   Nursing diagnoses likely to be made for clients who receive tamoxifen include the following:

> High risk for altered comfort: nausea and vomiting related to irritation secondary to tamoxifen therapy
> High risk for altered comfort: hot flashes related to vasomotor instability secondary to tamoxifen therapy
> High risk for altered comfort: pruritus vulvae and skin rash related to irritation and inflammation of tissues secondary to tamoxifen administration
> Knowledge deficit concerning antineoplastic therapy with the use of tamoxifen

Common collaborative problems that should be differentiated from the nursing diagnoses include

> Potential complication: thrombocytopenia and leukopenia
> Potential complication: visual impairment related to ophthalmic side effects of tamoxifen therapy

Planning Goals of nursing care include prompt detection and treatment of adverse drug reactions and education of the client about tamoxifen therapy.

Intervention During tamoxifen therapy, clients should be evaluated regularly for visual changes (especially papilledema), nausea, vomiting, hot flashes, rash, and pruritus. Laboratory reports of white blood cell and thrombocyte levels should be monitored. The physician should be notified of abnormal changes. The dosage of tamoxifen may be reduced or discontinued.

Client education. Clients should be taught the signs and symptoms of adverse reaction to tamoxifen and instructed to report these to the physician for adjustment in the drug regimen. Visual problems and unusual bleeding must be reported immediately.

Self-care measures to reduce nausea and vomiting should be explained to clients who experience these symptoms. The nurse may advise clients who have hot flashes to dress in layers to facilitate adjustments in clothing.

Evaluation Data required for evaluation include results of serial eye examinations, the incidence and severity of other adverse drug reactions, and the degree to which the client follows guidelines established during teaching sessions to manage the drug regimen.

Checklist of nursing actions

When tamoxifen is prescribed

☐ Assess visual function before drug therapy is initiated.

☐ Evaluate the client at each visit for adverse reaction to tamoxifen, particularly visual changes or bleeding.

☐ Monitor laboratory reports for leukopenia and thrombocytopenia.

☐ Report adverse reactions to the physician for adjustments in dosage or alternative treatment.

☐ Teach the client about tamoxifen therapy and its management.

Clomiphene

Pharmacodynamics. Clomiphene exerts both estrogenic and antiestrogenic effects. Its precise mechanism of action is unknown, but it appears to stimulate the release of pituitary gonadotropins. These compounds (follicle-stimulating hormone and luteinizing hormone) cause development and maturation of the ovarian follicle, ovulation, and development of the corpus luteum.

Pharmacokinetics. Clomiphene is administered orally and is absorbed readily from the GI tract. It circulates systemically but is rapidly disseminated from the blood without producing a high blood level. Studies suggest that it is stored in fat tissue and that it recycles through the enterohepatic circulation. Clomiphene is metabolized by the liver and is excreted slowly in feces through biliary elimination.

Therapeutic uses. Clomiphene is used to treat infertility caused by ovulatory dysfunction.

Adverse reactions. Adverse reactions to clomiphene include nausea, vomiting, CNS changes (dizziness, lightheadedness, fatigue), and abdominal discomfort: distention, bloating, and pain (especially at the time of ovulation). Jaundice and abnormal sulfobromophthalein retention have been reported.

Clomiphene can cause visual impairment characterized by intensification and prolongation of afterimages, blurring of vision, diplopia, scotomata, or photophobia. Visual changes are reversible and resolve within a few days or weeks after withdrawal of the drug.

Use of clomiphene results in an increased incidence of plural gestations (mainly twins, but including also births of 3 to 6 babies).

Precautions and contraindications. Before beginning a course of clomiphene therapy, clients should undergo a complete pelvic evaluation and assessment of visual function. Clomiphene should be discontinued and a complete ophthalmic evaluation performed if adverse visual signs or symptoms develop. Clients who receive the drug should be cautioned against performing hazardous tasks (such as operating powered machinery) that require mental alertness and physical coordination.

Contraindications for clomiphene therapy include presence of ovarian cysts, liver disease or a history of liver dysfunction, or abnormal uterine bleeding of unknown etiology.

Nursing management

Nursing implications

So-called "fertility" drugs such as clomiphene are usually not used until other causes of infertility are ruled out. Therefore, couples who resort to this therapy usually have experienced many months of testing and treatment in an effort to achieve pregnancy. For many, clomiphene therapy represents a final chance to have biologic children before resorting to adoption.

Nursing process

Assessment Each time a course of clomiphene therapy is planned, the client undergoes a complete pelvic evaluation. Visual function should also be tested to provide a baseline for comparison if changes occur during the course of treatment. The client's data base should include a complete reproductive and menstrual history, including specific information related to premenstrual syndrome, mittelschmerz, dysmenorrhea, pelvic disease, such as infection, ovarian cysts, or endometriosis, and prior use of contraceptives.

Nursing diagnosis Nursing diagnoses related to clomiphene therapy include the following:

> *Anxiety related to desire for children and to infertility*
> *Knowledge deficit concerning clomiphene and its use to stimulate ovulation*
> *Altered comfort: dizziness, lightheadedness, and fatigue related to CNS and visual changes secondary to clomiphene therapy*

A common collaborative problem that should be differentiated from the nursing diagnoses is

> *Potential complication: visual impairment related to ophthalmic side effects of clomiphene therapy*

Planning Goals of nursing care include reducing fear and anxiety, promptly detecting and treating adverse drug reactions, and teaching the client about clomiphene therapy.

Intervention Clients who resort to drugs to stimulate ovulation need considerable emotional support in their endeavor to achieve pregnancy. They and their spouses need reassurance that everything possible will be done to assist them. If several courses of treatment are followed without success, they may be advised to abandon their attempt and try adoption or adjustment to their present state. The nurse must be prepared to counsel them, or refer them for counseling, and, if they wish, to direct them to social agencies that handle adoption.

The nurse should assess the client at each visit for changes in vision or CNS function, as well as for signs and symptoms indicative of pregnancy. The drug should be discontinued and a complete ophthalmic examination arranged if visual changes develop.

Client education. The client should be informed about clomiphene, including the possibility of multiple births and adverse drug reactions. Any change in vision should be reported without delay to the physician. Other reactions should also be reported if they become severe. Clients should be cautioned against performing hazardous tasks (such as operating powered machinery) that require mental alertness and physical coordination while taking clomiphene.

Evaluation Data required for evaluation include reports or comments from the client that indicate emotional state, results of periodic assessments for visual and CNS changes, the incidence and severity of adverse drug reactions, and the degree to which the client follows the guidelines for drug management conveyed during teaching sessions.

Checklist of nursing actions

When clomiphene is prescribed
- [ ] Provide emotional support to couples who are undergoing treatment for infertility.
- [ ] Obtain a data base that includes visual function and a complete menstrual and reproductive history.
- [ ] Assess the client at each visit for signs and symptoms of pregnancy and adverse drug reaction.
- [ ] If visual changes develop, discontinue drug and contact the physician to arrange a complete ophthalmic evaluation.
- [ ] Teach the client the information necessary for proper management of clomiphene therapy.

Progestogens

Pharmacodynamics. Progesterone binds to a specific intracellular receptor protein. The progesterone-receptor complex then translocates to the nucleus, where it stimulates the synthesis of messenger RNA for ovalbumin, avidin, and other proteins. Because the number of progesterone cell receptor proteins fluctuates with estrogen levels, the effects of progesterone depend in part on adequate production of estrogen.

Progesterone is the natural hormone that protects the embryo and maintains pregnancy. During and after ovulation, its production by the follicle and corpus luteum promotes secretion by the mucous membranes of the fallopian tubes and endometrium. These secretions sustain the zygote should an ovum be fertilized. The hormone also changes the nature of endocervical secretion from the watery fluid that is characteristic of estrogenic stimulation to a scanty viscid material that forms the mucous plug of pregnancy. In the absence of fertilization, the abrupt decline of progesterone levels that follows degeneration of the corpus luteum precipitates menstruation. When pregnancy does occur, the corpus luteum maintains progesterone levels until the placenta develops, at which time hormone production is taken over by this organ. During gestation, progesterone suppresses uterine contractility and prevents immunologic rejections of the fetus by inhibiting the function of T lymphocytes. In conjunction with estrogen, this hormone stimulates proliferation of the acini of the breast in preparation for lactation. Both estrogens and progestogens inhibit the effects of prolactin, however, and lactation begins only after their levels drop after parturition.

Progesterone promotes a rise in body temperature of about 1°F during the secretory phase of the menstrual cycle. Detection of this change in basal temperature confirms ovulation and establishes the time of its occurrence. Progesterone increases renal sodium retention directly, but this effect is opposed by competitive inhibition of aldosterone, which results in a net effect of diuresis during short-term exposure. Progesterone tends to suppress pituitary gonadotropin production but does not prevent ovulation. It promotes tissue breakdown somewhat, having a catabolic effect similar to that of the glucocorticoids.

Pharmacokinetics. Natural progesterone is transported and metabolized at a rapid pace; its half-life in blood is only a few minutes. The chemical is held in tissue sites, where it continues to exert physiologic effects long after it has disappeared from the plasma. As compared to the low level of the follicular phase of the menstrual cycle, progesterone secretion and metabolism increases twofold to fourfold during the secretory phase of the menstrual cycle, and fiftyfold to seventyfold by the end of pregnancy. Levels drop precipitously at the times of menstruation and parturition.

Progesterone administered parenterally is rapidly absorbed and distributed in a manner similar to the handling of endogenous progesterone by the body.

Oral administration is much less effective than parenteral because progesterone is promptly transformed by the liver. The majority of such exogenous hormones are eliminated in the urine, but about one-tenth is excreted in the feces. The properties of synthetic and semisynthetic progestogens vary somewhat from those of progesterone. They are more effective when administered orally. Table 32-9 lists some of the progestogens used in practice.

Therapeutic uses. Progestogens are used therapeutically to terminate dysfunctional uterine bleeding, alleviate premenstrual tension and postpartum afterpains, suppress lactation, and prevent conception. They have been prescribed for toxemia in late pregnancy, for amenorrhea, and for the palliative treatment of some cancers. Progestogens help prevent abortion that is caused by inadequate luteal response to gonadotropin with inadequate progesterone secretion. This condition must be demonstrated by hormone assay, because the use of progestogens during

Table 32-9. Progestogenic drugs

Drug name	Preparations	Usual adult dosage
hydroxyprogesterone (Delalutin, Duralutin, Gesterol L.A., Hydrosterone, Hylutin, Hyprogest, Hyproval)	Solution in oil for IM injection	For the treatment of amenorrhea or abnormal uterine bleeding: 375 mg at 4-week intervals For the adjunctive and palliative treatment of advanced endometrial carcinoma: 1 g or more, 1–7 times weekly PC: X
medroxyprogesterone (Amen, Depo-Provera, Oragest, Provera)	Oral tablets Suspension for IM injection	For the treatment of amenorrhea or abnormal uterine bleeding: 5–10 mg/day, PO, for 5–10 days beginning on the 16th to 21st day of the menstrual cycle For the adjunctive and palliative treatment of endometrial or renal carcinoma: 400–1000 mg/week, IM PC: X
norethindrone (Norlutin)	Oral tablets	For the treatment of amenorrhea or abnormal uterine bleeding: 5–20 mg/day for 21 days (beginning on the 5th day of the menstrual cycle) PC: X
norethindrone acetate (Aygestin, Brevicon, Loestrin, Micronor, Minestrin, Noriday, Norinyl, Norlutate, Ortho, Ortho-Novum, Symphasic; *Can:* Norlestrin)	Oral tablets	For the treatment of endometriosis: 10–30 mg/day for 14 consecutive days (low dosages are used at first and may be increased with each cycle until maximum dosage is reached) For the treatment of amenorrhea or abnormal uterine bleeding: 2.5–10 mg/day for 21 days (beginning on the 5th day of the menstrual cycle) For the treatment of endometriosis: 5–15 mg/day for 14 consecutive days (low dosages are used at first and may be increased with each cycle until maximum dosage is reached) PC: X
norgestrel (Ovrette; *Can:* Ovral)	Oral tablets	For contraception: 0.075 mg/day PC: X
progesterone (Femotrone in Oil, Luteinol, Progelan in Oil, Progest 50 Oil, Progestaject-50, Progestosert)	Powder Solution in oil and suspension for IM injection	For treatment of amenorrhea: 5–10 mg/day for 6–8 days, beginning 8–10 days before the anticipated start of menstruation For the treatment of abnormal uterine bleeding: 5–10 mg/day for 6 days (sometimes preceded by 2 weeks of estrogen therapy) or a single 50–100-mg dose PC: X

KEY: PC = pregnancy category. (The validity of pregnancy risk categories has not been established; see Chapter 16, p 216.)
Can = Canadian trade name.

pregnancy poses a high risk of fetal anomalies. In combination with estrogens, progestogens are used to prevent conception, regulate erratic menstrual cycles, relieve dysmenorrhea, and induce regression of endometriosis. Such combinations administered cyclically produce an anovulatory cycle that more closely resembles the natural menstrual cycle than does that produced by estrogens alone.

In the past, progestogens were administered as a diagnostic test to establish pregnancy. In the absence of pregnancy, withdrawal of the progestogen is followed by menstrual flow. This use is presently obsolete and contraindicated; safer and more rapid tests are available.

Adverse reactions. The adverse reactions of progestogens are poorly differentiated from those of estrogens. Many studies that contribute to our understanding of these hormones involve combination contraceptives, and the individual effects of the two classes of hormones could not be distinguished. It is to be expected that the adverse reactions of these hormones overlap to some degree because their physiologic effects are similar in many respects. Both work in conjunction to regulate the menstrual cycle, promote fertility in the female, and prepare for lactation.

Progestogens, like estrogens, are teratogenic when administered during early pregnancy. Abnormalities in the fetus are more apt to affect the heart and limbs than with estrogens; genital malformations are less apt to occur. Progestogens, like androgens, cause masculinization of the female fetus. Because of these effects, progestogens are contraindicated during pregnancy, unless luteal production in response to gonadotropin is demonstrably inadequate.

Progestogens are more likely to induce irregularities in vaginal bleeding than estrogens. Breakthrough bleeding is a common problem and causes a high dropout rate among users of progestogen contraceptives (the "mini-pill"). Mood changes, especially lethargy, loss of initiative, and fatigue are more common with progestogens. Side effects related to sodium retention (hypertension, dizziness, weight gain) are less likely to occur than with estrogens but do develop with prolonged use of high doses. Breast engorgement and GI symptoms appear similar to those caused by estrogen.

Progesterone tends to increase a woman's energy needs slightly (by up to 16%) (Need for food, 1987). It has also been suspected of contributing to nausea of pregnancy which may be associated with transient hypoglycemia.

Precautions and contraindications. Progestogens, like estrogens, are generally contraindicated during early pregnancy, during lactation, and when a history of genital malignancy exists. Prolonged use should be avoided in clients with asthma, epilepsy, and migraine.

■ Summary

Progesterone is the steroid hormone produced by the corpus luteum and placenta that promotes maintenance of pregnancy and preparation of the breasts for lactation. Synthetic and semisynthetic preparations of progesterone are available for drug therapy. They are prescribed for contraception and for treating various medical problems related to the female reproductive system. The hormones are carcinogenic, teratogenic, and masculinizing. They are contraindicated during pregnancy and lactation and when a history of genital cancer exists.

Nursing management
Nursing implications

Progestogens have effects that resemble those of estrogens: they are teratogenic and can cause masculinization of a fetus. Birth defects that stem from exposure to progestogens are apt to affect the extremities, whereas those caused by estrogens usually affect the genitals. Accordingly, progestogens are contraindicated during pregnancy, unless luteal production in response to gonadotropins is demonstrably inadequate. Clients need a careful explanation of potential benefits and risks of drug therapy, as well as alternatives, to make an informed decision about treatment. The use of progestogens, like estrogens, is often elective. These drugs are used as components of oral contraceptives. Such combination contraceptives allow use of lower dosages of each active ingredient and may be administered in sequences that closely mimic the hormone fluctuations of normal menstrual cycles.

Nursing process

Assessment Before progestogen therapy is instituted, clients should be screened for contraindications for treatment and risk factors for adverse reaction to the hormones. The drugs are not usually prescribed for women with a history of genital malignancies. Pregnancy is also a contraindication unless the expectant mother is known to have a failure of corpus luteum production of progestogens. Women with histories of asthma, migraine, seizure disorders, and diabetes are at increased risk for complications.

Nursing diagnosis A nursing diagnosis likely to be made for clients who are receiving progestogens is:

Fluid volume excess related to sodium and water retention secondary to progestogen therapy

Common collaborative problems that should be differentiated from the nursing diagnosis include

Potential complication: seizures
Potential complication: hyperglycemia

Planning Goals for nursing treatment include preventing or alleviating fluid volume excess and maintaining blood glucose levels within normal limits.

Intervention. Diets offered to clients who receive progestogens should be low in sodium and limited in calories to the level required for maintaining lean body weight. Complex carbohydrates are preferable to refined sugars.

Client education. Clients should be fully informed of potential benefits and risks of progestogen therapy, as well as alternatives, to make an informed decision about treatment. Women who elect to receive the drugs should be taught the effects of the drugs, including the signs and symptoms of possible adverse reactions.

Fluid retention can be minimized if clients limit salt and sodium intake. Diabetic clients should be warned that progestogens can decrease glucose tolerance. The diabetic regimen should be followed conscientiously. Stress hormones have similar metabolic effects to those of progestogens; that is, they increase sodium and water retention and impair glucose tolerance. For this reason, clients should be taught stress management techniques.

When progestogen therapy is prolonged, the client should weigh herself at least twice a week and watch for signs of edema. Bloating, sudden weight gain, and frequent attacks of wheezing, headache, or seizures should be reported promptly.

The care of clients who receive oral contraceptives is discussed in detail in Chapter 38.

Evaluation Data required for evaluation include information that relates to fluid intake and output, tissue turgor, blood pressure, blood glucose levels, and reports from the client of feelings of bloating.

Checklist of nursing actions

☐ When clients are to receive progestogens, assess them for contraindications for treatment (pregnancy, lactation, history of genital cancer).

☐ Assess clients for the presence of medical conditions likely to be exacerbated by progestogen therapy (asthma, migraine, seizure disorder, diabetes mellitus).

☐ Explain the potential benefits and risks of progestogen therapy.

☐ Help the client develop health care practices that minimize the discomforts and risks of progestogen therapy.

Progesterone antagonists

The development of progesterone antagonists would provide physicians with agents that could alleviate symptoms of adverse responses to endogenous progesterone or terminate pregnancy. Some medical authorities theorize that premenstrual syndrome is caused by an allergy to progesterone, which reaches its highest levels (except for pregnancy) during this part of the menstrual cycle. A progesterone antagonist used experimentally to treat premenstrual syndrome is luteinizing hormone–releasing hormone agonist, known as LHRHa.

A second progesterone antagonist, mifepristone (RU486), is used clinically in France to induce abortion. When used in conjunction with prostaglandins, a success rate of 95% is claimed. The remaining 5% are surgically aborted (Palca, 1989). Considerable interest in this compound has arisen in the U.S., and the testing program required for approval by the FDA may be inaugurated soon.

References

Arrowsmith J, Dreis M. (1986). Thrombocytopenia after treatment with danazol (letter). *New Engl J Med, 315,* 585.

Bracken M, et al. (1990). A randomized, controlled trial of methylprednisolone or naloxone in the treatment of acute spinal-cord injury. *RN, 53*(7), 95.

Drug update: Flutamide. (1989). *Nursing 89, 19*(12), 62.

Forrest APM. (1989). Tamoxifen comes of age. *Br J Surg, 76,* 325.

Helfer E, et al. (1988). Side effects of spironolactone therapy in the hirsute woman. *J Clin Endocrinol Metab, 66,* 208–211.

More bad news on D.E.S. (1986). *Nursing 86, 16*(5), 23–24.

Need for food increases during menstrual cycle. (1987). *Tufts University Diet and Nutrition Letter, 5,* 1.

Palca J. (1989). The pill of choice? *Science, 245,* 1219.

Shag A, et al. (1987). Danazol and benign intracranial hypertension (letter). *Br Med J, 294,* 1323.

Slater J, et al. (1987). Recurrent anaphylaxis in menstruating women: Treatment with a luteinizing hormone releasing hormone agonist: A preliminary report. *Obstet Gynecol, 70,* 542.

Bibliography

*Donham JA. (1986). The weakness of steroids. *Am J Nurs, 86*(8), 917–919.

Edwards DD. (1985). The pill and breast cancer. *Science News, 128,* 293.

Ellsworth AJ, et al. (1987). A randomized trial of dexamethasone and acetazolamide for acute mountain sickness prophylaxis. *Am J Med, 83,* 1024.

Estradiol skin patch may relieve hot flashes. (1986). *Am J Nurs, 86*(11), 1215.

Estrogen effects assessed. (1989). *Science News, 136,* 86.

Fackelmann KA. (1990). Blocking breast cancer. *Science News, 137,* 296–297.

FDA panel questions drugs to stop milk. (1989). *RN, 52*(8), 99.

Garden J, Freinkel R. (1986). Systemic absorption of topical steroids. *Arch Dermatol, 122,* 1007–1010.

*Gever LN. (1987). Pharmacist on call: Sorting out the topical corticosteroids. *Nursing 87, 17*(9), 115.

Katzin L. (1989). Drug capsules: Hormone blocker for prostate cancer. *Am J Nurs, 89*(6), 796.

Katzin L. (1988). New drugs. *Am J Nurs, 88*(6), 837–838.

Lamb DR. (1984). Anabolic steroids in athletics: How well do they work and how dangerous are they? *Am J Sports Med, 12*(1), 31–38.

Lavin M, Rose G. (1986). Use of steroid eye drops in general practice. *Br Med J, 292*, 1414–1415.

Lebel MH, et al. (1988). Dexamethasone therapy for bacterial meningitis. *N Eng J Med, 319*, 964.

Lufkin E, et al. (1988). Estrogen replacement therapy: Current recommendations. *Mayo Clin Proc, 63*, 453–460.

Mrazik MJ, Mrazik T. (1989). Drug hot line: Induced menopause? *Nursing 89, 19*(9), 107.

Niculescu AM. (1986). Effects of *in utero* exposure to DES on male progeny. *J Obstet Gynecol Neonatal Nurs, 14*, 6.

*Orshan SA. (1988). The pill, the patient and you. *RN, 51*(7), 49–53.

Paganini-Hill A, et al. (1988). Postmenopausal oestrogen treatment and stroke: A prospective study. *Br Med J, 297*, 519–522.

Richman R, Kirsch L. (1988). Testosterone treatment in adolescent boys with constitutional delay in growth and development. *N Eng J Med, 319*, 1563–1567.

Roberts D. (1986). Steroids, the eye, and general practitioners. *Br Med J, 292*, 1414–1415.

Rodman MJ (1990). New drugs you're giving now: A topical steroid for skin disorders. *RN, 57*(3), 76.

Rodman MJ. (1987). A skin patch to ease menopause. *RN, 50*(1), 84.

Rusting R. (1990). Easing the trauma. *Scientific American, 262*(6), 34–37.

Steroids stir mental backlash. (1988). *Science News, 133*, 284.

Twelve-hour steroid aerosol. (1985). *Am J Nurs, 85*, 242.

*Ulmann A, et al. (1990). RUR 486. *Scientific American, 262*(6), 42–48.

Weiss R. (1990). "Abortion pill": New data, new markets. *Science News, 137*(6), 100.

Wolkowitz O, Rapaport M. (1989). Long-lasting behavioral changes following prednisone withdrawal (letter). *JAMA, 261*, 1731–1732.

*Recommended for further reading.

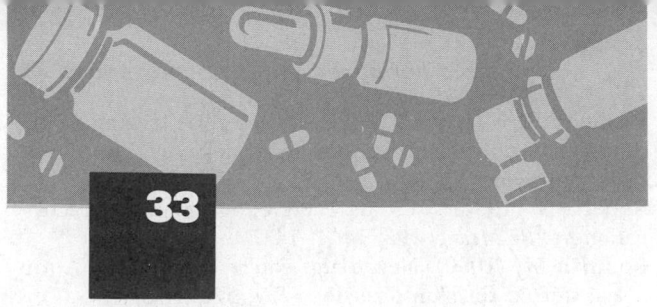

33

Protein hormones: insulin and other drugs that affect blood glucose

Nonsteroidal hormones are generally protein in nature. They may be simple proteins, complex combinations of proteins and other substances, or amino acid derivatives. Insulin, glucagon, parathormone, and some pituitary hormones are simple proteins composed of chains of amino acids joined by the peptide link. Sulfide or other bonds may connect different chains or parts of a single chain.

Pharmacodynamics. Most protein hormones do not appear to interact with the nuclei of body cells but, instead, interact with specific plasma membrane receptors linked with cellular enzymes (Fig. 33-1). The hormone-receptor complexes influence enzyme action and alter the synthesis of intracellular messenger proteins or electrolyte uptake. Because the primary site of action is the cytoplasm rather than the nucleus, these hormones act more rapidly than steroid hormones.

Pharmacokinetics. Since most protein hormones have numerous peptide linkages, they are destroyed by the peptidases in the digestive tract and cannot be administered orally. Many are effective when applied topically to mucous membranes, which absorb them readily, but administration by injection is often required. Natural hormones usually are mobilized, distributed, and broken down rapidly by the body; they have a short duration of activity. Analogues or modifications of the natural compounds that have been developed are absorbed and metabolized more slowly, providing a prolonged duration of therapeutic activity.

Protein hormones are degraded at the receptor site by the target tissue and also, to a large degree, by the liver and kidneys. Both hormones and their metabolites are excreted primarily in urine.

Insulin

Physiology. Insulin is secreted by the beta cells of the islets of Langerhans of the pancreas. Insulin is composed of two chains of amino acids held together by disulfide linkages. Like most proteins, it is a large molecule (MW 5734) compared with inorganic substances.

Pancreatic secretion of insulin is stimulated by a rise in blood sugar and inhibited by low blood sugar levels. Because the hormone's physiologic effect is to enhance body metabolism of glucose, thus lowering blood sugar, glucose-insulin interaction forms a stable negative feedback system that tends to return blood sugar levels to normal soon after the usual postprandial elevation.

Insulin appears to enhance both the enzyme reactions involved in glucose metabolism and the active transport system by which glucose crosses cell membranes. The hormone increases glucose use by most body tissues, increases glycogenesis in muscles and liver, promotes the oxidation of carbohydrates for energy by the muscles, and increases the synthesis of fats by adipose tissue. Under the influence of the hormone, gluconeogenesis and hepatic glycogenolysis decrease, and serum levels of sugar drop. Potassium and phosphate move from the serum into the cells, and an increase in protein and nucleic acid synthesis necessary for growth occurs. Because oxidation of fats for energy is minimized, ketosis is reduced or reversed. Insulin has a protein-sparing effect because of its enhancement of energy production from carbohydrates. Overall, insulin increases the movement of glucose

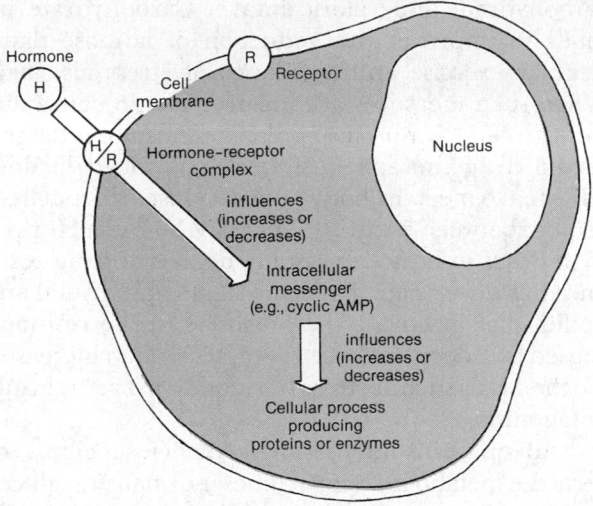

Figure 33-1. Mechanism of action of protein hormones. Protein hormones are believed to act in the cytoplasm (compare with Fig. 32-3).

from the blood to the intracellular compartment, where it is used for anabolic processes, energy production, or storage.

Blood sugar levels may be influenced by many substances other than insulin. Theoretically, fluctuations in serum glucose could result from changes in any of the following factors:

1. The rate of glycogenolysis or gluconeogenesis
2. Use of glucose by peripheral cells
3. The number of insulin receptors on these cells
4. Insulin antibody levels
5. The secretion of hormones that affect glucose metabolism, including insulin, glucagon, cortisone, epinephrine, and growth hormone

As yet, only a few substances have been identified as significant enhancers of glucose metabolism. Independent of insulin levels, vitamin C is known to increase tissue use of glucose, apparently by a direct effect on cellular metabolism. Chromium is suspected of enhancing glucose metabolism and lowering blood sugar. The effects of exercise, which increases glucose use by skeletal muscle, are mediated by changes in biochemistry that remain obscure. Further study may reveal other chemical agents that could be used to control blood sugar levels in people with metabolic disturbances such as diabetes mellitus or hypoglycemia.

Pathologic conditions. Derangements of insulin secretion may produce either excesses or deficiencies of the hormone. Hyperinsulinism is less frequent than hypoinsulinism, but it does occur intermittently in reactive hypoglycemia and chronically in insulin-secreting tumors (insulinomas). According to the thrifty gene theory of the etiology of diabetes mellitus, the

prediabetic period is characterized by some degree of hyperinsulinism, which promotes growth in immature subjects and fat production in adults. When pancreatic failure is impending, erratic insulin production may result in alternating hyperinsulinism and hypoinsulinism. These fluctuations and changes in levels of insulin antibodies are reflected in blood sugar levels.

Impairment of glucose metabolism is the major clinical feature of diabetes mellitus. This condition is not always caused by an absolute deficiency of insulin; it may be related to the presence of antibodies that interfere with hormone action, or it may be related to a reduction of insulin receptors in the target tissues. Contributing factors include stress, obesity, lack of exercise, and vitamin C deficiency. The stress hormones, epinephrine and cortisone, antagonize insulin. Obesity is associated with the impaired ability of tissues to properly use glucose.

Significant impairment of glucose metabolism leads to serious disruptions of chemical homeostasis in the diabetic. Blood sugar rises, increasing the osmotic pressure of body fluids. When the renal threshold is exceeded, glucose is excreted in urine, carrying with it large amounts of water. Concurrently, the body breaks down fats and proteins for energy metabolism, and the production of nitrogenous wastes increases. Blood lipids rise. Because fats cannot metabolize to completion in the absence of carbohydrate metabolism, intermediate products of fat metabolism (acidic ketone bodies) accumulate. The resulting dehydration, hyperosmolarity, and acidosis cause illness and, when progressive, coma and death. Diabetic ketoacidosis requires the administration of insulin, carbohydrates, fluids, and electrolytes to reverse the disease process.

Pharmacodynamics. Pharmacologically, insulin is an agonist that interacts with specific receptors on body cell membranes. Its presence on these receptors accelerates movement of glucose into the cells, use of glucose to produce energy, and storage of energy as glycogen and fat. Its physiologic effects include a lowering of extracellular glucose concentrations, increased energy production, increased glycogen storage, and proliferation of fatty tissues.

Insulin increases the total quantity of protein in the body by at least three mechanisms: increased active transport of amino acid into the cells, accelerated translation of messenger RNA code by the ribosomes to form increased quantities of protein, and increased transcription of DNA in the cell nuclei to form increased quantities of RNA. Because it enhances the production of energy from carbohydrates, insulin also decreases the metabolism of amino acids for energy. Insulin is required for normal growth and development during childhood.

Pharmacokinetics. Insulin cannot be administered orally because peptidases in the digestive juices destroy the protein molecule. Drug preparations may be administered by subcutaneous, intramuscular (IM), or intravenous (IV) injection. Because the onset and duration of action of plain (regular, crystalline) insulin are brief, the compound has been modified by reaction with other substances to form complexes that must be broken down by the body before absorption can occur (Table 33-1). This process delays onset and prolongs duration of action. Absorption may also be delayed or decreased by the presence of insulin-binding antibodies, which develop in people who receive exogenous insulin. Investigationally, insulin has been successfully administered topically by nasal spray (Clinical news: Insulin as a nasal spray, 1987) and by implantable pump (Point Study Group, 1988).

Commercially available insulin preparations are classified as short, intermediate, or long-lasting in action. After absorption, insulin is rapidly distributed throughout extracellular fluids. In healthy people, insulin has a plasma half-life of a few minutes; however, the biologic half-life may be prolonged in diabetic people, probably because of binding to antibodies. The hormone is rapidly metabolized, mainly in the liver but also in the kidneys and muscle tissue. The metabolites and a small fraction (less than 2%) of unchanged drug are excreted by the kidneys.

Therapeutic uses

Diabetes mellitus. Insulin is widely used in the treatment of diabetes mellitus, a disease characterized by an absolute or relative deficiency of insulin, which results in inadequate carbohydrate metabolism. When the pancreas is totally unable to produce insulin, affected people depend on exogenous supplies of insulin. This condition, called insulin-dependent (IDDM or type I) diabetes mellitus, usually develops during childhood. Some evidence suggests that the inability to secrete insulin is caused by degeneration of the islets of Langerhans after a viral infection. Some older diabetics develop insulin-dependent diabetes, indicating the pancreatic secretion of insulin has failed completely.

Non–insulin-dependent (type II) diabetes mellitus affects mostly older people and is milder than type I. These clients seem to produce insulin, but glucose metabolism is not maintained at a normal level. The mechanisms are not completely understood, but research indicates that the causes may be multiple. Insulin antibodies demonstrable in the serum of non–insulin-dependent diabetics may impair or block completely the action of endogenous hormone. Diabetics often have fewer insulin receptors on tissue cells, but the reason for their disappearance is not known. Inactivity, obesity, and low vitamin C levels further decrease the ability of body tissues to effectively use glucose.

Insulin therapy is not the preferred treatment for non–insulin-dependent diabetes mellitus. Some diabetics can maintain normal metabolism by reducing carbohydrate and caloric intake. Carbohydrate use tends to improve with reduction of adipose tissue. Regular exercise and avoidance of stress also help. When such measures are unsuccessful in controlling the signs and symptoms of diabetes, insulin is the preferred drug therapy. Insulin is prescribed in doses adjusted to meet the body's needs. Most diabetic clients require between 5 and 40 U per day. The need for very high doses indicates that some degree of drug resistance has developed. This may stem from insulin antibodies that inactivate the hormone, tissue resistance caused by a decrease in cell receptors, or an increase in biochemicals such as stress hormones that act as insulin antagonists.

Adequate insulin therapy in diabetes mellitus corrects the metabolic abnormalities, normalizing glucose use for energy production, tissue repair, and the formation of glycogen. Insulin therapy eliminates excessive ketogenesis (though some ketosis may develop in clients on weight-reduction diets) and corrects the negative nitrogen balance that occurs in ketoacidosis. The characteristics symptoms of type I diabetes mellitus (hyperglycemia, glycosuria, polyuria, polydipsia, polyphagia, muscle-wasting, weight loss, and susceptibility to infection) subside. Good control of glucose levels reduces but does not eliminate the risk of diabetic complications.

Acute ketoacidosis. Treatment of acute ketoacidosis (diabetic coma) requires intensive therapy with IV fluids and electrolytes, as well as regular insulin to correct body chemistry. Clients sometimes delay seeking treatment until metabolic acidosis is pronounced enough to cause lethargy or unconsciousness. Dehydration may be severe. Insulin, fluids, and electrolytes must be administered initially. IV infusions are usually required. Sodium bicarbonate is given to correct the acidosis. As the client responds to treatment, serum potassium levels may drop precipitously (Fig. 33-2). Additional potassium is added to the treatment regimen in accord with serial determinations of blood levels of the electrolyte. Other electrolytes are also administered as necessary to maintain normal levels.

Other uses of insulin. Insulin is occasionally used to stimulate the appetite in cases of malnutrition. A small dose (about 5 U) of regular insulin is administered 20 to 30 minutes before a meal. The hormone may also be required to control hyperglycemia in clients who receive large quantities of nutrients by IV, as in hyperalimentation procedures. Insulin was once used to induce hypoglycemic shock in treating psychosis, but this practice is now considered obsolete.

Drug preparations. Until recently, insulin used medicinally was derived solely from the pancreata of slaughtered cattle, pigs, and sheep. Animal insulin is not identical chemically to the human hormone but is physiologically active. Porcine insulin most nearly re-

(*Text continues on p. 774*)

Table 33-1. Insulin preparations

Drug Names	Appearance/preparations	Protein modifier	Time and route of administration	Approximate time of onset (hours)	Time of peak action (hours)	Duration of action (hours)	Time when glycosuria is most likely to occur	Time when hypoglycemia is most likely to occur	Pregnancy risk category*
Animal insulins									
Fast-acting									
insulin, regular insulin, crystalline zinc insulin, unmodified insulin (Actrapid, Iletin; Can: Insulin-Toronto, Velosulin)	Clear solution/pork insulin in concentrations of 40, 100, and 500 U/ml; beef insulin in concentration of 100 U/ml; mixed pork and beef insulins in concentrations of 40 and 100 U/ml	None	For treatment of ketoacidosis: IM injection or IV infusion as required For maintenance: 15–20 min before meals, subcutaneous	½–1	2–3	5–7	During sleep	2–3 h after the lightest meal (usually between 10 AM and noon if given before breakfast)	B
prompt insulin zinc (Semilente Insulin, Semilente Iletin, Semitard)	Cloudy suspension/beef insulin in concentration of 100 U/ml; pork insulin in concentration of 100 U/ml; mixed pork and beef insulins in concentrations of 40 and 100 U/ml	None	For maintenance: 30–45 min before a meal (usually before breakfast), subcutaneous	½–1	4–7	12–16	During sleep	Before meals, especially before lunch if given before breakfast	B
Intermediate-acting									
isophane insulin (NPH Iletin, Initard, Insulatard, Protaphane NPH)	Cloudy suspension/beef insulin in concentrations of 40 and 100 U/ml; pork insulin in concentration of 100 U/ml; mixed beef and pork insulin in concentrations of 40 and 100 U/ml	Protamine	For maintenance: 1 hr before a meal (usually before breakfast), subcutaneous	1–2	8–12	18–24	With daily doses, 5–6 h after administration (at lunch time if given before breakfast)	Before meals, 10 h after administration (before the evening meal if given before breakfast)	B

(Continued)

Table 33-1. Insulin preparations (Continued)

Drug Names	Appearance/ preparations	Protein modifier	Time and route of administration	Approximate time of onset (hours)	Time of peak action (hours)	Duration of action (hours)	Time when glycosuria is most likely to occur	Time when hypoglycemia is most likely to occur	Pregnancy risk category*
Animal insulins (cont.)									
insulin zinc (Lente Insulin, Lente Iletin)	Cloudy suspension/ beef insulin in concentrations of 40 and 100 U/ml; pork insulin in concentration of 100 U/ml; mixed beef and pork insulin in concentrations of 40 and 100 U/ml	None	For maintenance: 1 hr before a meal (usually before breakfast), subcutaneous	1–2	8–12	18–24	With daily doses, 5–6 h after administration (at lunch time if given before breakfast)	Before meals, 10 h after administration (before the evening meal if given before breakfast)	B
Long-Lasting protamine zinc insulin (Protamine, Zinc, Iletin, Protamine Zinc, Purified)	Cloudy suspension/ beef insulin in concentration of 100 U/ml; pork insulin in concentration of 100 U/ml; mixed beef and pork insulin in concentrations of 40 and 100 U/ml	Prot-amine	For maintenance: 1 hr before a meal (usually before breakfast), subcutaneous	4–8	14–20	36	With daily doses, after administration to 5–14 h later (lunch, supper, and bedtime specimens)	18–24 h after administration (between 2 AM and breakfast if given before breakfast)	B

772

| extended insulin zinc (Ultralente Insulin, Ultralente Iletin, Ultratard) | Cloudy suspension/beef insulin in concentration of 100 U/ml; mixed beef and pork insulin in concentrations of 40 and 100 U/ml | None | For maintenance: 1 hr before a meal (usually before breakfast), subcutaneous | 4–8 | 16–18 | 36 | With daily doses, after administration to 5–14 h later (lunch, supper, and bedtime specimens) | 18–24 h after administration (between 2 AM and breakfast if given before breakfast) | |

Human Insulins

Rapid-acting

| insulin human, regular rDNA (Humulin R) semisynthetic (Novolin R; *Can:* Novolin-Toronto, Velasulin Human) | Clear solution/recombinant DNA origin in concentration of 100 U/ml; semisynthetic in concentration of 100 U/ml | None | For treatment of ketoacidosis: IM injection or IV infusion as required For maintenance: 15–20 min before meals, subcutaneous | ½–1 | 2–3 | 5–7 | During sleep | 2 h after the lightest meal (usually between 10 AM and noon if given before breakfast) | B |

Intermediate-acting

| human insulin zinc suspension, rDNA (Humulin L), Semisynthetic (Novolin L) | Cloudy suspension/semisynthetic in concentration of 100 U/ml | None | For maintenance: 1 hr before a meal (usually before breakfast), subcutaneous | 1–2 | 8–12 | 18–24 | At lunch time if given before breakfast | Before the evening meal if given before breakfast | B |

| isophane insulin human, rDNA (Humulin N), semisynthetic (Novolin N, Insulatard NPH Human) | Cloudy suspension/recombinant DNA origin in concentration of 100 U/ml | Protamine | For maintenance: 1 hr before a meal (usually before breakfast), subcutaneous | 1–2 | 8–12 | 18–24 | At lunch time if given before breakfast | Before the evening meal if given before breakfast | B |

*The validity of pregnancy risk categories remains unproven; see Chapter 16, p 216.

KEY: *Can* = Canadian trade name.

Potassium shifts when *pH* is declining:

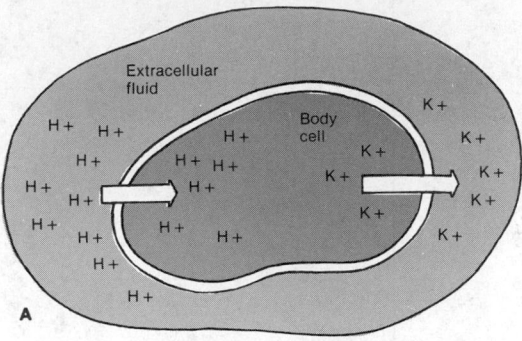

Potassium shifts when *pH* is rising:

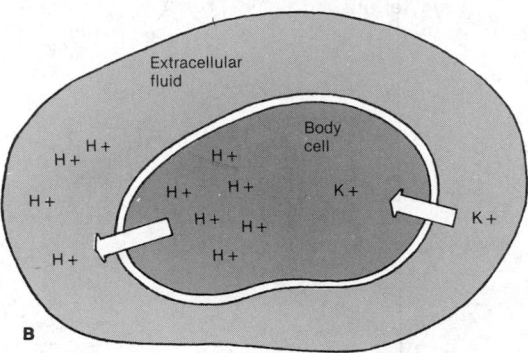

Figure 33-2. Mechanisms that affect potassium balance in ketoacidosis. **A.** In developing acidosis, hydrogen ions enter the intracellular space in larger than normal numbers. To maintain electrical balance, potassium ions migrate from cells to extracellular fluid. Serum potassium rises, and potassium is excreted in the urine. Blood levels of the electrolyte are high, but body supplies are declining. **B.** With correction of acidosis, hydrogen ions leave the cells and reenter the extracellular fluid. Potassium returns to the cell, lowering serum levels. Because the body potassium has been depleted, severe hypokalemia may develop.

sembles human insulin. A modified insulin, changed chemically to a form identical to endogenous human hormone, is presently available. Human insulin is also produced by bacterial cultures using recombinant DNA (rDNA) techniques. These newer drugs are relatively expensive (Berger, et al, 1989a, 1989b).

Although the purity of insulin preparations has improved in recent years, it is still measured in units according to bioassay. Current preparations are more stable than previous ones, and the drug no longer requires constant refrigeration. Heat, light, and agitation are to be avoided, because they destroy the drug.

In the past, insulin has been produced in several concentrations (20, 40, 80, 100, and 200 U/ml) with syringes calibrated in units for each concentration. The variety of solutions and syringes was confusing to some clients and predisposed to errors in dosage. As a result of the recommendation of the American Diabetes Association's Committee on the Use of Therapeutic Agents, U-100 is presently recommended as the single concentration for all types of insulin. Transition to this form is well advanced; U-100 is the predominant form of insulin prescribed for newly diagnosed diabetics. Insulin with 200 U/ml continues to be available for diabetics who require unusually large doses. U-500, which contains 500 U/ml of insulin, is useful when very large doses (200–500 U) are required. Syringes designed for use with U-100 insulin are scaled in units, with calibrations for every 1 to 2 U (Fig. 33-3). The system is compatible with the metric system, and a tuberculin syringe may be used for accurate measurement of doses. Each 1/100 ml calibration on the tuberculin syringe measures 1 U of U-100 insulin (Fig. 33-4). When very large doses of insulin are required, U-200 and U-500 insulin can be measured with a tu-

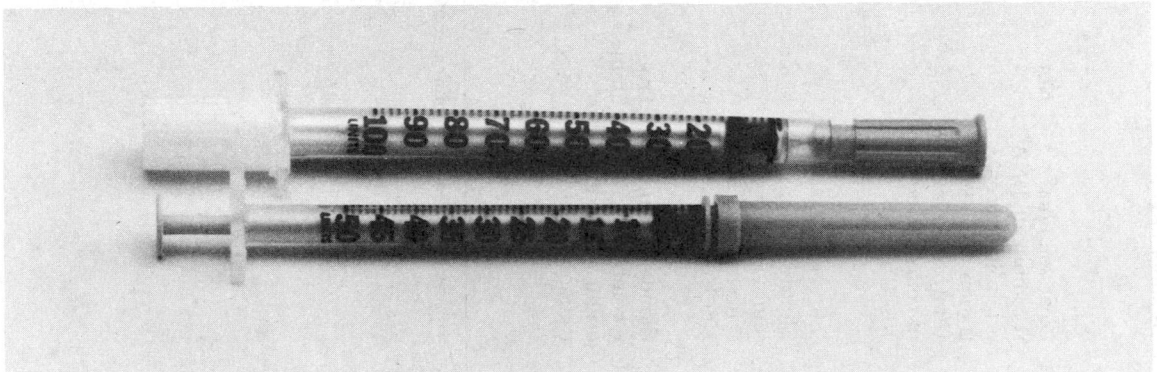

Figure 33-3. U-100 insulin syringes. The very short needle allows subcutaneous injection with a 90° angle of insertion. (*Top*) Single-use, 1-ml insulin syringe. Note that the scale is in units with gradations of 2 units (equal to 0.02 ml) each. Odd numbers cannot be measured with precision with this syringe. Compare with the 1/2-ml syringe below and the tuberculin syringe in Figure 33-4. (*Bottom*) Single-use, 1/2-ml insulin syringe. It has a narrower barrel and longer scale. Single-unit markings allow greater accuracy, but the capacity is 50 units. (Courtesy of Becton Dickinson and Company, Rochelle Park, NJ)

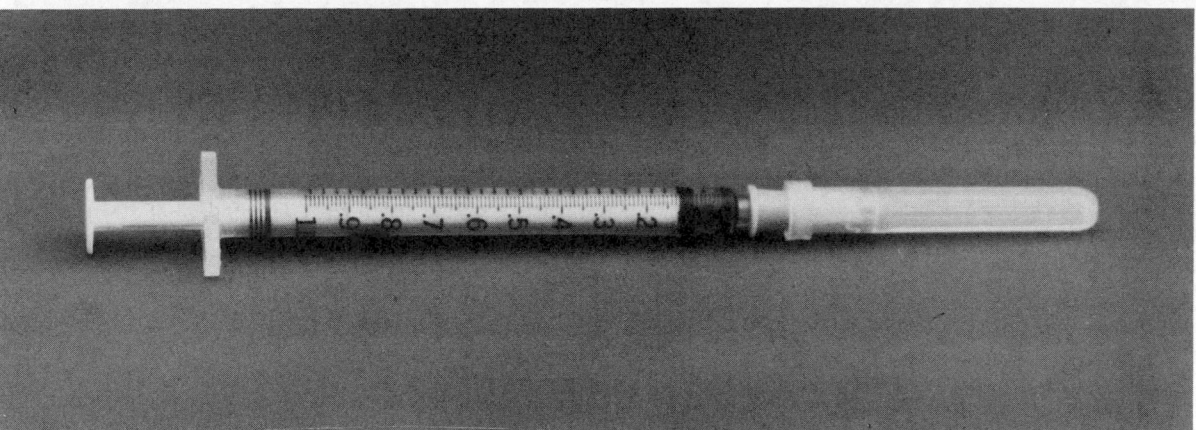

Figure 33-4. Tuberculin syringe. Note the scale graduated in hundredths of a milliliter. Insulin dosages of 1 unit to 100 units (of U-100 insulin) can be measured accurately, whether odd or even in number. (Courtesy of Becton Dickinson and Company, Rochelle Park, NJ)

berculin syringe; $1/100$ ml provides 2 U and 5 U, respectively, of these preparations.

Insulins are divided into three categories according to rapidity of action: fast-acting, long-acting, and intermediate-acting. Time of onset, time of peak action, and duration of action differ for each group (see Table 33-1 and Figs. 33-5, 33-6, 33-7).

Fast-acting preparation. Insulin injection (or *regular insulin*) is the only form of insulin suitable for IV administration. Its rapid action and prompt dissipation provide the most accurate control of blood sugar in labile clinical situations. Regular insulin dosage is often adjusted to the results of blood glucose levels or degree of glycosuria. When used in chronic management of the disease, it is administered about 20 minutes before each meal.

Long-acting preparation. *Protamine zinc insulin* is a compound prepared by the reaction of insulin and zinc with protamine, a basic protein. The resulting suspension is injected subcutaneously, where it is absorbed at a retarded but steady rate. This form of insulin is often combined with regular insulin to produce short-term and long-term insulin effect with a single injection.

Intermediate-acting preparation. Further modification of the protamine-insulin-zinc combination produced *isophane (NPH*) insulin*. This preparation has a fairly rapid onset and moderately prolonged duration of action.

Globin zinc insulin, a mixture of insulin, zinc, and the protein globin has properties similar to NPH insulin but is not widely used at present.

The *lente insulins* are prepared by precipitating insulin with zinc and resuspending the compound in an acetate buffer. The size of the crystals formed are influenced by the specific method of preparation; this in turn alters the duration and intensity of action. Extended (ultralente) insulin contains large particles and produces effects similar to protamine zinc insulin. Prompt (semilente) insulin contains smaller particles and has an action similar to regular insulin, but it is somewhat longer lasting. By mixing ultralente and semilente insulins, a preparation similar in effect to NPH insulin is produced (lente insulin). Lente insulins

---

*The letters *NPH* signify properties of the preparation and its origin: *N* denotes that the solution is neutral (*p*H 7.2); *P*, the protamine zinc content; and *H*, Hagedorn, the laboratory of origin.

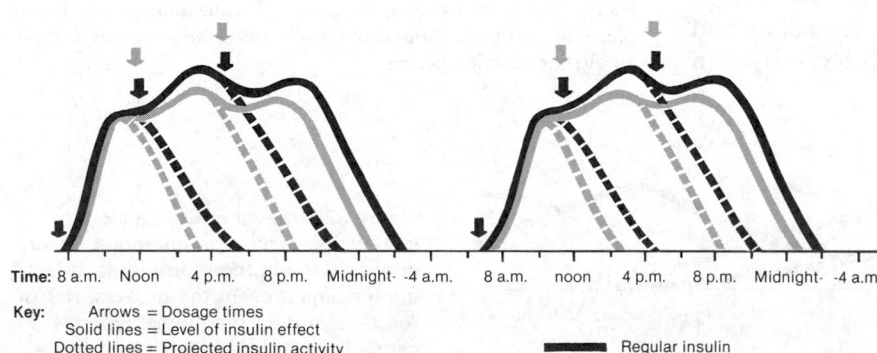

Time: 8 a.m. Noon 4 p.m. 8 p.m. Midnight 4 a.m.   8 a.m. noon 4 p.m. 8 p.m. Midnight 4 a.m.

Key: Arrows = Dosage times
Solid lines = Level of insulin effect
Dotted lines = Projected insulin activity
in absence of repeated doses

████ Regular insulin
████ Semilente insulin

Figure 33-5. Level of drug action in fast-acting insulin preparations. When used alone, short-acting insulins must be administered several times a day to provide adequate activity at meal times (compare with Figs. 33-6 and 33-7).

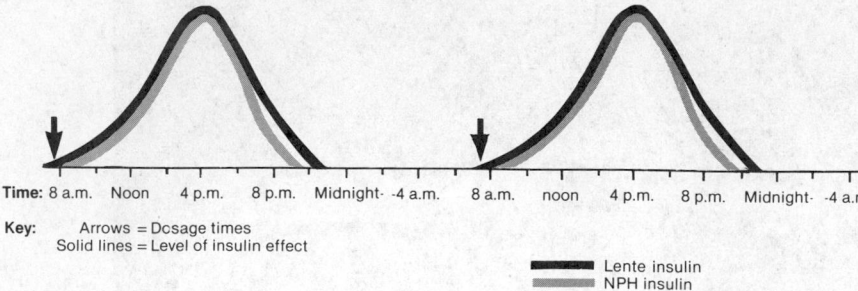

Time: 8 a.m. Noon 4 p.m. 8 p.m. Midnight -4 a.m. 8 a.m. noon 4 p.m. 8 p.m. Midnight -4 a.m.

Key: Arrows = Dosage times
Solid lines = Level of insulin effect

Lente insulin
NPH insulin

Figure 33-6. Level of drug action in intermediate-acting insulins. Reactions are most likely to occur in the late afternoon and early evening hours (compare with Figs. 33-5 and 33-7).

do not induce allergic sensitivity as often as other preparations (Steil & Deakins, 1990).

Dosage and administration. Since insulin usually is administered by injection, it is preferable to minimize the number of doses needed daily. Most clients can be maintained with one injection daily of a sustained-release insulin. This is usually administered in the morning, before breakfast. At present, isophane (NPH) insulin is prescribed most often. Lente insulins are especially useful when allergic hypersensitivity develops. Protamine zinc insulin and insulin combinations are used infrequently.

Insulin therapy can be tailored to meet individual needs by altering the time of administration or by mixing various types of insulin. Occasionally, long-lasting insulin is administered before the evening meal rather than in the morning. Regular insulin may be mixed with the long-lasting forms or may be administered separately. The various lente insulins may be mixed with each other. When used as the sole therapeutic agent, regular insulin must be administered before each meal.

Insulin can be administered subcutaneously, IM, or (if regular insulin) IV. The subcutaneous route is preferred when prolonged action is desired. IV administration is not as reliable as subcutaneous or IM injection, because the drug adheres to the surfaces of solution bottles and tubing, preventing total delivery of the prescribed dose to the client. It may be necessary to administer the drug IV, however, in diabetic ketoacidosis when the client is in circulatory shock.

Adverse reactions. When they contain foreign proteins, insulins can trigger antibody formation and allergic hypersensitivity (Box 33-1). Allergy is often manifested initially by urticaria and edema at the injection site. These phenomena tend to subside with continued treatment. Changing the insulin prescription to a less antigenic preparation (pure porcine, a lente insulin, or human insulin) may resolve the problem. Rarely, desensitization regimens may be needed. These are carried out by accelerated schedules (*rapid desensitization**) to prevent prolonged interference with treatment of the diabetes. Desensitization is required if anaphylaxis occurs. Insulin allergy is most likely to develop when hormone use is suspended for a period of time and then reinstituted. Diabetics who use an insulin preparation that contains protamine (NPH or PZI insulin) sometimes develop an asymptomatic allergy to protamine; this allergy causes an acute reaction to this substance when it is later used medicinally to neutralize heparin, as in hemodialysis.

Insulin exerts local effects at the site of injection that may cause lipodystrophy. Either atrophy (evidenced by pitting) or hypertrophy (manifested by swelling) may occur. The more frequently injections are administered in a given area, the more likely it is that lipodystrophy will develop. The injection of cold insulin also increases risk. The mechanisms that underlie lipodystrophy are poorly understood but are undoubtedly related to the influence of insulin on fat metabolism. Paradoxically, additional injections of a pure insulin directly into atrophic areas can sometimes restore the normal contours of the area.

*Rapid desensitization begins with administration of a minute dose of drug, followed at short intervals by progressively larger doses, until the therapeutic dose is achieved or the client experiences an allergic reaction. A course of rapid desensitization usually is completed in less than 24 hours but must be restarted at a minimal dose if an allergic reaction occurs.

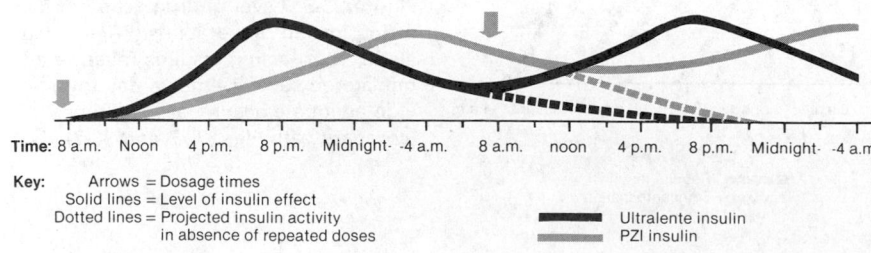

Time: 8 a.m. Noon 4 p.m. 8 p.m. Midnight -4 a.m. 8 a.m. noon 4 p.m. 8 p.m. Midnight -4 a.m.

Key: Arrows = Dosage times
Solid lines = Level of insulin effect
Dotted lines = Projected insulin activity
in absence of repeated doses

Ultralente insulin
PZI insulin

Figure 33-7. Level of drug action in long-acting insulin preparations. When administered in the morning, long-lasting insulins present the greatest risk of reactions during the night. Hyperglycemia is most likely after lunch (compare with Figs. 33-5 and 33-6).

Box 33-1. Insulin components and contaminants that act as allergens

Allergen

Insulin of animal origin

Porcine proteins (contaminants)

Escherichia coli polypeptides (contaminants that amount to <4 ppm)

Protamine (derived from salmon sperm)

Insulin Preparations

Bovine and porcine insulin

Semisynthetic human insulin

Biosynthetic human insulin (rDNA insulin)

NPH and PZI insulins

The institution of insulin therapy for the treatment of newly diagnosed diabetics may coincide with a period of persistent visual blurring. This disturbance is caused by the rapid changes in fluid and electrolyte levels as metabolism is restored to normal.

High blood levels of insulin contribute to the acceleration of vascular degeneration. Insulin excesses are characteristic of both the prediabetic stage of non–insulin-dependent diabetes and intensive insulin treatment for insulin-dependent diabetes. Cardiovascular degeneration is a frequent complication of diabetes mellitus, and, not infrequently, cardiovascular disease precedes the onset of frank diabetes (Reaven, 1988).

Toxicity. Whenever the body's insulin level exceeds metabolic needs, blood sugar tends to drop below normal. The brain is an obligate user of glucose for energy; an adequate supply is essential for normal function. Abnormally low blood sugar initially causes a sympathoadrenal discharge; symptoms of central nervous system (CNS) impairment follow. The more rapid the drop in blood sugar, the more severe the symptoms. Either hunger or nausea can occur.

In most people, a drop in blood glucose below 70 mg/dl results in typical signs and symptoms of sympathetic activity: perspiration, tachycardia, weakness, trembling, and anxiety. This release of catecholamines is compensatory, raising blood glucose by antagonizing the effect of insulin. If the response is pronounced, a paradoxical hyperglycemia and glycosuria can follow (the Somogyi effect). Usually, however, the hormone levels are inadequate to correct the hypoglycemia. Diabetics who use sympathetic blocking agents (eg, β-blocking drugs) do not exhibit these manifestations; in such clients, the onset of hypoglycemia is signaled by such symptoms as severe headache, epigastric pain, diarrhea, nausea, vomiting, dizziness, nocturnal sweating, lethargy, demoralization, and personality change.

As hypoglycemia progresses, the brain is deprived of its sole source of energy and cannot function normally. Headache, confusion, and incoherent speech often develop. The client may exhibit bizarre behavior that resembles drunkenness. If blood sugar drops further, convulsions, coma, and death ensue. Permanent brain damage can occur in people who survive severe insulin reactions. This can result in subsequent retardation, hemiparesis, ataxia, incontinence, aphasia, chorea, parkinsonism, or seizure disorder.

The antidote to insulin toxicity is the immediate administration of sugar. If the client is conscious, candy, sweetened orange juice, or some other rapidly absorbed sweet is given. Most candy (except for chocolate) is appropriate to use. If consciousness is lost, or if the client resists taking the sweet (as sometimes happens owing to brain malfunction), parenteral therapy is required. Either IV glucose or IM glucagon should be used. When consciousness returns, the client should be fed, because continuing insulin activity may cause hypoglycemia to recur after correction of the initial symptoms.

Insulin reactions develop much more rapidly than diabetic coma and are considered to be more dangerous. For this reason, labile diabetics are often advised to maintain a slight glycosuria (trace to +1 on urine tests, or 100–150 mg/d blood sugar) to guard against frequent episodes of hypoglycemia. Whenever it is unclear if the client is experiencing insulin reaction or hyperglycemia, sugar should be given. Sugar can prevent serious hypoglycemia and permanent brain damage. The relatively small amounts of glucose added to the body are unlikely to increase markedly the metabolic disturbance in hyperglycemia.

The administration of high doses of insulin to markedly malnourished individuals sometimes results in gross fluid volume retention and edema (Evans, et al, 1986).

Precautions and contraindications. No absolute contraindications to insulin therapy except hyperinsulinism exist. Hypersensitivity to the drug may be alleviated by using insulins with reduced antigenic properties or by rapid desensitization. Because insulin accelerates cardiovascular degeneration, and because hypoglycemia poses a serious risk of permanent brain damage, the minimum amount of drug needed to restore normal metabolism should be used. Clients who respond to dietary management should avoid insulin therapy as long as possible. The practice of increasing insulin intake to compensate for increased food intake is dangerous. Not only does this promote weight gain that tends to accelerate the progress of the diabetic condition, but it exposes the client to higher insulin doses than necessary, increasing the risk of vascular degeneration.

Once insulin therapy becomes necessary, treatment should be maintained without interruption.

Soon after insulin therapy is started, an improvement in the diabetic condition is often noted. This response is associated with the improvement in general condition and cellular nutrition, which improves beta cell function. The dosage of insulin is decreased to minimize the occurrence of hypoglycemic reactions but is not eliminated. In most cases, the improvement is temporary, with insulin needs rising after a short period of time. Interruption of insulin therapy during this temporary remission would increase the risk of hypersensitivity owing to antibody formation. Insulin may be discontinued when a marked decrease in obesity is followed by sustained improvement in the diabetes. These individuals are considered to have reverted to the latent phase of diabetes. Over time, they may again experience overt diabetes if the disease progresses, when infectious illness occurs, or if they again become obese.

Persistent hyperglycemia despite gradually increasing doses of insulin indicates the need for a careful evaluation for Somogyi effect. The client may be experiencing undetected insulin reactions that are followed by a rebound hyperglycemia. A reduction in insulin dosage may produce improvement in the blood test results.

■ Summary

Insulin is a hormone produced by the pancreas that promotes glucose use by most body cells. Its secretion is highest when blood sugar is elevated, and it functions to reduce blood sugar to normal fasting concentrations. Insulin also promotes lipogenesis and enhances body use of proteins for tissue building.

Learning experience 33-1

In a hospital or nursing home, examine the insulin preparations available for treating diabetic clients. Are these preparations stored under conditions that minimize the risk of medication errors? If the vials are refrigerated, are the solutions allowed to reach room temperature before doses are administered? What proportion of clients in the nursing unit are receiving long-term insulin therapy?

Diabetes mellitus is a disease characterized by inadequate insulin effect. Most body tissues are unable to use glucose adequately; serious metabolic disturbances ensue. The administration of exogenous insulin helps correct these physiologic aberrations and helps promote normal tissue nutrition.

Insulin has a relatively narrow safety margin. Inadequate dosage allows the pathology of diabetes mellitus to persist, whereas excessive dosage induces dangerous hypoglycemia. Because glucose metabolism is influenced by a number of extraneous factors, achieving and maintaining a relatively steady state requires skillful manipulation of diet, exercise, and general hygiene, in addition to control with medication.

Nursing management

Nursing implications: the critically ill diabetic client

Severe complications of diabetes mellitus frequently underlie critical illness of clients in acute care facilities. Diabetic coma and insulin reactions represent medical emergencies. The nurse must thoroughly understand the nature of the disease and the mechanisms that underlie its pathologic processes.

When a diabetic suddenly becomes ill or the condition of a hospitalized diabetic worsens, accurate identification of the cause is critical. Two common syndromes are hyperglycemia and hypoglycemia. Another condition that may complicate diagnosis is hyperventilation (Table 33-2). Hypoglycemia develops within a matter of minutes and must be treated immediately to avert serious consequences. Occasionally, hypoglycemia may be difficult to distinguish from hyperglycemia or hyperventilation syndrome. The nurse should be familiar with the signs and symptoms of all three conditions. Few distinctive features differentiate hypoglycemia from hyperventilation. Both syndromes are characterized by hyperirritability of the nervous system; however, the hyperventilating client exhibits rapid and deep breathing not seen in hypoglycemia. The differences between hypoglycemia and hyperglycemia are generally more pronounced, but it is important to remember that in some situations they may not be clear-cut.

When in doubt, the safest course is to treat for hypoglycemia. This treatment buys time for a definitive diagnosis of insulin reaction and poses no serious risk for clients with other conditions.

Moderate illness and diabetes. Diabetics may be admitted to general hospital units because of illnesses unrelated to the underlying metabolic condition or because of difficulty in maintaining metabolic balance. Any illness, including infectious processes, increases the secretion of stress hormones that tend to exacerbate diabetes. Careful assessment of glucose balance and the efficacy of the medical regimen is required. Diabetics who normally are well controlled with insulin therapy may require larger doses during an intercurrent illness. Those usually controlled by diet alone often exhibit hyperglycemia and glycosuria, and insu-

Table 33-2. Comparison of the clinical manifestations of hypoglycemia, diabetic ketoacidosis, and hyperventilation

	Hypoglycemia	Ketoacidosis	Hyperventilation
Usual history			
Onset	Sudden onset (within minutes)	Gradual onset (hours to days)	Sudden onset
Associated events (contributing factors)	Missed meal, unusual exertion, or (in labile diabetics and those patients who experience remission) none	Unusual stress, febrile illness, missed doses of hypoglycemic medication, gradual weight gain, or (when disease has worsened) none	Stressful episode that culminates in a panic reaction
Presenting symptoms			
Subjective feelings	Feeling of weakness, anxiety, jitteriness	Feeling of sluggishness	Feeling of nervousness, worry, jitteriness, and weakness
Behavior	Excited, "drunken," tremors	Lethargy, slowness	Excited, tremors
Headache	Present	Absent	Absent
Respirations	Normal to rapid and shallow; (in coma) stertorous	Kussmaul (rapid, deep), air hunger, acetone odor to breath	Rapid, deep breathing
Skin	Pale, cool, clammy	Warm, dry, flushed	Variable
Diaphoresis	Present (usually marked)	Absent	Variable, but rarely marked
Blood pressure	Normal to somewhat elevated	Low	Normal
Gastrointestinal	Hunger or (rarely) nausea	Nausea and vomiting	Nausea may occur
Central nervous system	Headache, hyperactive reflexes, increased alertness (before coma), demoralization, personality change, night sweats	Hypoactive reflexes, decreased level of consciousness	Increased alertness, hyperactive reflexes
Corroborating data			
Urine (fresh, double-voided specimen)	Negative for glucose	Strongly positive for glucose, low pH, positive for acetone	Usually positive for glucose, high pH
Blood	Low glucose	Elevated glucose	Glucose may be elevated

lin may be prescribed. Fasting may be imposed for diagnostic or surgical procedures, requiring modifications of the usual diabetic regimen. In such instances, insulin medication is usually delayed until just before the fast is broken. Regardless of the reason for hospitalization, diabetic control tends to be unstable in hospitalized clients and requires close monitoring.

Compliance. Compliance with insulin prescriptions can be a problem. Doses are not often omitted, but clients may take extra amounts of insulin to compensate for taking more food than prescribed in the diet. It should be noted that some physicians do allow a degree of flexibility and client control of diet and medication, especially in young insulin-dependent clients. The nurse should verify that the practice in question is indeed contrary to the prescribed regimen before attempting corrective action. Careful addition of balanced amounts of insulin and carbohydrates may not significantly alter glucose balance, but imbalance can result from this practice. The chief danger may be that the additional food and insulin promote weight gain and adiposity that eventually exacerbates the diabetic condition.

Nursing process

Assessment Whenever a client with diabetes mellitus needs health care, glucose balance should be determined and monitored. If blood glucose is within normal limits, no overt or laboratory evidence of hyperglycemia or hypoglycemia should be present.

Inadequate insulin (hyperglycemia) causes increased metabolism of fat and other tissues for energy. Ketoacidosis and significant dehydration develop. The client is likely to appear flushed and may be lethargic or stuporous. Blood pressure tends to be low ("sugar shock") and respirations rapid and very deep. Blood and freshly produced urine test positive for excessive glucose, and urine contains ketone bodies. If hyperglycemia (and hyperosmolarity) are severe, the client may exhibit confusion or other signs of CNS malfunction. Unless proper treatment is given, coma and death may ensue. Hyperglycemia and shock develop over a period of hours to days. They are more likely to develop in clients whose need for insulin has risen, owing to unusual stress, infection, or other illness, or to progressive reduction in endogenous insulin production or utilization.

Excessive caloric intake (more than can be metabolized by the insulin available to the client) produces a syndrome (nonketotic hyperosmolar hyperglycemia) somewhat different from that of insulin deficiency. In this condition, the client's insulin supply is adequate to meet basic needs for energy and growth. No reserve insulin, however, is available for tissue storage of excess calories, which are or tend to be converted to glucose. Blood glucose rises and body tissues become hyperosmotic. This condition is toxic to the tissues and stimulates osmotic diuresis and dehydration. The client with nonketotic hyperosmolar hyperglycemia exhibits signs and symptoms similar to those of insulin deficiency hyperglycemia, except that ketoacidosis does not develop.

Excessive insulin (hypoglycemia, insulin shock) progresses much more rapidly than does hyperglycemia. This condition develops after an inadvertent overdose of insulin, unusual exercise, or missed feedings. Blood sugar decreases rapidly, depriving the brain of its only energy source. The client experiences apprehension, tremors, excitation, bizarre behavior (or other manifestations of CNS malfunction), perspiration, and severe headache. Blood tests show abnormally low blood glucose; freshly produced urine tests negative for glucose. Clients may lose consciousness and suffer brain damage if hypoglycemia is not corrected promptly.

Hyperventilation causes body changes that mimic, in part, both ketoacidosis and hypoglycemia. Like the client with ketoacidosis, the hyperventilating client breathes rapidly and deeply. In this case, however, the respiratory pattern is the cause of the syndrome rather than one of its effects. Rapid respirations increase the rate of carbon dioxide loss from the blood; respiratory alkalosis follows. Some signs and symptoms of alkalosis (apprehension, irritability, and tremor) resemble insulin reaction. Headache is usually absent.

If a client complains of episodes of apprehension, trembling, perspiration, and headache but tests positive for excess glucosuria and hyperglycemia, the problem may be a Somogyi effect. These clients overreact to hypoglycemia by secreting excess glucagon, glucocorticoids, or epinephrine, all of which inhibit the effect of insulin and promote glycolysis and increased blood sugar. The Somogyi effect can be caused by excessive dosages of insulin, and it is exacerbated if insulin dosages are increased in response to the glucosuria and hyperglycemia

Clients who have hyperglycemia should be closely assessed for signs and symptoms of infection, which is more likely to develop when body fluids are rich in glucose.

Nursing diagnosis Nursing diagnoses likely to develop in diabetic clients include the following:

Fluid volume deficit related to osmotic diuresis secondary to a relative insulin deficiency
High risk for infection related to hyperglycemia and hyperosmolarity secondary to nonketotic hyperosmolar hyperglycemia
Altered nutrition: less than body requirements related to impaired glucose metabolism secondary to a relative insulin deficiency
High risk for impaired tissue integrity: decubitus related to impaired tissue secondary to ketoacidosis

Common collaborative problems that should be differentiated from the nursing diagnoses include

Potential complication: hypovolemic shock
Potential complication: metabolic acidosis
Potential complication: hypoglycemia
Potential complication: hyperglycemia

Diagnoses likely to develop in clients who are receiving exogenous insulin include the following:

Anxiety related to hypoglycemia secondary to insulin overdose (fasting, vigorous exercise)
Pain: headache related to hypoglycemia secondary to insulin overdose (fasting, vigorous exercise)
Altered thought processes: confusion, bizarre (aggressive) behavior, or coma related to hypoglycemia secondary to insulin overdose (fasting, vigorous exercise)

Most newly diagnosed diabetics and some clients with a longer history of the disease exhibit a knowledge deficit about diabetes mellitus and its treatment.

Planning Goals of nursing care include restoring homeostasis (normal blood levels of glucose, pH, osmolarity, and emergence from coma), promoting glucose metabolism, restoring tissue perfusion, preventing stroke due to hypoglycemia, alleviating anxiety due to sympathoadrenal discharge or alkalosis, alleviating hypoglycemic headache, preventing or promptly detecting and treating complications such as infection or decubitus, and eliminating knowledge deficit.

Intervention The initial nursing intervention for hypoglycemia is the immediate administration of sugar, orally if possible. One glass of orange juice to which 2 teaspoons of sugar have been added can be offered to the client. If this is not immediately available, candy or table sugar may be substituted. Chocolate candy should not be used. Some authorities recommend placing sugar or a sugar gel under the tongue of the comatose client in the belief that some of the nutrient will be absorbed by the sublingual vessels, decreasing the severity of the hypoglycemia. Positioning the client to prevent aspiration is particularly important if this is done.

If response to the sugar is good, the client should be given food that contains carbohydrate (preferably starch) and protein. These nutrients provide glucose over a period of time to counteract the continued action of insulin. The rise in blood glucose from refined sugar tends to be temporary, therefore hypoglycemia is apt to recur. More than one feeding may be necessary if the client is using a long-lasting insulin.

If the client refuses to take a sweet or is unconscious, parenteral treatment is required. Glucagon injections or IV infusions of dextrose are prescribed to correct serious hypoglycemia. Glucagon is administered IM. If response to the first dose is not satisfactory, a second may be given after 20 minutes. More than two doses is not recommended, because response to further medication is unlikely. Clients who fail to respond to glucagon may have deficient glycogen stores. IV dextrose elevates blood glucose levels and restores brain function. Most people who experience serious hypoglycemia are admitted to the hospital for 24 hours to observe for recurring hypoglycemia. If convulsions or coma have occurred, a careful assessment for CNS damage must be made.

Like hypoglycemia, severe diabetic ketoacidosis also represents a medical emergency. The client may be admitted in a profound coma and hypovolemic shock. Restoration of fluid, electrolyte, and acid–base balance is of primary importance. Blood is drawn for chemical studies, and IV therapy is begun. Initially, isotonic saline is infused rapidly to restore blood volume. Sodium bicarbonate is added to the IV solution as needed to offset the degree of acidosis. Insulin is administered IM or IV because subcutaneous injections are not absorbed efficiently during circulatory shock. As soon as a drop in blood glucose establishes response to the insulin, dextrose is added to the IV infusion; insulin is continued either by addition to the infusion solutions or by periodic IM injections. Electrolyte content of fluids is adjusted in response to laboratory data. As the acidosis is corrected, serious hypokalemia develops and potassium levels must be maintained to avoid life-threatening cardiac arrhythmia.

When the client's condition improves and glucose metabolism stabilizes, the usual diabetic regimen is reinstituted. The intercurrent illness may have altered the diabetic status, however, and this regimen may now be inappropriate. Often the diabetes has worsened, and a higher dose of insulin is necessary. Occasionally, the client's immune status has changed. If insulin antibody levels have dropped, a decrease in insulin is needed.

Clients hospitalized specifically for adjustment of the diabetic regimen to reestablish control over the disease have orders for varying amounts of medication and diet until a satisfactory response occurs. During this period, the client's living conditions should simulate the normal environment as closely as possible. Regular meal times and activity patterns should be maintained. Physiotherapy may be ordered to provide

exercise. Excessive stress should be avoided. Because all of these factors tend to alter insulin needs, the regimen established in the hospital will not prove satisfactory after discharge unless hospital conditions are comparable to those at home.

Insulin reactions can occur at any time but are more likely as the client's condition improves. The nurse must monitor clients for signs and symptoms of insulin reactions, particularly at times of peak action and when the client has not eaten for some time (see Table 33-1 and Figs. 33-5, 33-6, and 33-7). Clients who receive long-lasting insulin in the morning are prone to hypoglycemia during sleep, especially if a bedtime snack has been omitted. Diaphoresis may be the only clue to hypoglycemia during sleep. The nurse must awaken the client and administer sugar if excessive perspiration is noted.

In acute care settings, diabetics are routinely tested for blood glucose or urine sugar and acetone, usually before meals and at bedtime. Some chronic care agencies still use urine test for sugar and acetone. Urine tests are most reliable when double-voided specimens are collected. Ten to fifteen minutes after the bladder has been emptied, the client is asked to void and the second specimen is tested. Presumably this urine has been freshly excreted by the kidneys and represents the current metabolic status. Monitoring urine has largely been superseded by fingerstick tests for blood glucose. If tests indicate that the diabetic condition is stable, the usual diet and insulin regimen may be maintained. Monitoring should be continued, however, because changes of routine and the stress that hospitalization imposes make metabolic instability likely.

Often the hospitalized diabetic exhibits an elevated blood sugar and glycosuria. The physician may order regular insulin supplements to the medication regimen (termed *insulin coverage* or *sliding scale*). Typically, urine or blood is monitored regularly (every 4 hours, or before meals and at bedtime), and insulin is given according to the degree of glucose detected. Usually no insulin is given if urine tests show 0.25% glucose or less. For 0.5% glucose, 5 U of insulin are given, for 1% glucose, 10 U, and for 2% glucose, 15 U. When blood is monitored, coverage is about 1 U per 25 mg/dl glucose above 180 mg/dl. If the client is particularly unstable, long-lasting insulin may be discontinued temporarily and the client may be maintained entirely with regular insulin.

Insulin by continuous infusion may be ordered for the treatment of ketoacidosis or foot lesions. The inner surfaces of bottles and tubing absorb insulin. To ensure delivery of uniform dosages, tubing should be flushed with a medicated solution before being connected to the IV line. The nurse should prepare 125% of the prescribed solution, using the excess to flush the tubing (Newton, 1987). This practice tends to saturate the tubing surface, preventing a reduction in insulin concentration from the rest of the solution. In-line filters are not recommended for insulin infusions.

Client education. Except during episodes of critical illness, the teaching needs of the diabetic should be given high priority in nursing care. Comprehensive diabetic education is beyond the scope of this text except as it relates to insulin use. As always, sound teaching and learning principles must be applied in the teaching plan.

Insulin administration. In relation to insulin administration, the diabetic must be taught the following:

Proper injection technique

How to store and handle insulin

The signs and symptoms of insulin excess and deficiency

Monitoring techniques

How to treat insulin reactions

When to seek medical attention

Insulin is usually administered subcutaneously using specifically designed disposable plastic syringes. These syringes are designed for one-time use. Recent research data indicate that disposable syringes may be used up to seven times without increased danger of infection, provided the needle is wiped with alcohol after each use, recapped, and the syringe refrigerated. Reuse effectively reduces the cost of syringes by six-sevenths. With successive use, however, the needle becomes considerably duller and eventually causes pain on insertion. Also, the longer the interval between initial use and final use, the greater the theoretical risk of infection. Keeping a used syringe longer than 7 days is not recommended; some authorities limit use to three injections.

Good surgical asepsis must be observed when insulin is injected. Whether or not the injection site should be massaged is controversial, as massage causes local vasodilation and more rapid absorption. Diabetics are unusually prone to infection, and infection in turn disrupts glucose balance, causing a rise in blood sugar. Contaminated equipment, which would be harmless in people with normal metabolism, can cause abscesses in diabetics. If an order for 100 U insulin is for an odd number of units, syringes must have gradations on the scale for hundredths of a milliliter. Some insulin syringes and all tuberculin syringes allow accurate measurement of the medication. When preparing insulin injections, avoid air bubbles, because these alter the dose.

If insulin syringes with short needles are used for injections, the needle should be inserted at a 90° angle to the skin. A 90° angle may also be used by obese people when using ⅝-inch needles, but an oblique approach is necessary for thin clients. Aspiration to verify placement in subcutaneous tissue rather than in a blood vessel is recommended but is not always taught to children or adults who have difficulty mastering injection technique. If injection sites are properly chosen to avoid areas rich in blood vessels, inadvertent IV injection is unlikely. Clients who administer their own insulin are limited to injection sites within reach, mainly the arms, thighs, and abdomen (Fig. 33-8). When these clients are hospitalized, injections administered by the nursing staff should use posterior sites to allow the anterior sites a period of rest. At home, a family member may be taught to give injections to allow use of a greater range of sites. The newest recommendations for choosing injection sites are to use one anatomic region only (*eg*, the abdomen or the thighs) and to rotate sites within this region. This procedure provides a more uniform absorption of insulin. After injection, the site should be massaged to promote absorption.

When insulin prescriptions specify that a mixture of insulins is to be administered, special care must be taken in preparing doses. Commonly, regular insulin and a long-lasting insulin (such as PZI) are combined. When different types of insulin are mixed, they tend to interact to produce an effect somewhat different from the sum of their individual effects. For example, long-lasting preparations may contain an excess of material used to modify their molecules for slower absorption; these substances convert a portion of the regular insulin mixed with it to a long-lasting form. For consistency in effect, individual doses must be prepared in a regulated manner. The sequence for drawing up the drugs should be the same for each dose preparation. To preserve the purity of the regular insulin supply, the regular insulin is usually drawn up first, followed by the long-lasting insulin. The vial that contains the long-lasting preparation must contain positive pres-

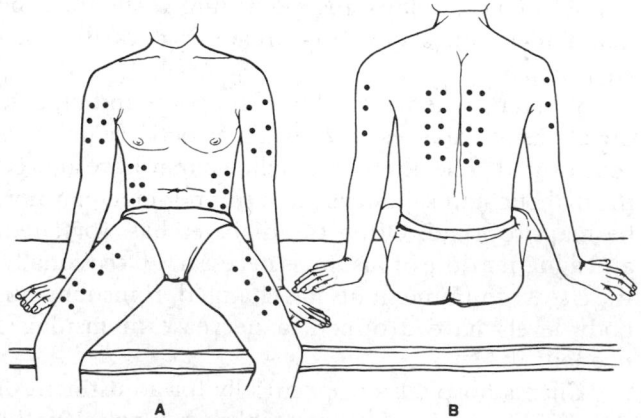

Figure 33-8. Sites of subcutaneous injections. **A.** Usual sites for self-administration are the outer aspects of the thighs. A systematic rotation of sites is important in insulin injections; it lessens irritation and improves absorption. **B.** Family members or hospital staff can use posterior sites for a wider variety of sites.

Box 33-2. Preparation of a mixed insulin injection

To prepare an injection that contains both long-lasting and regular insulin, roll both vials of insulin to distribute the drug evenly throughout the solution. Then, using sterile aseptic technique do the following:

1. Into the vial that contains the long-lasting insulin, inject a volume of air equal to the volume of long-lasting insulin required for the dose ordered.
2. Into the bottle that contains the regular insulin, inject a volume of air equal to the volume of the regular insulin required for the dose ordered; without withdrawing the needle, invert the vial.
3. Draw up the proper dose of regular insulin and withdraw the needle.
4. Invert the vial that contains the long-lasting insulin and insert the needle of the syringe through the rubber dam; do not allow the tip of the needle to protrude above the fluid level in the vial; allow the positive pressure in the vial to push the required volume of long-lasting insulin into the syringe.
5. Withdraw the needle from the vial. The volume in the syringe should be equal to the sums of the volumes of the two types of insulin ordered.

sure to eliminate any tendency toward suctioning of the regular insulin from the syringe into the vial.

Insulin deteriorates if exposed to excessive heat, light, or agitation. Constant refrigeration is not needed by the newer preparations, but clients should be instructed to refrigerate extra bottles until needed. Insulin must not be frozen. Insulin in current use should be kept at room temperature. Long-lasting insulins must be rolled to mix the suspension gently but thoroughly before drawing up the required dose. The bottle should never be shaken vigorously, because protein molecules are denatured by such whipping action. Frothing of the solution indicates the start of protein breakdown. All insulin should be protected from excessive heat or strong light. Travel is facilitated if insulin and equipment for administration are carried in a compact kit of some kind. Fitted containers are available commercially. Some kits have space for urine or blood testing equipment also.

Clients should be cautioned never to substitute one kind of insulin for another. The supply received from the pharmacist should conform exactly to that ordered by the physician. Substitution of a different concentration or type of insulin may cause errors in dosage and response. Because human insulin differs antigenic-

ally from animal insulins, it cannot be substituted for animal preparations unless the change is carefully supervised.

Hypoglycemia and hyperglycemia. Diabetics who receive insulin must be thoroughly familiar with the signs and symptoms of hypoglycemia and hyperglycemia. Many have developed hyperglycemia before the disease was diagnosed, and most experience one or more insulin reactions before a satisfactory medical regimen is achieved. The occurrence of such reactions provides a practical demonstration of the subjective symptoms of these conditions. The client should be instructed regarding the most likely times for hyperglycemia and hypoglycemia to develop and should be especially vigilant for symptoms at these times.

Because hypoglycemia may trigger socially unacceptable behavior, diabetics should always carry medical identification that indicates their disease and the hypoglycemia medication in use. If hypoglycemia is mistaken for drunkenness, the client is unlikely to receive timely treatment of this dangerous condition. Clients should also carry some form of sugar with them to take at the first sign of insulin reaction. Candy is a frequent choice, but cube sugar is preferable if the client craves sweets and is likely to eat the candy, a food allowed only in limited quantities by most diet prescriptions.

Monitoring glucose levels. Urine or blood testing is usually recommended for monitoring glucose balance. When renal threshold for glucose is normal, the occurrence and degree of hyperglycemia is reflected by the amount of glucose excreted in urine. Clients are usually instructed to test fasting urine or blood specimens before each meal and at bedtime. Urine tests are most reliable when double-voided specimens are used.

Testing is irrelevant if the client does not know what to do with the results. Sometimes the physician wants the record to be brought in to the office to guide decisions regarding insulin and diet prescription. The physician should always instruct the client about desired test results and abnormalities that should be reported promptly. Absence of hyperglycemia and glycosuria is desirable in adult onset diabetics who are relatively stable. The more closely blood glucose approaches normal levels in these clients, the less likely are complications to develop (although strict control does not always ensure that complications will not develop). In labile diabetics or those subject to frequent insulin reactions, some degree of hyperglycemia or glycosuria may be desirable to minimize the risk of serious hypoglycemia. Parameters for blood or urine glucose should be set by the physician. Urine tests of 0.25% or less are usually acceptable, but 0.5% or more glucose indicates poor control of blood sugar. If acetone is also present, ketoacidosis may have begun. (Positive acetone tests in the absence of glycosuria are normal in people on weight-reduction regimens.) Some clients have an abnormally low or high renal threshold to glucose. Because urine tests would not provide a reliable index to blood sugar levels, there is little purpose in monitoring the urine of these people. If weight is stable, acetone testing may furnish one indication of metabolic status. The substitution of fingerstick blood glucose tests for urine testing should be considered for these clients.

Ketoacidosis. Many clients omit insulin doses if they are unable to eat. This practice is logical but not advisable if the inability to eat is caused by nausea or other symptoms of illness. During illness, blood sugar levels tend to remain high despite fasting, probably because of the additional stress that affects the client. The regular dose of medication should be taken, and the physician should be consulted for treatment of the intercurrent illness. Nausea is one early sign of keto-acidosis, and many clients who are admitted to the hospital for treatment of this complication have omitted their regular dose of insulin, thus contributing to the severity of their condition (see Example of Nursing Process and Diabetes Maintenance).

Checklist of nursing actions

When insulin is prescribed

☐ Before drawing-up insulin into a syringe, rotate gently to mix.

☐ Exercise special care in preparing insulin to administer. Be sure the proper drug preparation is used. When possible, have the dosage checked for accuracy by another nurse.

☐ Rotate injection sites within a selected anatomic area according to a regular plan that allows at least 1 month between injections at any one site.

☐ Monitor urinary and or blood glucose to assess therapeutic response.

☐ Assess the client carefully for signs and symptoms of hyperglycemia and hypoglycemia.

☐ Administer sugar at the first sign of insulin reaction and when in doubt about the nature of a reaction in an insulin-dependent diabetic.

☐ Teach clients how to manage their diabetic regimens, including insulin medication; explain the factors that increase and decrease insulin requirement.

☐ Refrigerate stock supplies of insulin but protect from freezing; keep bottles in current use at

Learning experience 33-2

Care for a client with insulin-dependent diabetes. Assess the client for glucose balance. Plan and carry out nursing care designed to enhance therapeutic response and minimize adverse reactions to insulin.

room temperature and protect from heat and direct sunlight.

☐ Discard any insulin for which the expiration dates have passed or in which solid clumps or deposits have appeared.

☐ When preparing mixtures of regular and modified insulin, draw up the regular insulin first to avoid contamination of regular insulin vials with modified insulin.

☐ Delay administration of insulin if the client must fast for testing procedures.

Oral hypoglycemics

To date, only two classes of drugs other than insulin have been used therapeutically to control hyperglycemia, sulfonylureas and biguanides. Biguanides have been withdrawn from the market in the U.S. because they cause severe lactic acidosis. At present, sulfonylureas are the only oral hypoglycemics used to treat diabetes mellitus.

In 1942, researchers who investigated the treatment of typhoid fever with sulfonamides noted that one side effect of the drug *p*-amino-benzenesulfonamidoiso-propylthiadiazole was hypoglycemia. Several years later, a similar hypoglycemic effect was discovered in the antibacterial carbutamide. Modification of this compound produced tolbutamide, the first sulfonylurea. Several related drugs followed.

Sulfonylureas

These drugs are all arylsulfonylureas with substitutions on the benzene and urea groups. Recently, a new group of substances (so-called second generation sulfonylureas) has been under investigation. Two of these, glipizide and glyburide, are in clinical use. They are more potent than the first generation of sulfonylureas (Table 33-3).

Pharmacodynamics. Sulfonylureas stimulate the pancreas to secrete insulin. They exert no hypoglycemic effect in people who have an absolute deficiency of insulin due of pancreatectomy or total lack of insulin production. They are effective in lowering blood sugar in non–insulin-dependent adult-onset diabetes. These agents also inhibit the release of catecholamines and may enhance the metabolic effect of insulin by limiting the secretion of these insulin antagonists. Some investigators believe that prolonged use of the drugs results in an increase in the number of insulin receptors, thus increasing tissue sensitivity to the action of the endogenous hormone. Glyburide exerts a mild diuretic action and appears to inhibit platelet aggregation.

Pharmacokinetics. Sulfonylureas are well absorbed when administered orally. Onset of action, peak effect, and duration of effect vary with the preparation. The compounds that bind to serum proteins (tolbutamide,

Example of nursing process and diabetes maintenance

The client is an 18-year-old college woman with a 3-year history of insulin-dependent diabetes mellitus. At first, control of her blood sugar was difficult and required frequent doses of regular insulin before meals or at bedtime to lower glucose levels into the normal range. When she stopped growing, however, she was able to maintain good glucose control (blood levels below 180 mg/dl) with only rare supplements of regular insulin. Soon after the college term began, glucose metabolism again became more unstable and she is now taking regular insulin at least once a day. She has had no insulin reactions. She has come to the infirmary to find out what is wrong.

The nurse discusses with the client factors that may play a role in glucose instability, including diet, exercise, and stress. The client says dormitory menu offers enough variety so that she can easily choose foods suitable to her diet. She denies dietary noncompliance. Exercise has been somewhat erratic during the "settling in" period, because considerable walking was required to attend orientation sessions, but there were no regular physical education classes until recently. The client admits that college "is sure different" from high school but expresses doubt that stress could produce the hyperglycemia. She asks the nurse, "Could my diabetes be getting worse?"

Assessment data	Nursing diagnosis	Intervention	Goals and outcome criteria
Insulin-dependent diabetes mellitus	Altered health maintenance related to stress	**Explain** to the client the role stress and stress hormones play in body response to insulin.	Incidence or absence of preprandial hyperglycemia that requires supplemental doses of regular insulin will decrease.
Increased hyperglycemia since entering college		**Point out** the many changes in routine and environment to which the client must adjust in college; assist the client to identify stressors and plan changes that can reduce their number.	By the end of the first month of the semester, the client will require supplemental doses of insulin no more frequently than she did during her last year of high school.
Student's statement that "college is different" (elevation of stress hormones increases insulin resistance)		**Explore** stress management techniques the client has used in the past; teach the client new stress management techniques.	The client will not experience hypoglycemic reactions severe enough to cause CNS damage (*ie*, stroke).
(A decline in stress increases therapeutic action of insulin)		**Encourage** the client to continue to monitor blood glucose and take regular insulin in accord with the results.	
(Adaptation to change usually decreases stress)		**Reassure** the client that the stress of change is more likely to be the cause of hyperglycemia than a worsening of the disease.	
		Advise the client to avoid manipulation of dosage of long-acting insulin; recommend that she consult her physician if she continues to need insulin supplements after the first month of school.	
		Emphasize to the client that hypoglycemia is more likely to cause CNS injury than is hyperglycemia; positively reinforce compliance with treatment regimen.	

Table 33-3. Oral hypoglycemic drugs

Drug name	Approximate time of onset (hours)	Peak action (hours)	Plasma half-life (hours)	Duration of activity (hours)	Usual adult dosage	Pregnancy risk category*
Acetohexamide (Dymelor)	1	3	1.3 (4.5 for active metabolites)	12–24	250 mg–1.5 g daily, divided in 1–2 doses	D
Chlorpropamide (Diabinese)	1	3–6	36	24 +	100–500 mg daily, given as a single dose	D
Gliclazide† (Diamicron)	Not available	4–6	10.4	24	80–150 mg q12–24h	
Glipizide (Glucotrol)	0.5	1–3	3–4.7	24	*Initially:* 2.5–5 mg once daily; *maintenance:* 2.5–40 mg daily	C
Glyburide (Diabeta, Euglucon, Micronase)	0.5	1.5–3	1.4–1.8 (10 for active metabolites)	24	*Initially:* 1.25–5 mg daily, divided in 1–2 doses; *maintenance:* 1.25–20 mg daily, divided in 1–2 doses	B
Metformin† (Glucophage)	Relatively slow	Not available	Biphasic: 1.7–3 and 9–17	Not available	500 mg tid	
Tolazamide (Tolinase)	4–6	6–9	7	10	250 mg daily, divided in 1–2 doses	C
Tolbutamide (Orinase, Mobenol, Orinase)	1	5–8	7	6–12	1 g daily, divided in 2–3 doses	C

*The validity of pregnancy risk categories remains unproven.

†Not available in the U.S. at this time.

glipizide, and chlorpropamide) require several days of administration to achieve full effect. Elimination of the drugs is primarily through renal excretion, although metabolism by the liver is required for elimination of tolbutamide and glipizide and is involved in the action of acetohexamide and tolazamide by producing metabolites of varying physiologic potency. Chlorpropamide is excreted largely unchanged by the kidneys.

Therapeutic uses. For about 20 years, sulfonylureas were used as an alternative to insulin therapy in treating adult onset diabetes mellitus. Sulfonylureas help to control blood sugar levels and prevent ketoacidosis. In the last decade, however, evidence of adverse reactions from long-term therapy has induced caution; sulfonylureas are prescribed infrequently in current practice.

Adverse reactions. The overall risk of side effects from sulfonylureas is about 5%. Likelihood of adverse responses is related to potency, with reactions to chlorpropamide occurring four times more often than to tolbutamide. Some complications are most likely to occur within the first 2 months of treatment, whereas others develop only after prolonged treatment.

Because they stimulate endogenous insulin secretion, sulfonylureas can cause symptomatic hypoglycemia. Reactions tend to be less severe than with exogenous insulin but are more prolonged and may produce serious, even fatal, consequences. As with insulin, delayed meals or unusual exercise tend to precipitate such episodes. Hypoglycemia may occur at any time, even after months of trouble-free treatment.

Side effects include gastrointestinal (GI) distress, CNS malfunction, alcohol intolerance, skin eruptions, blood dyscrasias, jaundice, hepatitis (with glyburide), and inappropriate secretion of antidiuretic hormone (ISADH). Intestinal symptoms include heartburn, nausea, vomiting, abdominal pain, and diarrhea. CNS manifestations include confusion, vertigo, ataxia, paresthesia, weakness, tinnitus, headache, and visual impairment. A reaction that resembles that of disulfiram (Antabuse) may occur with alcohol intake. The most serious hematologic effect is agranulocytosis, but thrombocytopenia, pancytopenia, and hemolytic anemia also occur in rare instances. Jaundice is of the cholestatic type. Excessive antidiuretic hormone secretion may be associated with hyponatremia. Agranulocytosis and jaundice are most likely to develop within the first 2 months of treatment, but other complications may arise at any time.

Administering large doses of sulfonylureas to animals results in increased teratogenesis in the offspring. The drugs are not recommended for use in pregnancy.

A significant risk of earlier death from cardiovascular problems is associated with the use of oral hypoglycemics. At present, sulfonylureas are recommended only for use with people who have not responded to dietary treatment and weight loss and who are unwilling or unable to use insulin. It is considered a treatment of last resort that carries significant risk of shortened life expectancy.

Precautions and contraindications. Sulfonylureas are contraindicated in insulin-dependent diabetes, in the presence of serious hepatic or renal disease, and during pregnancy. They are not used for juvenile-type diabetes but are reserved for mild non–insulin-dependent diabetes with an onset at age 40 years or older.

Because liver and kidney functions influence the metabolism and excretion of these drugs, and because these functions may be impaired in older clients, high-loading doses are avoided. During the initial treatment, before the full effect of the drugs is achieved, insulin may be continued at reduced dosages, especially in people who require more than 20 U of insulin daily. Metabolic status must be monitored closely with urine and blood tests for sugar. Oral drugs often maintain normoglycemia in clients with otherwise stable health. However, stressors such as infection, fever, surgery, or trauma increase blood sugar, requiring additional exogenous insulin until the situation is resolved.

Drug interactions. Some sulfonylureas are highly bound to serum proteins. Concurrent administration of other protein-bound drugs (such as nonsteroidal, anti-inflammatory agents, oral anticoagulants, hydantoin, and sulfonamides) tends to alter serum drug levels and response to medication. Protein-bound drugs may enhance response to sulfonylureas, or their own action may be enhanced by sulfonylureas. In addition to its ability to displace sulfonylureas from plasma proteins, phenylbutazone also inhibits renal excretion of acetohexamide and the metabolism of tolbutamide. Other drugs that enhance hypoglycemic response include insulin, alcohol, and (for chlorpropamide and tolazamide) probenecid.

People treated with sulfonylureas may experience a disulfiram-like reaction (flushing, nausea, and vomiting) when drinking alcohol. The flush is particularly prominent with chlorpropamide. Chlorpropamide also prolongs the duration of barbiturate action.

When β-adrenergic blockers are administered concurrently with sulfonylureas, they tend to inhibit some diagnostic signs of hypoglycemia. The increases in pulse and blood pressure characteristic of sympathetic response to rapid decreases in blood sugar do not occur (see Focus on Sulfonylureas: Similarities and Differences).

■ **Summary**

Sulfonylureas act primarily by stimulating the secretion of endogenous insulin. They are effective only in mild adult onset diabetes. Because sulfonylureas may increase the death rate from cardiovascular disease, insulin therapy is preferable if feasible. In addition to the usual toxic effects of insulin, sulfonylureas can cause GI, CNS, skin, liver, and hematopoietic symptoms. Periodic use of insulin is often required to control glucose metabolism during intercurrent illness in clients normally controlled by sulfonylureas.

Nursing management

Nursing implications

Clients who receive oral hypoglycemics are likely to have had difficulty adjusting to the diabetic regimen, especially to insulin administration. They may need supervision and assistance.

Nursing process

Assessment Clients who receive sulfonylureas to treat diabetes mellitus must be monitored for glucose imbalance (hyperglycemia and hypoglycemia), just as clients who depend on diet alone or on diet combined with insulin. The nurse should also assess the client for adverse reactions to these drugs. During the first 2 months of treatment, any evidence of agranulocytosis or jaundice is particularly significant. Frequent sore throats or other infections must be reported to the physician. Periodic blood tests should be ordered to monitor for hematologic changes. The client should be observed for jaundice using natural sunlight or incandescent light. Fluorescent light that lacks yellow tones masks jaundice, even when it is quite pronounced. Ocular sclerae should be carefully examined for yellow discoloration to detect beginning jaundice. The client should be questioned about paresthesia, tinnitus, and visual changes to detect sensory-perceptual alterations.

In view of the evidence that sulfonylurea therapy increases the incidence of serious cardiovascular disease, clients who receive these drugs should be carefully assessed for the development of such pathology. Examination of the cardiovascular system should be carried out on a regular basis. The advisability of continued drug therapy should be critically reassessed if hypertension or cardiac arrhythmia develops.

Nursing diagnosis Nursing diagnosis likely to be made for clients who are taking sulfonylureas include the following:

Altered comfort: nausea, vomiting, abdominal pain secondary to sulfonylurea medication

Sulfonylureas: similarities and differences

Similarities	Differences

Similarities

Pharmacodynamics

These agents stimulate the release of endogenous insulin for the pancreas, lowering blood glucose levels.

Pharmacokinetics

These agents are rapidly and readily absorbed from the GI tract. They are distributed into the extracelluar fluid. They are metabolized by the liver and excreted by the kidneys.

Therapeutic uses

These agents are used to treat non–insulin-dependent diabetes mellitus.

Adverse reactions

These include: (CNS) headache, weakness, confusion, paresthesia, ataxia; (EENT) tinnitus, visual impairment; (GI) nausea, vomiting, GI distress, anorexia, abdominal pain, heartburn, jaundice, and altered liver function; (ENDO) hypoglycemia; (HEMA) blood dyscrasia, agranulocytosis, thrombocytopenia, hemolytic anemia, aplastic anemia and hyponatremia; (SKIN) urticaria, erythema, pruritus; (OTHER) disulfiram reaction, syndrome of inappropriate antidiuretic hormone (SIADH).

Contraindications

These agents are contraindicated for people with insulin-dependent diabetes mellitus (IDDM) and for those complicated with ketosis, acidosis, coma, or other acute complication, such as major surgery, severe infection, trauma, or burns. They are also contraindicated for people with severe hepatic or renal dysfunction and for those with a known hypersensitivity to sulfas, those who are pregnant, and those with nonfunctioning pancreatic beta cells.

Precautions

These agents should be used with caution in people with hepatic porphyria, in women of childbearing age, and people with impaired adrenal, pituitary, or thyroid function.

Differences

Pharmacodynamics

• **Chlorpropamide** has an antidiuretic action. • **Glyburide** exhibits mild diuretic action and appears to inhibit platelet aggregation.

Pharmacokinetics

• **Chlorpropamide** is excreted unchanged in the urine. • **Acetohexamide** has a half-life of 1 to 1.5 hours. • **Chlorpropamide** has an onset of 1 hour, peaking in 2 to 4 hours, with a duration of 24 hours and a half-life of 36 hours. • **Glypizide** has an onset of 15 to 30 minutes, peaking in 1 to 6 hours, with a duration of 24 hours and a half-life of 2 to 7 hours. • **Glyburide** has an onset of 15 to 60 minutes, peaking in 2 to 8 hours, with a duration of 24 hours and a half-life of 10 hours. • **Tolazamide** has an onset of 4 to 6 hours, with a duration of 10 hours and a half-life of 7 hours. • **Tolbutamide** has an onset of 30 to 60 minutes, peaking in 3 to 5 hours, with a duration of 6 to 12 hours and a half-life of 7 hours.

Adverse reactions

• **Tolbutamide, tolazamide**, and **chlorpropamide** may cause photosensitivity. • **Tolazamide** may also cause lethargy, dizziness, and vertigo.

Contraindications

• **Acetohexamide** is contraindicated in hyperglycemia and glycosuria with primary renal dysfunction. • **Chlorpropamide** is contraindicated for people with diminished thyroid function. • **Tolazamide** is contraindicated for people with uremia. • **Tolbutamide** is contraindicated for people with severe renal insufficiency.

Precautions

• **Chlorpropamide** should be used with caution in people with impaired cardiac function and fluid retention.

(continued)

Focus on

Sulfonylureas: similarities and differences (*Continued*)

Similarities	Differences
Nursing considerations	

Similarities

Nursing considerations

Instruct client in disease, treatment, drug therapy, regimen, adverse effects, and compliance; monitor blood glucose level and urine for glucose and ketones frequently; instruct client in how to check own glucose levels; administer 30 minutes before breakfast daily or 30 minutes before breakfast and dinner for BID regime; assess for signs and symptoms of hypoglycemia and hyperglycemia; instruct client in all aspects of diabetes, including diet; warn clients to avoid the intake of alcohol; assess clients for signs of infection or stress, which may necessitate dosage changes; monitor serum lab studies, including blood counts and bilirubin levels for changes.

Differences

When administering **chlorpropamide**, monitor fluid balance status closely; watch for signs of impending renal insufficiency, such as dysuria, anuria, and hematuria.

High risk for infection related to leukopenia secondary to bone marrow depression by sulfonylureas
Body image disturbance related to skin rash or jaundice secondary to adverse reaction to sulfonylureas
Fluid volume deficit related to inappropriate secretion of antidiuretic hormone secondary to adverse reaction to sulfonylureas
Impaired physical mobility: ataxia, vertigo, and weakness related to adverse reaction to sulfonylureas
Altered comfort related to disulfiram reaction to alcohol secondary to sulfonylurea medication

Common collaborative problems that should be differentiated from the nursing diagnoses include

Potential complication: hypoglycemia
Potential complication: anemia
Potential complication: bone marrow depression
Potential complication: cardiovascular degeneration
Potential complication: adverse reactions to sulfonylureas

Planning The goals of nursing care include maintenance of glucose balance, prevention of disulfiram-like reactions to ethanol, and prevention or prompt detection and treatment of adverse reactions to sulfonylureas.

Intervention Clients who are to receive hypoglycemic drugs must adhere to a health regimen like that required of other diabetics. To maintain glucose balance, they must comply with the prescribed diet and medication, they must maintain a regular schedule of rest and activity, they must avoid infection, and they must avoid high stress levels.

The nurse should assess the client regularly for signs and symptoms of adverse reactions to drugs. These should be reported to the physician for adjustment of the drug regimen.

The nurse should ensure that institutionalized clients who take sulfonylureas are not served alcoholic beverages and that medicinal preparations that contain alcohol are not administered to them.

Client education. Clients have the right to know that the use of oral hypoglycemics may pose an increased risk of early death from cardiovascular complications. In the absence of such information, consent for treatment is not valid, because it is not fully informed. Clients who wish to discontinue oral hypoglycemic therapy need considerable assistance in undertaking insulin treatment. If the physician changes the drug order, intensive nursing care should be available to help the client cope successfully with the new regimen.

Education is a cornerstone of treatment for all diabetics, but it is particularly important for the client who is receiving oral hypoglycemics. Control of diet and body weight are crucial to therapeutic outcome. Urine or blood glucose tests and monitoring for signs and symptoms of glucose imbalance are as important as for clients who take exogenous insulin.

Although many clients who receive sulfonylureas previously have not adjusted well to insulin therapy, the hormone may be needed periodically to maintain glucose balance during intercurrent illness. Either the client or someone in the family should be able to administer insulin if needed.

In addition to the usual instruction in the detection of hyperglycemia and hypoglycemia, clients must be taught the signs and symptoms of adverse reactions to sulfonylureas and must be urged to report these to their physicians. Blood dyscrasias and jaundice are particularly dangerous. The client should immediately report frequent infections, weakness, abnormal bleeding tendencies, or jaundice.

Additional prescriptions for interacting drugs should not be accepted without reminding the physician that sulfonylurea therapy is in progress. If such drugs are prescribed, the client should understand that the risk of side effects is increased, and self-monitoring is critical.

Nonprescription drugs that contain salicylates and alcohol should be avoided while sulfonylureas are in use. Drinking alcoholic beverages, if tolerated, increases the likelihood of hypoglycemic reactions.

The lay public sometimes applies the term "oral insulin" to these hypoglycemics. This term is not appropriate and may mislead clients about the nature of sulfonylurea actions. The drugs neither exert a hormone effect nor in any way replace insulin. Their stimulation of endogenous insulin secretion helps normalize glucose metabolism but appears to contribute to cardiovascular degeneration and may hasten pancreatic failure and create an insulin dependency.

Evaluation Data required for evaluation include serial blood glucose levels, presence or absence of signs of adverse drug reactions (such as depressed dehydration, blood cell counts, jaundice, infection), presence or absence of signs of cardiovascular degeneration, and statements by the client relating to sensory perception, discomfort, and self-concept (see Example of Nursing Process and Tolbutamide Therapy).

Checklist of nursing actions

When sulfonylureas are initially prescribed
☐ Review with the client the prescribed diabetic regimen, stressing the importance of diet control, regular exercise, good general hygiene, and monitoring practices.
☐ Provide the client with oral and written information about the sulfonylurea prescribed, including its action, toxic and side effects, and the amount and timing of the doses to be taken.

☐ Review all drugs used by the client to assess the risk of adverse drug interactions.

During the first 2 weeks of treatment
☐ Monitor closely for glucose imbalance.

During the first 2 months of treatment
☐ Monitor closely for frequent infections (especially sore throats) and jaundice.

Throughout treatment
☐ Analyze results of blood and urine tests to determine glucose balance.
☐ Assess client for symptoms of GI, CNS, hematopoietic, liver, and skin problems.
☐ Assess cardiovascular function regularly.
☐ Refer client to the physician for reassessment of the drug regimen when pertinent symptoms are found.
☐ Caution the client that use of alcohol may cause an unpleasant (disulfiram-like) reaction.

Hyperglycemics

Glucagon

Glucagon is a hormone secreted by the alpha cells of the islets of Langerhans of the pancreas. Glucagon's physiologic function is generally opposite to that of insulin. Glucagon, a protein hormone, is a single chain polypeptide made up of 29 amino acids.

Physiology. After secretion by the pancreas, glucagon enters the blood, where it circulates freely. Its plasma half-life (like insulin) is about 3 to 6 minutes. Peripherally, it increases blood sugar levels by stimulating glycogenolysis, exerts a positive inotropic and chronotropic effect on the heart, and relaxes the intestine. It is degraded at tissue-receptor sites and in the kidneys, liver, and plasma.

The main stimulus to glucagon secretion is a decrease in intracellular glucose concentrations, usually as a result of a drop in blood sugar. Increased intracellular glucose after a rise in blood sugar inhibits its production. Blood glucose and glucagon form a negative feedback mechanism that operates to restore blood glucose levels after a drop below normal, regardless of the cause. The effects of glucagon protect the body from tissue damage caused by inadequate supplies of readily available energy. Most importantly, glucagon functions to maintain a steady supply of energy to the brain, retina, and germinal tissue, which are obligate users of glucose. Just as insulin functions to promote the storage of energy nutrients in tissue depots, glucagon functions to mobilize stored energy when needed by the body. Insulin is most active when the body has ample supplies of nutrients; glucagon is most active during starvation states and after injury, when body requirements for energy are not met adequately by dietary intake. Glucagon secretion is the body's first line of defense against hypoglycemia.

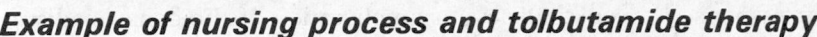

Example of nursing process and tolbutamide therapy

The client is an 80-year-old retired widowed printer who lives with his daughter, a part-time substitute teacher. Seven years ago, the client was told that he had adult onset non–insulin-dependent diabetes mellitus. The condition was controlled by diet until last year, when the client was hospitalized for treatment of a severe episode of ketoacidosis. Until that event, the client had lived alone in an efficiency apartment near his daughter.

After recovery from ketoacidosis, the client required insulin to control hyperglycemia. He was unable to learn injection technique, however, and tolbutamide 325 mg tid was prescribed. He came to live with his daughter, who supervises his diet. On days that she is called to work, the daughter leaves a cold lunch for the client in the refrigerator and his noon medication on the kitchen counter. When the public health nurse arrived for a visit at 2 PM today, she found the client wandering around the house, confused and incoherent. His lunch was still in the refrigerator, uneaten, but the medication container was empty.

Assessment data	Nursing diagnosis	Intervention	Goals and outcome criteria
Prescription for tolbutamide Confusion, incoherence	Potential complication: hypoglycemia*	**Prepare** a small glass of sweetened orange juice; using a quiet firm approach, try to persuade the client to drink it; if unsuccessful, call for emergency medical care. If the client drinks the orange juice and becomes more rational, **feed** him lunch.	The client's confusion will clear, he will become coherent and mentally alert.
Apparent ingestion of noon dose to tolbutamide Client's lunch had not been eaten	Impaired home maintenance mangement	**Inform** the daughter of the episode; suggest that she put the client's medication with his lunch to ensure that he will eat when he takes the drug.	Client will consistently take noon dose of tolbutamide with his lunch.
Client's failure to eat after taking hypoglycemic drug	Knowledge deficit related to oral hypoglycemic drug and its relation to diet in the treatment of diabetes mellitus	When the client is mentally alert, **explore** his knowledge about tolbutamide and its function in the control of diabetes mellitus. **Explain** that, although tolbutamide is not a form of insulin, it does increase the level of insulin in his blood and can cause hypoglycemia, just as exogenous insulin does; stress the importance of eating the meals prescribed for his diet.	The client will accurately repeat to the nurse (or to the daughter) the information conveyed during teaching. The client will eat all the meals prescribed for his diet.

*Although potential complications generally are not included in the Examples of Nursing Process, in this situation the identification of this collaborative problem is critical to the outcome for this client and illustrates the broad range of nursing responsibilities.

Pathology. Theoretically, disturbances in glucagon production could contribute to many problems in glucose metabolism. Inadequate glucagon response would cause an increase in the number and severity of hypoglycemic episodes in people subject to such reactions. This may be a factor in the reactive hypoglycemia of the late prediabetic state and in the frequent and severe hypoglycemic reactions in insulin-dependent diabetics. Excessive glucagon secretion tends to reduce the effectiveness of insulin, whether endogenous or exogenous. Such excesses could contribute to severe diabetes mellitus, stress-related hyperglycemia, and the Somogyi response to insulin reactions. Erratic glucagon response may be a factor in the pronounced blood sugar fluctuations of labile diabetes mellitus. At present, the degree to which glucagon imbalance is actually involved in these situations is not known. In clinical settings, the focus of medical treatment is the manipulation of insulin and glucose levels to achieve a metabolic equilibrium, with little attention paid to the possible roles of glucagon.

High levels of glucagon have been found in diabetics, but the cause–effect relationship of these two factors is unclear.

Pharmacodynamics. Glucagon stimulates the synthesis of cyclic adenosine monophosphate, especially in liver and adipose tissue. It promotes the breakdown of fuels stored in the tissues to meet the body's energy needs. Glycogenolysis and gluconeogenesis increase, and the glucose generated enters the blood, causing a rapid rise in blood sugar. (If blood sugar rises above the normal range, insulin secretion is stimulated.) In response to increased cyclic adenosine monophosphate, cardiac muscle contracts more strongly and more rapidly. The mechanism that underlies the hormone's relaxing effect on the intestinal musculature remains obscure.

Pharmacokinetics. Glucagon cannot be administered orally because it is destroyed by proteolytic enzymes in the digestive tract. After parenteral injection, maximum hyperglycemic effect occurs within 30 minutes; relaxation of GI smooth muscle develops within 15 minutes. Duration of action is about 1 to 2 hours for the hyperglycemic effect and about 30 minutes for GI relaxation.

The metabolic fate of glucagon is not known, but the drug is degraded in the liver and kidneys. It has a plasma half-life of 3 to 19 minutes.

Therapeutic uses. Glucagon is used to relieve hypoglycemia in clinical situations not amenable to the oral administration of sugar. It is useful in treating diabetics prone to rapidly developing insulin reactions in which unconsciousness occurs with little warning and in treating clients in whom hypoglycemia causes behavioral disturbances characterized by resistance to treatment. An initial dose of 1 U is administered by injection. Response to the drug as shown by a return of consciousness or amelioration of the behavior disturbance should be evident in 5 to 20 minutes. After 20 minutes, the dose may be repeated if necessary. More than two doses are not recommended since succeeding doses have not proved to be effective.

Glucagon is also used to induce intestinal relaxation before radiographic examination. It is sometimes administered to strengthen heart function as an adjunct in the treatment of shock.

Drug preparations. The structure of glucagon appears to be identical in many species. Human, porcine, and bovine hormone are alike in molecular makeup. The hormone has been synthesized and is available for therapeutic use. The drug is measured in both units and milligrams, with 1 mg equaling 1 U.

Glucagon for medicinal use is supplied as hydrochloride salt. It is dispensed as a dry powder in 1- or 10-U ampules with diluent sufficient to make a solution that contains 1 U/ml. The solution should be freshly prepared and refrigerated if not completely used. The usual dose is 1 U, administered subcutaneously, IM, or IV. The drug cannot be administered orally because it is destroyed by proteolytic enzymes in the digestive tract.

Adverse reactions. Glucagon is a relatively safe substance. Nausea and vomiting can occur, although these reactions can also be induced by hypoglycemia. The drug can produce a pronounced hyperglycemia, but this is usually transitory in nature because the glucagon is rapidly dissipated. Moreover, the rise in blood sugar stimulates insulin secretion in some clients, tending to correct the imbalance. In diabetics given the drug for insulin reactions, the hyperglycemia is also transitory, because continued insulin effect limits body response to glucagon and often induces a recurrent hypoglycemia. If glucagon is administered to a ketoacidotic diabetic, hyperglycemia increases in magnitude, accentuating the hyperosmolarity.

Large doses of glucagon have been administered experimentally in the treatment of cardiac disorders. Although such treatment has not been very effective, serious toxic or side effects from the glucagon were not reported.

Precautions and contraindications. No absolute contraindications for the use of glucagon exist. Because of its life-saving potential in the treatment of insulin reactions, it is recommended for use even when the diagnosis of hypoglycemia is not firmly established. Prompt recognition of failure to respond to the drug is important, however, so that other treatment can be instituted. If the client is not conscious and cooperative after the first half-hour of glucagon treatment, IV dextrose is needed.

■ **Summary**

Glucagon is a natural hormone secreted by the pancreas that mobilizes body stores of nutrient energy. Administered by injection, it causes a rapid but transitory hyperglycemia and is used most often for the initial treatment of acute hypoglycemia.

Nursing management

Nursing implications

Because glucagon is generally reserved for use when sugar cannot be administered to terminate a hypoglycemic reaction, it is often administered without the explicit consent of clients and sometimes in opposition to their immediate wishes. When a client is unconscious, the drug is clearly indicated as an emergency measure to terminate the coma. Questions of legal liability arise when the hypoglycemic client exhibits erratic behavior characterized by resistance to treatment. Because a biochemical glucose deficiency impairs brain function, the client is subject to a temporary delirium and is truly mentally incompetent, but there is no time to establish this in any legal sense. Hypoglycemia is a medical emergency; treatment must be carried out quickly to prevent permanent brain damage. The safest course is immediate administration of glucagon, by force if necessary. This action poses a dilemma for the nurse who is technically guilty of assault and battery if such a course is adopted. Clients who habitually exhibit resistive behavior while hypoglycemic should be asked to sign a statement granting prior permission for treatment in such situations. This provides a measure of legal protection for health care personnel.

When forcible administration of medications is necessary for the client's safety, sufficient personnel should be mobilized to nullify resistance and prevent or limit conflict. Serious injury to client or staff could result if a physical struggle develops. The staff should maintain an attitude of concern and helpfulness throughout the procedure. Successful treatment for the client is usually followed by a return to rational behavior.

Nursing process

Assessment   Glucagon is administered only when acute hypoglycemia does not respond to oral carbohydrates or when loss of consciousness precludes oral administration. Diabetic clients who receive insulin or oral hypoglycemics and other clients with excess insulin secretion (as in insulin-secreting tumors) should be monitored for signs and symptoms of low blood sugar: sympathoadrenal activity (apprehension, tachycardia, tremor, weakness, perspiration), bizarre behavior, and headache. Blood glucose levels may be tested by

fingerstick if the equipment is available. A blood glucose level of less than 60 mg/dl indicates hypoglycemia. (Symptoms of hypoglycemia also occur in clients who experience a sudden drop in blood glucose that is usually somewhat higher than normal, even though the drop may not depress glucose levels to 60 mg/dl.) Treatment should not be delayed if blood glucose cannot be tested promptly.

Nursing diagnosis   Nursing diagnoses likely in clients who are receiving glucagon include the following:

> *Altered thought processes related to hypoglycemia secondary to insulin or sulfonylurea toxicity, unusual exercise, or fasting (missed meal)*
> *Altered comfort: headache (perspiration, apprehension) related to hypoglycemia secondary to insulin or sulfonylurea toxicity, unusual exercise, or fasting (missed meal)*

Planning   The goal of nursing care is elimination of the signs and symptoms of hypoglycemia by restoration and maintenance of normal blood glucose levels.

Intervention   If the client is conscious and cooperative, sugar should be given orally. Sweetened orange juice, hard candy, or sugar cubes are usually effective. As soon as the acute symptoms have subsided and the client is more comfortable, a feeding should be given to prevent recurrent hypoglycemia.

If oral administration of carbohydrates is impossible, glucagon is usually administered. The medication must be reconstituted, using the diluent supplied in the package. The usual adult dosage is 0.5 to 1 mg (0.5–1 U) administered by IM or IV injection.

After glucagon is administered, the client should be observed carefully for response to the drug. A return to consciousness or rational behavior may occur quickly. If response is inadequate or incomplete at the end of 20 minutes, a second dose should be administered. At the same time, preparations should be made for immediate administration of IV dextrose in the event the second dose is also ineffective. If such treatment is not available, emergency medical care should be summoned immediately. No more than two doses of glucagon should be given for a single incident; response to further doses is unlikely, and alternative treatment is imperative.

After response to glucagon therapy, the client should be fed immediately. The effects of glucagon usually dissipate within 1 hour, and hypoglycemia is likely to recur. The nature and timing of feedings depend on the etiology of the hypoglycemia. If the client is receiving exogenous insulin, a combination of sugar and starches, such as bread and jelly, is administered to provide quickly assimilable sugar and more slowly metabolized caloric nutrients. If the insulin has a prolonged action, a protein food may also be needed to provide substrate for gluconeogenesis over a longer time period. Clients who suffer from reactive hypoglycemia (inappropriate surges of endogenous insulin secretion) should not be given sugar because it tends to stimulate repeated insulin hypersecretion. Protein foods such as meat, cheese, or peanut butter are more appropriate.

Clients who suffer from insulin-secreting tumors require feeding at short intervals around the clock to maintain blood glucose levels. Insulin secretion is maintained at a steady high rate, relatively independent of nutrient intake. Each feeding should include rapidly assimilable sugars as well as more slowly metabolized caloric nutrients. Because feedings may be required as often as every 2 hours, these clients tend to develop sleep deprivation unless rest periods are provided during the day.

Client education. Glucagon is used mainly to treat emergency situations. Because careful medical supervision is needed by clients subject to severe insulin reactions, the drug is not generally prescribed for use in the home by lay people. Glucagon could be useful, however, for the control of rapidly developing hypoglycemia characteristic of some juvenile diabetics. Relatives of insulin-dependent diabetics often learn to administer insulin injections; they could also learn to administer glucagon when necessary. Its use in the home for carefully selected clients could provide another resource in the therapeutic program and could possibly prevent serious damage during the interval required for obtaining emergency medical care for hypoglycemic reactions.

Clients who experience rapidly developing hypoglycemic reactions often have no memory of the episodes. Because brain function is impaired at the onset of the incident, they are aware only of a lapse in time followed by an awakening in the midst of physical ministrations by health care personnel. It is vital that the nature of these episodes be explained to the client and the importance of preventive measures be stressed.

It may be difficult for people who are suffering from secreting tumors to accept the reality of their illness. The high insulin levels, combined with some degree of overnutrition, promote anabolism, including muscle hypertrophy. These clients feel and look healthy. With no conscious recollection of the hypoglycemic attacks, their subjective perception does nothing to validate the information health care personnel give them about their condition. To ensure active participation in the treatment regimen, it is important to persuade these clients that their illness is both real and serious.

Evaluation Data required for evaluation include information that indicate that the hypoglycemia has resolved (return to consciousness, alleviation of the signs and symptoms of sympathoadrenal activity, resumption of normal behavior by the client), reports by the client that the headache and apprehension have ceased, and reports that he or she feels better.

Checklist of nursing actions

When hypoglycemia that cannot be treated by oral sugar is apparent
- ☐ Administer 1 U of glucagon IM immediately.
- ☐ Monitor closely for response to the drug.
- ☐ After 20 minutes, administer a second dose of glucagon if response to the drug is incomplete or inadequate. Immediately prepare for administration of IV dextrose, or summon emergency personnel who can do so.

After the client has responded to glucagon
- ☐ Promptly administer oral feedings appropriate to the type of hypoglycemia present.

When glucagon is prescribed
- ☐ Explore with clients their perceptions of the hypoglycemic episodes, explaining and clarifying as necessary.
- ☐ Obtain prior written consent for the administration of glucagon despite resistance from clients whose behavior while hypoglycemic makes medication difficult.

Miscellaneous hyperglycemic agents

Certain other drugs also act to elevate blood glucose. Many therapeutic agents cause hyperglycemia as a side effect. Of these, diazoxide and phenytoin have been prescribed therapeutically to control hypoglycemia caused by inappropriate endogenous insulin secretion. Both agents inhibit the secretion of insulin. Diazoxide also stimulates endogenous catecholamines, which further elevate serum glucose levels. These drugs are sometimes helpful in controlling hypoglycemia in clients with insulin-secreting tumors. (For more information on diazoxide, see Chapter 28; for phenytoin, see Chapter 25).

References

Berger W, et al. (1989a). Warning symptoms of hypoglycaemia during treatment with human and porcine insulin in diabetes mellitus. *Lancet, 1,* 1041.

Berger, et al. (1989b). Transferring diabetic patients to human insulin. *Lancet, 1,* 762.

Cactus that lowers blood sugar. (1988). *Am J Nurs, 88*(5), 634.

Clinical news: Insulin as a nasal spray. (1987). *Am J Nurs, 87*(8), 1011.

Cowen R. (1990). Seeds of protection: Ancestral menus may hold a message for diabetes-prone descendants. *Science News, 137,* 350–351.

Drugs that interfere with oral hypoglycemics. (1989). *RN, 52*(4), 50.

Evans D, et al. (1986). Insulin oedema. *Postgraduate Medical Journal, 62*, 665–668.

Gever LN. (1987). Drug dispatches: Human insulin: No more mixing. *Nursing 87, 17*(9), 94.

Newton M. (1987). When IV insulin isn't working. *RN, 50*(1), 81.

Point Study Group. (1988). One-year trial of a remote-controlled implantable insulin infusion system in type 1 diabetic patients. *Lancet, 2*, 866–869.

Reaven G. (1988). Role of insulin resistance and hyperinsulinemia in human disease. Presented at the 1988 American Diabetes Association Meeting, New Orleans.

Rotation of the anatomic regions used for insulin injections and day-to-day variability of plasma glucose in type 1 diabetic subjects. *JAMA, 263*, 1802.

Steil CF, Deakins DA. (1990). Today's insulins: What you and your patient need to know. *Nursing 90, 20*(8), 34–40.

Bibliography

*Atkinson MA, Maclaren NK. (1990). What causes diabetes? *Scientific American, 263*, 62–70.

Cohen MR, Wieland KK. (1988). Drug hot line: Mixing insulin: Safe storage. *Nursing 88, 18*(11), 119.

*Fackelmann KA. (1989). Hidden heart hazards: Do high blood insulin levels foretell heart disease? *Science News, 136*, 184–185.

Flavin K, Haire-Joshu D. (1986). The pharmacologic repertoire. *American Journal of Nursing, 86*, 1244–1250.

Hahn K. (1989). Think twice: . . . About insulin administration. *Nursing 89, 19*(4), 66–72.

Haire-Joshu D. (1986). CE: Diabetes: Controlling the insulin balance. *American Journal of Nursing, 86*(11), 1239–1255.

Haire-Joshu D, Flavin D, Clutter W. (1986). Contrasting type I and type II diabetes. *American Journal of Nursing,* 1240–1243.

*Haire-Joshu D, Flavin K, Santiago JV. (1986). Intensive conventional insulin therapy. *American Journal of Nursing, 86*, 1251–1255.

Herget MJ, Williams AS. (1989). New aids for low-vision diabetics. *American Journal of Nursing, 89*(10), 1219–1320.

*Hurxthal K. (1989). Quick! Teach this patient about insulin. *American Journal of Nursing, 89*(8), 1097–1100.

Krismer MK. (1989). Insulin shock pointers. *Nursing 89, 19*(11), 4.

*Lumley WA. (1989). Recognizing and reversing insulin shock. *Nursing 89, 19*(9), 34–41.

*Lumley W. (1988). Controlling hypoglycemia and hyperglycemia. *Nursing 88, 18*(10), 34–41.

McEvoy GK, ed. (1991). *Drug Information 91*, pp 1875–1908. Bethesda, MD: American Society of Hospital Pharmacists.

Nathan D, et al. (1988). Glyburide or insulin for metabolic control in non–insulin-dependent diabetes. *Ann Intern Med, 108*, 334–340

Newton M, Newton D. (1987). When IV insulin isn't working. *RN, 50*(1), 81.

Robertson C. (1989). The new challenges of insulin therapy. *RN, 52*(5), 34–38.

Robertson C. (1987). When the patient is also a diabetic. *RN, 51*(7), 33–35.

Thurkauf GE. (1988). How do you manage KDA with continuous insulin? *American Journal of Nursing, 88*(5), 727–732.

*Recommended for further reading.

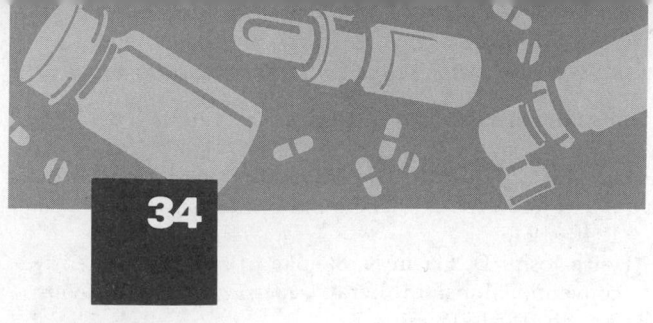

34

Thyroid, parathyroid, pituitary, and hypothalamic hormones

Proteinaceous hormones

The hormones discussed in this chapter are either proteins, polypeptides, or amino acid derivatives. Protein hormones do not enter the nuclei of target cells but occupy receptors on the cell membrane. The hormone-receptor complex then influences enzyme action in the cytoplasm, altering the synthesis of intracellular messenger proteins or the uptake of substances from the extracellular fluid (see Chapter 33).

Iodinated thyroid hormones

Physiology. Several related physiologically active hormones produced by the thyroid gland exert pronounced effects on body metabolism and energy production. Synthesized in the body by the conjugation of iodine and two molecules of tyrosine, these hormones are similar in molecular structure and physiologic effects. Iodinated thyroid hormones stimulate energy production, influence water and electrolyte balance, promote tissue growth and differentiation, and exert a sensitizing effect on the central nervous system (CNS) and the heart.

Pathology. Diseases caused by thyroid hormone imbalance are fairly common. Hyperthyroidism often affects young adults, causing signs and symptoms that reflect the stimulating properties of the hormones.

Body metabolism speeds up, producing nervousness, restlessness, and weight loss despite increased dietary intake. A rise in body temperature and increased perspiration occur. Prolonged thyroid hormone deficiency in adults (myxedema) is less common than excess. Thyroid hormone deficiency causes a slowing of mental and physical processes, including lethargy, sluggishness, memory defects, weight gain, dry skin, and intolerance to cold. Children who lack adequate thyroid hormone cannot develop normally; in the absence of treatment, they become mentally retarded dwarves (cretins).

Thyroid disorders are associated with enlargement of the gland (goiter).

Pharmacodynamics. Thyroid hormones enter the nuclei of many cells, binding to certain high-affinity sites where they influence cell function programmed in the genetic code. They stimulate the synthesis of many enzymes that affect protein synthesis. As a result, they promote tissue differentiation and growth. In the absence of sufficient thyroid hormone during childhood, body stature is stunted, axonal and dendritic networks in the brain are underdeveloped, and mental and physical development are significantly retarded.

Thyroid hormones increase the basal metabolic rate of all body cells. Energy use rises with a pronounced increase in heat production. This effect may be mediated by the mitochondria; high-affinity binding sites have been described in these structures. Thyroid hormones enhance lipolytic responses of fat cells to catecholamines and other hormones, stimulate metabolism of cholesterol to bile acids, and increase the metabolic rate of carbohydrates for the production of energy. Both nervous and cardiac tissues become more responsive to other stimuli, such as catecholamines and xanthines. Thyroid hormone inhibits pituitary production of thyrotropin, thus initiating a negative feedback system that normally maintains optimal levels of hormone in the body. Exogenous hormones share this effect, causing thyroid atrophy.

Pharmacokinetics. Although the intestinal absorption of thyroid hormones can vary, and a significant proportion of a given dose is lost in feces, oral doses of thyroid hormones are absorbed in sufficient quantity to be clinically effective. Parenteral forms of thyroid hormone may be administered subcutaneously, intramuscularly (IM), or intravenously (IV). After absorption, regardless of the route of administration, the drugs exhibit a latent period before effects are seen. Onset of action requires hours to days; peak effect occurs only after weeks or months of treatment. The drugs tend to be cumulative, and their effects persist for some time after administration is discontinued.

After entering the circulation, the hormones bind to certain plasma proteins and are distributed widely throughout the body. Less than 1% circulates in the free state, but this small proportion is responsible for the physiologic effects of the hormone. Certain factors can alter thyroid binding and the proportion of free hormone. For example, estrogen therapy or pregnancy elevates the concentration of thyroxine (T_4)-binding globulin and tends to lower the concentration of free hormone. The body compensates by increasing thyrotropin secretion and stimulating thyroid secretion. The net effects include enlargement of the thyroid gland and increases in total and bound thyroxine (the concentration of free T_4 remains relatively normal).

Thyroid hormone is degraded mainly in the liver by conjugation with glucuronic and sulfuric acids. These metabolites enter the enterohepatic circulation, where 60% to 80% of them are hydrolyzed and reabsorbed; the remainder is eliminated in feces.

Therapeutic uses. Thyroid hormone is used for replacement in deficiency states and to prevent and treat cretinism and correct myxedema. The drugs are administered to people with iatrogenic hypothyroidism caused by surgical removal of the thyroid or the pituitary gland or the destruction of these glands by radiation. Clients with mild hypothyroidism may benefit from treatment, and the hormones are also occasionally used for simple goiter that does not respond to iodine therapy.

Except in myxedema coma, when the hormones are administered IV, thyroid hormone is usually administered orally. In severe deficiency, the initial dose is small to prevent a sudden rise in metabolism, which can be dangerous. Full doses are usually attained by 2 to 4 weeks. Significant response may not be observed for weeks, and maximal effect develops over a period of months.

In the past, thyroid hormones have been used to treat obesity, though this treatment is no longer considered good medical practice. Only when the obese client exhibits other signs and symptoms of hypothyroidism is thyroid hormone therapy indicated. The use of thyroid combined with such medications as digitalis and amphetamines in weight reduction regimens has produced fatalities, usually from cardiac complications.

D-thyroxine has been used as an adjunct to dietary therapy to decrease elevated serum cholesterol and low-density lipoprotein concentrations in the treatment of primary hyperlipoproteinemia. It exerts a pronounced hypocholesterolemic effect with less metabolic stimulation than other thyroxine preparations.

Drug preparations. The first thyroid hormone used medicinally was made from dried animal thyroid glands. Taken orally, this drug has been used effectively for nearly a century to treat thyroid deficiencies. Refined and synthetic preparations that have been developed provide greater uniformity of dosage with decreased antigenicity (Table 34-1).

The standard for measuring the strength of thyroid preparations is iodine content. Some preparations are also subjected to bioassay and chromatographic analysis to ensure metabolic potency.

In some respects, the iodinated hormones resemble steroids more closely than protein hormones. Like most steroids, thyroid is not destroyed by the digestive process and is fully effective when taken orally. Its actions are not limited to cell membrane or cytoplasmic sites but involve some interaction with cell nuclei.

Adverse reactions. Toxic effects of the hormones mimic the signs and symptoms of endogenous hyperthyroidism as seen in toxic goiter. The skin is flushed, warm, and moist. Heat tolerance declines. Muscle fatigability and tremor develop. Blood pressure, pulse, and pulse pressure rise, and the heart beats more forcefully. Appetite increases, but the client tends to lose weight despite increased food intake. The client experiences increased alertness, difficulty in sleeping, nervousness, and fluctuations of emotional mood. Increased gastrointestinal (GI) motility may cause diarrhea. Blood sugar rises, and serum cholesterol drops. Women often experience menstrual irregularities. In severe toxicity, mental disturbances, cerebrovascular hemorrhage, or congestive failure may develop.

Long term L-thyroxine treatment is associated with decreased bone mass in both menopausal and premenopausal women (Paul, et al, 1988; Cooper, 1988).

Signs and symptoms of mild thyrotoxicosis have been reported after the consumption of ground beef that contains bovine thyroid tissue (Biomedicine: One hamburger . . . , 1986). Toxic reactions to thyroid hormone resolve slowly over a period of weeks because the body stores large hormone reserves in tissue depots.

Some thyroid preparations contain yellow dye #5 (tartrazine), which can trigger allergic reactions in people sensitive to aspirin.

Phenytoin affects thyroid hormone therapy by accelerating the catabolism of triiodothyronine (T_3) and T_4, reducing the effect of the hormone drugs as much as one-half. Lovastatin also increases the elimination of thyroid hormone and, additionally, interferes with its absorption (Demke, 1989). Thyroid dosages must be increased when either of these drugs is given with thyroid medication.

Therapeutic doses of thyroid enhance the physiologic effects of warfarin anticoagulants, apparently by increasing the catabolism of vitamin K-dependent clotting factors. The risk of bleeding increases, and anticoagulant drug dosages may have to be reduced. The hormones increase the insulin or oral hypoglycemic requirements of diabetic clients, and diabetes mellitus may first appear during thyroid hormone therapy. Thyroid hormone also accentuates the severity of hypoadrenalism and may precipitate an acute addisonian crisis in cortisone-deficient people.

Precautions and contraindications. Thyroid hormone is contraindicated for clients with a normal or excessive endogenous thyroid hormone production and for clients who have had myocardial infarction and uncorrected adrenal insufficiency. Thyroid hormones are not recommended for treating obesity in the absence of other thyroid deficiency. Caution must be exercised when the hormones are administered to people with a history of hypertension or cardiac disease. Clients who require warfarin anticoagulant or catecholamine therapy must be monitored closely and generally receive reduced doses of these drugs when thy-

Table 34-1. Thyroid hormone drug preparations

Drug name	Preparation	Usual adult dosage
levothyroxine sodium (Eltroxin, Synthroid, Levothroid)	Synthetic salt from the natural isomer of L-thyroxine (T_4) for oral use or injection	50–400 μg daily, depending on individual client requirements; for children, 8 μg/kg body weight/day PC: A
liothyronine sodium (Cytomel, Cynomel, Tyjodin)	Synthetic salt of L-triiodothyronine (T_3) for oral use	25–75 μg daily PC: A
liotrix (Euthroid, Thyrolar)	Mixtures of sodium salts of T_3 and T_4 (a pure mixture that resembles the natural secretion) for oral use	60–180 mg thyroid equivalent daily PC: A
thyroglobin (Proloid)	Extract from porcine thyroids for oral use	60–200 mg daily PC: A
thyroid (Thyrar, Thyroid P.D., Thyroteric, S-P-T)	Crude animal glands prepared by defatting and drying with alcohol for oral use	15–180 mg daily PC: A

KEY: PC = pregnancy risk category (The validity of pregnancy risk categories has not been established; see Chapter 16, p 216.)

roid is administered concurrently, because the other drugs are potentiated by thyroid therapy. Diabetics who receive thyroid hormone require close monitoring of glucose balance and may need increased doses of hypoglycemic medications.

Thyroid therapy is initiated with small doses that are gradually increased over a period of 2 to 4 weeks or more, especially in severe deficiencies, because sensitivity to the hormone is pronounced and the usual therapeutic doses are not well tolerated. Dosage should be reduced in elderly clients because the need for thyroid hormone appears to decrease with age.

Hormone replacement should be avoided if possible after partial thyroidectomy. Some degree of hypothyroidism is likely, but this often resolves itself spontaneously as the remaining gland hypertrophies under the influence of pituitary thyrotropin. Administering exogenous thyroid inhibits this pituitary response.

■ Summary

Thyroid hormones stimulate metabolism and promote growth and development. Drug preparations of the hormones are used for replacement therapy. They are administered orally over long periods of time. Response to treatment is slow, requiring weeks to months for full effect to appear. The drug is cumulative, and toxic states tend to resolve slowly. The signs and symptoms of toxicity include hyperactivity, muscle tremor, nervousness, intolerance to heat, and hypertensive cardiovascular disease.

Nursing management

Nursing implications

Nurses need to recognize the signs and symptoms of thyroid deficiency so that clients may be referred for diagnosis and treatment (Table 34-2). Special attention should be given to early manifestations of imbalance to facilitate timely treatment. Prompt diagnosis of deficiencies in infants is particularly crucial, because even a short delay in treatment is associated with some degree of permanent mental retardation. Routine blood tests for thyroid are the best screening procedure for infantile hypothyroidism. These tests allow diagnosis and treatment before significant irreversible pathology develops. Such tests are carried out routinely on all newborns in some medical centers. Nurses should support these programs and promote them where they have not yet been adopted.

Some elderly clients may require a higher level of serum T_4 and free thyroxine index (FT_4I) to sustain a euthyroid state. In one study, a large majority of elderly subjects with abnormally high levels of T_4 and FT_4I had no clinical signs or symptoms of thyrotoxicosis. Despite this apparent insensitivity to endogenous thyroid hormones, elderly clients appear to be

Table 34-2. Signs and symptoms of thyroid imbalance

Degree of imbalance	Hypothyroidism	Hyperthyroidism
Minimal	Fatigue, muscle cramps	Increased energy and alertness
	Constipation	Increased bowel motility
	Cold intolerance	Nervousness
	Paresthesia	
	Memory defects	
Moderate	Mental slowness and lethargy	Insomnia and a sense of nervous tension
	Loss of appetite and a tendency to gain weight	Increased food intake and a tendency to lose weight
	Thinning of the hair	Abundant hair growth
	Cold intolerance	Heat intolerance
	Increased acne despite a generally dry skin	Increased perspiration
	Fecal impactions	Diarrhea
	Increased sensitivity to depressant drugs	Increased sensitivity to stimulant drugs
	In diabetics, more numerous insulin reactions	Onset or increased severity of diabetes mellitus
	Hypercholesterolemia	Hypocholesterolemia
	Decreased protein-bound iodine	Increased protein-bound iodine
	Decreased response to stress	Tachycardia and palpitations
Marked	Emotional depression	Manic-type psychosis
	Weak cardiac contraction	Cardiac enlargement or congestive failure
	Enlarged tongue and periorbital edema (myxedematous facies)	Cerebrovascular hemorrhage
	Deafness (occasionally)	

unusually sensitive to exogenous hormones used to treat hypothyroidism. A possible explanation for this paradox is the development of autoimmune antibodies that inactive endogenous hormone but have no effect on exogenous hormones.

Nursing process

Assessment Risk factors for goiter and hypothyroidism include residence in inland upland regions, where soils are often deficient in iodine, exposure to ground water pollutants from coal mines (resorcinol, phthalates, dihydroxybenzoic acids, methoxyanthracene, and bromoform [Raloff, 1986a, 1986b]), consumption of goitrogens (see below), and a family history of thyroid disease.

Early signs and symptoms of hypothyroidism are often subtle and may easily be overlooked. In adults, as the condition progresses, the affected client becomes mentally as well as physically lethargic and apathetic. As a result of the disease process, the client may lack the initiative to seek medical care. Unless an outside agent intervenes, the condition may remain undiagnosed until a cardiac or respiratory emergency occurs. Thyroid-deficient infants who remain untreated develop into mentally retarded dwarves. Delayed treatment may result in normal physical maturation, but the mental retardation is irreversible. For these reasons, casefinding and referral for medical treatment is an important nursing function, especially among nurses who provide primary health care.

Signs and symptoms of adult hypothyroidism (myxedema) include sleepiness and lethargy, mental apathy, slowed speech, decreased appetite, weight gain despite decreased food intake, thinning of the hair, thickening and coarsening of the skin, a tendency toward constipation, enlargement of the tongue, periorbital and pretibial edema, sensitivity to cold, slow and weak pulse, and overreaction to depressant medication. Early manifestations include forgetfulness, a tendency to gain weight, and a decrease in energy. Infants deficient in thyroid hormone exhibit myxedematous facies (puffiness, especially around the eyes), excessive drooling, enlarged and protruding tongue, rough dry skin, coarse hair, potbelly, swayback, and an increased incidence of umbilical hernia.

Clients who receive thyroid replacement therapy should be assessed for excess hormone level as well as for deficiencies. Thyroid toxicity is characterized by restlessness, insomnia, tremor, fatigue, thickening of the hair, intolerance to heat, tachycardia, increased appetite, a tendency to lose weight despite increased food intake, a tendency toward diarrhea, and a feeling of nervous tension.

Because some thyroid preparations contain tartrazine (yellow dye #5), clients should be questioned about allergic sensitivity to this substance. Any client with a history of asthma associated with nasal polyps and aspirin allergy is at high risk for adverse reaction to tartrazine. Such a reaction could be difficult to treat, because thyroid hormone alters the body response to drugs used in the treatment of acute anaphylaxis, such as cortisone and Adrenalin.

Nursing diagnosis Nursing diagnoses for the thyroid-deficient client include the following:

> *Activity intolerance related to fatigue, secondary to hypothyroidism*
> *Sleep pattern disturbance: excessive sleepiness related to CNS depression, secondary to hypothyroidism*
> *Hypothermia related to deficient energy production secondary to hypothyroidism*
> *Altered thought processes: memory deficits and sluggishness of mental processes related to hypothyroidism*
> *Constipation related to intestinal atony secondary to hypothyroidism*
> *Decreased cardiac output related to cardiac weakness secondary to hypothyroidism*
> *Body image disturbance related to obesity and myxedema secondary to hypothyroidism*

Nursing diagnoses appropriate for hypothyroid infants include the following:

> *Fluid volume excess related to hypothyroidism*
> *Altered growth and development: physical and mental growth less than normal for the infant's age related to hypothyroidism*

Potential diagnoses for clients who receive thyroid hormone replacement include the following:

> *Sleep pattern disturbance: insomnia related to CNS stimulation secondary to thyroid toxicity*
> *Activity intolerance related to fatigue secondary to thyroid toxicity*
> *Anxiety related to CNS stimulation secondary to thyroid toxicity*
> *Altered comfort: heat intolerance related to hypermetabolism secondary to thyroid toxicity*
> *Diarrhea related to hypermotility of the gut secondary to thyroid toxicity*

A common collaborative problem that should be differentiated from the nursing diagnoses is

> *Potential complication: cardiac failure*

Many clients have a

> *Knowledge deficit related to hypothyroidism and its treatment*

Planning Goals for most clients who show signs and symptoms of hypothyroidism are definitive diagnosis and treatment. When hypothyroidism follows thyroid surgery or irradiation, the goal may be to stimulate gland function and avoid replacement hormone therapy. The goal for the client who receives hormone replacement therapy is to achieve or to remain in a euthyroid condition.

Intervention   The client who exhibits signs and symptoms of thyroid deficiency should be referred to an internist or endocrinologist for diagnosis.

The nursing needs of clients who receive thyroid hormone replacement vary, depending on the degree of the hypothyroidism. Severely deficient people are at high risk for serious complications. In such instances, treatment is begun in the hospital. The drugs may be administered IV, in which case only freshly prepared solutions should be used. The client should be watched closely for signs and symptoms of addisonian crisis (acute hypoadrenalism). Cortisone may be ordered to correct adrenal deficiencies before thyroid therapy is initiated. Many myxedematous clients are affected by cardiovascular disease characterized by a weakened myocardium and a tendency toward congestive failure. These clients are sensitive to thyroid hormones, and the heart can tolerate only small doses of the drugs at first. Dosages are advanced by small increments to promote strengthening of the heart before full dosages are administered.

Clients who are diagnosed in the early stages of myxedema do not exhibit advanced symptoms and may have little cardiovascular involvement. For these people, drug therapy may be carried out on an outpatient basis.

Treatment is needed for long periods of time, often for life. It is important that the client remain under medical supervision. Regular assessment for thyroid balance is important, because signs and symptoms of hypothyroidism and hyperthyroidism develop insidiously and may not be recognized by clients or their families, even when pronounced. Because the drug effects are delayed and cumulative in nature, day-to-day adjustment in dosage does not maintain hormone balance. It is important that the dosage be adjusted to the client's needs as closely as possible to prevent oscillations in hormone status.

The client should be assessed for evidence of diabetes mellitus, because the disease can develop during thyroid hormone therapy. Previously diagnosed diabetics find their conditions more difficult to control and may require additional hypoglycemic medication.

If anticoagulants are prescribed during thyroid hormone therapy, clients should be monitored closely for abnormal bleeding. Dosages of anticoagulants may have to be reduced, because the action of these drugs is increased by concurrent thyroid therapy.

A product that does not contain tartrazine should be obtained for clients allergic to this dye.

Client education.   The need for compliance to the drug regimen should be stressed. Obvious changes in body function or well-being do not occur when occasional doses are missed, and even complete omission of the drugs may not produce noticeable effects for a period of several weeks. Failure to correct the hormone deficiency adequately, however, increases the long-term risk of heart disease, because cholesterol levels in the blood rise and remain chronically elevated and because heart action weakens.

Thyroid hormones should be taken on an empty stomach. Most preparations may be stored at room temperature.

The client must understand the need for regular medical care while thyroid drugs are used. This can rarely be avoided because the drugs are limited to prescription use, and most physicians do not renew prescriptions repeatedly without reassessing the client. However, a client who does not accept the need for continued care is more apt to discontinue therapy and delay seeing the physician.

Clients should be taught the signs and symptoms of both hypothyroidism and hyperthyroidism and should be taught the need to report these to the physician. Manifestations of hypothyroidism should subside gradually but steadily during the first months of treatment. Thereafter, hormone balance should be maintained steadily. Symptoms of imbalance may develop after many months of uneventful treatment, because the body requirements for thyroid hormone fluctuate somewhat with the degree of stress and environmental temperatures to which the client is subjected. Because early manifestations of imbalance tend to be subjective, the client should watch for them and take care to communicate these clearly to the clinician.

Clients who experience temporary hypothyroidism after partial loss of the thyroid gland can be taught measures to promote gland hypertrophy and shorten the period of imbalance. Exercise and alternating hot and cold showers stimulate pituitary secretion of thyrotropin. As much as possible, high environmental temperatures should be avoided since these inhibit the trophic hormone. The client should dress in layered clothing and wear the minimum necessary to avoid chilling. The diet should be of high quality and should contain adequate iodine and protein for thyroid hormone production. The need for iodized salt should be carefully weighed. In inland upland areas the source of iodine may be needed to promote optimum thyroid function. However, in other areas, or when clients consume large amounts of seafood, iodized salt may raise intake of this mineral to levels that inhibit thyroid function.

Calorie intake should be limited to avoid weight gain, a task seldom difficult because most clients experience a loss of appetite. Excessive amounts of foods that contain substances that inhibit thyroid secretion should be avoided. The latter include turnips, rutabagas, cabbage, carrots, kale, soybeans, peanuts (especially the skins), peaches, peas, strawberries, spinach, mustard seed, radishes, milk from kale-fed cattle, and millet, especially that which has been allowed to stand

Example of nursing process and hypothyroidism

Betty M. is night charge nurse for a large unit in a skilled care facility. She is a long-time employee, respected as a good nurse. Lately, however, some of her colleagues have felt that she was becoming less productive. She accomplishes less work than usual and is "not on top of the work." Recently, they noticed that she has had to be reminded of events such as entertainment and outings that sometimes keep residents out of the home until after the night shift begins at 11 PM.

Last night, the night supervisor found Ms. M. bundled up in a heavy sweater, nodding in the nurses' station during her shift. In the conference room, Betty told the supervisor she didn't know what was wrong but she could not keep up with things at work or at home. Everything seems to be "speeding up," or she is "slowing down." She is sleeping long hours every day but always feels tired. She wonders if she is beginning early menopause; she is only 40, but her menses are irregular and her hair has "begun to fall out."

Assessment data	Nursing diagnosis	Intervention	Goals and outcome criteria
Staff reports that client's work pace is slowing	Activity intolerance related to reduced energy; hypothermia and altered role performance related to slowing of body processes; and body image disturbance related to thinning of hair; all possibly due to endocrine disorder such as thyroid deficiency	**Summarize** and discuss with Ms. M. her own and the staff's observations regarding recent changes in her behavior; point out the resemblance to endocrine disorder, particularly thyroid deficiency.	If endocrine disease is affecting the client, it will be diagnosed and treated.
Client's statement that she is "slowing down, . . . and can't keep up with things"			
Deterioration of work performance			
Irregular menses		**Recommend** that Ms. M. see an internist or endocrinologist for a diagnostic workup, either through referral from her own physician or by arrangement through the nursing home administration.	
Client wears heavy sweater at work in a well-heated nursing unit			
Client's hair is thinning			
Memory lapses			
Lengthened sleep time			

for several days after cooking (Raloff, 1986a). Drinking water contaminated by resorcinol or phthalates can also inhibit thyroid function (Raloff, 1986b).

Evaluation Data required for evaluation relate to thyroid balance or imbalance. Clients should be assessed regularly for signs and symptoms of hypothyroidism or hyperthyroidism (see Example of Nursing Process and Hypothyroidism).

Checklist of nursing actions

☐ Be alert to early signs and symptoms of hypothyroidism and refer affected clients for diagnosis and treatment.

When hormone therapy is instituted for severe deficiencies

☐ Prepare parenteral solutions immediately before use and discard unused preparations.

☐ Assess the client frequently for cardiac decom-

pensation and addisonian crisis; be especially alert for shock.

☐ Protect the client from stressors, including exertion.

When hormone balance is maintained by long-term therapy

☐ Teach self-monitoring for hormone imbalance.

☐ Stress the long-term benefits of compliance to the drug regimen.

When hormone deficiency is considered to be temporary

☐ Teach clients measures that stimulate thyroid function, as well as environmental factors that can inhibit it.

Antithyroid drugs

Substances that inhibit the production and use of thyroid hormone include propylthiouracil and related compounds and goitrogenic substances in water, food, and drugs. Chemicals may oppose or block the effects of thyroid hormone by reducing thyrotropin stimulation of the thyroid, interfering with thyroid hormone synthesis, blocking the release of thyroid hormone into the general circulation, altering the proportion of very active and less active forms of the hormone, or reducing their use by peripheral tissues. Most antithyroid chemicals exert their action directly on the thyroid gland. These substances cause levels of thyroid hormone to drop and a subsequent rise in pituitary production of thyrotropin. As thyrotropin concentrations rise, the thyroid hypertrophies, becomes more vascular, and increases its hormone production. A visible enlargement of the gland (goiter) develops. The increase in hormone production may be sufficient to maintain a euthyroid state, or some degree of hypothyroidism may occur. Whether or not the client becomes deficient in thyroid hormone, the gland may become large enough to be disfiguring and to exert pressure on the esophagus and trachea, causing dysphagia and dyspnea. These effects may occur secondary to dietary intake of goitrogens or as side effects of drug therapy for non–thyroid-related disease. A few antithyroid compounds stimulate autoimmune thyroiditis. All of these agents tend to reduce the physiologic effects of thyroid hormone (Box 34-1).

Thioamides

Antithyroid drugs used medicinally include methimazole and propylthiouracil. Thioamides interfere with the incorporation of iodine into tyrosyl residues of thyroglobulin and inhibit the coupling of these iodotyrosyl residues to form iodothyronine. In addition, propylthiouracil appears to reduce peripheral conversion of T_4 to the more potent T_3.

Pharmacokinetics. Antithyroid drugs are well absorbed by the GI tract. They are concentrated in the thyroid gland, where they exert their effects. However, they do cross the placenta and are secreted in breast milk. Although the drugs act promptly, clinical response is not evident for a few days to 2 weeks or more. Only when body stores of previously synthesized thyroid hormones have become depleted over time do signs and symptoms of hyperthyroidism subside. Duration of action varies with half-life and dosage (Table 34-3). Excretion of the drugs and their metabolites is mainly by the kidneys.

Therapeutic uses. Thioamides are used to treat and control hyperthyroidism. Administered alone over a period of months, they are a definitive treatment for thyroid toxicity, helping to maintain a normal metabolism until the natural course of the disease can produce a spontaneous remission. They also are used as adjuncts to radioiodine therapy to ameliorate the symptoms of thyroid toxicities until the effects of radiation are apparent. Antithyroid treatment before thy-

---

Box 34-1. Sources of goitrogenic substances

Foods

Foods that contain flavinoid pigments (red, yellow, blue)

Cabbage, turnips, rutabagas, peas, spinach, carrots, radishes

Soybeans, peanuts

Strawberries, peaches

Kale and milk from kale-fed cattle

Millet, especially cooked millet that has been stored for prolonged periods before consumption (Raloff, 1986b)

Contaminants in drinking water

Resorcinol

Phthalates (which are converted by bacteria to dihydroxy benzoin acids)

Methoxy anthracene and bromoform (which stimulate autoimmune thyroiditis) (Raloff, 1986a)

Drugs

Resorcinol, phenylbutazone, thiopental, dimercaptol, lithium

Analine derivatives (sulfonamides and salicylates)

Thioamides (methimazole and propylthiouracil)

---

roid surgery minimizes hormone toxicity and reduces the surgical risks posed by the toxic state. The drugs are also useful in the treatment of thyroid crisis, an acute and severe form of hyperthyroidism. Because of its additional peripheral action, propylthiouracil is the drug of choice for this condition.

Drug preparations. Propylthiouracil and methimazole (Tapazole) are the chief antithyroid drugs used in the U.S. They are marketed only as oral tablets. Carbimazole, which is widely used in Great Britain, is converted by body metabolism to methimazole.

Adverse reactions. Antithyroid drugs used to treat hyperthyroidism are relatively safe; the overall incidence of side effects varies from 3% to 7%. The most common reaction is skin rash; either a mild papular rash or urticaria can occur. Sometimes purpura and pruritus are features of the skin reaction. Skin complications often subside spontaneously, whether or not the drug is withdrawn.

Other side effects include nausea, vomiting, nasal

Table 34-3. Antithyroid thioamides

Drug name	Preparation	Usual dosage
methimazole (Tapazole)	Oral tablets	Adults: *Initial:* 15–60 mg/day, divided in 3 doses, administered q8h (depending on degree of thyroid toxicity); *maintenance* (after about 2 months of therapy): 5–30 mg/day
		Children: *Initial:* 0.4 mg/kg body weight/day; *maintenance:* 0.2 mg/kg body weight/day PC: D
propylthiouracil (Propyl-Thyracil)	Oral tablets	Adults: *Initial:* 300–1200 mg/day, divided in 3–6 doses, administered q4–q8h (depending on degree of thyroid toxicity); *maintenance:* (after about 2 months of therapy) 100–150 mg/day
		Neonates: 5–10 mg/kg body weight/day
		Children 6–10 yr of age: *Initial:* 50–150 mg/day
		Children 10 yr of age and older: *Initial:* 150–300 mg/day or 150 mg/m^2 body surface
		Maintenance dosage in children depends on response to therapy PC: D

KEY: PC = pregnancy category. (The validity of pregnancy risk categories has not been established; see Chapter 16, p 216.)

stuffiness, epigastric distress, arthralgia, myalgia, paresthesia, headache, drowsiness, neuritis, vertigo, loss of hair, and fading of skin pigmentation. Rarely, drug fever, hepatitis, and nephritis occur. The most serious but rare complication of antithyroid therapy is agranulocytosis. In most cases, recovery is spontaneous and complete, particularly when the dyscrasia is diagnosed early and the drug is discontinued immediately.

Antithyroid therapy tends to increase the vascularity and friability of the thyroid gland, an undesirable effect in clients about to have surgery. Propylthiouracil causes prothrombin deficiency and potentiates the effects of warfarin anticoagulants.

High doses of antithyroid drugs can induce hypothyroidism.

Precautions and contraindications. Antithyroid drugs are contraindicated during lactation and must be used with great caution during pregnancy. The drugs cross the placenta and suppress thyroid function in the fetus. They also are secreted in breast milk and affect the nursing infant. During gestation and for some time after birth, the brain normally grows rapidly. Thyroid deficiency during this critical stage of development causes retardation and permanently impairs intellectual capacity. When antithyroid therapy must be given to a gravid woman, thyroid hormone is also administered to prevent hormone deficiency in her and in her unborn child. Women who receive antithyroid drugs must not nurse their infants.

When skin eruptions caused by the drugs do not subside with continued therapy, the drug in question should be discontinued and a different antithyroid preparation prescribed. This switch is usually effective because cross-sensitivity is uncommon.

The development of agranulocytosis requires immediate drug withdrawal. This reaction usually develops during the first few months of treatment.

Clients who have received antithyroid drugs before surgical thyroidectomy are given iodine for 10 days to 2 weeks preoperatively to decrease the vascularity and friability of the gland induced by such treatment.

■ Summary

A number of chemicals found in drugs and foods inhibit synthesis of thyroid hormone and induce compensatory hypertrophy of the thyroid gland (goiter). Of these, thioamides (propylthiouracil and methimazole) are used therapeutically to treat hyperthyroid states. When administered orally over long periods of time, they control toxic symptoms and restore normal metabolism. Excessive dosage can cause hypothyroidism. An infrequent but serious side effect of antithyroid therapy is agranulocytosis. Withdrawal of the drug usually results in reversal of this life-threatening condition, particularly when detected in its early stages.

Nursing management
Nursing implications

Clients who show minimal signs and symptoms of thyroid imbalance, such as changes in body weight, may influence thyroid function and metabolism by altering their intake of goitrogenic chemicals. Clients who wish to increase thyroid function should avoid ingestion of food, water, and drugs that contain chemicals that inhibit the function of this gland (see Box 34-1). They should also avoid overheating the body. Alternating hot and cold showers may stimulate thyroid secretion.

Clients who experience nervous tension and other signs and symptoms of hyperthyroidism should increase their consumption of foods that contain inhibitors of thyroid secretion. They should also take care to keep the body warm; warm baths are recommended in preference to showers.

Teaching related to the prevention of goiter. Simple (euthyroid) goiter can be prevented by dietary measures. Factors that increase the risk of goiter are a vegetarian diet high in goitrogenic fruits and vegetables (listed above) and soy beans, very low or very high intake of iodine, use of milk from kale-fed cattle, and use of soy bean infant formulas. To maintain optimum thyroid function, the diet should contain adequate amounts of protein and iodine (substances used as substrate by the body in the production of thyroid hormone) and be free of excessive amounts of goitrogenic foods. A varied diet without excessive intake of any one kind of food should be recommended.

Nursing process

Assessment When antithyroid drugs are first prescribed, clients are usually overtly hyperthyroid, exhibiting varying degrees of hormone toxicity. Signs and symptoms may include increased alertness, hyperkinesis, weight loss despite an increased appetite, an increase in body temperature accompanied by perspiration and heat intolerance, hypertension, a wide pulse pressure, tachycardia, palpitation, and dyspnea. Cardiac enlargement and arrhythmia may be present. The client experiences a subjective feeling of nervous tension, irritability, and fluctuations in emotional mood. Hand tremor, clumsiness, and weakness are often present. The client tends to be unusually sensitive to stimulants such as pressor amines and caffeine. Women may complain of menstrual disturbances. An increased peristalsis or diarrhea is evident.

Nursing diagnosis Nursing diagnoses likely to be made for the hyperthyroid client include the following:

> *Activity intolerance related to fatigue secondary to hyperthyroidism*
> *Hyperthermia related to hypermetabolism secondary to hyperthyroidism*
> *Diarrhea related to hypermotility secondary to hyperthyroidism*
> *Anxiety related to CNS stimulation secondary to hyperthyroidism*
> *Sleep pattern disturbance: insomnia related to CNS stimulation secondary to hyperthyroidism*
> *Altered nutrition: less than body requirements related to hypermetabolism secondary to hyperthyroidism*
> *Body image disturbance related to thick hair growth, fatigue, and nervousness secondary to hyperthyroidism and hypermetabolism*

After antithyroid medication is initiated, clients are vulnerable to adverse reaction to these drugs, including the following:

> *Activity intolerance related to lack of energy secondary to inhibition of the thyroid*
> *Hypothermia related to hypometabolism due to inhibition of the thyroid*
> *Constipation related to hypomotility secondary to inhibition of the thyroid*
> *Altered thought processes: mental sluggishness related to CNS depression secondary to inhibition of the thyroid*
> *Altered nutrition: more than body requirements related to hypometabolism secondary to inhibition of the thyroid*
> *Self-esteem disturbance related to lack of energy, thinning of the hair, and mental sluggishness secondary to thyroid inhibition*
> *High risk for infection related to bone marrow depression secondary to antithyroid medication*

Most clients have a

> *Knowledge deficit related to hyperthyroidism and its treatment*

Planning Goals of treatment include eliminating the signs and symptoms of hyperthyroidism, increasing comfort, promoting normal bowel elimination, promoting positive self-image, promoting rest and sleep, preventing or promptly detecting and treating adverse reactions to antithyroid drugs, and teaching the client self-care measures necessary to promote optimal response to the drug regimen.

Intervention Because positive clinical response to the drugs cannot be expected for days to weeks, initially the client needs nursing care to minimize the toxic effects of hyperthyroidism.

If hyperthyroid clients are residents of health care institutions, they should be provided with light clothing and bed covers. The environment should be kept cool and relatively high in humidity. Health care personnel assigned to these clients should work efficiently but without haste.

Rest is important to conserve the client's energy and minimize fatigue. However, because of the high metabolic rate induced by the excess hormones, rest is difficult to achieve. The environment should be controlled to minimize stimuli. Elimination of noise and glare and the use of sedating or neutral colors (blues and greens) are helpful. Environmental temperatures should be relatively low. All possible measures to induce sleep should be used. The client is unduly stimulated by hurry and may become impatient with slow responses; therefore, people around the client should endeavor to maintain a calm but efficient manner.

Diet should be high in vitamins, minerals, and protein with adequate calories to prevent weight loss. Frequent feedings are usually needed. Coffee, tea, and cola drinks are contraindicated, and foods with a laxative effect should be avoided.

When the manifestations of thyroid toxicity subside, caloric intake should be reduced. If some weight gain is desired, this should be carefully controlled. A lean body build is desirable because the cardiovascular system may have been adversely affected by the toxic state.

The client should be monitored closely for hormone balance. When clinical manifestations of toxicity abate, the dose of antithyroid medication is decreased by as much as one-third. Assessment is particularly critical at this time; either hyperthyroidism or hypothyroidism may develop before the client is stabilized on a maintenance dose.

Should a client become pregnant, the physician must be notified at once. The drug therapy may be discontinued and alternative therapy (surgery) recommended. If the drugs are to be continued, thyroid hormone is added to the regimen, and the client is watched closely to detect any evidence of hypothyroidism that would be harmful to the fetus.

The nurse must monitor clients closely for signs of infection that could indicate leukocytopenia. Fever, sore throat, a head cold, or malaise are indications that the drug should be discontinued and immediate medical attention sought. Any existing infection needs vigorous treatment. Clients need protection from exposure to communicable diseases until their white blood cell counts return to normal. An alternative method of treating the hormone disturbance is substituted for the drug regimen.

Occasionally, an acutely ill client requires parenteral administration of antithyroid medication. Because parenteral solutions are not available commercially, they are prepared in the health care institution; quality controls may not approach the level of the drug factory. Such preparations are likely to contain pyrogens or antigens not found in commercial solutions. The client should be watched closely for fever, chills, allergy, or other adverse reactions.

To foster a positive self-image, nursing personnel should respond warmly to the client and should compliment the client whenever appropriate.

Client education. Most clients who receive antithyroid medication must take the drugs for long periods. After the initial few weeks, the toxic symptoms subside and clients feel well. They need a great deal of encouragement to continue with the drug treatment consistently when no evidence of illness is present. Interruption of therapy is likely to result in renewed symptoms and reduces the likelihood of permanent remission. Clients need assistance in developing an acceptable regimen that promotes a habit of regular and accurate medication.

Dosage of antithyroid drugs must be controlled to maintain optimum hormone balance. Too little medication prolongs the period of thyrotoxicity; too much can cause hypothyroidism. Clients and their families should understand the effects of thyroid hormone and the signs and symptoms of imbalance. After the latent period of initial treatment, manifestations of imbalance should be reported to the physician so that dosages can be adjusted.

Many clients affected by hyperthyroidism are young adults. Women should be taught the signs and symptoms of pregnancy and the need to report these promptly. Should pregnancy occur, the treatment regimen must be adjusted to protect the fetus. Because of the underlying endocrine imbalance, the client needs close supervision throughout the pregnancy.

Clients should be taught to report any intercurrent illness, especially infections, because these may be early indications of a drop in leukocyte count. Sore throat, enlarged lymph nodes, GI upsets, fever, rash, and jaundice are particularly significant. Periodic blood tests may be required also. Clients should understand the need for frequent medical follow-up throughout the lengthy treatment period.

Nutritional counseling includes explanation of the need for extra calories while hyperthyroidism persists. Calorie content should be reduced gradually as the symptoms of toxicity subside, a task not usually difficult for many clients since their appetites tend to decrease during this period. The diet should be high quality—high in protein, vitamins, and minerals—to meet the needs of the heightened metabolism and hormone production. To promote optimum gland function and resistance to infection, this quality should be maintained as the amounts of food are reduced. While the client remains toxic, no stimulants such as coffee, tea, chocolate, or cola drinks are allowed, and laxative foods should be avoided. These foods may be added gradually as toxicity subsides.

Clients should be cautioned against taking over-the-counter medications without their physician's knowledge and approval. Many nonprescription remedies contain pressor amines (decongestants) that are poorly tolerated by the hyperthyroid person. Diarrhea remedies that contain kaolin may absorb oral medications, reducing their absorption from the GI tract. These compounds could interfere with the effectiveness of the antithyroid drugs, causing recurrent toxicity. Remedies that contain aspirin delay clotting and should be avoided by clients who take propylthiouracil.

When methimazole is prescribed, the client should be cautioned to store the drug in its original container in a cool dark place.

Warfarin anticoagulants cannot be used in the

Example of nursing process and hyperthyroidism

The client is a part-time secretary, housewife, and mother, age 35. Ten weeks ago, she began treatment for hyperthyroidism with propylthiouracil 100 mg qid. She returns to the physician's office monthly for "check-ups." During her last visit 2 weeks ago, she complained to the nurse of a head cold that she could not get rid of. At that time, the nurse informed her that this could be a side effect of the antithyroid medication and cautioned her not to use over-the-counter decongestants, because hyperthyroidism causes sensitivity to their stimulant effects.

Today the client telephones the office and tells the nurse, "That head cold must be going down. I have a sore throat today."

Assessment data	Nursing diagnosis	Intervention	Goals and outcome criteria
Methimazole treatment for 10 weeks Complaint of sore throat	High risk for infection related to bone marrow depression secondary to antithyroid medication	**Remind** the client that a sore throat can signal adverse reaction to the medication she is taking. **Direct** the client not to take any more drug until she is seen by the physician; make an appointment for her to see the physician as soon as possible.	The client will not develop life-threatening irreversible bone marrow depression and aplastic anemia.

usual doses because of the potentiating effects of the antithyroid drugs. Phenylbutazone, thiopental, lithium, sulfonamides, and salicylates may increase the thyroid-inhibiting effect of thioamides.

Evaluation Data required for evaluation include evidence of thyroid imbalance, presence or absence of infection, patency of nasal airways, laboratory data on blood cell counts, number and consistency of stools, client comments and behavior indicative of self-concept, and client reports related to nervous tension and tolerance to changes in environmental temperature. Success of the teaching program is inferred by the ability of the client to manage the drug regimen and to repeat to the nurse information conveyed during teaching sessions (see Example of Nursing Process and Hyperthyroidism).

Checklist of nursing actions

☐ While the client remains hyperthyroid, prevent accidental injury, reduce environmental stressors, and promote rest.

☐ Encourage the client to take the drug as prescribed.

☐ Discontinue antithyroid medications and notify the physician at once if symptoms of infection occur.

☐ Teach the client to report any symptoms of infection to the physician immediately.

☐ Teach the client signs and symptoms of both hyperthyroidism and hypothyroidism; instruct the client to report their development to the physician.

☐ Emphasize the importance of follow-up care throughout the period of drug treatment.

☐ Store methimazole in light-resistant containers; warn the client to keep drugs in their original prescription containers.

Iodine

Pathophysiology. Iodine is an essential nutrient for proper thyroid function. When this mineral is deficient, the thyroid gland lacks sufficient substrate to produce hormone at the optimum level for body function. Lowered hormone levels cause a reduction in the inhibition of pituitary thyrotropin production. As thyrotropin levels rise, the thyroid gland hypertrophies and becomes more active in an attempt to produce more hormone, a condition known as *simple goiter*.

Goiter is prevalent in certain geographical areas, mainly inland upland areas (mountains or high plateaus). The soil in these "goiter belts" is subject to the leaching action of rain and fresh water drainage and tends to be deficient in trace minerals, including iodine. The crops and animals in such areas have low iodine content, and both animal and human populations tend to develop thyroid malfunction. (Pollutants from coal mines may include several antithyroid compounds that add to this effect.) A high incidence of goiter occurs unless supplementary iodine is provided in the diet. Other thyroid diseases, including thyrotoxicosis, myxedema, and cretinism, also develop more frequently than in populations with optimum iodine nutrition.

To be nutritionally complete, the diet must contain sufficient iodine to meet the thyroid's need for hormone production. From 35 to 150 µg daily are required, depending on the age, sex, and condition of the client. Infants need the lowest amounts, followed by nongravid women, and men, in that order. Pregnant and lactating women need the highest amounts of iodine. The mineral is found in abundance in saltwater fish, seaweed, and vegetables grown in iodine-rich soils (generally near the seacoast). The addition of iodine to the diet helps to reduce the incidence of thyroid disease associated with deficiencies of this mineral in inland areas. In the U.S., the addition of iodine to table salt is encouraged by a government subsidy that allows iodized salt to be produced and marketed at the same price as plain salt. Since iodized salt has become widely available, simple goiter and cretinism have become rare conditions in this country.

Pharmacodynamics. Iodine not only provides a substrate for thyroid hormone production but also promotes storage of this hormone and may antagonize the stimulating effect of thyrotropin on the gland. With prolonged administration, the follicular storage depots become saturated with hormone, excesses are released into the circulation, and blood levels return to a more normal level. In simple goiter, providing iodine in low doses is sufficient to correct the nutritional deficiency and restore thyroid hormone production to normal levels. The usual negative feedback mechanism that controls thyrotropin production is restored. Thyroid-stimulating hormone drops to normal levels, and the thyroid gland shrinks to its usual size.

In large doses, iodine has different effects. When plasma concentrations approach 100 times the normal levels and intracellular levels of the mineral reach a critical level, most thyroid gland activities are decreased. The rate of iodide trapping is reduced, the rate of thyroid hormone formation declines, the secretory activities of the thyroid cells are decreased, and the rate of thyroid release from the gland falls off. It is hypothesized that some of these effects are produced by direct inhibition of the thyroid-stimulating effects of thyrotropin, but this remains unproved. Some of the effects do not persist over time but subside after a period of a few weeks. Circulating hormone levels apparently rise when the storage depots of the thyroid follicles become saturated. Nevertheless, continued administration of high doses of iodine produces thyroid enlargement similar to the goiters induced by other thyroid inhibitors.

Pharmacokinetics. Iodine is well absorbed as iodides in the GI tract. It has an affinity for thyroid tissue and is taken up rapidly by this gland. Iodine is subsequently incorporated in the thyroid hormone molecules. It is stored for a time and is eventually secreted into the circulation. A portion is reused by the thyroid. The remainder, with other excess iodide, is eliminated by the kidneys.

Therapeutic uses. Iodine in small doses is used to supplement dietary sources in geographic areas where the soil is deficient in this mineral. Medicinal iodine preparations may be prescribed to treat simple goiter caused by dietary deficiency. For the prevention of this condition, the use of iodized salt is cheap and convenient. It is the most effective approach from the public health standpoint.

In the treatment of thyroid disorders, iodine is administered before surgery on the gland to reduce thyrotoxicity to a minimum and to induce involution of the gland. Usually Lugol's solution or saturated solution of potassium iodide is prescribed for a period of 10 days before the scheduled surgical date. The inhibitory effect of the mineral on the thyroid peaks at the end of 10 days to 2 weeks. At this time, thyrotoxicity is at its lowest, and the gland is smallest and least vascular and friable. If surgery is delayed more than 2 weeks after the initiation of iodine therapy, the effects dissipate. Blood levels of thyroid hormone rise to, and often above, previous levels. The beneficial effects of iodine are lost, and the client may be at greater risk for toxicity than before.

Before the development of thioamide drugs, iodine was the only drug available to decrease the severity of thyrotoxicity before thyroidectomy. Although improvement in metabolic state was apparent, toxicity was not eliminated, nor was metabolism restored to normal. Surgery remained hazardous. Present day regimens that use thioamide medication followed by preoperative iodine treatment achieve much more control over toxicity in the client scheduled for surgery. In most cases, a near normal metabolic state can be achieved before surgery, significantly reducing the risks of this type of surgery.

Iodides are also useful in the treatment of thyroid crisis ("thyroid storm"). They are administered in combination with thioamides, propanolol, and other drugs as needed to maintain vital functions and correct the serious pathologic features of this syndrome (Table 34-4).

Certain iodine compounds are used for other purposes in medicine. They are effective expectorants. They are occasionally used to promote resolution of granulomatous lesions, such as those that occur in leprosy, syphilis, and fungal infections. Iodine is a

Table 34-4. *Selected iodine preparations*

Drug name	Preparation	Medicinal use	Usual adult dosage
Iodized salt	1 part sodium or potassium iodine per 10,000 parts salt	Prevention of goiter	Add to food as ordinary salt
potassium iodine (Pima syrup, Iosol, Thyro-Block)	Solution (325 mg/5 ml or 1 g/ml) Oral tablets	Treatment of Graves' disease. Prevention of thyroid irradiation during radiation emergencies	60 mg tid 130 mg daily (Children younger than 1 year of age: 65 mg daily; children older than 1 year of age: 130 mg) PC: D
strong iodine solution (Lugol's solution, compound iodine solution)	Iodine (50 mg/ml) and potassium iodine (100 mg/ml) in aqueous solution for oral administration	Induction of thyroid involution before surgery of the glands; treatment of thyroid storm; control of hyperthyroidism	gtts iii-v q8h Neonates: gtt i q8h PC: D
saturated solution of potassium iodide (SSKI)	Solution that contains potassium iodide 1 g/ml	Control of hyperthyroidism, induction of thyroid involution before surgery on the gland Expectorant	50–100 mg daily or more, depending on individual client requirements PC: D 300–600 mg, qid
iodinated glycerol (Tussi-Organidin)	Oral solution that contains iodinated glycerol 60 mg/5 ml dose	Expectorant	60 mg, qid; dosage for children is one-half of this
tincture of iodine	Topical solution that contains 2% iodine and 2.4% sodium iodide in 46% ethyl alcohol	Topical antiseptic	Applied topically
povidone-iodine (Proviodine)	Detergent solutions, ointments, vaginal gel	Topical antiseptic	Strength and quantity vary with type of preparation
iopanoic acid (Telepaque)	Oral tablets that contain 500 mg of iopanoic acid	Radiopaque medium for cholecystography and cholangiography	3 g; for children, 50–150 mg/kg body weight
diatrizoate sodium (Hypaque)	Solution and powder for preparing solutions for oral or rectal use Solution for injection Sterile solution for urogenital instillation	Radiopaque medium for various diagnostic procedures	Varies, depending on procedure and individual client requirements

KEY: PC = pregnancy category. (The validity of pregnancy risk categories has not been established; see Chapter 16, p 216.)

component of many antiseptics used for the disinfection of utensils, linens, and the skin. Iodine is also used in contrast media necessary to many radiographic examinations. These uses of the element are not pertinent to its antihormone effects, except that people who have been exposed to iodine within these ancillary contexts may have become allergic to the element and may be at high risk for hypersensitive reaction to any iodide therapy.

Adverse reactions. Iodine administered orally is irritating to the gastric mucosa. The drug's expectorant properties are believed to derive in part from this effect, which initiates reflex stimulation of lung secretion. The drugs tend to produce anorexia, nausea and vomiting, diarrhea, and nasal congestion. Chronic administration, especially in large doses, is associated with a metallic or brassy taste in the mouth, malaise, and depression.

Allergic hypersensitivity to iodine is not uncommon. Reactions may be immediate or delayed. Allergic manifestations include the following:

- Angioedema (anaphylaxis)
- Multiple skin hemorrhages or purpura
- Skin rash including urticaria
- Reactions that resemble serum sickness with fever, arthralgia, lymph node enlargement, and eosinophilia
- Urticaria
- Thrombocytopenia
- Life-threatening periarteritis nodosa

Allergic reactions are more common and more serious when the drugs are administered parenterally than orally.

Toxicity in iodide therapy may be either acute or chronic. Acute iodism occurs primarily after accidental ingestion of iodine preparations by children. The victim complains of thirst, dizziness, and burning abdominal pain. Vomiting, diarrhea, and shock develop. The odor of iodine may be apparent in the emesis. If the substance ingested was an iodine solution, brown stains on the lips, tongue, and mouth, along with pain in these tissues, may be apparent.

Chronic iodism is also characterized by burning sensations in the mouth and throat. Additional symptoms are soreness of the gums and teeth, a brassy taste in the mouth, anorexia, and depression. Increased salivation, a productive cough, coryza, sneezing, eye irritation, and swelling of the eyelids may be present. Fever, pulmonary edema, and parotitis may develop.

Precautions and contraindications. Iodine therapy is hazardous to people who have become allergic to this substance. Adverse reactions are particularly likely when iodides are administered parenterally, as in the use of radiopaque contrast media and in the treatment of thyroid storm. When iodides are required for treatment despite a history of sensitivity, health care personnel must be prepared to treat allergic reactions such as anaphylaxis promptly and aggressively.

Enrichment experience 34-1

Study the labels of over-the-counter preparations that contain iodine (expectorant cough medicines and nutritional supplements that include kelp). Compare the amounts of iodine available in each. Which preparations supply maintenance doses of the mineral? Which contain therapeutic doses? Explain the potential effects on thyroid function for long-term use of each preparation.

Because of their ability to break down granulomatous lesions, iodides are contraindicated in clients with a history of tuberculosis. Dissolution of tubercles release tubercle bacilli within the body and reactivate the infection.

Any client who receives therapeutic doses of iodine over a period of time should be monitored for thyroid function, because hypothyroidism is likely to develop. The use of supplemental iodine (even iodized salt) may be detrimental in some clients with acne, since this condition is often exacerbated by the element.

■ **Summary**

Iodine is an essential nutrient required for normal thyroid function. In geographic areas where soils are deficient in this element, the use of iodized salt decreases the incidence of thyroid disease. Iodine and iodides are used medicinally as antiseptics, expectorants, radiopaque contrast media, and in the prevention and treatment of thyroid disorders. The drugs are used to reduce thyroid toxicity and to induce involution of the thyroid gland before thyroid surgery. Iodine is also used as an adjunct in the treatment of acute thyroid toxicity. Allergic anaphylaxis, the most dangerous adverse reaction to drugs of this class, is most likely to occur when the drugs are administered parenterally.

Nursing management

Nursing implications

Iodine antiseptics are frequently used in health care institutions for the disinfection of skin and utensils. For information about iodine radiopaque dyes, see Chapter 52.

Should iodine be ingested accidentally in poisonous amounts, immediate medical attention is required. Activated charcoal may be administered to adsorb the chemical. Gastric lavage is performed promptly to remove as much of the drug as possible before digestion can occur. Hospitalization is recommended to observe for and treat symptoms such as pulmonary edema and shock that arise from systemic absorption of toxic amounts. Iodine poisoning should be suspected when brown emesis has an odor of iodine. Nausea, vomiting, diarrhea, burning sensations in the mouth and throat, thirst, and abdominal pain are further clues of iodine poisoning.

Nursing process

Assessment   When iodine drugs are prescribed for a client, the drug history must include specific questions about previous tolerance to iodine. Use of iodine or iodides as topical antiseptics, nutritional supplements such as iodized salt, expectorants, radiographic contrast media, cold remedies, or prescription drugs (expectorants or antithyroid medications) should be explored. Adverse reactions associated with such use should be noted.

During the nursing history and physical examination, the client should be assessed for data that signify thyroid function or thyroid disease. The client should be asked if a personal or family history of goiter, Graves' disease, or autoimmune thyroiditis (Hashimoto's disease) exists. A tendency to lose (or gain) weight is also pertinent.

During the physical examination, the nurse should palpate the thyroid gland and note the presence or absence of signs of hyperthyroidism (thick hair, nervousness, restlessness, tremor, rapid pulse, warm moist skin, or exophthalmos) or hypothyroidism (thin brittle hair, puffiness of the face or anterior aspect of the tibia, lethargy, dry cool skin, or weak pulse).

Nursing diagnosis   Nursing diagnoses likely to be made for a client who is receiving iodine therapy include those that arise from thyroid imbalance, as well as the following:

> *Altered comfort: anorexia and nausea related to gastric irritation secondary to iodine therapy*
> *Ineffective airway clearance: airway congestion related to reflex stimulation of nasal and bronchial secretion secondary to iodine therapy*
> *Fluid volume deficit related to vomiting or diarrhea secondary to iodine therapy*
> *Sensory/perceptual alterations (gustatory): brassy taste related to iodine therapy*
> *Impaired tissue integrity: urticaria related to allergic reaction secondary to iodine therapy*
> *Knowledge deficit concerning iodine therapy*

Planning Goals for nursing care include prevention or prompt detection and treatment of adverse reaction to iodine (anorexia, nausea, vomiting, diarrhea, nasal congestion) and teaching the client to manage the iodine regimen.

Intervention The physician should be informed of any history of iodine allergy as early as possible so that the medical regimen may be modified if necessary. If a history of allergic hypersensitivity is elicited, the client should be monitored carefully while iodine is in use for skin rash, symptoms of serum sickness, and decreased peripheral circulation. If iodine compounds are to be administered parenterally, precautions should be taken to ensure prompt treatment of anaphylactic shock, should it develop.

When iodine or iodides are administered orally, they should be given after meals. They must be accompanied by ample fluids. As implied by their use as antiseptics, concentrated iodine solutions tend to damage cells. Ample dilution minimizes damage or irritation to the GI tract cells. Liquid preparations are diluted in milk or fruit juice and are administered through a straw to disguise the taste.

Iodine solutions are light sensitive and are dispensed in light-resistant containers. Doses are small, requiring the measurement of drops or minims when liquid preparations are used. When these drugs are poured, accuracy of measurement is crucial. Since iodides are poisons, they should be stored in secure areas where risk of accidental ingestion is minimal.

When iodine is prescribed to treat hyperthyroidism, sympathomimetic decongestants are contraindicated. Nasal stuffiness and bronchial congestion usually decreases in an environment with a high relative humidity. During the winter, containers of water may be placed on top of radiators, near heating units, or within hot air ducts. If discomfort persists, nasal irrigation with normal saline may alleviate some of the discomfort.

Clients should be monitored for vomiting or diarrhea. Foods known to be irritating should be excluded from the diet. Consumption of fluids up to 3 liters a day (for adults) should be encouraged.

Clients should be monitored for urticaria. If hives develop, iodine should be discontinued and the physician informed immediately. If the client has antiallergy medicine such as Benadryl, a dose may be taken. (If none has been previously prescribed, the physician is likely to order an antiallergen.) Tepid baths that contain either sodium bicarbonate or strained oatmeal gruel help reduce itching. The client should be kept comfortably cool and advised to press on any itching areas to suppress the sensation rather than to scratch.

Any adverse drug reaction that is severe or persistent should be reported to the physician for possible adjustment of the drug regimen. Clients with a history of iodine allergy should be advised to wear or carry a medical identification device that states the problem.

Clients who receive iodides for hyperthyroidism are likely to experience some signs and symptoms of thyrotoxicosis. They need rest, relief from stress, a high-quality high-calorie diet, and protection from undue stimulation. Their thyroid status should be monitored to assess response to medication. Clients scheduled for surgery need the usual preoperative preparation.

Clients in thyroid crisis require intensive nursing care to sustain vital functions and to control the severe physiologic disruptions characteristic of this condition: fever, hypertension, dehydration, and hypocorticism.

Client education. Nurses can do much to reduce the incidence and severity of thyroid disease by promoting adequate nutrition and early treatment of thyroid abnormalities. Adequate iodine intake is necessary for optimum thyroid function. If the diet includes foods from the sea (ocean fish, kelp, fruits and vegetables grown in coastal areas), iodine content is likely to be adequate. Nurses should promote the use of iodized salt in goiter belts known to have iodine-poor soils, particularly for families who raise much of their own food or who use local produce. In the continental U.S., iodine-poor soils are found in most inland areas, including the Great Lakes basin. Clients subject to acne should be referred to a physician for assessment of thyroid function before they are given iodine supplements, because excess iodine may exacerbate this skin condition.

Clients who exhibit goiter or signs and symptoms of thyroid imbalance should be referred promptly for a diagnostic workup. Early detection and treatment of such conditions often prevent the development of severe disease and complications. Adequate treatment of young women protects their future children also; the risk of cretinism rises if the mother-to-be has an iodine deficiency or other thyroid problems.

Clients who receive iodides in preparation for thyroidectomy need information about the side effects that may develop from their use. Skin rash, dyspnea, swelling or soreness of the parotid glands, fever, or irritation or swelling of the eyes should be reported promptly to the physician. Clients should be warned not to use over-the-counter cold remedies that contain stimulating pressor amines. It is best if no drugs are used without the knowledge and approval of the physician.

Compliance to the drug regimen should be stressed. Missed doses reduces the effect of the iodine and results in greater toxicity and higher surgical risks. The rate of complications is higher for such clients. Because timing in relation to surgery is critical, the client should inform the physician immediately if a circumstance arises that may require postponement of thyroid surgery.

Clients known to be allergic to iodine compounds should wear a medical identification device that warns of this condition.

Evaluation   Data required for evaluation relate to the presence or absence and severity of adverse drug reactions and, when iodides are ordered for home use, the ability of the client to manage the drug regimen.

Checklist of nursing actions

☐ Recommend the use of iodized salt to clients who live in goiter belts.

☐ Refer people with signs and symptoms of goiter or thyroid imbalance for diagnosis and treatment.

☐ Before administration of iodides, inquire specifically about adverse reactions to iodides (including radiopaque dyes).

☐ Protect iodine preparations from light and excessive heat.

☐ Store iodine preparations in secure areas.

☐ Monitor clients who receive iodine for symptoms of serum sickness syndrome, respiratory congestion, skin rashes, and thyroid imbalances.

☐ Recommend the use of a medical identification device to all clients with a history of hypersensitivity to iodides.

Radioiodine

Radioactive iodine is produced by subjecting the stable element to bombardment by high-velocity particles. The resultant material shares many properties with normal iodine but, in addition, emits nuclear particles, including α particles, β particles, τ-rays, and conversion electrons. Because it can be measured easily and can be readily distinguished from normal iodine in the body, radioiodine is useful for diagnostic, therapeutic, and research purposes. In large doses, it delivers radiation in therapeutic doses to thyroid tissue without obvious damage to other body tissues.

Radioactivity is measured by the curie (Ci), a unit that indicates the rate at which a given number of

Table 34-5. Radioactive iodine preparations

Drug name	Preparation	Half-life	Type of radiation
sodium iodide ^{131}I (Iodotope Therapeutic)	Solution for oral or IV administration; oral capsules	8 days	γ rays,* β particles
sodium iodide ^{123}I (for investigational use only)		13 hr	γ rays*

*Similar in effect to x-rays.

atoms disintegrate in a given period of time. As in other metric scales, one-thousandth of a curie is termed a *millicurie* (mCi); one-millionth of a curie, a *microcurie* (μCi); and one-trillionth of a curie, a *picocurie* (pCi).

Pharmacodynamics.   In small (tracer) doses, radioiodine has no discernible effect on cells or tissues. It is detectable with nuclear monitoring techniques and can be used to study the physiologic processes by which iodine is used by the body. Radioiodine can also monitor some aspects of thyroid function. In large doses, radioiodine damages thyroid tissue by delivering toxic doses of τ-rays that have an effect similar to that of x-rays. In the thyroid gland, pyknosis and necrosis of the follicular cells develop. The colloid disappears, and the gland becomes fibrous.

Pharmacokinetics.   Radioiodine is handled by the body in exactly the same way as the nonradioactive element. It is concentrated by the thyroid, incorporated into thyroid hormone molecules, and stored in the gland follicles. Later, it is released to the tissues and is subsequently excreted in urine.

Drug preparations.   Two radioactive isotopes of iodine are available for medicinal use (Table 34-5). To date iodine-131 has been used most widely. With a radiation half-life* of 8 days, the radioactivity of this preparation is 99% expended at the end of 56 days. Much of the drug has been excreted from the body before that time. Radioiodine may be administered orally or by IV injection.

Therapeutic uses.   Tracer doses of radioiodine (1–25 μCi) are used in diagnostic tests for thyroid function. The amount of radioiodine that enters the thyroid gland (radioactive iodine uptake or RAIU) provides an indirect measure of thyroid activity. A high RAIU is usually found in thyrotoxicity and a low RAIU in hypothyroidism. This test is not accurate if

*The half-life of radioactive elements is the time required for radioactivity to decline by one half.

iodine has been used in the diet or if antithyroid drugs are administered for medicinal purposes, because further iodine uptake is suppressed by these substances.

The pattern of iodine uptake (and metabolic activity) is revealed by scanning the thyroid for radioactive emissions after the administration of a tracer dose of radioiodine. Metabolically active tissue shows up as "hot spots" and inactive areas as "cold spots." Such areas often correspond to glandular lesions.

In therapeutic doses (1–200 mCi), radioiodine is used to treat thyrotoxicosis and selected thyroid malignancies. Both normal and malignant thyroid cells are destroyed by the drug, provided they are active and capable of concentrating iodine.

When partial destruction of the gland is desired, as in thyroid toxicity, doses range from 4 to 10 mCi. These doses err on the low side to avoid excessive destruction of the gland and subsequent hypothyroidism. As a result, therapeutic response is delayed and tends to be incomplete. If required, a second or even third dose can be given at 3-month intervals. During the period required for complete response to the drug, antithyroid medication may be given to control symptoms of thyrotoxicity.

Radioiodine is a valuable treatment for thyroid toxicity in clients older than age 50, especially those who are poor surgical risks, those with small glands or ectopic tissue, and those who experience exacerbations after completion of a course of antithyroid medication. Treatment may be carried out on an outpatient basis, avoiding the expense and trauma of surgery. The effect of radioiodine is fully evident about 8 to 10 weeks after administration.

Radioactive iodine is effective in treating thyroid cancer only when the malignant cells actively use iodine to produce hormone. Such tumors represent a small fraction of thyroid neoplasms. However, when cancers are radiosensitive, the drug is effective in treating metastases as well as the primary lesion. Large doses of 50 to 150 mCi are required to treat malignancies.

Radioiodine dosages are computed on the basis of gland size, RAIU, and the release rate of radioactive iodine from the gland. The amount of drug needed to deliver the required amount of irradiation also varies with the age of the medicinal preparation, because nuclear disintegration continues during storage time. The drug loses half of its radioactivity for each half-life period that occurs after its manufacture. The dose of isotope necessary to provide 7,000 to 10,000 rad/g of thyroid tissue is administered when a therapeutic effect is desired.

Adverse reactions. When used in tracer doses, radioiodine poses little radiation hazard. The dose of irradiation is extremely low and, alone, is of no physiologic significance. Like all exposure to radiation however, this dose adds to the total accumulated during a lifetime and should be administered only when a medical need exists.

Therapeutic treatment with radioiodine delivers toxic doses of irradiation to the thyroid gland but appears to present a relatively low risk of damage to other body tissues. Exposure of normal cells to irradiation is inversely proportional to the square of their distances from the thyroid follicles that comprise the tissue depots for iodine. Theoretically, a risk of increased mutation in exposed cells and an increased risk of malignancy at some time in the future exist. Significant increases in the incidence of cancer in throat structures have not been documented in the literature on radioiodine.

Radioactive iodine therapy is associated with increased risk of hyperparathyroidism at a later time. Excessive irradiation of the parathyroids could also cause a deficiency of parathormone.

Allergic reactions to radioiodine may develop in clients hypersensitive to iodine. Because the drug is usually administered orally, anaphylaxis is not likely. Skin reactions have occurred, sometimes involving small isolated areas rather than a generalized rash.

Though uncommon, tenderness and swelling of the gland have been reported. This symptom is more apt to occur with higher doses, as in cancer treatments.

The incidence of hypothyroidism after the use of therapeutic doses is relatively high. In treating cancer, when high doses are administered, this symptom may be an effect of the drug action. However, hypothyroidism may be the final manifestation of the hyperthyroid disease process. In Graves' disease, hypothyroidism is regarded by many authorities as a normal event in the final stage of the disease, regardless of the method of treatment. The incidence of eventual hypothyroidism in thyrotoxic clients who receive radioiodine correlates poorly with drug dosage.

Precautions and contraindications. Caution should be employed when radioiodine is used for diagnosis or treatment of people with a history of allergy to iodine. The health care team must be prepared to treat acute allergic reactions should they occur.

Because of the mutagenic and teratogenic potential of radioactive materials, therapeutic doses of radioiodine are relatively contraindicated for children and should be avoided in women of childbearing age. If radioactive drugs are used for lactating mothers, nursing must be discontinued until the substances are eliminated from the body.

The use of radioactive substances, including radioiodine, is restricted to personnel who are qualified by training and experience in the safe use and handling of radioactive pharmaceuticals. Radioactive therapy is available mainly in medical centers with departments of nuclear medicine. Special precautions are required to control radioactive emissions and to prevent undue exposure of personnel and clients to radiation hazards.

■ Summary

Radioactive iodine is used to diagnose thyroid disease and to treat selected cases of hyperthyroidism and thyroid malignancies. Tracer doses used for diagnostic studies are measured in microcuries and present no appreciable radiation hazard. Therapeutic (millicurie) doses deliver effective irradiation to the thyroid gland without obvious damage to other body tissues. Because of the theoretical risk of genetic damage and malignant change, the drug is not ordinarily used in these doses to treat children or women of childbearing age.

Radioiodine treatment offers significant advantages in terms of safety and economy. Treatment does not involve hospitalization and often eliminates the need for thyroid surgery. The drug may induce allergic reactions in iodine-sensitive clients or eventual iatrogenic hypothyroidism.

Nursing management

Nursing implications

Precautions to protect personnel and clients from undue exposure to irradiation are essential when radioactive substances are involved. Exposure is directly proportional to the time spent in proximity to the source of irradiation and inversely proportional to the square of the distance from the source. Personnel who work regularly in departments of nuclear medicine are subject to repeated exposure and must be trained in proper handling techniques to minimize irradiation. Rubber gloves are worn when handling radioactive drugs, and special care should be exercised to avoid spilling medication into the environment. Monitoring devices (dosimeters or film badges) are carried by personnel at all times to measure exposure to radiation. Maximum safe exposure levels are considered to be 20 mrem per day, 100 mrem (0.1 rem) per week, and 5 rem per year (Low-level radiation project: Radiation on the job, 1980). When exposure approaches these levels, personnel must be rotated to other areas of service until the designated period of time has elapsed.

Clients who receive radioactive substances are often fearful. The toxic effects of irradiation are well known to the lay public, and the precautions taken to minimize exposure of personnel serves to emphasize the risk. While the client who receives tracer doses of radioiodine is at minimal risk, the acknowledged aim of treatment with therapeutic doses is tissue destruction. Any person who receives a radioactive medication needs considerable emotional support.

After administration of radioiodine, clients are generally not considered to be sources of dangerous radioactivity. When therapeutic doses are administered, radioiodine is excreted in urine. Dilution in a municipal sewage system provides adequate protection; nevertheless, when clients are hospitalized for treatment, urinals and bedpans should be emptied promptly to eliminate this source of contamination from the immediate environment.

Nursing process

Assessment   Most clients who receive radioactive iodine are affected by an imbalance in thyroid hormones. Those who receive tracer doses may have either a deficiency or an excess of these hormones. Clients who receive therapeutic doses usually manifest thyrotoxicosis. Initial assessment should include an evaluation of thyroid function (see the earlier Nursing Process section for the assessment of clients who receive iodine). Laboratory tests for the thyroid hormones T_4 and T_3 are usually performed. Before the administration of radioiodine, a careful history should be taken relevant to treatment for thyroid malfunction. If antithyroid drugs have been prescribed, the date of the last dose must be determined. These drugs affect iodine uptake and may alter response to radioactive iodine. Thiouracil or iodine taken within the preceding week invalidate diagnostic tracer tests, as do potassium thiocyanate taken within the preceding month. Medication within these time spans also reduces the effectiveness of therapeutic doses of radioiodine and increases exposure of normal tissue to irradiation because the radioactive element is not taken up by the thyroid at the usual rate. The radioiodine continues to circulate in the bloodstream and appears in the urine in higher than normal concentrations.

The nurse should question the client specifically about adverse reaction to iodine or iodinated medications, including contrast media used for radiographic examination.

The nurse should determine the client's attitude toward and emotional response to the use of radioactive substances, response to previous exposure to iodine, and knowledge of thyroid imbalances and their treatment. In addition, the method used in the client's home for sewage disposal should be ascertained.

Nursing diagnosis   Diagnoses likely to be made for clients who are to receive radioactive iodine include the following:

Impaired tissue integrity: skin rash related to allergic reaction to iodine
Fear related to exposure to radiation secondary to use of radioactive iodine
Knowledge deficit concerning thyroid diseases and their treatment

A common collaborative problem that should be differentiated from the nursing diagnoses is

Potential complication: anaphylaxis

In addition, for clients who are to receive therapeutic doses of radioiodine, collaborative problems include

Potential complication: renal/urinary
Potential complication: metabolic

Planning Goals for nursing care include alleviating or eliminating fear and promptly detecting and treating allergic reaction to iodine, radiation injury, and parathyroid imbalance. Goals for the teaching plan are increased client knowledge about thyroid disorders and the use of radioiodine in their diagnosis and treatment.

Intervention The nurse should foster the client's trust in the health care personnel. Competent execution of medical procedures and expression of a warm concern for clients and their families establish initial trust. Honest explanations about the client's condition and the proposed treatment, including its risks, are essential. The nurse should clearly differentiate between a client's one-time or occasional exposure and the health care staff's cumulative exposure from daily contact with radioactive substances.

If the initial assessment of the client reveals previous allergic reaction to iodine, the nurse should immediately notify the physician. Before iodine administration, equipment, supplies, and trained personnel must be available to treat any allergic manifestation, including anaphylactic shock.

Before receiving any radioactive substance, clients should be as well hydrated as possible. This condition prevents undue concentration of radioiodine in body tissues and in the urinary tract.

Hyperthyroid clients require the same nursing care as any thyrotoxic person. After the administration of radioiodine, they are likely to receive antithyroid medication to suppress toxic symptoms until the effects of radioiodine are well established.

Clients should be monitored for symptoms of allergic reaction to iodine, especially if a history of past iodine treatment or hypersensitivity exists. Anaphylaxis is not likely to occur because the drug is administered orally. Skin reactions may develop and occasionally require symptomatic treatment. Long-term follow-up should include monitoring for parathyroid imbalance and for hypothyroidism.

Client education. Clients who receive tracer doses of radioiodine can be assured that the level of irradiation is extremely low and does not pose a significant health hazard. The precautions exercised in the nuclear medicine department may be compared to those practiced in the radiographic departments, where personnel must be protected from even low doses of irradiation because of the constant risk of exposure. After treatment, no special precautions need be taken by the client who receives low doses of radioiodine.

When therapeutic doses are administered, clients are often anxious. The nurse can explain that drugs potentially harmful to normal people are often helpful in disease conditions, that the client is exposed to radioactivity a limited number of times, whereas medical personnel are subject to repeated risk of exposure, and (when malignancy is not involved) that doses are computed to err on the side of undertreatment. Most clients experience no discomfort or other adverse reaction after receiving radioiodine.

If clients are treated as outpatients, the nurse should explore the plans for self-care to ascertain the need for special instructions. Clients should not live alone or be isolated from emergency medical care during the 3 months after therapy. Although rare, tissue destruction can release sufficient hormone to produce a thyroid crisis. Also infrequently, thyroiditis can occur, with subsequent swelling of the gland, pressure on the trachea, and an acute respiratory emergency. Should either situation arise, the client needs immediate medical treatment. For the first week after treatment, clients should remain in a setting served by a multiple-dwelling sewage system to avoid the concentration of radioactive wastes in a septic system.

Clients should be taught the signs and symptoms of hypothyroidism and parathyroid imbalance. For manifestations of hypothyroidism, see the assessment section of the Nursing Process regarding care of clients who receive iodine medications. Signs and symptoms of hyperparathyroidism include increased flexibility of joints, bone pain, emotional lability, and abdominal pain due to calcium renal stones. Parathormone deficiency causes muscle irritability, cramps, and tetany. Any of these symptoms should be reported promptly to the primary health care provider. Clients should be encouraged to remain under continued health supervision for monitoring of serum levels of thyroid hormone and calcium. These tests can alert the physician to abnormal changes before signs and symptoms of overt disease develop. Hypothyroidism or parathormone imbalance can develop years after the completion of radioiodine therapy.

Evaluation Data required for evaluation include the presence or absence of signs and symptoms of fear in the client, the incidence and severity of allergic reaction or bladder inflammation, the long-term incidence and severity of hypothyroidism or parathyroid imbalance, and long-term absence or occurrence of signs and symptoms of excessive exposure to irradiation in clients or their families. For short-term evaluation of the teaching plan, the client is questioned to test retention of material conveyed during teaching sessions.

Example of nursing process and radioiodine therapy

The client is a 45-year-old farm wife and writer who has come to the medical center for radioiodine therapy. She has previously undergone 2 years of propylthiouracil treatment and has had a subtotal thyroidectomy. After each treatment, she remained euthyroid for several months but toxicity gradually recurred.

Comments by the client indicate that she is well informed about health care. She understands that the proposed treatment involves exposure to ionizing radiation in relatively large doses, but she prefers not to undergo additional surgery.

Assessment data	Nursing diagnosis	Intervention	Goals and outcome criteria
Order for radioiodine therapy	Potential for impaired tissue integrity: dermatitis related to allergic reaction secondary to medication	**Ascertain** whether the client has a personal or family history of allergy, especially allergic reaction to iodine; report to the physician any positive findings. **Advise** the client to notify the physician's office promptly if skin rash develops after the radioiodine treatment.	The client will not develop allergic reaction to radioiodine; if such a reaction does occur, it will be detected and treated promptly.
Client's knowledge about health and health care related to previous therapies Rural residence	Possible knowledge deficit concerning some aspects of radioiodine therapy	**Explore** with the client her knowledge of radioiodine; ascertain her plans for care after the treatment. **Provide** the client with any information about radioiodine of which she is unaware; ensure that she knows she should remain in an area supplied with a central sewage plant for 1 week and should avoid living alone for 3 months after receiving the radioiodine.	The client will express confidence in relation to the radioiodine treatment. The client will make appropriate arrangement for aftercare.

Success over the long-term is implied by the client's maintenance of health care supervision and prompt reporting of abnormal signs and symptoms to the primary care provider (see Example of Nursing Process and Radioiodine Therapy).

Checklist of nursing actions

☐ Before administration of radioactive iodine, determine if the client has received antithyroid medication in the preceding month and if a history of iodine sensitivity exists. Report either finding to the physician.

☐ Assess the client for evidence of thyroid hormone imbalance.

☐ Explain the potential risks to clients in realistic terms.

☐ Handle radioactive substances with rubber gloves and minimize exposure to radiation by reducing the time spent in close proximity to the drugs.

☐ Provide emotional support to clients fearful of radiation injury.

When therapeutic dosages of radioiodine are prescribed

☐ Explain to clients the need for dilution of body wastes for 1 week after treatment.

☐ Monitor clients for allergic reaction to iodine; be prepared to treat anaphylactic shock, should it develop.

☐ Stress the need for long-term health care to detect thyroid and parathyroid imbalances, should they develop.

Calcitonin

A hormone with physiologic functions that oppose those of parathormone is produced by the parafollicular "C" cells of many animals. Depending on the species involved, these cells may be found in the parathyroid, thymus, or (in humans) thyroid glands. This hormone, called *calcitonin*, lowers calcium levels in the extracellular fluid by inhibiting bone resorption and altering absorption and excretion of calcium by the body. While calcitonin does not block the actions of parathormone, its effects tend to reverse those of parathormone.

Calcitonin is a single chain polypeptide composed of 32 amino acids with two disulfide linkages. Its molecular weight is about 3,600. The hormone is highly potent, producing pronounced effects in microgram doses. Its presence is determined by radioimmunoassay.

Preparations of salmon, porcine, and human calcitonin have been studied experimentally.

Pharmacodynamics. Calcitonin is believed to increase cyclic adenosine monophosphate (cAMP) in bone cells other than those affected by parathormone. It decreases the activity of osteoclasts and their formation from mesenchymal stem cells. Its immediate effect on osteoblasts is enhancement of their activity, although this declines with continued exposure. Calcitonin increases renal excretion of calcium, phosphorus, and sodium. Some evidence suggests that it may inhibit intestinal absorption of calcium. The hypocalcemic effect of calcitonin is rapid but transitory. Effects on bone metabolism are more long-lived.

Therapeutic uses. Calcitonin is useful in the treatment of hypercalcemia due to hyperparathyroidism, idiopathic hypercalcemia of infancy, vitamin D intoxication, osteolytic bone metastases, and hyperphosphatemia. Although it has been used experimentally for the treatment of postmenopausal osteoporosis, it appears to have minimal effects on this condition over the long term (Fatourechi, Heath, 1987). Calcitonin's major clinical use is the treatment of Paget's disease of the bone, a condition characterized by abnormal and increased bone formation and resorption that results in bone remodeling and abnormal bone structure. Long-term use in this disease tends to correct its characteristic physiologic abnormalities: elevated levels of blood alkaline phosphatase and urinary hydroxyproline and increased blood flow in the affected bone. The rate of bone turnover declines, and a more normal bone structure is restored.

Drug preparations. Two commercial preparations of calcitonin are available for clinical use: human calcitonin and salmon calcitonin (Table 34-6). When reconstituted, solutions must be refrigerated to maintain potency and should be used within 6 hours. The drugs are administered by injection.

Pharmacokinetics. Because its protein structure would be destroyed by digestive enzymes, calcitonin must be administered parenterally (subcutaneously, IM, or IV). When given IV, onset of action is immedi-

Table 34-6. Medicinal preparations of calcitonin

Drug name	Preparation	Therapeutic uses	Usual adult dosage	Additional information
calcitonin (human) (Cibacalcin)	Solution for injection	Paget's disease	SC: *Initially:* 0.5 mg/day; *maintenance:* up to 0.5 mg bid PC: C	Allergic hypersensitivity occurs infrequently.
calcitonin (salmon) (Calcimar)	Solution for injection	Paget's disease	SC: *Initially:* 100 IU/day; *maintenance:* 50 IU 3× weekly-100 IU/day	Allergic hypersensitivity to salmon calcitonin is more likely than to human calcitonin.
		Hypercalcemia	SC or IM: *Initially:* 4 IU/kg body weight q12h, increased to a maximum of 8 IU/kg body weight q6h when necessary	Calcium supplements are usually prescribed with calcitonin for the treatment of osteoporosis or osteogenesis imperfecta.
		Menopausal osteoporosis	100 IU/day	
		Osteogenesis imperfecta	2 IU/kg body weight 3× weekly PC: C	

KEY: PC = pregnancy category. (The validity of pregnancy risk categories has not been established; see Chapter 16, p 216.)

ate and duration of action is 30 minutes to 12 hours. After IM or subcutaneous administration, onset of action is 15 minutes, peak action is seen at 4 hours, and duration of action is 8 to 24 hours. Little is known about calcitonin's distribution. It is believed not to cross the placenta; endogenous calcitonin has been detected in human milk in concentrations 10 to 40 times that in serum. Calcitonin appears to be metabolized by the kidneys, in the blood, and in peripheral tissues. Its metabolites are excreted in urine (McEvoy, 1991).

Adverse reactions. Adverse reactions to calcitonin have been infrequent and mild; only occasionally have they been severe enough to require withdrawal of the drug. The administration of calcitonin can cause flushing, urticaria, diuresis, or nausea and vomiting. The volume and acidity of gastric secretion may decline. The drug can also cause tetany owing to a drop in blood calcium level. Continued use is often accompanied by swelling and tenderness of the hands. After several months of therapy, resistance to the drug characterized by antibody formation may be seen. Allergic reactions also can occur. High doses of calcitonin, or an exaggerated response to the drug, may precipitate acute hypocalcemia as well as nausea and vomiting.

Precautions and contraindications. Salmon calcitonin is contraindicated in pregnancy. Caution should be exercised with allergic people because hypersensitivity can develop, especially when salmon calcitonin is used. Before initiation of medication, a skin test for allergic hypersensitivity should be performed. During the initial period of calcitonin treatment, calcium solutions for injection should be available for parenteral administration to correct any significant hypocalcemia that may develop.

Clients who receive long-term therapy with calcitonin must be monitored and alternative treatment established if resistance to the hormone develops.

■ Summary

Calcitonin is a hormone with physiologic effects (hypocalcemia and decreased osteoclastic activity) that generally oppose those of parathormone. The drug is used mainly for the long-term treatment of Paget's disease of the bone. It is administered three to seven times a week by injection. Over time, immune bodies tend to develop, and the effectiveness of the drug declines.

Nursing management

Nursing implications

Calcitonin solutions are relatively unstable and must be protected from light and heat. They should be used within 6 hours of preparation.

Calcitonin therapy is relatively new and its long-term effects unknown. Clients should be regularly assessed for adverse reactions that have not previously been reported.

Resistance to the medication may develop due to antibody formation. Return of symptoms should be reported to health care personnel so that alternative treatment can be instituted.

Nursing process

Assessment Before administration of calcitonin, a broad data base should be established for comparison with the client's status during drug therapy. In addition, clients should be assessed for allergic tendencies, visible bone deformities, and signs and symptoms of hypercalcemia (increased formation of dental plaque, constipation, emotional lability, lethargy, calciuria, and abdominal pain caused by urinary calculi). The client's knowledge of and emotional reaction to the disorder and to the use of hormone medications should be ascertained.

Nursing diagnosis Nursing diagnoses likely to be made for clients who receive calcitonin therapy include the following:

> *Body image disturbance and self-esteem disturbance related to skeletal deformities caused by disorders of bone metabolism (osteoporosis, osteogenesis imperfecta, Paget's disease)*
> *Pain: abdominal pain related to urinary calculi secondary to hypercalcemia*

Nursing diagnoses that arise from calcitonin therapy include the following:

> *Altered comfort: nausea, vomiting, and abdominal discomfort related to adverse reaction to calcitonin medication*
> *Fluid volume deficit related to diuresis secondary to calcitonin therapy*
> *Potential for pain: tetany related to hypocalcemia due to calcitonin therapy*
> *Impaired tissue integrity: skin rash related to allergic hypersensitivity to calcitonin*

Common collaborative problems that should be differentiated from the nursing diagnoses include

> *Potential complication: tetany*
> *Potential complication: angioedema*
> *Potential complication: anaphylactic shock*
> *Potential complication: cardiac arrhythmia*

Most clients have a

> *Knowledge deficit concerning calcitonin therapy*

Planning Goals of nursing care are to improve self-concept and emotional stability, increase comfort,

Example of nursing process and calcitonin therapy

The client is a 41-year-old secretary who has just been informed that she has Paget's disease of the bones. The physician has ordered calcitonin (human) 0.5 mg IM daily. The client is to report daily to the office for the injections and for instruction in injection technique. When optimum dosage is determined, and the client is proficient in injection technique, the client will assume management of the regimen.

The client asks the nurse, "What is this calcitonin?"

Assessment data	Nursing diagnosis	Intervention	Goals and outcome criteria
New order for calcitonin medication	Knowledge deficit concerning calcitonin and its use in the treatment of Paget's disease	**Prepare** and implement a teaching plan that covers the nature of Paget's disease, the therapeutic effect of calcitonin, IM injection technique, toxic and side effects of calcitonin, as well as the need for continued supervision by health care professionals.	The client will demonstrate correct injection technique by self-injecting a dose of medication in the physician's office; she will be able to repeat to the nurse information conveyed during teaching.
Client's unfamiliarity with calcitonin			In the management of the drug regimen, the client will demonstrate behavior consistent with that recommended by health care personnel.

maintain normal fluid and electrolyte balance, and promptly detect and treat adverse drug reaction.

Intervention Because calcitonin therapy is relatively new, clients who receive the drug are maintained under close medical supervision. Injections are required three to seven times a week. When therapy is initiated in an acute care setting, the nurse administers the medication. Only fresh solutions (less than 6 hours old) should be used. The drug may be administered by IV infusion or by IM or SC injection. During initial treatments, calcium solutions for injection should be readily available in the nursing unit in case signs and symptoms of hypocalcemic tetany develop. These include numbness and tingling or carpopedal spasm when blood pressure cuff is applied.

Long-term treatment is carried out in the community. Client responses should be closely monitored to detect previously unrecognized effects of the drugs. These should be reported to the federal Food and Drug Administration (FDA; see Chapter 2 for reporting procedure). Specific responses to watch for include dehydration due to diuresis and loss of sodium and water, abnormal blood calcium levels, and signs and symptoms of allergy. Therapeutic response should be assessed at each nursing visit. A return of symptoms may indicate development of antibodies to the medication and should be reported to the physician so that alternative treatment can be instituted.

Skeletal deformities are not corrected by treatment. The nurse should reinforce client behavior indicative of a positive self-image. Clients should be praised and complimented for appropriate appearance and behavior whenever possible. The nurse's relationship to the client should be characterized by warm acceptance.

Client education. Clients who receive calcitonin should be taught to report their health status in detail to facilitate monitoring for hormone effects. They should know the identity of the drug they are receiving and also that calcitonin is a relatively new therapeutic agent.

Clients should be informed that skillful design and fit of clothing may camouflage skeletal changes. If the nurse is aware of local tailors or dressmakers who are adept at fitting clothes, the client may be referred to them.

Some clients administer their own drug therapy after dosage has been adjusted to individual needs. These clients need instruction in injection technique and in the specific signs and symptoms they should report to the physician. They must understand the general properties of the drug as well as the characteristics of the disease for which they are being treated. Regular medical supervision is needed indefinitely.

Evaluation Data required for evaluation include incidence and prevalence of behavior or comments by the client indicative of a positive (or negative) self-image, observed behavior or feelings reported by the client indicative of inappropriate emotional reactions, reports by the client that relate to comfort level, and incidence or absence of adverse drug reactions (GI upset, dehydration, muscle irritability, skin rash, or cardiovascular collapse). Short-term evaluation of the teaching program may include questioning the client about facts conveyed during teaching sessions and observation of the client's self-injection technique (see Example of Nursing Process and Calcitonin Therapy).

Checklist of nursing actions

When calcitonin therapy is initiated
☐ Administer drug doses IV, IM, or SC as ordered.
☐ Watch for nausea, vomiting, and tetany.
☐ Have parenteral calcium gluconate available for immediate administration should tetany occur.
☐ Report tetany immediately and assist in the administration of IV calcium.

When long-term calcitonin therapy is planned
☐ Teach the client how to administer parenteral medication.
☐ Teach the client signs and symptoms of adverse reactions to calcitonin, including diminution of therapeutic response.
☐ Caution the client to remain under medical supervision and to report significant changes in health status to the primary care provider.

Throughout calcitonin therapy
☐ Monitor the client for signs and symptoms of allergy to the hormone.
☐ Monitor the client for continued response to the drug. Should signs and symptoms of the disease process recur, refer to the physician for reassessment of the drug regimen and alternative therapy.

Whenever calcitonin is prescribed
☐ Watch the client for previously unrecognized effects of the drug; report these to the FDA to facilitate collection of data that relate to calcitonin's toxic and side effects.

Parathyroid hormone

Parathormone is a polypeptide composed of 84 amino acids arranged in a single chain. Its molecular weight is about 9,500. Preparations of bovine parathormone have only recently become available commercially. The drug is measured in biologic units, and its presence is determined by immunoassay techniques.

Physiology. Parathormone is produced by the parathyroid glands and acts to maintain adequate calcium levels in the blood. Stimulated by even small decreases in calcium ion concentration in the extracellular fluid, the chief cells of the parathyroids respond with increased secretion of this compound, which elevates blood calcium levels. Parathormone increases resorption of calcium from the bones, absorption of calcium and phosphorus by the gut, and reabsorption of calcium in the renal tubule. High levels of calcium in the extracellular fluid inhibit parathormone production.

Pathology. Pathologic conditions associated with parathormone imbalance include primary excesses of the hormone caused by hypertrophy of the glands, hyperparathyroidism secondary to pregnancy, lactation, rickets, or other hypocalcemic conditions, and iatrogenic hypoparathyroidism secondary to inadvertent surgical removal of the glands. Excesses of the hormone cause hypercalcemia, calciuria with formation of calcium stones in the urinary tract, and demineralization of the bones. When the hormone is deficient, calcium ion levels in the extracellular fluid drop, and tetany and cardiac arrhythmia ensue.

Pharmacodynamics. Parathormone causes an immediate activation of previously formed osteoclasts by increasing cAMP in these cells. Formation of new osteoclasts from mesenchymal stem cells is stimulated, and the conversion of osteoclasts to osteoblasts is delayed. These effects cause a temporary decrease in osteoblastic activity at the same time that osteoclastic activity is enhanced. Concurrently, renal tubular reabsorption of phosphorus, sodium, potassium, and amino acid ions is inhibited, and reabsorption of calcium, magnesium, and hydrogen ions is enhanced. Intestinal absorption of calcium and phosphorus also increases.

With continued exposure to the hormone, as seen in hyperparathyroidism, osteoblastic activity recovers somewhat as large numbers of osteoclasts are converted to osteoblasts. The bones can become significantly demineralized, however, with abnormal mobility of the joints and increased plasticity of the bones. Permanent skeletal deformities tend to develop.

Pharmacokinetics. Because the hormone is destroyed by peptidases in the intestinal tract, parathormone cannot be administered orally. When injected, its effect is not immediate, requiring about 4 hours for onset and lasting about 24 to 36 hours. Relatively little is known about its metabolic fate, although it appears to be degraded by the liver and kidneys.

Drug preparations. Parathormone is no longer available commercially for clinical use. Synthetic (bovine) parathormone is available for investigational purposes.

Therapeutic uses. Parathormone is not used frequently in the treatment of clinical conditions. It is sometimes administered initially to treat acute hypoparathyroidism, but the chronic condition is better managed by the prescription of large doses of vitamin D, which has a physiologic effect similar to that of the hormone.

Parathormone is also used in a diagnostic test for pseudohypoparathyroidism.

Adverse reactions. Subcutaneous injections of parathormone often produce local inflammation. Allergic hypersensitivity accentuates this response. Because drug preparations of the hormone are of animal origin and differ somewhat in molecular structure from the human hormone, immune bodies tend to develop, and allergy is not uncommon. Administration of large doses of the drug produces anorexia, vomiting, diarrhea, and weakness.

Because the drug is not used for long-term therapy, chronic toxicity is not seen as an iatrogenic condition. However, people with hyperparathyroid conditions tend to develop cardiac, GI and urinary tract, skeletal, and emotional pathology. Hypercalcemia promotes systolic contraction of the heart and shortened diastole, reducing cardiac output. Cardiac arrhythmia may develop. Anorexia, constipation, and a metallic taste in the mouth frequently occur. Peptic ulcers are seen in one-fifth of the clients. Kidney stones are common. Bony deformities and pathologic fractures can develop, as can mental lethargy, weakness, fatigue, and emotional depression or irritability.

Precautions and contraindications. Parathormone is contraindicated in hypercalcemia. It must be used with caution in renal or cardiac disease. Before administration, a skin test should be made for sensitivity, especially if the client is known to have received the drug in the past. When the drug is administered IV, epinephrine must be available for the treatment of anaphylactic or other allergic reactions.

■ **Summary**

Parathormone is a relatively new hormone drug agent with limited clinical usefulness. It is sometimes used in a diagnostic test for pseudohypoparathyroidism. Investigation continues for the purposes of clarifying its pharmacokinetics and for developing further therapeutic uses.

Nursing management

Nursing implications

Parathormone is used only for the diagnosis of pseudohypoparathyroidism, a condition in which the target tissues for parathormone (mainly bone) are unresponsive to the hormone. The drug is administered to determine whether it will trigger a rise in serum calcium level. Failure of response indicates tissue refractoriness to the hormone. This procedure is not likely to produce adverse reaction unless the recipient is allergic to the hormone.

Nursing process

Assessment When parathormone is to be used, the client should be questioned about previous use of the drug or previous episodes of hypocalcemia during which the hormone may have been used. If previous exposure to the hormone is suspected, a skin test for allergic hypersensitivity is performed.

Clients with suspected pseudohypoparathyroidism are likely to have a low serum calcium level. They should be assessed for signs and symptoms of pretetany (facial fasciculations where the skin over the facial nerve is tapped or carpopedal spasm on inflation of a blood pressure cuff on the arm). Hypocalcemia is also associated with nerve irritability; clients may be apprehensive and manifest nervous tension.

Nursing diagnosis Nursing diagnoses likely to be made for clients who undergo a parathormone test include the following:

Pain: nerve and muscle irritability related to hypocalcemia secondary to pseudoparathyroidism
Knowledge deficit concerning hypoparathyroidism and the diagnostic use of parathormone

A common collaborative problem that should be differentiated from the nursing diagnoses is

Potential complication: tetany

Planning Goals of nursing care are to promptly detect and treat hypocalcemic tetany (should it develop), increase the client's comfort, and teach the client about pseudoparathyroidism and the diagnostic test to be performed.

Intervention Clients who experience paresthesia and muscle and nerve irritability owing to a low serum calcium level should be given a paper bag and instructed to breathe in and out of the bag several times in a row. Bag rebreathing increases the carbon dioxide load of the blood and lowers its pH. This effect increases the ionization and physiologic action of the calcium present in the blood, temporarily alleviating the signs and symptoms of calcium deficiency and delaying the onset of tetany. Bag rebreathing is also used to ameliorate tetany when it develops.

The nurse may be responsible for coordinating the services required for accurate diagnostic testing. Blood tests for serum calcium are required before and at timed intervals after the administration of parathormone. If the drug is given IV or subcutaneously, the nurse may also be responsible for administering the hormone. Adrenalin should be available for treating acute allergic reaction to the drug, should it occur.

The site of hormone injection should be monitored for local inflammation, an indication of possible allergy. Because parathormone is a relatively new drug, the nurse should also watch for any unusual response by the client. This should be recorded and reported (see Chapter 2 for reporting procedure) to facilitate identification of previously unrecognized drug effects.

Client education. Clients should be informed about the test, expected responses, and the need to report any unusual symptoms that occur during the procedure. The client is unlikely to experience recognizable changes when the drug is administered. Clients who do respond may experience alleviation of nerve and muscle irritability as serum calcium level rises. This effect rules out pseudohypoparathyroidism.

Clients should be informed that they are receiving parathormone and should be advised to report this fact to health care personnel, particularly in situations when a repetition of the test is considered. Each exposure to the hormone increases the likelihood of allergic hypersensitivity.

Evaluation Data required for evaluation include the presence or absence of muscle fasciculations and tetany and client reports of changes in comfort level. Teaching may be evaluated by the client's ability to anticipate and adapt to procedures required for the diagnostic test.

Checklist of nursing actions

When parathormone is to be used as a diagnostic tool
☐ Ask the client about previous exposure to parathormone and susceptibility to allergic hypersensitivity; if allergic reaction is likely, arrange for a skin test to determine sensitivity to parathormone before the diagnostic test is performed.
☐ Have epinephrine available at the bedside for treatment of allergic reaction, should it occur; obtain an "as circumstances may require" (prn) order for its use.

During the test
☐ Monitor the client closely for anaphylaxis, nausea, weakness, and irregular heart rate.
☐ If anaphylaxis occurs, administer epinephrine immediately and summon medical help.
☐ Observe recipient for any unusual change in status; record and report any changes because they may indicate previously unrecognized effects of parathormone.

When hypocalcemic tetany occurs
☐ Immediately institute paper bag or glove rebreathing to lower body pH.

If tetany does not respond to rebreathing
☐ Prepare for the administration of IV medications, such as calcium.

Adenohypophysial hormones and related substances

The anterior pituitary produces a number of protein hormones that regulate the activity of various target tissues in the body. Hormones identified to date include growth hormone, prolactin, two gonadotropins, thyrotropin, and corticotropin. Similar protein hormones are produced by the human placenta. Some of these proteins closely resemble each other in structure (Table 34-7) and a few share physiologic properties to some degree.

Because of their protein structure, pituitary tropic hormones are not effective when administered orally, and they are not routinely used for hormone replacement in deficiency states. Instead, oral hormone preparations normally produced by the target glands (corticosteroids, and thyroid and sex hormones) are prescribed to maintain normal body function. Notable exceptions are growth hormone, which is the only agent effective in the treatment of pituitary dwarfism, and the gonadotropins, which are sometimes effective in restoring fertility to people with pituitary hypofunction. Some anterior pituitary hormones are used in diagnostic tests to differentiate between primary and secondary failure in relation to thyroid gland or adrenal cortex production. One tropic hormone, corticotropin, is used as a pharmaceutical agent in the treatment of certain progressive degenerative diseases.

Corticotropin

Physiology. Corticotropin is a protein hormone produced by the chromophobic cells of the anterior lobe of the pituitary gland. Its function is the control of steroid hormone production by the adrenal cortex. The hormone is a vital link in the mechanism of stress adaptation by which an organism maintains the heightened circulation and energy production required for resistance to environmental stressors. This response begins when sensory impulses stimulate the brain. Excitation of the anterior hypothalamus causes increased production of corticotropin-releasing factor. Itself a protein hormone, this chemical is conveyed to the adenohypophysis (anterior pituitary), where it stimulates the tissues to produce corticotropin. In the adrenal cortex, corticotropin stimulates production of steroid hormones, most notably the glucocorticoids. Undue fluctuations in hormone response to stress are prevented by a negative feedback system that involves inhibition of corticotropin production in the anterior pituitary by the glucocorticoid hormones themselves.

Pathology. Overproduction of corticotropin can arise from a secreting tumor of the pituitary. When

Table 34-7. Properties of the protein hormones of the human adenohypophysis and placenta

Hormone	Molecular weight	Peptide chains	Amino acid residues	Carbohydrate	Additional information
Group 1					
growth hormone (GH)	22,000	1	191	0	Human GH, Prl, and PL have con-
prolactin (Prl)	23,000	1	198	0	siderably less homology of amino
placental lactogen (PL)	22,000	1	191	0	acid sequence, in contrast to the striking degree observed in other species.
Group 2					
luteinizing hormone (LH, ICSH)	30,000	2	α-89 β-115	16%	Glycoproteins with nonidentical subunits (α and β); biologic specificity is in β subunit.
follicle-stimulating hormone (FSH)	32,000	2	α-89 β-115	18%	The α subunits of LH, FSH, TSH, and CG are nearly identical and interchangeable.
thyrotropin (TSH)	28,000	2	α-89 β-112	13%	FSH-α and FSH-β are similar in amino acid composition.
chorionic gonadotropin (CG)	38,000	2	α-92 β-145	31%	FSH-β and TSH-β share a sequence of 49 amino acid residues, whereas FSH-β and LH-β share a sequence of 39-residues.
					Residues 1 to 115 of CG-β have about 80% homology with the β subunits of LH, FSH, and TSH.
					Data suggest heterogeneity, even within each hormone.
Group 3					
corticotropin	4500	1	39	0	This group of peptides is derived from a common precursor.
α-Melanocyte-stimulating hormone (α-MSH)	1650	1	13	0	Group shares a common heptapeptide: Met-Glu-His-Phe-Arg-Trp-Gly
β-Melanocyte-stimulating hormone (β-MSH)	2100	1	18	0	Corticotropin (1–13) = α-MSH
β-Lipotropin (β-LPH)	9500	1	91	0	β-LPH (1–58) = λ-Lipotropin
γ-Lipotropin (γ-LPH)	5800	1	58	0	β-LPH (41–58) = β-MSH

(Gilman AG, Goodman LS, Rall TW, Murad F. [1985]. *Goodman and Gilman's The pharmacological basis of therapeutics*, 7th ed., p 1364. New York: Macmillan.)

adrenal function is normal, such excesses lead to hypercorticism, a condition called *Cushing's disease*. This condition is always characterized by excess production of glucocorticoids, often accompanied by excess adrenal androgens. Treatment of Cushing's disease is aimed at correcting the pituitary pathology.

Corticotropin deficiency, a feature of panhypopituitarism, causes adrenal atrophy and corticosteroid deficiencies. In this condition, the most convenient treatment is replacement of hormones by the administration of oral corticoids. Simultaneous replacement of other deficient hormones such as thyroid and sex hormones is also necessary to restore health. Of course, if an underlying progressive pituitary problem exists, this must also be treated.

Pharmacodynamics. Corticotropin reacts with a specific hormone receptor on adrenal cell membranes, causing an increase in cAMP in these cells. The availability of cholesterol substrate for steroid synthesis increases, and the initial reaction in steroidogenesis is stimulated by an increase in cholesterol binding to cytochrome P-450. Cholesterol esterase activity also increases. The cells of the zona reticularis, which produces glucocorticoid hormones, are most strongly affected. A weaker stimulation occurs in the zona fasciculata in which adrenal sex hormones are produced. The effect on the zona glomerulosa, which produces mineralocorticoids, is weakest of all, but it does serve to enhance response of this part of the cortex to the primary stimuli of hyperkalemia and hypovolemia. Total absence of corticotropin produces partial atrophy of the zona glomerulosa and almost total atrophy of the remainder of the cortex. Thus, corticotropin is a necessary factor for normal adrenal production of corticosteroids. Given adequate adrenal function, the level of glucocorticoid production is directly proportional to corticotropin levels.

Pharmacokinetics. As a protein substance, corticotropin is destroyed by digestive enzymes and is not effective when administered orally. It is rapidly absorbed parenterally and may be administered IM, SC, or IV. Like other protein hormones, corticotropin appears to be degraded by the tissues; the hormone does not appear in appreciable amounts in urine or other body excreta. Its half-life in plasma is 15 minutes, and the effects of a single dose are largely dissipated after 6 hours. Because repeated administration of the hormone produces hypertrophy of the adrenal cortex, increased secretion of corticosteroids continues for a time after tropic hormone levels have returned to normal.

Therapeutic uses. Corticotropin is medicinally useful in selected clinical situations. It is used diagnostically in corticosteroid deficiency states to determine the functional capacity of the adrenal cortex to respond to stimulation. If corticosteroid levels rise after administration of corticotropin, adrenal dysfunction is ruled out as a causative condition, and a search for pituitary pathology is begun. Failure of the adrenals to respond to stimulation indicates the likelihood of primary adrenal pathology, rather than pituitary disease. The test involves measurement of 17-hydroxycorticoid levels in the urine over a 24-hour period, before and after the administration of corticotropin by IV infusion for 2 or 3 consecutive days. Production of 17-hydroxycorticoids should increase threefold if adrenal function is normal. In primary adrenal corticoid deficiency, steroid production rises slightly on the first day, with no increase thereafter. In secondary insufficiency, steroid production rises higher with each succeeding dose of corticotropin.

Limited courses of corticotropin therapy also are used to produce temporary hypercorticism, with the aim of inducing remissions in certain progressive degenerative diseases. Therapeutic administration of corticotropin appears to be most useful in conditions that respond to glucocorticoid therapy, such as rheumatic disease, autoimmune conditions, myasthenia gravis, and multiple sclerosis. Theoretically, conditions characterized by remissions and exacerbations are most likely to benefit from corticotropin therapy. While these conditions do improve when treated by glucocorticoids, long-term therapy involves the risk of serious complications caused by the hormone drugs. Withdrawal of steroids produces a relative hypocorticism during which an exacerbation of the disease condition is likely. Administration of corticotropin increases endogenous steroid production, ameliorates symptoms, and may induce a lasting remission without the risk of significant hypocorticism when the drug is withdrawn.

Drug preparations. Medicinal preparations are produced mainly from the pituitaries of slaughtered animals, but some synthetic hormone is also available. Animal hormones differ from the human type by substitution of different amino acid residues at three positions on the protein chain. Animal hormones are physiologically effective in humans, however. Most drug preparations of corticotropin are standardized by bioassay techniques that measure the depletion of adrenal ascorbic acid in hypophysectomized rats in response to specific doses. (Ascorbic acid is required for the production of cortical steroids and is assumed to disappear in proportion to hormone synthesis within the gland.) Animal preparations of corticotropin are measured in these biologic units. The synthetic preparation is measured in milligrams, with a dose of 0.25 mg equivalent in action to 25 U of natural hormone.

Medicinal preparations of corticotropin include aqueous solutions for IV infusion and suspensions and gelatin solutions for IM or subcutaneous administration (Table 34-8). The latter are absorbed by the body at relatively slow rates and provide longer periods of therapeutic effectiveness per dose.

Table 34-8. Drug preparations of corticotropic hormone

Drug name	Preparation	Usual adult dosage
corticotropin injection (Acthar, ACTH, Cortrophin)	Lipophilized powder for reconstitution for injection	40 U daily PC: C
repository corticotropin (H.P. Acthar Gel, Cortigel, Corticotrophin Gel, Cortropic-Gel)	Highly purified corticotropin in gelatin solution for IM or subcutaneous injection	40 U daily PC: C
corticotropin zinc hydroxide suspension (Cortrophin-Zinc)	Purified corticotropin absorbed on zinc hydroxide, for IM injection	40 U daily PC: C
cosyntropin for injection (Cortrosyn)	Synthetic peptide with 24 amino acid residues that comprise the active portion of the corticotropin molecule for IV or IM administration	0.25 mg (equivalent to 25 U) used for diagnostic testing PC: C

KEY: PC = pregnancy risk category. (The validity of pregnancy risk categories has not been established; see Chapter 16, p 216.)

Adverse reactions. Corticotropin therapy is seldom continued over a long period; hence, hypercorticism is rare. Continued administration of the drug can produce iatrogenic Cushing's syndrome, indistinguishable clinically from the naturally occurring condition. This state is characterized by glucocorticoid toxicity and by masculinization in the female. Although full-blown Cushing's syndrome is not seen in short-term corticotropin therapy, there is a tendency toward sodium retention, potassium depletion, hypervolemia, hypertension, ketosis, lipolysis, immunosuppression, and mood elevation. Acne may also appear. Most of these side effects also develop during glucocorticoid therapy. The dermal atrophy that may occur when steroids are given is not a feature of corticotropin therapy, presumably because of the anabolic effects caused by increased androgen secretion.

Immediately after administration of corticotropin, blood sugar is depressed; later, insulin resistance and a tendency toward hyperglycemia are apparent. When administered to people capable of adrenal cortex response, corticotropin is both diabetogenic and ulcerogenic.

Allergy to animal preparations of corticotropin is not uncommon. Reactions vary from mild fever to anaphylaxis. Though allergy to synthetic preparations is less likely, it does occur. The usual dosage schedules, short terms of intensive therapy separated by long periods of drug withdrawal, favor the development of antibodies.

Precautions and contraindications. When a history of previous exposure to corticotropin or adverse reaction to it exists, precautions should be taken to prevent or treat allergic reactions. Rapid desensitization may be attempted before the therapeutic regimen is begun. Drugs and equipment necessary for treatment of anaphylaxis should be available before administering the tropic hormone.

Antituberculosis drugs are frequently prescribed for the period of therapy for clients with a history of this disease. Any concurrent infection should be aggressively treated with an appropriate anti-infective, because the body's immune and inflammatory response is suppressed during corticotropin therapy.

■ **Summary**
Corticotropin is a protein hormone normally produced by the pituitary gland that stimulates the adrenal cortex to produce glucocorticoids and enhances production of mineralocorticoids and adrenal sex hormones. Because it can be administered only by injection, corticotropin is not used for replacement therapy in hypopituitarism. Instead, the cortisol normally secreted by the target glands is prescribed. Corticotropin is used diagnostically to differentiate

between adrenal and pituitary etiology of hypocorticism. It is also administered in therapeutic doses for short periods of time to induce remissions in certain progressive degenerative diseases. Allergic reactions are the most common adverse reactions to such therapy. Continued administration can produce signs and symptoms of Cushing's syndrome.

Nursing management

Nursing implications

Clients who undergo diagnostic procedures that involve corticotropin administration are usually deficient in steroid hormones. They exhibit various features of hypocorticism characteristic of Addison's disease. These include lack of energy, emotional depression, and a tendency toward shock. Their ability to adapt to stress is significantly diminished. The period required for diagnosis is particularly trying because the nature of the underlying problem is unknown, and, regardless of the specific disease process, the hormone deficiency is likely to be chronic in nature. Therefore, the signs and symptoms of corticosteroid deficiency are likely to be unusually pronounced.

Clients who receive therapeutic doses of corticotropin usually have normal corticosteroid levels, but they commonly suffer from exacerbation of chronic progressive degenerative diseases. The nursing care required by clients during such a period of acute symptomatology varies, depending on the underlying condition, but invariably clients require careful monitoring of the physiologic condition, continuing rehabilitative therapy, and considerable emotional support. These basic needs must be met consistently and concurrently with drug therapy aimed at inducing remission.

Corticotropin therapy may be carried out in the hospital to facilitate IV therapy, or it can be given on an outpatient basis when the IM route is used. Medication is given daily or several times a week until symptoms subside or it is apparent that response will not occur.

Nursing process: care of the client who receives diagnostic doses of corticotropin

Assessment Clients for whom diagnostic procedures using corticotropin are scheduled should be assessed for signs and symptoms of adrenal insufficiency. These include a tendency toward salt and water depletion, hypotension, and hypoglycemia. Sensory perception may be acute, and the client may be especially sensitive to noxious stimuli, such as noise and glaring lights. Emotional outlook may be characterized by depression and dysphoria. Individuals with normal pituitary function but with corticosteroid deficiency may also exhibit a bronzing of the skin that resembles a deep even tan.

The client's emotional reaction toward the illness and diagnostic procedure should be determined. Knowledge about the suspected illness and the hormone therapy used to treat it should also be explored.

Nursing diagnosis Nursing diagnoses likely to be made include the following:

> High risk for fluid volume deficit related to salt and water depletion secondary to corticosteroid deficiency
> High risk for pain related to enhancement of sensory stimuli secondary to glucocorticoid deficiency
> Body image disturbance related to hyperpigmentation secondary to corticosteroid deficiency
> Altered thought processes related to depression secondary to glucocorticoid deficiency
> Anxiety related to the diagnostic procedure and the conditions it is designed to diagnose
> Knowledge deficit concerning corticosteroid deficiency and the diagnostic use of corticotropin

Planning Goals of nursing care include maintenance of blood volume, reduction of noxious stimuli, enhancement of body image, and amelioration of psychological depression. The goal of the teaching plan is to reduce the clients' anxiety by informing them about the suspected hormone abnormality and the procedure planned to diagnose it.

Intervention When preparing corticotropin medication, care should be taken to avoid rough handling. Proteins are degraded by agitation, and the potency of the medication can be impaired by shaking or repeated bubbling of air through the solution. The recommended solvent must be used when reconstituting powders. Vials may be rolled gently to accelerate dissolution. Drug preparations should be protected from excessive heat and freezing temperatures.

Care should be taken to reduce environmental stressors, particularly noxious stimuli such as pain, noise, and bright lights. When the IV infusion is begun, care should be taken to minimize the trauma of injection as much as possible. Use of a heparin lock eliminates the need for repeated insertions of needles and facilitates treatment should the client become hypotensive during the procedure. Vital signs should be monitored frequently, and the client should be assessed carefully for adverse reactions.

When the client is allowed oral intake, ample fluids and foods that contain sodium should be provided. Foods high in sodium (*eg*, ham, bacon, pickles) are helpful when included in the diet. The client should be

cautioned that increased need for sodium is probably temporary, since hormone replacement restores the body's ability to conserve sodium and water.

Vital signs should be monitored at regular intervals and the client assessed for weakness, faintness, or other symptoms of hypovolemic shock.

The nurse should praise and compliment the client whenever appropriate. A warm acceptance by the nurse helps increase the client's self-esteem. The client also requires considerable emotional support until a definitive diagnosis is made and treatment initiated.

Client education. Clients who undergo diagnostic procedures that involve corticotropin need careful explanations of the procedure to minimize the stress imposed by the test.

The nature of the corticotropin test for adrenal function should be carefully explained. Twenty-four-hour urine specimens are collected before and during the period of corticotropin dosage. Clients must understand the need to collect all urine produced during the testing period; loss of a part of the specimen invalidates the test.

Clients should be advised to drink ample fluids and increase sodium intake temporarily. The need for increased sodium is eliminated when the hormone deficiency is treated. Until that time, reduction of stressors and management of stress levels may be critical in the prevention of hypovolemic shock. The nurse should teach stress management techniques. The ability to control stress also enhances the client's response to hormone replacement therapy if this is prescribed.

Clients may be assured that definitive diagnosis of their condition can lead to effective treatment.

Evaluation Data required for evaluation include serial measurements of vital signs, especially pulse, blood pressure, and respirations, client reports about comfort level and emotional affect, and incidence and frequency of positive vs. negative comments by the client relating to self-image. Short-term evaluation of the teaching plan requires observation of the client's ability to accept and adapt to the diagnostic procedure.

Nursing process: care of the client who receives therapeutic doses of corticotropin

Assessment Clients who receive corticotropin therapy usually have normal corticosteroid levels, but they commonly suffer from exacerbation of chronic progressive degenerative diseases. They should be assessed for signs and symptoms of the underlying illness. The data base should include a complete history of the disorder, with a detailed description of the course over recent weeks or months.

Before administration of corticotropin, the nurse must carefully assess the client for infection, peptic ulcer disease, diabetes mellitus, and allergic sensitivity to corticotropin. These conditions are likely to increase in severity when corticotropin is given. The client should be questioned specifically about exposure to or history of tuberculosis.

The client's adequacy of adrenal response to stress as shown by the ability to maintain blood volume and adequate circulation under conditions of stress should also be determined. Any tendency toward hypotension may indicate a reduced adrenal reserve. Hypertension may indicate an already high output of corticosteroids.

The client should be questioned about previous exposure to corticotropin and reaction to such exposure. The susceptibility of the client to allergic reactions may be determined by gathering a personal and family history of allergic conditions.

Nursing diagnosis Nursing diagnoses likely to be made for clients who receive therapeutic doses of corticotropin include diagnoses appropriate for exacerbation of the underlying disorder as well as

Altered tissue perfusion related to hypotension secondary to reduced adrenal reserve and high stress levels

Common collaborative problems that should be differentiated from the nursing diagnosis include

Potential complication: renal impairment
Potential complication: hypovolemic shock

After corticotropin therapy is established, the client may have the following diagnoses:

High risk for infection related to immunosuppression secondary to high levels of corticosteroids
Altered thought processes: euphoria related to CNS stimulation secondary to excess glucocorticoids
Impaired tissue integrity: inflammation related to allergic reaction to corticotropin

Some clients may have a

Knowledge deficit concerning the underlying disease and to corticotropin therapy to induce remission

Common collaborative problems that should be differentiated from the nursing diagnoses include

Potential complication: peptic ulcer
Potential complication: thrombi
Potential complication: hyperglycemia

Planning Nursing goals for the client who receives corticotropin therapy include achievement of a remission of the underlying disease and prevention or prompt detection and treatment of adverse drug reactions, including infection, peptic ulcer, diabetes mellitus, intravascular coagulation, and acute allergic reaction. Client teaching should provide the client with information about corticotropin, signs and symptoms of adverse reaction to corticosteroids, procedures for monitoring urinary or blood glucose levels, and methods for stress management useful to prevent overproduction of corticotropin. A final nursing goal is maintenance of the client's motivation to participate in the treatment and rehabilitation regimen.

Intervention If a history of allergic reaction to corticotropin is elicited, or if a strong personal or family history of allergic illness exists, the client should be skin tested for allergic hypersensitivity to corticotropin. Rapid desensitization may be carried out to reduce the allergic response before therapeutic doses of corticotropin are administered. The health care team must be prepared to treat promptly any allergic reaction that may occur, including anaphylaxis.

Corticotropin therapy may be carried out in the hospital to facilitate IV therapy or it can be given on an outpatient basis when the IM route is used. Medication is given daily or several times a week until symptoms subside or it is apparent that a response will not occur.

When preparing corticotropin medication, care should be taken to avoid rough handling. Proteins are degraded by agitation, and the potency of the medication can be impaired by shaking or repeated bubbling of air through the solution. The recommended solvent must be used when reconstituting powders. Vials may be rolled gently to accelerate dissolution. Drug preparations should be protected from excessive heat and freezing temperatures.

Clients who receive therapeutic doses of corticotropin must be protected from exposure to contagious disease. Ambulation should be encouraged to promote circulation and decrease the risk of clot formation and phlebitis. To minimize the tendency toward diabetes, a diet low in concentrated carbohydrates, moderate in protein, and limited in calories to the level necessary to maintain a lean body weight is required. Clients known to react allergically should be protected against exposure to any substances that trigger the reaction, because allergic reaction to one allergen lowers the threshold for allergic response to another (in this case corticotropin).

Clients who receive repeated doses of corticotropin should be monitored for signs and symptoms of Cushing's syndrome, especially if the course of treatment is prolonged. They must be assessed regularly for pain and suppuration, which may be the only signs of infection owing to the anti-inflammatory action of glucocorticoids. Urine or fingerstick tests for increased glucose levels should be performed regularly. Clients must also be monitored for signs and symptoms of hyperacidity, peptic ulcer disease, and thromboembolic phenomena. These adverse drug reactions should be promptly reported to the physician so that corrective therapy may be instituted.

Anti-infectives may be prescribed to control infection or prevent a recurrence of tuberculosis if a history of this condition exists. Medications to control ulcer disease (histamine$_2$ receptor antagonists or antacids) may be ordered also. If the client develops hyperglycemia, insulin injections may be required.

Client education. Clients who receive corticotropin therapy need explanations of the rationale for using the drug and instructions regarding its side effects. During and after the course of treatment, clients should avoid exposure to infection, to which they are unusually vulnerable. The signs and symptoms of hypercorticism should be explained, and clients should be cautioned to report any evidence of hypertension, increase in symptoms attributable to peptic ulcer or diabetes mellitus, or infection. Because the inflammatory response is suppressed by glucocorticoids, some of the usual warning signs of infection, such as fever, redness, and swelling, may be absent. Pain and loss of function may be the only indications of infection, and these should be promptly reported. Infections tend to progress rapidly when adrenal cortex function is high; prompt treatment is essential.

The client should understand that the feeling of well-being produced by increased blood levels of corticosteroids is drug-induced and may not correspond to the degree of remission induced. This euphoria must not be allowed to interfere with motivation to participate in the treatment and rehabilitation regimen.

Clients should avoid severe stressors. These can limit the degree of response to the course of corticotropin and reduce the chances of a full or lasting remission. If remission is achieved, subsequent exacerbations are more likely to occur when stress levels exceed the adaptive capacity of the client, producing a relative hormone deficiency state. This physiologic state predisposes to exacerbation of the underlying disease. The nurse who works with clients to help develop their skills in the management of stress and coping strategies can make a real contribution to client welfare.

Evaluation Data required for evaluation relate to the amelioration or elimination of signs and symptoms of the underlying disease, absence or incidence and severity of adverse reactions to corticotropin, increased knowledge of corticotropin therapy by the client, and increased ability of the client to manage stress (see Example of Nursing Process and Corticotropin Therapy).

Checklist of nursing actions

☐ Before beginning treatment, assess clients carefully for the presence of infection and history of tuberculosis, peptic ulcer disease, diabetes mellitus, and allergic sensitivity to corticotropin. Take preventive action to minimize complica-

tions that relate to such conditions during hormone therapy.

When corticotropin therapy is prescribed
☐ Protect corticotropin solutions from heat, freezing, and agitation to prevent denaturing of the drug's protein molecule.
☐ Continue treatment of the client's underlying condition during corticotropin therapy.
☐ Monitor clients for evidence of hypercorticism.
☐ Teach clients to report symptoms that indicate infection, peptic ulcer disease, glucose imbalance, or hypercorticism.
☐ Teach clients techniques of stress management to promote long-term remission.

Growth hormone

The hormone produced most abundantly by the anterior pituitary is growth hormone (somatotropin). This protein hormone is necessary for normal growth and development of the immature organism. In adults, it appears to play a role in the adaptive response to stress, especially during the fasting state, and in the maintenance of muscle mass and strength (Fackelmann, 1990).

Somatotropin is produced by specific acidophilic cells in the anterior pituitary known as *somatotrophs*. Secretion is not steady but tends to be intermittent or sporadic. In prepubertal children, somatotropin production is highest during sleep, especially the deep sleep stage, lending credence to the folk saying that children grow most rapidly during sleep. somatotropin production at all ages is stimulated by emotional excitement, exercise, hypoglycemia, and other stressors.

Pathology. Abnormalities of growth hormone production produce several disease conditions. During childhood, excessive production of somatotropin causes excessive growth or gigantism, whereas hormone deficiencies impair growth, producing dwarfism characterized by delayed maturation and inadequate though symmetrical growth. In the adult, somatotropin deficiencies appear to be rare but may underlie weakness in bones, muscles, and the heart. Excesses cause a thickening of bony and soft tissue structures, a condition known as *acromegaly*. At any age, excesses of growth hormone eventually lead to musculoskeletal disorders and diabetes mellitus, while deficiencies predispose to hypoglycemia and reduce the hyperglycemic response to stress.

Pharmacodynamics. The specific mechanisms by which somatotropin stimulates cellular division and differentiation are unknown, but the hormone induces many metabolic changes that are supportive of these processes. Body levels of electrolytes such as sodium, chlorine, potassium, phosphorus, and calcium

Example of nursing process and corticotropin therapy

The client is a 31-year-old housewife and mother of two with a 5-year history of multiple sclerosis. At the time of diagnosis, she was pregnant; termination of the pregnancy produced a remission. She had no symptoms until yesterday, when she experienced difficulty walking due to significant weakness in the left leg. The exacerbation coincided with a record-breaking heat wave.

The client has been admitted to the local hospital for intensive treatment with IV corticotropin in an attempt to produce another remission. The client appears tense and apprehensive. She expresses fear that the treatment "won't work" and states that she "hates needles."

Assessment data	Nursing diagnosis	Intervention	Goals and outcome criteria
Diagnosis of multiple sclerosis Weakness of the left leg Recent heat wave (increased stress can precipitate an attack of multiple sclerosis)	Impaired physical mobility related to demyelinization secondary to multiple sclerosis	**Administer** IV corticotropin as ordered. **Eliminate** stressors that impinge on the client as much as possible. **Suggest** to the physician that the client receive physiotherapy while in the hospital. **Ensure** a comfortably cool environment for the client during her hospital stay.	Before leaving the hospital, the client will be able to walk with a normal gait.
Need for administration of medication by injection Client's statement that she "hates needles"	Fear of pain related to IV therapy venipuncture required for treatment of multiple sclerosis	**Explore** with the client previous experience with venipuncture; ascertain any special problems that relate to this procedure (*eg*, "poor veins") and relay this information to the person responsible for starting the IV infusion. **Request** special precautions to facilitate venipuncture (*eg*, use of topical nitroglycerin to dilate the vein in which the needle is inserted, use of a topical anesthetic to prevent pain from penetration of the skin, use of a heparin lock.) **Inform** the client of measures taken to decrease the discomfort of venipuncture.	The client will state that the intravenous procedure was not as painful as she expected.
Corticotropin therapy, involving stimulation of glucocorticoid secretion (glucocorticoids act as immunosuppressants) IV therapy	High risk for infection related to impaired skin integrity secondary to venipuncture and immunosuppression	**Maintain** strict sterile asepsis in relation to venipuncture, heparin lock, and IV infusion. **Caution** the client not to touch the infusion site or to get it wet.	The client will not develop redness, swelling, or pain at the site of injection or at the intubated vein. She also will not have chills and fever indicative of septicemia.

(Continued)

Example of nursing process and corticotropin therapy (Continued)

Assessment data	Nursing diagnosis	Intervention	Goals and outcome criteria
Client statement that she is afraid the treatment "might not work" Muscular tension and fearful facial expression	Fear of continued or progressive disability	**Acknowledge** that multiple sclerosis sometimes progresses rapidly and can cause severe disability; stress that sometimes it remains arrested for years and causes little disability, and that occasionally the disease will not recur at all after one or two acute episodes. **Inform** the client of measures she can take to reduce the risk of exacerbation (*eg*, management of stressors and prevention of high levels of stress, avoidance of acute infection). **Teach** the client stress management techniques or refer her to a clinic or independent practitioner where instruction in stress reduction is offered.	The client will appear more relaxed. Client comments will indicate that she "feels better" or feels "more in control" in relation to her disease.
Heat wave coinciding with exacerbation of MS (Increased stress can precipitate an attack of MS)	Possible knowledge deficit concerning relation of stress to exacerbation	**Explore** with the client her knowledge concerning the effects of stress on MS. Identify heat as a stressor likely to precipitate an exacerbation. Discuss with the client measures she can take to reduce the stress of high temperature (fans, air conditioning)	The client will not experience exacerbations during future periods of hot weather.

rise. All of these, except calcium, are reabsorbed by the kidneys at higher levels than normal; renal excretion of calcium increases but is offset by a distinct increase in calcium absorption by the gut. The body's lipid energy reserves are mobilized, and levels of circulating free fatty acids rise. Energy production is switched from carbohydrate to fat fuel sources, and blood sugar levels rise. Growth hormone has anabolic effects similar to those of insulin but opposes the hypoglycemic action of insulin by decreasing tissue sensitivity to it. As would be expected when tissue growth is accelerated, the transport of amino acids into tissue cells and their incorporation into protein are increased. The production of urea and other nitrogenous wastes declines, and a positive nitrogen balance is established.

The metabolic effects of somatotropin appear not only to enhance tissue growth in immature organisms but also to protect people of all ages from tissue breakdown during states that require increased use of stored energy because of stress or fasting. Somatotropin appears to reverse some of the effects of aging; it is known to increase muscle mass, increase bone strength, decrease fat deposits, and increase skin thickness in the elderly (Amato, 1990; Cueno, et al, 1989).

Pharmacokinetics. As a protein substance, somatotropin is degraded by proteases in the digestive tract and cannot be administered orally. It has been administered only by injection. Once absorbed, somatotropin moves rapidly into the cells. It affects all tissues by mechanisms that, in most cases, are still obscure. It is known that in the liver, kidneys, and other tissues, it stimulates the production of somatomedins, substances that stimulate the incorporation of sulfate into tissues such as cartilage. Although the serum half-life of somatotropin is only about 20 minutes, the effect of a given dose lasts at least a week.

Therapeutic uses. Somatotropin is indicated for the treatment of pituitary dwarfism. In usual dosages (thrice weekly IM injections of 0.1 mg/kg body weight), it stimulates normal proportional growth in dwarves without inducing sexual maturity, disproportionate growth of skin or bones, or other symptoms of hormone excess. Growth may be tripled the first year of treatment and doubled subsequently (Rodman, 1986). Treatment is aimed at producing a height of at least 5 feet, considered the minimum necessary for normal function in modern society.

Until recently, the only source of the hormone was human pituitaries removed at autopsy. Animal hormones are not effective because this hormone is species specific. Cadaver tissues are no longer used because they have been implicated as carriers of Creutzfeldt-Jakob disease, a fatal degenerative neurologic condition, and as possible transmitters of human immunodeficiency virus, the cause of AIDS. At present, two forms of biosynthetic human growth hormone are available for therapeutic use: somatrem (Protropin) and Humatrope. Both are products of recombinant DNA processes.

Somatotropin may prove of use in the future to maintain muscle and cardiac strength in the aged, to maintain body tissues under conditions of weightlessness (in which muscles and bones atrophy), and possibly as an adjunct in the treatment of obesity.

Adverse reactions. In the dosages used therapeutically to date, somatotropin toxicity has not been reported. High doses are likely to produce symptoms characteristic of gigantism: too rapid growth, development of heavy disproportionate bones, soft tissue hypertrophy, and hyperglycemia. Theoretically, somatotropin could increase the growth rate of malignant tumors; it has been reported to increase the risk of leukemia twofold (Weiss, 1988). It is known to be diabetogenic.

Precautions and contraindications. Clients who receive the drug should be monitored carefully in relation to growth and maturation. If sexual immaturity persists as height approaches adult proportions, replacement therapy with appropriate sex hormones may be needed.

▣ Summary

Somatotropin is the anterior pituitary hormone responsible for normal growth and development. It is approved for use as a drug only as replacement therapy for people deficient in this hormone (pituitary dwarfs).

Growth hormone antagonist

A mutant bovine hormone similar to somatotropin in structure has been reported to antagonize growth hormone (Weiss, 1990). Its action may be that of competitive inhibition for cell receptors that normally respond to somatotropin. This substance may prove useful in the treatment of gigantism (excess of somatotropin during childhood), acromegaly (excess of somatotropin in adults), or diabetic retinopathy (which appears to improve or stabilize when the pituitary is destroyed and endogenous somatotropin eliminated; Amato, Raloff, 1989).

Thyrotropin

Thyrotropin is a glycoprotein produced by basophilic cells in the anterior pituitary. The rate of its production is inversely proportional to circulating thyroid hormone levels, a negative feedback system that normally maintains thyroid hormone production within a narrow normal range.

Pharmacodynamics. Thyrotropin increases cAMP levels in thyroid cells. As a result, all phases of thyroid hormone synthesis and release are stimulated: iodine uptake, iodine organification, hormone synthesis, and endocytosis and proteolysis of colloid. The pituitary hormone increases vascularity in the thyroid and produces glandular hypertrophy and hyperplasia.

Pharmacokinetics. Little information is available concerning the distribution or elimination of thyrotropin. As a protein substance, it must be administered by injection.

Therapeutic uses. Thyrotropin is administered only for the purpose of differentiating between primary thyroid hypofunction and hypothyroidism due to deficiency of pituitary thyrotropin. To carry out this diagnostic test, 10 U of thyrotropin are administered IM followed 18 to 24 hours later by a tracer dose of radioiodine (iodine-131). After another 24-hour interval, radioactive iodine uptake (RAIU) is measured and compared with the client's baseline RAIU. If uptake has increased significantly, thyroid gland response to thyrotropin is demonstrated and a pituitary hypofunction is indicated. This diagnostic test may eventually be replaced by direct measurement of endogenous thyrotropin levels by radioimmunoassay.

Drug preparations. Bovine thyrotropin is available for medicinal use under the trade name Thytropar.

Adverse reactions. Thyrotropin has caused cardiac arrhythmia (tachycardia, auricular fibrillation), GI problems (nausea, vomiting), headache, fever, and menstrual irregularities. Allergic manifestations that have been reported include urticaria and anaphylaxis. In high doses, the drug can cause thyroid enlargement.

Precautions and contraindications. Clients in an advanced state of myxedema can tolerate only minute increments of thyroid hormone, and a thyrotropin diagnostic test could induce cardiac failure. Definitive diagnosis should be delayed until the acute hormone deficiency has responded to carefully graduated doses of thyroid hormone.

■ Summary

Thyrotropin is the protein hormone of the anterior pituitary that stimulates the thyroid gland to produce thyroid hormone. It is used medicinally in a diagnostic test to differentiate between pituitary and thyroid etiology of hypothyroidism.

Nursing management

Nursing implications

Clients who undergo thyrotropin diagnostic tests are deficient in thyroid hormone. They may exhibit various levels of thyroid deficiency and require the usual nursing care for this condition. If frank myxedema or cardiac malfunction is apparent, the diagnostic test may be postponed until the client has received some thyroid hormone therapy and is in better condition to withstand the test.

Hypothyroid clients experience cold intolerance and should be kept warm. They also have impaired adaptive responses and should be protected from stressors. These clients tend to be overweight and physically and mentally sluggish. They need considerable physical and emotional supportive care.

When preparing thyrotropin doses, the vial must be handled gently. Bubbling air through the solution or shaking the vial may cause breakdown of the protein molecule, reducing the preparation's potency. The hormone should be stored in a part of the refrigerator that does not drop below freezing.

Nursing process

Assessment   The signs and symptoms of hypothyroidism include intolerance to cold, physical and mental lethargy, weight gain despite reduced food intake, decreased mobility, a weakened heart, and the development of typical myxedema facies (thin brittle hair, puffiness around the eyes, and enlarged tongue). The client should be evaluated for these manifestations. In addition, the nurse should determine clients' knowledge of and emotional reaction to their condition. (Clients may not be able to communicate well if they have severe hormone deficiency; ability to do so improves as they respond to hormone treatment.)

Nursing diagnosis   Nursing diagnoses related to diagnostic use of thyrotropin include

> *Decreased cardiac output related to thyroid hormone stimulation secondary to TSH administration*

Diagnoses related to thyroid deficiency include the following:

> *Altered comfort: intolerance to cold related to decreased metabolism secondary to hypothyroidism*
> *Activity intolerance related to obesity and weak heart action secondary to thyroid deficiency*
> *Body image disturbance related to obesity and impaired mobility*

Most clients have a

> *Knowledge deficit concerning hypothyroidism and the diagnostic use of thyrotropin*

Planning   Goals for nursing care include prevention or prompt diagnosis and treatment of heart failure, increase in client comfort, promotion of a positive self-image, and teaching the client about hypothyroidism and the provocative test for its diagnosis.

Intervention   To prevent congestive heart failure, the client must be treated as other clients with weak hearts and little cardiac reserve. Physical care should be carried out by the health care staff. Because myxedematous clients are often obese, nursing care is physically demanding. Care should be administered by teams of two or more nurses, and clients should not be allowed to turn themselves or exert themselves in any way until the heart has been strengthened by a gradual return toward thyroid balance.

Warm clothing and a warm environment should be provided for the client. When the metabolic rate is very low, the body does not produce enough heat to maintain optimum temperature. The client should not become cold. Shivering imposes an added work load on the heart and could precipitate congestive failure.

When myxedema is severe, mental processes are sluggish, and clients often do not make comments or use body language to express feelings. As the metabolism begins to rise, the ability to communicate improves. The nurse should encourage ventilation of negative feelings about body image and self-concept. Negative feelings are frequently related to obesity, lack of energy, sluggish mental processes, poor memory, and impaired mobility. The health care staff should accept the client warmly and explain that the physical and mental changes are due to disease and that these situations will be reversed with successful treatment. The staff should praise and compliment the client whenever possible.

Client education.   Client teaching at first should be limited to the facts needed for the client's cooperation in the nursing regimen and to refute the client's negative self-image. Before the diagnostic test, the procedure should be explained to the client with simple instructions for participation. When memory and mental functioning improve, a teaching program appropriate for the definitive diagnosis can be carried out.

Evaluation Data required for evaluation include signs and symptoms indicative of cardiac function (color, pulse, blood pressure, respirations, warmth of extremities), absence or incidence of shivering, absence or incidence of complaints by clients that they feel cold, body temperature, and the number of positive and negative comments about self. At first, teaching is evaluated by the client's participation in the medical and nursing regimen and by the client's responses to the nursing staff's praise and compliments. Later, the client's ability to manage self-care and the prescribed regimen after discharge from the acute care facility implies success of the teaching program.

Checklist of nursing actions

☐ Provide nursing care appropriate to hypothyroidism to clients who are undergoing a thyrotropin diagnostic test.

☐ Before the test, assess the degree of hormone deficiency and cardiac status. Report frank myxedema or evidence of cardiac disease to the physician promptly.

☐ To preserve drug potency, protect thyrotropin solutions from heat, freezing, and agitation.

☐ Provide physical and emotional support to the client who is undergoing diagnostic testing.

Hypothalamic hormones

Within recent decades it has been discovered that a portion of the brain, the hypothalamus, produces hormone substances that control secretions of tropic hormones by the anterior pituitary. The hypothalamus also produces the hormones previously believed to have been synthesized in the posterior pituitary. The hypothalamus is situated in close proximity to the pituitary and is connected to it by a major vascular pathway by which the brain hormones are transported to the gland.

Releasing and inhibiting factors that control anterior pituitary function include thyrotropin-releasing hormone (TRH), corticotropin-releasing factor (CRF), growth hormone-releasing factor (GHRH), growth hormone-release inhibiting factor (GHRIH, or somatostatin), and various factors that control the release of pituitary gonadotropins (Table 34-9). The properties of these substances and their potential value for drug therapy are the subject of intense research activity. They are not available for therapeutic use, although nurses involved in research may encounter them in investigational procedures.

Two hormones long known to enter the blood from the posterior pituitary, antidiuretic hormone (ADH) and oxytocin, are actually synthesized by nerve bodies of the supraventricular or paraventricular nuclei of the hypothalamus. In normal people, these chemicals are transported to the neurohypophysis, where they are stored until they are subsequently released into the bloodstream. People whose pituitaries have been damaged or destroyed by disease or trauma may retain adequate production of these hormones provided the adjacent hypothalamic structures have escaped injury.

Antidiuretic hormone

Physiology. ADH (vasopressin) is a protein hormone produced in the hypothalamus and stored in and released by the posterior pituitary. Its function is to maintain normal osmotic pressure and extracellular fluid volume by regulating water reabsorption in the renal distal tubule. Osmoreceptors and vascular baroreceptors in the higher cerebral centers react to increased osmolarity in the blood and reduced extracellular fluid volume by stimulating ADH production by the hypothalamic neurosecretory cells. Other factors that stimulate ADH secretion include decreased plasma volume, pain, stress, sleep, exercise, positive pressure ventilation, and certain drugs (*eg*, nicotine, morphine, barbiturates, some anesthetics, vincristine).

Table 34-9. Hypothalamic hormones that control the release of pituitary hormones

Releasing hormone or factor	Abbreviations	Structure
Corticotropin-releasing factor	CRF	Peptide (41 residues)
Thyrotropin-releasing hormone	TRH	Tripeptide
Luteinizing-hormone–releasing hormone and follicle-stimulating hormone–releasing hormone (gonadotropin-releasing hormone)	LHRH, FSHRH, GnRH	Decapeptide
Growth hormone release–inhibiting hormone	GHRIH, somatostatin	Peptides (14 and 28 residues)
Growth hormone releasing factor	GHRF; GRF	Peptides (40 and 44 residues)
Prolactin release–inhibiting hormone	PRIH	Probably dopamine
Prolactin-releasing factor	PRF	Unknown
Melanocyte-stimulating hormone release–inhibiting factor	MIF	Tripeptides
Melanocyte-stimulating hormone release factor	MRF	Unknown

(Gilman AG, Goodman LS, Rall TW, Murad F. [1985]. *Goodman and Gilman's The pharmacological basis of therapeutics*, p 1382. New York: Macmillan.)

Released into the bloodstream, ADH promotes reabsorption of water in the medullary portion of the collecting duct of the nephron. This action tends to correct hyperosmolarity and inadequate extracellular fluid volume.

Pathology. Hyposecretion of ADH is the disease and syndrome known as diabetes insipidus. The deficiency may arise spontaneously as an idiopathic disease state or may occur as a result of brain trauma. After head injury or cranial surgery, diabetes insipidus tends to be a temporary malfunction that improves spontaneously as healing proceeds and brain function improves.

Excessive ADH is sometimes secreted by clients with a variety of tumors or head injuries, meningitis or encephalitis, pulmonary infections, and other diseases. Excess ADH may be produced by secreting tumors or by drugs such as vincristine or cyclophosphamide, which stimulate endogenous production. Hypersecretion of ADH causes water retention and pronounced dilutional hyponatremia.

Pharmacodynamics. As with many protein hormones, the effects of ADH appear to be mediated by an increase in cAMP in the target cells. In the kidney, ADH is bound by receptors on the cell surfaces of the collecting duct. As a result, cortical and medullary segments of the collecting duct become more permeable to water, and the water then diffuses passively across the membrane at a more rapid rate. High concentrations of ADH stimulate contraction of the vasculature, producing a vasopressor effect and an increase in blood pressure. The net effect partially depends on the reactivity of baroreceptor reflexes. When the efficiency of a baroreceptor reflex is impaired (*eg*, during anesthesia), small amounts of hormone elicit significant responses. Normally, such effects are not seen because the doses necessary for them are in excess of those required to maintain water balance.

Pharmacokinetics. Drug preparations may be given by injection or topical intranasal spray. The plasma half-life of some preparations is as short as 10 minutes. Some of the hormone is destroyed by blood peptidases and some binds to receptors on smooth muscle, but one-third to one-half of a given dose reaches the receptors of the renal distal tubule, where it stimulates water reabsorption. Most of the hormone is degraded by target tissues with less than 20% eliminated unchanged in urine.

Therapeutic uses. ADH is prescribed for hormone replacement in clients affected by diabetes insipidus. Treatment is short-term for clients who experience transient diabetes insipidus as a result of head injury or surgery but is lifelong for clients with idiopathic hormone deficiencies. The drugs of choice for

chronic deficiency are desmopressin and inpressin, which are administered intranasally two to four times a day in accordance with the degree of polyuria. When these drugs are not effective or cannot be used, vasopressin tannate is prescribed. This preparation is administered every 2 to 3 days. Dosage schedules are flexible and are determined by duration of response to a given dose. When urine production rises above normal, another dose is administered.

Vasopressin is sometimes used to control hemorrhage by vasoconstriction or to elevate blood pressure in people who suffer from vasogenic hypotension. It is also used in a diagnostic procedure to determine the ability of the kidneys to concentrate urine.

Drug preparations. Medicinal preparations of ADH include solutions (in both water and oil) of animal pituitary extracts and synthetic preparations (Table 34-10).

Adverse reactions. ADH is irritating to the tissues and can cause redness, swelling, and burning pain at the injection site. Nasal congestion and inflammation or itching can follow intranasal administration. Systemic effects of the medication include headache, nausea and vomiting, flushing or pallor, abdominal cramps and an urge to defecate, uterine cramps and vulval pain, and cardiovascular changes (angina pectoris, increased blood pressure). Large doses can produce hyponatremia and water intoxication, bradycardia, premature atrial contractions, heart block, myocardial infarction, and peripheral vascular collapse.

Allergic hypersensitivity to the hormone can develop regardless of the route of administration. Allergic reactions range from local inflammation in the nose when intranasal preparations are used to urticaria and anaphylaxis. Drug resistance may also develop.

Vasopressin tannate administration may result in sterile abscesses at the injection site. Large doses can produce peripheral vasoconstriction sufficient to cause gangrene.

Precautions and contraindications. Clients who suffer from cardiovascular disease, especially coronary artery disease, should not receive vasopressin, except in minimal doses if required for the control of diabetes insipidus. Increased angina, decreased cardiac output, and increased peripheral resistance may precipitate serious cardiac complications, including arrhythmia and congestive heart failure. The heart action of clients who receive IV infusions of ADH should be continually monitored.

When ADH is administered to clients who do not have diabetes insipidus, fluid intake should be restricted to prevent water intoxication. Vital signs, urine volume, and urine specific gravity should be monitored.

Table 34-10. Medicinal preparations of antidiuretic hormone

Drug name	Preparation/Concentration	Uses	Usual dosage
desmopressin acetate (DDVAP)	Clear liquid solution of synthetic peptide for intranasal administration; 100 μg/ml	Agent of choice for control of diabetes insipidus	Adults: 10–40 μg daily, divided in 2–4 doses Children: 0.05–0.3 ml daily, divided in 2–4 doses
	Solution for IV and subcutaneous injection; 4 μg/ml	Control of diabetes insipidus	Adults: 10–40 μg daily, divided in 2–4 doses Children: 0.05–0.3 ml daily, divided in 2–4 doses Management of excessive bleeding
2–4 μg daily, in accordance with response (divided in 2 doses) PC: B			
lypressin (Diapid)	Solution for injection; 4 μg/ml Solution for intranasal administration; 185 μg/ml	Control of diabetes insipidus	1–2 sprays (7–14 μg) each nostril 4 times daily PC: B
vasopressin injection (Pitressin, Pressyn)	Aqueous solution of synthetic vasopressin for injection; 20 pressor U/ml	Treatment of diabetes insipidus	Adults: 0.25–0.5 ml q6–12h PRN PC: B
vasopressin tannate (Pitressin Tannate)	Peanut oil suspension of water-insoluble tannate of antidiuretic principle; 5 pressor U/ml	Second choice agent for the control of diabetes insipidus	Adults: 0.3–1 ml every 2–3 days Children: 0.25–0.5 ml every 2–3 days PC: B

KEY: PC = pregnancy risk category. (The validity of pregnancy risk categories has not been established; see Chapter 16, p 216.)

Intranasal preparations should not be inhaled. The effect of a given dose in this form may be reduced by nasal congestion and hypersecretion because absorption is impaired. Until the rhinitis subsides, dosages should be increased as required by frequency of micturition.

ADH should be used with caution in treating diabetes insipidus in children. The drug should be administered intranasally. Special care should be taken to prevent water intoxication, which is likely to cause seizures in children.

ADH is contraindicated for people who are allergic to it and for those affected by type IIB or platelet-type von Willebrand's disease.

Several drugs interact with ADH. Lithium, demeclocycline, heparin, alcohol, and large doses of epinephrine decrease its physiologic effect. Chlorpropamide, urea, fludrocortisone, and clofibrate enhance its action.

■ Summary

ADH is a protein normally produced by the hypothalamus that acts to control osmolarity and volume of extracellular fluid by moderating water reabsorption in the renal distal tubule. Injectable or intranasal preparations are used to control the symptoms of diabetes insipidus and to treat shock caused by vascular hypotonicity or hemorrhage. Side effects of the drug include mild discomforts, such as intestinal hyperactivity or uterine cramps, and more serious complications, such as congestive heart failure and peripheral vascular insufficiency. The drug is rarely given to clients with cardiovascular disease.

Nursing management

Nursing implications

As with all protein preparations, ADH solutions must be protected from heat, freezing, and agitation. However, vasopressin tannate in oil must be warmed by immersion in heated water before it can be drawn up in a syringe. At room temperature, the solution is too viscid to pass through the bore of an IM needle.

Nursing process

Assessment Before administration of vasopressin, the fluid and electrolyte balance and cardiac status of the client should be carefully assessed. Clients with chronic deficiencies of ADH are relatively dehydrated despite intake of large amounts of fluids. Serum levels of sodium are likely to be elevated. Dehydration usually is not found in clients treated for vasogenic shock but may be apparent in clients affected by hemorrhage.

Client knowledge about and emotional reaction to

the diagnosed medical condition and the use of vasopressin in its treatment should be explored.

Nursing diagnosis A nursing diagnosis likely to be made for the client who is receiving vasopressin is

> *Fluid volume deficit related to inadequate reabsorption of water by the kidney secondary to ADH deficiency*

A common collaborative problem that should be differentiated from the nursing diagnosis is

> *Potential complication: vasogenic shock*

When vasopressin is administered for pharmacologic effect, diagnoses include the following:

> *Fluid volume excess: hyponatremic water intoxication related to excessive reabsorption of water by the kidneys secondary to vasopressin medication*
> *Knowledge deficit concerning the diagnosed illness and the use of vasopressin in its treatment*

A common collaborative problem that should be differentiated from the nursing diagnoses is

> *Potential complication: cardiovascular*

Planning Goals of nursing care include maintenance of fluid balance, restoration of tissue perfusion (by arresting hemorrhage, reversing excessive vascular dilation, or restoring fluid volume), and prompt detection and treatment of adverse drug reactions. The goal of the teaching program for clients with hemorrhage or vasogenic shock is to supply the client with specific information needed for cooperation with the treatment regimens. Clients with chronic hormone deficiency need a comprehensive teaching program designed to provide the knowledge and skills required to maintain hormone balance and fluid balance over the long-term through the use of endogenous hormone. Most clients need instruction in injection technique.

Intervention ADH preparations may be administered by SC, IM, or IV injection or nasal spray. Intranasal administration is preferred for the control of diabetes insipidus; for clients who cannot tolerate this form of medication, vasopressin tannate is usually prescribed.

Before using the nasal spray, the condition of the nasal membrane should be assessed. Redness, swelling, and discomfort or itching can develop. One or two sprays are administered, with subsequent doses used as needed (usually qid). If frequency of micturition is not controlled, individual doses should not be increased; rather, the interval of time between doses should be reduced.

To assess response to therapy, fluid balance must be monitored carefully. Inadequate hormone replacement causes excessive production of dilute urine and a return of the symptoms of diabetes insipidus. Excessive dosage causes fluid retention and dilution of electrolytes in body fluids. To prevent fluid and electrolyte imbalances, clients must be watched for low specific gravity of urine, polyuria and polydipsia (which denote ADH deficiency), high specific gravity of urine, and oliguria (which denotes ADH excess). Sudden changes in weight and blood pressure indicate serious fluid imbalance.

When vasopressin is used for purposes other than hormone replacement, clients should be closely watched for signs and symptoms of water intoxication or cardiovascular malfunction. Vital signs and urine osmolality should be monitored regularly. Fluid intake should be carefully controlled. When vasopressin is administered IV, clients should be placed on cardiac monitors, and peripheral circulation should be assessed frequently. Injection sites used for administration of vasopressin should be watched for signs of inflammation.

Client education. Clients who suffer from chronic diabetes insipidus face a lifetime of hormone therapy and may require considerable support to accept the treatment regimen. They must be taught techniques for administration of the prescribed drug. Either intranasal spray or IM injections may be used. Dosage must be adjusted in accordance with the degree of polyuria. Clients should be taught the signs and symptoms of allergic reactions and cautioned to report these promptly.

Evaluation Data required for evaluation of the care of clients treated for diabetes insipidus include information pertinent to fluid balance (tissue turgor, urinary frequency, urine volume and osmolality, thirst, and serum osmolality) and the absence or incidence of drug toxic or side effects. Evaluation of clients who receive vasopressin for pharmacologic effect requires data that relate to circulation (vital signs, color, warmth of extremities), intestinal motility, blood loss from hemorrhage, and absence or incidence of adverse drug reactions.

Checklist of nursing actions

*When vasopressin is used
for hormone replacement*

☐ To preserve potency of drug preparations, protect solutions from excessive heat, freezing, and agitation.

☐ Assess clients for local and systemic allergic reactions.

☐ Teach clients with chronic diabetes insipidus to administer their own drugs and adjust dosage regimens in accordance with volume of urinary output.

☐ Support client acceptance of lifelong drug therapy.

*When vasopressin is used for purposes
other than hormone replacement*

☐ Monitor clients closely for water intoxication and cardiovascular complications (angina, myocardial infarction, cardiovascular collapse, impaired peripheral circulation).

☐ Monitor injection sites for inflammatory changes.

Oxytocin

Oxytocin, another hormone produced by the hypothalamus, is involved in the stimulation of labor and postpartum lactation. It is used pharmacologically to induce labor. Because deficiency of this hormone is not recognized as a clinical problem, it is not used for replacement therapy. Oxytocin is discussed in detail in Chapters 16 and 38.

References

Amato I. (1990). Growth-hormone levels plummet in space. *Science News, 138*, 134.

Amato I, Raloff J. (1989). Chemistry: Pediatric peptide spurs growth hormone. *Science News, 136*, 252.

Biomedicine: One hamburger, hold the hormones. (1986). *Science News, 129*, 26.

Cooper D. (1988). Thyroid hormone and the skeleton: A bone of contention (editorial). *JAMA, 259*, 3175.

Cueno RC, et al. (1989). Cardiac failure responding to growth hormone. *Lancet, 1*, 836.

Demke DM. (1989). Drug interaction between thyroxine and lovastatin. *N Engl J Med, 321*(19), 1341.

Fackelmann KA. (1990). Hormone may restore muscle in elderly. *Science News, 138*, 23.

Fackelmann KA. (1989). Pygmy paradox prompts a short answer. *Science News, 136*, 22.

Fatourechi V, Heath H. (1987). Salmon calcitonin in the treatment of postmenopausal osteoporosis. *Ann Intern Med, 107*, 923–925.

Low-level radiation project: Radiation on the job, p 11. (1980). San Francisco: Coalition for the Medical Rights of Women.

McEvoy GK, ed. (1991). *Drug information 91*, p 1909. Bethesda, MD: American Society of Hospital Pharmacists.

Orreago H, et al. (1987). Long-term treatment of alcoholic liver disease with propylthiouracil. *N Engl J Med, 317*(23), 1421.

Paul T, et al. (1988). Long-term L-thyroxine therapy is associated with decreased hip bone density in premenopausal women. *JAMA, 259*, 3137–3141.

Raloff J. (1986a). Geologically induced goiters. *Science News, 129*, 18.

Raloff J. (1986b). Goiter? Do you eat millet? *Science News, 129*, 18.

Rodman MJ. (1986). What's new in drugs: A synthetic hormone helps growth disorders. *RN, 49*(2), 83.

Weiss R. (1988). Human growth hormone treatment-leukemia link reported. *Science News, 133*, 308.

Bibliography

Erickson D. (1990). Science and business: Big-time orphan: Human growth hormone could be a blockbuster. *Scientific American, 263*(3), 164–166.

Geologically induced goiters. (1986). *Science News, 129*, 18.

Hussar DA. (1990). New drugs: Nafarelin acetate. *Nursing 90, 20*(12), 49.

Kortbawi P. (1990). Nursing consult: Myxedema coma: Causes and symptoms. *Nursing 90, 20*(8), 90.

Langreth RN. (1990). Milk from engineered hormone: Udderly safe. *Science News, 138*, 372.

Mercer ME. (1990). Myths and facts: About diabetes insipidus. *Nursing 90, 20*(5), 20.

Underwood LE, ed. (1987). *Human growth hormone: Progress and challenge*. New York: Marcel Dekker, Inc.

Weiss PL. (1990). Growth-gene mickey makes mice mini. *Science News, 138*, 20.

Drugs affecting the immune system

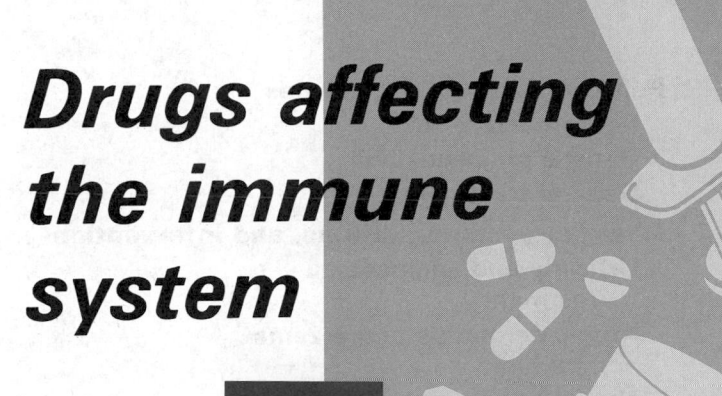

9

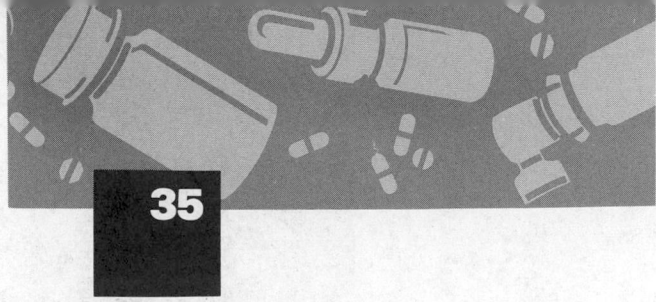

35

Drugs used in the treatment of allergy

Pathophysiology of allergies
Background review

In 1905, Bella Schick and Von Pirquet observed that some people who received injections of horse serum against infectious diseases developed what was called *serum sickness*. The reaction occurred 8 to 12 days after the injection and was manifested by neutropenia, enlarged lymph nodes, fever, urticaria, arthralgia, and edema. These symptoms disappeared after a few days, leaving the person fully recovered. The two researchers named this reaction *allergy*. Today, the term *immune-complex disease* has replaced serum sickness. The reaction may be due not only to the serum but also to the presence of a sufficient number of antibodies that unite with antigens in the person's circulation and interstitial fluids.

Circulating immune complexes are associated with more than 100 human disorders. More than 40 assays are being developed for their detection, but many are not yet considered accurate enough for absolute identification in every instance.

Immune complexes (antibodies plus antigens) are usually taken up by the reticuloendothelial system and rendered harmless. However, some complexes too large to be inactivated by the reticuloendothelial system may be deposited in the joints, glomeruli, arteries, or heart valves, causing an inflammatory reaction. This can lead to autoimmune diseases (rheumatoid arthritis, systemic lupus erythematosus) and hemolytic anemia, including Rh incompatibility, as well as some kidney and infectious diseases. Current investigation of these disorders is directed toward discovering a cure based on manipulation of the immune system rather than on treatment of symptoms.

Minimal immune complexes form if the antigen concentration is low or of limited duration. Exogenous antigens (those that come from outside the body) result in acute transient disease, as in single immunizations. Chronic human immune-complex disease is associated with on-going viral or bacterial infections, or with autogenous antigen (from within the body) that causes autoantibodies to form. A close relationship between immunology and allergy exists (see Chapter 36).

Immunoglobulins offer protection against foreign substances in the body. Some individuals react to allergens present in their bodies with increased levels of a particular immunoglobulin known as *IgE*. Some immunodeficiency diseases result from an excessive production of IgE and may be difficult to differentiate from allergic or other disorders. For example, the Wiskott-Aldrich syndrome in children causes a dermatitis similar to atopic eczema and can result in a positive response to skin tests with food or inhalant allergens. Another disorder, hyper-IgE syndrome, causes skin infections and furunculosis that can resemble atopic dermatitis.

Usual allergic reactions result from the introduction of a foreign substance (antigen or allergen) to which the body subsequently reacts. This process is commonly referred to as a *type 1 sensitivity* and may manifest itself as a localized reaction (hives, rhinitis, dermatitis, asthma, respiratory distress, or gastrointestinal [GI] symptoms) or as a severe bodily reaction that may be life-threatening, leading to cardiovascular or respiratory collapse (anaphylaxis; Box 35-1 lists steps in an allergenic reaction).

Mast cells that have been actively or passively sensitized release several substances, including amines, proteins, peptides, enzymes, polysaccharides, and histamine on contact with an antigen. The activated mast cells also generate potent vasoactive, bronchospastic, and chemotactic substances (Wasserman, 1986).

Basophils and platelets, which also contain histamine, probably act in a similar manner as they circulate in the peripheral blood. *Histamine* causes an increase in vascular permeability, as well as contractions of the bronchioli and other smooth muscle. *Antihistamines* block these actions, reducing the chance of an allergic reaction (see Box 35-1).

Genetic predisposition

Genetic predisposition plays a role in allergic reactions. When one parent is allergic, the child has a 25% to 40% chance of developing an allergy. If both parents have allergies, the child has a 40% to 65% chance of developing allergies. If no history of family allergies exists, the child has about a 16% chance of developing an allergic reaction at some point. The allergy may show up as a rash (including eczema), diarrhea, vomiting, coughing, wheezing, tearing, itching or swelling of the eyes, itchiness of the ears, or a runny nose (clear, nonirritating fluid), sneezing, and nasal stuffiness. Anaphylaxis is also possible in children and should be considered

---

Box 35-1. The sequence of an allergic reaction

1. Linking of an antigen with a specific antibody, which excites the cell membrane receptor.
2. Adsorption of antibody to the specific receptor, which is thought to exist on most cells.
3. Release of histamine, serotonin, slow-reacting substance, and kinin-forming enzymes. These require esterase, calcium, and energy, moderated by cyclic nucleotides.

---

before administering vaccines or allergenic medications to children with a familial history of allergies.

General treatment

Allergic reactions may be prevented if contact with allergens is eliminated or minimized. Drugs used for treatment include corticosteroids (to suppress the allergic response and inflammation), antihistamines (to ameliorate the signs and symptoms), and other palliative drugs, depending on the tissues and organs affected. In selected cases, *hyposensitization* or *desensitization* can increase tolerance to exposure to the offending allergen.

Allergens, manifestations, and intervention

Urticaria and angioedema

Urticaria (hives) appears as an erythematous, sometimes pruritic, skin elevation that blanches with pressure, whereas angioedema results in a swollen area with the skin appearing normal.

Urticaria and angioedema occur in about 15% to 20% of the population. Both conditions may appear in acute (self-limiting) or chronic (lasting longer than 6 weeks) forms. If an allergen has been inhaled, it can be expected to cause respiratory symptoms, whereas allergens that are ingested usually lead to urticaria, angioedema, or GI symptoms. Skin contact can cause urticaria, although internal symptoms, such as rhinitis or asthma, may be manifested.

Drug reactions are commonly responsible for allergic responses, which can occur at the time of administration or become apparent up to 2 weeks later (Cullen, Araujo, 1987). Some reactions can last for weeks and produce symptoms that resemble those of immune-complex disease: neutropenia, eosinophilia, enlarged lymph nodes, fever, urticaria, arthralgia, and edema. Clients who have a history of urticaria associated with multiple medications should consider that the reaction may be caused by a common ingredient or activity in all the drugs and that all other similar substances should be avoided. Over-the-counter drugs used by the client should be included in the history, since they may contain, or act synergistically with, substances related to the allergic reaction (Cullen, Araujo, 1987).

Foods, additives, or some natural substances, such as salicylates, may also result in allergic reactions. Other causative factors include cold (including the holding or eating of cold substances), heat, pressure, the sun, water, or heredity. Most food allergies in children result from cow's milk, soybeans, wheat, peanuts and other nuts, and hen's eggs. Cutaneous reactions to drugs are presented in Table 35-1.

Table 35-1. Cutaneous reactions to drugs

Disorder	Usual precipitating drug	Appearance
Urticaria	Acute form: penicillin, sulfa, diuretics, sedatives, laxatives Chronic form: aspirin	Transient wheals, reddened papules
Angioedema	As above	
Maculopapular (exanthematous eruptions)	Varies with medication	Possible vesicles; toxic epidermal necrolysis (life-threatening)
Erythema multiforme	Sulfonamides, phenytoin barbiturates	Macules, papules, vesicles, bullae, target lesions on palms; 6–8 weeks to resolve
Toxic epidermal necrolysis	Allopurinol, sulfonamides, penicillin, phenylbutazone, anticonvulsants, barbiturates	Facial puffiness, bullae with yellow fluid; malaise, anorexia; 4 weeks to heal; 50% morbidity regardless of treatment
Fixed drug eruption	Tetracycline, phenolphthalein	Occurs at same site(s) as previous reactions (lips, genitalia, sacral area, palmar or plantar areas), pruritus, burning
Photosensitivity reactions	Thiazides, phenothiazines, psoralens, chlorpromazine	Urticaria; burning or tingling
Acneiform eruptions	Halogens, corticosteroids, iodine, testosterone, anticonvulsants, bromides	Comedones, papules, pustules, cysts
Pigmentary changes	Oral contraceptives, arsenic, phenothiazides	Hyperpigmentation or hypopigmentation
Allergic purpura	Sulfa drugs, penicillin, barbiturates, anticonvulsants	Palpable purpuric papules
Temporary burning sensations	Alcohol, as found in Rhus Tox antigen injection, used in the treatment and prophylaxis of dermatitis caused by poison ivy, oak, and sumac	No change

Treatment

Treatment of urticaria and angioedema is usually managed by removing the offending substance, whether it is a material with which the client has contact (*eg*, feathers, wool, dust), a food, or a drug substance. Antihistamines or corticosteroids may help treat some allergies. Injections for hyposensitization to pollen may be beneficial for some clients.

To relieve severe urticaria, with or without angioedema, epinephrine (0.1–0.5 ml of 1 : 1000 solution) can be injected. Antihistamines such as chlorpheniramine 2 to 4 mg three times a day, diphenhydramine 25 to 50 mg three or four times a day, or hydroxyzine 25 mg four times a day are used to follow-up. The condition is usually cleared within 24 to 48 hours. Chronic urticaria usually responds to antihistamines, given in the dosage already described. Topical corticosteroids are ineffective for urticaria. If symptoms are severe, systemic steroids may be beneficial but should not be used unless absolutely necessary. Treatment may require prednisone at 5 to 60 mg a day for a short time, then reduced to every other day at the same dose. The dose should then be tapered down to the lowest possible amount to prevent symptoms. Periodically, attempts to discontinue the drug should be made, because spontaneous remissions, which eliminate the need for medication, do occur. Cimetidine 300 mg intramuscularly (IM) lessens itching and reduces wheal intensity but does not result in as much sedation as an equivalent amount of diphenhydramine.

Atopic dermatitis and eczema

Eczema manifests itself by erythema and vesiculation of the skin in the acute stages and by scaling and thickened skin in the chronic stages. *Atopic eczema*, also called *atopic dermatitis*, is a pruritic form of eczema, frequently associated with asthma and allergic rhinitis. About 40% to 65% of clients with this disease have family histories of allergies. Most of them react to many common food and inhalant allergens by producing IgE antibodies.

Atopic eczema is found in children primarily on the cheeks or the antecubital or popliteal fossae, and in adults as a response to harsh chemicals or scratching. In adults, it is called *neurodermatitis*.

Infantile atopic dermatitis can start at 4 to 6 months and disappear between 3 and 5 years. It sometimes continues as childhood atopic dermatitis, beginning at 2 to 4 years, disappearing at age 10, or continuing into adulthood, with lesions on the forehead, wrists, feet, and sides of the neck, with lichenification of flexural surfaces.

Extreme pruritus is present in all phases of eczema, possibly becoming worse on contact with rough fabrics or when the person is under stress.

Treatment does not seem to shorten the duration of atopic eczema, but seasonal variations can exist.

About 60% of children are free of symptoms by 6 years, with 40% then developing bronchial asthma and 50% allergic rhinitis. Adults with the milder form of the disease are usually symptom free by 20 to 30 years of age, but some may continue to experience symptoms at age 45 years or older. About 30% of clients with the severe form have a remission in a 20-year period. Increased IgE levels are found in about 80% of clients, with a questionable tie between serum level and severity.

Treatment

Treatment of eczema focuses on topical therapy, including such measures as wet dressings of Burrow's solution or tap water, topical steroid creams or lotions, and coal tar products. In the chronic form, steroid ointments and emollients counteract dermatitis and loss of skin moisture.

Noneczematous dermatitis

Noneczematous dermatitis can be caused by allergic or nonallergic contact with a variety of substances. It may occur in clients with atopic eczema and is diagnosed by clinical judgment rather than tests, although patch tests may be used when allergies are suspected. Poison ivy, sumac, or oak are common examples of environmental allergens. Other causative substances include topical medications, dyes, formaldehyde, rubber, epoxy glues, cosmetics, perfumes, and antimicrobial agents.

Treatment

Treatment focuses on preventing future contact with the offending substance (allergen) and on treating the area.

If systemic corticosteroids are administered for any reason, they should be used for the shortest time possible. Topical corticosteroids (in the form of creams or lotions) are useful when the dermatitis is mild. In chronic cases, petrolatum-base ointments counteract the dryness and fissures. Topical antihistamines are generally ineffective and should not be used. Hyposensitization seems to be of limited value.

Pharmacodynamics. Corticosteroids suppress inflammatory response and the production of antibodies.

Pharmacokinetics. Corticosteroids are absorbed through normal intact skin. Absorption increases in the presence of inflammation, disease, or occlusive dressings.

Corticosteroids are bound to plasma proteins, metabolized in the liver, and excreted by the kidneys and sometimes in bile.

Adverse reactions. Clients who undergo unusual stress may require a temporary increase of fast-acting corticosteroids to be administered before, during, and after the situation.

Corticosteroids may produce a reversible hypothalamic-pituitary-adrenal (HPA) axis suppression, Cushing's syndrome, hyperglycemia, and glycosuria. Clients who take corticosteroids should be tested periodically for HPA axis suppression with urinary-free cortisol test and corticotropin stimulation tests. If positive, the drug should be carefully withdrawn.

Precautions and contraindications. When corticosteroids are applied topically to the perineal area, plastic or tight fitting diapers or pants should not be used (see Chapter 32 for a detailed discussion of corticosteroids).

Drug reactions

Five percent of clients are hospitalized because of adverse drug reactions, whereas 10% of hospitalized clients experience at least one adverse drug reaction. Not all reactions are allergic in nature. Some may be due to a deliberate (suicide attempt) or inadvertent overdose or to personal idiosyncrasy not related to immunologic factors (such as hemolytic anemia caused by primaquine; Box 35-2.) Others are side effects of drugs (such as drowsiness caused by antihistamines and hair loss from some antineoplastic drugs).

Clinical manifestations

Allergic reactions to drugs may or may not result in specific antibodies or sensitized lymphocytes. For this reason, the recognition of clinical manifestations is of

---

Box 35-2. Drug reactions

I. Overdose
  A. Deliberate overdose (suicide attempt or belief that "more" increases effectiveness)
  B. Inadvertent overdose
    1. Lack of compliance (poor client education)
    2. Potentiation of drug (synergism with another drug; client's age or condition)
II. Idiosyncrasy (unexpected personal reaction)
  A. Anaphylactic shock from penicillin
  B. Anaphylactic shock from radiopaque substance
III. Adverse reactions (known possible reactions)
  A. Drowsiness from antihistamines
  B. Dry mouth and throat from antihistamines
IV. Secondary effects (known possible reactions)
  A. Hair loss from antineoplastic drugs
  B. Inaccurate allergy skin tests unless drug is discontinued 4 days before testing.

the utmost importance. Some adverse reactions to drugs are presented in Table 35-2.

Anaphylactic shock

The most serious manifestation of drug reaction is anaphylactic shock, with acute cardiovascular collapse and hypotension that usually occur within 5 to 30 minutes. At the most extreme level, death from anaphylaxis may ensue within minutes. In its less severe form, anaphylaxis may cause malaise, vertigo, nausea, vomiting, hives, itching, or diffuse erythema. Bronchospasm, laryngeal edema, and hyperperistalsis may also occur. Cardiac arrhythmia is another possible reaction, which can lead to myocardial infarction and sudden cardiac arrest.

The medication that causes anaphylactic reaction most frequently is penicillin. Other drugs implicated in anaphylactic shock include local anesthetics, streptomycin, tetracycline, cephalosporins, dextrans, heroin, and radiopaque organic iodides. No drug should be considered totally safe from this potential.

Hematologic problems

Some drug reactions result in hematologic manifestations. Thrombocytopenia (with hemorrhage and petechiae and possibly accompanied by fever and arthralgia) is a common reaction to quinidine and quinine, chloramphenicol, sulfonamides, and their derivatives—thiouracil, meprobamate, and phenylbutazone. When the offending drug is withdrawn, bleeding usually ceases within a week.

Agranulocytosis has resulted from aminopyrine, thiouracil, anticonvulsants, phenothiazine, tolbutamide, sulfonamides, and chloramphenicol. Once the causative drug is discontinued, improvement usually occurs within 1 to 2 weeks. However, reexposure to the offending drug generally leads to another episode of agranulocytosis.

Severe anemia can also be caused by an immunologic reaction; chloramphenicol may lead to aplastic anemia, whereas acetophenetidin, para-aminosalicylic acid (PAS), quinine, Mesantoin, and penicillin can cause hemolytic anemia.

Vascular reactions to drugs may be localized or generalized, involving many organs (kidneys, skin, joints, coronary arteries, GI tract). Penicillin, sulfonamides, tetracycline, pyrazoline derivatives, thiazide, quinidine, allopurinol, and thiouracil are the drugs most commonly associated with severe vasculitis. Hydralazine therapy may lead to a syndrome resembling rheumatoid arthritis or systemic lupus erythematosus.

Liver damage

Liver damage from drugs may lead to intrahepatic biliary obstruction or hepatocellular damage and necrosis. The former is associated with chlorpromazine, thiouracil, propylthiouracil, and methyltestosterone. The latter usually results from the use of sulfonamides, erythromycin estolate, PAS, halothane, phenylbutazone, nitrofurantoin, and indomethacin. Accompanying the hepatocellular damage are other symptoms, such as fever, lymphadenopathy, skin rash, blood eosinophilia, and infiltration of the liver with eosinophils, lymphocytes, or plasmacytes.

Fever

Fever is also associated with drug allergies. The usual offending drugs are sulfonamides, streptomycin, pen-

Table 35-2. Adverse reactions to drugs

Condition	Usual causative agents
Anaphylactic shock	Penicillin, local anesthetics, streptomycin, tetracycline, cephalosporins, dextrans, heroin, radiopaque organic iodides
Thrombocytopenia	Quinidine, quinine, chloramphenicol, sulfonamides, thiouracil, meprobamate, phenylbutazone
Agranulocytosis	Aminopyrine, thiouracil, anticonvulsants, phenothiazines, tolbutamide, sulfonamides, chloramphenicol
Aplastic anemia	Chloramphenicol
Hemolytic anemia	Acetophenetidin, PAS, quinine, mesantoin, penicillin
Severe vasculitis	Penicillin, sulfonamides, tetracyclines, pyrazolone derivatives, thiazides, quinidine, allopurinol, thiouracil
Syndrome that resembles rheumatoid arthritis or SLE	Hydralazine
Intrahepatic biliary obstruction	Chlorpromazine, thiouracil, propylthiouracil, methyltestosterone
Hepatocellular damage and necrosis	Sulfonamides, erythromycin estolate, PAS, halothane, phenylbutazone, nitrofurantoins, indomethacin
Elevated fever levels	Sulfonamides, streptomycin, penicillin, quindine, iodine, thiouracil, antithyroid drugs, anticonvulsants, procainamide, PAS, mercurial diuretics
Rebound effect (nasal mucosa)	Phenylephrine HC$_1$, oxymetazoline HC$_1$, chlorpheniramine maleate, pseudoephedrine
Excitability (especially in children)	β_2-agonists, methylxanthines

icillin, quinidine, iodine, thiouracil, antithyroid drugs, as well as anticonvulsants, procainamide, PAS, and mercurial diuretics.

Drugs involved in allergic responses

The drugs most likely to cause an allergic response are penicillin (urticaria, anaphylactic shock), tetracycline (phototoxic skin reaction), chloramphenicol (delayed skin allergy, urticaria, anaphylaxis, aplastic anemia), streptomycin (delayed type anaphylactic shock), sulfonamides (fever, skin reaction), aspirin (urticaria, asthma), and derivatives of aminopyrine, phenacetin, and pyrazoline (skin, systemic, blood dyscrasias). These drugs are listed in Table 35-3.

Sulfiting agents

Sulfiting agents, used as preservatives for such foods as fruit juices, wines, beers, soft drinks, potato chips, dried vegetables and fruits, and many commercially prepared or restaurant foods, can cause severe reactions, including airway constriction. At highest risk are asthmatics.

As of June 1987, the federal Food and Drug Administration (FDA) required that the physician package insert for prescription drugs that contain sulfites include a warning about possible allergic reactions. However, injectable sulfite-containing epinephrine has an alternate warning: epinephrine should still be used in the treatment of serious allergic or other emergency situations even for sulfite-sensitive individuals, since the benefits outweigh the disadvantages (Warning for prescription drugs containing sulfites, 1987).

Insect bites

The bites of yellow jackets, bees, wasps, and hornets are also potential causes of allergic reaction, responsible for 50 to 100 reported deaths a year. Most of the victims are younger than 20 years of age, and males are twice as likely to be affected, possibly because more are likely to be exposed while involved in outdoor work or recreation. Reactions are more frequent when the stings occur around the head and neck, but reactions can occur from bites in other areas as well. The reactions can range in severity from acute anaphylactic shock (usually within 15 minutes) to a transient swelling, pain, and redness. The peak of the reaction can be expected to appear within 48 to 72 hours and may last for a week. Neurologic or vascular reactions or immune-complex disease may also be seen. Severe edema of the pharynx, epiglottis, and trachea is the major cause of death in sensitive people.

Treatment

The best treatment for people allergic to insect stings is prevention, with precautions to avoid stings. When stings do occur, prompt medication is required.

A systemic injection of epinephrine 0.1 to 0.5 ml of 1 : 1000 solution should be given immediately. It can be given IM or, in potentially fatal situations, diluted to 1 ml of 1 : 10,000 solution and administered intravenously (IV). If the results are not satisfactory, the injections should be repeated every 10 to 15 minutes. In addition, 50 mg of diphenhydramine (an antihistamine) should be administered IV. Laryngeal obstruction may require tracheostomy and oxygen. Bronchospasm requires IV use of 200 to 500 mg aminophylline in a drip. IV saline may be needed to increase hydration, and cardiopulmonary resuscitation may be needed if cardiac arrest occurs. Other drugs that are helpful include antihistamines, oxygen, vasopressors, and, if the reaction is of long duration, steroids.

Learning experience 35-1

You are planning a picnic with a friend who is allergic to bee stings. What precautions would you urge your friend to take before setting out for the day?

Hyposensitization should be considered for adults who have had a systemic allergic reaction to a sting or for children who have had a severe systemic reaction not limited to the skin. In a study completed in 1990, it was found that most children did not require the injections, since second insect bites did not cause a more severe reaction (Injections for stings, 1990).

Nasal hypersensitivity

Environmental contaminants in inspired air may contain antigens that cause reactions in sensitive people. The function of the nasal mucosa is to remove large particles, such as pollens, dust, chemicals, and noxious gases from the inspired air, then to humidify and warm the air as it travels to the lower respiratory tract. The mucosa has a complex nervous system (a factor in its ability to sense odors) and a rich blood supply. Just

Table 35-3. Drugs most likely to cause an allergic response

Drugs	Allergic responses
Penicillins	Urticaria, anaphylactic shock
Tetracycline	Phototoxic skin reaction
Chloramphenicol	Delayed skin allergy, urticaria, anaphylaxis, aplastic anemia
Streptomycin	Delayed-type anaphylactic shock
Sulfonamides	Fever, skin reaction
Aspirin	Urticaria, asthma, rhinitis, nasal polyposis
Aminopyrine, phenacetin, and pyrazolone derivatives	Skin reaction, systemic reaction, blood dyscrasia

as inhalants expose the nose to external allergens, the rich vascular bed in the nose exposes it to ingested allergens, hormones, and other products carried to it by the circulatory system. Abnormal or excessive stimuli to the parasympathetic and sympathetic pathways of the nasal neurogenic system can cause allergic reactions.

Allergic rhinitis

Allergic rhinitis (also known as hay fever) occurs in about 5% to 10% of the population on a seasonal basis, coinciding with the presence of specific pollens or mold spores. This exposure may result in sneezing, congestion, or nasal itching and may be accompanied by tearing and itching of the eyes, as well as itching of the throat and ears. Probably 15% to 30% of the population has a chronic form of (perennial) allergic rhinitis that is associated with dust, feathers, animal dander, or other antigens. It has been shown that genetic factors play a part in transmitting a predisposition to these allergic reactions. The latest research shows that peptide leukotrienes are produced as a reaction of the body's immune defense system to the allergenic substance, resulting in the runny nose and eyes, sneezing, swelling, and itchiness. Antihistamines have been used to lessen the symptoms but have not been too effective, because they are incapable of blocking the effects of leukotrienes. Continuing development of drugs for this purpose should result in effective treatment over the next few years. One such experimental drug, zileuton, is being tested for its ability to control hay fever symptoms in those allergic to grasses and ragweed and for asthma induced by breathing cold air. The drug interferes with 5-lipoxygenase, an enzyme necessary for the production of leukotrienes. Zileuton does not appear to cause side effects. Another experimental drug, venzair, is used to prevent exercise-induced asthma. It, too, appears to be safe (Test drugs, 1990).

Treatment

Therapy is used to relieve symptoms rather than to prevent the linkage of the antigen with the antigen-specific antibody found on the mast cells. Having the client avoid the offending substance is the preferred method of management. If that is impossible, medications may be necessary. Antihistamines are frequently used and are available in three major types of compounds: ethanolamine (diphenhydramine), ethylenediamine (tripelennamine), and alkylamines (chlorpheniramine).

Using antihistamines to counteract allergies started in 1942, with the development of phenbenzamine, followed soon by pyrilamine, diphenhydramine, and tripelennamine. Symptomatic relief usually begins within 15 to 30 minutes after oral administration, lasting 3 to 6 hours.

Rebound phenomenon

The excessive use of topical decongestants may lead to a "rebound phenomenon" in about 3% of the population. This results in a temporary decongestion followed by increased congestion that is more severe than the original problem.

Atropine, decongestants, and corticosteroids have also been used to relieve symptoms. After they have been used for a period, they appear to be less effective. Cromolyn sodium is used as a nasal solution, one spray in each nostril every 3 to 4 waking hours, because it is not absorbed well when administered orally. When symptoms are less severe, administration can be decreased to every 5 to 6 waking hours.

Immunotherapy

Clients who are allergic primarily to inhalants may be treated with allergen immunotherapy, also referred to as *desensitization* or *hyposensitization*. Because the treatment is based on clinical empirical evidence, it varies from practitioner to practitioner. Most allergen immunotherapy includes ragweed, grass, and tree pollen allergens, as well as antigens from mold spores and house dust. Treatment is started by administering small doses of antigen subcutaneously in weekly injections that contain gradually increasing amounts of the antigen until a maintenance dose is reached, usually about 2500 protein nitrogen units (0.15 mg protein). The dosage schedule is then reduced to one injection every 2 weeks, later to one injection every 3 weeks, and finally to one every 4 weeks, which is usually continued for 3 to 4 years. Immunotherapy may be limited to weekly or biweekly injections during or before the season in which the allergenic agent, such as pollen, is present.

The principal problems with injections for immunotherapy are the cost of the multiple visits to the physician, the inconvenience, including the possible loss of income while keeping medical appointments, and the physical dangers, which include local reaction, malaise after injection, nasal symptoms, bronchospasm, or anaphylactic shock that leads to death.

Antihistamines

Pharmacodynamics. Antihistamines compete with histamine for cell receptor sites on effector cells. They alleviate the discomforts of seasonal allergic and vasomotor rhinitis, allergic conjunctivitis, urticaria, rashes, and other allergic symptoms.

Other actions of antihistamines are effectiveness against motion sickness and vestibular system disorders, as well as anticholinergic actions that decrease rigidity and extrapyramidal reactions.

Pharmacokinetics. Antihistamines can be administered orally as tablets, capsules, or elixirs. They are also available as topical ointments, nasal sprays, and injectables. After absorption, they attach to cell receptor sites on effector cells. They are degraded in the liver and are almost completely excreted through the kidneys within 24 hours. Antihistamines have not been proved safe in pregnancy or during lactation.

Therapeutic uses. Antihistamines may be prescribed or purchased as over-the-counter preparations to ease allergic reactions to food, inhalants, or contact allergens. They may be used to treat the rigidity of parkinsonism or the extrapyramidal symptoms caused by some psychotropic medications. Some effectively treat motion sickness and vestibular disorders. Antihistamines may be combined with decongestants to dry secretions in the respiratory tract.

Adverse reactions. Antihistamines can cause skin reactions (urticaria, photosensitivity), GI disturbances (nausea, diarrhea, constipation, epigastric distress), urinary and reproductive system disturbances (urinary frequency or retention, early menses), respiratory reactions (thickening of bronchial secretions, wheezing, nasal stuffiness), cardiovascular problems (hypotension, headaches, palpitations, extrasystole), or hematologic disorders (hemolytic anemia, thrombocytopenia, agranulocytosis). They frequently cause sleepiness and decrease alertness. Other central nervous system (CNS) manifestations include inability to concentrate, dizziness, sedation, disturbed coordination, blurred vision, convulsions, or excitation.

Precautions and contraindications. Antihistamines should be avoided by anyone with a history of bronchial asthma, cardiovascular disease, increased intraocular pressure or narrow-angle glaucoma, hyperthyroidism, hypertension, stenosing peptic ulcer, pyloroduodenal obstruction, symptomatic prostatic hypertrophy, or bladder-neck obstruction. They should not be used by people who take monoamine oxidase inhibitors.

Since the possibility of an additive effect exists, clients who take antihistamines should be made aware of the possibility of CNS depression and should not operate dangerous equipment or perform functions that require alertness. Antihistamines should not be used during pregnancy or lactation (see Focus on Antihistamines: Similarities and Differences).

Allergic ocular disorders

Allergies can effect the eyes, causing itching, redness, and tearing. As with other allergies, the ideal situation is prevention by avoidance of the catalysts. When that is not possible, a 4% optic solution of cromolyn sodium can be used, instilling 1 to 2 drops in each eye 4 to 6 times a day or, when less serious, one drop in each eye four times a day.

Table 35-4 compares antiallergy drugs used in the treatment of allergic rhinitis and ocular allergies.

Bronchial asthma

It is estimated that at least 12 to 15 million adult asthmatics live in the United States, and about 40 million have additional allergies. About 3,760 asthmatics die after attacks yearly. Those in the 10- to 14-year age range have had the greatest increase in death rates, whereas those older than 45 years (who also have heart or lung diseases) have the highest percentage of asthma-related deaths (Shute, 1987).

The paroxysmal wheezing and dyspnea of bronchial asthma result from reactions in the trachea and bronchi, which lead to bronchospasm, edema of the mucosa, and excessive production of mucus. This condition differs from emphysema, in which the resultant bronchial obstruction is irreversible. In status asthmaticus, asthma's most severe manifestation, death can ensue.

In asthma, the bronchi have been sensitized by allergens and, in the first phase of the attack, go into spasms triggered by any number of causes (Table 35-5). In the early response, the mast cells release histamine, causing the bronchial muscles to contract and the airway linings to become swollen. At the same time, thick and sticky mucus is secreted into the bronchi, clogging the airway. Air is trapped in the air sacs of the lungs, keeping the carbon dioxide there and making exhalation difficult. The bronchi vibrate as the air is forced out, causing the wheezing sound. This reaction usually ends within 90 minutes.

A second phase, the late response, occurs within 3 to 4 hours, lasting up to 12 hours or even longer. Other cells join the mast cells, in particular eosinophils, which enter the muscular bronchial wall. They send forth substances (*eg*, prostaglandins, leukotrienes) that normally help provoke inflammatory reactions and promote immunity. The lungs also release substance P and calcitonin. All of this action results in a sustained inflammation of the airway lining and makes the tissue hyperresponsive to the original offending substance. Each subsequent exposure to an allergen intensifies the early and late responses. An inhaled β_2-agonist should be used for an acute attack (Altman, 1991).

Clients self-administer the β_2-agonists by using a metered-dose inhaler (Fig. 35-1). The typical dose is 2 puffs every 4 to 6 hours, with the drug delivered directly to the bronchi. Clients usually experience an improvement in breathing within a few seconds to 30 minutes, which may encourage them to use higher amounts in search of even greater relief. In addition, clients may overuse the drug as symptoms of the disease process escalate. Some allergists suggest that use of β_2-agonists be limited to no more than once or twice a day to prevent overuse (Meier, 1991).

Excessive use of β_2-agonists are being studied as a possible factor in an increased number of fatal or near-

Antihistamines: similarities and differences

| Similarities | Differences |

Similarities

Pharmacodynamics

These agents compete with histamine for H_1 receptor sites on effector cells.

Differences

• **Diphenhydramine** inhibits the action of acetylcholine; it suppresses the cough reflex directly by its effect on the cough center. • **Dimenhydrinate**, **diphenhydramine**, and **promethazine** diminish vestibular stimulation and depress labrynthine function; they may also affect the chemotrigger zone for their antiemetic effect.

Pharmacokinetics

These agents are administered topically, nasally, or parenterally. They are well absorbed after oral or parenteral administration. They have an onset of action of 15 to 30 minutes, peaking in 1 hour, with a duration of 3 to 6 hours. They are well distributed with highest concentrations in the lungs and lower concentrations in the spleen, kidneys, brain, muscles, and skin. They are metabolized by the liver and excreted in the urine as metabolites.

• **Astemizole** is excreted unchanged. • **Astemizole** and **terfenadine** do not distribute into the CNS; small amounts are distributed into breast milk. Half-life varies: **astemizole** has a half-life of 1.5 days; **azatadine** has a half-life of 12 hours; **brompheniramine** has a half-life of 25 hours; **carbinoxamine** has a half-life of 10 to 20 hours; **chlorpheniramine** has a half-life of 21 to 27 hours; **diphenhydramine** has a half-life of 1 to 4 hours; **terfenadine** has a half-life of 3 hours. • **Dimenhydrinate** IM has an onset of 20 to 30 minutes; rectally, it has an onset of 30 to 45 minutes. • **Clemastine** has a duration of 12 hours; **pyrilamine** has a duration of 8 hours; **tripelennamine** has a duration of 4 to 6 hours; **azatadine** has a duration of 12 hours; **cyproheptadine** has a duration of 8 hours; **terfenadine** has a duration of more than 12 hours.

Therapeutic uses

These agents are used in the symptomatic relief of allergy and as adjunctive therapy in anaphylaxis and laryngeal edema. They are also used in the management of nasal allergies, rhinitis, common cold, allergic dermatoses, and for the symptomatic treatment of chronic idiopathic urticaria.

• **Dimenhydrinate**, **diphenhydramine**, and **promethazine** are used in the treatment and prevention of nausea, vomiting, and vertigo of motion sickness. • **Diphenhydramine** is used as a night-time sleep aid and for the symptomatic treatment of parkinsonian and extrapyramidal reactions. • **Diphenhydramine** and **tripelennamine** are used topically for the temporary relief of pruritus and pain of minor skin conditions.

Adverse reactions

These include: (CNS) headache, sleepiness, decreased alertness, inability to concentrate, dizziness, sedation, incoordination, excitation; (CV) hypotension, palpitations, tachycardia; (RESP) thickening of bronchial secretions, wheezing, nasal stuffiness; (EENT) blurred visions; (GI): nausea, diarrhea, constipation, epigastric distress, dry mouth, cholestatic jaundice; (GU) urinary frequency, retention; (ENDO) early menses; (SKIN) urticaria; (HEMA) hemolytic anemia, thrombocytopenia, agranulocytosis; (OTHER) photosensitivity.

• **Promethazine** may cause transient myopia. • **Trimeprazine** and **methdilazine** may cause extrapyramidal reactions, postural hypotension, tonic-clonic convulsions, and electrocardiographic changes. • **Diphenhydramine** may cause hallucinations, fever, chest tightness, and anaphylaxis. • **Terfenadine** does not cause drowsiness. • **Astemizole** may cause weight gain and arthralgia. • **Cyclizine** may cause tinnitus and dysuria. • **Cyproheptadine** and **dexchlorpheniramine** may cause appetite stimulation, visual hallucinations, ataxia, and weight gain.

(continued)

fatal asthma attacks (see Chapter 22 for a detailed discussion of sympathomimetic β_2-agonists).

The inflammatory response in asthma is considered more damaging than the bronchospasm, since it can eventually cause structural changes in the lungs. Prophylactic use of cromolyn sodium and the administration of steroids during an attack help lessen the inflammation (Altman, 1991).

Nocturnal symptoms are noted in up to 90% of people with asthma; they usually occur between 3 and 5 AM. Close to 80% of asthmatic respiratory arrests occur between midnight and 6 AM. Normally, a lessen-

Focus on

Antihistamines: similarities and differences (Continued)

Similarities	Differences

Similarities

Contraindications

These agents should be used with caution in people with hypersensitivity and in people who are having an acute asthmatic attack.

Differences

• **Tripelennamine**, **methdilazine**, **diphenhydramine**, dexchlorpheniramine, **cyproheptadine**, **clemastine**, **chlorpheniramine**, **carbinoxamine**, **brompheniramine** and **azatadine** are contraindicated for people who have taken monoamine oxidase inhibitors in the preceding 2 weeks and in breast-feeding or pregnant women. • **Dimenhydrinate** is contraindicated for people sensitive to theophylline. • **Trimeprazine**, **promethazine**, and **methdilazine** are contraindicated in the acutely ill or debilitated children. • **Trimeprazine** and **promethazine** are contraindicated for people with bone marrow depression, epilepsy, or coma and in neonates. • **Tripelennamine** is contraindicated on breast-feeding women.

Precautions

These agents should be used cautiously in people with increased intraocular pressure, hyperthyroidism, cardiovascular or renal disease, diabetes, hypertension, asthma, urinary retention, prostatic hypertrophy, bladder neck obstruction or stenosis, peptic ulcer disease, closed angle glaucoma, and in the elderly.

• **Cyclizine** and **dimenhydrinate** should be used with caution in people with GI obstruction. • **Dimenhydrinate** should be used with caution in people with seizure disorders. • **Methdilazine**, **promethazine**, and **trimeprazine** should be used with caution in children with history of sleep apnea, sudden infant death syndrome, or Reyes syndrome. • **Promethazine** and **trimeprazine** should be used with caution in people with acute or chronic respiratory dysfunction.

Nursing considerations

Instruct client in disease, treatment, drug therapy, regimen, adverse effects, and compliance; assess cardiopulmonary status and vital signs frequently; institute safety measures to prevent injury; caution client about activities that require mental alertness until drug effects are known; administer with food or milk to prevent GI upset; institute measures to relieve dry mouth, such as hard candy, ice chips; monitor blood studies for abnormalities; instruct client to avoid alcohol; do not crush extended release tablets; evaluate for effectiveness of therapy.

Administer **chlorpheniramine** IV slowly over 1 minute, do not give parenteral form intradermally. Instruct client that **buclizine** and **meclizine** tablet may be chewed, swallowed whole, or dissolved in water. Do not mix **cyproheptidate**, **diphenhydramine**, **promethazine**, or **dimenhydrinate** parenteral solutions with other solutions; they may be incompatible; administer 30 minutes before travelling for motion sickness and before meals and bedtime; undiluted IV solutions are irritating and may cause sclerosing. Rotate **promethazine** and **diphenhydramine** injection sites to prevent irritation; inject IM deep into large muscle. Protect IV **promethazine** from light; do not give subcutaneously because it may cause necrosis.

---

ing of airflow occurs during sleep. Those with asthma tend to have this condition to a greater degree; as many as 60% wake with wheezing, coughing, and shortness of breath. One theory is that a gastroesophageal reflux occurs while the client is lying flat; hydrochloric acid from the stomach stimulates the vagus nerve endings in the esophageal lining and the lungs, causing the bronchi to constrict (Nocturnal asthma, 1990).

Diagnosing asthma may be difficult if the client does not have the usual clinical symptoms of wheezing, decreased pulmonary function, or coughing. Usually, an increased blood eosinophil count is found, and, if sputum is present, eosinophils appear in the sputum (Parsons, 1986). Methacholine, a bronchoconstrictor,

can be used in a challenge test when a differential diagnosis is necessary to determine whether the individual has asthma or another pulmonary disorder. A positive test demonstrates hyperreactivity of the airways.

Pulmonary function tests (PFTs) are carried out before the methacholine challenge test. If the PFT is normal, a four-step test is carried out. If the PFT is abnormal, the challenge test requires nine steps, with smaller amounts of drug administered over a longer span of time. Either test starts with the inhalation of a small dose of methacholine, which causes bronchoconstriction in asthmatic individuals by stimulating the parasympathetic nervous system. A forced vital capacity is taken after each dose of methacholine is inhaled, and if no reaction is noted, the concentration of methacholine is increased. The process is repeated until the client has a 20% drop in the PFT, is short of breath, starts wheezing (all diagnostic of asthma), or has reached the upper limit of the methacholine dosage ordered. A bronchodilator (Alupent) reverses the symptoms of asthma and usually returns the PFT to normal within 10 minutes (Scherer, 1987).

Bronchospasm can occur with exposure to a variety of medications. Aspirin sensitivity may be deceptive since wheezing may not occur for several hours after its ingestion. The client history may elicit the aspirin triad: aspirin-induced asthma, nasal polyps, and perennial asthma (Parsons, 1986). β-Blocking agents are also widely recognized as catalysts or perpetrators of asthmatic reaction in susceptible individuals. Even nonsteroidal anti-inflammatory drugs, sulfites, sodium salicylate, and acetaminophen

Table 35-4. Antiallergy drugs for allergic rhinitis and ocular allergies

Drug	Purpose	Adverse side effects/additional information
Antihistamines		
chlorpheniramine (Chlor-Trimeton,* Deconamine)	Block histamine effects	Drowsiness; ineffective with prolonged use
		Use caution with narrow angle glaucoma, stenosing peptic ulcer, prostatic hypertrophy, bronchial asthma, and chronic pulmonary disease. PC: C
diphenhydramine (Benadryl*)		PC: B
Terfenadine (Seldane)	Blocks histamine effect without crossing the blood–brain barrier	Does *not* cause drowsiness PC: C
astemizole (Hismanal)	Treatment of seasonal allergic rhinitis	Weight gain for 4% of clients
		Use caution with lower airway disease (asthma) and hepatic and renal impairment.
		Efficacy drops 60% when taken with food. PC: C
Decongestants		
Nasal sprays	Relieve nasal stuffiness and eustachian tube congestion	Rebound congestion may occur if used more than twice a day or for more than 3 consecutive days.
		Insomnia, nervousness
		Decongestants may cause excessive dryness of mucous membranes (mouth, nose, vagina.)
Oral		
pseudoephedrine (Eltor, Novafed, Sudafed*)		Ephedrine-like reactions include tachycardia, headache, dizziness, nausea, anxiety, tremor.
		Clients older than 60 years may exhibit hallucinations, convulsions.
		Contraindicated in severe hypertension, severe coronary artery disease, monoamine oxidase inhibitor therapy, and for children younger than 12 years of age. PC: C
Combination decongestant plus antihistamine		
(Actifed,* Brexin)	Relieve nasal congestion, tearing, itching	May react to either component as above.
		Impairment of mental and physical abilities.

(Continued)

Table 35-4. Antiallergy drugs for allergic rhinitis and ocular allergies (Continued)

Drug	Purpose	Adverse side effects/additional information
Inhibitor of sensitized mast cell degranulation		
	Inhibits release of mediators histamines and leukotrienes from mast cells	Throat irritation and dryness, bad taste, cough, wheeze, nausea, bronchospasm
cromolyn sodium (Intal inhaler, Nasalcrom nasal spray)	Preventive action—especially helpful before exercise or exposure to allergen (animal, cold, and so forth)	Noncompliance with overuse common Administer 10–60 min before exposure. PC: B
(Opticrom eye gtt) (Vistacrom)	Relieve redness, itching, tearing	
Immunotherapy		
	Build up allergen antibodies	May require 100 or more injections over 3 years Possibility of anaphylaxis
Corticosteroid nasal spray		
(Beconase, Nasalide)	Relieve allergic rhinitis without side effects of oral corticosteroids	Tables 5–7 days to take effect

*Over-the-counter (OTC)

KEY: PC = pregnancy category. (The validity of pregnancy risk categories has not been established; see Chapter 16, p 216.)

should be administered cautiously to clients who are aspirin sensitive, because some clients may demonstrate sensitivity to these drugs also (Incaudo, Gershwin, 1986).

Asthma is the most common chronic childhood disease. About 80% of children who develop asthma are affected before starting school (Zamula, 1990). Childhood asthma is one of the 60 diseases that most frequently results in death in the U.S. At highest risk are those children who have had recurring episodes of severe asthma and those with early onset asthma. Other risk factors include dependence on corticosteroids, overuse of adrenergic inhalers, or unwillingness to obey medical regimens.

Children with mild intermittent wheezing can be expected to recover spontaneously, in contrast to children with chronic asthma, which will probably persist into adulthood.

Table 35-5. Risk factors in asthma

Asthma precipitants	Observable effects	Treatments
Hereditary (genetic) factors	Familial allergies	Elimination of known allergens
Environmental exposure Inhaled allergens: Pollens, dust, dander, feathers, molds, cigarettes, perfume, pollutants	Laboratory findings (elevated IgE levels, increased blood eosinophils in sputum if productive cough)	Remove allergenic substances from environment, absolute cleanliness of surroundings, remove animals if active allergens
Ingested allergens: Foods, drugs, molds, dander	Bronchospasm, dermatitis, ocular reaction, rhinitis; laboratory findings as above	Check food and medication labels and reject those that contain allergens
Temperature: Cold, heat, humidity	Bronchospasm, dermatitis	Avoid temperature extremes; medicate
Exercise	Bronchospasm, dyspnea	Cromolyn within an hour before, as a preventive
Respiratory infections	Wheezing with upper respiratory infection, bronchospasm	Avoid exposure to upper respiratory infection, antibiotics as ordered
Medication reaction	ASA triad, isoproterenol, or other drug	Absolute compliance with medication regimen as ordered
Emotional stress	Bronchospasm	Avoidance of stressful situations

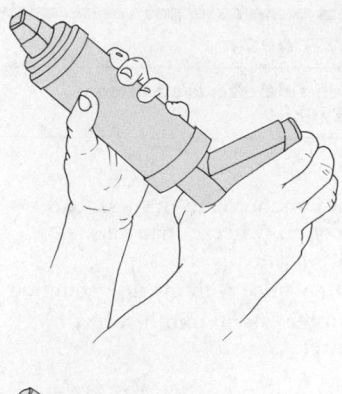

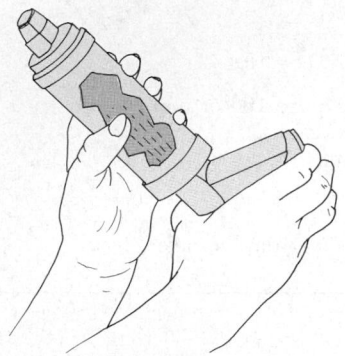

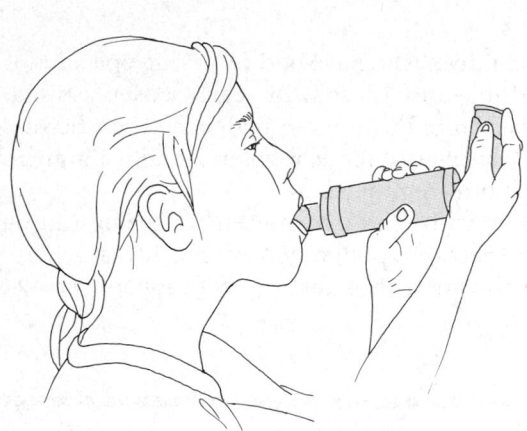

Figure 35-1. Metered-dose inhaler with AeroChamber. To use the AeroChamber the client follows this procedure: (1) Remove caps; (2) Visually check the AeroChamber for foreign objects and make sure that the one-way valve is secured; (3) Insert inhaler into AeroChamber; (4) Shake vigorously 3 or 4 times; (5) Place AeroChamber mouthpiece in mouth and close lips; (6) Spray one puff from the metered-dose inhaler into the Aero-Chamber; (7) Breathe in slowly and deeply through the mouth. Whistle should sound only when inhaling too quickly; (8) Hold breath for 5-10 seconds; (9) Repeat steps 4 to 8 as instructed by a physician. (Redrawn; original art and instructions courtesy Forest Pharmaceuticals, Inc./UAD Laboratories, New York, NY.)

Treatment

Cromolyn

Cromolyn sodium (Intal) is useful as a preventive but must be used before an attack begins. It is of no value during an asthma attack. Cromolyn sodium makes the airways less vulnerable to allergens and also prevents the release of histamine from the mast cells, lessening the inflammatory process. It is not a bronchodilator, and benefit may not be noted for 2 to 4 weeks after it has been incorporated into the daily antiasthma routine.

Adrenergic bronchodilators are the drugs of choice for treating bronchial asthma. Their use dates back to 1910, when injections of epinephrine and adrenergic drug with both α- and β-stimulant properties were found to be effective. The first drug to be used orally for asthma was ephedrine in 1924. Subsequently, β-adrenergic drugs were used because they were more specific in their effects as bronchodilators. In 1941, isoproterenol was used as an inhalant, without the α-adrenergic side effects associated with epinephrine. Isoproterenol and epinephrine are both sympathomimetic amines (*ie*, they mimic action of sympathetic nervous system).

By 1961, metaproterenol, a noncatechol adrenergic bronchodilator with a longer effective action time than isoproterenol, was developed for oral use. Drugs aimed at having greater selectivity for β_2-receptors were then produced, lessening the systemic side effects (primarily tachycardia, palpitations, and tremor) associated with epinephrine. These drugs include terbutaline, fenoterol, albuterol, and carbuterol (Table 35-6).

Tolerance to oral or inhaled β-adrenergic agonist drugs causes a decrease in the peak as well as the duration of bronchodilation after each dose. This reaction usually reaches its height within 2 weeks after

Table 35-6. β-Adrenergic drugs frequently used as bronchodilators

Drug name	Route of administration	Additional information
albuterol (Proventil, Ventolin)	Oral, metered-dose inhaler	Long-acting, effective bronchodilation. Prevents EIA* 6 h
		Low incidence of cardiac stimulation in usual doses
bitolterol mesylate (Tornalate)	Inhalation	Prevents EIA 45 min
		Greater accumulation in lungs than heart, therefore may minimize potential cardiac effects
		Use caution with cardiovascular disease, diabetes mellitus, and hyperthyroidism
cromolyn sodium (Intal, Vistacrom)	Metered-dose inhaler / Nebulizer / Turbo-inhaler (spinhaler)	Preventive when used before exposure to allergen or exercise; turbo-inhaler or spinhaler used with powder form; compressor driven nebulizer or metered-dose inhaler with liquid form
epinephrine (catecholamine) (ANA-Kit, Bronkaid, Vaponefrin)	Parenteral, subcutaneous	Includes α- and β-adrenergic actions, therefore the drug of choice for anaphylactic reactions; limited duration
		For small children with bronchoconstriction, inject 0.25 mg epinephrine or 0.01 mg/kg at 15- to 30-min intervals
ephedrine (Efedron)	Oral	First oral adrenergic bronchodilator to be used effectively. Not used often because newer β-$_2$- agonists are more effective, with fewer side effects
ephedrine with theophylline	Oral	Used in fixed combination for patients who require a mild bronchodilator effect
		Contraindicated for cardiovascular disease, hypertension, hyperthyroidism, prostatic hypertrophy PC: B
fenoterol (Berotec)	Inhalation	Prevents EIA 4 h
ipratropium bromide (anticholinergic) (Atrovent)	Inhalation (aerosol)	Maintenance treatment for chronic obstructive pulmonary disease (for local effect only)
		Contraindicated for those with atropine hypersensitivity
isoetharine (catecholamine) (β$_2$-Bronkometer, Bronkosol)	May cause severe allergic reaction in sensitive clients	
	To avoid overstimulation, do not administer with epinephrine	
isoproterenol (catecholamine) (Isuprel, Norisodrine)	Metered-dose inhaler	Effective relief within 5 min but action declines quickly—ineffective in about 2 h. Increased dosage may cause cardiac stimulation.
		Use caution with diabetes mellitus and hyperthyroidism PC: C
metaproterenol (noncatecholamine) (Alupent, Metaprel)	Oral, metered-dose inhaler	Longer duration with parenteral route than in oral or aerosol forms. Increased dosage may cause cardiac stimulation. Prevents EIA 30 minutes PC: C
terbutaline (noncatecholamine) (Brethaire, Brethine)	Oral, parenteral, subcutaneous	Used to treat bronchospasm associated with chronic obstructive pulmonary disease
		Equal or more effective bronchodilation than epinephrine, but increase in side effects of cardiac stimulation and tremor. Prevent EIA 1 h
		Use caution with monoamine oxidase inhibitors or tricyclic antidepressants

*EIA: Exercise-induced asthma
KEY: PC = pregnancy category. (The validity of pregnancy risk categories has not been established; see Chapter 16, p 216.)

initiation and may occur with all β-adrenergic drugs rather than be limited to the drug that causes the tolerance. IV administration of adrenal corticosteroids can reestablish the effectiveness of β-adrenergic agonists within an hour.

Combining β-adrenergic agonists and theophylline increases bronchodilation, allowing a lesser amount of each drug to be used, thereby decreasing the possibility of side effects that may occur with the larger dose required by either drug used alone (Sly, 1986).

Aerosols result in fewer side effects than oral or parenteral drugs (Table 35-7).

Table 35-7. Drugs commonly used for aerosol-bronchodilator delivery (metered-dose inhalers)

Drug	Dose	Additional information
Anticholinergics		
ipratropium bromide (Atrovent)	2 puffs qid	Dry mouth and throat, cough. Not as effective as β_2 agonists. Can cause tachycardia.
β-Agonists (sympathomimetics, anticholinergics)		Can cause tachycardia; affect smaller airways; relax smooth muscles
metaproterenol sulfate (Alupent, Metaprel)	2 puffs q 3–4 h	
terbutaline sulfate (Brethaire, Brethine)	2 puffs q 4–6 h	
albuterol (Proventil, Ventolin)	2 puffs q 4–6 h	
Corticosteroids		
triamcinolone acetonide (Azmacort, Aristocort, Aristo-Pak)	2 puffs tid or qid	Reverse persistent inflammation of bronchi; fewer systemic effects than oral steroids; may cause oral symptoms (hoarseness, dry mouth, irritated throat, oral candidiasis). Follow use with water or mouthwash rinse to prevent oral fungus infection.
Mast cell inhibitors		
cromolyn sodium (Intal, Vistacrom)	2 puffs before exercise to prevent EIA*	Not for use during an acute attack.
	2 puffs qid	Takes 2–4 weeks to see effect
epinephrine (AsthmaHaler, Bronkaid, Primatene, AsthmaNefrin, Vaponefrin)		Over the counter. Should not be used without physician's recommendation for asthma. Can cause tachycardia.

*EIA = Exercise-induced asthma.

Methylxanthines

Methylxanthines are thought to act by interfering with the sequestration of calcium in bronchial smooth muscle, thus preventing bronchoconstriction. One of the most commonly used methylxanthines is aminophylline (theophylline ethylenediamine). Aminophylline is 80% theophylline base. The dose varies widely among clients and must be individualized, preferably by serum concentration monitoring.

Theophylline seems to be most effective when serum concentrations are maintained in the 10- to 20-μg/ml range. Low doses should be administered initially, increasing to full therapeutic effect within 7 to 10 days. Slow release (sustained-release) preparations are widely used because of more convenient dosage regimens (Table 35-8).

Combining β-adrenergic agonists and theophylline prevents the release of histamine from human peripheral leukocytes, which is induced by the antigen. These agents, as well as certain prostaglandins,

Table 35-8. Selected commonly used theophylline preparations

Drug name	Preparations	Amount of theophylline present
aminophylline		
(Phyllocontin)	Sustained-release tablet (225 mg)	178 mg
(Somophyllin)	Oral solution (105 mg/5 ml)	90 mg/5 ml
(Somophyllin Rectal Solution)	Rectal solution (60 mg/5 ml)	51 mg/5 ml
(Aminophyllin)	Tablets (100 mg, 200 mg)	79 mg, 158 mg
theophylline anhydrous		
(Constant-T)	Sustained-release tablet	200 mg, 300 mg
(Slo-Phyllin)	Syrup (80 mg/15 ml)	80 mg/15 ml
	Tablet (100 mg, 200 mg)	100 mg, 200 mg
(Theo-Dur)	Sustained-release tablet (100 mg, 200 mg, 300 mg)	100 mg, 200 mg, 300 mg
oxtriphylline		
(Choledyl)	Oral solution (100 mg/5 ml)	64 mg/5 ml
	Tablet (100 mg, 200 mg)	64 mg, 128 mg
(Choledyl SA)	Sustained-release tablet (400 mg, 600 mg)	256 mg, 384 mg

may act as mediators in inhibiting the degranulation of primary mast cells, which leads to allergic reactions.

Theophylline interacts with other drugs. The actions of theophylline and any other drug given at the same time must be monitored. It has a synergistic bronchodilator action with β-agonists and can also increase the chance of adverse reactions. Theophylline serum concentrations can increase when given with allopurinol, furosemide, cimetidine, propranolol, erythromycin, and oral contraceptives. Even dietary considerations are important in client education: high-carbohydrate low-protein diets, caffeine, and other dietary xanthines increase serum levels, whereas high-protein low-carbohydrate diets decrease serum levels (Sly, 1986).

Serum levels can decrease if theophylline is given with phenytoin or phenobarbital. Cigarette and marijuana smoking also increase metabolism of theophylline, resulting in lower serum theophylline concentrations. Theophylline may also lower phenytoin levels, decreasing the anticonvulsant effect of the drug.

In an acute asthmatic attack, when the client is unable to use a metered-dose inhaler, one treatment is a subcutaneous injection, usually 0.3 to 0.5 ml of 1:1000 epinephrine. This is repeated two or three times after 15 or 30 minutes have elapsed, if needed. If this is not successful, aminophylline should be administered IV in an individualized dose. This treatment is followed by a course of oral bronchodilators and an increased dose of corticosteroids if the client is already taking them.

The combination of β-agonists and aminophylline in the treatment of status asthmaticus or severe acute asthma has been clinically more effective than epinephrine alone. In addition, inhalation of β-adrenergic medications appears to be as effective for acute asthma as drugs given by injection.

If IV aminophylline is used in the treatment of status asthmaticus, it should be maintained at a specific blood level (10–20 μg/ml). The client may also require oxygen therapy and IV fluids to maintain hydration. Treatment of any associated illness or disorder, including heart failure or respiratory infections, is mandatory. A close watch of blood gases and *p*H determinations is also imperative, so that treatment can be modified as needed.

Corticosteroids

Many physicians feel that systemic corticosteroids should be limited to those asthmatic clients who cannot be controlled by immunology or other medications. When necessary, prednisone should be used, preferably at moderate to low levels, 0.5 mg/kg body weight daily or 0.75 mg/kg body weight every other day, to control asthma. The dose should be tapered slowly, until 30 mg are given on alternate days; after that, the dose should be tapered even more slowly to reach the minimal dose necessary to prevent acute or chronic asthmatic episodes. Corticosteroids eliminate inflammation of the airways and reduce airway irritability, swelling, and production of mucus. For this reason, some physicians regard inhaled corticosteroids as the treatment of choice for asthma.

It takes several hours before systemic corticosteroids become clinically effective, with even more time for maximum level. Despite the possibility of adverse side effects, the use of corticosteroids to relieve airway obstruction in status asthmaticus reduces morbidity and, at maintenance levels, permits clients to live more comfortably. Intermittent short courses of corticosteroids, as in alternate-day therapy, appear to produce few adverse responses. At times of exacerbation, higher doses may be reinstituted and used until symptoms are again under control. A short-acting corticosteroid should then be used, lengthening the time between doses.

Clients who receive systemic corticosteroids must be watched carefully for complications and be instructed about such possibilities. Among these are obesity and cushingoid facies, hyperglycemia, suppression of linear growth, hirsutism, thinning of the skin, and delayed sexual maturation.

The effectiveness of steroids is diminished when barbiturates, phenytoin, or rifampin are used. Corticosteroids increase the bronchodilator action of adrenergic agents. Again, clients who receive drugs that interact must be monitored.

Topical corticosteroids, such as beclomethasone dipropionate, when given by inhalation may allow for the discontinuation or reduction of systemic prednisone. Oral use of prednisone can be reinstituted when needed (see Chapter 32 for a detailed discussion of corticosteroids).

Hypersensitivity pneumonitis

When sensitized people inhale organic dusts or animal proteins, hypersensitivity pneumonitis may occur. It is frequently found in farmers, pigeon breeders, and people in contact with drugs or certain low-molecular-weight industrial chemicals. Preventing sensitization depends on preventing inhalation of the antigen by wetting composts before handling or grinding, sterilizing organic dust fibers, cleaning and changing the water of air humidifier units, using appropriate indoor ventilation systems, or supplying workers with protective face masks and clothing covers during work periods. Corticosteroids (usually given every other day) may be required by workers habitually exposed to antigens.

Testing for allergies

Some clinical tests are helpful in the diagnostic evaluation of allergic disorders. However, the tests themselves are not free of adverse effects, such as sensitization or even fatal anaphylaxis. To prevent the misuse of allergy testing, The American College of Physicians set new guidelines in 1989, recommending that testing be limited to the verification of diagnoses already determined by the client's history and symptoms. Before these guidelines, clients were subjected to testing that included multiple skin pricks with a wide range of extracts, inhalation or ingestion of suspected allergens, and blood tests. Many of the tests were overused or misused, resulting in diagnostic errors and treatment for allergies that were nonexistent. The FDA removed more than 300 of the extracts from the market, labeling them as ineffective or even unsafe. The 1989 guidelines suggest the tests described in the following sections.

Skin tests

The advantage of skin testing is that it is simple, allows many substances to be tested simultaneously, and provides immediate results. Two techniques are available: *intradermal skin tests* or *prick tests*. Intradermal tests should be 2 to 3 inches apart so that reactions do not overlap. A small bleb can be observed with the use of 0.02 to 0.05 ml of the extract, which produces a visible wheal and erythema after 15 to 20 minutes. If a negative reaction occurs, higher concentrations of the extract are given until a positive reaction is reached or until the highest concentration produces no observable reaction. If the initial test proves positive, serial dilutions are used to determine the weakest dilution that produces a 2^+ reaction (21–30 mm erythema or 5–10 mm wheal).

The prick test is carried out by placing a drop of extract on the skin, then pricking the skin with a needle. After about 1 minute, the extract is wiped off, and the area is observed for a wheal and flare in about 15 minutes. The concentration of extract used for the prick test must be about a thousand times greater than that used for the skin test to correlate the results of the techniques. In either test, false positives may occur in response to the trauma of the needle or to the diluent that transports the concentrated extract. False negative responses may be due to poor technique, deteriorating or incorrect extracts, or to reduced sensitivity caused by medication (*eg*, antihistamine) taken by the client. One way of checking the responsiveness of the client's skin is to conduct a skin or prick test with a histamine solution as a positive control.

In the rare instance when a generalized reaction to skin testing occurs, a tourniquet should be placed on the extremity above the test site and 1:1000 aqueous epinephrine given immediately.

Although hundreds of allergens are still approved by the FDA, fewer than 50 should be needed in tests for a given client. They are highly specific when used correctly and are economical, relatively safe, and comfortable to use.

The titration test should only be used to determine the safe dose of antiallergy medication that can be employed initially to start a course of treatment. To carry out this test, gradually increasing concentrations of the allergen are injected subcutaneously into the client until a positive skin reaction is noted. That level becomes the starting dose for treatment, a fact that is particularly important when the allergen is the venom of a stinging insect. A false reading can be obtained if too large a dose of the allergen is used.

The patch test, in which an absorbent pad that contains the allergen is taped to the client's back, is primarily used to diagnose allergies to substances that can cause cutaneous reactions, such as cosmetics, dyes, ointments, costume jewelry, or fabrics.

Provocation tests

In the bronchial provocation test, the suspected allergen is inhaled in an attempt to produce the adverse reaction, such as sneezing, stuffy nose, coughing, or wheezing. This test is expensive, uncomfortable, and dangerous because it bears the small risk of causing a severe asthma attack.

For the oral provocation test, foods are removed from the diet until symptoms disappear or ease, then are reintroduced until the symptoms reappear. The test must be carefully administered and analyzed to avoid misinterpretation.

Other tests

Allergic responses can also be tested by determining the level of the immunoglobulin IgE in the blood serum. Two of these tests are radioimmunoassays: the competitive radioimmunosorbent test (competitive RIST) and the noncompetitive radioimmunosorbent test (noncompetitive RIST). The third test is a double antibody radioimmunoassay. The interpretation of any of these tests is difficult and varies with the client's age and genetics and the influence of parasites on IgE levels. Some of the newer laboratory tests to identify allergies are able to measure the primary reaction of antibody and antigen as they bind (equilibrium dialysis, Farr test, radioimmunoprecipitation, affinity chromatography) or to measure the secondary reactions, which include precipitation (quantitative precipitin reaction), agglutination, complement fixation, enzyme immunoassay, enzymatic radioimmunoassay, immunofluorescence, immunoelectron microscopy, and radioallergosorbent testing (RAST), which may be performed with an enzyme instead of a radioactive substance.

The ability to identify specific allergens has increased during the last decade. Allergens can be isolated in serum, saliva, hair, dander, and the pelts of dogs and cats. Horse and bovine allergens can be found in their amniotic and allantoic fluid, hair, and dander. Insects carry allergens in their venom. House dust can contain dander, mites, fibers, and chemicals in mixtures that make it difficult to isolate the offending substance.

■ Summary

Allergic reactions may be due to environmental factors (pollens, dust, industrial pollutants), foods (cow's milk, wheat, eggs), drugs (penicillin, tetracycline, chloramphenicol, aspirin), or insect bites.

The body reacts to an allergen by producing specific antibodies that excite the membrane receptors on mast cells. This process leads to the release of histamine, serotonin, and other substances that also may be involved in the physical reactions recognized as allergic responses. Stress intensifies these responses.

Treatment of allergies includes removal of the offending substance when possible, as well as desensitizing procedures (allergen immunotherapy), preventive use of cromolyn, and symptomatic treatment with antihistamines, β-adrenergic agonists, atropine decongestants, and corticosteroids.

Nursing management

Nursing process

Assessment The medical diagnosis of allergy should be made from the client's history or clinical observation verified by specific allergy testing. Nurses play a vital role in initial casefinding. The history should include known and suspected allergens and the nature of allergic reactions.

Allergic reactions may involve any tissue or organ; therefore, their manifestations are varied. These may include such symptoms as headache, indigestion, or joint pain as well as the more common dermatitis, rhinitis, and wheezing. Allergic symptoms often accompany an acute illness such as cold or bronchitis. However, when symptoms such as cough persist after the resolution of the illness, the possibility of allergy should be considered.

Triggers for allergic reactions also are manifold. In addition to chemical allergens such as drugs and foods, heat, cold, and sunlight can cause them. In the hospital, molds from air conditioners, other volatile substances in the air, plastics, and latex rubber may also act as allergens.*

* In 1991, several clients died from anaphylactic reactions induced by allergies to the latex cuffs on enema tips, which were then recalled by the FDA. Professionals have also reported personal reactions to latex products, possibly due to repeated exposure to proteins in latex. For those who suspect sensitivity, or for those who have had an allergic reaction, plastic devices should be substituted for latex. Severe reactions to latex (or any other product, drug, or biologic substance) should be reported to the FDA Problem Reporting Program at 800-638-6725.

Asthmatic symptoms (dyspnea, cough, and wheezing) may appear in children about 5 minutes after heavy exercise and last from 20 minutes to several hours. Adults with asthma can also be prone to bronchoconstriction after exercise. It is more common for adults to associate their symptoms with inhaled substances (pollens, spores, house dust). Perennial symptoms tend to recur with environmental factors such as seasonal pollens. Foods, particularly eggs, nuts, and fish, may cause a violent reaction, possibly including diarrhea, vomiting, cramps, and urticaria. Occupational allergens include fumes, dust, wood pulp, pharmaceuticals, chemicals, printed matter, and foods. Other harmful substances are solvent odors, tobacco smoke, and chlorine in swimming pools. Drugs that induce asthma include aspirin, some nonsteroidal anti-inflammatory drugs, and β-blockers.

When treatment is initiated, the nurse should assess the client's knowledge of the allergy and its treatment. Since the tendency to have allergic reactions is inherited and related people tend to have similar reactions, the client may be familiar with the particular condition (asthma, hay fever) but may not have accurate or complete information about it.

After treatment is begun, the nurse must ascertain the number and severity of recent allergic attacks, current dosage of anti-allergy drugs, therapeutic response to the drugs, adverse reactions to the drugs, and the client's general level of stress.

Nursing diagnosis Nursing diagnoses may include the following:

> High risk for impaired tissue integrity (eg, dermatitis, rhinitis) related to exposure to allergens (eg, pollens, dust, drugs)
> High risk for ineffective airway clearance, ineffective breathing pattern, impaired gas exchange related to bronchospasm and inflammation secondary to asthma
> Sleep pattern disturbance related to CNS stimulation secondary to therapy with β_2-agonists or corticosteroids
> Pain: stomach cramps related to oral theophylline therapy
> Knowledge deficit concerning allergy or its treatment

Planning Long-term goals of nursing care include decreasing the number and severity of allergic reactions and early detection and treatment of adverse reactions to treatment. Some short-term goals are resolution of acute allergic reactions, minimization of client exposure to allergens, prompt detection and resolution of adverse drug reactions, assistance to reduce stress levels and integrate treatment into personal lifestyles, and education about allergy and its treatment.

Intervention A history of allergic reactions should be brought to the attention of the health practitioner, including specific circumstances. Information about offending foods, fabrics, detergents, animals, insect stings, and the timing of reactions (time of day, date, season) should be relayed. Clients may be referred to their personal physicians or to allergists.

Minimizing exposure to allergens. Exposure to allergens may occur by skin contact, inhalation, ingestion, or injection (*eg*, insect stings). Avoidance precautions must be tailored to specific allergens that affect individual clients. Thus, offending foods are removed from the diet; allergenic fabrics, plastics, or cosmetics are replaced by hypoallergenic substitutes; inhaled allergens are eliminated from the home; and offending drugs are discontinued. Specific measures can be taken by individuals allergic to insects to prevent stings (see Client Education below). Pets are a special problem because many people react to their danders. Birds, horses, cats, and dogs are frequent offenders. Fish and short-haired dogs are least likely to cause reactions. Weekly bathing of cats and dogs removes dander and reduces their antigenicity.

Clients prone to asthma who experience nocturnal acid reflux should limit food intake before bedtime, take antacids, and elevate the head of the bed (Hoffmann, 1991). They may also need to increase antiasthma medication at night (Nocturnal asthma, 1990).

Clients should be questioned carefully about a history of allergies before being given a β-blocker for angina, hypertension, or any other disorder, since they would be at high risk for allergic reaction, including possible anaphylaxis, when exposed to an allergen. β$_2$-Agonists, the usual treatment for such reactions, would likely be antagonized by the β-blocker. Allergy testing for individuals who receive oral or topical β-blockers should be limited to *in vitro* RAST. When the allergies are relatively benign, clients who take β-blockers should be treated with drugs rather than immunotherapy, except for clients with bee sting allergy, since immunotherapy provides the only effective preventive treatment. These individuals should be switched to a non–β-blocker before they receive Hymenoptera venom immunotherapy.

Breast-feeding for at least the first 4 to 6 months is believed to reduce the risk of allergy in the baby if the mother avoids allergenic foods in her diet. Solid foods should be introduced cautiously into the baby's diet after 6 months of age, with only one new food offered at a time and at least 1 week passing before another food is given, to allow for a potential reaction.

Resolution of acute allergic reactions. The most critical allergic reaction, anaphylaxis, requires immediate intervention. Epinephrine is the treatment of choice. It can be administered by injection or aerosol inhalation. The medications in bee-sting kits are epinephrine dispensed in a special syringe and an oral antihistamine. The epinephrine syringe is designed for repeated administration of fractional parts of the contents. If an initial dose (0.1 to 0.5 ml of 1 : 1000 solution) is not effective within 10 to 15 minutes, it should be repeated and the antihistamine administered. Successive doses should be administered as needed every 10 to 15 minutes. Emergency medical help should be summoned as cardiopulmonary resuscitation may be required if cardiac arrest occurs.

Anaphylaxis that occurs in clients who are taking β-blockers may require prolonged and aggressive treatment, with prompt administration of epinephrine plus an injectable H$_1$ antihistamine. If bronchospasm is noted, treatment can be either with albuterol by inhalation or, if unresponsive, with atropine by inhalation. Additional treatment may include respiratory support, IV fluids, or even the use of shock trousers. If bronchospasm is persistent, IV isoproterenol or dopamine, possibly with a dose up to 80 times normal, may be necessary to overcome β blockade (see Table 35-5; Toogood, 1987).

Acute attacks of asthma are usually treated by β$_2$-agonist inhalations. These drugs usually relieve dyspnea within 30 minutes. This prompt effect may encourage clients to use higher amounts in search of even greater relief. In addition, clients may overuse the drug as symptoms of the disease process escalate. Some allergists suggest that use of β$_2$-agonists be limited to no more than once or twice a day to prevent overuse (Meier, 1991). Clients can have difficulty using inhalers, or they may abuse the metered-dose inhalers. Combining topical and systemic medication is helpful (Box 35-3). Figure 35-2 shows a metered-dose inhaler with mask attachment, making administration easier for children, the infirm, or the elderly.

Refractory asthma (status asthmaticus) requires treatment in an acute care institution, preferably in an intensive care setting. Treatment usually involves IV therapy and assisted respirations.

Exercise induced asthma can be controlled by using a bronchodilator (aerosol or orally) or by inhalation of cromolyn sodium prophylactically, which prevents the release of chemical mediators, whether allergen or nonallergen induced.

Acute dermatitis is usually treated with topical corticosteroids. Ointments should be applied sparingly in a thin layer because the active ingredients are absorbed readily by inflamed skin. Skin areas touched by poison ivy, sumac, or oak should be washed with cool water as quickly as possible. This action inactivates urushiol, the oily agent that causes the itching rash and blisters. Soap should not be used since it may spread the oil to other skin areas. Use of rubbing alcohol after the water helps remove oil absorbed by the skin. Steroids (oral or injected) can be helpful if administered before the blisters form.

Allergic optic disorders are controlled with cromolyn eye drops. Soft contact lenses should not be

Box 35-3. Proper use of metered-dose inhaler

Follow directions for the use of the specific metered-dose inhaler (MDI) ordered for the client, since brands may differ. The usual directions are as follows:

1. The client should shake the canister for 30 seconds. This action mixes the drug and the propellant.
2. The client should remove the cap from the mouthpiece.
3. The client then inhales deeply through his or her nose, exhales completely but gently through the mouth, to begin the treatment.
4. The client holds the mouthpiece about 1.5 inches from the mouth, which must be open for the treatment.* The index finger should be at the top of the canister, and the thumb on the bottom.
5. The client then inhales through the mouth while simultaneously depressing the top of the canister. This delivers a metered dose into the mouth.†
6. The client must close his or her mouth after the inflow of the medication, hold his or her breath for the count of 10, then exhale gently through pursed lips.
7. The client must wait 2 to 5 minutes, then repeat for a second puff if ordered. The client should be cautioned not to use more than the prescribed amount of drug, nor increase the frequency of administration without the physician's permission.
8. Remove the metal MDI canister from the inhaler.
9. The inhaler should be cleaned daily with warm soapy water, rinsed under warm running water, and then dried completely. It can then be reconnected to the MDI canister to be available when needed.

*Controversy exists about whether the mouth should be open during inhalation or closed around the mouthpiece. However, it has been found that twice as much drug is available to the bronchial tree when the mouth is open (Newhouse, 1986).

†Some clients have difficulty in coordinating inhalation and drug delivery from the MDI. Spacers can be attached to the MDI; these help to get the drug to the bronchi (see Fig. 35-2).

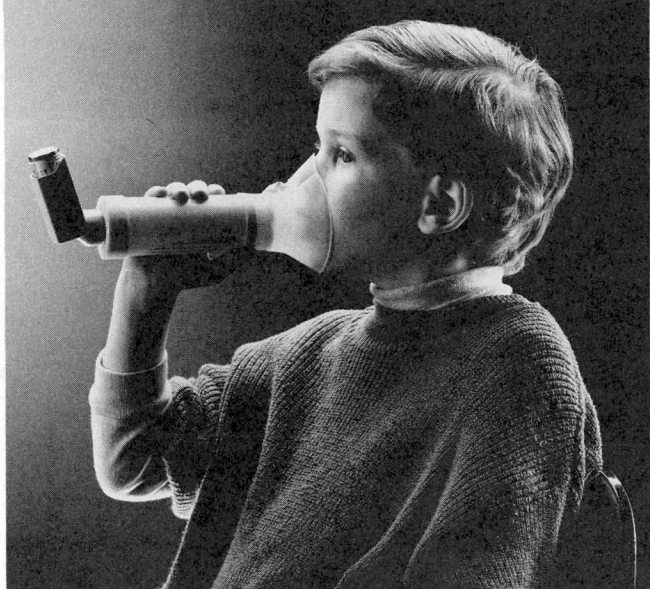

Figure 35-2. Metered-dose inhaler with AeroChamber with mask. (Courtesy Forest Pharmaceuticals, Inc./UAD Laboratories, New York, NY.)

reactions, allergic clients need to develop stress-management skills. Measures to minimize stressors that impinge on institutionalized clients should be taken by the nurse.

Monitoring drug therapy. The nurse should evaluate the client for both therapeutic and adverse responses to the drug regimen. Signs and symptoms of adverse drug reactions should be recorded and reported promptly to the physician.

Asthmatic clients who require β-blockers for the treatment of nonallergic conditions may not respond therapeutically to β₂-agonists. The physicians who prescribe these drugs should be informed of the client's allergy so that a blocker least likely to antagonize the allergy medications, such as metoprolol, can be prescribed and its dosage carefully titrated to determine the minimal effective dosage. The physician who treats the allergy must also be informed of the β-blocker medication.

Client education. Many allergic individuals are unaware of basic ways to avoid allergens. People allergic to pollens should be advised to stay in air-conditioned rooms or vehicles, with windows closed and air conditioning on between 4 and 10 AM, since pollen counts are highest during those hours. Air conditioner filters should be kept clean, in good repair, and replaced when necessary to decrease both the pollen and

worn during the treatment period because one of the drug ingredients, benzalkonium chloride, is contraindicated in the presence of soft lenses.

Maintenance therapy. Recurrent asthma attacks can be minimized by long-term systemic theophylline or inhalant cromolyn therapy (see Chapter 37 for a detailed discussion of respiratory drug regimens).

Management of stress. Because stress is associated with exacerbations of allergy and increased severity of

Learning experience 35-2

How would you make a bedroom as free of allergens as possible for a 5-year-old child?

mold particles (from the air conditioner) in the atmosphere of the room or vehicle. High-efficiency particulate air filters help remove up to 90% of airborne allergens but are ineffective against dust mites, which cling to fabrics or carpeting.

Cleaning chores should be carried out by others when possible, and silicone-coated dust cloths should be used to cut the circulation of dust particles in the air. The client who is unable to delegate these tasks should wear a dust mask while cleaning to lessen dust inhalation. Dust mites can be kept out of bedding by the use of plastic cases for the mattress and pillows and by laundering covers, blankets, and pillows frequently. Feather pillows, a source of dander, should be replaced with fiberfill or foam pillows that are machine washable.

Clients with dust allergies should avoid rugs, choosing hardwood or other floor coverings without pile. If carpets are used, they should have the shortest pile possible and should be vacuumed frequently, should be machine washable, and washed often to get rid of dust mites and dried thoroughly. Room temperature should be below 70°F and humidity below 50% to provide an environment inhospitable to the mites, which are microscopic (7,000 can fit on a dime).

Dogs and cats are responsible for much of the dander found in homes. For those who cannot accept the thought of removing pets, limitations should be set as to where they may roam in the home. Whenever possible, pets should be banned from the bedroom and should not be permitted to stay on furniture with fabrics likely to harbor dander or on carpeting with a pile.

Clients who use β$_2$-agonists must be warned to employ them cautiously and to follow their physicians' advice as to use, since twice the recommended daily dosage may contribute to doubling the risk of fatal or near-fatal attacks. β$_2$-Agonists can increase blood pressure, result in an irregular or rapid heartbeat, and cause nervousness, dry mouth, and difficulty in urination.

Clients who are allergic to insect stings should be taught to dress for the out-of-doors with long pants and sleeves, using perfume-free cosmetics, wearing drab or dark colors, and using insecticides and insect repellents when necessary. They should be instructed in the use of bee-sting kits and should carry one with them at all times. When traveling in an automobile, windows should be adjusted so that they do not "scoop" air into the car, as this can propel insects into the car.

Clients who are allergic to sulfites must usually restrict their diets to fresh foods and be certain that medications intended to lessen allergic reactions do not contain sulfites. Sulfiting agents include sodium sulfite, potassium or sodium bisulfite, sulfur dioxide, and potassium or sodium metabisulfite. Sulfites also form naturally in wines, reaching high concentrations. Sulfites help keep foods looking fresh and prevent deterioration, thus reducing waste. The FDA has prohibited adding sulfites to fresh fruits and vegetables. It has also ordered the listing of sulfites on labels of canned, prepared, or frozen foods when the concentration exceeds 10 parts per million (Shultz, 1986). However, allergically sensitive people have to question the contents in restaurants or other places where food is prepared. Very sensitive people should carry epinephrine (Adrenalin) with them for treatment of severe respiratory emergencies.

Clients who use cromolyn should be cautioned to use this drug as prescribed, without interruption, as its action is preventative and it is ineffective if an allergic reaction is allowed to develop. Long-term theophylline regimens should also be maintained without interruption.

Clients who take drugs by inhalation need specific instruction in the use of their devices. The mists from metered-dose inhalers must be actively inhaled into the lungs to prevent deposition on the oral and pharyngeal surfaces. If the medication contains a corticosteroid, clients should be cautioned to rinse their mouths with water or mouthwash after use of the inhaler to prevent oral fungus infections from developing.

Evaluation Data required for evaluation relate to the incidence and severity of allergic reactions, the absence or incidence of adverse drug reactions and the speed with which they are resolved, and the knowledge and skill with which clients manage their regimens and integrate them into their lifestyles (see the Example of Nursing Process and Chemical Allergy).

Checklist of nursing actions

☐ Assess clients carefully for signs and symptoms of allergic reaction; list in the history specific substances associated with them.

When caring for clients with allergies

☐ Remove from the environment those specific substances associated with their allergic reactions.

☐ Have epinephrine readily available for treatment should anaphylaxis occur.

☐ Minimize stressors that impinge on clients; assist them to manage stress levels.

☐ Monitor closely clients who experience severe or prolonged allergic reactions.

☐ Apply topical corticosteroid preparations sparingly to minimize absorption of the hormone.

When teaching clients regarding allergy and its treatment

☐ Warn clients on long-term cromolyn or theophylline therapy not to omit or discontinue doses without the advice of their physicians.

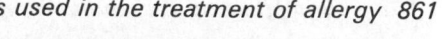

Example of nursing process and chemical allergy

The client is a 33-year-old woman who has had eczematous lesions on the fingertips and palmar surfaces of both hands for 10 years. Prior testing resulted in a medical diagnosis of allergic dermatitis, which has been kept under control with twice daily applications of a topical corticosteroid. She is allergic to soaps, detergents, cleaning agents, and many household chemicals and avoids chores that involve their use. Her husband is very supportive and does the household cleaning to lessen her exposure to allergenic substances. She has been told to continue the medication and to undergo periodic testing for possible hypothalmic-pituitary-adrenal (HPA) axis suppression, which is negative at present.

Assessment data	Nursing diagnosis	Intervention	Goals and outcome criteria
Eczematous lesions on fingertips and palmar surfaces of both hands; topical application of ointment that contains corticosteroids	High risk for impaired tissue integrity: delayed healing of eczematous lesions related to excessive absorption of corticosteroids through damaged skin	**Teach** the client to apply a thin coat of ointment to the lesions; caution client to avoid occlusive dressings, which tend to increase absorption of the drug. **Warn** the client that overmedication retards healing of lesions.	The client will demonstrate proper technique for applying the ointment.
As above Periodic testing for HPA axis suppression	Knowledge deficit concerning reversible HPA axis suppression, Cushing's syndrome, and other symptoms related to excessive absorption of corticosteroid drugs	**Teach** the client proper application and use of corticosteroid ointment as above. **Stress** the importance of periodic tests for adrenal function.	The client will not develop severe HPA axis suppression: if suppression does develop, it will be promptly reversed without causing symptoms of corticosteroid deficiency.

- ☐ Advise clients of measures to minimize their contact with allergenic substances.
- ☐ Teach clients about adverse reactions to their drugs, including criteria for consulting the physician for a change in medication.
- ☐ Warn clients to clean air conditioners frequently to minimize microbial growth within its mechanisms.
- ☐ Warn clients not to increase their dosages of medication (especially β₂-agonists) without consulting their physicians.
- ☐ Instruct clients in the proper use of inhalers.

References

Altman L. (1991, February 6). More vigilance urged in treating asthmatics. *The New York Times*, p A12.

Cullen SI, Araujo OE. (1987). Is that rash drug induced? *Diagnosis*, Apr, 38–45.

Hoffmann S. (1991). Asthma, Part 1. *Harvard Health Letter, 16*(7), 5–7.

Incaudo G, Gershwin ME. (1986). Aspirin and related non-steroidal anti-inflammatory agents, sulfites, and other food additives as precipitating factors in asthma. In Gershwin ME, ed. *Bronchial asthma*, 2nd ed. Orlando: Grune & Stratton.

Injections for stings may not be necessary. (1990, December 11). *The New York Times*, p 9.

Meier, B. (1991, August 8). Company tells of dangers in overusing asthma drugs. *The New York Times*, p A14.

Newhouse M, Dolovich M. (1986). Control of asthma by aerosols. *N Engl J Med, 315*, 870–874.

Newman A. (1987). Pain pills may damage kidney. *Johns Hopkins Magazine, 39*(4), 16.

Nocturnal asthma. (1990). *New Directions, 19*(2), 5.

Parsons GH. (1986). Treatment of asthma in adults. In Gershwin ME, ed. *Bronchial asthma*, 2nd ed. Orlando: Grune & Stratton.

Scherer P. (1987). New drugs. *American Journal of Nursing, 87*, 646.

Shultz C. (1986). Sulfite sensitivity. *American Journal of Nursing, 86*, 914.

Shute S. (1987). Stop sneezing, stop wheezing. *American Health, 6*(6), 85–94.

Sly RM. (1986). Treatment of asthma in children. In Gershwin ME, ed. *Bronchial asthma*, 2nd ed. Orlando: Grune & Stratton.

Test drugs raise hope of preventing asthma (1990, December 20). *The New York Times*, p B20.

Toogood J. (1987). Beta-blocker therapy and risk of anaphylaxis. *Can Med Assoc J*, May 1, 929–933.

Warning for prescription drugs containing sulfites. (1987). *FDA Drug Bulletin, 17*, 1,2.

Wasserman SI. (1986). The pathophysiology of mediators in asthma. In Gershwin ME, ed. *Bronchial asthma*, 2nd ed. New York: Grune & Stratton.

Zamula E. (1990). More than snuffles, childhood asthma. *FDA Consumer, 24*(6), 10–13.

Bibliography

Ritter C, et al. (1990). IgE hidden in immune complexes with anti-IgE autoantibodies in children with asthma. *J Allergy Clin Immunol, 88*(5), 793–801.

Shapiro G, et al. (1991). Cromolyn vs. triamcinolone acetonide for youngsters with moderate asthma. *J Allergy Clin Immunol, 88*(5), 742–748.

Venge P, et al. (1991). Eosinophils in exercise induced asthma. *J Allergy Clin Immunol, 88*(5), 699–704.

Williams R. (1991). How to take your medicine, adrenergic bronchodilators. *FDA Consumer, 25*(5), 30–31.

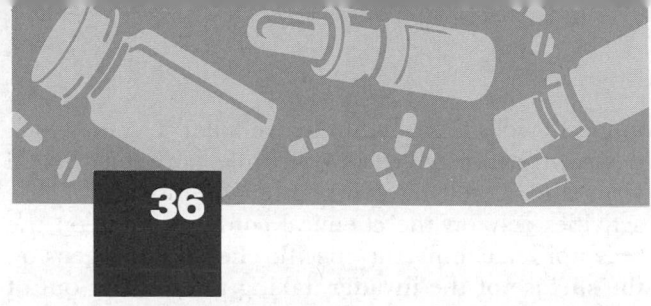

Drugs used to moderate the immune system

The presence of an immune response in the human body was recognized in the 18th century. Much more has been learned since then. In 1798, Edward Jenner differentiated reactions of people who had received primary smallpox vaccinations from reactions of those who had acquired immunity through the disease or previous vaccination. In 1890, Robert Koch described the skin reaction (induration and swelling) that resulted from the subcutaneous injection of tuberculin into persons who had previously contracted tuberculosis. By 1919, this procedure, called the *Mantoux test*, was used for diagnostic purposes. It is discussed later in this chapter.

Immunity

The body's immune response is its third line of defense against microorganisms (the first includes the mechanical barriers of skin, mucous membranes, body hair, and body secretions; the second includes inflammation and phagocytosis). Immunity to disease exists when the body is able to produce specific substances (antibodies) that combat infectious agents (antigens) to which it is exposed. Invading organisms contain proteins and polysaccharides that act as antigens. The antigens stimulate the body's reticuloendothelial and lymphoid tissues to produce protein gamma globulins (protective antibodies). Interferon, an antiviral protein, is produced by the body's nonlymphoid cells. These antibodies defend the body by binding with and incapacitating microorganisms. This mechanism is specific (*ie*, antibodies will bind only with the particular antigens that stimulated their formation). Figure 36-1 indicates sites where antibodies are produced.

Protein gamma globulins are also called *immunoglobulins*. Immunoglobulins, no matter how they are acquired, cause the body to react to foreign substances by challenging antigens that might otherwise prove harmful. One way this occurs is when the body's antibodies link with the invading antigens to trigger the host defense system. This process activates the phagocytic or cytoxic K cells (nonphagocytic monocytes), eventually destroying the antigen. Another way the body controls foreign substances is by preventing toxins or viruses from binding with the host cells by neutralizing them, which interferes with the linkage of the foreign substance to the epithelial cells.

Newborn immunity

Antibodies transmitted through the placenta protect newborns against certain diseases to which their mothers have immunity. Thus, most infants are born with some natural immunity acquired from their mothers through an immunoglobulin (IgG). Additional protection is afforded by breast-feeding because another specific immunoglobulin (IgA) found in colostrum can be absorbed through the newborn's intestinal tract. However, immunoglobulins must be given

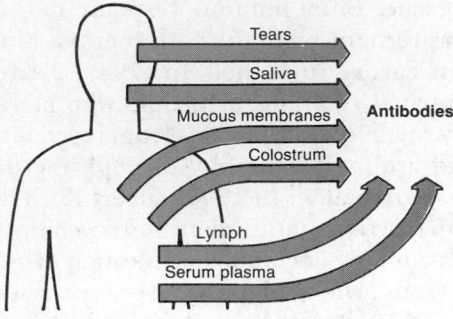

Figure 36-1. Body structures and sites in which antibodies are produced.

to the child on a regular basis until the body's own defense system is activated, usually between 16 and 30 months of age. Some infants who are born without or with insufficient built-in protection (agammaglobulinemia or hypogammaglobulinemia) lack protective responses to bacterial or viral invaders. Agammaglobulinemia is an abnormality characterized by the absence of gamma globulins in the body. Persons who suffer from this condition cannot produce antibodies and are highly susceptible to infections. Persons with hypogammaglobulinemia produce antibodies but in insufficient amounts. Because their resistance is lower than usual, they do not readily recover from infections.

Cell-mediated immunity

The body's defense or immune system is activated when foreign materials (viruses, bacteria, allergens, or foreign tissue) invade the body. When the invader is a virus, it is engulfed by a microphage. Antigens, composed of viral protein, travel from inside the microphage to its surface, where they unite with a major histocompatability complex molecule.

The major histocompatability complex with the antigen acts as a marker so that the body's thymus-derived lymphocytes (T cells) recognize the invaders and differentiate the friendly from the harmful ones. Incorrect recognition may prevent the production of protective antibodies within the host, leading to infection or disease, whereas overproduction may lead to autoimmune disorders. When working properly, the system turns itself on and off at the proper times. To do this, some T cells (helper T cells) have receptors consisting of two linked chains of amino acids (alpha and beta) capable of bolstering the activity of bone-marrow-derived lymphocytes (B cells). Other T cells (suppressor T cells) stop that action when it is no longer needed. Their proper relationship is necessary to balance the immune system.

The helper T cell receptors can recognize the invading antigens, increasing the activity of B cell receptors, which then produce antibody-forming plasma cells that attack the foreign substance: B cells are derived from and matured in the bone marrow. The

helper T cells then manufacture killer T cells, which destroy the infected cell. Meanwhile, both the original virus and T cell have replicated themselves. These activities rely on the chemical configurations on the receptors matching the specific chemical antigens on the surface of the invader, taking the invader out of circulation. Future attacks by that or similar invaders will result in a rapid immunologic response to prevent infection. This response takes place whether the original episode was due to illness or to use of a vaccine.

Each T or B cell contains only one kind of antigen receptor, and will recognize only that antigen. There may be millions of variations of the receptors, any of which can replicate itself many times, creating a memory of the invader. Thus, any future meeting with that antigen will result in more immediate reaction (Benderly, 1988).

Lymphokines

T cells also produce lymphokines, substances capable of activating other immune cells in the body. They are useful in stimulating cytotoxic activity in lymphocytes and are sometimes helpful in tumor regression. One form of lymphokine is interleukin-2, which is a genetically engineered drug administered to a cancer client intravenously. The lymphocytes that the client produces are removed from his or her blood by leukopheresis and are incubated with additional interleukin-2, causing the cells to reproduce more quickly. These cells are then referred to as lymphokine-activated killer cells and are reinjected into the client through a central venous catheter or large peripheral vein in the hope that tumor regression will follow. The FDA has approved this treatment for clients with metastatic kidney cancers and melanomas, which generally have been incurable. Further experimentation is now being carried out for clients with non-Hodgkin's lymphoma and colorectal cancer. The side effects of this therapy include fever, fluid retention, irregularities in cardiovascular and kidney function, and even death (Sticklin, 1987).

Interferon is another member of the lymphokine family, produced by using recombinant gene cloning. It is composed of three types of protein: alpha, beta, and gamma. Each differs somewhat from the others in its actions. Alpha interferon has both antiviral and antineoplastic properties. The action of beta interferon is similar but somewhat weaker. Gamma interferon primarily activates macrophages.

Immune system moderators

The healthy immune system balances the recognition of foreign invaders (which occurs through the body's major histocompatibility complex) and the ability to repel them, with mediation of that response when continuation would be inappropriate or injurious to the body. Drugs that moderate the immune system include both immunopotentiating agents and immunosuppressive agents.

Pathophysiology of the immune system

Deficiencies

Deficiencies of the immune system can be hereditary or acquired. Children may be born with genetic immunodeficiencies of varying severity. The most serious of these is severe combined immune deficiency. One example of an hereditary partial immunodeficiency is chronic granulomatous disease. Acquired deficiencies may be caused by infection such as the human immunodeficiency virus (HIV) that causes acquired immunodeficiency syndrome. The acquired immunodeficiency syndrome virus destroys T4 lymphocytes, rendering the body unable to fight various infections and malignant growths.

Inappropriate activities

Inappropriate activity of the immune system is the cause of allergies, autoimmune disease, and transplant rejection.

Allergy

In allergy, the immune system misidentifies substances such as pollen, foods, or other (usually innocuous) substances as harmful to the body. Antibodies produced in response to this "threat" combine with the antigens, stimulating local production of histamine and leukotrienes which, in turn, cause inflammation. The type of allergic reaction produced is dependent, in part, on the location of this reaction. For example, in asthma the lungs are affected, and inflammation and bronchospasm produce dyspnea. Skin reactions are characterized by rash. The nose, eyes, and nasopharynx are affected in hay fever. Allergy causes chronic illness and certain reactions (such as anaphylaxis and status asthmaticus) can be fatal. (See below and Chapters 35 and 37 for discussion of these conditions.)

Autoimmune disease

Misidentification of the body's own tissues as foreign "threats" can also lead to a another serious, even deadly reaction: that of autoimmune disease. It is believed that the autoimmune process is triggered by a change in certain body cells (sometimes caused by an infectious agent such as a virus) that alters its antigenic properties. The immune system then attacks the affected tissues, causing chronic inflammatory changes and destruction of tissue. The autoimmune process is believed to be involved in such chronic disabling diseases as arthritis, rheumatic fever, sarcoidosis, diabetes mellitus, and scleroderma.

Transplant rejection

The introduction into the body of organs and tissues that differ genetically in any way from the recipient's tissues affects the immune system like any other "foreign body." If left to proceed uninterrupted, this *rejection* reaction will cause cell death, necrosis of the transplanted tissue, and failure of the transplant.

Transplanted bone marrow is not rejected because the recipient's immune system is destroyed prior to the transplant. However, the immune cells produced by the transplanted marrow can attack the tissues of the recipient (*graft versus host* disease or GVHD) causing widespread damage throughout the body (Benderly, 1989). In most cases, organ and tissue transplants cannot succeed unless immune system function is suppressed.

Immune system modifiers

Immunosuppressants

Treatment of autoimmune disorders

Immunosuppressant drug agents have been employed recently to treat several autoimmune disorders. Among the agents employed are cortisone and antineoplastic drugs such as methotrexate. (See Chapters 4 and 32 for discussion of these agents.)

Three main immune system antibodies have been found in the blood of potential diabetics before overt diabetes has appeared. Islet cell antibodies have been discovered in 75% of those who will develop diabetes. Insulin autoantibodies have appeared in 100% of those children who will develop diabetes before age 5. The most important immune system antibody discovered to date is 64 K (glutamic decarboxylase), which is found in the blood of 70%–80% of potential diabetics. The 64 K antibody is produced in response to islet cell protein. It appears as early as 7 years before the overt onset of diabetes, and is an excellent predictive marker of diabetes. Although no immunosuppressants specific to these antibodies have yet been developed, in Copenhagen, experiments are under way to develop a "poison pill" to destroy the 64 K antibodies but spare the rest of the immune system.

Immunosuppressants such as azathioprine (AZA), glucocorticosteroids, or Imuran are being tested to prevent destruction of beta cells before diabetes actually surfaces. However, long-term preventative treatment with these agents poses high risks of infection. Immunosuppressants also are used to suppress rejection of pancreatic transplants. (See discussion of transplant rejection later in this chapter).

An experimental treatment for scleroderma involves the removal from the body of white blood cells (leukopheresis) and subsequent exposure of these cells to ultraviolet light and 8-methxypsoralen, an antineoplastic drug used in the treatment of lymphoma. The theory is that the exposure to ultraviolet light injures the rapidly dividing immune system cells, thereby interfering with the autoimmune disease process. This procedure is twice as effective as, and produces fewer side effects than, the standard treatment, D-penicillamine.

Certain forms of arthritis have been shown to benefit from the immunosuppressive drugs cortisone and methotrexate. Cyclophosphamide or other antisuppressive agents may be administered if these agents are ineffective. A newer approach to arthritis is the use of biologicals (body chemicals) to block the release of inflammation-provoking cytokines, including interleukins, tumor necrosis factor, and gamma interferon (Lewis, 1991).

It is possible to produce a monoclonal antibody that kills T cells, thus acting as an immunosuppressant. (See discussion of monoclonal antibodies below.) In clinical trials, these antibodies have been combined with a toxin that kills the T cells and have been used to treat rheumatoid arthritis when other treatments were ineffective. The reduction in T cells was temporary, returning to normal after 10 to 14 days. There was no apparent increased risk of infections.

Prevention and treatment of transplant rejection

Presently, immunosuppressant drugs are the treatment of choice to protect transplanted tissue. They include cyclosporine, azathioprine, and glucocorticosteroids.

Cyclosporine

Cyclosporine is a cyclic polypeptide immunosuppressant consisting of 11 amino acids.

Pharmacodynamics. Cyclosporine's mechanism of action is obscure; it must always be used in conjunction with corticosteroids.

Pharmacokinetics. Cyclosporine is incompletely absorbed from the gastrointestinal tract, with peak concentrations occurring in blood and plasma at about 3.5 hours. Cyclosporine is concentration-dependent in the blood, with its uptake by leukocytes and erythrocytes at high concentrations. In plasma, about 90% is bound to proteins. It has a half-life of about 19 hours, and is extensively metabolized by the liver, with elimination primarily biliary. Only 6% is excreted in urine. The injectable form is reserved for clients unable to take the oral forms (oral solution or soft gelatin capsules) because of the risk of anaphylaxis thought to be caused by the polyoxyethylated castor oil used as the vehicle for the intravenous formulation.

Therapeutic uses. Cyclosporine is used for the prophylaxis of organ rejection in human kidney, liver, and heart allogeneic transplants. It can be used to treat chronic rejection of transplanted organs in clients treated previously with other immunosuppressive agents.

Adverse reactions. Cyclosporine's immunosuppressive action increases the client's risk of infection and the possible development of lymphomas and other malignancies, particularly of the skin. Tremor, hirsutism, and gum hyperplasia are common side effects. Hepatotoxicity, as evidenced by elevations of hepatic enzymes and bilirubin, has been noted in fewer than 7% of transplantation clients. It has usually occurred during the first month of therapy when high doses of cyclosporine were administered, and subsided when the dose was reduced.

Nephrotoxicity has been associated with 25% of renal transplants, 38% of cardiac transplants, and 37% of liver transplants. Mild nephrotoxicity has been noted 2 to 3 months after transplantation, receding with cyclosporine dosage reduction. More overt nephrotoxicity, occurring most often during the first 6 months after transplantation, is similar to episodes that characterize graft rejection, particularly of renal transplants. It is important to differentiate between nephrotoxicity and graft rejection since treatment differs. Laboratory tests for blood urea nitrogen and creatinine, kidney biopsies, and various radiologic tests aid in the differentiation. To add to the difficulty, nephrotoxicity and graft rejection may occur simultaneously. Nephrotoxicity usually responds to reduction in the dosage of cyclosporine or a switch to other immunosuppressive therapy. Severe and unremitting rejection may necessitate removal of the transplanted kidney.

Cyclosporine may have to be reduced or discontinued if the client develops a syndrome that combines thrombocytopenia and microangiopathic hemolytic anemia, possibly resulting in graft failure or rejection.

The client receiving intravenous cyclosporine is at high risk for anaphylaxis for the first 30 minutes after the start of the infusion. If it should occur, cyclosporine should be discontinued immediately, and an aqueous solution of epinephrine administered immediately. Oxygen may also be required.

Cyclosporine does not appear to be mutagenic or teratogenic. However, embryotoxicity and fetotoxicity has been demonstrated in animals. In humans, prematurity, malformations, and neonatal complications have been observed. It has been classified in pregnancy category C.

Precautions and contraindications. Oral cyclosporine should not be used by clients hypersensitive to it. Its injectable form should not be used by clients sensitive to cyclosporine or polyoxyethylated castor oil.

Clients with malabsorption may not achieve therapeutic levels with oral administration of cyclosporine.

The client's blood pressure should be monitored during cyclosporine therapy. Hypotension is a common side effect, but hypertension is also a possibility, with mild or moderate elevation decreasing over time. Antihypertensive therapy may be required using any of the common agents (see Chapter 28) but potassium-sparing diuretics should not be used since cyclosporine may cause hyperkalemia.

Drug interactions

The use of calcium antagonists may require cyclosporine dosage adjustment since they interfere with cyclosporine metabolism and increase its presence in the blood. Blood levels of circulating cyclosporine levels are essential to determine the effects on those levels caused by other drugs. Increases in cyclosporine levels can result from administration of drugs such as nicardipine, verapamil, ketoconazole, bromocriptine, erythromycin, and methylprednisolone. A decrease in cyclosporine levels may be found in clients receiving rifampin, phenobarbital, phenytoin, and carbamazepine. Clients receiving prednisolone, digoxin, lovastatin, and nifedipine may demonstrate a reduced clearance of these drugs while on cyclosporine. As a result, severe digitalis toxicity has occurred within days after cyclosporine therapy has been instituted, myositis has occurred in clients on lovastatin, gingival hyperplasia in clients on nifedipine, and convulsions in clients on high-dose methylprednisolone. Vaccinations may be less effective when the client is receiving cyclosporine. The use of live vaccines should be avoided.

Breast-feeding is not recommended because the drug is present in mother's milk.

■ Summary

Cyclosporine is a cyclic polypeptide used with adrenal corticosteroids for the prophylaxis of organ rejection in clients who have received human kidney, liver, or heart allogeneic transplants. Side effects include the increased risk of neoplastic disease and the possibility of life-threatening infections.

Nursing management

Nursing implications

The use of any immunosuppressive therapy must be evaluated carefully for the risk versus value factors. Adverse reactions most commonly seen are renal dysfunction, tremor, hirsuitism, hypertension, and gum hyperplasia. The client must be watched for signs of hepatotoxicity, nephrotoxicity, and graft rejection. Differentiation between nephrotoxicity and renal graft rejection is difficult, particularly in cases where they appear simultaneously.

Blood levels of cyclosporine and any other drugs administered concurrently (particularly digoxin) must be monitored carefully to determine any need for dosage adjustments.

Nursing process

Assessment   Pertinent client information includes a history of hypersensitivity to cyclosporine or polyoxyethylated castor oil. Other factors to explore are whether the client is pregnant or has a condition requiring medication that may cause adverse reactions when administered concurrently with cyclosporine. A complete drug history should be taken.

Nursing diagnosis   Nursing diagnoses likely to be made for clients receiving cyclosporine therapy include the following:

> High risk for infection related to immunosuppression
> Impaired tissue integrity: gum hyperplasia secondary to cyclosporine therapy
> Body image disturbance related to hirsutism and gum hyperplasia secondary to cyclosporine therapy
> Knowledge deficit concerning expected benefits of and possible adverse reactions to prescribed medication

Common collaborative problems that should be differentiated from the nursing diagnoses include

> Potential complication: renal
> Potential complication: hepatic
> Potential complication: anaphylaxis

Planning   Goals of nursing care are to reduce the risk of, detect, treat, and report reactions to cyclosporine; to enhance body image; and to teach the client about the drug regimen and its effects.

Intervention   Careful checks of the client for adverse reactions include inspection for gum hyperplasia, changes in blood pressure levels, signs of hepatotoxicity, signs of nephrotoxicity or renal graft rejection, and signs of reactions to cyclosporine or drugs administered concomitantly. Differentiation between nephrotoxicity and renal graft rejection is particularly important.

Client education.   Clients should be made aware of the possibility of infections and neoplasms when immunosuppressive therapy is administered. They should be taught the specific signs and symptoms that should be reported to the health care practitioner. The rationale and need for dosage changes for drugs they may be taking that react with cyclosporine should be explained.

Mouth care should be stressed (brushing, flossing, massaging) to prevent and treat gum hyperplasia. The client be may taught to bleach or remove unwanted hair. The fact that frequent blood tests will be required to monitor liver enzymes, and blood urea nitrogen and creatinine levels should be discussed with the client. The possibility of fetotoxicity and embryotoxicity related to cyclosporine should also be shared with the client.

Evaluation   Careful records should be kept of the incidence or absence, and reporting of any adverse reactions to cyclosporine or other drugs administered concurrently. The adjustment in dosage of any of the drugs should be recorded, and any changes (positive or negative) in the client's status should also be reported and recorded.

Checklist of nursing actions

☐ Inform clients of expected beneficial and adverse reactions before starting cyclosporine therapy.

☐ Take a careful history to determine the presence of allergies to cyclosporine or polyoxyethylated castor oil.

☐ List all drugs the client is taking; identify any that may interact with cyclosporine; report these to the physician.

☐ Notify the physician if the client is pregnant or breast-feeding.

☐ Advise the client of signs and symptoms of adverse reactions to cyclosporine; specify those that should be reported to health care personnel.

☐ Observe the client for signs of hepatotoxicity, nephrotoxicity, and graft rejection.

Azathioprine

Azathioprine is an immunosuppressant antimetabolite derived from 6-mercaptopurine.

Pharmacodynamics. Azathioprine is used to suppress renal homograft rejection. Although the mechanisms of this action are obscure, its use is well established. Suppression of cell-mediated hypersensitivities and variable alterations in antibody production are known to occur when AZA is given at the time of engraftment or in the presence of an antigenic stimulus. It is not effective in treatment of secondary responses, or when established grafts undergo rejection.

Azathioprine is also used for clients with severe, active, and erosive rheumatoid arthritis unresponsive to conventional management (rest, aspirin, nonsteroidal anti-inflammatory drugs, nursing comfort measures). Its use is combined with rest, physiotherapy, and salicylates. If corticosteroids are in use, reduction in dosage should be considered.

Pharmacokinetics. Azathioprine is absorbed well when administered orally. Its effectiveness depends on the thiopurine nucleotide levels in tissues rather than in the blood levels, which are low. It is moderately bound to serum proteins (30%), and is undetectable in urine after 8 hours. Azathioprine is partially dialyzable. It is rapidly eliminated from blood, and is oxidized in erythrocytes and the liver.

Therapeutic uses. Azathioprine is used as an adjunct for the prevention of rejection of renal homografts. This use provides a 5-year survival rate of 35%–55% that is also dependent on other variables (donor, match for HLA antigens).

Azathioprine is also used in the treatment of autoimmune disease. At this writing, this use is restricted to adults with severe rheumatoid arthritis that is unresponsive to conventional treatment.

Adverse reactions. Chronic immunosuppression with AZA increases the risk of neoplasia in humans. Severe leukopenia and/or thrombocytopenia, as well as macrocytic anemia and severe bone marrow depression, may occur in clients receiving AZA. Adverse gastrointestinal reactions such as nausea and vomiting may occur within the first few months of AZA therapy. These reactions can be reduced by administering the drug in divided doses or after meals. If gastrointestinal hypersensitivity occurs, there may be severe nausea vomiting, diarrhea, rash, fever, increase in liver enzymes, myalgias, malaise, and hypotension. These problems are reversible when the drug is discontinued. If a single dose of AZA is administered as a rechallenge, the symptoms may recur within an hour.

Serious, even fatal, fungal, viral, bacterial or protozoal infections can occur during therapy with AZA, and should be treated vigorously (see Chapter 43). The AZA dosage may have to be reduced or even discontinued.

Drug interactions

Azathioprine is degraded through conversion to inactive 6-thiouric acid by xanthine oxidase. Since allopurinol inhibits this conversion, the dose of AZA must be reduced for clients concurrently receiving allopurinol.

Precautions and contraindications. Azathioprine has been shown to be mutagenic in animals and humans; therefore, it should not be used during pregnancy. Since AZA is considered to be slow-acting, with effects persisting after discontinuation, delay of pregnancy should be considered until no remnants of the drug are found in the system. Azathioprine is listed in pregnancy category D. It is not recommended for nursing mothers.

Baseline blood counts should be performed before initiation of therapy with AZA. Blood counts should be monitored throughout therapy. Unusual bleeding or bruises and signs or symptoms of infection should be reported to the physician immediately.

Since AZA is dialyzable, clients on dialysis should receive the drug after dialysis is completed. Those with oliguria may have delayed clearance and, therefore, require a lower dose of AZA.

Maintenance of AZA should be at the lowest effective dose to lessen the risks of adverse reactions. This is accomplished by reducing the top dose 0.5 mg/kg or approximately 25 mg daily every 4 weeks until the lowest effective dose is attained.

■ Summary

Azathioprine is an immunosuppressive antimetabolite used to prevent renal homograft rejection, and for the suppression of severe adult rheumatoid arthritis unresponsive to conventional treatment. Side effects include the increased risk of neoplastic disease, gastrointestinal and/or hematologic disorders, and the possibility of life-threatening infections.

Nursing management

Nursing implications

The use of any immunosuppressive therapy must be evaluated carefully for the risk versus value factors. Although the specific mechanism of action is unknown, the use of AZA to prevent renal homograft rejection is almost universal. On the other hand, the use of AZA for the treatment of severe adult rheumatoid arthritis is restricted to those clients for whom conventional treatment has been unsuccessful.

Adverse reactions include nausea, vomiting, pancreatitis, leukopenia, and neoplasias. Infections may be life-threatening, and must be treated with appropriate medications.

Nursing process

Assessment   Pertinent client information includes a history of previous use of AZA, hypersensitivity to the drug, and the possibility of pregnancy. Clients with a history of previous treatment with alkylating agents (cyclophosphamide, chlorambucil, melphalan) may have a prohibitive risk of neoplasia if treated with AZA.

Nursing diagnosis   Nursing diagnoses likely to be made for clients receiving AZA include the following:

> High risk for infection secondary to immunosuppressive therapy
> Altered nutrition, less than body requirements, related to nausea and vomiting secondary to azathioprine therapy
> Diarrhea related to azathioprine therapy
> Impaired tissue integrity: bruises related to azathioprine therapy
> Knowledge deficit concerning expected benefits of, and possible adverse reactions to, azathioprine

Planning   Goals of nursing care are to reduce the risk of, detect, report and treat adverse reactions to AZA therapy, and to teach the client about the drug regimen.

Intervention   The environment should be kept as infection-free as possible when the client is on immunosuppressive therapy. Personnel and visitors with signs or symptoms of any infection should not be permitted near the client. Check the client carefully for adverse reactions; include assessing for bleeding or bruises (hematologic), severe nausea, vomiting, diarrhea, abnormal liver enzymes (gastrointestinal), urinary problems (rejection of renal graft, use of al-lopurinol), elevated fever, respiratory congestion, localized redness, and swelling (infection).

Client education.   Clients must be informed of the importance of protecting themselves against infection by self-care techniques including proper washing of hands, and avoiding contact with infected others or contaminated foods. They should be taught the signs and symptoms of infection, and told to report them immediately. Clients should be advised to report signs of bleeding (mouth, gums, tarry stools, bruises) immediately.

Clients should be informed of the mutagenic or teratogenic dangers of AZA therapy during pregnancy. They should be taught early the signs and symptoms of malignant neoplasms that should be reported to the health care professional.

Evaluation   Data required for evaluation include incidence or absence of adverse reactions to AZA, and the speed with which they are detected and resolved. Client teaching may be assessed by questioning the client about the content that was taught.

Checklist of nursing actions

☐ Take a careful client history to determine if the client has previously been treated with AZA or alkylating agents, and whether an allergic reaction to AZA occurred.

☐ Ascertain whether clients are presently using allopurinol, angiotensin-converting enzyme inhibitors, or drugs affecting leukocyte production.

☐ Determine whether female clients are pregnant or nursing a baby, and inform them of AZA effects on these conditions.

☐ Advise clients about dangers of infection while receiving AZA therapy; teach clients how to avoid infections.

☐ Reduce incidence of nausea and vomiting by administering AZA in split doses or after meals.

☐ Observe the client for signs and symptoms of infection, tumors, and bone marrow depression.

Immunosuppressant regimens

The prevention and suppression of transplant rejection with minimal toxicity requires the use of more than one agent, and different drugs have been shown to be effective for different transplanted organs. For example, cortisone is usually prescribed when cyclosporine is administered. Recipients of liver transplants are most commonly treated with cyclosporine A, corticosteroids, AZA, monoclonal antibodies (OK T3), and FK 506 (Whiteman, 1990). Clients who have had kidney transplants demonstrate fewer acute rejection episodes, fewer infections, and fewer readmissions when the synthetic prostaglandin misoprostol (Cytotec) is added to cyclosporine and prednisone. Because it enhances the anti-rejection actions, it must be added during the first 12 weeks after surgery (Altman, 1990).

The rejection of transplanted hearts is reversed through the use of steroids, antithymocyte serums or globulins, or muromonab-CD3 (Orthoclone OKT3) to block the regeneration and functioning of the T3 complex of human T lymphocyte cells (Dault, 1989). Unfortunately, antibody development to OKT3 has appeared within 2–3 weeks of treatment in 80% of the clients in one study, with the possibility that the drug would be useless in future rejection episodes (Scherer, 1987).

The newest drug used for immunosuppression is FK 506, a peptid from Japan, derived from a soil fungus. It has been found to be 100 times more powerful than cyclosporine with few side effects. It has been used successfully for multi-organ transplants by Dr. Thomas Starzl at the University of Pittsburgh as well as by the Diabetic Research Institute of the National Institute for Health (Edison, 1991).

FK 506 is also being used experimentally for the treatment of new onset type I diabetes mellitus at the University of Pittsburgh. The clients must have started insulin therapy no more than 7 days prior to this treatment, while they presumably still have some islet cells capable of producing insulin. At this early point of treatment, the researchers believe that some of the beta cells stop functioning due to high acidity and blood sugar levels. These levels drop to a more normal range once insulin therapy begins. At this point, the nonfunctioning beta cells, which have not been destroyed, begin to produce insulin, and will continue to do so unless eventually killed by the disease process. FK 506, given within the first week of insulin therapy, prevents the immune system from attacking and destroying those beta cells that are still functioning (Marino, 1991).

Clients receiving any immunosuppressant therapy are at high risk for life-threatening infections, particularly from herpes simplex and cytomegalovirus. They are also vulnerable to *Staphylococcus epidermidis* and *Pneumocystis carinii*. Even minor infections can escalate to major problems because the client lacks the ability to manufacture sufficient disease-fighting antibodies.

Immunopotentiators

Acquired immunity
The production or transfer of antibodies, which results in immunity, is called *acquired immunity*. Acquired immunity is further defined as *active acquired* and *passive acquired* immunity. Figure 36-2 and the following text describe these different types of immunities.

Active acquired immunization
Repeated exposures to the same antigens result in their linking with specific antibodies already developed by the body. Previously acquired immunity

thereby prevents reinfection. This is called *naturally active acquired immunization*. However, it is not necessary to develop a clinical or even subclinical infection to acquire active immunity to a disease. Instead, the person at risk can be given antigens that have been deprived of their pathogenic activity. These antigens are taken from living or dead microorganisms, their toxins, or from bacterial extracts. By giving clients at risk such antigens, it is possible to stimulate their production of antibodies without exposing them to the dangers of the disease process. This *artificially acquired active immunity* is retained indefinitely, resulting in antibody production whenever reexposure to the same antigen occurs. This immunity is reinforced with the administration of "booster" doses at periodic intervals. Artificial active agents, then, are dead (extract) vaccines, attenuated viruses, and toxoids. Following active immunization, the number of antibodies rises relatively quickly and reaches a peak in 10–14 days. This type of immunity lasts for a long time (years to lifetime).

Passive acquired immunization
Passive immunity is the transferral of antibodies formed in a human or animal to a susceptible person. Passive acquired immunization can be obtained naturally by children from their mothers because antibodies cross the placenta and are also present in colostrum. Passive acquired immunization can also be obtained artificially through antiserum, antitoxin, and gamma globulin.

In an emergency, immunity can be conferred passively by giving immune serum to the previously unexposed person. This substance is acquired from a human or animal already actively immunized against the organism in question. For example, gamma globulin is given to persons exposed to infectious hepatitis. The antibodies in the transferred serum temporarily provide the same protection afforded by an actively acquired immunity. However, unlike the continuing protection provided by active immunity, passively acquired immunity is lost within a few weeks as the antibodies break down and are discharged from the body.

Treatment of immunodeficiency
Clients with hereditary or acquired immunodeficiency do not develop active immunity in response to vaccines and toxoids. They must be protected from infection by providing passive immunity (after exposure to infection); replacement of deficient immune mediators; or by administration of bactericidal anti-infective agents (after infection is established.) Agents that provide passive immunity include gamma globulin, antisera, and antitoxin (see above). One immune mediator, a genetically engineered form of gamma interferon, has been approved by the FDA for treatment of chronic granulomatous disease, a hereditary form of immunodeficiency (Gamma interferon for immune disor-

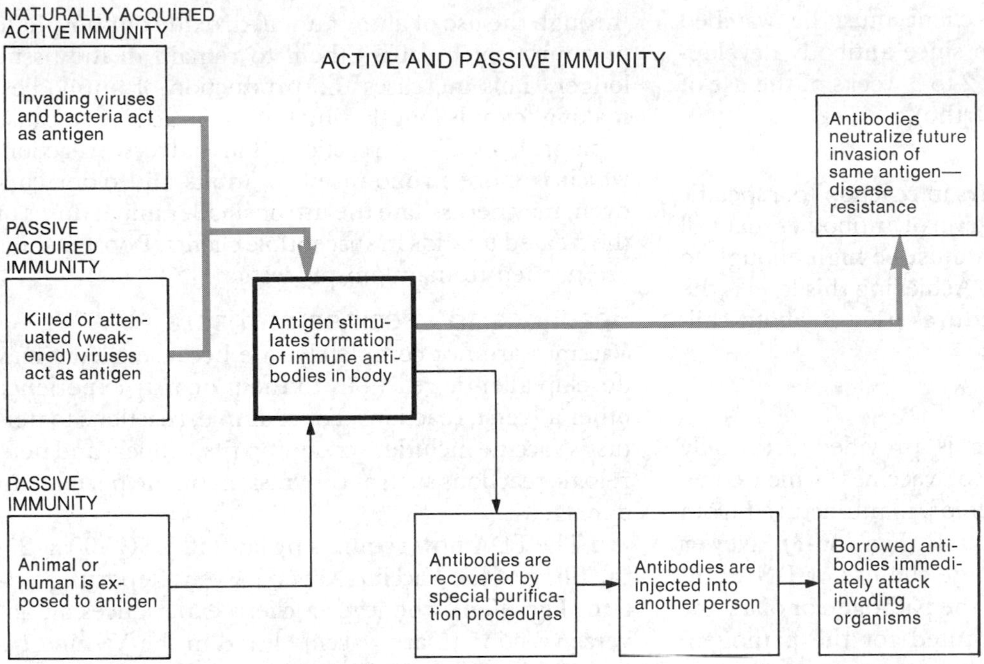

ACTIVE AND PASSIVE IMMUNITY

NATURALLY ACQUIRED
ACTIVE IMMUNITY

Invading viruses
and bacteria act
as antigen

PASSIVE
ACQUIRED
IMMUNITY

Killed or atten-
uated (weak-
ened) viruses
act as antigen

Antigen stimu-
lates formation
of immune anti-
bodies in body

Antibodies
neutralize future
invasion of
same antigen—
disease
resistance

PASSIVE
IMMUNITY

Animal or
human is ex-
posed to antigen

Antibodies are
recovered by
special purifica-
tion procedures

Antibodies are
injected into
another person

Borrowed anti-
bodies immedi-
ately attack
invading
organisms

Figure 36-2. Active and passive immunity.

der, 1991). Bacteriostatic anti-infective agents cannot effectively treat infection in immunodeficient individuals because they only prevent multiplication of pathogens, relying on the recipient's immune response to eradicate them.

Clients with weak immune systems may be treated with agents such as bacillus Calmette-Guérin that provide a general stimulus to the immune system.

Monoclonal antibodies

Scientists can produce monoclonal antibodies (MoAbs) in the laboratory to meet the needs of clients unable to produce sufficient specific antibodies of their own. One example of this procedure is the genetic fusing of disease cells with healthy cells, making hybrid cells (hybridomas) that are capable of unlimited reproduction and of producing a perpetual supply of a specific antibody.

Mice are used in the preparation of most MoAbs, presenting the possibility of allergic responses to mouse protein, a risk that increases with each MoAb administration.

MoAbs are usually administered by slow IV infusion over 1 to 2 hours. Allergic reactions are most likely to occur within 30 to 60 minutes after the IV is started. Vital signs should be checked every 15 minutes during the first hour and then every 30 minutes thereafter. Fever, hypotension, or an increase in heart rate or respirations may be the first side effects noted. Milder reactions (hives, urticaria) can be treated with 25 to 50 mg of diphenhydramine IV. For more serious responses (hypotension, bronchospasm, anaphylaxis, or anaphylactoid reactions), MoAb infusion must be discontinued immediately and an IV of normal saline started. It also may be necessary to administer epi-

nephrine, diphenhydramine, and hydrocortisone. Resuscitation may be necessary if anaphylaxis occurs.

Because MoAbs are a new type of therapy, their side effects are not yet fully known. The client must, therefore, be observed closely for any adverse reactions, which should then be reported and documented. Hypersensitivity may eventually be eliminated when MoAbs are manufactured from human rather than mouse cells (Rieger, 1987, pp 470–473).

MoAbs can also be tailored to attack T cells, thus becoming immunosuppressant in their action. One such MoAb (muromonab-CD3) has been approved for treating acute renal transplant rejection. It acts by specifically attacking all forms of the body's T cells, whether juvenile or mature, helper or suppressor. The antibody attaches itself to the renal-graft T-cell antigen, stopping the T cells from functioning at that time and moderating their future response so that they no longer try to reject the graft. This reversal has been found effective in 94% of the transplants compared to 75% success with high-dose steroids, with graft survival in the MoAb group at 62% versus 45% in the steroid group.

Although this treatment suppresses only the T cells rather than the entire immune system, the risk of infection is equal to that of high-dose steroids. Therefore, infection control is necessary. It is also important to prevent fluid overload prior to or during treatment because of the danger of pulmonary edema.

Frequent side effects that occur with the initial IV injection include fever, chills, dyspnea, tremor, and, less often, chest pain, nausea, vomiting, and wheezing. The symptoms usually occur within 45 to 60 minutes and are alleviated with corticosteroids, antihistamines, and acetaminophen. There is usually better tolerance of subsequent doses. The client must be watched closely for signs of rejection since antibody development has been noted within 2 to 3 weeks of the use of muromonab-CD3 (OKT3-Ortho).

Immunization

The antibody response occurs in reaction to a specific antigen. For this reason, the level of antibodies that will react to an invading antigen must be high enough to cause a response in the host. Achieving this level is the goal of immunization procedures used for both children and adults.

Vaccines and toxoids

Active immunity to disease is provided artificially through the administration of vaccines, which come from microorganisms, or toxoids, manufactured from the poisons of some bacteria (Fig. 36-3). Newer methods of production include the use of DNA and the alteration of the genes of the pathogen or of a safer organism that can be substituted for the pathogen. This leads to greater quantity of a purer product.

Some vaccines are made from viruses, bacteria, or rickettsia that have been inactivated ("killed") by chemicals. Others are made from live microorganisms that have been treated to reduce their pathogenic activity. Both kinds of vaccines will stimulate antibody production without, in most instances, inducing the disease. However, there has been some virulence with type 3 live polio vaccine. Vaccines are available for the prevention of 18 communicable diseases (Amler, 1983). These vaccines differ in their methods of preparation, recommendations for use, routes of administration, and conditions for storage. Immunity attained through the administration of live vaccines is longlasting because it is similar to the immunity acquired by a natural infection.

Toxoids, like vaccines, stimulate antibody production for longlasting immunity without causing disease. During the preparation of toxoids, the toxin's pathogenic quality is destroyed but its antigenic quality remains. Some toxoids are precipitated or absorbed

through the use of aluminum hydroxide or phosphate or alum, which causes them to remain in the tissue longer. This increases the production of antibodies, making toxoids long-lasting but the practice can cause a painful, localized reaction. This adverse reaction, which is more pronounced in adults and older children, may necessitate the use of smaller initial doses of the treated toxoids in susceptible clients. Booster shots are needed to maintain protection.

Reactions to vaccines and sera

Vaccines are not completely safe because clients may develop allergic reactions to them or may experience other adverse reactions. For example, reactions to pertussis vaccine include "screaming fits," shock, and neurologic reactions such as convulsions but no permanent damage.

The FDA now requires by law (42 USC 300aa-25) the filing of the Vaccine Adverse Event Reporting System (Fig. 36-4) whenever a client experiences an adverse reaction to any vaccine listed in the Vaccine Injury Table (Table 36-1). Low-grade allergic responses occur when a vaccine has been made from killed bacteria that used artificial media for growth. Viruses grown in living animal tissues cause a higher rate of allergic reactions. This happens because it is nearly impossible to remove all the foreign protein needed for viral growth, no matter whether the vaccine is made from a live or "dead" virus. For this reason, vaccine made from the live virus may be safer for allergic recipients because they may obtain immunity after a single dose instead of requiring several doses.

Some immune animal sera are used for their antitoxin or antivenom effects. These products may cause allergic reactions, ranging from general discomfort to anaphylactic shock. Usually, the serum has been obtained from horses. For this reason, before administration, the client should be questioned about any previous reaction or exposure to horse serum. If the serum must be used, even when lack of previous serum sensitivity has been established, it is necessary to have epinephrine, corticosteroids, antihistamines, and oxygen available to manage any possible allergic response.

Hypersensitivity is the abnormally high sensitivity of a person to allergens (antigens that cause allergic reactions). In hypersensitive clients, antibodies irritate some body cells and destroy some tissue. *Delayed hypersensitivity* is part of the technique used in the Mantoux tuberculin skin test (Fig. 36-5). In this test, the skin reacts after 24 to 48 hours but this reaction only occurs after preimmunization or an active bout of the disease.

There has been a shortage of vaccines for rubeola, mumps, rubella, pertussis, and haemophilus influenza because drug manufacturers are fearful of product liability lawsuits resulting from repeated adverse reactions. The Federal government has interceded, and now accepts responsibility under the National Childhood Vaccine Injury Act of 1986. Presently, Merck,

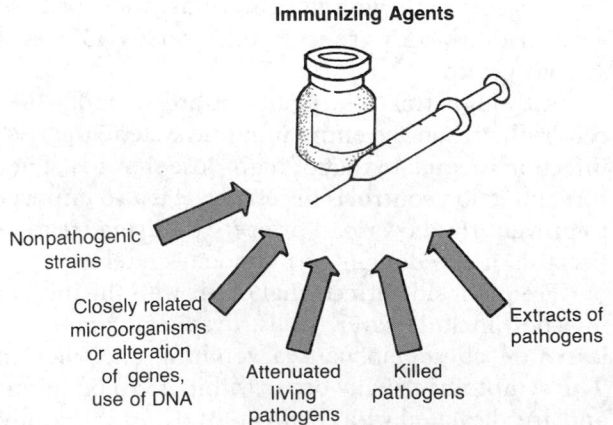

Immunizing Agents

Nonpathogenic strains

Closely related microorganisms or alteration of genes, use of DNA

Attenuated living pathogens

Killed pathogens

Extracts of pathogens

Figure 36-3. Variety of sources of immunizing agents.

VACCINE ADVERSE EVENT REPORTING SYSTEM

24 Hour Toll-free information line 1-800-822-7967

VAERS

Patient identity kept confidential

For CDC/FDA Use Only
VAERS Number _____
Date Received _____

Patient Name:	Vaccine administered by (Name):	Form completed by (Name):
_____ Last First M.I. Address _____ _____ _____	_____ Responsible Physician _____ Facility Name/Address _____ _____ _____	_____ Relation to ☐ Vaccine Provider ☐ Patient/Parent Patient ☐ Manufacturer ☐ Other Address *(if different from patient or provider)* _____ _____ _____
City State Zip	City State Zip	City State Zip
Telephone no. (_____)_____	Telephone no. (_____)_____	Telephone no. (_____)_____

1. State	2. County where administered	3. Date of birth ___/___/___ mm dd yy	4. Patient age	5. Sex ☐ M ☐ F	6. Date form completed ___/___/___ mm dd yy

7. Describe adverse event(s) (symptoms, signs, time course) and treatment, if any	8. Check all appropriate:
	☐ Patient died (date ___/___/___) ☐ Life threatening illness mm dd yy ☐ Required emergency room/doctor visit ☐ Required hospitalization (_____days) ☐ Resulted in prolongation of hospitalization ☐ Resulted in permanent disability ☐ None of the above

9. Patient recovered ☐ YES ☐ NO ☐ UNKNOWN	10. Date of vaccination	11. Adverse event onset
12. Relevant diagnostic tests/laboratory data	___/___/___ mm dd yy Time _____ AM PM	___/___/___ mm dd yy Time _____ AM PM

13. Enter all vaccines given on date listed in no. 10

	Vaccine (type)	Manufacturer	Lot number	Route/Site	No. Previous doses
a.	_____	_____	_____	_____	_____
b.	_____	_____	_____	_____	_____
c.	_____	_____	_____	_____	_____
d.	_____	_____	_____	_____	_____

14. Any other vaccinations within 4 weeks of date listed in no. 10

	Vaccine (type)	Manufacturer	Lot number	Route/Site	No. Previous doses	Date given
a.	_____	_____	_____	_____	_____	_____
b.	_____	_____	_____	_____	_____	_____

15. Vaccinated at: ☐ Private doctor's office/hospital ☐ Military clinic/hospital ☐ Public health clinic/hospital ☐ Other/unknown	16. Vaccine purchased with: ☐ Private funds ☐ Military funds ☐ Public funds ☐ Other /unknown	17. Other medications

18. Illness at time of vaccination (specify)	19. Pre-existing physician-diagnosed allergies, birth defects, medical conditions (specify)

20. Have you reported this adverse event previously?	☐ No ☐ To doctor	☐ To health department ☐ To manufacturer	*Only for children 5 and under*
			22. Birth weight _____ lb. _____ oz.	23. No. of brothers and sisters

21. Adverse event following prior vaccination (check all applicable, specify)				*Only for reports submitted by manufacturer/immunization project*

	Adverse Event	Onset Age	Type Vaccine	Dose no. in series	24. Mfr. / imm. proj. report no.	25. Date received by mfr. / imm. proj.
☐ In patient	____	____	____	____		
☐ In brother	____	____	____	____	26. 15 day report?	27. Report type
or sister	____	____	____	____	☐ Yes ☐ No	☐ Initial ☐ Follow-Up

Health care providers and manufacturers are required by law (42 USC 300aa-25) to report reactions to vaccines listed in the Vaccine Injury Table.
Reports for reactions to other vaccines are voluntary except when required as a condition of immunization grant awards

Form VAERS -1   P

Figure 36-4. Sample Vaccine Adverse Event Reporting System form.

Table 36-1. Reportable events following vaccination

Vaccine/toxoid	Event	Interval from vaccination
DTP, P, DTP/Polio Combined	A. Anaphylaxis or anaphylactic shock	24 hours
	B. Encephalopathy (or encephalitis)*	7 days
	C. Shock-collapse or hypotonic-hyporesponsive collapse*	7 days
	D. Residual seizure disorder*	See aids to interpretation*
	E. Any acute complication or sequela (including death) arising from above events	No limit
	F. Events in vaccinees described in manufacturer's package insert as contraindications to additional doses of vaccine† (such as convulsions)	See package insert
Measles, Mumps, and Rubella; DT, Td, Tetanus Toxoid	A. Anaphylaxis or anaphylactic shock	24 hours
	B. Encephalopathy (or encephalitis)*	15 days for measles, mumps, and rubella vaccines; 7 days for DT, Td, and T toxoids
	C. Residual seizure disorder*	See Aids to Interpretation*
	D. Any acute complication or sequela (including death) of above events	No limit
	E. Events in vaccinees described in manufacturer's package insert as contraindications to additional doses of vaccine†	See package insert
Oral Polio Vaccine	A. Paralytic poliomyelitis in a nonimmunodeficient recipient; in an immunodeficient recipient; and in a vaccine-associated community case	30 days / 6 months / No limit
	B. Any acute complication or sequela (including death) of above events	No limit
	C. Events in vaccinees described in manufacturer's package insert as contraindications to additional doses of vaccine†	See package insert
Inactivated Polio Vaccine	A. Anaphylaxis or anaphylactic shock	24 hours
	B. Any acute complication or sequela (including death) of above event	No limit
	C. Events in vaccinees described in manufacturer's package insert as contraindications to additional doses of vaccine†	See package insert

* **Aids to interpretation**: Shock-collapse or hypotonic-hyporesponsive collapse may be evidenced by signs or symptoms such as decrease in or loss of muscle tone; paralysis (partial or complete); hemiplegia; hemiparesis; loss of color or turning pale white or blue; unresponsiveness to environmental stimuli; depression of or loss of consciousness; prolonged sleeping with difficulty arousing; or cardiovascular or respiratory arrest.

Residual seizure disorder may be considered to have occurred if no other seizure or convulsion unaccompanied by fever or accompanied by a fever of less than 102°F occurred before the first seizure or convulsion after the administration of the vaccine involved, AND, if in the case of measles-, mumps-, or rubella-containing vaccines, the first seizure or convulsion occurred within 15 days after vaccination OR in the case of any other vaccine, the first seizure or convulsion occurred within 3 days after vaccination, AND, if two or more seizures or convulsions unaccompanied by fever or accompanied by a fever of less than 102°F occurred within 1 year after vaccination.

The terms seizure and convulsion include grand mal, petit mal, absence, myoclonic, tonic-clonic, and focal motor seizures and signs. Encephalopathy means any significant acquired abnormality of, injury to, or impairment of function of the brain. Among the frequent manifestations of encephalopathy are focal and diffuse neurologic signs, increased intracranial pressure, or changes lasting at least 6 hours in level of consciousness, with or without convulsions. The neurologic signs and symptoms of encephalopathy may be temporary with complete recovery, or they may result in various degrees of permanent impairment. Signs and symptoms such as high-pitched and unusual screaming, persistent unconsolable crying, and bulging fontanel are compatible with an encephalopathy, but in and of themselves are not conclusive evidence of encephalopathy. Encephalopathy usually can be documented by slow wave activity on an electroencephalogram.

† The health care provider must refer to the Contraindication section of the manufacturer's package insert for each vaccine.

From *FDA Drug Bulletin*, October, 1990.

Sharp, and Dohme has agreed to develop and market vaccines in the United States.

Research is now focusing on genetic engineering techniques to develop a new type of recombinant vaccine based on bacillus Calmette Guérin that could be administered with one injection at birth, and would protect a child against 12 or more diseases. This would be particularly valuable in areas where health care is not easily accessible, as in developing nations. It would also eliminate the need for boosters, and bring the price down to as little as $.06 per dose (Angier, 1991).

Special concerns

There has been a resurgence of measles throughout the United States, in large part due to the ineffectiveness of the vaccine administered prior to 1957. In 1990, 26,500 cases were reported, with more children dying than any year since 1971. The American Nurses' Association urges nurses to establish local efforts for the promotion of immunizations, particularly for infants and young children, as well as for health workers exposed to the measles virus (ANA urges nurses to promote immunization standards, 1991).

The public, and in particular health professionals (because of their exposure to contaminated blood, fecal and other sources of the disease), should be alerted to the seriousness of hepatitis B infections, and to the importance of preventative vaccinations.

The recommendation has been made that neonates at high risk for hepatitis B (those living in households with an infected person, children born of drug abusers or to immigrants from endemic areas such as

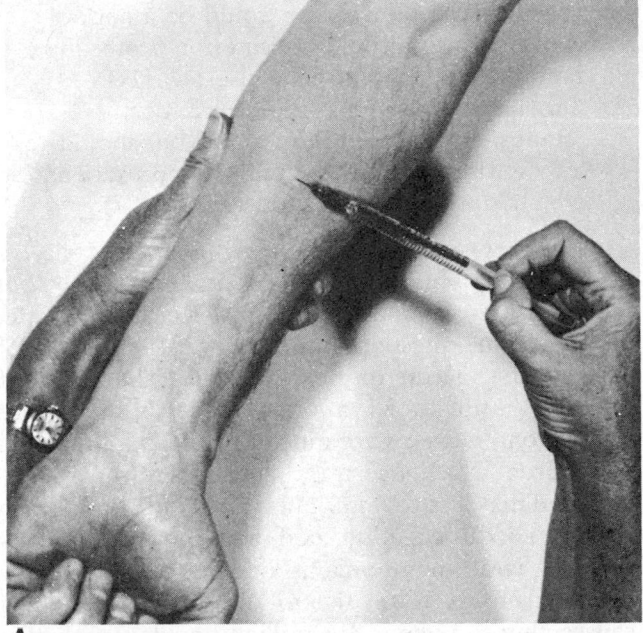

A

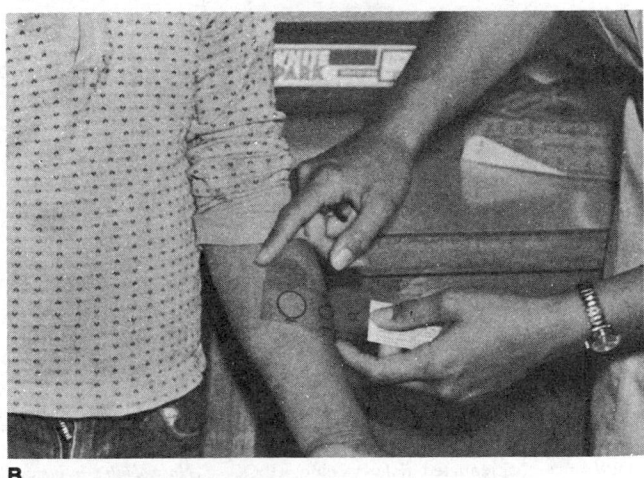

B

Figure 36-5. The Mantoux intracutaneous test to detect persons with the tubercle bacillus. A. A tuberculin syringe and a subcutaneous needle, with the bevel up, are used to inject purified protein derivative (PPD) into the skin of the forearm to form a wheal. B. Interpretation of the Mantoux test. The test is read 48–72 hours after injection because tuberculin skin tests are tests of delayed hypersensitivity. The area of induration (not erythema) is measured most accurately with the aid of a plastic ruler containing concentric circles of specific diameters. (Courtesy of American Lung Association)

Alaska, Southeast Asia, the Pacific Islands, China) be given HBV (Recombivax HB, Engerix B) at birth. Up to 50% of children infected with hepatitis B before their fifth birthday will become chronic carriers of the disease. Of those infected at birth, 90% will become chronic carriers.

To counteract the reluctance of adults to be immunized against hepatitis B, the Immunization Practices Advisory Committee of the Public Health Service has recommended that children receive the hepatitis B vaccine at 2, 4, 6, and 15 months. This is suggested despite the fact that those affected by the disease are usually teenagers or adults. It is the first time that a program to prevent illness and possibly death in adults is being directed toward children. The effectiveness will not be apparent until the vaccinated children reach their teens or adulthood.

Selection of an immunization program

The selection of a proper immunization program for the client is determined to some extent by genetic considerations. For example, some infants are found to have agammaglobulinemia or hypogammaglobulinemia. Research now underway demonstrates that immune system response requires the presence of two distinct genes, which are expressed by the actions of the thymus-derived (T) lymphocytes and the bone marrow-derived (B) lymphocytes.

Two committees review data on immunizations, give recommendations on immunization programs, and publish revised information. They are the Committee on Infectious Diseases appointed by the American Academy of Pediatrics (AAP) and the Public Health Service Advisory Committee on Immunization Practices (ACIP), under the Centers for Disease Control (CDC). The American Academy of Pediatrics and its newsletters are concerned with pediatric and general practice in conjunction with public health. Therefore, there may be some differences between its recommendations and those of the ACIP in its *CDC Morbidity and Mortality Weekly Report*.

Enrichment experience 36-1

You are speaking to a group of new mothers who question the need for routine immunization. What information would you provide to convince them of the value of this protection?

Schedule for infants and children

The usual schedule for active immunization of infants and children is given in Table 36-2. The recommendation has been made that a new conjugate vaccine, *Haemophilus influenzae* vaccine (HbOC), available since 1990, be given to all children.

The ACIP has listed the following guidelines for immunizations of children infected with HIV.

Table 36-2. Active immunization schedule for infants and children

Age	Immunization
2 months	DPT, OPV (earlier in high endemic areas, HBV, HbOC
4 months	DPT, OPV, HBV, HbOC
6 months	DPT, OPV (may be given if desired, as in southwest United States), measles vaccine in epidemic areas, HbOC
12 months	Measles vaccine in epidemic areas (omit at 15 months)
15 months	HbOC, MMR
18 months	DPT, OPV
4–6 years	DPT, OPV; MMR before entry to school
11–12 years	MMR
14–16 year	Td and every 10 years thereafter
College	Measles if newer vaccine was not used previously

DPT = diphtheria and tetanus toxoids and pertussis vaccine combined; OPV = oral attenuated polio vaccine; HbOC = *Haemophilus influenza B* conjugate vaccine; HBV = hepatitis B vaccine; MMR = measles, mumps, rubella; and Td = adult-type combined tetanus and diphtheria toxoids, containing a smaller diphtheria compound than TD.

Immunization with VZIG (varicella-zoster immune globulin) should be considered for immunocompromised children or other children at high risk.

Updated from the 1982 Report of the Committee of Infectious Diseases of the American Academy of Pediatrics.

Children with symptomatic HIV infections

1. Inactivated polio vaccine replaces the oral polio vaccine. Do not administer mumps-measles-rubella vaccine, bacillus Calmette Guérin vaccine, or other live vaccines.
2. The following inactivated vaccines should be given, although the immunization may be less effective than in immunocompetent children: diphtheria-pertussis-tetanus vaccine, *Haemophilus influenzae* type B (HbOC) vaccine and, as previously noted, inactivated polio vaccine.
3. Annual immunizations with inactivated influenza vaccine are recommended for children over 6 months of age; one-time administration of pneumococcal vaccine is recommended for those over 2 years of age.
4. Passive immunization with immune globulin or varicella-zoster immune globulin should be administered to any immunocompromised child who has had significant exposure to measles or varicella. These children are at increased risk of developing serious complications from either disease.

Children with previously diagnosed asymptomatic HIV infection

1. Mumps-measles-rubella should be administered, watching for possible adverse reactions, as well as for the disease itself, since effectiveness may be less than for uncompromised children.

2. Inactivated polio vaccine would be a better choice than oral polio vaccine for protecting family members who may also have HIV.
3. Other immunizations (diphtheria-pertussis-tetanus, *Haemophilus influenzae* type) should follow ACIP recommendations (Immunizations for US children with HIV infections, 1987).

The newest vaccine for chickenpox is varicellazoster immune globulin (VZIG). Clinical trials show that varicellazoster immune globulin is effective and safe. There is some question, however, over the wisdom of offering the vaccine to the public since the length of immunity is not known, and the severity of the disease and its complications are much greater in adults than in children. The concern is that children who are immunized may lose that immunity in later life and catch chickenpox during adulthood, with the chance of developing viral pneumonia as a consequence.

Chickenpox is related to the herpes virus and causes illness in about 3½ million people a year. It is usually a highly contagious, benign disease for children under 15 years of age. However, some children develop complications, including encephalitis and viral pneumonia, and about 100 die from varicella each year. There are situations when it can become life-threatening, as in immunocompromised children, newborns infected transplacentally just before birth, bone marrow recipients, persons with neoplastic diseases, exposed infants or adults over 30 years of age, and pregnant women. When contracted during pregnancy, chickenpox can cause fetal death. If the fetus is infected and survives, there is the possibility that the baby will suffer brain damage and be mentally retarded.

The chickenpox virus remains in the body for life, entering nerve cells and migrating to the nerves in the spine. If the immune system is weakened later in life, the virus may emerge to cause shingles, a painful inflammation of a nerve that produces a rash along the nerve pathway on the skin. Pain occurs along the nerve endings in the area of the rash, usually lasting for a short time but sometimes lasting for years (postherpetic neuralgia). Shingles on the upper half of the face can involve the cornea (zoster keratitis), which can lead to blindness unless treated.

Immunocompromised children are at risk for serious complications from chickenpox. The vaccine has been given to 400 children with leukemia, of whom 60 were exposed to chickenpox in their families. Of those, 85% did not develop the disease, and the other 15% had only mild cases. One concern about using this attenuated live virus is that it can cause shingles in these children to about the same extent that it occurs after a bout of the natural disease. In addition, about 5% of the children developed the chickenpox rash. They were treated with acyclovir, which prevented the virus from replicating. Research is now underway to determine whether acyclovir will shorten the length of illness in otherwise healthy children (Kolata, 1987).

Immunization of adults

Some adults have been improperly or never immunized against vaccine-preventable diseases and may not have been exposed to these diseases as children. Therefore, medical histories taken from adults should include this information with the idea of offering them a program of immunization, particularly if they are in a high-risk group (Table 36-3) or pregnant (Table 36-4).

It has been recommended that persons born after 1956 should be required to have proof of live measles vaccination on or after the first birthday or documentation of having had physician-diagnosed measles. Those who cannot provide this information should be vaccinated unless they are likely to have an anaphylactic reaction related to egg ingestion, they have been immunocompromised, or they are receiving corticosteroids, alkylating drugs, antimetabolites, or radiation (Amler, 1983).

Immunization for adults should be determined on an individual basis, taking age, physical status, and possible allergic reactions into account. Pertussis immunization is inappropriate because the risk of reactions to the vaccine outweigh the protection needed, particularly in elderly clients.

Immunologic agents

Table 36-5 provides information about the usual methods of administration and doses of immunologic agents. See Box 36-1 for general considerations for immunization.

Rho(D) isoimmunization

The immune system sometimes miscalculates when trying to protect the individual, as when antibodies to an Rh-positive fetus develop in an Rh-negative mother. The fetus is perceived as an invader to be destroyed, a process that can be prevented or stopped with proper treatment.

Prophylaxis to prevent isoimmunization resulting from a mother with negative Rhesus (Rh) factor, (an antigen system in which the D antigen is of primary importance) bearing an Rho(D)-positive fetus, involves administration of Rho(D) immune globulin by intramuscular injection within 72 hours after delivery. This helps prevent sensitization of the mother by fetal blood cells that may enter her blood, leading to her production of anti-D antibodies. If antibodies are produced by the mother, they can cross the placenta and cause agglutination of the fetal red blood cells. This process may lead to hemolysis and loss of erythrocytes, with the possibility of fetal anemia, heart failure, and hydrops.

Rho(D) immune globulin should also be given to any Rh-negative woman within 72 hours after a termination of pregnancy, a transfusion of Rh-positive blood, a chorionic villus biopsy, or an amniocentesis, particularly if the needle has gone through the placenta. Research is now underway to determine whether the Rh-negative newborn of an Rh-positive mother should also be given Rho(D) immune globulin,

---

Table 36-3. Suggested immunizations for unimmunized adults

Disease	Agent	Comments
Influenza	Inactivated virus vaccine	Annual vaccination for those over 65 or at high risk
	Live virus vaccine in nose drops or spray (under development)	
Diphtheria Tetanus	Combined tetanus and diphtheria toxoids	Two doses 4 weeks apart
		Third dose 6–12 months after second dose
		Booster every 10 years
Measles	Live virus vaccine	One dose for those born after 1956; important for those attending college
Mumps	Live virus vaccine	One dose; important for postpubertal males to prevent orchitis associated with mumps
Rubella	Live virus vaccine	One dose; important for nonpregnant women of childbearing age to prevent fetal abnormalities associated with rubella during pregnancy
Poliomyelitis	IPV (inactivated polio vaccine) OPV (live virus trivalent oral polio vaccine)	For inadequately immunized adults in contact with children being vaccinated with OPV
		IPV preferred: three doses, 4 weeks apart, then fourth dose 6–12 months after third dose
		OPV—3 doses
		Single dose of IPV or OPV can be administered to adults with documentation of previously completed primary series.
Varicella-zoster	Varicella-zoster immune globulin	For immunocompromised children or the elderly at risk of zoster, as well as persons receiving corticosteroids

Table 36-4. Vaccination during pregnancy

	Vaccine	Indications for vaccination during pregnancy
Live virus vaccines		
Measles Mumps Rubella	Live-attenuated	Contraindicated
Yellow fever	Live-attenuated	Contraindicated except if exposure is unavoidable
Poliomyelitis	Trivalent live-attenuated (OPV)	Persons at substantial risk of exposure may receive live-attenuated virus vaccine
Inactivated virus vaccines		
Hepatitis B	Plasma derived or recombinant produced purified hepatitis B surface antigen	Pregnancy is not a contraindication
Influenza	Inactivated type A and type B virus vaccines	Usually recommended only for patients with serious underlying disease. It is prudent to avoid vaccination during the first trimester. Consult health authorities for current recommendations.
Poliomyelitis	Killed virus (IPV)	OPV not IPV, is indicated when immediate protection of pregnant females is needed.
Rabies	Killed virus Rabies IG	Substantial risk of exposure
Inactivated bacterial vaccines		
Cholera Typhoid	Killed bacterial	Should reflect actual risks of disease and probable benefits of vaccine
Plague	Killed bacterial	Selective vaccination of exposed persons
Meningococcal	Polysaccharide	Only in unusual outbreak situations
Pneumococcal	Polysaccharide	Only for high-risk persons
Toxoids		
Tetanus-diphtheria (Td)	Combined tetanus-diphtheria toxoids, adult formulation	Lack of primary series, or no booster within past 10 years. It is prudent to avoid vaccination during first trimester.
Immune globulins, pooled or hyperimmune		
	Immune globulin or specific globulin preparations	Exposure or anticipated unavoidable exposure to measles, hepatitis A, hepatitis B, rabies, or tetanus

to prevent sensitization due to an inadvertent transfer of maternal blood to the fetus during labor and delivery.

A supplement to the protocol has been developed using prenatal administration of Rho(D) immune globulin. This is particularly helpful if, for any reason, the Rho(D)-negative woman develops anti-D antibodies during the pregnancy. Because isoimmunization is unlikely to occur before the third trimester, the Rho(D) immune globulin is usually administered during the 28th week of gestation and again within 72 hours after delivery if the fetus is Rho(D) positive. Maternal reactions to the immune globulin are infrequent and usually localized. The prenatal use of Rho(D) immune globulin is expensive but it is estimated that it lowers maternal sensitization rates from

15% of all untreated women at risk to 1.5%–2% for those treated.

Antibody testing of women who are already immunized should be done monthly through the 28th week of pregnancy and then twice a month. After the 22nd week of pregnancy, amniocentesis should be done if the antibody level is higher than 1.0 μg/ml. Exchange transfusions are ordered for the fetus when appropriate (Filbey, 1987, p 15).

Viral flu vaccines

Flu vaccines have presented difficulties because a specific vaccine had to be developed for each different influenza virus. Again, past vaccines were not without risk, as was shown in the mass vaccination program against swine flu in 1976. Some recipients developed

Table 36-5. Immunologic agents

Agent	Methods of administration	Doses	Comments
BCG	Intradermal	0.1 ml	Provides active immunity against tuberculosis in those with negative skin test
cholera vaccine	SC, IM	Two doses of 0.5–1 ml, 7–28 days apart	Revaccinate with 0.5 ml every 6 months for those at risk
diphtheria and tetanus toxoids, pertussis vaccine	SC	Three doses of 0.5–1 ml, 4–6 weeks apart; one dose 1 year later	
influenza vaccine (various strains)	SC	Two injections of 0.5 ml at least 2 months apart	May be replaced by modified live virus nasal spray
measles virus vaccine (live, attenuated)	SC	1 vial (1,000 TCID*)	
mumps virus vaccine (live, attenuated)	SC	1 vial (5,000 TCID*)	
Poliomyelitis vaccine	SC, O	SC: three injections of 1 ml 4–5 weeks apart, 1 ml at least 7 months later; O (trivalent): dose depends on concentration used; 3 doses are given at 8-week intervals	
pneumococcal vaccine, polyvalent (Pneumovax 23)	SC, IM	0.5 ml	Protects against lobar pneumonia and bacteremia caused by 23 types of pneumococci
Rocky Mountain spotted fever vaccine	SC	1 ml for three doses 7–10 days apart	
rubella virus vaccine (live, attenuated)	SC	1 vial (1,000 TCID*)	For children and nonpregnant women of childbearing age
typhoid and paratyphoid vaccines	SC	0.5 ml for two doses, 28 days apart	For travelers who may be in contact with disease
typhus vaccine	SC	1 ml for two doses, 28 days apart	For travelers who may be in contact with disease
Yellow fever vaccine	SC	0.5 ml	For travelers who may be in contact with disease
Hepatitis B vaccine (from recombinant DNA)	SC	Dose amounts and schedule not yet established	For clients who are on hemodialysis; those with hemoglobinopathies or clotting disorders who receive frequent transfusions; those with an immune deficiency; oncology and transplant clients; men in military service; spouses of carriers and children of carrier mothers; those living or traveling in endemic areas; health care professionals working in high-risk practices; others at risk due to special situations (drug addicts, institutionalized clients, homosexual men, and prostitutes)
Agents given following exposure			
Botulism antitoxin (passive immunizing agent)	IM, IV	10,000–50,000 U	Also given prophylactically in dose of 2,500 U
Hepatitis B immune globulin, human	IM	0.06 ml/kg	Administer as soon as possible after exposure
Rabies vaccine, human diploid cell	IM	Single-dose vial	First dose is given as soon as possible after exposure; an additional dose is given on days 3, 7, 14, and 28 after the first dose
Tetanus antitoxin (passive immunizing agent)	IM, SC	3,000–50,000 U	
Tetanus immune globulin (passive immunizing agent)	Im	250 U or more	Preferred to tetanus antitoxin because it does not cause allergic reactions and has a longer duration of action

*TCID = tissue culture infectious doses.

Adapted from Hoffman CP, Lipkin GB. (1981). *Simplified nursing*, 9th ed. Philadelphia: JB Lippincott.

Box 36-1. General considerations for immunization

1. Immunizations may be started at any age. If an immunization program is not begun in infancy, a slightly different schedule may be followed, depending on the age and the prevalence of specific infections at the time.
2. An interrupted primary series of immunizations need not be restarted; it need only be continued, regardless of the length of time that has elapsed.
3. The immunoresponse is limited in a significant proportion of young infants, and the recommended booster doses are designed to ensure and maintain immunity.
4. A time lapse of 8 weeks is recommended between the first three DPT injections for desirable maximum effects.
    a. The combination of depot antigens is preferred because it is more immunogenic.
    b. Because of the increased risk of possible reactions to either diphtheria or pertussis antigen, Td (adult-type tetanus and diphtheria toxins) is recommended for children over 6 years of age.
    c. For contaminated wounds, a booster dose of tetanus should be given if more than 5 years have elapsed since the last dose.
5. Pertussis
    a. Protection of infants against pertussis should begin early.
    b. In newborn infants, the best protection against pertussis is avoidance of household contacts by adequate immunization of siblings.
6. Tuberculin test
    a. It is recommended that the tuberculin test be given before or simultaneously with the measles vaccine.
        1. The measles vaccine may invalidate the tuberculin test, giving a false-negative finding, if given within 6 weeks after measles immunization. Theoretically, measles vaccine could activate latent tuberculosis.
    b. Frequency of repeated tuberculin testing depends on the following:
        1. Risk of exposure to the child
        2. Prevalence of tuberculosis in the population group
        3. High-risk situations; intervals between routine testing should not exceed 6 months.
7. Measles vaccine is most effective when given at about 12–15 months of age. At this age, all maternal transplacental antibody has been catabolized. Measles vaccine may be administered at 6 months of age when child is at a high risk of contact with natural measles. A

second dose should be given 12–15 months of age if the original vaccine was given prior to 1 year of age, since the rate of seroconversion before 1 year of age is variable. A third dose should be given prior to starting school.
8. Live trivalent oral polio virus vaccine is preferred to the inactivated form because administration is easier, and the immunologic effects are broader and longer.
9. Mumps vaccine—all preadolescent or older males who have not had mumps should be immunized.
10. Rubella vaccine
    a. Live vaccine is recommended for boys and girls between 1 year of age and puberty.
    b. Children in kindergarten should be given priority because they are the major source of viral dissemination.
    c. A history of rubella illness is not reliable enough to exclude children from immunization.
    d. Nonimmunized, nonpregnant women of childbearing age should be vaccinated.
11. Immunizations should be deferred if child has an acute febrile infection or illness. The common cold, without fever, is not a contraindication to immunization.
12. Contraindications to receiving measles-mumps and rubella vaccines include the following: pregnancy; generalized malignancy; cell-mediated immunodeficiency disorders; current immunosuppressant therapy; sensitivity to animal species used in vaccine preparation; transfusion of immune serum globulin, plasma, or blood. If any of these contraindications exist, immunizations may be temporarily deferred or an alternative vaccine preparation may be used.
13. Smallpox vaccination
    a. No longer recommended in the United States.
    b. Where indicated (*ie,* while traveling), initial smallpox vaccine may be given at any time between 12 and 24 months of age (after age 12, it may be given every 3–10 years).
14. A good nursing history will include determining whether or not the child has been exposed to or has experienced any communicable disease. Surveillance in this area will prevent unnecessary disease and allow for proper immunization for the child and family.
15. Strict adherence to the manufacturer's storage recommendations is vital. Failure to observe these precautions and recommendations may reduce the potency and effectiveness of the specific vaccine.

Adapted from Hoffman CP, Lipkin GB. (1981). *Simplified nursing,* 9th ed. Philadelphia: JB Lippincott.

Guillain-Barré syndrome with paralysis, and some people even died. It is important to evaluate the medical risk for the client before administering the vaccine. Because the aged and infirm are usually at greater risk, it is suggested that they be given the vaccine appropriate for the prevalent flu virus.

A safer, more durable influenza vaccine is now available because of new methodology. A live virus vaccine, made harmless through modification of its genes in the laboratory, is given by nose drops or nasal spray. This technique appears to offer greater immunity to influenza for the recipient than injections of vaccines made from killed viruses. It also results in a significant reduction of the amount of flu viruses shed into the air by the client after exposure to the disease-causing flu viruses.

The use of this new virus, harmless in itself, results in stimulation of the client's immunity. Because the live virus can be manipulated within a laboratory setting, it is conceivable that vaccines could be developed quickly to meet the challenge of rapidly changing influenza viruses. In addition, the public is likely to accept vaccine administered in nose drops or sprays more readily than that given by injection. Live virus vaccines increase antibodies in the respiratory tract and blood and also stimulate cell-mediated immunity. Dead virus vaccines lead to higher antibody levels mostly limited to the blood and, therefore, are not as effective.

Future developments

Research is now being directed at developing a vaccine against malignant melanoma. This cancer of the melanocytes is the result of unprotected overexposure to sunlight. If a melanoma is removed surgically when it is less than 0.75 mm thick, there is an almost 100% cure rate.

However, if it is thicker than one-eighth of an inch, it has probably metastasized, and has become difficult to treat. Immunotherapy is now being used since there are a high number of antigens on the melanoma's surface that would be easy targets for this treatment. Presently, a harmless version of the vaccinia virus has been placed in the melanoma cell taken from a client, and the membranes of the infected cell then pulverized, leaving a combination of vaccinia particles and melanoma antigens. This mixture has then been injected into the client, with 80% surviving for 2 years without a recurrence. In time, the vaccine should be available to inoculate those at high risk as a preventative before the formation of the tumor.

Another approach is the use of interleukin-2 and interferon to stimulate the production of immune cells. The use of either drug in infusions has resulted in marked regressions from several months to over 5 years. More testing will take place to determine the full effectiveness of these drugs.

Human gene therapy was approved by the FDA in 1991 for experimental treatment of advanced melanoma. Tumor-infiltrating lymphocytes from the client will be combined with the gene for tumor necrosis factor and grown in media for 4–6 weeks. The altered cells will then be returned to the client in a transfusion. Tumor necrosis factor cuts off the developing blood supply in tumors but can cause shock and body wasting if left in the body too long. The tumor-infiltrating lymphocyte cells will carry the tumor necrosis factor directly to the tumor, which should maximize the benefits and minimize toxicity to the rest of the body.

In the underdeveloped, nonindustrialized nations, tuberculosis, typhoid, diphtheria, pertussis, tetanus, and measles are the most prevalent life-threatening diseases. As vaccines are introduced into these countries to prevent death from childhood diseases, there will be an increased need for the development of protective vaccines against the parasites and other diseases common among adolescents in these nations.

In the future, there may be vaccines available for protection against syphilis, dental caries, acquired immunodeficiency syndrome, and other infections. The National Institute of Allergy and Infectious Diseases is presently supporting projects that splice genes to design new vaccines for influenza, hepatitis, chickenpox, herpes, gastroenteritis, gonorrhea, respiratory illnesses, and childhood diarrhea.

■ Summary

Immunity to infectious diseases can be provided through the use of immunizing agents to persons who have not been previously exposed. This immunity can be acquired passively on a temporary basis through immune sera. Active immunity can be acquired by vaccines made from live or killed viruses, or from toxoids, which are manufactured from the poisons of some bacteria.

Nursing management

Nursing implications

Immunization is usually considered a safe procedure; in most cases, reactions are minor and pass in a few days. However, because there are some risk factors, such as allergies and adverse reactions, vaccinations should always be given with caution.

Adverse reactions to usual immunization procedures commonly include low-grade fever, swelling, and soreness at the site of injection. On rare occasions, anaphylaxis occurs, usually immediately after administration of the antigen. Mild reactions occur 12 to 24 hours after immunization.

Prospective travelers should contact their local health department for current information about immunizations needed for international travel. The requirements vary from time to time and from country to country. The requirements sometimes change because a particular disease has been eradicated in a certain country (see Chapter 44).

Monoclonal antibodies present a new set of challenges for nurses. Since they have been used for a short time only, it is likely that there are potential problems that have yet to surface. It is, therefore, imperative that any adverse reactions, expected or not, be reported and documented immediately.

Immunosuppressive drugs can result in serious infections because of the body's inability to protect itself. To compensate for this, strict reverse isolation techniques may be necessary, including the screening of visitors with communicable diseases (including the common cold). Opportunistic infections can kill the immunocompromised patient. MoAbs may cause, among other things, chills with fevers of 104° F (40° C), nausea, vomiting, and chest pains. Some reactions can be checked with corticosteroids, antihistamines, or acetaminophen. More serious side effects may require immediate termination of treatment, and the start of normal saline IV. Drugs such as epinephrine, diphenhydramine, or hydrocortisone may be required. Resuscitation may be necessary if anaphylaxis occurs.

Nursing process

Assessment   An assessment of all pertinent client information enables the nurse to set priorities for care. A complete immunization history, including reactions to any previous vaccinations, information about allergies (particularly to eggs and horse serum), and the present health status of the client, will help determine the immunization schedule that should be followed. Health personnel must be especially careful in taking histories to determine if the client has any allergies. This care may prevent a fatal reaction to a vaccine, antiserum, or gamma globulin. The possible medical risks must be weighed against the expected benefits of vaccination.

If the vaccine is derived from chicken embryo, antibiotics, or another inorganic material, the client may be allergic to the vaccine. Package inserts should be consulted for a list of the vaccine's components before inoculation. This information should be compared with the client's history to determine if the vaccine is contraindicated. Further questioning should be continued if there is even a possibility that the client may have allergies to any of the substances in the vaccine.

For women of childbearing age, reproductive status must be determined. Live virus vaccines are contraindicated for pregnant women or when pregnancy is a possibility or for immunocompromised individuals, including those with the HIV virus. It is safe, however, to immunize the child of a pregnant woman because the vaccine virus is not communicable (See Table 36-5).

Nursing diagnosis   Nursing diagnoses likely to be made for clients receiving immunizations include the following:

> *High risk for altered body temperature related to response to immunizing antigens*
> *High risk for altered tissue integrity related to inflammatory response secondary to immunizing antigens*
> *Knowledge deficit concerning immunization*

A common collaborative problem that should be differentiated from the nursing diagnoses is

> *Potential complication: anaphylactic shock*

Planning   Goals of nursing care are to prevent severe reactions to immunizing medications, alleviate or eliminate fever and inflammation, maintain vital functions during anaphylactic reactions, and teach the client (and public) about immunization.

Intervention   No matter what the reason for vaccination, it is important to check the potency of the vaccine and be aware of how long it is expected to confer immunity. Vaccines must also be stored properly, according to the manufacturer's instructions, to ensure potency, and they must be used within the time limit set by the manufacturer and according to the manufacturer's specific recommendations.

When assessment of the client reveals contraindications for immunization, the nurse should alert the physician to the situation. Following administration of the antigen, clients should be monitored for at least 30 minutes for immediate reaction such as anaphylaxis.

Emergency equipment and medications, such as epinephrine and antihistamines, must always be available for managing an anaphylactic reaction.

The health care worker should keep accurate immunization records in the health care center and give one to the client or, in the case of children, to parents. Adverse reactions should be documented in both records and adverse reactions to vaccines listed on the Vaccine Injury Table reported as required by law.

Client education.   Before giving immunizations, nurses should inform parents and clients of expected beneficial and possible adverse reactions. If a health care facility requires parents to sign informed consent papers, the nurse should tell parents and clients not to be unduly alarmed.

Clients should be advised to observe for adverse reactions and to contact their physician if they occur (see Table 36-1). Children should be instructed not to scratch or rub the site of an injection. Such an action may cause autoinoculation. To reduce itching, parents may apply cold compresses and instruct the child to

Example of nursing process and MoAb therapy

The client is a 30-year-old woman who had a kidney transplant about 6 months prior to the present hospital admission. Her progress following surgery was slow, with poor food intake, episodes of edema, and extreme fatigue. Her recent laboratory studies, x-rays, and antibody levels all indicated that her body was rejecting the kidney. The physician decided to administer a MoAb, muromonab-CD 3, which has been approved for treatment of acute renal transplant rejection.

Assessment data	Nursing diagnosis	Intervention	Goals and outcome criteria
Diagnosis of kidney transplant rejection	Hopelessness related to dependence on transplanted kidney, which may be rejected	**Explain** to the client the MoAb treatment that has been ordered. **Remind** the client that dialysis or another kidney transplant are still viable treatments.	The client will express a realistic appraisal of prognosis.
Inadequate function of transplanted kidney	Fluid volume excess: hypervolemia related to oliguria due to kidney failure	**Limit** fluids before and during treatment.	The client will not develop swelling of peripheral tissues or dyspnea due to pulmonary edema.
Treatment involving immunosuppression	High risk for infection related to immunosuppression	**Institute** reverse isolation. **Exclude** persons with communicable diseases from the client's room.	The client will remain free of signs and symptoms of infection such as fever and pain.
Rejection of the transplanted kidney will be life-threatening unless another transplant can be performed or the client goes on regular dialysis	Anxiety related to threat of rejection	**Provide** information about the procedure; stress the high (96%) success rate. **Teach** the client relaxation techniques and imagery	The client will be relaxed and hopeful of successful treatment.
Bed rest required for MoAb procedure	Impaired physical mobility related to requirement of bed rest for 1–2 hours during treatment	**Place** belongings and call bell within reach **Answer** call bell promptly	The client will state, when questioned, that she has no unmet needs.
MoAb treatment ordered (Side effects of MoAb treatment include fever, pain, nausea, and wheezing)	Altered comfort: fever, pain, nausea, or wheezing	**Monitor** the client for signs and symptoms of adverse reaction to MoAb treatment. **Administer** analgesic or antihistamine medication as ordered by the physician.	If signs and symptoms of adverse reaction develop, they will be promptly identified and alleviated.

press on the affected area. Acetaminophen may be recommended to control fever.

At the community level, nurses are actively involved in educating the public to the benefits and risks of immunizations. To do so, they must remain aware of changes in the agents employed and recommendations for their use as they evolve from new research findings.

Evaluation Data required for evaluation include immunization records of clients and populations, the occurrence or absence of adverse reactions to immunizations, and the speed and effectivenes of treatment for adverse reaction.

(See the accompanying Example of Nursing Process and MoAb Therapy.)

Checklist of nursing actions

☐ Inform clients or parents of expected beneficial and possible adverse reactions before starting immunization.

☐ Take a careful client history to determine if any allergies are present that may be affected by the immunization.

☐ Check for history of conditions that contraindicate use of vaccines or MoAbs (*ie*, pregnancy, immunocompromised individuals, cardiac status).

☐ Before giving immunizations, consult package inserts for vaccine ingredients that may cause allergic reactions; administer drugs according to the specific recommendations.

☐ Store vaccines properly to ensure potency.

☐ Give vaccines in the proper doses and according to the correct schedule.

☐ Do not give live virus vaccines to pregnant women, women who may be pregnant, or to children or adults with HIV or who are otherwise immunocompromised.

☐ Immunize the child of a pregnant woman if a current immunization is needed.

☐ Have clients or parents sign an informed consent if this is the procedure of the health care facility.

☐ Have the client remain in the office for about half an hour after immunization so that you can observe for systemic reactions.

☐ Keep emergency equipment and medications available.

☐ Keep accurate immunization records in the health care facility and give a copy to the client.

☐ Advise clients or parents to observe for adverse reactions and report these to physicians if they do occur.

☐ Report adverse reactions to vaccines listed on the Vaccine Injury Table as required by law.

☐ Advise clients to treat minor adverse reactions with antipyretics and cold compresses.

☐ Advise children not to scratch or rub the site of an injection.

☐ Advise clients who plan to travel to contact the local health department for current immunization requirements for the country they wish to enter.

References

Altman L. (1990). Help for patients with new kidneys. *The New York Times, April 26*, p A11.

Amler RW, et al. (1983). Measles on campus. *J Am Coll Health, 32*, 58.

ANA urges nurses to promote immunization standards. (1991). *Capitol Update, 9(2)*, 5, 6.

Angier N. (1990). Girl in gene therapy test raises hope for technique. *The New York Times, December 14*, p B1.

Angier N. (1991). Scientists struggle to undo tanning's deadly damage. *The New York Times, June 6*, p A23.

Benderly B. (1988). The immune system: Your body's department of defense. *FDA Consumer, 22(2)*, 22–25.

Blakeslee S. (1990). Human genes turn plants into factories. *The New York Times, January 16*, p 19.

Cherry J. (1990). Pertussis vaccine encephalopathy (editorial). *JAMA, 263*, 1679–1680.

Dault L, et al. (1989). Reversing cardiac transplant rejection with Orthoclone OKT3. *American Journal of Nursing, 89(7)*, 953–955.

Doner K. (1989). Who will get diabetes? *Countdown, 10(3)*, 10–17.

Dworetzky T. (1991). A bold step in preventing diabetes. *Countdown, 12(1)*, 31–39.

Edison L. (1991). Progress in diabetes treatment and technology. *Countdown, 12(1)*, 28–29.

Experimental gene therapy for cancer (1991). *FDA Consumer, 25(2)*, 4.

Fass, S, Defeating immune rejection in the thymus. *Countdown 12(3)*, 26–29.

Filbey D. (1987). A management program for Rh alloimmunization during pregnancy. *Early Human Development, 15(1)*, 11–20.

Gamma interferon for immune disorder (1991). *FDA Consumer, March 1991*, 4.

Hood LE. (1987). Interferon. *American Journal of Nursing 87*, 459–464.

Immunizations for US children with HIV infections. (1987). *FDA Drug Bulletin, 17(2)*, 23–24.

Kolata G. (1987). Chicken pox vaccine appears safe, effective. *The New York Times, December 22*, p C3.

Kolata G. (1991). In the war on cancer, a new kind of weapon. *The New York Times, May 7*, pp C1, C10.

Lewis R. (1991). Arthritis. *FDA Consumer, 25(6)*, 19–21, 24–25.

Marino J, (1991) Sheltering beta cells from a hostile immune system. *Countdown, 12(3)*, 6–8.

Peebles JM. (1900). *Vaccination: A curse and a menace to personal liberty, with statistics showing its dangers and criminality.* Battle Creek, MI: Temple of Health.

Pollack A, (1990). A rich new biotech frontier. *The New York Times, January 10*, pp 29, 34.

Pollack A. (1990). Two drugs in a new class pass a major FDA hurdle. *The New York Times, December 15*, pp 19, 20.

Rieger PT. (1987). Monoclonal antibodies target specific magic bullets. *American Journal of Nursing, 87*, 469–473.

Rosenthal E. (1990). Patient's marrow emerges as key cancer tool. *The New York Times, March 27*, pp C1, C8.

Rosenthal E. (1991). Camouflaged donor tissue holds transplant promise. *The New York Times, June 21*, p A10.

Scherer P. (1987). New drugs. *American Journal of Nursing, 87*, 448–454.

Scolnick EM, et al. (1984). Clinical evaluation in healthy adults of a hepatitis B vaccine made by recombinant DNA. *JAMA, 251(21)*, 2812.

Seagram WE. (1987). Immunomodulation, in Sites DP, Stobo JD, Wells JV. (eds): *Basic and clinical immunology*, 6th ed. Norwalk, CT: Appleton & Lange.

Sharts-Engel N. (1990). Pertussis vaccine: Safety update. *MCN, 15, September/October*, 293.

Stehlin D. (1990). Living with lupus. *FDA Consumer, 23(10),* 8–12.

Sticklin LA. (1987). Interleukin-2 and killer T cells. *American Journal of Nursing, 87,* 468–469.

Stobo JD. (1987). Lymphocytes, T cells, in Sites DP, Stobo JD, Wells JV. (eds): *Basic and clinical immunology,* 6th ed. Norwalk, CT: Appleton & Lange.

The arthritis you never hear about. (1991). *Arthritis Today, 5(1),* 40–42.

Whiteman K, et al. (1990). Liver transplantation. *American Journal of Nursing, 90(6),* 68–72.

Winkle T. (1990). Marrow transplant today and tomorrow. *American Journal of Nursing, 90(5),* 48–86.

Bibliography

Sites DP, Stobo JD, Wells JV. (1987). *Basic and clinical immunology,* 6th ed. Norwalk, CT: Appleton & Lange.

Theofilopoulos AN. (1987). Autoimmunity, in Sites DP, Stobo JD, Wells JV. (eds): *Basic and clinical immunology,* 6th ed. Norwalk, CT: Appleton & Lange.

Drugs affecting other body systems

10

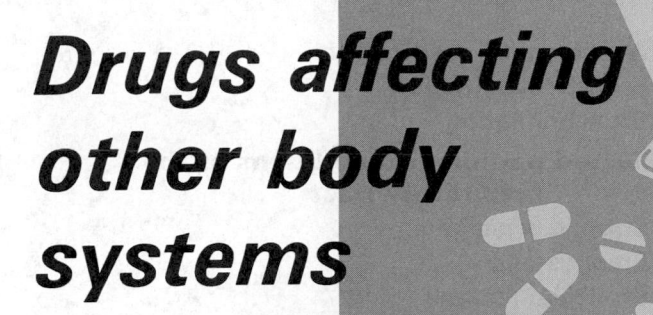

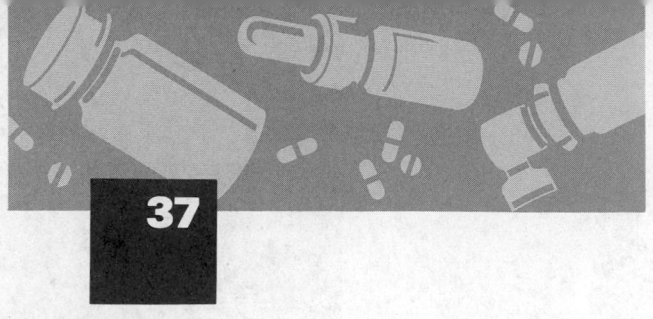

37

Drugs that affect the respiratory tract

A functioning or intact respiratory system is vital to sustain life; a patent airway is the highest priority in nursing care (with the possible exception of caring for terminally ill clients). Yet, the incidence of people who suffer from respiratory disease continues to rise with the result that more nursing functions are necessary to provide respiratory supportive care. Large medical centers have established separate respiratory intensive-care units, with members of various disciplines working as a team to administer care. This team helps clients and their families adjust to the changed lifestyle imposed by chronic lung disease and promotes optimal levels of functioning for the client. The nurse plays an important role in the team. Smaller centers often have respiratory clinical nurse specialists responsible for working with nurses and agency personnel to manage the care of the client with respiratory disease.

With the shift in health care from acute care centers to the community, it is not unusual to see people with severe respiratory disease cared for in the home, requiring the use of oxygen therapy and ventilatory support mechanisms such as respirators. The processes involved with the pathologic conditions in respiratory disorders are complicated, diverse, and difficult to understand. Many factors are interrelated. For clients and their families, respiratory distress and failure are extremely frightening. The client who experiences air hunger is often at the panic stage of anxiety. This places an added burden on the client and increases the demand for oxygen. The situation may be life-threatening, and the nurse must respond quickly in a calm, efficient manner. Psychological care for these clients is as important as physical care.

Although it is fortunate that most cases are not so extreme, the nurse still has many responsibilities. Nursing care can make a great deal of difference in helping clients manage their disease, improve their quality of life, and lead productive lives.

An analysis of nursing practice demonstrates that many general nursing measures apply to respiratory care.

It is beyond the scope of this chapter to discuss respiratory care in depth; the bibliography at the end of the chapter lists nursing and medical texts devoted to the subject. This chapter specifically addresses the pharmacologic treatment and essential nursing management required for clients with airway obstruction (the characteristic physiologic abnormality shared by chronic bronchitis, emphysema, and asthma). The effort or cost of breathing is directly related to the elastic properties of the lung, the anatomy of the thorax, diaphragm, and abdomen, and the degree of pathology or resistance to air flow throughout the respiratory tract. This chapter presents the basic information the nurse needs to know about the pharmacologic treatment and supportive respiratory care for clients diagnosed with chronic bronchitis, emphysema, or asthma with the use of bronchodilators, expectorants, mucolytic agents, antitussives, aerosols, and oxygen therapy. (The following drugs may also be used in the treatment of certain types of respiratory disease but are covered elsewhere in the text: antihistamines, corticosteroids, antibiotics, narcotics, muscle relaxants, and respiratory stimulants.)

Physiology of respiration

To understand the principles behind the pharmacologic treatment of respiratory disease, it is necessary to review the anatomy and physiology of the body's respiratory and immunologic systems. (For an in-depth discussion, consult a physiology textbook, such as Guyton [1991], or a pharmacology text, such as Gilman, et al [1990]. It is also helpful to read the chapters in this book about the autonomic nervous system and allergic and immune responses, Chapters 22, 35, and 36, respectively.)

To function, the human body requires a constant source of energy. The energy comes from chemical reactions that require oxygen. A normal healthy respiratory system is necessary for this process. Oxygen in the air is transported to tissue cells, and carbon dioxide is transported from the cells out of the body. This process, the exchange of oxygen and carbon dioxide between the outside atmosphere and the cells of the human body, is referred to as *respiration*.

The goal of respiration is to provide oxygen to the tissues and to remove carbon dioxide from the tissues.

Air is made up of varying concentrations of different gases. Each gas has molecules that collide with molecules of other gases, and each gas exerts its own pressure on the remaining molecules. This pressure is called *partial pressure*. It is expressed as P. Other designations used in respiratory care are partial pressure of oxygen (Po_2), partial pressure of carbon dioxide (Pco_2), partial pressure of arterial oxygen (Pao_2), partial pressure of arterial carbon dioxide ($Paco_2$), and several others.

The respiratory system consists of the organs involved in respiration; it is divided into the *upper airway*, which consists of the nose, mouth pharynx and larynx, and the *lower airway*, or tracheobronchial tree, which comprises the trachea and bronchial airways, respiratory airways, and alveoli (Box 37-1).

The trachea and tracheobronchial tree consist of a series of bifurcating tubes of various sizes that become smaller as they near the alveoli, or tiny pocket-like air sacs (Fig. 37-1). The bronchi and the respiratory tract are lined with a fine membrane and cilia. The cilia bring mucus and secretions up the tree toward the nasopharynx, where secretions can be expectorated or swallowed (Fig. 37-2). Goblet cells that lie within the membrane (epithelium) continually produce mucus, which keeps the respiratory tract moist (Fig. 37-3).

Mucus consists of at least 84% and as much as 94% water and other constituents, such as carbohydrates, lipids, and protein components. The glycoproteins of respiratory tract mucus are secreted mainly from submucosal bronchial glands, which have acini that contain mucus and serous cells in tubules. The glands are supplied by cholinergic, adrenergic, and peptidergic innervation (Ziment, 1987).

Normally, adults produce about 100 ml of mucus a day. The mucociliary system refers to the cilia as well as mucus secretions. The control mechanism of the cilia is not fully known. Cilia beat at a rate set by their metabolic state, not under the control of the nervous system but affected by hormones and metabolic regulators. It is partially determined by the supply of adenosine triphosphate (ATP) (Ziment, 1987).

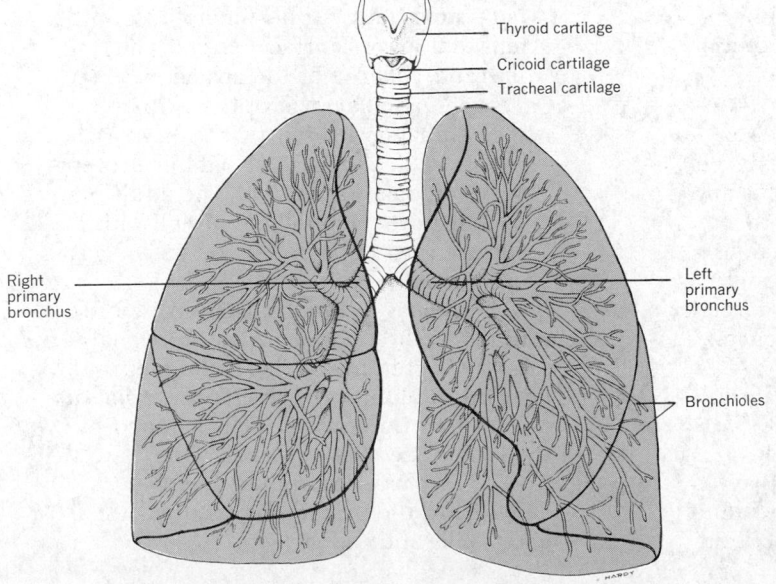

Figure 37-1. Anterior view of the larynx, trachea, and bronchial tree.

Thyroid cartilage
Cricoid cartilage
Tracheal cartilage
Right primary bronchus
Left primary bronchus
Bronchioles

Box 37-1. Organs of the respiratory system

I. Upper airway

Air from the atmosphere first enters the upper airway through the nose (*ie*, the beginning of the respiratory tract).

A. *Nose:* Passage for air; opens into the nasopharynx. The nose has important functions: filtering, warming, humidifying, and moisturizing air. After air passes through the nose, the inspired air temperature approximates body temperature with a relative humidity of 75% to 80%. The nasal hairs filter out particles larger than 10 μm. Air passes through the nose to the pharynx, then to the larynx, trachea, and bronchi to the lungs.

B. *Pharynx:* After entering the nose, inspired air next passes through the pharynx, which is made up of three sections: the nasopharynx, the oropharynx, and the laryngeal pharynx. The pharynx is a common passage for both food and air. Air goes to the trachea. (The muscles of the oropharynx help propel food from the mouth to the esophagus during swallowing.) Directly anterior to the laryngeal pharynx is the epiglottis (see below).

C. *Larynx:* The larynx lies between the base or root of the tongue and connects the pharynx to the trachea. The larynx is the area that connects the upper and lower airways. The larynx is in the middle of the neck, composed of nine cartilages connected by ligaments and moved by muscular action. Some of the cartilages, such as the cricoid and thyroid cartilages, are already familiar and serve as landmarks in health assessment. The larynx is called the organ of the voice or voice box, because it contains mucous membranes made into folds. These vocal folds and the space between them are referred to as the *glottis*. The epiglottis is made up of elastic cartilage covered by mucous membrane and forms the superior portion of the larynx. The epiglottis guards the glottis during swallowing. The larynx separates food and air. It is also involved in the initiation of a cough and in the production of speech. Coughing is an important protective mechanism of the lung, and a cough is often referred to as the "watch dog" of the lung. The cough reflex is stimulated by secretions or foreign material in the upper airways or bronchi.

II. Lower airway

A. *Trachea:* The first-generation respiratory passageway; this membrane is a cartilaginous, cylindrical tube lined with mucous that contains goblet cells. It is about 12 cm in length and 2 cm in diameter and extends vertically from the cricoid cartilage of the larynx into the thorax, where it divides into two main stem bronchi. This point is called the *carina*.

B. *Bronchi and lungs:* The bronchi continue to break up into branches, becoming subsegmental bronchi, bronchi, terminal bronchi, bronchioles, terminal bronchioles, and the right and left bronchi, second generation. There are 20 to 25 generations before the air reaches the alveoli.

Bronchial tree: This refers to the branching of the bronchi of the lungs. It is considered a structural unit. As the bronchi become smaller, the structural rigidity or cartilage disappears, and the patency of the airway is then subject to the elastic recoil and action of smooth muscle.

C. *Lungs:* Considered the organs of respiration. They are porous, spongy, and cone-shaped, and they fill the lateral aspects of the thoracic cavity. The lung consists of bronchial tubes and terminal dilations, blood vessels, lymphatics, nerves, and elastic connective tissue. Each lobe of the lung is composed of lobules, where the bronchiole enters and then divides into alveoli or air cells.

D. *Alveoli* (gas-exchanging units): These are distal to the bronchi and are the units in which the gases are exchanged. The alveolar wall forms part of the barrier known as the alveolar capillary membrane, where the exchange of gases for respiration takes place.

Three distinct types of cells are found in the alveoli:

Type 1—Alveolar epithelial cells: basic structures that form pulmonary surface epithelium and form the alveolar wall where gas exchange takes place.

Type 2—Large cells that produce pulmonary surfactant, a phospholipid lipoprotein that lowers surface tension and prevents collapse of the alveoli.

Type 3—Alveolar macrophages, that ingest phagocytize particles, microorganisms, or debris and are vital in preventing pulmonary infection. The adult lung contains over 300 million alveoli with a surface area of 70 to 80 meters for gas exchange.

E. *Pleura:* This is a thin, transparent, moist serous membrane that forms two clonal sacs, the right and the left. The pleura envelop the lungs and line the interior surface of the thoracic cavity invaginated by the lung. The *visceral* pleura adheres to the lung. The *parietal* portion is loosely attached to the underlying tissue of the chest walls and diaphragm.

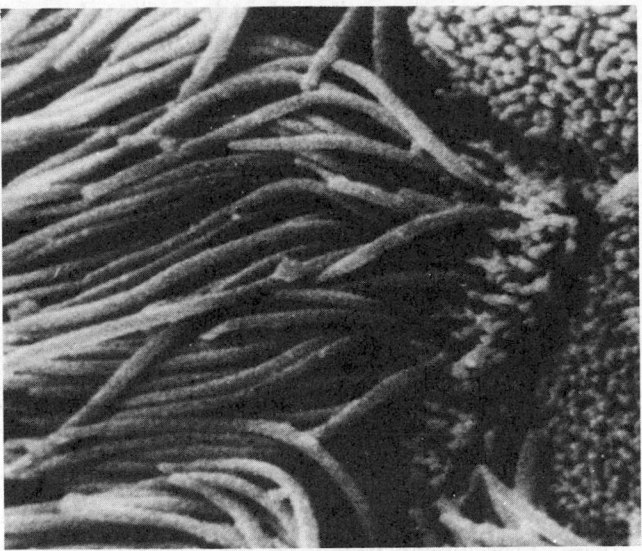

Figure 37-2. Scanning electron micrograph that shows cilia (longer projections) that are in constant motion, moving the mucociliary blanket upward in a conveyor fashion toward the pharynx. The small flat clusters are the microvilli, which transport fluid across the bronchial lining. (Courtesy of Janice Nowell, University of California, Santa Cruz)

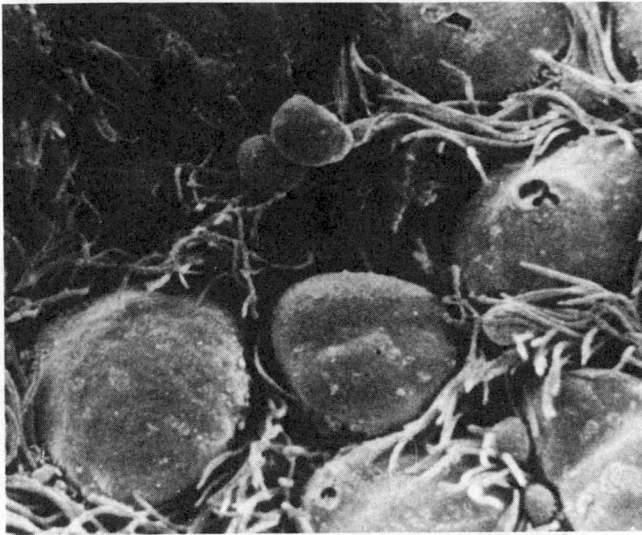

Figure 37-3. Scanning electron micrograph of the small round goblet cells that secrete mucus. (Courtesy of Janice Nowell, University of California, Santa Cruz)

A layer of mucus covers the upper and lower airway as far as the terminal bronchiole. The mucus blanket that is formed is composed of two layers: a *sol* layer and a *gel* layer. The blanket lines the trachea, bronchi, and larger bronchioles. The deeper sol layer is watery and has a low viscosity through which cilia move freely, propelling material up to the overlying or surface gel layer. This layer is viscous. The cilia only briefly touch the gel layer, which protects the cilia from dehydration, particles, and toxic gases (Guyton, 1991; Traver, et al, 1991). Smoke, infection, and pollutants decrease mucociliary transport, however.

The diffusion of the gases occurs in the alveoli through the alveolar-capillary membrane. While oxygen passes through the membrane to the blood, waste carbon dioxide diffuses out, leaves the blood, and crosses in the opposite direction. Most of the time, respiration is passive and occurs involuntarily through pressure changes in the thoracic cavity, which allow air to enter and leave the respiratory tract with diffusion across the alveolar-capillary membrane. There is a balance in the amount of oxygen consumed by the cells to meet energy demands and the amount of carbon dioxide given off by the cells. However, if the body's oxygen requirements change, an adjustment is made in the amount of oxygen supplied. If forceful active inspiration and expiration are required to meet increased demands placed on the body, this requirement is met. Respiratory action, therefore, can also be active and voluntary.

The human body adjusts readily to increasing or decreasing demands for oxygen. During exercise or other physiologic states that increase metabolic activity, the respiratory system responds by increasing the quantity of oxygen available to the tissues and by removing increased quantities of carbon dioxide. The body is able to adjust to external environmental changes (such as higher altitudes with less oxygen available) and internal changes in the chemical composition of the blood that correspond to energy demands. Although the exact mechanism is not fully known, the respiratory center in the brain stem is able to adjust the rate of alveolar ventilation almost exactly to the demands placed on it. The respiratory center located in the medulla oblongata and pons is sensitive to changes in the concentration of hydrogen ions (acidity) of the fluid that bathes it and to changes mainly in the concentration of carbon dioxide, and in oxygen to a lesser degree. This center determines the depth and frequency of respiration. Chemoreceptors in the carotid and aortic bodies are sensitive mainly to changes in the amount of oxygen and also to carbon dioxide circulating in the blood. They transmit signals to the respiratory center. Stretch reflexes (Hering-Breuer) in the lung regulate the degree of inflation of the lungs. Because of signals from the respiratory center, alveo-

---

Learning experience 37-1

At rest, sing a song with which you are familiar. Exercise vigorously for 10 to 15 minutes—running or jogging—to stimulate sympathetic activity. Stop and try to sing the same song. Stop and cough. Do you notice any difference in your ability to sing and how it feels? Do you notice any difference in your respiratory secretion?

lar ventilation adjusts to meet varying demands for oxygen consumption and carbon dioxide disposal.

For respiration to occur, the respiratory, neuromuscular, and circulatory systems must all be intact and able to interact. In addition, hemoglobin must be sufficient to carry the oxygen. When disease strikes the respiratory system, the body's ability to maintain a supply of oxygen to meet the demand may be impaired. The result could be *hypoxia* (decreased amount or availability of oxygen to the cells or tissues of the body) or *hypoxemia* (reduced oxygen in the body fluids, especially in the arterial blood). Disease may also affect the ability of the respiratory system to remove carbon dioxide, resulting in *hypercapnia* (elevated levels of carbon dioxide in the body fluids in particular at the cellular level). Much of respiratory therapy is directed at improving the exchange and movement of air by bronchodilation.

Bronchoconstriction

The walls of the bronchi are mainly composed of smooth muscle, and the walls of the bronchioles are almost entirely smooth muscle. Under normal conditions, air flows easily through the respiratory tree and through the bronchi and bronchioles to the alveoli with little resistance. Direct control of the bronchioles by sympathetic nerve fibers is weak; however, the bronchial tree is exposed to circulating norepinephrine and epinephrine. These are released by sympathetic stimulation of the adrenal medullae and result in bronchial dilatation (Guyton, 1991). Some parasympathetic nerve fibers are present in the lung parenchyma and secrete acetylcholine. When these nerves are activated, mild to moderate bronchial constriction occurs. Histamine and slow-reactive substance of anaphylaxis (SRS-A) are also formed in the lungs themselves and cause bronchoconstriction (Guyton, 1991).

Irritants such as smoke, dust, smog and sulfur dioxide can activate parasympathetic nerve reflexes and cause bronchoconstriction in airways (Guyton, 1991). Certain respiratory diseases cause bronchoconstriction. Airway flow resistance can increase as small bronchioles become occluded, and they constrict easily because they contain a high percentage of smooth muscle. In addition, bronchoconstriction is frequently seen in a disease such as asthma.

Bronchial asthma frequently occurs in people allergic or hypersensitive to a particular foreign substance (*eg*, ragweed pollen). The person forms an abnormal type of antibody (a protein, such as IgE) in response to the antigen (foreign substance). The antibodies attach themselves to mast cells found just beneath the bronchial epithelium in close association with the bronchioles and small bronchi. They are abundant in the lung just beneath the basement membrane of the airways, near blood vessels in the submucosa, adjacent to submucous glands, throughout

muscle bundles, in the bronchial lumen, and in the intra-alveolar septa (Guyton, 1991). When the antigen reacts with the antibody through a degranulation process, swelling within the cell occurs, and a rupture leads to a release of several substances. histamine and slow-reacting substance of anaphylaxis (SRS-A) are released. Bradykinin, acetylcholine, serotonin, and prostaglandins are also all released and lead to bronchoconstriction. SRS-A produces prolonged contraction of the smooth muscle in the bronchi. Histamine leads to bronchospasm, a significant increase in the production of mucus, and localized bronchial swelling and edema (Guyton, 1991; Wade, 1977). SRS-A is composed of cysteinyl-containing leukotrienes (LTC_4, LTD_4, and LTE_4), of which LTD_4 is a potent bronchoconstrictor (Wyngaarden, Smith, 1985). The leukotrienes are far more potent than histamine in producing bronchoconstriction (Guyton, 1991). All of these body responses lead to impairment of respiratory function.

Bronchodilation

Bronchial smooth muscle tone is controlled by the tonic cholinergic (vagal) and the inhibitory (sympathetic) systems. A third system, a noncholinergic nonadrenergic one called a *purinergic* system, also mediates bronchial muscle relaxation (Rakel, 1984). The sympathetic nervous system plays a major role in determining the diameter of the bronchi. Sympathetic nerve endings secrete synaptic neurotransmitter substances. Those endings that secrete norepinephrine are said to be adrenergic. (Drugs that mimic the action of sympathetic activity are called *sympathomimetic* or *adrenergic* drugs or *catecholamines*.) Adrenergic activity affects two types of receptors: α and β. Two types of β-adrenergic receptors exist: β_1 and β_2. β_1-adrenergic receptors act chiefly at cardiac sites. β_2 receptors are present in the glands and smooth muscle and mucosal vessels of the bronchial tree. Adrenergic stimulation of β_2 receptors results in bronchodilation.

Stimulation of α receptors produces vasoconstriction, smooth muscle contraction, intestinal relaxation, pilomotor contraction, and iris dilation. Stimulation of β receptors leads to vasodilation in the muscles, cardioacceleration (β_1), increased myocardial strength (β_1), myometrial relaxation (β_2), and most importantly, bronchial relaxation.

Adenyl cyclase is an enzyme present in the β_2 receptor membrane. When stimulated by adrenergic drugs, adenyl cyclase catalyzes the conversion of ATP to cyclic $3',5'$ adenosine monophosphate (cyclic AMP; Fig. 37-4). Cyclic AMP (cAMP) is an intracellular hormonal mediator. It is sometimes called the second messenger for hormone mediation, the first being the original stimulating hormone (Guyton, 1991). cAMP (SMRS, smooth muscle-relaxing substance) results in bronchodilation. Specific receptors for the pharmacologic

Adrenergic Regulation of cAMP:

Adenosine triphosphate (ATP) → Adenyl cyclase → Cyclic adenosine monophosphate (cAMP)

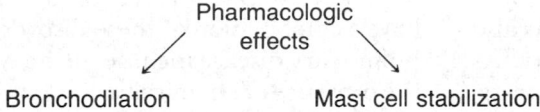

Pharmacologic
effects

Bronchodilation   Mast cell stabilization

Cholinergic Regulation of cGMP:

Guanosine triphosphate (GTP) → Guanylate cyclose → Cyclic guanosine monophosphate (cGMP)

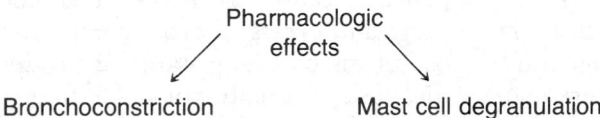

Pharmacologic
effects

Bronchoconstriction   Mast cell degranulation

Figure 37-4. Autonomic control of bronchial smooth muscle tone. (Diagram created by Vincent P. Gotz, M.S., R.Ph.)

mediators have been postulated as being attached to surface enzymes, namely, adenyl cyclase, phosphodiesterase, and prostaglandin synthetase (Segal, MacDonnell, 1977). cAMP destruction leads to bronchoconstriction. If phosphodiesterase is inhibited, it effectively alters histamine release by delaying cAMP degradation, leading to bronchodilation (MacDonnell, Segal, 1977). β_2 Receptors mediate the inhibition of bronchiolar smooth muscle contraction by β agonists, producing bronchodilation by means of the cAMP mechanism (MacDonnell, Segal, 1977). The vagal effects are mediated by cyclic cytidine monophosphate (CMP), whereas sympathetic effects are mediated by cAMP. The release of factors or mediators are decreased by high intracellular levels of cAMP. The converse is true if high levels of cyclic guanosine monophosphate (cGMP) exist within cells (Rakel, 1984).

In short, either the stimulation of cAMP production or the decrease and prevention of the destruction of cAMP is the major principle behind effective bronchodilation therapy.

Recently, interest in bronchial smooth muscle control by the cholinergic (or parasympathetic) nervous system has been renewed (see Fig. 37-4). Blockage of the cholinergic system by means of anticholinergic agents (*eg*, atropine) results in stabilization of the mast cells and bronchodilation. In the past, atropine had been used to treat asthma; however, its use was limited by unpleasant adverse reactions and the belief of some physicians that the inhibition and drying of secretions in the upper and lower respiratory tract was potentially dangerous for clients with chronic bronchitis and emphysema. Continuing research has found that the bronchodilatory effect of inhaled or intravenous (IV) anticholinergics (atropine) is equal to and in some cases better than that of β adrenergics in chronic obstructive pulmonary disease (COPD) and some types of asthma. Glycopyrrolate has fewer side effects, especially when administered through inhalation therapy (Slovis, et al, 1987). Atropine and ipratropium bromide block the vagally mediated production of cGMP and thus reduce bronchial tone. A congener of methylatropine, ipratropium bromide is as effective as the β_2-adrenergic agonist albuterol in clients with chronic bronchitis, but albuterol is more effective in bronchial asthma.

Selected pathologic conditions of the respiratory tract

Clients are diagnosed as having respiratory failure if they are unable to maintain adequate oxygenation of their blood and tissues or are unable to prevent undue retention of carbon dioxide. In respiratory failure, the PaO_2 falls below 55 to 60 mm Hg. The $PaCO_2$ may be normal, or it may be elevated above 50 mm Hg. The *p*H may be less than 7.25; however, this level may be misleading because kidney compensation in clients with long-standing lung disease may increase the *p*H. Client symptoms may or may not correlate with blood gas levels. If the PaO_2 is lowered, the client becomes hypoxic. The symptoms of moderate hypoxia include irritability, hostility, headache, and change in mentation. If the condition continues to deteriorate, tachycardia, dyspnea, muscle weakness, double vision, judgmental errors, loss of coordination, and cyanosis occur. With low levels of oxygen, cardiac arrhythmia may develop, and the client may become apneic and co-matose (Bryan, Taylor, 1973).

The symptoms of increasing levels of carbon dioxide may be difficult to differentiate from low levels of oxygen. Carbon dioxide is a potent vasodilator, and the client's skin may assume a reddish hue. Clients also complain of headache, insomnia, and irritability. As the $PaCO_2$ rises, the client is unable to concentrate, develops drowsiness, may appear to be intoxicated, and ultimately may become comatose.

Respiratory disease and failure may occur as a result of various pathologic conditions. In some cases, inadequate ventilation of the alveoli occurs. Other diseases prevent the diffusion of gases across the respiratory membrane. If the movement of the lungs and thorax is impeded, the condition is referred to as *restrictive lung disease*. Clinical manifestations or signs and symptoms of respiratory disturbance and failure may include restlessness, confusion, tachycardia, diaphoresis, headache, hypotension, labored breathing, dyspnea, cough, sputum production, rales, rhonchi, and cyanosis. Expiratory air flow can be limited by three main causes:

1. *Airway resistance*, which can occur from an inflammatory process or mucus gland hyperplasia seen in bronchitis
2. *Collapse of airways* after bronchial muscle spasm as seen in asthma, with narrow and collapsing peripheral airways trapping large volumes of air
3. *Decrease or loss of elastic recoil of the lung* as seen in emphysema (Menkes, et al, 1984)

Dyspnea (or difficult breathing) is a common complaint in chronic respiratory disease. It is different for each person and does not always correlate with pulmonary function tests or the ability to carry out the activities of daily living. Research shows that the sensation of dyspnea may represent conscious awareness of outgoing motor commands to respiratory muscles based on changing muscle tension and muscle length. It is the "sensing" of respiratory effort (Mahler, 1987).

Chronic obstructive pulmonary disease

Chronic obstructive pulmonary disease (COPD) occurs when the outflow of air from the lungs or the exchange of gases at the alveolar level is impeded. Obstruction can occur as a result of pathologic changes in the airways, spasm within the airways, changes in the amount and viscosity of the mucus secretions, or any combination of these factors. Paralysis of nerves that innervate the respiratory tract also leads to failure, but that discussion is not within the scope of this chapter. This chapter discusses respiratory failure that results from increased airway resistance, increased tissue resistance, and decreased lung compliance.

Three common serious obstructive pulmonary diseases are chronic bronchitis, pulmonary emphysema, and bronchial asthma. Bronchitis (with thick secretions, infections, and bronchospasms) or emphysema (with overinflation of the lungs, collapse of airways, and dyspnea) rarely occurs singly. Most people have a combination of these disorders. Risk factors for pulmonary disease include the heavy use of cigarettes, the presence of chemical pollutants in industrial urban areas, cold damp climates, and an increase in life expectancy, which prolongs the life-time exposure to environmental pollutants.

Chronic bronchitis

In chronic bronchitis, the expiratory air flow is impeded because of airway obstruction from mucus plugs and excessive production of mucus. The client complains of a long-standing productive cough (the diagnosis is usually not made unless the person has complained of cough with increased sputum production for at least 3 months of the year over a period of at least 2 years). Hypertrophy of the mucus glands occurs with excessive mucus production as a result of infection or irritation from chemicals. Chronic inflammation with cell infiltration and swelling of the bronchial mucosa is present. In addition, the movement of the cilia is slowed and loss of cilia occurs, decreasing the client's ability to eliminate secretions. Clients may develop bronchospasm from smoke, chemical irritants, dust, fumes, or cold air. Acetylcholine, serotonin, and histamine may also lead to bronchospasm. Therapy is directed at removing the irritants, including cigarette smoking, and the provision of rest, proper hydration, antibiotics, bronchodilation, expectorants, and pulmonary toilette.

Emphysema

The word *emphysema* originates from Greek and means "to puff up." In emphysema, the air spaces distal to the terminal bronchioles are enlarged from dilatation, and alveolar wall destruction occurs. The etiology of emphysema is not fully known, but the predisposing factors previously mentioned do contribute to its development. Destruction of elastic tissue in the alveolar walls leads to loss of elastic recoil, loss of tone, and hyperinflation of the affected alveoli, impeding inspiratory and especially expiratory air flow. Air is trapped, and lung size increases as the residual volume increases. Affected clients have a barrel chest, use pursed-lip breathing, and are dyspneic. They use accessory muscles for inspiration, and decreased movement of the chest and diaphragm is seen. Clients may be cyanotic and have clubbing of the fingers.

Pulmonary hypertension with cor pulmonale may develop and lead to symptoms of congestive heart failure. Hemoglobin and hematocrit levels may rise in a compensatory mechanism as the PaO_2 decreases and the $PaCO_2$ increases. Therapy is palliative and is aimed at improving respiratory function by relieving the obstructed air flow, by correcting the infection, and by making the respiratory effort more effective.

The therapy for COPD includes the removal of respiratory tract irritants, including cigarette smoke, and improvement of respiratory function by bronchodilator therapy and removal of secretions. The latter is accomplished in several ways. Clients are instructed in proper coughing techniques, and secretions are modified by proper hydration of the client. Physical therapy for the chest with percussion and vibration may be necessary, as well as treatment with expectorant, mucolytic, and proteolytic agents. These agents may be administered by aerosol and intermittent positive-pressure breathing (IPPB) therapy. Any superimposed infection must be treated. For those clients with severe disease who have continual hypoxemia and little physical energy and reserve, both morbidity and mortality improve with *controlled* oxygen enrichment of inspired air, continuously for 24 hours rather than administered intermittently.

Bronchial asthma

Asthma is a common disease that affects 5% to 10% of the population. Ten million people have this disease in the United States, and African Americans are twice as likely to be hospitalized with asthma (Guidelines, 1991). It is currently considered the most commonly occurring chronic illness in children. Despite significant advances in treatment and therapy, morbidity and mortality from asthma is rising and is unacceptably high. From 1980 to 1987, the prevalence of asthma in the United States increased 29%, and the death rate for asthma as the first listed diagnosis increased 31% (Guidelines, 1991), suggesting that current treatment modes may be inadequate or are not being used optimally (Barnes, 1989a).

Bronchial asthma is a clinical syndrome characterized by increased responsiveness of the airways to various stimuli. This leads to a distressing frightening type of dyspnea and wheezing resulting from recurrent generalized airway obstruction that is paroxysmal and reversible at least initially. Bronchial hyperactivity occurs with contractions of bronchial muscle, or bronchospasm. Subepithelial edema is present, along with thick tenacious mucus that results from an increase in the number of goblet cells and mucus glands. Until recently, pharmacologic therapy for asthma has been directed at bronchoconstrictor mechanics and abnormalities in the smooth muscles of the airway. Bronchodilators were the mainstays of therapy. In the last few years, though continued research is necessary, it has become accepted that chronic asthma involves a late-phase inflammatory response (Barnes, 1989a, 1989b; Rumbak 1991; Guidelines, 1991). Therapeutic implications of this are important. Pharmacologic agents directed at the inflammatory response play an important role in treating asthma in addition to drugs that affect smooth muscles in the airway. The inflammatory response is also present in clients with mild asthma. Bronchial tissue biopsy in asthma clients reveals inflammatory cell infiltration, especially eosinophils and lymphocytes and epithelial shedding. An increased proportion of inflammatory cells is also evident in bronchoalveolar lavage (Barnes, 1989a).

Classification

Extrinsic and intrinsic asthma

The disease may be classified according to precipitating factors and is frequently described as either extrinsic or intrinsic. *Extrinsic* (allergic) *asthma* is usually caused by an inhaled, ingested, or injected allergen. Often, a family history of asthma exists, and the person has elevated levels of immunoglobulin E (IgE), positive skin tests for an external allergen, and sputum eosinophils.

In *intrinsic asthma*, or nonallergic asthma, the pathologic condition within the bronchial tree originates from within the person as a result of an infection or from a toxic material. It generally occurs in older people. The IgE is normal or low and therefore no clear-cut immune response. This form is often continuous, more chronic, and more resistant to therapy. Spontaneous remissions are unlikely, and the disease may be more severe and progressive. With some clients, aspirin sensitivity triggers the attack; this action is more prevalent in females. Nasal polyps are usually also present. When assessing these clients, the nurse should look for sensitivity to codeine, morphine, and aminopyrine. Psychogenic factors may be important in clients with intrinsic asthma.

Extrinsic atopic and nonatopic asthma

Extrinsic atopic asthma is mediated by a reaginic antibody (IgE). With some clients, a more delayed type of asthma, the type III asthma reaction (Pepys or Arthus), occurs. This is more common in adults and is also known as *extrinsic nonatopic asthma*. This condition is usually mediated by circulatory antibodies IgE, IgA, and IgM.

Mixed allergic–nonallergic asthma

In many clients, the type of asthma cannot be classified as allergic or nonallergic. They may follow the pattern of both or may start with a classic or typical allergy-induced asthma and then show the characteristics of nonallergic asthma (Menkes, et al, 1984).

Exercise-induced (cold air) asthma

Many people with asthma wheeze, are dyspneic, and experience bronchospasm after exercise, especially if it takes place in cool dry air.

Phases

The intermittent wheezing, cough, and dyspnea characteristic of asthma is a result of narrowing of the pulmonary airways. This airway obstruction is reversible, and between attacks, clients often have symptom-free periods. Current research demonstrates that obstruction to air flow is only part of the picture and that, in effect, the reaction takes place in three phases.

The first phase occurs within 20 to 30 minutes. An inhaled allergen triggers immediate bronchoconstriction. Mast cell degranulation and bronchospastic mediators are released. Airways may return to normal during the next 2 hours. Mediators released from the mast cells attract other inflammatory cells with an increase in the number of eosinophils. The second phase peaks about 6 to 8 hours after exposure and represents an eosinophilic inflammatory response in the bronchi. This phase moves into the third phase, which may last up to 3 to 4 weeks. This phase correlates with the severe inflammatory response. Eosinophils cause airway injury. Mediators are released; neutrophils, macrophages, basophils, and lymphocytes are present. Cells release platelet-activating factor (PAF), leading to eosinophilic chemotaxis. During this phase, the airways are more responsive to nonspecific irritants, including cigarette smoke, aerosols, dust, dander, mites, and other elements in the environment. A viral respiratory infection may provoke or alter the asthmatic response and produce further epithelial damage. This damage in turn can produce specific IgE antibodies directed against the viral antigens, further enhancing the release of mediators. Airway hyperresponsiveness may be evident for weeks beyond the initial infection (Rumback, 1991; Guidelines, 1991).

Pathophysiology of late-phase reaction

Bronchial hyperresponsiveness with an exaggerated bronchoconstrictor response to many different stimuli is a key characteristic of asthma. In moderate and severe asthma, bronchial reactivity increases, and airway narrowing worsens gradually over time in spite of therapy and may persist despite therapy.

The mechanisms that contribute to the response and to the inflammation of the airway are multiple and result from complex interactions among inflammatory cells, mediators, and cells and tissues present in the airways (Guidelines, 1991). Figure 37-5 shows some of these mechanisms and the sequences in which they are believed to develop.

An initial trigger leads to a release of inflammatory mediators from bronchial mast cells, macrophages, and epithelial cells that are present in the airways. These then activate other inflammatory cells (eosinophils, leukotrienes, and neutrophils) that change epithelial integrity, alter autonomic neural control of airway tone, affect mucociliary function, and increase airway smooth muscle responsiveness. Epithelial injury leads to a loss of ciliated cells and complete denudation of the epithelium (Guidelines, 1991).

■ Summary

Until recently, the pharmacologic therapy for asthma has been directed predominantly at the airway obstruction that results from spasm of the smooth muscle, with bronchodilation as the major goal. Increased attention is now being focused on the pathogenesis of asthma, partly in response to increasing morbidity and mortality. Because the pathogenesis of asthma includes microvascular leakage and bronchial hyper-responsiveness in addition to bronchoconstriction, treatment must be directed at bronchodilation as well as reduction of the inflammatory response.

Management includes the identification of the causes, which may be allergy, exercise, cold, or sensitivity to viruses and bacteria in the airways. Present therapy includes the use of cortisone for anti-inflammatory effect, β-adrenergic agonists and theophylline for bronchodilation, and cromolyn sodium to prevent mast cell activation.

Research for new asthma drugs is moving toward the development of agents to alter specific components of the complex pathophysiology of asthma. This research may find drugs to alter eosinophils and lymphocytes or to block PAF, neurogenic inflammation, or the production of leukotrienes.

Bronchodilators

The two classes of drugs used predominantly to produce bronchodilation are *sympathomimetics* and *methylxanthines*. These drugs are effective because they imitate or alter sympathetic activity. The methylxanthines and β-adrenergic agonists are effective in improving air flow by combating muscular bronchospasm and in improving mucociliary clearance (Petty, et al, 1982). *Bronchodilators* act by reversing the smooth muscle airway contraction and include β-adrenergic agonists, theophylline, and anticholinegics. β-Adrenergic agonists are effective in preventing the immediate bronchoconstrictor response to challenge by allergens.

Inhaled β-adrenergic agonists are used for the short-term relief of bronchoconstriction and are the treatment of choice for acute exacerbations. They are also used for exercise-induced asthma. Inhaled selective β_2-adrenergic agonists (albuterol, terbutaline, fenoterol, and bitolterol) have a rapid onset of action and are effective for 3 to 6 hours. Formoterol and salmeterol are longer acting and are presently undergoing clinical trials. Salmeterol may be effective for more than 12 hours and therefore useful in the treatment of nocturnal symptoms.

The oral route is used less frequently because of the increased incidence of side effects, but slow-release

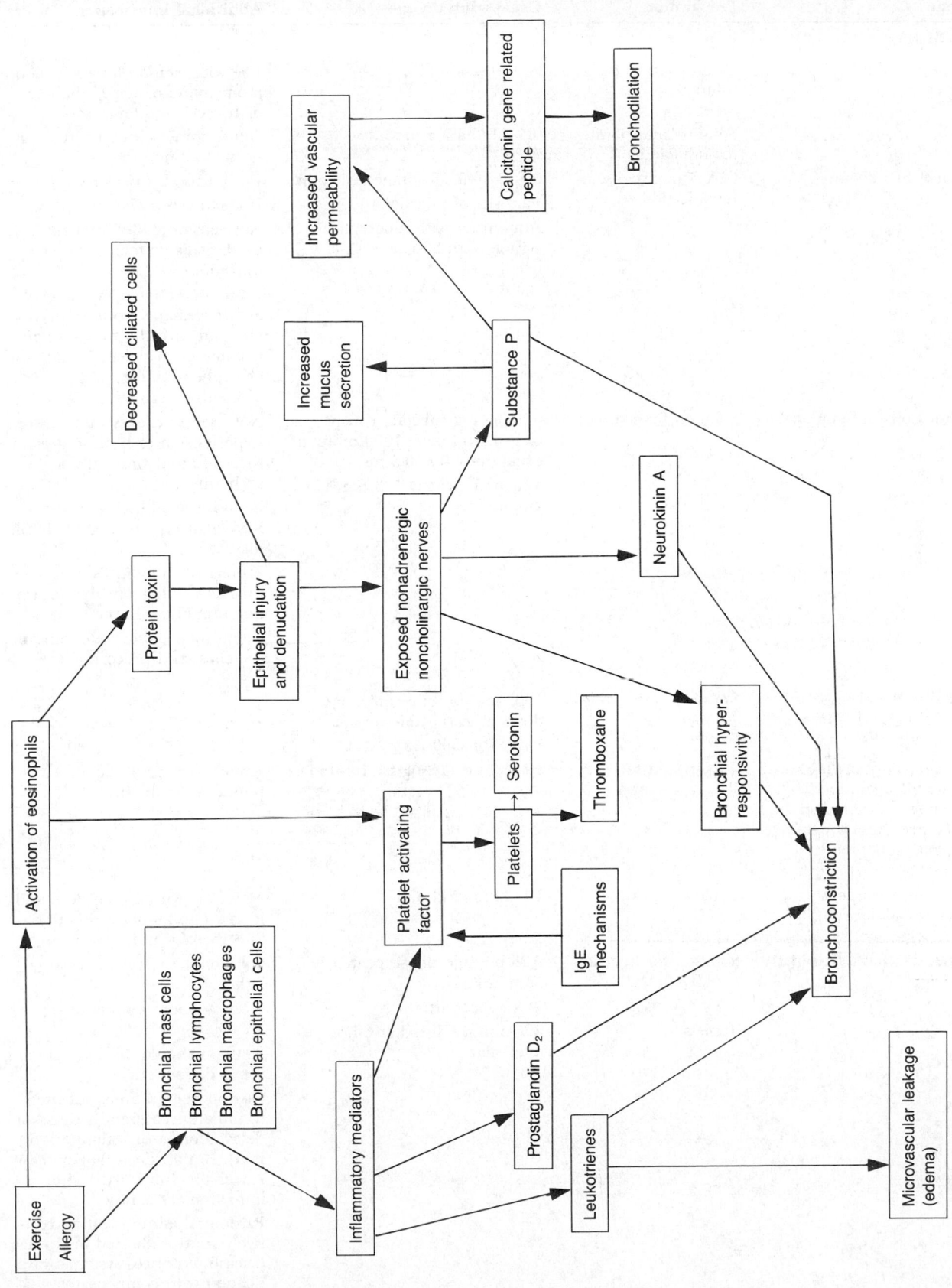

Figure 37-5. Pathologic processes that contribute to asthma. New drugs might interrupt processes by blocking inflammatory mediators, prostaglandin D_2, platelet-activating factor, protein toxin, substance P, or neurokinin A.

Table 37-1. Representative oral or parenteral sympathomimetic bronchodilators*

Drug name	Preparation	Usual adult dosage	Additional information
Bronchodilators			
albuterol, salbutamol (Proventil, Ventolin)	Oral tablets and solution	2–4 mg, tid-qid	Use with caution for patients on monoamine oxidase inhibitors or tricyclic antidepressants.
	Solution and powder for inhalation	0.5 ml (0.5% solution) PC: C	Dilute spray solution with 3 ml normal saline
epinephrine (Sus-Phrine)	Glycerin suspension for injection	0.1–0.3 ml subcutaneously q6h	Do not use if discolored.
		Vary site of injection	It is not given IV.
		Administer with tuberculin syringe with 26-gauge ½-in needle	Not recommended if client is on digitalis or mercurial diuretics.
			Effect potentiated by tricyclic antidepressants, sodium thyroxine, and with the following antihistamines: tripelennamine, chlorpheniramine, and diphenhydramine.
(Adrenalin, EpiPen, Simplene)	Solution for injection	0.1–0.5 mg subcutaneously (0.1–0.5 ml of 1 : 1000 dilution) usual dose: 0.3–0.5 ml	Not used in clients with severe hypertension or a pulse greater than 140 and with cardiac arrhythmia.
		May be repeated 2–3 times at 20-min intervals	Do not use with clients who have glaucoma or organic brain disease.
			Protect from light. Do not use if brown or has precipitate. Do not administer in the buttocks.
			Client may exhibit pounding in the chest and precordial distress.
(Asthmahaler, Bronitine Mist, Bronkaid Mist, Epinephrine Mist, Primatene Mist)	Spray for inhalation	160–250 µg (once only, or 2 doses at least 1 minute apart) *Via IPPB:* 300 µg	
isoproterenol, isoprenaline, isopropylnoradrenaline, isopropylarterenol (Aludrin, Isuprel, Isuprel-Neo Misthaler, Medihler-Iso, Neoepinine, Norisodrine)	Tablets, glossets	10–20 mg sublingual, tid–qid	Similar feelings to above with pounding in chest.
metaproterenol (Alupent, Orciprenaline, Metaprel)	Tablets	10–20 mg, tid–qid	May start with 10-mg dose and increase to 20-mg dose after 2–3 weeks if indicated.
terbutaline (Brethine, Bricanyl)	Solution for injection	0.25 mg injection repeated in 15 min PRN	Solution is sensitive to heat, light.
		May repeat after 4 h	Store at room temperature: 15°–30°C.
	Tablets	2.5–5 mg, tid–qid at 6-h intervals	Solution should be clear. Do not use if discolored.
			Give in deltoid area, not used to initiate treatment because of delayed onset of action (30–60 min). But action is longer than Adrenalin and is used after improvement is noted.
			Parenteral administration relatively contraindicated in cardiac disease. Produces systemic vasodilation with compensatory tachycardia.

(Continued)

Table 37-1. Representative oral or parenteral sympathomimetic bronchodilators* (Continued)

Drug name	Preparation	Usual adult dosage	Additional information
			Store at room temperature. Tremors are a common adverse reaction.
Combination products			
Bronkotabs ephedrine 24 mg guaifenesin 100 mg theophylline 100 mg phenobarbital 8 mg	Tablets	1 tablet q3–4h	May cause drowsiness. Ephedrine may cause urinary retention in clients with partial obstruction. Ephedrine may cause palpitations.
Tedral ephedrine 24 mg theophylline 130 mg phenobarbital 8 mg	Tablets	1–2 tablets po q3–4h	Use with caution in client with glaucoma and prostatic hypertrophy. Monitor urinary output in elderly males.

* Use with caution in clients who suffer from cardiovascular disease, hypertension, hyperthyroidism, diabetes. Adverse reactions include palpitations, tremor, nervousness, tachycardia, nausea, vomiting, diaphoresis, anxiety, insomnia.

KEY: PC = pregnancy category. (The validity of pregnancy risk categories has not been established; see Chapter 16, p 216.)

tablets may be used to prevent nocturnal asthma. Isoproterenol and other nonselective β-adrenergic agonists are used infrequently because of their high incidence of cardiovascular side effects.

Sympathomimetics

Sympathomimetic drugs stimulate the action of the autonomic nervous system (Tables 37-1 and 37-2).

Pharmacodynamics. Sympathomimetics are also known as catecholamines. Differences in actions of the sympathomimetics occur because of the two main types of adrenergic receptors, α and β. Norepinephrine, epinephrine, and isoproterenol are catecholamines used in bronchodilation. They act at the different receptor sites. Norepinephrine stimulates α receptors predominantly; isoproterenol stimulates both β receptors; and epinephrine stimulates α, $β_1$, and $β_2$ receptors. The degree to which they are stimulated is dose related or drug related, because some sympathomimetic drugs are more $β_2$ related. The latter is desirable because activation of β receptors within smooth muscle leads to relaxation. Since norepinephrine stimulates α receptors, norepinephrine has little effect in bronchial air flow, because receptors in bronchial smooth muscle are largely $β_2$ type (Gilman, et al, 1990), and norepinephrine mainly stimulates α receptors.

Epinephrine and isoproterenol are potent bronchodilators because of their β-receptor activity. $β_2$ Receptors produce bronchodilation by the cAMP mechanism (MacDonnell, Segal, 1977). $β_1$ Receptors mediate the stimulation of cardiac muscle; this results in increased cardiac output, increased pulse, and palpitation. β-Adrenoreceptor stimulants are direct smooth muscle relaxants and activate cell adenylate cyclase to convert ATP to cAMP. The $β_2$ stimulants cause fewer $β_1$ effects.

Epinephrine

Epinephrine (Adrenalin) is a powerful bronchodilator, especially when bronchoconstriction occurs in asthma, because epinephrine inhibits the antigen-induced release of histamine. Epinephrine is also a potent vasopressor through direct $β_1$ myocardial stimulation, with positive inotropic effects leading to enhanced force of myocardial contraction and positive chronotropic action causing increased heart rate. The action of epinephrine on α receptors produces vasoconstriction in many vascular beds; this can relieve congestion within the bronchial mucosa. Epinephrine must be stored in tight light-resistant containers. Freezing should be avoided. Oxidation occurs if air is introduced into vials, turning the drug pink and rendering it unusable. Epinephrine should also not be used if a precipitate is evident. Epinephrine increases glycogenolysis in the liver, reduces glucose uptake in tissues, and inhibits insulin release in the pancreas. As a result, hyperglycemia may occur (AHFS drug information, 1991).

Therapeutic uses. Epinephrine is used to relieve respiratory distress due to bronchospasm. It is also effective for rapid relief from hypersensitivity reactions.

Dosage and administration. Epinephrine is not given orally because it is rapidly conjugated and oxidized in the gastrointestinal (GI) tract and liver and metabolized by catechol-o-methyl transferase (COMT). Norepinephrine and epinephrine are both destroyed by COMT, mainly in the liver (Guyton, 1991).

Epinephrine injection 1 : 1000, a sterile solution in

Table 37-2. Representative adrenergic (sympathomimetic) bronchodilators*

Drug name	Preparation	Usual adult dosage	Additional information and adverse reactions
albuterol, salbutamol (Proventil, Ventolin)	Metered-dose inhaler	2 inhalations (180 μg) q4–6h over 5 min	Similar adverse reactions to Alupent listed below
	Aerosol (0.5%)	0.5 ml (with 3 ml normal saline) PC: C	Lasts 5–6 h
			Antagonized by β-adrenergic blocking agents such as propranolol.
epinephrine bitartrate (Medihaler-Epi)	Metered-dose inhaler	1 inhalation (160 μg) Repeat once after 2 min PRN, give q4h	Rinse mouth with water after inhalation.
			Tremulousness, tachycardia.
			Use with caution if client has hypertension, hyperthyroid disease, or cardiovascular disease.
			Use with caution in client with tuberculosis.
racemic epinephrine (equivalent to 2.25% epinephrine) (Vaponefrin)	Solution for inhalation	2–3 inhalations Rest 5 min if needed, take 2–3 more inhalations Use 4–6 times a day PC: C	Nervousness, bronchial irritation, insomnia.
			Do not use if client has hypertension, heart disease, hyperthyroidism, or diabetes.
			Do not use if the solution is brown or contains a precipitate.
isoetharine (Bronkometer)	Metered-dose inhaler	1–2 inhalations (340–680 μg) qid PC: C	Wait 1 min between inhalations.
			Headache, tachycardia, palpitation, restlessness, tremor, weakness, nausea, dizziness.
(Bronkosol, Dey-Lute)	Solution for inhalation	*Hand nebulizer:* 4 inhalations, undiluted *IPPB:* 0.5 ml with 1–3 ml normal saline for 15–20 min, qid	Loses effectiveness with use.
			Do not administer with other sympathomimetic drugs.
			Adjust dosage if client has hypertension, hyperthyroid disease, cardiac asthma, coronary artery disease.
isoproterenol hydrochloride, phenylephrine bitartrate (Duo-Medihaler)	Metered-dose inhaler	1–2 inhalations at 4–6 h intervals PC: C	Tachycardia, palpitations, flushing, anginal pain, cardiac arrhythmia, dizziness, diaphoresis, nausea.
			Do not use in patients with cardiac arrhythmia.
			Excessive use may lead to loss of effect.
			Do not use with epinephrine.
			Caution in clients with cardiovascular disease, coronary insufficiency, diabetes, hyperthyroidism.
isoproterenol sulfate (Medihaler-Iso)	Metered-dose inhaler	1–2 inhalations (80–160 mg) repeated at 3–4 h intervals PC: C	Change in blood pressure, tachycardia, palpitation, vertigo, tremors, headache, insomnia, nausea, CNS excitation.
			Increased use leads to loss of effectiveness.
			Do not use if client exhibits cardiac arrhythmia.

(Continued)

Table 37-2. Representative adrenergic (sympathomimetic) bronchodilators* (Continued)

Drug name	Preparation	Usual adult dosage	Additional information and adverse reactions
metaproterenol (Alupent, Metaprel)	Metered-dose inhaler	2–3 inhalations (1.3–1.95 mg) qid over 5 min	Caution clients with diabetes, cardiovascular disease, hypertension, hyperthyroidism. Hypertension, tachycardia, palpitations, nervousness, tremor, vomiting, bad taste in mouth.
		Hand nebulizer: 10 inhalations of an undiluted 5% solution	Do not administer with another sympathomimetic agent.
		IPPB: 0.3 ml with 2.5 ml normal saline, qid	Administer with caution in client with hypertension, hyperthyroidism, diabetes, congestive heart failure, coronary artery disease.
	Solution for inhalation	0.5 ml (with 3 ml normal saline) PC: C	

*Used in aerosols or nebulizers. Drugs used for reversible bronchospasm and chronic asthma; may also be used for COPD.
KEY: PC = pregnancy category. (The validity of pregnancy risk categories has not been established; see Chapter 16, p 216.)

water, is used for parenteral injection. The usual adult dose is 0.1 to 0.5 ml (0.1–0.5 mg) subcutaneously. If symptoms do not abate in 15 to 20 minutes, another injection of the same dose may be repeated. It can also be administered slowly and with caution IV.

Sus-Phrine is an aqueous 1:200 suspension of crystalline epinephrine. It has a prolonged duration of action because of low solubility. The dose is 0.1 ml to a maximum of 0.3 ml subcutaneously. Do not repeat before 6 hours have elapsed, and do not give the drug IV.

Epinephrine inhalation is a 1% aqueous solution that may be used in nebulizer, aerosol, or IPPB form. This 1:100 solution is not to be confused with the 1:1000 solution.

Epinephrine nasal solution is used in 1:50,000 to 1:2000 solutions for nasal spray to constrict vessels of nasal mucosa or for abraded skin areas.

Adverse reactions. Many toxic and adverse reactions are associated with this drug. Signs and symptoms of toxicity include fear, anxiety, restlessness, tension, tremor, palpitation, throbbing headaches, pallor, ventricular arrhythmia, and tachycardia. Epinephrine increases rigidity and tremors in clients with Parkinson's disease. Nausea, vomiting, sweating may also occur. Epinephrine has been known to cause syncope and loss of consciousness. Repeated injections can cause necrosis at the vascular site as a result of vascular constriction. Tissue necrosis may also occur in the extremities, kidneys, and liver. Injections should not be given in the buttocks. Gas gangrene may occur. A possible rationale is that epinephrine-induced vasoconstriction reduces tissue oxygen tension, then enabling anaerobic *Clostridium welchii*, possibly present on the buttocks from the client's feces, to multiply (AHFS drug information, 1991).

Bronchial irritation and edema may result from oral inhalation of epinephrine. In some clients, rebound bronchospasm may also occur. Dryness of the pharyngeal membranes occurs from oral inhalation. (Rinsing the mouth with water after inhalation may prevent drying.)

Precautions. Caution should be used if the drug is administered to clients with hyperthyroidism, hypertension, diabetes mellitus, cardiovascular disease (coronary artery disease [angina pectoris, myocardial infarction] and tachycardia), or susceptibility to adverse pressor reactions.

Isoproterenol

Isoproterenol (Isuprel) provides powerful β_2 stimulation, leading to relaxation of the bronchial tree.

Pharmacodynamics. Isoproterenol is the strongest sympathomimetic drug that acts almost exclusively on β receptors. The actions of isoproterenol include increased cardiac output, lowered peripheral vascular resistance, relaxation of smooth muscle, and inhibition of antigen-induced release of histamine. Isoproterenol is used as a cardiac stimulant and as a bronchodilator to relieve bronchoconstriction.

Dosage and administration. The drug is given parenterally or as an aerosol. It is metabolized in the liver by COMT. Duration of action is about 1 hour.

Isoproterenol (Isuprel) can be given parenterally as a sterile injection: 1:5000 equals 0.2 mg/ml. The infusion must be given slowly.

Isoproterenol hydrochloride inhalation, an aqueous solution available in 1:100 or 1:200 solutions, may be administered in 1:200 strength by hand nebulizer or IPPB machine. It is usually used to relieve bronchoconstriction (as in asthma). A dose of 0.5 ml of

1 : 200 solution diluted with 2.5 ml isotonic saline or water for 10 to 20 minutes is given qid with an IPPB machine. If administered by hand-bulb nebulizer, the usual dose is 5 to 15 deep inhalations using 1 : 200 solution (see Nursing Management sections for client instruction on the proper use of the nebulizer).

Isoproterenol metered-dose aerosols are available in solutions of 0.25%. To administer, the client is instructed to hold the aerosol unit in the inverted position and to close the teeth and lips securely around the mouthpiece. The client should exhale fully and then inhale while pressing down on the canister that activates the mechanism. The client should hold his or her breath a few seconds before exhaling. The client should wait a few minutes before repeating this once. One application is about equal to five to seven inhalations from the hand-held nebulizer. This dose may be repeated up to five times daily at intervals of 3 to 4 hours. Initially, clients may complain of a sore throat from the alcohol content, but this symptom tends to disappear.

Drug tolerance may occur. These drugs are used less frequently because of the adverse reactions.

Adverse reactions. The toxic and adverse reactions of isoproterenol include palpitation, tachycardia, flushing of the skin, headache, tremor, anginal pain, nausea, dizziness, weakness, diaphoresis, and cardiac arrhythmia.

Precautions. It is important to take the apical and radial pulse and to observe the electrocardiogram on the monitor when treating a client with isoproterenol.

Isoetharine

Because of β_1 stimulation with resultant adverse reactions, effort has been made to use drugs with more selective β_2-adrenergic stimulant action (agonists). Isoetharine is such an example. It is available as a solution for nebulization (Bronkosol) and as a metered aerosol (Bronkometer). It is used for bronchodilation. The duration of action is longer, lasting for 2 hours, but the onset of action is slower. Adverse reactions include tachycardia, nausea, anxiety, and restlessness.

Other β_2 stimulants

Also available for bronchodilation are other selective β_2 stimulants that are not catecholamines and therefore less subject to COMT inactivation. Examples of these are metaproterenol (Alupent, Metaprel), terbutaline (Brethine, Bricanyl), and albuterol (Ventolin, Proventil). These also may be administered orally. The duration of action is 3 to 6 hours. These drugs are useful in the treatment of bronchial asthma and reversible bronchospasm associated with bronchitis or emphysema. These drugs reduce airway resistance, and pulmonary function studies reveal a significant improvement in forced expiratory volume in 1 second (FEV_1).

Metaproterenol

Metaproterenol is an effective bronchodilator whether given by inhalation or the oral route. With a single oral dose of 20 mg, significant improvement of airway function lasts about 4 hours. (Dosage and administration are indicated in Table 37-3). The effect is more variable if inhaled, but duration of action may be 5 hours or longer. Adverse reactions include tachycardia, increased blood pressure, tremor, palpitation, nervousness, and nausea and vomiting. These adverse reactions seem to be less frequent than those seen with catecholamines. Metaproterenol should be used with caution in clients who also suffer from coronary artery disease, congestive heart failure, hypertension, diabetes, and hyperthyroidism.

Terbutaline sulfate

Terbutaline sulfate, a synthetic sympathomimetic agent, is a selective β_2-agonist. It is an effective bronchodilator. (Dosage and administration are given in Table 37-4). Adverse reactions include nervousness, muscle tremor, palpitation, tachycardia, diaphoresis, and nausea and vomiting. Effects usually are mild and often decrease as therapy is continued. If given orally, the onset of action occurs within 1 hour, but the effect lasts 4 to 8 hours. If given subcutaneously, the onset of action is 5 to 15 minutes with peak action at $^1/_2$ to 1 hour, and the duration is 4 hours. The onset of action for the inhaled product is more rapid with a similar duration of effect, but the duration of action is only 3 to 4 hours. Especially important to note, however, is that if given subcutaneously, the selectivity of β_2 receptors diminishes, and cardiovascular adverse reactions are more frequent. The drug may also lower the diastolic blood pressure.

Albuterol

Albuterol (Ventolin, Proventil) has been available in Europe and Canada and is now approved for use in the United States. Similar to the preceding drugs, it ap-

Table 37-3. Dosage and administration of metaproterenol

Preparations	Dosage	Age
Tablets	20 mg, PO, tid or qid	Adult dose
Syrup		
(10 mg)	10 mg = 5 ml	
	10 mg tid if less than 27 kg	Pediatric dose 6–9 yr of age
(20 mg)	20 mg tid or qid if larger than 27 kg	9 yr and older
Inhalation metered	0.65 mg nebulized dose	
	Administer 2–3 deep inhalations; repeat q4h	
	No more than 12 inhalations a day	

Table 37-4. Dosage and administration of terbutaline sulfate (Bricanyl, Brethine)

Route	Dosage	Additional information
Oral	2.5–5 mg, PO, tid-qid (6-h intervals)	If adverse reactions present, give 2.5 mg Tablets available 2.5 and 5 mg
Subcutaneous	0.25 mg; repeat after 15–30 min if no significant improvement	Do not exceed 0.5 mg in 4 h Available in 1 mg/1 ml solution

pears to induce less angina in asthmatics who have ischemic heart disease. Albuterol may also be given either by inhalation or by mouth. Adverse reactions are similar to those of the other sympathomimetic agents. Though less common, the reactions include tachycardia, palpitation, tremor, nervousness, nausea, vomiting, muscle cramps, angina, headache, vertigo, insomnia, and, rarely, dizziness. Blood pressure may increase or decrease. Some people complain of an unusual taste in the mouth and of oropharyngeal symptoms such as cough, irritation, and dryness. This drug is also used cautiously in clients with hyperthyroidism, diabetes mellitus, hypertension, and cardiovascular disease. One puff of albuterol via a metered-dose inhaler, drug powder inhaler, or jet nebulizer is reported to be about three times as potent as each puff (650 µg) of metaproterenol. Albuterol is about two times more potent than each puff (225 µg) of terbutaline (Ahrens, 1991).

Overuse of albuterol is suspected of contributing to increased mortality from asthma. At this writing, reports in the news media indicate that use of more than one container of albuterol metered-dose inhalant per month is associated with a significant increase in the death rate.

Antimuscarinics and anticholinergics

Research continues on the use of anticholinergic drugs in the mediation of bronchial tone in treating asthma and bronchitis. Because of their adverse reactions and the advent of effective sympathomimetic agents, these drugs are used infrequently today. This use could change in the future, however, because of increased knowledge about the pathophysiology of asthma, especially with respect to neurogenic vagal reflexes and imbalances between the inhibiting (cAMP) and excitatory (cGMP) mediators. A derivative or congener of atropine (ipratropium) that has also been developed is effective as a bronchodilator and free of many of the detrimental effects.

These drugs inhibit the action of acetylcholine or autonomic effects innervated by postganglionic cholinergic nerves. They antagonize cholinergic stimuli at muscarinic receptors and inhibit vagal cholinergic tone, resulting in bronchodilation. They block cholinergic reflex constriction. Although these drugs are used as antispasmodics, this section only addresses their actions on the respiratory tract. These drugs reduce the volume of secretions from the nose, mouth, pharynx, and bronchi. Most important, they reduce airway resistance by relaxing bronchial smooth muscle. Atropine and ipratropium are potent bronchodilators, especially in the large bronchial airways. They are effective if bronchoconstriction is the result of parasympathetic stimulation. They are effective in treating COPD and less effective in chronic asthma. Atropine can be administered orally, but for respiratory effect, it is usually administered parenterally or by oral inhalation. The effect is similar to that of isoproterenol. Onset of action is slower than orally inhaled isoetharine, but the duration of action is longer. Adverse reactions of atropine include dry mouth, blurred vision, tachycardia, urinary hesitancy, and constipation. Some clients complain of dizziness, weakness, nervousness, nausea, vomiting, and insomnia. Urticaria, rashes, and anaphylaxis have been reported. These reactions are less frequent when the drug is administered by inhalation, although the drying of secretions has been a serious problem for people with COPD. Ipratropium is only available for oral inhalation. It has few of the adverse reactions of atropine and is as effective as terbutaline. These drugs are effective in treating exercise-induced bronchospasm.

Ipratropium does not appear to affect the volume or viscosity of sputum. The drug is available but is not yet widely used. Dosage is between 20 and 80 mg by inhalation. Atropine sulfate is given 1.0 mg orally, 0.4 to 0.6 mg subcutaneously, or by inhalation 0.8 to 1 mg in 2-ml saline. Onset of action occurs in 30 minutes and lasts 2 to 3 hours.

Xanthines

Another major class of drugs used to produce bronchodilation and treat bronchitis, emphysema, and asthma is the xanthine group. In fact, they have been referred to as the cornerstone of therapy in clients who suffer from bronchospasm (MacDonnell, Segal, 1977). Theophylline, caffeine, and theobromine are closely related alkaloids chemically defined as methylated xanthines. Theophylline and various derivatives come in many preparations (Table 37-5), such as aminophylline, oxtriphylline, and theophylline sodium glycinate. Dyphylline is structurally and pharmacologically similar to theophylline but chemically distant. Tolerance to these drugs rarely occurs. These drugs can be used with the sympathomimetic agonists because they have different modes of action. Adrenergic drugs directly increase cAMP.

Table 37-5. Availability of theophylline preparations

Drug name	Preparation	Strengths
aminophylline U.S.P.	Solutions for injection	250 mg/10 ml or 500 mg/20 ml IV or 500 mg in 2 ml
	Rectal suppository	250 mg, 500 mg
theophylline (Corfilamin, Corophyllin, Ethophylline Palaron, Phyllocontin)	Tablets/capsules	50 mg, 100 mg, 125 mg, 200 mg, 225 mg, 250 mg, 300 mg
	Elixir	80 mg/15 ml, 100 mg/15 ml, 250 mg/15 ml
	Solution for rectal use	60 mg/ml, 100 mg/ml
	Sustained-release	50 mg, 65 mg, 100 mg, 200 mg, 250 mg, 300 mg

Theophylline

Pharmacodynamics. Theophylline directly relaxes smooth muscle of the bronchi and pulmonary blood vessels by competitively inhibiting phosphodiesterase, resulting in an increase of cAMP. The latter inhibits the release of the SRS-A and histamine. (Phosphodiesterase degrades or breaks down cAMP.) Bronchodilation occurs if it results from bronchospasm. Other pulmonary effects include central respiratory stimulation, reduction in pulmonary hypertension and alveolar carbon dioxide tension, and increase in pulmonary blood flow. Nonpulmonary effects include stimulation of the central nervous system (CNS), promotion of diuresis, increased secretion of gastric acid, and inhibition of uterine contractions. Cardiovascular effects include weak positive chronotropic and inotropic effects.

It is postulated that intracellular translocation of ionized calcium is responsible for the neuromuscular and cardiovascular effects (Gilman, et al, 1990).

Theophylline has many effects on the respiratory tract, making it useful in treating obstructive airway disease. In combination with other respiratory drugs, it is very effective. Theophylline increases respiratory muscle strength, strengthens diaphragmatic contractions, and delays diaphragmatic fatigue (Aubier, 1987). These characteristics are especially effective in clients with chronic lung disease who retain carbon dioxide. Theophylline stimulates ciliary motility in the proximal portion of the respiratory tree, and, with the increased bronchodilation, increased mucociliary clearance occurs, improving pulmonary ventilation (Ziment, 1987; Phillips, 1990).

In addition to its bronchodilator effect, theophylline enhances mucociliary clearance. It is also a respiratory stimulant and increases the strength of diaphragmatic contraction (Phillips, 1990).

Theophylline also enhances cardiovascular performance in clients with COPD. Theophylline improves both right and left heart systolic pump function and lowers pulmonary artery pressure and pulmonary vascular resistance (Matthay, 1987).

Recent research suggests another important action of theophylline in treating clients with asthma and COPD. Theophylline appears to inhibit airway inflammation (Pauwels, 1987). This action is relevant to late-phase response seen in people with asthma.

Theophylline is used with β_2-agonists in treating respiratory clients. These two classes of drugs are the main agents in therapy. Long-acting theophylline agents produce a relatively constant effect, and theophylline is effective in reducing the increased airway responsiveness seen in asthma. This effect may occur because theophylline is a direct competitor antagonist with the adenosine receptor. β-Agonists have a shorter duration of action, and long-acting theophylline covers the time period at the end of the duration of a dose of β_2-agonist and before the next dose, reducing disease symptoms that occur as a result of troughs (Ahrens, 1991).

Until recently, this drug has been the first choice of therapy, although its mechanism of action is not fully understood. Initially, its action was thought to be the result of inhibition of the production of phosphodiesterase, thereby increasing the concentration of intracellular cAMP that results in bronchodilation. The amount of drug required to do this exceeds the therapeutic range. Current proposed modes of action include antagonism of adenosine receptors or inhibition of the intracellular release of calcium and stimulation of catecholamine release (Barnes, 1989a). Theophylline may have anti-inflammatory action, however, and does have a synergistic effect with β-adrenergic agonists. Slow release preparations given in the evening help prevent nocturnal asthma.

Although further research is needed, reports indicate that therapy that combines theophylline and β_2-agonists induces greater bronchodilation than when either drug is used alone (Jenne, 1987).

Pharmacokinetics. Theophylline is well absorbed after oral administration. Food does not affect the drug's bioavailability, although it may slow absorption of the drug. If taken with a high-protein diet or with a large volume of fluid, absorption is accelerated. The oral route is preferred, because rectal absorption from suppositories is erratic and slow. However, if necessary or indicated, rectal solutions by retention enemas are more rapidly absorbed.

Enteric-coated tablets and sustained-release dosage capsules may be absorbed unreliably. Each person must be monitored closely and tested with the same preparation until the desired level is reached. The serum concentration necessary to produce bronchodilation is 10 to 20 μg/ml. The dose needed to achieve this level differs from person to person. Newer continuous-release products have produced desirable drug serum levels, and client compliance has increased as the interval between doses has increased. Once a person's dose is stabilized, serum levels tend to remain constant with the same dose.

Absorption is fastest after IV theophylline and aminophylline administration, with the desired level being achieved in 1/2 hour. After each administration (tablet, capsule, liquid), the serum concentration is reached in 1 to 2 hours. Enteric-coated theophylline tablets produce variable serum concentrations and require 5 hours to peak. Single-dose extended-release capsules or tablets produce peak serum levels within 4 hours. Retention enemas reach the desired level in 1 to 2 hours, and suppositories require 3 to 5 hours (AHFS Drug Information, 1986). Distribution is widespread but not into fatty tissue. Theophylline does cross the placenta and is present in breast milk.

Theophylline is metabolized in the liver and is essentially excreted by the kidneys. Many factors affect the elimination of theophylline, however, and it varies greatly from person to person. In adult nonsmokers, the plasma elimination half-life averages 7 to 9 hours, whereas it is 4 to 5 hours in adult smokers. In children, the drug's half-life is reduced to 3 to 5 hours, and for premature infants, it requires 20 to 36 hours. Decreased plasma clearance also occurs in people with heart failure, liver disease, pulmonary edema, and COPD. Prolonged high fever may decrease elimination, and various drugs affect clearance. Smokers, therefore, may require a larger dose, and the interval between doses may be shorter, because smoking induces the hepatic metabolism of theophylline (Box 37-2).

The dosage of theophylline is highly individualized. It depends on the client's clinical response and requires monitoring of desired serum levels. For the client with liver disease, congestive heart failure, pulmonary infection, and pulmonary edema, the duration of action may be much longer, whereas with a smoker, it may be much shorter. The age, weight, and degree of illness are all considered. Serum concentration is the determining factor and should be between 10 and 20 µg/ml. New methods for determining serum levels are being developed, and accurate accu-level finger prick methods exist. In addition, the various theophylline salts and derivatives differ in content and are not equivalent by weight (Table 37-6). Current treatment aims for serum levels between 10 and 15 µg/ml.

The margin of safety with theophylline is narrow, and the potential for toxicity is high, especially if administered too rapidly by IV. However, it is an extremely useful drug that is used extensively. If properly monitored, it provides many people with relief.

Adverse reactions. Adverse reactions are not common with serum theophylline levels below 20 µg/ml. At levels above this, 75% of clients report GI symptoms such as nausea, vomiting, and diarrhea, in addition to irritability, headache, and insomnia. At levels above 30 to 35 µg/ml, tachycardia, cardiac arrhythmia, hypotension, seizures, brain damage, and death may occur.

In general, symptoms can be related to every organ system. Additional GI problems include dyspepsia, epigastric pain, rectal irritation if administered PR, intestinal bleeding, and reactivation of peptic ulcers.

CNS irritability, especially in children, may be observed, and restlessness, lightheadedness, muscle toxicity, depression, speech disturbances, and hyperactivity may be seen. Occasionally, renal problems such as proteinuria and urinary retention occur in males with prostate enlargement. Theophylline interacts

---

Box 37-2. Considerations in theophylline therapy

1. Special precautions for the nurse
   a. Half-life is shortened in clients who smoke.
   b. Half-life is prolonged in clients with alcoholism, congestive heart failure, and in clients using the following antibiotics:
      (1) Erythromycin
      (2) Troleandomycin
   c. Prolonged high fever decreases elimination of the drug.
2. Therapeutic serum level: Between 10 and 20 µg/ml
3. Adverse reactions: Correlate with serum concentration. More prevalent if level is greater than 20 µg/ml.
   a. Early signs and symptoms: Nausea, restlessness, insomnia, vomiting, anorexia, ventricular arrhythmia, and convulsions
   b. Other symptoms: Epigastric pain, hematemesis, diarrhea, headache, irritability, muscle twitching, palpitations, tachycardia, flushing, circulatory failure, and convulsions

---

Table 37-6. Comparison of various theophylline salts and derivatives

Drug name	Percentage of theophylline	Equivalent dose
theophylline anhydrous	100%	100 mg
theophylline monohydrate	91%	110 mg
aminophylline anhydrous	86%	116 mg
aminophylline dihydrate	79%	127 mg
oxtriphylline	64%	156 mg
theophylline sodium glycinate	49%	204 mg
theophylline calcium salicylate	48%	208 mg

with many medicinal drugs, resulting in changes in the level of action of theophylline or the interacting drug (Box 37-3).

Precautions. It is helpful to administer oral theophylline with meals to avoid gastric irritation and GI upset. If the client is nauseated, give the drug after the meal. The sustained-release preparation and the enteric-coated tablets must not be chewed.

Careful administration of IV aminophylline and careful attention to rate is required. If the drug is administered too rapidly, a fatal reaction may occur.

These drugs are most effective in providing relief for bronchial constriction; however, serum concentrations must be monitored closely, and the client must be evaluated for adverse reactions. These drugs are frequently given in conjunction with the sympathomimetic drugs and steroids. Clients with COPD frequently exhibit gastroesophageal reflux, which, it is believed, contributes to their disease. Theophylline can relax the lower esophageal sphincter; consequently, theophylline therapy may contribute to chronic respiratory disease as well as produce heartburn. This symptom can be lessened if people do not sleep flat in bed.

Another problem associated with asthma is also gastroesophageal reflux as a result of high negative intrapleural pressures generated during an asthmatic attack (Mansfield, 1989). In asthmatic clients, an increase in bronchial reactivity may occur in response to acid in the esophagus. This effect is often observed during the night in asthma clients, as the asthma often occurs early in the morning when acid enters the esophagus as a result of sleeping in a supine position (Mansfield, 1989). Bronchodilators may also predispose clients to gastroesophageal reflux, as theophylline, β-adrenergic stimulating agents, and anticholinergic medicines can cause relaxation of the lower esophageal sphincter (Mansfield, 1989).

It is recommended that antireflux therapy be instituted or theophylline stopped if symptoms of gastroesophageal reflux occur (Berquist, et al, 1981; Mansfield, 1989).

Dosage and administration. Dosages of theophylline are individualized, because the amount required to achieve a therapeutic serum level (between 10 and 20 μg/ml) varies from one client to another. The dose is adjusted based on monitoring serum results and clinical response (Table 37-7). For faster absorption, the drug is taken with a glass of water on an empty stomach (30 minutes to 1 hour before meals or 2 hours after a meal). If the person complains of GI irritation, theophylline may be given with meals. Capsules, enteric-coated tablets, and sustained-release tablets must not be crushed or chewed. Parenterally, theophylline is *not* administered intramuscularly. For IV administration, 25 mg/ml injection is used and may be further diluted with IV fluids. The medication must be administered slowly (no faster than 20 to 25 mg/minute) to prevent hypotension and peripheral circulatory collapse. To initiate therapy, a larger loading dose is given, which then is followed by maintenance doses (Box 37-4; see also Focus on Xanthines: Similarities and Differences).

Other drugs for asthma

Corticosteroids

Corticosteroids, discussed in Chapter 32, are also used to treat clients with asthma. Several halogenated corticosteroids on the market can be given by inhalation. They provide selective topical effects, leading to improvement in the client's respiratory status with minimal absorption in the blood. Inhalation helps avoid the associated adverse reactions of steroids and does not appear to suppress adrenal function. Corticosteroid aerosols for the treatment of asthma include beclomethasone dipropionate (Vanceril, Beclovent), dosage: 2 inhalations [84 μg], tid–qid; triamcinolone acetonide (Azmacort), dosage: 4 inhalations [200 μg], tid–qid; and flunisolide (AeroBid), dosage: 2 inhalations [500 μg], bid. Any orally administered steroid does essentially the same thing. Recent research indicates that the systemic administration of corticosteroids improves air flow in respiratory failure in clients

---

Box 37-3. Drug interactions with theophylline

- Phenobarbital increases theophylline metabolism.
- Charcoal-broiled food increases theophylline elimination.
- Drugs that increase the effect of theophylline (increasing serum levels by decreasing hepatic clearance):
    Cimetidine
    Erythromycin
    Influenza virus vaccine
    Troleandomycin
    Allupurinol
    Furosemide
    Propranolol
- Theophylline increases the effects of other drugs:
    Enhances sensitivity to digitalis
    High doses may increase the effect of anticoagulants
    Excessive CNS stimulation with sympathomimetic drugs
- Theophylline decreases the effect of phenytoin.
- Theophylline increases excretion of lithium carbonate and may reduce its therapeutic effect.
- Avoid the use of theophylline with halothane and ketamine.

Table 37-7. Selected xanthine preparations*

Drug name	Preparation	Usual adult dosage	Additional information
aminophylline (Aminodur)	Sustained-release tablet 300 mg (Duratab)	300 mg q12h	30 minutes before eating.
aminophylline	Solution for injection	*Loading dose:* 5–6 mg/kg IV over 20 min (250–500 mg in 100 ml–200 ml D5W) Then 0.2–0.7 mg/kg/hr	Omit loading dose if patient is on theophylline preparation. IV alone—less effective in initial therapy of acute attack than either inhaled or parenteral subcutaneous sympathomimetics, but the combination is effective.
oxtriphylline (Choledyl)	Tablets 100 mg 200 mg Elixir 100 mg/5 ml Syrup 50 mg/5 ml	200 mg, qid	
theophylline (Constant-T)	Sustained-release tablets 200 mg 300 mg	200–300 mg, q12h	Do not crush or chew. Keep tightly closed. Store at room temperature (60°–80° F).
theophylline (Elixophyllin)	Capsules 100 mg 200 mg Elixir 80 mg/15 ml	*Initially:* 16 mg/kg/day or 400 mg/day in divided doses every 6–8 h	
dyphylline (Lufyllin)	Tablets 200 mg 400 mg	1–2 tablets q6h (up to 15 mg/kg)	Give on an empty stomach.
ephedrine 25 mg theophylline 130 mg hydroxyzine 10 mg (Marax)	Tablets	1 tablet, 2–4 times daily	Administer after meals. Drowsiness may occur.
theophylline 150 mg guaifenesin 90 mg (Quibron)	Capsules	1–2 capsules q6–8h	
theophylline (Slo-Phyllin)	Tablets 100 mg 200 mg Syrup 80 mg/15 ml	1–2 tablets 3 mg/kg q8h	Give with food.
aminophylline 105 mg/ 5 ml (Somophyllin)	Oral liquid	13 mg/kg/day or 900 mg/day; give at 6 h–8 h	
theophylline (Theodur)	Sustained-release tablets 100 mg 200 mg 300 mg	200–300 mg, q12h	Do not chew or crush. Keep tightly closed. Store at room temperature (60°–80° F).

* With all preparations, the maintenance dose is adjusted to maintain serum concentrations between 10 and 20 μg/ml. Nausea, vomiting, and cardiac dysrhythmia are more common if the serum concentration is greater than 20 μg/ml.

β-adrenergic blockers may antagonize action of methylxanthines.

with COPD (Petty, et al, 1982). Short-term use of high doses of steroids, referred to as a "burst of steroids," includes doses of 100 to 200 mg a day, or treatment may include 7 to 10 days of high doses such as 40 to 80 mg/day of prednisone with subsequent tapering. Some clients with severe uncontrolled asthma require chronic treatment with oral steroids. Corticosteroids suppress inflammation and block the steps necessary for late-phase reactions by inhibiting arachidonic acid metabolism. Until recently, corticosteroids were used when other bronchodilators were ineffective. Inhaled corticosteroids, which have fewer systemic side effects, may be used more frequently in the future to prevent late-phase reactions (Kaliner, 1987).

With the current view that a chronic inflammatory process plays a central role in the pathophysiology of asthma, anti-inflammatory agents will be used far more frequently in practice. Clients will also be given them sooner. Corticosteroids are effective in suppressing the inflammatory effect and are also used prophylactically to prevent an inflammatory response. Their action inhibits the release of mediators from eosinophils and macrophages. When given over a longer period of time (2 to 3 months), they also reduce bronchial hyperresponsiveness, especially if administered by inhalation. Steroids that are given over a period of time also prevent exercise-induced asthma, reduce the response to allergens, reduce the numbers of mast cells in the airways, and reduce the formation of certain cytokines (Barnes, 1989a).

Until recently, steroids were administered after β-adrenergic agonists or theophylline were used without sufficient relief. Steroids were given orally with systemic side effects. Steroid inhalants are now available as "high dose" (200 μg of steroid per puff) and "low dose" (50 μg/puff) inhalers. The different steroid inhalers are similar in effectiveness. They are effective when given twice a day, and this dosage improves compliance. Some individuals require therapy four times a day, however (Barnes, 1989a). Systemic steroids given orally may be indicated during periods of exacerbation. Oral steroids may be given 5 to 10 days until peak expiratory flow rates are stable or approach the client's best or predicted values. Inhaled steroids are safe and reduce the need for the chronic use of oral steroids.

Adverse reactions. Adverse reactions to corticosteroid aerosols include sore throat and oropharyngeal and laryngeal infection with *Candida albicans*. Strict oral hygiene must be instituted, and proper inhalation techniques must be taught. Antifungal medication may be necessary. Instruct clients to rinse the mouth with water after inhalation therapy with steroids. They may also need to rinse and gargle with an antifungal agent such as nystatin if fungal infections occur in the oral cavity.

Cromolyn sodium

Another useful drug for treating asthmatics is cromolyn sodium, or disodium cromoglycate (Intal). A synthetic substance, cromolyn is an antiasthmatic, antiallergenic, and a mast cell stabilizer. While it is not an antihistamine, anti-inflammatory agent, bronchodilator, or steroid, it has enabled some people to decrease their use of steroids.

Pharmacodynamics. Cromolyn sodium appears to act by stabilizing the cell membranes of mast cells, thereby preventing the release of asthmatic mediators that occur when an allergen combines with IgE fixed to the cell surface. The precise action is not fully understood, but cromolyn indirectly blocks the calcium channels in mast cells and prevents mast cell degranulation by blocking phosphorylation of a membrane protein (Kaliner, 1987). Cromolyn interferes, therefore, with the release of allergic mediators from bronchial mast cells. It is used prophylactically to prevent the secretion and release of histamine and SRS-A, therefore reducing the stimulus for bronchospasm. This drug prevents immediate and late-phase allergic reactions. Cromolyn prevents the late response seen in asthma and bronchial hyperresponsiveness. Cromolyn may also act on macrophages and eosinophils.

Pharmacokinetics. Cromolyn is poorly absorbed from the GI tract. It is not metabolized and is excreted essentially unchanged.

Dosage and administration. Cromolyn sodium is inhaled because it is poorly absorbed orally. It is available as a dry powder, 20 mg in a gelatin capsule. The drug has not shown the promise hoped for, however, because it is impractical to take and must be used four times a day. Cromolyn sodium is delivered through a spinhaler device. Because client compliance with this drug has not been good, a solution has been newly formulated (20 mg/2 ml) for nebulization. Perhaps this new formulation will improve acceptability of this drug. Bronchospasm has been a repeated problem, even though it is minimized somewhat by concurrent administration of an adrenergic bronchodilator. Cromolyn sodium is available in an ophthalmic solution for

Focus on

Xanthines: similarities and differences

Similarities	Differences

Similarities

Pharmacodynamics

These agents competitively inhibit phosphodiesterase, resulting in an increase in cAMP. They are also believed to alter smooth muscle calcium ion concentration, inhibit the effects of adenosine receptors, and inhibit the release of histamine from the mast cells. They also directly stimulate the medullary respiratory center and directly relax smooth muscle of the respiratory tract. They also stimulate the vasomotor and vagal centers, relax all smooth muscles with the respiratory smooth muscles as the most sensitive, and cause coronary vasodilation and cardiac, cerebral, and skeletal smooth muscle stimulation.

Pharmacokinetics

These agents are well absorbed after oral administration; absorption varies with the form used, and the rate of absorption varies with the size of the dose. These agents are rapidly distributed to the extracellular fluid and body tissues; they are also found in breast milk. They are converted to theophylline and metabolized in the liver to inactive compounds. They are excreted in the urine as theophylline and its metabolites. The half-life in adult nonsmokers is 7 to 9 hours.

Therapeutic uses

These agents are used as bronchodilators in symptomatic treatment of acute and chronic asthma and reversible bronchospasm.

Adverse reactions

These include: (CNS) restlessness, irritability, muscle twitching, headache, insomnia, dizziness, convulsions, reflex hyperexcitability; (CV) hypotension, palpitations, arrhythmia, ventricular tachycardia, sinus tachycardia; (RESP) tachypnea, respiratory arrest; (GI) nausea, vomiting, loss of appetite, diarrhea, dyspepsia; (GU) urinary retention, frequency; (HEMA) elevated aspartate aminotransferase; (DERM) urticaria

Contraindications

These agents are contraindicated in people who are taking other xanthines; those sensitive to theophylline, caffeine, or theobromine; and those with preexisting cardiac arrhythmia.

Differences

• **Dyphylline** has only one-tenth of the bronchodilator effect of other drugs of this class.

Enteric and extended-release forms of **aminophylline**, **oxtriphylline**, and **theophylline** are unreliably absorbed. • **Dyphylline** is rapidly absorbed, is not metabolized to **theophylline**, is excreted unchanged in the urine, peaking within 1 hour, with a half-life of 2 to 2.5 hours; the half-life in smokers is 4 to 5 hours; in children, it is 3 to 5 hours, and in premature infants, it is 20 to 36 hours. • **Theophylline** (IM) is incompletely and slowly absorbed. • **Theophylline** in oral and retention enema form peaks in 1 to 2 hours; enteric-coated **theophylline** peaks in 5 hours; extended-release **theophylline** peaks in 4 to 7 hours.

• **Aminophylline** and **theophylline** are used in the treatment of neonatal apnea and Cheyne-Stokes respirations, and to relieve periodic apnea and increase arterial blood *p*H.

• **Aminophylline** (rectal) can cause rectal irritation. Rapid IV administration of **aminophylline** can cause syncope, precordial pain, flushing, profound bradycardia. IM **aminophylline** can cause local pain and tissue sloughing at the injection site. • **Dyphylline** can cause hyperglycemia.

• **Aminophylline** is contraindicated in people hypersensitive to ethylenediamine.

(*continued*)

Focus on

Xanthines: similarities and differences (Continued)

Similarities	Differences

Precautions

These agents should be used with caution in young children and people older than age 55, neonates, and people who are undergoing influenza immunization or those with active influenza infection; with people with cardiac failure, COPD, cor pulmonale, renal or hepatic dysfunction, peptic ulcer, hyperthyroidism, glaucoma, diabetes, severe hypoxemia, hypertension, compromised cardiac or circulatory function, angina pectoris, or acute myocardial injury.

Some **theophyllines** contain sulfites and should be used with caution in people sensitive to sulfites.

Nursing considerations

Instruct client in disease, treatment, drug regimen, adverse effects, and compliance; administer with meals if GI irritation occurs; otherwise administer on an empty stomach with a full glass of water; monitor vital signs, especially pulse and blood pressure; assess pulmonary status, including respiratory rate and breath sounds; monitor serum levels of the drug and be alert for signs of toxicity; monitor intake and output; encourage fluids to liquify secretions; institute safety precautions, especially for the elderly, if dizziness occurs; warn client about the use of over-the-counter drugs, which may contain ephedrine and cause excessive CNS stimulation.

Warn clients not to crush, dissolve, or chew extended-release preparations of **theophylline**; administer "sprinkles" with soft food to children who are unable to swallow. Dilute IV **aminophylline** with dextrose and water to prevent burning and do not mix with any other drugs; administer IV push slowly at a rate of 25 mg/min. When administering **aminophylline** suppositories, give after the client has a bowel movement and instruct to remain recumbent for 15 to 20 minutes after insertion. Protect **dyphylline** from light and give only by the IM route. Administer **oxtriphylline** after meals and at bedtime; protect elixir from light and protect tablets from moisture.

use in allergic conjunctivitis and in an oral preparation for use in food allergy. However, the latter form still lacks Food and Drug Administration approval and is not for sale in the United States.

In emphysema and bronchitis, bronchodilators are used to provide symptomatic relief. Because current therapy for asthma is changing with respect to the order in which drugs are administered, two examples of step-approach are outlined here (Boxes 37-5 and 37-6).

Adverse reactions. Adverse reactions to cromolyn sodium include bronchospasm, wheezing, cough, nasal congestion, and pharyngeal irritation. Though rare, other effects that may occur are dizziness, dysuria, joint swelling, pain, nausea, headaches, rash, and, rarely, laryngeal edema, angioedema, urticaria, and anaphylaxis. If the client develops eosinophilia pneumonitis, the drug should be discontinued.

Precautions and contraindications. Cromolyn sodium is not used in acute attacks of asthma. It is only effective given prophylactically to prevent asthmatic attacks.

■ **Summary**

Drugs that affect the respiratory system achieve their beneficial effects through different mechanisms. Adrenergic drugs act by direct stimulation of cAMP through adenyl cyclase. Xanthine drugs act indirectly by inhibiting phosphodiesterase and may also act on bronchial smooth muscle by calcium sequestration. Steroid drugs act through a variety of possible mechanisms. Cromolyn, although not a bronchodilator, acts prophylactically by stabilizing the membrane of the mast cells. In the future, prostaglandins may be used in therapy.

Expectorants and mucolytic agents

Expectorants and mucolytic agents are another group of drugs used to treat respiratory disease. These drugs affect mucus or the mucous blanket either by direct action on the mucus or by increasing the secretion of mucus. The term *mucous blanket* refers to the mucous layer that covers the tracheobronchial tree in a contin-

Box 37-5. Overview of asthma therapy*

Aim of therapy

Optimum medication needed to maintain control with minimal risks and few adverse effects

Mild to episodic: β_2-agonist

Moderate: Add additional therapy
  Anti-inflammatory: cromolyn sodium, inhaled cortocosteroid
  Bronchodilation: inhaled β_2-agonist, oral theophylline, oral β_2-agonist

Severe: Add oral corticosteroid

Treatment

Mild: Asymptomatic, symptoms last less than 2 hours, and attacks occur one or two times a week: β_2-agonist by inhalation, 1 to 2 puffs prn. If used more than 3 to 4 times a day, additional therapy is needed.

If the person is symptomatic, use inhaled β_2-agonist, 2 puffs every 3 to 4 h for duration of episode.

Chronic moderate disease: Symptoms occur more than 1 to 2 times a week: use inhaled β_2-agonist prn or tid, qid. Add anti-inflammatory medication: inhaled corticosteroids, 2 to 4 puffs bid, or cromolyn sodium 2 puffs qid. If symptoms persist, add sustained release theophylline and/or oral β_2-agonist.

Severe asthma: Inhaled medication, β_2-agonist, required qid and inhaled corticosteroid, 2 to 6 puffs bid–qid with or without cromolyn sodium 2 puffs qid. Add theophylline if nocturnal asthma is present. May need to use burst oral corticosteroid: prednisone 40 mg every day, single dose or divided dose for 1 week and taper for 1 week.

Acute life-threatening asthma: Immediate therapy is aimed at bronchodilation. Selective β_2-agonist are used: albuterol, metaproterenol, and terbutaline all have similar profiles. Albuterol and metaproterenol are administered by inhalation, terbutaline by subcutaneous route or Medihaler. Epinephrine may also be given subcutaneously. The use of epinephrine depends on the severity of the bronchospasm or the onset and risk of cardiac effects. If it is used, it is administered and followed by another dose in 15 minutes for 3 more times, then once an hour. The use of IV aminophylline is considered by some physicians to be controversial. If it is used and if the person is not already taking theophylline, a loading dose of 6 mg/kg is administered over 30 minutes, then infusion rates are as follows:

Adults: 0.6 mg/kg/h
Youth: 0.9 mg/kg/h
Elderly: 0.4 mg/kg/h
CHF, liver disease: 0.2 to 0.3 mg/kg/h†

Treatment for children

Moderate disease: Use inhaled β_2-agonist prn to tid or qid; cromolyn sodium as anti-inflamatory: 2 puffs bid or qid or 1 capsule.

Severe asthma: β_2-agonist in nebulizer before age 5, or 2 puffs with inhaler or dry powder capsule in spinhaler qid. Anti-inflammatory: inhaled corticosteroid, 2 to 4 puffs bid to qid with β_2-agonist with or without cromolyn.

Therapy for asthma in children

Children younger than age 5 are unable to use metered-dose inhalers. Children older than age 5 can use them. Use nebulizers or spacers with children ages 3 to 5.

*Guidelines for the diagnosis and treatment of asthma. (1991). National Heart, Lung, and Blood Institute. National Asthma Education Program Expert Panel Report. *J Allergy Clin Immunol*, *88*(Suppl. 2), p. 425.

†Dellinger RP. (1991). Acute life-threatening asthma. *Postgrad Med*, *90*(3), 63.

uous manner and is moved up the tree by the motion of the cilia that line the respiratory tract (see Fig. 37-2).

Ciliary function depends on the moisture and viscosity of mucus:

The mucous blanket rests upon a clear serous fluid of low viscosity that bathes and surrounds the cilia. It is upon this fluid that the mucous blanket floats. . . . Dehydration and lack of humidification deplete the fluid upon which the mucous blanket floats and increases the viscosity of mucus itself (Morrison, 1979).

The word *expectorant* is derived from Latin and means "out of the chest." It refers to those drugs that *increase* the amount of sputum. If the drug also stimulates mucus production, it is called *bronchomucotropic*. These drugs are administered either systemically or by inhalation. In other cases, it may be necessary to *decrease* the amount of mucus produced; drugs that inhibit the production of respiratory tract fluid are called *antibronchomucotropic* agents.

Mucolytic agents

Mucolytic agents act directly on mucus. These drugs are useful in breaking down tenacious viscid secretions. Their action disrupts chemical bonds that hold segments of mucoproteins together. They are effective

Box 37-6. Pharmacologic therapy for asthma*

Step approach

Step 1 β-adrenergic stimulants, *eg*, albuterol (Proventil, Ventolin)
β$_2$ selective agonists
Inhaled delivery: metered-dose inhaler or spacer or rotohaler. Use as required

Step 2 Inhaled anti-inflammatory (best as initial therapy)
Corticosteroids or cromolyn sodium
Steroid drug of choice
Beclomethasone dipropionate (Beclovent, Vanceril) 2 puffs bid; if persistent and nocturnal, 4 puffs qid
or may use flunisolide (Aerobid) or triamcinolone acetonide (Azmacort)
In children, use cromolyn sodium first

Step 3 Inhaled steroid high dose; use spacer with any dose greater than 500 μg/day
or
use inhaled ipratropium bromide (Atrovent)

Step 4 Add oral β$_2$-agonist or methylxanthine (not preferable as first line treatment)
Single dose or sustained release
Oral albuterol at night for nocturnal asthma
Twice daily sustained release may be necessary

Step 5 Oral steroids; short course: prednisone 30–60 mg
Continue until peak expiratory flow rate is reached
Continue full dose 2 days, then half-dose is given

Step 6 Maintain on oral steroids; given daily or on alternate days

*Rumbak MJ. (1991). New concepts in the treatment of chronic persistent asthma. *Postgrad Med, 90*(3), 81.

---

in loosening secretions and in enabling clients to raise sputum. See Table 37-8 for a variety of selected mucolytic agents. Although it is irritating to tissue, acetylcysteine is the only true mucolytic drug available in the United States.

Pharmacodynamics. Acetylcysteine (Mucomyst) is a sulfhydryl compound that liquefies mucus and DNA through the process of mucolysis by breaking disulfide bonds of mucus protein. This compound also decreases the viscosity of mucus and is one of the most effective mucolytic agents. Liquefaction occurs within minutes after administration. The maximum effect occurs within 5 to 10 minutes.

Dosage and administration. Acetylcysteine is available in a 10% or 20% solution. A dose of 1 to 10 ml of 20% or 2 to 20 ml of 10% tid or qid may be given undiluted by hand nebulizer, aerosol, or IPPB machine. The usual dose is 3 to 5 ml of 20% solution or 6 to 10 ml of 10% solution. Occasionally, it is administered directly into the trachea through an endotracheal tube or tracheostomy tube in doses of 1 to 2 ml of 10% to 20% solution.

Adverse reactions. The nurse must watch closely for bronchospasm. Because of this possibility, the drug is often administered in conjunction with or immediately after a bronchodilator. Should bronchospasm occur, the drug should be discontinued.

Adverse reactions include a burning sensation in the back of the throat, stomatitis, nausea, rhinorrhea, and epistaxis. This drug has an unpleasant odor, similar to rotten eggs, which could be offensive to the client.

Precautions. Acetylcysteine should not be put in a heated nebulizer nor should it come in contact with iron, copper, or rubber, since these may affect the concentration. The drug is stored in the refrigerator and must be used within 96 hours. The bottle should be dated, timed, and initialed when opened.

Expectorants

Drugs that stimulate the production of respiratory secretions are known as expectorants. Guaifenesin (Robitussin) in Table 37-9 and potassium iodide in Table 37-8 are examples of expectorants.

Saturated solution of potassium iodide stimulates respiratory mucosal glands by reflex stimulation of the gastric mucosa. Adverse reactions to the drug include GI upset with nausea, vomiting, and epigastric pain. The client may complain of a metallic taste, and skin rashes sometimes occur. Potassium iodide should not be used in clients with known allergies to iodine or in clients who suffer from hyperthyroidism. It is administered diluted in a glass of water and given orally, 300 to 650 mg, three or four times a day. Enteric-coated tablets are also available; dosage is 1 to 2 tablets, tid.

Guaifenesin (Robitussin), formerly called glyceryl guaiacolate, is a frequently used expectorant. It is thought to stimulate secretions. It also inhibits platelet function in these doses and should be used with caution in clients who receive anticoagulant therapy. The usual dosage is 200 to 400 mg (10–20 ml), four times a day. The drug has been used as a mucolytic agent, but this action has not been adequately demonstrated. Although the drug is widely used, with few adverse reac-

Table 37-8. Representative mucolytic agents*

Drug name	Preparation	Usual adult dosage	Additional information
Mucolytic agents			
acetylcysteine alone or with isoproterenol (Mucomyst)	Solution 10% undiluted 20% undiluted	6–10 ml of 10% tid or qid 3–5 ml of 20% tid or qid	Observe for bronchospasm, stomatitis, rhinorrhea. If epistaxis occurs or bronchospasm, discontinue the drug. If bloody secretions, discontinue. Store in refrigerator. *Use within 96 hours.* May corrode metal.
Expectorants			
potassium iodide	Tablets, solution Saturated solution (1 g/ml)	300–600 mg 5–10 drops if saturated solution	Observe for gastric distress, headache, acneiform skin rash. Use with caution in client with thyroid disease. Do not use if client is sensitive to iodine products. Administer solutions well diluted in water or preferably in fruit juice.
theophylline 120 mg/15 ml iodinated glycerol 30 mg/15 ml, and alcohol 15% (Theo-Organidin)	Elixir	15–30 ml, q6–8h	May cause drowsiness, rash. Use care with client with thyroid disease and sensitivity. Caution when used with other xanthine drugs.
iodinated glycerol 30 mg/5 ml, codeine 10 mg/5 ml (Tussi-Organidin)		5–10 ml every 4 h	

* To decrease viscosity of secretions to liquefy tenacious sputum. Used in clients who have pulmonary disease, cystic fibrosis, COPD, and atelectasis from mucus obstruction.

Table 37-9. Representative cough suppressants

Drug name	Preparation	Usual adult dosage	Additional information
diphenhydramine 12.5 mg/5 ml (Benylin Cough Syrup)	Syrup	10 ml, q4h	Use with care in clients with narrow-angle glaucoma, stenosing peptic ulcer disease, prostatic hypertrophy, bladder neck obstruction. Observe for rash, drowsiness, increased viscosity, bronchial secretions, GI disturbance.
brompheniramine 2 mg/5 ml (Dimetane)	Elixir	10 ml, q4h	Same as above
hydrocodone 5 mg/5 ml, homatropine 1.5 mg/5 ml (Hycodan)	Syrup	5–15 ml, q4h	Take after meals. Observe for sedation, nausea, vomiting, constipation. CNS depression. Clients should not drive or operate dangerous machinery.
codeine 10 mg/5 ml, pseudoephedrine 30 mg/5 ml, chorpheniramine 2 mg/5 ml, alcohol 5% (Novahistine DH)	Liquid	10 ml, q4–6h	Caution in clients with coronary artery disease, hypertension, glaucoma, urinary tract obstruction, diabetes mellitus. All the same potential adverse reactions as sympathomimetics.
guaifenesin 100 mg/5 ml (Robitussin)	Liquid	10–20 ml	

tions, little objective evidence proves that it in fact produces bronchorrhea (Morrison, 1979).

Water and saline have also been used as agents to affect mucus through dilution, which is the most important means of thinning excretions. Water, which is hypotonic, must be used with caution, however, because mucosal edema can occur. Saline is effective, and clients find relief after aerosol therapy with it; 2 to 3 ml is administered by IPPB machine or nebulizer three to four times a day. In addition to the water used in nebulizers and IPPB machines, water taken systemically acts as an expectorant; clients are urged to drink at least 2 to 3 quarts of water a day unless they have congestive heart failure.

■ Summary

Expectorants and mucolytic agents affect mucus or the mucous blanket. Expectorants reduce the viscosity of mucus and aid in removing it from the respiratory tract. Mucolytic agents work directly on mucus.

Antitussive drugs

Antitussives are drugs used to control or bring relief from coughs. They are used to treat dry nonproductive coughs. The agents used as antitussives affect the cough control center in the medulla and suppress the cough reflex. Both narcotic and non-narcotic preparations are used as cough remedies. Some of the preparations include combinations of antihistamines or sympathomimetic agents in addition to the antitussive. Ingredients must be checked carefully for each antitussive, and adverse reactions should be assessed for each client (see Table 37-9).

Codeine is an effective narcotic cough suppressant. Antitussives that contain codeine are usually obtained by prescription. The adult dose varies between 10 and 30 mg, but 15 mg four times a day is frequently used. (The adverse reactions to codeine are discussed in Chapter 24.)

An equally effective but non-narcotic drug is dextromethorphan. It is widely used in over-the-counter preparations. Adverse reactions are rare, although occasional GI distress and drowsiness have been reported. The dose is 15 to 30 mg qid.

Aerosols and nebulizers

Some drugs are given topically by deposition in the respiratory tract. Some of the newer drugs (*eg*, metaproterenol, albuterol, and terbutaline) produce adverse reactions if absorbed through the GI tract and are better administered through aerosol or nebulization therapy. Nebulization is derived from the Latin word *nebula*, meaning cloud. Aerosol is from the Greek *aero*, meaning air, and *sol*, meaning solution. Aerosols

refer to relatively stable particulate suspensions of liquids or solids in air or in gases. Fog and mist are used synonymously; nebulizer and aerosol are used interchangeably.

Briefly, humidification therapy occurs in two ways:

1. A humidifier that, through vaporization, converts water to a gaseous state
2. A nebulizer that delivers medication in droplet form (Fig. 37-6)

The size of the particles and droplets is important in determining where they are deposited in the tracheobronchial tree and alveoli.

The droplets produced are measured in microns (μ; $1 \mu = \frac{1}{25,000}$ of an inch). Nebulization that uses a system of baffles removes large particles from the mist that cannot penetrate deeply. The smaller the particle, the deeper the penetration, unless the particle is smaller than 1μ. The nose filters particles larger than 5μ. Particles of 2 to 5μ deposit in the bronchi, trachea, and pharynx. Particles between 1 and 2μ tend to be deposited deep in the alveoli, especially if inhaled through the mouth. Medications used in nebulizers and aerosols include bronchodilators, mucolytic agents, corticosteroids, and antibiotics.

Some therapists believe that aerosols are of little benefit, because if used improperly, little or none of the drug reaches deep into the respiratory tract. Therefore, it is important to supervise the client while the treatment is being administered and to assess whether the desired effect is occurring. Proper inhalation technique is discussed under Nursing Management.

Oxygen therapy

Oxygen is found freely in the earth's atmosphere. At sea level, air contains 20.95% oxygen. Oxygen is an odorless, tasteless, and invisible gas. It supports com-

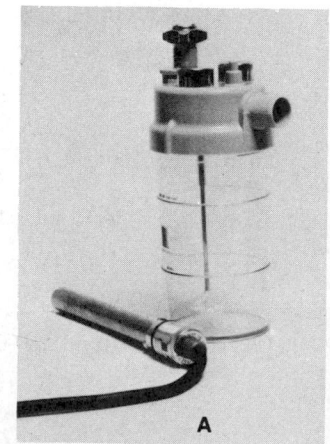 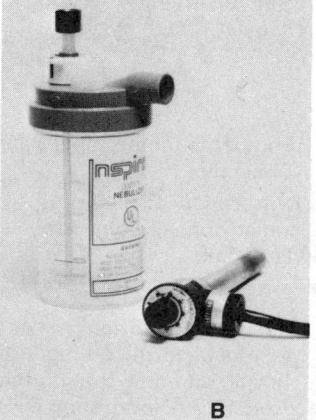

Figure 37-6. Jet nebulizers. (*A*) Nondisposable model with reusable heater. (*B*) Disposable model with reusable heater.

bustion and increases the rate of incineration. Oxygen is essential to life. The CNS is susceptible to damage by a lack of oxygen, and the heart, kidneys, liver, and adrenal glands are also compromised quickly in the presence of low oxygen.

Oxygen is considered a drug when it is used in the management of respiratory diseases. The aim of therapy is to restore and maintain a normal PaO_2 (up to 100 mm Hg) with an oxygen saturation of greater than 80%. Body tissues require a PaO_2 of at least 25 mm Hg (40% saturation), assuming that the person has a normal hemoglobin and cardiac output. Oxygen is administered at the lowest inspired PO_2 that produces an PaO_2 between 60 and 90 mm Hg and that provides adequate tissue oxygenation. Oxygen must be administered with extreme caution to clients with severe long-standing pulmonary disease who retain carbon dioxide, because their respiratory drive is based on low oxygen levels.

Oxygen is not without danger. Although oxygen is essential for life, high concentrations are toxic to tissue. Consequently, many nursing implications are involved in its use.

Therapeutic uses. Oxygen plays an important role in the therapy of clients with respiratory disease, cardiac disease, and other diseases. It is also vital in situations in which blood–gas documentation indicates that the client has a low PaO_2. Oxygen may be given to reduce strain on another organ (*eg,* after heart surgery). Oxygen occasionally is used to treat decubiti and anaerobic infections.

Indications for therapy

Oxygen therapy is indicated when a diagnosis of hypoxia and hypoxemia is made. The nurse must assess clients for symptoms of decreased oxygen, dyspnea, tachypnea, and a drop in blood pressure. Cardiac arrhythmia may exist, and the client may appear cyanotic (often a late sign). The client may be anxious and complain of a headache. Irritability, hostility, restlessness, clipped speech, poor judgment, drowsiness, and inability to perform intellectual skills may all be symptoms of low oxygen reserve. Signs of increased intracranial pressure may also be evident. The nursing history, laboratory blood results, and a nursing assessment that describes these signs and symptoms all contribute to the nursing diagnosis of respiratory impairment with a need for oxygen therapy.

Administration. Oxygen can be administered to clients in a variety of ways. A physician's order should specify the concentration of oxygen to be administered (*ie,* the fraction of inspired oxygen, FIO_2) and the type of therapy (how it is to be administered). The duration of administration may also be indicated. Before the therapy is initiated, it is important to explain fully to the client what will be done, why it is necessary, what is expected of the client, and what the client may feel.

Oxygen may be administered by nasal catheters, nasal cannula, face tents, or masks. Oxygen tents or croupettes may be used. It may be necessary for a support system such as a respirator to be used.

Listed below are some methods, their advantages and disadvantages, and approximate concentrations of oxygen that the various methods can deliver. The concentrations of oxygen cited for the different masks vary. Approximate concentrations have been listed, and it is always important to determine the concentration of oxygen delivered to each client by measuring the inspired air with an oxygen analyzer; for example, nasal prongs are not exact.

Oxygen dries the mucous membranes; therefore, humidification is a consideration in oxygen therapy.

Nasal catheters

Nasal catheters can deliver a concentration of 25% to 40% O_2 at a flow rate of 4 to 8 liters/min (Fig. 37-7). Nasal catheters are not very comfortable. The nurse must also assess the client for gastric dilatation. Nasal catheters are not used often, but they are effective even in mouth breathers. The nasopharynx is enriched by the nasal entraining mechanism (Petty, 1982). Final tracheal concentration of oxygen depends on the oxygen liter flow, minute ventilation, and the pattern and depth of breathing.

Nasal cannulae

Nasal cannulae are either single or double short soft prongs that insert into the clients' nostrils 5/8 inch (Fig. 37-8). At flows of 1 to 10 liters/min, they deliver 23% to 40% oxygen. Nasal cannulae are used more frequently than nasal catheters and allow the client more freedom. Clients can talk and eat without removing them; they are able to cough and still leave them in place. Nasal cannulae are easily and quickly applied, are com-

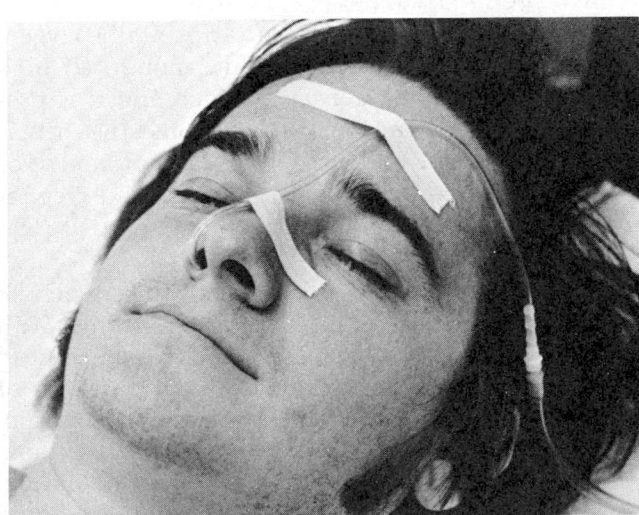

Figure 37-7. This client is receiving oxygen through a nasal catheter. The catheter is taped in place and should be changed every 8 hours.

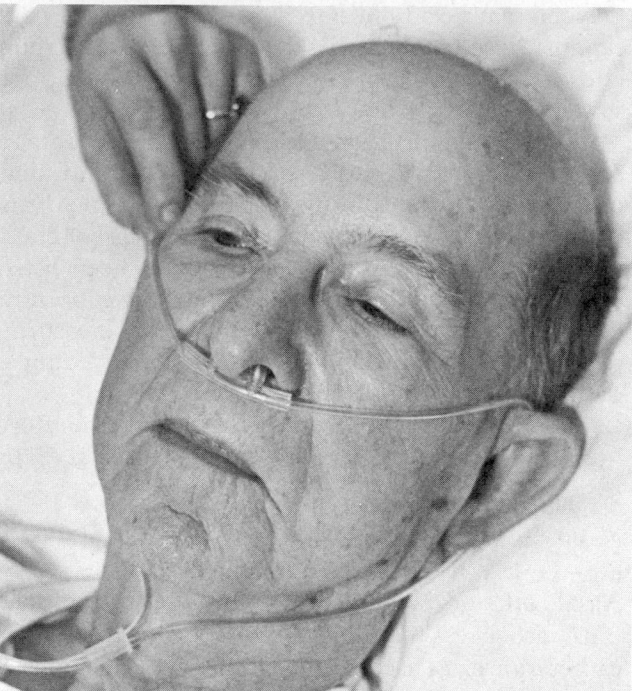

Figure 37-8. This client is receiving oxygen through a nasal cannula. The nurse is adjusting the elastic headband for comfort.

fortable for the client, and are low in cost. The nurse must assess if the client has sinus discomfort, nasal–pharyngeal irritation, or sore red eyes and drying of the nasal membranes. Pressure irritation may develop from the plastic tubing on the ears and under the nose.

Face tents

Face tents are useful in clients who are mouth breathers or whose respiratory secretions are very dry. They can deliver 25% to 50% oxygen at flow rates of 5 liters/min.

Oxygen masks

Oxygen masks can deliver from 24% to 100% oxygen. They cover both the nose and the mouth. (If high concentrations of oxygen are needed and it is projected this will be true for a period of time, the client is usually intubated and placed on a respirator.) For short-term therapy and for clients not in acute respiratory failure, the following masks may be used (Fig. 37-9).

Simple masks are useful for delivering moderate amounts of oxygen for a short period of time. With proper adjustment of the metal clips across the nose to secure a tight fit, they can deliver concentrations of 35% to 55% oxygen run at a flow of 6 to 12 liters/min.

Partial rebreathing masks have reservoirs that hold 1500 ml and can deliver 40% to 60% or 70% oxygen when run at 8 to 15 liters/min. The reservoir should deflate slightly when the client inspires.

Nonbreathing masks fit tightly over the face and also have a reservoir. The client breathes pure oxygen (100% oxygen). These can deliver concentrations of

60% to 90% using a flow rate of 10 to 15 liters/min. The flow is adjusted to keep the reservoir bag fully inflated. Masks of this type are frequently used with clients who suffer from smoke inhalation or pulmonary edema.

For those clients for whom it is important to deliver exact concentrations of oxygen and low flow concentrations (*eg*, clients with chronic pulmonary disease), *Venturi masks* are used. The concentration of oxygen depends on the flow of oxygen and the size of the orifice in the mask, which is color coded for concentration and clearly indicates oxygen flow rates. Oxygen may be delivered at concentrations of 24%, 28%, 35%, or 40%.

Clients may also receive oxygen delivered through a *transtracheal catheter*. This requires a minor surgical procedure for placement and care of the catheter. It can afford the client greater flexibility and the desired oxygen concentration may be reached with lower flow rates of oxygen. A smaller portable system can be used and eventually costs may be lower.

Adverse reactions. When oxygen is delivered at high concentrations, the nurse should assess the client for the following signs and symptoms: tearing, redness, pain, and edema of the eyes, burning substernal chest pain, nasal congestion and sinus pain, retrolental fibroplasia, sore throat and pharngeal irritation, tracheal irritation, severe coughing, anorexia and nausea, and tingling and paresthesia.

Toxicity

Oxygen has the potential to damage all body tissues. The eye of the neonate is especially susceptible, but so are the CNS and the lungs. Even though the mechanism of oxygen toxicity is unknown, high concentrations of oxygen over a period of time lead to a serious

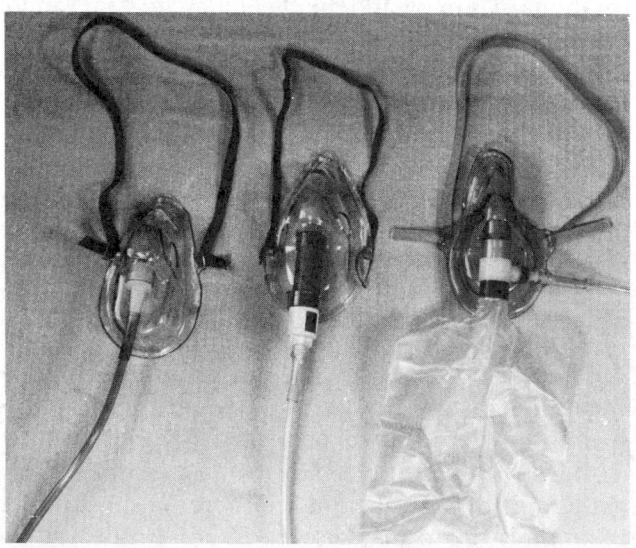

Figure 37-9. The three most common face masks used to administer oxygen. (*Left*) Simple mask. (*Center*) Venturi-type mask. (*Right*) Partial rebreathing or reservoir mask. All are disposable. (Photo by Paul Montague)

condition in which the lung becomes heavy, boggy, and edematous. Lung compliance decreases, and a vicious cycle begins, in that the clinical picture deteriorates, respiratory failure progresses, and more oxygen and higher concentrations of oxygen are required.

Two types of oxygen toxicity exist, *acute* and *chronic*. Chronic toxicity is seen with low-dose oxygen. Acute toxicity develops in two phases. The initial phase is the *exudative phase* and is characterized by "atelectasis and alveolar interstitial edema which leads to intra-alveolar hemorrhage. . . . Protein and fibrin exudation, along with cellular debris coalesces to form prominent hyaline membrane with destruction of capillary and endothelium and alveolar lining cells, type I pneumocytes. This phase occurs within four days" (Baldwin, 1977). The *proliferative* phase that ensues if the process is not stopped is most prominent in 12 days. This phase is characterized by "prominent hyperplasia of Type II pneumocytes, fibroplastic proliferation, and scattered regions of early fibrosis leading to cellular swelling that results in a markedly thickened blood air barrier" (Baldwin, 1977). The chronic form of oxygen toxicity resembles the proliferative phase of acute injury with hyperplasia of type II pneumocytes and fibrosis.

The results of the tissue injury are an abnormal vital capacity and poor compliance. Gas exchange is decreased, alveolar hypoventilation occurs, and respiratory failure increases. The aim of therapy is to prevent these events. Oxygen is delivered using the lowest concentration possible to provide adequate tissue oxygenation.

For the client on a respirator, periodic sighing may help prevent toxicity. Placing the client on positive end expiratory pressure or continuous positive airway pressure may also help. Careful assessment and monitoring of clients for early detection are also important.

Precautions and contraindications. Smoking is prohibited when oxygen therapy is instituted. Smoking materials should be removed, and signs must be clearly displayed that indicate oxygen is in use (Fig. 37-10). No oil, grease, alcohol, or other combustible materials should be near the oxygen. If tanks or cylinders are used rather than wall outlets, they must be secured so that they cannot fall. The nurse must also check to see how full the tanks are and whether an adequate supply of oxygen exists (Fig. 37-11). The tanks should not be placed near heat sources. Electrical equipment must be inspected for damage, and all equipment should be grounded.

Oxygen must be administered with *extreme caution* to clients with COPD. These people adjust to lower levels of oxygen and may do poorly when given oxygen, especially people who retain carbon dioxide and increase their carbon dioxide levels. With long-standing lung disease, oxygen is administered to bring a PaO_2 up to 50 to 60 mm Hg. If oxygen is administered, the client must have arterial blood gases monitored

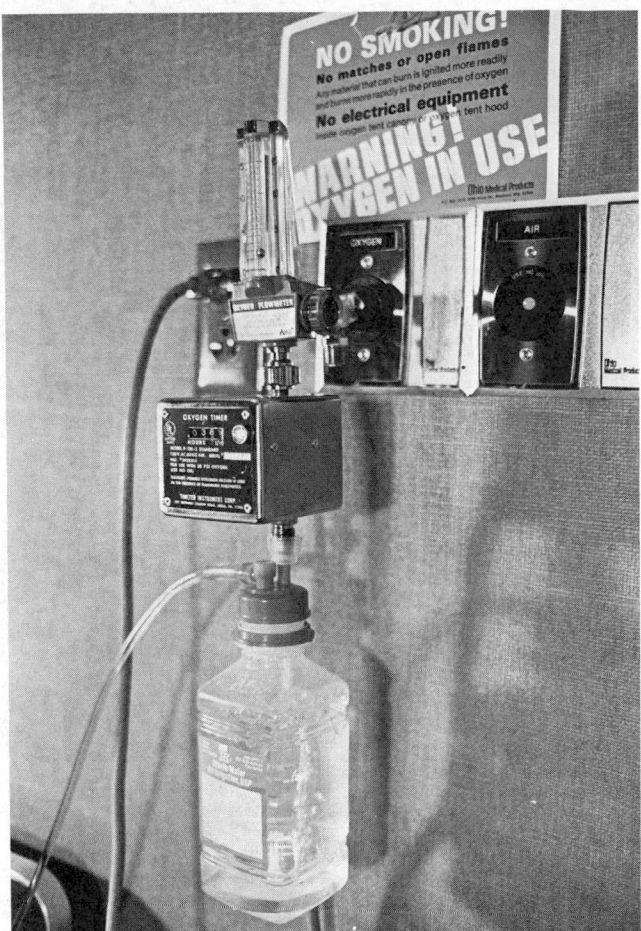

Figure 37-10. Piped-in oxygen equipment. The flowmeter or regulator determines the rate of flow of the oxygen that is bubbled through the humidifier bottle and passes through the plastic tubing to the client. A sign that indicates the use of oxygen is placed at bedside and on the door to the client's room.

and must be observed for apnea. Ventilatory assistance must be available.

■ Summary

Oxygen is considered a drug and is useful when correctly administered to clients unable to oxygenate their tissues sufficiently to support life. It may be given to reduce strain on an organ, for example, after heart surgery. Improper administration may lead to complications; therefore, oxygen should be administered with care and should not be given indiscriminately.

Nursing management

Nursing implications

Respiratory clients present a challenge to the nurse. Clients with chronic respiratory diseases frequently are hostile, uncooperative, anxious, dependent, rest-

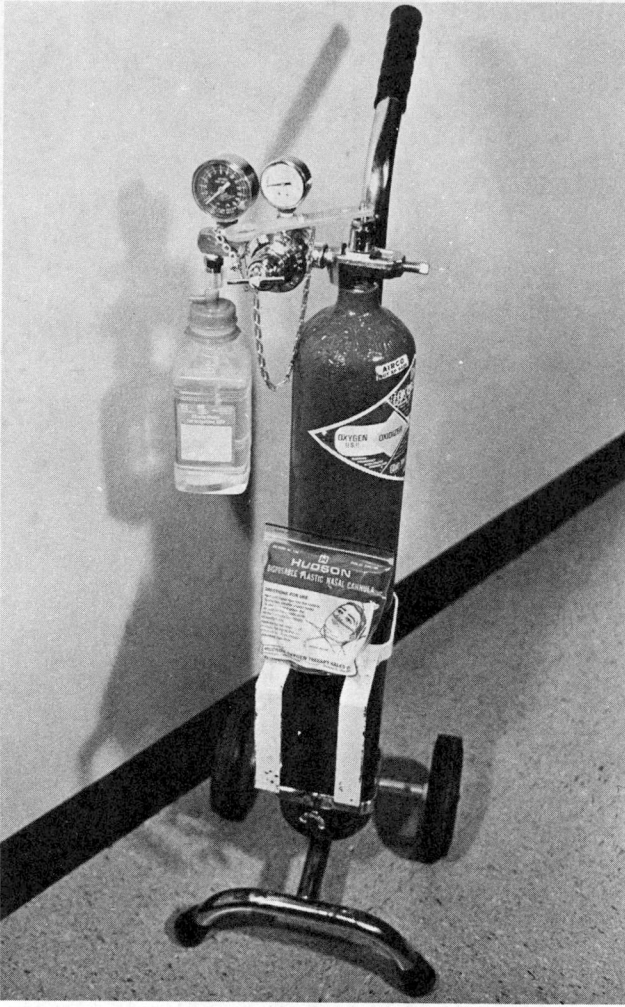

Figure 37-11. A small cylinder of oxygen is in readiness for an emergency. The regulator and humidifier bottle are attached and ready for use.

less, and irritable. In spite of this fact, the nurse must remain calm, often in a situation that is an emergency. The nurse must stay with the client who is having respiratory difficulty and keep the client informed of what will be done and what is expected of him or her. Most clients are unable to talk much at this time. The nurse must second guess many needs while assisting with proper breathing, coughing, and positioning. The client's respiratory status must be assessed continually.

Clients and their families are important members of the team; without their cooperation, health goals will not be attained. The aims of therapy include the following:

- Improvement of respiratory function
- Relief from anxiety
- Promotion of rest and preservation of energy
- Prevention of further complications
- Restoration to optimal level of functioning

Respiratory function can be improved by the following:

- Establishing a patent airway
- Providing oxygen therapy when indicated
- Providing mechanical ventilatory support when indicated
- Improving gas distribution
- Providing adequate hydration and humidification
- Decreasing airway resistance through relief of bronchospasm, removal of secretions, reduction in the viscosity of secretions, and control of bronchial secretions through the use of expectorants
- Decreasing anxiety
- Teaching coughing, deep breathing, and new breathing patterns
- Preventing or curing superimposed respiratory infections

Some of these aims constitute the medical regimen; however, the nurse is involved in administering the therapy and in evaluating the client response.

Nursing process

Assessment Nursing measures related to data collection for clients with respiratory disorders must be comprehensive. Begin with the health history and determine the client's smoking habits; degree of fatigue; symptoms of cough; whether the cough is constant; intermittent; or related to time of day; and whether it is productive or not. Inquire if allergic stimuli or environmental pollutants were present. Identify whether evidence of weight loss, anorexia, or a history of peptic ulcer disease is present. Determine the medications being used and determine efficacy of what the client says provides relief. If sputum is present, determine quantity, color, viscosity, and history of recent changes in character. Determine if the client has ever required ventilatory support.

Then inspect or observe the client for the ability to speak in full sentences (difficult in compromised respiratory status). Determine the level of consciousness or mentation; is the person irritable and confused? Ascertain if the client has a headache. Observe the client's position. Is he or she sitting, leaning forward? Is the client using accessory muscles for breathing? Is breathing labored? Is there evidence of pursed-lip breathing, flaring of the nostrils, intercostal or sternal retractions? Are there signs of congestive heart failure? What is the inspiratory–expiratory ratio? What is the pulse rate, respiratory rate, and depth of respirations? Is chest expansion or chest excursion symmetrical? Is there a barrel chest? Is there digital clubbing? Other information that must be determined includes evidence of cyanosis of the lips, nostrils or tip of the nose, or, in a dark-skinned person, evidence of cyanosis in the cheeks or oral mucosa.

The nurse must also percuss and auscultate the chest to determine presence of breath sounds, fine or coarse rales, rhonchi, or wheezes. Finally, the nurse must collect data on the client's blood gases, cultures, blood counts, and radiographic findings.

Nursing diagnosis Clients with respiratory disease such as asthma or bronchitis and emphysema experience the following:

> *Impaired gas exchange related to airway obstruction which may result from bronchospasm, bronchoconstriction, (or increased secretions)*
> *Ineffective breathing pattern related to decreased lung compliance*
> *Ineffective airway clearance related to copious secretions or inability to expectorate*
> *Anxiety*
> *Fear*
> *Social isolation related to decreased energy, immobility, or activity intolerance*
> *Impaired home maintenance management*
> *Self-care deficit*
> *Altered tissue perfusion (cardiopulmonary)*
> *Decreased cardiac output*
> *Impaired verbal communication related to impaired gas exchange*
> *Altered thought processes related to impaired gas exchange*
> *Fluid volume deficit related to increased perspiration secondary to increased work of breathing*
> *High risk for infection*
> *Sleep pattern disturbance related to CNS stimulation secondary to sympathomimetic and methylxanthine drug use*
> *Altered comfort: nausea, vomiting, cramping, palpitations, nervousness, dizziness, anginal pain, and tremor related to the use of stimulant drugs*
> *High risk for ineffective management of therapeutic regimen related to knowledge deficit*

Clients and families may also have

> *Knowledge deficit concerning the condition, drug therapy, and treatment regimen.*

Planning Goals of treatment are to improve client's aeration, maintain tissue oxygenation, reduce airway resistance, prevent or cure infection, alleviate anxiety and fear, improve coughing and breathing techniques, reduce adverse reactions, reduce secretions and viscosity, improve hydration and nutrition, and ensure compliance with therapy.

Intervention
Airway patency. To implement the first goal (improve respiratory function), the nurse must improve airway patency. In fact, the nurse's first priority is to maintain a patent airway for the client. This goal can be accomplished by placing the client in a semi-Fowler's position and by turning the head to the side or by hyperextending the neck if the client is drowsy and cannot be aroused. The client should be turned from side to side every 2 hours. If the client can tolerate it, the swimmer's position should be used two to three times a day. Proper coughing and deep breathing improve oxygen and carbon dioxide exchange. Respiratory status must be continually observed, and emergency measures must be instituted for clients with respiratory failure.

Breathing techniques. Instructing the client to take slow deep breaths is essential if he or she is dyspneic and breathing in a rapid, shallow, and ineffective manner. The client should be urged to take at least six to eight deep breaths an hour. Clients should learn how to breathe diaphragmatically. This type of breathing can be practiced by placing hands on the chest or abdomen and inhaling in such a way that the hands rise as the chest or abdomen expands. Another method is for the client to place hands on the rib cage, take a deep breath, and try to move the hands out by lateral chest expansion. The client should inhale slowly through the nose, hold his or her breath 1 to 3 seconds, and then exhale slowly through the mouth. The client with severe COPD may need to do pursed-lip breathing, in which air is exhaled slowly through pursed lips. The diaphragm is exercised if the client sniffs through the nose in short quick sniffs and exhales through the nose the same way.

Coughing. Proper coughing is most important in clearing the airway. An effective cough begins with a slow deep inspiration through the nose. A cough consists of three phases. First, the client must inhale deeply. Then, pressure behind the air must be built up by the client contracting the abdominal, accessory, and thoracic muscles that build up pressure when the glottis is closed and traps the air. Once the intrapulmonary pressure is increased, the client then exhales forcefully, opening the glottis. The air is then expelled at the speed of sound, carrying with it sputum and respiratory secretions. The cough may be more effective if the client first takes several slow deep breaths before the cough. These enable maximum buildup of intrathoracic pressure during inspiration followed by a deep forceful cough or coughs on expiration. It may also help to instruct the client to give several coughs from one deep breath. The cough is most effective if the client is in a position that allows for free movement of the chest wall. The client should be assisted to a sitting position and instructed to lean slightly forward.

Modifying secretions. Respiratory function is also improved if the tracheobronchial tree is free of excessive secretions; therefore, it may be necessary to modify the client's secretions. If the mucus or sputum is loose and watery, it is easier for the client to expectorate it. Assess whether the client is dehydrated. Test the skin turgor, and measure the intake and output and weight of the client. Evaluate the sputum for viscosity, and auscultate the chest. Measure the amount of sputum, and check the color. Seek data on whether the client has a productive cough. If the client is dehydrated, increase the amount of fluids up to 3 to 4 liters/day (for adults). Continue to evaluate the state of hydration and the nature of the secretions. If the client's secretions are thick and inspissated, instruct the client not to drink milk or have many milk products, because these adversely affect viscosity. Tea, coffee, and other caffeine-containing beverages should be avoided, because they all act as diuretics, which promote further dehydration.

Adjusting humidity. Assess the room environment to determine whether the humidity is too low. Room humidifiers and vaporizers can be ordered for the client. It may be necessary to administer increased humidity directly to the respiratory tract with an aerosol or a nebulizer. Again, proper instruction is important. Teach the client to exhale fully before starting the treatment. If the nebulizer is hand-driven, ask the client to inhale deeply as the mechanism is pumped. Then the client should hold his or her breath for 1 to 3 seconds, allowing the nebulization or drug to be deposited properly. The client should repeat these steps until the solution is used up. The client should know that it is better to perform the treatment fully as prescribed by the physician rather than to take frequent short puffs throughout the day. Because most clients awake in the morning with congestion, the first treatment should be on arising. IPPB machines are also used for aerosol therapy in those clients who require high inspiratory pressures.

Administration of drugs. Many nursing implications are involved in the administration of drugs to respiratory clients. It is important for the nurse to have baseline data on the client's respiratory status and vital signs. The nurse must be familiar with the client's history and have knowledge of other diseases that may contribute to complications (*eg*, diabetes, thyroid disease, and cardiovascular problems). When the drugs are first administered, the nurse must stay with the client and ascertain whether adverse reactions are occurring. The presence of adverse reactions does not necessarily mean that the drug is to be stopped, but in some cases, it may be discontinued. The proper storage of medications is also important.

In general, these medications are stopped if the client develops a tachyarrhythmia that continues or if ventricular arrhythmia, such as frequent premature ventricular contractions, occurs, especially with the use of isoproterenol. Serum theophylline concentrations must be watched closely, and the dose must be reduced if it is near the toxic level of 20 μg/ml. Any chest pain and bronchospasm must be detected immediately, and emergency measures must be instituted. These symptoms may indicate that the drug should be discontinued and therapy with another drug instituted. For bronchodilation, the newer β_2-adrenergic stimulants seem to offer promise with fewer and less severe adverse reactions. (For specific nursing precautions, review Tables 37-1 to 37-4.)

Mucolytic agents. Expectorants and mucolytic agents are ordered if the client has scant inspissated secretions with mucus plugs and atelectasis. These medications should be added to the nebulizer immediately before the client receives the treatment. After the medication is administered, the nebulizer should be thoroughly washed and aired to dry. In some hospitals, respiratory therapists administer these treatments, but the nurse must see that the treatment is administered and then evaluate the response to therapy. Do not let the client use only some of the medication, leave it, and return to use what remains later. If the client has bloody secretions and is taking acetylcysteine, stop the treatment and report the symptoms to the physician.

Bronchodilators. If the client suffers from bronchospasm, bronchodilators are administered to reduce the airway resistance. It cannot be overemphasized that the nurse must instruct the client in the proper use of inhaling aerosols. The metered-dose inhaler is the most common method of administering an inhaled bronchodilator.

Methods of inhalation

Metered-dose inhaler. Medication and a gas propellant are used to deliver bronchodilators by inhalation; anticholinergic drugs and antiinflammatory drugs, such as corticosteroids and cromolyn sodium, are used.

Small-volume jet nebulizers. A compressed gas–air source with a side stream method of nebulization should be used. The medication and diluent is placed in a small reservoir; then the air is driven by a small electric compressor to deliver the medication.

Spacers. For young children, older clients, and others, even after demonstration and practice, a spacing device is necessary to deliver medication by the inhalation route. It takes coordination to use a metered-dose inhaler; the client must start to inhale, then activate the device while continuing to inhale. When this action is not possible, spacer devices are used. In these, the medication is deposited in a reservoir by activating the inhaler; the client then inhales the medication from the reservoir. Slow deep inspirations are still necessary.

Spinhalers and rotohalers. Some medications are prepared as capsules that contain the medication in powder form, such as cromolyn sodium and albuterol. A spinhaler is a device that punctures the capsule, allowing the medication to be inhaled by the client. This device may be used more frequently in the future for environmental reasons if the Freon used in aerosols becomes banned.

It is extremely important that the clients receive instruction on the use of these devices. All too frequently, they are given a prescription with no education as to why or how to take the medication. Inhalation is the preferred route but inhalers require instruction plus guided practice. In a study reported by Jones (1989), only 54% of clients used an inhaler correctly, whereas 77% used the dry powder spinhaler device correctly. Surprisingly, only 37% used a large volume spacer device correctly. New devices are appearing on the market, such as a breath-activated aerosol inhaler (Aerolin Auto) and a new one referred to as BAI. In these devices, a lever applies pressure to the canister spring, but the drug is released only when the person inhales (Jones, 1989).

Inhalation technique. Clients should be instructed in the proper use of inhaling medications. The first step is to shake the medication by shaking the inhaler. The client then is instructed to breathe in and out slowly and normally. The client should follow the directions given by their health care provider or those on the medication canister as to whether they should use the open-mouth or the closed-mouth technique. If the open-mouth method is used, the client should tilt the head back slowly and hold the inhaler 2 inches away from the mouth. For the closed-mouth method, again the head is tipped back, and the client should place the mouthpiece between the teeth, over the tongue, and close the lips tightly around the mouthpiece. Then the client should begin to inhale slowly, activate the chamber, and continue to inhale to the maximal or deepest inhalation possible. At this point, the client should hold his or her breath so that the medication is deposited deep in the airways. It is desirable to hold the breath for 10 seconds, if possible. The client should wait several minutes before taking another puff. The medication is deposited in the mouth if the inhalation technique is not followed as described.

Pulmonary hygiene. Percussion, vibration, and bronchial drainage may be ordered to further loosen secretions if the client is unable to move and expel them through coughing. These treatments are referred to as pulmonary hygiene or toilet. The order and sequence of these treatments is important. Bronchodilators and mucolytic agents must be given before chest physical therapy or percussion, vibration, and drainage are performed. Along with vibration, the client does expulsive coughing. The procedure should be as follows:

1. Bronchodilators (if ordered)
2. Mucolytic agents (if ordered)
3. Moisture through aerosol or nebulization
4. Expulsive coughing

The client routine might be aerosol treatment for 10 to 15 minutes, followed by chest physical therapy for 10 to 20 minutes. If the client has an order for a steroid or anti-infective agent to be inhaled, this drug should be administered after the therapeutic treatments. This procedure seems so obvious that it does not warrant mentioning; however, often the hours ordered for these latter medicines are in conflict with the pulmonary toilet and too often the clients eliminate the medication by coughing because the timing was incorrect. Because coughing triggers the gag reflex and vomiting may occur, these treatments must be administered before meals. Coughing and mobilization of the person through proper positioning, ambulation, and exercise produces the greatest effect on mucus clearance.

Oxygen therapy. If oxygen is needed, the safety precautions mentioned earlier must be instituted. In addition, the client should be evaluated for desired versus adverse reactions.

The nurse should know the type of oxygen and the percentage ordered. The nurse should assess the client for labored breathing and should determine whether the client's color is improving and if the respiratory effort is becoming more effective. The nurse should know the latest blood–gas data on the client and should know if improvement has occurred. The nurse should make sure that a low-flow oxygen device is being used for oxygen delivery below 6 liters/min. It is important to remember that carbon dioxide narcosis is a potential complication if the client has high $PaCO_2$ concentration.

Promotion of rest and preservation of energy. All of the procedures described require energy on the clients' part, and this is a scarce commodity for them. It is important for the nurse to promote rest and to preserve the client's energy, a task not easily accomplished. The need for rest must be emphasized to clients and their families. Clients with severe respiratory difficulties expend all their energy on breathing, especially if they are using accessory muscles, retracting, and demonstrating air hunger. These clients must be helped to establish a schedule of eating, performing daily activities, doing chest physical therapy, and resting. Uninterrupted rest and sleep periods are an important part of therapy. For the client in the hospital, the nurse needs to coordinate treatments, laboratory tests, radiographs, and meals so that constant interruptions do not occur. Nutrition is important to build up energy, because respiratory clients are frequently anorexic from both the disease process and the medications; frequent small meals may be the answer to nutritional problems.

Relief of anxiety. A therapeutic nurse–client relationship and respiratory improvement after the previously described nursing measures should lead to a reduction in anxiety. Anxiety increases the client's oxygen need; it is important to reduce the stressors on the client. The nurse should stay with clients while treatments are being performed and while clients are in distress. Clients should be urged to change breathing patterns. Brief and concrete explanations should be given so clients know what is expected of them. The family should be kept informed as to what is occurring. The nurse should not deny that respiratory problems are a frightening experience but should give reassurance that the client will not be left alone and that help is always available. Because some of the adverse reactions from the medications resemble symptoms of anxiety, the nurse must assess precipitating factors in anxiety.

Prevention of complications. Prevention of further complications is another nursing goal. Scrupulous aseptic technique is a necessity, and clients should be instructed in the proper disposal of their secretions. Clients should also be instructed to avoid drafts and people with infections and colds. Dehydration should be prevented; all respiratory irritants, such as dust, smoke pollutants, and allergenic materials, should be removed.

Client education. Chronic respiratory conditions impose severe chronic disabilities in affected clients and force clients to adopt a changed lifestyle. For example, clients who suffer from chronic bronchitis and emphysema can anticipate a long downhill course. The disease usually is not cured, but clients can be restored to an optimal level of functioning and can be helped to live productive lives with the disease. Client and family education by the nurse can make a difference and can help people make decisions regarding their lives, aspirations, and health goals. Respiratory clients need to establish a regimen that includes treatments that may be necessary for the rest of their lives. Motivation is a major factor; client compliance plays a large role in therapeutic success.

Box 37-7 lists elements to be incorporated in teaching plans. The nurse needs to decide which points are appropriate to cover with clients. Much material needs to be covered, requiring careful planning of time and teaching goals. Demonstrations and return demonstration by the client's family must be included in the teaching strategy. The client's intellectual capacity is often impaired if oxygen levels are disturbed; the nurse must take this fact into consideration when developing the teaching plan.

Evaluation Data required for evaluation reflect attainment of the goals or outcomes established. Are secretions decreased, are they thinner? Are laboratory tests such as hematocrit and hemoglobin levels nor-

---

Box 37-7. Elements to incorporate in teaching plans

The nature of the disease and the pathologic process

The need to control pulmonary irritants and to refrain from smoking

Deep breathing and coughing techniques

Breathing exercises; when and how to do them

When to call the physician (increased shortness of breath, fever, increased cough, change in color and amount of sputum, change in condition)

The need to avoid drafts, irritants, people with colds

Proper inhalation technique (aerosol, humidifier)

Indication, use, care, and cleaning of equipment

Chest physical therapy (*ie*, bronchial drainage with percussion and vibration)

The order of therapies for maximum value

The need for fluids; the amount and type required

Understanding of medications (types, action, dose, timing, adverse reactions, special precautions, such as protection from light and heat)

Drug interactions and precautions

Pertinent disease conditions that affect the medication or interact with it adversely

Contraindications of narcotics and sedatives

Precautions with oxygen

Safety precautions with the drugs; how to reorder the medicines

---

mal? Are cultures negative? Is the white blood cell count normal? When the chest is auscultated, are breath sounds present and adventitious sounds absent? Does the client report that dyspnea is reduced and that anxiety and fear have decreased? The presence or absence of adverse drug reaction directs the nurse about whether to continue therapy as indicated. Client education is evaluated by the demonstration of compliance with therapy, by proper order of drug administration, and by inhalation, breathing, and coughing techniques (see Example of Nursing Process and Aminophylline Therapy).

Clients with respiratory diseases present a challenge to the nurse. The nurse is instrumental in helping clients and their families adjust to their changed lifestyle, which may include a change in the client's occupation. Through proper referrals and concerned help, people with COPD can lead quality lives.

Example of nursing process and aminophylline therapy

The client is a 64-year-old man who has smoked three packs of cigarettes a day for 40 years. He is restless, hostile, and breathing heavily. His color is flushed and he exhibits air hunger and pursed-lip breathing. He has a cough productive of green sputum. His chest is barrel-shaped. Vital signs are BP 162/95, P. 132 irregular, R. 32-grunting, T. 37.4°C. Blood gases ph. 7.47, PaO_2 50, $PaCO_2$ 95, AB. 31. On auscultation, there is a prolonged expiratory wheeze and decreased breath sounds, with rales noted at the lung bases.

   The physician orders Aminophylline IV 0.6 mg/kg/ml, Bronkosol 0.5 ml in 1.5 ml normal saline in IPPB and nasal O_2 1–2 L/min.

Assessment data	Nursing diagnosis	Intervention	Goals and outcome criteria
History of emphysema	Impaired gas exchange related to inadequate air flow in and out of alveoli secondary to poor lung compliance	**Administer** oxygen as ordered.	Client's color will become less cyanotic and more pink.
Decreased breath sounds and rales at lung bases		**Monitor** respiratory rate and blood gases.	Depth of respiration will increase.
Prolonged expiratory wheeze		**Monitor** vital signs.	Rate of respiration will decrease.
Barrel chest		**Administer** medications as ordered.	Adverse reaction from medication will not develop.
Pursed-lip breathing		**Identify** if client is taking a drug that interacts with methylxanthine or sympathomimetic drugs.	
Air hunger			
Abnormal blood gases		**Instruct** patient in proper respiration techniques.	
Thick inspissated, greenish mucus	Ineffective airway clearance related to increased thick secretions	**Perform** percussion and vibration, followed by suction.	Secretions will be thinner.
Decreased breath sounds and rales at lung bases		**Observe** for adverse reactions.	Amount of secretion will decrease.
		Monitor for therapeutic level of aminophylline.	
		Instruct the client in coughing technique.	
		Position client to promote respirations.	
Hostility	Anxiety related to decreased air exchange and poor aeration	**Remain** with client.	The client will appear more relaxed.
Restlessness		**Instruct** client in breathing and relaxation techniques.	The frequency and intensity of hostile behavior will decline.

Checklist of nursing actions

- ☐ Remain calm, especially in emergencies.
- ☐ Remain with client in respiratory distress and keep client informed of procedures and expectations.
- ☐ Accept clients and family members as part of the health care team.
- ☐ Assess respiratory status and vital signs continually.
- ☐ Strive to reach goals for respiratory care of clients.
- ☐ Maintain a patent airway for client.
- ☐ Assess client for dehydration.
- ☐ Assess room environment for humidification.
- ☐ Provide pollutant-free environment and advise client to refrain from smoking.
- ☐ Establish (and inform others of) sequence of planned routine.
- ☐ Coordinate treatments and tests so client has rest periods.
- ☐ Measure amount and color of sputum.
- ☐ Observe for adverse reactions to drugs.
- ☐ Teach proper use of inhaled medications.
- ☐ See that nebulizations are administered properly and evaluate response to treatment.

- [ ] After each use, wash nebulizer and air dry.
- [ ] Administer expectorants before meals.
- [ ] Ensure an adequate supply of oxygen.
- [ ] Secure oxygen cylinders so they will not fall.
- [ ] Check electrical equipment and do not place oxygen supply near heat.
- [ ] Prohibit smoking when oxygen is being administered. Signs should be evident on doors and at the client's bedside.
- [ ] Perform percussion, vibration, and drainage as ordered.
- [ ] Promote rest for the client.
- [ ] See that the client has proper nutrition.
- [ ] Prevent further complications, especially from infectious diseases and colds.
- [ ] Plan teaching situations carefully.
- [ ] Instruct client in breathing techniques and help him or her carry these out.
- [ ] Teach the client to cough properly.
- [ ] Instruct client on beverages to avoid when he or she is dehydrated.
- [ ] Help client and family plan for productive lives.

References

Ahrens RC. (1991). On comparing inhaled beta adrenergic agonists. *Annals of Allergy, 67*(3), 296–298.

Ahrens RC, Milavets G, Joad J. (1987). The effect of theophylline and B₂ agonists on airway reactivity. *Chest, 92*(Suppl. 1), 15s–21s.

Aubier M. (1987). Effect of theophylline on diaphragmatic muscle function. *Chest, 92*(Suppl. 1), 27s–31s.

Baldwin GR. (1977). Oxygen: Therapeutics, toxicity, advances. In MacDonnell KF, Segal MS (eds): *Current respiratory care*, pp 191–228. Boston: Little, Brown.

Barnes PJ. (1989a). A new approach to the treatment of asthma. *N Engl J Med, 321*(22), 1517–1527.

Barnes PJ. (1989b). New concepts in the pathogenesis of bronchial hyperresponsiveness and asthma. *J Allergy Clin Immunol, 83*(6), 1013–1026.

Berquist WE, Rachelefsky GS, Kadden M, et al. (1981). Effects of theophylline on gastroesophageal reflux in normal adults. *J Allergy Clin Immunol, 67*, 402–411.

Bryan CP, Taylor JP. (1973). *Manual of respiratory therapy*, pp 1–3. St. Louis: CV Mosby.

Chanez P, et al. (1988). Increased eosinophil responsiveness to platelet activating factor in asthma. *Clin Sci, 75*, 5.

Crofton EH, Douglas A. (1975). *Respiratory diseases*, 2nd ed, pp 435–438. London: Blackwell Scientific Publications.

Dellinger RP. (1991). Acute life-threatening asthma. *Postgrad Med, 90*(3), 63–77.

Fuller RW, et al. (1986). Prostaglandin D₂ potentiates airway responses to histamine and methacholine. *Am Rev Respir Dis, 133*, 252–254.

Green GM, Ball WC. (1984). Respiratory and non-respiratory functions of the lung. In Harvey AM (ed): *The principles and practice of medicine*, 21st ed. Norwalk, CT: Appleton-Century-Crofts.

Guidelines for the diagnosis and management of asthma. (1991). National Heart, Lung, and Blood Institute. National Asthma Education Program Expert Panel Report. *J Allergy Clin Immunol, 88*(Suppl. 2), 425–533.

Guyton AC. (1991). *Textbook of medical physiology*, 8th ed. Philadelphia: WB Saunders.

Jenne JW. (1987). Theophylline as a bronchodilator in COPD and its combination with inhaled beta-adrenergic drugs. *Chest, 92*(Suppl. 1), 7s–14s.

Jones K. (1989). New delivery systems for asthma drugs. *The Practitioner, 233*, 265–267.

Kaliner MA. (1987). The late-phase reaction and its clinical implications. *Hosp Pract, 22*(10), 73–83.

Larsen GL. (1985). Late-phase reactions: Observations on pathogenesis and prevention. *J Allergy Clin Immunol, 76*(5), 665–669.

MacDonnell KF, Segal MS, eds. (1977). *Current respiratory care*. Boston: Little, Brown.

Mahler DA. (1987). The role of theophylline in the treatment of dyspnea in COPD. *Chest, 92*(Suppl. 1), 2s–6s.

Mansfield LE. (1989). Gastroesophageal reflux and asthma. *Postgrad Med, 86*(1), 265–269.

Matthay RA. (1987). Favorable cardiovascular effects of theophylline in COPD. *Chest, 92*(Suppl. 1), 22s–26s.

McEvoy GK, ed. *AHFS drug information 91*. Bethesda: American Society of Hospital Pharmacists.

Menkes HA, et al. (1984). Obstructive pulmonary disease. In Harvey AM (ed): *The principles and practices of medicine*, 21st ed, pp 391–393. Norwalk, CT: Appleton-Century-Crofts.

Minette P, et al. (1988). Is there a defect in inhibitory muscarinic receptors in asthma? *Am Rev Respir Dis, 137*(Suppl.), 239.

Morrison ML. (1979). *Respiratory intensive care*, 2nd ed. Boston: Little, Brown.

Pauwels R. (1987). The effects of theophylline on airway inflammation. *Chest, 92*(Suppl. 1), 32s–37s.

Petty TL, et al. (1982) *Intensive and rehabilitative respiratory care*, 3rd ed, pp 223–227; p 391. Philadelphia: Lea & Febiger.

Phillips B. (1990). Chronic obstructive lung disease. In Rakel RE (ed): *Conns' Current Therapy*, pp 145–150. Philadelphia: WB Saunders.

Rakel RE. (1984). *Textbook of family practice*, 3rd ed. Philadelphia: WB Saunders.

Rumbak MJ. (1991). New concepts in the treatment of chronic persistent asthma. *Postgrad Med, 90*(3), 81–90.

Segal MS, MacDonnell KF. (1977). Therapeutic aerosols. In MacDonnell KF, Segal MS (eds). *Current respiratory care*. Boston: Little, Brown.

Sexton DL. (1981). *Chronic obstructive pulmonary disease: Care of the adult and child*. St. Louis: CV Mosby.

Slovis CM, Daniels GM, Wharton DR. (1987). Intravenous use of glycopyrrolate in acute respiratory distress due to bronchospastic pulmonary disease. *Ann Emerg Med, 16*(8), 898–900.

Stechschute DJ. (1990). Leukotrienes in asthma and allergic rhinitis. *N Engl J Med, 323*(25), 1769–1770.

Traver GA, Mitchell JT, Flodquist-Priestley G. (1991). *Respiratory care: A clinical approach*. Gaithersburg, MD: An Aspen Publication.

Wade JF. (1977). *Respiratory nursing care: Physiology and technique*, 2nd ed. St. Louis: CV Mosby.

Wyngaarden JB, Smith LR. (1985). *Cecil-Loeb textbook of medicine*, 7th ed. Philadelphia: WB Saunders.

Ziment I. (1987). Theophylline and mucociliary clearance. *Chest, 92*(Suppl. 1), 38s–43s.

Bibliography

Ahrens RC, Milavets G, Joad J. (1987). The effect of theophylline and B$_2$ agonists on airway reactivity. *Chest, 92*(Suppl. 1), 15s–21s.

Aubier M. (1987). Effect of theophylline on diaphragmatic muscle function. *Chest, 92*(Suppl. 1), 27s–31s.

Bleeker ER, Smith PL. (1986). Obstructive airway disease. In Barker LR (ed): *Principles of ambulatory medicine*, pp 637–669. Baltimore, MD: Williams & Wilkins.

Crompton G, Duncan J. (1989). Clinical assessment of a new breath actuated inhaler. *Practitioner, 233*, 260–269.

de Shazo RD. (1987). Introduction: Update on allergy. *Postgrad Med, 82*(5), 152–153.

Dolovich I, Hargreave, FE. (1987). The late-phase reaction: Something for the clinician. *Hosp Pract, 22*(10), 13–19.

Driscoll CE, Bope ET, Smith CW, Carter BL. (1986). *Handbook of family practice*. Chicago: Year Book Medical Pub.

Facts and Comparisons, p. 178. (1985). St. Louis: JB Lippincott. Pub.

Foresi A, Mattoli S, Corbo GM, et al. (1986). Late bronchial response and increase in methacholine hyperresponsiveness after exercise and a distilled water challenge in atopic subjects with asthma with dual asthmatic responses to allergen inhalation. *J Allergy Clin Immunol, 78*, 1130–1139.

Frank WO. (1986). Safety: Cimetidine and concomitant theophylline or warfarin: Drug interactions and their implications. *Clin Ther, 8*(A), 57–68.

Gilman AG, et al, eds. (1990). *Goodman and Gilman's the pharmacological basis of therapeutics*. New York: Pergamon Press.

Griffin JP. (1986). *Hematology and immunology*. Norwalk, CT: Appleton-Century-Crofts.

Jenne JW. (1987). Theophylline as a bronchodilator in COPD and its combination with inhaled beta-adrenergic drugs. *Chest, 92*(Suppl. 1), 7s–14s.

Kaliner MA. (1987). The late-phase reaction and its clinical implications. *Hosp Pract, 22*(10), 73–83.

Kesten S, et al. (1991). A three-month comparison of twice daily inhaled formoterol versus four times daily inhaled albuterol in the management of stable asthma. *Am Rev Respir Dis, 144*(3), 622–625.

Larsen GL. (1985). Late-phase reactions: Observations on pathogenesis and prevention. *J Allergy Clin Immunol, 76*(5), 665–669.

Li JTC. (1989). Five steps toward better asthma management. *Am Fam Physician, 40*(5), 201–210.

Lopez M, Salvaggio JE. (1987). Bronchial asthma: Mechanisms and management of a complex obstructive airway disease. *Postgrad Med, 82*(5), 177–190.

Mahler DA. (1987). The role of theophylline in the treatment of dyspnea in COPD. *Chest, 92*(Suppl. 1), 2s–6s.

Matthay RA. (1987). Favorable cardiovascular effects of theophylline in COPD. *Chest, 92*(Suppl. 1), 22s–26s.

Nakamira T, Morita V, Kuriyama M, et al. (1987). Platelet-activating factor in late asthmatic response. *Int Arch Allergy Appl Immunol, 82*, 57–61.

Patterson R, Greenberger P, Patterson D. (1991). Potentially fatal asthma: The problem of noncompliance. *Ann Allergy, 67*, 138–142.

Pauwels R. (1987). The effects of theophylline on airway inflammation. *Chest, 92*(Suppl. 1), 32s–37s.

Respiratory care handbook. (1989). Springhouse, PA: Springhouse Corporation.

Rice KL, Leatherman JW, Duane PG, et al. (1987). Aminophylline for acute exacerbations of chronic obstructive pulmonary disease. *Ann Intern Med, 107*(3), 305–309.

Rumbak MJ. (1991). New concepts in the treatment of chronic persistent asthma. *Postgrad Med, 90*(3), 81–90.

Slovis CM, Daniels GM, Wharton DR. (1987). Intravenous use of glycopyrrolate in acute respiratory distress due to bronchospastic pulmonary disease. *Ann Emerg Med, 16*(8), 898–900.

Soto-Aguilar MC, de Shazo RD, Waring NP. (1987). Anaphylaxis: Why it happens and what to do about it. *Postgrad Med, 82*(5), 154–170.

Spector SL. (1991). Common triggers of asthma. *Postgrad Med, 90*(3), 50–59.

Ziment I. (1987). Theophylline and mucociliary clearance. *Chest, 92*(Suppl. 1), 38s–43s.

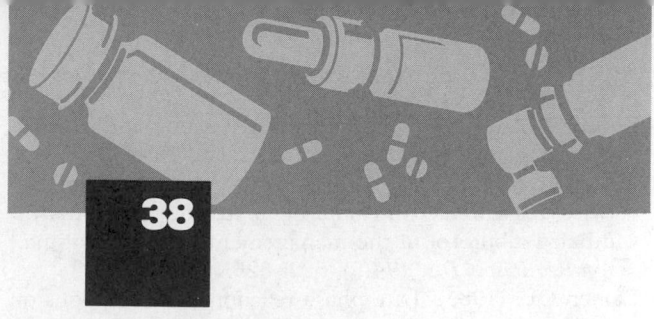

38

Drugs that affect the reproductive systems and sexuality

Reproductive systems

Sperm fertilize ova in the outer third of the fallopian tube, and their genetic information is integrated in the fertilized ova. New research indicates the presence of a substance in the fluid that surrounds the ripe ovum that may attract sperm, leading to fertilization. At the moment of fertilization, the blood type and tissue type, the hair color and eye color, and the general characteristics and body build of the person are established. The initial information about the baby's sex is also determined, depending on whether an X or Y chromosome is received from the sperm cell.

Despite the genetic input concerning gender that is present at fertilization, each human embryo starts life as a female. Males require the addition of fetal androgens to complete the process of sex determination. Even in the uterus, the presence or absence of sex hormones makes a difference.

Once the baby is born, it relies on its own endocrine system to produce the hormones that add to gender identification. However, the effects of maternal estrogens are still visible in some newborns. The baby's breasts may be enlarged and may even produce a white discharge called "witch's milk." Some female infants may have vaginal bleeding, referred to as "vicarious menstruation." These discharges disappear as the maternal estrogen in the newborn dissipates.

As children reach puberty, the effects of the hormones they produce become recognizable. Estrogens, progestogens, and androgens are produced by both sexes but in different quantities. Androgens are associated with the development of the penis and testes and the greater muscle mass and bone structure of males, whereas estrogens lead to the growth of female sex organs, breasts, and other secondary female sexual characteristics. (Hormone production is discussed in detail in Chapters 32 and 34.)

Physiology and hormones of the reproductive systems

The growth and state of the reproductive systems of both sexes are affected by many factors: nutrition (from infancy through adulthood), general physical status and health, environmental conditions (pollutants), health habits (rest, recreation, drug abuse, cigarette smoking), work environment (exposure to teratogens, abortifacients, substances that lead to carcinogenesis or mutagenesis), and emotional status (ability to cope with stress).

Females and hormonal factors

Maturation

At puberty, the pituitary gonadotropins stimulate the follicular hormone in the ovaries, resulting in the maturation of female sex organs. The uterus lengthens to about 7.5 cm, and the labia minora, the labia majora, and the clitoris enlarge. In addition, the secondary sex characteristics (voice pitch, pubic and axillary hair distribution, breast size, and skin texture) evolve. Estrogens cause the cells of the myometrium and endometrium to multiply rapidly during the menstrual cycle. Estrogens also influence height by their effect on the growth and development of the body's long bones. The increase in estrogens at puberty results in epiphyseal closure and the end of further endochondral bone formation and transformation of cartilage into bone.

Rigorous sports activity may delay menarche or cause menstrual irregularities, particularly in girls younger than age 16. A 17% level of body fat must be present for menarche to occur, and 22% fat must be present for maintenance of regular cycles. This level is affected by exercise as well as caloric intake.

Delay of menarche is not considered serious if breast development and the appearance of pubic and axillary hair have started by the age of 14 years. Investigation should be instituted if menstruation has not occurred by age 16, with treatment indicated if it has not started by age 18.

Hypoestrogenic amenorrhea is a frequent diagnosis when menarche is delayed, usually resulting from excess exercise, disease, or severe dieting. It may be complicated by bone loss, leading to osteoporosis and possible fractures, especially when amenorrhea is accompanied by cigarette smoking and high caffeine or alcohol intake.

Birth control pills may be prescribed, since the combination of estrogen and progesterone helps convert the endometrium into a mature structure. The estrogen content in oral contraceptives also increases the body's ability to reabsorb dietary calcium from the intestinal tract before it is lost through the kidney tubules. This reabsorption decreases calcium loss from the bones, lessening the chance of osteoporosis and bone fractures, which may occur even in the young (see later discussion of calcium needs).

Estrogen storage in fat tissue makes osteoporosis less likely in overweight women. Another protective factor in their favor is the increase in weight bearing on their bones. Thinner women can stress their bones effectively by lifting weights.

Immediately after menopause, and for the next 5 years, rapid bone loss occurs, particularly in the vertebrae and pelvic bones, because of lowered estrogen levels. After 5 years, bone loss levels off to a slower constant rate.

Hormones in the menstrual cycle

As the levels of hormones and other chemicals shift during the menstrual cycle, the female body is subjected to a series of changes. The sequence of the changes depends on the interactions of several hormones, the levels of which vary during different phases of the cycle. These changes are illustrated in Figure 38-1 and Table 38-1. Just as important to the client are the mood shifts that may occur with phases of the cycle.

The anterior lobe of the pituitary gland produces several hormones in the female. One of these is the *follicle-stimulating hormone* (FSH), which initiates the development of the graafian follicle in the ovary. A second hormone, the *luteinizing hormone* (LH), is also known as the *interstitial cell-stimulating hormone*. Both FSH and LH stimulate the graafian follicle to mature and to produce estrogen. These effects result in ovulation and in the formation of the corpus luteum.

The follicular hormone produced by the graafian follicle cells and the luteal hormone made by the corpus luteum are ovarian hormones or estrogens. They must exist in proper proportions for the normal development and activity of the reproductive system. Their production depends on the presence of their precursors, the hormones produced by the anterior lobe of the pituitary.

If pregnancy occurs, a third hormone, *luteotropic hormone* (LTH), also called *lactogenic hormone* or *prolactin*, activates secretory activity in the corpus luteum, resulting in the production of progesterone. Without LTH, the corpus luteum disintegrates and does not supply progesterone. Luteal phase defects are discussed on p. 965 (see "Progesterone").

Whether or not pregnancy occurs, the estrogen levels before ovulation can be expected to increase as the ovarian follicle develops. After ovulation, if fertilization and implantation of the ovum have not occurred, estrogen levels drop slightly, remaining at that level for over a week. During the last week of the cycle, estrogen levels drop precipitously. The deprivation caused by the withdrawal of estrogen results in menstruation.

Pregnancy and lactation

The production of progesterone by the corpus luteum is essential in preparing and maintaining the uterine lining during pregnancy. Progesterone secreted during pregnancy also suppresses ovulation and enhances

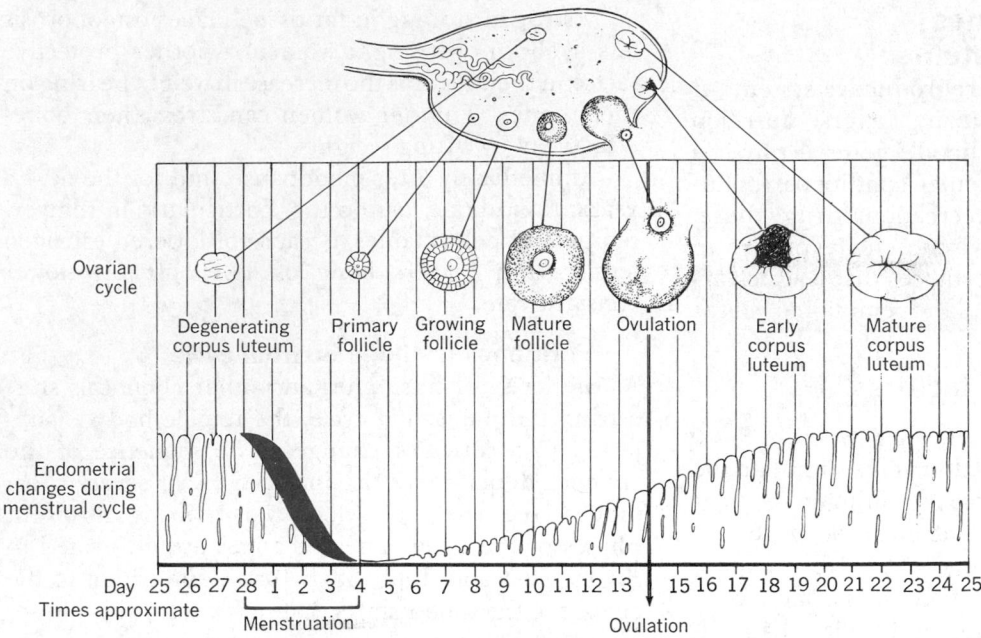

Figure 38-1. Schematic representation of one ovarian cycle and the corresponding changes in the thickness of the endometrium. The endometrium is thickest just before the onset of menstruation and thinnest just as menstruation ceases (compare with Table 38-1).

breast development, including the secretory action of the mammary glands in preparation for breast-feeding after the child is born.

The uterus has to expand in many directions to supply room for the fetus and placenta as well as the amniotic fluid and umbilical cord. Maintenance of pregnancy depends on good muscle tone; this is helped by the presence of estrogens, which stimulate protein synthesis in the uterus, and by androgens, which are involved in the production of proteins used in the development of muscles. The placenta produces a high level of estrogens in the maternal circulation during pregnancy, nurturing the fetus. Through another action of estrogen, serum levels of prothrombin and of clotting factors VII, VIII, IX, and X increase progressively, providing protection against severe hemorrhage at parturition. Ironically, these factors also increase the risk of thromboembolic disease, par-

Table 38-1. Correlation of hormonal activities with ovarian and uterine changes

Phase	Menstrual	Follicular	Ovulation	Luteal	Premenstrual
Days	1 2 3 4 5 6 7 8	9 10 11 12 13 14	15 16 17 18	19 20 21 22 23 24	25 26 27 28 1 2
Ovary	Degenerating corpus luteum; beginning follicular development	Growth and maturation of follicle	Ovulation	Active corpus luteum	Degenerating corpus luteum
Estrogen production	Low	Increasing	High	Declining, then a secondary rise	Decreasing
Progesterone production	None	None	Low	Increasing	Decreasing
FSH production	Increasing	High, then declining	Low	Low	Increasing
LH production	Low	Low, then increasing	High	High	Decreasing
Endometrium	Degeneration and shedding of superficial layer; coiled arteries dilate, then constrict again	Reorganization and proliferation of superficial layer	Continued growth	Active secretion and glandular dilatation; highly vascular; edematous	Vasoconstriction of coiled arteries; beginning degeneration

(Chaffee EE, Lytle IM. [1980]. *Basic physiology and anatomy*, 4th ed, p 559. Philadelphia: JB Lippincott)

ticularly during the postpartum period (see Chapter 16). *Human chorionic gonadotropin* (hCG) is the luteotrophic hormone produced by the placenta; it is not influenced by the pituitary. It apparently intensifies the action of the corpus luteum early in pregnancy, strengthening fetal and placental growth.

Toward the end of pregnancy, the uterine contractions that mark labor may be stimulated by an increased production of *prostaglandins* in the body. *Oxytocin*, a hormone produced by the posterior pituitary, is also involved in the onset and effectiveness of the uterine contractions by acting on the myometrium.

Breast-feeding, in a supplementary action, stimulates the uterus to contract through the release of neurohypophysial oxytocin. Therefore, the uterus goes through involution more quickly. Oxytocin continues to be released during the postpartum period when the nursing mother sees or hears her newborn's demands for feeding. This release results in the so-called milk let-down, a conditioned reflex in which smooth muscle in the breast contracts, releasing milk (Fig. 38-2).

Drug use during pregnancy and lactation is discussed in Chapter 16.

Menopause

The decrease in serum levels of estrogens at menopause may lead to the development of osteoporosis, the

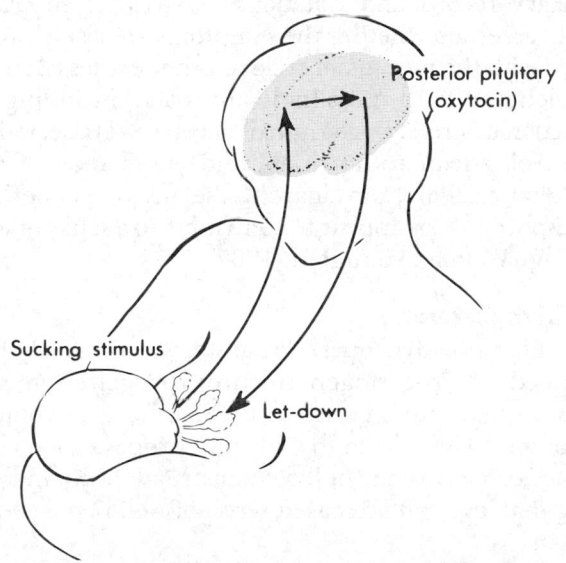

Figure 38-2. Diagrammatic representation of the basic features of the let-down reflex. The sucking stimulus arrives at the hypothalamus, which promotes the release of oxytocin from the posterior pituitary. Oxytocin stimulates contraction of the myoepithelial cells around the alveoli in the mammary glands. Contraction of these muscle-like cells causes the milk to be propelled through the duct system and into the lactiferous sinuses, where it becomes available to the nursing infant. (Worthington B. [1977]. Lactation, human milk and nutritional considerations. In Worthington B, Vermeersch J, Williams IR [eds]: *Nutrition in pregnancy and lactation.* St. Louis: CV Mosby)

loss of bone density, causing the so-called dowager's hump that results in the pronounced loss of height seen in older women. Other manifestations of estrogen deficiency are senile vaginitis, with lack of lubrication during sexual stimulation, a burning sensation during intercourse, and even dyspareunia (painful intercourse), as well as hot "flashes" (or "flushes"). The breasts also diminish in size. Women with greater fat deposits appear to have higher estrogen levels, as well as greater susceptibility to uterine cancer, after menopause. Loss of estrogen also seems to be responsible for an increase in atherosclerosis in older women.

Males and hormonal factors

As a boy reaches puberty, additional androgens are produced, leading to sexual development. The testes and phallus enlarge, and secondary sex characteristics become apparent, stimulated by the presence of hCG. Bone and muscle masses increase, the voice lowers, the beginnings of a beard appear, a growth spurt usually occurs, nocturnal emissions may take place, and penile erections may be difficult to control.

Testosterone is the most powerful androgen, yet it is similar to progesterone in its chemical structure. Its production depends on stimulation by FSH of the anterior lobe of the pituitary. The action of FSH on the seminiferous tubules leads to the production of spermatozoa. The LH acts on the interstitial cells of the testes, stimulating the production of androgen. When a high blood level of androgens is reached, feedback to the anterior lobe of the pituitary inhibits the production of FSH and LH. As a result, sperm formation stops.

Sperm production is affected by the general level of the man's health, nutrition, immunology, various drugs and toxins, testicular temperature, endocrine factors, and age.

As men grow older, testosterone levels can be expected to decrease, leading possibly to difficulty in initiating and maintaining an erection. The quantity of ejaculate may be smaller and propelled with less force. For some men, these changes may lead to a fear of failure in sexual performance, with resultant sexual and emotional problems. Some respond well to the knowledge that the increased time needed for arousal permits more stimulation of the woman, with greater vaginal lubrication possible. The increased foreplay time may, in effect, be mutually advantageous.

Male impotence can be due to a variety of factors. If its onset is recent, the history should include information about any newly started drugs. Medications have been implicated in about 25% of impotency cases.

Anabolic steroids have been misused and abused by athletes who try to develop bigger muscles. These drugs can lead to death from hepatorenal failure or may cause other reactions, including cancer, increased cholesterol levels (with lower high-density lipoprotein levels), heart disease, hirsutism and male pattern baldness in women, enlargement of the penis and prostate, priapism, sterility, fetal damage, and testicular atrophy.

Drugs and the reproductive systems

Estrogens and progestogens are discussed in detail in Chapter 32.

Prophylactic uses of estrogens

A relative lack of estrogen can cause delayed sexual development, prolonged growth (leading to excessive height), and thinning of the bones. High doses of estrogen have been used prophylactically in an attempt to prevent some tall girls from reaching a predicted height of over 6 feet. Ethinyl estradiol (Estinyl) has been used to retard growth, administered in daily doses from 0.25 mg to 1 mg in cycles of 3 weeks, followed by 1 week without the medication. Monitoring of serum antithrombin levels in necessary to lessen the risk of thrombosis. Cigarette smoking, surgery, infection, and prolonged immobilization are examples of contraindications to this therapy (Blomback, et al, 1983).

In 1990, the Third International Symposium on Osteoporosis recommended 800 mg of calcium as the minimum daily adult intake, with an increase to 1200 mg for menopausal and postmenopausal women, since their bodies have a decreased ability to absorb calcium. The Symposium also recommended estrogen therapy in addition to exercise and calcium supplement to prevent bone loss after menopause or when ovarian function is ineffective. Combined estrogen–progestin administered after menopause has been shown to lower the risk of hip fracture by 60% over the following 10 years. This regimen is contraindicated for women at risk for breast cancer, those who smoke, or those at risk for thromboembolic disease.

Drugs for premenstrual symptoms

Women react differently to menses. For many, the cycle passes without symptoms or difficulty. However, some women suffer from premenstrual symptoms that range from mild to incapacitating. In the past, most women believed they had to bear their discomfort in silence. They were often made to feel that their complaints were based on emotional factors. Although emotional factors may account for the symptoms some women experience, more recent research has demonstrated that premenstrual syndrome (PMS) has its basis in physiologic considerations. One study has demonstrated the secretion of a lowered level of melatonin, a hormone secreted at night by the pineal gland in the brain. This reduced level is associated with premenstrual depression.

PMS includes mood swings, irritability, a feeling of being bloated, fluid retention, sore breasts, migraine-type headaches, anxiety, depression, loss of concentration, fatigue, food cravings, backache, lethargy, dizzi-ness, heaviness in the legs, acneiform skin disorders, and general aches and pains. These symptoms may escalate under stress and seem to be associated with the decrease in progesterone that occurs during the final week of the menstrual cycle.

The major diagnostic factor in PMS is that the symptoms present themselves in a recurrent pattern after ovulation, occurring 1 to 14 days before or during the first few days of menstruation. The symptoms may even occur after a hysterectomy if the ovaries have not been removed, ending finally only after ovarian function ceases.

PMS tends to affect women in their 30s and 40s; it is sometimes triggered by hormonal changes that develop after childbirth, after the discontinuation of oral contraceptives, after tubal ligation, or after removal of an ovarian cyst. (PMS may be present on alternate months if only one ovary is affected.) There are different reactions to the syndrome, such as depression, anxiety, or anger. Mood swings are absent in 40% of women with PMS; 50% have mild mood swings, and 10% have moderate to severe problems.

Treatment for PMS varies and may include progesterone (Dalton, 1984), psychotherapy, mild diuretics 5 to 10 days before menses, oral contraceptives to prevent ovulation, Vitamin B_6 (up to 500 mg daily) exercise, and high-protein snacks. Education and awareness appear to be helpful. Charting the menstrual cycle and distressing symptoms and keeping a dietary record and notations of stressful situations help ascertain whether the symptoms are really associated with the menstrual cycle or other causes (Bender, Kelleher, 1986). A wellness approach, including reduction in stress, a program of aerobic exercise, weight control, adequate nutrition, and elimination of salt, alcohol, caffeine, and cigarettes, seems to be beneficial. Support groups appear to contribute to a sense of well-being (Walton, Youngkin, 1987).

Progesterone

Pharmacodynamics. Progesterone is usually prescribed as Progestogen (medroxyprogesterone acetate) when used to treat PMS. The syndrome is thought to be related to a drop in progesterone levels that normally occur before menstruation. By increasing that level, an increased sense of well-being should occur.

Progesterone, when administered orally to women with adequate endogenous estrogen, transforms proliferative endometrium tissue into secretory tissue. When given parenterally, in addition to the above action, progesterone inhibits gonadotropin production, which then prevents follicular maturation and ovulation.

Pharmacokinetics. Progesterone may be administered orally or intramuscularly (IM). It affects many organs throughout the body, although the effects of prolonged use on pituitary, ovarian, adrenal, hepatic, or uterine functions remain under study. In a small number of cases, when given in combination with estrogen as in oral contraceptives, it has been linked to a decrease in glucose tolerance. It is degraded by the liver and excreted by the kidneys.

Congenital anomalies, including heart defects and limb reduction defects, are associated with progesterone administered during pregnancy, an indication that it crosses the placenta. Detectable amounts have also been found in breast milk.

Therapeutic uses. Progesterone is used orally to treat secondary amenorrhea, for abnormal uterine bleeding not associated with organic pathology, and for PMS. It is often administered in combination with estrogen, primarily in oral contraceptives. It is also used in the adjunctive or palliative treatment of inoperable, recurrent, and metastatic endometrial or renal carcinoma.

Dosage and administration. Oral doses vary from 2.5 mg to 10 mg. A description of doses when used in conjunction with estrogen is included in Table 38-9. The IM dose varies from 100 to 400 mg/ml.

Adverse reactions. Progesterone should never be used during pregnancy because of the possibility of fetal congenital defects. Nursing mothers should avoid progesterone since it is secreted into breast milk. The drug has been associated with thromboembolic episodes and pulmonary emboli. Progesterone may cause fluid retention, which might adversely affect clients who suffer from epilepsy, migraine, asthma, or cardiac or renal dysfunction. Some skin reactions may occur: urticaria, pruritus, generalized rash, acne, alopecia, and hirsutism. The client should be aware of the possibility of break-through bleeding, changes in menstruation with the possibility of amenorrhea (immediate check for pregnancy should take place), weight changes, cholestatic jaundice, pyrexia, insomnia, nausea, somnolence, and depression.

Precautions and contraindications. Before using progesterone, a thorough physical examination with emphasis on breast and pelvic areas should be carried out, including a Papanicolaou smear and, if indicated, a pregnancy test. The drug should not be used if pregnancy or organic pathology are present. It is important that pelvic examinations be carried out at frequent intervals to make certain that pregnancy has not occurred. Undiagnosed vaginal bleeding should be investigated immediately.

Clients with any condition that might be affected by fluid retention should be watched carefully. Diabetic women may have a decrease in their glucose tolerance while on estrogen–progestin therapy and therefore, must be followed carefully. Those with a history of depression should be observed carefully; if an exacerbation occurs, the drug should be discontinued. The drug should also be stopped at any sign of a thrombotic disorder.

Progesterone is contraindicated for anyone who demonstrates or who has a history of thrombophlebitis, thromboembolic disorders, cerebral apoplexy, liver dysfunction or disease, known or suspected breast or genital malignancy, undiagnosed vaginal bleeding, missed abortion, or known sensitivity to the drug. It should not be used as a test for pregnancy, because it may cause severe defects to the fetus.

Drugs for dysmenorrhea

Dysmenorrhea, which may be severe for some women, appears to be due to the release of prostaglandins in the uterus during menstruation. Aspirin has inhibitory effects on prostaglandin production and is helpful when mild cramps occur, especially if taken before the pain begins. If more pronounced cramps are present, several other drugs that prevent the action and production of prostaglandins are available. These include ibuprofen (Motrin) and mefenamic acid (Ponstel), which are taken only when pain is present. Ibuprofen and mefenamic acid infrequently cause a delay of up to 2 weeks in menstruation, as well as dysfunctional uterine bleeding. These side effects are reversible when the medication is stopped (Halbert, 1983).

Drugs used in menstrual symptoms are discussed in Table 38-2.

Drugs for menopause

Estrogen and transdermal 17β-estradiol

See Chapter 32 for general information on estrogens.

Estrogen-replacement therapy has been used widely for relief of symptoms during menopause, including vasomotor symptoms and vaginal atrophy. It helps prevent osteoporosis secondary to menopause. Also, estrogens have been shown to have a positive effect on lipid status by making the ratio of high-density to low-density lipoprotein cholesterol levels more favorable. This action is associated with a lesser incidence of ischemic heart disease. In late 1975, estrogens were implicated in the fivefold increase in the incidence of endometrial carcinoma. As a result, the National Institute of Health recommended that estrogen-replacement therapy (ERT) be used only for women with severe postmenstrual symptoms and for the shortest possible time. The organization cautioned that local applications of estrogenic creams and suppositories were easily absorbed into the bloodstream and were equal in potency to oral doses.

More recent studies indicate that endometrial cancer is slow growing and can be easily diagnosed and cured before it causes a serious health threat. The risk of endometrial cancer is therefore considered low; it can be reduced and possibly eliminated if ERT is prescribed in cycles of 3 weeks on and 1 week off, and if

Table 38-2. Drugs for premenstrual and menstrual symptoms

Drug name	Usual adult dosage	Effect	Additional information
acetaminophen (Tylenol, Tempra, Datril)	325–650 mg, q4–6h, up to 3900 mg/day PC: B	Pain relief	Excessive use may lead to liver damage, particularly in alcoholics.
aspirin (Bufferin, Empirin)	325–650 mg, q4h, up to 3900 mg/day PC: C (D in 3rd trimester)	Inhibits prostaglandin production; decreases mild dysmenorrhea	Give with milk or food to lessen GI side effects; should be taken before pain begins; do not use if sensitive to aspirin.
ibuprofen (Motrin, Nuprin, Advil)	400 mg, q4–6h, up to 2400 mg/day PC: B (D in 3rd trimester)	Inhibits prostaglandin production; decreases moderate to severe dysmenorrhea	Give with milk or food to lessen GI side effects; take only when pain is present; do not give to clients who have asthma or nasal polyps or cardiac decompensation. Should not be used by pregnant or lactating women.
mefenamic acid (Ponstan, Ponstel)	500 mg to start, then 250 mg q6h, generally given for only 2 to 3 days, not to exceed 1 week PC: C	Inhibits prostaglandin production; decreases moderate to severe dysmenorrhea in pregnant or nursing women	Give with milk or food to lessen GI side effects. May cause dizziness or headache. Should not be used by lactating women or pregnant women, particularly in the last trimester; may prolong prothrombin time.
naproxen sodium (Anaprox, Naprosyn)	550 mg to start, then 275 mg q6–8h PC: B (D in 3rd trimester)	Inhibits prostaglandin production; decreases moderate to severe dysmenorrhea	Give with milk or food to lessen GI side effects; take only when pain is present; do not give to clients who have asthma or nasal polyps or cardiac decompensation. Should not be used by pregnant or lactating women.
progestins (various)	Varies PC: X	Increases level of progesterone that may be responsible for dysmenorrhea	Do not give to patients who have thromboembolic disorders, missed abortion, breast cancer, or abnormal vaginal bleeding.
estrogen with progestogen	See Table 38-9 for dosage PC: X	Increases the level of progesterone that may be responsible for dysmenorrhea	Same as for progesterone; in addition, educate client on importance of taking as directed.

KEY: PC = pregnancy category. (The validity of pregnancy risk categories has not been established; see Chapter 16, p 216.)

the drug is combined with progesterone during the last 7 to 13 days of each cycle.

A study reported in 1991 indicated many positive effects of ERT if the estrogen dose is maintained at 0.625 mg and it is taken daily for many years. It was shown to prevent fractures, strokes, heart disease, and menopausal symptoms. Users outlived nonusers by 1.2 years, a span that increased to 2.5 years with long-term use. In addition, the report stated that the overall death rate from all cancers for the 9,000 women who were studied for more than 7 years was no higher for the estrogen users than for nonusers. However, a precautionary note was added, reminding women to be aware of possible signs of cancer, including breast lumps and unexplained uterine bleeding. The Food

and Drug Administration (FDA) has approved the use of oral estrogens to retard bone loss in postmenopausal women.

In September 1986, the FDA approved Estraderm (Estradiol Transdermal System) for ERT. It is a skin patch that delivers 17β-estradiol into the circulatory system at a constant level (Fig. 38-3). The transdermal patch is about the size of a silver dollar and is prescribed to control the symptoms of menopause, including hot flashes, night sweats, and vaginal dryness. The patches have four separate layers: an impermeable backing, a reservoir that contains the estradiol, a porous membrane to control the drug's release, and a nonallergenic adhesive to keep the unit on the skin. Application is made twice weekly to a nonoily, dry,

Should postmenopausal women receive estrogen replacement therapy?

Pros	Cons
Estrogens relieve vasomotor symptoms and vaginal atrophy in postmenopausal women.	The risk of endometrial cancer may be increased.
They help prevent osteoporosis by enhancing absorption of calcium.	Breast tenderness may occur.
A positive effect on high-density to low-density lipoprotein cholesterol levels is found.	Skin irritation may develop from application of transdermal patches.
Women who receive estrogens appear to have increased feelings of well-being.	Increased risk for high blood pressure and thromboembolic disease exists, especially in smokers, users of alcohol, and inactive women.
	Breakthrough bleeding may occur.
	The risk of gallbladder disease is increased.

hair-free skin area, preferably the abdomen, never the breasts or genitalia. It may remain in place while bathing.

The replacement site should be rotated, and a minimum of a week should be allowed before reusing the same site. The patches are replaced every 3½ days (twice weekly) and are usually on a cyclic schedule. The usual starting dose is 0.05 mg, with adjustment possible to 0.1 mg. The 17β-estradiol is the same form of estrogen produced by premenopausal women. The most commonly reported adverse reaction to the patch is irritation and redness (17%); in 2% of women, it is serious enough to cause therapy to be discontinued (Estraderm [Estradiol] transdermal system: Prescribing information], 1986).

Pharmacodynamics. The use of a transdermal patch to deliver 17β-estradiol permits a steady administration of the hormone, with raised serum levels of estradiol occurring within 4 hours of application. Levels of estrone also increase slightly, remaining rather constant. Serum and urinary levels of estradiol conjugates appear to be typical of the early follicular phase found in premenstrual women.

Pharmacokinetics. ERT may be carried out orally or by using a transdermal patch. The patch must be applied to intact skin and left in place on the trunk of the body, preferably on the abdomen, and replaced every third day.

Transdermal ERT has a range of serum levels of estradiol 24 hours after administration similar to oral ERT. However, a significant increase in estrone levels is noted after oral administration, with signs of estrogen retention after only three doses of oral estrogens (Powers, et al, 1985).

Oral estrogens are initially metabolized within the gut wall, with the conversion of estradiol to estrone. They are carried to the liver through the portal circulation. Further metabolism then occurs, with estrone broken down to estrone sulfate and estrone glucuronide. Potentially high levels of antithrombin III and renin substrate could increase the risk of hypertension and thrombosis in predisposed people. This metabolic process is avoided with the transdermal patch, which delivers drug directly to the blood, elim-

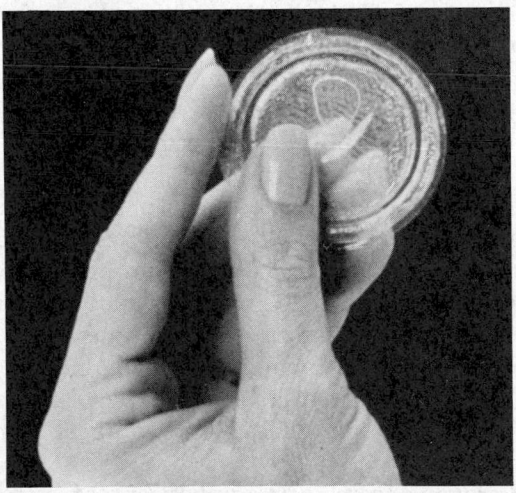

Figure 38-3. This low-dose estrogen skin patch, marketed under the brand name Estraderm (Estradiol Transdermal System), is transparent and about the size of a silver dollar. It contains 17β-estradiol, which is identical to the estrogen produced naturally before menopause. In releasing small amounts of estrogen at a relatively constant and controlled rate directly into the bloodstream, the patch is the first pharmaceutical product to closely mimic the natural levels of estrogen produced in premenopausal women.

inating first pass through the liver (Padwick, et al, 1986). Pretreatment levels of estradiol and estrone are attained within 24 hours of removing the transdermal patch.

Therapeutic uses. Estrogen is given as a replacement for low estrogen levels in postmenopausal woman. It is used to lessen the flashes and sweating that cause discomfort to some postmenopausal women, to lessen the symptoms caused by vaginal atrophy (burning and pain during intercourse), and to prevent osteoporosis and possible bone fractures. It also enhances the sense of well-being and lessens such psychologic symptoms as difficulty in concentrating, anxiety, and forgetfulness (Padwick, et al, 1986). Oral estrogen has to be given in large amounts to provide relief, producing higher than physiologic concentrations of estrone. This dose may result in endometrial proliferation, possibly leading to endometrial carcinoma. Therefore, cyclic administration is ordered, with 12 days of progestogen therapy used to prevent endometrial hyperplasia.

ERT is also used to enhance the absorption of calcium in postmenopausal women, decreasing the possibility of osteoporosis and subsequent bone fractures. The increase in calcium intake without concurrent estrogen replacement has proved ineffective in preventing bone loss associated with aging. ERT to prevent bone loss should be started as soon as possible after menopause and continued for at least 7 to 10 years. It may be recommended throughout life for those women at high risk for osteoporosis based on family history, small bone structure, corticosteroid medications, or heavy use of cigarettes or alcohol.

Dosage and administration. Oral preparations are conjugated equine estrogens (Premarin; 0.625 or 1.25 mg/day) or a micronized form of 17β-estradiol (Estrace). A transdermal 17β-estradiol patch (0.025, 0.05, or 0.1 mg/day) is applied as directed and left in place until changed, every third day.

Although the doses of estradiol in the transdermal patches are lower than those given orally, 12 days of norethindrone may be ordered to prevent endometrial hyperplasia or the recurrence of menopausal symptoms during treatment-free times. Low-dose progestogens produce a more acceptable bleeding pattern, ridding the uterus of the hyperplastic endometrial lining, regardless of the route of estrogen administration.

Estrogens from local applications of estrogenic creams and suppositories are absorbed into the bloodstream. Vaginal use of conjugated estrogen cream in low-dose dilution (0.1 mg) seems superior to higher doses (1.25 mg) and has a beneficial carry-over effect that lasts 3 weeks, which is not evident with the higher dose. This dose may enable the client to gain relief while limiting the application to only 1 or 2 weeks each month, thereby reducing the possible dangers.

Adverse reactions. The patch may cause topical side effects, such as itching, redness, rash, swelling, or dermatitis. Usually, these symptoms are mild to moderate and are transitory. However, the patch should be discontinued if reactions are severe. Other symptoms, such as breast tenderness and break-through bleeding, are expected reactions to estrogen, regardless of the route of administration. Endometrial hyperplasia can also develop. Observation of women in a clinical trial over a 3-week period did not demonstrate an accumulation of estradiol or estradiol conjugates in the body.

Precautions and contraindications. Regardless of the estrogen source for ERT, women should have semiannual checkups, including breast and pelvic examinations. Endometrial biopsies are recommended by some health care providers before ERT, to determine the risk factor for endometrial carcinoma, as well as to ascertain the optimal dosage of progestin (Padwick, et al, 1986). Estrogen therapy is contraindicated in women with a history of endometrial or breast cancer, blood clots, strokes, coronary artery disease, severe migraine headaches, liver disease, or unexplained vaginal bleeding. Those on ERT are at higher risk for gallbladder disease, elevated blood pressure, and blood clots. Cigarette smoking, alcohol intake, and physical inactivity negate some of the benefits of hormone therapy.

Calcium

Menopausal women may be at an increased risk for osteoporosis because of a calcium deficiency. Osteoporosis is a serious problem that affects about 20 million Americans (80% are women), with 1.3 million osteoporosis-related fractures occurring annually. Of these, about 20% of those who develop hip fractures will die from complications within 12 months of occurrence. It may be necessary to prescribe calcium in addition to the exercise to increase the bone mass (see later discussion of calcium needs).

Adequate calcium intake, 800 mg daily in childhood, 1200 mg from ages 11 to 24 and for pregnant or lactating women, and 800 mg daily for adults over 25, can result in a peak bone mass at maturity. Information on calcium-rich foods should be included in health teaching. If the dietary intake is insufficient, a calcium supplement, such as Ca-Plus with 280 mg per tablet, may be required. (For more information on calcium, see the section on minerals in Chapter 50.)

The effects of toxic materials

The number of women in the labor force is increasing yearly, particularly in jobs linked to exposure to toxic materials. Some of these women may be pregnant, and many are of reproductive age.

In a 1975 report for the Department of Health, Education and Welfare, a need was expressed for "more detailed information by occupation . . . on a continuing basis if efficient monitoring procedures are to be developed for evaluating the health of the fetus in the work place." Because of federal antidiscriminatory legislation, it is illegal to bar women from any occupation even though the occupation may lead to biologic risks for a fetus. However, the employer must make employees aware of those risks, with no assurance of job protection for those who decide the dangers are too great.

Employees are supposed to be made aware of substances known to be teratogens or abortifacients, as well as substances that lead to carcinogenesis or mutagenesis. Nurses, particularly those who work in operating rooms or radiology, oncology, or hematology departments, are at high risk because of their exposure to toxic substances. They often place the client's care ahead of their own well-being, such as when nurses risk being contaminated by remaining with clients who have radium implants.

Little has been done to identify substances that interfere with fertility. One substance, carbon disulfide, used in the production of viscose, has been documented as a cause of menorrhagia, amenorrhea, and sterility in women. Other industrial environments or wastes (*eg*, pesticides, mercury, polychlorinated biphenyl) are suspected of having caused infertility in men and women or of having caused damage to fetuses. However, documentation remains scarce.

People with cancer, leukemia, or one of the lymphomas may become sterile by surgery or radiation. Anyone on psychotropic drugs or with a pathologic condition that affects the reproductive system may find various aspects of sexual functioning affected. In addition, environmental factors such as toxic wastes found in industry, the air, or polluted waters may have an effect on the reproductive system.

Fetuses may be at greater risk than mothers when exposed to toxic materials, because their tissues are more sensitive to substances that may be teratogenic at an early stage of fetal development or carcinogenic at a later point. One example is the synthetic hormone diethylstilbestrol (DES), which was used by women with threatened abortions. Daughters born to women who took DES during pregnancy are at high risk for vaginal adenosis and cancer and must be followed carefully during and after adolescence. Studies also show a higher than statistically expected number of varicoceles and epididymal cysts in males exposed prenatally to DES. They demonstrate a significantly lower sperm count and potential for decreased fertility. There is also the possibility of eventual malignancies, based on findings that males exposed to DES have an increased incidence of cryptorchidism and hypoplastic testes, which has been correlated with adult testicular carcinomas (Niculescu, 1985).

In recent years, episodes of toxic shock syndrome have occurred; the syndrome is usually associated with highly absorbent tampons and possibly diaphragms, cervical sponges, and cervical caps. The causative organism is *Staphylococcus aureus*. Early medical intervention is necessary to prevent serious illness.

The risk of developing toxic shock syndrome is increased by 37% for each 1-g increase in the absorbency of the tampon. A labeling system indicates the degree of tampon absorbency (Farley, 1990).

■ Summary

The level of female reproductive hormones depends on several aspects of the client's lifestyle. Education as to the importance of positive health habits (proper weight maintenance, nutrition, exercise), as well as the elimination of negative environmental factors are important. The client's emotional status also requires evaluation as one possible aspect of her desire or ability to comply with the suggested health regimes. The addition of calcium or estrogen and the elimination of cigarette smoking and alcohol may be necessary for proper maintenance of her reproductive system, as well as prevention of bone loss.

Many women suffer from various premenstrual and menstrual symptoms. Premenstrual symptoms include mood swings, a feeling of being bloated, sore breasts, and migraine-type headaches. Stress further accentuates the symptoms. Treatments differ and may include progesterone, vitamin B_6, diet, exercise, psychotherapy, and relief from stress. Dysmenorrhea appears to be due to the release of prostaglandins during menstruation. The use of nonsteroidal anti-inflammatory agents, which inhibit prostaglandin synthesis, is usually effective in relieving dysmenorrhea. Estrogen as a therapy for menopausal women is constantly under study, with attention given to the 17β-estradiol skin patch currently favored for ERT, as well as for the prevention and treatment of osteoporosis.

With the increase of women in the job market and the increase of environmental pollutants, the possibility of women becoming infertile, or aborting or experiencing sexual dysfunction is rising.

Nursing management

Nursing implications

The women's movement has not only raised the sense of female consciousness, it has also awakened in women a responsibility toward themselves regarding their sexuality. Positive ideas and information on sexuality from nurses can reinforce "good" feelings, including respect for female bodily functions.

Society's emphasis on thinness has resulted in an

A 17-year-old female is distressed that menarche has not occurred. She is 5'6" tall and weighs 95 pounds. What information about her health habits would you anticipate while gathering data for your nursing assessment? Include a discussion of the causes of hypoestrogenic amenorrhea that are related to delayed menarche.

obsessive reliance on dieting and exercise among many women. Carried to an extreme, the combination may lead to amenorrhea and bone damage because of insufficient estrogen and calcium levels, as well as lowered resistance to disease due to negative changes in the immune system (see section on Estraderm).

Nursing process

Assessment Assessment through a history and physical examination is important in care that involves the reproductive systems. When physical findings and laboratory tests are normal, the history may provide important clues to these problems. These clues may involve any of the factors mentioned at the beginning of the chapter and may include such small items as excessive coffee drinking preceding the menstrual period.

Recent findings have disclosed that premenstrual problems have a physical basis. Therefore, women who suffer from premenstrual symptoms no longer need to feel they "have to suffer in silence" each month. They should be made aware of medications and other measures that may help alleviate symptoms. Before drugs are ordered or administered, a nursing history should be taken and include questions about the presence of allergies to aspirin or other drugs, the existence of thromboembolic disorders, breast cancer, or abnormal vaginal bleeding, and the possibility of pregnancy.

The client's physical appearance may present valuable information. She may be thin to the point of emaciation, listless, fatigued without exertion, and pale. Borborygmi may be heard frequently, and she may rub her abdomen in reaction to hunger pangs. Her history may include information about infections, colds, and fractures, indicating changes in health maintenance and comfort levels. Women need a 22% body fat level to maintain regular menstrual cycles. Estrogens cannot be manufactured or stored properly without this fat level.

Nursing diagnosis Nursing diagnoses likely to be made for excessively thin female clients with inadequate hormones include the following:

Altered nutrition: less than body requirements to maintain sufficient fat storage for estrogen production

High risk for injury related to loss of bone mass and osteoporosis
High risk for sexual dysfunction: change in sexual function related to altered body image as weight increases
Noncompliance with dietary regimen related to desire to maintain thin body
Noncompliance with medication regime: taking less than therapeutic dosages of hormones related to fear of cancer

Diagnoses likely to be made for women with PMS may include the following:

Body image disturbance associated with irritability and weight gain
Altered nutrition: more than body requirements related to craving for carbohydrates secondary to PMS
Fluid volume excess related to sodium retention secondary to PMS
Impaired social interaction (role performance, parenting, family process) related to irritability
Ineffective individual coping related to emotional changes secondary to PMS

Pregnancy, lactation, and menopause present other types of hormonal changes that can cause the following:

Body image disturbance
Altered role performance
Altered family processes secondary to PMS

At any stage of development, clients may exhibit the following:

Anxiety related to changes in sexuality
Knowledge deficit related to self-care practices and sexuality

Planning Goals for care vary with the problems presented by the client. Regardless of the diagnosis, the nurse's ability to work with the client in establishing goals will affect compliance.

Most hormonal changes have common components for which similar goals are appropriate. Reduced anxiety and stress, attention to nutrition and self-care, better coping mechanisms, and improved self-concept and sexuality patterns are goals in the treatment of hormonal problems. Improved comfort levels in the face of hormonal changes should be sought whether the hormonal level is increasing (menarche, pregnancy), shifting (lactation), or decreasing (menopause).

Goals for excessively thin women may include increased daily caloric intake, increased body fat, increased bone density, and restoration of normal menstruation.

An appropriate goal for many clients is increased knowledge about sexuality, the causes and effects of hormone changes, and self-care practices.

Intervention Whenever her body undergoes hormonal changes, the client may need a variety of interventions, including diet, relaxation techniques, mental health counseling, exercise, and adherence to medication as ordered (diuretics, oral contraceptives, prenatal or postpartum medications). Acceptance of bodily changes may be one of the most important areas of nursing intervention, whether for the young adolescent just developing physically, the pregnant client with her enlarging breasts and abdomen, or the middle-aged or elderly woman who sees herself as losing attractiveness.

The underweight client requires knowledge of the dangers to her reproductive and skeletal systems that result from deficiencies in estrogen and calcium. She should be given information on the effects of insufficient fat deposits in her body and the resultant inability of the body to produce and store estrogen for a proper menstrual cycle as well as maintain bone mass.

The emotional component in remaining underweight requires as much nursing intervention as the actual dietary aspects of care. It is important to recognize the happiness that the client may feel with her thin body. It may have taken great strength of character to give up eating normally, to reject "treats," and to exercise daily, regardless of the elements or her physical status. She may get a "high" from the endorphins released in her brain by the exercise and may be reluctant to give up that feeling. The client may have received positive input from peers regarding her ability to remain so thin, for maintaining her strict diet, and for exercising so conscientiously. She requires an equal substitute for those positive elements to make it worthwhile to give up her present behavior. It is helpful to stress that her hunger pains and borborygmi will disappear, that she will have more energy, that her color will improve, that her bones will stop aching, and that she will have increased resistance to upper respiratory infections and other infections.

Meal planning should include three small meals plus small between-meal snacks until stomach capacity increases. Food should be high in calories and calcium and be easily digestible.

The client needs support as she changes her lifestyle and cuts back on excessive physical activity. A slight weight gain may be unacceptable to her, and she may not want to comply. Although she may accept the need to gain weight intellectually, she may not be able to do so emotionally.

Use of birth control pills supplies the necessary estrogen and progesterone for the endometrium to become mature. Estrogen also helps absorb dietary calcium. The importance of compliance with the regimen that has been ordered must be stressed as a health care, not a contraceptive, factor.

Client education. Education should begin with premenstrual girls. Counseling preteens in normal anatomy and physiology, helping them and their parents to understand developing sexuality, dispelling myths and misinformation by providing the correct facts, and conveying an attitude of positive acceptance are ways to achieve this goal.

Education continues through the help the nurse gives to women with premenstrual or menstrual symptoms and to women during menopause. Often, simple comfort measures alleviate such problems.

Some women find that relief and comfort may be provided by dietary changes, such as limiting sodium and carbohydrates to lessen fluid retention. Breast swelling may be eased by the elimination of caffeine (coffee, tea, chocolate, cola, and even other supposedly decaffeinated drinks) from the diet.

Alternatives to estrogens during the climacteric are based on comfort measures. These include wearing layers of clothing so that the outer layers can be removed if hot flashes occur, drinking cold fluids to cool the body, using water-soluble vaginal lubricants (K-Y jelly) as an aid during sexual intercourse, and regulating weight through diet and exercise. Vaginal atrophy seems to be slowed when women engage in frequent sexual activity. The greatest relief is provided when ERT is used. However, a careful health history and examination must precede such treatment, to rule out the presence of breast or endometrial carcinomas. Annual checkups are a necessity during ERT.

Women who work in areas polluted by environmental contaminants should be made aware of their possible effects on sexual function, fertility, or the fetus. Nurses who work in operating rooms or who care for clients with radium implants are in this high-risk group.

The underweight client requires education about the need for adequate body fat. If a nutritionist is not available, the nurse must be able to explain how to prepare small meals that are high in calories and calcium (at least 1,000 mg daily), along with nutritious snacks. Since the client has kept her food intake at a low level for a prolonged time, she will probably be unable to eat more than small amounts at a time as she increases her intake.

Evaluation Some of the evaluations made (stress and anxiety reduction, adherence to the medical regimen, self-acceptance) depend on the client's perceptions. Other factors (dietary regimen, follow-up with mental health counseling, control of edema, coping) can be evaluated through direct observation or reports from family members or other professionals involved in client care.

For the underweight client, weight gain takes place slowly, since only small feedings are tolerated. In time, the hunger pangs, borborygmi, pallor, bone pain, and lowered resistance disappear. The menstrual cycle will most likely produce only slight bleeding at first, increasing as the endometrium matures over a period of months (see the Example of Nursing Process and Menopause).

Example of nursing process and menopause

The client complains of PMS symptoms that have occurred for the past year, with emotional lability and headaches being the most prominent problems. She is now 45 years old and is experiencing some discomforts of approaching menopause. She has nightly hot flashes, dyspareunia, and the beginning of senile vaginitis. Her periods are irregular and often painful, beginning on 1/2, 2/27, 4/30, 5/15, with a sparse flow. She is divorced and has varied postmarital activities from abstinence to being sexually active, depending on her feelings at the moment. She speaks of this time of her life as causing many of the same feelings that she had during puberty, including difficulty in accepting bodily changes. Her physician states that she cannot receive hormonal therapy because of a history of a breast cancer that resulted in a right mastectomy 3 years ago. Her treatment will, therefore, have to rely primarily on nursing concepts. She takes acetaminophen for headaches.

Assessment data	Nursing diagnosis	Intervention	Goals and outcome criteria
Difficulty in accepting bodily changes related to menopause	Self-esteem disturbance related to discomforts and irregular menses during menopause	**Help** client increase self-esteem by encouraging a wider range of nonsexual activities and by positive reinforcement of admirable attributes.	The client will express positive feelings more often than negative feelings about herself.
Emotional lability	Ineffective individual coping related to changes of menopause	**Explore** with the client incidents of emotional upset, identifying common factors associated with their onset.	The client will report fewer emotional upsets and more appropriate response to situations that stimulate them.
		Help the client to plan alternative responses to stimuli that cause emotional upset.	The client will report a decrease in stress levels.
		Teach the client techniques for minimizing stress levels.	
Headaches	Pain: headache	**Encourage** the client to continue use of acetaminophen for headaches.	The client will report that the headaches become less intense or cease after employing self-care techniques.
		Advise the client about self-care practices that help to alleviate headaches, such as cold applications to the head, reducing noxious stimuli such as bright lights, and increased rest or sleep.	
Dyspareunia	Pain: dyspareunia related to vaginal atrophy and decreased secretions	**Advise** the client to use a water-soluble lubricant such as surgical jelly before intercourse.	The client will report that discomfort associated with intercourse has decreased or ceased.
Hot flashes	Altered comfort: hot flashes related to hormone imbalance due to menopause	**Advise** the client to dress in multiple layers of clothing, some of which may be removed when hot flashes occur.	The client will report that hot flashes are less discomfiting when clothing can be adjusted to compensate for them.
		Reassure the client that hot flashes tend to decrease and disappear as the body adjusts to altered hormone levels.	The client will state that knowing the temporary nature of hot flashes makes them more bearable.

(Continued)

Example of nursing process and menopause (Continued)

Assessment data	Nursing diagnosis	Intervention	Goals and outcome criteria
Emotional reaction to menopause perceived by the client as being similar to that experienced during puberty	Body image disturbance related to physical changes attributable to menopause	**Explain** the nature of menopause and the usual progression, stressing that it is a natural process and part of normal adult development. **Help** the client identify positive aspects of menopause (*eg*, freedom from fear of pregnancy, absence of menses, relief from dysmenorrhea or premenstrual syndrome).	The client will become more relaxed when discussing menopause. The client will make statements that indicate acceptance of the changes associated with menopause.

Checklist of nursing actions

☐ Help clients have respect for themselves as women and have positive thoughts about their bodily functions.

☐ Educate premenarchal girls in the anatomy and physiology of their bodies and help them have respect for themselves as people.

☐ Make a careful assessment through a history, physical examination, and laboratory tests.

☐ Educate women on how pollutants in their environment could affect sexual function and reproduction.

☐ Take a careful history to justify a diagnosis of PMS and give information about available treatment.

☐ Give the client alternatives to estrogens if she is in her climacteric and unable to be treated with ERT.

When caring for underweight clients

☐ Inform them of expected benefits of proper weight maintenance.

☐ Evaluate physical and psychosocial aspects of underweight condition.

☐ Keep accurate records that pertain to compliance with regimen as noted in weight gain, regularity of menstrual cycle, and number of recommended doses actually taken by client.

Sexuality and sexual behavior

Sexual behavior depends on the interweaving of many factors—physical, social, cultural, and emotional. Libido (erotic desire and the ability to enjoy sexual intercourse) is only one aspect of sexual behavior. The physiologic response (in men, erection, orgasm, and ejaculation; in women, lubrication of the vagina, tumescence and orgasm) is another. Some pathologic conditions that affect other systems of the body seem insignificant to sexual behavior, but they are important factors (Table 38-3).

Sexually transmitted diseases

A number of diseases are transmitted primarily by sexual intercourse. With the exception of AIDS, infection with *Chlamydia trachomatis* and condylomata acuminata (also known as human papilloma virus or HPV) are the most common sexually transmitted diseases (STDs). HPV causes genital warts that may be visible to the eye or are detected by colposcopy and is thought to be a precursor to cancer of the cervix and penis (Table 38-4). Herpes simplex, which was the first of the heavily publicized less familiar STDs, can now be treated, although chronic cases are still considered to be incurable. Other STDs include syphilis, gonorrhea, candidiasis (yeast infection), trichomoniasis, infection with *Gardnerella vaginalis*, and hepatitis B.

Syphilis, once one of the most feared STDs because of its chronic effects (dementia, stillbirths), appeared to be under control until recently, when the number of reported cases increased sharply. It has reached epidemic proportions in New York, where testing is carried out on all clients between 15 and 45 years of age who are admitted as inpatients or who receive emergency treatment. In other states, pregnant women are routinely tested. Nationally, about 50,000 cases were expected in 1990, with the highest risk among those with multiple sex partners (including prostitutes), intravenous (IV) drug abusers, and those with other STDs. (Drugs used for the treatment of STDs are discussed in Chapters 41–44.)

One of the most serious threats to worldwide public health is acquired immunodeficiency syndrome (AIDS). It was first noted in the United States in 1981, primarily in male homosexual and bisexual populations and among IV drug users (Koop, 1987). Since

Table 38-3. Pathologic conditions that affect the reproductive system

Systemic illness	Anticipated problems
AIDS	Weakness, debilitation, death
Alcoholism	Impotence with heavy use; fetal alcohol syndrome
Anorexia nervosa and bulimia	Amenorrhea; fetus size small for gestational age
Cardiovascular disorders	Angina during and after intercourse; impairment of orgasmic response due to anxiety, depression, antihypertensive medications, or other prescribed drugs; effects of decreased maternal oxygenation on fetal development
Connective tissue disorders	Possibility of lupus erythematosus in offspring
Diabetes mellitus	Impotence caused by peripheral neuropathy that affects erection; impairment of orgasmic response due to neuropathy; effects of maternal diabetes on fetal development
Endometriosis	Pelvic pain; infertility
Infectious diseases	See Table 38-4
Sexually transmitted diseases	Transmission of infection to fetus if acquired during pregnancy; fetal defects may occur; hydrocephalus, chorioretinitis, intracranial calcifications, microophthalmia, deafness; disease may not appear until infancy, childhood, or adulthood
Congenital toxoplasmosis	
Kidney disease and dialysis	Impotence due to arteriosclerotic changes in penis and pelvis; debilitation may preclude interest or ability to perform sexually; effects of maternal kidney disease on fetal development
Liver disease	Impotence that results from neutralization of androgens due to insufficient conjugation of estrogen; debilitation may lead to diminished desire or performance
Neurologic disorders	
Brain	Sensations may be decreased for some; debilitation or confusion may lead to diminished desire or performance; effect of maternal anticonvulsive medication on fetal development
Peripheral nerves	Pain, urinary bladder or rectal difficulties, or alcoholic neuropathy may cause impotence or orgasmic problems; debilitation or paralysis of lower neural structures, particularly those that affect genital reflexes, leading to impotence and lack of orgasm
Oncologic diseases	Debilitation or pain may lead to avoidance of intercourse; impairment of orgasmic response due to anxiety, depression, physical state, chemotherapy, radiation therapy, or extensive surgery; effect of maternal oncology treatments on fetus; infertility
Endocrine disorders	
Diabetes mellitus	See above
Thyroid deficiencies	May cause infertility in either sex; effect of maternal deficiency or medications on fetal development
Estrogen deficiency in females	Menopausal symptoms; atrophic vaginitis that causes dyspareunia; infertility
Testosterone deficiency in males or females	Loss of libido in both sexes; decreased penile erection or vaginal lubrication; decreased orgasmic response; infertility

then, more than 100,000 people have died of AIDS, and more than 1,000 new cases are being diagnosed each month. The number of new cases doubles every 8 months, with a projection that there will be an estimated total of 390,000 to 480,0000 Americans with AIDS and 285,000 to 340,000 deaths from AIDS by the end of 1993.

AIDS is caused by at least two human immunodeficiency viruses, HIV-1 and HIV-2, both retroviruses (previously designated as HLTV-III). It is anticipated that additional viruses will be identified as the disease spreads geographically. Although no cure has been found, one drug, zidovudine triphosphate, also known as azidothymidine (AZT or Retrovir), appears to forestall the disease's progress.

Drugs useful in the treatment of HIV/AIDS infection

The most commonly administered drug for the treatment of AIDS is zidovudine. It is not a cure, nor does it reduce the transmission of the infection. However, it does appear to slow the progression of the disease process.

Children with AIDS whose immune systems have not been severely weakened have been shown by the National Institute of Health to benefit from monthly doses of IV immunoglobulin (IVIG). The monthly administration of IVIG curtails infections such as pneumonias, sepsis, meningitis, and sinusitis and is given in addition to zidovudine and drugs to prevent

Table 38-4. Sexually transmitted diseases

Disease	Cause	Problems	Treatment
AIDS	Human immunodeficiency virus (HIV), a retrovirus	At increased risk of infection: Men with homosexual contacts since 1977; those who share needles while injecting drugs; those with symptoms of AIDS or AIDS-related illness (or their sexual partners); male or female prostitutes and their sexual partners; those with hemophilia who have received clotting factor products; infants of high-risk or infected mothers or their breast-feeding infant Those who receive contaminated blood, plasma, sperm, or other body tissues or organs Health care professionals in contact with blood or other secretions of infected clients	Zidovudine (Retrovir, formerly called AZT) 200 mg q4h around the clock inhibits replication of HIV. Has reduced mortality and risk of opportunistic infections; increased ability to perform activities of daily living and maintain body weight Potential antiviral agents (under investigation): Ribavirin, DDC (Dideoxycytidine), HPA-23, AL 721, Ansamycin, UA 001 Potential immunomodulating agents (under investigation): Alpha interferon, Ampligen, AS 101 Anti-alpha interferon serum, Gamma interferon, Immune globulin IG-IV, Imreg-I, Interleukin II, Isoprinosine, Thymopentin, Thymostimuline, Methionine-enkephalin A vaccine is now undergoing early clinical trials, with little likelihood of early licensing.
Infection with *Chlamydia trachomatis*	Intracellular parasite Gram-negative bacteria	Female: Infertility, ectopic pregnancy, recurrent cervicitis, urethritis, pelvic inflammatory disease Male: Nongonococcal urethritis	Tetracycline 500 mg, po, qid, minimum 7 days 500 mg, po, qid, 10–14 days 500 mg, po, qid, 7 days
Types D to K Types LI to LIII		Genital infections Lymphogranuloma venereum	As above
Gonorrhea	*Neisseria gonorrhoeae*	Pelvic inflammatory disease, infertility, arthritis, meningitis, chronic pelvic pain, urethritis, discharge Penicillin resistance; tetracycline resistance	Ampicillin 3.5 g, po, or amoxicillin 3 g po, plus probenecid 1 g, po, plus doxycycline 100 mg po, bid Cephalosporin (Cefoxitin 2 g, IM); ceftriaxone 250 mg IM, single dose Norfloxacin (Noroxin) 1200 mg in 2 equal doses PO, 4 h apart Spectinomycin (Trobicin) 2 mg IM, single dose
Syphilis	Spirochete *Treponema pallidum*	Dementia, bone and nerve degeneration, congenital syphilis, abortion, stillbirth; promotes spread of AIDS	Benzathine penicillin G 2.4 mU IM
Genital herpes	Herpes simplex virus	Pain, chronic infection, neonatal infection, cervical cancer	Acyclovir (Zovirax) Initial infection: 200 mg q4h when awake, to 5 caps, qd for 10 days (50 cap) Chronic infection: 200 mg tid, up to 6 months Intermittent therapy: 200 mg q4h when awake, to 5 cap qd for 5 days (25 cap)
Condylomata acuminata (human papilloma virus [HPV])	Papillomavirus	Infection and necrosis of lesions, obstruction of vaginal outlet, infection of neonate	Topical agents: 5-Fluorouracil (5-FU) cream, 5-day course or once a week for 10 weeks CO_2 laser; interferon alpha injected into tissues twice weekly for 8 weeks

(Continued)

Table 38-4. Sexually transmitted diseases (Continued)

Disease	Cause	Problems	Treatment
Candidiasis (vulvovaginal)	*Candida albicans* and other candida (yeastlike fungus)	Vaginal discharge, itching, pain Thrush in neonate; possible precursor of genital cancer	Clotrimazole vaginal 　Mycelex-G 500 mg single dose 　Gyne-Lotrimin vag. tab., insert 2 for 3 nights, or 1 for 7 nights 　Gyne-Lotrimin vag. cream. Applicator full (5 g) 7–14 nights
Trichomoniasis	*Trichomonas* organisms	Cervicitis, endocervicitis, discharge	Metronidazole 　Flagyl vag. tab. 2 g as single or divided dose in 1 day, or 250 mg tid for 7 days
Infection with *Gardnerella vaginalis*	*Gardnerella vaginalis*	Discharge	Sulfathiazole, sulfacetamide, sulfabenzamide and urea in vag. cream 　Sultrin vag. cream 1 applicator full bid, 4–6 days 　Sultrin vag. tab. 1 vag. tab. bid (1 in morning, 1 at night) for 10 days Metronidazole 500 mg vag. bid for 7 days
Chancroid	*Haemophilus ducreyi*	Promotes sexual spread of AIDS	Erythromycin 1 g/day in 3–4 doses, administered at equal time intervals

Pneumocystis carinii infection. For more information on anti-infectives used to treat STDs, see Unit 11, Chapters 41 to 44.)

Considerable research is under way to find better ways to treat AIDS. Among those showing promise are flutathione, N-acetylcysteine, heme, and BI-RG-587.

Didanosine (DDI) has been approved as a treatment for AIDS even though it was found to be a possible cause of pancreatitis and peripheral neuropathy. Efficacy has not been studied as yet. DDI has been used primarily by clients unable to continue zidovudine because of adverse reactions or those who were not improving (Kolata, 1991b).

Learning experience 38-1

Identify anxieties you may have about caring in the labor and delivery area for clients diagnosed as having AIDS. Include information on precautions that you should take to protect yourself when caring for the mother and the newborn. Discuss these with classmates or instructors.

Health care workers and HIV infection

The United States Public Health Service (USPHS) has stated that health care workers are at risk of acquiring the HIV virus and should therefore be aware of postexposure management. The source person should be tested (if willing) for any evidence of HIV infection. If seropositive, the worker should then be tested to obtain baseline information. If seronegative, the worker should then be retested periodically for at least 6 months after the exposure. Workers who develop any acute illness, especially one that includes fever, rash, myalgia, fatigue, malaise, or lymphadenopathy, should be evaluated immediately for the possibility of an acute HIV infection. Seroconversion is most likely to occur during the first 6 to 12 weeks after exposure.

The Public Health Service recommends that health care workers should receive information about postoccupational exposure treatment during job orientation and ongoing educational programs. Information should be included about the efficacy, safety, and toxicity of zidovudine use for prophylaxis after occupational exposure to HIV. Opinions as to the wisdom of its use differ. Issues relating to pros and cons of prophylactic zidovudine therapy appear in the accompanying display. Zidovudine dosages vary with the institution, perhaps 200 mg every 4 hours (six times daily) for 6 weeks, or 200 mg every 4 hours (five times daily) for 4 weeks, or some other regime. Some institutions begin prophylaxis within 1 hour after exposure. To date, information is insufficient to determine which schedule is most effective. Regardless of the decision, any exposed worker should be counseled to follow Public Health Service recommendations for preventing transmission of HIV (refraining from blood, semen, or organ donation; abstaining from or using measures to prevent HIV transmission during sexual intercourse; abstaining from breast-feeding by women who have been exposed; PHS statement pamphlet, 1990).

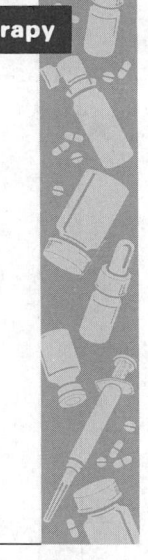

Should health care workers who may have been exposed to HIV infection receive prophylactic ziduvodine?

Pros	Cons
At present, AIDS is considered to be an incurable (eventually) fatal disease.	Whether or not ziduvodine can prevent the development of AIDS is unknown.
At present, ziduvodin is the drug of choice to use for AIDS.	Ziduvodine has known toxic effects.
The antiviral effect of ziduvodine has been documented.	The potential of ziduvodine to cause adverse reactions when administered to noninfected individuals is unknown.
The known toxic effects of ziduvodine are reversible after short-term use.	Optimum schedules for a preventative regimen with the use of ziduvodine have not been established.

Drugs that affect sexual behavior

Libido and sexual response may be affected by drugs that alter the way sex centers of the brain function or by medications that act on the peripheral nerves or blood vessels of the genitalia.

Some agents are used to produce a direct modification of sexual behavior. More often drugs are used for other medical purposes and influence sexual behavior only as a side effect (Table 38-5).

Aphrodisiacs

Aphrodisiacs are drugs used to stimulate the sex centers of the brain. Most substances used for this purpose are pharmacologically inactive but seem to have a placebo effect when used in a sexually provocative situation. Historically, such substances have had symbolic significance based on male dominance and have included drugs made from rhinoceros horns and powdered penises of lions.

Alcohol, frequently used as an aphrodisiac, acts on the brain centers in a sequence that first increases libido by lessening inhibitions. However, if intake of alcohol continues, it begins to act as a general central nervous system (CNS) depressant, interfering with sexual performance. In fact, heavy or chronic use of alcohol may lead to sexual dysfunction. Therefore, clients who seek sexual therapy are told to decrease alcohol consumption to lessen its debilitating neurologic effects, which interfere with sexual activity.

Marijuana (pot, grass) has an active ingredient, tetrahydrocannabinol (THC), that also seems to affect male sexual response in two phases. THC enters the bloodstream rapidly, with an almost immediate effect on the testes. This effect leads to instant testosterone production, with an increase in sexual arousal during and after smoking. In high doses, THC also results in an increase in LH manufactured by the pituitary. This increase occurs at the same time that testosterone is being produced by the testes, bypassing the usual sequence in which LH is produced by the pituitary about 20 minutes after sexual stimulation. Normally, LH would travel to the testes, where it is a factor in testosterone production. However, the testosterone level in the smoker's blood is higher than normal. This level causes a shutdown in the further production of testosterone, and the blood level is rapidly depleted to below normal within 20 minutes, decreasing sexual drive and, in heavy marijuana users, suppressing testicular activity. The resultant lowered levels of testosterone lead to chronic reduction of sexual drive. As with alcohol, limited use of marijuana may lead to increased arousal and stronger muscular contractions during orgasm. However, extended heavy use has the same negative effect as alcohol, with a resultant decrease in sexual function.

Other hallucinogens have an effect on the general nervous system, including the brain's sexual centers. Hallucinogens cause the user to undergo intensified mental as well as an auditory and visual awareness. Intercourse under these circumstances reportedly leads to a longer orgasmic response. Amphetamines and cocaine stimulate the brain centrally and are said to increase sexual drive and performance. Either drug may lead to habituation or addiction, with the probability that sexual drive and ability will eventually decrease significantly.

Androgen (the male sex hormone) increases sexual drive by acting directly on the brain's sex centers and is used by men and women. However, it has undesirable side effects, such as an exacerbation of prostatic cancer in men, acne and hirsutism in women, and the

(*Text continues on p. 950*).

Table 38-5. Effects of drugs on sexual response

Drug name	Therapeutic use	Pharmacodynamics	Phase of sexual response affected		
			Desire	Excitement	Orgasm
Sedative-hypnotics					
alcohol and nontoxic doses of barbiturates and other similar agents (eg, ethchlorvynol, chloral hydrate, and methaqualone)	Insomnia and anxiety states	General CNS depression. Effects are dose related. In general, the higher the dose, the more interference with sexual performance. All of these drugs affect the central state. Set and setting are very important. Expectation can override or alter pharmacologic effect. Most of these drugs potentiate one another. Alcohol with CNS depressants leads to greater CNS depression. In low doses, desire may be increased by reducing inhibition. In higher doses all phases of sexual response are inhibited. Chronic alcoholism may result in permanent neurologic damage and consequent impaired genital functioning.	Increased(?) in low doses in presence of inhibition; expectation may play a major role on this parameter; decreased in high doses	With low doses, excitement may be prolonged due to decreased sensitivity or to intimacy and shared feelings; impotence with high chronic intake of alcohol and barbiturates	Delayed in high doses
Antianxiety drugs					
Benzodiazepines (diazepam, chlordiazepoxide, chlorazepate), meprobamate	Anxiety states, muscle tension, convulsive states	Action on limbic system and on internuncial neurons in the spinal cord	May enhance desire slightly if inhibited or avoided due to anxiety; diminished in high doses	None reported	No effect in usual doses; in very high doses orgasm may be delayed
Narcotics					
morphine, codeine paragoric, D-propoxyphene, and methadone	Analgesia (pain relief); control of diarrhea, coughing, and narcotic withdrawal (methadone)	General depression of CNS and possible direct depression of sex centers; alteration of normal balance of biogenic amines in CNS	Absent in high doses	Impotence in high doses	Inhibited by high doses

Antipsychotic agents	Psychosis	Probably have no direct effect on the brain's sex centers (with the possible exception of haloperidol, which may affect the sexual response directly); may affect sexuality indirectly because of their favorable effects on the psychic state; in addition, some agents infrequently are reported to cause erectile and ejaculatory difficulties probably because of their mild antiadrenergic or anticholinergic or antidopamine effects	Decreased desire reported only in very high doses	Impotence reported with some agents (rare)	Inhibition of ejaculation reported with thioridazine (Mellaril)
Phenothiazines (Stelazine, Mellaril, Thorazine)	Psychiatric disorders; antiemetic	Sexual response may be improved as by-product of recovery from mental illness; "dry" ejaculation may be caused by effects of internal vesical sphincter paralysis, causing semen to empty into bladder; often seen with thioridazine (Mellaril)			
Butyrophenones (Haldol)	Gilles de la Tourette's syndrome, schizophrenia	Reported to reduce libido and potency and cause retarded ejaculations in some clients; mechanism unknown—may involve central or peripheral antiadrenergic or antidopamine activity	May be decreased	Impotence reported with some agents (rare)	None reported
Antidepressants Tricyclics, monoamine oxidase inhibitors	Depression	No direct effects on sexuality; sex drive and performance may improve as depression lifts; the antidepressants have some peripheral autonomic effects that rarely cause some potency and ejaculatory problems in men	Probably none	None	Some females report delay of orgasm

(Continued)

Table 38-5. Effects of drugs on sexual response *(Continued)*

Drug name	Therapeutic use	Pharmacodynamics	Phase of sexual response affected		
			Desire	*Excitement*	*Orgasm*
Tricyclics (Elavil, Tofranil) Monoamine oxidase inhibitors (Nardil, Marplan, Norpramin)		Anticholinergic side effects	Probably none	None	
lithium carbonate	Manic states and possible prevention of depression in bipolar illness	No reported effects on the sexual response, except that sexual urgency may diminish manic activities	Urgency or desire may be reduced	None	None
Stimulants					
cocaine	Local anesthetic	General CNS stimulant; augments sympathetic CNS function	Reported to be enhanced	Reported to be enhanced; high doses may cause impotence	May be enhanced; high doses may interfere with orgasm, more so in females
Amphetamines	Stimulant, appetite suppressant, minimal brain damage in children; narcolepsy	General brain stimulation; in acute cases, reported to enhance libido; in chronic cases, diminishes libido and sexual functioning as well as causes general debility	Reported to be enhanced at low doses; diminished at high doses	Decreased in chronic doses	May be enhanced; high doses may interfere with orgasm, more so in females
Hallucinogens					
LSD (lysergic acid diethylamide)	Methysergide (LSD analog) used in prophylaxis of migraine headaches; no medical use for LSD except for experimental purposes	Vasoconstrictor; may be a central inhibitor of 5-hydroxytryptamine (5-HT); serotonin	Mixed effects reported	None	Physiologically none; altered experience reported
DMT (Dimethyltryptamine), mescaline (trimethoxyphenylethylamine)		Disrupt neurotransmission in limbic system; reported by some to enhance libido and orgasm, by others to have no effect, while some users report impaired sexuality	Mixed effects reported	None	Mixed effects reported
THC (tetrahydrocannabinol)		May have some effects on muscle contractions; some reports of enhanced erotic feelings (?)	Mixed effects reported	Mixed effects reported	Enhanced orgasm reported (?)

Miscellaneous CNS agents

L-dopa	Parkinson's disease	Increased levels of dopamine centrally	Reports of increased desire in elderly male patients	None	None
p-CPA (parachlorophenylalanine)	Carcinoid syndrome	Inhibitor of serotonin synthesis	Reports of increased desire		
Hormones		Presumably stimulate the sex centers of the CNS and so increase the libido and the genital response; also maintain the genital organs in a functional state			
Androgens (eg, testosterone)	Impotence, as replacement therapy, anabolic agent; low libido states	Stimulate sex centers of both genders; fetal androgen causes gender differentiation of behavior; also act on periphery to enhance the growth, development, and functioning of the male genitals and of the clitoris	Stimulates sexual desire in both sexes	In males, may increase ability to have an erection in testosterone-deficient states	In males, volume of ejaculate may be increased
Estrogens (estriol, estradiol, estrone)	Oral contraceptive; replacement therapy in postmenopausal women; prostatic cancer; mature uterine lining in clients with anorexia	Do not increase libido, in fact, may decrease sexual interest; act on the cells of the female genitalia to enhance their growth, development, and functioning	In men, may decrease desire; in women, variable responses reported, increased desire may be due to decreased fear of pregnancy	May cause impotence in males	Ejaculatory delay; volume of ejaculate decreased
Progesterones (physiologic precursors to testosterone)	Endometriosis; component of some oral contraceptives		Probably none	Probably none	Probably none
thyroxine	Hypothyroid states; depression	Increased motor activity and augmented sympathetic nervous system activity; may decrease depression	Enhanced desire reported		
cyproterone acetate	Experimental; employed in treatment of compulsive sexual disorders	Antagonizes testosterone	Loss of libido in both genders	Impotence in males	In males, volume of ejaculate may decrease; ejaculatory delay
Adrenal steroids	Addison's disease; allergic and inflammatory disorders	Mechanisms unknown	May decrease libido in high doses		

(Continued)

Table 38-5. Effects of drugs on sexual response (Continued)

Drug name	Therapeutic use	Pharmacodynamics	Phase of sexual response affected		
			Desire	Excitement	Orgasm
Antihypertensives					
Centrally acting (eg, alphamethyl dopa)	Hypertension	Block adrenergic nerves and innervated structures in periphery, causing disturbances in the hemo-dynamics of erection by various mechanisms; occasional inhibition of emission	Decreased	Decreased; impotence is major problem	May be inhibited
Diuretics					
Thiazides	Hypertension, edema	Dilate blood vessel walls; decrease circulating fluid volume; disturb penile blood pressure	None	May cause impotence	None
spironolactone	Hypertension, edema, hypokalemia	May block binding of testosterone at receptor site; gynecomastia due to action on breast tissue	Occasional loss of libido	May cause impotence	None
Ganglionic blockers					
Quaternary ammonium compounds	Hypertension	Block postganglionic nerves and innervated structures; disturb penile blood pressure; may inhibit sympathetic mediation of emission	None	Often causes impotence	May be inhibited
General antiadrenergic drugs					
phentolamine; phenox-ybenzamine; ergot alkaloids	Pheochromocytoma; migraine headaches				
α-Blockers (eg, clonidine)	Hypertension; narcotic withdrawal	Blocks α-adrenergic receptors–central and peripheral action	None	None	Block emission in males—dose related
Sympathoplegic drugs (eg, guanethidine, bretylium)		Deplete adrenergic nerves of norepinephrine		Often cause impotence	May be inhibited
β-blockers (eg, propranolol)	Hypertension; angina; migraine prophylaxis	Blockade of β-adrenergic receptors of heart–central and peripheral action	Sometimes decreased	Sometimes decreased	None reported

Anticholinergic drugs					
Banthine, Pro-Banthine, atropine, scopolamine, Cogentin	Peptic acid disease; GI irritability; alleviation of extrapyramidal effects of phenothiazines	Block the nerves that control the smooth muscles and blood vessels of the genital organs that are involved in the sexual responses; inhibit the action of acetylcholine on structures innervated by postganglionic parasympathetic nerves; also have central anticholinergic action	None	May rarely cause impotence	None
Aphrodisiacs					
Spanish fly (cantharides), amyl nitrite	Poisonous—no medical indications; vasodilator, angina pectoris	Irritates genitourinary tract—causes priapism; enhances vascular response of genitals (?); reported to improve orgasm (?)	None	Priapism, organic impotence	None
Miscellaneous drugs					
disulfiram (Antabuse)	Alcohol abuse		None	Occasional impotence reported	Delay of ejaculation
tryptophan		Increased CNS concentration of serotonin	Decreased	Decreased	
ephedrine	Antiasthmatic agent	α-Adrenergic stimulator			Treatment of failure to ejaculate
cimetidine	Peptic ulcer	Inhibits H$_2$ receptors; may cause lowered sperm count	Loss of libido and impotence have been reported		
Neurotoxic agents					
Halogenated aromatic hydrocarbons	No medical indications; agricultural fungicides	Neuropathy	Decreased	Decreased	
carbon disulfide	No medical indications; industrial exposure	Neuropathy and premature arteriosclerotic changes due to hyperlipidemia	Decreased	Decreased	

(Adapted from Kaplan HS. [1979]. *Disorders of sexual desire*. New York: Brunner/Mazel. The original table was prepared in collaboration with David Benjamin, Ph.D.)

possibility of cerebral or cardiovascular problems in either sex (see Chapter 32).

Cantharides (Spanish fly) acts as an irritant to the bladder and urethra of the male, resulting indirectly in sexual excitement and priapism (continuous penile erection). Its continued use may lead to permanent penile damage and impotence.

Antianxiety, antidepressant, and antipsychotic drugs may act as aphrodisiacs by lessening the person's negative self-image, thereby enhancing sexual interest and performance. However, their action is general and such drugs are not specific for sexual problems.

Anaphrodisiacs

Anaphrodisiacs are drugs that impair sexual function. They include drugs that depress the action of the CNS (alcohol in large doses, barbiturates, hypnotics, sedatives, narcotics). Other drugs manifest anaphrodisiac actions because of their peripheral effect on the genitalia, influencing either erectile or ejaculatory responses. Hormones such as estrogen and hormone analogues such as leuprolide acetate (Lupron acetate) used in the treatment of some breast and prostate cancers can adversely affect sexual functioning.

Drugs that act on the nervous system

Anticholinergic drugs, used to treat gastrointestinal (GI) and psychiatric disorders, may block the parasympathetic nerves that normally increase genital vascularization, thereby impeding erection.

Antiadrenergic drugs (β-blockers, α-blockers), used to treat hypertension, may block the nerves of the sympathetic division of the autonomic nervous system, leading to difficulty in ejaculation. Libido is not directly affected by either anticholinergic or antiadrenergic medications. However, repeated inability to respond favorably during sexual performance may lead to inhibitions and eventual withdrawal from sexual activity.

Some psychotropic drugs act as anaphrodisiacs. Haloperidol (Haldol), an antipsychotic drug used to treat Gilles de la Tourette's syndrome, lessens libido and potency through a direct effect on the brain's sex centers. Lithium, an antidepressant used to treat bipolar depression, calms the manic phase and effectively lowers sexual activity.

Drugs used in the treatment of sexual problems

Monoamine oxidase inhibitors are mood regulators sometimes used to treat premature ejaculation (see Chapter 26). These drugs help prevent panic attacks in clients with phobias concerning sexual activity. The person is usually more amenable to psychotherapeutic intervention after treatment.

Cyproterone acetate is an experimental antiandrogen used to treat people with compulsive sexual disorders. Researchers continue to hope for other drugs that may be similarly specific in treating sexual disorders. Antiandrogens lessen libido in either sex by antagonizing testosterone. Their use produces impotence in males and leads to a reduction in the amount of ejaculate.

Because of the positive emotional responses they induce, some psychotropic drugs affect sexual response favorably. However, some of these drugs may also cause difficulties in erections or ejaculation because of their antiadrenergic or anticholinergic actions. Phenothiazines may improve sexual function as the mental state becomes healthier. However, one of these, thioridazine (Mellaril), may paralyze the internal vesical sphincter, causing semen to empty into the urinary bladder instead of being propelled through the penis. The possibility of a "dry" ejaculation should be explained to clients who take this drug.

■ Summary

Many factors (physical, social, cultural, and emotional) influence sexual behavior. Response may be affected by drugs that alter the function of the brain's sex centers, act on peripheral nerves, or act on genital blood vessels. Some drugs are used specifically for modifying sexual behavior; others are used for other medical purposes, resulting in altered sexual behavior as a side effect. Aphrodisiacs are drugs that stimulate sex centers of the brain, whereas anaphrodisiacs impair sexual functioning.

Nursing management

Nursing implications

The subject of sexuality has been mired in privacy and secrecy and has developed many related taboos. Even political and religious implications are involved in discussions of pregnancy and childbearing and the medications and techniques used to affect their outcomes. Small wonder that clients often hesitate to tell health care providers about changes in their sexual feelings that may be drug related.

Nurses who feel comfortable with their own sexuality are probably going to seem more approachable to clients with sexual problems. Accessibility is important if nurses are to help clients voice sexual concerns.

Clients with STDs may be reluctant to discontinue or change sexual or drug behaviors regardless of the risks to themselves or their partners. It is more helpful to suggest safer alternate practices than to demand cessation.

Contagious diseases, including STDs, can be contracted by health care personnel. Measures to protect against AIDS cannot be emphasized strongly enough. With proper and reasonable precautions, however, the risk to health care personnel of contracting AIDS is negligible.

Health care workers have contracted AIDS primarily through injuries to themselves (*eg,* needle pricks) from infected needles. Contact through broken skin (as in a rash) or exposed mucous membrane (the open mouth) may be all that is necessary for the virus to enter the body. The following practices are recommended to protect nurses who care for clients who may have AIDS.

1. Wear latex gloves and additional protective clothing as needed when exposed to clients known to have AIDS or when health information about the client is unavailable. Precautions should be taken (gowns, masks, and even goggles for extensive contact) when handling body fluids, mucous membranes, and tissue during surgery or deliveries, or when a chance of being splashed or aerosolized during contact exists.
2. Take precautions when caring for an unbathed neonate.
3. Needles should not be broken, cut, recapped, or removed from syringes by hand, because of the danger of needlestick or other injury. They should be disposed of with care in puncture-resistant containers.
4. Exercise extreme caution when handling, cleaning, or disposing of any sharp instruments, or when caring for specimens, soiled dressings, body excretions, or secretions.
5. Hand-washing is important to protect both the client and the staff.
6. Be aware of symptoms of contamination: viral-like illness with malaise and fever, erythematous rash, lymphadenopathy, cough, decreased white blood cell count, weight loss, diarrhea, or oral candidiasis. HIV antibody tests with an inverted ratio of T helper/T suppressor cells (normal is greater than one) indicate infection. The usual tests include the Western Blot, the enzyme-linked immunosorbent assay (ELISA), and a radioimmunoprecipitation assay (AIDS nursing update statement, 1987; Bennett, 1986; Boland, Klug, 1986).

Nursing process

Assessment As noted in the first part of this discussion, sexual behavior is not an isolated issue. Sexual dysfunction may be affected by the client's physical status, emotions, or other factors, including medications. The nursing history should include inquiries about any drugs taken that may affect libido, performance, or orgasm. These include prescribed medications as well as self-administered preparations or recreational drugs.

Medications can directly or indirectly affect sexual response. Some drugs are used specifically to enhance or diminish erotic behavior, while others do so as a side effect. For example, some cardiac, psychiatric, or GI drugs may cause changes in libido or performance levels.

STDs require astute observation and history-taking by the nurse. Clients may deny the presence of STDs or not share information about sexual behaviors that may contribute to STD development, especially clients initially infected with AIDS, particularly if it is asymptomatic, as it may be for several years. Although the HIV test may be negative, it is not an absolute. Seroconversion may not occur for several years.

Nursing diagnosis Case finding is an important nursing function in relation to STDs. The nurse may make the initial diagnosis of probable infection related to various symptoms or unsafe sexual practices.

This diagnosis should be confirmed by the appropriate specific diagnostic tests. Further diagnoses depend on any infection that is present and its symptoms. A diagnosis appropriate for most clients is knowledge deficit related to STDs and their treatment.

A careful analysis of the data obtained during the assessment process may indicate the reason for sexual problems. If the client is receiving medications that affect sexual ability or thinking, a drug change should be considered. If this is not possible, the nursing diagnoses may include the following:

> *Ineffective individual coping*
> *Hopelessness related to sexual dysfunction*
> *Knowledge deficit related to alternative methods of sexual expression*
> *Body image disturbance (if the sense of self is tied into sexual performance)*
> *Self-esteem disturbance*
> *Impaired social interaction related to feelings of sexual inadequacy*

Planning The major goal for clients with sexual problems should be increased self-esteem and self-acceptance, regardless of the level of sexual performance, with separation of social identity from that of sexual performance. Compliance with the medication regimen is another important goal, as are increased coping skills, return to a normal sense of power and hope, increased social interaction, and acceptance of sexuality with the ability to attain and give sexual satisfaction in ways other than intercourse.

For clients with STDs other than herpes or AIDS, the goal of treatment is elimination of the infection. For those affected by herpes or AIDS, nursing goals depend on the client's reaction to the diagnosis and treatment regimen.

Intervention Nursing intervention should encourage self-esteem by helping the client develop a realistic appraisal of self, including abilities that are not sexually oriented. This would include relationships with others, work or study successes, bonds with family members, and an interest in the outside world. The intervention should include encouragement in learning how to receive gratification from a loving relationship, with caressing, kissing, and touching rather than intercourse, and an interest in meeting the needs of lovers.

Clients with STDs need support in preventing transmission to others by abstention or the use of preventive measures. These may require unwanted changes in relationships or activities and the implementation of practices (safer sex, nonsharing of drug-taking equipment) that the client considers unnecessary or bothersome.

Client education. Clients should be alerted if medications ordered for physical or emotional disorders may as a side effect alter sexual response. Clients who take medications to combat alcoholism or obesity probably may not realize that these drugs can cause temporary impotence; however, clients have the right to know of this side effect.

Clients should be made aware of the effects on their sexual feelings not only by prescribed medications but also by over-the-counter preparations. Compliance with medication routines may be rejected if clients unexpectedly find themselves sexually uncomfortable.

Clients may also be unaware of the ability of self-prescribed substances to potentiate or lessen the effects of medications ordered for sexual therapy. For instance, clients who take monoamine oxidase inhibitors for treatment of premature ejaculation and who use over-the-counter cold remedies or who eat foods high in tyramine or tryptophan may suffer extremely dangerous side effects. The nurse who understands the emotional consequences of premature ejaculation is more helpful to the client than one who appears annoyed or angry that the client is using substances that interact with the medication. Basically, the nurse should keep in mind that the client may not want to lose his symptoms (premature ejaculation) if the result is a more threatening problem (closeness in a relationship), even though he has agreed to take the medication.

Client education for those with STDs should include information on the proper use of latex condoms prelubricated with nonoxynol-9 and the use of additional lubricant with nonoxynol-9 before every involvement in vaginal or rectal intercourse. Cunnilingus should not be performed without protection (dental rubber or latex dam). Fellatio should not take place without a condom. IV drug use should be discouraged since it may result in the contraction of AIDS through the use of shared equipment. Clients who refuse or are unable to abstain from drug abuse should be warned against the sharing of equipment and instructed to clean their own syringes and needles with soap, running water, and bleach.

Evaluation The client should accept sexual limitations without losing sight of other aspects of life. There should be gratification from a loving relationship and an acceptance of self, with an increase in self-esteem. There should be a willingness to comply with the medical regimen, despite its effect on sexual performance, with the realization that sexuality and self are separate entities.

Checklist of nursing actions

☐ Become comfortable with your own sexuality and be accessible to clients who wish to discuss sexuality and sexual problems.

☐ Include information about drugs that affect sexuality in the nursing history.

☐ Become familiar with sexual behavior affected by various medications.

☐ Inform clients who are taking medications that will affect their sexual behavior.

☐ Inform clients about the sexual side effects of over-the-counter drugs.

☐ If a medication that affects sexuality must be taken, inform the clients of alternative methods of lovemaking (see the Example of Nursing Process and Oral Contraception).

☐ Inform clients of their responsibility to protect themselves and others from STDs

Contraceptives

A variety of contraceptives have been used since ancient times. Some methods have been more acceptable than others. Many factors influence the selection: religious beliefs, political influence, economic power, cultural outlooks, age, ignorance, education, convenience, and so forth. Contraceptive techniques also vary in effectiveness and safety. Figure 38-4 illustrates a variety of methods.

Male contraceptive measures

Condoms are 90% effective in preventing pregnancy. Additional protection can be attained by applying nonoxynol-9 cream, jelly, or foam to the exterior of the condom before actual intercourse. This spermicidal agent, as well as benzalkonium chloride (presently available in Europe), appears to deactivate HIV, offering additional protection against AIDS (Brody, 1987b).

Drugs under investigation for their usefulness as contraceptives for males include the following:

▪ Gossypol, a cotton-seed derivative used in China, reduces sperm formation and motility. Side effects include nausea, fatigue, decreased libido, hypokalemia, and high levels in the liver. Twenty-five percent of the long-term users did not become fertile after discontinuance.

Example of nursing process and oral contraception

A 22-year-old woman has come to the clinic for her annual gynecologic checkup. Last year, she decided to take oral contraceptives, and after a thorough history and examination to rule out any contraindications, she received a prescription for a 28-day combination of estrogen and progestin. She returned to the clinic three times during the year, stating that she was taking the pills daily and offering no complaints. At the current examination, she stated that she had ended her relationship with her original boyfriend and was now taking the pills only when she was sexually active.

A review of the initial educational program demonstrated that at that time, she appeared to understand the need to take the pills consistently for efficacy. However, she saw no reason to continue them when she no longer was sexually active. Without seeking medical advice, she resumed their use when she developed another relationship. At this point, she was no longer consistent in her regimen, since her sexual activity was not as intense, and she assumed she did not require as much protection. She also resisted the use of condoms, saying they interfered with her pleasure and that she did not want her new friend to feel that she suspected him of having any STDs.

A new educational program was instituted so that the client would thoroughly understand the need for compliance to prevent pregnancy. Condoms were also discussed as a necessity so long as she did not have a monogamous relationship and had no assurance that neither she nor her partner had any STD.

Assessment data	Nursing diagnosis	Intervention	Goals and outcome criteria
Inconsistent use of oral contraceptive medication	Knowledge deficit concerning oral contraceptive regimen	**Explore** the client's knowledge about the drug regimen; provide additional information and correct misinformation as required. **Stress** the need for consistency in dosage to achieve the desired result—suppression of ovulation.	The client will not become pregnant.
Nonuse of condoms Termination of original sexual relationship and subsequent intermittent sexual activity	High risk for infection: sexually transmitted disease related to intercourse unprotected by condoms	**Explore** with the client her present sexual practices to determine whether multiple partners are involved; if so, advise client of the increased risk of infection. **Explore** the client's knowledge related to sexually transmitted disease; provide additional information and correct misinformation as required. **Caution** the client that there is no vaccine for AIDS, which is believed to be 100% fatal. **Assist** the client in reassessing her sexual pattern and alternatives, such as abstinence and use of condoms. **Teach** the client signs and symptoms of sexually transmitted infection and caution her to report these promptly to her primary health care provider, so that she may be treated promptly.	The client will adopt sexual practices more likely to protect her from infectious disease. If infection develops, it will be promptly detected and treated.

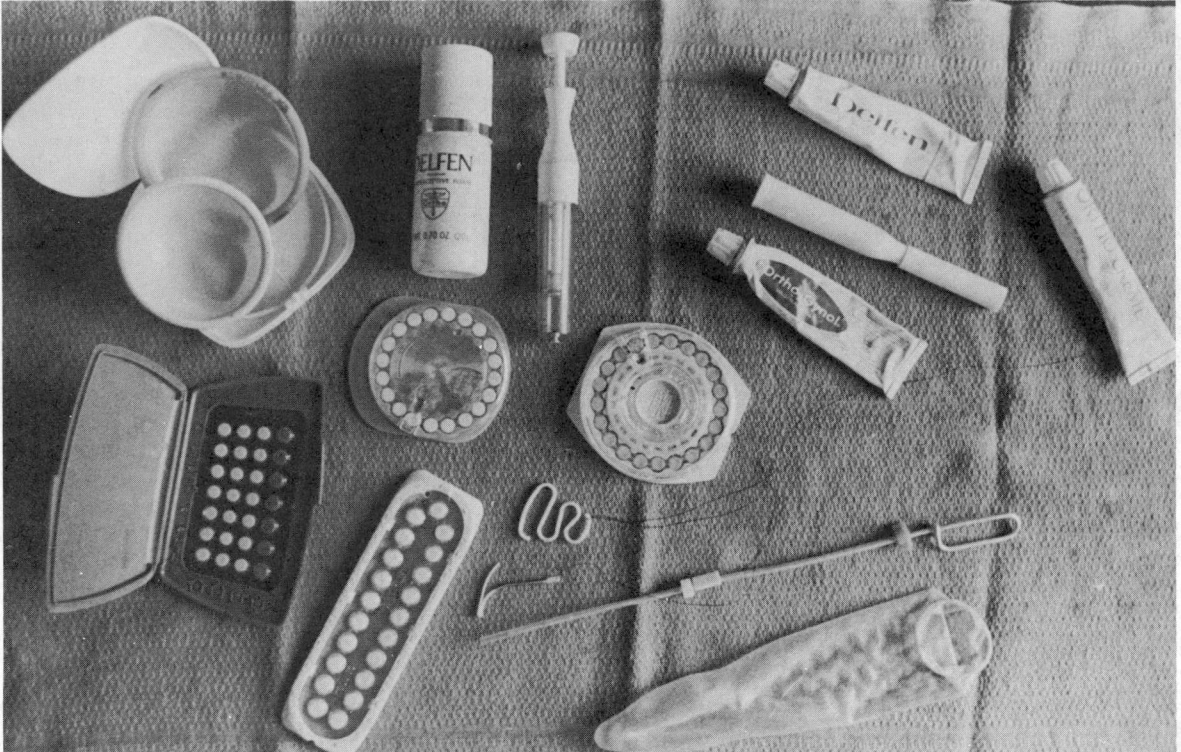

Figure 38-4. Common devices used for contraception.

- Sulfasalazine lessens sperm motility and density while increasing the percentage of abnormal sperm.
- Phenoxybenzamine causes azoospermia by paralyzing the ejaculatory system.
- Tolnizamine interferes with the maturation of sperm. Evidence of toxicity in the kidneys and marked reduction in testicular size in laboratory rats have been found. It is hoped that changing the dosage may lessen the side effects without decreasing efficacy.

It is important that clients understand that condoms tend to provide "safer" rather than "safe" sex; they do not guarantee absolute safety whether used as a contraceptive device or in the prevention of the transmission of STDs.

Permanent male contraception can be provided through a *vasectomy*. In this procedure, an incision is made through the scrotum, and each of the two tubes that carry sperm from the testes to the penis is cut, tied, or coagulated, preventing sperm from going through the vas deferens.

A vas deferens intraluminal device, which blocks the passage of sperm through the vas on a temporary basis, is available. It can then be removed when a pregnancy is desired (Table 38-6).

The World Health Organization is supporting research on the development of a birth control injection for men using a synthetic form of testosterone. The drug is being tested with weekly injections that keep the client's testosterone level at a high enough level to interfere with the pituitary gland's production of LH and FSH. This interference effectively stops the body's normal production of testosterone, preventing the production of sperm by the testes. A second synthetic testosterone would require injections only once every 3 months and would therefore be more acceptable. It is hoped that this method will have a lower failure rate than the present 17% for condoms (Paulsen, 1987).

Female contraceptive measures

The contraceptive measures available for females are summarized in Table 38-7. In addition to abstinence and tubal ligation, female contraceptive methods include nonpharmacologic (natural), chemical, mechanical, and hormonal means. Nonpharmacologic methods include those making use of fertility awareness: basal body temperature method, cervical mucus method, and monoclonal antibody test. Mechanical methods include the use of the diaphragm, intrauterine device (IUD), cervical cap, contraceptive sponge, and most recently, the vaginal sheath (female condom). The discussion in this chapter focuses on the chemical and hormonal agents women can use (Figs. 38-5 to 38-8).

Chemical methods

Chemical contraceptives are made up of two basic ingredients: a relatively inert vehicle that forms a barrier to delay progress of sperm and an active spermicidal agent that immobilizes or destroys the sperm bio-

Table 38-6. Male contraceptive measures

Method	Rate of pregnancy	Advantages	Disadvantages
Coitus interruptus	20%	Inexpensive; requires no preliminary actions; acceptable to most religions; available at any place or time	Requires absolute control; some ejaculate may enter vagina before withdrawal
Condom	10% (5% when used with spermicide)	Easy availability; external application; helps protect males and females from diseases sexually transmitted through genital or anal intercourse	Requires proper application (before leakage of semen, with ½ in of space at tip to collect ejaculate); must be hole-free; must be removed properly; cannot be reused
Vasectomy	0.15%	Permanent male contraception	Possibility of negative physical effects due to sperm destruction in body; difficult to restore fertility

Table 38-7. Female contraceptive measures

Method	Rate of pregnancy	Advantages	Disadvantages
Fertility awareness			
Calendar method	21%	Inexpensive; acceptable to all religions	Ovulation may not occur on projected date
Basal body temperature	7%	Inexpensive; acceptable to all religions	Determines when ovulation has occurred, but does not provide information in advance; requires time for taking temperature on awakening in morning
Monoclonal antibodies test	Informational only (would have to abstain or use contraceptives to be effective)	Over-the-counter availability Predicts ovulation 12–44 h in advance	Must be used for 12 days for 90% accuracy (67% for 6 days; 80% for 9 days)
Spermicides	20%–25%	Easily available	Must be reintroduced before each attempt at intercourse; coital position may cause leakage from vagina; usage varies according to type and manufacturer's instructions
Diaphragm	10.3%–57%	No systemic reaction	Must fit and be inserted properly; should be used with spermicidal cream or jelly; recurrent cystitis, allergy to latex; prolonged retention may increase risk of *Staphylococcus aureus* in lower genital tract (possible toxic shock syndrome)
Cervical cap	8.1%–17.4%	Adheres to cervix by suction, can be left in place for 36 h	Requires proper fitting; need for manual dexterity to replace; should be used with spermicidal jelly or cream; expensive; holds secretions against cervix as long as cap is in place, with possible relationship to toxic shock syndrome and abnormal Pap smears; vaginal odor
Polyurethane sponge with nonoxynol-9 (Today vaginal contraceptive sponge)	17%	Easy to insert; over-the-counter; lasts 24 h	Possibility of toxic shock syndrome; possible carcenogenicity of polyurethane; possible teratogenicity; allergic reactions; cost (about $1 per sponge)
Intrauterine device (IUD)	5%	Convenient; high degree of effectiveness	Limited availability because of possibility of uterine perforation, with complications (*eg*, infection, intestinal obstruction); may cause ectopic pregnancy
Oral contraceptives ("the pill")	4%–10%	High degree of effectiveness; useful for women with hypermenorrhea or endometriosis	Missing doses lessens effectiveness; possibility of thromboembolic disorders, gallbladder disease, mental depression, vaginal bleeding, visual disturbances, increase in size of fibroid tumors, infertility after discontinuation, cessation of milk supply during lactation, birth defects if used during pregnancy

(Continued)

Table 38-7. Female contraceptive measures (Continued)

Method	Rate of pregnancy	Advantages	Disadvantages
Danazol	Experimental	Minimal side effects	Not always effective; breakthrough bleeding; occasional development of facial hair
Injectable contraceptives—medroxy-progesterone (Depo-Provera)	0.7%	Injectable every 1–3 months	Same disadvantages as pill; need for injection every 3 months, weight gain; irregular vaginal bleeding
Implantable contraceptive (Norplant, with 35 mg levonorgestrel)	0.5%–2.6%	Protection after 24 h, lasting up to 5 yr Removal takes only about 15 min	Must be inserted beneath skin of forearm, upper arm, or scapular area; can be felt and sometimes seen; initial irregular vaginal bleeding; headaches, breast tenderness, mood changes, infection at implantation site; user must weigh <150 lb
Postcoital diethylstilbestrol (DES)	Only useful if used within hours of intercourse	Undesirable pregnancy (*eg*, rape, incest) can be aborted	Side effects may be severe (*eg*, nausea, vomiting, headache, dizziness, abdominal pain); chance of thromboembolic disease; if already pregnant, may lead to vaginal adenosis in female offspring or epididymal anomalies in male offspring
Postcoital Ovral (estradiol and progesterone)	Investigational	Can abort undesired pregnancy; easy to use (2 tablets in morning, 2 tablets 12 h later)	Must start within 24 h; nausea, vomiting
Mifepristone (RU486)	7%–15%	Eliminates need for surgical procedure in 60%–95% of cases	Legal concerns where abortions are illegal; at this writing is not available in U.S.; may need follow-up surgical procedure
Silastic vaginal ring	3.5%		
High dosage		Eliminates ovulation; can leave in place for 3 wks	Must be removed after 3 weeks and replaced to prevent pregnancy; can be expelled spontaneously; may develop noninfectious discharge and/or vaginal erosion; irregular vaginal bleeding
Low dosage		Makes cervical mucus impermeable to sperm; can leave in place for several months	
Tubal obstruction—silicone injected through uterus to block tubes	Experimental	Nonsurgical; 50%–80% chance of reversibility	Sometimes not reversible
Sterilization—banding or clipping of fallopian tubes	Almost 100%	50%–80% chance of reversal with microsurgery and drugs to prevent adhesions	May not be reversible

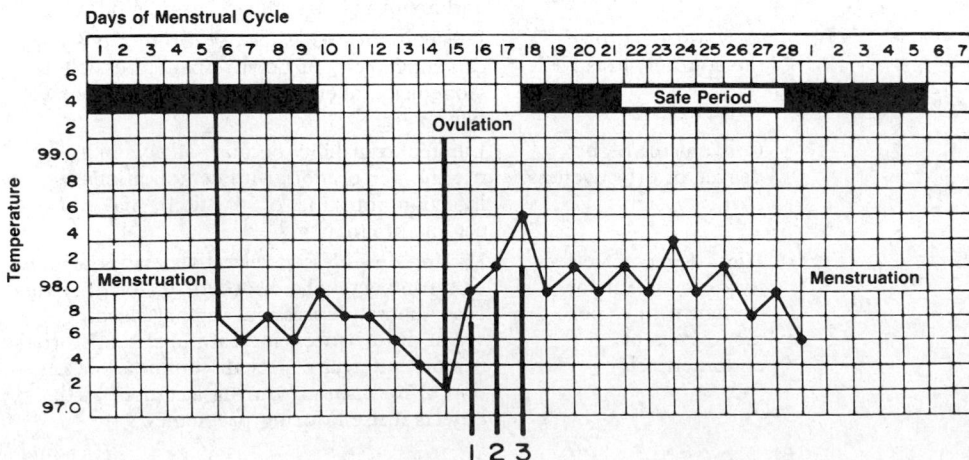

Figure 38-5. Basal body temperature chart.

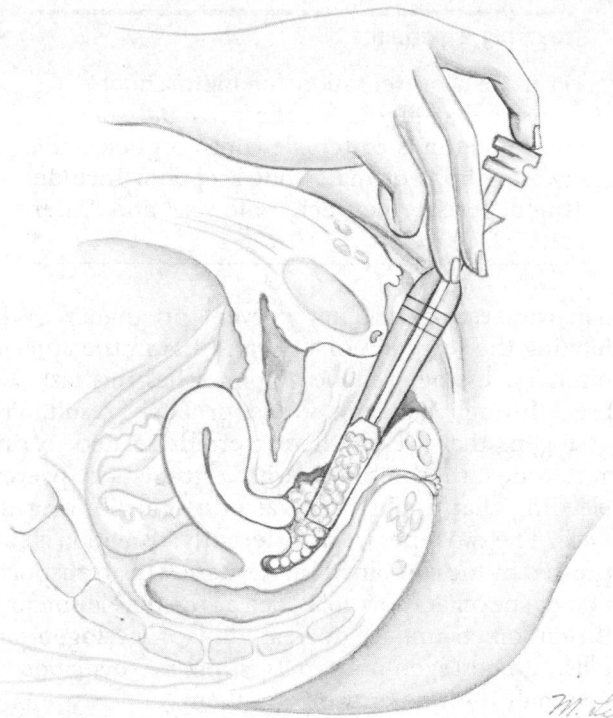

Figure 38-6. To apply the contraceptive foam, the client lies on her back, inserts the applicator, and applies the foam high in the vaginal vault, covering the cervix.

chemically (Hafez, 1980). These ingredients are presented in Table 38-8.

Spermicides are available as creams, jellies, foams, foaming tablets, and suppositories. High failure rates are probably due to inconsistent or improper use. Spermicides must be used each time intercourse is to occur, even if intercourse is repeated within a time lapse of a few minutes. Products must be inserted high in the vaginal vault next to the cervix. Suppositories depend on body heat to melt them and to permit their spread over the cervix. Tablets require sufficient vaginal moisture to foam properly. To be effective, all spermicides must cover and remain in contact with the cervix during intercourse. Coital positions that result in leakage from the vagina may lead to contraceptive failure.

Hormonal methods

Oral contraceptives

Oral contraceptives, commonly referred to as "the pill," provide the greatest effectiveness, with about a 4% to 10% pregnancy rate for the combination of estrogen and progestogen and a 5% to 10% pregnancy rate for progestogen alone, known as the "mini-pill."

Skipping pills, particularly around the time of

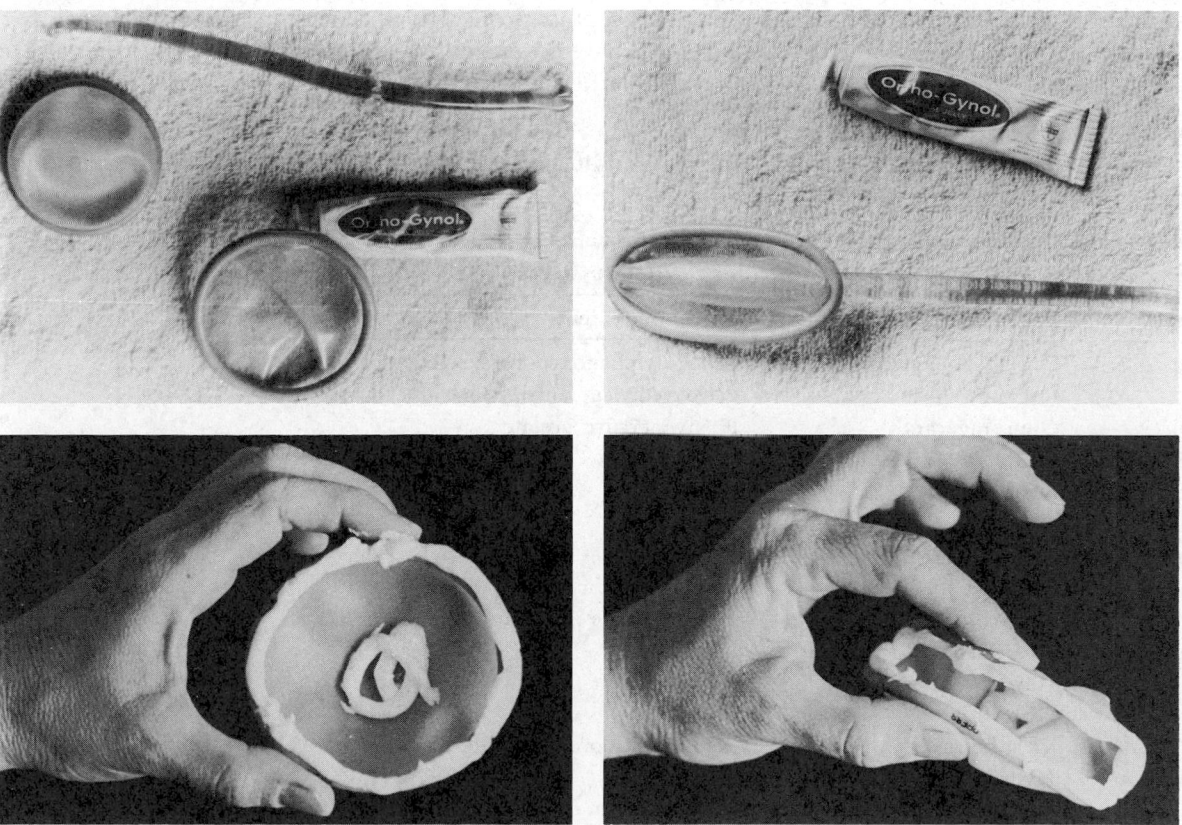

Figure 38-7. (*Top, left to right*) Diaphragms, spermicidal jelly, and inserter. Diaphragm in position on inserter. (*Bottom, left to right*) Diaphragm with spermicidal cream applied. Diaphragm compressed and ready for manual insertion.

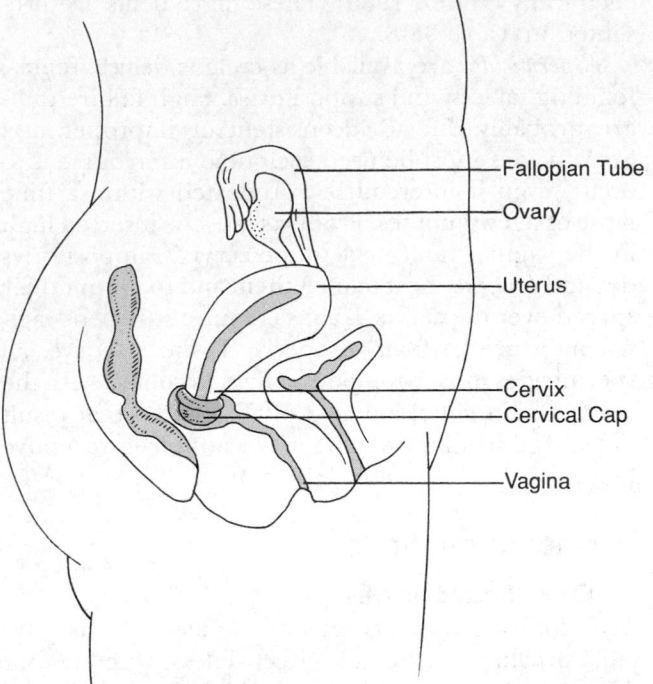

Figure 38-8. Placement of the cervical cap.

ovulation, decreases the effectiveness of the method, as does vomiting or diarrhea or the use of certain drugs. Other contraceptives should be added at such times. Missing three pills makes the method unreliable, and additional measures should be employed through the rest of the cycle.

Pharmacodynamics. Oral contraceptives contain either progestogens alone or progestogen in combina-

Learning experience 38-2

Prepare a presentation for high school seniors that highlights the pros and cons of three methods of female contraception and two methods of male contraception. Include the difference between "safe sex" and "safer sex."

tion with estrogen. They prevent pregnancy by inhibiting the secretion of FSH and LH in the anterior pituitary. Estrogen alone accomplishes this task, but breakthrough bleeding would probably result. Progestogens that are synthetic steroids related to progesterone are combined with estrogen to prevent bleeding that might occur at odd times during the cycle. The two types work differently: ovulation is suppressed by the combined pills, whereas the transportation of sperm and ovum as well as the development of the endometrium are decreased by progestogen-only pills. Progestogen-only pills suppress ovulation in only half the women who use them.

Fluctuating progesterone levels. The newer combined pills have fluctuating progesterone levels, thereby lowering unnecessary exposure to higher levels of progesterone throughout the menstrual cycle. They contain a higher level of progesterone to coincide with the expected time of ovulation, offering greater contraceptive protection at that time. These pills appear to have fewer side effects but offer a slightly lower level of efficacy. Oral contraceptives are listed in Table 38-9.

Therapeutic uses. In addition to being used as an oral contraceptive, the pill has proved particularly

Table 38-8. Composition of vaginal chemical contraceptives

Type of product	Base materials	Active ingredients
Jellies and pastes	Polyethylene glycol	Diisobutylphenoxypolyethoxyethanol
	Gelatin	Polyoxyethylenenonylphenol
	Gum tragacanth	Phenylmercuric acetate
Creams	Stearates	Nonoxynol-9
	Stearic acid	
	Glycerin	
Suppositories	Cocoa butter	Nonoxynol-9
	Soap	Phenylmercuric borate
	Glycerin	Polysaccharide-polysulfuric acid ester
Foam tablets	Bicarbonate of soda	Nonoxynol-9
	Polyethylene glycol	Polysaccharide-polysulfuric acid ester
	Glycerin	Chloramine
	Tartaric acid	Sodium dichlorosulfamidobenzoate
Foam aerosol	Hydrocarbon and freon	Nonoxynol-9
	Polyethylene glycol	Benzethonium chloride
	Glycerin	

(After Population Reports. [January 1975]. Series 4, No. 4. Population Information Program. The Johns Hopkins University, Baltimore. Also published in Hafez ESE. [1980]. *Human reproduction: Conception and contraception, 2nd ed.* Hagerstown: Harper & Row.)

Table 38-9. Most currently available combination and microdose of progestin oral contraceptives

Product	Manufacturer	Type	Estrogen	Progestin	Inert
Ortho-Novum 1/35–21	Ortho	Comb	0.035 mg ethinyl estradiol	1 mg norethindrone	
1/35–28	Ortho	Comb	0.035 mg ethinyl estradiol	1 mg norethindrone	7
1/50–21	Ortho	Comb	0.05 mg mestranol	1 mg norethindrone	
1/50–28	Ortho	Comb	0.05 mg mestranol	1 mg norethindrone	7
2 mg	Ortho	Comb	0.10 mg mestranol	2 mg norethindrone	
Norinyl 1 + 35–21	Syntex	Comb	0.035 mg ethinyl estradiol	1 mg norethindrone	
1 + 35–28	Syntex	Comb	0.035 mg ethinyl estradiol	1 mg norethindrone	7
1 + 50–21	Syntex	Comb	0.05 mg mestranol	1 mg norethindrone	
1 + 50–28	Syntex	Comb	0.05 mg mestranol	1 mg norethindrone	7
2 mg	Syntex	Comb	0.1 mg mestranol	2 mg norethindrone	
Ovulen-21	Searle	Comb	0.1 mg mestranol	1 mg ethynodiol diacetate	
Ovulen-28	Searle	Comb	0.1 mg mestranol	1 mg ethynodiol diacetate	7
Norlestrin-21 1/50	Parke-Davis	Comb	50 mcg ethinyl estradiol	1 mg norethindrone acetate	
-28 1/50	Parke-Davis	Comb	50 mcg ethinyl estradiol	1 mg norethindrone acetate	7
Fe 1/50	Parke-Davis	Comb	50 mcg ethinyl estradiol	1 mg norethindrone acetate + 75 mg ferrous fumarate	
-21 2.5/50	Parke-Davis	Comb	50 mcg ethinyl estradiol	2.5 mg norethindrone acetate	
Fe 2.5/50	Parke-Davis	Comb	50 mcg ethinyl estradiol	2.5 mg norethindrone acetate + 75 mg ferrous fumarate	
Nordette-21	Wyeth	Comb	0.03 mg ethinyl estradiol	0.15 levonorgestrel	
-28	Wyeth	Comb	0.03 mg ethinyl estradiol	0.15 levonorgestrel	7
Ovral-21	Wyeth	Comb	0.05 mg ethinyl estradiol	0.5 mg norgestrel	
-28	Wyeth	Comb	0.05 mg ethinyl estradiol	0.5 mg norgestrel	7
Demulen-1/50–21	Searle	Comb	50 mcg ethinyl estradiol	1 mg ethynodiol diacetate	
-1/50–28	Searle	Comb	50 mcg ethinyl estradiol	1 mg ethynodiol diacetate	7
-1/35–21	Searle	Comb	0.035 mg ethinyl estradiol	1 mg ethynodiol diacetate	
-1/35–28	Searle	Comb	0.035 mg ethinyl estradiol	1 mg ethynodiol diacetate	7
Brevicon-21	Syntex	Comb	0.035 mg ethinyl estradiol	0.5 mg norethindrone	
-28	Syntex	Comb	0.035 mg ethinyl estradiol	0.5 mg norethindrone	7
Loestrin-21 1/20	Parke-Davis	Comb	20 mcg ethinyl estradiol	1 mg norethindrone acetate	
-Fe 1/20 28	Parke-Davis	Comb	20 mcg ethinyl estradiol	1 mg norethindrone acetate + 75 mg ferrous fumarate	7
-21 1.5/30	Parke-Davis	Comb	30 mcg ethinyl estradiol	1.5 mg norethindrone acetate	
-Fe 1.5/30 28	Parke-Davis	Comb	30 mcg ethinyl estradiol	1.5 mg norethindrone acetate + 75 mg ferrous fumarate	7
Lo/Ovral-21	Wyeth	Comb	0.03 mg ethinyl estradiol	0.3 mg norgestrel	
-28	Wyeth	Comb	0.03 mg ethinyl estradiol	0.3 mg norgestrel	7
Modicon-21	Ortho	Comb	0.035 mg ethinyl estradiol	0.5 mg norethindrone	
-28	Ortho	Comb	0.035 mg ethinyl estradiol	0.5 mg norethindrone	7
Ovcon-35–21	Mead Johnson	Comb	0.035 mg ethinyl estradiol	0.4 mg norethindrone	
-35–28	Mead Johnson	Comb	0.035 mg ethinyl estradiol	0.4 mg norethindrone	7
-50–21	Mead Johnson	Comb	0.05 mg ethinyl estradiol	1 mg norethindrone	
-50–28	Mead Johnson	Comb	0.05 mg ethinyl estradiol	1 mg norethindrone	7

Progestogens

Micronor	Ortho	Prog		0.35 mg norethindrone	
Nor-Q.D.	Syntex	Prog		0.35 mg norethindrone	
Ovrette	Wyeth	Prog		0.075 mg norgestrel	

Fluctuating progesterone levels

Ortho-Novum 7/7/7–21	Ortho	Comb	0.035 mg ethinyl estradiol	7–0.5 mg, 7–0.75 mg, 7–1 mg norethindrone	
7/7/7–28	Ortho	Comb	0.035 mg ethinyl estradiol	7–0.5 mg, 7–0.75 mg, 7–1 mg norethindrone	7

(Continued)

Table 38-9. Most currently available combination and microdose of progestin oral contraceptives (*Continued*)

Product		Manufacturer	Type	Estrogen	Progestin	Inert
	10/11–21	Ortho	Comb	0.035 mg ethinyl estradiol	10–0.5 mg, 11–1 mg norethindrone	
	10/11–28	Ortho	Comb	0.035 mg ethinyl estradiol	10–0.5 mg, 11–1 mg norethindrone	7
Tri-Norinyl-21		Syntex	Comb	0.035 mg ethinyl estradiol	7–0.5 mg, 9–1 mg, 5–0.5 mg norethindrone	
	-28	Syntex	Comb	0.035 mg ethinyl estradiol	7–0.5 mg, 9–1 mg, 5–0.5 mg norethindrone	7
Triphasil-21		Wyeth	Comb	6–0.03 mg, 5–0.04 mg, 10–0.03 mg ethinyl estradiol	6–0.05 mg, 5–0.075 mg, 10–0.125 mg levonorgestrel	
	-28	Wyeth	Comb	6–0.03 mg, 5–0.04 mg, 10–0.03 mg ethinyl estradiol	6–0.05 mg, 5–0.075 mg, 10–0.125 mg levonorgestrel	7

advantageous to women with hypoestrogenic amenorrhea, hypermenorrhea, or endometriosis. It also seems to provide some protection against ovarian cysts, ovarian and uterine cancers, and benign breast disease. It provides the greatest safety when used by young white women who are healthy, do not smoke cigarettes, and who limit use to 5 years.

Dosage and administration. The mini-pill is taken continuously, without interruption, whereas the combined pill may be taken in a 21- or 28-day series. Women who use the 21-day series can expect menses to start within 2 to 7 days after taking the last pill in the series. They are usually told to start a new pack on the fifth day, whether or not they are still bleeding, or to wait for a week before starting a new series. Those on the 28-day series start a new pack as soon as the present pack is finished. (The additional pills are placebos, but they prevent the break in the daily pill-taking routine.) Forgotten doses should be taken as soon as remembered.

Adverse reactions. The pill remains controversial because it poses severe risks to the user. The biggest danger is increased mortality from thromboembolic disorders (Vessey, et al, 1986). Other potential problems include an increase in migraine headaches, mental depression, hypertension, disturbances in carbohydrate metabolism, elevated serum lipids, gallbladder disease, vaginal bleeding, visual disturbances, impaired fertility after discontinuation, discolored skin areas, and an increase in the size of fibroid tumors. After discontinuation of the pill, the risk of cerebrovascular disease may persist for 6 years and that of myocardial infarction for 9 years.

Precautions and contraindications. Women who smoke more than 15 cigarettes a day or who have vascular disease, cardiac problems, diabetes mellitus, breast or reproductive carcinoma, liver disease, hypertension, obesity, or who are older than 35 years of age should not use the pill. Others who should seek different contraceptive methods are those with folic acid deficiency, epilepsy, fibrocystic breasts, infrequent or scant menses, or varicose veins. Using the pill during pregnancy is contraindicated because it may cause birth defects, and use during lactation may cause a cessation of the milk supply. The effects on the infant of hormonal contraceptives used by the nursing mother have not been fully documented. Therefore, hormonal contraceptives should not be used during lactation.

Certain medications have been reported to interfere with the efficacy of oral contraceptives. Among these are the antituberculous drug rifampin (breakthrough bleeding and increased risk of pregnancy); anticonvulsants, including phenytoin, phenobarbital, and primidone; some antibiotics (ampicillin, tetracycline); analgesics (phenacetin); and the psychotropic drugs chlordiazepoxide and meprobamate. Clients who take anticoagulants may develop a higher circulating level of some clotting factors, particularly factor VII. Slower excretion of caffeine, diazepam, and prednisone may occur for women who take the pill. Vitamin plasma levels may also change, with an increase in vitamin A and decreases in vitamins B_2, B_{12}, and C, as well as folic acid. Dietary increases or supplements may be needed for women at risk, that is, those who recently gave birth or who want to become pregnant shortly, adolescents, or those with poor diets (Stoehr, White, 1983).

Manufacturers have voluntarily withdrawn pills that contain more than 50 mg estrogen to increase the safety of the method.

Devices used with hormonal methods

The Silastic vaginal rings combine the convenience of a mechanical method with the greater efficacy of a hormonal contraceptive. They are available in two strengths, with differing actions. The high dose ring contains 250 to 280 µg levonorgestrel with 180 µg estradiol. It acts by eliminating ovulation. It must be removed after 3 weeks and replaced a week later to prevent pregnancy. It can be expelled spontaneously, interfering with efficacy. It may cause a noninfectious vaginal discharge or a vaginal erosion, as well as irregular bleeding. It releases a high level (180 µg) of estradiol. The low-dose ring releases only 20 to 50 µg levonorgestrel and no estrogen. Ovulation, therefore, occurs. The low-dose ring is effective because it makes the cervical mucus impermeable to sperm. It can remain in place for several months.

Implantable hormones

Levonorgestrel (Norplant) capsules are implanted during menstruation in a fanlike pattern in the medial aspect of the upper arm or in the scapular area (Fig. 38-9). The procedure is carried out under local anesthesia by a physician. The capsules release 36 µg of levonorgestrel and are effective after 24 hours for 5 years, with a failure rate of 0.5% to 2.6%. They can be removed (again, under local anesthesia) at any time. Although the initial expense is greater, the fact that no other contraceptive products need to be purchased equalizes the cost over time. Disadvantages include irregular vaginal bleeding that diminishes over time; ovarian cysts in 10% of the users, usually regressing within 6 weeks without intervention; irregular menstrual cycles, acne, headaches, breast tenderness, infection at the insertion site; and weight must be under 150 lb. Cosmetically, the capsules can be felt and sometimes seen. They should not be used for women with acute liver disease or liver tumors, unexplained vaginal bleeding, breast cancer, or thrombophlebitis.

Postcoital contraceptive

In emergency situations in which unprotected intercourse may lead to an undesirable pregnancy (rape, incest), a postcoital contraceptive may be the method of choice. DES is used to prevent (not terminate) a pregnancy by interfering with implantation of the fertilized ovum.

A 25-mg tablet is given orally twice each day for 5 days. To be effective, the treatment should begin within 24 hours after intercourse and must be completed despite possible nausea, vomiting, headache, dizziness, abdominal pain, or other side effects. Initiating treatment later than 72 hours after intercourse is probably ineffective.

DES must not be administered if the client is already pregnant, because it may lead to vaginal adenosis or cervical cancer in female offspring or to epididymal anomalies in male offspring. If possible, a blood test to quickly determine if the client is pregnant should be carried out before the administration of the first dose. If the client is already pregnant, it is extremely unlikely that she ovulated again, and therefore DES is unnecessary. The treatment should be terminated if any signs of thromboembolic disease are present, because this condition can lead to death.

■ Summary

Contraceptive choices are influenced by the client's religious beliefs, knowledge, and socioeconomic level and by the method's effectiveness, esthetics, and safety, as well as by other factors. Before choosing a method, couples must consider mutual comfort and motivation for success, as well as each partner's physical and emotional status.

Aside from abstinence or tubal ligation, oral contraceptives are the most effective female measure. However, the dangers of a thromboembolic incident have led many women to seek other methods. The IUD is infrequently prescribed because of physical dangers. Fertility awareness, diaphragms, and condoms are being used more widely because of safety factors.

Men have fewer contraceptive choices. Researchers are questioning the sustained effects of vasectomies, leaving a vas deferens intraluminal device, abstinence, coitus interruptus, or condoms as alternatives. Experiments with contraceptive drugs are under way.

Nursing management

Nursing implications

Opportunities and responsibilities that allow professional nurses to respond creatively to the expanding field of women's health care have increased in current nursing practice. These include counseling and instruction in contraceptive practices. Although both

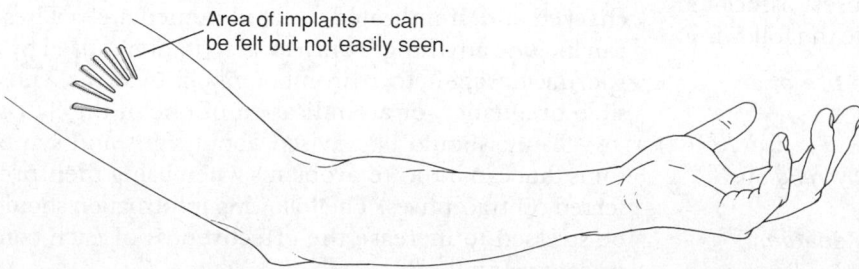

Area of implants — can be felt but not easily seen.

Figure 38-9. Six Norplant silicone rubber capsules that contain synthetic progestin implanted in medial aspect of the upper arm. A low dose of hormone is released steadily into the bloodstream within 24 hours after insertion for the next 5 years, providing contraceptive protection.

men and women should be provided with sufficient information concerning available contraceptive measures, in today's society, women still have the major responsibility for using contraception.

Sex is a very natural thing. If nurses can accept themselves as sexual beings and are comfortable with discussing sexual matters, they can better serve their clients. It is particularly important for nurses who work in obstetrics, gynecology, and pediatrics (in hospitals, clinics, and doctors' offices), in community health fields, or in family-planning clinics to be comfortable and skilled in discussing family-planning practices. However, all nurses probably will be asked some questions concerning sex and contraceptive measures, because most people are concerned about sexuality, sexual problems, family size, and family welfare. Contraceptive counseling requires knowledge, communication skills, and an ability to evaluate client and partner backgrounds (religious, cultural, ethnic).

The decision to prevent pregnancy is easy for some clients and difficult for others. The use or availability of contraceptives implies that sexual intercourse is anticipated. For some, acknowledgment of anticipated intercourse is too painful emotionally or too embarrassing, so unprotected intercourse becomes preferable. Men or women may spend a great deal of time rationalizing why they will or will not use specific contraceptive measures.

The most important objective in family planning is finding a method that will be used. The "safest" methods are not "safe" if the client consciously or unconsciously wants to become pregnant.

Nursing process

Assessment A history, physical examination, and lab work are important first steps in family planning. Discussions with client and partner provide information that pertains to lifestyle, values, priorities, religious and cultural feelings, and knowledge of and attitudes about the body and contraceptive measures. Some methods may be eliminated as a result of this discussion, either for physical or personal reasons. Each method has some drawbacks, and these should be discussed completely and honestly, along with the advantages. Only after open discussion of the facts can the couple make an intelligent choice about the method they prefer and the one with which they can comply.

Nursing diagnosis Nursing diagnoses associated with contraceptive selection may include the following:

> *Altered sexuality patterns related to use of a mechanical contraceptive device*
> *Spiritual distress related to use of contraceptives that are proscribed by religious beliefs*
> *Knowledge deficit related to genital anatomy or use of contraceptives*

Planning The goal is to present knowledge to prevent pregnancy, including making certain that the client knows how to use contraceptive methods correctly and is motivated to use them consistently. No side effects should be present, or, if they are, they should be corrected immediately, usually by selecting another method. If pregnancy occurs, contraceptive methods should be discontinued immediately, particularly if oral contraceptives have been used. The goal for using condoms may be the prevention of the spread of STDs. Again, to be effective, condoms must be used consistently and properly.

Intervention Selection of a contraceptive method should include information about possible circumstances that would prohibit the use of certain types of contraceptives. For example, clients with physical disorders that might be affected by fluid retention (migraine, renal problems) or clients with a history of cancer or thromboembolic episodes should not consider oral contraceptives. Clients with pelvic abnormalities may not be able to be fitted properly for a diaphragm or cervical cap. Men with premature ejaculation may not be able to use a condom effectively.

Oral contraceptives should be prescribed by the practitioner only after a complete evaluation of the client's physical status. Oral contraceptives are used most safely by young, healthy, white women who do not smoke cigarettes and who limit their use of the drugs to 5 years.

Client education. Education that pertains to the reproductive systems, sexuality, and family planning should begin early so children learn it from a reliable source rather than from "the street." It can be carried out at home, in school, in private practice, or in clinics. It may be taught or discussed in a group situation or on a one-to-one basis. Films, models, and other audiovisual equipment should be used.

After the choice of contraception for the sexually active client is made, the nurse is responsible for giving further instruction on its use. This may include illustrations, models, demonstrations, and actual practice by the client. It may involve proper fitting, as with diaphragms, or advice on where to buy supplies, such as monoclonal antibody tests for ovulation and thermometers and graphs on which to record information.

It is important for the client to be taught to recognize any untoward or abnormal signs or symptoms related to the contraceptive method and to have them checked and, if indicated, treated immediately. These can include anything from a local irritation caused by a spermicidal agent to a thromboembolic incident, a possible pregnancy, or an indication of one of the STDs.

Clients should be advised about signs and symptoms that can indicate problems when using their preferred contraceptives. The following information should be stressed to increase the effectiveness of each contraceptive method.

If lubrication is desired when condoms are used, only a spermicide or a water-based product (such as K-Y Jelly) should be used. Products with an oil base (petroleum jelly, cold cream, A and D Ointment) may weaken the condom.

Client education is an important part of a successful fertility-awareness program. The woman is unlikely to succeed if her cycles are irregular or if she or her partner is not motivated enough to remain abstinent during ovulation. Effectiveness increases when all four methods of ovulatory detection are used simultaneously.

Spermicidal jellies, creams, foams, vaginal suppositories, or foaming tablets, with or without concurrent use of a condom, diaphragm, contraceptive sponge, or cervical cap, all require proper application and timing according to manufacturers' instructions. Instructions for each type of spermicidal preparation must be read and followed carefully. Differences in insertion techniques, the time interval needed between application and intercourse, and the period of effectiveness exist. The client must check the product expiration date and store any remaining spermicide as directed by the manufacturer.

Cans of foam must be shaken well before the contents are used, and suppositories or tablets must be removed from their wrappers before insertion. Using either of these methods requires some time, but not as much time as needed to insert a diaphragm. Spermicides can be adapted to foreplay and lovemaking.

Proper placement of a diaphragm requires instruction and supervised practice. Two teaspoonfuls of spermicide should be placed inside the diaphragm dome; an additional amount of spermicide should be used to cover the rim before insertion. The device may be inserted vaginally as much as 6 hours before intercourse, with the flexible rim seated firmly from above the symphysis pubis over the cervix to the rear vaginal wall. Additional applications of spermicide may be advisable if more than 2 hours pass before intercourse or when intercourse is repeated. The diaphragm must remain in place for 6 to 8 hours after intercourse occurs. The diaphragm should be inspected for holes or tears, particularly under the rim, before and after each use. It should not be used if any holes or tears are found.

To be effective, condoms must cover the erect penis completely before insertion into the vagina. Condoms with holes or weak spots should not be used. Air must be removed from the condom before it is applied, and a half-inch space must be left at the tip to act as a reservoir for semen. The condom must be held firmly at the base of the penis during its withdrawal after the act, before the erection ends, to prevent leakage of the ejaculate into the vagina. Condoms are not reusable and should be discarded immediately after use.

Women who take oral contraceptives should be warned that breakthrough bleeding may occur, particularly during the first six cycles. The importance of reporting the following symptoms immediately should be stressed: abdominal pain (possible ectopic pregnancy); numbness, pain in legs (thromboembolic disorder); pressure or pain in chest, shortness of breath (embolus); visual disturbances with blurred vision, flashing lights, blind spots (cerebrovascular accident); two consecutive missed periods (pregnancy). Clients should also be aware of possible changes in libido and of intolerance to contact lenses. Appetite or weight changes as well as vaginal candidiasis may occur. Clients should be encouraged to have annual gynecologic examinations as well as Pap smears at prescribed intervals to detect any problems as quickly as possible.

Clients should be encouraged to take oral contraceptives as advised, recognizing that missing a dose lessens the effectiveness of the contraceptives. Missed doses must be taken as soon as possible. If three or more pills are missed, the rest of the packet should be discarded and another method of contraception substituted entirely. A new pack of pills should be started on the fifth day of menstruation.

Women who receive oral contraceptives or progesterone should be cautioned against cigarette smoking, because cigarette smoking increases the risk of thromboembolic problems. Clients should be alerted to signs and symptoms of possible side effects of oral contraceptives (see Example of Nursing Process and Oral Contraception).

Evaluation Efficacy can be evaluated according to success: no pregnancy for the sexually active individual who uses contraception consistently during every sexual encounter. If condoms are used to prevent the transmission of STDs, the evaluation should include testing for those diseases, with none present as an indication of success.

Checklist of nursing actions

- [ ] Become comfortable with your own sexuality and that of your client.
- [ ] Develop a knowledge base concerning reproductive systems, sexuality, and all matters that pertain to contraceptive methods.
- [ ] Become skillful in being communicative with your clients.
- [ ] Take a careful history, include the results of a physical examination and do lab work on your client before discussing a suitable contraceptive method.
- [ ] Develop an ability to assess, evaluate, and accept other backgrounds, lifestyles, and values.
- [ ] Learn everything you can about each method of contraception so you can present it factually, discuss it honestly, and provide precise instructions on its use.
- [ ] Become adept at using models and audiovisual material in presenting methods.

☐ Provide your client with handout material and advice on signs and symptoms of adverse reactions.

Infertility and fertility drugs

A diagnosis of infertility is made when couples who have engaged in frequent unprotected intercourse around the time of ovulation have not conceived in a year or longer. Multiple factors are present in 35% of the cases, with problems present in either partner. Treatment is based on the findings.

Some of the treatment regimens currently available are cytotoxic therapy (in clients with certain autoimmune disorders) and immunization with vaginal suppositories derived from cell-free seminal plasma (in women with inappropriate alloimmune response to the fetus). Heparin and aspirin (in women with primary antiphospholipid antibody syndrome) are being investigated for their effectiveness in dissolving or preventing the formation of placental clots. Other techniques showing promise are intrauterine insemination (IUI), gamete intrafallopian transfer (GIFT), in vitro fertilization (IVF), and tubal ovum transfer.

Male infertility

The inability of the male to procreate may be complicated by impotence, which is the inability to attain or maintain an erection firm enough for intercourse. Several factors have been implicated in impotence. A detailed history and physical examination must, therefore, be carried out to determine the course of treatment.

Occasionally, the history indicates a need for client education about male sexuality. Timing of intercourse may have an effect on ability to perform, since higher levels of testosterone occur on awakening. The suggestion might be made that intercourse be carried out then. Age is another factor, bringing with it a slowdown in the ability to have an erection, to ejaculate, and to have additional orgasms, indicating a need to space sexual activities further apart and to dedicate more time to foreplay for stimulation. Sensate focus exercises may also be helpful (Renshaw, 1987).

Physical causes may be the basis for impotence, including atherosclerotic deposits that interfere with adequate circulation to the penis and prevent an erection, diabetes mellitus that results in damaged erectile nerves as well as atherosclerotic damage (perhaps before the diabetes is diagnosed), hormonal imbalances, side effects of medications taken for other conditions that may lead to noncompliance in the face of the impotence, excessive and prolonged use of alcohol that leads to liver damage, and changes in sex hormone levels. Nicotine from cigarette smoking can cause constriction of penile blood vessels and interference with the metabolism of sex hormones by the liver. Drug abuse can cause impotence (from use of marijuana) and inhibited ejaculation and orgasm (from cocaine use).

Other factors that affect potency include spinal cord injuries, surgical removal of the entire prostate, radiation to the prostate, medication to shrink the prostate, neurologic disorders such as multiple sclerosis, elevations in testicular temperature, obesity, and psychological considerations. Simple health measures may have an effect on some aspects of potency, including better nutrition and weight control, elimination of drug and cigarette abuse, and reduction of stress and reactions to it. One simple measure to reduce testicular temperature is to wear boxer shorts rather than close fitting underwear. More severe cases may require the use of a Testicular Hypothermia Device, which lowers scrotal temperature about 2°C, with a resultant improvement in the quality of the semen (count, motility, and morphology; Zorgniotti, Plawner, 1987).

Various medications have been used to overcome infertility in men. Testosterone may be helpful to men unable to produce it on their own. Tricyclic antidepressants may help reverse nerve damage to the penis caused by diabetes. Zinc supplements (100 mg daily) are needed for replacement for men who are undergoing kidney dialysis. Papaverine is no longer recommended for self-injection directly into penile erectile tissue because there are serious side effects, including priapism for up to 2 days. Occasionally, the reaction has been severe enough to require surgical intervention and has resulted in blood vessel scarring. Another medication under investigation is yohimbine hydrochloride (Yocon), 18 mg taken daily. This drug may also lower blood pressure and lessen depression. Some of its ability to cause an erection may be due to its placebo effect rather than to the drug itself.

Menotropins

Menotropins (Pergonal) are being used to treat infertile men diagnosed as having hypogonadotropic hypogonadism. This condition is thought to affect 1 in 25,000 men in the reproductive age range. It causes a low sperm count due to inadequate pituitary secretion of the hormones LH or FSH, both of which are needed for normal sperm production.

In men, LH controls the testosterone-producing cells, whereas FSH is needed to transport testosterone to the sperm-producing cells. Inadequate amounts of either hormone interfere with the production of adequate numbers of sperm.

IM injection of menotropins stimulates testosterone production, leading to an increase in the sperm count. The injections may be given for 6 months to several years before pregnancy occurs in the treated male's partner.

Multiple births are not associated with Pergonal when it is administered to the male. Temporary breast enlargement has been the only side effect noted to date.

Female infertility

Ovulatory stimulants

Although most drugs that affect ovulation are used for contraceptive purposes, some are used to treat infertility caused by anovulation. The exact cause of this problem must be determined before proper treatment can be started. Fertility stimulants must be administered under the direction of a practitioner.

Thyroid and adrenal gland activity may contribute to the lack of ovulation. Thyroid preparations to control hypothyroidism or hyperthyroidism may be appropriate. Cortisone, which increases the level of human gonadotropic hormones through suppression of the production of androgens and estrogens by the adrenals, is used in cases of adrenal dysfunction.

Menotropins

Menotropins are natural human gonadotropic hormones obtained from the urine of postmenopausal women. Both LH and FSH, in equal proportions, are present in menotropins.

Pregnancy occurs in about 20% to 45% of the women who receive menotropins within six series of treatments. Of these, about 25% of the clients abort and 17% to 50% have multiple births.

Dosage and administration. LH and FSH, 75 IU of each, are given IM for 9 to 12 days to increase the growth and maturation of the graafian follicles. On the day after the last injection of LH and FSH, 10,000 U of hCG are injected to induce ovulation. In some instances, the doses of LH and FSH are doubled during the course of treatment.

Adverse reactions. Several uncomfortable side effects accompany administration of menotropins: fever, nausea, vomiting, diarrhea, and flatulence. More serious signs of adverse reactions include ascites, pleural effusion, hypercoagulation, oliguria, hypotension, and ovarian enlargement. If ovarian cysts rupture, intraperitoneal hemorrhage may occur, requiring abdominal surgery.

Human chorionic gonadotropin

Luteinized unruptured follicle syndrome is one of the ovulatory failures not commonly recognized. Diagnosis is made on the basis of low peritoneal fluid assays of progesterone and estradiol when other tests (serum progesterone, endometrial dating, and basal temperatures) appear to be normal after presumed ovulation. Ultrasound reveals this syndrome by showing a luteinized follicle that has not ruptured. Treatment is hCG, 5,000 U given IM in the presence of a mature follicle. The follicle can be expected to mature within 24 to 36 hours (LeMaire, 1987).

Bromocriptine mesylate

Bromocriptine mesylate (Parlodel) is used for infertility associated with amenorrhea in the presence of hyperprolactinemia not caused by a pituitary tumor (Forbes-Albright syndrome). It is given during the follicular phase and the preovulatory period to normalize prolactin levels, in the hope that it will lead to spontaneous ovulation (Lee, 1987).

One 2½-mg tablet is given at mealtime on the first day. The dosage is increased to 2 or 3 tablets per day at mealtimes within the first week. Mechanical contraception should be used until normal cycles are established, and then contraception should be discontinued. The medication should be discontinued if menstruation does not occur within 3 days of the expected date, and a test for pregnancy should be performed. This drug should not be used once the client is pregnant.

Progesterone

Luteal phase defects are suspected when infertility is unexplained and when single or serial progesterone assays or endometrial biopsies carried out in two cycles during the midluteal phase of the menstrual cycle demonstrate low progesterone levels. Decreased progesterone has been implicated in repeated early miscarriages. Progesterone in the form of vaginal suppositories (25 mg twice a day) or IM injections (12.5 mg) has been therapeutically successful. Dihydrogesterone (Duphaston) is also under study for treatment of early miscarriage (Lee, 1987).

Danazol

One percent to three percent of women in their childbearing years are afflicted with endometriosis. It may cause pain during menstruation, defecation, or intercourse and may be responsible for abnormal menses or hematuria. If extensive, it can cause ovarian adhesions that impede the release of ova, press against the fallopian tubes, preventing the ovum and sperm from meeting for fertilization, or block the passage of the embryo through the tubes to the uterus for implantation.

Diagnosis of endometriosis may be made by noninvasive tests (sonography or magnetic resonance imaging) but is usually made definitively through surgery, using a laparoscope. The degree of involvement is classified in stages, with I and II being milder. Stages III and IV are considered serious, since they may interfere with fertility. Surgery to remove the areas of abnormal endometrial implantation may use electric or laser cautery via laparoscopy. The surgery is usually followed by a course of hormone therapy. Young women usually receive continuous low-dose oral contraceptives (referred to as a pseudopregnancy regimen) over several months.

Norethynodrel with mestranol (Enovid) may be used, beginning on the 5th day of the menstrual cycle, starting with 5 to 10 mg/day for 2 weeks. This dosage is increased by 5 to 10 mg every 2 weeks up to 20 mg/day, for 6 to 9 months. If this treatment is ineffective or if the client is an older woman, danazol (Danocrine), an oral androgen, may be prescribed.

Danazol (Danocrine) is used to inhibit the output of gonadotropins from the pituitary. The usual dosage is 400 mg bid, starting during menstruation and continuing without interruption for 3 to 6 months. It can be extended to 9 months. If symptoms recur within a year, treatment can be restarted. This drug should not be used during pregnancy (Speroff, 1983). Danazol may cause weight gain, decreased breast size, hot flashes, muscle pains, changes in libido, or acne in about 85% of the women to whom it is administered. A new drug, nafarelin, is under investigation and seems likely to become the drug of choice, with fewer side effects. It is administered as a nasal spray. It decreases estrogen production to cause a temporary menopause. Endometrial growth stops, and a regression of endometrial implants may occur. It has side effects that mimic menopause (hot flashes, vaginal dryness, changes in libido, and about a 5% loss of existing bone mass), all of which end when the nafarelin is withdrawn. Endometriosis usually is no longer a problem at menopause. If symptoms are unbearable before then, a complete surgical menopause may be suggested.

Clomiphene citrate

Clomiphene citrate (Clomid), another ovulatory stimulant, is a synthetic agent that resembles the synthetic estrogen chlorotrianisene (TACE). Its mode of action is not understood, but it seems helpful in treating amenorrhea that originates in the pituitary. Pregnancy occurs in 25% to 30% of the women who receive this drug, with multiple births occurring in 10%.

Clomiphene is usually started on the 5th day of the menstrual cycle, increasing the gonadotropins, hoping to produce one oocyte. (If *in vitro* fertilization is planned, clomiphene is started earlier so that more than one oocyte is available.) Dosage must be clinically tailored to the woman's needs, based on evidence of ovulation (temperature chart, endometrial biopsy), ovarian enlargement, and side effects. The FSH level should increase, stimulating normal follicular development with adequate LH receptors on granulosa cells. This process seems to promote an adequate luteal phase.

Clomiphene citrate may cause minor side effects, including nausea, vomiting, and hot flashes. Of greater concern is the possibility of ovarian enlargement or ovarian cysts and the possibility of teratogenic effects on the fetus if the client is pregnant.

■ Summary

Fertility stimulants provide help for the infertile client. The drugs are used to stimulate ovula-

tion or sperm production. Clients must be aware of possible adverse effects or side effects.

Nursing management

Nursing implications

Infertility is a field of health care in itself. Those who deal with it are specialists. However, nurses may help clients initially by recognizing problems of infertility, making assessments, and suggesting referrals to specialists. Any preliminary information the nurse can give the specialist is helpful.

The tests used to determine the cause of infertility and the treatments are time consuming, expensive, and, in some cases, painful or embarrassing. Many times, a definite cause cannot be determined and when intervention begins, no guarantee can be made that the woman will become pregnant. The entire experience is an emotional and (possibly) financial drain on the family. Emotional support should be extended to the entire family, but especially to the woman who is undergoing assessment and treatment.

Women treated for infertility tend to be fairly depressed through the months of the treatment cycles. The injections are painful and expensive and the chance of success is less than 50%. In addition, sexual activity is determined by ovulation; therefore, sexual intercourse loses spontaneity.

Nursing process

Assessment Determining the causes of infertility requires a complete history, including the timing of sexual intercourse against the time of ovulation. Monoclonal antibody tests help couples anticipate this more accurately than previous dependence on temperature charts. Completion of the sex act with deposit of semen at the cervical orifice is important. Examinations of the semen to determine sufficient sperm motility and evaluation of the cervical environment are also necessary.

The histories of both partners must be examined to determine whether either has a physical condition or is taking medications that may interfere with initiating a pregnancy. Illicit drugs or alcohol may interfere with sperm production, while douching may render the environment of the vagina detrimental to sperm.

Nursing diagnosis Nursing diagnoses likely to be made for clients who are undergoing treatment for infertility may include the following:

Sexual dysfunction related to changes in sexual practices secondary to the infertility treatment regimen
Altered family processes related to the precedence given to the requirements of the infertility treatment regimen

Self-esteem disturbance related to failure to conceive

Hopelessness related to repeated failures to achieve pregnancy

Many clients with fertility problems have difficulty in coping with the extreme pressure of regulating sexual activity to coincide with ovulation. The self-concept of each partner tends to go through extreme swings: up before each attempt to start a pregnancy, and down to the point of grieving if the attempt proves unsuccessful. Sexual dysfunction may result as each partner feels a sense of failure. Sexual avoidance may occur at the time of ovulation to avoid another defeat.

Planning The reality of infertility treatment is that the rate of failure is high. Treatment may be required for many months, or even years, without a promise of success. It is therefore important for the goal to be realistic. The primary goal is to attain pregnancy, but the important secondary goal is for the couple to retain a loving, trusting, supportive relationship that will survive the pressures of the testing and treatment process.

Intervention The couple needs help in maintaining a sense of priorities through the time of testing and treatment. They need to be encouraged to continue with other enjoyable activities to lessen the tension of the fertility program. Their other health needs should not suffer as they use time, energy, and often a great deal of money to achieve a pregnancy. Other avenues should also be explored: insemination with donor sperm, adoption, and, if no other choices are available, the possibility of surrogate parenthood or remaining childless.

Evaluation The ideal outcome is a successful pregnancy that leads to a healthy child and healthy parents. If that is not possible, an outcome that results in a continuation of a good marriage with the acceptance of adoption or childlessness should be regarded as a success.

References

AIDS nursing update statement, 1(1). (1987). Los Angeles: UCLA AIDS Clinical Research Center.

Airman L. (1991,) Growth of AIDS virus is suppressed in research. *The New York Times*, p A10.

Altman L. (1991,). A simpler way to employ RU-486 is reported. *The New York Times*, p B6.

Barrick B. (1990). Light at the end of a decade. *American Journal of Nursing, 90*(11), 37–40.

Bender S, Kelleher K. (1986). *PMS: A positive program to gain control.* Tucson, AZ: The Body Press, HP Books.

Bennett J. (1986). AIDS: What precautions do you take in the hospital? *American Journal of Nursing, 86*(9), 952–953.

Boland MG, Klug RM. (1986). AIDS: The implications for home care. *MCN*, 404–411.

Bourcier KM, Seidler AJ. (1987). Chlamydia and con-dylomata: An update for the nurse practitioner. *J Obstet Gynecol Neonatal Nurs*, 17–22.

Couzinet B, et al. (1986). Termination of early pregnancy by the progesterone antagonist RU486 (mifepristone). *N Engl J Med, 87*, 1565–1570.

Dunkin MA. (1991). Delivering hope. *Arthritis Today, 5*(3), 20–24.

Estraderm (Estradiol transdermal system: Prescribing information). (1986). Summit, NY: CIBA Pharmaceutical Co.

Farley D. (1990). Preventing TSS. *FDA Consumer, 24*(1), 6–9.

FDA Drug Bulletin. (1987). 17(3), 27–28.

Florida's top ranking in syphillis cases is linked to use of drugs. (1987, May 26). *The New York Times*, p A19.

Franklin D, Podolsky DM. (1987). Miracles in your medicine cabinet. *American Health, VI*(92), 92.

Kolata G (1991b,). US weighs early release of experimental AIDS drug. *The New York Times*, p A14.

Koop CE. (1987). *Surgeon General's report on acquired immune deficiency syndrome.* Washington, DC: U.S. Department of Health and Human Services.

Kugel C, Verson H. (1986). Relationship between weight change and diaphragm size change. *J Obstet Gynecol Neonatal Nurs*, 123–129.

Larson E, Ropka M. (1991). An update on nursing research and HIV infection. *Image, 23*(1), 4–12.

Lee CS. (1987). Infertility: Luteal phase defects. *Obstet Gynecol Surv, 42*(5), 267–274.

LeMaire GS. (1987). The luteinized unruptured follicle syndrome: Anovulation in disguise. *J Obstet Gynecol Neonatal Nurs*, 116–120.

Maugh TH II. (1987). Fighting the plague: 27 new drugs to stop a killer. *American Health, VI*(5), 73–84.

Monier M, Laird M. (1989). Contraceptives: A look at the future. *American Journal of Nursing, 89*(4), 497–499.

Nettina S. (1990). Syphilis: A new look at an old killer. *American Journal of Nursing, 90*(4), 68–70.

Niculescu AM. (1985). Effects of *in utero* exposure to DES on male progeny. *J Obstet Gynecol Neonatal Nurs*, 468–470.

Padwick ML, Pryse-Davies J, Whitehead MI. (1986). A simple method for determining the optimal dosage of progestin in postmenopausal women receiving estrogens. *N Engl J Med, 315*, 930.

Papazian R. (1991). Osteoporosis treatment advances. *FDA Consumer, 25*(3), 29–32.

Paulsen CA. (1987, February 24). Interview on birth control injections for men. *The New York Times*, p C4.

Public Health Service statement on management of occupational exposure to human immunodeficiency virus, including considerations regarding zidovudine postexposure use. (1990). *MMWR*, Centers for Disease Control.

Randal J. (1991). Trying to outsmart infertility. *FDA Consumer, 25*(4), 20–29.

Remington K, et al. (1987). Effect of the Today contraceptive sponge on growth and TSS toxin-1 production by *S. aureus. Obstet Gynecol*, 563–569.

Renshaw D. (1987). Management of impotence. I. Psychological considerations. *Clin Ther, 9*(2), 142–148.

Return to fertility for anejaculatory men. (1991). *American Journal of Nursing, 91*(4), 18.

Rinzler CA. (1987). The return of the condom. *American Health*, *July*, 97.

Segal M. (1991). Norplant: Birth control at arm's reach. *FDA Consumer*, *25*(4), 9–11.

Segal M. (1988). Cervical cap: Newest birth control choice. *FDA Consumer*, *22*(7), 32–34.

Suida S. (1990). The pill: 30 years of safety concerns. *FDA Consumer*, *24*(10), 8–11.

US syphilis cases rise 23%. (1987, July 3). An Associated Press Release. *The New York Times*, p A10.

Vessey M, et al. (1986). Oral contraceptives and venous thromboembolism: Findings in a large prospective study. *Br Med J*, *292*, 526.

Walton J, Youngkin E. (1987). The effect of a support group on self-esteem of women with premenstrual syndrome. *J Obstet Gynecol Neonatal Nurs*, 174–178.

Zorgniotti AW, Plawner J. (1987). Testicular hypothermia for male infertility. *Medical Aspects of Human Sexuality*, *21*(1), 23–27.

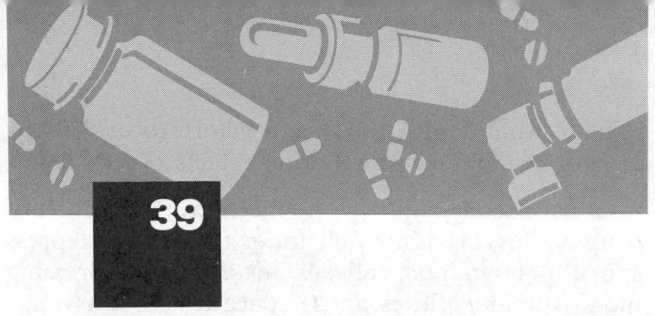

39

Drugs that affect the musculoskeletal system: skeletal muscle relaxants and antispasmodic agents

Physiology

Muscle tissue is characterized by contraction and relaxation, a process that moves bones around joints for locomotion and other body movements. The body contains more than 600 skeletal muscles, which, together with skeletal bones, support and move the body. Skeletal muscles are called voluntary, because they can be controlled by conscious commands, in contrast to car- diac muscles and visceral muscles, which are involuntary (not commanded by conscious thought).

Muscle fibers can contract (shorten), relax (elongate), or be at rest (Fig. 39-1). Resting muscles are in a semicontracted state and are always ready for action.

When a muscle contracts, a nerve impulse is sent from the brain and spinal cord through a motor neuron to a muscle cell membrane at a communication point called the *motor endplate* (Fig. 39-2). The stimulus alters the permeability of the membrane to various ions, generates an action potential, and releases calcium ions. The localized increase of calcium causes an interaction between myosin and action in the sarcomeres, which results in contraction. Conversely, as the calcium is removed from the sarcomeres, the muscles relax.

Pathophysiology
Peripheral muscle spasms

Injury to peripheral muscle system structures, such as muscles, joints, tendons, or ligaments, can cause involuntary muscle contractions or spasms. Spasms are sudden, violent, painful, and involuntary.

The injured muscle part sends sensory impulses to the spinal cord, which are passed by one or more connecting interneurons to the spinal motor neurons. The excessive number of motor impulses that pass to the periphery from the spinal cord causes the muscle spasm; the original pain can also trigger additional spasms. Specific conditions that cause muscle spasms include whiplash injuries, cervical root syndromes, herniated discs, lower back syndromes, bursitis, myositis, neuritis, dislocations and fractures, muscle strains from excessive stretching or overuse, and sprains from wrenched joints with stretched or torn ligaments.

Spasticity from central nervous system damage

Spasticity occurs in a variety of neurologic conditions. It can result from damage within the central nervous system (CNS) rather than in the peripheral structures. It can be caused by injury to nerve cells at any of the various CNS centers that control muscle tone and coordinate complex movements. Spasticity requires a period of time to develop after neural injury and varies in its severity during different stages of recovery from injury or during the progression of a disease. Nevertheless, spasticity is permanent and frequently leads to disabling contractures.

Spasticity can result from either an increase in excitatory influences or a decrease in inhibitory influences. As a result, the stretch reflex is augmented, and the imbalance causes muscle fibers to stretch in an exaggerated way. Other proprioceptive reflexes may also be hyperactive. Specific conditions that cause spasticity include cerebral palsy, multiple sclerosis, polio-

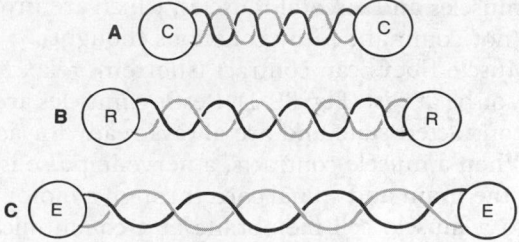

Figure 39-1. Sarcomeres perform the contraction and elongation of muscles. (*A*) Muscle fibers shorten as they contract. (*B*) Muscle fibers at rest in a semicontracted state in which they are ready for action. (*C*) Muscle fibers lengthen as they relax.

myelitis, hemiplegia, quadriplegia, paraplegia, spinal tumors, and tetanus. Once muscle tissue (such as nervous tissue) has been injured, repair occurs only with difficulty or not at all. Damaged tissue frequently is replaced by scar tissue.

Drugs used to relax skeletal muscles and treat spasticity

Different kinds of drugs are capable of relaxing skeletal muscles and treating spasticity. These include neuromuscular-blocking agents, local anesthetics, and spinal and general anesthetics (see Chapter 24). This chapter discusses skeletal muscle relaxants that have a more selective action than many agents included in the other classes of drugs that can relax muscle spasms and spasticity. For example, these agents do not depress consciousness to the degree that a general anesthetic does. Because of its other actions and mode of administration, a general anesthetic is not clinically useful in managing spasms caused by whiplash or paraplegic spasticity.

No completely satisfactory therapy for alleviating skeletal muscle spasticity exists. Several drugs provide varying relief, depending on circumstances, but negative effects on ambulation, sedation, and a variety of other adverse reactions minimize their overall usefulness. In some situations, it cannot be determined whether the benefits of a drug come primarily from its muscle-relaxing properties or from its sedative effect.

Skeletal muscle relaxants

Mephenesin (Tolseram) is the oldest drug among skeletal muscle relaxants. It is not discussed here because it is the prototype for the centrally acting drugs, but it is no longer used clinically.

The muscle relaxants that are similar to mephenesin include carisoprodol, chlorphenesin, chlorzoxazone, metaxalone, and methocarbamol (Table 39-1). The selection of one of these preparations over another is a subjective decision, because no well controlled studies compare the relative safety and efficacy of these compounds. In addition, it is difficult to deter-

mine to what degree the beneficial effects of therapy are attributable to the sedating effects of the drugs.

Pharmacodynamics. The mechanism of action of drugs in this class is not well understood. They depress spinal polysynaptic reflexes instead of depressing monosynaptic reflexes, and they are described as interneuronal-blocking agents. They also depress facilitative and inhibitory neuronal activity that affects muscle stretch reflexes, primarily in the lateral reticular area of the brain. The drugs cause drowsiness, possibly reflecting depression of neuronal activity in the medial reticular ascending system that is needed for wakefulness (Department of Drugs, 1990).

Therapeutic uses. The therapeutic uses for this class of drugs include relief of pain and increase in the mobility of affected muscles in acute musculoskeletal disorders. They are used in conjunction with rest, analgesics, and physical therapy. They are not used for spasticity of upper motor neuron lesions, cerebral palsy, multiple sclerosis, and spinal cord trauma.

Carisoprodol, chlorphenesin, chlorzoxazone, metaxalone, and methocarbamol

The dosage and administration and most adverse reactions for these drugs are covered in Table 39-1.

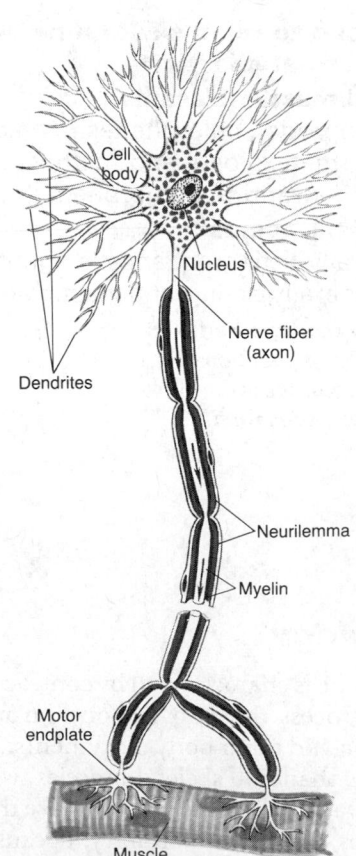

Figure 39-2. A typical motor neuron.

Table 39-1. Skeletal muscle relaxants

Drug name	Preparation	Usual dosage	Adverse reactions
carisoprodol (Carisoma, Rela, Sanoma, Soma, Soma Compound [carisoprodol and aspirin], Soma Compound with Codeine [carisoprodol, aspirin, and codeine])	Oral tablets	Adult: 350 mg qid Child: not recommended PC: C	Drowsiness, dizziness, headache, hypersensitivity reactions, paradoxic reactions (*eg*, stimulation, nervousness, insomnia), idiosyncratic reactions
chlorphenesin carbamate (Maolate, Mycil)	Oral tablets	Adult: *Initially*, 800 mg tid; *maintenance*, 400 mg qid Child: not recommended PC: C	Drowsiness, dizziness, headache, hypersensitivity reactions, GI disturbances, paradoxic reactions, reactions to FD&C yellow #5 component
chlorzoxazone (Oxyren, Paraflex, Parafon Forte [chlorzoxazone and acetaminophen])	Oral tablets and caplets	Adult: 250–750 mg tid or qid Child: 125–500 mg tid or qid PC: C	Drowsiness, dizziness, headache, GI disturbances, rarely GI bleeding, hypersensitivity reactions
metaxalone (Skelaxin)	Oral tablets	Adult: 800 mg tid or qid Child: not established	Drowsiness, dizziness, headache, GI disturbances, paradoxic reactions
methocarbamol (Delaxin, Robaxacet, Robaxin, Robaxisal [methocarbamol and aspirin], *Can:* Tresortil)	Oral tablets and solutions for IM and IV injection	Adult: *Initially*, orally, 1.5–2 g qid for 48–72 h; *maintenance:* 1 g qid; IV, 1–3 g qd at rate of 3 ml/min; IM, 500 mg q8h Child: not established PC: C	Dizziness, drowsiness, headache, anorexia, nausea, rarely skin eruptions, signs of nephrotoxicity; after IV use metallic taste, diplopia, hypotension, bradycardia
cyclobenzaprine hydrochloride (Flexeril)	Oral tablets	Adult: 10 mg tid; maximum dosage: 60 mg qd PC: B	Drowsiness, dryness of mouth, dizziness, blurred vision, arrhythmia, urinary retention, constipation, unpleasant taste
orphenadrine citrate (Norflex, Norgesic, Norgesic Forte [orphenadrine, aspirin, caffeine])	Oral tablets, prolonged-release tablets, and solutions for IM and IV injection	Adult: orally, 100 mg bid; IM or IV, 60 mg bid PC: C	Dryness of mouth, blurred vision, drowsiness, dizziness, tachycardia, urinary retention, constipation

KEY: PC = pregnancy category. (The validity of pregnancy risk categories has not been established; see Chapter 16, p 216.)

Can = Canadian trade name.

Carisoprodol is chemically related to meprobamate. In addition to its other adverse reactions, it has been responsible for idiosyncratic reactions occasionally after initial administration (*eg*, extreme asthenia, transient quadriplegia, dizziness, ataxia, diplopia, agitation, confusion, disorientation). In addition, it is contraindicated in clients with acute intermittent porphyria.

Chlorphenesin contains F D and C yellow #5 dye, (containing tartrazine); tartrazine has produced allergic reactions in asthmatics and especially in those who exhibit asthmatic symptoms when they are allergic to aspirin.

Chlorzoxazone is a benzoxazole derivative and, thus, is chemically distinct from others in this class. Hepatotoxic symptoms have been reported, but a causal relationship has not been established. Clients who receive this drug should be monitored closely for signs of liver damage; it should be used cautiously in clients with a history of liver disease. The symptoms resemble a viral hepatitis.

Chlorzoxazone may discolor urine orange or purple-red.

Metaxalone should not be administered to clients with a tendency toward drug-induced, hemolytic, or other kinds of anemia. It is contraindicated in clients with liver disease or impaired renal function. Liver function tests should be ordered periodically while this medication is being administered.

Methocarbamol may be given intramuscularly (IM), although this route is uncommon. IM injections may be uncomfortable or painful.

Intravenously, methocarbamol may be administered undiluted directly into the vein at a maximum rate of 300 mg (3 ml) per minute. It may also be administered as an IV infusion of 0.9% sodium chloride solution or 5% dextrose solution (1 g diluted in 250 ml). When injected, methocarbamol has caused a metallic taste in the mouth, diplopia, hypotension, and bradycardia. The injectable form should not be administered to clients with known or suspected renal pathology, because of the polyethylene glycol 300 in the vehicle. Polyethylene glycol 300 by itself has been known to increase preexisting acidosis and urea retention in clients with renal impairment. If methocarbamol is used parenterally for more than 3 days, even if no known or suspected renal pathology exists, renal function should be monitored because of the nephrotoxicity of the polyethylene glycol 300.

The injectable form is also not recommended for epileptics, because the onset of seizures during IV administration has been reported.

Care should be taken to avoid extravasation of the hypertonic solution, which may result in thrombophlebitis. The client should be in a recumbent position for 10 to 15 minutes after the injection to reduce the likelihood of fainting, syncope, or hypotension.

Methocarbamol may darken urine that has stood for a period to brown, black, or green.

Cyclobenzaprine and orphenadrine

These two drugs are somewhat pharmacodynamically different from others in the skeletal muscle relaxant class, but the therapeutic uses are basically the same. The pharmacokinetics, dosage and administration, and adverse reactions are reviewed in Table 39-1.

Cyclobenzaprine is structurally related to the tricyclic antidepressants (amitriptyline). Its antidepressant effects are thought to be minimal. It acts neither at the neuromuscular junction nor directly on skeletal muscle. It acts at the level of the brain stem rather than the spinal cord, and it reduces motor neuron efferent activity.

One study showed that clients with fibrositis who took cyclobenzaprine experienced a significant decrease in the severity of pain, the total number of areas of tenderness, and muscle tightness. They also showed a significant increase in the quality of sleep (Bennett, et al, 1988). The fibrositis–fibromyalgia syndrome is a common form of nonarticular rheumatism. Unlike other rheumatic diseases, symptoms have not been shown to be very responsive to analgesics, nonsteroidal anti-inflammatory drugs, or even corticosteroids.

Orphenadrine is an analog of diphenhydramine. It may reduce skeletal muscle spasm through action in the cerebral motor centers or medulla. It does not have direct skeletal muscle relaxant activity.

The adverse reactions for cyclobenzaprine and orphenadrine are mainly due to their anticholinergic properties. Therefore, they should be used cautiously in clients with angle-closure glaucoma or prostatic hypertrophy. Cyclobenzaprine is contraindicated during the recovery from myocardial infarction because of certain cardiotoxic effects that have been identified.

Cyclobenzaprine may interact with monoamine oxidase inhibitors. It may enhance the effects of alcohol, barbiturates, and other CNS depressants.

A few instances of tremors, confusion, and anxiety have been reported when orphenadrine and propoxyphene have been used together. Hypoglycemic reactions have developed when propoxyphene or a phenothiazine was given concomitantly.

Learning experience 39-1

Interview a client who is receiving a skeletal muscle relaxant on a regular basis. Determine what methods of pain relief the client uses in addition to the medication prescribed. Carry out a pain assessment before the next ordered dose of medication and reassess the client's pain about 1 to 2 hours after medication. Write your assessments and prepare conclusions about the medication's effectiveness with this client.

Antispastic agents

Centrally acting antispastic agents

Baclofen

Pharmacodynamics. Gamma-aminobutyric acid (GABA) is an inhibitory neurotransmitter. Baclofen (Lioresal) is a derivative of GABA, and its mechanism of action is not completely understood. It does not have a direct effect on the neuromuscular junction. Research indicates that two GABA receptors exist (GABA-A and GABA-B). Baclofen may act as an agonist at GABA-B (bicuculline-insensitive) receptors found in the CNS and in the spinal cord. Its major site of action appears to be the spinal cord; it diminishes the transmission of monosynaptic extensor and polysynaptic flexor reflexes in the spinal cord. Among other actions, it may inhibit the release of excitatory transmitters, glutamic and aspartic acids, from primary afferent fibers.

Pharmacokinetics. The onset of this drug is variable; peak action is at 2 hours; duration of action is between 6 and 8 hours; and the half-life is 3 to 4 hours. This agent is excreted in the urine and feces.

Therapeutic uses. It relieves some of the components of spinal spasticity: involuntary flexor and extensor spasms and resistance to passive movements. It is useful in multiple sclerosis and in traumatic lesions of the spinal cord (paraplegia). It is not useful with spasms that follow cerebrovascular accidents or that occur with Parkinson's disease or Huntington's disease.

It has been used with clients with focal dystonic movements, including torticollis (wryneck). It has been used in Miege's syndrome (blepharospasm–oromandibular dystonia) and in stiff-man syndrome and Moersch-Woltmann syndrome. The latter syndrome is characterized by muscular rigidity, predominantly in men, that is accompanied by paroxysmal painful spasms precipitated by physical and emotional stimuli.

Diaphoresis and tachycardia accompany the spasms. The sensory system and intellect are not affected.

Intrathecal infusion has been studied for long-term treatment of clients whose spasticity is not adequately controlled by oral administration (in multiple sclerosis and with spinal cord traumatic lesions). A surgically implanted pump has been used to deliver the baclofen.

It is considered by some as the drug of choice in the treatment of trigeminal neuralgia (Fromm, 1990).

Hiccups are abrupt involuntary contractions or spasms of the diaphragmatic muscles. It has been found that baclofen is effective in the treatment of intractable hiccups that have proven unresponsive to more conventional therapy (Burke, White, 1988).

Adverse reactions. The adverse reactions are outlined in Table 39-2.

Baclofen is poorly tolerated by the elderly. The threshold for seizures may be lowered by baclofen in epileptics; reports have been conflicting on this point.

Asymptomatic increases in aspartate aminotransferase (AST), alanine aminotransferase (ALT), and alkaline phosphatase and serum glucose levels have occurred.

The drug reduces the rigidity of flexor muscles. At the same time, however, it lessens extensor muscle spasticity of the lower limbs. The loss of this reflex response can reduce some clients' ability to walk, because they have greater difficulty balancing themselves while standing. Thus, the drug should be used with caution when spasticity actually appears to sustain posture, balance, or function.

Low doses should be used for those with impaired renal function. The effects of baclofen may intensify the effects of CNS depressants, such as alcohol and barbiturates.

To discontinue, the drug's dosage should be reduced gradually over 1 to 2 weeks. Sudden or abrupt withdrawal after long-term administration causes a rebound increase in number of flexor spasms. Also, auditory and visual hallucinations, paranoid ideation, agitated behavior, and seizures (especially in clients with cerebral lesions) have occurred with abrupt withdrawal.

Benzodiazepines

This group of drugs includes diazepam (Valium). These drugs are discussed in detail in Chapters 25 and 26. Diazepam has an antispastic action in addition to its antianxiety and convulsant properties. It depresses the CNS, probably by potentiating GABA or GABA-mediated presynaptic inhibition. It probably produces skeletal muscle relaxation by inhibiting spinal polysynaptic afferent pathways. It also depresses neurons in the reticular ascending system that mediate wakefulness.

Therapeutic uses. Diazepam has been administered for a wide variety of musculoskeletal problems that involve pain and muscle spasm. It has been used with spasticity caused by upper motor neuron disorders, such as spinal cord lesions, multiple sclerosis, and cerebral palsy.

Unlike dantrolene, it does not relax peripheral muscles and cause weakness, so it may be appropriate for clients with borderline muscle strength.

Its central side effects (*eg*, drowsiness, lethargy) may make it less useful in certain clients with spasticity. It has been used in stiff-man syndrome, but it often produces sedation at the doses required.

When given IV, it is a useful adjunct in muscle spasms caused by tetanus toxin or strychnine. Its

Table 39-2. Antispastic agents

Drug name	Preparation	Usual dosage	Adverse reactions
Centrally acting antispastic agent			
baclofen (Liovesal, *Can:* Alpha-Baclofen)	Oral tablets and capsules	Adult: *Initially*, 5 mg bid; dose increases made every 3 days based on client response; maximum dosage: 20 mg qid Child: 1–1.5 mg/kg qd PC: C	Drowsiness, insomnia, dizziness, weakness, ataxia, confusion, fatigue, nausea
Peripherally acting antispastic agent			
dantrolene (Dantrium)	Oral capsules, suspension, and solutions for IV injection	Adult: *Initially*, 25 mg qd; dose increases made every 4 to 7 days based on client response; maximum dosage: 400 mg qd Child: 0.5 mg/kg bid; increased to a maximum of 3 mg/kg qid PC: C	Weakness in nonspastic muscles, drowsiness, dizziness, malaise, fatigue, diarrhea, hepatotoxicity, anorexia, nausea, vomiting, acne-like rash

KEY: PC = Pregnancy category. (The validity of pregnancy risk categories has not been established; see Chapter 16, p 216.)
Can = Canadian trade name.

anticonvulsant property has made it useful in status epilepticus.

Valium is available as 2-mg, 5-mg, and 10-mg tablets; in 2-ml and 10-ml ampules for injection; and in 15-mg slow-release capsules (Valrelease). The pharmacokinetics, dosage and administration, adverse reactions, and nursing implications of the benzodiazepines are discussed in Chapter 26.

Peripherally acting antispastic agents

Dantrolene

Dantrolene (Dantrium), unlike the drugs discussed earlier in this chapter, exerts its effects directly on skeletal muscle tissue.

Pharmacodynamics. Dantrolene does not change the electric properties of skeletal muscle membranes, nor does it block the transmission of spinal motor nerve impulses at the myoneural junction in skeletal muscles. However, it produces skeletal muscle relaxation by acting directly on excitation–contraction coupling within each muscle fiber. It is thought to inhibit the release of calcium ions from the sarcoplasmic reticulum. The release of calcium is the fiber's usual response to excitation by nerve impulses and is necessary in activating the contractile response. Thus, dantrolene prevents activation of the contractile apparatus and diminishes the mechanical force of contraction.

Pharmacokinetics. The onset of action of this drug is 1 hour; peak action is at 4 hours; duration of action is about 8 hours; and the half-life is 9 hours. About 15% to 25% of this drug is excreted in the urine.

Therapeutic uses. Clients whose functional rehabilitation is retarded by spasticity may benefit from dantrolene. It has significantly reduced spasticity and has sustained this reduction for the majority of paraplegic and hemiplegic clients who have taken it. Mass reflex movements and abnormal resistance to passive stretch are reduced. About half of the clients with athetoid cerebral palsy and some with multiple sclerosis have also improved with dantrolene therapy. Tolerance to dantrolene's therapeutic effect has not been noted.

Some of the manifestations of improved function that result from dantrolene therapy are a greater ability to carry out the activities of daily living (washing, dressing, or feeding oneself), to exercise, to maintain posture and balance, and to use braces, all of which lessen the need for nursing care.

Dantrolene does produce a generalized weakness. In some clients, the ability to stay upright and to maintain balance actually depends on certain muscles remaining in a spastic state. Therefore, dantrolene's major usefulness may be with the more nonambulatory client with spasticity.

Dantrolene has also been effective in treating malignant hyperthermia. It may even be used prophylac-

tically in clients if this disorder is anticipated. Malignant hyperthermia is a genetically determined rare syndrome usually precipitated by the administration of neuromuscular-blocking agents and inhalation anesthetics during surgery. This syndrome is recognized by the presence of rapid and dangerous increase in body temperature, tachycardia, tachypnea, metabolic acidosis, skeletal muscle rigidity, cyanosis, mottling of the skin, and signs and symptoms of renal failure. Apparently, the symptoms are caused by an excessive release of calcium ions from the sarcoplasmic reticulum.

The increase in calcium activates acute catabolic processes. Dantrolene may interfere with the release of calcium from the sarcoplasmic reticulum to the myoplasm to reverse or attenuate the crisis situation. Before dantrolene was used for this condition, the mortality rate for malignant hyperthermia was 50% to 70%.

Dantrolene has been used on an investigational basis in neuroleptic malignant syndrome, heat stroke, and muscle rigidity from toxicity from cocaine and carbon monoxide. It should not be used in clients with amyotrophic lateral sclerosis because these clients have a low tolerance for the muscle weakness that dantrolene produces.

Dosage and administration. Dantrolene is available for oral use in capsules and as a suspension. It is available for IV use in vials that contain 20 mg dantrolene and 3,000 mg mannitol to be reconstituted with 60 ml sterile water for injection.

For the client with spasticity, when dantrolene is used orally, a general guideline mandates that, if benefits are not evident within 60 days, dantrolene should be discontinued.

For the client who experiences malignant hyperthermia, dantrolene is given by continuous rapid IV push. The beginning dose is 1 mg/kg body weight, and the administration is continued until symptoms subside or the maximum dose (10 mg/kg) has been reached. Oral administration of dantrolene (1–2 mg/kg four times a day) may be necessary for 1 to 3 days to prevent recurrence of the symptoms.

Adverse reactions. The adverse reactions are outlined in Table 39-2.

Adverse reactions are commonly seen with dantrolene therapy. One of the main problems is that dantrolene may cause persistent weakness in nonspastic muscles, resulting in slurring of speech, drooling, and enuresis. This weakness is probably an extension of its effect on skeletal muscle.

Diarrhea may be severe enough to require treatment, dose reduction, or even cessation of therapy. A gradual increase in dosage may help keep this and other adverse reactions under control.

Dantrolene may compound the effects of alcohol, barbiturates, and other CNS depressants.

Hepatotoxicity is a potential adverse reaction to dantrolene. Symptomatic hepatitis (fatal and nonfatal) has occurred. The incidence is greater in clients who take doses higher than 300 mg/day, in females, in clients older than 35 years of age, and in clients who are taking other medications (such as estrogens). Hepatotoxicity occurs most frequently between 3 and 12 months after initiation of therapy. Baseline data about liver function (AST, ALT, and alkaline phosphatase) should be obtained and the studies repeated periodically during dantrolene therapy.

Quinine

The bark of the cinchona tree contains more than 20 alkaloids, chief among which is quinine. The cinchona tree is found in certain regions of South America. The first written record of cinchona use appeared in 1633.

Pharmacodynamics. Quinine acts on skeletal muscle by increasing its refractory period through direct action on the muscle fiber, decreasing the excitability of the motor endplate region and affecting the distribution of calcium within the muscle fiber. It also has analgesic, antipyretic, and oxytocic effects.

Pharmacokinetics. Quinine is readily absorbed when given orally. Peak plasma concentrations occur within 1 to 3 hours, and the half-life is 4 to 5 hours. The subcutaneous and IM routes of administration are contraindicated because of the likelihood of local tissue damage (*eg*, pain and sterile abscesses).

Quinine is metabolized largely in the liver, and the metabolites are excreted mainly in urine. Small amounts are excreted in feces, bile, gastric juice, and saliva. If urine is acidic, renal excretion is twice as rapid as when urine is alkaline. Urinary alkalizers may increase quinine blood levels and cause toxicity.

Therapeutic uses. Until the 1930s, cinchona alkaloids were the only agents used for the specific treatment of malaria. Today, synthetic antimalarial drugs are available that are less toxic and more effective. Quinine is still needed, however, to treat resistant strains of plasmodia. It is used as an adjunct with pyrimethamine and sulfadiazine or tetracycline to treat chloroquine-resistant *Plasmodium falciparum.*

Quinine is also prescribed for clients who experience nocturnal leg cramps, including those associated with arthritis, diabetes, varicose veins, thrombophlebitis, arteriosclerosis, and certain foot deformities. These cramps occur at night when clients are recumbent. Some clients require only a brief period of quinine therapy to achieve long periods of freedom from leg cramps. However, in some cases, even large doses of quinine do not give relief.

Dosage and administration. For clients who experience nocturnal leg cramps, the quinine dose is 260 to 300 mg before bedtime. This dosage may be increased if needed by adding one dose after the evening meal.

For clients with chloroquine-resistant malaria, the usual oral dosage is 650 mg every 8 hours for 10 to 14 days. It is taken with food or after meals to decrease gastric irritation. The pregnancy category for quinine is X (see Chapter 16).

Adverse reactions. Quinine produces many different side effects. However, if only one or two tablets are used daily, as with nocturnal leg cramps, these manifestations are unlikely to occur unless the person is hypersensitive to the drug. For example, in a hypersensitive client, as little as 300 mg of quinine may produce tinnitus or other evidence of hypersensitivity. Other common signs and symptoms of hypersensitivity include extreme cutaneous flushing accompanied by intense pruritus, fever, gastric distress, dyspnea, and visual difficulties.

When quinine is given in full doses or over a period of time or when plasma levels exceed 10 to 12 g/ml, a cluster of symptoms called *cinchonism* occurs. The syndrome includes a variety of signs and symptoms, including tinnitus and decreased auditory acuity, headache, visual disturbances, nausea, diarrhea, and other signs of gastrointestinal (GI) irritation, hematologic changes, and evidence of neurotoxicity. These signs and symptoms usually subside when the drug is discontinued.

Interactions. Quinine has been identified as interacting with digoxin, digitoxin, aluminum-containing antacids, neuromuscular-blocking agents, warfarin, and urinary alkalinizers.

■ Summary

No completely satisfactory therapy for relaxing skeletal muscles or treating spasticity exists. Sometimes with some of the drugs, it cannot be determined whether relief is provided through their muscle-relaxing properties or through their sedative effects. Skeletal muscle relaxants include mephenesin and related drugs (carisoprodol, chlorphenesin, chlorzoxazone, metaxalone, methocarbamol), orphenadrine, and cyclobenzaprine. Antispastic agents include centrally acting agents (baclofen and benzodiazepines) and peripherally acting agents (dantrolene and quinine).

Nursing management

Nursing implications

Clients who receive antispastic agents frequently require long-term nursing care and support.

Nursing process

Assessment Nurses should assess clients for underlying conditions that may create problems when taking skeletal muscle relaxants or antispastic agents. For example, metaxalone and parenteral methocarbamol should not be administered to clients with known renal pathology. Chlorzoxazone, metaxalone, and dantrolene are not advised for clients with known hepatic impairment. Epilepsy is a contraindication for use of parenteral methocarbamol. Angle-closure glaucoma or prostate hypertrophy are contraindications for cyclobenzaprine and orphenadrine.

Nurses should assess clients for a history of sensitivity to medication, because allergic reactions have occurred with carisoprodol, chlorphenesin, and chlorzoxazone.

Cyclobenzaprine may interact with monoamine oxidase inhibitors, and death has occurred. Therefore, nurses should be certain that clients who are taking cyclobenzaprine have not taken a monoamine oxidase inhibitor within 14 days before initiation of cyclobenzaprine and that the concurrent use of these agents is not planned.

When conducting the physical examination, nurses should assess the neuromuscular function of clients who are taking any skeletal muscle relaxants (*eg*, gait, muscle coordination and strength, areas of spasticity, posture, and ability to carry out activities of daily living).

Nursing diagnosis   Many clients who receive skeletal muscle relaxants or antispastic agents are being treated for herniated lumbosacral disc, multiple sclerosis, or paraplegia. Nursing diagnoses that may apply include the following:

> Constipation
> Altered urinary elimination
> Impaired physical mobility
> Self-care deficit
> Impaired skin integrity
> Self-esteem disturbance
> Altered sexuality patterns
> Ineffective individual coping
> Ineffective family coping
> Impaired home maintenance management

Planning   In preparing a plan of client care, the nurse should set goals to eliminate constipation, attain urinary continence, achieve maximum physical mobility, perform self-care activities within physical limitations, maintain skin integrity, adapt to changes in body function and level of independence, perceive self as sexually adequate and acceptable, use effective coping skills, and reduce pain.

Interventions   Clients require extra supervision because of the drowsiness and dizziness that may occur when several of these agents are being taken concurrently. If the client is in a wheelchair, the nurse should provide adequate body support or use restraining methods to prevent the client from falling from or tipping the wheelchair.

When methocarbamol or dantrolene is administered IV, the nurse should be aware of the special instructions to follow to avoid extravasation of the drug into subcutaneous tissues.

When methocarbamol is administered IV, the nurse should advise the client to remain in a recumbent position for 10 to 15 minutes after the injection to reduce the likelihood of fainting, syncope, or hypotension. The client should be assisted with ambulatory activities (as allowed) for at least 2 hours after IV administration. If CNS effects are severe, the client should remain recumbent until the effects decrease.

If dry mouth is an adverse reaction to the agent being administered (such as with cyclobenzaprine), relief may be obtained by sips of water, ice chips, chewing gum, or hard candy.

Liver function tests (AST, ALT, and alkaline phosphatase) are performed before onset of therapy with chlorzoxazone, metaxalone, and dantrolene and periodically thereafter during treatment. The nurse should monitor the results for evidence of hepatotoxicity.

Quinine may be given with the evening meal and a bedtime snack to minimize any GI upset. Capsule contents should not be emptied or tablets crushed and added to food, because the drug has a bitter taste and is irritating to the stomach. An oral suspension is available if there is difficulty in swallowing the capsule or tablet.

Client education.   Mephenesin-related drugs, cyclobenzaprine, baclofen, and dantrolene are capable of causing drowsiness and dizziness. Nurses should tell clients about these effects and advise against driving a motor vehicle or performing potentially hazardous tasks, such as operating machinery, if such reactions occur. These effects should pass after the client has become accustomed to the medication.

Methocarbamol, cyclobenzaprine, baclofen, and dantrolene may compound the effects of alcohol, barbiturates, and other CNS depressants. Clients should be advised to avoid such combinations, including the use of nonprescription preparations (*eg*, liquid cough medications) that contain alcohol.

Since clients who receive quinine may experience nausea, vomiting, and epigastric pain, the nurse should suggest that the medication be taken with food.

Sudden withdrawal of baclofen after prolonged administration may cause hallucinations and exacerbate spasticity. Therefore, if it has been determined that the drug should be discontinued because of its limited efficacy, the drug's withdrawal should be gradual.

Because some clients experience continued relief from nocturnal leg cramps after only a short period of treatment with quinine, it may be appropriate to discuss the possibility of a quinine-free period with the physician and client as part of the program evaluation.

Example of nursing process and treatment for spasticity

The client is a 24-year-old man who 2 years ago sustained a complete spinal cord transection at T9–10. Over the last 2 months, he has had increased difficulty with spasticity in his legs, to the degree that it disrupts his exercise program and daily living. He has been receiving baclofen 15 mg three times a day, which is now being discontinued gradually.

He has a neurogenic bladder and has been practicing intermittent self-catheterization every 6 hours. Now he has developed symptoms of a urinary tract infection (UTI). He is admitted to the hospital for treatment of the UTI and for a trial with a different antispastic medication.

It is August, and the client was scheduled to begin community college in September. He is irritable and expresses anger at the staff. He speaks briefly about having "no control" over his situation and about being frustrated about his inability to perform previously mastered activities.

Before hospitalization, he had been receiving Mandelamine 1 g four times a day and Dulcolax rectal suppositories every other morning. The Mandelamine is temporarily discontinued when he enters the hospital. A urine specimen is obtained for culture, and he is started on ampicillin 500 mg IV by saline lock every 6 hours, pending results of the culture.

Assessment data	Nursing diagnosis	Intervention	Goals and outcome criteria
Complete transection of spinal cord at level T9–10 2 years ago	High risk for injury: development of contractures related to immobility of joints	**Avoid** stimulation of extremities (*eg*, avoid loud noises or sudden movements near client, avoid touching client when he is asleep, do not jar bed).	The client will maintain normal range of motion.
Increased spasticity in legs over last months		**Position** lower extremities in extension if client can tolerate.	The client will resume exercise program.
Exercise program and daily activities disrupted		**Administer** baclofen as follows: day 1, 10 mg tid; day 2, 10 mg bid; day 3, 5 mg tid; day 4, 5 mg bid; and day 5, 5 mg.	The client will participate as possible in self-care.
Receiving baclofen 15 mg tid		**Exercise** legs (support extremities thoroughly, perform all movements slowly and smoothly, and do this after nighttime stiffness has loosened up).	
		Start dantrolene 25 mg tid on day 6 and observe for drowsiness, dizziness, weakness, malaise, fatigue, and diarrhea.	
Irritable	Powerlessness related to hospitalization due to complications of spinal cord transection	**Encourage** verbalization of concerns about feelings of powerlessness.	The client will participate in decision-making about care.
Expresses anger at staff		**Provide** situations in which client can succeed and experience control.	The client will participate as possible in self-care.
Speaks of having "no control" over his situation and of frustration about inability to perform previously mastered activities		**Provide** positive reinforcement and acknowledgment for active participation in own care.	The client will resume optimal level of psychological control.
		Sensitize staff and significant others to the importance of their reaction to client's situation.	

(Continued)

Example of nursing process and treatment for spasticity (*Continued*)

Assessment data	Nursing diagnosis	Intervention	Goals and outcome criteria
Neurogenic bladder from spinal cord transection Self-catheterization program every 6 hours Use of Mandelamine before admission Current UTI symptoms	Altered urinary elimination related to neurogenic bladder and UTI symptoms	**Administer** ampicillin 500 mg IV every 6 hours. **Monitor** for therapeutic and adverse effects. **Force** fluids (240 ml) each hour between 7 AM and 7 PM. **Reinforce** previous teaching about technique during self-catheterization. **Assist** with perineal care every shift and after each bowel movement. **Maintain** acidic urine by encouraging client to increase intake of foods and fluids that form an acid ash (*eg*, cranberry and prune juice, poultry, fish, grapes) and decrease intake of foods that tend to alkalinize urine (*eg*, milk, carbonated beverages, many fruits and vegetables). **Administer** ascorbic acid as ordered.	The client will no longer exhibit UTI symptoms, as evidenced by clear urine, no unusual odor to urine, absence of frequency of urination, absence of chills and fever, absence of bacteria and white blood cells in urine, and negative urine culture.

Evaluation The nurse must evaluate the client to determine drug efficacy and to observe for evidence of adverse reactions. It is important to establish whether real benefit has been achieved. Data that indicate drug efficacy include client statements about pain relief, decreased frequency or severity of spasms, increased mobility, increased ability to carry out daily activities, decreased flexor spasms and muscle rigidity on physical examination as compared with data base, increased range of motion, decreased intensity or degree of nursing care required, and increased ease of positioning client's extremities properly.

Checklist of nursing actions

☐ When mephenesin-related drugs, cyclobenzaprine, orphenadrine, baclofen, or dantrolene are prescribed, advise clients about the possibility of drowsiness and dizziness, as well as the necessity of avoiding potentially hazardous tasks.

☐ Assess clients for underlying conditions that may create problems with the administration of mephensin-related drugs, cyclobenzaprine, orphenadrine, baclofen, or dantrolene.

☐ Watch for idiosyncratic reactions during the early period of carisoprodol therapy.

☐ Watch for allergic reactions with carisoprodol, chlorphenesin, and chlorzoxazone.

☐ Check that liver function tests are performed periodically during chlorzoxazone, dantrolene, and metaxalone therapies.

☐ Take special precautions when assisting with IV administration of methocarbamol and dantrolene to avoid extravasation of the drug into subcutaneous tissues.

☐ Teach the client the benefits to expect from the drugs and the adverse reactions that may occur (see Example of Nursing Process and Treatment for Spasticity).

References

Bennett RM, Gatter RA, Campbell SM, Andrews RP, Clark SR, Scarola JA. (1988). A comparison of cyclobenzaprine and placebo in the management of fibrositis. *Arthritis Rheum, 31*(12), 1535–1542.

Burke AM, White AB. (1988). Baclofen for intractable hiccups. *N Engl J Med, 319*, 1354.

Department of Drugs, Division of Drugs and Toxicology.

(1990). *Drug Evaluations Annual*. Milwaukee, WI: American Medical Association.

Fromm GH. (1990). Clinical pharmacology of drugs used to treat head and face pain. *Neurol Clin, 8*(1), 143–151.

Bibliography

Basmajian JV. (1989). Acute back pain and spasm. *Spine, 14*(4), 438–439.

Davidoff RA. (1985). Antispasticity drugs: Mechanisms of action. *Ann Neurol, 17*, 107–116.

Drug Facts and Comparisons. (1991). St. Louis: Facts and Comparisons Division, JB Lippincott.

Gilman AG, et al, eds. (1990). *Goodman and Gilman's the pharmacological basis of therapeutics*, 8th ed. New York: Pergamon Press.

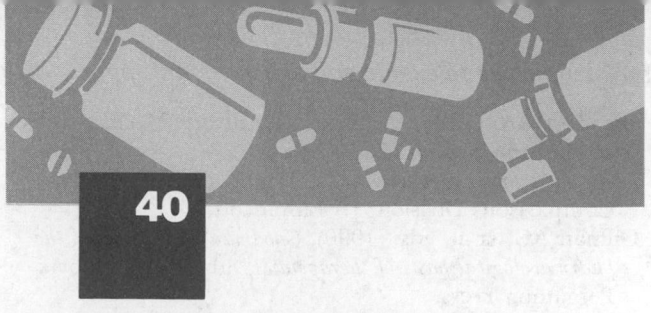

40

Drugs that affect the kidneys: diuretics

Diuretics are drugs that induce loss of body fluid by increasing the production of urine by the kidneys. Because the body's fluid balance is affected significantly by sodium ions, losing fluid usually involves increasing the kidney's excretion of sodium; thus sodium loss is the primary mechanism by which many diuretics act.

Although diuretics have a long history of effectively treating edema, many of the drugs presently used were unknown a generation ago. These newer drugs, which are more potent and generally safer than older preparations, have replaced the early diuretics.

Physiology of the kidneys

The urinary tract is the system responsible for maintaining chemical homeostasis of the blood. The kidneys eliminate excess fluids, electrolytes, and nitrogenous wastes, as well as toxins that find their way into the body. By selectively excreting unneeded chemicals, the kidneys keep the body's blood chemistry properly balanced.

The functional unit of the kidney is the nephron. The nephron is composed of a glomerulus, which filters fluid from the blood, and a tubule, in which the filtrate is converted into urine (Fig. 40-1). Blood enters the glomerulus through the afferent arteriole. As the blood passes through the capillaries, hydrostatic pressure causes fluid to filter into Bowman's capsule. This filtrate resembles interstitial fluid; it contains electrolytes and other solutes but normally has little protein and no red blood cells. As it moves through the tubule, it is separated from the blood by only two membranes, the tubular membrane and the vascular membrane. By selective movement of molecules across the tubular membrane, chemicals required by the body are reabsorbed, and waste products and toxins are concentrated in the tubule, transforming filtrate into urine.

Mechanisms of absorption and secretion in the tubule are complex and incompletely understood. However, they are known to differ in various segments of the tubule, correlating with the anatomic structure of the membrane. These segments and their physiologic function are outlined in Box 40-1. Molecules may be reabsorbed by either passive diffusion or carrier-mediated transport mechanisms. Secretion is accomplished by active transport processes. Tubule function is influenced by the hormones aldosterone and antidiuretic hormone and by the enzyme carbonic anhydrase (CAH).

Factors that influence the production of urine include glomerular filtration (which depends on hydrostatic pressure of the arteriolar blood), tubular reabsorption (which is affected by the rate of fluid flow through the tubule), and tubular secretion. The production of urine, therefore, can be altered by drugs that influence blood pressure, tubular active transport mechanisms, and tubular flow rate. Most diuretic drugs decrease reabsorption, increase fluid flow rates in the tubule, or do both.

Pathophysiology

Several pathologic conditions are characterized by excessive retention of sodium and fluid in the body. No matter what its etiology, fluid overload may result in

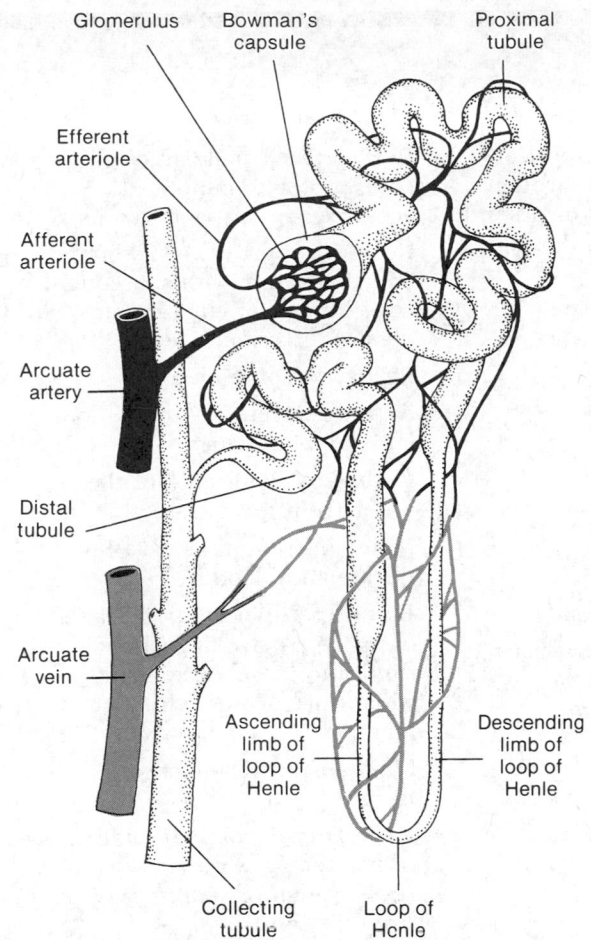

Glomerulus Bowman's Proximal
capsule tubule

Efferent
arteriole

Afferent
arteriole

Arcuate
artery

Distal
tubule

Arcuate
vein

Ascending Descending
limb of limb of
loop of loop of
Henle Henle

Collecting Loop of
tubule Henle

Figure 40-1. The nephron, the functional unit of the kidney.

hypervolemia, hypertension, and movement of fluid from the vascular network to interstitial spaces. As a result, the work load of the heart increases, tissue perfusion decreases, and the functioning of the organ systems (*eg*, lungs, gastrointestinal [GI] tract, liver, kidneys) may decline.

Heart disease

The most frequent life-threatening disease characterized by edema is heart disease. In this condition, fluid retention may result from several mechanisms: increased hydrostatic pressure in the vascular system (arterial or venous hypertension), increased secretion of glucocorticoid stress hormones that foster sodium and water retention, and excessive aldosterone production in response to cardiogenic shock. Kidney function is often compromised by hemodynamic changes: reduced hydrostatic pressure and reflex constriction of the afferent arterioles in cardiac shock impair glomerular filtration. A reduced tubular flow rate promotes the reabsorption of electrolytes and water in the kidney. Reversing fluid retention and reducing edema dramatically relieve symptoms and reduce some of the heart's work load. Diuresis may be directly responsible

for saving the life of a client in congestive heart failure, especially when pulmonary edema is present. For this reason, diuretics are used in the treatment of both acute and chronic cardiac conditions.

Nephrosis and hepatic cirrhosis

Although the edemas of nephrosis and hepatic cirrhosis are primarily due to depletion of serum proteins and the resulting loss of vascular oncotic holding power, sodium retention stimulated by reduced blood volume also plays a causative role. For this reason, diuretics are helpful in these conditions.

Other conditions

Other conditions in which diuretics may be beneficial include water retention associated with premenstrual syndrome, hypertension, obesity, and asthma. The prevention of fluid retention is important in controlling epilepsy (since edema in the brain can stimulate seizure activity) and in adrenal steroid therapy. Diuresis is also useful in conditions associated with increased intracranial or intraocular pressure, because general reduction of body fluid levels are reflected in these compartments of the body.

Drugs used as diuretics

Many substances increase urine production by the normal kidney, including dietary components such as water, osmotically active salts and sugars, and xanthines (caffeine, theobromine). Drugs used therapeutically include CAH inhibitors, osmotic diuretics, thiazides, a hormone antagonist, and several other compounds. They are best classified in relation to their predominant effects on kidney function.

Most diuretics act by decreasing reabsorption of electrolytes or water in the renal tubule. The resulting increase in tubular fluid flow rate further interferes with salt reabsorption by reducing tubular transit time (Fig. 40-2). A general principle in diuretic therapy, therefore, is that certain chemicals, in addition to water, are lost by the body. Many of the serious adverse effects of diuretic therapy are related to electrolyte imbalance.

Agents that increase glomerular filtration
Fluids

When kidney function is impaired owing to hypovolemic shock, the administration of fluids may raise the hydrostatic pressure in the glomerulus and restore function by promoting glomerular filtration. The subsequent dilution of urine in the tubule also helps protect the renal tissues from chemical damage sometimes caused by very concentrated urine. Fluids are chosen to correct electrolyte imbalances that may be present.

Overhydration also increases glomerular filtration

Box 40-1. Physiologic segments of the renal tubule

Segment	Characteristics	Effects on filtrate
Proximal tubule (from the glomerular membrane to the thin portion of the loop of Henle)	Capable of active transport of many substances (reabsorption of nutrients and electrolytes and secretion of hydrogen ions and drugs) Freely permeable to water	Reabsorbs virtually all of glucose, protein, amino acids, acetoacetate ions, and vitamins Reabsorbs part of the sodium and potassium, with subsequent reabsorption of chloride ions by passive diffusion Reabsorbs some urea Actively secretes hydrogen ions and common drugs Reabsorbs about 65% of the water from the filtrate Maintains isotonicity between filtrate and blood
Descending portion of the thin segment of the loop of Henle	Highly permeable to water Moderately permeable to ions such as sodium and urea	Produces a hypertonic filtrate owing to passive diffusion of fluid into the hypertonic interstitial fluid of the kidney medulla
Ascending portion of the thin segment of the loop of Henle	Less permeable to water and urea than descending portion	Maintains hypertonicity of filtrate
Distal tubule diluting segment (from the thick portion of the ascending loop of Henle to about the midpoint of the distal convoluted tubule)	Capable of active transport of chloride ions Relatively impervious to water	Actively transports chloride ions out of tubule (with subsequent reabsorption of sodium by passive diffusion) Renders the filtrate hypotonic
Late distal tubule (from the midpoint of the distal convoluted tubule to the collecting tubule)	Capable of actively reabsorbing sodium and secreting potassium in response to the hormone aldosterone	Adjusts concentration of sodium and potassium ions in the filtrate
Collecting tubule	Variably permeable to water, depending on the presence of antidiuretic hormone (ADH)	Concentrates urine

in normal people. The administration of fluids in excess of homeostatic needs increases fluid flow in the tubule, decreases required tubule transit time, and reduces overall reabsorption of electrolytes. Because of this secondary depletion of electrolytes, fluid loss tends to exceed intake, resulting in a net loss of both fluids and electrolytes.

Fluid diuresis is contraindicated in people with hypervolemia and edema. It is not used therapeutically except for the administration of fluids to correct hypovolemic shock. Fluids used for this purpose may include sodium solutions, which are contraindicated in most clinical situations that require diuresis.

Xanthines

Xanthines (theophylline, theobromine, caffeine) induce diuresis by several mechanisms. Their cardio-tonic and vasopressor effects increase blood flow and glomerular filtration. They also reduce sodium and chloride reabsorption in the proximal tubule. The diuretic effect of xanthines is not pronounced, and their usefulness is limited because of their stimulant actions on the central nervous system (CNS). The diuretic effect of xanthines, although weak, may be additive with that of other diuretics. Xanthine drugs are discussed in more detail in Chapters 23 and 37.

Osmotic diuretics

A number of substances can increase water excretion by osmotic action. To be useful, these agents must be freely filterable in the glomerulus, not readily reabsorbed by the renal tubule, and otherwise pharmacologically inert.

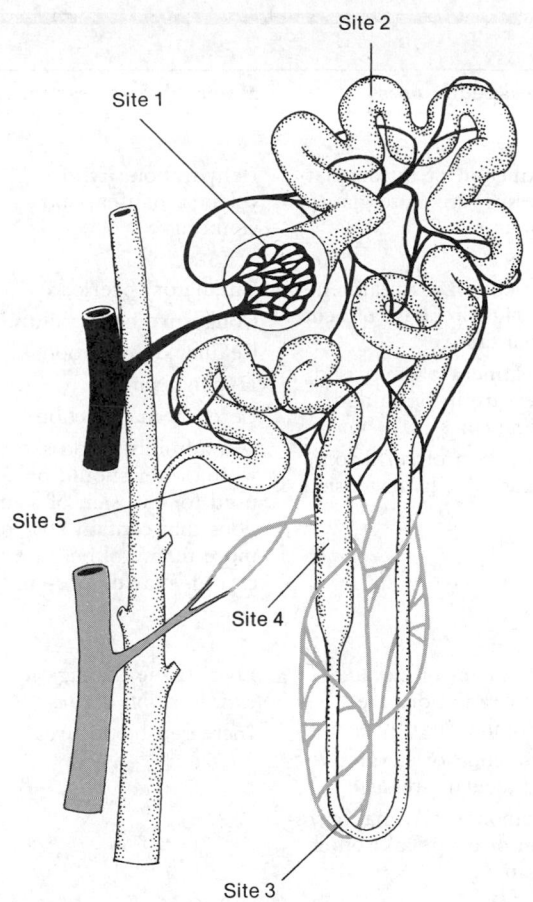

Figure 40-2. Sites of diuretic action. (*Site 1*) Renal vasculature. Agents that increase renal blood flow or renal artery hydrostatic pressure also increase glomerular filtration rate. (*Site 2*) Proximal tubule. Agents that decrease electrolyte reabsorption in the proximal tubule allow a large volume of filtrate to pass through to the distal tubule. (*Site 3*) Loop of Henle. High-ceiling diuretics reduce electrolyte reabsorption in the ascending loop of Henle. (*Site 4*) Diluting segment. Agents that decrease chloride reabsorption in the diluting segment allow both sodium and chloride to pass through to the distal tubule. (*Site 5*) Distal tubule. Drugs may interfere with sodium reabsorption or may block the effects of aldosterone at this site.

Pharmacodynamics. A high concentration of solute molecules in the renal tubule increases osmotic pressure within the tubule, inhibiting diffusion of water from the tubule to the blood vessels of the nephron. This action increases the volume of fluid in the tubule and accelerates fluid flow. Reabsorption of electrolytes is reduced secondarily. Osmotic diuretics also dilute the waste products in urine, which may damage the kidney due to excessive concentration.

Pharmacokinetics. Osmotic diuretics may be administered orally or intravenously (IV). After absorption into the bloodstream, they filter freely through the glomerulus and are excreted in urine.

Therapeutic uses. Osmotic diuretics are used to prevent acute renal failure during prolonged surgery or trauma; to prevent increased cerebral, cerebrospi-

nal, or intraocular pressures during surgery, trauma, or disease; and to reduce intraocular pressure rapidly in acute glaucoma.

Osmotic preparations in common use are glycerol (glycerin) and mannitol (Table 40-1). Glycerol is given orally just before eye surgery to decrease intraocular pressure. While in the blood vessels, glycerol's osmotic holding power promotes water movement into the intravascular space. By this mechanism, water is removed from the vitreous fluid of the eye. Although a part of the glycerol is metabolized by the body as calories, some is excreted, carrying water with it. Mannitol is the osmotic diuretic most commonly used to prevent renal failure. It is usually administered by IV infusion.

Adverse reactions. Osmotic diuretics tend to induce nausea and vomiting and produce headache, water intoxication, and electrolyte imbalance. Pulmonary edema or intraocular hemorrhage can occur. When administered IV, they tend to cause phlebitis because they are irritating; if allowed to infiltrate, they produce pronounced tissue edema and may cause sloughing.

Mannitol can accumulate if kidney function is not restored. Mannitol toxicity is characterized by cellular dehydration, extracellular fluid overload, and hyponatremia. Pulmonary edema, congestive heart failure, and significant cerebral dysfunction can develop.

Precautions and contraindications. Because osmotic diuretics temporarily increase blood volume, they cannot be used in impaired cardiac function or congestive heart failure. They are also contraindicated in active intracranial hemorrhage and severe dehydration.

Administration of mannitol should be preceded by a test dose for oliguric clients to determine whether the kidney is capable of responding to the drug. The test dose should raise the urinary output to about 30 ml/h. Therapeutic infusions should be adjusted to maintain a urinary output of about 100 ml/h. Mannitol cannot be given to clients with kidney failure (anuria), pulmonary edema, dehydration, or intracranial hemorrhage. The drug should be discontinued if renal function continues to decline or if heart failure or pulmonary edema develops. Removal of the drug by hemodialysis may be necessary.

Agents that act on the proximal tubule
Diuretics that act primarily on electrolyte reabsorption in the proximal tubule include xanthines and CAH inhibitors.

Carbonic anhydrase inhibitors
CAH is an enzyme that catalyzes the breakdown of carbonic acid into carbonate and hydrogen ions. These ions play a role in the excretion by the kidney of acid

(Text continues on p. 987)

Table 40-1. Representative diuretics

Drug name	Preparations	Usual dosage	Therapeutic uses	Major adverse reactions
Osmotic diuretics				
glycerin (Osmoglyn, Glyrol)	Oral solution	1–1.5 g/kg body weight once (or repeated at intervals of at least 5 h) PC: C	Reduction of intraocular pressure in acute glaucoma or before eye surgery	Dehydration, hypovolemia, nausea, and vomiting
mannitol (Isotol, Osmitrol, Resectisol)	Solutions for IV administration	Adults: Initial dosage for oliguria: 200 mg/kg body weight of 12.5 g as a 15% or 20% solution infused over 3–5 min; to prevent acute renal failure, 50–100 g, administered initially as a 15% or 20% solution and followed by a 5% or 10% solution Children: Dosage has not been established PC: C	Prevention or treatment of oliguric phase of acute renal failure Treatment of increased pressure in brain and spinal cord Reduction of refractory intraocular hypertension	Circulatory overload Congestive heart failure Cellular dehydration Hyponatremia Cerebral malfunction (An administration set with a filter should be used for infusion of solutions that contain 20% or more mannitol because crystals may be present)
urea (Ureaphil)	Solutions for IV administration Crystals for preparing IV solutions	500 mg–1.5 g/kg body weight/day administered as a 30% solution in dextrose or invert sugar solution PC: C	Treatment of elevated intracranial or cerebrospinal fluid pressure Reduction of elevated intraocular pressure Promotion of renal excretion of drugs and other toxins	Local tissue damage if extravasation occurs Increased blood urea nitrogen
Carbonic anhydrase inhibitor				
acetazolamide (AK-Zol, Diamox, Glaupax, Novozolamide, Oedemin, Storzolamide)	Oral tablets and extended-release capsules Solution for injection	Adults: 250–1000 mg daily, divided in 1–4 doses Children: 8–30 mg/kg body weight/day, divided in 3 doses PC: C	(As an adjunct) treatment of glaucoma and edema secondary to congestive heart failure, prevention of seizures during the premenstrual period in epileptics	Metabolic acidosis GI disturbance (nausea, vomiting, dry mouth, diarrhea or constipation, altered taste) CNS disturbances (confusion, depression, excitement, dizziness)
dichlorphenamid (Oratrol)	Oral tablets	Adults: 50–100 mg bid-tid PC: C	(As an adjunct) treatment of glaucoma	Same as above
methazolamide (Neptazane)	Oral tablets	100–300 mg daily, divided in 2–3 doses PC: C	Reduction of intraocular pressure in chronic simple glaucoma	Teratogenesis Bone marrow depression Paresthesia
Loop (high-ceiling) diuretics				
bumetanide (Bumex, Burimex)	Oral tablets Solutions for IM or IV injection	Adults: *Oral:* 0.5–2 mg; *Parenteral:* 0.5–1 mg q2–3h Maximum daily dosage: 10 mg Maintenance: 1–2 mg/day Children: 0.015 mg/kg body weight on alternate days—0.1 mg/kg body weight/day PC: C	Rapid diuresis in the treatment of edema when furosemide is contraindicated	Fluid and electrolyte depletion Ototoxicity

(Continued)

Table 40-1. Representative diuretics (Continued)

Drug name	Preparations	Usual dosage	Therapeutic uses	Major adverse reactions
ethacrynic acid (Edecrin, Hydromedin, Reomax, Taladren)	Oral tablets Solution for IV injection	Adults: *Oral:* 50–200 mg daily, divided in 1–2 doses; *IV:* 50–100 mg as a single dose PC: D	Rapid diuresis in the treatment of edema and as an adjunct in the treatment of hypertension	Fluid and electrolyte depletion Ototoxicity
furosemide (Furomide, Fursemide, Lasilix, Lasix, Novosemide, Seguril, Uritol)	Oral tablets Solutions for IM or IV injection	Adults: 20–600 mg daily, divided in 1–4 doses PC: C	Rapid diuresis in the treatment of edema and as an adjunct in the treatment of hypertension	Fluid and electrolyte depletion Deafness
Thiazide and related diuretics			Long-term therapy for chronic renal or hepatic disease, chronic congestive heart failure, and hypertension	Hypokalemia Hyperuricemia Hyperglycemia
bendroflumethiazide (Aprinox, Berkozide, Centyl, Naturetin, Neo-Naclex, Sodiuretic)	Oral tablets	Adults: 2.5–20 mg/day, divided in 1–2 doses Children: 0.05–0.4 mg/kg body weight or 1.5–12 mg/m² body surface/day, divided in 1–2 doses PC: B		
benzthiazide (Aquapres, Aquatag, Exna, Marazide, Proaqua, Urazide, Urease)	Oral tablets	Adults: 25–200 mg/day, divided in 1–2 doses Children: 1–4 mg/kg body weight or 30–120 mg/m² body surface/day, divided in 3 doses PC: D		
chlorothiazide (Chlotride, Diurigen, Diuril, Saluric)	Solution for IV injection Oral tablets and suspension	Adults: 500 mg–2 g daily, divided in 1–2 doses Children: 20–22 mg/kg body weight or 600 mg/m² body surface/day divided in 2 doses PC: D		
chlorthalidone (Bigroton, Chloride, Digroton, Hygroton, Novothalidone, Saluretic)	Oral tablets	Adults: 25–100 mg daily in a single dose Children: 2 mg/kg body weight or 60 mg/m² body surface, 3 times weekly PC: D		
cyclothiazide (Anhydron)	Oral tablets	Adults: *Initially:* 1–2 mg/day; *maintenance:* 1–2 mg, 2–3 times weekly Children: 0.02–0.04 mg/kg body weight or 0.6–1.2 mg/m² body surface/day, in a single dose		
hydrochlorothiazide (Apo-Hydro, Aquazide-H, Chlorzide, Diaqua, Direma, Diuchlor, Esidrix, Fluvin, Hydro-D, Hydro-Diuril, Hydromal, Hydro-Saluretic, Hydro-Z, Hydrozide, Hyperetic Lexor, Manuril, Mictrin, Momaril, Neo-Codena, Novohydrazide,	Oral tablets	Adults: 25–100 mg daily, divided in 1–3 doses Children: 2–2.2 mg/kg body weight or 60 mg/m² body surface/day, divided in 2 doses PC: D		

(Continued)

Table 40-1. Representative diuretics (Continued)

Drug name	Preparations	Usual dosage	Therapeutic uses	Major adverse reactions
Oretic, SK-Hydro-chlorothiazide, Thiuretic, Zide)				
hydroflumethiazide (Diucardin, Hydrenox, NaClex, Saluron)	Oral tablets	Adults: 25–200 mg/day in 1 or 2 doses Children: 1 mg/kg body weight or 30 mg/m² body surface/day, in a single dose PC: B		
methyclothiazide (Aquatensen, Diuretic, Enduron)	Oral tablets	Adults: 2.5–10 mg/day, in a single dose Children: 0.05–0.2 mg/kg body weight or 1.5–6 mg/m² body surface/day, in a single dose PC: D		
metolazone (Diulo, Mykrox, Zaroxolyn)	Oral tablets	Adults: 2.5–10 mg/day as a single dose PC: D		
polythiazide (Dren-usil, Nephril, Renese)	Oral tablets and capsules	Adults: 1–4 mg daily in a single dose Children: 0.02–0.08 mg/kg body weight or 2 mg/m² body surface/day in a single dose PC: D		
quinethazone (Hydromox)	Oral tablets	Adults: 50–100 mg/day, divided in 1–2 doses PC: D		
trichlormethiazide (Aquazide, Diurese, Metahydrin, Naqua, Trichlorex)	Oral tablets	Adults: 1–4 mg/day, divided in 1–2 doses Children: 0.07 mg/kg body weight or 2 mg/m² body surface/day, in single or divided doses PC: D		
Indolines				
indapamide (Lozide, Lozol, Natrilix)	Oral tablets	Adults: 2.5–5 mg/day as a single dose PC: B	Treatment of edema and hypertension	Hypokalemia Hyperuricemia Hypochloremic alkalosis
Potassium-sparing diuretics				
amiloride (Arumil, Colectril, Midamor, Modaide, Nilurid)	Oral tablets	Adults: 5–10 mg/day Children: 0.625 mg/kg body weight/day (safety and efficacy in children have not been established) PC: B	Treatment of steroid-induced edema, edema in which hypokalemia poses unusual risks, and edema associated with excessive aldosterone secretion	Hyperkalemia Hypotension Spironolactone can cause estrogen- or androgen-like side effects
spironolactone (Aldactone, Novospiroton)	Oral tablets	Adults: 100 mg daily, divided in 2–4 doses Children: 3.3 mg/kg body weight daily PC: D		
triamterene (Dyrenium, Dytac, Jatropur)	Oral capsules	Adult: *Initial maintenance:* 100 mg bid; 100 mg qd to qid Children: Dosage has not been established PC: D		

KEY: PC = pregnancy category. (The validity of pregnancy risk categories has not been established; see Chapter 16, p 216.)

urine and the reabsorption of sodium and potassium ions.

Three CAH inhibitors are available for use as diuretics (see Table 40-1). Acetazolamide is discussed as the prototype of this class.

Acetazolamide

Pharmacodynamics. Acetazolamide (Diamox) promotes sodium, potassium, and bicarbonate excretion by inhibiting the action of CAH, an enzyme vital for the active transport of ions across the proximal tubular membrane during reabsorption. Normally, CAH carries sodium, potassium, and bicarbonate ions across the membrane, picking up hydrogen ions on its return to the kidney tubule. Inactivation of the enzyme enhances excretion of electrolytes, secondarily reduces water reabsorption, and tends to lower the *p*H of body fluids. Inhibition of CAH is not limited to the renal tissues but occurs in other tissues, including the eyes, where it reduces the formation of vitreous humor.

Pharmacokinetics. Acetazolamide is administered orally, intramuscularly, or IV. It is well absorbed from the GI tract. After absorption, it is widely distributed throughout the tissues, especially the erythrocytes, plasma, kidneys, liver, muscles, eyes, and CNS. The drug is believed to cross the placenta and to be distributed into breast milk. Acetazolamide is secreted unchanged by the kidney tubule. Some is reabsorbed and redistributed in the blood. An average of 90% is eliminated within 24 hours of administration.

Therapeutic uses. CAH inhibitors have proved useful in controlling glaucoma, edema of congestive heart failure, and acute mountain sickness. In epilepsy, a moderate metabolic acidosis helps suppress seizures.

Adverse reactions. Inhibition of CAH reduces the kidneys' ability to excrete hydrogen ions. An inevitable side effect is some degree of metabolic acidosis. Other adverse reactions affect the GI system (anorexia, nausea, vomiting, diarrhea), the CNS (drowsiness, headache, confusion, depression, malaise, irritability, nervousness, excitement, dizziness, seizures, peripheral paresthesia, and signs of impaired innervation of the muscles), hematopoietic system (agranulocytosis, aplastic anemia, thrombocytopenia, leukopenia, hemolytic anemia), and renal system (dysuria, crystalluria, renal colic, and renal lesions). Uric acid excretion may be reduced, and gout may be exacerbated. Allergic reactions to acetazolamide include fever, rash, skin eruptions, urticaria, and pruritus.

Drug interactions. Acetazolamide increases excretion of lithium. Because it renders urine alkaline, it reduces the rate of excretion of some drugs (amphetamines, procainamide, quinidine, tricyclic antidepressants) and increases excretion of weak acids (phenobarbital and salicylates). Drugs that require an acid urine to be effective (methenamine compounds) may be ineffective when used concurrently with acetazolamide. CAH inhibitors may also augment the effects of other diuretics, possibly by displacing the drugs from binding sites. Because hypokalemia sometimes develops, acetazolamide may also interfere with the hypoglycemic response to insulin and oral antidiabetic agents and predispose to digitalis toxicity. Acetazolamide may hasten bone demineralization and accentuate impaired metabolism of calcium.

Precautions and contraindications. Electrolyte and acid–base balance and hematologic status should be monitored in clients who receive CAH inhibitors. Bicarbonate and potassium levels are of particular concern. Caution should be exercised when these drugs are used in respiratory conditions that predispose to respiratory acidosis and in diabetes mellitus. If blood dyscrasia develops, the drugs must be discontinued and appropriate treatment instituted. CAH inhibitors are contraindicated for people with hepatic disease, electrolyte (sodium and potassium) deficiencies, adrenal insufficiency, metabolic acidosis, or severe renal disease. They are not recommended for use during pregnancy.

Loop diuretics

Diuretics that act in the loop of Henle include furosemide, ethacrynic acid, and bumetanide.

Pharmacodynamics. The mode of action of the loop diuretics has not been clearly defined. They inhibit the reabsorption of sodium and chloride and decrease the absorption of other electrolytes in the ascending loop. They also increase potassium excretion by the distal tubule. Because of their powerful effects on fluid and electrolyte balance, these drugs are known as *high-ceiling diuretics*. Diuretic response is independent of acid–base balance.

Pharmacokinetics. Loop diuretics may be administered either orally or parenterally. They are well absorbed from the GI tract. Information on their distribution is incomplete. Ethacrynic acid may accumulate in the liver. The extent to which it crosses the placenta or appears in the milk of lactating mothers is unknown. Furosemide is about 95% bound to plasma proteins. These diuretics are concentrated and partially excreted by the kidneys. About 50% of ethacrynic acid is excreted in bile. Furosemide can also be metabolized by the liver when renal excretion is impaired. Bumetanide and its metabolites are excreted primarily in urine. After oral administration, these drugs act within 30 minutes to 1 hour, peak in about 2 hours, and have a duration of action of 6 to 8 hours.

Therapeutic uses. Loop diuretics are used in the treatment of edema associated with congestive heart failure, especially severe left-sided heart failure. They are also used in the treatment of edema associated with nephrotic syndrome or hepatic cirrhosis and ascites. Loop diuretics function as adjuncts in the treatment of renal failure and hypertension. Furosemide and ethacrynic acid have been also used to treat hypercalcemia.

Adverse reactions. Loop diuretics can cause rapid fluid and electrolyte depletion and metabolic alkalosis. Sodium, chlorine, potassium, calcium, magnesium, and phosphate deficiencies may develop. Hypovolemia may cause hypotension. Other adverse reactions include GI upset and ototoxicity. Deafness (either temporary or permanent) may occur. A variety of reactions that involve the hematopoietic system, CNS, liver, skin, and glucose balance have also been reported.

Furosemide can decrease the serum level and effectiveness of theophylline when the two drugs are used concurrently. Furosemide also raises blood levels of uric acid and increases the risk of acute gout, especially in elderly women.

Precautions and contraindications. Contraindications to the use of high-ceiling diuretics include anuria, severe renal disease, hepatic coma, pregnancy, and allergic hypersensitivity to individual drugs in this group. Because they have powerful effects on fluid and electrolyte balance, treatment is usually initiated in the hospital, where the client can be closely observed for toxicity. Initial doses are small and are increased gradually to optimal levels.

For clients who receive furosemide, blood levels of uric acid should be monitored. If theophylline and furosemide are used concurrently, blood levels of theophylline should also be monitored.

Diluting segment diuretics

Thiazides

Pharmacodynamics. Thiazide diuretics act by decreasing the reabsorption of sodium, chloride, potassium, and bicarbonate ions in the diluting segment of the ascending loop of Henle and in the distal tubule (see Fig. 40-2, site 4). They also increase the excretion of magnesium, phosphate, bromide, and iodide. They act independently of shifts in acid–base balance (see Focus on Thiazides: Similarities and Differences).

Pharmacokinetics. Thiazides are absorbed rapidly from the GI tract; chlorothiazide can also be administered IV. Renal response is apparent within 1 to 2 hours, and peak action occurs about 4 to 6 hours after administration. Duration of action varies with the individual thiazide but may persist up to 24 hours. Thiazides cross the placenta and are secreted in the milk of lactating mothers. They are actively secreted by the proximal tubule of the kidney and are excreted in urine.

Therapeutic uses. Thiazides are frequently used to control edema and hypertension in clients who require long-term therapy. They are useful in treating edema associated with chronic congestive heart failure, chronic renal or hepatic disease, pregnancy, and as drug therapy with glucocorticoids. They are sometimes used to treat bromide poisoning.

A potentially useful side effect of thiazide diuretics is the inhibition of calcium excretion. One study reported a decrease in the incidence of hip fracture in recipients of these drugs (Help for hip fractures, 1990).

Adverse reactions. The most frequent serious adverse reaction to thiazide therapy is potassium deficiency. Deficiencies of other electrolytes and minerals may also be harmful. Other undesirable side effects that may be clinically significant include an increase in blood uric acid concentrations that may precipitate gout in susceptible people, an increase in the incidence of cholelithiasis in nonobese women, increased blood levels of cholesterol and lipids, decreased cell response to insulin, and an increase in the severity of diabetes mellitus (Pollaire, et al, 1990). Cholestatic hepatitis may also occur. Glomerular filtration may be decreased by thiazides, particularly when administered IV. Like sulfonamides, thiazides can precipitate hypersensitivity reactions characterized by purpura, bone marrow depression, and necrotizing vasculitis. Dermatitis from exposure to ultraviolet light may also develop (Addo, et al, 1987).

Precautions and contraindications. Thiazide diuretics must be used with caution when treating debilitated or elderly clients. Clients who receive concurrent therapy with digitalis, corticosteroids, or estrogens are especially vulnerable to potassium loss and for this reason must be watched closely for signs of hypokalemia. Potassium supplements should be prescribed for such clients unless they are also receiving a potassium-sparing diuretic, such as spironolactone (Aldactone). Thiazides must be used with extreme caution in clients with impaired renal function, advanced cirrhosis, or a history of allergic hypersensitivity to these drugs.

Some authorities believe that thiazide diuretics should not be prescribed for individuals with insulin resistance and high blood insulin levels (Weiss, 1989).

Indolines

The first in a new class of diuretics known as indolines is indapamide (Lozol).

Pharmacodynamics. Indapamide exerts a diuretic action identical to that of the thiazide diuretics. It enhances excretion of sodium, chloride, and water by interfering with the transport of sodium ions across the epithelium of the diluting segment of the renal tubules. In addition, it exerts a direct vascular effect that lowers blood pressure. The mechanism for this action is unknown, but it may include calcium channel blocking with subsequent vasodilation.

Focus on

Thiazides: similarities and differences

Similarities

Pharmacodynamics

These agents decrease the reabsorption of sodium, chloride, potassium, and bicarbonate ions in the diluting segment of the ascending loop of Henle and in the distal tubule. They also increase the excretion of magnesium, phosphorus, bromide, and iodide. They also decrease extracellular fluid volume, plasma volume, and cardiac output, and they directly cause arteriolar dilation.

Pharmacokinetics

These agents are absorbed rapidly and by varying degrees from the GI tract. When administered orally, they have an onset of action within 2 hours, peaking in 3 to 6 hours. They are distributed into the extracellular space, cross the placenta, and are in breast milk. They are excreted unchanged in urine.

Therapeutic uses

These agents are used to treat edema and hypertension.

Adverse reactions

These include: (CNS) dizziness, vertigo, paresthesia, headache, weakness, muscle spasms; (CV) orthostatic hypotension, volume depletion, dehydration; (RESP) respiratory distress; (GI) nausea, vomiting, cramps, diarrhea, jaundice, pancreatitis; (GU) allergic interstitial nephritis, reversible renal failure, nephrolithiasis; (MET) hypochloremic acidosis, hyperglycemia; (HEMA) hypokalemia, dilutional hyponatremia, hypercalcemia, hyperuricemia, elevated serum cholesterol, leukopenia, thrombocytopenia, agranulocytosis; (SKIN) rash, urticaria, photosensitivity.

Contraindications

These agents are contraindicated for people with anuria and known hypersensitivity.

Differences

IV **chlorothiazide** has an onset of 15 minutes, peaking in 30 minutes. • **Bendroflumethiazide** peaks in 6 to 12 hours, with a duration of greater than 18 hours and a half-life of 8.5 hours. • **Chlorothiazide** has a duration of 6 to 12 hours and a half-life of 1 to 2 hours. • **Chlorthalidone** has a duration of 24 to 72 hours and a half-life of 30 to 50 hours. • **Cyclothiazide** peaks in 7 to 12 hours with a duration of 18 to 24 hours. • **Hydrochlorothiazide** has a duration of 6 to 12 hours and a half-life of 5 to 15 hours. • **Hydroflumethiazide** has a duration of 18 to 24 hours. • **Methyclothiazide** has a duration of greater than 24 hours. • **Metolazone** has a duration of 12 to 24 hours with a half-life of 14 hours. • **Polythiazide** has a duration of 24 to 48 hours, and small amounts are excreted in feces. • **Quinethazone** has a duration of 18 to 24 hours. • **Trichlormethiazide** has a duration of greater than 24 hours.

• **Metolazone** also may cause abdominal bloating, palpitations, chest pain, and chills. • IV **chlorothiazide** may cause hematuria. • **Hydrochlorothiazide** may cause pulmonary edema and allergic pneumonitis.

• **Metolazone** is contraindicated for people with hepatic coma or precoma states.

(continued)

Focus on

Thiazides: similarities and differences (Continued)

Similarities	Differences
Precautions	
These agents should be used with caution in people with severe renal disease, impaired hepatic function, progressive liver disease, and in the elderly or debilitated.	Some preparations of **bendroflumethiazide**, **benzthiazide**, and **trichlormethiazide** contain **tartrazine** and should be used with caution in people who are sensitive. Some preparations of **hydrochlorothiazide** contain sulfites and should be used with caution in people sensitive to sulfites.
Nursing considerations	
Instruct client in disease, treatment, drug therapy regimen, adverse effects and compliance; assess cardiopulmonary status and vital signs for changes; monitor fluid and electrolytes frequently for changes; check daily weights for significant increases or decreases; assess extremities and abdomen for presence and amount of edema; measure abdominal circumference; monitor serum electrolytes for imbalances; check renal function studies, including serum blood urea nitrogen, creatinine, and uric acid levels; assess client for signs and symptoms of hypokalemia; administer in the morning with foods; institute diet teaching, including low sodium and high potassium foods; monitor blood sugars for signs of hyperglycemia; instruct client to use sunblock when going outside; institute safety measures to prevent injury; caution client to change position slowly and dangle feet before getting out of bed; discontinue drug before any parathyroid function tests; instruct client to check with physician before taking any over-the-counter medications.	Do not administer **chlorothiazide** (the only injectable thiazide) subcutaneously or IM; reconstitute with sterile water for injection and administer as an infusion; use the IV route only in emergencies or when the oral route is unavailable; monitor IV site for infiltration and pain.

Pharmacokinetics. Indapamide is lipophilic and well absorbed when administered orally, in both the fasting and nonfasting state. The drug distributes widely, especially to the red blood cells, in which it competitively and reversibly binds to CAH. Protein binding is about 71% to 79%. No data are available on distribution across the placenta or into breast milk. Indapamide is metabolized in the liver and excreted in urine. One-sixth to one-quarter of the drug is excreted in feces, probably through biliary elimination. Elimination half-life is 14 to 18 hours.

Therapeutic uses. Indapamide is used in the management of edema caused by congestive heart failure and renal or hepatic disease. It is also used in the initial treatment of hypertension.

Adverse reactions. Indapamide has a low incidence of adverse effects. It does, however, share many of the toxic potentials of thiazide diuretics, including electrolyte disturbances (hypokalemia, hypochloremic alkalosis, and hyponatremia), increased serum creatinine, increased blood urea nitrogen, and hyperuricemia. The drug has occasionally increased serum cholesterol and serum glucose. Other adverse reactions include CNS effects (headache, dizziness, fatigue, weakness, lethargy, muscle cramps, paresthesia, tension, anxiety, irritability, and agitation), GI upset (anorexia, nausea, vomiting, gastric irritation, abdominal pain, constipation or diarrhea), skin disorders (rash, urticaria, pruritus, and vasculitis), cardiovascular changes (orthostatic hypotension, premature ventricular contractions, irregular heart beat, and palpitations), renal changes (frequency, nocturia, and polyuria), and sexual dysfunction (impotency, decreased libido). Rhinorrhea, flushing, dry mouth, weight loss, and hepatitis may also occur.

Precautions and contraindications. Clients who receive indapamide should be monitored for blood glucose and electrolyte imbalances, especially hypokalemia. The drug should be used with caution in clients with severe renal diseases, impaired hepatic function, and parathyroid or thyroid disorders. Indapamide is contraindicated for clients with anuria and for those with allergic hypersensitivity to sulfonamide derivatives.

Agents that act on the distal tubule

Potassium-sparing diuretics

A few diuretics conserve potassium in the body while increasing sodium excretion. This class includes amiloride, spironolactone, and triamterene (see Focus on Potassium-Sparing Diuretics: Similarities and Differences).

Pharmacodynamics. Spironolactone (Aldactone) acts by antagonizing aldosterone. Its usefulness depends on significant aldosterone secretion. Other diuretics of this class do not normally affect hormone action but do inhibit sodium–potassium exchange in the distal tubule, which is controlled by aldosterone.

Pharmacokinetics. Potassium-sparing diuretics are administered orally. In the absence of loading doses, spironolactone does not achieve maximum effect for 2 to 3 days. Diuresis persists for a comparable period after discontinuation. The onset of action of both amiloride and triamterene occurs within 2 to 4 hours. Both amiloride and triamterene cross the placenta in mammals. Small amounts have been detected in breast milk. Both drugs are excreted primarily in urine. Spironolactone crosses the placenta and is distributed into breast milk. It is transformed by the body to an active metabolite, canrenone, that is subsequently excreted by both the liver and kidneys.

Therapeutic uses. Potassium-sparing diuretics are frequently used as adjuncts with potassium-wasting diuretics to treat edema and hypertension. Potassium imbalance may be avoided by careful titration of the respective dosages.

Adverse reactions. The most serious adverse reaction to these drugs, hyperkalemia, is most likely to occur when the drugs are used alone without concurrent administration of potassium-wasting diuretics. Spironolactone can also cause GI upset (anorexia, nausea, vomiting, diarrhea), CNS effects (headache, drowsiness, ataxia, confusion), and sexual changes (gynecomastia, decreased libido and impotence in males; breast soreness and menstrual irregularities in females).

Precautions and contraindications. Potassium-sparing diuretics are contraindicated for clients with limited renal reserve who cannot easily correct high potassium levels in the blood. These diuretics are not prescribed for clients with elevated blood urea nitrogen levels or those in acute renal failure. Blood urea nitrogen and electrolyte levels should be monitored at regular intervals during therapy.

Drugs that produce diuresis as a side effect

Certain other drugs can be said to have a diuretic action although they have no direct effect on kidney function. For example, the "diuretic" effect of digitalis derives from its cardiotonic action, which improves cardiac output, increases kidney perfusion, and generally improves kidney function. The drug does not directly influence tubular reabsorption.

When used to treat clients with glomerulonephritis, glucocorticoids may be said to induce diuresis. Normally, these drugs are antidiuretic because they increase sodium reabsorption by the kidneys. In the client with glomerulonephritis, however, the glucocorticoid's anti-inflammatory effect improves glomerular function sufficiently to produce a net increase in water and salt excretion. This secondary diuretic effect outweighs the primary antidiuretic action of glucocorticoids.

■ **Summary**

Diuretics are drugs that promote urine production. Most act by interfering with electrolyte reabsorption in the tubules of the kidney. They are prescribed to reduce edema caused by heart disease, nephrosis, hepatic cirrhosis, and other conditions that involve sodium and water retention, such as hypertension.

Drugs used as diuretics include osmotic diuretics, CAH inhibitors, high-ceiling diuretics (furosemide, bumetanide, and ethacrynic acid), and potassium-sparing agents. Drugs used to improve circulation or kidney function, such as digitalis and glucocorticoids, often produce a secondary diuresis.

Nursing management

Nursing implications

Diuretics exert many adverse effects on physiology, including excessive diuresis, increased blood uric acid levels, and increased blood glucose. Fluid and electrolyte imbalances are likely to develop, and gout and diabetes mellitus may increase in severity.

Hypokalemia. Hypokalemia poses a particular risk for clients who receive digitalis because adequate levels of potassium are necessary to prevent digitalis toxicity. Pharmacologically, potassium does not influence serum digitalis levels; it decreases the physiologic effect of digitalis. A client with hypokalemia may develop symptoms of digitalis overdose in the absence of

Focus on

Potassium-sparing diuretics: similarities and differences

Similarities

Pharmacodynamics

These agents act on the distal renal tubule, blocking sodium exchange for potassium and resulting in an increased secretion of water and sodium and retention of potassium.

Pharmacokinetics

These agents are incompletely absorbed. They are metabolized by the liver and excreted in urine and feces. They cross the placenta and small amounts are found in breast milk.

Therapeutic uses

These agents are used to treat edema.

Adverse reactions

These include: (CNS) headache, weakness, fatigue, confusion, ataxia, dizziness; (CV) cardiac arrhythmia, orthostatic hypotension; (RESP) cough, dyspnea; (GI) nausea, vomiting, bowel disturbances, diarrhea, abdominal pain; (MET) hyperkalemia; (SKIN) photosensitivity, rash.

Contraindications

These agents are contraindicated for people with serum potassium above 5.5 mEq/L, for those who are receiving other potassium-sparing diuretics or potassium supplements, and for those with anemia, acute or chronic renal insufficiency, diabetic neuropathy, and known hypersensitivity.

Precautions

These agents should be used with caution in people with severe hepatic insufficiency and diabetes.

Differences

• **Spironolactone** competitively inhibits aldosterone and it also has an antiandrogenic effect.

• **Amiloride** and **triamterane** cross the placenta.
• **Spironolactone** is well absorbed after oral administration.
• **Amiloride** is not metabolized and is excreted only by the kidneys. • **Amiloride** has an onset of 2 hours, peaking in 6 to 10 hours, with a duration of 24 hours and a half-life of 6 to 9 hours. • **Triamterene** has an onset of 2 to 4 hours, peaking in 1 to 3 days, with a duration of 7 to 9 hours and a half-life of 90 to 120 minutes. • **Spironolactone** has a slow onset, peaking in 3 days, with a duration of 2 to 3 days and a half-life of 13 to 24 hours.

• **Amiloride** and **spironolactone** are used to treat mild to moderate hypertension. • **Spironolactone** is used to diagnose primary hyperaldosteronism.

• **Amiloride** may cause impotency. • **Triamterene** may cause megaloblastic anemia. • **Spironolactone** may cause hyponatremia, transient rise in blood urea nitrogen and acidosis, gynecomastia in males, and menstrual disturbances and breast soreness in females.

(continued)

any increase in absolute serum levels. This client is caught in a vicious cycle that tends to be self-perpetuating; common symptoms of *early* digitalis toxicity are anorexia and nausea. Food intake, the chief source of potassium, is interrupted. Potassium levels drop more rapidly, accentuating the toxic symptoms.

An important influence on potassium levels is the amount of stress imposed on the client, because stress stimulates cortisone secretion. Two effects of cortisone on the kidneys are increased potassium excretion and sodium retention. Stress, therefore, not only increases the risk of hypokalemia but reduces the therapeutic

Focus on

Potassium-sparing diuretics: similarities and differences (Continued)

Similarities

Nursing considerations

Instruct client in disease, treatment, drug therapy regimen, adverse effects, and compliance; assess cardiopulmonary status and vital signs for changes; monitor intake and output and daily weight for signs of fluid imbalance; check serum electrolyte levels frequently; assess client for signs and symptoms of hyperkalemia; assess heart rate and rhythm for irregularities; administer in the morning with meals; institute safety measures to prevent injury; warn client to change positions slowly and dangle feet before getting out of bed; make sure that urinal, bedpan, or commode are within client's reach; discontinue if serum potassium level is 6.5 mEq/l or greater.

Differences

Protect **spironolactone** from light.

effect of the prescribed diuretics. Nursing measures to reduce client stress are critical to treatment.

Hyperkalemia. Although relatively rare, hyperkalemia poses a danger for the client who receives potassium-sparing diuretics, particularly if this is the only diuretic prescribed. Hyperkalemia, which may develop quickly, predisposes the client to fatal cardiac arrhythmia, and the electrolyte imbalance requires early diagnosis and prompt corrective action.

Sodium balance. Most clients under treatment for fluid retention are on sodium-restricted diets. The degree of restriction varies with the severity of the edema, the type of diuretic used, and the physician's preference. Usually 500 to 2000 mg of sodium are allowed.

Intensive diuresis may precipitate sodium and water depletion, a syndrome that resembles heat exhaustion. The signs and symptoms of this condition depend on the relative proportions of the two substances lost. If water and sodium are excreted in equal proportions, isotonic dehydration develops; if more sodium than water is lost, hypotonic dehydration occurs (Table 40-2). These conditions are more apt to occur in hot humid weather when large amounts of salt water are lost through perspiration.

Diuresis and intercurrent chronic disease. Diuresis may increase the symptoms of clients with diabetes mellitus and gout. Some diuretics increase blood sugar levels and predispose to ketoacidosis. Clients may need an increased dose of hypoglycemic drugs or an adjustment in diet. Many of these clients have crystalline insulin prescribed in accordance with the results of these tests. If the diuretic is reduced in dose or discon-

tinued without an adjustment of the diabetic regimen, the client may experience hypoglycemic reactions. Certain diuretics cause a rise in the blood levels of uric acid. Clients subject to gout are likely to experience an attack of arthritic symptoms when they receive large doses of these drugs.

Nursing process

Assessment Before diuretic therapy is initiated, baseline data are needed for parameters likely to change with diuresis. These include body weight, signs and symptoms of fluid balance, and serum levels of electrolytes, glucose, and uric acid. Peripheral edema should be assessed and ankle circumference measured. If ascites is present, circumference of the abdomen should be measured.

Nursing diagnosis Nursing diagnoses likely to be made when clients receive diuretics include the following:

Fluid volume excess related to sodium and water retention secondary to congestive heart failure (renal failure, hepatic impairment)
Fluid volume excess related to hypoproteinemia secondary to renal dysfunction (hepatic impairment)
Altered urinary elimination: polyuria related to increased excretion of electrolytes secondary to diuretic therapy
Body image disturbance related to tissue wasting that becomes apparent after loss of edematous fluid with diuresis

(Text continues on p. 996)

Table 40-2. Signs and symptoms of common electrolyte disturbances in clients who take diuretics

Electrolyte problem	Symptoms		Underlying mechanisms
	Early	*Late*	
Hypokalemia			
General effects	Malaise, apathy, weak, flabby muscles, speech changes, decreased reflexes, shallow respirations	Muscle paralysis, absent reflexes, apnea,* respiratory arrest,* flat cadaverous posture	The concentration of potassium ions within cell membranes are insufficient to support depolarization and impulse transmission in some tissues.
Smooth muscle changes	Anorexia, vomiting, distention, postural hypotension	Paralytic ileus Hypotensive shock	Decreased impulse transmission in smooth muscle reduces peristalsis and vasoconstriction.
Effects of metabolic alkalosis	Irritability (muscular and neurologic), fasciculations, tremors, paresthesia, muscle pain, and tenderness	Confusion Tetany	Potassium migrates from the intracellular space to the extracellular space. To maintain electrical balance in the cells, hydrogen ions migrate to the intracellular fluid. The resulting metabolic alkalosis reduces calcium solubility and ionization, thereby enhancing impulse transmission in some tissues.
Influence on the heart	Increased cardiac contractility Cardiac arrhythmia Decreased intensity of heart sounds, weak pulse, decreased blood pressure	Heart block Ventricular fibrillation (cardiac arrest in systole), degeneration of myocardium	Disruption of calcium–potassium balance in heart muscle causes prolongation of systole and shortening of diastole.
Electrocardiogram changes	Prolonged PR interval, depressed ST segment, prominent U waves, flat T waves	Inverted T waves	
In clients taking digitalis, symptoms of digitalis toxicity	Anorexia Bradycardia Visual disturbances Nausea/vomiting Cardiac arrhythmia	Tachycardia (over 100, cardiac arrest)	The calcium–potassium imbalance enhances the physiologic activity of a given dose of a digitalis drug.
Renal effects	Low specific gravity of urine Polyuria, nocturia, polydipsia, and thirst		Renal tubule damage impairs concentrating ability of kidneys.
Effects of prolonged deficiencies	Delayed healing	Impaired growth	New cells cannot be produced without sufficient potassium for the formation of intracellular fluid.
Hyperkalemia			
Effects on nerve and muscle	Irritability	Weakness and flaccid paralysis Difficulty in phonation Difficult respirations	High potassium ion levels within cells initially enhance depolarization and impulse transmission; eventually extracellular potassium levels become high enough to inhibit depolarization.
Smooth muscle changes	Nausea Cramping colic	Diarrhea	High potassium levels stimulate smooth muscle contraction.

(Continued)

Table 40-2. Signs and symptoms of common electrolyte disturbances in clients who take diuretics (Continued)

Electrolyte problem	Symptoms		Underlying mechanisms
	Early	*Late*	
Cardiac muscle changes	Slow weak pulse	Ventricular fibrillation (cardiac arrest in diastole)*	Disruption of normal calcium–potassium balance in heart muscle prolongs diastole and weakens and shortens systole. Impulse transmission in the heart is slowed or prevented by excess potassium.
Electrocardiogram changes		P waves disappear Fusion of QRS complex; RS-T segment and T waves	
Renal effects	Oliguria	Anuria	Cardiogenic shock reduces renal perfusion.
Acid–base changes	Metabolic acidosis		Potassium migrates from the extracellular space to the intracellular space, forcing hydrogen ions to leave the cell and enter the extracellular fluid, which lowers its pH.
Hyponatremia, isotonic			
Effect on fluid balance	Poor tissue turgor Dull sunken eyes Low blood pressure Increased pulse rate Vertigo, fainting, especially on rapid changes in posture Oliguria	Vasomotor collapse Hypotension Rapid thready pulse Cold clammy skin Cyanosis Anuria	Reduced sodium levels in the intravascular space decrease osmotic holding power, decrease blood volume, and cause postural hypotension. Shock impairs circulation and reduces tissue perfusion. Decreased blood volume stimulates aldosterone secretion, which increases sodium (and water) reabsorption by the kidney. Hypotension reduces glomerular filtration in the kidney.
Hyponatremia, hypotonic			
Effect on smooth muscle	Abdominal cramps	Diarrhea	The migration of potassium from the intracellular space to the extracellular space that accompanies dilutional hyponatremia causes a transitory hyperkalemia.
Connective tissue changes		Fingerprinting over the sternum	Fluid shifts from the extracellular space to the intracellular space increases "plasticity" of soft tissues, which tend to retain any deformity that results from pressure.
Skeletal muscle changes	Weakness	Paralysis	Decreased sodium ions outside cell membranes inhibit depolarization and impulse transmission.

* A common cause of death.

Pain related to hyperuricemia secondary to diuretic medication

Impaired tissue integrity: skin rash related to inflammation secondary to photosensitive drug reaction

Altered thought processes: confusion related to edema and electrolyte imbalance secondary to diuretic therapy

Knowledge deficit related to edema and diuretics used in its treatment

High risk for ineffective management of therapeutic regimen possibly related to knowledge deficit, powerlessness, or lack of perceived benefits

A common collaborative problem that should be differentiated from the nursing diagnoses is

Potential complication: cardiac arrhythmia

Planning Nursing goals include promotion of sodium and water excretion, assistance with the client's adaptation to urinary frequency, elimination of fear, promotion of a positive self-image, promotion of normal potassium balance, alleviation of abdominal discomfort, alleviation of joint pain, maintenance of normal sodium balance, and prompt detection and treatment of adverse drug reactions, including skin rash and confusion. Goals for the teaching plan include client involvement in the management of the drug regimen and proper management of the regimen by the client after discharge from the acute care facility.

Intervention Whenever possible, diuretics should be administered early in the day so that the drug can be dissipated before bedtime, when the client's sleep would be interrupted by the need to urinate. Oral medications that irritate the GI mucosa are usually administered with meals to provide maximum dilution.

Parenteral diuretics should be administered by infusion. Unless fluids are severely restricted, intermittent doses may be diluted in 50 to 100 ml of parenteral solution and infused over 30 to 60 minutes. Bolus administration markedly increases the risk of adverse reactions, including that of ototoxicity in the case of Lasix (Gever, 1987).

Mannitol solutions that contain crystals must be warmed by placing them in hot water; a microwave oven should never be used because the containers may explode. Shaking the bottles occasionally hastens dissolution (Gever, 1985). One or two test doses of mannitol (200 mg/kg body weight each, infused over 3 to 5 minutes) are administered before the therapeutic infusion is started to verify the capacity of the kidneys to respond to the drug. Mannitol is usually not given if urinary output is less than 30 ml/h in response to test doses, because hypervolemia can cause hypertension, pulmonary dysfunction, cerebral dysfunction, and congestive heart failure. The flow rate of therapeutic doses of mannitol is adjusted to achieve a urinary output of about 100 ml/h.

If clients who receive diuretics are acutely ill or debilitated, the nurse should be available to assist them to the bathroom without delay. Clients who are unable to ambulate need a bedpan or urinal readily available.

Promoting salt and water loss. Most clients who receive diuretics are on sodium-restricted diets. The nurse should be thoroughly familiar with the diet ordered and should monitor the tray sent to the client to ensure that the foods are appropriate. Herbs and flavorings may help improve the taste of food. Seasonings that contain sodium, such as garlic salt, are not allowed, although the pure herb would be permissible. A nutritionist should be consulted if the nurse has any doubt about the suitability of specific substances.

The nurse should take measures to reduce stressors on the client. Noxious stimuli, including noise and glaring lights, should be minimized. The lower the client's stress levels, the lower the level of corticoid hormones. The action of diuretics is inhibited by these hormones, which favor sodium retention, and control of stress promotes a therapeutic response to these drugs.

Failure to respond to treatment. Urine output must be monitored. If the client fails to respond to medication with a measurable diuresis by 24 hours, the physician must be notified promptly. The nurse should reassess sodium intake, because excessive sodium can interfere with diuresis. An inadequate or poor response may also result from poor circulation, which reduces renal blood flow, or from impaired drainage (venous or lymph), which traps fluid in various tissues.

Promoting a positive self-concept. Clients who respond well to diuretic therapy may be distressed by their appearance as the abnormal fluid is lost. While edema is present, the body contours are well rounded. As the edema subsides, any tissue wasting that has occurred is revealed. Emotional support is critical at this stage of treatment. The nurse should acknowledge the client's changed appearance and encourage the client to ventilate feelings about it. Hope of improvement should be promoted. If consistent with the client's condition, the nurse may reassure the client that improved health will result in weight gain and regrowth of healthy tissue. Garments that cover the extremities make tissue wasting less obvious. The nurse should promote good grooming and use of cosmetics and toiletries to enhance appearance and scent. Whenever appropriate, the client should be complimented on appearance and physical attractiveness.

Preventing potassium imbalance. Nurses can do much to prevent potassium deficiency. The physician may be asked if a potassium supplement should be ordered for the client who is receiving potassium-wasting diuretics. Foods rich in potassium should be offered to the client. Common sense and individual preference should influence selection. A seriously ill client may well prefer orange juice to a banana or dried apricot. Tea and coffee are significant sources of potassium if allowed in the diet.

Whenever liquid potassium supplements are administered, they should be well diluted. Parenteral solutions must be administered slowly. High concentrations of this electrolyte in body fluids can cause smooth muscle spasm and a weak heart action. IV infusions that contain potassium can cause vasospasm that compromises the IV line. More seriously, rapid IV administration can precipitate ventricular fibrillation.

High potassium concentrations in the intestinal tract can also produce serious GI effects. Rapid absorption into intestinal blood vessels promotes vasospasm that can compromise the circulation of the area, producing infarctions. Solid forms of potassium are specially formulated to release the drug gradually as it passes through the intestinal tract. However, liquid forms are also marketed, and it is vital that these medications be well diluted before administration.

If potassium deficiency develops despite all precautions, it is vital that the condition be detected as early as possible. The signs and symptoms of hypokalemia are outlined in Table 40-2. The nurse should assess the client regularly for early signs and symptoms of hypokalemia. These reactions often appear before blood chemistry reports for hypokalemia are obtained. The laboratory data only confirm what should have been detected earlier by the nursing staff.

Clients who receive only a potassium-sparing diuretic are at risk for the development of hyperkalemia. They should reduce their intake of potassium. Foods rich in this mineral (orange juice, bananas, apricots, water in which vegetables are cooked, and foods of animal origin) should be taken in moderate amounts only. Coffee, tea, and chocolate also contain significant amounts of potassium and should be limited.

Alleviating discomfort. Abdominal discomfort and intestinal upset should be reported to the physician. These problems are likely to be adverse reactions to the diuretic, to digitalis in a potassium-deficient client, or to renal calculi. Joint pains due to acute gout are also drug related. Informing the physician usually prompts alteration in the drug regimen to correct the underlying cause of these complications.

A history of gout should alert the nurse to take measures to prevent this complication. The physician who is aware of this risk may order antigout medication before symptoms develop. The nurse can modify the diet to exclude foods rich in purine, which tends to elevate further the body's production of uric acid. Foods rich in purine include meat extracts (gravies, bouillon), organ meats, and legumes.

Preventing hyponatremia. Excessive diuresis, especially if fluid intake is ample, can lead to hyponatremia and water intoxication. Clients should be monitored for this development, especially if the environment is hot, causing further loss of salt through perspiration (see Table 40-2 for signs and symptoms of hypotonic hyponatremia).

Correcting drug-induced complications. Diuretic therapy sometimes is continued for long periods. One study found that indefinite diuretic therapy may be unnecessary after recovery from acute congestive heart failure (Portnoi, Pawlson, 1981). It was found that withdrawal of diuretics was well tolerated provided clinical signs and symptoms had subsided. Nurses caring for the chronically ill should request a trial withdrawal of diuretics. Nursing measures to relieve leg edema (elevation of the legs, avoidance of prolonged sitting or standing in one place) due to local causes should be instituted. Withdrawal of diuretics often results in resolution of chronic complaints that were adverse drug reactions but had not been recognized as such.

Nurses should be alert to adverse reactions characteristic of the specific diuretic ordered. Signs and symptoms should be listed in the client's nursing care plan. All diuretics can cause confusion owing to electrolyte imbalance, and all can cause allergic reactions, including skin rash. Diabetics should be monitored closely to facilitate control of hyperglycemia, which can increase when diuretics are used. Clients with gout should also be monitored for signs and symptoms of exacerbation. Gout may appear in clients who have previously been free of it.

Every client who receives long-term diuretic therapy should be reviewed periodically by the staff for indications of drug-induced complications, and the nursing staff should work closely with the physician to develop an individualized drug regimen with optimal effect. Clients on intensive diuretic therapy in the hospital setting require close monitoring to detect early adverse reactions and toxicity. An accurate record of intake and output is essential. Measurements that are often ignored in monitoring fluid balance must be included in the record. For example, if the client is taking ice chips, the amount of fluid ingested in this way should be recorded accurately.

Daily body weights are the most sensitive measure of diuresis. To be reliable, weights must be taken at the same time each day, under standard conditions, using the same scale. Commonly, in the hospital, weights are recorded before breakfast, after the client has voided. The client should wear the same clothing at each weighing. If clients are unable to stand alone, they may be weighed on a bed scale. Clothing and linens should be similar for each weighing to avoid distortion of weight changes. Alternatively, the weight of the linens may be subtracted from the reading of the scale and the client's actual weight (as if nude) is recorded. A loss of 1 kg (2.2 lb) of body weight represents a loss of 1 liter of fluid.

Client education. Clients who receive diuretics for the first time should be warned that they will urinate in amounts greater than normal. Losses in weight should be presented as a desirable therapeutic result so that clients are not concerned about the rapid changes that can occur. Clients should be instructed to report dizziness, weakness, and other subjective symptoms of adverse reactions to the drugs.

Clients should be warned that they may appear abnormally thin when the edema has resolved. This state is partly due to the contrast between the contours of edematous and normal tissues (although some tissue wasting often accompanies the diseases that underlie sodium and fluid retention). The nurse should assist the client to maintain a presentable appearance throughout the period of physical changes.

Clients who become sensitive to light while taking thiazide diuretics should be advised to use a broad-spectrum sun block when outdoors.

Clients who take diuretics on a prolonged basis at home must be taught how to assess their response to the medication. They must be taught the signs and symptoms that should be reported to their physicians. They should be urged to take the drug regularly as ordered because some clients tend to reduce the dose, taking the "water pill" only when they notice visible edema. If clients have more than one physician, it is essential that all physicians be fully informed about all medical orders.

Clients should also be advised to maintain complete drug profiles at the pharmacy where they purchase most of their drugs. Pharmacists are now taking an active role in monitoring drug regimens for incompatibilities, drug interactions, and other drug-related problems. Clients who receive diuretics on a continuing basis often receive several other drugs also. Selected clients should be seen periodically by a public health nurse or private nurse practitioner so that the effectiveness of the medical regimen can be evaluated.

Evaluation Therapeutic response is evaluated by urinary output as compared to fluid intake, serial weights, and reduction of edema (as measured by serial ankle or abdominal circumferences). Other data required for evaluation include relaxation of the client and adaptability to the treatment; reports by the client that he or she feels more comfortable, less anxious or fearful, or "feels better about things"; the number of positive and negative comments that relate to self-image; laboratory data and physical evidence that relate to electrolyte balance; and the incidence or absence of signs and symptoms of adverse drug reaction, such as rash and confusion (see the Example of

Nursing Process and Hypokalemia Due to Diuretic Therapy).

Checklist of nursing actions

When diuretics are prescribed

☐ Question the client about previous experience with drugs of this type; carefully assess fluid and electrolyte status.

☐ Whenever possible, administer diuretics early in the day to minimize their effects during sleeping hours.

☐ Advise the client that urine output will increase noticeably after diuretic therapy is begun.

☐ Monitor fluid status of acutely ill clients by keeping accurate intake and output records and daily weight charts.

☐ Unless clients are receiving potassium-sparing diuretics, encourage clients to eat potassium-rich foods to prevent hypokalemia.

☐ Control stressors that impinge on clients and teach them techniques to manage stress.

☐ Consult with the physician for a change in medication if the expected diuretic response to treatment fails to occur.

☐ Monitor clients closely for signs and symptoms of electrolyte imbalance and other adverse reactions specific to the drugs given.

☐ If signs and symptoms of hypokalemia develop, consult with the physician about the use of potassium supplements or a reduction in diuretic dosage.

☐ Dilute liquid potassium medications well before administering them.

☐ Monitor food offered to the client to make sure that it conforms to the prescribed sodium intake; consult with the dietitian about client preferences in food selection.

☐ Monitor diabetic clients who receive thiazide diuretics for glucose imbalance.

☐ Encourage clients who receive thiazide diuretics who have a history of gout to reduce dietary intake of purine.

☐ Give emotional support to the client in whom

Learning experience 40-1

When caring for an acutely ill client who is receiving diuretics, review the chart carefully to ascertain: 1) changes in urinary output in response to the medication, 2) changes in serum electrolyte levels as diuresis progresses, and 3) laboratory reports indicative of side effects of the diuretic.

Example of nursing process and hypokalemia due to diuretic therapy

The client is a 66-year-old retired railroad engineer admitted to the hospital a week ago for acute congestive heart failure. He has improved with a regimen of low sodium diet, digoxin, and furosemide. For the last 2 days his vital signs have been normal. There is no visible edema except for swollen ankles in the afternoon and evening. He is presently on maintenance doses of digoxin and furosemide.

Because he lives alone and has become increasingly disabled by osteoarthritis, admission to a health-related facility is planned.

When the client's medications are brought to him this morning, he complains of weakness and dizziness on arising. He moves listlessly, and his abdomen appears distended. The client states that he could not eat all of his breakfast because he "just didn't have any appetite." Pulse is 56. Serum electrolytes tested 2 days ago show low normal sodium and potassium.

Assessment data	Nursing diagnosis	Intervention	Goals and outcome criteria
Weakness	Potential complication: cardiac arrhythmias*	**Withhold** the digoxin and furosemide.	The client will state that he feels less weak and dizzy and is more interested in eating.
Postural hypotension		**Offer** the client a glass of orange juice, cup of decaffeinated coffee, or other beverage that contains potassium.	Serum electrolytes will rise gradually; sodium will reach minimal limits of normal and potassium will rise above minimal normal limits.
Restricted sodium intake			
Digoxin and furosemide medications			
Anorexia		**Consult** with the physician for possible change in medications.	
Bradycardia			The client's abdominal girth will decrease.
Abdominal distention		**Evaluate** the client for stress; reduce stressors and assist the client in managing stress levels.	The client will not experience cardiac arrest.
		Monitor serum electrolytes.	If cardiac arrest occurs, it will be detected and treated promptly.
		Monitor abdominal girth.	
		Monitor the client's pulse for irregularity or sudden rise above normal levels (>100/min).	
		Be prepared to initiate cardiopulmonary resuscitation if cardiac arrest occurs.	

* Although potential complications generally are not included in the Examples of Nursing Process, in this situation the identification of this collaborative problem is critical to the outcome for this client and illustrates the broad range of nursing responsibilities.

Learning experience 40-2

Compare the charts of several chronically ill clients who are receiving diuretics. What specific diuretics are prescribed for individual clients? Can you determine why? Assess one or more clients who are receiving diuretics for adverse reactions to these drugs. What, if any, precautions are taken to prevent deficiencies of electrolytes such as potassium?

reduction of edema produces upsetting changes in appearance.

When long-term diuretic therapy is planned

☐ Teach clients how to assess their responses to medication.

☐ Teach clients the signs and symptoms to report to their physician.

☐ Stress the importance of taking diuretics regularly as ordered.

☐ Advise clients to inform *all* physicians of current medical orders.

☐ Advise clients to maintain complete drug profiles at their pharmacy.

☐ Stress the importance of continued regular medical supervision.

References

Addo H, et al. (1987). Thiazide-induced photosensitivity: A study of 33 subjects. *Br J Dermatol, 116*, 749–760.

Carpentiere G, Marino S, Castello F. (1985). Furosemide and theophylline (letter). *Ann Intern Med, 103*, 957.

Gever LN. (1987). Consultation: Lasix: How much, how fast? *Nursing 87, 17*, 87.

Help for hip fractures. (1990). *Nursing 90, 20*, 126.

Pollaire T, et al. (1990). Doctors reveal downside to hydrochlorothiazide. *RN, 53*, 128.

Portnoi V, Pawlson L. (1981). Abuse of diuretic therapy in nursing homes. *J Chronic Dis, 345*, 363–365.

Weiss R. (1989). Hypertension, heart disease and diuretics. *Science News, 136*, 254.

Bibliography

Blake G. (1990). Pharmacist on call: Furosemide for pulmonary edema. *Nursing 90, 20*, 108.

Gilman AG, Goodman LS, Rall TW, Murad F (eds). (1985). *Goodman and Gilman's The pharmacological basis of therapeutics*, 7th ed, pp 897–925. New York: Macmillan.

Guyton AC. (1986). *Textbook of medical physiology*, 7th ed, pp 393–437. Philadelphia: WB Saunders.

*Hill MN. (1987). Diuretics for mild hypertension: Still the best choice? *Nursing 87, 17*, 62.

Kakar F, Weiss NS, Strite SA. (1986). Thiazide use and the risk of cholecystectomy in women. *Am J Epidemiol, 124*, 428–433.

Koegel L. (1985). Ototoxicity: A contemporary review of aminoglycosides, loop diuretics, acetylsalicyclic acid,

Langford H, et al. (1987). Is thiazide-produced uric acid elevation harmful? *Arch Intern Med, 147*, 645–649.

Maggini R (ed). (1985). *Drug interaction facts*, p 573. St. Louis: JB Lippincott.

* Recommended for further reading.

Drugs used for inflammations and infections

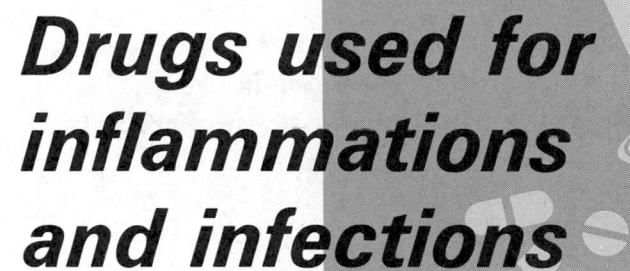

11

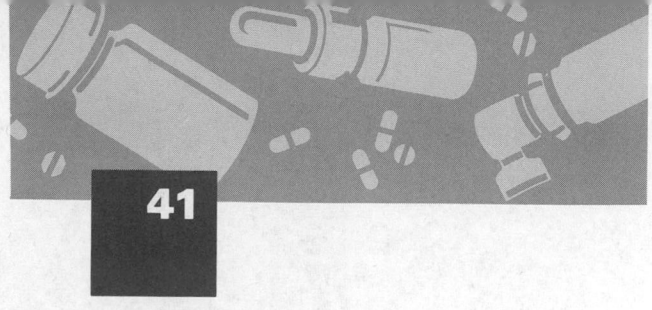

41

Major antimicrobial drugs

Introduction to anti-infectives

Infection, or invasion of the body by a parasitic organism, has been a major cause of sickness and death since the beginning of humanity. In fact, many life forms cannot thrive except by preying on other living organisms. Humans are susceptible to attack by such smaller organisms as lice, worms, mites, amoebae, fungi, bacteria, and viruses. These agents settle in preferred locations on or within the body, drawing from it the substances necessary for their survival and reproduction. By injuring cells, removing nutrients, and producing toxins, they cause illness and often the death of their host (Fig. 41-1).

Until the mid-19th century, little could be done to help victims of infection except to provide general supportive care during the body's struggle against the invading pathogen. Young people were particularly vulnerable, and deaths from contagious illnesses were a major factor in keeping the average life expectancy low. Epidemics decimated whole communities, leaving too few survivors even to bury the dead properly. The rapid increase in life expectancy enjoyed by most societies in the last century has been largely due to the control of contagious diseases.

Once the discovery of microorganisms revealed the true nature of infection, the way was open to develop effective means of combating infectious illnesses. The first efforts attempted to prevent infection, either by eliminating the infectious agent before it could enter the body or by strengthening people's defenses against the pathogen. Antiseptics, disinfectants, and sanitizers reduced the number of organisms in the environment. Vaccines were administered to induce

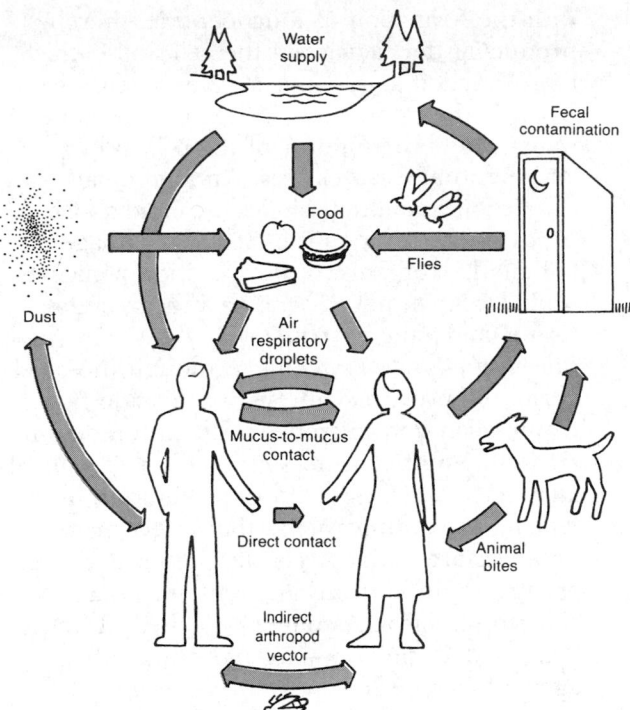

Figure 41-1. Modes of disease transmission. Inanimate materials and living hosts, including humans, serve as reservoirs of infectious organisms. Agents of infection leave their hosts through excretions and secretions (urine, feces, mucus). They are sometimes carried by insect vectors or fomites. They gain entry to new hosts through the skin, mucous membranes, and open wounds. Whether or not the invading organism can live and grow in the new host depends on the strength of that host's resistant mechanisms.

the development of active immunity in susceptible persons. Eventually, chemical agents were developed that could selectively inhibit or destroy pathogens within the body without harm to the host. In the mid-20th century, well organized wide-ranging research produced a large number of such drugs. We now have agents effective against most bacterial pathogens. The number of systemic drugs available to combat fungal and protozoan infections is more limited, and antiviral agents are rare and of limited usefulness. Research efforts continue, however, and hope for the future remains high. The effort is a competitive one—an attempt to develop weapons in the fight against infection faster than pathogens can adapt through mutation to their presence.

Unlike most medicinal drugs, many anti-infective drugs are truly curative in that they correct the cause of the disease by killing or inhibiting the growth of pathogens. Most drugs are unable to cure in this sense but instead alleviate symptoms, reverse pathologic processes, or support the body in its recuperative process.

Introduction to antimicrobials

When it became widely accepted that microorganisms cause disease, medical scientists began searching for a "magic bullet"—a substance that would be lethal to pathogenic microorganisms without affecting the health of the host. They believed that for each disease a chemical exists that would selectively destroy the causative microbe. (Although antitoxins do possess this kind of specificity, their usefulness is limited by their antigenicity as foreign proteins. Vaccines and antitoxins are discussed in Chapter 36.) Selectivity in antimicrobials depends on differences in structure and function between host and pathogen cells. Because most living organisms share the same basic characteristics, these differences are not sufficient to provide complete safety when antimicrobial chemotherapy is used. However, drugs have been found that exhibit both effectiveness and an acceptable therapeutic index. Early investigators did not live to see the outcome of the research they had launched, but the world of the mid-20th century has seen the development of many treatment agents that, although not without risk, are true cures of infections.

Characteristics of the ideal antimicrobial

A perfect anti-infective chemotherapeutic agent would destroy pathogens without harming host cells. It would be effective against large numbers of infectious organisms and lose none of its action in the presence of such materials as exudates or tissue enzymes. The ideal anti-infective would not promote the development of resistance by pathogens. It would distribute rapidly to all body fluids and tissues and remain in the body for relatively long periods of time.

Realistically, this ideal will probably never be achieved. Indeed, some of the characteristics of the ideal anti-infective agent tend to be mutually exclusive. For example, a selective agent probably could not affect a wide variety of pathogens. Because pathogens vary in their characteristics, an agent chemically suited to damage a particular microorganism would affect similar organisms but not others that differ in nature. Other problems exist as well. The ability to affect a wide variety of pathogens is in itself a double-edged sword. Treatment agents with a broad spectrum of activity are apt to reduce the natural microscopic flora of the body to such a degree that the host is rendered vulnerable to superinfection or overgrowth of fungi and protozoa that is normally suppressed by this flora.

Probably no chemical exists to which resistance cannot be developed. It has been discovered that microorganisms use several mechanisms to transfer the ability to resist a particular chemical agent. The rapid rate of reproduction of these small life forms favors the emergence of mutant strains. Microbes can transfer genetic material from one to another, a process that allows those individual organisms that happen to be resistant to a drug to transfer their resistance to a large percentage of a pathogenic population. It is not surprising, therefore, that with prolonged use, antimicrobials tend to become less effective because susceptible pathogens have been replaced by resistant ones. Because they interact with living matter, antimicrobials also combine with many biochemical materials of the host. This fact decreases the therapeutic activity of the antimicrobials. Rapid penetration and prolongation of an antimicrobial's therapeutic effect can increase the severity and duration of adverse reactions if these occur. Finally, even if the treatment agent were inert in its effect on host cells, allergic reactions or other adverse reactions in sensitive clients could occur.

Despite the problems inherent in the development of antimicrobial agents, scientists have developed an arsenal of treatment agents that provide adequate protection against most nonviral pathogens at this time. The value of antimicrobial drugs in medical treatment is inestimable. Not only are they used to cure the acute and chronic infections that have been responsible for much death and illness throughout history, but when prescribed with discrimination, they also provide the margin of protection necessary for successful immunosuppression, antineoplastic chemotherapy, and surgery in high-risk clients.

The use of antimicrobials

Pharmacodynamics

The best anti-infectives interfere with metabolic or growth processes that are specific to pathogenic microorganisms and not characteristic of host cells (Box 41-1). These mechanisms include the following:

- *Inhibition of bacterial cell wall synthesis.* Bacterial cell walls are generally thicker and more rigid than the membranes of mammalian cells. One important molecule responsible for this rigidity is mucopeptide. Certain antimicrobials interfere

---

Box 41-1. Actions of antimicrobial drugs

Mechanisms by which drugs affect microorganisms include the following:

- Inhibition of bacterial cell synthesis
- Inhibition of protein synthesis
- Interference with the cell membrane
- Interference with energy metabolism
- Interference with nucleic acid metabolism

---

with the formation of mucopeptide, thereby producing deficiencies in the cell walls, which then function as semipermeable membranes. Because the interior of the cell is hypertonic, water enters the interior of the cell, swells it, and eventually causes lysis. Antimicrobials with this action are all antibiotics (*ie,* a metabolic product of one organism that can damage or kill another organism); they include penicillin, cephalosporin, novobiocin, bacitracin, cycloserine, and vancomycin.

- *Inhibition of protein synthesis.* Although the mechanism for protein synthesis is similar in both mammalian and microbial cells, differences in ribosomal number and structure do permit relative selectivity in inhibiting protein synthesis. Among the antimicrobials that affect protein synthesis are aminoglycoside, the tetracycline, erythromycin, lincomycin, gentamicin, and chloramphenicol. As might be expected, these drugs—all antibiotics—are more toxic than agents that interfere with a system unique to pathogens.

- *Interference with the cell membrane.* Certain compounds attack microbial cell membranes by binding to the cell wall. Because the permeability of the membrane is thereby increased, assorted electrolytes and sugars leak from the cytoplasm. Examples of this type of antimicrobial are the polymyxins, nystatin, colistin, and amphotericin. The difference in ratios between sterol and phospholipid contents in mammalian and microbial cell membranes appears to be the basis for the selectivity of these agents.

- *Interference with metabolism.* Bacteria that cannot use preformed folic acid, as mammalian cells do, synthesize it by using para-aminobenzoic acid (PABA) as the substrate. Antimicrobials, such as the sulfonamides, trimethoprim, and para-aminosalicylic acid (PAS) function as competitive analogues of PABA in the synthesis of folic acid. Because the molecules of folic acid that incorporate these drugs do not perform their metabolic function, the pathogen develops folic acid deficiency. Because various microbes use different biochemical pathways in producing folic acid, these antimetabolites have differing spectra of activity. A pathogen sensitive to one of the group may not respond to the others.

- *Interference with nucleic acid production.* Agents that block nucleic acid synthesis prevent reproduction of microbial cells. Rifampin, nalidixic acid, other quinolones, and griseofulvin appear to use this mechanism.

The mode of action of some antimicrobials remains unknown. Continued research in microbiologic pharmacology may reveal the mechanisms involved. Such knowledge will provide clues to changes in molecular structure likely to help the pharmaceutical chemist in developing new drugs.

Antimicrobials may either inhibit the growth of pathogens (bacteriostatic) or kill pathogens (bactericidal). Bacteriostatic agents rely on host defenses to eliminate pathogens. Treatment of infection in clients with inadequate resistance to infection requires bactericidal drugs.

Spectra of activity

A drug's *spectrum of activity* refers to the number and type of organisms vulnerable to its action. Broad-spectrum antimicrobials injure a wide variety of pathogens, and narrow-spectrum drugs affect only a few. Antimicrobials tend to affect pathogens with similar biochemical characteristics. One of the methods used to distinguish various microorganisms is to stain them with certain laboratory dyes. The characteristic ways organisms take the stain are associated with chemical differences in the cell membrane or intracellular components. Pathogens with similar staining properties tend to be sensitive to the same antimicrobials. A drug's spectrum of activity, therefore, may be described in terms of its effectiveness against gram-positive, gram-negative, or acid-fast bacilli. Morphology also influences efficacy because drugs vary in their effects on such groups as cocci, rods, spirochetes, and fungi. The spectra of some drugs appear to be unrelated to the ordinary systems of classification, and microbial strains susceptible to their action are listed individually.

Bacterial resistance

One factor that limits the usefulness of antimicrobial agents is the propensity of pathogens to develop resistance to a drug's action. Resistance is the ability of a microorganism to live and grow in the presence of an anti-infective substance, which usually exerts a bactericidal or bacteriostatic action on organisms of its species. Resistance, arising from chance mutation in one or more cells, allows the cell to survive in the presence of the antimicrobial. This capacity may subsequently spread throughout the bacterial population by the mechanisms of selected reproduction (survival and multiplication of more resistant cells than nonresistant), transduction (transfer of genetic material from one microbe to another through a bacteriophage viral transducer), transformation (incorporation by one pathogen of genes from another that have been released into the environment), or conjunction (a flow of cytoplasmic genes from one organism to another through a corridor that connects two cells in conjugation). The mutant strain may produce an enzyme that breaks down the chemical structure of the drug. The cell wall may be so altered that it is less permeable to the drug, an increased production of an endogenous antagonist to the drug may occur, or the critical target or receptor on the cell may be so altered that the drug cannot function.

The likelihood of drug resistance varies from microbe to microbe and from drug to drug. Whether or not resistance develops is also directly related to whether an organism is exposed to nonlethal doses of the drug in question. The staphylococcal species has been notoriously proficient in developing resistance to penicillin by the production of the enzyme penicillinase. A common inhabitant of skin and environmental surfaces, resistant strains of this microbe often develop in health care institutions, where antimicrobials are in common use. Nosocomial infections result, and these can be difficult to eradicate. Not only are clients vulnerable, especially those who are debilitated or who have wounds, but infections due to resistant strains are an occupational hazard for health care employees and their families.

Adverse reactions

Antimicrobials are potentially harmful to the recipient, who can develop allergic sensitivity to the treatment agent, alterations of body functions, or toxic tissue changes. The drug may damage body tissues or organs and interfere with absorption or use of necessary nutrients. Disruptions of the normal microscopic flora in the body may precipitate infection by nonsusceptible organisms.

Allergy

Every antimicrobial has the ability to stimulate antibody production in some people. The frequency of sensitivity varies greatly from one drug to another, depending on the antigenic properties of the chemical and how frequently the population is exposed to it. People who have never received drug therapy may have become allergic to antimicrobials owing to exposure to environmental contamination that results from agricultural or industrial use of the chemicals. Reactions vary from minor to catastrophic, and succeeding reactions tend to increase in severity. A personal or family history of atopic allergy indicates increased susceptibility to allergic drug sensitivity. The topical use of antimicrobials (especially application to open wounds) appears to stimulate antibody production and increase the incidence of allergy. Reactions are most likely if a drug is initially applied topically and then subsequently administered systemically. For this reason, topical agents are prepared from antimicrobials, such as bacitracin, that are not generally suitable for systemic use. Allergic responses to injected drug doses are generally more severe than to drugs given orally.

Toxicity

Theoretically, harmful effects on host cells should correspond to the drug's mechanisms of action. For example, rapidly dividing cells would more likely suffer toxic effects from chemicals that interfere with nucleic acid formation and protein synthesis because these two processes proceed at a rapid rate during reproduction. Clinical data indicate that drugs that affect nucleic acid production do not seem to damage rapidly dividing mammalian cells, whereas those that interfere with protein synthesis do. In other categories, the relationship between biochemical action and toxic effects seems obscure, probably because we still lack essential knowledge of biology at the molecular and chemical levels to explain them.

Antimicrobials can damage any part of the body. Symptoms of toxicity range from the trivial to the serious and vary depending on the therapeutic agent in use. Nausea, vomiting, and diarrhea are fairly frequent. Liver malfunction, kidney damage, bone marrow depression, degeneration of nerves, and teeth and bone defects can occur. Damage to the rapidly dividing cells of the body causes symptoms related to alterations of bone marrow and intestinal mucosa. Leukopenia and agranulocytosis are usually reversible if detected early and drug treatment is discontinued. If the damage is allowed to progress to pancytopenia and aplastic anemia, it may be irreversible and fatal. Lesions of the gastrointestinal (GI) tract cause nausea and vomiting. Ulcerations may develop throughout the tract, and fulminating colitis can ensue.

The liver and kidneys are subject to damage by certain agents, especially when these organs are involved in the degradation and excretion of the drugs. The sulfonamides, which tend to crystallize in the urine, cause mechanical damage to the kidneys. Other agents precipitate renal shutdown, especially when administered concomitantly with diuretics. The kidneys are the major avenue for elimination of most antimicrobials. Fortunately, many drug agents produce few or no toxic effects on this organ. Initially, altered liver function may be characteristic of cholestasis. Symptoms of hepatitis may occur. Some antibiotics affect both organs, placing the recipient in double jeopardy.

Manifestations of damage to the central nervous system (CNS) include nervousness, convulsions, paresthesia, ataxia, neuropsychiatric episodes, photosensitivity, peripheral neuritis, insomnia, encephalopathy, temporary blindness, and eighth cranial nerve toxicity. Fortunately, most of these effects are relatively rare. The most common is acoustic nerve damage with initial symptoms of tinnitus, decreased perception of high tones, and eventual deafness. In some cases, loss of hearing is temporary, but in most it is permanent.

Bone and tooth defects occur primarily from tetracycline therapy. The drug is deposited in developing teeth, producing permanent discoloration. The rate of bone growth is also affected by the drug. Owing to these effects, the tetracyclines are not administered to clients during pregnancy or early childhood.

Superinfection

Decimation of large numbers of normal microbial inhabitants of the body may so alter the environment that the uncontrolled growth of nonsusceptible organisms becomes possible. Such an infection, superimposed on the original infection being treated, is called a *superinfection*. For example, yeasts and molds normally present in certain tissues do not reproduce at a rapid rate because their growth is inhibited by bacteria also present in the normal flora. If the inhibiting bacteria are eliminated by an antimicrobial drug, these fungi can then multiply rapidly and cause symptoms of an infection, such as inflammation of oral, vaginal, anal, and other tissues. Concomitant administration of an antifungal, such as nystatin, is frequently necessary to suppress such opportunistic mycotic infections in clients who receive antimicrobial drugs.

Any organism present in the body that is not susceptible to the systemic anti-infective administered may produce a superinfection. Common offenders are fungi of the *Candida* genus, which produce localized infections in the mouth and vagina; resistant strains of staphylococci, which can cause severe diarrhea; and gram-negative *Pseudomonas* organisms, which can cause the most serious superinfections. Such infections occur most frequently in clients who receive broad-spectrum antibiotics and are most dangerous in debilitated clients or those who receive corticosteroids or antineoplastic treatments, which reduce the body's inflammatory or immune responses.

The development of superinfection may require the administration of one or more anti-infectives in addition to the primary treatment agent prescribed to treat the original infection. The use of multiple drugs increases the risk of serious adverse reactions. In spite of vigorous treatment, iatrogenic superinfection causes illness in some clients treated with anti-infectives and can cause death.

Treatment failures

A successful outcome of treating infection with drugs depends on the susceptibility of a pathogen to the action of the antimicrobial and the host's response to both the treatment agent and the invading organism. A number of factors may interfere with recovery of the client treated for infection (Box 41-2).

An adequate concentration of the drug in tissue fluids is necessary for effective treatment. If the prescribed dose is too low or some doses are omitted, drug concentration is inadequate.

Client noncompliance may be due to difficulty in remembering to take the correct number of doses at designated times, lack of money to purchase the prescribed amount, unwillingness to use limited funds for medication, unhappiness with side effects, or lack of information about the drug's importance. If medication is taken in liquid form, it should be measured with a special medicine spoon available at the pharmacy. If taken in a glass of liquid, the client should be reminded to drink the entire amount (even adding more liquid if any adheres to the glass) to be certain to obtain the full dose. Poor absorption and rapid metabolism or excretion of the drug by the recipient also depress blood levels. Drug therapy may be discontinued before the infection is completely resolved if the physician underestimates the time required for treatment, if severe adverse reactions occur, or if the client stops taking the drug before completing the prescribed regimen. If the infection affects parts of the body with a poor blood supply, drug levels in these tissues may be inadequate to eliminate the microorganisms, despite a high blood level.

The antimicrobial chosen for therapy must be capable of inhibiting or killing the microorganism involved. Culture and sensitivity tests of tissue specimens, which must be completed for definitive identification of infecting organisms and appropriate drug agents, require 2 to 3 days. (Specimens for cultures must be taken before anti-infective therapy is begun.) In the interim, drugs are ordered in accordance with the initial diagnosis, based on clinical signs and symptoms. If the causative agent is misdiagnosed or the strain of organism that is causing the illness is resistant to the drug prescribed, initial therapy will be ineffective.

Combination drug therapy is required to delay development of drug resistance in certain pathogens. Use of a single agent in these situations results in rapid desensitization of the infecting organism and failure of therapy.

Delays in treatment allow large populations of pathogens to establish themselves. Overwhelming infections tend to deplete the host's defenses, that is, inflammatory response, antibody levels, numbers and activity of white blood cells, and the integrity of membrane barriers, such as skin and mucosa. Reduced resistance to infection may also be due to genetic defects, malnutrition, general debility, medical suppression of the immune response, or stress. Defenses fluctuate during the client's life cycle, with increased susceptibility to infection in the very young, the very old, individuals under severe stress, and during pregnancy.

If a drug antagonistic to an antimicrobial is present in the body of the host, the effectiveness of the antimicrobial is reduced. For example, bacteriostatic anti-infectives reduce the susceptibility of microorganisms to bactericidal drugs by slowing the rate of reproduction. Bactericidal drugs are most toxic to rapidly dividing organisms. Moreover, they are not very effective when used with or immediately after administration of a bacteriostatic agent. A drug that is compatible with the residual drug should be used.

■ Summary

Antimicrobials are valuable agents for preventing and treating infections. They kill or inhibit the growth of pathogens with minimal risk to the host. Adverse reactions to these drugs include allergic reactions, damage to specific organs, and overgrowth of opportunistic organisms in the normal flora of the body.

Widespread use of antimicrobials has resulted in the emergence of resistant strains of pathogens, especially in health care institutions. Resistant infections are a hazard for clients and staff in affected agencies.

Nursing management
Nursing implications: prevention

Given the real dangers of anti-infective therapy, the nurse's first obligation is to prevent the need for its use, whenever possible. This prevention requires nursing care designed to protect vulnerable clients from exposure to infectious agents and to maintain and increase their resistance to these pathogens.

Risk factors. Individuals at risk for bacterial infections include people whose normal body defenses against infection are impaired. The very young and the very old are not capable of the vigorous inflammatory and immune responses characteristic of young and middle-aged adults. Malnourished or debilitated clients also have reduced resistance. Their depleted resources are inadequate to support the production of white blood cells, antibodies, and other body constituents needed to eliminate pathogens. Surgical incisions or traumatic wounds offer additional portals of entry for infection. Certain methods of treatment (immunosuppressive therapy, cancer chemotherapy, irradiation), which impair the immune response, place the client at risk. In addition, any client subjected to prolonged or severe stress is likely to have reduced resistance owing to hormone response (chiefly cortisone secretion) during the alarm and the subsequent exhaustion stages of stress adaptation. The nurse must identify the client at risk and assess the need for additional protection.

Aseptic measures. The general measures of cleanliness and hygiene adequate to control healthy clients' exposure to pathogens in the community environment are not sufficient in health care institutions. The client population in hospitals and nursing homes is generally at high risk for existing illness, wounds, and high levels of stress. The setting also is likely to contain a higher concentration of dangerous organisms than that of the general community. Infected clients are a prime source of pathogens. In addition, the normal microscopic flora in institutional environments are more likely to be resistant to antibodies than are organisms that inhabit the community at large. For these reasons, special measures must be used to reduce the number and mobility of pathogens in health care institutions.

In addition to environmental and personal hygiene, barrier techniques to restrict mobility of pathogens must be employed. Housekeeping routines have been developed to control the level of infective microorganisms in the institutional environment. Medical and surgical asepsis are routinely used to reduce or eliminate the introduction of pathogens to individual clients. Specific techniques are beyond the scope of this discussion; the student is referred to texts that deal with basic nursing skills for details. Special isolation techniques are employed to confine particularly dangerous or abundant pathogens that affect individual clients. The aim of these procedures is to prevent the pathogens from escaping into the general environment in large numbers. Reverse isolation is employed to protect particularly vulnerable clients from the pathogens present in the normal institutional environment. Both regular and reverse isolation are adapted to the requirements of the specific situation, the special needs of the individual client to be protected, and the characteristics of the pathogen. These may range from the simple use of masks to elaborate sterile life-island environments.

The initiation of special aseptic techniques is a nursing function. Institutional policy should grant authority to the nurse to order isolation procedures when appropriate. The decision to continue such measures should be a collaborative decision shared by the nurse and the physician.

Nursing process

Assessment The institution of systemic anti-infective chemotherapy imposes many responsibilities on the nurse. Nursing management must be directed toward achieving optimum therapeutic efficacy with the least risk to the client and others.

A careful drug history is essential to help prevent harmful drug reactions. Sensitivities and allergies should be noted conspicuously on the exterior of the chart to alert physicians as to which drugs are to be avoided or used only with special precautions. Any client who develops sensitivity to a drug agent should be fully informed of the significance of this problem and of what specific chemicals to avoid in the future. Adverse reactions to drugs are increasing in incidence and in severity as examples of iatrogenic illness.

The most critical factor is careful assessment of the client's response to medication. Physicians need to know if and how much their clients are improving to guide their choice of drug agents and dosage. Adverse reactions must be detected early so that protective measures can be taken. If serious or life-threatening reactions appear likely and unavoidable, special preparations must be made for prompt and effective treatment.

Nursing diagnosis Nursing diagnoses usually relate to signs and symptoms of infection, to reactions to the anti-infective drugs, and other aspects of care and may include the following:

> *Diarrhea related to effects of antibacterial medications*
> *Altered nutrition: less than body requirements related to diarrhea secondary to antibacterial medications*
> *Altered oral mucous membrane related to candidiasis, secondary to antibacterial medications*
> *High risk for infection (stomatitis, glossitis, vaginitis, colitis) related to alteration in normal flora secondary to antibacterial medication*
> *Noncompliance related to dislike of side effects or cost of medication*
> *Knowledge deficit concerning proper timing of drug administration and need to complete therapeutic regimen*

Planning Goals of treatment include alleviation or elimination of the signs and symptoms of infection, prevention of adverse drug reactions, client compliance with the regimen, and prompt detection and treatment of adverse reaction, should one occur.

Intervention Drugs must be administered accurately and skillfully. Timing is particularly important, because serum drug concentrations must be maintained at therapeutic levels. Anti-infectives given intravenously (IV) must be administered slowly to prevent irritation of the vein and possible phlebitis. Clients who receive parenteral drugs are particularly vulnerable to severe and rapidly developing systemic reactions and should be observed closely. Oral anti-infectives are usually given between meals to prevent delays or decreases in absorption due to the drug's interaction with food.

Care must be exercised to minimize environmental dispersion of anti-infectives, which promotes the development of resistant strains of microorganisms. Wasted drugs should be incinerated to destroy the chemical. Disposal in hoppers or toilets increases contamination of natural water reservoirs. When handling solutions with syringes, draw up the exact dose before removing the syringe from vial or bottle to avoid ejecting excess solution into the environment.

Whenever both cultures and anti-infective drugs are ordered for a client with an infection, drug administration must be delayed until the culture is obtained. Cultures taken after initiation of therapy may fail to reveal the pathogen or reflect an altered microbial population. Drug therapy must not be delayed beyond this minimal period, however, as pathogen populations increase enormously within a short period of time. For example, waiting until morning to start drug therapy ordered in the evening or night hours can be disastrous for the client.

When anti-infectives are ordered before laboratory data are available to identify the pathogen and its drug sensitivity, the physician is likely to order a broad-spectrum drug known to be effective in illnesses that resemble the client's clinical picture. If the client responds well, this drug may be continued even after lab data are available, or therapy may be altered to a more specific agent for the particular organism isolated. Should the client's clinical response be inadequate, however, the test data are crucial for selecting the specific drug agent most suitable for the client's condition. In such circumstances, the drug order will be changed about the third day after cultures have been taken, when the sensitivity reports become available. Nurses should report the laboratory results to the physician promptly to facilitate adjustments in the treatment regimen.

Anti-infective drugs should be administered consistently and at intervals that ensure maintenance of a therapeutic blood level. Recommendations regarding the use of these drugs (*eg*, to be given on an empty stomach) must be followed. Hours for scheduling the administration of anti-infectives should be selected with these objectives in view. Drugs ordered several times a day (bid, tid, qid) are usually administered at equal intervals (q12h, q8h, q6h).

Nurses should watch for adverse reactions that are common to the drug in use, but they must also be alert for responses that are unusual to that agent. Of particular significance are skin rashes, intestinal upsets, and allergic reactions. Unless the drug regimen is considered as a possible cause, these reactions are likely to be attributed to the client's illness, environmental antigens, general stress, or other factors. Failure to identify the problem as a drug reaction often results in inadequate treatment and prolonged or progressive symptoms in the victim.

Use of general supportive measures are important to promote increased resistance to infection in the client. Adequate nutrition and rest are critical for maintaining immune and inflammatory responses. Promotion of wound healing restores the normal barrier to entrance of pathogens. It is particularly important that general stress be reduced for the institutionalized client. For the client subject to unavoidable sources of stress, nursing interventions to promote progression from the alarm to the resistance phase of adaptation reduce hormonal responses detrimental to resistance.

Client education. Educating the public in the proper use of anti-infectives is crucial in preventing overuse of these drugs. The client with a cold who pressures a physician to prescribe an antibiotic may succeed, despite the physician's knowledge that such drugs are not effective against viral agents. Prophylactic use is rarely justified. The exercise of discriminating professional judgment is necessary if the effectiveness of our present treatment agents is to be enhanced and prolonged and the development of resistant pathogens delayed. The client needs education about the specific medication, its administration for optimal effect, and the need for compliance.

Individuals who have experienced allergic reactions to antimicrobial drugs should be advised to wear a medical identification device that lists the substance to which they are hypersensitive.

Evaluation Criteria for evaluation relate to signs and symptoms of infection and adverse drug reactions, as well as to compliance.

Checklist of nursing actions

☐ Inform clients of the expected beneficial and adverse reactions before implementation of the drug regimen.

☐ Take a careful client history to determine the presence of allergies or other conditions that may interfere with the effectiveness of the particular medication or pose a high risk of adverse reaction to it.

☐ Check for use of other medications that may be affected by this drug, and determine the need for any modification of dosage.

Major antimicrobial drug families

Sulfonamides

The first effective systemic antimicrobial was a sulfonamide developed in Denmark and Germany in the 1930s. As a result of research that involved coal tar aniline compounds, Prontosil, a bright red dye, was found to produce dramatic improvement in clients who suffered from certain bacterial infections. This compound and its derivative, sulfanilamide, were used in the successful treatment of coccal infections, such as pneumonia, meningitis, and puerperal sepsis. In the absence of other effective treatment agents, use of the sulfonamides mushroomed, despite their relatively high cost. During World War II, "sulfa" powder sprinkled over the wounds of injured soldiers was credited with saving innumerable lives by suppressing infection.

Sulfonamides are structural analogs of PABA, a substance required by many microorganisms for the production of folic acid. They are weak acids that are generally insoluble in water; most sodium salts of the drugs are strongly basic and readily soluble in water but deteriorate rapidly in solution (Table 41-1).

Modification of the sulfonamide drugs has resulted in the development of several other useful therapeutic drug agents. These include the antituberculosis drug PAS, sulfones used to treat leprosy, carbonic anhydrase inhibitor diuretics, sulfonylurea hypoglycemics, and thiouracil antithyroids. The last three of these exploit side effects of the original sulfonamide group.

Pharmacodynamics. The sulfonamides are bacteriostatic rather than bactericidal. They prevent the growth of microorganisms by inhibiting the production of folic acid in bacterial cells through competition with PABA. Host cells (in mammals) are unaffected because they cannot synthesize folic acid but use the preformed vitamin.

Pharmacokinetics. Most sulfonamides (except sulfapyridine and sulfasalazine) are absorbed readily from the GI tract. Absorption from other mucous membranes and abraded skin is unreliable, but enough drug may reach the circulation to induce allergic hypersensitivity. Absorbable sulfonamides are lipid soluble and distribute readily into body tissues and fluids, including the cerebrospinal fluid, as well as the pleural, peritoneal, and synovial spaces. Most sulfonamides readily cross the placenta and are distributed in breast milk. Penetration is poor into the bile, saliva, or prostatic fluid. Sulfonamides bind loosely to serum albumin and, to a lesser degree, serum globulin. Within the body they are metabolized by acetylation and glucuronidation, mainly in the liver. Metabolites are inactive; the acetylated form is less soluble than the unchanged drug, particularly in acid media. Excretion is mainly through the kidneys. Solubility of these drugs in the urine and the rate of excretion are enhanced by alkalinization of the urine.

The poorly absorbed sulfonamides remain in the GI tract and are eliminated in feces.

Therapeutic uses. Sulfonamides remain the agents of choice for the treatment of urinary tract infection and are useful secondary drugs for many other conditions, including shigellosis, nocardiosis, trachoma, and toxoplasmosis. In combination with trimethoprim, sulfamethoxazole is used to treat typhoid fever, *Pneumocystis carinii* infections, and brucellosis. Sulfasalazine is used in the treatment of chronic ulcerative colitis. The drugs have a wide range of activity against both gram-positive and gram-negative organisms. Sulfonamides are also used in the prophylaxis of traveler's diarrhea and otitis media.

Adverse reactions. Because early sulfonamide preparations were poorly soluble, they tended to crystallize in the kidneys, causing serious renal impairment. Renal toxicity in present-day preparations is less likely, because more soluble salts have been developed and less soluble salts are used in combinations that allow a lower dose of each component (Box 41-3). Some potential for kidney damage remains, however.

Adverse reactions to sulfonamides tend to be allergic in nature. Most common are skin rashes and fever. Anaphylaxis, aplastic anemia, hemolytic anemia, and Stevens-Johnson syndrome are seen rarely but can be life-threatening. Sensitivity is most likely to develop in people with a history of topical treatment with sulfonamides.

The emergence of resistant strains of pathogens has limited the usefulness of sulfonamides. Other newer antimicrobials have superseded them in treating many infections caused by organisms likely to be insensitive.

Long-term sulfonamide therapy can produce vitamin K deficiency because of inhibition of microorganisms that normally synthesize this vitamin within the intestine. This can lead to hypoprothrombinemia and bleeding tendencies.

Occasionally, sulfonamides cause hypoglycemia as a result of the stimulation of insulin release by the pancreas. The drugs can also suppress production of thyroid hormone, impair liver function, and reduce fertility in males. Sulfonamides increase the anticoagulant effects of warfarin and may cause bleeding when the drugs are used concurrently. When applied to denuded areas, sulfonamide creams cause a burning sensation. High doses of sulfasalazine may cause subclinical folate deficiency in individuals with chronic colitis.

Table 41-1. Sulfonamide preparations

Drug name	Preparations	Usual dosage	Additional information
mafenide (Marfanil, Napaltan, Sulfamylon)	8.5% Topical cream	q.s. to cover the affected area to a depth of ¹/₁₆ inch PC: C	Used to prevent infection in the treatment of burns
silver sulfadiazine (Flamazine, Silvadene, SSD Cream)	1% Topical cream	q.s. to cover the affected area to a depth of ¹/₁₆ inch PC: C	Used to prevent infection in the treatment of burns
sulfacetamide sodium (AK-Sulf, Bleph-10, Cetamide, Sulamyd, Sulfair, Sulfamide, Sulfex, Sulf-O)	Ophthalmic solution (10%, 15%, and 30%) Ophthalmic ointment (10%)	*Ointment:* 1.25–2.5 cm ribbon q2–3h *Solution:* gtt i–2 ql–2h PC: C	Used in the treatment of superficial eye infections
sulfadiazine (Microsulfon, Sulfadets)	Oral tablets	Adults: 2–4 g/day, divided in 3–6 doses Children older than 2 mo: 150 mg/kg body weight/day, divided in 4–6 doses PC: B (D if near term)	Rapidly absorbed by the GI tract; rapidly excreted; less soluble than sulfisoxazole
sulfamethizole (Microsul, Proklar, Thisulfil, Thiosulfil Forte, Ultrasul, Urifon, Urobiotic, Urolucosil)	Oral tablets	Adults: 1.5–4 g/day, divided in 3–4 doses Children older than 2 mo: 30–45 mg/kg body weight/day, divided in 4 doses PC: C (Not to be used at term)	Rapidly excreted; use limited to treatment of urinary tract infections
sulfamethoxazole (Gantanol, Methoxanol, Urobak; *with trimethoprim:* Bactrim, Septra)	Oral tablets and suspension	Adults: 2–3 g/day, divided in 2–3 doses Children: 50–60 mg/kg body weight/day, divided in 2 doses PC: B (D if near term)	More slowly absorbed and excreted, and less soluble than sulfisoxazole
sulfapyridine (Dagenam)	Oral tablets	Adults: 0.5–2 g/day, divided in 1–4 doses	Used for the treatment of dermatitis herpetiformis when sulfones are contraindicated
sulfasalazine (Azaline EC, Azopyrin, Azulfidine, S.A.S.-500, Salazopyrin, Sulfadyne)	Oral tablets and suspension	Adults: 1–4 g/day, divided in 1–4 doses Children older than 2 mo: 30 mg/kg body weight/day, divided in 4 doses PC: B (D if near term)	Poorly absorbed in the GI tract; administered for local effect in the gut; used in the treatment of ulcerative colitis, regional enteritis, granulomatous colitis
sulfisoxazole (Gantrisin, Gantrisona, Koro-Sulf, Novosoxazole, Pediazole, SK-Soxazole, Sulfizin, Sulfasin)	Oral tablets Vaginal cream	Adults: 4–8 g/day, divided in 4–6 doses Children older than 2 mo: 150 mg/kg body weight/day, divided in 4–6 doses *Vaginal infection:* 2.5–5 ml 10% cream placed in vagina bid PC: B (D if near term)	Highly soluble; rapidly absorbed from the GI tract; rapidly excreted
sulfisoxazole acetyl (Erizole, Oral Suspension, Gantrisin Pediatric, LipoGantrisin)	Oral suspension or flavored syrup	Adults: 4–8 g/day, divided in 4–6 doses Children: 150 mg/kg body weight/day, divided in 4–6 doses PC: B (D if near term)	Same as above

KEY: PC = pregnancy category. (The validity of pregnancy risk categories has not been established; see Chapter 16, p 216.)

Precautions and contraindications. Because sulfonamides easily cross the placenta and are excreted into breast milk, caution must be exercised when they are used during pregnancy and lactation. Sulfonamides are not used to treat newborns, because they displace bilirubin from protein-binding sites, increasing the risk and severity of kernicterus.

Sulfonamide therapy is contraindicated by a history of allergic reaction or anuria after use of a drug from this group. When these drugs are used concurrently with warfarin, the dose of anticoagulant should be decreased.

Before ophthalmic use of sulfonamides, crusts or discharge should be removed from the eyes with a new

Box 41-3. Combination drugs that contain two or more sulfonamides

Drug names	Preparations
Trisulfapyrimidines, a combination of sulfadiazine, sulfamerazine, and sulfamethazine (Triple Sulfa [suspension], Neotrizine, Sulfaloid, Sultrin, Terfonyl)	Tablets and suspension for oral use
Sulfadiazine, sulfamethizole, and phenazopyridine (Suladyne)	Tablets for oral use
Sulfabenzamide, sulfacetamide, and sulfathiazole (Sultrin, Triple Sulfa, Trysul)	Tablets for oral use Vaginal cream

cotton ball and clean hands. Drops or ointment should be stored at room temperature and applied as prescribed, preventing contact between the dropper or tube tip and the eye. Clients with an infection should not use eye cosmetics nor share towels or washcloths.

■ **Summary**

The sulfonamides are bacteriostatic antimicrobials that act by competitive inhibition of folic acid synthesis in the microbial cell. They are effective agents for the treatment of urinary tract infections and useful adjuncts in the treatment of many other infections. Their clinical usefulness is somewhat reduced by the development of drug-resistant strains of pathogens and allergic sensitivity in recipients. The sulfonamides have the potential to cause crystalluria-induced nephrotoxicity.

Nursing management

Nursing process

Assessment A careful history should be taken before sulfonamide therapy is begun. Pregnancy, lactation, and the recent use of PABA (a sulfonamide antagonist) should be ruled out. The nurse should question clients about their previous use of sulfonamides, any adverse reactions to these drugs that may have occurred (specifically skin rashes, reduction in urinary output, or kidney problems), and personal or family history of allergy to them.

Nursing diagnosis Diagnoses may concern the risk of adverse reaction to sulfonamide preparations or the risk of recurrent infection amenable to sulfonamide therapy, such as cystitis.

Nursing diagnoses likely to be made for clients who are receiving sulfonamides may include the following:

Altered nutrition: less than body requirements related to abdominal discomfort secondary to sulfonamide medication
Diarrhea related to sulfonamide medication
Noncompliance: discontinuation of medication before full course is completed
High risk for infection by sulfonamide-resistant pathogens related to failure to complete course of medication
Knowledge deficit related to effects of medication and need for compliance
Pain related to cystitis or to kidney damage secondary to adverse reaction to sulfonamide medication

A common collaborative problem that should be differentiated from the nursing diagnoses is

Potential complication: renal

Planning Treatment goals include promoting resistance to infection, reducing the risk of recurrent infection that requires multiple courses of drug therapy, reducing the risk of adverse reaction to sulfonamides, and prompt detection and treatment of adverse reactions, should they occur.

Intervention Oral sulfonamide preparations should be administered with ample fluids (a full glass for adults, proportionate amounts for children). Intake and output should be recorded, and the level of hydration and renal function should be carefully appraised. Ample hydration must be maintained.

Nursing measures that minimize the recurrence of infection should be instituted. For example, clients with a history of frequent urinary tract infections sometimes are placed on long-term therapy with sulfisoxazole or sulfamethoxazole. Often, the cycle of recurrent infection can be interrupted by removing retention catheters, instituting hygienic measures to minimize urethral contamination by intestinal organ-

Example of nursing process and sulfonamide therapy for cystitis

The client is a 31-year-old mother of two who has had three episodes of cystitis within the past 2 years. All have been treated successfully with sulfisoxasole medication. The client is known to have a cystocele (a predisposing factor for cystitis). She has a history of hay fever and asthma. No adverse reaction to previous courses of sulfonamides occurred.

Assessment data	Nursing diagnosis	Intervention	Goals and outcome criteria
Recurrent episodes of cystitis treated with sulfonamides	Possible knowledge deficit related to cystitis and its prevention	**Prepare** and implement a plan to teach the client hygienic measures to reduce the risk of recurrent cystitis; the plan should cover (1) the need for ample hydration (3 liters of fluid daily), (2) proper removal and application of perineal pads, (3) cleaning the perineum from front to back to prevent transfer of intestinal organisms from the anus to the urinary meatus, and (4) avoidance of detergent additives to bath water (*eg*, bubble bath or bath salts).	Within the next 2 years, the client will experience fewer than three episodes of cystitis.
History of asthma and hay fever	High risk for impaired tissue integrity: rhinitis and bronchial inflammation related to antigen–antibody reaction secondary to allergy to sulfonamides	**Inform** the client of the risk of allergic hypersensitivity in response to intermittent drug use.	If adverse reaction to sulfisoxasole occurs, it will be treated within 12 hours of onset.
		Warn the client to maintain ample hydration during sulfonmide therapy. Teach her the signs and symptoms of adverse reactions to sulfonamides and urge her to report them promptly, should any occur.	

isms, and maintaining ample hydration. General supportive measures to enhance the host's resistance to pathogens also reduce the incidence of infection and the need for drug therapy.

Burn victims who receive sulfonamide creams should be warned that the medication may cause discomfort (temporary burning and stinging sensations) when first applied. Analgesic drugs should be administered before applying the antimicrobial.

Client education. Clients who receive sulfonamides should be advised to drink plenty of fluids (200 to 300 ml/day for adults). They should also be told to report promptly any reduction in urine output, blood in the urine, flank pain, and symptoms of allergic reaction, such as skin rash.

Evaluation Data required for evaluation include decreases in the signs and symptoms of infection (indications of a therapeutic response) and signs and symptoms of adverse reaction to the antimicrobial drugs. Intake and output should be recorded and the level of hydration and renal function carefully appraised. Skin rash or flank pain may signify adverse drug reaction (see Example of Nursing Process and Sulfonamide Therapy for Cystitis).

Checklist of nursing actions

☐ Assess the risk of sulfonamide therapy by taking a careful history from the client before drug administration is begun.

☐ Teach clients with recurrent infections hygienic measures to reduce the incidence of infection.

☐ Whenever possible, substitute nursing management of urinary incontinence for the use of retention catheters.

☐ Maintain ample hydration in clients who receive sulfonamides.

☐ Observe clients who receive sulfonamides for early signs and symptoms of allergic reactions and renal impairment. Report these promptly.

☐ Administer analgesics to burn victims before administering topical sulfonamides.

β-Lactam antibiotics

Two major antibiotic families, penicillins and cephalosporins, share a common structural component, the β-lactam ring:

$$-CH-CH-$$
$$O=C-N-$$

The significance of this common structure is unclear, since antibiotic and pharmacokinetic properties appear to vary as functions of adjacent rings or side chains. The fact that penicillins and cephalosporins exhibit some cross-sensitivity (*ie*, individuals allergic to penicillin are likely to exhibit allergic sensitivity to some cephalosporins) indicates that the shared component is clinically important. Drugs from both families are inactivated by an enzyme, β-lactamase, which is produced by some resistant pathogens.

Penicillins

The era of antibiotic chemotherapy began with the development of penicillin during World War II. This natural product of a blue-green bread mold was remarkably effective in treating a wide range of infections. Although many pathogens have developed resistance to some penicillins, this family of drugs remains a valuable therapeutic agent for treating a wide range of infections.

Pharmacodynamics. Penicillins interfere with a number of microbial enzymes involved in processes such as cell division and synthesis, as well as maintenance of cell walls. As a result, organisms fail to reproduce, and some die from cell lysis. Penicillins, therefore, are both bacteriostatic and bactericidal.

Pharmacokinetics. Many forms of penicillin are destroyed in the digestive tract. Other preparations are acid-resistant and consequently are unaffected by digestion.

Penicillin is widely distributed in the body, but concentrations are highest in the plasma, where much of it is reversibly bound to plasma albumin. Protein-binding provides some prolongation of biologic half-life but can cause interactions with other protein-bound substances owing to competitive displacement. Most preparations penetrate the blood–brain barrier poorly, except when the meninges are inflamed or fever is present.

Penicillin is excreted from the body largely unchanged by metabolic processes. Most of the drug is eliminated by the kidneys, where it is actively secreted by the tubule. Urinary excretion of the drug may be inhibited by the concurrent administration of probenecid, resulting in higher plasma concentrations. Some drug is eliminated in the bile and other body secretions.

Therapeutic uses. Penicillin is one of the most important classes of antibiotics. Its derivatives are used in the treatment of many common infections. Penicillins have been used successfully against infections caused by such penicillin-sensitive organisms as streptococci, staphylococci, pneumococci, *Corynebacterium diphtheriae, Bacillus anthracis, Clostridium* organisms, *Actinomyces bovis, Streptobacillus moniliformis, Listeria monocytogenes, Leptospira* organisms, *Neisseria gonorrhoeae*, and *Treponema pallidum*. The most recently developed penicillins are effective against an even wider range of organisms.

An upsurge in virulent and sometimes fatal streptococcal infections, including strep throat, rheumatic fever, and streptococcal pneumonia, has occurred. Immediate and accurate diagnosis is important so that proper treatment can be instituted without delay. A strep antigen test provides a diagnosis within a half-hour. If positive, treatment is begun immediately. However, if the result is negative (possibly falsely so), a throat culture is done, with a more accurate diagnosis available in a day. Treatment with antibiotics is necessary to prevent the body's immune system from acting in error against its own tissue, leading to possible permanent damage to the heart valves and kidneys. The treatment is usually a 10-day course of penicillin (or penicillin alternative), which must be completed to prevent a recurrence of the infection.

Drug preparations. Preparations of penicillin suitable for oral, IV, and intramuscular (IM) administration are available for clinical use (Table 41-2). IV (aqueous) solutions and IM suspensions must not be confused; the suspensions must never be administered IV. Topical applications and inhalation therapy are not recommended because they are not very effective, and they often induce allergic sensitivity.

Adverse reactions. Some strains of microorganisms (notably staphylococci) readily develop resistance

Table 41-2. Penicillin preparations

Drug name	Preparations	Usual dosage
amoxicillin (Amoxil, Larotid, Novamoxin, Polymox, Robamox, Sumox, Trimox, Utimox, Wymox)	Capsules, suspensions and chewable tablets for oral administration	Adults and children who weigh 20 kg or more: 750 mg–1.5 g/day, divided in 3 doses, administered at equal time intervals Children who weigh less than 20 kg: 20–40 mg/kg body weight/day, divided in 3 doses administered at equal time intervals PC: B
amoxicillin and potassium clavulanate (Augmentin)	Tablets, chewable tablets, and suspension for oral administration	Adults: "250" or "500" coated tablet every 8 hours. Note: Each "250" or "500" tablet contains same amount of clavulanic acid (125 mg as potassium salt); therefore, do not substitute two of "250" tablets for one "500" tablet; "125" or "250" chewable tablet every 8 hours; "125" banana-flavored or "250" orange-flavored suspension PC: B
ampicillin (Amcap, Amcill, Ampicin, Ampilean, D-Amp, Nu-Ampi, Penbristol, Pfizerpen A, Polycillin, Principen, SK-Ampicillin, Supen, Totacillin, Unasyn)	Capsules and suspensions for oral administration Vials that contain powder for reconstitution for IM or IV administration	Adults: 1–2 g/day, divided in 4 doses, administered at equal time intervals Children: 24–50 mg/kg body weight/day, divided in 4 doses, administered at equal time intervals For severe infection, larger doses may be required PC: B
azlocillin sodium (Azlin)	Vials and infusion bottles that contain powder for reconstitution for IV administration	Adults: 100–300 mg/kg body weight/day, divided in 4–6 doses, administered at equal time intervals Children: 450 mg/kg body weight/day, divided in 3–6 doses, administered at equal time intervals Maximum dosage: 24 g/day Not recommended for newborns PC: B
bacampicillin (Penglobe, Spectrobid)	Tablets and suspension for oral administration	Adults and children who weigh 25 kg or more: 800–1600 mg/day divided in 2 doses, administered at equal time intervals Children who weight less than 25 kg: 25 mg/kg/day, divided in 2 doses, administered at equal time intervals PC: B
carbenicillin disodium (Anabactyl, Geopen)	Vials that contain powder for reconstitution for IM or IV administration	Varies with the nature and severity of infection Adults: 250–500 mg/kg body weight/day administered by continuous IV infusion or divided in 4–6 doses Children: 250–500 mg/kg body weight/day, depending on age, divided in 4–6 doses
carbenicillin indanyl sodium (Geocillin, Pyopen)	Oral tablets	Adults: 1.5–3.0 g/day, divided in 4 doses PC: B
cloxacillin sodium (Cloxapen, Tegopen)	Capsules and solution for oral administration	Adults and children who weigh 20 kg or more: 1–2 g/day, divided in 4 doses, administered at equal time intervals Children who weigh less than 20 kg: 50–100 mg/kg body weight/day, divided in 4 doses PC: B

(Continued)

Table 41-2. Penicillin preparations (Continued)

Drug name	Preparations	Usual dosage
cyclacillin (Cyclopen)	Tablets and suspension for oral administration	Adults: 1–2 g/day, divided in 4 doses, administered at equal time intervals Children: 50 mg/kg/day, divided in 4 doses, administered at equal time intervals
dicloxacillin sodium (Diclocil, Dycill, Dynapen, Pathocil)	Capsules and suspension for oral administration	Adults and children who weigh 40 kg or more: 0.5–1 g/day, divided in 4 doses, administered at equal time intervals Children who weigh less than 40 kg: 12.5–25 mg/kg body weight/day, divided in 4 doses PC: B
methicillin sodium (Celbenin, Dimocillin-RT, Penistaph, Staphcillin, Syntricillin)	Vials that contain powder for reconstitution for IM or IV administration	Adults and children who weigh 20 kg or more: 4–6 g/day, divided in 4–6 doses, administered at equal time intervals Children who weigh less than 20 kg: 100 mg/kg body weight/day divided in 4 doses, administered at equal time intervals (for severe infections, larger doses may be required) PC: B
mezlocillin sodium (Mezlin)	Vials and infusion bottles that contain powder for reconstitution for IM or IV administration	Adults: 100–300 mg/kg body weight/day, divided in 4–6 doses, administered at equal time intervals Children 1 mo–12 yr of age: 300 mg/kg body weight/day, divided in 6 doses Neonates over 7 days old: 225–300 mg/kg body weight/day, divided in 3–4 doses, administered at equal time intervals Neonates 7 days or younger: 150 mg/kg body weight/day, in 2 doses, administered at equal time intervals PC: B
nafcillin sodium (Nafcil, Nallpen, Unipen)	Capsules, solution, and tablets for oral administration Vials that contain powder for reconstitution for IM or IV administration	Adults: 1–6 g/day, divided in 4–6 doses Children (depending on the age of the child and the route used): 20–50 mg/kg body weight/day, divided in 4–6 doses PC: B
oxacillin sodium (Bactocill, Bristopen, Penstapho, Prostaphlin, Resistopen)	Capsules and solution for oral administration Vials that contain powder for reconstitution for IM or IV administration	Adults and children who weigh 40 kg or more: 2–3 g/day, divided in 4–6 doses Children who weigh less than 40 kg: 50 mg/kg body weight/day, divided in 4 doses PC: B
penicillin G, benzathine (Bicillin, Extenilline, Megacillin, Neolin, Penidural, Permapen, Tardocillin)	Tablets for oral administration Suspensions for IM injection in multiple dose vials, prefilled cartridges and disposable syringes	*Oral:* Adults: 1,200,000–3,600,000 U/day, divided in 4–6 doses; children: 25,000–90,000 U/kg body weight/day, divided in 3–6 doses *IM:* 300,000–2,400,000 U (dosage varies with the indications) PC: B
penicillin G, potassium (Forpen, Ka-Pen, M-cillin, NovoPen, Pentids, Pfizerpen G, SK-Penicillin, Sugracillin)	Tablets and solution for oral administration Vials that contain powder for reconstitution for IM or IV administration	Varies with age of recipient and severity of infection *Oral:* Adults and children more than 12 yr of age: 1,200,000–2,000,000 U/day, divided in 3–4 doses; children less than 12 yr of age: 25,000–90,000 U/kg body weight/day, divided in 3–6 doses

(Continued)

Table 41-2. Penicillin preparations (Continued)

Drug name	Preparations	Usual dosage
		Parenteral: Adults: 5,000,000–20,000,000 U/day; children: 30,000–50,000 U/kg body weight/day, divided in 4–6 doses (dosage varies greatly with indication and severity of infection)
penicillin G, procaine (Ayercillin, Bicillin, Crysticillin, Duracillin, Pfizerpen-AS, Wycillin)	Suspensions for IM injection in multi-dose vials, prefilled cartridges, and disposable syringes	Adults and children more than 12 yr of age: 600,000–9,800,000 U/day Children (depending on size): 50,000–300,000 U/day, given in a single dose (dosage varies greatly with indications) PC: B
penicillin V potassium, (Beepen-VK, Betapen, Betapen-VK, Cocillin, Deltapen-VK, Ledercillin, Ledercillin-VK, Penapar-VK, Pen-Vee K, Pfizerpen VK, Repen, Repen-VK, Robicillin, SK-Penicillin VK, Suspen, Uticillin VK, V-Cillin K, Veetids)	Tablets and solutions for oral administration	Adults and children more than 12 yr of age: 0.25–2 g/day, divided in 2–4 doses Children less than 12 yr of age: 15–62.5 mg/kg body weight/day, divided in 3–6 doses PC: B
piperacillin (Pipracil)	Solutions for IM or IV injection	Adults: 6–18 g/day, divided in 4–6 doses Maximum adult dose: 24 g/day Children: 50–100 mg/kg body weight/day divided in 6 doses, administered at equal time intervals PC: B
ticarcillin (Ticar)	Vials that contain powder for reconstitution for IM or IV administration	Adults and children: 200–300 mg/kg body weight/day, divided in 4–8 doses PC: B
ticarcillin disodium and clavulanate potassium (Timentin)	Vials that contain powder for reconstitution for IV administration by direct infusion over 30 min or piggyback (discontinue other drugs temporarily during infusion)	Varies with weight of recipient, type and severity of infection Adults (>60 kg): moderate gynecologic infection–200 mg/kg/day (3.1-g vial) divided in 6 doses; severe gynecologic infection–300 mg/kg/day divided in 6 doses Adults (<60 kg): 200–300 mg/kg/day, divided in 4–6 doses PC: B

KEY: PC = pregnancy category. (The validity of pregnancy risk categories has not been established; see Chapter 16, p 216.)

to penicillin. One form of resistance is the ability to produce an enzyme (penicillinase) that chemically degrades the penicillin molecule. When penicillinase-susceptible drugs are prescribed to treat infections caused by pathogens with this type of resistance, therapeutic response is absent or inadequate. Immunity to drugs caused by this or other inheritable traits can be transferred from one organism to another by several mechanisms that involve exchange of chromosomal material.

Allergic reactions to penicillin are frequently seen in clinical practice. Initially, penicillin sensitivity may be manifested by local erythema and itching at the site of parenteral injection. Skin rashes, especially urticaria with pruritus, are common and occur after oral, as well as parenteral, administration. Anaphylactic shock, a rapidly developing syndrome characterized by dyspnea and hypotension, may occur and can be fatal. When penicillin is combined with procaine, adverse reaction to the procaine component may take the form of a violent psychotic reaction. These reactions tend to be short-lived and resolve in 15 to 30 minutes.

Other adverse reactions to penicillin include neutropenia, hemolytic anemia, bleeding stemming from platelet malfunction, adult respiratory distress syndrome, superinfection, and CNS changes (seizures, psychoses). Superinfection tends to cause intestinal symptoms (sore mouth, nausea, diarrhea). Seizures are most likely in recipients with meningitis, because inflammation of the meninges allows the drug to penetrate the blood–brain barrier in large amounts.

Penicillin interacts with several drugs. It is known

to reduce the effectiveness of oral contraceptives. Both natural and semisynthetic penicillins deactivate aminoglycosides. A drop in serum levels of atenolol has been reported when ampicillin is administered concurrently with this β-blocker (Shafer-Korting, et al, 1983).

Precautions and contraindications. Owing to the dangerous nature of some allergic reactions to penicillin (anaphylaxis), any indication of developing sensitivity is reason for caution. Use of the drug is avoided if possible when a history includes respiratory distress, shock, or anaphylaxis after administration of penicillin. If penicillin is prescribed for high-risk clients, rapidly eliminated forms of the drug are preferred. Rapid desensitization with oral doses should be attempted if penicillin therapy is required for allergic individuals. Doses are administered at 15-minute intervals, starting with very small doses and doubling the dose with each succeeding administration.

When penicillin is prescribed for women who are taking oral contraceptives, an alternate method of contraception should be used for the duration of antibiotic therapy. The oral contraceptive regimen should be continued at the same time to preserve the anovulatory cycle.

■ Summary

Penicillin and its derivatives are reliable agents for the treatment of many common infections. They exert primarily bactericidal effects on pathogens. Their action can be prolonged by the concurrent administration of probenecid. Allergic sensitivity can cause dangerous reactions to these drugs.

Nursing management

Nursing implications

To reduce the incidence of antibiotic nosocomial infection, it is vital to reduce the resident population of microorganisms, minimize contact between microbes and antibiotics, and eliminate the transmission of microorganisms from infected victims and carriers to healthy people. To accomplish these tasks, rigorous environmental cleanliness, careful handling of antibiotic drugs, and good medical asepsis is required.

Although environmental cleanliness in health care institutions is the responsibility of the housekeeping staff, the nurse shares responsibility for environmental safety. Staff should be summoned promptly when infectious material escapes into the environment. The nursing staff should work with the housekeeping staff to ensure adequate sanitary cleanliness.

Exposure of environmental microbial inhabitants to penicillin occurs in two ways. Because the drug is present in the urine of clients who undergo treatment,

it can reach the environment if excreta are not properly handled. When penicillin solutions are mixed and measured, they are often spilled on surfaces in the medication room. It has been common practice, for example, to eject excess drug from the syringe into the sink. This practice adds to environmental contamination. Instead, any excess should be burned by placing it in a flame, an oven, a microwave, or even under a hot iron. The more penicillin ordered and administered to clients, the greater the potential for environmental contamination. Although physicians now exercise greater discrimination in prescribing penicillin as a means of controlling hospital infection, corresponding efforts by nurses have been slower to take hold. Careless handling of antibiotic solutions is still prevalent in nursing practice.

Transmission of infection can be minimized by rigorous aseptic precautions. The need for tight isolation technique and medical asepsis is verbally acknowledged in medical institutions. However, assessment of actual practices usually uncovers many breaches of technique. One factor may be the use of a high proportion of paraprofessionals on the staff. Aides and orderlies often begin work with a minimum of training. Turnover may be high, and a qualified staff with adequate preparation is hard to maintain. Trained staff must recognize the part played by their poor example and failure to maintain high standards.

Reaction to penicillin therapy must also be closely monitored by the nurse. When a potassium penicillin is administered parenterally, a risk of acute hyperkalemia exists. Excessive blood potassium can precipitate cardiac arrest. To prevent this problem, IV potassium salts should be administered no faster than 5 mEq/h.

Because penicillin inactivates aminoglycosides, when both drugs are prescribed, they should be administered at different times, at least 1 hour apart.

Anaphylactic reactions to penicillin require immediate treatment. Antiallergenic measures include administration of epinephrine, antihistamines, and a corticosteroid. These drugs should be readily available when penicillin therapy is initiated.

Nursing process

Assessment Whenever penicillin therapy is contemplated, the nurse must take a careful history to assess the risk of allergic reaction. The client should be questioned specifically about previous use of penicillin and any adverse reaction to it. Of particular significance are urticaria, skin rash, itching, or inflammation at sites of penicillin injection. Other drugs may be chosen if hypersensitivity to penicillin is present.

Nursing diagnosis Diagnoses are concerned primarily with responses to the drug regimen (therapeutic or adverse) and may include the following:

Pain: abdominal discomfort related to antimicrobial medication

Diarrhea related to antimicrobial medication

High risk for impaired skin integrity: rash related to allergic reaction to amtimicrobial medication

Noncompliance: stopping medication before full course of medication has been related to discomfort of adverse reaction to the drug, or omission of the drug related to inability to pay for the prescription

Knowledge deficit related to antimicrobial drugs and the regimens for their administration

Planning Goals of treatment are to promote recovery from the infection and to reduce the risk and severity of adverse drug reactions.

Intervention Because clients may become sensitized to penicillin through environmental exposure, all clients who receive penicillin should be monitored for signs and symptoms of allergic reaction (skin rash, urticaria, dyspnea). Epinephrine should be readily available for treating serious reactions (anaphylaxis). Particular penicillins require additional information for clients. They should be warned not to drink acidic beverages for an hour after taking penicillin G, or the effectiveness will be lessened. Some penicillins (particularly amoxicillin and clavulanate, azlocillin, mezlocillin, oxacillin, piperacillin) occasionally cause abdominal pain, dark urine, or jaundice, which should be reported to the physician immediately. Other penicillins (ampicillin, bacampicillin, or penicillin V) may interfere with the effectiveness of birth control pills that contain estrogen, requiring additional contraceptive measures.

Client education. Some form of lactobacilli (yogurt, buttermilk, or Bacid capsules) may be administered to help maintain a normal intestinal flora and reduce the risk of superinfection. These inoculants should not be administered for at least 1 hour after the oral dose of penicillin, so that they are not inactivated by the drug. If white patches are seen on the tongue or oral mucosa (indicating a possible infection with a *Candida* organism), the physician should be asked to prescribe an antifungal drug, such as nystatin.

Clients who react allergically to penicillin must be informed that they are hypersensitive to such drugs. A medical identification device that lists this allergy should be recommended.

When penicillin is prescribed for clients outside health care agencies, the importance of completing the treatment regimen should be stressed. Many clients discontinue medication as soon as they feel well. Residual pathogens may cause a later recurrence. Owing to their exposure to the antibiotic, the surviving organisms are more likely to be resistant and the recurring infection more difficult to treat. Interruption of therapy also increases the risk of developing an allergy.

Evaluation Facts required for evaluation include therapeutic response to the antibiotic regimen and signs and symptoms of adverse reaction to the prescribed drug (see Example of Nursing Process and Penicillin Therapy for Pneumonia).

Checklist of nursing actions

☐ When taking drug histories from candidates for penicillin therapy, ask specifically about previous exposure to penicillin and adverse reactions to it, such as urticaria or skin rash.

☐ Avoid spilling penicillin solutions into the environment.

☐ Monitor clients who are receiving penicillin for signs and symptoms of allergic reaction.

☐ Advise clients who are allergic to penicillin to wear a medical identification device with this information.

☐ Caution clients who are receiving penicillin to complete the course of treatment or (if adverse reaction occurs) to contact the physician for alternative therapy.

Cephalosporins

The first cephalosporins were produced by an organism cultured from sea water collected near a sewer outlet off the coast of Sardinia. Like penicillin, these compounds (and their semisynthetic derivatives) contain a β-lactam structure in their molecules. Mechanism of action, renal excretion, and allergenicity resemble those of penicillin, and some cross-sensitivity exists between the two groups of drugs. Penicillin-resistant organisms that produce β-lactamase also tend to be resistant to many cephalosporins.

The cephalosporins have been altered chemically to produce many different molecules with antibiotic properties. These are classified into three "generations" according to when they were developed and their characteristics (Table 41-3). Each generation exhibits slightly different spectra of activity and susceptibility to enzymes produced by resistant organisms.

Pharmacodynamics. The cephalosporins exert primarily bactericidal effects by inhibiting enzymes necessary to mucopeptide synthesis in bacterial cell walls. As a result, defective cell walls are formed, and autolysis causes cell death.

Pharmacokinetics. Cephalosporins can be administered orally, IM, or IV. Individual preparations vary in the extent to which they are absorbed from the intestinal tract, in their degree of plasma binding, and in their metabolism. After absorption, they are widely

Example of nursing process and penicillin therapy for pneumonia

The client is a 4-year-old girl who is receiving penicillin for lobar pneumonia. Vital signs are temperature 39.1°C (102°F), pulse 105/min, respirations 34/min, blood pressure 130/74 mm Hg; she has a productive cough. She clings to her mother, cries easily, and withdraws when approached by most members of the health care staff.

Assessment data	Nursing diagnosis	Intervention	Goals and outcome criteria
Fever, tachycardia, tachypnea, productive cough	Anxiety related to illness and hospitalization	**Assist** the mother in her role as supportive haven for the child.	Signs and symptoms of anxiety will gradually subside.
Diagnosis of pneumonia	High risk for noncompliance related to anxiety	**Promote** the development of a trusting therapeutic relationship between the child and one member of the staff on each of the work shifts; the personnel chosen should not be involved in painful procedures but should comfort the child after such treatments.	Vital signs will gradually return to normal.
Withdrawal from health staff members			Frequency of cough will decrease.
(Stress is known to impair the body's immune response. Ample hydration assists the body to eliminate metabolic products of infectious processes. The need for vitamin C is increased during infection.)		**Offer** fluids rich in vitamin C frequently.	
		Encourage consumption of a nutritious diet.	
		Promote adequate rest.	
		Administer penicillin as ordered.	
		Monitor the child for signs and symptoms of adverse reaction to penicillin.	

distributed except in the CNS; only a few penetrate the blood–brain barrier sufficiently to deliver therapeutic concentrations to the cerebrospinal fluid. Cephalosporins cross the placenta, as well as the synovial and pericardial membranes. They penetrate the bile and aqueous humor but not the vitreous humor. Binding by serum proteins ranges from 6% to 86%, depending on the specific drugs being used.

The cephalosporins and their metabolites are excreted by the kidneys, with the same tubular secretory mechanism as penicillin. As with penicillin, their elimination can be inhibited by probenecid. Serum half-lives range from 21 to 132 minutes, depending on the specific preparation.

Therapeutic uses. The cephalosporins are used for the treatment of septicemia and infections that involve the skin, soft tissues, bones, joints, and urinary and respiratory tracts caused by susceptible organisms, including streptococci, staphylococci, *Escherichia coli*, *Proteus mirabilis*, and *Shigella* organisms.

First-generation cephalosporins exhibit good activity against gram-positive organisms but only moderate activity against gram-negative organisms. Second-generation cephalosporins are more effective against gram-negative organisms. Third-generation drugs of this family are the most active against gram-negative organisms but are less effective than the first-generation drugs against gram-positive organisms.

Adverse reactions. The most common adverse reactions to the cephalosporins are nausea, vomiting, and diarrhea after oral administration, phlebitis in veins used for injection, pain with IM injection, superinfection, and allergic reactions. Kidney damage, bone marrow depression, prolongation of prothrombin time, mild hepatotoxicity, and acute colitis have also been reported. Intrathecal administration can result in CNS toxicity (hallucinations, nystagmus, and seizures).

Allergic hypersensitivity to the cephalosporins resembles that to penicillin. It is manifested by a mac-

Table 41-3. Cephalosporins

Drug name	Preparations	Usual dosage	Therapeutic uses and additional information
First-generation			
cefadroxil (Duricef, Ultracef)	Capsules, suspensions, and tablets for oral use	Adults: 1–2 g/day, divided in 2 doses Children: 30 mg/kg body weight/day, divided in 2 doses PC: B	Treatment of susceptible infections caused by gram-positive cocci (staphylococci, streptococci) and some strains of gram-negative bacteria (*Klebsiella organisms*)
cefazolin (Ancef, Kefzol, Zolicef)	Vials that contain powder for reconstitution for IM or IV administration	Adults: 750 mg/kg/day, divided in 3–4 doses (maximum daily dosage: 12 g) Children aged 1 mo or older: 25–50 mg/kg body weight/day, divided in 3–4 doses PC: B	Treatment of serious susceptible infections of the biliary tract, bones, joints, and respiratory tract
cephalexin (Biocef, Keflex, Losporal, Novalexin)	Capsules, suspension, and tablets for oral use	Adults: 1 g/day, divided in 4 doses Children: 25–50 mg/kg body weight/day, divided in 4 doses PC: B	Treatment of serious susceptible infections of the bones, respiratory tract, urinary tract, and skin
cephalothin (Keflin, Seffin)	Vials that contain powder for reconstitution for IM or IV administration	Adults: 2–6 g/day, divided in 4–6 doses (maximum daily dosage: 12 g) Children: 80–160 mg/kg body weight/day, divided in 4–6 doses PC: B	Treatment of susceptible infections caused by gram-positive and gram-negative bacteria Perioperative prophylaxis in contaminated or potentially contaminated surgery Drug of choice for treatment of serious staphylococcal infections
cephapirin (Cefadyl)	Vials that contain powder for reconstitution for IM or IV administration	Adults: 2–6 g/day, divided in 4–6 doses (maximum daily dosage: 12 g) Children aged 3 mo or older: 40–80 mg/kg body weight/day, divided in 4 doses PC: B	Treatment of serious susceptible infections, including septicemia, endocarditis, and osteomyelitis Dosage adjustment required for clients with renal dysfunction
cephradine (Anspor, Sefril, Velosef)	Capsules, suspension, and tablets for oral use Vials that contain powder for reconstitution for IM or IV administration	Adults: 2–4 g/day, divided in 2–4 doses (maximum daily dosage: 8 g) Children aged 9 mo or older: 25–100 mg/kg body weight/day, divided in 2–4 doses (maximum dosage: 4 g)	Treatment of susceptible infections, including otitis media and infections of the respiratory tract Dosage adjustments required for clients with renal dysfunction
Second-generation			
cefaclor (Ceclor)	Capsules and suspension for oral use	Adults: 0.75–1.5 g/day, divided in 3 doses (maximum daily dosage: 4 g) Children aged 1 mo or older: 20–40 mg/kg body weight/day, divided in 3 doses (maximum daily dosage: 1 g) PC: B	Treatment of susceptible infections caused by gram-positive cocci (staphylococci, streptococci), some strains of gram-negative bacteria (*Klebsiella organisms* and *H. Influenzae*)
cefamandole (Mandol)	Vials that contain powder for reconstitution for IM or IV administration PC: B	Adults: 1.5–6 g/day, divided in 4 doses (maximum daily dosage: 12 g) Children aged 1 mo or older: 50–150 mg/kg body weight/day, divided in 3–4 doses	Treatment of serious susceptible infections of the bones, joints, respiratory tract, biliary tract, as well as peritonitis and septicemia
cefmetazole sodium (Zefazone)	Sterile powder for IV use; reconstituted drug may be diluted in 0.9% normal saline, 5% dextrose solution, or lactated Ringer's solution	Adults: 2g/day divided in 2–4 doses for 5–14 days PC: B	Treatment of susceptible infections caused by aerobic and anaerobic organisms, gram-positive and gram-negative organisms Resistant to β-lactamases Treatment of lower respiratory tract, skin, urinary tract, and intra-abdominal infections, prophylactically before some surgeries

(Continued)

Table 41-3. Cephalosporins (Continued)

Drug name	Preparations	Usual dosage	Therapeutic uses and additional information
Second-generation			
cefonicid (Monocid)	Vials that contain powder for reconstitution for IM or IV administration	Adults: 500 mg–2 g/day, given as a single dose PC: B	Treatment of lower respiratory, skin, bone, joint, and urinary tract infections and septicemia; perioperative prophylaxis
ceforanide (Precef)	Vials that contain ceforanide and lysine powder for reconstitution for IM or IV administration	Adults: 1–2 g/day, divided in 2 doses Children aged 1 yr or older: 20–40 mg/kg body weight/day, divided in 2 doses PC: B	Treatment of lower respiratory, skin, bone, joint, and urinary tract infections, septicemia, and endocarditis; perioperative prophylaxis
cefoxitin (Mefoxin)	Vials that contain powder for reconstitution for IM or IV administration	Adults: 3–8 g/day, divided in 3–4 doses (maximum daily dosage: 12 g) Children aged 3 mo or older: 80–160 mg/kg body weight/day, divided in 4–6 doses PC: B	Treatment of serious susceptible infections, including bone and joint infections, lung abscess, pelvic inflammatory disease, and septicemia
cefuroxime (Kifurox, Zinacef)	Vials that contain powder for reconstitution for IM or IV administration	Adults: 2.25–4.5 g/day, divided in 3 doses Children older than 3 mo of age: 50–100 mg/kg body weight/day, divided in 3–4 doses PC: B	Treatment of lower respiratory, skin and genitourinary infections, septicemia, and meningitis; perioperative prophylaxis
Third-generation			
cefoperazone (Cefobid)	Vials that contain powder for reconstitution for IM or IV administration Frozen solutions for IV infusion	Adults: 2–4 g/day, divided in 2 doses (maximum daily dosage: 12 g) Children: 50–200 mg/kg body weight/day, divided in 2 doses PC: B	Treatment of serious susceptible infections, including pelvic inflammatory disease, peritonitis, and septicemia
cefotaxime (Claforan)	Vials that contain powder for reconstitution for IM or IV administration Frozen solutions for IV infusion	Adults: 3–8 g/day, divided in 3–6 doses (maximum daily dosage: 12 g) Children aged 1 mo to 12 yr: 50–180 mg/kg body weight/day, divided in 4–6 doses PC: B	Treatment of serious susceptible infections caused by gram-negative bacteria (*E. coli, Klebsiella, Proteus, Shigella, Acinetobacter, Neisseria, Serratia*, and *Providencia* organisms) Dosage adjustment required for clients with renal dysfunction
cefotetan (Cefotan)	Vials that contain powder for reconstitution for IM or IV administration	Adults: 2–4 g/day, divided in 2 doses Children: 40–60 mg/kg body weight/day, divided in 2 doses Safety and efficacy in children is not established PC: B	Treatment of respiratory, urinary, skin, bone, joint, gynecologic, and intra-abdominal infections; perioperative prophylaxis
ceftazidime (Fortaz, Tazicef)	Vials that contain powder for reconstitution for IM or IV administration Frozen solutions for IV	Adults: 2–3 g/day, divided in 2–3 doses Children: aged 1 mo–12 yr: 90–150 mg/kg body weight/day, divided in 3 doses Maximum daily dosage: 6 g PC: B	Treatment of lower respiratory, skin, urinary tract, bone, joint, gynecologic, central nervous system, and intra-abdominal infections; treatment of septicemia After reconstitution, solutions generate carbon dioxide gas and must be vented before use
ceftizoxime (Cefizox)	Vials that contain powder for reconstitution for IM or IV administration	Adults: 2–6 g/day, divided in 2–3 doses (maximum daily dosage: 12 g) Children aged 6 mo or older: 150–200 mg/kg body weight/day, divided in 3–4 doses PC: B	Treatment of serious susceptible infections, including those of the respiratory tract, urinary tract, and skin, including septicemia Dosage adjustment required for clients with renal dysfunction

(Continued)

Table 41-3. Cephalosporins (*Continued*)

Drug name	Preparations	Usual dosage	Therapeutic uses and additional information
Third-generation			
ceftriaxone (Rocephin)	Vials that contain powder for reconstitution for IM or IV administration	Adults: 1–2 g/day, given in 1–2 doses (maximum daily dosage: 4 g) Children aged 12 yr or older: 50–75 mg/kg body weight/day, divided in 2 doses (maximum daily dosage: 2 g) PC: B	Treatment of lower respiratory, skin, bone, joint, urinary tract and intra-abdominal infections; treatment of septicemia, meningitis and gonorrhea; perioperative prophylaxis
moxalactam (Moxam)	Vials that contain powder for reconstitution for IM or IV administration	Adults: 2–4 g/day, divided in 2–3 doses (maximum daily dosage: 12 g) Children: 50–200 mg/kg body weight/day, divided in 2–4 doses PC: C	Treatment of serious susceptible infections, including septicemia, central nervous system infections, and bone and joint infections Dosage adjustment required for clients with renal dysfunction

KEY: PC = pregnancy category. (The validity of pregnancy risk categories has not been established; see Chapter 16, p 216.)

ulopapular rash, sometimes associated with fever; eosinophilia; and lymphadenopathy. Less commonly, anaphylaxis, bronchospasm, urticaria, or blood dyscrasia occurs.

Precautions and contraindications. The cephalosporins should not be used for the treatment of clients with a history of a recent, severe, immediate reaction to either penicillin or cephalosporins. The drugs are used with caution if previous reactions have been mild or far removed in time. Epinephrine should be available for emergency use, should an acute reaction develop.

To prevent phlebitis and the need for frequent changes of parenteral administration sites, cephalosporin solutions should be infused into veins slowly. Either continuous, slow drip, or intermittent infusion is recommended. Bolus medication, if required, should be administered over a period of several minutes.

Because they are potential nephrotoxins, the cephalosporins should not be used concurrently with other nephrotoxic drugs. They should be used with caution in clients with a history of renal pathology, especially if kidney function is less than optimal (see Focus on Cephalosporins: Similarities and Differences).

■ **Summary**

The cephalosporins are similar to penicillin in their mechanism of action, their toxicity, and some aspects of their molecular structure. They are sometimes effective against pathogens resistant to penicillin. Adverse reactions include allergic reactions, superinfections, and occasionally, nephrotoxicity.

Nursing management

Nursing implications

Solutions of cephalosporins for parenteral use should be freshly prepared. If solutions must be stored, they should be refrigerated. The labeling information packaged with each preparation provides data on stability and storage requirements.

Nursing process

Assessment Clients who are candidates for cephalosporin therapy should be screened for renal impairment and allergic sensitivity to either cephalosporins or penicillins.

Nursing diagnosis Diagnoses concern both therapeutic and adverse responses to medication. They may include the following:

Altered nutrition: less than body requirements related to nausea and vomiting
Diarrhea
Knowledge deficit related to drug regimens necessary for effective anti-infective treatment
Noncompliance related to knowledge deficit or to cost of drug prescriptions

A common collaborative problem that should be differentiated from the nursing diagnoses is

Potential complication: renal

Planning Goals of treatment are to resolve the infectious process, reduce the risk of adverse reaction to the antibiotics, and promptly detect and treat any adverse reaction, should one occur.

Intervention IV doses must be infused slowly, preferably over a period of at least 30 minutes. Rapid

Focus on

Cephalosporins: similarities and differences

Similarities

Pharmacodynamics

These agents exert bactericidal action by inhibiting mucopeptide synthesis in the bacterial cell wall. They bind with enzymes in the bacterial cytoplasmic membrane, interfering with cell wall synthesis.

Pharmacokinetics

These agents are absorbed in varying degrees, depending on how they are administered (PO, IM, or IV). Absorption is delayed in the presence of food. They are widely distributed to tissues; distribution to cerebrospinal fluid varies; they readily cross the placenta and are found in low concentrations in breast milk. The serum half-life ranges from one-half to 2 hours, peaking in one-half to 1 hour. They are primarily excreted by the kidneys.

Therapeutic uses

These agents are used for the treatment of a wide range of infections. They are active against many gram-positive aerobic bacteria, some gram-negative aerobic bacteria, and some anaerobic bacteria.

Adverse reactions

These include: (CNS) dizziness, headache, malaise, fatigue, vertigo; (GI) nausea, vomiting, diarrhea, abdominal pain, glossitis, dyspepsia, tenesmus; (GU/REPRO) vaginitis; (HEME) eosinophilia, elevated liver enzymes, neutropenia, positive direct and indirect Coomb's test; (SKIN) urticaria, pruritus, rash; (OTHER) hypersensitivity reaction, fever, pain, tenderness, and irritation after IM injection, bacterial or fungal superinfection, thrombophlebitis after IV injection.

Contraindications

These agents are contraindicated in people with a history of recent severe immediate reaction to penicillin or cephalosporins and in those who are taking other nephrotoxic drugs.

Differences

• **Cefamandole**, **cefazolin**, **cefonicid**, **cefoperazone**, **ceforanide**, **cefotaxime**, **ceftazidime**, **ceftizoxime**, **ceftriaxone**, **cefuroxime**, **cephalothin**, and **cephapirin** are not absorbed from the GI tract and are given parenterally. • **Cefaclor**, **cefadroxil**, **cefuroxime**, **cephalexin**, and **cephadrine** are well absorbed from the GI tract. • **Cefuroxime's** absorption is increased with food. • **Cefotaxime**, **ceftazidine**, **ceftizoxime**, **ceftriaxone**, **cefuroxine**, and **moxalactam** are distributed into the cerebrospinal fluid. Half-lives include: 3.5 to 5.8 hours for **cefonicid**; 2.6 to 3.3 hours for **ceforanide**; 5.4 to 10.9 hours for **ceftriaxone**. Peak times include: 1.5 to 2 hours for **cefadroxil** (PO); .2 hours for **cefamandole** (IV) 1 to 2 hours for **cefazolin** (IM); .1 hour for **cefazolin** (IV), **cefoxitin** (IV), **cefonicid** (IV), **ceftizoxine** (IV), and **cephradine** (IV); .3 to .5 hours for **cefoxitin** (IM); 2 hours for **ceftriaxone** (IM); .25 hours **cefuroxine** (IV); .25 to .5 hours for **cephalothin** (IV); 1 to 2 hours for **moxalactam.**

First generation drugs have the highest activity against gram-positive organisms; second generation have enhanced activity against gram-negative organisms; third generation drugs are active against wider spectrum of gram-negative organisms. • **Cefamandole**, **cefozolin**, **cefonicid**, **ceforanide**, **cefotaxime**, **cefotetan**, **cefoxitin**, **ceftriaxone**, **cefuroxime**, **cephalothin**, and **cephapirin** are used in the prophylactic treatment of perioperative infection.

• **Cefamandole**, **cefoperazone**, **moxalactam**, **cefonicid**, and **cefotetan** may cause a disulfiram reaction if taken with alcohol. • **Cefaclor** may cause hyperactivity, nervousness, insomnia, confusion, and hypertonia. • **Cephradine** (IM, PO, IV) may cause chest tightness and paresthesia. • **Cephradine**, **cefamandole**, **cefoperazine**, **cefotetan**, and **moxalactam** may cause bleeding and hypoprothrombinemia.

(continued)

Focus on

Cephalosporins: similarities and differences (*Continued*)

Similarities

Precautions

These agents should be used with caution in people with renal problems and those with a history of GI disease.

Nursing considerations

Instruct client in disease, treatment, drug regimen, adverse reactions, and compliance; obtain specimens for culture and sensitivity testing before starting therapy; instruct client to notify physician if rash develops; tell client to continue taking drug as ordered even if he or she feels better and to finish the entire prescription; administer PO 1 hour before meals or 2 hours after meals for maximum absorption; refrigerate oral suspensions and shake well before administering; administer IM deep into large muscle mass and rotate injection sites; do not add or mix parenteral preparations with other drugs; rotate IV infusion sites frequently to prevent vein irritation; monitor vital signs, especially temperature for signs of improvement of infection; encourage fluids and use antipyretics as necessary to alleviate fever of infection; encourage use of yogurt or buttermilk to diet to prevent superinfection that results from suppression of normal intestinal flora; teach client regarding signs and symptoms of possible superinfections; watch for possible false-positive urinary glucose results when using copper sulfate reagents, such as clinitest.

Differences

• **Cefamandole**, **cefoperazone**, **cefotetan**, and **moxalactam** should be used with caution in people with bleeding disorders.
• **Cefoperazone** should be used cautiously in people with impaired liver function.

Keep in mind that vitamin K may be ordered prophylactically for clients who are taking **cefotetan**, **cefamandole**, **cefoperazone**, and **moxalactam**. Administer **cefadroxil** and **cephalexin** with food to minimize GI upset. Be aware that **moxalactam** does not interfere with urinary glucose determinations.

---

injection causes pain and irritation of the vein. Pain at the site of IM injection may be minimized by applying ice packs to the site before and after the injection.

If cephalosporins are prescribed for clients in renal failure, the dose is reduced. Because the drugs are removed from the body by dialysis, they should be administered after each treatment.

If cephalosporins are prescribed for clients with a history of allergy to either these drugs or penicillin, an acute reaction could occur. Epinephrine should be available for emergency treatment.

Clients should be monitored closely for signs and symptoms of superinfection: diarrhea, sore mouth, and vaginal itching or drainage. Diarrhea, the main sign of intestinal superinfection, is most common when oral preparations are used. Women sometimes develop vaginal yeast infections, manifested by itching, inflammation, and increased vaginal drainage. If signs and symptoms of superinfection develop, consult the physician about the need for antimycotic medication.

Before cephalosporin therapy is begun, the physician should be informed of any history of allergic reaction to either penicillin or cephalosporin drugs.

Clients should be cautioned not to discontinue medication prematurely, even though the signs and symptoms of infection have resolved completely. Adverse reactions, including sore mouth, diarrhea, vaginal irritation, or signs and symptoms of renal malfunction should be reported to the physician promptly. An alternate antibiotic may be substituted to complete the antibiotic regimen. Clients who experience an allergic reaction to cephalosporins should be informed that they are sensitive to these drugs. A medical identification device should be recommended.

Example of nursing process and oral cephalosporin treatment

Oral cephalosporin has been prescribed to treat infection in a surgical wound after surgical repair of a serious hand injury. The client, a 71-year-old woman, is to be treated as an outpatient. She lives in a rural area 25 miles from the nearest hospital; the local emergency medical unit is 15 minutes away from her residence.

The client has a history of severe generalized skin rash during oral penicillin therapy.

Assessment data	Nursing diagnosis	Intervention	Goals and outcome criteria
Order for cephalosporin for infected hand	High risk for altered tissue perfusion related to vasodilation secondary to allergic reaction to cephalosporin drug therapy	**Inform** the physician of the client's history of generalized allergic reaction to penicillin, as well as the inaccessibility of prompt emergency care in the area in which she lives.	The client will not suffer an allergic reaction to cephalosporin drugs (because an alternate drug was substituted).
History of severe generalized allergic reaction to oral penicillin	Self-care deficit related to inability to use injured hand	If the antibiotic order is not changed to a non-β-lactam drugs, **advise** the client of emergency measures that may be needed should an allergic reaction occur (*eg*, cardiopulmonary resuscitation by a member of the family or neighbor and emergency medical personnel).	Should an allergic reaction to cephalosporin occur, the risk of permanent harm will be minimized by prompt emergency treatment.
(People with penicillin allergy are also likely to be allergic to cephalosporins, which are related drugs.)		**Teach** the client one-handed techniques for self-care	Good hygiene and grooming will be maintained throughout the period of disability.
Client's residence is 15 minutes or more from emergency medical care.		**Teach** a family member or significant other how to assist the client in self-care	

Client education. Oral cephalosporins should be taken on an empty stomach, not with meals. The client's diet should contain a minimum of foods that irritate the intestinal tract. The timing of meals and medicines can be a problem. The drug must be taken at least 2 hours after food intake, and food may not be taken for 1 hour after medication. Four doses of cephalosporins are usually ordered daily. To maintain a fairly normal schedule of meals, the first dose of medication should be taken before breakfast.

Clients may need assistance in planning a schedule of meals and medication to maintain proper nutrition and accommodate the required drug regimen. The nurse may suggest the following routine:

6 to 7 AM: first dose of medicine

Breakfast between 8 and 9 AM

11 AM: second dose of medicine

Lunch between noon and 2 PM

5 PM: third dose of medicine

Dinner between 6 and 7 PM

If taken, bedtime snack before 9 PM

11 PM: fourth dose of medicine

The use of buttermilk or yogurt with every meal should be recommended to prevent intestinal superinfection.

Evaluation Data required for evaluation include signs and symptoms that indicate resolution of the infectious process and indications of adverse reactions to the drug regimen. Clients should be monitored for GI upset, vaginitis, and renal impairment, neutropenia, impaired clotting, or renal dysfunction (see Example of Nursing Process and Oral Cephalosporin Treatment).

Checklist of nursing actions

☐ Before initiating cephalosporin therapy, take a complete drug history to rule out allergic hypersensitivity to penicillin or cephalosporins.

☐ Assess the client for renal dysfunction and history of kidney disease.

☐ Use fresh solutions for administration by injection.

☐ Administer IV cephalosporins slowly.

☐ Teach the client who receives oral cephalosporins to schedule doses at least 1 hour before and 2 hours after meals.

☐ Recommend buttermilk or yogurt with each meal during cephalosporin treatment.

☐ Monitor clients who receive cephalosporins for signs and symptoms of superinfection or renal impairment.

☐ If cephalosporins are prescribed for clients with a history of allergy to these antibiotics or penicillin, have epinephrine available for emergency treatment, should an acute reaction occur.

Miscellaneous β-lactam antibiotics

Two β-lactam antibiotics that are neither penicillins nor cephalosporins have been developed.

Imipenem resembles the penicillins in therapeutic action but is resistant to β-lactamases. It must be administered parenterally because it is not absorbed by the GI tract. Because it is rapidly hydrolyzed in the proximal tubule of the kidney by an enzyme, dehydropeptidase, drug preparations of imipenem (Primaxin) also contain a dehydropeptidase inhibitor, cilastin. Nausea and vomiting are the most common adverse reactions to Primaxim.

Aztreonam (Azactam) is effective against Enterobacteriaceae and *Pseudomonas aeruginosa* but not against most anaerobic and gram-positive organisms. Aztreonam's main advantage is that it does not affect the normal flora of the intestinal tract.

β-Lactamase inhibitors

Certain chemicals bind to and inactivate β-lactamases, thus reducing drug resistance of β-lactamase–producing pathogens. One of these, clavulanic acid, has been combined with oral amoxicillin and parenteral ticarcillin in preparations used to treat resistant infections. Such combinations have a synergistic effect, attacking both the bacteria and the β-lactamase enzyme produced by those bacteria that are resistant to antimicrobials. Adverse GI effects have been noted in some children when the proportion of clavulanic acid has been increased. The chemical sulbactam may be administered concurrently with β-lactam antibiotics to increase their efficacy in treating resistant pathogens.

Aminoglycosides

The first antibiotic to join penicillin and sulfanilamide in the struggle against infection was an aminoglycoside, streptomycin. Streptomycin was the first systemic antimicrobial effective against gram-negative pathogens. It was an excellent complement to penicillin, and combined therapy with the two drugs was often employed to achieve a broader spectrum of efficacy.

Pharmacodynamics. Aminoglycosides contain two or more amino sugars in glycoside linkage with a hexose nucleus. They act as bactericidal agents against susceptible organisms by binding irreversibly to ribosomal subunits within the pathogens, thus preventing protein synthesis.

Pharmacokinetics. Aminoglycosides are highly polarized molecules that are poorly absorbed by the GI tract. They are rapidly absorbed from IM sites, producing a peak action in 30 to 90 minutes if tissue perfusion is good. After systemic administration, aminoglycosides are widely distributed in the extracellular fluid, accumulating in high concentrations in the renal cortex and the perilymph of the inner ear. They do not cross the blood–brain barrier when administered in therapeutic amounts. They do bind to plasma proteins (in the case of streptomycin about 35% is so bound).

Aminoglycosides are not metabolized and are excreted unchanged in the urine primarily by glomerular filtration. Although the drugs do enter the enterohepatic cycle, this is not an important route for elimination. Plasma half-life is 2 to 4 hours in normal adults. The drugs are readily removed by hemodialysis and, to a lesser extent, by peritoneal dialysis. When given orally, kanamycin and neomycin are excreted in feces.

Therapeutic uses. Aminoglycosides are valuable therapeutic agents for the control of aerobic gram-negative bacterial infections.

When administered by IM injection or IV infusion, aminoglycosides are effective against infections in most tissues except the CNS and the eye. Intrathecal administration is required for CNS conditions. The drugs are also administered orally to reduce the microscopic flora within the intestinal lumen preoperatively, in acute intestinal infections, and in the treatment of hepatic encephalopathy. The drugs are sometimes nebulized and administered by inhalation and applied topically to the eyes.

Drug preparations. The aminoglycoside group includes streptomycin, gentamicin, tobramycin, kanamycin, neomycin, netilmicin, and amikacin (Table 41-4). Each drug varies somewhat in its properties and has advantages in certain clinical situations.

(Text continues on p. 1030)

Table 41-4. Aminoglycoside antibiotics

Drug name	Preparations	Usual dosage	Additional information
amikacin sulfate (Amikin)	Solutions for IM and IV injection	15 mg/kg body weight/day, divided in 2–3 doses Maximum daily dosage: 1.5 g Desired peak serum concentrations: 15–30 µg/ml Desired trough serum concentrations: 10 µg/ml PC: D	Monitor for ototoxicity and nephrotoxicity Dosage adjustment required for clients with renal dysfunction
gentamicin sulfate (Apogen, Garamycin, G-Myticin)	Solutions for IM or IV injection Preservative-free solutions for intrathecal or intraventricular injection Ointments and creams for topical application Ointments and solutions for ophthalmic use	Adults: 3–5 mg/kg body weight/day, divided in 3–4 doses, administered at equal intervals Children: 6–7.5 mg/kg body weight/day, divided in 3 doses, administered at 8–h intervals Desired peak serum concentration: 4–10 µg/ml Desired trough serum concentration: 2 µg/ml *Ophthalmic ointment:* 1 cm ribbon bid-tid *Ophthalmic solution:* gtt i–ii q4h PC: C (Can cause deafness in child exposed *in utero*)	Dosage adjustment required for clients with renal dysfunction Inactivated by carbenicillin if mixed in same solution Sometimes administered intrathecally for treatment of gram-negative meningitis Monitor for ototoxicity and nephrotoxicity
kanamycin sulfate (Kantrex, Klebcil)	Capsules for oral use Solutions for IM or IV administration	15 mg/kg body weight/day, divided in 2–3 doses administered at equal intervals Maximum daily dosage: 1.5 g Oral dose to "sterilize" gut: 1 g every hour for 4 doses, then every 6 h for 36 to 72 h; 8–12 g/day, in divided doses for treatment of hepatic encephalopathy Desired peak serum concentrations: 15–30 µg/ml Desired trough serum concentrations: 5 µg/ml PC: D	Oral preparations used for preoperative "sterilization" of the gut and in the treatment of hepatic encephalopathy; 1% solutions administered as retention enemas Rarely used IV; ineffective against *Pseudomonas* organisms Used to treat gram-negative urinary tract infections and tuberculosis resistant to other therapeutic agents Monitor for toxicity and nephrotoxicity Dosage adjustment required for clients with renal dysfunction
neomycin sulfate (Myciguent, Neobiotic, Neosporin, Mycifradin)	Oral tablets and solutions for ophthalmic and otic use Ointments and creams for topical application Sterile solution for preparation of irrigating solutions Powder for reconstitution for IM injection	Adults: 4–12 g daily, divided in 4 doses Children: 88 mg/kg body weight divided in 6 doses, administered at equal intervals PC: C	Often combined with other antibiotics Rarely administered by injection due to marked ototoxicity Used as an adjunct in the treatment of hepatic encephalopathy Monitor for ototoxicity and nephrotoxicity Dosage adjustment required for clients with renal dysfunction

(Continued)

Table 41-4. Aminoglycoside antibiotics (Continued)

Drug name	Preparations	Usual dosage	Additional information
netilmicin (Netromycin)	Solutions for IM or IV administration	Adults: 4.0–6.5 mg/kg body weight/day, divided in 2–3 doses Infants and children aged 6 wk–12 yr: 5.5–8.0 mg/kg body weight/day, divided in 2–3 doses Neonates: 4.0–6.5 mg/kg body weight/day, divided in 2 doses PC: C Desired peak serum concentrations: 4–12 µg/ml Desired trough serum concentrations: 4 µg/ml PC: D	Monitor for ototoxicity and nephrotoxicity Dosage adjustment required for clients with renal dysfunction
paromomycin (sulfate (Humatin)	Oral capsules	25–35 mg/kg body weight/day, divided in 3 doses	Used as an adjunct in the treatment of hepatic coma Also used in the treatment of intestinal amebiasis Monitor for ototoxicity and nephrotoxicity
streptomycin sulfate (Stepolin)	Vials that contain powder for reconstitution for IM administration	Adults: 1–2 g/day, divided in 2–4 doses, administered at equal intervals Children: 20–40 mg/kg body weight/day, divided in 2–4 doses, administered at equal intervals Desirable peak serum concentrations: 5–25 µg/ml Desirable trough serum concentrations: 5 µg/ml PC: D	Used in the treatment of serious infections that do not respond to other treatment agents, such as bacterial endocarditis, tularemia, plague, and brucellosis; sometimes used in combination with penicillin or other antibiotics Monitor for ototoxicity and nephrotoxicity Rarely administered IV because of ototoxicity Dosage adjustment required for clients with renal dysfunction Used in treating mycobacterial infections, tuberculosis (in combination with one or more other drugs), and leprosy
tobramycin sulfate (Nebcin)	Vials that contain powder for reconstitution for IM or IV administration Ophthalmic ointments and solutions	3 mg/kg body weight/day divided in 3 doses, administered at 8-h intervals Desired peak serum concentrations: 4–10 µg/ml Desired trough serum concentrations: 2 µg/ml *Ophthalmic ointment:* 1 cm ribbon bid–tid *Ophthalmic solution:* gtt i–ii q4h PC: B	Ineffective against mycobacteria; very effective against *Pseudomonas* organisms Monitor for ototoxicity and nephrotoxicity Dosage adjustment required for clients with renal dysfunction

KEY: PC = pregnancy category. (The validity of pregnancy risk categories has not been established; see Chapter 16, p 216.)

Adverse reactions. As often happens with new treatment agents, the dangers of the aminoglycosides were not recognized at first. Streptomycin was regarded as nontoxic until it was employed for intensive therapy for tuberculosis, when its toxic properties became apparent. Ototoxicity and nephrotoxicity are the most serious adverse reactions to aminoglycosides. These effects are most often seen in the elderly, clients with preexisting renal dysfunction, and in those who are receiving concurrently other drugs capable of producing ototoxicity and nephrotoxicity.

The aminoglycosides can cause irreversible eighth cranial nerve damage. Therapy that involves large doses or prolonged periods of treatment permanently damages hearing. Acoustic nerve irritation is first indicated by abnormal (often ringing) sensations in the ear. Both vestibular and auditory functions are affected. Hearing loss begins with reduced perception of high tones, which can seriously impair comprehension of speech, even though deafness is not apparent. Nerve cell death is irreversible, and hearing loss is permanent.

Peripheral nerve toxicity is further manifested by neuromuscular blockade, which sometimes occurs when aminoglycosides are administered to clients immediately after surgery. The drugs appear to interact with general anesthetics or muscle relaxants that remain in the tissues to produce this effect. When administered to neonates with high serum magnesium levels, respiratory arrest can (rarely) occur.

Aminoglycosides can induce acute tubular necrosis in the kidney. Nephrotoxicity appears to be related to the high concentrations of drug that develop in the renal cortex. Kidney damage has been reported after intracavity injection and topical application to abraded surfaces, as well as parenteral administration.

Although only small amounts of the aminoglycosides are absorbed from the GI tract, oral administration can produce systemic toxicity in clients with poor kidney function in whom the drugs accumulate. Superinfections sometimes develop during therapy.

Aminoglycosides exhibit little allergic potential. However, allergy to these drugs may produce rash, urticaria, stomatitis, pruritus, generalized burning, fever, and eosinophilia. Agranulocytosis and anaphylaxis have rarely occurred. Individuals who develop allergic sensitivity to one aminoglycoside sometimes exhibit cross-sensitivity to other drugs of this class.

Bacterial strains resistant to the action of the aminoglycosides arise when organisms acquire the ability to produce enzymes that break down the aminoglycoside molecule. Traits such as a cell transport mechanism less accepting of the aminoglycosides and ribosome structure with less affinity to the drug molecules can also cause resistance. Organisms resistant to one aminoglycoside are not necessarily resistant to all drugs of this class.

Precautions and contraindications. Kidney function in clients who receive aminoglycosides should be monitored closely. Doses of aminoglycosides must be reduced in clients with kidney damage to maintain serum concentrations below the toxic level. Drug serum levels should be monitored and dosage controlled to prevent excessively high peak and trough serum concentrations.

Aminoglycoside therapy is contraindicated for clients with a history of toxic or hypersensitive reaction to aminoglycosides. Oral doses are contraindicated in clients with intestinal obstruction. The drugs should be discontinued if tinnitus, hearing loss, oliguria, azotemia, or respiratory paralysis develop. Periodic audiometric and caloric stimulation tests are advisable for clients who receive aminoglycosides over a long period of time.

Aminoglycosides should not be administered concurrently with other ototoxic, neurotoxic, or nephrotoxic drugs, general anesthetics, muscle relaxants, and diuretics such as ethacrynic acid, furosemide, urea, and mannitol. Sequential use is also to be avoided, because residues of the first drug employed may increase the toxicity of succeeding agents. Oral aminoglycosides potentiate the action of oral anticoagulants (warfarin) by decreasing bacterial synthesis of vitamin K within the intestine. The dose of anticoagulant should be reduced initially when these antibiotics are prescribed and prothrombin time closely monitored (see Focus on Aminoglycosides: Similarities and Differences).

■ **Summary**

The aminoglycosides are the major antibiotics for use in gram-negative infections. When administered orally, they exert a local effect on the GI tract; systemic effects depend on administration by injection. The aminoglycosides are often used in combination with other antibiotics to achieve a broad spectrum of activity and to minimize the development of resistant strains. These drugs are ototoxic and nephrotoxic but not markedly allergenic.

Nursing management

Nursing implications

Aminoglycoside solutions are relatively unstable and should be used promptly. Solutions that must be stored should be refrigerated. Specific data regarding stability are available in the labeling information that accompanies the drug. Before the administration of each dose, the solution's expiration date should be checked.

Nursing process

Assessment The renal function and hearing of clients about to receive aminoglycosides must be care-

Aminoglycosides: similarities and differences

Similarities

Pharmacodynamics

These agents are bactericidal and appear to inhibit protein synthesis by irreversibly binding to the ribosomal subunits in susceptible bacteria.

Pharmacokinetics

These agents are rapidly absorbed after IM administration, and they are absorbed in significant amounts by body surfaces. They are poorly absorbed from the GI tract after oral administration. They are widely distributed into body fluids, primarily extracellular, and they diffuse poorly into the cerebrospinal fluid after IM or IV administration. They readily cross the placenta, and small amounts are found in bile, saliva, sweat, tears, sputum, and milk. The elimination half-life ranges from 2 to 4 hours in clients with normal renal function. They are not metabolized, and they are excreted unchanged in the urine.

Therapeutic uses

These agents are used in the short-term treatment of serious infections by gram-negative bacteria. They are also active against aerobic gram-negative and some aerobic gram-positive bacteria. They are also used in the treatment of serious recurrent urinary tract infections caused by gram-negative bacteria.

Adverse reaction

These include: (CNS) peripheral neuropathy, eighth cranial nerve damage, vertigo, ataxia, paresthesia, headache, tremors, lethargy, numbness, tingling, muscle twitching, neuromuscular blockade; (CV) tachycardia, hypotension, myocarditits; (EENT) ototoxicity, nystagmus; (GI) nausea, vomiting, diarrhea; (GU) nephrotoxicity; (HEME) hemolytic anemia, transient neutropenia, leukopenia, thrombocytopenia; (OTHER) hypersensitivity, vein irritation, phlebitis, sterile abscess at injection site.

Differences

• **Kanamycin**, **paromomycin**, and **neomycin** also inhibit ammonia-forming bacteria in the GI tract.

• **Gentamicin** (intrathecal) has a half-life of 5.5 hours. • **Amikacin** peaks in 45 minutes to 2 hours (IM) and over 1 hour (IV infusion). • **Gentamicin** and **tobramycin** (IM and IV infusion) peak in 30 to 90 minutes. • **Kanamycin** (IM and IV infusion) peaks in 1 hour. • **Netilimicin** (PO and IM) peaks in 30 to 60 minutes; IV infusion peaks within 30 minutes. • **Streptomycin** (IM) peaks in 1 to 2 hours. • **Neomycin** (PO) is excreted unchanged in feces. • **Neomycin** and **gentamicin** administered topically are best absorbed when the cornea is abraded (ophthalmic) and are readily absorbed through denuded areas of skin or through skin that has lost its keratin layer. • **Neomycin** is also rapidly absorbed from the peritoneum, draining wounds, sinuses, and surgical sites.

• **Paromomycin**, active against protozoa, is used to treat intestinal amebiasis. • **Streptomycin** is active against mycobacterium. • **Gentamicin** is used intrathecally or intraventricularly to supplement IM or IV administration in the treatment of CNS infections. • **Clindamycin**, in conjunction with an IM or IV aminoglycoside, is used for the treatment of mixed aerobic–anaerobic infections. • **Gentamicin** and **neomycin** topical are used to treat superficial eye and skin infections and bacterial ocular infections. • **Neomycin** topical is used to treat otitis externa, and it is combined with **polymyxin B** for urinary tract irrigation to prevent bacteremia and bacteriuria from use of an indwelling catheter. • **Gentamicin** and **clindamycin** are used to treat pelvic inflammatory disease. • **Kanamycin**, **neomycin**, and **paromomycin** (PO) are used as a retention enema as an adjuvant treatment for hepatic encephalopathy. • **Kanamycin** and **neomycin** are used in combination for preoperative intestinal antisepsis. • **Neomycin** (PO) is used as an adjunct for fluid and replacement treatment for severe diarrhea caused by *Escherichia coli.*

• **Gentamicin** (opthalmic) may cause transient irritation burning or stinging. • **Neomycin** (topical) may cause local irritation, dermatitis, erythema, rash, urticaria, and photosensitivity.

(continued)

Focus on

Aminoglycosides: similarities and differences (Continued)

Similarities

Contraindications

These agents are contraindicated in people with history of toxicity or hypersensitivity and in those who are receiving other ototoxic, neurotoxic, or nephrotoxic drugs.

Precautions

These agents should be used cautiously in people with neuromuscular disorders, such as parkinsonism and myasthenia gravis, in premature and full term neonates less than 6 weeks of age, in those with impaired renal function, and in the elderly.

Nursing considerations

Instruct client in disease, treatment, drug regimen, adverse reactions, and compliance; obtain specimens for culture and sensitivity before initiating therapy; monitor vital signs, especially temperature and pulse for changes that indicate improvement of infection; assess renal function studies, such as specific gravity, blood urea nitrogen, and creatinine levels before and periodically after the start of therapy for changes; encourage fluids and monitor intake and output for changes; assess client's hearing before and periodically during therapy for changes; assess client for signs of hearing difficulties; obtain serum peak and trough levels and report abnormalities to physician; do not mix with other drugs when giving parenterally; stop IV infusion of aminoglycoside if other drugs must be given and flush tubing with normal saline or dextrose and water afterward; administer IM deep into large muscle and rotate injection sites to prevent tissue injury; instruct client in signs and symptoms of possible superinfection and toxicity.

Differences

• **Neomycin**, **kanamycin**, and **paromomycin** (PO) are contraindicated in people with intestinal obstruction. • **Streptomycin** is contraindicated in people with labyrinthine disease.

When giving **neomycin** preoperatively, administer a low-residue diet and cathartics as ordered. IM **neomycin** is not recommended because of the possibility of ototoxicity and nephrotoxicity. When given for tuberculosis, discontinue **neomycin** when client's sputum is negative. Watch for respiratory depression in clients with renal disease, hypocalcemia, and neuromuscular disease. Administer **neomycin** (otic) to a clean dry ear canal. Administer **neomycin** as a GU irrigant through a three-way indwelling catheter. Apply **gentamicin** or **neomycin** ophthalmic ointment to the conjunctival sac; apply topical ointment or cream gently to the clean affected area and cover with a sterile gauze; protect hands when applying because drug is irritating.

---

fully evaluated before drug therapy is begun. If these functions are marginal, alternative treatment may be considered.

Nursing diagnosis Diagnoses relate to both therapeutic and adverse responses of the client to aminoglycoside therapy. They may include the following:

High risk for injury related to nephrotoxicity or ototoxicity of anti-infective drugs
Sensory/perceptual alterations related to loss of auditory input secondary to ototoxicity of drugs
Knowledge deficit concerning need for compliance with regimen and recognition of adverse effects

Noncompliance with medication regimen related to discomforting adverse reactions or inability to pay for prescriptions

Common collaborative problems that should be differentiated from the nursing diagnoses include

Potential complication: renal toxicity
Potential complication: ototoxicity

Planning Goals of treatment are to support the client's resistance to infection, reduce the risk of adverse drug reaction, and detect and promptly treat any adverse reaction that may occur.

Example of nursing process and antibiotic therapy for treatment of endocarditis

The client is a 67-year-old woman who has developed endocarditis after successful replacement of a defective mitral valve. She is also receiving a nonsteroidal anti-inflammatory drug (Naprosyn) for long-term treatment of a subacute rheumatoid arthritis. She experiences occasional tinnitus, which subsides when one or two doses of the antirheumatic drug are omitted. Gentamicin has been ordered for treatment of the endocarditis.

Assessment data	Nursing diagnosis	Intervention	Goals and outcome criteria
Long-term use of Naprosyn for treatment of arthritis History of tinnitus Order for gentamicin therapy (Gentamicin and Naprosyn are both ototoxic and nephrotoxic drugs.)	Knowledge deficit concerning the possible ototoxic and nephrotoxic effects of the drug regimen	Before initiation of gentamicin therapy, the physician should be informed (or reminded) that the client is taking one ototoxic and nephrotoxic drug and that she has intermittent tinnitus. **Inform** the client that she should report to the physician any signs and symptoms of renal or hearing impairment (change in urinary excretion, tinnitus, or vertigo) as soon as they develop. If the antibiotic order is not changed to one that is less apt to cause ototoxicity and nephrotoxicity, **advise** the client to consult with her rheumatologist for a possible change in antirheumatic medication. This change should be followed until after the antibiotic has been completely eliminated (at least 72 hours after the final dose of medication) **Remind** the client to report regularly for the laboratory tests that are required by the protocols for monitoring clients who receive nonsteroidal anti-inflammatory drugs for arthritis.	The client will not develop permanent renal or hearing impairment during or after the completion of antibiotic therapy.

Intervention Nursing interventions include implementing measures to enhance resistance to infection, administering the antibiotics, monitoring for response to treatment, and consulting with the physician when no therapeutic response or adverse reaction occurs.

Client education. Clients should be taught hygienic practices to enhance the therapeutic regimen and the signs and symptoms of adverse drug reactions that should be reported to the physician.

Evaluation Data required for evaluation include signs and symptoms of infection and signs and symptoms of adverse drug reaction (see Example of Nursing Process and Antibiotic Therapy for Treatment of Endocarditis).

Checklist of nursing actions

☐ Before administering the initial dose of aminoglycoside drugs, evaluate the client for renal dysfunction, hearing loss, allergy to aminoglycosides, and concurrent use of other ototoxic or nephrotoxic drugs.

☐ Verify that the client has been informed of the risks of treatment, especially the risk of hearing loss.

☐ Use only fresh solutions of aminoglycosides.

☐ Monitor clients who are receiving aminoglycosides for early signs and symptoms of ototoxicity or nephrotoxicity, such as ringing or a sense of fullness in the ears and changes in urinary excretion.

☐ Monitor respiratory status of clients who receive aminoglycosides concurrently with neuromuscular blocking agents.

Tetracyclines

Tetracyclines are derivatives of the polycyclic chemical naphthacenecarboxamide obtained from cultures of *Streptomyces* organisms. They exhibit a wide range of activity against both gram-positive and gram-negative bacteria and other microorganisms not responsive to other drugs. A variety of preparations are available for clinical use (Table 41-5).

Pharmacodynamics. Like the aminoglycosides, tetracyclines interfere with protein synthesis by microbial ribosomes. Unlike the aminoglycosides, these compounds gain access to the interior of the cell by more than one mechanism, including passive diffusion. They affect only multiplying organisms but are both bacteriostatic and, in high concentrations, bactericidal.

Pharmacokinetics. Although not completely absorbed by the GI tract, tetracyclines produce adequate blood levels when given orally, the usual route of administration. Because the drugs react with polyvalent cations (calcium, magnesium, aluminum, and iron), foods or medicines that contain these minerals chelate the tetracyclines and prevent absorption if ingested at the same time. Although they can be administered parenterally, tetracyclines are rarely injected. IM injection, which produces intense pain, is not recommended.

Tetracyclines are widely distributed in body tissues. They cross the blood–brain barrier gradually but do reach therapeutic concentrations in the CNS. The ability of individual drugs to bind to plasma protein varies, ranging from 20% to 95%. Tetracyclines localize in and form stable complexes at sites of new bone and tooth formation. They readily cross the placenta and are distributed into breast milk in concentrations similar to maternal serum concentrations.

Both the liver and kidneys excrete tetracyclines, eliminating the drugs in both urine and feces. A considerable part of drugs secreted in the bile is reabsorbed, contributing to their tendency to persist in the body. Tissues that store the drugs in significant amounts include the liver, spleen, bone marrow, bone, and dentin.

Therapeutic uses. Tetracyclines are useful therapeutic agents in the treatment of infections caused by rickettsiae (Rocky Mountain spotted fever, Q fever), bacteria (brucellosis, tularemia), some *Mycoplasma* organisms that cause pneumonia, and *Chlamydia* organisms (lymphogranuloma venereum, psittacosis, trachoma). They also are used in the management of acne and amebiasis. Since their introduction, many pathogenic strains have developed resistance to the tetracyclines, and their clinical use has diminished accordingly. Tetracyclines remain important agents for the treatment of serious infections resistant to other antibiotics. Doxycycline is the drug of choice for treating uncomplicated *Chlamydia trachomatis*, a prevalent sexually transmitted disease.

Adverse reactions. Tetracyclines irritate the GI mucosa. When taken orally, nausea, vomiting, abdominal distress, distention, and diarrhea are common during treatment. Esophageal ulcers have been reported. These signs and symptoms are improved somewhat if the drugs are taken with food. However, many foods form inactive complexes with the drug, and tetracyclines are usually taken on an empty stomach.

Preparations administered IV are highly irritating to the veins and frequently cause phlebitis and thrombosis. IM injections are painful. The drugs are never injected intrathecally.

If administered during the period of tooth formation, tetracyclines permanently discolor the teeth. Initially, the color changes to yellow, but with aging, permanent browning of the enamel develops. Minocycline colors not only teeth, but also bones, skin, fingernails, and the thyroid gland.

Allergic reactions are rare but can be serious. They include skin manifestations (rash, urticaria, fixed eruptions), asthma, fever, angioedema, and anaphylaxis. Cross-sensitivity is the rule; recipients allergic to one tetracycline usually react allergically to all.

Superinfections may develop owing to alteration of the normal microbial flora. Enteritis caused by tetracycline-resistant bacteria can be life-threatening. Mycotic infections can affect the mouth, throat, or vagina. Even systemic infections can develop in immunosuppressed recipients and diabetics.

Adverse reactions, which vary with individual drugs, include phototoxicity, liver and kidney damage, and vestibular malfunction. The drugs exert a catabolic effect, producing a tendency toward negative nitrogen balance and weight loss. Blood dyscrasia and

Table 41-5. Tetracycline preparations

Drug name	Preparations	Usual dosage
demeclocycline (Declomycin, Ledermycin, Tollerclin)	Tablets and capsules for oral use	Adults: 600 mg daily, divided in 2–4 doses Children: aged 8 yr or older: 6.6–13.2 mg/kg body weight/day, divided in 2–4 doses PC: D
doxycycline (Bio-Tab, C-Pak, Doryx, Doxy-Caps, Doxycin, Doxychel, Doxy-Lemmon, Doxy-Tabs, Vibramycin Vibra-Tabs Vivox)	Tablets, capsules, and suspensions for oral use Vials that contain powder for reconstitution for IV administration	Adults and children aged 8 yr or older: 100–200 mg/day, divided in 1–2 doses PC: D
methacycline (Rondomycin)	Capsules for oral use	Adults: 600 mg daily, divided in 2–4 doses Children: aged 8 yr or older: 6.6–13.2 mg/kg body weight/day, divided in 2–4 doses
minocycline (Minocin, Min-Ovral, Vectrin)	Tablets and capsules for oral use Vials that contain powder for reconstitution for IV administration	Adults: 200 mg daily, divided in 2–4 doses, administered at equal intervals Children aged 8 yr or older: 2 mg/kg body weight/day, divided in 2 doses, administered at 12-h intervals PC: D
oxytetracycline (Abbocin, E. P. Mycin, Imperacin, Oxlopar, Oxymycin, Terramycin, Urobiotic)	Tablets, capsules, and suspensions for oral use Vials that contain powder for reconstitution for IV administration)	*Oral:* Adults: 1–2 g daily, divided in 4 doses Children aged 8 yr or older: 25–50 mg/kg body weight/day, divided in 4 doses *IM:* 250–300 mg daily, divided in 1–3 doses PC: D
tetracycline (Achromycin, Achromycin V, Apo-Tetra, Bristacycline, Brodspec, Cycline, Cyclopar, Deltamycin, Desamycin, G-Mycin, GT-250, Hosta Cyclin, Kesso-Tetra-M, M-Tetra, Mysteclin-F, Nor-Tet, Novotetra, Panymycin, Tetracyn, Tetralan)	Tablets, capsules, and suspensions for oral use Ointment and suspension for ophthalmic use Vials that contain powder for reconstitution for IM administration Vials that contain powder for reconstitution for IV administration Powder for preparing topical solutions	*Oral:* Adults: 1–2 g daily, divided in 2–4 doses Children aged 8 yr or older: 25–50 mg/kg body weight/day, divided in 2–4 doses *IV:* Adults: 500 mg–1 g daily, divided in 2 doses, administered at equal intervals Children aged 8 yr or older: 10–20 mg/kg/day *IM:* Adults: 250–300 mg/day Children aged 8 yr or older: 15–25 mg/kg/day PC: D

KEY: PC = pregnancy category. (The validity of pregnancy risk categories has not been established; see Chapter 16, p 216.)

increased intracranial pressure have also developed during therapy.

As they age, tetracyclines tend to be degraded and become more toxic. Outdated preparations have been reported to cause photosensitivity; a lupoid lesion of the face; and a form of Fanconi's syndrome, which is evidenced by nausea, vomiting, polyuria, polydipsia, proteinuria, acidosis, glycosuria, and aminoaciduria.

Precautions and contraindications. Tetracyclines are contraindicated in pregnancy because of their potential for discoloring the developing teeth of the fetus and because gravid women are highly susceptible to tetracycline-induced hepatic damage. These drugs are not recommended for nursing mothers or children younger than 8 years. Most are also contraindicated in renal insufficiency.

Because they are irritating to tissues, tetracyclines are rarely administered by injection. If IV use cannot be avoided, the drug should be well diluted and infused by slow continuous drip.

Diarrhea that occurs during tetracycline therapy must be carefully evaluated to rule out enteritis due to superinfection. When this condition, which is life-threatening, is suspected, tetracycline therapy should be discontinued. To minimize GI irritation, oral doses of the drugs may be administered with food, provided it does not contain polyvalent cations. Milk must be avoided because of its calcium content.

If tetracyclines are administered for a long period of time, periodic laboratory tests should be carried out to screen for blood dyscrasia and liver or kidney damage. Clients with a history of allergy should be monitored for indications of hypersensitivity. Emergency treatment for severe reactions, such as anaphylaxis, must be available.

■ Summary

Tetracyclines are used to treat serious infections caused by strains of organisms that are resistant to other drugs but are susceptible to tetracyclines. They are usually administered orally. They are accompanied by many adverse reactions, the most serious of which are liver and kidney damage and life-threatening enteritis. Fetuses and young children under age 7 develop permanent brown discoloration of the teeth when exposed to tetracyclines. The drugs should not given to pregnant or nursing women or to children under age 8.

Nursing management

Nursing implications

The expiration date of solutions for parenteral injection should be checked before administration. Outdated preparations must never be used because the drugs are prone to degradation and may cause toxic reactions. Preparations marketed as sterile powders should be used promptly after reconstitution. IV solutions must be well diluted and administered by continuous slow drip. Orders for IM injections should be questioned because this route is not generally recommended.

Nursing process

Assessment
Clients who are to receive tetracycline drugs should be screened for allergic hypersensitivity to these drugs, renal impairment, pregnancy, and lactation. The age of children should be ascertained. Tetracyclines are not appropriate for pregnant or nursing women, children under age 8, or older children who show delayed or arrested growth and development.

Nursing diagnosis
Diagnoses consider the client's response to drug therapy, including therapeutic effects and adverse reactions. They may include the following:

> Altered urinary elimination related to adverse reaction to anti-infective medication
> High risk for fluid volume deficit related to increased need for fluids to prevent drug toxicity
> Diarrhea related to adverse reaction to tetracyclines
> Altered nutrition: less than body requirements related to diarrhea secondary to tetracycline medication
> Noncompliance related to discomforting adverse reactions to medication or to inability to pay for prescriptions
> Knowledge deficit concerning anti-infective medications, their adverse effects, and the regimens required for their effectiveness

Planning
Goals of treatment are to promote therapeutic response to the antibiotics and to reduce the risk of adverse drug reactions.

Intervention
Oral preparations of tetracycline should be administered with ample fluids (2 to 3 liters for adults). To prevent esophageal irritation and possible ulcer formation, the dose must be propelled into the stomach. This fact is particularly important for clients with a history of hiatal hernia, who may have a malfunctioning cardiac sphincter of the stomach.

If oral tetracyclines cause epigastric or abdominal distress, they can be administered with food, provided no milk or milk products are given. Drugs that contain calcium, magnesium, aluminum, or iron prevent absorption of these antibiotics and should not be administered at the same time.

Orders for tetracyclines for children younger than age 8, for pregnant or lactating women, and for IM injection are rarely appropriate and should be questioned. If IM administration is necessary, ice should be applied to the injection site to minimize discomfort.

Clients who receive tetracyclines should be monitored for signs and symptoms of adverse drug reaction, including intestinal upset, allergy, diarrhea, renal or hepatic impairment, and vestibular impairment.

Client education.
A program for teaching recipients about their drugs should be planned and implemented. Clients often need assistance in establishing a regimen that will provide optimal drug absorption with the least irritation to the intestinal tract. If the drugs are well tolerated, they should be taken on an empty stomach. If the client experiences epigastric or abdominal discomfort, the antibiotics may be taken with selected food. The client should be instructed not to ingest milk or milk products or drugs that contain

Example of nursing process and tetracycline therapy for acne

The client is a 17-year-old married female who is under treatment with tetracycline for acne. Drugs the client takes include occasional doses of acetaminophen for headaches, a multivitamin daily, and an oral contraceptive.

Assessment data	Nursing diagnosis	Intervention	Goals and outcome criteria
Prescription for tetracycline for treatment of acne Use of oral contraceptive (Tetracycline drugs damage and discolor developing tooth enamel in fetuses and children younger than 8 years of age.)	Knowledge deficit concerning the effects of tetracycline on the teeth of a fetus exposed to it *in utero*	**Ask** the client the purposes for which the oral contraceptive has been prescribed. If the client is sexually active, **explain** to her the effect tetracycline has on the teeth of the fetus *in utero*; caution the client to consult her dermatologist for a change in medication before attempting conception and to request alternative treatment for acne should accidental pregnancy develop.	The client will not discontinue contraceptive medication without consulting her dermatologist for a change in medication. Should conception occur, the client will discontinue tetracycline immediately and consult her dermatologist for an alternative treatment for acne. If the client becomes pregnant, the child's deciduous teeth will be free of the yellow-brown discoloration characteristic of tetracycline exposure during tooth development.

calcium, iron, magnesium, or aluminum with the antibiotic. Stools may become somewhat looser during the drug regimen. The client should be cautioned to report true diarrhea (liquid or loose stools accompanied by gripping or cramping pain) to the physician.

Clients should understand that exposure of young children to tetracyclines permanently discolors their teeth. The drugs can also cause hypersensitivity to sunlight, especially in individuals with lightly pigmented skin.

Prescription drugs should never be given to anyone other than the client for whom they were prescribed, particularly with tetracyclines, which are contraindicated for pregnant or nursing women and young children. Unless the medication is discontinued by the physician, all of the prescribed dose should be taken. If the physician advises that the drug be stopped, remaining doses should be discarded, preferably by burning.

Clients should be taught to report any unusual signs and symptoms to the physician, particularly diarrhea characterized by watery stools.

Evaluation Data required for evaluation include signs and symptoms that indicate reduction and elimination of infection and absence or incidence of adverse reaction to the anti-infective drug (see Example of Nursing Process and Tetracycline Therapy for Acne).

Checklist of nursing actions

☐ Screen clients for pregnancy, lactation, incomplete skeletal development, renal or liver impairment, and allergic hypersensitivity before initiating tetracycline therapy.

☐ Administer oral tetracyclines with ample fluids (an 8-oz glass of water for adults).

☐ Use only fresh solutions for parenteral injection.

☐ Monitor clients for signs and symptoms of liver or renal malfunction, enteritis, superinfection, and bone marrow depression.

☐ If clients have a history of allergy, be prepared to give emergency care should an acute reaction occur.

☐ Do not give milk, milk products, or drugs that contain polyvalent cations with oral tetracyclines. Nonmilk foods may be given with the drugs if they cause intestinal discomfort.

☐ Warn clients not to take outdated tetracyclines nor to "share" their prescriptions with other people.

☐ Instruct clients to report adverse reactions, especially diarrhea, to the physician.

Erythromycins

Erythromycin is a macrolide produced by *Streptomyces erythraeus*. It acts as a bacteriostatic but kills highly susceptible organisms, especially when used in large doses. This drug category includes not only the parent compound but also derivatives that were developed in attempts to alter properties of the drug (Table 41-6).

Pharmacodynamics. Erythromycin is bacteriostatic in action. It inhibits protein synthesis in susceptible organisms by binding to ribosomal subunits, thereby inhibiting polypeptide synthesis. Other drugs that bind to these receptors on the ribosomal units include oleandomycin, troleandomycin, clindamycin, lincomycin, and chloramphenicol. Because they compete for the sites of action, these drugs should not be used together.

Erythromycin penetrates the cell wall of gram-positive organisms readily. It is effective against some gram-negative organisms (cocci and bacilli). Other gram-negative organisms (*Escherichia coli, Enterobacter, Klebsiella, Proteus, Pseudomonas, Salmonella*, and *Shigella* organisms) as well as viruses, yeasts, and fungi are resistant to this drug.

Pharmacokinetics. Erythromycin drugs are administered most frequently by mouth. They are absorbed in the duodenum. Gastric acidity partially destroys the drug; oral preparations must be enteric coated or buffered. The drug should be given a half-hour before or 2 hours after a meal; enteric-coated tablets can be taken with meals. Binding to serum proteins ranges from 73% to 93%. The drug is partially metabolized by the liver, and a portion enters the enterohepatic circulation. Serum levels of the drug are not significantly reduced by hemodialysis. The drug does not cross the blood–brain barrier readily.

Therapeutic uses. Erythromycin is used in the treatment of mild to moderately severe streptococcal infections, especially in individuals for whom penicillin is contraindicated. It is also used in the treatment of impetigo contagiosa caused by group A β-hemolytic streptococci and *Staphylococcus aureus*. It is considered to be the antibiotic of choice for the treatment of diphtheria. Erythromycin may also be used in the treatment of primary atypical pneumonia due to *Mycoplasma pneumoniae*.

Erythromycin ophthalmic ointment is used to prevent chlamydial conjunctivitis in neonates born to women who harbor *Chlamydia trachomatis* in the genital tract. It also prevents neonatal gonococcal ophthalmia. In addition, it is used as a topical solution in the treatment of acne vulgaris.

Adverse reactions. The most common side effects of systemic erythromycin therapy are abdominal pain and cramping. Nausea, vomiting, and diarrhea also occur, especially when large doses are used. Stomatitis, heartburn, anorexia, melena, and pruritus ani have been reported.

Allergic manifestations include skin rashes and (rarely) anaphylaxis. Erythromycin estolate may also cause reversible cholestatic hepatitis.

Erythromycin lactobionate has caused transient deafness, which is most likely to occur in individuals with renal impairment.

IM injection of erythromycin ethylsuccinate is painful and may result in abscess or local necrosis of tissue. Pain and thrombophlebitis may occur after IV administration.

Precautions and contraindications. Erythromycin estolate is contraindicated in clients with hepatic disease or malfunction. Other erythromycins should be used with caution in clients with liver or biliary disease. Hepatic function should be monitored when large doses of the antibiotic are required.

Erythromycin is contraindicated for clients with a history of allergic reaction to this class of drugs. Safe use in pregnancy has not been determined.

■ Summary

Erythromycin is an antibiotic with primarily bacteriostatic action used in the treatment of mild to moderate infection. It is especially useful in the treatment of clients who are allergic to penicillin and in chemotherapy of diphtheria.

Erythromycin is considered a drug of relatively low toxicity among antibiotics, but it can cause GI upset, skin rashes, and cholestatic hepatitis.

Nursing management

Nursing process

Assessment Before erythromycin therapy is initiated, clients should be assessed for previous allergic response to this or other antibiotics, liver or biliary disease, and pregnancy.

Nursing diagnosis Diagnoses address response to drug therapy, both therapeutic and adverse. They may include the following:

Altered nutrition: less than body requirements related to nausea and vomiting secondary to anti-infective drug therapy
Diarrhea related to superinfection secondary to anti-infective drug therapy
Impaired tissue integrity (rash, pruritus ani) related to adverse reaction to anti-infective therapy
Pain related to abscess or local necrosis secondary to IM injection of erythromycin ethylsuccinate

Table 41-6. Erythromycin preparations

Drug name	Preparations	Usual dosage	Therapeutic uses
erythromycin (Delta-E, Dowmycin, Eryc, E-Mycin, EryDerm, EryGel, Ery-Tab, Erythromid, Erythromycin Base Filmtabs, Ilotycin, Ophthalmic ointment, PCE Dispertab, Pediazole Robimycin)	Capsules, tablets, and enteric-coated tablets for oral administration Ophthalmic ointments	Adults: 1 g/day, divided in 3–4 doses, administered at equal time intervals Children: 30–50 mg/kg body weight/day, divided in 4 doses PC: B	Treatment of syphilis, gonorrhea, chlamydial infections during pregnancy, pertussis, and legionnaires' disease and pneumonia caused by *Mycoplasma pneumoniae* Alternative to penicillin in the prevention of streptococcal infections
erythromycin estolate (Ilosone)	Capsules, suspension, tablets, and chewable tablets for oral administration	Adults: 1 g/day, divided in 4 doses, administered at equal time intervals Children: 30–50 mg/kg body weight/day, divided in 4 doses PC: B	Treatment of syphilis, gonorrhea, chlamydial infections during pregnancy, pertussis, and legionnaires' disease and pneumonia caused by *Mycoplasma pneumoniae* Alternative to penicillin in the prevention of streptococcal infections
erythromycin ethylsuccinate (E.E.S., E-Mycin E, EryPed, Erythrocin, Eryzole, Pediamycin, Wyamycin E)	Suspensions, tablets, and chewable tablets for oral administration	Adults: 1.6 g/day, divided in 4 doses, administered at equal intervals Children: 30–50 mg/kg body weight/day, divided in 4 doses PC: B	Treatment of syphilis, gonorrhea, chlamydial infections during pregnancy, pertussis, and legionnaires' disease and pneumonia caused by *Mycoplasma pneumoniae* Alternative to penicillin in the prevention of streptococcal infections
erythromycin gluceptate (Ilotycin)	Vials that contain powder for reconstitution for IV administration	Adults and children: 15–20 mg/kg body weight/day, usually given by continuous slow IV infusion PC: B	Treatment of syphilis, gonorrhea, chlamydial infections during pregnancy, pertussis, and legionnaires' disease and pneumonia caused by *Mycoplasma pneumoniae* Alternative to penicillin in the prevention of streptococcal infections
erythromycin lactobionate (Erythrocin Lactobionate)	Vials that contain powder for reconstitution for IV administration	Adults and children: 15–20 mg/kg body weight/day, given as a continuous IV infusion, or divided in 4 intermittent infusions PC: B	Treatment of syphilis, gonorrhea, chlamydial infections during pregnancy, pertussis, and legionnaires' disease and pneumonia caused by *Mycoplasma pneumoniae* Alternative to penicillin in the prevention of streptococcal infections
erythromycin stearate (Bristamycin, Eramycin, Erypar, Erythrocin Stearate, Ethril, Pfizer-E, SK-Erythromycin, Wyamycin-S)	Tablets for oral administration	Adults: 1 g/day divided in 4 doses, administered at equal time intervals Children: 30–50 mg/kg body weight/day, divided in 4 doses PC: B	Treatment of syphilis, gonorrhea, chlamydial infections during pregnancy, pertussis, and legionnaires' disease and pneumonia caused by *Mycoplasma pneumoniae* Alternative to penicillin in the prevention of streptococcal infections

KEY: PC = pregnancy category. (The validity of pregnancy risk categories has not been established; see Chapter 16, p 216.)

A common collaborative problem that should be differentiated from the nursing diagnoses is

Potential complication: deafness

Planning Goals of treatment are to promote natural resistance to infection, to reduce the risk of adverse drug reactions, and to promptly detect and treat adverse reaction, should one occur.

Intervention Because erythromycin is usually administered orally, orders for administration by other routes should be questioned. Clients who receive erythromycin should be monitored for signs and symptoms of GI upset, skin rash, and hepatic impairment. Because the drugs are frequently prescribed for clients with allergies to other antibiotics, recipients are often prone to allergic responses and should be monitored for signs and symptoms of developing allergy.

Client education. Client teaching should include cautions to report to the physician: persistent abdominal discomfort, skin rash, yellowing of the skin or eyeballs, and signs and symptoms of allergic reaction. If erythromycin lactobionate is prescribed, changes in hearing should also be reported.

Evaluation Data required for evaluation are the signs and symptoms of therapeutic or adverse reactions to antibiotic therapy.

Checklist of nursing actions

☐ Assess clients who receive erythromycin antibiotics for liver disease or impairment and allergic hypersensitivity to these drugs.

☐ Monitor clients who receive erythromycin for signs and symptoms of GI irritation, skin rash, and liver impairment.

☐ Teach clients the symptoms of adverse reactions to erythromycin antibiotics and caution them to report their occurrence.

Chloramphenicol

Chloramphenicol is a broad-spectrum antibiotic originally produced by a strain of *Streptomyces* organisms but now produced synthetically. Its molecular structure is unique among antibiotics; it contains a nitrobenzene structure.

Pharmacodynamics. Chloramphenicol inhibits protein synthesis by ribosomes of bacterial cells by binding to ribosomal subunits that catalyze peptide bond formation. Its action is usually bacteriostatic, but in high concentrations and against highly susceptible organisms, it does act as a bactericidal agent.

Pharmacokinetics. Chloramphenicol salts must be hydrolyzed to free chloramphenicol before it can exert its pharmacologic action. When administered orally, hydrolysis occurs within the GI tract; after IV administration, hydrolysis occurs in the plasma. After absorption, the drug is widely distributed to most body compartments, including the cerebrospinal fluid. Plasma proteins bind about 60% of the drug. Chloramphenicol readily crosses the placenta and is secreted in breast milk.

Chloramphenicol is primarily deactivated by glucuronidase in the liver. The unchanged drug, as well as the inactive metabolites, are excreted in urine. A small fraction is eliminated in the bile and feces after oral administration. Plasma half-life in normal adults is 1.5 to 3.5 hours. It is greatly prolonged in individuals with immature or inadequate liver function, reaching 24 hours or longer in neonates.

Therapeutic uses. Because chloramphenicol causes serious and potentially fatal adverse reactions, and because few organisms have developed resistance to it, the drug is recommended as one of last resort for the treatment of life-threatening infections that are resistant to other antibiotics. The medical profession has proposed a policy of reserving systemic use for treatment only in serious infections for which other treatment agents are ineffective. This policy is expected to reduce the incidence of serious toxicity and also to delay the development of resistance to chloramphenicol in virulent pathogens, thus prolonging the drug's usefulness.

Chloramphenicol is active against most gram-positive and gram-negative bacteria, and *Rickettsia, Chlamydia,* and *Mycoplasma* organisms. It is inactive against fungi. Chloramphenicol is administered topically to treat eye and external ear infections.

Among the diseases for which this drug is used systemically are ampicillin-resistant typhoid fever, influenzal meningitis, pelvic and brain abscesses caused by anaerobic organisms, brucellosis, rickettsial disease in clients for whom the tetracyclines are contraindicated, and bacteremia caused by organisms resistant to other antibiotics. It is the drug of choice for the treatment of typhoid fever (Table 41-7).

Adverse reactions. The most important and serious adverse reaction to chloramphenicol is bone marrow depression. Two forms of bone marrow depression exist. The first is non–dose-related and is irreversible, leading to aplastic anemia, with a mortality rate of 50% or more. This reaction may be a form of allergic hypersensitivity. A genetic predisposition to this type of bone marrow depression appears to exist; it is quite rare, with estimates of the incidence being 1 in 40,000 or more courses of therapy. The more common type is dose-related and is usually reversible once the drug is discontinued. This type is seen frequently with plasma chloramphenicol concentrations of 25 μg/ml or more or when adult dosage exceeds 4 g daily. Neonates and recipients with hepatic dysfunction are at high risk, probably owing to inadequate metabolism of the drug by their liver microsomal enzymes.

Table 41-7. Chloramphenicol preparations

Drug name	Preparations	Usual dosage	Therapeutic uses
chloramphenicol (Amphicol, Chloracol, Chloromycetin, Chloroptic, Econochlor, Ophthochlor)	Capsules for oral use, 0.5% ophthalmic solution, 1% ophthalmic ointment, 0.5% otic solution	50 mg/kg body weight/day, divided in 4 doses (dosage should be kept as low as possible and must be reduced for clients with hepatic dysfunction) *Ophthalmic ointment:* small amount in lower conjunctival sac q3–6h *Ophthalmic solutions:* gtt i–ii q3–6h *Otic solution:* gtt ii–iii tid PC: C (Can cause gray syndrome in premature infants and normal neonates)	Treatment of active typhoid fever; treatment of meningitis, bacteremia, or other serious infections caused by organisms resistant to other antibiotics Treatment of superficial eye infections and otitis externa
chloramphenicol palmitate (Chloromycetin Palmitate)	Suspension for oral use Ophthalmic ointment and solutions Otic solution	50 mg/kg body weight/day, divided in 4 doses (dosage should be kept as low as possible and must be reduced for clients with hepatic dysfunction) *Ophthalmic ointment:* small amount in lower conjunctival sac q3–6h *Ophthalmic solutions:* gtt i–ii q3–6h *Otic solution:* gtt ii–iii tid PC: C (Can cause gray syndrome in premature infants and normal neonates)	Treatment of active typhoid fever; treatment of meningitis, bacteremia, or other serious infections caused by organisms resistant to other antibiotics Treatment of superficial eye infections and otitis externa
chloramphenicol sodium succinate (Mychel-S)	Powder for preparing solutions for IV administration Ophthalmic ointment and solutions Otic solution	50 mg/kg body weight/day, divided in 4 doses (dosage should be kept as low as possible and must be reduced for clients with hepatic dysfunction) *Ophthalmic ointment:* small amount in lower conjunctival sac q3–6h *Ophthalmic solutions:* gtt i–ii q3–6h *Otic solution:* gtt ii–iii tid PC: C (Can cause gray syndrome in premature infants and normal neonates)	Treatment of active typhoid fever; treatment of meningitis, bacteremia, or other serious infections caused by organisms resistant to other antibiotics Treatment of superficial eye infections and otitis externa

KEY: PC = pregnancy category. (The validity of pregnancy risk categories has not been established; see Chapter 16, p 216.)

Less serious allergic reactions to chloramphenicol include macular or vesicular skin rashes, fever, and angioedema. All are uncommon. Other adverse reactions include nausea and vomiting, diarrhea, perineal irritation, and an unpleasant taste in the mouth after oral doses. Optic neuritis, superinfection, and inhibition of microsomal enzymes have also been reported.

Premature and newborn infants exposed to chloramphenicol *in utero* and infants who receive chloramphenicol therapy may develop a type of circulatory collapse known as the gray syndrome. Symptoms include failure to feed, abdominal distention, vomiting, pallor, cyanosis, and vasomotor and respiratory collapse. The syndrome usually develops 2 to 9 days after exposure to the drug. Death may occur within a few hours; however, the process may reverse completely if

chloramphenicol is discontinued immediately when early symptoms appear. Lack of enzymes for metabolizing the antibiotic and accumulation of drug to excessive blood levels is believed to be the cause of this toxic reaction. Inactive metabolites of chloramphenicol accumulate in the tissues of clients with renal insufficiency. The toxic potential of these substances is unknown.

Precautions and contraindications. Systemic administration of chloramphenicol is contraindicated if alternative agents are available for the effective treatment of the infection. The drug is contraindicated for neonates and for individuals with a history of allergic hypersensitivity to it. Chloramphenicol therapy should be avoided in individuals with anemia and during pregnancy and lactation. Reduced doses must be given to newborns, to clients with impaired hepatic function, and to those who receive concomitant treatment by drugs that inhibit the liver microsomal enzymes. Complete blood counts should be carried out regularly to monitor bone marrow function during treatment. Prolonged therapy should be avoided.

Chloramphenicol may inhibit biotransformation and prolong the plasma half-lives of chlorpropamide, dicumarol, phenytoin, and tolbutamide; dosages of these drugs may need to be reduced during concomitant chloramphenicol therapy.

■ Summary

Chloramphenicol is a drug of last resort for the treatment of serious infections that cannot be treated with other antibiotics. The most serious adverse reaction to this drug is bone marrow depression, which can lead to fatal aplastic anemia.

Nursing management

Nursing process

Assessment Clients who are to receive chloramphenicol should be screened for a personal or family history of allergic hypersensitivity to the drug, impairment of liver function, and the recent use of drugs that inhibit the liver microsomal enzymes.

Nursing diagnosis Nursing diagnoses address reactions to the drug, both therapeutic and adverse. They include the following:

> *Knowledge deficit concerning symptoms of adverse reactions to anti-infective therapy*
> *Noncompliance related to inability to pay for drug prescriptions*

Common collaborative problems that should be differentiated from the nursing diagnoses include

> *Potential complication: hematopoietic*
> *Potential complication: immune*

Planning Goals of treatment are to promote the client's resistance to infection, to reduce the risk of adverse reaction to drug therapy, and to detect and treat adverse drug reaction promptly, should it occur.

Intervention When preparing chloramphenicol medications, environmental contamination should be avoided so as to prevent the development of resistant strains of microorganisms. Orders for systemic chloramphenicol that appear to be frivolous should be questioned. The drug is recommended only for the treatment of serious infections that cannot be treated by other agents. Clients who receive systemic chloramphenicol are usually acutely ill and under close medical

supervision. They should be informed of the risk involved in treatment with this drug before giving consent to it. Throughout their course of treatment, clients should be closely monitored for signs and symptoms of bone marrow depression and visual changes. Complete blood cell counts should be carried out at regular intervals.

Clients who receive topical preparations of chloramphenicol for outpatient use should be instructed to destroy unused medication after completing the course of treatment, preferably by burning to minimize environmental pollution. They should also be informed about symptoms of adverse reactions.

Evaluation Data required for evaluation are the signs and symptoms of therapeutic or adverse reactions to antibiotic therapy.

Checklist of nursing actions

☐ Screen clients for a personal or family history of chloramphenicol allergy, impaired liver function, pregnancy and lactation, anemia, and the use of drugs that reduce activity of liver enzymes before initiating systemic chloramphenicol therapy.

☐ Verify that the client has been informed of the risks of chloramphenicol treatment before initiating systemic chloramphenicol therapy.

☐ During treatment with systemic chloramphenicol, monitor blood counts for decreased levels of blood cells.

☐ Question orders for systemic chloramphenicol that do not appear justified. This drug should be used as a treatment of last resort.

☐ Avoid environmental contamination by chloramphenicol preparations.

☐ Monitor clients who are receiving systemic Chloromycetin for signs and symptoms of bone marrow depression, such as decreased white blood cell counts, decreased red blood cell counts, or intercurrent infections, such as sore throat.

Quinolones

Quinolones are synthetic broad-spectrum antibacterial drugs. Three of them, nalidixic acid, norfloxacin, and cinoxacin, are limited to treatment of urinary tract infections (see Chapter 42). The fourth, ciprofloxin hydrochloride, has much broader application and is discussed below in detail.

Quinolones may cause CNS stimulation that results in tremor and (rarely) convulsions. They may also cause lightheadedness and confusion. Anaphylaxis has occurred after the first dose, requiring epinephrine and other emergency measures (Table 41-8).

Table 41-8. Quinolone derivatives

Drug name	Preparation	Usual adult dosage	Additional information
ciprofloxacin (Cipro)	Oral tablets	250–750 mg q12h PC: C	Excretion is reduced by about 50% when given with probenecid.
			If a skin rash develops, the drug should be discontinued.
			Do not take with polyvalent cations (aluminum, calcium, iron, zinc).
			Recipients should avoid activities that require mental alertness or coordination.
norfloxacin (Noroxin)	Oral tablets	400 mg bid (maximum dosage: 400 mg bid) PC: C	Norfloxacin is not used to treat children.
			Caution should be exercised with recipients who have CNS disorders.
			Doses should be taken with liberal fluids, 1 h ac or 2 h pc.
			Antacids should not be taken within 1 h before and 1 h after taking norfloxacim.

KEY: PC = pregnancy category. (The validity of pregnancy risk categories has not been established; see Chapter 16, p 216.)

Ciprofloxacin hydrochloride

Ciprofloxacin hydrochloride (Cipro) is a synthetic broad-spectrum oral antibiotic derived from fluoroquinolone. It is supplied as 250-mg, 500-mg, and 750-mg tablets. It does not cross react with β-lactams, aminoglycosides, or other antimicrobials. It is generally well tolerated.

Pharmacodynamics. Ciprofloxacin HCl interferes with DNA gyrase, an enzyme needed to synthesize bacterial DNA, and is, therefore, bactericidal.

Pharmacokinetics. Ciprofloxacin HCl is available as the monohydrochloride monohydrate salt. When administered orally, it is well absorbed from the GI tract, with 40% to 50% unchanged in urinary secretion after 24 hours, and 20% to 35% recovered from the feces within 5 days. Another 15% appear as four metabolites in human urine. Serum proteins bind 20% to 40% of the drug. The serum half-life is about 4 hours. It is widely distributed throughout the body in body secretions, lymph, peritoneal fluid, cerebrospinal fluid, skin, bone, muscle, cartilage, and fat, and is excreted in urine.

Therapeutic uses. Ciprofloxacin HCl is used to treat infections caused by susceptible organisms. It is active against a wide range of gram-negative and gram-positive organisms. It is used to treat infections of the lower urinary and respiratory tracts, skin and skin structures, bones and joints, and infectious diarrhea. Dosage for most infections is 500 mg every 12 hours; mild to moderate urinary tract infections require 250 mg every 12 hours. Severe or complicated respiratory infections, or those of the skin, bone, or joints require 750 mg every 12 hours.

Adverse reactions. Ciprofloxacin HCl may cause mild to moderate symptoms that abate without treatment soon after discontinuation. These include GI symptoms (pain, nausea, vomiting, discomfort), headache, and restlessness. Photosensitivity, flushing, pruritus, and urticaria may occur, as well as disturbed vision, and renal problems (nephritis, polyuria, urinary retention, renal failure). Rare (< 1%) adverse reactions include cardiovascular symptoms (palpitations, atrial flutter, syncope, myocardial infarction, cardiopulmonary arrest) and respiratory symptoms. Since ciprofloxacin causes arthropathy in immature animals, it should not be used during pregnancy or lactation or in children.

Precautions and contraindications. Ciprofloxacin HCl should not be used during pregnancy or lactation or for children. It should be used with caution for clients with CNS disorders. Clients should not use machinery or be involved in activities that require alertness since they may suffer from lightheadedness or confusion. All clients should be observed for signs of sensitivity to the drug.

Norfloxacin

Norfloxacin is much like ciprofloxin but is limited to treatment of urinary tract infections. It is effective against both gram-negative and gram-positive aerobic bacteria (see Table 41-8). Norfloxacim is not approved for use in children and should be used with caution in clients who have CNS disorders. It increases the effects of xanthines (theophylline and caffeine), predisposing the client to seizures.

■ Summary

Ciprofloxacin HCl is increasingly used as a wide-spectrum antibiotic that is safe for most clients. Adverse reactions usually disappear when the drug is discontinued. Norfloxacin is similar to ciprofloxacin but is usually used only to treat urinary tract infections.

Nursing management

Nursing process

Assessment Clients who are to receive ciprofloxacin HCl should be screened for a personal or family history of allergic hypersensitivity to the quinolones. Check for concurrent administration of theophylline, since it may cause elevated plasma concentrations of theophylline and prolongation of its elimination half-life. Antacids that contain magnesium hydroxide or aluminum hydroxide should be avoided since they interfere with the absorption of ciprofloxacin HCl or may increase the risk of crystalluria. Probenecid interferes with the renal tubular secretion of ciprofloxacin HCl, thereby increasing the serum level of ciprofloxacin HCl.

Nursing diagnosis Nursing diagnoses address reactions to the drug, both therapeutic and adverse. They may include the following:

Altered nutrition: less than body requirements related to nausea, vomiting, and abdominal discomfort secondary to anti-infective therapy
Urinary retention related to ciprofloxin therapy
High risk for injury related to lightheadedness or confusion secondary to anti-infective therapy
Knowledge deficit related to the need for compliance (symptoms related to adverse reactions to drugs)

Planning Goals of treatment are to promote the client's resistance to infection, reduce the risk of adverse reaction to the drug therapy, and detect and treat any adverse drug reaction, should one occur.

Intervention Ciprofloxacin may be taken with or without meals, but preferably 2 hours after a meal. Fluids should be taken liberally throughout the course of treatment. Sodium bicarbonate and antacids should be avoided for 2 hours after each dose. Children and pregnant women should not receive ciprofloxacin. Clients should be monitored for any adverse reactions due to ciprofloxacin HCl.

Client education. Clients need to understand the importance of compliance with the regime for taking ciprofloxacin HCl, including the proper dose and length of time to be taken. Most infections require the drug to be taken for 7 to 14 days or longer for severe infections. Therapy for bone and joint infections may be continued for 4 weeks or more. Clients should be aware of signs and symptoms of adverse reactions.

Evaluation Data required for evaluation are the signs and symptoms of therapeutic or adverse reactions to antibiotic therapy.

Enrichment experience 41-1

Interview an ambulatory client, relative, or friend to determine what antibiotics have been used in the past and the responses to the therapy. Did the client take the medicine as ordered? Was the course of treatment completed as ordered? Did the infection resolve? Did any allergic symptoms or other adverse reactions occur? Was the education of the client sufficient to ensure understanding of the regimen and the importance of compliance?

Checklist of nursing actions

☐ Inform clients of expected beneficial reactions and possible adverse reactions.
☐ Take a careful client history to determine if concurrent administration of any drugs that may cause an adverse reaction (theophylline, antacids with magnesium hydroxide or aluminum hydroxide, probenecid) exists.
☐ Make certain that the client is not pregnant or breast-feeding, since ciprofloxacin has been shown to cause arthropathy in immature animals and may do the same in humans.

References

Schafer-Korting M, Kirch W, Axthelm T, Kohler H, Mutschler E. (1983). Atenolol interaction with aspirin, allopurinol, and ampicillin. *Clin Pharmacol Ther, 33,* 283–288.

Bibliography

Brody J. (1990, November 17). Resurgence of rheumatic fever puts focus on treatment of strep throat. *The New York Times*, p B7.
Gilman AG, Goodman LS, Rall TW, Murad F, eds. (1985). *Goodman and Gilman's The pharmacological basis of therapeutics, 7th ed*, pp 1066–1198. New York: Macmillan.
Kurtzweil P. (1991). How to take your medicine: Erythromycin. *FDA Consumer, 25*(3), 36–37.
McEvoy GK, ed. (1987). *Drug information 87*, pp 20–66, 81–312, 379–390. Bethesda, MD: American Society of Hospital Pharmacies.
Snider S. (1990). How to take your medicines: Penicillins. *FDA Consumer, 24*(6), 29–31.

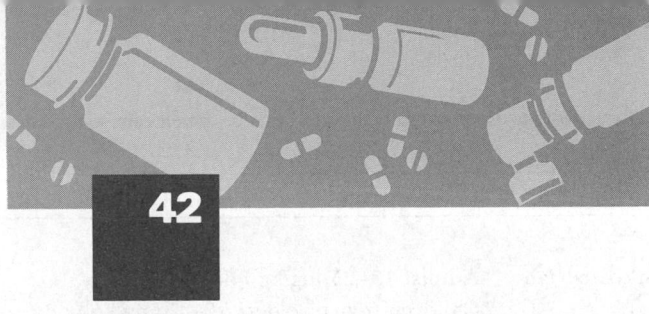

42

Antimycobacterial agents, miscellaneous antimicrobials, and urinary tract antiseptics

Antimycobacterial agents
  Streptomycin
  Ethambutol hydrochloride
  Isoniazid
  Rifampin
  Para-aminosalicylic acid
  Capreomycin sulfate
  Cycloserine
  Ethionamide
  Pyrazinamide
  Dapsone
  Sulfoxone sodium
  Clofazimine
  Nursing management
    Nursing implications
    Nursing process
      Client education
Miscellaneous antimicrobials
  Aztreonam
  Bacitracin
  Clindamycin
  Colistin
  Lincomycin
  Nitrofurazone
  Novobiocin
  Polymyxin B
  Spectinomycin
  Troleandomycin
  Vancomycin
  Sugar

Nursing management
  Nursing implications
  Nursing process
    Client education
Urinary tract antiseptics
  Methenamine
  Nalidixic acid
  Nitrofurantoin
  Phenazopyridine
  Trimethoprim
  Urine acidifiers
  Nursing management
    Nursing process
      Client education

Antimycobacterial agents

Several antibiotics and synthetic anti-infectives are used in treating infections caused by organisms of the genus *Mycobacterium*. Diseases treated with these drugs include tuberculosis, leprosy, and a variety of lesser known mycobacterial infections (atypical mycobacterial infections). The drugs most effective and least toxic (the primary antituberculosis agents) are isoniazid (INH), ethambutol, rifampin, and streptomycin. Other more toxic and less effective agents include *p*-aminosalicylic acid, capreomycin, cycloserine, ethionamide, kanamycin, and pyrazinamide (Table 42-1).

Mycobacterium tuberculosis has the ability to develop resistance readily against anti-infective drugs. For this reason, single agents are never employed for the treatment of active disease; at least two or three drugs are administered concurrently to achieve rapid clinical improvement, to eliminate infectiousness, and to delay or prevent emergence of resistant organisms. Therapy with a single drug (usually isoniazid) is used, however, to prevent active disease in asymptomatic patients.

Tuberculosis therapy is often long term, traditionally requiring 18–24 months of medication. Newer treatment regimens for uncomplicated tuberculosis using INH and rifampin for 9 months are acceptable alternatives to more prolonged regimens. Clients may be hospitalized initially and given three treatment agents, one of which is administered parenterally. When sputum cultures become negative, the parenteral drug is discontinued, and the client is discharged from the hospital on a drug regimen of two or more oral agents. Many clients are treated with oral drugs solely on an outpatient basis. Clients must be monitored throughout the course of treatment because antituberculosis drugs can be quite toxic. Notwithstanding such treatment difficulties, anti-infective drugs have revolutionized the treatment of this serious

Table 42-1. Antimycobacterial agents

Drug name	Preparations	Usual dosage
Primary antituberculosis agents		
ethambutol (Etibi, Myambutol)	Tablets and film-coated tablets for oral use	Adults: 15–25 mg/kg body weight/day Children 6 yr or older: 10–15 mg/kg body weight/day PC: B
isoniazid (Armazide, Cotinazin, Ditubin, INH, Isotamine, Izonid, Laniazid, Niconyl, Nydrazid, Panizid, Pycazide, Pyryzidin, Tisin, Tubizid)	Oral tablets Powder Solution for IM injection	Adults: *treatment:* 5–10 mg/kg body weight/day; *prophylaxis:* 300 mg/day (maximum daily dosage: 300 mg) Infants and children: *treatment:* 10–20 mg/kg body weight/day (maximum daily dosage: 500 mg); *prophylaxis:* 10 mg/kg body weight/day (maximum daily dosage: 300 mg) PC: C
rifampin (Rifadin, Rifamate, Rimactane, Rofact)	Oral tablets	Adults: 600 mg/day Children older than 5 yr: 10–20 mg/kg body weight/day (maximum daily dosage: 600 mg) PC: C
Secondary antituberculosis agents		
capreomycin sulfate (Capastat)	Vials containing powder for reconstitution for IM administration	Adults: 15 mg/kg body weight/day (maximum daily dosage: 20 mg/kg body weight/day) Safe use in children has not been established PC: C
cycloserine (Closina, Oxamycin, Serociclina, Seromycin, Setavax, Tysomycin)	Oral capsules	Adults: 500 mg–1 g/day, divided in 2 doses (maximum daily dosage: 1 g) Children: 10 mg/kg body weight/day, divided in 2 doses (maximum daily dosage: 500 mg) (However, safe use in children has not been established.) PC: C
ethionamide (Trecator S.C., Trescatyl)	Oral tablets	Adults: 500 mg–1 g/day, divided in 1–3 doses (maximum daily dosage: 1 g) Children: 12–15 mg/kg body weight/day, divided in 3–4 doses (maximum daily dosage: 750 mg) PC: D
para-aminosalicylic acid/aminosalicylate sodium (PAS, Teebacin)	Oral tablets Powder	Adults: 10–12 g/day, divided in 2–3 doses Children: 200–300 mg/kg body weight/day, divided in 3–4 doses
pyrazinamide	Oral tablets	Adults: 20–35 mg/kg body weight/day divided in 3–4 doses (maximum daily dosage: 2 g) PC: C
Antileprosy agents		
clofazimine (Lamprene)	Oral capsules	Adults: for dapsone-resistant leprosy: 100 mg/day with meals, combined with one or more antileprosy drugs for 3 years, then 100 mg/day For erythema nodosum leprosum reactions, 200 mg/day, taper to 100 mg/day PC: C
dapsone (Avlosulfon, Disulone, Udolac)	Oral tablets	Adults: 50–100 mg/day Children: 1–1.5 mg/kg body weight PC: A
sulfoxone (Diasone)	Enteric-coated tablets for oral use	Adults: 330–660 mg/day Children 4 yr of age or older: 165–330 mg/day PC: C

KEY: PC = pregnancy risk category. (The validity of pregnancy risk categories has not been established. See Chapter 16, p 216.)

disease. Prior to their development, the prognosis of clients suffering from active tuberculosis was not hopeful. Treatment required institutionalization (legally enforced in many jurisdictions) and isolation for months or years.

In 1991, a more virulent form of tuberculosis, unresponsive to present treatment modalities, was noted in several prisons, affecting prisoners and guards. Tuberculosis is also noted among clients with acquired immunodeficiency syndrome. This has caused an increase in the statistics for tuberculosis, reversing the downward trend. New treatments are now being studied.

Leprosy is similar to tuberculosis in that it is caused by a mycobacterium, it is a chronic illness requiring years of treatment, and the causative organism tends to become resistant to therapeutic drugs. Although optimum drug combinations and dosages for the treatment of leprosy are yet to be determined, 3–5 years of treatment are recommended for active disease, with maintenance drugs given for life to many clients. Medical supervision is required indefinitely to verify that the disease has not become reactivated.

Other mycobacterial infections tend to follow the patterns of tuberculosis and leprosy. As a class, these diseases are difficult to treat, often require combination drug therapy, tend to persist in an inactive state in the body after active signs and symptoms of infection subside, and may reactivate later when the host's defenses are depleted.

Clients receiving antimycobacterial drugs face a prolonged therapeutic regimen, a high risk of adverse reactions to the drugs, and indefinite supervision to guard against recurrence of the disease.

Streptomycin

The aminoglycoside streptomycin is often used in the initial treatment of tuberculosis in acute-care settings. A detailed discussion of streptomycin can be found in Chapter 41.

Ethambutol hydrochloride

Ethambutol is a primary antituberculosis agent (see Table 42-1).

Pharmacodynamics. Ethambutol's exact mechanism of action is unknown but it appears to impair cell metabolism and arrest replication. It is bacteriostatic, exhibiting activity against dividing cells. Ethambutol is highly specific, acting only against mycobacteria.

Pharmacokinetics. Following oral administration, ethambutol is well absorbed from the gastrointestinal (GI) tract. It is widely distributed into most body tissues and fluids, including the cerebrospinal fluid (CSF). The drug is secreted in breast milk but it is not known whether it crosses the placenta.

Ethambutol is partially inactivated in the liver,

with the unchanged drug and its metabolites excreted in the urine. Unabsorbed ethambutol remaining in the GI tract is excreted in feces. The drug is dialyzable.

Therapeutic uses. Ethambutol is used to treat active tuberculosis. It is especially useful for treating individuals who may have contracted a resistant strain of *Mycobacterium* and for re-treating clients whose initial course of medication did not fully arrest the disease.

Adverse reactions. The most important adverse reaction to ethambutol is optic neuritis resulting in impaired vision. This reaction is related to both dose and duration of drug treatment. When detected early, the reaction is usually reversible if the drug is discontinued.

Other adverse effects of ethambutol include skin rash, neurotoxicity, GI upset, gout, transient liver impairment, peripheral neuritis, and anaphylactoid reactions.

Precautions and contraindications. Visual testing should be performed monthly during ethambutol therapy for clients receiving greater than 15 mg/kg body weight daily. Renal, hepatic, and hematopoietic function must also be monitored. The drug must be used with caution in individuals with ocular defects and impaired renal function. Optic neuritis and allergic hypersensitivity are contraindications for the drug. Safety during pregnancy has not been established.

Isoniazid

Isoniazid (INH) is a primary antituberculosis agent (see Table 42-1).

Pharmacodynamics. INH is bacteriostatic or bactericidal in effect, depending on the concentration of the drug and the susceptibility of the pathogen. The exact mechanism of action is unknown but it appears to interfere with bacterial metabolism. It changes the acid-fast characteristic of the bacteria, apparently by inhibiting mycolic acid synthesis. The drug is active only against dividing cells. It is highly specific and active only against organisms of the genus *Mycobacterium*.

Pharmacokinetics. INH is administered both orally and by intramuscular injection. Following absorption, it is distributed into all body tissues and fluids. Concentrations in the CSF reach levels 90%–100% of concurrent plasma levels. INH readily crosses the placenta and appears in breast milk in concentrations similar to maternal plasma levels.

INH is inactivated in the liver primarily by acetylation, a process that is genetically determined. Slow inactivation is an autosomal recessive trait that appears in approximately 50% of whites and blacks; it is relatively uncommon among Mongolian populations.

Most of the drug is excreted in urine, with small amounts appearing in saliva, sputum, and feces. INH is removed by both peritoneal dialysis and hemodialysis.

Therapeutic uses. INH is used for the treatment of clinical tuberculosis and for the prevention of disease in individuals at risk.

Adverse reactions. INH causes a relative deficiency of pyridoxine, evidenced most often by peripheral neuritis. Concurrent use of pyridoxine (vitamin B$_6$) can prevent or relieve the syndrome. It is seen most often in malnourished individuals, alcoholics, and diabetics. Optic neuritis has been reported in recipients of INH. The drug can also reduce serum levels of vitamin D.

Other adverse effects include liver impairment, allergic hypersensitivity (fever, rashes, lymphadenopathy), vasculitis, hematologic reactions, and syndromes resembling systemic lupus erythematosus and rheumatic arthritis. Dry mouth, GI upset, hyperglycemia, metabolic acidosis, urine retention, and gynecomastia in males have also been reported.

INH prolongs the degradation of valium and carbamazepine; concurrent use with either of these drugs may require a reduction in their dosage.

Precautions and contraindications. Visual function and liver function should be monitored regularly during INH therapy. Safe use during pregnancy has not been established. The drug should be used with caution in patients with underlying liver dysfunction and in those receiving other neurotoxic or hepatotoxic drugs.

Rifampin

Rifampin is a primary antituberculosis agent (see Table 42-1).

Pharmacodynamics. Rifampin may be bacteriostatic or bactericidal, depending on the concentration of the drug and the susceptibility of the pathogen. It acts by inhibiting RNA synthesis in susceptible bacteria. It is most active against dividing cells but has some effect during the resting stage. Rifampin has a wide spectrum of action and is active against mycobacteria and many gram-positive and gram-negative bacteria.

Pharmacokinetics. Rifampin is administered orally. It is widely distributed into most body tissues and fluids, including the CSF. The drug crosses the placenta and is secreted into breast milk.

Rifampin is metabolized in the liver. The drug and its metabolite are excreted mainly in the bile. Unchanged drug is reabsorbed, but the metabolite does not complete the enterohepatic cycle and is excreted in the feces. Dialysis does not remove appreciable amounts of the drug.

Therapeutic uses. Rifampin is used in the treatment of active tuberculosis and other mycobacterial diseases, including leprosy.

Adverse reactions. Gastrointestinal disturbances are the most frequent adverse reactions to rifampin. Symptoms of neurotoxicity, nephrotoxicity, and liver impairment can also occur. Allergic reactions are characterized by a flulike syndrome. Skin rash, sore mouth, sore tongue, and conjunctivitis have also occurred.

Drug interactions. Rifampin induces liver enzymes and tends to increase dosage requirements of therapies involving methadone, oral hypoglycemics, corticosteroids, dapsone, oral anticoagulants, digitoxin, quinidine, verapamil, and estrogens.

Side effects. Rifampin imparts its orange-red color to body fluids, including sweat, urine, feces, saliva, tears, and CSF. Clients should be cautioned not to wear contact lenses since these may become discolored by the orange tears.

Precautions and contraindications. Clients receiving rifampin should be monitored for impaired liver function and symptoms resembling viral hepatitis. It is important that the daily dosage regimen be maintained, because the drug is not as effective when administered intermittently. Allergic hypersensitivity to rifampin or to any of the rifamycins is a contraindication for use of the drug.

Para-aminosalicylic acid

Pharmacodynamics. Para-aminosalicylic acid (PAS) is a synthetic drug with a structure similar to that of aminobenzoic acid. It competes with aminobenzoic acid in the metabolism of mycobacteria and prevents the synthesis of folic acid by susceptible organisms. Its bacteriostatic action may be partially inhibited by aminobenzoic acid. The drug is a highly specific agent, acting only against *Mycobacterium tuberculosis*.

Pharmacokinetics. Para-aminosalicylic acid is absorbed from the GI tract and distributed widely throughout the body. It does not cross the blood–brain barrier unless the meninges are inflamed, when CSF levels may reach 10%–50% of serum concentrations. Small amounts of the drug are distributed into breast milk. It is not known if it crosses the placenta.

Acetylated by the liver and intestinal mucosa, the unchanged drug and its metabolites are eliminated in urine by glomerular filtration and tubular secretion.

Therapeutic use. Para-aminosalicylic acid is used only in the treatment of clinical tuberculosis.

Adverse reactions. The most frequent adverse reactions to PAS are GI in nature (nausea, vomiting, diarrhea, anorexia, abdominal pain). Other less frequently observed complications include peptic ulcer, malabsorption, allergic reactions (fever, rash, joint pain, reduced blood cell counts, hepatitis, Löffler's syndrome,* and psychotic reaction), hemolytic anemia, and goiter.

Precautions and contraindications. Caution must be exercised when the drug is given to individuals with renal or hepatic impairment or gastric ulcer. Paraaminosalicylic acid contains considerable sodium and may not be tolerated by clients with congestive heart failure or other conditions requiring reduced sodium intake. Allergic hypersensitivity is a contraindication for its use.

Drug interactions. Probenecid inhibits the renal excretion of PAS and its concurrent use may result in toxic blood levels of the latter unless dosages are reduced. The action of oral anticoagulants may be enhanced by this anti-infective.

Capreomycin sulfate

Capreomycin is a polypeptide antibiotic derived from a strain of *Streptomyces*.

Pharmacodynamics. The drug exerts a bacteriostatic action by an unknown mechanism. Its spectrum of activity includes *Mycobacterium tuberculosis, M. bovis, M. kansasii, M. avium*, and some gram-positive and gram-negative bacteria.

Pharmacokinetics. Because it is not absorbed well from the GI tract, capreomycin is administered intramuscularly. No information is available on its distribution in body tissues. It is not known if it is secreted in breast milk or if it crosses the placenta. The drug is eliminated unchanged in the urine by glomerular filtration.

Therapeutic uses. Capreomycin is used in the treatment of clinical tuberculosis and other mycobacterial diseases.

Adverse reactions. The most serious adverse reactions to capreomycin are nephrotoxicity and ototoxicity. Both the auditory and vestibular portions of the eighth cranial nerve are affected. Prompt discontinuation of medication upon appearance of signs and symptoms of toxicity usually results in reversal of these effects, but permanent deafness and fatal toxic nephritis have occurred. Local reaction at the site of injection may include pain, induration, bleeding, and sterile abscess. Allergic reactions (urticaria, photosensitivity, and maculopapular rash) are rare. Abnormal liver function and partial neuromuscular blockade have been reported.

Precautions and contraindications. Caution should be exercised when administering capreomycin to cli-

ents with renal insufficiency or auditory impairment. Renal, auditory, and vestibular function should be monitored before and at regular intervals during therapy. Reduced dosage is required for clients with impaired renal function. Capreomycin is contraindicated for clients who are allergic to it; caution should be used in clients with a history of allergic reaction, especially to drugs. Safe use in children has not been established.

Drug interactions. Nephrotoxic or ototoxic effects of capreomycin could be enhanced by other drugs. The concurrent or sequential use of this drug and aminoglycosides, colistin, polymyxin B, and vancomycin should be avoided.

Cycloserine

Cycloserine is a derivative of *Streptomyces* cultures and is also produced synthetically.

Pharmacodynamics. Cycloserine acts both as a bacteriostatic and bactericidal agent by competing with D-alanine for incorporation into bacterial cell walls, thus inhibiting cell wall synthesis. Its spectrum of activity includes several strains of mycobacteria, including the organism causing tuberculosis, as well as some gram-positive and gram-negative bacteria.

Pharmacokinetics. Cycloserine is well absorbed from the GI tract, is widely distributed into body tissues and fluids (including the CSF), and is excreted in the urine. About a quarter of all oral doses appear to be metabolized to unidentified metabolites. The drug readily crosses the placenta and appears in breast milk. Excretion is mainly renal, with smaller amounts eliminated in feces.

Therapeutic uses. Cycloserine is used in the treatment of active tuberculosis and a number of other mycobacterial diseases. It is also used in the treatment of selected urinary tract infections (UTIs) caused by susceptible bacteria when other more effective and less toxic agents are contraindicated.

Adverse reactions. Cycloserine is toxic to the central nervous system. Central nervous system reactions occur most frequently and include drowsiness, dizziness, headache, lethargy, depression, tremor, dysarthria, hyperreflexia, paresthesia, nervousness, anxiety, vertigo, confusion, disorientation, memory loss, weakness, seizures, and coma. Ingestion of alcohol increases the risk of these adverse reactions. Psychosis has also been reported.

Allergic reactions (rash and photosensitivity) have occurred on rare occasions with cycloserine. Cardiac arrhythmias and congestive heart failure can also occur. Liver impairment and nutritional deficiency (vitamin B_{12}, folic acid) have been reported.

Precautions and contraindications. Dosage should be reduced or the drug discontinued if symptoms of

---

*A syndrome resembling infectious mononucleosis.

neurotoxicity appear. Administration of pyridoxine (100–300 mg) may prevent or alleviate these adverse reactions. Sedatives and anticonvulsants are useful in treating toxicity.

Cycloserine is contraindicated for individuals with a history of mental depression, psychosis, anxiety reactions, or seizures. It should not be administered to persons who frequently drink alcohol, those with severe renal disease, and those who have an allergic hypersensitivity to it.

Ethionamide

Ethionamide is a derivative of isonicotinic acid and is produced synthetically. It should be administered with at least one other effective antituberculosis drug.

Pharmacodynamics. Ethionamide appears to inhibit peptide synthesis in mycobacteria, the only organisms it is known to affect. Depending on the concentration attained at the site of infection and the susceptibility of the organisms, the drug may be bacteriostatic or bactericidal.

Pharmacokinetics. Ethionamide is administered orally and is rapidly absorbed from the GI tract. It is widely distributed into body tissues and fluids, producing concentrations in the CSF equal to concurrent plasma levels.

Ethionamide is extensively metabolized, probably in the liver, to both active and inactive metabolites. Both drug and metabolites are excreted in urine.

Therapeutic uses. Ethionamide is used in the treatment of tuberculosis, leprosy, and other mycobacterial infections.

Adverse reactions. Gastrointestinal disturbances are the most frequent adverse effects of ethionamide and are dose-related. Reducing dosage, changing the time of administration, or giving the drug with food may alleviate these reactions. Neurotoxic effects include dizziness, weakness, changes in levels of activity, peripheral neuritis, paresthesia, tremor, seizures, optic neuritis and other changes in vision, olfactory disturbances, and hallucinations. These may be prevented or relieved by the administration of pyridoxine hydrochloride.

Hepatotoxic reactions include transient increases in hepatic enzymes and hepatitis. Hepatotoxicity is generally reversible if drug therapy is suspended immediately.

Allergic reactions, which are uncommon, include rash, stomatitis, photosensitivity, thrombocytopenia, and purpura.

The management of diabetes mellitus may be more difficult when ethionamide is prescribed because the drug sometimes causes hypoglycemia. Other rare reactions include gynecomastia, impotence, menorrhagia, joint pain, acute rheumatic symptoms, and acne.

Precautions and contraindications. Liver function should be monitored before ethionamide treatment is begun and regularly checked during treatment. The drug is contraindicated for clients with severe liver impairment and for those who are allergic to it. Safe use during pregnancy and in children has not been established.

Pyrazinamide

Pyrazinamide is a synthetic compound derived from niacinamide.

Pharmacodynamics. The mechanism of action of pyrazinamide is not known. It acts only against *Mycobacterium tuberculosis* and may be either bacteriostatic or bactericidal, depending on the concentration at the site of infection and the susceptibility of the bacilli.

Pharmacokinetics. Pyrazinamide is administered orally and is well absorbed from the GI tract. The drug is widely distributed into body tissues and fluids and produces concentrations in the CSF approximately equal to serum levels. It is not known whether the drug crosses the placenta or appears in breast milk.

Therapeutic uses. Pyrazinamide is used in the treatment of active tuberculosis.

Adverse reactions. Hepatotoxicity, the most frequent adverse effect, occurs in about 15% of patients receiving maximum doses of pyrazinamide. This adverse reaction appears to be dose-related and may occur at any time during treatment. Acute yellow atrophy of the liver and death have occurred.

Acute gout may develop because pyrazinamide inhibits renal excretion of urates. Allergic reactions include maculopapular rash, arthralgia, fever, and photosensitivity with reddish-brown discoloration of the exposed skin. Acne, porphyria, dysuria, nausea, vomiting, anorexia, and blood dyscrasias have also occurred. Some recipients have exhibited increased serum iron-binding capacity and serum iron levels.

Precautions and contraindications. Liver function tests and uric acid levels should be monitored before pyrazinamide therapy is begun and periodically during treatment. Caution should be used when the drug is administered to clients with renal failure, history of gout, porphyria, or diabetes. Severe hepatic impairment is a contraindication for the drug.

Dapsone

Dapsone is a synthetic sulfone.

Pharmacodynamics. Although the mechanism of action of dapsone is not fully understood, it appears to resemble the action of sulfonamides, which inhibit folic acid synthesis in susceptible organisms. It exerts a bacteriostatic effect.

Pharmacokinetics. Dapsone is well absorbed from the GI tract. It is distributed to most tissues and enters the enterohepatic cycle. It does not penetrate the eye well, a matter of concern since eye lesions can occur in leprosy—a disease for which it is used. The drug is secreted in breast milk.

Therapeutic uses. Dapsone is active against the organisms causing leprosy and tuberculosis. It is the drug of choice for the treatment of leprosy, in conjunction with rifampin or clofazimine. It is also administered to individuals at risk for developing leprosy because of their close, prolonged contact with patients with lepromatous leprosy. Other therapeutic uses for dapsone are palliative treatment of dermatitis herpetiformis, malaria (in conjunction with pyrimethamine), and diseases characterized by bullous eruptions or mucocutaneous lesions, such as lupus erythematosus.

Adverse reactions. Adverse reactions to dapsone range from hemolytic anemia and methemoglobinemia to skin rash, peripheral neuropathy, GI upset, hepatotoxicity, renal toxicity, and two types of reactional states in leprosy patients: *erythema nodosum* and reversal reaction, in which the skin lesions become erythematous, swollen, and ulcerated. Dapsone has also caused malignant tumors in experimental animals.

Precautions and contraindications. Pretreatment with ascorbic acid, folate, and iron helps prevent blood changes caused by the drug. If a reactional state is severe or accompanied by neuritis, the client is hospitalized and given corticosteroids. *Erythema nodosum leprosum* reactions are treated with analgesics, steroids, and (in countries where the drug is approved) thalidomide. Dapsone is contraindicated in individuals who are allergic to the drug or to other dapsone derivatives (*eg*, sulfoxone sodium).

Dapsone should not be used during pregnancy and lactation because it crosses the placenta and is secreted into breast milk.

Drug interactions. Oral probenecid decreases urinary excretion of dapsone and its metabolites; when the two drugs are administered concurrently, the dosage of dapsone should be reduced to avoid toxicity. Rifampin increases metabolism of dapsone in the liver and thereby decreases serum concentrations of the drug. Larger than usual doses of dapsone may be required.

Sulfoxone sodium

Sulfoxone sodium is a synthetic sulfone that is converted to dapsone in the GI tract. About half of the dapsone so formed is absorbed. Each 165-mg enteric-coated tablet of sulfoxone is approximately equal to 25 mg of dapsone.

Sulfoxone is used in the treatment of leprosy and dermatitis herpetiformis in individuals who cannot tolerate dapsone. Adverse reactions resemble those of dapsone, and can include allergic reactions as well.

Clofazimine

Pharmacodynamics. Clofazimine is an antileprosy agent that inhibits mycobacterial growth and binds to mycobacterial DNA. Its precise mechanisms of action are unknown.

Pharmacokinetics. Clofazimine is retained in the human body for a long time (about 70 days), tending to be deposited in fatty tissue and cells of the reticuloendothelial system. It does not show cross-resistance with dapsone or rifampin.

Therapeutic uses. Clofazimine is useful in treating lepromatous leprosy, including that which is dapsone-resistant. Clofazimine is also used for lepromatous leprosy complicated by erythema nodosum leprosum, but not for any other leprosy-associated inflammatory reaction.

Combination drug therapy is recommended for initial treatment of multibacillary leprosy to prevent the development of drug resistance.

Adverse reactions. Severe abdominal symptoms have resulted in exploratory laparotomies. There have been rare instances of splenic infarction, bowel obstruction, and GI bleeding, and some reports of death due to clofazimine deposits in tissues, including the intestinal mucosa, liver, spleen, and mesenteric lymph nodes. Clofazimine discolors skin (reddish brown to black.) This discoloration may be so extreme that the client becomes depressed, even suicidal. Discoloration of urine, feces, sputum and sweat may also occur. Coloration may take months or years to disappear after therapy ends. Other side effects include ichthyosis and dryness, rash and pruritus, nausea, vomiting, and elevated blood sugar and erythrocyte sedimentation rate (ESR).

Precautions and contraindications. The client should be monitored for depression if skin discoloration occurs. It may take months or years before discoloration disappears.

Drug interactions

Concurrent administration of dapsone may inhibit the anti-inflammatory activity of clofazimine. Nevertheless, treatment by both drugs should continue.

■ Summary

Antimycobacterial anti-infectives are the first effective agents for controlling mycobacterial diseases, such as tuberculosis and leprosy. Some of these agents are highly specific for mycobacteria and are not useful in treating other infections. To prevent resistance from developing in mycobacterial pathogens, the drugs are usually used concurrently in combinations of two or more. Antimycobacterial drugs are relatively toxic and may impair hearing or vision, and cause hepatotoxicity, nephrotoxicity, and central nervous system changes.

Nursing management

Nursing implications

Antibiotic treatment of acute tuberculosis is often initiated in an acute-care setting, where the client can be isolated until the sputum becomes noninfectious. Parenteral drugs are sometimes prescribed in conjunction with oral drugs, which are continued after discharge. The client may neither expect nor wish to be hospitalized. Successful treatment often hinges on the client's willingness to comply with a lengthy, strict treatment regimen of polypharmacy and hygiene.

Nursing process

Assessment Before antimycobacterial therapy is initiated, clients should be screened for contraindications for using these drugs. A complete history should be taken and physical examination performed. Particular attention should be given to factors indicating renal or liver impairment, gout, cardiovascular disease (especially congestive failure), gastric ulcer, loss of hearing or vision, vestibular disturbances, electrolyte imbalances, abnormal blood cell levels, neuromuscular disorders, epilepsy, mental illness, chronic alcohol use, or severe allergy to drugs. If women are of childbearing age, reproductive status (pregnancy or lactation) should be determined. This information will help the physician select the safest agents for the drug regimen.

A complete drug history must be taken, with specific attention given to any previous antimycobacterial therapy and to the client's response to those drugs. All drugs currently used, including social drugs such as alcohol and nicotine, should be listed. Many medications interact with the antimycobacterial drugs. Smoking is harmful to clients being treated for tuberculosis because of its toxic effect on the lungs, which are the organs most often affected by the disease. Alcohol impairs liver function and will potentiate the hepatotoxic and neurotoxic effects of some antimycobacterials. In the author's experience, clients affected by tuberculosis often have a history of poor self-care practices, including malnutrition and use of nicotine and alcohol.

The social circumstances of the client's life should also be evaluated. Treatment of mycobacterial infections generally requires lengthy therapy using multiple drugs. Consequently, the more stable the client's lifestyle, the more likely it is that the therapy will be successful. Many people suffering from tuberculosis are among the homeless or disadvantaged; conditions of poverty contribute to active infection, reactivation of arrested infections, and treatment failure in both tuberculosis and leprosy. For some, cost of medications may be a barrier to treatment.

The nurse should also explore the client's knowledge of and psychological reaction to the diagnoses.

Nursing diagnosis Diagnoses for clients receiving antimycobacterial treatment relate to both therapeutic and adverse responses to the drug regimen. They may include the following:

Altered nutrition, less than body requirements: pyridoxine deficiency related to INH, ethambutol, or ethionate therapy
Body image disturbance related to skin discoloration secondary to clofazimine therapy
Noncompliance with the drug regimen related to the complexity of the drug regimen, including the need for multiple doses (or to limited funds to pay for medication)
Knowledge deficit related to tuberculosis and its treatment
Anxiety related to the prognosis and to the adverse effects of the drug regimen

Common collaborative problems that should be differentiated from the nursing diagnoses include

Potential complication: auditory impairment
Potential complication: visual impairment

Planning Treatment goals are to support and enhance clients' natural resistance to infection, to assist them in carrying out the therapeutic regimen accurately, to reduce the risk of adverse reaction to medications, and to detect and treat adverse drug reactions promptly.

Intervention Nursing measures used to build natural resistance to infection include hygienic practices that support and enhance functioning of the immune system (*eg*, good nutrition, ample rest, and reduced stress). Clients should be monitored for signs and symptoms of adverse drug reactions. The physician may need to be consulted to tailor the treatment regimen to the client's needs. Many clients may also need the support services of a social worker or social service agency to obtain the necessities for healthy living (*eg*, food, clothing, shelter).

Clients suffering from mycobacterial infections need a great deal of emotional support during the treatment period. Many are frightened by the diagnosis. Throughout history, leprosy has been considered an incurable and loathsome disease. Many older Americans remember when tuberculosis was a scourge that killed or incapacitated people of all ages, particularly young adults. Although other mycobacterial infections may be lesser known, their prognoses are generally similar to that of tuberculosis. Although the antimycobacterials have greatly improved the outlook for these conditions, treatment requires years of medication, and a return to health is not called "cure" but "arrest" of the disease. The microorganisms often remain in the body, sealed off and inactive, but capable of causing renewed infection should the host's defenses be depleted. When clients are hospitalized, anxiety is heightened, especially if isolation precautions are imposed. It is imperative that stress levels be controlled, because undue stress causes impairment of the immune and inflammatory responses. The nurse must maintain an optimistic outlook. It is important to listen to clients as they voice their concerns and assist them to control their levels of stress.

Hospitalized patients are likely to be receiving parenteral drugs. Intravenous (IV) infusions should be closely regulated to control the rate and prevent rapid administration. Intramuscular injections are likely to cause acute discomfort at the site. Ice packs may be applied to prevent and relieve the pain. (Prolonged cold has a numbing effect.)

Administration of specific drugs requires special consideration. For example, PAS should be given with food to minimize GI side effects. Parenteral solutions of INH should be warmed to room temperature before administering to redissolve crystals that may form at low temperatures.

During treatment, clients must be closely supervised. Assessment for adverse reactions, including certain laboratory tests (depending on the drug), is required approximately every 2 weeks.

If INH is prescribed without supplementary pyridoxine, the client should be monitored for early signs and symptoms of vitamin B_6 deficiency (*eg*, leg pains), and the physician should be consulted if supplementation is required.

Client education.
Most clients will need careful instruction to properly manage their therapeutic regimens. When developing a teaching plan, the nurse should consider the client's knowledge of, and psychological reaction to, the diagnosis. Misconceptions should be corrected, and an improved outlook should be stressed.

The need for drug regimen compliance must be emphasized. Interrupting or discontinuing drug dosage is likely to result in the development of drug resistance in the pathogen, making successive treatment difficult. The nurse should assist the client in devising a system for maintaining the medication regimen. (Many clients pour all the drugs required for the day's medication in the morning and check at night to be sure all have been taken.) Whatever system is used, the drugs must be secured against accidental ingestion by others, particularly children.

If cost is a problem the client should be referred to social service for assistance. Many people are reluctant to take this step and clients may need some persuasion to accept this kind of help. The nurse should point out that successful treatment of the infection as early as possible will shorten the time of dependence on financial aid.

Clients should be taught the signs and symptoms of adverse reactions to the specific drugs. These should be listed in writing, with specific instructions for alleviating symptoms, and for consulting a physician. Clients receiving rifampin should be warned that the drug may color body excretions red-orange and be reassured that this is harmless.

Host resistance is a critical factor in treating mycobacterial infections. The nurse should explore clients' health habits and assist them in planning and carrying out measures that will enhance resistance. Particular attention should be paid to nutrition, rest, and stress management.

Therapeutic response must be evaluated to determine whether the prescribed drugs are effective. Compliance with the drug regimen should also be determined because it is critical in the successful treatment of mycobacterial diseases.

Evaluation
Information required for evaluation includes changes in the signs and symptoms of inflammation and infection, the signs and symptoms of adverse reactions to the prescribed drugs, acuity of vision and hearing, and the client's knowledge of and compliance with requirements of the self-care drug regimens.

(See the accompanying Example of Nursing Process and Pyridoxine Deficiency From Isoniazid Therapy.)

Checklist of nursing actions

When antimyobacterial drugs are to be used
☐ Screen clients for contraindications for drug therapy and conditions that could increase the risk of adverse reactions.

During antimycobacterial therapy
☐ Assess clients frequently for therapeutic and adverse reactions; outpatients should be evaluated at least every 2 weeks.
☐ Monitor laboratory data for adverse drug effects; notify the physician promptly when these occur.
☐ When drugs are administered IV, maintain a slow infusion rate.
☐ When drugs are administered intramuscularly, apply an ice pack to the site before and after the injection.
☐ Caution the client to take all drugs as ordered; assist clients in devising a system for ensuring compliance.

Example of nursing process and pyridoxine deficiency from isoniazid therapy

The client is a 45-year-old female secretary. A month prior to this visit, she had been placed on a preventive regimen of isoniazid because of a known exposure to active tuberculosis and a positive tine test. (A tine test performed 5 years earlier had a negative result.)

The client is knowledgeable about tuberculosis and the hygienic measures necessary to support and enhance natural resistance to infection. She has had no signs or symptoms of active tuberculosis (cough, purulent sputum, fevers, fatigue).

The client has had some unusual sensations in her legs (prickling, mild pain), especially on weekends when it is her custom to take long walks.

Assessment data	Nursing diagnosis	Intervention	Goals and outcome criteria
Isoniazid therapy Leg pain and paresthesias	Altered comfort: leg pain and paresthesia related to pyridoxine deficiency secondary to isoniazid therapy High risk for altered health maintenance related to lack of knowledge of the tuberculosis disease process and the therapeutic regimen required to treat it	**Inform** client that leg pains could be an adverse reaction to the isoniazid medication; advise her to report this symptom to her physician. **Inform** client that isoniazid can cause such a reaction because it increases the body's need for pyridoxine (vitamin B$_6$). **Advise** client that pyridoxine supplements are usually prescribed to alleviate this type of reaction to isoniazid; recommend that she take additional vitamin B$_6$ while on isoniazid medication. **Teach** the client the nature of tuberculosis, the benefits of drug therapy, and the importance of compliance. **Explain** the adverse reactions that may occur, stressing the signs and symptoms that should be reported to the health care provider. **Assist** the client to develop a drug dosage schedule that fits into her lifestyle.	Within 1 month the client will no longer experience abnormal sensations, since additional B$_6$ will alleviate pyridoxine deficiency. The client will remain free of signs and symptoms of tuberculosis.

- [ ] Provide encouragement and emotional support throughout the long period of treatment.
- [ ] Teach clients to recognize adverse reactions to the drugs and when to report these to the physician.
- [ ] Teach clients measures to improve nutrition, promote rest, and manage stress, all aimed at improving systemic resistance.

Miscellaneous antimicrobials

The drugs discussed in this section are not used routinely because most are relatively toxic; newer drugs are more effective; or they are unsuitable for oral administration. They are useful drugs for treating infections when the causative organisms are resistant to other less toxic agents, or when the affected client is allergic to the usual treatment agents (Table 42-2).

Table 42-2. Miscellaneous antimicrobials

Drug name	Preparations	Usual dosage	Therapeutic uses and additional information
bacitracin (Baciguent, Baci-IM, Basitin, Topitracine)	Vials containing powder for reconstitution for IM administration	Adults: *IM:* 40,000–100,000 U/day, divided in 4 doses Infants weighing 2.5 kg or less: 900 U/kg/day, divided in 2–3 doses Infants weighing more than 2.5 kg: 1,000 U/kg/day, divided in 2–3 doses PC: C	Treatment of pneumonia and empyema in infants caused by susceptible staphylococci Antisepsis of the intestinal tract (using the oral route) Treatment of superficial wounds (applied topically)
clindamycin (Cleocin)	Capsules and solution for oral use Solution for IM or slow IV injection	Adults: *Oral:* 400–1800 mg/day, in divided doses Children over 1 mo of age: 15–40 mg/kg body weight/day divided in 3–4 doses PC: C	Treatment of septicemia, intra-abdominal infections, pelvic infections, serious infections affecting the skin, soft tissues, and respiratory tract, and bone and joint infections caused by susceptible anaerobes and staphylococci
colistin (Coly-Mycin)	Solution for topical use Suspension for oral use Vials containing powder for preparing solutions for IM injection	Apply topically 2.5–5 mg/kg body weight/day, divided in 2–4 doses (maximum daily dosage: 5 mg/kg)	Treatment of acne vulgaris Treatment of infections caused by susceptible strains of gram-negative bacteria when other anti-infectives are contraindicated or ineffective Dosage adjustment required for clients with renal dysfunction
lincomycin (Lincocin, Mycivin)	Oral capsules Solution for IV infusion	Adults: *Oral:* 1.5–2 g/day, divided in 3–4 doses; *IM:* 0.6–1.2 g/day, divided in 2–3 doses Children older than 1 mo: *Oral:* 30–60 mg/kg body weight/day, divided in 3–4 doses; *IM:* 10–20 mg/kg body weight/day, divided in 1–2 doses; *IV:* 10–20 mg/kg body weight/day, divided in 2–3 doses PC: B	Treatment of serious respiratory tract, skin, and soft tissue infections caused by susceptible cocci when other less toxic drugs are contraindicated
nitrofurazone (Furacin)	Cream, solution, and ointment for topical use	Apply intermittently PC: C	Second- and third-degree burns (as an adjunct) and skin grafts and donor sites (prophylactically)
novobiocin (Albamycin, Cardelmycin, Cathomycin)	Oral capsules	Adults: 1–2 g/day, divided in 2–4 doses (maximum daily dosage: 2 g) Children: 15–45 mg/kg body weight/day, divided in 2–4 doses	Susceptible strains of *S. aureus,* when other less toxic drugs are contraindicated
polymyxin B sulfate (Aerosporin, Pediotic Suspension, Polysporin Ophthalmic Ointment)	Solution for injection Solution for urogenital irrigation	Adults and children aged 2 yr or older: *IV:* 15,000–25,000 U/kg body weight/day, divided in 2 doses; *IM:* 25,000–30,000 U/kg body weight/day, divided in 4–6 doses Maximum daily dosage for infants: 40,000 U/kg body weight/day Maximum daily dosage for adults: 2,000,000 U PC: B	Infection causes by organisms resistant to other less toxic drugs Dosage adjustment required for clients with renal dysfunction
spectinomycin (Trobicin)	Vials containing powder for reconstitution for IM administration	Adults: 2 g as a single dose Children younger than 8 yr: 40 mg/kg body weight as a single dose PC: B	Treatment of uncomplicated gonorrhea when penicillin and tetracycline are contraindicated and when resistant strains of pathogens fail to respond to other drugs

(Continued)

Table 42-2. Miscellaneous antimicrobials (Continued)

Drug name	Preparations	Usual dosage	Therapeutic uses and additional information
troleandomycin (Cyclomycin, TAO)	Capsules and suspension for oral use	Adults: 1–2 g/day, divided in 4 doses Children: 0.5–1 g/day, divided in 4 doses	Respiratory tract infections caused by susceptible staphylococci or streptococci when erythromycin is contraindicated or ineffective
vancomycin (Vancocin, Vancoled, Vancor IV)	Capsules and solutions for oral use Vials containing powder for reconstitution for IV administration	Adults: 2 g/day, divided in 2–4 doses Children: 40 mg/kg body weight/day, in divided doses Newborn infants: 20 mg/kg body weight/day, in divided doses PC: C	Treatment of staphylococcal and other infections caused by susceptible organisms which cannot be treated by other less toxic drugs Treatment of necrotizing enterocolitis caused by *Clostridium difficile* Dosage adjustment required for clients with renal dysfunction, those who are elderly, or young infants Use cautiously for hearing impaired or those on other ototoxic drugs
sugar (dextrose)	Ordinary table sugar	Sufficient granules to fill the wound	Treatment of infected wounds

KEY: PC = pregnancy risk category. (The validity of pregnancy risk categories has not been established. See chapter 16, p 216.)

Aztreonam

Aztreonam is the forerunner of a new class of synthetic antibiotics called monobactams.

Pharmacodynamics. Aztreonam is effective against a variety of gram-negative bacteria, including some that are resistant to penicillin, aminoglycosides, and cephalosporins.

Pharmacokinetics. Aztreonam is administered by IV infusion or deep intramuscular injection. Dosage varies from 1 to 8 g a day, depending on the severity of the infection and its location.

Therapeutic uses. Aztreonam is used in the treatment of septicemia and skin infections, lower respiratory infections, and intra-abdominal infections caused by gram-negative bacteria.

Adverse reactions. To date, adverse reactions have been reported in fewer than 2% of the recipients. Because the drug is chemically related to penicillins and cephalosporins, some cross-sensitivity (allergy) can be anticipated. The drug does not appear to cause ototoxicity or nephrotoxicity.

Precautions and contraindications. Caution should be used when aztreonam is administered to individuals with a known allergic hypersensitivity to penicillins or cephalosporins. Dosage must be reduced and renal function monitored when it is used for clients with renal impairment.

Solutions are reconstituted immediately before administering them. They must be used within 48 hours. When diluted, the drug must be shaken vigorously.

Because this is a new drug, health care personnel should be alert to detecting previously unrecognized adverse reactions, should they develop.

Bacitracin

Bacitracin is an antibiotic produced by *Bacillus subtilis* with a polypeptide structure.

Pharmacodynamics. The action of bacitracin is bactericidal or bacteriostatic, depending on the concentration of the drug and the susceptibility of the pathogen. It inhibits bacterial cell wall synthesis, probably by interfering with the final dephosphorylation step in the phospholipid carrier cycle involved in the transfer of mucopeptide to the growing cell wall. Bacitracin also damages the bacterial plasma membrane. It is active against many gram-positive organisms and some gram-negative pathogens. Resistance to bacitracin seldom occurs in susceptible bacteria.

Pharmacokinetics. Bacitracin is not absorbed from the GI tract. Following intramuscular injection, it is widely distributed to body organs and fluids, including ascitic and pleural fluids. Only traces cross the blood–brain barrier, unless the meninges are inflamed. Following oral administration, bacitracin is excreted in the feces. After parenteral injection, most of the dose cannot be accounted for and may be destroyed in the body. About 10% to 40% is excreted in the kidneys by glomerular filtration.

Therapeutic uses. Systemic bacitracin can be used to treat infants with pneumonia and empyema caused by susceptible staphylococci that are resistant to penicillin. However, penicillin-resistant penicillin and cephalosporins are equally effective and less toxic. The drug is also used orally as an intestinal antiseptic.

Bacitracin ointment is marketed over-the-counter for use in treating superficial wounds.

Adverse reactions. The most serious toxic effect of bacitracin is renal tubular and glomerular necrosis. This reaction occurs less often in infants than in older individuals. Pain and induration may occur at the site of injection. Gastrointestinal upset, superinfection, and respiratory paralysis have occurred. Allergic reactions include urticaria, fever, blood dyscrasias, eosinophilia, and anaphylaxis.

Precautions and contraindications. Renal function should be assessed before beginning parenteral bacitracin therapy and regularly during treatment. The drug is contraindicated for individuals with renal impairment and should be discontinued if renal toxicity develops. Myasthenia gravis, pregnancy, and allergic sensitivity to bacitracin are other contraindications for using the drug. Clients receiving bacitracin should be kept well hydrated and urine pH should be kept at or above six to decrease renal irritation.

Concurrent use of neuromuscular blocking agents should be avoided. Bacitracin is not administered IV because it causes severe thrombophlebitis. Because of stability problems, bacitracin powder should be kept refrigerated.

Clindamycin

Clindamycin is a semisynthetic derivative of lincomycin.

Pharmacodynamics. Clindamycin appears to bind to 50S ribosomal subunits and inhibit peptide bond formation and protein synthesis. It is bacteriostatic or bactericidal, depending on the concentration of drug at the site of infection and the susceptibility of the pathogen involved. This drug is effective against most aerobic gram-positive cocci and several anaerobic and microaerophilic gram-negative and gram-positive organisms. Natural and acquired resistance to clindamycin and cross-resistance between clindamycin and lincomycin have been demonstrated.

Pharmacokinetics. Clindamycin is well absorbed from the GI tract. The presence of food may delay but does not appreciably decrease absorption. The drug is distributed into many body tissues and fluids but does not readily cross the blood–brain barrier, even when the meninges are inflamed. Clindamycin is distributed to synovial fluid and bone. It readily crosses the placenta and is distributed into breast milk.

Clindamycin is partially metabolized in the liver to both active and inactive metabolites. Excretion of metabolites and active drug is primarily through the kidneys, with a small fraction eliminated in the feces. The drug is not dialyzable.

Therapeutic uses. Clindamycin is used to treat septicemic disease and serious infections caused by susceptible organisms, including those found in skin and soft tissue, in the respiratory system, and in the intra-abdominal system. It is also used as an adjunct in the treatment of chronic bone and joint infections and acute hematogenous osteomyelitis caused by staphylococci.

Adverse reactions. Adverse GI reactions to clindamycin (nausea, vomiting, diarrhea, abdominal pain) frequently occur and may be severe enough to require termination of drug therapy. This reaction occurs with parenteral and oral administration of the drug. Fatal colitis has occurred.

Allergic reactions include generalized rash (the most common adverse reaction), fever, hypotension, polyarthritis, and anaphylaxis. A syndrome resembling Stevens-Johnson syndrome has also occurred.

Clindamycin is an irritating substance and can cause tissue damage when administered parenterally. Other adverse reactions include hepatotoxicity, blood dyscrasias, and superinfection.

Precautions and contraindications. Clindamycin should be used with caution in clients with a history of intestinal disease, especially colitis. Renal and hepatic function should be monitored before and during therapy with the drug.

Clindamycin should be used with caution in clients with a history of atopic allergy; the drug is contraindicated for clients with a history of allergy to this drug. Clindamycin has neuromuscular blocking properties and caution should be used when the drug is administered to clients with myasthenia gravis. Safe use of clindamycin during pregnancy has not been established.

Drug interactions. Because of its nephrotoxic, neurotoxic, and neuromuscular blocking properties, the use of clindamycin with other drugs with these properties should be avoided.

Colistin

Colistin (also known as polymyxin E) is an antibiotic produced by a variety of *Bacillus polymyxa*.

Pharmacodynamics. Colistin acts as a cationic detergent. It damages the bacterial cytoplasmic membrane, causing leakage of essential intracellular metabolites and nucleosides. It is active against many gram-negative bacteria. The action of the drug is bactericidal.

Pharmacokinetics. Colistin is poorly absorbed from the GI tract, skin, and mucous membranes. It must be administered parenterally. Following intramuscular or IV injection, colistin is widely distributed into body tissues. It is not distributed appreciably into synovial, pleural, or pericardial fluids. The drug tends to remain in body organs and muscles.

Colistin and its metabolites are eliminated primarily by the kidneys. The drug is not dialyzable.

Therapeutic uses. Colistin is used in the treatment of gram-negative infections when other more effective and less toxic anti-infectives are ineffective or contraindicated. It is useful in treating UTIs caused by *Pseudomonas aeruginosa* that are not susceptible to aminoglycosides. The drug has been used to treat intestinal infections caused by *Escherichia coli* and *Shigella*.

Adverse reactions. The most serious toxic reactions to colistin are nephrotoxicity and neurotoxicity. Nephrotoxicity is usually reversible with discontinuation of the drug; reducing the dosage of this antimicrobial may relieve the signs and symptoms of neurotoxicity.

Other adverse reactions include rash, fever, GI upset, dysphonia, leukopenia, granulocytopenia, superinfection, and hepatotoxicity. Neuromuscular blockade with apnea can occur.

Colistin may cause pain at the site of injection. Resistance to colistin rarely develops during therapy.

Precautions and contraindications. Renal function should be monitored in clients receiving colistin. Dosage must be reduced for clients with renal dysfunction. When neurotoxicity occurs during therapy, the dosage should be reduced and the client observed closely. Clients should be warned that the drug may impair their ability to carry out activities requiring alertness or physical coordination. Colistin should be avoided in individuals with myasthenia gravis. Should apnea occur during therapy, respiration must be assisted mechanically.

Safe use of colistin in pregnancy has not been established.

Drug interactions. Concurrent use of colistin and other nephrotoxic or neurotoxic drugs should be avoided. Colistin also increases the effects of neuromuscular blocking agents.

Lincomycin

Lincomycin is an antibiotic produced by a variant of *Streptomyces lincolnesis*.

Pharmacodynamics. Lincomycin inhibits protein synthesis by binding to 50S ribosomal subunits. It is bacteriostatic or bactericidal, depending on the concentration of drug at the site of infection and the susceptibility of the pathogen. Its spectrum of activity is similar to that of clindamycin.

Pharmacokinetics. Lincomycin can be administered orally, although only 20%–30% of the drug is absorbed from the GI tract, and the presence of food both delays and decreases its absorption. The drug is also administered IV and intramuscularly. Distribution into body tissues and fluids is widespread. The drug diffuses into peritoneal fluid, pleural fluid, synovial fluid, bone, bile, and the aqueous humor of the eye but it crosses the blood–brain barrier only when the meninges are inflamed, and then only in low concentrations. Distribution into bone also is poor. Lincomycin readily crosses the placenta and appears in breast milk.

Lincomycin is partially metabolized by the liver. The drug is excreted in both urine and feces. A portion of drug is unaccounted for and may be destroyed in the body.

Therapeutic uses. Lincomycin is used to treat serious coccal infections in individuals for whom less toxic antimicrobials, such as penicillin or erythromycin, are contraindicated.

Adverse reactions. Adverse reactions to lincomycin resemble those to clindamycin. The drug has also caused hypotension and cardiac arrest.

Precautions and contraindications. Lincomycin should be used with caution in clients with a history of GI disease (especially colitis), renal impairment, atopic allergy, and liver impairment. It is contraindicated in individuals with allergy to either lincomycin or clindamycin. Safe use during pregnancy has not been established. The drug is presently not recommended for use in infants.

Lincomycin has neuromuscular blocking properties and caution should be exercised when it is used to treat clients with myasthenia gravis.

Drug interactions. The use of lincomycin with other drugs with neuromuscular blocking properties should be avoided.

Concurrent use of kaolin with lincomycin interferes with absorption of the anti-infective. Absorption may be reduced to as little as 10% of a given dose.

Nitrofurazone

Nitrofurazone is a synthetic nitrofuran derivative.

Pharmacodynamics. The mechanism of action of nitrofurazone is unknown. The drug appears to impair carbohydrate metabolism, probably by inhibiting bacterial enzymes involved in carbohydrate metabolism. The drug is effective against a wide variety of gram-positive and gram-negative bacteria but does not inhibit fungi or viruses.

Pharmacokinetics. Nitrofurazone is absorbed from the denuded skin. It is not known if the drug is secreted in breast milk. Nitrofurazone is excreted by the kidneys.

Therapeutic uses. Nitrofurazone is used topically as an adjunct in the treatment of second-degree and third-degree burns and in the prevention of infection in skin grafts and donor sites. It is especially useful when resistance to other antimicrobials is likely.

Adverse reactions. Allergic dermatitis occurs in approximately 1% of the clients treated with nitrofurazone. Because signs and symptoms of allergy (redness, itching, or burning) resemble those of skin infection, this reaction may be confused with the condition under treatment.

The vehicle used in nitrofurazone ointment may impair kidney function when absorbed from the topical site of application. Superinfection by nonsusceptible organisms may occur.

Precautions and contraindications. Wounds to which nitrofurazone is applied must be debrided because organic matter inhibits the antimicrobial action of the drug. The drug should be used with caution in individuals with renal impairment. Therapy should be discontinued if progressive renal dysfunction or rash develops. The drug is contraindicated for individuals known to be allergic to it.

Safe use during pregnancy and lactation has not been established.

Novobiocin

Novobiocin is an antibiotic produced by *Streptomyces niveus* or *S. speroides*.

Pharmacodynamics. Novobiocin appears to interfere with bacterial cell wall synthesis and to inhibit protein and nucleic synthesis in pathogens. It is usually bacteriostatic in action. It is active against some gram-positive cocci and bacilli and certain gram-negative bacteria. Resistant strains can develop rapidly during therapy.

Pharmacokinetics. Novobiocin is well absorbed from the GI tract. Concentrations in pleural, synovial, and ascitic fluids are usually lower than concurrent serum concentrations. The drug does not cross the blood–brain barrier in significant amounts even when the meninges are inflamed. Highest concentrations of novobiocin are found in the liver, small intestines, and bile. The drug is excreted primarily in bile and feces with a small fraction eliminated by the kidneys.

Therapeutic uses. Novobiocin is presently used only when other less toxic agents are ineffective or contraindicated. It has been used to treat infections caused by *Staphylococcus aureus* and *Proteus*.

Adverse reactions. Allergic reactions occur frequently in clients receiving novobiocin. Gastrointestinal reactions also occur but are rarely severe. Other adverse effects include hematologic changes, hepatotoxicity, and dizziness, drowsiness, and lightheadedness. Superinfection can also occur.

Precautions and contraindications. Hepatic and hematologic systems should be assessed before and at regular intervals during novobiocin therapy. The drug should be discontinued if impairment of either system develops. It is contraindicated for individuals who are allergic to the drug. Because the drug tends to cause hyperbilirubinemia, its use is contraindicated in neonates. Safe use during pregnancy has not been established.

Polymyxin B

Polymyxin B is an antibiotic produced by various strains of *Bacillus polymyxa*.

Pharmacodynamics. Polymyxin B binds to phosphate groups in the lipid portion of bacterial membranes. Acting as a detergent, it breaks down the membrane barrier, allowing leakage of essential macromolecules from the cell. The drug's spectrum resembles that of colistin. Bacterial resistance to polymyxin B seldom develops.

Pharmacokinetics. Except in infants, polymyxin B is not appreciably absorbed from the GI tract, mucous membranes, or skin. For this reason, it is usually administered by intramuscular or IV injection. Following absorption, the drug is widely distributed into body tissues. It does not appear in the CSF, even when the meninges are inflamed, and does not cross the placenta or appear in synovial fluid or aqueous humor. Although the drug is not highly bound to serum proteins, about 50% of a dose is reversibly bound to phospholipids of tissue cell membranes.

Polymyxin B is excreted primarily unchanged in the urine by glomerular filtration. Unaccounted for is about 40% of a dose. Infants excrete the drug faster than adults. Polymyxin B is not dialyzable.

Therapeutic uses. Polymyxin B is useful in treating serious infections caused by pathogens resistant to other more effective and less toxic agents. In the past, it has been administered orally to treat GI infections but oral dosage forms are no longer available.

Adverse reactions. Adverse reactions to polymyxin B resemble those to colistin, primarily nephrotoxicity and neurotoxicity. This drug is not highly allergenic when applied topically but other drugs administered in combination with it may induce allergy.

Precautions and contraindications. Polymyxin B is contraindicated in individuals with a history of allergy to any of the polymyxins. Before therapy is begun, clients should be screened for renal impairment. During therapy, renal function should be monitored frequently. Safe use during pregnancy has not been established.

Drug interactions. Concurrent or sequential use of nephrotoxic, neurotoxic, or neuromuscular blocking agents with polymyxin should be avoided.

Spectinomycin

Spectinomycin is an antibiotic produced by *Streptomyces spectabilis*.

Pharmacodynamics. Spectinomycin appears to bind to 30S ribosomal subunits, thereby inhibiting bacterial protein synthesis. It acts against a wide variety of gram-positive and gram-negative bacteria but it is used almost exclusively in the treatment of gonorrhea caused by penicillinase-producing strains of cocci. Drug resistance has been reported.

Pharmacokinetics. Spectinomycin is not absorbed from the GI tract. The drug is administered intramuscularly. It is unknown whether spectinomycin crosses the placenta or distributes into breast milk. Spectinomycin and its active metabolites are primarily excreted in the urine by glomerular filtration.

Therapeutic uses. Spectinomycin is used in the treatment of uncomplicated gonorrhea as an alternative to penicillin.

Adverse reactions. The most frequent adverse effect of spectinomycin is pain at the injection site. Nephrotoxic, hepatotoxic, hematologic, and allergic reactions have been reported. Severe reactions are infrequent, however, and the drug is usually well tolerated.

Precautions and contraindications. Before initiating spectinomycin therapy for gonorrhea, clients should be screened for syphilis. The drug is not an effective treatment for syphilis and may mask its symptoms. If syphilis is present, another agent effective against both diseases must be used.

Spectinomycin should be used with caution in clients with a history of allergies; hypersensitivity to the drug is a contraindication for its use. Safe use of spectinomycin during pregnancy or in infants and children has not been established.

Troleandomycin

Troleandomycin is an antibiotic produced by *Streptomyces antibioticus*. It is a macrolide antibiotic related to erythromycin.

Pharmacodynamics. Troleandomycin is deacetylated in the body to oleandomycin. This metabolite inhibits protein synthesis by binding to 50S ribosomal subunits. It is active against gram-positive cocci and some gram-negative bacilli. Resistance does develop and cross-resistance between oleandomycin and erythromycin sometimes occurs.

Pharmacokinetics. Troleandomycin is administered orally and is rapidly absorbed from the GI tract. After absorption, it is metabolized to oleandomycin and is widely distributed. The drug diffuses poorly into the CSF. Troleandomycin is excreted primarily by the liver, with lesser amounts eliminated by the kidneys.

Therapeutic uses. Troleandomycin is used in treating infections when other less toxic antimicrobials are ineffective or contraindicated.

Adverse reactions. Adverse reactions to troleandomycin are manifested most frequently as GI symptoms, such as nausea, vomiting, intestinal cramping, diarrhea, esophagitis, and rectal burning. Allergic reactions to the drug include rash, cholestatic hepatitis, and anaphylaxis. Superinfection also can occur.

Precautions and contraindications. Reducing dosage sometimes relieves the GI effects of troleandomycin. The drug should be used with caution in individuals with impaired hepatic function. Liver function should be monitored during therapy. The drug is contraindicated for individuals allergic to it. Safe use during pregnancy has not been established.

Drug interactions. Troleandomycin should not be used concurrently with ergotamine because it increases the toxicity of that drug, apparently by reducing its detoxification by the liver. When used with theophylline or carbamazepine, the dosage of these drugs may need to be reduced because troleandomycin interferes with their hepatic metabolism.

Vancomycin

Vancomycin is a tricyclic glycopeptide antibiotic derived from nocardia orientalis.

Pharmacodynamics. Vancomycin does not appear to be metabolized by the body. It is approximately 55% serum protein bound. It acts through inhibition of cell-wall biosynthesis and alterations in bacterial cell membrane permeability and RNA synthesis. It is active against staphylococci, streptococci, *Clostridium difficile*, and diphtheroids. There is no cross-resistance to other antibiotics.

Pharmacokinetics. Because it is poorly absorbed by the GI tract, vancomycin is administered orally only for treatment of staphylococcal enterocolitis and antibiotic-associated pseudomembranous colitis. It is administered IV for any other systemic infections. In the first 24 hours, about 75% is excreted in urine by glomerular filtration but that percentage may be reduced in the elderly. It diffuses poorly across normal meninges into CSF but does penetrate when the meninges are inflamed. Doses for young infants or low birth weight infants must be lowered to prevent ototoxicity and nephrotoxicity.

Therapeutic uses. Vancomycin is used in treating serious or severe infections caused by beta-lactam resistant staphylococci for penicillin-allergic clients, or for clients with infections unresponsive to other antimicrobials. It can be used in combination with an aminoglycoside for synergistic action against early onset prosthetic valve endocarditis caused by *S. epidermidis* or diphtheroids.

Adverse reactions. Adverse reactions to vancomycin include transient or permanent ototoxicity, mostly in clients receiving excessive doses; those who have an underlying hearing loss; or those who are being treated with another ototoxic agent. Reversible neutropenia may occur.

Precautions and contraindications. Vancomycin should be used with caution in clients with renal insufficiency or renal dysfunction. The risk of thrombophlebitis can be minimized by slow administration and rotation of infusion sites. Acuity of hearing should be tested regularly, especially if other ototoxic drugs are administered concurrently.

Vancomycin is contraindicated for clients with a known hypersensitivity to this antibiotic. Intravenous administration must take place over not less than 60 minutes, using a dilute solution. Rapid infusion may result in sudden, profound hypotension, accompanied by an erythematous maculopapular rash (red man's syndrome) that is not an allergy. Too rapid administration may also lead to cardiac arrest. During infusion, blood pressure should be monitored. Renal function and hearing should be checked serially for those on prolonged vancomycin therapy. Pain and necrosis may result from extravasation. Therefore, IV routes must be secure.

Drug interactions. Because of its ototoxicity, caution should be exercised when vancomycin is administered concurrently with other ototoxic drugs, such as the aminoglycosides.

Sugar

Sugar has been used empirically in treating infected wounds (Sweethearts resist infection, 1985). The wound is filled with dry sugar and the packing and dressing changed several times a day.

Pharmacodynamics. The mechanism by which sugar affects infectious pathogens is unknown. It has been suggested that the high osmotic pressure exerted by sugar dehydrates bacterial cells, and that the material blocks access to other nutrients.

Pharmacokinetics. Sugar acts locally when administered topically.

Therapeutic uses. Sugar has been used to treat infected wounds, including postsurgery chest wounds, burns, lacerations, amputations, gunshot wounds, and decubiti. It may be used in combination with povidone iodine.

Adverse reactions. Adverse reactions to topical sugar have not been reported.

■ **Summary**
The miscellaneous drugs discussed here are agents that are used when primary drugs are not effective or cannot be used for some reason. They generally are more toxic than the primary agents.

Nursing management

Nursing implications

Reconstituted oral solutions of clindamycin should not be refrigerated because they thicken when chilled.

Nursing process

Assessment Because most of the drugs discussed above are relatively toxic, clients about to receive them should be screened carefully for allergic sensitivity to related drugs and for any organ impairment (especially renal impairment), which can increase the risk of drug accumulation and toxic reaction.

Nursing diagnosis Diagnoses for clients receiving these drugs may include the following:

> *Impaired gas exchange related to neuromuscular blockade secondary to anti-infective therapy*
> *Pain: at drug injection sites; nausea, vomiting, abdominal pain secondary to use of oral anti-infective drugs; neuritis secondary to colistin therapy*
> *Nutrition less than body requirements related to diarrhea secondary to anti-infective therapy*
> *Impaired skin integrity: rash related to anti-infective therapy*
> *High risk for infection related to changes in normal body flora secondary to anti-infective therapy*
> *Knowledge deficit related to anti-infective therapy*

Common collaborative problems that should be differentiated from the nursing diagnoses include

> *Potential complication: hepatotoxicity*
> *Potential complication: ototoxicity*
> *Potential complication: cardiovascular*
> *Potential complication: respiratory*

Planning Goals of treatment include supporting and enhancing natural resistance to infection; reducing the risk of adverse reaction to the prescribed drug; and promptly detecting and treating an adverse drug reaction should one occur. An important goal is an increase in the client's knowledge about infection and its treatment.

Intervention Nursing actions include consulting with the physician about client response to medication

Example of nursing process and severe pain from polymyxin B therapy

The client is a 62-year-old man admitted to the hospital for treatment of a deep sacral decubitus, which developed in a nursing home where he has lived since suffering a paralyzing stroke. The decubitus is infected with a gram-negative bacillus. The organism is sensitive to polymyxin B, which has been ordered for treatment. After receiving his first dose of polymyxin B, the client complains of severe pain in the injection site.

Assessment data	Nursing diagnosis	Intervention	Goals and outcome criteria
Polymyxin B therapy Complaint of pain at injection site	Pain related to inflammation at the injection site secondary to polymyxin B therapy	**Apply** an ice pack to the injection site for 5–10 minutes before administering the injection and again for 5–10 minutes after administering the injection.	The client will report that the pain has been eliminated or reduced when ice is used to anesthetize the site because ice causes a numbing sensation.

(*ie*, lack of therapeutic response, adverse drug reaction). Because these drugs are frequently used in acute-care settings, administration is often the responsibility of the nurse. Most drugs of this class are irritating to the tissues. Injection sites will be painful and may be inflamed. Ice should be applied to the site before and after injections.

All possible nursing measures that support and enhance natural resistance to infection should be implemented (*eg*, good nutrition, ample hydration, adequate rest, and reduction of stress).

Clients must be monitored closely for response to treatment. Frequent laboratory tests are performed; the results of these tests should also be monitored.

If clients have undergone previous treatment with primary antimicrobials, they may be discouraged by the failure of these agents. Emotional support should be given to assist them through the prolonged period of therapy.

When ototoxic drugs are administered, serial tests of auditory function should be used to detect early loss of hearing while it is reversible.

Client education. Clients should be taught the drug regimen, including possible adverse reactions and expected therapeutic response. Care should be taken to maintain a hopeful outlook, stressing that symptomatic treatment or a change in drug dosage or drug agent should resolve any problems that may arise. (See Chapter 42-17 for other areas of client education).

Evaluation Data required for evaluation include the client's response (therapeutic or adverse) to the drug regimen, the resolution of adverse reactions should they occur, and the client's knowledge and under-

standing of the drug regimen. (See the accompanying Example of Nursing Process and Severe Pain From Polymyxin B Therapy.)

Checklist of nursing actions

☐ Monitor clients receiving miscellaneous antimicrobials carefully for adverse reactions because these drugs are relatively toxic.

☐ Before administering injections of these drugs, numb the site by applying ice. Reapply the ice after injection to maintain comfort.

☐ Maintain a hopeful outlook and provide emotional support for the client receiving these drugs, particularly when other drugs have been unsuccessful in resolving the infection.

☐ Teach clients what symptoms to report to health care personnel.

☐ Teach clients to manage the drug regimen and self-care practices that promote recovery from infection.

Urinary tract antiseptics

Urinary tract antiseptics are a group of disinfectants given systematically for their local effect in the urinary tract. These drugs cannot be administered in large enough doses to produce therapeutic concentrations in the general circulation. They become concentrated in the kidneys and reach antibacterial concentrations only in the urinary tract. Their use, therefore, is limited to infections in this system (Table 42-3).

Methenamine

Methenamine is a synthetic chemical that decomposes in acid solution.

Table 42-3. Urinary tract antiseptics

Drug name	Preparations	Usual dosage	Summary of pertinent information
cinoxacin (Cinobac)	Oral capsules	Adults: 1 g/day, divided in 2 doses PC: B	Not recommended for use by prepubertal children
methenamine (Hiprex, Mandelamine, Mandelets, Urised, Uro-Phosphate)	Tablets, enteric-coated tablets, and suspensions for oral use	Adults: 4 g/day, divided in 4 doses, administered pc and hs Children: 6–12 yr of age: 50 mg/kg body weight/day, divided in 3 doses Children less than 6 yr old: 75 mg/kg body weight/day, divided in 4 doses PC: C	Releases formaldehyde in acid urine
nalidixic acid (NegGram, Nogram, Wintomylon)	Tablets and suspension for oral use	Adults: 4 g/day, divided in 4 doses Children 3 mo–12 yr of age: 55 mg/kg body weight/day, divided in 4 doses PC: B	Kills urinary tract pathogens by inhibiting DNA synthesis
nitrofurantoin (Chemiofuran, Furadantin, Furalan, Furan, Furanex, Furanite, Furantoin, Furaton, I Dantin, Ituran, Macrodantin, Nephronex, Nitrex, Nitrofan, Parfuron, Sarodent)	Tablets and suspension for oral use	Adults: Oral 200–400 mg/day, divided in 4 doses Children older than 1 mo: 5–7 mg/kg body weight/day, divided in 4 doses PC: B	Rarely induces resistance in susceptible pathogens Antiseptic action enhanced in an acid urine Turns urine brown Take with food or milk to reduce GI upset
trimethoprim (Proloprim, Trimpex)	Tablets for oral use	Adults: 200 mg/day, divided in 1–2 doses The prophylactic dosage is 100 mg/day, administered hs PC: C	Safety and efficacy in children younger than 12 years of age has not been established Dosage adjustment required for clients with renal dysfunction.
co-trimoxazole-sulfamethoxazole-trimethoprim combination (Abactrim, Bactramine, Bactrim, Bactrimel, Bethaprim, Comoxol, Cotrim, Novotrimel, Protrim, Roubac, SMZ-TMP, Septra, Sulfatrim, Sulfa-Trimethoprim)	Tablets and suspension for oral use Solutions for dilution for IV infusion	The drug combination is prepared in a fixed ratio of 5 mg of trimethoprim to 25 mg of sulfamethoxazole Adults: For prophylaxis: 40–80 mg of trimethoprim (as co-trimoxazole) up to 7 times weekly *For treatment:* 320 mg/day of trimethoprim (as co-trimoxazole), divided in 1–2 doses Children 2 months of age or older: 15 mg of trimethoprim (as co-trimoxazole)/kg body weight/day, divided in 2 doses PC: C (D if near term)	See previous information for individual drugs Dosage varies with type and severity of disease Up to 720 mg/day may be used to treat severe infections in adults Dosage adjustment required for clients with renal dysfunction

* Level of formaldehyde, the active metabolite.

KEY: PC = pregnancy risk category. (The validity of pregnancy risk categories has not been established. See Chapter 16, p 216.)

Pharmacodynamics. In acid urine, methenamine generates formaldehyde, an effective anti-infective, in therapeutic concentrations.

Pharmacokinetics. Methenamine is administered orally. It must be protected from decomposition in the acid gastric juice by enteric coating. In the blood and in body tissues whose pH levels are above 7.0, little methenamine breakdown occurs. The drug acts primarily within the urinary tract. Its efficacy depends on the pH of urine, which must be maintained at an acid level.

Therapeutic uses. Methenamine is used to suppress chronic UTI.

Adverse reactions. Formaldehyde is irritating to tissues, and irritation of the urinary tract may develop. Methenamine's chemical reaction releases ammonia as a by-product. This ammonia may increase chemical imbalance in clients with hepatic impairment.

Precautions and contraindications. Methenamine cannot be used for clients with hepatic insufficiency. High doses given for initial treatment should be reduced when the urine becomes sterile to avoid irritation of the urinary tract.

Drug interactions. Methenamine is antagonistic to sulfonamide drugs and is not used in combination with them.

Nalidixic acid

Nalidixic acid is a synthetic naphthyridine derivative which is structurally related to oxolinic acid. It is one of the quinolones.

Pharmacodynamics. Nalidixic acid is believed to inhibit microbial DNA synthesis.

Pharmacokinetics. Nalidixic acid is well absorbed from the GI tract. Except for serum proteins, to which the drug is highly bound, nalidixic acid does not accumulate in the tissues. It does not cross the blood–brain barrier but does cross the placenta and is secreted in breast milk. Nalidixic acid is partially metabolized by the liver and kidneys and is excreted in the urine.

Therapeutic uses. Nalidixic acid is used in treating UTIs caused by susceptible gram-negative organisms.

Adverse reactions. Nalidixic acid is more toxic than other urinary antiseptics. Adverse reactions include GI irritation, behavioral changes indicative of central nervous system damage, reduced blood cell levels, altered liver function, and allergic reactions.

Precautions and contraindications. Clients receiving nalidixic acid must be monitored closely for adverse reaction.

Drug interactions. Nalidixic acid tends to displace warfarin from serum protein-binding sites and thus enhances the effects of this oral anticoagulant. When the drug is administered concurrently with warfarin, the dosage of anticoagulant should be reduced.

Nitrofurantoin

Nitrofurantoin is a synthetic compound.

Pharmacodynamics. Nitrofurantoin appears to inhibit several bacterial enzyme systems. It may be bacteriostatic or bactericidal, depending on concentration in the tissues.

Pharmacokinetics. Nitrofurantoin is readily absorbed from the GI tract. Macrocrystal preparations are absorbed more slowly than microcrystal preparations. Binding to plasma proteins ranges from 20% to 60%. The drug crosses the placenta and is distributed into breast milk and bile.

Therapeutic uses. Nitrofurantoin is used in treating UTIs caused by susceptible organisms. Its spectrum of activity includes many gram-negative and gram-positive organisms.

Adverse reactions. Nitrofurantoin frequently causes GI upset (nausea, vomiting, and anorexia). Serious potential complications include neuropathy and hepatotoxicity (which are not dose-dependent), allergic pulmonary reactions, hemolysis, and reduced blood cell levels. Nitrofurantoin may cause superinfection, especially *Pseudomonas* overgrowth.

Precautions and contraindications. Because serious adverse reactions to nitrofurantoin develop insidiously, clients receiving the drug should be monitored closely for signs and symptoms of drug reaction. The drug should be discontinued at the first sign of pulmonary reaction or neurotoxicity. Caution should be used when the drug is prescribed for clients with renal impairment, asthma, diabetes mellitus, electrolyte imbalance, vitamin B deficiency, or general debility. It is contraindicated in infants younger than 1 month and in pregnant women at term.

Phenazopyridine

Phenazopyridine is an azo dye that exerts weak antiseptic and effective analgesic actions within the urinary tract.

Pharmacodynamics. The exact mechanism of action of phenazopyridine is unknown. Although the drug acts as a weak inhibitor of the growth of microorganisms, it is most valued for its effect as a local anesthetic on the urinary tract mucosa.

Pharmacokinetics. The pharmacokinetic properties of phenazopyridine have not been determined. It is believed to cross the placenta. Metabolism probably occurs in the liver and other tissues. The drug is excreted mainly by the kidneys.

Therapeutic uses. Phenazopyridine is used as an adjunct with other, more effective urinary tract antiseptics for relief of the symptoms of UTI (pain, burning, urgency, and frequency).

Adverse reactions. Adverse reactions to phenazopyridine are relatively infrequent. Headache, vertigo, and mild GI upsets are seen occasionally. More rarely, methemoglobinemia, hemolytic anemia, skin pigmentation, jaundice, hepatitis, crystalization in the urine, and transient acute renal failure develop. Most effects are dose-related. Individuals with renal impairment are at high risk.

Precautions and contraindications. Phenazopyridine is contraindicated in glomerulonephritis, severe hepatitis, uremia, pyelonephritis during pregnancy, or impaired renal function.

The client should be advised that phenazopyridine produces an orange to red color in the urine. Stains on fabrics can be removed by soaking in a 0.25% solution of sodium dithionate or sodium hydrosulfite. If the skin or sclerae become discolored (yellow), the drug is accumulating in the tissues and should be discontinued.

Trimethoprim

Trimethoprim is a synthetic compound that acts as a folate antagonist.

Pharmacodynamics. Trimethoprim inhibits bacterial enzymes of the folic acid pathway. It is slowly bactericidal.

Pharmacokinetics. Trimethoprim is used in treating initial episodes of acute UTI caused by susceptible pathogens.

Adverse reactions. The most frequent adverse reactions to trimethoprim are skin rash and pruritus. Less frequently, hematologic changes, fever, nephrotoxicity, and hepatotoxicity are seen. The incidence and severity of drug reactions are dose-related and may subside with a reduction in dosage. When administered IV, solutions of trimethoprim-sulfamethoxazole tend to precipitate as solids in the tubing.

Drug interactions. When combined with sulfamethoxasone, additional adverse reactions are seen. These include pancreatitis, jaundice, psychosis, fixed genital drug eruption, and aseptic meningitis.

Precautions and contraindications. Caution must be exercised when trimethoprim is prescribed for clients with impaired renal or hepatic function, or with a folate deficiency. The drug is not recommended for clients with creatinine clearances of less than 15 ml/min. The drug is contraindicated for clients with allergic hypersensitivity to the drug.

Urine acidifiers

Lowering the *p*H of urine inhibits the growth of most common pathogens involved in UTI. Poorly metabolized acids used to accomplish this include mandelic acid, hippuric acid, ascorbic acid, and sodium biphosphate. The same effect can be accomplished by administering acid-ash foods, such as cranberries, plums, and prunes. When acidification of the urine is desired, the client should not be given large amounts of alkali-ash foods (most fruits and vegetables).

■ Summary

Urinary tract antiseptics are given systemically for their local effect and are excreted by the kidneys. Phenazopyridine is most valuable for its analgesic property; it relieves itching, burn-

ing, and cramping. Clients should be warned that their urine will turn a bright orange or red-orange color with this drug. Urine acidifiers are used to lower *p*H and inhibit the growth of pathogens in the urinary tract. Acid-ash foods can be given, whereas alkali-ash foods are to be avoided. Methenamine, although not a primary drug for acute infection of the urinary tract, is useful in chronic suppressive treatment. Nalidixic acid is effective against gram-negative bacteria. It is more toxic than the other urinary antiseptics. Nitrofurantoin is used against *E. coli* and other susceptible organisms. Clients should be warned that it turns urine brown.

Nursing management

Nursing process

Assessment Urinary tract infections tend to recur in susceptible individuals. Women are especially vulnerable because of the comparative shortness of the urethra and its proximity to the vaginal and rectal orifices. A careful history of such infections and the anti-infective drugs used to treat them is needed before therapy begins. A complete history of other drugs is also required. The clients' reaction to the diagnosis should be assessed. If they have experienced repeated episodes of UTI, they may be discouraged.

Nursing diagnosis Nursing diagnoses for clients receiving medication for UTIs may include the following:

Altered comfort: bladder spasms, frequency, urgency, burning on urination or flank pain related to UTI
Altered comfort: headache and vertigo secondary to anti-infective therapy
Altered comfort: abdominal distress secondary to nalidixic acid (phenazopyridine) therapy
Impaired skin integrity: rash related to trimethoprim therapy
Altered comfort: pruritus related to trimethoprim therapy
Knowledge deficit concerning UTI measures to reduce the risk of UTI, treatment regimes for UTI
Fear of kidney failure related to repeated UTIs and courses of anti-infectives that are potentially nephrotoxic

A common collaborative problem that should be differentiated from the nursing diagnoses is

Potential complication: renal

Planning Treatment goals are to reduce the risk of recurrent infections, alleviate the signs and symptoms of inflammation, and reduce the risk of adverse drug

Example of nursing process and methenamine treatment for pyonephritis

The client is a 33-year-old married woman with a 5-year history of paraplegia. She has two children at home.

The client has controlled urinary retention with intermittent self-catheterization. She has been hospitalized for treatment of pyonephritis. Within the last 3 years, the client has experienced four episodes of cystitis.

During this hospitalization, the client has been treated with nalidixic acid. She is to be discharged on a maintenance regimen of methenamine.

The client understands her vulnerability to urinary tract infections and the prognosis if repeated infections occur.

Assessment data	Nursing diagnosis	Intervention	Goals and outcome criteria
Urinary retention	High risk for infection: recurrent urinary tract infection related to intermittent catheterization secondary to urinary retention	**Review** with client the technique for self-catheterization. Suggest improvements that might reduce risk of further infection.	The client will not experience another episode of pyonephritis. Recurrences of cystitis will decrease in frequency or disappear.
Regimen of self-catheterization			
History of recurrent urinary tract infection		**Explain** function of methenamine in the control of recurrent urinary tract infections.	
(Kidney disease secondary to infection is a leading cause of death among individuals with neurological problems that require catheterization.)	Knowledge deficit concerning self-catheterization, medication therapy, and measures to minimize urinary tract infections	**Recommend** that the client use a method of promoting formation of acid urine (use of large doses of ascorbic acid, cranberry juice, and acid ash foods such as plums and prunes).	
		Recommend a daily intake of 3,000 ml fluid daily to promote flushing of microorganisms from the urinary tract and to dilute the urine to minimize irritation by the methanamine.	
		Caution the client to maintain good perineal hygiene, especially prior to intercourse, which tends to introduce microbes mechanically into the urinary meatus.	

reaction. Prompt detection and treatment is also desired in the event of a drug reaction.

Intervention Nursing actions include measures to support and enhance normal resistance to infection (good nutrition, ample hydration, rest, and reduction of stress), monitoring for response to the drug regimen, and administration of the ordered drugs. When trimethoprim-sulfamethoxazole is administered IV, the tubing should be thoroughly flushed following each dose to prevent precipitation.

Risk factors for UTI should be reduced as much as possible. The nurse may recommend acid-ash foods to lower the pH of urine. Bladder training programs should be instituted so that retention catheters can be discontinued. A bowel program can reduce fecal incontinence, which increases the number of pathogens on the skin in the perineal area.

Overhydration is helpful if tolerated by the client. Volumes of fluid moving through the urinary tract wash out pathogens and reduce their population. For most normal adults, a goal of 3,000 ml fluid intake daily is appropriate. Amounts for children or adults with a reduced body mass should be adjusted accordingly. "Forcing" fluids to this degree may be difficult to accomplish and should not be left to chance. A glass of fluid, offered hourly between meals during waking hours, will usually be sufficient. An accurate record of fluid intake and output should be maintained.

Genitalia should be cleaned frequently, using techniques designed to reduce the transfer of organisms to the urethral orifice. Perineal hygiene and cleansing should proceed from front to back; perineal pads should be applied and removed with similar precautions, always moving pads in a front-to-back direction.

Client education. Client instruction should include information about the drug regimen and the hygienic measures that reduce the risk of repeated UTI. Clients should be taught proper perineal hygiene. When washing the genitals, the urinary meatus should be cleansed first, and washing action should proceed outward from this area. Women should be instructed to cleanse from front to back with toilet tissue. Detergent substances (bubble bath, bathing salts) should be avoided because they increase penetration of bath water into the urinary meatus. To minimize transfer of microorganisms into the urethra, women should void before and immediately after intercourse.

Clients at risk for UTIs should be counseled about the importance of hydration. Specific instructions should be given on the appropriate amounts and types of liquids to take. Acid-ash fruit juices (cranberry and prune) are usually preferable to citrus and vegetable juices that are alkaline-ash. (If a UTI is associated with renal stones composed of acidic materials such as oxalic acid, alkaline-ash foods are preferred to increase solubility of the stones in the urine.) Some clients do not tolerate the caffeine in tea, coffee, and soft drinks. For others, sugar or carbonated beverages are contraindicated. The characteristics of specific beverages, as well as personal preference, must be considered. Plain water is probably the most appropriate drink. If the quality of local water is poor, a little lemon juice may improve the taste, or bottled water may be recommended.

When phenazopyridine or nitrofurantoin is prescribed, the client should be warned about the innocuous change in urine color.

Evaluation Data required for evaluation include information relating to changes in the signs and symptoms of UTI, the signs and symptoms of adverse drug reaction, and the rate of UTI recurrence. In making their evaluation, nurses should also consider the extent to which the client is able to understand and repeat back the content of the treatment program.

(See the accompanying Example of Nursing Process and Methenamine Treatment for Pyonephritis.)

Checklist of nursing actions

- [ ] Teach clients at high risk for UTIs proper perineal hygiene to reduce the risk of infection.
- [ ] Counsel clients regarding food and fluid intake that will enhance hydration and maintain the desired urinary *p*H.
- [ ] When urinary antiseptics are ordered, warn clients of changes in urine color that will occur as a result of medication.
- [ ] Use all possible nursing measures to avoid the use of catheters for continuous urinary drainage.
- [ ] Monitor clients receiving urinary tract antiseptics for adverse reactions.

Enrichment experience 42-1

In a hospital or nursing home, determine the clients who receive urinary antiseptics. How many of these clients have indwelling urinary catheters? How many are monitored for fluid intake? Plan and carry out a nursing care conference to review care plans, with the objective of reducing to a minimum the need for antiseptic medication among these clients.

References

Sweethearts resist infection. (1985). *Science News, 128,* 125.

Bibliography

Antonow D. (1986). Acute pancreatitis associated with trimethoprim-sulfamethoxasole. *Ann Intern Med, 104,* 363–365.

Biosca M, De La Figura M, Garcia-Bragado FM, Sampol G. (1986). Aseptic meningitis due to trimethoprim-sulfamethoxazole (letter). *J Neurol Neurosurg Psychiatry, 49,* 332–333.

*Broad spectrum UTI agent. (1987). *American Journal of Nursing, 87,* 113.

*Drugs commonly used to treat TB. *RN, 47(9),* 52–57.

Gilman AG, et al, eds. (1990). *Goodman and Gilman's The pharmacological basis of therapeutics*, 8th edition, p 1095–1114, 1199–1218. New York: Pergamon Press.

Mermel L. (1986). Acute psychosis in a patient receiving trimethoprim-sulfamethoxazole intravenously. *J Clin Psychiatry, 47,* 269–270.

O'Neil TJ, Manipon N, Avery BJ. (1985). Problems with trimethoprim-sulfamethoxasole regimen for oropharyngeal gonorrhea. *Milit Med, 150(1),* 47.

Rahn K, Mooy J, Bohm R, Vet A. (1985). Reduction of bio-availability of verapamil by rifampin (letter). *N Engl J Med, 312,* 920–921.

Seaman J, Goble M, Madsen L, Steigerwald JC. (1985). Fasciitis and polyarthritis during antituberculosis therapy. *Arthritis Rheum, 28,* 1179–1184.

*Recommended for further reading.

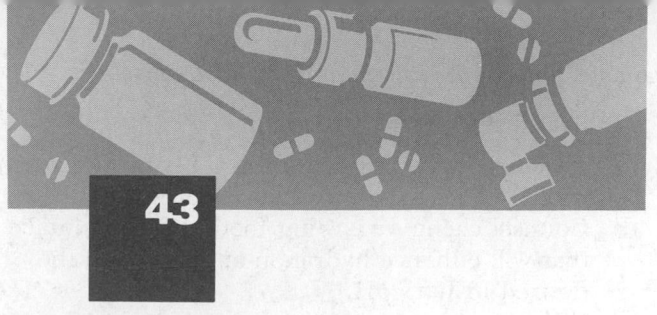

43

Drugs used to treat infections caused by viruses and fungi

Infections caused by viruses and fungi do not respond well to antimicrobial drugs. Viruses penetrate the cells of their hosts, where they complete the reproductive phase of their life cycles. Their intracellular location protects them from many anti-infective agents. Drugs capable of affecting viruses tend to be harmful to host cells. Fungi possess a rigid cell wall in some stage of the life cycle. Not only are they unaffected by most antimicrobial drugs, but the elimination of a host's natural microbial flora by broad spectrum anti-infectives also allows them to grow without restraint. Fungi are often responsible for superinfection secondary to antimicrobial therapy. Both viral and fungal infections are relatively difficult to treat with medication.

Fungal infections may be topical, affecting the superficial tissues, or systemic, involving vital organs such as the lungs. Because methods of treatment and agents used for the two types of illness differ, they will be discussed separately in this chapter.

Pathophysiology of viral infections

Viruses are little more than strands of ribonucleic or deoxyribonucleic acids wrapped in protein envelopes. They share some of the attributes of pure chemicals (they can be prepared in crystalline form) and of life forms (they can reproduce). Unlike other organisms, they do not have cellular structures, nor do they take in nutrients, produce and use energy through metabolism, excrete wastes, or propel themselves through the environment. Their reproduction is a parasitic process by which they use the mechanisms in a living cell to replicate themselves.

The methods of viral replication are not yet fully understood. One strategy is for the virus to copy and incorporate within itself a gene that governs part of the host's immune system. The virus can then deactivate the host's immune cells that would fight the viral infection. At the same time, the host's cell can be transformed into a factory that quickly produces viral proteins and offspring, allowing rapid multiplication of the virus. Researchers are now studying the possibility of aiming effective medications at receptors on the affected cells, which would then be a new way to fight infection.

The search for chemicals that are selectively toxic to viruses requires an understanding and exploitation of the differences between the replicative cycles of the viruses and that of the cells they invade. As yet, no safe, broad-spectrum antiviral drug has been discovered. However, we are not completely defenseless. A limited number of compounds have been developed that are helpful in selected situations, and some substances under investigation show promise of broader usefulness. Moreover, immunizing vulnerable populations against disease with vaccines and sera has done much to reduce the ravages of viral parasites (Table 43-1).

Table 43-1. Antiviral drugs

Drug names	Actions or clinical uses	Drug names	Actions or clinical uses
Vaccines*		**Anti-inflammatories**	
smallpox†	Stimulates formation of antibodies against cowpox virus, which also act against the smallpox virus	glucocorticoids	Suppress the inflammatory process; used for palliation of life-threatening infections
varicella‡	Stimulates formation of antibodies against chickenpox virus	**Antibacterials**	
rabies	Stimulates formation of antibodies against rabies virus; normally administered only after infected or suspicious animal bites	sulfonamides	Treatment of trachoma, inclusion blennorrhea, some strains of lymphogranuloma venereum
poliomyelitis (Poliovirus)	Stimulates formation of antibodies against three strains of poliomyelitis virus	tetracyclines	Treatment of trachoma, inclusion blennorrhea, lymphogranuloma venereum, and psittacosis
rubella‡	Stimulates formation of antibodies against German measles virus	chloramphenicol	Treatment of trachoma, inclusion blennorrhea, and lymphogranuloma venereum
rubeola‡	Stimulates formation of antibodies against measles virus	**Antimetabolities**	
infectious parotitis‡ (Mumpsvax)	Stimulates formation of antibodies against mumps virus	acyclovir	Treatment of herpes simplex, varicella-zoster, Epstein-barr virus, herpes simplex virus (B), and cytomegalovirus infections
influenza§	Stimulates formation of antibodies against one or more strains of influenza virus		Treatment of viral infections in immunosuppressed individuals
hepatitis B (Hepatavax-B, Recombivax)	Stimulates formation of antibodies against serum hepatitis virus		Treatment of genital herpes
		amantadine	Prevention and treatment of influenza A_2
Sera (immune globulins)		zidovudine	Treatment of AIDS and ARC
immune globulin	Provides passive resistance (already formed antibodies) against a number of infections	idoxuridine	Treatment of herpes simplex keratitis and herpes genitalis
hepatitis B immune globulin	Provides antibodies against hepatitis B virus	vidarabine	Treatment of herpes simplex encephalitis (systemic) and herpes simplex keratitis and keratoconjunctivitis (topical)
rabies immune globulin	Provides antibodies against rabies virus		
Inducers of general resistance			
interferon‡	Appears to prevent virus particles from replicating		
poly I:C§	Induces interferon production		
statalon§	Induces interferon production		
vitamin C	Clinical usefulness is controversial		

Measles, mumps, and rubella virus vaccines are combined in MMRII, a mixture of live, attenuated viruses.

*See chapter 36 for more details about vaccines.

†Smallpox vaccination is no longer recommended because the disease appears to have been eradicated.

‡Considered experimental and not available for general use at this writing.

§Multiple vaccines specific to individual viruses.

Agents that stimulate, simulate, or inhibit host responses to viruses

Vaccines and sera

The most successful approach to combating viral infections has been to prevent their development. Vaccines have been developed to stimulate active immunity to a number of diseases: smallpox, rabies, poliomyelitis, rubella, rubeola, mumps, and serum hepatitis. A vaccine against chickenpox/shingles, originally developed in Japan, should be available for use in the United States soon. Vaccines against the influenza virus have a limited period of usefulness because this organism mutates rapidly, and new strains are not inactivated by the antibodies of people previously immunized. Agents for immunization against rotavirus (a cause of many childhood diarrheas), herpes, and acquired immunodeficiency syndrome (AIDS) are in the process of development. As yet, no immunizing agents have been developed against the adenoviruses causing the common cold.

Traditional techniques for developing vaccines are fairly well developed but they involve a tedious search for methods to attenuate (inactivate or weaken) organisms without altering their antigenicity. Application of genetic recombinant techniques to the production of vaccines promises a more rapid development in the future. However, it will still be impossible to produce new vaccines on demand. New vaccines must be tested for harmful effects first in animals and then in humans. In addition, a process is needed for safe production of vaccines in large quantities. Developing and marketing a new vaccine usually requires from one to several years. When the public feels threatened by a given disease, it may generate pressure to speed up this process. On at least two occasions, yielding to this pressure has proved disastrous.

When the development of the first poliomyelitis vaccine was announced by Jonas Salk in the early 1950s, public clamor for immunization was intense. The vaccine was rushed into production in an attempt to immunize as many people as possible before the next polio "season" during the summer months. Cases of fully developed paralytic disease developed in recipients of the drug. The outbreak was attributed to faulty production techniques that released at least one batch of insufficiently attenuated vaccine for public use. Quality control was tightened, and the Salk vaccine continued to be used successfully until the advent of the Sabin oral poliomyelitis vaccine.

In the late 1970s, a strain of influenza called "swine flu" seemed to pose the threat of an epidemic similar to the pandemic that occurred in 1918. Fearing a high death toll, the United States government pressed for the rapid development of an immunizing vaccine. Drug companies were reluctant to begin volume production before extensive testing. To obtain a sufficient quantity of the drug for widespread use before the disease became epidemic, the federal government assumed liability for its use. After the immunization campaign, the vaccine was found to produce a serious paralytic neurologic disorder, Guillain-Barré syndrome, in a few recipients. In retrospect, some medical authorities claim that mortality and morbidity from the vaccine may have equaled or exceeded that which would have occurred from the disease itself, which proved to be milder than expected. Suits against the federal government stemming from this incident are still in litigation.

It is clear that violation of proven guidelines for developing and testing new drugs is risky. Caution must temper enthusiasm for new, untried vaccines.

The public is currently pressing for development of a vaccine against AIDS. Research is progressing at a measured pace but scientists warn that it will probably be several years before a safe, effective vaccine is available for general use. The first completed clinical study of a potential human AIDS vaccine, recombinant gp160, was announced in January 1991, and has proven to be safe and well-tolerated.

A sudden increase in a strain of raccoon-borne rabies along the east coast of the United States has resulted in several new approaches to that disease, including a new test that detects the rabies virus within 4 days, rather than the 30 days previously required, and a genetically engineered vaccine that can be placed in food and used for mass animal immunization. This method is speedier than the present method of injecting each animal individually, is safer, and is less costly than human vaccination.

Human immune globulin

Human immune globulin, a serum derived from human blood, contains antibodies (which provides temporary, passive immunity) against various endemic diseases. It can be used to prevent the onset of viral diseases in people who have been exposed or to ameliorate the symptoms resulting from the disease. Because the immunity that is conferred is passive, the protective effects of human immune globulin last for only a short period. Although human immune globulin is in limited supply and is relatively expensive, supplies are adequate to treat people known to have been exposed

---

Enrichment experience 43-1

Interview a client who has received human immune globulin as a prophylactic measure to prevent development of a viral infection, such as hepatitis. Determine the client's response to the drug, including discomfort from the injections and emotional reaction to the threat of illness. Is the client in favor of such preventive measures?

to serious contagion. Sera of proven potency against individual diseases are available. Sera cannot be substituted for active immunization by vaccines, which provide continuous protection for long periods. (See Chapter 36 for a detailed discussion of vaccines and sera, including current recommendations for their use.)

Inducers of general resistance

Interferon and interferon inducers

On interacting with viruses, animal cells produce *interferon*, a carbohydrate-containing protein that apparently prevents the virus particles from replicating in body tissues. This compound is species-specific; interferon from lower animals will not inhibit viruses in human hosts and vice versa. Until recently, the supply of interferon was inadequate to allow extensive experimentation but the development of production techniques using tissue cultures has increased the pace of research. The dose of interferon varies, depending on the disease to be treated, the route of administration, and the amount of endogenous interferon being produced by the host. Because exogenous interferon is broken down or removed from the blood stream quickly, it is necessary to administer the drug at least once a day. Clinical trials indicate that the drug may be helpful in treating both RNA and DNA viruses including influenza, rhinoviruses, rubella, hepatitis B, cytomegalovirus, herpes, varicella, and vaccinia. It is best given early in the course of the disease, and prophylactic use is even more effective. Interferon can be given concurrently with vaccines to provide protection while active immunity is developing. Interferon has also been used with some success in neoplastic diseases such as Hodgkin's disease, non-Hodgkin's lymphoma, hairy cell leukemia, and osteogenic sarcoma. In one study, the drug is believed to have reduced the number and severity of acute attacks in relapsing-remitting multiple sclerosis (Benowitz, 1985).

Interferon is not without side effects. It has caused fever, nausea, hair loss, and white cell depression.

In another attempt to exploit the advantages of interferon's effects, researchers are looking for substances that will induce interferon production in an infected host. Two such compounds, poly I:C (a synthetic polymer that resembles RNA) and statalon (a substance extracted from fungi), show promise of being helpful in treating respiratory viral infections, although neither has been proven safe or effective enough for clinical use.

Interferon and interferon inducers remain experimental and are not yet available for general use. However, they are potentially valuable in the future treatment of contagious and neoplastic disease.

Vitamin C

Vitamin C's effectiveness in preventing and treating viral infections remains controversial. The noted biochemist, Linus Pauling, believed that large doses of vitamin C increase the body's resistance to viruses and can prevent the common cold. Many medical authorities refute this. It is agreed that the body's need for this compound increases substantially when infection is present. However, the role of vitamin C in preventing or curing infection remains controversial.

Whether self-administered or prescribed by a physician, vitamin C used to combat viral infections is taken in doses of grams per day. Because the minimum daily requirement of this vitamin is 40 to 50 mg, these doses are approximately 100 times the usually recommended maintenance dose. Although ascorbic acid has a wide safety margin, such large doses can cause undesirable effects in the body. (See Chapter 50 for a detailed discussion of vitamin C.)

Anti-inflammatories

Glucocorticoids

Although usually contraindicated in infections because of their immunosuppressant effect, corticosteroids (*eg*, cortisone) are sometimes employed to control serious complications of viral infections caused by inflammation. The drug may be ordered to prevent orchitis in adult men suffering from infectious parotitis (mumps). It is used to control intracranial pressure in measles encephalitis and to prevent fibrosis during healing. In carefully selected cases, cortisone is also helpful in mononucleosis. Any client treated with cortisone while harboring an infection requires close observation to monitor the progress of recovery. Wherever possible, anti-infective chemotherapy specific to the organism involved is used concurrently. (See Chapter 32 for a detailed discussion of corticosteroids.)

Antiviral compounds

In selected cases, antibacterials have proved effective against viruses (see Table 43-1). These drugs are discussed in Chapters 41 and 42.

A major research program to discover or develop specific drugs to combat virus growth has already produced a limited number of useful compounds (Table 43-2). Most of the chemicals are antimetabolites or are related to the antimetabolites used in treating malignant tumors; they are most harmful to rapidly dividing cells. These drugs tend to be toxic, and their usefulness is limited to carefully selected clinical situations. Clients receiving these drugs must be carefully monitored for adverse effects, as well as for therapeutic responses.

Acyclovir

Acyclovir (Zovirax) is a synthetic purine nucleoside analogue.

Pharmacodynamics. Acyclovir acts as an antimetabolite and suppresses viral replication by inhibiting DNA and polypeptide synthesis. It is effective

Table 43-2. Antiviral anti-infective drugs

Drug names	Preparations	Usual dosage/PC	Precautions and contraindications
acyclovir (Zovirax)	Oral capsules Sterile powder for reconstitution into intravenous infusion Topical ointment	Adults and children aged 12 years or older: 15–30 mg/kg body weight/d, divided in 3 doses Children aged 12 years or younger: 750 mg/m²/d, divided in 3 doses PC: C	Dosage must be decreased for individuals with renal impairment.
amantadine (Symmetrel)	Solution and capsules for oral administration	Clients aged 10–64: 200 mg/d, divided in 1–2 doses Children aged 1–9 years: 4.4–8.8 mg/kg body weight/d, divided in 1–2 doses Maximum daily dosage: 150 mg PC: C	Dosage must be decreased for those receiving other antiparkinsonian agents, those with seizure disorders, the elderly, and those with renal impairment. The drug should be stored in tightly closed containers at 15°–30°C.
idoxuridine (Dendrid Herplex, IDU Stoxil)	Ophthalmic solution Ophthalmic ointment	One drop q1–2h Apply q4h IA PC: C	Improvement should occur within 7–8 days. Normal course of treatment is 21 days.
ribavarin (Virazole) trifluridine (Viroptic)	Powder reconstituted for oral or nasal inhalation Ophthalmic solution	Continuous inhalation for 12–16 hr/d for 3–7 days PC: X One drop q2h IA (maximum daily dose: 9 drops) PC: C	Inhalation therapy requires hospitalization. Cardiac and cardiovascular function must be monitored. Treatment should be discontinued if no improvement has occurred after 7 days, or if complete re-epithelialization has not occurred after 14 days. Treatment should be limited to 21 days to avoid ocular toxicity. Dosage must be decreased for clients with renal impairment. Use with caution in individuals susceptible to fluid overload or cerebral edema. Monitor recipients for adverse hematologic or CNS reactions.
vidarabine (Vira-A)	Ophthalmic ointment Concentrated sterile solution diluted for IV infusion	1 cm q3h for 5 days 10–15 mg/kg body weight/d for 5–10 days	Dosage must be decreased for clients with renal impairment.
zidovudine (Azidothymidine, AZT, Retrovir, Zovirax)	Tablets and extended-release capsules for oral use Sterile powder reconstituted for IV infusion or IM injection	Adults: 1 g/d, divided in 2–4 doses PC: C	Monitor recipients for bone marrow depression. Observe for and report previously unknown adverse reactions to the drug.

KEY: PC = pregnancy risk category. (The validity of pregnancy risk categories has not been established. See Chapter 16, p 216.)

against varicella-zoster virus, Epstein-Barr virus, cytomegalovirus, and various herpes viruses. Resistant strains of viruses do develop following exposure to the drug.

Pharmacokinetics. Acyclovir is administered by oral, topical and intravenous (IV) routes. Gastrointestinal (GI) absorption is reported to range from 15% to 30%. After absorption, acyclovir is widely distributed in body tissues and fluids, including the cerebrospinal fluid (CSF). About 9% to 33% of the drug is bound to plasma proteins. Acyclovir does cross the placenta; it is not known whether the drug or its metabolites are distributed into breast milk. Excretion is primarily in urine by filtration and tubular secretion using the same mechanism as penicillin. The drug is removed by hemodialysis.

Therapeutic uses. Acyclovir is used parenterally for treating initial and recurrent infections caused by susceptible viruses in immunocompromised adults and children. It is considered the drug of choice for treating chicken pox. Oral acyclovir is used for suppressing genital herpes; topical ointment is applied to mucocutaneous lesions of herpes simplex.

Adverse reactions. The most common adverse effects of parenteral acyclovir are local reactions at the injection site. These reactions are dose-related and may include phlebitis, erythema, pain, and inflammation. Renal impairment occurs in 5% to 10% of recipients. Rapid administration of the drug increases the risk of nephrotoxicity. Central nervous system toxicity (lethargy, tremors, confusion, hallucinations, seizures, and coma) may also occur. Other less frequent adverse reactions include rash, GI upset, and bone marrow abnormalities.

The drug has a low order of toxicity when applied topically. The most frequent reaction following topical use of the drug on ulcerated genital lesions is mild pain, which may include burning and stinging.

Drug interactions. Acyclovir interacts with interferon and the antifungal drugs amphotericin B and ketoconazole to produce additive or synergistic anti-infective effects. Concurrent administration of probenecid inhibits renal excretion of acyclovir and prolongs the drug's effects.

Precautions and contraindications. Clients receiving parenteral acyclovir must be well hydrated, especially during the peak action of the drug (for 2 hours following injection). The drug must not be administered intramuscularly (IM), subcutaneously, or topically to the eye. Intravenous dosages must be infused slowly. Acyclovir should be used with caution in persons with renal impairment or underlying neurologic abnormalities, or in those receiving other nephrotoxic drugs. Caution should also be exercised when the drug is given to clients with previous neurologic reactions to

cytotoxic drugs and to those receiving interferon or intrathecal methotrexate concurrently. Extended prophylactic use is not advisable because resistant strains of viruses are likely to develop.

Acyclovir is contraindicated for individuals with allergic sensitivity to the drug. Safety during pregnancy and lactation has not been established.

Amantadine

Amantadine (Symmetrel) is a synthetic amine with a structure unrelated to any other antimicrobial agent.

Pharmacodynamics. The exact mechanisms of amantadine's action are unknown. The drug exerts both antiviral and dopaminergic effects. It has been theorized that amantadine inhibits the uncoating of virus particles, thereby preventing penetration of viruses into host cells. This would leave viruses stranded on the cell surface, where they are vulnerable to attacks by host antibodies. Amantadine is effective against influenza A and C, but not influenza B, rhinoviruses, or respiratory syncytial viruses.

In the nervous system, amantadine may act by stimulating postsynaptic receptors, releasing catecholamines from peripheral nerve storage sites, and blocking reuptake of dopamine into presynaptic neurons of the basal ganglia.

Pharmacokinetics. Amantadine is administered orally and is well absorbed by the GI tract. Animal studies indicate that the drug distributes into saliva, nasal secretions, and milk, and that concentrations in the lungs may exceed those in the blood. Human distribution is not well understood but the drug is known to penetrate the blood–brain barrier and be distributed in breast milk. Amantadine is eliminated unchanged in the urine. It is only minimally dialyzable. Its half-life has been reported to range from 9 to 37 hours.

Therapeutic uses. Amantadine is used to prevent and treat respiratory infections caused by influenza A virus. It is also used in the symptomatic treatment of all forms of parkinsonism.

Dosage and administration. Amantadine (Symmetrel) is available in oral capsules and solution. For both antiviral and antiparkinsonian effect, the adult dosage is 100 mg twice daily. Dosage must be reduced for clients who are very young or elderly, those with renal impairment, and those with seizure disorders.

Adverse reactions. Adverse reactions to amantadine include disturbances to the central nervous system: nervousness, irritability, fatigue, mental depression, decreased alertness, incoordination, ataxia, slurred speech, psychoses, anxiety, insomnia, visual oculogyria, confusion, forgetfulness, and convulsions; to the cardiovascular system: congestive heart failure, orthostatic hypotension; to the hematopoietic system:

leukopenia and neutropenia; to the skin: rash, eczema, bluish mottling, photosensitization; and to the GI system: anorexia, nausea, vomiting, abdominal discomfort. Anticholinergic effects include dry mouth, constipation, and urinary retention. Dyspnea and urinary frequency may also occur. The anticholinergic effects of amantadine are additive to those of other anticholinergic drugs. Amantadine also increases adverse reactions of other antiparkinsonian drugs when used concurrently. Resistance to amantadine does develop in viruses exposed to it repeatedly or over a long term.

Precautions and contraindications. Amantadine should be administered with caution in persons with liver disease, eczema, uncontrolled psychosis or severe psychoneurosis, seizure disorders, congestive heart failure, peripheral edema, orthostatic hypotension, and to those receiving treatment with other antiparkinsonian drugs. Dosage may need to be reduced when the drug is used to treat persons with renal impairment. When amantadine is used to treat Parkinson's disease, it should not be discontinued abruptly because symptoms may recur in an exaggerated form (parkinsonian crisis). This syndrome is manifested by confusion, rigidity, urine retention, and bulbar palsy. Safety and efficacy have not been established in children younger than 1 year of age. Use during pregnancy and lactation is not recommended.

Zidovudine

Zidovudine (formerly referred to as azidothymidine), is also known as AZT and Retrovir. It is a thymidine analogue that shows promise of prolonging the lives of individuals with AIDS. The drug does not, however, cure the disease.

Pharmacodynamics. AZT competes with thymidine* for incorporation into DNA or RNA molecules synthesized by the retrovirus responsible for AIDS. The presence of zidovudine (AZT) along the virus strand not only prevents reproduction of the retrovirus but destroys it as well.

Pharmacokinetics. AZT is known to cross the blood–brain barrier, a capability that increases its effect on the AIDS retrovirus, which resides in the brain.

Therapeutic uses. Zidovudine is approved for use only in treating AIDS patients with opportunistic infections such as *Pneumocystis carinii* pneumonia and people with AIDS-related complex.

Adverse reactions. Zidovudine (AZT) is known to suppress bone marrow production in some recipients.

Precautions and contraindications. Although Zidovudine has been approved for use, it was developed

---

*Thymidine is one of the bases incorporated in the structure of nucleic acid.

and released for general use more rapidly than normal in an effort to provide some relief for those afflicted with AIDS. Recipients should be monitored carefully for both their therapeutic response and their adverse reaction to the drug. Data on client response should be submitted to the government agency charged with compiling such information. (See Chapter 2 for more information about drug reaction reports.)

Idoxuridine

Idoxuridine (Herplex, Stoxil) is a halogen and pyrimidine derivative.

Pharmacodynamics. The exact mechanism of action of idoxuridine is unknown. It is believed that the drug inhibits replication of DNA-type viruses because it is incorporated into DNA in place of natural pyrimidine nucleotides, resulting in abnormal DNA, which is susceptible to breakage. The drug also appears to inhibit cellular metabolism in host cells.

Pharmacokinetics. Idoxuridine is poorly absorbed when administered topically. Absorption is inversely related to the concentration of the drug. It is believed that tissue uptake is a function of cellular metabolism, which may be inhibited by the drug.

When administered IV, idoxuridine is rapidly degraded to inactive metabolites, which are eliminated in urine.

Therapeutic uses. Idoxuridine is used for treating herpes infections of the eye. It has also been used to treat herpes genitalis with some success. Administration is limited to topical use.

Adverse reactions. Idoxuridine can cause eye irritation, pain, pruritus, inflammation, and edema of the eyelids. Photophobia sometimes develops. Not all types of infection respond equally well to therapy; total healing or improvement does not always occur, even when the infection appears to be superficial. The drug may delay healing.

Studies show that idoxuridine is relatively toxic if administered parenterally. Adverse reactions include liver function abnormalities, as well as severe leukopenia and thrombocytopenia.

Viruses commonly develop resistance to idoxuridine.

Precautions and contraindications. Idoxuridine should be used only under the supervision of an ophthalmologist. The recommended dosage should not be exceeded, and prolonged administration should be avoided.

Boric acid solutions and idoxuridine must not be applied to the eyes concurrently because the combination is irritating to the eyes.

Ribavirin

Ribavirin is a synthetic nucleoside whose structure resembles that of guanosine.

Pharmacodynamics. The exact mechanism of ribavirin's action is unknown. The drug is believed to interfere with RNA, DNA, and protein synthesis by inhibiting enzymes necessary to these processes.

Ribavirin has a wider spectrum of action than other currently available antiviral drugs. It is active against both RNA and DNA viruses.

Pharmacokinetics. Ribavirin is usually administered by inhalation. When this route is used, concentrations of the drug are higher in respiratory secretions than in the plasma. Ribavirin administered orally is rapidly absorbed. The drug tends to concentrate in vascular tissue such as skeletal muscle, blood cells (mainly red), and the liver. It distributes slowly into the CSF. It is not known whether ribavirin crosses the placenta or distributes into breast milk in humans.

In a process believed to be essential to antiviral activity, ribavirin is phosphorylated by the liver and red blood cells. The drug and its metabolites are excreted mainly in urine. Ribavirin tends to persist in red blood cells, remaining in the body for weeks or longer after its use has been discontinued.

Therapeutic uses. Ribavirin is administered by inhalation in treating severe lower respiratory infections caused by respiratory syncytial virus and pneumonia caused by adenovirus, as well as for preventing and treating influenza A and B viral infections.

Oral ribavirin has been used experimentally to treat infections such as Lassa fever, measles, herpes simplex types 1 and 2, and hepatitis A. Parenteral preparations have been used to treat other serious viral infections, such as Crimean-Congo hemorrhagic fever. Herpes zoster infections (shingles) have been treated with ribavirin topical ointment.

Ribavirin is available commercially as a sterile powder, which is used in preparing solutions for inhalation only. The drug is usually administered continuously for 12–18 hours daily for 3–7 days.

Adverse reactions. When administered by inhalation, ribavirin rarely produces any adverse effects. However, reactions to the drug can be life-threatening. They include worsening of respiratory function, cardiac arrest, hypotension, and (in individuals using digitalis) digitalis toxicity. Dyspnea, chest soreness, and anemia can also develop. The mist is irritating and can cause rash, erythema of the eyelids, and conjunctivitis. Oral or parenteral administration may cause transient changes in liver function tests.

Ribavirin is considered to be mutagenic, teratogenic, and tumorigenic. It is toxic to lactating animals and their offspring. Toxic effects, which can be fatal, include anorexia, vomiting, diarrhea, muscle weakness, lethargy, prostration, and intestinal hemorrhage.

Precautions and contraindications. Ribavirin is used only to treat severe infections in high-risk clients. Its use is limited to hospital settings because respiratory and cardiovascular function must be monitored carefully during the course of treatment. When therapy is extended beyond 1 or 2 weeks, clients should be monitored for anemia. The drug is contraindicated for pregnant or lactating women.

Vidarabine

Vidarabine is a purine nucleoside produced by *Streptomyces antibioticus*.

Pharmacodynamics. The exact mechanism of action of vidarabine is unknown. The drug is believed to inhibit viral DNA polymerase. Vidarabine is active against herpes simplex virus types 1 and 2, varicella-zoster, cytomegalovirus, vaccinia, and hepatitis B virus. Epstein-Barr virus, rhabdoviruses, and oncornaviruses are also affected by the drug. Vidarabine is not effective against adenovirus, variola major (smallpox virus), bacteria, and fungi.

Pharmacokinetics. Vidarabine is administered by IV infusion. It is poorly absorbed by other routes (PO, IM, SC). The drug and its metabolite, arahypoxanthine, are widely distributed into body tissues and fluids. They readily cross the blood–brain barrier and the placenta. It is not known whether the drug distributes into breast milk. Protein binding is 20%–30% for vidarabine and 0%–3% for arahypoxanthine. Vidarabine and its metabolite are excreted mainly in the urine. Plasma half-lives are 1.5 hours and 3.3 hours, respectively. Allopurinol may interfere with the metabolism of vidarabine.

Therapeutic uses. Vidarabine is used in treating cytomegalovirus infections in infants and immunosuppressed individuals. It is an alternative to acyclovir treatment of varicellazoster and herpes simplex infections.

Adverse reactions. Gastrointestinal reactions (anorexia, nausea, vomiting, diarrhea) are the most common adverse effects of vidarabine. Pain and thrombophlebitis at the infusion site also occur. These adverse effects tend to subside with continued therapy. Nervous system reactions (malaise, weakness, dizziness, tremor, ataxia, confusion, hallucinations, and psychosis), which are seen occasionally, are dose-related and usually reversible when the drug is withdrawn. Other adverse reactions include altered liver function tests, bone marrow depression, and inappropriate antidiuretic hormone secretion.

Vidarabine is considered to be mutagenic, carcinogenic, and teratogenic.

Drug interactions. Adverse reactions are more frequent in individuals receiving allopurinol therapy.

Precautions and contraindications. During vidarabine therapy, clients should be monitored for fluid overload, which can occur because of the large volumes of solvents required to administer vidarabine.

The drug should be used with caution in those clients with impaired liver or kidney function and in those susceptible to fluid overload. Vidarabine is contraindicated for pregnant women or nursing mothers.

■ Summary

The search for chemotherapeutic agents to combat viral infection has produced only a few compounds with limited applications. Most antiviral drugs have a narrow margin of safety. Because experience with these drugs is limited, knowledge of their side effects and long-term toxicity is incomplete. Intensive research continues, and new antiviral substances will probably emerge in the near future, including biologic response modifiers. These may include colony-stimulating factors such as granulocyte colony-stimulating factors and granulocyte macrophage colony-stimulating factors.

Nursing management

Nursing implications

Because there are no safe drugs for treating most viral infections, prevention remains of primary importance. The best prevention of contagious diseases is eliminating contact between host and parasites. The nurse must be thoroughly familiar with the sanitary, hygienic, and aseptic measures needed to reduce infections and infestations. Cleanliness alone may not be sufficient. Because many viruses are airborne, infected individuals must be isolated from those who are susceptible.

Resistance to infection can be promoted by good general hygiene, as well as a nutritious diet, adequate rest, and avoidance of excessive stress. Vaccines can be used to stimulate active immunity. Cleanliness and the avoidance of unnecessary contact with persons suffering from viral infections reduce the likelihood of illness. If susceptible clients are known to have been exposed, the use of sera to confer temporary passive immunity may prevent active infection.

Parents should be encouraged to immunize their children against the viral diseases for which we have reliable vaccines. They should also be taught the importance of general health measures, to maintain the general resistance that helps to control the severity of viral illnesses when they occur. Susceptible persons of all ages should obtain immunization against viral pneumonia and influenza.

Following exposure to viral hepatitis, clients should be urged to obtain preventive injections of human immune globulin. Preparations certified to contain antibodies for specific diseases, such as rubella (German measles), should be recommended to exposed clients for whom a viral infection could be hazardous.

Treatment of viral infections relies heavily on general supportive measures to assist the body in overcoming the pathogenic agents. Hydration is critical; fluid intake should be ample (up to 3 liters a day for most adults) but not excessive. Intravenous infusions of antiviral drugs require considerable dilution, and recipients of these preparations must be monitored for fluid overload. Foods rich in vitamin C should be encouraged. In addition, nurses should advise rest and control of stress.

Clients receiving antiviral medications should be monitored closely for adverse reactions. Careful records should be kept of side effects and allergic reactions. These should be reported to the Division of Epidemiology and Drug Experience of the Food and Drug Administration (see Chapter 2, Standards and Controls). Nurses involved in clinical studies of experimental drugs must keep detailed records of the administration of drugs and the subjects' responses.

The nurse should verify that subjects participating in drug studies have been informed of the experimental nature of the study and the risks involved. Clients should be told that consent to such experimentation is completely voluntary and may be withdrawn at any time.

Nursing process

Assessment   Because antiviral drugs are toxic, clients for whom they are prescribed tend to have serious infections or predisposing factors that reduce their natural defenses against infection. Before drug therapy is initiated, the client should be carefully assessed to determine resistance to infection, general state of health (nutrition, rest, ability to manage stress), and understanding of the infection (including possible sequelae and prognosis). Women of childbearing age should be screened for pregnancy and lactation. Renal and hepatic function, as well as fluid and electrolyte balance should also be evaluated. Clients' knowledge of their illnesses and proposed treatments, and their emotional reaction to these should be assessed.

Nursing diagnosis   Diagnoses are related to altered tissue integrity due to inflammation related to the viral infection, risk of or actual adverse reaction to the antiviral drugs, and knowledge deficit regarding the infection or the drug regimen.

Drug-related diagnoses may include the following:

> *Pain related to phlebitis at site of infusion, secondary to IV administration of antiviral medication*
> *High risk for fluid volume deficit related to increased need for hydration during acyclovir therapy*
> *Fluid volume excess: water intoxication related to syndrome of inappropriate antidiuretic*

hormone secretion secondary to vidabarine therapy

Impaired skin integrity: rash secondary to amantidine therapy

Anxiety related to viral infection and its treatment

Fear of adverse reactions to relatively new, relatively toxic antiviral drugs

Common collaborative problems that should be differentiated from the nursing diagnoses include

Potential complication: hepatic

Potential complication: renal

Potential complication: respiratory

Potential complication: cardiovascular

Potential complication: hematopoietic

Interventions   Nursing care should include all possible measures to increase the clients general resistance to infection. This includes good hygiene and a reduction in stress, which suppresses the immune system.

The nurse is responsible for monitoring the client for responses (both beneficial and detrimental) to the drug regimen. Any signs and symptoms of serious adverse reactions to the treatment regimen should be reported to the physician, who may modify the drug regimen. An accurate record of fluid intake and output should be kept, and evaluated regularly for imbalance. Fluid intake should be encouraged except in the client receiving vidarabine who begins to retain fluid.

To relieve the pain of phlebitis, either cold or warmth may be applied to the site. If clients receiving amantidine develop a rash, cold applications may relieve discomfort. These clients need reassurance and support, especially if discoloration of the skin develops. The rash should subside when the drug is withdrawn.

Most lay people understand that viral infections are not as readily cured with medication as are microbial diseases. Therefore, clients with severe viral infections are likely to be anxious or fearful, especially those who are immunocompromised (*eg,* people with AIDS or organ transplants.) They should receive consistent, personalized emotional support.

Client education.   An important nursing intervention is the development and implementation of a teaching plan to assist the client to understand the disease process and treatment regimens. The nurse can reassure clients that the treatment of viral infections has improved in recent times, and that ongoing research continues to develop new treatment agents. Clients should be informed of the therapeutic effects of their drugs, as well as their adverse effects. They should be told in specific terms which signs and symptoms of drug response to report to health care personnel.

Inform the client of expected beneficial effects of the medication, and of possible adverse reactions.

Warn the client of any possible interactions between this medication and others taken for this or additional conditions.

Inform the client of the importance of drinking 2,000–3,000 ml of fluid daily while medications are being administered. Warn the client not to engage in activities requiring alertness if medication results in confusion or inability to concentrate.

Evaluation   Data required for evaluation include the signs and symptoms of infection and of adverse drug reaction, and a demonstrated ability by the client to understand the material covered in the teaching plan.

(See the accompanying Example of Nursing Process and Ribavirin Treatment for Viral Pneumonia.)

Checklist of nursing actions

☐ Urge parents to immunize their children against viral diseases, as recommended by public health authorities.

☐ Encourage good hygiene to promote general resistance.

☐ Give good supportive care to clients with active viral infections.

☐ Maintain appropriate fluid intake (up to 3,000 ml daily for adults) in clients with viral infections.

☐ For susceptible clients exposed to hazardous viruses, recommend human immune globulin injections for passive immunity, or available vaccines for active immunity.

☐ Inform the client of the importance of hydration.

☐ Report adverse reactions to new or experimental antiviral drugs.

☐ Inform the client of the expected benefits of medication, as well as the adverse reactions that could occur.

☐ Counsel subjects in experimental clinical studies about giving informed consent.

Antifungal drugs for superficial fungal infections

Fungi attacking the skin and mucous membranes tend to be opportunists, thriving in moist, warm environments and subsiding when conditions are not conducive to growth. Once a fungus becomes established, it usually remains part of the natural flora of the skin or mucous membrane, ready to seize the opportunity for renewed growth when conditions are favorable. For this reason, many fungal conditions tend to recur periodically. The incidence of fungal infections appears to be high, although accurate statistics are difficult to obtain. Many, if not most, victims treat themselves, using nonprescription, over-the-counter drugs. Only

Example of nursing process and ribavirin treatment for viral pneumonia

The client is a 38-year-old man who developed pneumonia while receiving chemotherapy for acute lymphoma. A sputum culture and sensitivity failed to produce a bacterial growth, and a diagnosis of viral pneumonia has been made. Antineoplastic therapy has been suspended.

    The client has been hospitalized for a course of ribavirin treatments. Vital signs on admission are T: 38.3°C (101°F); P: 110/min; R: 29/min; B/P: 135/80. The client complains of dyspnea; color is flushed, with slight cyanosis of the nail beds.

Assessment data	Nursing diagnosis	Intervention	Goals and outcome criteria
Respirations: 29/min Pulse: 110/min Cyanosis of nail beds Diagnosis of viral pneumonia Order for ribavirin therapy (Ribavirin can cause further respiratory impairment, cardiac arrest, and hypotension.)	Altered tissue integrity related to inflammation secondary to nonbacterial pneumonia Potential complication: adverse reaction to systemic antiviral medication*	**Use** all possible nursing measures to support natural resistance to infection. Encourage fluid intake of 3,000 ml/d and consumption of a high vitamin, high calorie, light diet; promote rest; assist the client in decreasing his level of stress. **Monitor** vital signs and peripheral circulation closely. **Question** the client regularly about such symptoms as dyspnea, pain, stress, and lightheadedness. Monitor blood cell counts for red and white cell counts. **Place** the client in reverse isolation to protect him from contact with further infections, until his immune system recovers from the suppressant effect of his antineoplastic chemotherapy. Be prepared to initiate resuscitation if cardiac arrest occurs. **Report** any deterioration in pulmonary or cardiovascular function to the physician promptly.	After initiation of ribavirin therapy, client's respiration will decrease to 18–22/min; pulse will decrease to 70–90; temperature will decrease to 37.8°C (100°F) or less; blood pressure will remain above 100/60 mm Hg; cyanosis will disappear. The client will state that breathing is easier. The client will not develop cardiac arrest or hypotension. If respiratory impairment increases, or hypotension or cardiac arrest occurs, it will be detected and treated promptly

* Although potential complications generally are not included in the Examples of Nursing Process, in this situation the identification of this collaborative problem is critical to the outcome for this client and illustrates the broad range of nursing responsibilities.

when an eruption fails to respond to these remedies, or when the infection is detected during medical appraisal for another condition, are these infections likely to be seen by the physician.

    Common fungal diseases are caused by members of the genera microsporum, trichophyton, epidermophyton, and candida. They include ringworm, athlete's foot, "jock itch," thrush, and diaper rash (Fig. 43-1). Over-the-counter remedies for these conditions use a variety of chemicals: astringents, keratolytic agents, the salts of fatty acids, and antiseptics. Antibiotic antifungals, which are generally available only by prescription, are often prescribed by the physician when a client seeks medical care.

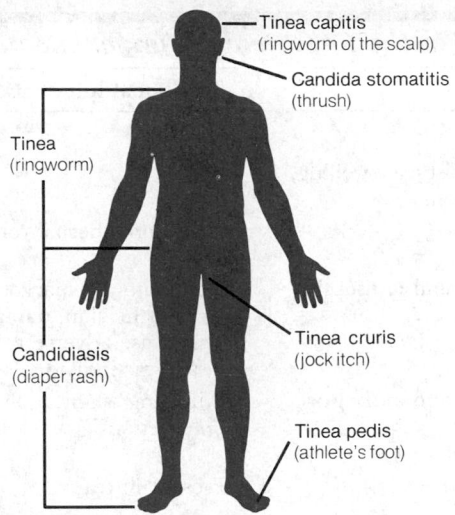

Figure 43-1. Common fungal diseases.

Labels in figure:
- Tinea capitis (ringworm of the scalp)
- Candida stomatitis (thrush)
- Tinea (ringworm)
- Candidiasis (diaper rash)
- Tinea cruris (jock itch)
- Tinea pedis (athlete's foot)

Astringents

Pharmacodynamics. Astringents act by precipitating proteins at the surface of the cell, reducing the permeability of the membrane without killing the cell. Secretions are inhibited and the local inflammatory response reduced.

By reducing moisture in a local area, astringents make the local conditions less conductive to fungal growth. In addition, alcohol and the metallic salts, which are antiseptic in nature, have a direct, antifungal effect.

Preparations. The metallic salts are marketed as antiperspirants in the form of sprays, powders, pads, creams, liquids, and semisolids. Alcohol is a common ingredient in proprietary lotions and liquids marketed for the treatment of athlete's foot. Tannic acid, in the form of tea, is a traditional home remedy for many skin problems. The solution acts as an astringent but it is rarely effective by itself in relieving the symptoms of fungal infections. Tannic acid is sometimes included as an ingredient in over-the-counter skin products.

Pharmacokinetics and therapeutic uses. Astringents are applied topically to suppress perspiration for fungal infections. They are not absorbed in appreciable amounts. They may be used alternately with body powders to keep the skin dry.

Adverse reactions. Aluminum compounds tend to hydrolyze in aqueous solution, producing acids that can irritate the skin and damage fabrics contacting the treated skin. Allergic reactions frequently develop in sensitive persons. If open lesions are present on the feet, alcohol will sting when it is applied. Repeated applications of alcohol preparations help suppress the growth of fungi but will not eliminate them from the skin.

Precautions and contraindications. Aluminum antiperspirants are contraindicated for persons with an allergic sensitivity to them. The use of aluminum compounds is also under question because of a possible relationship between their use and the aluminum tangles found in the brain tissue of clients who have died of Alzheimer's disease. Of the zirconium salts, only the hydroxychloride is suitable for use; other salts have been associated with granulomas of the skin (Gilman, et al, 1990).

Keratolytic agents

Fungi that cause common skin infections have the ability to burrow down to the base of the keratin layer, where they are relatively protected from contact with topical medications. Keratolytic agents remove some fungi and aid in the penetration of other drugs.

Pharmacodynamics. Keratolytic agents act by softening keratin and loosening cornified epithelium. This promotes desquamation of the stratum corneum, exposing the lower layers of the skin.

Preparations. The most common keratolytic agents are topical salicylates and benzoic acid. Whitfield's ointment contains salicylic acid and benzoic acid in an ointment base (Table 43-3).

Therapeutic uses. Keratolytic agents are used to soften and remove corns and as an adjunct in the treatment of superficial fungal infections. Salicylanilide in a 5% ointment is applied to the scalp to treat tinea capitis. Whitfield's ointment is used to treat epidermophytosis.

Adverse reactions. Keratolytic agents can cause swelling and softening of viable cells, leading to breaks in the skin and the risk of secondary infection.

Precautions and contraindications. Keratolytic agents are contraindicated for use by clients with diabetes mellitus and others prone to infection.

The salts of fatty acids

Because of their antifungal activity, fatty acids and their salts are used as inhibitors of mold growth. Among these compounds are sodium propionate, undecylenic acid, and zinc undecylenate (Table 43-4). They are used primarily for the treatment of tinea pedis.

Antiseptics

Most antiseptic dyes are fairly good antifungal compounds. They have been used for years to prevent or treat skin infections, despite their undesirable staining properties. Crystal violet, gentian violet, methyl violet, brilliant green, fuchsin, and potassium permanganate are among the chemicals of this class (see Box 43-1).

Other antiseptics useful in treating fungal infections include various phenols (resorcinol, thymol, chlo-

Table 43-3. Topical astringents and keratolytic agents used in the treatment of fungal infections

Drug name	Uses and preparations	Properties	Additional information
Astringents			
		Reduce moisture, swelling, and secretions	
witch hazel	Over-the-counter preparations for hemorrhoids	Astringent	Traditional herbal remedy
metallic salts (zinc, aluminum, zirconium)	Antiperspirants—sprays, powder, pads, creams, liquids, ointments	Astringent and antiseptic	Dominate the market; many irritate the skin, damage fabrics; cause adverse reactions in allergic individuals
alcohol	Ingredient in many over-the-counter lotions and liquids for athlete's foot	Astringent and antiseptic	Will sting when applied to open lesions
tannic acid	Ingredient in many over-the-counter skin remedies	Astringent	Present in tea
Keratolytic agents			
		Remove fungi and dead tissue; aid in penetration of other drugs	Contraindicated in those prone to infection
salicylanilide	Ointment (5%) for tinea capitis		
salicylic acid (Acnex)	2% solution for acne		
Keralyt	6% gel for hyperkaratotic skin		
Salac	2% cleanser for acne		
Sebcur	4% shampoo for seborrheic dermatitis (dandruff) and cradle cap		
Trans Ver Sol	15% solution soaked pads for wart infections		
X Seb	4% shampoo for seborrheic dermatitis (dandruff) and cradle cap		
salicylic acid and benzoic acid (Whitfield's ointment)	Ointment for epidermophytosis		

rothymol, phenol), sulfur compounds, acetic acid, and iodine.

Pharmacodynamics. The exact mechanism of the antiseptic action in these dyes is unknown. They may act as protoplasmic poisons. Many also act as astringents.

Pharmacokinetics. Antiseptic dyes are applied topically and are not absorbed to any great degree.

Therapeutic uses. Diluted solutions of antiseptic dyes (usually potassium permanganate) have been used as foot dips in gymnasium dressing rooms for years to prevent transmission of fungi. The dyes are also sometimes painted on the affected skin to combat fungal infections.

Adverse reactions. Foot dips are of questionable efficacy. Antiseptic dyes discolor skin, as well as linens.

Skin pigmentation is usually temporary, although permanent tattooing may occur when gentian violet is applied to granulation tissue.

The drugs may cause irritation; mucous membranes sometimes ulcerate when exposed to these compounds. Allergic hypersensitivity may develop in some recipients.

Precautions and contraindications. Antifungal use of antiseptic dyes has declined with the advent of newer, more effective antifungal agents. When used, dyes should be applied according to label instructions. Application should be limited to the skin, with care taken to avoid contact with mucous membranes. Clients using these agents on the face should be cautioned against swallowing the drugs, for example, by licking areas around the lips which have been treated. Gentian violet should not be applied to open lesions.

Table 43-4. Salts of fatty acids used as antifungals

Drug name	Additional information
sodium propionate	Used as an ingredient of proprietary antifungals
	Added to doughs to retard spoilage in baked goods
undecylenic acid (Desenex)	Marketed as powders, creams, lotions, topical aerosols, and ointments
zinc undecylenate	Combines the astringent action of zinc with the antifungal properties of fatty acid

Antifungal antibiotics

Various antifungals are in general use for the treatment of superficial fungal infection. The major drugs are nystatin, griseofulvin, clotrimazole, miconazole, and ketoconazole. Each has a distinct spectrum of activity and specific therapeutic uses (Table 43-5).

Clotrimazole

Clotrimazole (Lotrimin, Myclex) is a synthetic antifungal imidazole derivative.

Pharmacodynamics. Clotrimazole binds with phospholipids in the fungal cell membrane, increasing permeability and causing loss of potassium and other cellular constituents. It inhibits or kills many genera of fungi, including yeasts and dermatophytes.

Pharmacokinetics. Clotrimazole's primary action is local; it binds to tissues in the skin or mucous membranes from which it is released gradually. Only small amounts of the drug are absorbed systemically. Following systemic absorption, clotrimazole is metabolized by hepatic microsomal enzymes.

Therapeutic uses. Clotrimazole is used for the topical treatment of candidiasis, including oral, skin, and vaginal infections. Systemic administration of clotrimazole remains experimental.

Adverse reactions. Clotrimazole is usually well tolerated when administered topically, although local reactions (erythema, edema, blistering, pruritis, burning, stinging, peeling, urticaria, skin fissures, and general irritation) have occurred. When administered intravaginally, local irritation can occur, as can abdominal cramps and bloating, intercurrent cystitis, and burning or irritation in the sexual partner.

Oral lozenges produce some systemic absorption of clotrimazole. Minimally elevated liver enzymes have been reported in approximately 15% of the clients receiving this form of the drug. Nausea and vomiting also occur in a small proportion (5%) of recipients. Clotrimazole is embryotoxic in rats.

Precautions and contraindications. Oral lozenges of clotrimazole must be dissolved slowly in the mouth to maximize the local effect while minimizing the rate of systemic absorption. When this form of the drug is used, liver function tests should be conducted periodically, especially in clients with pre-existing hepatic impairment.

Clotrimazole should be avoided during the first trimester of pregnancy, regardless of the route of administration. Safe use in children younger than 3 years of age has not been established.

Griseofulvin

Griseofulvin is an antibiotic effective against a variety of topical mycoses. It is produced by one strain of *Penicillium*.

Pharmacodynamics. Griseofulvin is fungistatic rather than fungicidal. It arrests cell division by disrupting mitotic spindle structure and also, possibly, by causing production of defective DNA. Only young, active cells are killed by the drug; older, more dormant cells are not affected. The presence of the drug in keratin makes the tissues resistant to fungal invasion. As nails and hair grow out, new growth becomes free of disease-producing organisms. Fungal cells are depleted as older growth is shed or cut off. Thus, griseofulvin eradicates from the body the reservoirs of infectious cells harbored at the base of the keratin layer (Table 43-6).

Box 43-1. Antiseptics used as antifungals

Antiseptic dyes (many also act as astringents)

crystal violet

gentian violet

methyl violet

brilliant green

fuchsin

potassium permanganate

Phenols

resorcinol

thymol

chlorothymol

phenol

Sulfur compounds

Acetic acid

Iodine

Table 43-5. Antifungals used in the treatment of superficial infections

Drug name	Preparations	Usual dosage/PC	Therapeutic uses
clotrimazole (Canestan, Clotrimaderm, Gyne-Lotrimin, Lotrimin, Mycelax, Myclex, Myclo, Trimysten)	Oral lozenges Creams, solutions, vaginal cream, and vaginal tablets for topical use	Lozenges: one 5 times daily for 14 days Skin cream and solution: apply bid Vaginal cream or tablets: 100 mg qd for 7 days or (for nonpregnant women) 200 mg qd for 3 days PC: B	Treatment of oropharyngeal candidiasis, dermatophytoses, superficial mycoses, cutaneous candidiasis, and vulvovaginal candidiasis
griseofulvin (Fulvicine, Grifulvin, Grisactin, Grisovin, Gris-PEG, Likuden)	Oral tablets in two formulations: microsize and ultramicrosize	Varies with requirements and responses of the client Adults: microsize formulation: 500 mg–1 g/d; ultramicrosize formulation: 250–600 mg/d Children: microsize formulation: 10 mg/kg body weight/d; ultramicrosize formulation: 5.5–7.3 mg/kg body weight/d Duration of therapy: 2 weeks–3 months PC: C	Treatment of infections of hair, skin, and nails caused by tinea and susceptible species of *Trichophyton, Microspira,* and *Epidermophyton*
ketoconazole (Nizoral)	Oral tablets	Adults: 200–400 mg/d, given in a single dose Children weighing less than 20 kg: 50 mg/d Children weighing 20–40 kg: 100 mg/d Children weighing more than 40 kg: 200 mg/d Duration of therapy: 1–12 mo PC: C	Treatment of infections of hair, skin, and nails caused by tinea and susceptible species of *Trichophyton, Microspira,* and *Epidermophyton* Treatment of systemic coccidioidomycosis, histoplasmosis, chromomycosis, and candidiasis
miconazole (Monistat)	Solution for IV infusion Creams, lotions, vaginal cream, and vaginal suppositories for topical use	*IV:* adult: 0.2–3.6 g/d, divided in 3 doses; children: 20–40 mg/kg body weight/d, divided in 3 doses (dosage varies with the susceptibility of the infecting organism) *Skin cream or lotion:* apply qd–bid *Vaginal cream or suppository:* 100 mg/d for 7 days PC: C	Treatment of severe systemic fungal infections and fungal meningitis Treatment of dermatophytoses, superficial mycoses, cutaneous candidiasis, and vulvovaginal candidiasis
nystatin (Candex, Moronel, Mycostatin, Mycolog, Mytrex, Nadostine, Nilstat, Nyaderm, PMS Nystatin)	Suspensions and tablets for oral use Solutions, creams, powders, ointments, and vaginal suppositories for topical use	Adults: 1,500,000–2,400,000 U/d, divided in 2–4 doses Infants: 400,000–800,000 U/d, divided in 3–4 doses Duration of therapy: until 48 hr after symptoms disappear PC: B	Treatment of candida infections: stomatitis (thrush), vaginitis, diaper rash

KEY: PC = pregnancy risk category. (The validity of pregnancy risk categories has not been established. See Chapter 16, p 216.)

Table 43-6. Duration of griseofulvin treatment required to eliminate fungal infection

Area of body affected	Time required
Soles of the feet, palms of the hands	4–8 weeks
Fingernails	4 months
Toenails	6 months

Pharmacokinetics. Griseofulvin is administered orally. Ultramicrosized formulations are almost completely absorbed, whereas microsized formulations are erratically and unpredictably absorbed. Its systemic absorption is enhanced by the presence of fat in the intestinal tract. From the blood, the drug migrates to the skin, where it is deposited in keratin precursor cells. It has a special affinity for diseased skin but is also found in liver, fat, and skeletal muscle tissues. Griseofulvin is partially metabolized by the liver; excretion is mainly by the kidneys but appreciable fractions are eliminated in feces and perspiration. Elimination half-life is 9–24 hours.

Therapeutic uses. Griseofulvin is used for the treatment of superficial fungal infections caused by susceptible organisms not responsive to topical treatment. Although griseofulvin therapy is not appropriate for mild, intermittent skin infections, it is a valuable drug for the relief of severe or refractory disease. Symptomatic relief usually appears after 2–4 days of treatment. The drug must be continued until the infected structures are eliminated. The length of time required varies with the structure involved (see Table 43-6) but it is frequently many weeks or even months.

Adverse reactions. Although multiple adverse reactions have been reported, these tend to be minor. Nervous system manifestations include headache (which can be severe), neuritis, lethargy; confusion, fatigue, syncope, vertigo, blurred vision, and transient macular edema. Dry mouth, thirst, angular stomatitis, heartburn, flatulence, nausea, vomiting, diarrhea, and black, furred tongue are common GI side effects. Transient leukopenia, neutropenia, monocytosis, skin eruptions, itching, and photosensitivity also can occur. Hepatotoxicity and renal impairment have been observed.

Drug interactions. Griseofulvin interacts with several drugs, including alcohol, phenobarital, and warfarin. It potentiates the effects of alcohol. The therapeutic effectiveness of griseofulvin is diminished by phenobarbital, either by impairing absorption or inducing hepatic microsomal enzymes. Griseofulvin appears to accelerate metabolic breakdown of warfarin; clients on maintenance doses of coumarin anticoagulants experience a decrease in prothrombin time when the antifungal is added to the drug regimen.

Precautions and contraindications. Griseofulvin is contraindicated in porphyria and hepatocellular failure. It should not be given to clients with a history of allergic reaction to the drug. Safe use during pregnancy and in children under the age of 2 years has not been established.

Combined use of griseofulvin and alcohol, phenobarbital, and warfarin should be avoided. When the antifungal must be used with the latter two, adjustments of dosage may be required.

Blood studies should be carried out weekly during the first month of treatment to detect changes in hematopoietic function.

Ketoconazole

Ketoconazole is a synthetic antifungal closely related to miconazole and clotrimazole.

Pharmacodynamics. The action of ketoconazole is usually fungistatic, but fungicidal effects have been demonstrated *in vitro*. The drug blocks metabolic processes vital to cell membrane synthesis in fungi. The altered membrane cannot transport purines into the cell, and replication cannot proceed.

Pharmacokinetics. Oral doses of ketoconazole react with hydrochloric acid in the stomach to form a hydrochloride salt that is subsequently absorbed. Absorption is impaired when the gastric pH is elevated. Plasma proteins bind 84%–99% of the drug. Serum levels decline in a biphasic manner, with half-lives varying from 2 hours at peak levels to 8 hours when blood levels are minimal. The drug is partially metabolized in the liver.

The major pathway for elimination is the biliary tract to the feces, although smaller fractions are excreted in the urine.

Therapeutic uses. Ketoconazole is useful in the treatment of infections caused by most pathogenic fungi, including dermatophytes. It is effective against superficial and some systemic infections. It has had little effect against aspergillosis. Investigation continues to determine its specific spectrum of activity and therapeutic effectiveness.

Adverse reactions. The most frequent adverse reactions are GI (nausea, vomiting, abdominal pain, constipation, flatulence, GI bleeding, and diarrhea). Hepatotoxicity may occur, especially in children. Gynecomastia has been reported. Preliminary reports indicate the drug may decrease serum cholesterol and depress serum testosterone concentrations. Relatively rare adverse reactions include anaphylaxis, arthralgia, chills and fever, dyspnea, tinnitus, abnormal dreams, impotence, photophobia, and changes in patterns of perspiration. Ketoconazole interacts with warfarin to enhance the latter's anticoagulant effect.

Precautions and contraindications. Clients receiving ketoconazole should be monitored for hepatotoxicity and the drug discontinued if changes in laboratory values are substantial, or if signs and symptoms of hepatic malfunction develop.

Because animal studies indicate the drug may be teratogenic, and it is not known whether the drug appears in breast milk, ketoconazole is not used to treat pregnant or nursing women.

The drug is contraindicated for clients with a history of allergic hypersensitivity to it.

Miconazole

Miconazole is a synthetic antifungal imidazole derivative related to clotrimazole.

Pharmacodynamics. At fungistatic concentrations, miconazole thickens fungal cell membranes and inhibits purine transport. At higher concentrations, it interferes with peroxisomal enzymes and causes necrosis of intracellular constituents, apparently because of peroxidase accumulation within the cell.

Pharmacokinetics. Absorption of miconazole varies, depending on the route of administration. About 50% is absorbed from the GI tract. Only small amounts are absorbed when the drug is applied to the vaginal mucosa, and none appears to be absorbed from the skin.

Following absorption, miconazole is widely distributed into body tissues and fluids, including inflamed joints, the vitreous humor of the eye, and the peritoneal cavity. Little drug is found in sputum or saliva. It is not known whether the drug crosses the placenta or is distributed into breast milk in humans. Distribution into the CSF is unreliable, and the drug must be administered intrathecally to treat meningitis.

Miconazole is 91% to 93% bound to plasma proteins. The drug is metabolized by the liver and excreted in urine. Plasma concentrations decline triphasically, with sequential biologic half-lives of 0.4, 2.1, and 24.1 hours.

Therapeutic uses. Miconazole is used topically in the treatment of infections caused by susceptible fungi, including candidiasis, superficial mycoses, and dermatophytoses. It is also administered systemically in the treatment of serious systemic fungal infections, including meningitis.

Adverse reactions. When applied topically, miconazole occasionally causes irritation and burning.

When administered systemically, miconazole has a lower order of toxicity than the systemic antifungal amphotericin B. The most common adverse reactions to IV administration are phlebitis and pruritus, with or without skin eruptions. Anaphylaxis has been reported following IV administration. Other adverse effects include GI disturbances, fever, drowsiness, dizziness, anxiety, increased libido, headache, dryness of the eyes, and bitter taste.

Because miconazole is a relatively new drug, there may be other adverse effects that remain undetected.

Drug interactions. Miconazole enhances the anticoagulant effect of warfarin and delays metabolism of phenytoin.

Precautions and contraindications. Miconazole administered systemically should be used with caution for individuals with hepatic insufficiency. Clients are hospitalized for initiation of systemic miconazole therapy. Hematocrit, hemoglobin, electrolytes, and lipids should be monitored regularly throughout the period of drug therapy.

To reduce the risk of phlebitis, a central venous line may be used for administration. Treatment should be discontinued if severe skin problems develop. Other adverse reactions can be ameliorated by reducing the dose of drug, slowing infusion rates, avoiding doses at mealtimes, or administrating antihistamine or antiemetic drugs. Caution must be exercised when the drug is given to clients with hepatic insufficiency. If coumarin is administered concurrently, prothrombin time must be carefully monitored, and the dose of anticoagulant adjusted accordingly.

Allergic hypersensitivity is a contraindication for use of miconazole. Safe use of the drug during pregnancy and in children less than 1 year of age has not been established. Miconazole is contraindicated for those exhibiting allergic hypersensitivity to it.

Miconazole preparations should not be allowed to come in contact with the eyes.

Nystatin

Nystatin (Mycostatin) is an antifungal antibiotic produced by a strain of *Streptomyces*.

Pharmacodynamics. Nystatin is both fungistatic and fungicidal. It acts by binding to sterols in the fungal wall, interfering with the integrity and function of the membrane. Loss of potassium and other intracellular constituents causes cell death.

Pharmacokinetics. Nystatin is poorly absorbed from the GI tract, skin, or mucous membranes. Whether taken orally or applied topically, it is used for local effect only. The drug passes through the GI tract unchanged and is eliminated in the feces. The drug is not absorbed from the intact skin or mucous membranes. Topical preparations are sloughed off from the surface.

Therapeutic uses. Nystatin is the main therapeutic agent for the prevention and control of infections caused by *Candida albicans*, including thrush (stomatitis) and diaper rash in children. Although thrush can be a mild, self-limiting condition, severe candida infections can occur, and nursery epidemics are considered serious. Candida infection in adults primarily affects persons rendered susceptible by debility or by treatment with broad-spectrum antibiotics or immunosuppressants. Stomatitis and vaginitis are the most common manifestations.

Adverse reactions. Adverse reactions to nystatin are rare and generally mild and transitory. Nausea, vomiting, and diarrhea occasionally develop from oral doses. Allergic hypersensitivity is rare but is a contraindication for continued use of the drug.

■ **Summary**

The risk of localized fungal infections is greatest when the surface is moist and warm. Astringents and metallic antiperspirants are useful in reducing moisture on the skin. Two antibiotics (nystatin and griseofulvin) and three related synthetic antifungals (clotrimazole, miconazole, and ketoconazole) are used to treat superficial fungal infections. Nystatin is used topically, in the form of ointments, suppositories, and suspensions. It is relatively free of adverse effects. Griseofulvin and ketoconazole are administered orally over long periods of time to eliminate residual reservoirs of infection. Clotrimazole and miconazole are applied topically for relatively short periods of therapy.

Nursing management

Nursing implications

Fungal infections can be a serious problem in hospital settings, particularly in nurseries. Because candida often is part of the normal flora of the vagina, the newborn is likely to acquire the organism during the birth process. Babies are highly susceptible to this organism, and epidemics develop quickly in the nursery if the infection is introduced. The first evidence often is the appearance of white patches on the tongue and mucous membranes of the baby's mouth (thrush). These patches resemble a thin layer of milk but they are adherent to the membrane and are not easily dislodged. The infection can spread to the skin, usually involving the diaper area. The affected skin becomes bright red, resembling the first-degree burns of a scald. Mothers of nursing infants with thrush often develop candida infection, manifested by sore or

---

Enrichment experience 43-2

Interview an infection control nurse in a hospital or nursing home to determine the incidence and severity of fungal superinfection in clients receiving systemic anti-infectives. What antifungal treatment agents are employed in the care of these clients? Have any of the recipients of these antifungal drugs exhibited adverse reactions?

---

fissured nipples. Nurseries in which the spread of the infection cannot be stemmed may be quarantined or closed.

Nursing process

Assessment Risk factors for tinea infection include the use of occlusive clothing that prevents the evaporation of perspiration or other secretions. Hot, humid weather increases the risk. Once tinea are established, they may remain part of the skin's flora unless a long-term course of griseofulvin medication is completed. Individuals who have had an acute fungal outbreak are at increased risk of recurrences. This is particularly true of tinea pedis (athlete's foot).

In addition to newborns and nursing mothers, candida infections affect persons made vulnerable by debility or treatment with broad-spectrum antibiotics or immunosuppressants. The fungus grows when the host's natural defenses are deficient, or when the normal flora changes, due to administration of antibiotics, such as the penicillins, cephalosporins, or tetracyclines. Extension of the infection into the intestinal tract can occur in susceptible clients, such as those with diabetes or leukemia, or in recipients of corticosteroid therapy.

Clients at risk for fungal infection should be assessed for skin lesions (rough, itchy patches on the scalp or arms, itching and cracks between the toes, sore and reddened areas, sore and fissured nipples), mucous membrane lesions (white adherent plaques, sore and reddened areas), and abnormal drainage (thick, frothy vaginal drainage).

When clients experience chronic skin irritations, a history should be taken to determine what cleansers, cosmetics, or other preparations have been applied to the skin. Chemicals used on clothing should also be listed because they can cause skin problems when allergic hypersensitivity has developed to laundry detergents, stain removers, bleaches, or softeners.

Nursing diagnosis Drug-related diagnoses may include the following:

High risk for impaired skin integrity: rash related to adverse reaction to antifungal medication
Body image disturbance related to rash secondary to superficial antifungal medication
Altered comfort: headache, itching related to adverse reaction to griseofulvin medication
Altered comfort: joint pains, nausea, vomiting, abdominal pain related to adverse reaction to antifungal medication
High risk for altered body temperature: fever related to adverse reaction to ketoconazole medication
Knowledge deficit related to fungal infections

and the regimen required to treat them, and to prevent their recurrence

Common collaborative problems that should be differentiated from the nursing diagnoses include

Potential complication: phlebitis
Potential complication: anaphylaxis

Planning Goals of care include reducing inflammation, reducing the risk and alleviating the symptoms of adverse drug reactions, and instructing the client about medications and self-care measures to reduce the incidence and severity of fungal infections.

Intervention If skin rash is suspected as an allergic reaction, a change in detergents, cosmetics, or other chemicals contacting the skin or clothing may resolve the problem. If the offending preparation is an aluminum antiperspirant, the client may be advised to use a mixture of cornstarch and soda bicarbonate as a deodorant. Because this mixture will not reduce perspiration, the client may need to wash more frequently and protect clothing from underarm perspiration with shields.

If thrush is detected among nursery newborns, vigorous measures should be taken to prevent contagion. The infection is less likely to develop in babies whose mouths are cleaned of milk following feeding. This can be accomplished by rinsing the infant's mouth with water after every feeding. If any oral lesions appear, 1 ml of nystatin should be applied to them by dropper for a full 2 weeks, continuing to do this as directed, even if the lesions disappear before then.

Nursing mothers of babies with thrush may prevent the development of sore nipples by applying nystatin ointment to the nipple and areola following each feeding (Lawrence, 1989). If thrush spreads to the skin, the physician should be consulted for an antifungal ointment prescription. Clients subject to fungal infections should be instructed in special techniques of skin care that will reduce the recurrence of active infection. Because the pathogens are usually part of the normal flora of the skin in such clients, it is crucial to prevent the moist, warm conditions that favor fungal growth. To suppress athlete's foot, for example, the feet should be kept clean and dry. Daily washing followed by thorough drying and the application of an astringent lotion or antifungal foot powder may be recommended. Care should be taken to distribute the medication to all areas, especially between the toes. Because conditions are ideal for fungal growth in intertriginous areas, lesions are most common there. Clients should be advised to avoid shoes made of plastics or synthetics in favor of materials such as leather and cotton or wool cloth, which allow perspiration to evaporate. Socks should be changed daily and shoes rotated so that they dry thoroughly between wearings.

If an active fungal infection is present on the feet, socks should be boiled between wearings to destroy residual fungi. The use of tea on the infected areas is not harmful but rubbing alcohol may be as effective and does not stain. Alcohol should not be applied to broken skin areas because it causes considerable pain.

Oily preparations should never be applied to the feet if a fungal infection is suspected. By preventing evaporation of perspiration, oils promote fungal growth and may increase the irritation.

When nystatin is ordered for fungal stomatitis, administration by "swishes" is usually specified. The required dose of nystatin suspension is measured, then diluted with enough water to produce about 20 ml of fluid. Clients should rinse the mouth thoroughly with the dose, gargle if necessary, then swallow it. This technique provides a direct topical application of the drug to the affected area plus a prophylactic effect on the rest of the GI tract.

Clients receiving griseofulvin should have periodic blood tests to detect changes in their differential count. Leukopenia may necessitate discontinuing the medication. Because griseofulvin treatment requires months to years of medication, clients need support and encouragement to persist in following the regimen.

Clotrimazole, miconazole, and ketoconazole are relatively new drugs and not yet fully understood. Clients receiving these drugs should be assessed carefully for signs and symptoms indicating adverse reactions that may have remained undetected in the past. Before these drugs are administered to women of childbearing age, pregnancy and lactation should be ruled out. To facilitate absorption, ketoconazole should be administered with fruit juice to lower gastric *p*H.

Drug interactions. Clients receiving antifungal drugs should be instructed to report serious adverse reactions to the physician. When nystatin is ordered, simple measures to minimize intestinal irritation (bland food and avoidance of irritating drugs such as aspirin) may control the reaction. Allergic phenomena (skin eruptions and jaundice) should be reported and the drug discontinued until the physician is consulted. Clients receiving griseofulvin should report malaise, changes in urinary excretion, and photosensitivity or other neurologic symptoms: They should avoid the use of ingested alcohol. During the first month of treatment with this agent, the client will need to report for weekly blood tests. The importance of completing the course of therapy should be stressed.

Diabetic clients should be warned not to use keratolytic preparations because these can damage the skin and lead to ulcers, especially when used on the feet.

Evaluation Data required for evaluation include signs and symptoms of inflammation; incidence or absence of signs and symptoms of adverse drug reac-

Example of nursing process and treatment of fungal foot infection

The client is a 16-year-old female student who complains of burning and itching of the feet, especially of the toes and intertriginous areas. The affected area appears red but the skin is unbroken, even between the toes.

  The client has used hand lotion on her feet in an attempt to relieve the symptoms. She wears plastic shoes most of the time. Her walking shoes are made of cloth with rubber soles. She wears nylon socks much of the time and likes panty hose when "dressing up."

Assessment data	Nursing diagnosis	Intervention	Goals and outcome criteria
Burning and itching of the feet Redness of affected area Skin remains unbroken	Altered comfort: itching and burning of the feet related to inflammation probably secondary to a fungal infection	**Apply** rubbing alcohol to the affected area. **Advise** the client to leave the feet uncovered until thoroughly dry, then dress them in cotton socks and cloth, leather, or well-ventilated slippers or shoes.	The client will state that the itching and burning have decreased.
Use of nonporous hose and shoes Use of hand lotion to relieve itching and burning	Knowledge deficit concerning fungal infections and self-care measures to control them	**Prepare** and implement a teaching plan for the hygienic care of the feet and use of over-the-counter preparations for the treatment of a fungal foot infection. Content covered should include: techniques for keeping the feet clean, dry, and cool (using leather or cloth shoes when possible, airing the feet periodically, alternating shoes to allow them to dry thoroughly, changing socks daily, and boiling them between wearings. **Advise** client to use liquid foot care preparations containing alcohol on all areas of the feet except where the skin is broken, and antifungal medication foot powders (especially between the toes) to keep the skin dry; oily lotions or ointments should be avoided, and absorbent hose (cotton or wool) should be substituted for nylon whenever possible.	On subsequent nursing visits, the client will be able to repeat to the nurse information conveyed during the teaching sessions. On subsequent visits, the client will be wearing absorbent shoes and hose, and she will report that she is using alcohol or alcohol-based lotions on her feet. The redness and itching of the feet will continue to improve. Open skin lesions of the feet will not develop.

tion; the client's ability to repeat information conveyed during teaching sessions; the client's observed behavior in carrying out self-care measures; and the incidence or absence of recurrent infection.

  (See the accompanying Example of Nursing Process and Treatment of Fungal Foot Infection.)

Checklist of nursing actions

☐ Teach clients subject to fungal infections to keep their skin clean, cool, and dry.

☐ Recommend leather or cloth shoes instead of plastic or synthetic shoes.

- [ ] Monitor newborns for signs and symptoms of candida infection. Institute early treatment and isolation to prevent epidemics in the nursery.
- [ ] When administering nystatin for candida stomatitis, instruct clients to dilute the suspension as directed, and rinse their mouths with the suspension before swallowing.
- [ ] Monitor white blood cell counts of clients receiving griseofulvin.
- [ ] Inform clients of beneficial effects and adverse reactions that can occur.
- [ ] Instruct clients receiving griseofulvin to report signs and symptoms of liver or renal impairment.
- [ ] Warn clients receiving griseofulvin to reduce alcohol consumption.
- [ ] Warn diabetic clients not to use keratolytic preparations on the skin.

Antifungal drugs for systemic fungal infections

Although systemic fungal diseases are serious, life-threatening conditions, most escaped notice until relatively recently because of misdiagnosis. The lung diseases, blastomycosis, coccidioidomycosis, and histoplasmosis mimic tuberculosis so closely that they were not differentiated from that condition. When effective tuberculosis chemotherapy was developed, some "tuberculosis" clients who failed to respond to the new drugs were found to be suffering from entirely different diseases—the fungal infections. Definitive diagnosis of such lung disorders is made by skin testing for antibodies against each organism. Fungi can affect tissues other than the lungs, causing pleural, peritoneal, ocular, urinary, and meningeal infections. Systemic disease must be treated by systemic antifungals: amphotericin B, ketoconazole, miconazole, and flucytosine (Table 43-7).

Amphotericin B

Amphotericin B is an antifungal antibiotic. It is effective against fungi and other organisms containing sterols in the cell membrane. It is not effective against bacteria, rickettsiae, or viruses.

Pharmacodynamics. Amphotericin B is usually fungistatic in action. As a result of its binding with sterols in the cell membrane, the drug destroys the selectivity of the membrane. Subsequent loss of intracellular constituents such as potassium may kill the organism.

Pharmacokinetics. Because amphotericin B is poorly absorbed from the GI tract, it must be given parenterally. It is administered IV and (less frequently) intrathecally, intraventricularly, or intra-articularly. Distribution is poorly understood but appears to be multicompartmental, although concentrations in many compartments such as the cerebrospinal, pleural, pericardial, and synovial fluids and aqueous humor are low. Cross-placental transport has been reported. Most of the drug (90% to 95%) binds to serum lipoproteins. The metabolic fate of amphotericin B is unknown. An elimination half-life of 24 hours has been reported. Because plasma levels tend to persist, the drug can be detected in the urine for up to 8 weeks following cessation of therapy. Urinary excretion is the main pathway for elimination. Amphotericin B is not removed from the blood by dialysis.

Therapeutic uses. Amphotericin B is used for the treatment of severe, life-threatening systemic infections caused by susceptible fungi and protozoa (Box 43-2). It is the drug of choice for systemic fungal disease.

Adverse reactions. Most clients receiving amphotericin B experience adverse reactions. The most common include headache, chills, fever, malaise, joint pain, anorexia, dyspepsia, cramping, epigastric pain, nausea, vomiting, anemia, and some degree of kidney malfunction. Hypokalemia develops in many clients and may account for the muscle weakness that commonly occurs. Although rare, anaphylaxis, cardiovascular toxicity, blood dyscrasias, pruritic rash, gastroenteritis, neurologic symptoms (including seizures), and acute hepatic failure have been reported. Pain in the injection site, phlebitis, and thrombophlebitis are common.

Precautions and contraindications. Because the incidence of adverse reactions is high and reactions tend to be serious, use of amphotericin B is limited to the treatment of clients with a confirmed diagnosis of a progressive and potentially fatal fungal infection susceptible to the drug. Clients receiving the drug are hospitalized. During therapy, kidney and cardiovascular function must be monitored closely. Concurrent use of other nephrotoxic drugs is contraindicated. Corticosteroids may alleviate some of the side effects of the drug, but they will exacerbate the hypokalemia many clients experience and should be used cautiously. Renal function, potassium, magnesium, hemoglobin, and hematocrit require close monitoring during amphotericin B therapy.

Flucytosine

Flucytosine (Ancobon, 5-FC) is a chemical relative of the antineoplastic drug fluorouracil.

Pharmacodynamics. Within fungal cells, flucytosine is deaminated to fluorouracil, acting as an antimetabolite and competing with uracil in the cell processes producing RNA and proteins.

Pharmacokinetics. Unlike amphotericin B, flucytosine is well absorbed and can be given by mouth. It

Table 43-7. Antifungals used in the treatment of systemic infections

Drug name	Preparations	Usual dosage	Therapeutic uses
amphotericin B (Amphozone, Fungilin, Fungizone)	Powder for preparing solutions for IV injection Capsules and suspensions for oral use	Varies with severity of infection and tolerance of recipient Low dosages are given initially and increased gradually to 1 mg/kg body weight/d or 1.5 mg/kg q2d (IV) Duration of therapy: 6wk–4 mo PC: B	Treatment of severe systemic infections caused by susceptible strains: aspergillosis, blastomycosis, candidiasis, coccidioidomycosis, cryptococcosis, histoplasmosis, phycomycosis, and leishmaniasis
flucytosine (Ancoban, Ancobon, Ancotil)	Oral capsules	50–150 mg/kg body weight/d, divided in 4 doses, administered at equal intervals Duration of therapy: several months PC: B	Treatment of severe systemic infections caused by susceptible strains: candidiasis, cryptococcosis

KEY: PC = pregnancy risk category. (The validity of pregnancy risk categories has not been established. See Chapter 16, p 216.)

readily penetrates the blood–brain barrier to reach therapeutic levels in the CSF. Flucytosine is minimally bound to plasma proteins (2%–4%). The drug's half-life is 2.5–6 hours in clients with normal renal function. Flucytosine is only minimally metabolized and is excreted almost entirely unchanged in the urine. The dosage of flucytosine must be reduced for clients with renal insufficiency.

Therapeutic uses. Flucytosine is used only for the treatment of severe fungal infections caused by susceptible strains of *Candida* or *Cryptococcus.*

Adverse reactions. Adverse reactions to flucytosine are similar to those to fluorouracil (see Chapter 48). It tends to cause bone marrow depression and GI symptoms (nausea, vomiting, and diarrhea). It raises the level of hepatic enzymes and can cause symptoms of CNS toxicity. Adverse reactions are more frequent when azotemia is present.

Ketoconazole and miconazole

Ketoconazole and miconazole are discussed in the previous section on antifungals that are used in treating superficial infections. These two agents are usually considered secondary to amphotericin B, which is the drug of choice for most systemic fungal infections.

■ **Summary**
Amphotericin B, ketoconazole, miconazole, and flucytosine are drugs used to treat systemic fungal infections. Amphotericin B must be administered by injection. Because these drugs are relatively toxic, hospitalization is usually required for treatment.

Nursing management

Nursing implications

Clients receiving treatment for systemic fungal infections are seriously ill. These diseases can be life-threatening. Good supportive nursing care is essential to promote recovery by increasing general resistance to the pathogens.

Treatment may require 6 weeks to 3 or 4 months when amphotericin B is administered. This drug is administered every day to every 2 days, usually by IV infusion.

Clients receiving flucytosine with amphotericin B are at high risk for bone marrow depression and liver damage. Gastrointestinal symptoms are likely to be severe. In addition, symptoms of central nervous system irritation, such as confusion, hallucinations, headache, sedation, and vertigo may develop.

Clients with systemic fungal diseases face a difficult and sometimes lengthy course of treatment. Not only is drug treatment uncomfortable and risky, but many clients with lung disease also eventually require surgery to remove infected tissue. The systemic antifungals have improved the prognosis and shortened the recovery period but successful therapy requires highly supportive care.

Box 43-2. Infections treated by amphotericin B therapy

aspergillosis	histoplasmosis
blastomycosis	leishmaniasis
candidiasis	phycomycosis
coccidioidomycosis	sporotrichosis
cryptococcosis	

Nursing process

Assessment Data required for assessment include a history of the client's illness; signs and symptoms indicative of the client's current condition; a full assessment of general health, particularly cardiovascular, neurologic, and renal function; information about the specific disease that has been diagnosed; an assessment of the client's emotional status; and information about the drugs prescribed for treatment.

Nursing diagnosis Diagnoses may include

*Impaired tissue integrity related to
inflammation secondary to fungal infection
Anxiety concerning the prognosis or drug
regimen
Knowledge deficit concerning the disease or its
treatment*

Drug related diagnoses may include the following:

*Altered comfort: chills, fever, joint pain,
epigastric pain, nausea, malaise, itching,
headache related to adverse reaction to
amphotericin B medication
Altered comfort: Nausea and vomiting related
to adverse reaction to flucytosine medication
Hopelessness resulting from severe adverse
reactions to drugs
Ineffective individual coping due to severity
of the illness
Ineffective family coping related to disabling
severity of the client's illness
Knowledge deficit regarding the systemic
fungal disease, its treatment, and possible
effects of the drug regimen*

Common collaborative problems that should be differentiated from the nursing diagnoses include

*Potential complication: anaphylaxis
Potential complication: phlebitis
Potential complication: hepatic
Potential complication: bone marrow
depression
Potential complication: adverse reaction to
medication for systemic fungal infection*

Planning Goals of treatment include recovery of tissue integrity by lessening or eliminating inflammation and infection; reduction of the risk of adverse drug reactions; prompt detection and treatment of adverse drug reactions should they occur; alleviation of client anxiety; and increased client awareness about the disease and its treatment.

Intervention Before initiating drug therapy, clients should be warned that drugs can cause adverse reactions that may require changes in the treatment regimen. They should be instructed to report any unusual signs and symptoms to the health care team. A teaching program to inform the client about the disease and its treatment should be developed and implemented. (See Chapter 2 for patient information.)

In the hospital setting, the nurse is responsible for administering the prescribed drugs. Amphotericin B is most often given by IV infusion. When a solvent is added to the powdered drug, the vial should be rolled until the suspension is clear; vials containing particulate matter should be discarded. If an in-line filter is used during administration, its mean pore diameter must be at least 1 micron to allow passage of the drug. Infusion should be slow; a flow control device should be used to control the rate of infusion. If an acute reaction occurs, the rate should be reduced to one tolerated by the client. Because the drug is irritating, infusion may be difficult to maintain.

Institution policy may require shielding amphotericin B suspensions from light. The drug is light-sensitive but chemical breakdown is slow and usually does not occur during the treatment interval. Only fresh solutions should be infused.

The client should be monitored carefully for signs and symptoms of adverse drug reaction, specifically for allergic reactions (including anaphylaxis) and renal or liver impairment. During treatment, the blood is tested frequently for evidence of complications such as hypokalemia, anemia, leukopenia, and azotemia. Laboratory reports should be monitored by the nurse and deviations from normal reported promptly to the physician. The nurse must be prepared to give emergency care for anaphylaxis, and seizure precautions should be instituted. Because hypokalemia often develops, foods high in potassium should be encouraged. Adequate sodium intake should also be maintained; sodium depletion increases the risk of renal toxicity.

General supportive measures (adequate diet and rest, management of stress levels) are important in promoting the client's natural resistance to infection and ability to heal damaged tissue.

Client education. Both amphotericin B and flucytosine are toxic drugs; clients may become more ill when therapy is established. They need good, supportive care to alleviate the physical symptoms (anorexia, nausea, vomiting, chills and fever, headache, and pain) and emotional support to persevere through the course of treatment. Although the alternative to treatment is progressive, illness and death, the duration of treatment (which may last for months), and the severity of adverse reactions make the period of treatment extremely stressful.

Before administering drugs to treat systemic fungal infections, the client should be informed about the expected beneficial and possible adverse reactions.

Clients should be provided with information about adverse reactions, and how to contact the physician if any occur. In addition, clients treated with experimen-

Example of nursing process and reaction to amphotericin B

The client is a 63-year-old man who has been receiving hyperalimentation through a central venous catheter as part of his treatment for a debilitating intestinal condition. A candida septicemia has been diagnosed and intravenous amphotericin B prescribed.

Within a half-hour following initiation of the IV antifungal agent, the client complains of feeling cold and begins to shiver.

Assessment data	Nursing diagnosis	Intervention	Goals and outcome criteria
Amphotericin B therapy Shaking chills	Altered comfort: shaking chills related to fever secondary to intravenous administration of amphotericin B	**Spread** extra blankets on the client's bed to assist him in conserving body heat. **Slow** the flow of the intravenous antifungal to a keep-open rate until the chill ends. Monitor vital signs. Notify the physician of the client's condition. **Consult** with the physician for a change in the flow rate of the intravenous medication to one that is tolerated by the client without repeated episodes of chills and fever. (The rate of flow may be halved initially, then gradually increased in subsequent treatments as the client's tolerance rises.) When the chill ends, **adjust** the number of blankets to whatever keeps the client warm enough not to shiver. **Administer** any antipyretic drug the physician orders to control the client's fever. **Administer** any anti-inflammatory drug the physician may order. Consult with the physician regarding the need to add an anti-inflammatory steroid to subsequent bottles of amphotericin B.	Within a half-hour of initiating treatment, the client's shivering will stop, and he will state that he is more comfortable. Within an hour of administering an antipyretic, the client's temperature will decrease. During subsequent infusions of amphotericin B, chills and fever will not develop.

tal drugs must have full knowledge about the dangers involved. They may be required to sign an informed consent. They should be informed of their right to stop treatment at any time that they wish.

Clients should receive information on adequate dietary measures while on the medication, with particular instruction on replacing substances that may be depleted by the treatment, as with sodium depletion caused by amphotericin B.

Evaluation Data required for evaluation include evidence that the inflammation and infection have been reduced or eliminated; adverse drug reactions and the time required to detect and treat them; the client's subjective assessment of anxiety during the treatment phase; and the ability of the client to repeat to the nurse information included in the teaching plan.

(See the accompanying Example of Nursing Process and Reaction to Amphotericin B.)

Checklist of nursing actions

☐ Question clients who are about to receive amphotericin B therapy to determine if there is a history of convulsive disorders. Take seizure precautions for all clients treated with this drug.

☐ Assess clients completely on admission and periodically during treatment to detect adverse drug reactions promptly.

☐ Monitor clients receiving amphotericin B for allergic hypersensitive reactions.

☐ Be prepared to administer emergency treatment should an anaphylactic reaction occur.

☐ Control IV infusions of amphotericin B with infusion control devices or pumps.

☐ Monitor clients receiving either amphotericin B or flucytosine for bone marrow depression and renal or liver impairment.

☐ Monitor clients receiving flucytosine for confusion, hallucinations, or other signs and symptoms of CNS impairment.

☐ Encourage high dietary potassium intake while systemic antifungals are in use; monitor serum potassium levels.

☐ Provide good supportive nursing care to increase general resistance to the fungal infection.

References

Benowitz SI. (1985). Interferon may reduce MS attacks. *Science News, 126,* 231.

Gilman AG, et al, eds. (1990). *Goodman and Gilman's the pharmacological basis of therapeutics*, 8th ed, pp 949–952, 1219–1239. New York: Pergamon Press.

Lawrence R. (1989). *Breastfeeding. A guide for the medical profession*, 3rd ed., p 392. St Louis: CV Mosby Co.

Bibliography

Angier N. (1991). Gene that checks cell growth may be key to many cancers. *The N.Y. Times, April 23,* 140, C9.

Another role for TNF/cachectin. (1986). *Science News, 130,* 328.

Benowitz SI. (1984). More kudos for interferon. *Science News, 126,* 294.

Chee M, et al. (1990). Human cytomegalovirus encodes 3 G protein-coupled receptor homolologues. *Nature, 344,* 774–777

*Gever LN. (1984). Giving amphotericin B for systemic fungal infections. *Nursing 84, 14(7),* 8.

Gilman AG, et al, eds. (1990). *Goodman and Gilman's the pharmacological basis of therapeutics*, 8th ed, pp 949–952, 1219–1239. New York: Pergamon Press.

Glaberson W. (1991). A tide of anxiety over rabies sweeps the N.Y. region. *The N.Y. Times, May 6,* 140, B1.

*Good news—at last—for herpes patients. (1985). *American Journal of Nursing, 85,* 355.

*Help for herpes. (1986). *Nursing 86, 16(7),* 19.

Hepatotoxic potential of ketoconazole under investigation. (1987). *FDA Drug Bulletin, 12(2),* 11.

McEvoy GK, ed. (1987). *Drug Information 87*, pp 67–80, 348–355. Bethesda: American Society of Hospital Pharmacists.

Okino K, Weibert R. (1986). Warfarin-griseofulvin interaction. *Drug Intell Clin Pharm, 20,* 291–293.

*Raloff J. (1985). A cure for the common cold? *Science News, 127,* 292.

Rosenberg S, et al. (1990). Gene therapy for gene transfer into humans-immunotherapy with advanced melanomas using tumor-infiltrating lymphocytes modified by retroviral gene transduction. *N Engl J Med, 323(9),* 570–578.

Silberner J. (1986). AIDS drug: Not cure, but hope. *Science News, 130,* 196.

*Silberner J. (1987). AIDS drug approval recommended. *Science News, 131,* 56.

*Recommended for further reading.

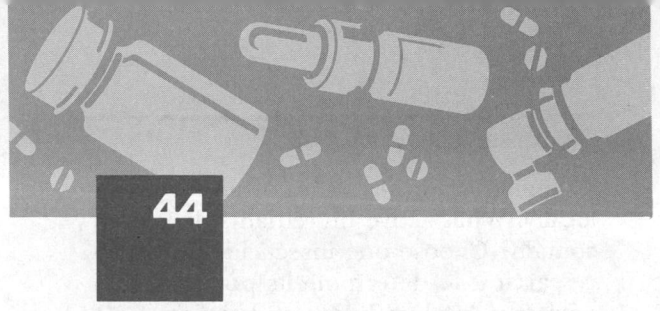

44

Drugs used to control vector-borne diseases and protozoan, helminthic, and ectoparasitic infections

Vector-borne diseases

Rickettsial diseases

Rickettsiae, rod-shaped to round microorganisms found in the tissue cells of lice, fleas, ticks, and mites, are transmitted to humans by bites. They are smaller than bacteria and cause many diseases that affect humans (Box 44-1). These diseases generally cause fever and rash and may progress to bronchopneumonia or cause other potentially fatal complications.

The best way to control rickettsial diseases is to suppress the animals and insects that serve as reservoirs of infection. The illnesses are uncommon in environments where good public sanitation is consistently maintained. Not only must the insects be combated, but also the mammals that harbor these insects, such as rats and mice. A crucial factor in maintaining sanitary environments is the destruction of rodents' and insects' habitats. Simple cleanliness and physical barriers that exclude these pests from human dwellings are important measures. Encouraging the natural enemies of these pests also helps to reduce their populations. For examples, frogs, toads, and birds eat large numbers of insects; snakes and large birds prey on rodents.

When natural controls and cleanliness are inadequate and dangerous numbers of disease-carriers de-

---

Box 44-1. Diseases caused by rickettsiae

- The spotted fever group (Rocky Mountain spotted fever, boutonneuse fever, rickettsial pox)
- The typhus group (typhus fever, murine typhus, recrudescent epidemic typhus [Brill's disease])
- Scrub typhus
- Q fever
- Trench fever

---

velop, other measures must be taken to control rickettsial diseases. This development is most likely to occur during civil disruption or serious damage to the environment, as in war, floods, and other disasters. In such cases, the incidence of disease can be reduced by the judicious use of rodenticides and insecticides or by immunization against diseases such as typhus fever and Rocky Mountain spotted fever. Active cases of disease are treated with antimicrobial drugs.

Antibiotic therapy

The drug of choice for treating rickettsial illnesses is tetracycline. This antibiotic produces striking clinical improvement within 24 hours after that initiation of treatment. It shortens the duration of the disease and lowers the incidence of relapses and complications. When tetracycline is inappropriate because of a client's sensitivity, pregnancy, age, or impaired renal function, chloramphenicol is used. These drugs are discussed in Chapter 41.

Vaccination

Vaccines are available to prevent Rocky Mountain spotted fever and typhus fever. Vaccines are discussed in Chapter 36.

■ Summary

Rickettsial diseases in humans are often serious and potentially fatal. They are best controlled by suppressing the animals and insects that

---

Enrichment experience 44-1

Examine warfarin rodenticides offered for sale in local stores. Compare preparations of pure drugs with those that contain bait. If possible, evaluate the odor and appearance of the compounds. Are they likely to be attractive to children? Do the directions for use on the labels specify safety measures to prevent accidental ingestion by animals and humans?

Enrichment experience 44-2

Examine liquid pesticides offered for sale locally. What active ingredients does each contain? Choose one insecticide and research it to determine its potential for environmental pollution and toxicity.

---

serve as carriers. Rodenticides and insecticides used to reduce populations of these pests are themselves poisons that can cause health problems in desirable animals and humans. Guidelines for safe use must be followed closely. The drugs of choice for treating rickettsial diseases are the tetracyclines.

Nursing management

Nursing implications

Because of the difficulty in treating rickettsial infections and their potential for causing serious disease, it is important to maintain environmental sanitation to prevent infection. The elimination of rodents and insect carriers from the immediate environment is of great concern to nurses, particularly those in the public health field.

Caution must be used when poisons are employed to eliminate the animal and insect carriers of disease. Directions and precautions for the use of rodenticides and insecticides must be followed. Improper use or accidental exposure can lead to poisoning in humans.

Nursing process

Assessment Data required for assessment include signs and symptoms of rickettsial disease, information about drugs prescribed for the treatment of these infections, client knowledge of rickettsial disease and its transmission and treatment, and client knowledge and practices regarding control of disease vectors (rodents and insects).

Nursing diagnosis Nursing diagnoses for clients who have contracted a rickettsial disease are likely to include the following:

> High risk for altered body temperature: fever secondary to infection
> High risk for diarrhea secondary to infection
> Knowledge deficit concerning rickettsial diseases, their prevention, transmission, and treatment
> Knowledge deficit related to the safe use of pesticides and insecticides

Planning Goals of treatment are to eliminate the signs and symptoms of infection, to prevent (or promptly detect and treat) adverse drug reactions, and

Example of nursing process and control of rodent infestation

The clients are a 19-year-old mother and her 2-year-old daughter, who has just recovered from a rat bite to her right big toe.

    The family has recently moved into an apartment in a public housing area. The mother has taken no measures to control pests on the premises, although she sees a rat somewhere in the building almost every day. The mother states that she remembers her mother setting spring traps for mice, but she knows no other methods of rodent control.

Assessment data	Nursing diagnosis	Intervention	Goals and outcome criteria
Statement by the client that she knows of no ways to control rats Visible rats on the premises History of rat bite to child	Knowledge deficit concerning measures to control rodents in living area	A teaching plan should be developed and implemented that will cover the following: (1) the role home construction and repair plays in controlling ingress of rodents into residential buildings; (2) the importance of storing garbage properly (in metal containers with tight-fitting covers) to decrease the food available to sustain rodent populations; (3) safe use of rodenticides (placing poisoned bait in areas that are inaccessible to pets or children); (4) procedures for reporting to the housing authority conditions (broken doors or windows, presence of pests) that need to be corrected; and (5) suggestions for enlisting the help of neighbors in a concerted effort to control rodents.	After control measures are taken, rodents will no longer be readily visible in the residences; injuries and illness attributable to rodents will no longer occur; adverse reaction to rodenticides will not occur.

to teach the client about rickettsial diseases, their transmission and treatment, and methods to prevent their occurrence.

Intervention Nursing measures to alleviate symptoms of disease and to support natural resistance to infection are appropriate. Clients must be monitored for adverse drug reaction.

    Client education. Educate clients about rickettsial diseases, their transmission and treatment, and methods to prevent their occurrence. Clients need to be taught about the prescribed medication, the expected beneficial effects, and possible adverse reactions. They also need to be taught to protect themselves from the effects of pesticides and rodenticides.

Evaluation Data required for evaluation include signs and symptoms of infection, signs and symptoms of adverse drug reaction, the client's subsequent practices for preventing rickettsial disease, and the incidence of recurrent infection (see the Example of Nursing Process and Control of Rodent Infestation).

Checklist of nursing actions

- ☐ Teach clients techniques for avoiding contact with carriers of rickettsial diseases.
- ☐ Help clients learn nonpharmaceutical methods for controlling rodents and insects.
- ☐ Caution clients to follow directions for using rodenticides and insecticides.

☐ Warn clients to avoid unnecessary exposure to pesticides.

☐ Take a careful history from clients affected by rickettsial infections to determine the means of exposure.

Lyme disease

Lyme disease was first recognized in the United States in 1975, when an outbreak occurred in the small Connecticut town for which it was named. Since then, the disease has proliferated to the point at which cases have been reported on three continents and in 45 of the contiguous states in this country. The heaviest outbreaks have been in southern New England, Suffolk county of eastern Long Island, NY, and in Georgia.

Lyme disease is caused by the bite of several different ticks, including *Ixodes dammini, I. scapularis,* and *I. pacificus,* all of which can transmit the spirochete *Borrelia burgdorferi* at any time during their 2-year life cycle. Prompt tick removal helps prevent transmission of the disease. Lyme disease usually occurs during the late spring and early summer, when the tick transmits the spirochete from its host (deer, mouse, bird, or other animal) to humans.

The disease process parallels the stages of untreated syphilis, also a spirochete disease. It starts with a rash (in this case a bull's eye pattern about 4 inches in diameter) and possibly flulike symptoms (mild, if at all), which disappear. In some instances, neither the rash nor any other symptoms appear, making diagnosis difficult. Within weeks to months, arthritis, cardiac, or neurologic symptoms appear. As with syphilis, treatment at the onset of Lyme disease usually prevents the complications.

Diagnosis of Lyme disease is difficult to determine because no national reference standard for a laboratory test exists, the symptoms vary considerably, and even the rash, if present, is inconsistent in appearance. Therefore, Lyme disease is not diagnosed in some clients, who then do not receive proper treatment, while other cases may have a false positive diagnosis, causing clients to be treated for nonexistent disease. Prevention of chronic arthritis depends on proper treatment with antibiotics within the first 6 weeks after the infection develops. Clients in endemic areas are urged to save ticks for identification, thus speeding the diagnostic procedure.

Prevention of Lyme disease has centered on limited use of insect repellents that contain *N* diethylmeta-toluamide (DEET), protective clothing (long sleeves and pants), as well as the use of insecticides on lawns in areas where the ticks are prevalent. If lawns are sprayed, care should be taken to protect human and pet populations by keeping them out of the areas being sprayed. Planting chrysanthemums, which appear to have a natural tick repellent, may also help.

Ivermectin has been given to deer to kill the ticks feeding on them, and deer have also been killed to lessen the tick population. Natural methods of tick control have included the introduction of a small wasp that is an enemy of the tick, but does not sting humans, and the use of pheromones that attract ticks to insecticide traps. A gene-engineered vaccine has been developed to protect mice against Lyme disease and may lead to a vaccine for humans.

Antibiotic therapy

The drugs used to treat Lyme disease are doxycycline, tetracycline, amoxicillin, or ampicillin. If started promptly, these oral antibiotics usually shorten the period that symptoms are present and prevent cardiac, neurologic, and arthritic problems in the future. These drugs are discussed in Chapter 41.

Enrichment experience 44-3

You have been invited to spend a spring weekend in a rustic area of Suffolk County on Long Island, NY, where outbreaks of Lyme disease have occurred. Describe the clothing you would wear while outdoors. Your hosts have three young children, a dog, and two kittens in their home. What precautions would you advise your hosts to take when county pesticide spraying takes place?

■ **Summary**

Lyme disease is difficult to diagnose; therefore, the initiation of proper treatment may be delayed or, in some cases, unnecessarily instituted. Methods of reducing the tick population must be carried out so as not to endanger humans or the environment. The risk of tick bites can be reduced through the use of protective clothing when outdoors in endemic areas.

Nursing management

Nursing implications

Because of the difficulty in making a prompt and accurate diagnosis of Lyme disease, it is important to prevent the infection from occurring. After outdoor activities, the skin should be searched, and any ticks should be carefully removed. If a bite has been sustained, the tick should be saved to facilitate diagnosis.

Nursing process

Assessment Data required for assessment include signs and symptoms of Lyme disease, identification of the tick if possible, and information about the drugs prescribed for treatment. An evaluation should be made of client knowledge of Lyme disease and its transmission and treatment and client knowledge and practices regarding control of disease vectors and their hosts (deer, mice, birds).

Nursing diagnosis Nursing diagnoses for clients who have (or have the potential to develop) Lyme disease are likely to include the following:

Altered comfort: joint pains, fatigue, and malaise secondary to infection
Altered family processes related to inability of affected person to maintain family role function
Knowledge deficit related to Lyme disease and its prevention and treatment
Knowledge deficit regarding safe use of insecticides
Potential for impaired tissue integrity secondary to adverse reactions to anti-infective treatment

Common collaborative problems that should be differentiated from the nursing diagnoses include

Potential complication: cardiovascular
Potential complication: musculoskeletal

Planning Goals of treatment are to alleviate the initial discomfort caused by the infection, prevent its progression to the stage of chronic arthritic, cardiac, or neurologic problems, and assist the family to adjust to altered role function of the affected member. Other goals include prevention, detection, and treatment of any adverse drug reactions and education of the client and family about Lyme disease, its prevention, transmission, and treatment.

Intervention Nursing measures to alleviate symptoms of the disease and to support natural resistance to infection are appropriate. The nurse may use crisis intervention techniques to assist family adjustment; a referral for family counseling may be appropriate. The client must be monitored for adverse drug reactions.

Client education. A teaching plan should be developed and implemented to inform the client about Lyme disease, its prevention, transmission, and treatment. This should include methods of controlling disease vectors (deer, mice, birds) as well as ways to protect self and others from the effects of pesticides.

Clients must be educated to wear protective clothing when outdoors in endemic areas. Appropriate clothing includes hats, pants, and shirts that cover the body and extremities, with cloth of sufficient thickness to prevent ticks from reaching the skin.

Insecticides may be applied to exposed skin and clothing. DEET is applied to clothing or directly to the skin. Permethrin is applied to clothing. These agents should be use sparingly, since they may cause toxic encephalopathy.

If a tick bite does occur, the tick should be removed with tweezers, at a 45° angle, to reduce the risk of injection of the spirochete into the tissues. The tick should be saved for identification, especially if a bite has occurred.

Evaluation Data required for evaluation include signs and symptoms of infection, the quality of family interactions, and the client's subsequent practices for preventing Lyme disease.

Checklist of nursing actions

☐ Employ nursing measures to relieve clients' discomfort and support their resistance to infection.
☐ Assist the family to adapt to the client's disability; refer for family counseling if appropriate.
☐ Monitor client's responses to the treatment regimen.
☐ Teach clients techniques for avoiding contact with the carriers of Lyme disease.
☐ Caution clients to follow directions when using insecticides.
☐ Warn clients against unnecessary exposure to pesticides.
☐ Teach clients the techniques for removing and preserving the tick for identification when tick bites occur.

Protozoan infections

Protozoa are among the most important causative agents of parasitic diseases. A warm climate, unsanitary conditions, and overcrowding favor their transmission. Especially prevalent in the underdeveloped tropical areas of the world, protozoa affect a large proportion of the world's population and are a major cause of morbidity and mortality. Vector control and improved sanitation seem to be the most reliable methods of eradicating or controlling these illnesses. However, even massive international campaigns have been unsuccessful in achieving this goal. In some areas of the world, protozoan infections have been controlled for a time only to recur at a later date. With modern rapid transportation, spread of the disease from reservoirs of infection is likely, even when great distances are involved. Obviously, as long as these protozoan diseases remain epidemic or endemic in large areas of the world, chemotherapy for their treatment is important.

The agents being used to treat protozoan diseases are not ideal drugs. In many cases, organisms have become resistant to previously effective drugs. Continued research is needed to discover and develop more effective drugs that are less toxic and less likely to induce the emergence of resistant disease strains.

Although many of the diseases discussed here are rarely seen in developed countries, it is important for all nurses to have a basic understanding of them. Nurses should also be aware of methods for controlling their spread and the medical treatment of victims. A small number of cases do occur in people who have returned from abroad and in populations exposed to overcrowding and unsanitary conditions. The danger of epidemics or the re-establishment of diseases previously eradicated from a territory is always present. The World Health Organization reports that nearly one of every ten people in the world suffers from a tropical disease. Yearly, malaria infects 270 million, schistosomiasis infects 200 million, and lymphatic filariasis infects 90 million.

Tourists from the U.S. have become more adventurous and increasingly travel to areas where tropical diseases are rampant. Many health professionals are unfamiliar with these diseases, are unable to diagnose them, and do not know the most effective treatments for them. Travelers are therefore at risk of not receiving proper information to safeguard their health while traveling and of placing the population at-large at risk of contracting tropical diseases that they may bring back to this country. To meet this need, travel medicine clinics are opening throughout the U.S. to counsel those who are going to areas where unfamiliar diseases may prevail.

Travel medicine clinics not only advise clients about health problems in the areas to be visited but are authorized to administer yellow fever vaccinations that are required for entry into some countries. Clients should be given information as to the location of the clinics or directed to tropical disease centers, epidemiology departments of hospitals, or state health agencies that can provide the information.

Enrichment experience 44-4

Contact the local health department to determine the prevalence of malaria in the local community. Is the disease considered to be endemic? If not, what factors are associated with occurrence of the disease? What therapeutic agents are used most commonly by local physicians to treat malaria?

Malaria
Malaria causes an estimated 2 million deaths each year. It is still prevalent in many lands and infects many people. About 80% of the imported malaria cases reported by U.S. travelers during 1980 to 1988 were acquired in sub-Saharan Africa, with 27 fatal infec-

tions. Backpackers or adventure travelers are probably at higher risk than tourists in air-conditioned hotels.

The oldest treatment for malaria was ingestion of a tea made from the bark of the cinchona tree of South America. The infusion contained several alkaloids, one of which (quinine) eliminated the symptoms of the disease. Until the third decade of the 20th century, quinine was the only available effective antimalarial agent. In 1930, the first antimalarial synthetic drug, quinacrine (Atabrine), was introduced. For a brief period it was the official drug for the treatment of malaria. During World War II, quinacrine was produced on a large scale by the Allied Nations to replace quinine, which was still in short supply. However, because of its relative toxicity and therapeutic limitations, further research developed newer more improved agents.

Malarial strains that are resistant to all of these newer agents have emerged. In fact, resistance frequently develops to one of the most effective drugs, chloroquine. As research continues, newer and better drugs may displace present drugs, especially those to which the malaria organism has become resistant. Drugs most frequently used are listed in Tables 44-1 and 44-2.

Pathophysiology
The action of antimalarial drugs and the rationale that underlies treatment is best understood in relation to the biologic nature of the malarial infection. Four species of the genus *Plasmodium* cause malaria in humans; their characteristics are listed in Table 44-3.

Humans are infected by carrier mosquitoes, usually of the anopheles type. (Occasionally, malaria transmission is via blood transfusion or congenitally from mother to fetus). The cycle is shown in Figure 44-1. Malarial sporozoites, present in the saliva of the mosquito, are deposited under the skin, and travel through the circulation to the parenchymal cells of the liver and other tissues, where they undergo asexual cell division and reproduction, forming spores called *merozoites*. During this pre-erythrocyte phase of the disease, the victim remains free of symptoms. On reaching maturity, the merozoites rupture the cells in which they were formed and are released into the circulation. Most enter erythrocytes to start the blood cycle of the disease. In all forms of malaria except infection with *Plasmodium falciparum*, some of the merozoites infect more tissue cells, a stage of the disease (*exoerythrocytic cycle*) that may continue for several years, causing relapses in the infected person. The merozoites that infect red blood cells develop and divide asexually, eventually bursting from the ruptured red cells. The liberated spores invade still more erythrocytes, reproducing once again. After several such cycles, the number of organisms is sufficient to destroy large numbers of red blood cells each time a new generation of merozoites is produced. The release of swarms of malarial organisms and of large amounts of cellular

Table 44-1. Drugs used in the prophylaxis of malaria

Drug	Adult dose	Pediatric dose
chloroquine phosphate (Aralen)	300 mg base (500 mg salt) orally, once/week	5 mg/kg base (8.3 mg/kg salt) orally, once/week, up to maximum adult dose of 300 mg base
hydroxychloroquine sulfate (Plaquenil)	310 mg base (400 mg salt) orally, once/week	5 mg/kg base (6.5 mg/kg salt) orally, once/week, up to maximum adult dose
mefloquine (Lariam)	228 mg base (250 mg salt) orally, once/week*	15–19 kg: ¼ tab/week* 20–30 kg: ½ tab/week* 31–45 kg: ¾ tab/week* >45 kg: 1 tab/week*
doxycycline (Vibramycin)	100 mg orally, once/day	>8 years of age: 2 mg/kg of body weight orally/day up to adult dose of 100 mg/day
proguanil (Paludrine)	200 mg orally, once/day in combination with weekly chloroquine	<2 years: 50 mg/day 2–6 years: 100 mg/day 7–10 years: 150 mg/day >10 years: 200 mg/day
primaquine	15 mg base (26.3 mg salt) orally, once/day for 14 days	0.3 mg/kg base (0.5 mg/kg salt) orally once/day for 14 days

*The dose (250 mg for an adult) should be taken once each week for 4 weeks, followed by one dose every other week, as indicated in Figure 44-1.

debris produces the chills and fever that mark the beginning of an exacerbation of the disease.

Some of the merozoites that invade erythrocytes fail to follow the asexual pattern of reproduction. Instead, they form male and female gametocytes, which develop no further in the human host. However, when a victim is bitten by a carrier mosquito, these sexual forms are ingested by the insect. In the gut of the mosquito, the gametocytes unite to produce a zygote that subsequently develops into an oocyte in the gut wall. Oocytes eventually give rise to the infective sporozoite, completing the life cycle of the parasite.

Choice of therapy

During the past 10 years, the malaria parasite has learned to outwit the drugs that have been used in its prevention and cure. Even chloroquine, once thought to be the ultimate drug of choice, is no longer reliable. Chloroquine resistance is common in all malarious areas except Haiti and Central America north of the Panama Canal. Alternative drugs, although available, are not fully effective, require difficult schedules, cause serious side effects, or are too expensive; for example, mefloquine costs more than $5 per capsule. After only a year of use, strains of malaria resistant to its action were reported. Two newer drugs, halofantrine and artemisinin, have also proved to induce the rapid emergence of resistant strains. Another drug, fansidar has been resisted by 30% of the various malarial strains. It has also caused some rare but life-threatening reactions. Quinine, used for centuries in South America as an antipyretic, is also ineffective

Table 44-2. Drug used in the presumptive treatment of malaria

Drug	Adult dose	Pediatric dose weight (kg): tablet(s)
pyrimethamine-sulfadoxine (Fansidar)	3 tablets (75 mg pyrimethamine and 1,500 mg sulfadoxine), orally as a single dose	5–10:½ 11–20:1 21–30:1½ 31–45:2 >45:3

Chemoprophylaxis should continue during travel in the malarious areas and for 4 weeks after a person leaves the malarious areas (except for mefloquine, for which two tablets after the end of exposure are adequate). *For travel to areas of risk where chloroquine-resistant* P. falciparum; *has NOT been reported*, once-weekly use of chloroquine *alone* is recommended. Chloroquine is usually well tolerated. The few people who experience uncomfortable side effects may tolerate the drug better by taking it with meals or in divided twice-weekly doses. As an alternative, the related compound hydroxychloroquine may be better tolerated. Chloroquine prophylaxis can begin 1 to 2 weeks before travel to malarious areas. (Health Information for International Travel. (1990). HHS Pub. No. (CDC) 90-8280.)

Table 44-3. Malaria-causing plasmodia

Species	Form	Additional information
Plasmodium falciparum	Malignant tertian* malaria, a frequently fatal form of the disease	Attacks are acute and severe and may lead to kidney failure, coma, and death.
Plasmodium vivax	Benign tertian* malaria	This species produces milder clinical attacks than those of *P. falciparum*, but with a greater tendency to recur after treatment.
Plasmodium malariae	Quartan (4-day cycle) malaria	Common in localized areas in the tropics.
Plasmodium ovale	A rare mild form of tertian* malaria	More readily cured than *P. vivax*.

*Tertian refers to the cycle characteristic of attacks, in which chills and fever occur at 3-day intervals.

against many malarial strains, and must be taken for 7 days with another drug to be at all useful. This resistance to drugs has resulted in an increase in cases as well as more serious cases.

Researchers are also finding a multiple drug resistance gene in resistant malaria parasites. The gene seems to act in concert with a special gene that makes the parasite invulnerable to chloroquine. If this proves to be so, drugs to stop or block resistance to chloroquine could be developed to treat clients whose disease is due to resistant strains of malaria.

A new synthetic vaccine under study takes a twofold approach to the malaria parasite. It involves the use of a previously known malaria protein that induces antibody response, in combination with a newly discovered malaria protein or antigen, a natural killer cell that induces an immune cell (cytotoxic lymphocyte) response. The immune cells are able to seek out and destroy infected cells. The vaccine is being used successfully to protect mice against malaria and appears to be promising for the development of an antimalarial vaccine for humans (Box 44-2). Until such time as newer drugs or a vaccine become available, the following drugs are being used for chemoprophylaxis.

Quinine

An alkaloid derived from cinchona bark, quinine is the antimalarial drug with the longest history of use. The study of quinine has provided the background necessary for the development of more effective and less toxic synthetic antimalarials.

Pharmacodynamics. A potent schizonticide, quinine is effective both as a suppressive drug and in the control of clinical attacks. It acts by interfering with the function of plasmodial DNA. It destroys the gametocytes of *Plasmodium vivax* and *P. malariae* but not those of *P. falciparum*. It is neither a true causal prophylactic agent, nor is it effective against sporozoite or pre-erythrocytic tissue forms.

Quinine also inhibits skeletal muscle fiber response to tetanic stimulation. It has limited analgesic and antipyretic effects.

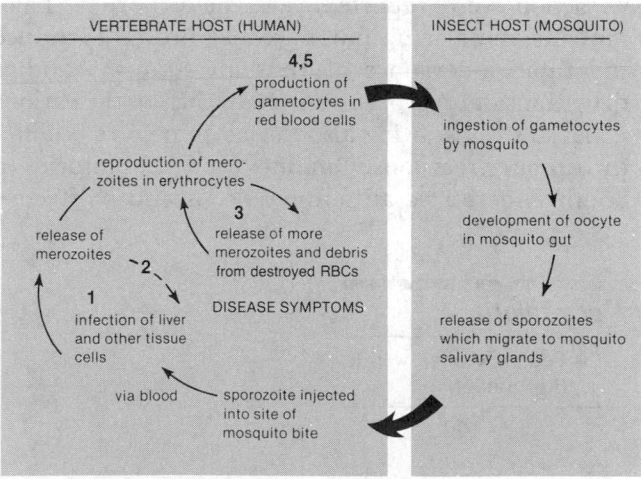

Figure 44-1. Life cycle of the malarial parasite. Points numbered on the illustration indicate the location in the malarial life cycle where specific drugs might be effective. (*1*) Chlorguanide, pyrimethamine, and primaquine used for causal prophylaxis. (*2*) Primaquine used to prevent relapses. (*3*) Agents against the erythrocytic phase: potent action—chloroquine, amodiaquine, quinine; limited action—pyrimethamine and chlorguanide. (*4*) Gametocidal drugs: primaquine. (*5*) Gametocyte sterilizing drugs: chlorguanide, pyrimethamine.

Box 44-2. Classification of antimalarial chemotherapy

- *Causal Prophylaxis:* Administering an agent that prevents infection and further transmission of malaria
- *Suppressive Treatment:* Using a drug that inhibits the erythrocytic stage of development, which produces symptoms
- *Clinical Cure:* Using schizonticides to terminate the clinical attack by interrupting erythrocytic schizogony
- *Radical Cure:* Eradicating both the erythrocytic and the exoerythrocytic parasites of an established infection
- *Suppressive Cure:* Completely eliminating malarial parasites from the body by suppressive treatment, which continues longer than the life span of the infection
- *Gametocidal Therapy:* Administering gametocides, which interrupt the disease cycle by preventing the reinfection of mosquitoes

Pharmacokinetics. Because quinine is absorbed well by the GI tract, it is administered orally. Quinine is 70% bound by plasma proteins and has a half-life of 4 to 5 hours. About 95% of the drug is degraded by the liver and other tissues. The drug is excreted primarily by the kidneys. Renal excretion is enhanced when the urine has an acidic *p*H.

Therapeutic uses. Quinine is used therapeutically in conjunction with primaquine for the radical cure of relapsing *Plasmodium vivax* malaria and for the treatment of strains of *P. falciparum* resistant to other antimalarials. It has long been used indiscriminately by the lay public for fevers, although it has little effect on nonmalarial fevers. Quinine has also been used for the management of nocturnal leg cramps (myoclonus).

Adverse reactions. Because quinine is irritating to the tissues, it can cause gastric pain, nausea, and vomiting on ingestion, pain and sterile abscesses on injection into tissues, and thrombosis when given intravenously (IV). Renal concentrations may reach toxic levels, causing tubular damage.

Cinchonism may occur with excessive doses of quinine. This syndrome is manifested by tinnitus, headache, nausea, and visual disturbances.

Precautions and contraindications. Quinine cannot be used for clients who suffer from myasthenia gravis because it decreases the excitability of the motor endplate region, so that responses to repetitive nerve stimulation and to acetylcholine are reduced; serious respiratory distress and dysphagia can occur. Extreme caution must also be exercised if the client has previously taken mefloquine prophylaxis since they are pharmacologically similar and show similar cardiovascular and neurologic toxicity.

Mefloquine

Mefloquine is recommended for use in areas where chloroquine-resistant *Plasmodium falciparum* exists. It has caused minor side effects at prophylactic levels (GI upset and dizziness) and hallucinations and convulsions at the higher treatment dosages. It is not recommended for those with a known sensitivity to it, for children under 15 kg (30 lb), pregnant women, those using β-blockers or other drugs that prolong or alter cardiac conduction, those involved in tasks that require fine coordination or special discrimination, or those with a history of epilepsy or psychiatric disorder.

Synthetic antimalarials

Although most of the synthetic antimalarials share some similarities in chemical structure with quinine, they are classified as 4-aminoquinoline derivatives (chloroquine and hydroxychloroquine), 8-aminoquinoline derivatives (primaquine), 2,4-diaminopyrimidines (pyrimethamine), and biguanides (chloroguanide). Each drug has particular advantages and disadvantages (Table 44-4).

Chloroquine. Chloroquine is highly effective in terminating acute attacks of *Plasmodium vivax* malaria and is an effective suppressant agent. It is administered in the form of medicated table salt for large-scale prophylaxis in remote areas of South America, although its value when used in this way has been questioned. Given by mouth and by injection, chloroquine is generally well tolerated; its chief adverse reactions are pruritus and GI discomfort. The most serious adverse effect of chloroquine therapy is dose-related retinopathy. It is also toxic to the eight cranial nerve. Because the drug is concentrated in the liver, it should be used with caution when hepatic disease is present. Resistance to chloroquine has developed in some strains of *P. falciparum*. The related drug, amodiaquine, is often active in these resistant infections.

Hydroxychloroquine. Hydroxychloroquine, like chloroquine, is a blood schizonticidal agent and is active against the asexual erythrocytic forms of most strains of *Plasmodium malariae*, *P. ovale*, *P. vivax*, and many strains of *P. falciparum*. The drug is not effective against pre-erythrocytic or exoerythrocytic forms of the *Plasmodia* organism or the gametocytes of *P. falciparum*. It is gametocidal for *P. malariae* and *P. vivax*.

In doses administered orally for the treatment of malaria, adverse effects of hydroxychloroquine are usually mild and reversible. The drug is used in high dosages and for prolonged periods for the treatment of autoimmune diseases (rheumatoid arthritis and lupus erythematosus), and under these circumstances, serious and irreversible toxicity including retinopathy may develop.

Like chloroquine, hydroxychloroquine tends to concentrate in the liver and should be used with caution in clients with hepatic disease or alcoholism and in clients who receive other hepatotoxic drugs.

Primaquine. Primaquine is the drug of choice for prevention of relapses of infection with *Plasmodium vivax* and *P. ovale*. It is the only agent that can eliminate the infection in the late tissue stages of relapsing malaria. Although it is fairly innocuous when given to most whites, the drug causes hemolytic reactions in some blacks and in certain white ethnic groups (Sardinians, Sephardic Jews, Greeks, and Iranians). These populations are deficient in glucose-6-phosphate dehydrogenase, a condition that also causes favism (intolerance of broad beans). Although resistant strains of malaria have been produced in the laboratory, no significant resistance seems to exist among disease strains at present.

Pyrimethamine. Pyrimethamine is generally used with sulfadoxine to treat uncomplicated chloroquine-resistant *Plasmodium falciparum* infections. The low doses of each drug used in combination therapy are believed to be less conducive to the development of resistance in the malaria organism. Pyrimethamine is

Table 44-4. Antimalarial drugs

Drug name	Preparations	Spectrum of activity	Therapeutic uses and additional information
Single agents			
chloroquine (Aralen, Avloclor, Quinachlor)	Medicated table salt (not available in the U.S.) Oral tablets Vials that contain solution for IM injection PC: C	Active against the asexual erythrocytic forms of plasmodia Effective against *E. histolytica* in extra-intestinal tissues	Used for large-scale prophylaxis in areas where malaria is endemic Treatment, suppression, and prevention of malaria (primaquine must be used concomitantly if infecting plasmodia are *P. ovale* or *P. vivax*) Treatment of extra-intestinal amebiasis Adjunct in the treatment of rheumatoid arthritis, lupus erythematosus Ototoxic Optic effects, including retinopathy, are most serious toxicity
hydroxychloroquine (Plaquenil, Tenecridine)	Oral tablets PC: C	Similar to chloroquine (see above)	Alternative when chloroquine is not available (chloroquine is considered the drug of choice)
mefloquine (Lariam)	Oral tablets PC: C	Similar to quinine Treat and prevent *P. falciparum* and *P. vivax*	Effective newer drug; some resistance noted; may cause extra systoles, neuropsychiatric disturbances, convulsion, and coma
primaquine	Oral tablets PC: C	Active against the pre-erythrocytic and exo-erythrocytic forms of *P. ovale, P. vivax, P. falciparum,* and *P. malariae*	Prevention of delayed primary attacks and relapses of malaria caused by susceptible plasmodia Radical cure of *P. vivax* or *P. ovale* malaria after a confirmed clinical attack (chloroquine or other schizonticidal agent must be used concomitantly)
pyrimethamine (Daraprim)	Oral tablets PC: C	Schizonticidal Active against the asexual erythrocytic forms of plasmodia Arrests sporogony in mosquitoes	Suppression or prevention of malaria caused by chloroquine-resistant plasmodia, especially infections caused by chloroquine-resistant *P. falciparum* Treatment of uncomplicated attacks of chloroquine-resistant *P. falciparum* malaria Causes hemolytic reactions in recipients subject to favism
quinacrine (Atabrine, Tenicridine)	Oral tablets PC: C	Active against the asexual erythrocyte forms of plasmodia Gametocidal for *P. malariae* and *P. vivax* Effective against *Giardia lamblia*	Drug of choice for treatment of giardiasis in children Suppression or prevention of malaria caused by *P. malariae* and *P. vivax* Drug of choice for suppressive treatment of malaria caused by susceptible strains

(Continued)

Table 44-4. Antimalarial drugs *(Continued)*

Drug name	Preparations	Spectrum of activity	Therapeutic uses and additional information
quinine (Coco-Quinine, Novaquinine, QM-260 Quinamm, Quine, Quiphile, Quinite, Strema)	Capsules, suspensions, and tablets for oral use IV preparation available in the U.S. only from the Parasitic Diseases Division of the Centers for Disease Control, Atlanta, GA PC: X	Schizonticidal Active against the asexual erythrocytic forms of *P. falciparum, P. malariae, P. ovale,* and *P. vivax* Gametocidal for *P. malariae* and *P. vivax*	Suppression or prevention of malaria caused by susceptible plasmodia Especially useful for infections caused by *P. falciparum* resistant to both chloroquine and pyrimethamine-sulfadoxine Treatment of uncomplicated attacks of chloroquine-resistant *P. falciparum* malaria Treatment of nocturnal leg cramps The natural alkaloid of the cinchona bark Ototoxic
Combination preparations			
chloroquine phosphate with primaquine phosphate (Aralen Phosphate with Primaquine Phosphate)	Oral tablets	Active against all stages of human malarial parasites except for certain strains of chloroquine-resistant *P. falciparum*	Prevention of malaria, regardless of species, in areas where the disease is endemic.
pyrimethamine and sulfadoxine (Fansidar)	Oral tablets	Synergistic activity against susceptible plasmodia	Drug of choice for treatment, suppression, and prevention of malaria caused by chloroquine-resistant *P. falciparum*

KEY: PC = pregnancy category. (The validity of pregnancy risk categories has not been established; see Chapter 16, p 216.)

also used as a prophylactic and suppressive agent in weekly doses. Few adverse reactions are reported when recommended dosages are not exceeded. Larger doses may produce a megaloblastic anemia that resembles that caused by folic acid deficiency. Strains of *P. falciparum* have become resistant to the drug in certain geographic areas after drug programs for mass suppression of malaria.

Quinacrine. Quinacrine is a synthetic acridine derivative structurally related to primaquine. Its mechanism of action against *Plasmodium* species is unknown. It is believed that the drug acts by combining with nucleic acid in the organism or by inhibiting digestion of hemoglobin by the parasite. It is active against the asexual erythrocytic forms of *P. malariae, P. vivax,* and *P. falciparum.* It is also gametocidal for *P. malariae* and *P. vivax* but not for *P. falciparum.* It is not active against pre-erythrocytic or exoerythrocytic forms of plasmodia.

Quinacrine is administered orally and is widely distributed into body tissues, tending to concentrate in the liver and other vascular tissue, such as bone marrow, spleen, erythrocytes, and skeletal muscle. Quinacrine crosses the placenta freely.

Adverse reactions to quinacrine include headache, dizziness, and GI upset. The drug imparts a pronounced yellow color to urine and skin, especially in children. This color change is a benign condition not related to jaundice. Central nervous system changes and skin rashes may occur. Prolonged administration may cause retinopathy. The drug can cause a disulfiram-like reaction when used with alcohol. Quinacrine is teratogenic in animals. It should be used with caution in people who have renal or cardiac diseases, those with a history of psychosis, and in the very young and in the elderly. Visual function should be monitored regularly during therapy. Quinacrine is contraindicated for people with psoriasis or porphyria and for pregnant women.

Antibacterial agents

The sulfonamides, tetracyclines, and chloramphenicol have been shown to be active against malaria. Although not as effective as other drugs, they are useful when administered in combination with either quinine or pyrimethamine to treat drug-resistant strains of malarial parasites. These antibacterial agents are discussed in Chapter 41.

Doxycycline. Doxycycline is used as an alternative when mefloquine cannot be tolerated or is contraindicated. Prophylaxis for malaria can begin 1 to 2 days before travel to malarious areas and should be continued daily while there and for 4 weeks after leaving the area. The client may develop photosensitivity while taking the drug, usually appearing as an exaggerated sunburn reaction. To lessen this possibility, the client should be cautioned against prolonged direct exposure to the sun. The client should also use sun screens that absorb long-wave ultraviolet radiation and should take the drug in the evening. Other side effects include nausea or vomiting (less when the drug is taken with meals) and monilial vaginitis. It is contraindicated in pregnancy and children younger than 8 years of age.

■ Summary

Antimalarial drugs used today include the natural alkaloid quinine and the synthetic drugs primaquine and chloroquine. Certain systemic antibacterials with antimalarial properties are used as adjuncts in the treatment of malaria. Regimens for their use and objectives of treatment vary, depending on the status of the disease in the client and whether or not malaria is endemic. Quinine and chloroquine are ototoxic. The synthetic antimalarials may cause respiratory depression and shock, especially in children. Chloroquine and quinacrine can cause retinopathy and visual impairment.

Many drugs used in the past are no longer effective because of resistance developed by the malaria strains. Even the newer drugs are rendered ineffective by some strains. Work is being aimed at developing a vaccine to replace the drugs. Prevention of infection is presently the most important weapon against the disease.

Nursing management

Nursing implications

Control of malaria requires control of mosquitoes, the vectors necessary to complete the life cycle of the *Plasmodium* species. Mosquito reproduction may be suppressed by draining watery lands and stagnant pools or by adding enough oil to stagnant pools to form a thin layer on the surface. Such environmental changes are no longer considered desirable. Wetlands are in short supply as breeding grounds for water fowl, and their elimination or contamination with noxious chemicals is no longer approved. In some areas mosquito fish (*Gambusia affinis holbrooki*) have been introduced to eat the larvae deposited in water by mosquitoes. The fish are about 1½ inches long and ecologically acceptable.

In areas that contain numerous mosquitoes, especially those known to carry disease, precautions should be taken to reduce contact between insects and people. Houses that are tightly constructed with screens at doors and windows help to exclude insects from living areas. Damp areas in basements should be treated to eliminate moisture; mosquitoes often breed in these areas and gain access to living areas through (usually unscreened) cellar doors. Lawns should be kept clipped, because long grass traps moisture and provides a good environment for mosquitoes to breed. If mosquitoes cannot be completely eliminated from indoors, canopies of netting should be installed around the beds to prevent their biting during sleep. Outdoor clothing should cover as much of the skin as possible and fit snugly at the wrists and ankles. Oil of citronella or other insect repellents may be applied to exposed areas. A minimum of repellent should be used because these chemicals may also be toxic.

Nursing process

Assessment Clients who are to receive antimalarial medication should be assessed for contraindications and risk factors for adverse drug reactions. These reactions include visual impairment from retinal damage, hearing impairment indicative of eighth cranial nerve damage, myasthenia gravis, alcoholism, liver impairment, favism, and anemia (common in those infected with malaria). A careful assessment of general health is also required. (Over a long term, malaria is a debilitating disease.) The circumstances that mandate malaria treatment (existing disease, expectation of exposure, latent disease) should be delineated.

Nursing diagnosis Nursing diagnoses likely to be made for clients infected with malaria include the following:

> *Ineffective thermoregulation: intermittent high fevers secondary to malaria*
> *Altered comfort: shaking chills and drenching perspiration secondary to malaria*
> *High risk for fluid volume deficit related to excessive perspiration*
> *Potential for ineffective breathing pattern related to neuromuscular-blocking action of antimalarial medication*
> *Impaired physical mobility related to weakness secondary to malaria exacerbations*
> *Knowledge deficit concerning malaria, its prevention, control, and treatment*

Common collaborative problems that should be differentiated from the nursing diagnoses include

> *Potential complication: renal*
> *Potential complication: tinnitus and hearing impairment related to ototoxic effects of antimalarial medication*

Planning Goals of treatment are to alleviate client discomfort, reduce or eliminate signs and symptoms of malaria, prevent adverse drug reactions, detect and treat adverse drug reactions should they occur, and teach the client about malaria, its control, and its treatment.

Intervention Nursing measures to promote comfort and resistance to infection (ample fluids, a good diet, adequate rest, and reduced stress) are basic. Measures to prevent exposure to mosquitoes must be taken. If malaria is endemic to the area, the client could be infected by more than one strain of the *Plasmodium* species, making the infection more difficult to treat. If malaria is not endemic to the area, it could be established in the mosquito population if the infected client is bitten.

Antimalarial drugs must be secured to prevent accidental ingestion by children. Fatalities due to shock and respiratory arrest from antimalarial poisoning have been reported in children who are particularly susceptible to the hypotensive and depressive effects of the drugs.

Clients should be taught to identify the early signs and symptoms of adverse drug reactions. Of particular concern are eighth cranial nerve damage and renal impairment. The client should report unusual auditory sensations (ringing or roaring noises and a sense of fullness in the ears). Changes in urinary output should also be reported. Shock and respiratory depression can occur; these conditions require immediate medical attention.

Malaria tends to be a chronic disease. Treatment may be long-term or recurrent. Because antimalarial agents cause discomfort and are somewhat hazardous, clients need a great deal of encouragement to comply with their medication regimen. The nurse should point out improvements and stress the benefits of suppressing or eradicating the disease. Clients should be informed that missed doses of medication may jeopardize the therapeutic result and may induce resistance in the malarial parasites. Clients may require assistance in developing a system of compliance to minimize missed doses of medication.

If the client is acutely ill, treatment is likely to take place in an acute-care setting. The nurse is responsible for administering the medications, which may be given parenterally at first. Quinine is usually given by mouth, although it can be administered IV. When given parenterally, quinine should be well diluted and administered by slow infusion. Because the drug is irritating to the veins, the injection site should be inspected regularly for signs of phlebitis.

Clients must be assessed regularly for adverse reactions to antimalarial drugs. Laboratory tests that indicate renal function should be monitored.

Client education. Teaching plans should be developed and implemented for each client under treatment for malaria. The client should be taught self-care techniques to support and enhance natural resistance

to infection and to ameliorate the debilitating effects of the illness. Clients should also be taught measures required to prevent transmission of malaria to others and to prevent recurrences of active infection.

Clients must learn to identify the early signs and symptoms of adverse reactions to prescribed drugs. They should be given specific directions regarding data that should be reported promptly to the physician.

Evaluation Data required for evaluation include the absence or presence of signs and symptoms of malarial infection and adverse drug reaction, as well as the client's ability to relate material conveyed during teaching sessions to carry out the drug regimen (see the Example of Nursing Process and Treatment of Malaria).

Checklist of nursing actions

☐ Teach safe and effective techniques for controlling populations of mosquitoes.

☐ Monitor clients who receive quinine or chloroquine for eighth cranial nerve irritation.

☐ Monitor clients who receive synthetic antimalarial drugs or IV quinine for hypotension and respiratory depression.

☐ Monitor urinary output of clients who receive quinine.

☐ Dilute quinine solutions for IV use and administer by slow infusion.

☐ Encourage clients who receive antimalarial medication to comply with drug regimens.

☐ Warn clients that antimalarial drugs must be secured to prevent accidental ingestion by children.

☐ Clients should be informed that there is a 24-hour telephone information service available with detailed recommendations for the prevention of malaria. The Centers for Disease Control Malaria Hotline number is (404) 332-4555.

Amebiasis

Mode of transmission and pathophysiology

The causative organism in amebiasis is the protozoan *Entamoeba histolytica*. The parasite enters the body as a cyst, a nonvegetative inactive form that is resistant to adverse environmental conditions. The mode of its transmission is by the anal to oral route—cysts voided in the feces of hosts enter the environment and are ingested through contaminated food or water or are contracted from unclean hands (Fig. 44-2). Once they are inside the intestinal tract, the organisms become active and produce daughter cells called *trophozoites*, which feed, multiply, and move about. Trophozoites can penetrate tissue, causing irritation and ulceration of the colon's mucosa and inducing diarrhea. If they

Example of nursing process and treatment of malaria

The client is a 40-year-old Vietnam veteran who has experienced an exacerbation of malaria caused by *Plasmodium malariae*. Chloroquine has been prescribed.

The client first contracted malaria during his service in Vietnam. He had one recurrence of symptoms 5 years ago, which was successfully treated with chloroquine.

No history of renal or hepatic impairment exists. The client was treated 9 months ago for retinitis of unknown etiology.

The client is presently unemployed, and he and his wife are living in a beach house on a lake. The house is run down and poorly screened. Family income is limited to what the client and his wife can earn doing odd jobs.

Assessment data	Nursing diagnosis	Intervention	Goals and outcome criteria
History of retinitis Order for chloroquine therapy Family has limited income. House is unscreened.	Potential complication: optic toxicity*	**Inform** the physician of the client's history of retinitis, so that the order may be changed to a drug less likely to damage vision.	The client will not experience an adverse drug reaction that impairs vision.
	High risk for infection: transmission of malaria to others related to exposure of the client to mosquitoes	**Explore** with the client and his wife their options regarding housing. **Refer** to social services for assistance in either repairing their current home or moving to another. **Explore** with the client and his wife their ability to obtain the food he needs during convalescence. If needed, and acceptable to them, refer to social services for financial assistance.	By the time the client is cdischarged, he and his wife will have a home that is screened to exclude insects, including mosquitoes. By the time the client is discharged, the couple will have adequate resources to supply them both with an adequate diet.

* Although potential complications generally are not included in the Examples of Nursing Process, in this situation the identification of this collaborative problem is critical to the outcome for this client and illustrates the broad range of nursing responsibilities.

enter the blood stream (commonly through the portal vein), they can migrate to the liver, lungs, heart, and eventually to the brain. In the tissues, the parasite forms potentially fatal abscesses. The infection may be active in an acute or chronic form or harbored by carriers who remain asymptomatic.

Although amebiasis occurs throughout the world, it is found mainly in the tropics, where 50% of the population may be affected, and in institutions for mentally retarded and elderly persons, where the disease tends to be spread by direct contact with fecal matter that contains the parasite. More than 10% of the world's population is said to be infected; the incidence in the U.S. is estimated to be between 2% and 5%.

Agents used for treatment

Before the mid-20th century, agents used for treating amebiasis were effective against either the intestinal or tissue organisms, but not both. To effect a cure, both kinds of drugs had to be used, and repeated courses were often necessary. Metronidazole, introduced in 1955, was the first agent effective against the parasite both within the gut and in extraintestinal tissues. Today, this compound is considered the drug of choice to treat the infection, although older agents are still used in certain situations. Metronidazole has recently been found to produce cancers in experimental animals and to induce mutation in microbial cultures. Concern over these findings has spurred further research to develop

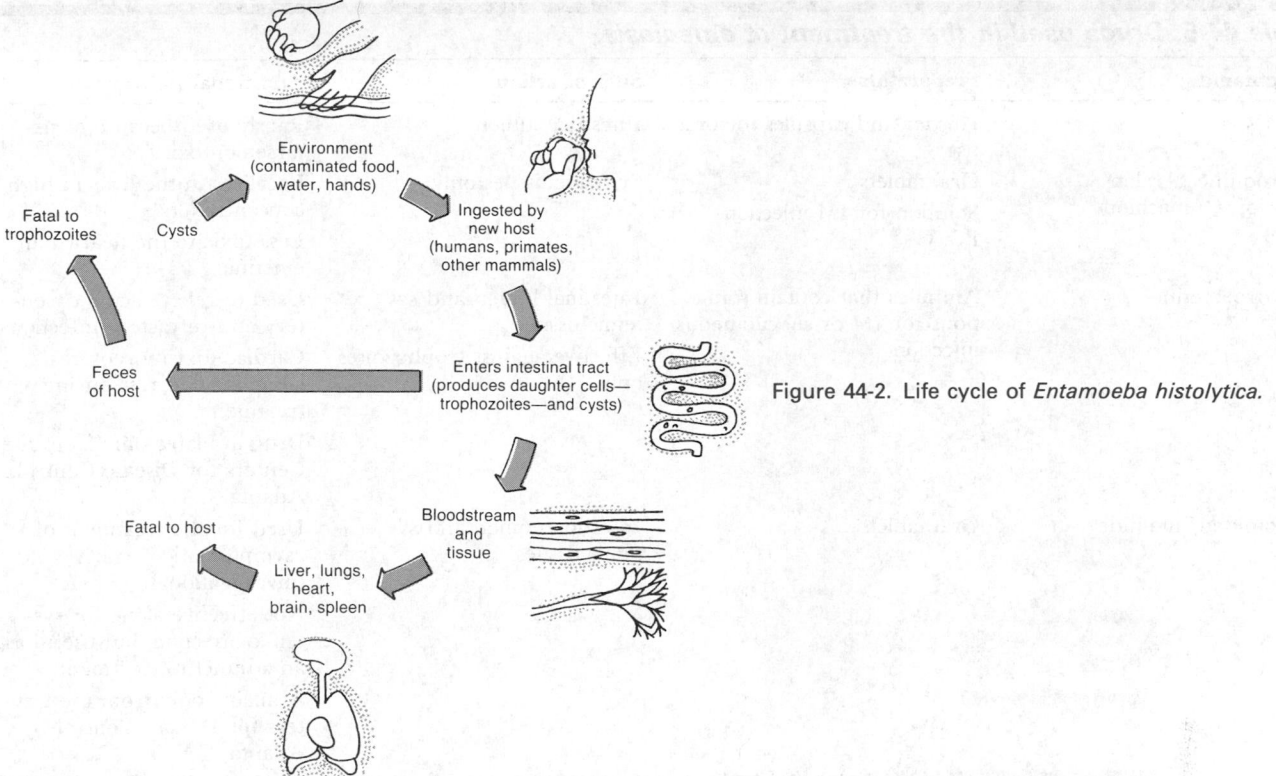

Figure 44-2. Life cycle of *Entamoeba histolytica*.

better treatment agents (drugs presently used in the treatment of amebiasis are listed in Table 44-5).

Carbarsone

Carbarsone is an organic arsenical compound that contains about 29% arsenic.

Pharmacodynamics. Carbarsone's amebicidal activity is apparently due to inhibition of sulfhydryl enzymes necessary for metabolism. It is not known why its toxicity is selective, affecting protozoa more than the cells of the host. The drug is believed to be active against the trophozoite but not against the encysted form of *Entamoeba histolytica*.

Pharmacokinetics. Carbarsone is readily absorbed from the GI mucosa. Distribution and metabolism are poorly understood, but the arsenicals in the drug appear to be converted partly to methylarsonates. Excretion is in the urine. Because elimination is slow, accumulation may occur.

Therapeutic uses. Carbarsone is rarely used because of its toxicity. However, it may be used alone in the treatment of mild cases of amebiasis and in the elimination of the carrier state in asymptomatic individuals. In combination with a tissue amebicide (metronidazole, chloroquine, or emetine), it is used in the treatment of acute or severe forms of amebiasis.

Adverse reactions. Carbarsone may cause arsenical toxicity, manifested by sore throat, edema of the ankles, knees, and wrists, pruritic skin eruptions, enlargement of the spleen, and a wide range of GI symptoms. Other adverse reactions include hepatotoxicity, neurotoxicity, nephrotoxicity, agranulocytosis, and pulmonary congestion. Convulsions have been reported. Fatalities from exfoliative dermatitis, liver necrosis, and hemorrhagic encephalitis occur rarely.

Precautions and contraindications. Carbarsone should be discontinued when any evidence of intolerance to the drug exists. Because the drug is eliminated slowly, serious problems develop if toxicity is allowed to progress beyond the early stages. Carbarsone is contraindicated for individuals with liver or kidney disease, known allergic hypersensitivity to arsenic, or visual impairment (*ie*, contracted visual or color fields). Safe use during pregnancy has not been established.

Chloroquine

Chloroquine is an antiprotozoan drug used in the treatment of malaria as well as amebiasis. See the previous section on synthetic antimalarials for further discussion of this drug.

Diloxanide furoate

Diloxanide furoate is effective against cysts and is considered by some to be the drug of choice for treating an asymptomatic carrier. It is of no value in the treatment of invasive or extraintestinal amebiasis. Treatment must be carried out for 10 days, twice the required time for paromomycin. Diloxanide furoate appears to be nontoxic; only mild GI symptoms and increased

Table 44-5. Drugs used in the treatment of amebiasis

Drug name	Preparations	Sites of action	Additional information
carbarsone	Powder and capsules for oral use	Intestinal lumen	Rarely used because of its (arsenic) toxicity
chloroquine (Aralen, Avloclor, Quinachlor)	Oral tablets Solution for IM injection PC: C	Systemic tissues only	Localizes in the liver in high concentrations Less toxic to the heart than emetine
dehydroemetine	Ampules that contain solutions for IM or subcutaneous injection	Intestinal lumen and systemic tissues Effective against trophozoites only	Used to relieve acute dysentery and refractory infections Cardiac toxicity requires complete bed rest during treatment Drug available only from the Centers for Disease Control, Atlanta, GA
diloxanide (Entamide)	Oral tablets	Intestinal lumen and systemic tissues	Used for the treatment of asymptomatic carriers (investigational) Not effective alone for systemic infection, but useful as an adjunct to treatment Available only from the Centers for Disease Control, Atlanta, GA
emetine	Ampules that contain solutions for IM injection PC: X	Intestinal lumen and systemic tissues Effective against trophozoites only	Used to relieve acute dysentery and refractory infections Cardiac toxicity requires complete bed rest during treatment Oral doses not retained Too toxic to be given IV
iodoquinol (Amequin, Diodoquin, Diquinol, Floraquin, Moebiquin, Panaquin, Vytone, Yodoxin)	Oral tablets and capsule PC: C	Intestinal lumen only Effective against both trophozoites and cysts	May cause myelo-opticneuropathy and blindness in the malnourished Not recommended for clients hypersensitive to iodine
metronidazole (Apo-Metronidazole, Clont, Flagyl, Metric 21 Tablets, Metizol, Metrogel, Neo-Metric, Novonidazol, PMS-Metronidazole, Prostat, Trichazol, Trikacide, Trikamon)	Oral tablets Parenteral solution for IV infusion PC: B	Intestinal lumen and systemic tissues Effective against both trophozoites and cysts	Drug of choice to treat amebiasis Useful for the treatment of giardiasis and anaerobic bacterial infections Aspiration of amebic abscesses possibly required May cause a disulfiram reaction May turn urine reddish-brown
paromomycin (Humatin)	Oral capsules PC: C	Intestinal lumen only	Not well absorbed by the intestinal tract Course of treatment shorter than that with other amebicides

KEY: PC = pregnancy category. (The validity of pregnancy risk categories has not been established; see Chapter 16, p 216.)

flatulence have been reported. The drug is available only by special request from the Centers for Disease Control in Atlanta, Georgia.

Emetine
Emetine was first used as an amebicide in 1912, when the drug was shown to kill ameba *in vitro*.

Pharmacodynamics. Emetine acts as a general protoplasmic poison and interferes with the multiplication of trophozoites.

Pharmacokinetics. Emetine and dehydroemetine (an investigational analogue available from the U.S. Centers for Disease Control) are administered by deep intramuscular (IM) injection. They are not administered orally because they are highly irritating to the GI tract. After absorption, the drugs spread quickly throughout the tissues, with high concentrations in the liver. They are excreted slowly by the kidneys and tend to accumulate in the tissues.

Therapeutic uses. Emetine and dehydroemetine are used to treat clients with severe dysentery who require quick relief of symptoms, those with refractory infections, and those with extraintestinal infections. Because it is toxic, emetine should not be used to treat mild or asymptomatic amebiasis. These drugs are effective against amebic hepatitis and amebic liver abscess but not against amebic cysts. Treatment by emetine must be supplemented by a concurrent course of metronidazole, tetracycline, or another drug effective against cysts.

Adverse reactions. Both emetine and dehydroemetine are toxic, and clients must be hospitalized during treatment. The drugs can cause severe cardiovascular toxicity (*eg*, arrhythmia, hypotension, chest pain, congestive heart failure, cardiac arrest). Gastrointestinal reactions are seen in up to 50% of treated clients and include diarrhea, abdominal cramps, nausea, and vomiting.

Precautions and contraindications. During treatment, recipients of emetine therapy are kept on bed rest and must be closely monitored for signs and symptoms of cardiac malfunction. The drug must be used with extreme caution in the elderly and in those with underlying cardiovascular or renal disease.

Iodoquinol
Iodiquinol is a synthetic 8-hydroxyquinoline with amebicidal properties. It contains about 64% iodine.

Pharmacodynamics. The precise mechanism of action of iodoquinol is unknown. It acts primarily against amebae in the intestinal lumen.

Pharmacokinetics. Iodoquinol is poorly absorbed from the GI tract and acts primarily within the lumen. Elimination is mainly in feces. The fate of absorbed drug is not fully understood. One study reported that, after distribution to the tissues, iodine appears in the urine. The drug was conjugated to glucuronide and sulfate.

Therapeutic uses. At one time 8-hydroxyquinolines were sold over the counter and widely used to treat travelers' diarrhea. Because of a serious side effect (optic neuropathy) detected in Japan, distribution in the U.S. is now limited to prescription use.

Iodoquinol is used in the treatment of intestinal amebiasis. It is considered the drug of choice for the treatment of asymptomatic cyst carriers.

Adverse reactions. The most serious adverse effect of iodoquinol is neurotoxicity, particularly optic neuritis, optic atrophy, and peripheral neuropathy. Children and poorly nourished individuals are at increased risk. In Japan, where serious visual problems that stemmed from use of the drug were first reported, the reaction took the form of subacute myelo-opticoneuropathy, which resulted in blindness.

Other adverse reactions that have been observed include chills, fever, dermatitis, anal irritation and itching, abdominal discomfort, diarrhea, and headache. A generalized furunculosis is apparently caused by the drug's high iodine content, which can also precipitate reactions in iodine-sensitive people, cause thyroid enlargement, and interfere with thyroid function tests for many weeks after the completion of a course of therapy.

Precautions and contraindications. Iodoquinol should be administered with caution to malnourished individuals, children, and those with thyroid disorders. Clients who receive the drug should be advised to notify their physician if skin rash occurs. Iodoquinol should be discontinued if allergic symptoms develop.

Iodoquinol is contraindicated for individuals with hepatic or renal impairment, optic neuropathy, or known allergy to iodine or 8-hydroxyquinolines.

Safe use during pregnancy and lactation has not been established.

Metronidazole
Metronidazole (Flagyl), originally introduced for treatment of infection with *Trichomonas vaginalis*, another protozoan infection, was soon recognized as a superior agent for the treatment of amebiasis.

Pharmacodynamics. Metronidazole is bactericidal and trichomonacidal, as well as amebicidal. The mechanism of action of this drug has never been fully explained. The drug is known to disrupt DNA and inhibit nucleic acid synthesis. It is equally effective against dividing and nondividing cells.

Pharmacokinetics. Taken by mouth, metronidazole is about 80% absorbed. Residues that remain in the intestinal tract eradicate the trophozoites that reside in the large bowel. For these reasons, the drug is effective in treating both intraluminal and extraluminal amebae.

After absorption, metronidazole is widely distributed into body tissues and fluids, including the cerebrospinal fluid and cerebral and hepatic abscesses. Protein binding is less than 20%. The drug readily crosses the placenta and is distributed in breast milk.

Plasma half-life of metronidazole is between 6 and 8 hours in normal adults. Plasma half-life is not prolonged by renal impairment but is by hepatic impairment. The drug is metabolized by the liver and excreted in both urine and feces. Metronidazole is removed by hemodialysis but not by peritoneal dialysis.

Therapeutic uses. Metronidazole is used in the treatment of trichomoniasis, amebiasis, giardiasis, and anaerobic bacterial infections. It is also used to prevent postoperative anaerobic bacterial infections in people who are undergoing intestinal surgery, in which contamination of the operative field by anaerobic bacteria is likely.

Adverse reactions. Metronidazole is relatively nontoxic. Even in large doses, it does not affect the cardiovascular or respiratory systems. Gastrointestinal symptoms (nausea, anorexia, diarrhea, epigastric distress) are the most common adverse reactions. Disturbances of the nervous system may occur, including peripheral neuropathy, dizziness, vertigo, and, rarely, incoordination and ataxia. The compound may produce an effect like disulfiram (*ie*, it causes unpleasant symptoms when alcohol is ingested). Neutropenia has been observed in some clients who receive treatment. The urine of some recipients turns a reddish-brown color, because metronidazole contains metabolites that are water-soluble pigments. Metronidazole is considered to be carcinogenic and mutagenic in some animal species. Superinfection by *Candida* organisms may occur.

Precautions and contraindications. Caution should be used when metronidazole is administered to individuals with blood dyscrasia or hepatic impairment. White blood cell counts should be monitored before and during therapy. If abnormal neurologic symptoms occur during therapy, withdrawal of the drug should be considered. When metronidazole and warfarin are administered concurrently, prothrombin times must be closely monitored and the anticoagulant dosage adjusted accordingly.

Metronidazole is contraindicated in individuals with a history of allergic sensitivity to this and related drugs.

Paromomycin

Paromomycin is an aminoglycoside antibiotic with amebicidal properties.

Pharmacodynamics. Paromomycin exerts amebicidal effects against both the trophozoite and encysted forms of *Entamoeba histolytica*. The exact mechanism of action is unknown, but aminoglycosides appear to inhibit protein synthesis in susceptible organisms by binding to 30S ribosomal subunits.

Pharmacokinetics. Paromomycin is administered orally for its local effect on the GI tract. While the drug is poorly absorbed from the tract, significant amounts may be absorbed if intestinal motility is impaired or if open lesions are present in the tract. Drug absorbed systemically is eliminated slowly in the urine, and accumulation can occur in people with renal impairment.

Therapeutic uses. Paromomycin is used in the treatment of intestinal amebiasis. It is used alone to treat mild cases and asymptomatic carriers and in conjunction with other amebicides in acute or severe forms of the disease. Paromomycin is not effective against extraintestinal forms of amebiasis.

Because of its relative nontoxicity, paromomycin is particularly useful in the treatment of nondysenteric amebiasis in uncooperative clients.

Adverse reactions. Paromomycin is relatively nontoxic. Adverse reactions are chiefly GI and include anorexia, nausea, vomiting, epigastric burning and pain, abdominal cramps, diarrhea, and pruritus ani. The drug can cause malabsorption similar to that caused by neomycin.

Superinfection with *Candida* organisms can develop during paromomycin treatment. Like other aminoglycosides, paromomycin has the potential for causing nephrotoxic, ototoxic, and neuromuscular-blocking effects.

Allergic reactions include rash, eosinophilia, and exanthema.

Precautions and contraindications. Paromomycin is administered with caution to clients with ulcerative bowel lesions because the drug may be absorbed in large amounts. High doses of or prolonged therapy with the drug should be avoided.

Paromomycin is contraindicated for individuals allergic to it and for those with impaired renal function or intestinal obstruction.

■ Summary

Drugs used to treat amebiasis (metronidazole, emetine, chloroquine, and others) are quite toxic. Clients require close monitoring and good supportive care. Because emetine is cardiotoxic, clients who receive this drug are hospitalized. The choice of drugs and regimen for treatment depend on the client's general condition, the previous course of the disease, and whether the infection involves extraintestinal tissues.

Nursing management

Nursing implications

Clients who receive emetine or dehydroemetine are hospitalized for treatment. Because both drugs are toxic to the heart, clients must be on complete bed rest for the duration of treatment (10 days for adults and 4–6 days for children). The drugs tend to accumulate in the tissues, and the risk of serious toxicity increases as treatment progresses. Frequent electrocardiograms are taken, and therapy is discontinued if abnormalities appear, especially when heart rates exceed 110/min. Because clients who are not acutely ill have difficulty accepting that cardiac risk may be present, maintaining bed rest can be a nursing challenge. Quiet diversions must be provided to prevent boredom and maintain intellectual stimulation.

Nursing process

Assessment Clients who are to receive amebicides should be screened before treatment is begun for risk factors that could influence the choice of a treatment agent. The nursing history should include specific information about nutritional status, kidney, liver, or cardiac impairment and hypersensitivity to iodine. In women of childbearing age, pregnancy should be ruled out.

The client's general condition should be carefully assessed. Amebiasis can be debilitating, and poor physical condition increases the risk of drug therapy. Signs and symptoms of amebiasis should also be determined. The client's knowledge about amebiasis and its treatment should be assessed.

Nursing diagnosis Diagnoses are related to the signs and symptoms of amebiasis, risk of adverse reaction to amebicides, signs and symptoms of adverse drug reaction, and knowledge deficit related to amebiasis and its treatment. They include the following:

> *Altered nutrition: less than body requirements related to diarrhea secondary to amebiasis*
> *Diarrhea related to amebiasis (or related to adverse reactions to antiamebiasis medication)*
> *Pain: abdominal cramps related to adverse reaction to antiamebiasis medication (or secondary to the disease process)*
> *Self-care deficit: inability to perform routine self-care activities related to cardiotoxicity of antiamebiasis drugs*
> *Knowledge deficit concerning amebiasis, its prevention, control, and treatment*

A common collaborative problem that should be differentiated from the nursing diagnoses include

> *Potential complication: cardiac*
> *Potential complication: optic toxicity*

Planning Goals of treatment include reducing the signs and symptoms of amebiasis, preventing or promptly detecting and treating adverse drug reactions, and teaching clients about amebiasis and its treatment.

Intervention Nursing measures to support and enhance natural resistance to infection are essential. Because most amebicides cause anorexia, nausea, vomiting, and epigastric and intestinal distress, clients do not feel like eating. Good nutrition, however, is important, because many clients have become debilitated by the amebic infection. The nurse, therefore, must employ every means available to provide inviting meals and to make mealtime an enjoyable occasion. The nurse should also take measures to promote rest and reduce stress.

Emetine is administered by deep IM injection. Care must be taken not to inject the drug IV; the drug is too toxic to be given by this route. An ice pack should be applied to the injection site to minimize the pain from tissue irritation caused by the drug.

Clients who receive emetine must be monitored for functional impairment of the liver, kidneys, and muscles, as well as the heart. Visual function should be tested periodically when either chloroquine or an 8-hydroxyquinoline drug is prescribed, because these drugs can damage the optic nerve. Because clients who receive metronidazole may experience neutropenia, their white blood cell counts must be monitored.

Client education. Clients who receive metronidazole must be instructed to avoid alcohol, because the drug can cause a reaction like that with disulfiram. They should also be warned that their urine may turn a reddish-brown color. This color comes from pigmented metabolites in the drug and is no cause for alarm.

Clients hospitalized for emetine treatment should be carefully prepared for the period of bed rest required by the treatment. They must be instructed about the precautions required and the need to request assistance rather than exert themselves. After completing the course of treatment, activity must be increased gradually, over a period of weeks. Specific instructions about activity should be given in accordance with the physician's recommendations.

All clients who receive amebicides should be warned that nausea, vomiting, diarrhea, and intestinal discomfort are likely. They should be cautioned to eat a nourishing diet during the period of treatment to maintain general resistance to infection.

Evaluation Data required for evaluation include information about changes in the signs and symptoms of amebiasis, incidence of adverse reaction to drug therapy, and the client's knowledge about amebiasis and its treatment.

Checklist of nursing actions

☐ Screen clients who are to receive amebicides for malnutrition, major organ impairment, hypersensitivity, and pregnancy.

☐ Administer emetine by deep IM injection. Apply an ice pack to the injection site.

☐ Maintain cardiac precautions for clients who receive emetine.

☐ Monitor clients who receive emetine for kidney, liver, and muscle impairment.

☐ Monitor clients who receive 8-hydroxyquinoline or chloroquine for visual impairment.

☐ Maintain good nutrition in clients treated for amebiasis.

☐ Teach clients about amebiasis and the prescribed treatment regimen.

☐ Instruct clients who receive metronidazole to avoid alcoholic beverages.

☐ Reassure clients who receive metronidazole that the reddish-brown discoloration of their urine is a normal and harmless result of the drug treatment.

☐ Stress the importance of maintaining good nutrition during treatment for amebiasis.

Miscellaneous protozoan infections

Of the remaining protozoan diseases, trypanosomiasis (African sleeping sickness and Chagas' disease) and leishmaniasis (kala-azar) are not found in the U.S. Information about treatment of these infections can be obtained by writing to the Parasitic Disease Drug Service 8, Centers for Disease Control, Atlanta, GA 30333. Four protozoan infections commonly seen in the U.S. and drugs for treatment are shown in Table 44-6.

Giardiasis

Giardiasis is an intestinal infection characterized by diarrhea, malabsorption, and epigastric distress. It occurs frequently among people who travel abroad but is also seen in parts of the U.S. where the infection is endemic. As in amebiasis, the organism is transmitted as a cyst by the anal to oral route. However, it does not invade extraintestinal tissues. Once diagnosed, the disease should be treated whether or not the client is experiencing symptoms. One course of metronidazole is effective in most cases. If necessary, a second course, or quinacrine, can be given.

Trichomoniasis

Trichomoniasis is commonly manifested as a vaginitis. The organism is often carried by infected males, most of whom are asymptomatic. Transmitted during sexual intercourse, the organism causes inflammation, itching, and burning of the vaginal mucosa and produces a greenish-yellow discharge. Metronidazole by mouth is effective in most cases. Both sexual partners must be treated at the same time. Refractory cases of vaginitis may be treated topically by vaginal suppository.

Toxoplasmosis

Toxoplasmosis is a protozoan infection transmitted to humans from cats, which excrete the organism in their feces. Infection in the adult generally produces few if any symptoms, but transmission from an infected mother to an infant *in utero* or at birth can severely damage the child's CNS. Recommended treatment in-

Table 44-6. Treatment for four miscellaneous protozoan infections

Infection	Route of transmission	Drug	Additional information
Giardiasis (intestinal)	Cyst by anal–oral route	One course of metronidazole; if necessary, a second course, or quinacrine	The disease should be treated whether or not the client is experiencing symptoms.
Trichomoniasis (vaginitis)	Sexual intercourse (partner often is asymptomatic)	Oral metronidazole	Both sexual partners must be treated at same time. Refractory cases of vaginitis may be treated topically by vaginal suppository.
Toxoplasmosis	From cat feces to humans	Pyrimethamine and sulfisoxazole given simultaneously	Produces few, if any, symptoms in adults; danger is in transmission from infected mother to fetus *in utero* or at birth
Infection with *Pneumocystis carinii* (pneumonia)	Protozoal	Co-trimoxazole, zidovudine (AZT), pentadine isothionate, Bactrim, Septra (trimethoprim plus sulfamethoxazole), steroids	Opportunistic infection seen in immunosuppressed hosts

cludes pyrimethamine and sulfisoxazole given simultaneously.

Pneumocystis carinii

Pneumocystis carinii is an opportunistic protozoan that causes pneumonia in people whose immune response is depressed from debility, acquired immunodeficiency syndrome (AIDS), or immunosuppressant therapy. Co-trimoxazole has been used to treat *Pneumocystis carinii* pneumonia (PCP), but its side effects, including severe renal impairment, blood dyscrasia, and Stevens-Johnson syndrome, lessened its choice for treatment of PCP. Pentamidine isethionate (Pentam) has been approved in the aerosol form by the FDA for prevention of PCP. This inhaled form of the drug rarely causes side effects more serious than a cough. Pentamidine isothionate has also been used effectively for mild pneumonia but may fail to be helpful in more advanced pneumonia. Pentamidine is used IV to treat established PCP but may result in severe side effects, particularly blood dyscrasia. Pentamidine methanesulfonate is another form of the drug not yet available for general use. The two forms differ in labeling and dosage. The isothionate form reflects the combined weight of base and salt, while the methanesulfonate form reflects the weight of the base alone. The dosages of the two drugs are therefore not equivalent when prescribed for PCP. The dose for pentamidine isothionate is usually 4 mg/kg/day, while for pentamidine methanesulfonate, it is usually 2.3 mg/kg/day. Recent studies have demonstrated that trimethoprim plus sulfamethoxazole (Bactrim, Septra) are effective in controlling PCP, given three times a week, at a cost of $7 a year!

Helminthic infestations

Infestation by parasitic worms is the most common disease in the world. Its victims are estimated to number a billion or more. The incidence is rising with the increase in cultivated land and artificial irrigation. There is also a tendency toward a wider distribution of parasites because of easy, rapid, long-distance travel and the mobility of migrating populations. As with other contagious diseases, helminthiasis is most common in areas with overcrowding, poverty, poor sanitation, and inadequate control of intermediate hosts.

Worm parasites may be classified according to zoologic species, mode of transmission, distribution within the body, or the pharmacologic agents used for treatment (Table 44-7 and Fig. 44-3). Most are visible to the eye in their adult form but are transmitted as ova or larvae of microscopic size. Effects on the host vary from minimal symptoms to lethal damage to vital organs. Many victims develop general debility, often with a severe anemia. Because they lower the energy level of affected populations (up to 90% of a given population

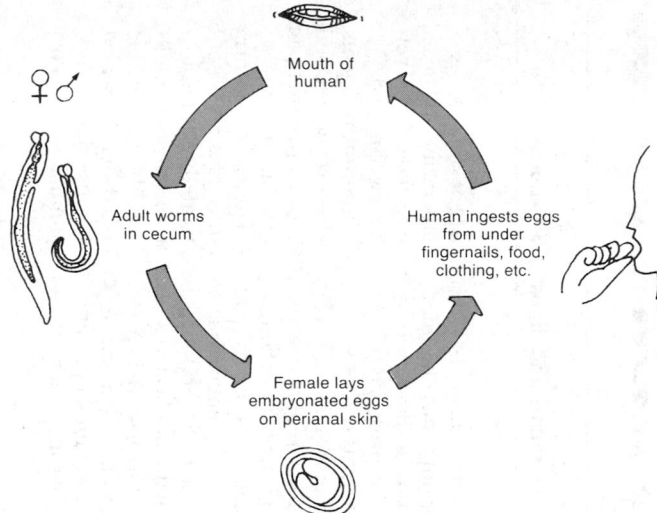

Figure 44-3. Life cycle of *Enterobius vermicularis*. (Redrawn from Armed Forces Institute of Pathology, Neg No. 75-10881-13)

may be infested), helminth infections are a serious impediment to economic and cultural development.

Agents used for treatment

The older, less efficient, and more toxic anthelminthics have been discarded in favor of newer agents that are more active and less toxic (Table 44-8). Treatment has become considerably more simplified, as fewer agents are required and dosage schedules tend to be shorter. Although newer treatment agents tend to be less toxic than older drugs, many are still debilitating, and the client must be carefully supported during the treatment period. Often, the victim's general condition must be improved before anthelminthic agents can be administered with safety. Because drug treatment is specific to the species involved, it varies with different classes of infection. A definitive diagnosis, therefore, is required before rational treatment can be prescribed. Anthelminthics should never be used merely on the basis of a suspected infection.

Piperazine

Pharmacodynamics. Piperazine blocks the effects of acetylcholine at the neuromuscular junction of ascarids, producing paralysis of the worms. Normal peristalsis then eliminates the live parasites from the GI tract. This feature is desirable, because killing the parasites induces tissue reactions in response to the absorption of foreign protein.

Pharmacokinetics. Piperazine is administered orally and is readily absorbed from the GI tract. Systemically, some of the drug is metabolized, probably in

(Text continues on p. 1118)

Table 44-7. Characteristics of selected helminth infections

Class or subclass/genus or species	Synonym/distribution	Method of transmission	Preventive measures	Distribution within the body	Symptoms and signs	Treatment
Nematoda						
Ascaris lumbricoides	Roundworms are found worldwide, especially where sanitation is poor; infestation is common in indigent children in the southern U.S.	Anal–oral route; ova shed in feces of human or animal hosts reach manured fields and ground water, contaminating water and food. Pets transmit infections to humans, especially children.	Purification of water; thorough cleaning of food, especially vegetables; composting of manure before use as fertilizer; careful hand-washing after toileting and handling of animals.	Ingested eggs hatch into larvae in the small intestine, then migrate to the lungs. Later, the larvae migrate back into the stomach and intestine and grow to adult size. The infection remains intraintestinal unless perforation occurs as a complication.	Many clients have no symptoms; the infection is discovered by the presence of the worms in the stool. Early signs and symptoms resemble a respiratory infection; later, abdominal pain and distention may occur. Several intestinal complications (eg, obstruction) may occur when worms are stimulated into migratory activity.	Agent of choice is piperazine. In mixed infections that involve hookworms and roundworms, agents effective against both, such as pyrantel pamoate, are recommended. Hookworm infections must not be treated with tetrachlorethylene until roundworm is either ruled out or treated, because this agent stimulates migratory activity in roundworms.
Necator americanus and Ancylostoma duodenale	New World and Old World hookworms ("miner's disease" and "tunnel disease") are most common between latitudes 30° south and 40° north. The organisms are found in mines and large mountain tunnels farther north.	Anal–percutaneous route; ova shed in feces of hosts hatch into larva in the soil. Larva burrow through the skin (usually of the foot) to reach the bloodstream	Proper disposal of fecal wastes; wearing of shoes.	Larvae that enter the skin are carried by the bloodstream to the lungs. They propel themselves up the trachea, are swallowed, and reach the intestines as adult worms. There they attach themselves to the intestinal mucosa and live on blood sucked from the host.	Fatigue and apathy due to iron deficiency anemia; fluid and electrolyte disturbances.	Agents of choice are bephenium or thiabendazole. Fluid and electrolyte solutions to restore physiologic balance must precede the use of anthelminthics. Iron salts or transfusion are given to correct the anemia. Bephenium and thiabendazole are also effective against any coexisting roundworm infection. Tetrachlorethylene must not be used unless roundworm has been ruled out or eliminated.
Strongyloide stercoralis	Threadworms are most common in the tropics and southern U.S.; occasionally they are found in	Anal–percutaneous route; larvae in soil enter the skin, usually the soles of the feet.	Proper disposal of fecal wastes; wearing of shoes.	Worms burrow beneath the mucosa of the small intestine. The female lays many eggs that hatch into	Lightly infested victims may show no symptoms. Abdominal tenderness, epigastric pain similar to	Agents of choice are thiabendazole or pyrvinium pamoate. All people whose stools are found to contain

	mines, even in temperate zones.		larvae able to penetrate to all parts of the body.	that of peptic ulcer, and diarrhea that resembles that of ulcerative colitis may occur. Extraintestinal effects depend on the area of the body invaded and may include bronchopneumonia or lung abscess.		threadworm larvae should be treated to prevent the serious effects of the disease.
Dracunculus species	Guinea worm disease, primarily in Nigeria, also in Africa, India, Pakistan.	Drinking water contaminated with worm larvae.	Ingested larvae released into abdomen of host, where they mate. Males die; females travel to host's legs or feet, grow to length of 2 to 3 feet.	After a year, mature worm travels to skin surface, secretes a poison that causes blister or abscess. To relieve pain, victim soaks it, usually in area's water supply. Worms release hundreds of thousands of new larvae into water supply.	Use of nylon filters through which water is poured. Forbid soaking blisters or abscesses in area's water supply.	Treat client for malnutrition. Teach clients to pour water through nylon filter to remove larvae. Treat blisters or abscesses for pain symptomatically. Do not allow soaking in area's water supply. Pyrantel pamoate is effective against threadworms.
Enterobius vermicularis	Pinworm is the most common cause of helminthiasis among American school children	Anal–oral route; ova shed in feces of infected hosts dry, becoming light enough to move easily in air currents. Ova are found in the dust of the environment where infected hosts live; ova under nails after scratching the pruritic anus may be ingested.	Ova ingested travel to the large intestine, where they hatch into larvae. Worms migrate through the anus, especially at night, and may reach the genital tract in females.	Pruritus of the perianal and perineal regions is most common. Secondary infection, caused by scratching, may occur. Salpingitis or peritonitis are occasional complications in females.	Careful hand-washing; wet mopping and disinfection of bathroom and bedroom floors; disinfection of toilet seats; fingernail care, including close trimming.	Agent of choice: pyrantel pamoate. To achieve a high proportion of cures, rigid standards of personal hygiene must be enforced. Nails are trimmed short, handwashing before meals is emphasized, undergarments are changed twice a day. Thorough cleaning and disinfection of bathroom and bedroom floors and toilets are also important. Children should be given a shower in the morning to wash away any ova deposited in the anal area during the night.

(Continued)

Table 44-7. Characteristics of selected helminth infections *(Continued)*

Class or subclass/ genus or species	Synonym/distribution	Method of transmission	Preventive measures	Distribution within the body	Symptoms and signs	Treatment
Trichinella spiralis	Pork roundworm is worldwide in distribution, frequent in North America and Europe; most common in areas where pigs are fed raw cabbage.	Ingestion of rare or raw meat from infected animals that contain encysted larvae.	Thorough cooking of meats (animals other than pigs can carry the disease); cooking of garbage used for feeding domestic animals; frequent thorough cleaning of utensils used to process raw meat or to prepare it for cooking.	Ingested larvae reach maturity in the intestinal tract. Fertilized females deposit larvae in the intestinal mucosa. Carried by the bloodstream throughout the body, the larvae penetrate skeletal muscles and other organs, evoking inflammatory reactions.	Skeletal muscle pain is common. Effects of damage to internal organ depend on the body areas involved and include pneumonia, heart failure, and encephalitis.	No effective anthelminthic is yet available. Thiabendazole appears to kill some but not all of the parasites in tissues. Corticosteroids are helpful in reducing the inflammatory reaction. Otherwise, treatment is symptomatic.
Wuchereria bancrofti	Filariasis ("elephantiasis") is common in central Africa, southwest Pacific, eastern Asia; also occurs in the West Indies and tropical South and Central America.	Transmission by flies, mosquitoes, and mites.	Control of intermediate hosts.	Larvae deposited in the skin by mosquito or other intermediate hosts develop into adults. Microfilariae produced by fertilized females migrate to the lymphatics and bloodstream and develop into worms, which lodge in lymphatic vessels and nodes.	Signs and symptoms of inflammation wherever living or dead worms are present—inflammation of the lymph nodes with temporary swelling in the affected area, red streaks along the extremity, pain, and tenderness. Obstruction of the lymphatic system leads to gross enlargement of the extremities, scrotum, or breast by edema.	Varies, depending on the particular filariae involved. Antihistamines and corticosteroids are used to alleviate allergic reactions to debris from killed worms.

Cestoda

Organism	Distribution	Transmission	Prevention	Pathology	Symptoms	Treatment
Taenia saginata	Beef tapeworm is found worldwide.	Ingestion of raw or inadequately cooked meat from infected animals.	Thorough cooking of meat before tasting.	Most tapeworms remain intraintestinal. The scolex, or head, attaches itself to the intestinal wall and grows a variable number of segments, which may produce a worm several yards long. Segments of the worm break off and are passed in the feces. Pork tapeworm produces larvae capable of extraintestinal invasion. They are carried by the bloodstream to muscles, liver, or brain.	Mild abdominal symptoms and weight loss are common. Discovery of worm segments in the stool often frightens the victim into seeking treatment. Symptoms are signs of extraintestinal pork tapeworm infection vary with tissues involved.	Agents of choice: dichlorophen, niclosamide, or paramomycin. If pork worm is involved, treatment must be followed by a purgative to remove worm segments before they can be digested, releasing the ova that can cause extraintestinal invasion.
Taenia solium	Pork tapeworm is found worldwide.					
Diphyllobothrium latum	Fish tapeworm is common in Europe, the Near East, Siberia, northern Manchuria, Japan, and the lake regions of North America.					

Trematoda

Organism	Distribution	Transmission	Prevention	Pathology	Symptoms	Treatment
Schistosoma haematobium, Schistosoma mansoni	Blood flukes, schistosomiasis, or bilharziasis are widespread throughout Africa and Brazil; some foci occur in Near East and West Indies.	Transmission from snail to man by way of contaminated bathing water.	Control of snails (the intermediate host); avoiding contact with contaminated water. Avoid fresh water swimming; add iodine or chlorine to water; filter water with paper coffee filters to remove cercariae from bathing water.	Larvae that enter the skin penetrate to the bloodstream or lymphatics. They move first to the lungs, then to the liver, where they mature in the portal veins. The mature adult worms mate and move to areas of the large and small intestines and bladder, producing eggs that are eliminated in feces and urine.	A pruritic rash, called *swimmer's itch*, develops as a reaction to larvae which die in the skin. About 1 to 2 months later, fever, chills, headache, and other allergic and inflammatory symptoms may occur. Heavy infestations cause abdominal pain and diarrhea. Engorgement of vital organs occurs from venous obstruction in chronic infections.	Drug choice depends on type of fluke involved. No available drugs are known to be effective for chemoprophylaxis.

Table 44-8. Representative drugs used in the treatment of helminth infestations

Drug name	Preparations	Susceptible organisms	Additional information
mebendazole (Pantelmin, Telmin, Vermox)	Oral chewable tablets PC: C	Whipworm, pinworm, hookworm, roundworm	Is teratogenic and embryotoxic in animals
piperazine (Antepar, Entracyl, Perin, Vermisol, Vermizine)	Tablets, powders, and solutions for oral use PC: B	Roundworm, pinworm	Causes flaccid paralysis of organisms, which are subsequently expelled from the body in the feces
			Does not require fasting or catharsis before treatment
pyrantel pamoate (Antiminth, Conbantrin)	Suspensions for oral use PC: C	Hookworm, roundworm, pinworm	Causes spastic paralysis of organisms, which are subsequently expelled from the body in the feces
			Does not require fasting or catharsis before treatment
pyrvinium pamoate (Molevac, Poquil, Povan, Vanquin)	Oral tablets	Pinworm, threadworm	Colors stools and emesis red and may stain materials
quinacrine (Atabrine)	Oral tablets PC: C	Tapeworm	Imparts a yellow color to urine and skin
			Can precipitate acute attacks of psoriasis in individuals affected by the disease
tetrachlorethylene	Soft gelatin capsules for oral use	Hookworm	Cannot be given in mixed infections before treatment for roundworm infestation
			Cannot be given before correction of anemia and fluid and electrolyte imbalances
			Should not be given with dietary fat or alcohol, which enhance absorption
thiabendazole (Mintezol, Minzolem)	Suspensions and chewable tablets for oral use PC: C	Pinworm, threadworm, roundworm, hookworm	Is given after a meal
			May impair alertness and coordination due to CNS effects
			Sometimes causes Stevens-Johnson syndrome

KEY: PC = Pregnancy category. (The validity of pregnancy risk categories has not been established; see Chapter 16, p 216.)

the liver, and the remainder is excreted unchanged by the kidneys.

Therapeutic uses. Piperazine is used in the treatment of enterobiasis (pinworm infestations) and ascariasis (roundworm infestations). Piperazine is administered orally. It is used to treat all members of an exposed group simultaneously, whenever possible. Rigorous sanitary measures are also carried out to rid the environment, as well as the victims, of the contagion.

Adverse reactions. When given orally, piperazine has a wide safety margin, and few adverse reactions occur. Clients who receive piperazine may experience nausea and vomiting, abdominal pain, diarrhea, or headache. Vertigo, weakness, lethargy, and blurred vision also occur. Skin reactions take the form of urticaria or erythema multiforme. Neurotoxic effects are seen primarily in clients with renal dysfunction, whose excretion is impaired.

Precautions and contraindications. Caution should be used when piperazine is administered to malnourished or anemic individuals and those with a history of neurologic disturbances, including epilepsy. Pro-

longed treatment and high doses are to be avoided. The drug is contraindicated in individuals who are allergic to piperazine or its salts. If renal function is impaired, the drug is likely to accumulate in the tissues.

Safe use during pregnancy has not been established, although the drug has been used successfully during the last trimester.

Piperazine and pyrantel pamoate should not be given concurrently, because their actions are mutually antagonistic.

Pyrantel pamoate

Pharmacodynamics. Pyrantel pamoate exerts a persistent nicotinic activation and inhibition of cholinesterase that causes a spastic paralysis in parasitic worms.

Pharmacokinetics. Pyrantel pamoate is given orally and is poorly absorbed by the GI tract. Most of the dose remains in the GI tract and is eliminated in the feces. Drug that is absorbed is partially metabolized in the liver and excreted by the kidneys.

Therapeutic uses. Pyrantel pamoate is considered a broad-spectrum anthelmintic because it is effective against hookworms as well as roundworms and pinworms.

Adverse reactions. Although pyrantel pamoate has a wide safety margin, GI upset and CNS reactions are occasionally reported. Elevations in liver enzymes have also occurred.

Precautions and contraindications. Caution should be exercised when pyrantel pamoate is used to treat individuals with liver dysfunction, malnutrition, or anemia. Safe use during pregnancy and in children younger than 2 years of age has not been established. The drug is contraindicated for individuals with allergic hypersensitivity to it.

Pyrantel pamoate and piperazine should not be given together, because their actions are mutually antagonistic.

Pyrvinium pamoate

Pharmacodynamics. Pyrvinium pamoate inhibits oxygen uptake in aerobic parasites and prevents the use of carbohydrates by helminths.

Pharmacokinetics. Pyrvinium pamoate is not absorbed by the GI tract in significant amounts. It acts within the tract and is eliminated in the feces.

Therapeutic uses. Pyrvinium pamoate is used to treat pinworm infestation. It has also been used to treat threadworm infestation.

Adverse reactions. The adverse effects of pyrvinium pamoate are confined to the GI tract and usually are mild. The drug does color both stools and vomitus red and can stain most materials. Allergic reactions may include photosensitivity and Stevens-Johnson syndrome.

Precautions and contraindications. Pyrvinium pamoate is contraindicated for individuals who are allergic to it, as well as for individuals with inflammatory bowel disease or other conditions that might increase absorption from the GI tract. Safe use during pregnancy and for children who weigh less than 10 kg has not been established.

Thiabendazole

Thiabendazole belongs to a class of drugs known as substituted benzimidazoles, which are among the most potent anthelminthics known.

Pharmacodynamics. The exact mechanism of action of thiabendazole is unknown. The drug does inhibit the helminth-specific enzyme, fumarate reductase. In animals, the drug has anti-inflammatory, antipyretic, and analgesic effects.

Pharmacokinetics. Thiabendazole is administered orally and is readily absorbed from the GI tract. In the body, it is metabolized to 5-hydroxythiabendazole and is subsequently excreted in the urine as glucuronide or sulfate conjugates. A small amount (5%) is excreted in the feces.

Therapeutic uses. Thiabendazole is used in the treatment of pinworms, threadworms, roundworms, and hookworms. Although it does not eradicate the disease, it is the only drug that appears to alleviate the symptoms of trichinosis (*eg*, fever, tenderness, muscle pain).

Adverse reactions. Adverse reactions to thiabendazole resemble those to piperazine. Clients may experience anorexia, nausea, vomiting, diarrhea, abdominal distress, headaches, dizziness, drowsiness, malodorous urine, lethargy, or pruritus. Liver function tests may become transiently elevated. Allergic reactions include fever, facial flush, chills, skin rashes, and Stevens-Johnson syndrome. CNS effects may impair alertness and coordination.

Precautions and contraindications. Caution should be exercised when thiabendazole is used to treat individuals with hepatic or renal dysfunction, those with malnutrition or anemia, and those for whom vomiting may be dangerous. The drug is contraindicated in clients who are allergic to it. Safe use during pregnancy and lactation and for children who weigh less than 15 kg has not been established.

Mebendazole

Mebendazole is structurally related to thiabendazole. It differs in action, however; mebendazole inhibits the uptake of glucose and other nutrients by susceptible helminths. Mebendazole has a broad spectrum of activity, including whipworms, pinworms, roundworms, and hookworms. The drug is relatively nontoxic, with adverse reactions limited mainly to mild GI symptoms and allergic reactions. It has been reported to cause damage to the fetuses of experimental animals and is contraindicated for pregnant women.

Traditional anthelminthics

Some traditional anthelminthics previously used to treat helminth infections have become obsolete, whereas others are still used in selected cases. Oleoresin of aspidium, gentian violet, and quinacrine are seldom used, having been replaced with more effective less toxic compounds. Hexylresorcinol and the trivalent antimony compounds are still used to treat certain fluke diseases.

Hexylresorcinol is most effective when the intestinal tract is empty (see Box 44-3 for the recommended treatment regimen). When hexylresorcinol is administered, the gelatin-coated pills must be swallowed without breaking because the drug is corrosive to the mouth. Excoriation of the perianal region may occur from fecal elimination of the medication.

Tetrachlorethylene was introduced to replace carbon tetrachloride, which it resembles. Both are effective anthelminthics, but tetrachlorethylene is safer,

---

Box 44-3. Recommended regimen for hexylresorcinol treatment

1. Give a saline purgative the evening before treatment.
2. Allow no food from the time the purgative is taken until treatment is completed.
3. Administer a single dose of drug in the morning.
4. Give another saline purgative 2 to 4 hours later.

---

probably because it is not absorbed as completely as carbon tetrachloride. Most effective against hookworms, tetrachlorethylene is given orally after the restoration of fluid and electrolyte balance and correction of anemia. Before administration, alcohol should be eliminated and fat reduced in the diet to control systemic absorption of the drug. Adverse reactions include GI and CNS symptoms. The drug is contraindicated in debilitated or alcoholic clients and those with GI inflammation. It must not be given to those who also harbor a roundworm infection until this disease has been treated, because tetrachlorethylene stimulates migratory activity in roundworms and may cause serious complications. With the introduction of safe broad-spectrum anthelminthics, the use of tetrachlorethylene has declined.

Drugs used as adjuncts in the treatment of helminth infections, but without specific anthelminthic effects, include corticosteroids, antihistamines, and analgesics; in addition, antipruritics, fluids, electrolyte solutions, blood, vitamins, and iron are given to improve the client's general condition. Insecticides and poisons are also widely used to control intermediate hosts and vectors in the environment. All of these agents are discussed elsewhere in the text.

■ Summary

Both helminth infestations and the drugs used in their treatment are debilitating. Clients in need of treatment may require supportive care to build up their general condition before anthelminthics can be administered.

Among the anthelminthics are piperazine, pyrantel pamoate, thiabendazole, tetrachlorethylene, and pyrvinium pamoate. Special precautions specific to the agent used are often required during the treatment regimen.

Nursing management

Nursing implications

Before anthelminthic therapy is begun, clients must be carefully evaluated to determine if their general condition is sufficiently good to withstand treatment. Ane-

mia, fluid and electrolyte imbalances, and malnutrition as a result of the infestation are frequently present. A period of general supportive care may be needed before treatment.

The causative organisms must be identified before treatment agents can be selected. If the infestation involves more than one organism, the order of treatment may be crucial. Roundworms are generally treated first, because some drugs used to treat other types of worms irritate roundworms, causing them to migrate actively from the intestines. Invasion of the bile ducts and liver, intestinal obstruction, or intestinal perforation may result.

Because killing roundworms within the body leads to absorption of toxic materials, drugs used for these organisms paralyze rather than kill them. The worms expelled in the feces, therefore, are alive. They need no special treatment before they are discarded with the feces, because they cannot survive unaided outside the body. However, the feces, which also contain the infectious ova, must be disposed of in proper toilet facilities.

Pinworm infestations usually affect all members of a common household. For this reason, treatment of this infestation involves corresponding medication for all family members. Hygienic measures to eliminate the cysts from the environment are critical to prevent reinfestation. These cysts are light, move freely in the air, and permeate dust; hence, a thorough housecleaning is in order.

Nursing process

Assessment The client's general condition should be carefully assessed. Debilitated clients are at high risk for adverse reaction to anthelminthic drugs. Of particular concern are fluid and electrolyte imbalances, renal function, anemia, and malnutrition. Before piperazine is administered, seizure disorders and renal impairment should be ruled out. The nurse should question the client specifically about epilepsy, "fits," "blackouts," or "absence" episodes. The drug is contraindicated in epilepsy. If renal function is inadequate, the drug is likely to accumulate in the tissues.

Nursing diagnosis Nursing diagnoses for clients with helminth infestations may include the following:

> *Altered nutrition: less than body requirements related to infestation with helminths (or related to anthelminthic medications)*
> *Impaired tissue integrity: erosions of the mouth and/or perianal tissues related to hexylresorcinol medication*
> *Knowledge deficit concerning helminth infestations and their prevention, control, and treatment*

Planning The objective of treating helminth infestations is not always the elimination of the organism. If the client's general health does not allow vigorous treatment, or if reinfestation appears inevitable, treatment is limited to reducing the population of organisms. The number of organisms does not increase unless more ova reach the host from the environment, because the life cycle of the organisms requires a period of time outside the host. Goals of treatment also include preventing or promptly detecting and treating any adverse reaction to prescribed anthelminthics, as well as teaching the client about helminth infestations and their treatment.

Intervention Clients treated for helminth infestations require supportive care to maintain vital functions and enhance natural resistance to disease. They are often debilitated by the disease, a condition which anthelminthics can intensify.

Specific measures to reduce the risk of adverse drug reaction vary with the drugs used. For example, when tetrachlorethylene is prescribed, dietary fat must be controlled. Tetrachlorethylene can be absorbed in toxic amounts when fat and alcohol are present. The client is given a low-fat meal the evening before treatment. No food is given on the morning of the treatment. After the administration of a single dose of tetrachlorethylene, the client is kept in bed and observed closely for adverse reactions for 2 to 4 hours. Dizziness, drowsiness, nausea, and vomiting may occur. One week after treatment, the stools are examined for ova and the treatment repeated if necessary.

Before administering anthelminthics, the nurse should verify that conditions that contraindicate the use of the specific drug have been ruled out. For example, piperazine should not be used for clients with a history of seizure disorders or renal disease. Tetrachlorethylene must not be administered in the presence of roundworm infestation.

The client should be monitored carefully for adverse reactions to the prescribed drug. Among the signs and symptoms that may develop are GI upsets (nausea, vomiting, abdominal pain, and diarrhea), weakness and lethargy, blurred vision, CNS reactions, elevations in liver enzymes, pruritus, and other allergic reactions. Clients with impaired renal function are at high risk for adverse drug reactions.

Client education. A teaching plan should be developed and implemented that covers precautionary measures to reduce the risk of serious adverse reactions to the prescribed drug. Signs and symptoms of adverse drug reaction should be reported promptly to the health care staff. During convalescence, the client must be informed about measures to prevent reinfestation.

Because the client may remain a carrier after treatment, education is essential to prevent continued contamination of the environment and reinfestation. The ability to follow these recommendations depends on the client's resources. Referral to social service agencies for assistance may be needed. Specific instructions should be given about measures to prevent environmental contamination and reinfestation.

In some clients, during administration of thiabendazole, metabolites eliminated in the urine impart an odor similar to that caused by ingestion of asparagus. Clients should be prepared for this fact. Clients should also be advised against performing hazardous activities that require mental alertness (*eg*, operating power machinery) during therapy, because drowsiness, giddiness, and headache occur frequently.

Evaluation Data required for evaluation include changes in the signs and symptoms of helminthiasis, any signs and symptoms of adverse drug reaction, the degree of the client's compliance with the therapeutic regimen, and the ability of the client to relate accurately the material covered by the teaching plan.

Checklist of nursing actions

- [ ] Before anthelminthic therapy, evaluate the client's fluid, electrolyte, and nutritional status.
- [ ] Verify the causative organisms through the laboratory reports.
- [ ] Recommend corresponding treatment for all family members affected by pinworms.
- [ ] Rule out epilepsy before administering piperazine.
- [ ] Warn clients who receive hexylresorcinol not to chew or break the gelatin tablet when swallowing it.
- [ ] Rule out roundworm infestation before administering tetrachlorethylene.
- [ ] Restrict fat and alcohol in the diet of clients treated with tetrachlorethylene.
- [ ] Maintain clients who receive tetrachlorethylene at bed rest throughout the treatment and for several hours after treatment is completed.
- [ ] Instruct clients in measures to break the chain of reinfestation.

Ectoparasitic infestations

Modes of transmission and pathophysiology

Ectoparasitic diseases are those caused by parasites attached to the outer surface or situated beneath the skin of the host. Strictly speaking, the term encompasses fungal infections of the skin as well as infestations by lice and mites. In practice, it refers only to lice and mites.

The two most common ectoparasite infestations are scabies and pediculosis. Scabies is a highly communicable skin disease caused by a mite that burrows in the skin to reproduce (Fig. 44-4). Warm intertriginous

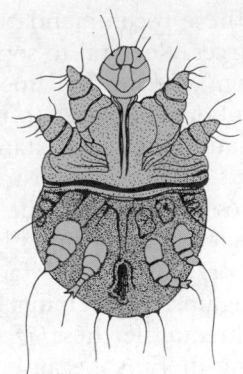

Figure 44-4. The scabies mite burrows in the skin to reproduce (not drawn to scale). (Thomas CL [ed]. [1985]. *Taber's cyclopedic medical dictionary*, 15th ed. Philadelphia: FA Davis.)

areas are most commonly affected. Pediculosis is an infestation caused by lice that live on the surface of the body and bite or suck blood to obtain nourishment from the host (Fig. 44-5). Both pediculosis and scabies are characterized by itching and scratching that often result in secondary skin infections. Both diseases occur more frequently and persist for longer periods under conditions of overcrowding and poor hygiene, although they also occur in affluent communities. The scabies mite causes world-wide epidemics that usually last about 15 years, with another epidemic starting 15 years later. However, the present epidemic started in the late 1960s and has not abated.

Pediculosis has increased in recent years, particularly among the homeless and other groups who have difficulty carrying out personal hygiene. Scabies is a frequent cause of epidemics in institutions, such as nursing homes and schools for the mentally retarded. Residents of economically depressed areas (especially alcoholics) are also prone to both conditions. These infestations can and do spread to any exposed person, but they are more apt to be treated early and their severity limited in people who practice good hygiene. Treatment involves elimination of the secondary infec-

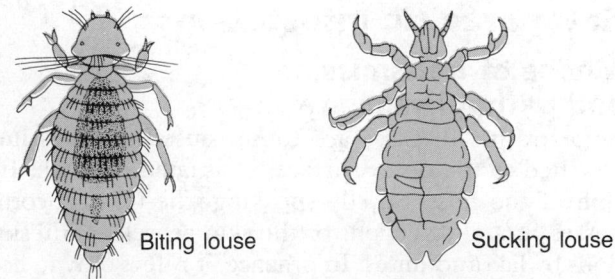

Biting louse   Sucking louse

Figure 44-5. Two types of lice that live on the surface of the skin (not drawn to scale). (Thomas CL [ed]. [1981]. *Taber's cyclopedic medical dictionary*, 14th ed. Philadelphia, FA Davis.)

tions that may be present, as well as the parasite. Insecticides applied to the skin, often in a single application, are effective. They penetrate the exoskeleton of the organism and cause nervous system hyperactivity. By rendering the neuron or membrane unstable, these insecticides are toxic to animals, including humans; for this reason, caution should be exercised in their use. Because insecticides provide no residual protection, reinfestation can be prevented only by disinfecting bedding and clothing through laundering or dry cleaning. Because insecticides are toxic to humans, exposure of clients and health care personnel should be kept to a minimum. The emergence of parasite strains resistant to most insecticides is common. To delay this process, these compounds should be used only when necessary, and dispersal into the environment should be avoided.

Insecticides used for treatment

Agents used to treat ectoparasitic infestations are listed in Table 44-9.

Benzyl benzoate
Benzyl benzoate is an ester of benzoic acid.

Pharmacodynamics. The mechanism of benzyl benzoate is unknown. It is toxic to *Sarcoptes scabiei* (the causative organism of scabies), *Pediculosis capitis* (head louse), and *Phthirus pubis* (pubic or "crab" louse).

Pharmacokinetics. Whether benzyl benzoate is absorbed by humans when applied topically is unknown.

Therapeutic uses. Benzyl benzoate is used for the topical treatment of scabies. It is recommended by the manufacturer for the treatment of head and crab lice, but its effectiveness in these conditions is unproved.

Adverse reactions. When applied topically, benzyl benzoate is not highly toxic. Local irritation and allergic skin reaction may occur. Repeated use may cause contact dermatitis. Oral ingestion of benzyl benzoate causes CNS impairment: incoordination, excitation, and seizures that can be fatal.

Precautions and contraindications. Benzyl benzoate should not be applied to inflamed or raw skin areas. Contact with the face, eyes, and mucous membranes should be avoided. The drug should not be used by individuals who have allergic hypersensitivity to it.

Crotamiton
Crotamiton is a synthetic compound.

Pharmacodynamics. Crotamiton's mechanism of action is unknown.

Pharmacokinetics. It is unknown whether crotamiton is absorbed systemically after topical applications.

Table 44-9. Agents used in the treatment of ectoparasitic infestations

Drug name	Preparation	Usual dosage	Additional information
Scabicides			
benzyl benzoate (Scabanca)	Lotion for topical application	Two applications of 20–30 ml of 28% lotion PC: C	The lotion should be spread thinly over the entire skin (except the face). The second layer is applied as soon as the first layer has dried. Second and third treatments may be administered on successive days if necessary. The drug should be removed by bathing 24–48 hours after treatment.
crotamiton (Eurax)	Cream and lotion for topical application	20–30 g of cream or lotion PC: C	The cream or lotion should be spread thinly over the entire skin (except the face). The treatment is repeated once, 24 hours after the first application. Treatment may be repeated 7–10 days later if mites or new lesions develop. The drug should be removed by bathing 48 hours after the last application.
permethrin (Elmite, Nix)	5% cream for topical application	One application of 30 g PC: B	Massage into skin from head to soles of feet. Remove in bath or shower after 8–14 hours. Infants should be treated on scalp, temple, and forehead.
Delousing agents			
lindane (Kwell, gBH, Hexit, Kwelada, NCP Linane Shampoo, PMS Lindane)	Cream, lotion, and shampoo for topical use	20–30 g of cream or lotion PC: C	The cream or lotion should be spread thinly over the entire skin (except the face). The drug should be removed by bathing 8–12 hours after treatment. The drug is removed by shampooing 10 minutes after application. Treatment may be repeated 7–10 days later if necessary.
pyrethrins with piperonyl butoxide (A-200 Pyrenate, Blue Gel, Pyrinal, Pyrinyl, R & C Shampoo, A & C Spray, RID, Tisit, Triple X)	Gel, shampoo, cream, lotion, and solution for topical use	20–30 g of cream or lotion PC: C	The drug should not be allowed to contact the eyes, mucous membranes, or denuded areas of the skin.

KEY: PC = pregnancy category. (The validity of pregnancy risk categories has not been established; see Chapter 16, p 216.)

Therapeutic uses. Crotamiton is used for the topical treatment of scabies.

Adverse reactions. Adverse reactions resemble those of benzyl benzoate. Information about crotamiton's effects when ingested is not available.

Precautions and contraindications. Like benzyl benzoate, crotamiton should not be applied to inflamed or raw skin areas. Contact with the face, eyes, and mucous membranes should be avoided. The drug should not be used by individuals with a history of allergic reaction to it.

Lindane

Lindane (gamma benzene hexachloride; Kwell) is a chlorinated hydrocarbon originally developed as an agricultural insecticide. On absorption by insects through the exoskeleton, lindane stimulates the CNS, causing seizures and death.

Pharmacokinetics. Lindane is absorbed directly through the exoskeleton of susceptible insects and circulates systemically.

It is absorbed slowly through the intact mammalian skin (when applied topically), from the GI tract (when ingested), and from the mucous membranes (when inhaled). It is stored in body fat, metabolized by the liver, and excreted in urine and feces.

Therapeutic uses. Lindane is used for the topical treatment of scabies and pediculosis. Many clinicians consider it the agent of choice for treatment of these conditions in older children, men, and nonpregnant and nonlactating women.

Adverse reactions. When used appropriately, topically applied lindane appears to be nontoxic. Skin irritation and rash may occur, and contact dermatitis frequently develops with repeated use.

Inhalation of lindane vapors produces more serious reactions. Acute exposure may cause headache, nausea, vomiting, and irritation of the eyes, nose, and throat. Chronic exposure may result in hematologic disorders, including fatal aplastic anemia. (These adverse effects have not been reported after use of 1% lindane, the preparation usually used therapeutically.)

Systemically absorbed lindane, whether ingested or absorbed through the skin, can cause serious CNS, hepatic, and renal toxicities. Initial stimulation of the CNS results in vomiting, restlessness, muscle spasms, ataxia, and (possibly) seizures. Subsequent depression may cause respiratory failure and coma; death may occur within 24 hours. Other adverse reactions to ingested lindane include cardiac arrhythmia (*eg*, bradycardia, sinus arrhythmia, ventricular fibrillation), pulmonary edema, hepatitis, microscopic hematuria, and bladder irritation.

Precautions and contraindications. Lindane should never be applied to the face, eyes, mucous membranes, urethral meatus, or abraded or inflamed skin. If the eyes are accidentally contaminated, they should be flushed immediately with copious amounts of water.

If irritation or allergic reaction develops, the drug should be removed with soap and water.

Lindane should be used with caution in infants, small children, and pregnant or nursing women. Studies in mice indicate that the substance may be carcinogenic.

Lindane is contraindicated for individuals with a history of allergic hypersensitivity to it. Some resistance to the drug by lice and mites has been found, in which case permethrin may be more effective.

Permethrin

Permethrin is a pyrethroid compound.

Pharmacodynamics. Permethrin acts on the nerve cell membrane to disrupt the sodium channel current that regulates the polarization of the membrane. This disruption delays repolarization and paralyzes the pests.

Pharmacodynamics. Permethrin is rapidly metabolized by ester hydrolysis to inactive metabolites that are excreted primarily in the urine. Studies have not determined the exact amount absorbed, but it appears to be 2% or less of the amount applied.

Therapeutic uses. Permethrin is used for topical treatment of scabies.

Adverse reactions. Permethrin may temporarily exacerbate the pruritus, edema, and erythema caused by the scabies. Mild burning or stinging may also occur

after the application. Pruritus may continue for 2 to 4 weeks after application.

Precautions and contraindications. Permethrin may be mildly irritating to the eyes. If contact takes place, the eyes should be flushed with water immediately. Permethrin should not be used by those with a hypersensitivity to it or by nursing mothers.

Pyrethrins with piperonyl butoxide

Pyrethrins are purified derivatives of pyrethrum flowers (*eg*, chrysanthemums). Piperonyl butoxide is a synthetic piperic acid derivative. These two components are combined with petroleum distillate in the combination product.

Pharmacodynamics. Pyrethrins block nerve impulse transmission, causing paralysis and death. Piperonyl butoxide potentiates the action of pyrethrins by inhibiting hydrolytic enzymes that catalyze the degradation of pyrethrins. This product is effective in treating all three types of lice.

Pharmacokinetics. Pyrethrins are absorbed through the intact skin when applied topically. Piperonyl butoxide is poorly absorbed transcutaneously. Information on distribution and elimination of the two drugs in humans is not available. Pyrethrins are normally metabolized rapidly to water soluble inactive compounds. When administered to animals orally, piperonyl butoxide is excreted in feces.

Adverse reactions. When used in appropriate doses, this preparation usually causes only mild skin irritation, although the drug can cause itching and inflammation. Corneal erosion and stromal edema may also occur.

When ingested accidentally, pyrethrins produce CNS symptoms: excitation, incoordination, tremors, seizures, and death. Piperonyl produces GI symptoms (nausea, vomiting, diarrhea, hemorrhagic enteritis) and CNS depression.

Precautions and contraindications. Contact of the drug with face, eyes, mucous membranes, and inflamed or raw surfaces should be avoided. If the drug contacts the eyes, the eyes should be irrigated with copious amounts of water. The drug should not be used for individuals with an allergic hypersensitivity to it. If marked inflammation or allergic reaction develops when the drug is applied, it should be removed by bathing, and a physician should be consulted.

■ Summary

Scabies and lice are the most prevalent ectoparasites that require treatment. The chemicals used to treat these infestations are toxic insecticides. A single treatment often eliminates the mites or lice. Some drug agents can be absorbed systemically, either transcutaneously or by inhalation. Unnecessary exposure should be avoided. These preparations should not be applied to the face, eyes, mucous membranes, or inflamed raw skin areas.

Nursing management

Nursing implications

Nurses must be alert to diagnose infestations of mites and lice. Affected clients should be isolated from others free of the infestation until treatment is completed, especially in institutions where infestations can rapidly reach epidemic proportions. When many individuals are affected, treatment should be simultaneous.

Clients are often ashamed of harboring the scabies mite or lice. These feelings are exacerbated by the use of protective equipment, which impedes direct contact between nurse and client. The nurse must be sensitive to the client's reaction. Care should be exercised to display no revulsion while treating the client. The nurse's attitude should be matter-of-fact and warmly accepting.

Nursing process

Assessment The nurse is often the health care professional who first diagnoses cases of ectoparasitic infestation. Lice may be detected by inspecting the hair and scalp. If only a few lice are present, they probably are not visible. However, hair infestation may be assumed if nits (eggs) are found on hair shafts. Nits have the appearance of dandruff, but they surround a hair shaft and adhere tenaciously. Nits are often thickest in the hair near the base of the skull.

Mites are barely visible to the eye. As with lice, scabies is rarely diagnosed by identification of the ectoparasite. Typical lesions in scabies are abrasions in the area of the wrists or ankles. These are caused by scratching where the mites burrow. Secondary infection may develop, and the lesions may spread beyond the areas initially affected.

Nursing diagnosis Diagnoses related to the symptoms include

Altered comfort: itching
Altered tissue integrity: inflammation
Infection, secondary, from the burrowing or bites of ectoparasites
Knowledge deficit concerning ectoparasite infections, and their prevention, control, and treatment

Planning Immediate goals of treatment are to eliminate the ectoparasites, promote healing of skin lesions, and prevent adverse reaction to the scabicides and pediculicides used for treatment. Education of the client regarding ectoparasite infestations and their prevention, control, and treatment is the major long-term goal.

Intervention Individuals with whom the affected person has frequent or close contact should be assessed for infestation. All affected people should be treated simultaneously. Clothing and bedding should be disinfected by dry cleaning or washing with hot water, followed by drying in a hot dryer. After treatment is completed, the drug is removed by bathing or shampooing.

Client education. Clients who are willing to carry out the treatment should be instructed in the proper technique for using insecticides. Directions for application and duration of treatment must be followed accurately. Clients should be cautioned to avoid excessive exposure to the drugs; the importance of good ventilation and body areas to be avoided when applying the medication should be specifically explained. When the medication is removed, freshly cleaned clothing should be worn. After treatment for head lice, the hair should be combed with a fine-tooth comb to remove nits.

Clients should be instructed in specific measures for preventing reinfestation. Clothing and personal items, such as combs, should not be shared. Cleanliness reduces the risk of infestation but cannot prevent it. Head lice are often a chronic problem in public schools, making avoidance of reinfestation difficult. Short hair and daily applications of ordinary hair spray are simple but effective ways to reduce the risk of reinfestation.

The client should be reassured that ectoparasitic infestation is a contagious condition "caught" from others and not the result of lack of cleanliness or "bad" behavior.

Evaluation During treatment, clients should be observed for signs and symptoms of adverse drug reaction (marked irritation of the skin, irritation of the eyes). After treatment, clients should be monitored for new lesions or other evidence of reinfestation for a period of 1 to 2 weeks.

Client teaching may be evaluated by questioning the client regarding content that has been taught. The absence of recurrent infestation is the most desirable evidence of effective teaching (see the Example of Nursing Process and Treatment for Head Lice).

Checklist of nursing actions

☐ Obtain prompt treatment for clients affected by ectoparasites.
☐ Avoid unnecessary exposure to drugs used to treat ectoparasitic infestations.
☐ Teach clients to avoid sharing clothing and personal items to reduce the risk of reinfestation.

Example of nursing process and treatment for head lice

The clients are a family of five: the parents, a boy aged 12, and two girls aged 9 and 7. The children have experienced several episodes of head lice within the past year and a half, which occur during the school term. The children are again complaining of itching scalps. One daughter found a louse in her hair yesterday, and nits are visible in the hair at the back of her head.

The girl has never had her hair cut; it reaches almost to her waist. The boy's hair is collar length. Neither parent has signs or symptoms of infestation.

The mother is disheartened by the perception that she has failed to "keep the kids' heads clean." She has been using an over-the-counter preparation but is not sure that all lice have been eliminated. She asks if there is anything she can do to get rid of the lice and prevent reinfestations.

Assessment data	Nursing diagnosis	Intervention	Goals and outcome criteria
Complaints by the children of itching scalps	Altered comfort: itching related to inflammation secondary to recurring head lice	The nurse may recommend that the mother consult a physician to obtain a prescription for lindane, an effective pediculocide.	After treatment, the children's hair will appear clean and free from lice or nits.
Live louse and nits found in hair of one daughter			Reinfestation will not recur.
		Work with the mother as she follows the treatment regimen, complimenting her on aspects of the treatment that are carried out properly. If errors in technique (*eg*, not allowing enough time for the pediculocide to work) become evident, explain and demonstrate the correct method.	
		After the pediculocide has been removed from the children's heads, a fine-tooth comb should be used to remove any nits from the hair.	
		The nurse should advise the mother to discuss with the children ways in which lice can be contracted (*eg*, sharing combs, brushes, hats, or other personal items used in the hair) and precautions that help reduce the risk of reinfestation. The mother may be informed that, although it may be easier to care for short hair, it is not necessary to cut the children's hair to prevent reinfestation.	
		The nurse should suggest the daily use of hair spray on all of the children's hair, to act as an insect repellant.	

☐ When repeated reinfestation with head lice is a problem, recommend the daily use of hair spray as a louse repellent.

☐ Be accepting of clients and understand the guilt and shame that they may feel.

Nursing management of clients with infections or infestations
Nursing implications

Prevention. The best prevention of contagious disease is to eliminate contact between host and parasites. The nurse must be thoroughly familiar with the sanitary, hygienic, and aseptic measures needed to reduce infections and infestations. Cleanliness alone may not be sufficient. Sharing personal care items and clothing tends to spread scabies and pediculosis. Inadequate sanitation, improper handling of human waste, water and food pollution, and overcrowding contribute to the spread of contagion. The nurse must be knowledgeable in preventative measures to educate people in self-care, to protect clients in health care settings, and to advise community authorities about public health measures.

Waste disposal. Proper disposal of human waste is of primary importance. Excreta must be confined until disinfected, to prevent the dispersion of contagion into the environment by physical means or through intermediate hosts. Traditional systems for handling sewage in liquid form are under scrutiny because of the difficulty in purifying the effluent, which must be returned to ground water supplies. Systems for composting wastes on residential premises are offered as alternatives to this inefficient process. One such system, the *clivus multrum* (How the clivus system works, 1972) mixes paper, vegetable, and other organic materials along with excreta in a closed system built within the home. Over a period of time (2 or more years), bacterial action and chemical breakdown eliminate pathogens in the waste pile and produce a powdery material used as fertilizer. Some heat is produced by the process. The system is constructed to prevent contact between wastes and vectors capable of carrying disease. Present equipment is vented to remove the methane gas formed by the process; recovery of this methane for use as a fuel has been proposed. No matter how human wastes are treated, sewage must be protected from access by flies, snails, or other disease carriers, and pathogens must be destroyed before the wastes are dispersed into the environment.

Control of vectors. To eliminate disease carriers from the immediate environment, physical barriers are important. Rat-proof construction and tight screening help eliminate rodents and insects from buildings. Encouraging natural predators (birds, frogs, toads, snakes, and cats) also reduces vector populations. Alleviating crowded living conditions and promoting good personal hygiene also help reduce contagion. General improvement of living conditions is associated with a reduction in infectious disease.

Safe use of pesticides. When diseases transmitted by intermediate hosts are not adequately controlled by barrier techniques, the use of pesticides to control vector populations may be necessary. These toxic chemicals often disturb the ecology, poison beneficial life forms, and threaten human welfare. Wherever possible, natural predators or diseases should be used to combat the pests. In some cases, the release of sterilized males has reduced the natural reproduction of insects by interfering with fertilization of the females.

When poisons must be used as a last resort, handlers of the chemical must protect themselves from contamination. Inhalation, ingestion, and skin contact are to be avoided. Food should not be exposed to contamination. After application of the pesticide, the handler should remove clothing and shower. The clothes must not be worn again until cleaned. Certain toxic chemicals are reserved for use by specially trained and licensed applicators. Others, however, are freely available to the public. Use of these chemicals in or around the home often violates the principles outlined previously.

Vaccines. Vaccines are sometimes used to prevent outbreaks or epidemics of infectious disease. When normal sanitation is disrupted by natural disaster or civil disturbance, it is assumed that contagious diseases are likely to occur. Mass immunizations (*eg*, against typhus) are often used to forestall a potential epidemic. The nurse must be proficient in administering these drugs, because this is usually a nursing task, whether the medicines are given in a clinic or in a private office setting.

Casefinding. The nurse must be thoroughly familiar with the disease—its geographic distribution, environmental conditions associated with increased incidence, personal risk factors, and the signs and symptoms of illness—to identify victims of infection in the early stages. Particular attention must be paid to early signs and symptoms if the client is to be referred for treatment when the cure is easiest to accomplish and the disease is least serious. It is important that the nurse give accurate information about methods of treatment used locally. Clients have many questions about the treatment recommended. If the nurse does not have reliable knowledge, consultation with public health nurses, public health authorities, or local physicians may provide the needed information.

Maintaining the client's dignity. Many of the diseases discussed in this chapter carry a stigma because of their association with poverty and poor health practices. Nurses must be nonjudgmental in their approach to both victims and contacts if they want them to comply with their recommendations. It should be remembered that living conditions are not always a matter of choice and that contagious illness can and does occur in every level of society. Care must be taken to respect the dignity of the client, particularly when contagious illness occurs. Known or suspected carriers need encouragement because they are not ill and derive no personal benefit from treatment, except the knowledge that they are no longer capable of spreading the illness.

Support. Some victims of contagious disease are debilitated or acutely ill. They may need considerable supportive care to improve their condition before treatment can be initiated. Some, but not all, are hospitalized during this period. The nurse must appraise the condition of the client at every phase of treatment, because medication can be dangerous. Toxic drugs are administered cautiously to such clients. In some conditions, particularly systemic fungal or fluke infections, the prognosis may not be favorable. The nurse should strive to foster hope but avoid overly optimistic reassurances.

Client education. While undergoing active treatment for disease, victims of contagion need help in managing their drug regimens. Specific instructions for administering the drug must be given. Any special precautions should be clearly described. Clients must be informed of adverse reactions to their medications and should know when to contact the nurse, pharmacist, or physician for additional advice or treatment. Victims of known cases of disease must be advised about preventive measures and be referred for treatment.

After successful treatment for contagious conditions, some measures to prevent recurrence are usually needed. If the infectious agent can be eliminated from the environment, the client can be taught sanitary or hygienic measures to prevent reinfection. When the infection has been arrested or suppressed, clients must be instructed about the signs and symptoms of recurrence, so that they secure prompt medical attention when needed.

A variety of toxic insecticides are used in the home; for this reason, clients should be cautioned against practices that expose humans to these chemicals. Garden sprays may also be toxic and should be used with great caution to protect the public, particularly children. Sprays should be used indoors only when the area to be treated can be evacuated. The rooms should be cleaned immediately afterward to remove dead insects and pesticide residues. Pesticides should never be used in food preparation areas; residues can be found in the food in measurable amounts

when this happens. As new chemicals are developed, they are marketed with specific directions for handling and recommended doses. These must be carefully followed. All toxins should be kept under lock and key, whether used by commercial firms or private citizens.

Travelers abroad often need to take special precautions to remain well. Immunization is usually recommended against diseases that are either epidemic or endemic to the area. Suppressant medication to prevent malaria is prescribed for those planning to visit malarial areas. Clients should be advised to avoid outdoor bathing where flukes are a problem. Precautions for avoiding contaminated food and water are often advisable. For example, tap water may be unsafe to drink in cities such as Paris, with its aging sewer and water systems. Breaks in pipes or conduits often lead to cross contamination. In countries with poor sanitation or where fresh human wastes are used as fertilizer, fresh fruits and vegetables often carry disease. Hot food, which has been thoroughly cooked, is usually safe; rare meat may transmit worms. Blanket prescriptions are to be avoided. Instruction should be specific about problems in the regions the traveler visits. If unnecessary precautions are advised, the traveler may lose confidence in the advice given and abandon all precautions. Moreover, unnecessary anxiety and restrictions on activities interfere with the pleasure anticipated by the ordinary tourist.

The future. In all probability, it will not be possible to eliminate infectious disease from the Earth. Until recently, we have not been successful in eradicating any single disease. Claims have been made, however, that smallpox in its natural state has disappeared. This disease is peculiar in that no natural reservoir of infection outside of human victims seems to exist. Moreover, it has taken a concerted worldwide effort to suppress smallpox to the point at which it appears to have been conquered. It is much more difficult to eliminate contagions that affect other species or are carried by intermediate vectors. Although we have many new chemical weapons against contagion, these drugs not only are not without risk, but they also often become ineffective as resistance to them develops in pathogens. The prevention and treatment of contagion continues to be important in health care. The ability to use chemicals in these endeavors remains an important nursing skill.

References

How the clivus system works. (1972). *Organic Gardening and Farming, 19,* 47.
Miller JA. (1986). Malaria vaccine tests under way. *Science News, 129,* 232.
Raloff J. (1986). Infant dioxin exposures reported high. *Science News, 129,* 264.

Bibliography

Agranulocytosis associated with the use of amodiazine for malaria prophylaxis. (1986). *MMWR, 35,* 165–166.

Altman L. (1990, October 23). Tiny mite causes overwhelming itch: Elusive scabies. *The New York Times,* p B6.

Altman L. (1990, July 3). Genetic factor emerges as key to onset of Lyme disease. *The New York Times,* p C1.

Brooke J. (1991, April 19). Cholera kills 1100 in Peru and marches on, reaching the Brazilian border. *The New York Times,* p A3.

Gever LN. (1986). Pentamidine: Treatment for A.I.D.S. complications. *Nursing 86, 16(9),* 92.

Gilman AG, et al, eds. (1990). *Goodman and Gilman's the pharmacological basis of therapeutics,* 8th ed, pp 977–979, 1004–1065. New York: Pergamon Press.

Glaberson W. (1991, May 6). A tide of anxiety over rabies sweeps the N.Y. region. *The New York Times,* p B1.

*Insecticides growing in trees. (1985). *Science News, 128,* 168.

McEvoy GK, ed. (1987). *Drug Information 87,* pp 31–49, 1881–1885. Bethesda: American Society of Hospital Pharmacists.

Meinking TL, Taplin D, Kalter DC, Eberle MW. (1986). Comparative efficacy of treatments for pediculosis capitis infestations. *Arch Dermatol, 122,* 267.

Miller JA. (1986). Malaria vaccine tests under way. *Science News, 129,* 232.

Nash N. (1991, February 17). A model hospital in Peru is hard-pressed by a growing cholera epidemic. *The New York Times,* p Y3.

A new rinse for head lice. (1986). *RN, 49(8),* 69.

Okino K, Weibert R. (1986). Warfarin-griseofulvin interaction. *Drug Intell Clin Pharm, 20,* 291–293.

Paparone. (1990). The summer scourge of Lyme disease. *American Journal of Nursing, 90,* 44–47

*Raloff J. (1986). Infant dioxin exposures reported high. *Science News, 129,* 264.

Rosenberg S, et al. (1990). Gene therapy for gene transfer into humans: Immunotherapy with advanced melanomas using tumor-infiltrating lymphocytes modified by retroviral gene transduction. *N Engl J Med, 323(9),* 570–578.

Rosenthal E. (1991, May 9). Hope of a human malaria vaccine is offered as mice are innoculated. *The New York Times,* p B9.

Rosenthal E. (1991, February 12). Outwitted by malaria, desperate doctors seek new remedies. *The New York Times,* p B5.

Serious problems with antimalarial drugs (editorial). (1986). *J Infect, 13,* 1–4.

Shlian K, Goldstone J. (1986). Toxicity of butylated hydroxytolulene (letter). *N Engl J Med, 314,* 648–649.

*Recommended for further reading.

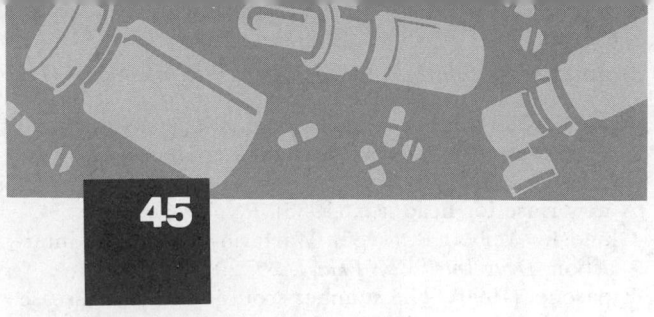

45

Antipyretics

Certain drugs are capable of reducing the abnormally high temperatures characteristic of febrile illnesses. Their use requires an understanding of the body's thermostatic control.

Under normal circumstances, the body's temperature remains in a relatively narrow range between 98.0°F and 100°F (36.5°C and 37.5°C). This range represents a dynamic equilibrium between the heat produced by cell metabolism and muscle activity and the heat lost by radiation, conduction, convection, and evaporation. Body temperature is regulated by a neuronal mechanism located in the hypothalamus, which adjusts heat-producing and heat-dissipating functions in response to changes in blood temperature.

Fever

Pathophysiology of fever

Fever is an increase in body temperature above the normal range. This may result from the impairment of normal temperature-regulating mechanisms of the body or from factors that influence the hypothalamic "thermostat." When the heat-dissipating mechanisms do not function adequately, body temperature rises and may reach extreme levels.

Certain chemicals, characterized by large molecules, are capable of influencing the temperature-regulating mechanism. Those that increase body tem-

perature, including proteins, protein breakdown products, and polysaccharides, are called *pyrogens*. Disease states characterized by fever are believed to cause a release of autogenous pyrogens. Therapeutic agents, such as intravenous (IV) solutions, may cause fever because they contain contaminants that act as pyrogens. Injections of killed typhoid bacilli also raise body temperature and have been administered in the past to induce a therapeutic increase in temperature.

When the hypothalamic thermostat is reset at a higher level through the influence of pyrogens, heat-dissipating mechanisms are inhibited, and heat-producing mechanisms are activated. Peripheral blood vessels constrict, perspiration decreases, and muscle tone increases. The affected person experiences a subjective feeling of cold and shivers uncontrollably. The skin is pale and dry. This syndrome, called a *chill*, will persist until body temperature rises to the level dictated by the new thermostatic setting. At this point, the normal balance of control mechanism is restored, and the person feels comfortably warm and moist, and shivering disappears.

The resolution of fever may follow one of two patterns, *crisis* or *lysis*. In crisis, the hypothalamic thermostat reverts suddenly to a normal setting in response to a change in the disease process (Fig. 45-1). Heat-dissipating mechanisms are stimulated. The person feels hot, and the skin is flushed and wet from perspiration. Body temperature drops rapidly to a normal level. Lysis is characterized by a more gradual decline in temperature than that which occurs in crisis (Fig. 45-2). In lysis, the thermostatic setting is readjusted by repeated small changes, causing a more erratic course in temperature declines.

Protective and detrimental effects of fever

Fever is a defensive response of the body that can generate both protective and harmful effects (Table 45-1).

The protective effects of fever include the impairment and destruction of certain pathogenic organisms in the body and the stimulation of the body's production of cellular immune substances that defend it against bacterial invasion. Fever also promotes rest, because the discomforts associated with it are less severe when activity is decreased. An elevation in body temperature appears to be especially helpful during acute infectious illnesses, where complete suppression of fever is usually not desirable.

In the years prior to the use of antibiotics, induction of fever was used to treat some illnesses (syphilis, gonorrhea). Today, local hyperthermia may be combined with chemotherapy to suppress the proliferation of some cancer cells.

Harmful effects of fever include increased stress on the heart, tissue damage, and nutritional depletion. Increased heat production is accomplished by an excessive consumption of calories. If nutritional intake is

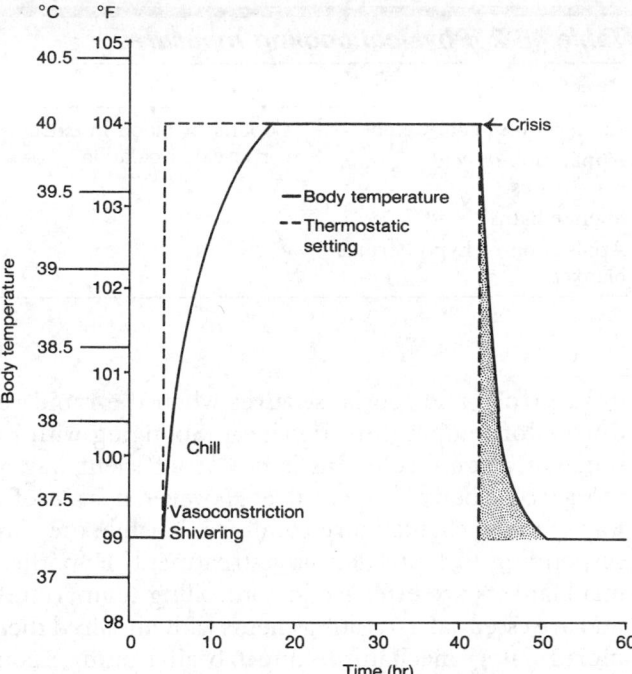

Figure 45-1. Temperature changes during a febrile illness that resolves by crisis. Crisis is characterized by a rapid return of body temperature to normal, accompanied by peripheral vasodilation (flushing), perspiration, and a sensation of being hot.

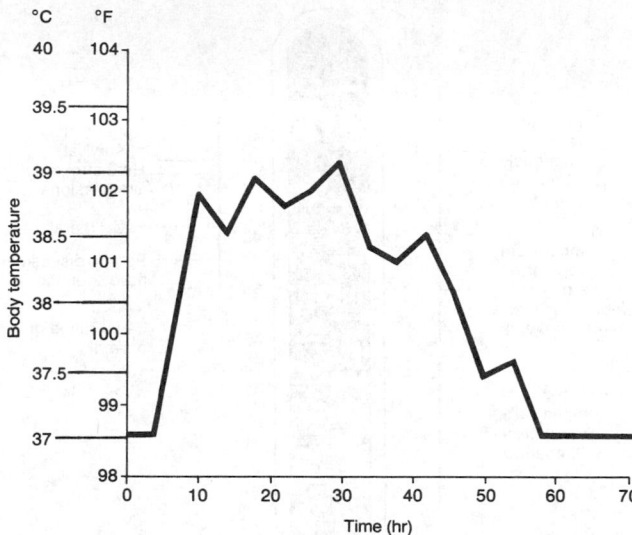

Figure 45-2. Typical temperature changes during a febrile illness that resolves by lysis. This pattern is seen more commonly than crisis, especially when febrile infections are treated with antimicrobial drugs.

inadequate to meet the need for calories, body tissue will be broken down, causing the tissue wasting that is characteristic of febrile states. Very high temperatures may be life-threatening. Rapid rises of temperature in children often induce grand mal seizures. In adults, delirium is not uncommon. Prolonged or extremely high fever may produce severe dehydration. Very high temperatures (above 41°C [106°F]) appear to break down the body's enzyme systems and also seem to interfere with many critical life processes. Permanent brain damage, including the body's mechanism for temperature regulation, can occur (Fig. 45-3). For these reasons, very high or prolonged fevers must be controlled to prevent serious injury.

Because body temperature is considered one of the cardinal signs of general physiologic status, it is used as an important diagnostic factor. Suppression of fever before diagnosis can make a definitive diagnosis difficult. For this reason, measures to reduce fever are often delayed or restricted until the basic pathologic process and appropriate therapy are determined.

Defining and diagnosing fever

Normal temperature varies from individual to individual and from time to time. It is ususally higher in younger people and in those with a relatively higher metabolic rate. Vigorous exercise produces a rise in temperature, as can emotional excitement. In women, normal temperatures rise at the time of ovulation, an increase usually sustained until just before menstruation. For these reasons, the presence of fever can be determined with certainty only after a client's normal range of temperature has been established. Averaging a number of temperature readings taken under similar conditions provides a base for assessing subsequent temperatures. For example, a number of early morning temperatures taken before arising from bed (and before eating) can be averaged to produce an average basal temperature. The nurse must bear in mind that average temperature levels later in the day are higher in most clients. When interpreting and using such

Table 45-1. Effects of fever

Beneficial	Detrimental
Promotion of rest in response to discomfort and weakness	Discomfort—headache, photophobia, malaise, muscle and bone soreness
Impairment or destruction of pathogens (*eg*, organisms that cause syphilis and brucellosis)	Increased work load on the heart
	Losses of water and sodium
Increased production of immune substances	Constipation
	Anorexia
Improvement of inflammatory changes (*eg*, in uveitis, rheumatoid arthritis)	Loss of body mass consumed for the production of energy—negative nitrogen balance
	Stimulation of seizures
	Tissue damage
	Local hemorrhage, parenchymal degeneration of cells

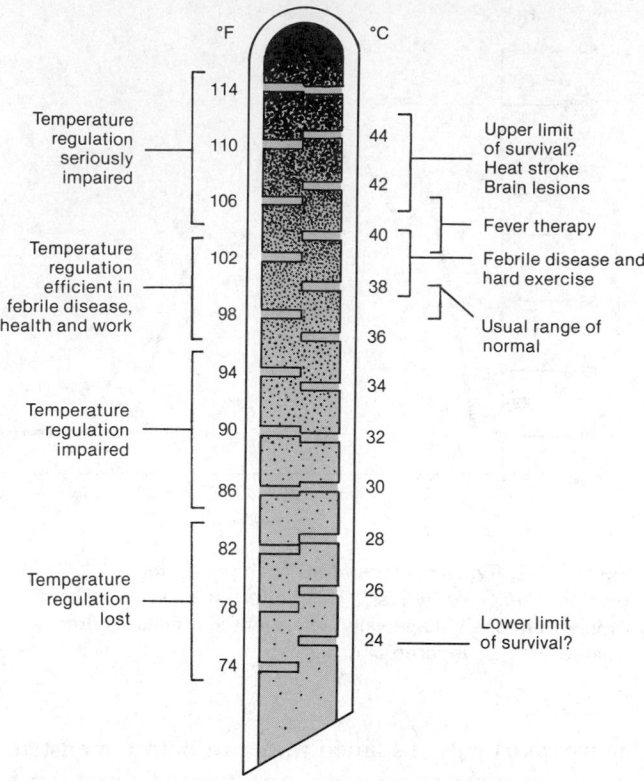

Figure 45-3. Body temperatures under different conditions. (Dubois EP. [1948]. *Fever and the regulation of body temperature*. Springfield, IL: Charles C Thomas.)

averages, the nurse must also consider such factors as the menstrual cycle, exercise, eating, and emotional stimulation.

Fever is considered to be present whenever temperature is 1° or 2° above the expected reading. Despite individual differences, fever is also considered to be present whenever oral temperature exceeds 37.8°C (100°F), or rectal temperature exceeds 38.4°C (101°F).

Therapeutic management of fever

The aim of therapeutic measures to reduce fever is to prevent serious injury to affected clients and to reduce their discomfort without eliminating any of the beneficial effects of the temperature elevation associated with fever and without obscuring diagnosis (Box 45-1). Medication is only one of several methods used to reduce temperature (Table 45-2). Immersion is useful

---

Box 45-1. Aim of therapeutic measures in fever:

- To prevent serious thermal injury to client
- To reduce discomfort
- To maintain the benefits of temperature elevation
- To avoid obscuring the diagnosis

Table 45-2. Physical cooling measures

Direct cooling	Indirect cooling
Immersion in cool water	Cooling of blood in extra-corporeal circulation
Application of cold compresses	
Sponge baths	
Application of hypothermia blanket	

in sunstroke and febrile seizures when the rapid reduction of temperature is critical. Sponging with ice water or alcohol solutions is not an efficient way to reduce core body temperature. However, it is a useful way to make clients more comfortable while they are responding to more definitive treatment. Hypothermia blankets are effective in controlling temperature and are essential in treating clients with impaired thermoregulatory mechanisms due to brain trauma, a condition in which antipyretic drugs are of no value.

Drugs used to control fever

Drugs that directly influence the pyrogenic process include quinine, dantrolene sodium (a muscle relaxant), the glucocorticoids, and various anti-inflammatory analgesics (Table 45-3).

Quinine is of interest because it was the first antipyretic drug. An effective antimalarial, it was at first believed to be useful in many febrile conditions. In fact, the drug has a weak antipyretic action; its efficacy in malaria stems mainly from its specific effects on the plasmodia. Although quinine is no longer used in medical therapy to reduce fever, it may still be valued for this purpose by advocates of folk or herbal medicine.

Most of the drugs presently used to control fever belong to the class of nonopioid analgesics. They include the salicylates and other nonsteroidal anti-inflammatory drugs (*eg*, phenylbutazone, indomethacin, ibuprofen, sulindac). Because they are effective and relatively safe, acetylsalicylic acid (aspirin) and acetaminophen (Tylenol) are most commonly used.

Pharmacodynamics. The glucocorticoids effectively reduce fever that stems from infection or inflammation by suppressing the inflammatory response.

Dantrolene sodium interferes with the release of calcium from the sarcoplasmic reticulum to the myoplasm. This interference may prevent the increase in myoplasmic calcium, which activates acute tissue breakdown in the skeletal muscle in malignant hyperthermia.

The nonopioid analgesics appear to antagonize the effect on the hypothalamus of endogenous pyrogens derived from leukocytes. By interacting with

Table 45-3. Antipyretic drugs

Drug name	Preparations	Usual dosage/PC	Adverse reactions
Traditional			
quinine (Coco-Quinine, Novo-quinine, QM-2 Quinamm, Quine, Quinite, Quiphile, Strema)	Cinchona bark infusion Capsules and tablets for oral use	Frequent small amounts of cinchona bark tea until the temperature declines or until tinnitus develops PC: X	Tinnitus, dizziness, tremor, palpitations (in therapeutic doses) Hearing impairment (in toxic doses)
Glucocorticoids			
dexamethasone (AK-Dex, Decadron, Deconil, Dexameth, Dexasone, Dexone, Gammacorten, Hexadrol, Maxidex, Oradexon, PMS-Dexamethasone, Spersadex)	Tablets and solutions for oral use Solution for injection and inhalation	Adults: Initially, 10 mg; thereafter, 4 mg–6 mg q6h Children: Initially, 0.5 mg–1.5 mg/kg body wt; thereafter, 0.05 mg–0.8 mg/kg body wt q6h PC: C	Hypercortism Symptoms of toxicity rarely seen because drug is used for short terms Signs and symptoms of inflammation useful for definitive diagnosis are suppressed
Hydantoin derivative			
dantrolene sodium (Dantrium)	Oral capsules, sterile powder for preparing solutions for IV administration	Adults: For treatment of malignant hypertension, 1 mg/kg body wt, repeated as necessary to a maximum total dose of 10 mg/kg body wt; for prevention of malignant hypertension, 1 mg/kg body wt tid or qid for 1 day–2 day preoperatively PC: C	Nervous system changes: muscle weakness, fatigue, drowsiness, dizziness, visual disturbances, change in taste, depression, confusion, hallucinations, nervousness, seizures Gastrointestinal disturbances: anorexia, nausea, vomiting, diarrhea, constipation, GI bleeding, hepatotoxicity Genitourinary changes: dysuria, retention, crystaluria, hematuria Cardiovascular changes: erratic blood pressure, phlebitis
Salicylates			
aspirin (Alka Seltzer, Arthritis Pain Formula, A.S.A., Ascriptin, Aspergum, Bayer Aspirin, Bufferin, Cama, Easprin, Empirin, Measurin, Zorprin)	Chewing gum Capsules, powder, tablets, and enteric-coated tablets for oral use Rectal suppositories In combination with other drugs, such as phenacetin and codeine	Not recommended for fever of viral etiology Adults: 300 mg–600 mg q4h–q6h for temperature >37.4°C (101°F); maximum daily dosage: 4 g Children: Depending on age, up to 480 mg q4h–q6h for temperature >39.4°C (103°F); maximum daily dosage: 5 doses PC: C (D in last trimester)	Gastric irritation, increased risk of peptic ulcers Tinnitus and hearing impairment Asthma Mucosal ulcerations from use of suppositories Anticoagulation and increased bleeding tendency
Para-aminophenol derivatives			
acetaminophen (Abenol, Aceta, Acetagesic, Actimin, Anicin-3, Anaphen, Apo-Acetaminophen, Atasol, Calpol, Children's Anicin-3, Dapa, Datril, Dolonex, Exdol, Liquiprin, Panadol, Paralgin, Pedric, Phenaphen, Robigesic, Rounex, SK*Apap, Tempra, Tylenol, Tralgon, Valadol, Valorin)	Powder, tablets, and liquid for oral use Rectal suppositories In combination with other drugs, such as codeine	Adults and children older than 11 yrs of age: 300 mg–600 mg q4h–q6h; maximum daily dosage: 4 g Children: Depending on age, up to 480 mg q4h–q6h PC: B	Kidney and liver damage (in toxic doses, severe liver damage)
phenylbutazone (Apo-Phenylbutazone, Azolid, Butazolidin, Ecobutazone, Intrabutazone, Novobutazone, Phenbuff)	Capsules and tablets for oral use	Adults: 300 mg–600 mg once a day PC: C	Nausea, vomiting Increased risk of peptic ulcers Blood dyscrasias Skin reactions Visual and hearing impairment

(Continued)

Table 45-3. Antipyretic drugs (Continued)

Drug name	Preparations	Usual dosage/PC	Adverse reactions
Indoleacetic acid derivative			
indomethacin (Amuno, Apo-Indomethacin, Indocid, Indocin, Indomee, Metacen)	Capsules for oral use	Adults: 25 mg bid or tid; maximum daily dosage: 200 mg Children: 2 mg–4 mg/kg body wt daily, divided in 2–3 doses; maximum daily dosage: 150 mg PC: B	Central and peripheral nervous system toxicity (headache, dizziness, ataxia, insomnia, hallucinations, and depression) Gastrointestinal upset (nausea, vomiting, abdominal pain, diarrhea, and increased risk of peptic or intestinal ulcers

receptor sites in the thermoregulating centers of the hypothalamus, such fever-inducing chemicals cause the control level to shift to a higher temperature. By interfering with this agonistic action on the body thermostat, antipyretics lower fever of inflammatory origin. They reduce abnormally high temperatures but do not lower normal body temperature. Nonsteroidal anti-inflammatory drugs inhibit prostaglandin synthase and, in so doing, interfere with the redness, swelling, heat, and pain exhibited when tissue injury occurs.

Pharmacokinetics. Most antipyretic drugs are administered orally or rectally. However, the glucocorticoids can be injected, and dantrolene sodium can be administered IV. For distribution, metabolism, and excretion of these drugs, see the appropriate sections in Chapters 32, 39, 47, which discuss these drugs in detail.

Therapeutic uses. Antipyretic drugs are used to prevent or reduce dangerously high temperatures, which are capable of causing serious physiologic damage. These drugs also are used to moderate temperatures in febrile illness after a firm diagnosis and an appropriate treatment have been established. The therapeutic goal is usually not to restore temperatures to normal levels, but to reduce the discomfort and physiologic depletion characteristic of prolonged or pronounced fever.

The use of dantrolene sodium is limited to preventing and treating malignant hyperthermia. This anesthesia-induced condition is a familial disease associated with musculoskeletal abnormalities and high blood levels of the creatinine-phosphokinase. It is manifested by high fever, tachycardia, irregular pulse, and rapid shallow breathing.

Cortisol is sometimes used to suppress life-threatening manifestations of inflammatory disease when diagnosis cannot be established or when no response to other therapy, such as antibiotics, can be achieved.

Dosage and administration. Corticosteroids may be administered by mouth or by injection (intramuscular or IV). Dosage requirements for glucocorticoids are influenced by the degree of stress that affects the client and by endogenous hormone production. Because they vary widely, these dosages are determined by clinical response of the individual client (see Chapter 32).

To treat malignant hyperthermia, dantrolene sodium is administered by rapid IV in doses of 1 mg/kg body weight. The dose may be repeated up to a maximum total dose of 10 mg/kg body weight. To prevent malignant hyperthermia crisis, 1 to 2 mg/kg body weight may be administered orally three or four times a day for 1 to 2 days preoperatively.

Antipyretic dosages for aspirin and acetaminophen are similar. Adults receive 300 to 600 mg every 3 to 4 hours; children receive 65 mg/kg body weight per day, divided in 4 to 6 doses (or 10 to 20 mg/kg body weight/dose). These drugs are administered orally or, if nausea or vomiting occur, rectally.

Adverse reactions. The side effects and toxic effects that can occur are those characteristic of the drugs employed. The reader is referred to the detailed discussions of glucocorticoids in Chapter 32, dantrolene sodium in Chapter 39, and aspirin and acetaminophen in Chapter 47.

Precautions and contraindications. The use of antipyretics may obscure diagnostic signs and symptoms by suppressing the body's response to the underlying disease process. The administration of these drugs, therefore, should be delayed until diagnosis can be established, unless temperature elevations reach dangerous levels.

The use of corticosteroids to suppress the dangerous effects of generalized inflammation is an extreme measure and places the client at high risk. Because such therapy usually does not continue for long periods, Cushing's syndrome (which results from prolonged excessive intake of glucocorticoids) commonly does not develop. However, the suppression of symptoms makes definitive diagnosis difficult and evaluation of subsequent therapy uncertain. Moreover, although the client appears improved clinically, infection may continue to progress rapidly, as body defenses against the infectious process are suppressed by the drug. In this situation, the client requires careful monitoring and intensive supportive care.

Liver, cardiac, and pulmonary functions should be monitored in clients who receive dantrolene sodium.

Before giving aspirin, the client's tolerance for the drug should be ascertained. Aspirin should not be administered by any route to a client with a history of a previous allergic asthmatic response to the drug. Aspirin should not be given to children or adolescents with chicken pox or flu symptoms, since this administration has been associated with the development of Reye's syndrome, a serious and sometimes fatal illness. Aspirin should also be withheld from anyone with bleeding or bleeding tendencies or anyone who is taking anticoagulant drugs, because aspirin interferes with blood clotting by inhibiting platelet aggregation. Aspirin should not be used by anyone with nasal polyps, as polyps indicate aspirin hypersensitivity.

Clients who experience gastric distress after ingesting aspirin may tolerate buffered preparations, enteric-coated tablets, or rectal suppositories. Because intolerance to acetaminophen appears to occur less frequently, this drug is commonly used for clients for whom aspirin is contraindicated.

The reader is referred to Chapters 32, 39, and 47 for drug interactions that involve the glucocorticoids, dantrolene, and aspirin and acetaminophen (see Focus on Salicylates: Similarities and Differences).

■ Summary

Antipyretics are drugs that reduce abnormally high body temperatures by suppressing inflammation or resetting the hypothalamic thermostat toward normal levels. They include corticosteroids and nonsteroidal anti-inflammatories such as aspirin and acetaminophen. These drugs are used to prevent serious damage characteristic of extremely high temperatures and to ameliorate the discomforting and debilitating effects of prolonged or pronounced fevers. Premature suppression of fever may obscure diagnosis and delay definitive treatment of the underlying disease.

Learning experience 45-1

Prepare a table that lists the therapeutic effects of the antipyretic drugs, aspirin, acetaminophen, and corticosteroids. Then contrast the adverse reactions to these same drugs. For each drug, delineate the clinical circumstances in which it would be preferred over the others.

Nursing management
Nursing process

Assessment The assessment of fever requires accurate and consistent monitoring of body temperature. A variety of techniques is available for this purpose. Thermometers may be made of glass (the classic mercury thermometer) or plastic and metal (electronic thermometers). Some electronic monitors have probes that remain in place for prolonged periods, providing a continuous record of temperature fluctuations. Thermosensitive tapes applied to the skin indicate gross changes in temperature but generally do not provide a sufficiently accurate measurement for professional use. A device used in pediatrics is a urine receptacle that immediately measures the temperature of urine voided into it. A pacifier designed to change color at a critical temperature level has proved to be unreliable (Wong, 1989).

Procedures used for measuring temperature should include safeguards against the generation of spurious data due to temporary modification of temperature at the site monitored. For example, oral temperatures taken immediately after the ingestion of very warm or very cold foods or beverages do not accurately reflect the actual body temperature. Similarly, rectal temperatures should not be taken immediately after the administration of enemas.

Records of body temperature should denote the body site where the temperature was measured and the type of instrument used, as well as the time of the measurement. Temperatures vary at different sites; on the Fahrenheit scale, rectal temperatures are generally 1° higher and axillary temperatures 1° lower than oral temperatures. The temperature record must be interpreted in the light of environmental influences, as well as the client's normal baseline data and rhythmic patterns.

The nurse should also keep in mind the antipyretic and anti-inflammatory properties of cortisol. Clients under prolonged or extreme stress may have high circulating levels of these hormones. In such clients, slight elevations of temperature may be highly significant. These clients often harbor active infections without exhibiting inflammatory changes.

Nursing diagnosis Nursing diagnoses for clients with hyperthermia may include the following:

Altered nutrition: less than body requirements related to increased need for calories secondary to fever
Potential for fluid volume deficit related to profuse perspiration secondary to fever
Altered oral mucous membrane: dryness related to dehydration
Altered role performance: inability to carry out

Salicylates: similarities and differences

Similarities

Pharmacodynamics

These agents inhibit the activity of the enzyme cyclooxygenase to decrease formation of precursors of prostaglandins and thromboxanes from arachidonic acid. They act peripherally by blocking pain impulse generation and centrally in the hypothalamus by inhibiting prostaglandin synthesis. They may produce antipyretic effect by acting centrally on the heat-regulating center of the hypothalamus.

Pharmacokinetics

These agents are rapidly and completely absorbed after oral administration. Food decreases the rate but not the extent of absorption. Absorption is delayed after rectal administration. These agents are distributed throughout the extracellular fluid and most tissues, highest being in the liver and kidneys. They are metabolized by the liver, peaking in 1 to 2 hours, and excreted by the kidneys.

Therapeutic uses

These agents are used in the treatment of mild to moderate pain, especially low-intensity pain of nonvisceral origin, such as headache, myalgia, and neuralgia. They are also used to relieve mild to moderate postoperative pain, dysmenorrhea, and other visceral pain. They are also used to reduce fever and as the initial and long-term symptomatic treatment of inflammatory conditions, such as rheumatoid arthritis, osteoarthritis, polyarthritic conditions, and systemic lupus erythematosus, and in the treatment of rheumatic fever.

Adverse reactions

These include: (EENT) tinnitus, hearing loss; (GI) dyspepsia, heartburn, epigastric distress, nausea, vomiting, anorexia, abdominal pain, occult GI bleeding; (GU) reduced creatinine clearance, albuminuria, proteinuria; (HEMA) leukopenia, pancytopenia, agranulocytosis, elevated liver enzymes, aplastic anemia; (OTHER) acute reversible hepatotoxicity.

Contraindications

These agents are contraindicated in children or teen-agers with chicken pox or flu because of the association with Reye's syndrome. They are also contraindicated in people who are hypersensitive or those with GI ulcers or bleeding.

Differences

• **Aspirin** interferes with platelet aggregation.

The half-life of **aspirin** ranges from 15 to 20 minutes. Extended-release, suppositories, or chewing gum preparations are incompletely absorbed. • **Aspirin** peaks in 30 to 60 minutes. • **Salsalate** has a plasma half-life of 1 hour. • **Diflusinal** peaks in 2 to 3 hours, with a half-life of 2 to 3 hours.

• **Diflusinal** does not have any antipyretic properties. • **Aspirin** is also used to prevent arterial and venous thrombosis and in the treatment of Kawasaki syndrome, in the treatment of prophylaxis of platelet hyperaggregation such as in coronary artery disease, myocardial infarction, and postoperative deep vein thrombosis.

• **Diflusinal** may cause dizziness, somnolence, headache, fatigue, palpitations and syncope, stomatitis, dry mouth, dysuria, renal impairment, chest pain, dyspnea, peripheral edema, and muscle cramps. • **Sodium salicylate** (IV) may cause thrombophlebitis and tissue sloughing if extravasation occurs.

• **Aspirin** is contraindicated in people sensitive to tartrazine dye and those with hemophilia.

(continued)

Focus on

Salicylates: similarities and differences (*Continued*)

Similarities	Differences
Precautions	
These agents should be used cautiously in people with hypoprothrombinemia, vitamin K deficiencies, bleeding disorders, and liver or renal dysfunction and in pediatric clients who are dehydrated.	• **Diflusinal** should be used cautiously in clients with impaired cardiac function.
Nursing considerations	
Instruct in disease, treatment, drug regimen, adverse reactions, and compliance; administer with food or meals, milk, or antacids to minimize GI upset; encourage client to take with a full glass of water and remain sitting for 15 to 20 minutes afterward to ensure passage into the stomach; do not crush enteric-coated tablets; crush or combine tablet with soft food or mix with liquid if client has difficulty swallowing; monitor vital signs, especially temperature; assess for signs and symptoms of possible masking of infection; assess client's pain level before administering the drug; evaluate drug's effectiveness; monitor lab studies, such as complete blood cell count, platelets, and renal and liver function studies for changes; assess for signs of hearing impairment and notify physician; watch for signs of possible bleeding, such as bruising, petechiae, and tarry stools; instruct client in use of over-the-counter medications and possible interactions.	Stop **aspirin** 1 week before elective surgery. Institute safety measures for clients on **diflusinal** if CNS effects occur; monitor weights and presence and amount of peripheral edema; check intake and output. Administer **aspirin** delayed release whole. Dilute injectable form of **sodium salicylate** in 1 liter of normal saline or lactated Ringer's solution and administer slowly over 4 to 8 hours; check IV site frequently for signs of infiltration; monitor serum salicylate levels for toxicity. Assess clients who receive **sodium salicylate** for signs and symptoms of fluid retention.

---

usual work (family, school) tasks related to
fatigue secondary to fever
*Knowledge deficit related to the effects of fever
and its treatment*

Common collaborative problems that should be differentiated from the nursing diagnoses include

Potential complication: seizures
Potential complication: delirium
*Potential complication: adverse reaction to
antipyretic drugs*

Planning Goals of treatment include alleviating discomfort, preventing impairment of tissue integrity, reducing body temperature to the appropriate range, and promptly detecting and treating adverse reactions to antipyretic drugs, should any occur, as well as teaching the client about antipyretic drugs. Orders for antipyretic drug therapy commonly include the drug name, dose, route, and the temperature at which the drug order is to be activated, for example, aspirin

suppository (650 mg) for temperature of 39.4°C (103°F) or higher.

If the physician has not designated a temperature below which the client is to be maintained, the nurse should establish one. In most situations, clients' baseline temperatures are not known because their fevers are established before they enter the health care system. The nurse should consider the client's age when determining probable norms. In children, temperatures of 39°C may be acceptable, because they normally have higher temperature peaks than adults. However, a child with a history of febrile seizures requires maintenance at a lower temperature to avoid triggering seizure activity. Clients or their relatives may know what the normal temperatures are. Clients who suffer from hormonal abnormalities may also have baseline temperatures that differ from expected levels. Often, in the absence of unusual factors that affect temperature, antipyretic drugs are administered when the temperature in adults reaches 37.8°C (101°F) and in children, 39.4°C (103°F). It is usually not desirable to lower temperature to normal ranges, because this action deprives the client of the beneficial effects of fever and makes it more difficult to determine the remission of the febrile illness.

Intervention Clients who receive antipyretic drugs should be observed closely and assessed carefully. Not only their fever but also the inflammation and pain that accompany the febrile illness are suppressed by these drugs. The recovery process is more difficult to monitor in them. When receiving analgesic antipyretics, clients feel better than they actually are. It may be more difficult to prevent overexertion or inappropriate activity. Temperature should be checked for response 1 hour after antipyretic medication has been administered.

All clients should be monitored for adverse reactions to antipyretics as well as other drugs used such as antibiotics. Corticosteroids are powerful hormones capable of producing many toxic effects. Therapy with these drugs usually is short-term, and Cushing's syndrome does not commonly develop. However, the suppression of symptoms makes diagnosis difficult and the evaluation of subsequent therapy uncertain. Moreover, although the client appears improved clinically, the disease process continues to progress, often rapidly, because body defenses are suppressed by the drug. Minor changes in vital signs and symptoms may be highly significant.

Aspirin and acetaminophen are commonly administered orally or rectally. The consumption of milk or antacids with the oral dose may prevent gastric irritation. If the oral route is specified and nausea or vomiting develops, the physician should be consulted. A change in order is required before the nurse may administer drugs by an alternate route. More important, the physician should be apprised of the change in the client's condition.

The erosive effect of aspirin on the gastric mucosa is widely known among health care personnel. That it has a similar effect on the rectal mucosa when administered by suppository may be overlooked. Clients who receive aspirin suppositories frequently, or over a prolonged period of time, should be carefully assessed for signs and symptoms of rectal erosion. Clients who develop this reaction require a change of medication or an alternate approach to the control of their fever.

Client education. Clients must be informed of both the beneficial and the harmful effects of antipyretic drugs. Aspirin and acetaminophen are commonly used over-the-counter preparations. As such, they are not regarded as dangerous by the lay public. Yet, clients must be taught how to detect harmful reactions to these drugs and to know when such reactions should be reported to a health care professional. Clients should also be taught the importance of seeking medical help without delay when simple remedies do

not produce prompt and lasting improvement. A temperature above 38.5°C (102°F) or an elevation that persists for more than 48 hours should be evaluated by a health care professional.

Clients who are treated as outpatients may discontinue medication prematurely as symptoms subside. They should be cautioned to adhere to the prescribed drug regimen throughout their recovery phase, to prevent relapses due to inadequate treatment. Clients who have taken these drugs in the past without ill effect can usually continue to take them unless an allergic response develops. Acetaminophen may be recommended for clients who react adversely to aspirin, provided that liver function is normal. Clients should be warned not to increase the dose of antipyretic analgesics above the recommended levels because toxicity may develop. If the febrile illness does not respond to treatment as expected, the physician should be consulted. A change in therapy may be needed.

Devotees of herbal medicine who employ quinine for its antipyretic effect should be instructed in the relative merits of available antipyretics. Care must be taken to present information in a form that can be usefully integrated into the client's value system. The nurse could encourage the use of willow bark infusion, which contains salicylates instead of cinchona bark, which contains quinine, for antipyretic purposes. The importance of a daily intake of at least 3,000 ml (for adults) should be stressed to prevent dehydration.

Evaluation Data required for evaluation include the client's perception of comfort or discomfort, the presence or absence of seizures or other evidence of impaired tissue integrity related to hyperthermia, signs and symptoms of adverse reaction to antipyretic drugs, changes in vital signs, especially temperature, and evidence that the client understands the material included in the teaching plan (see the Example of Nursing Process and Antipyretic Treatment).

Checklist of nursing actions

☐ Before administering antipyretic drugs, assess the client for previous tolerance to the drug ordered.

☐ When antipyretic drugs are ordered, monitor the client's condition closely.

☐ Administer antipyretic medications to maintain body temperature within the desired therapeutic range.

☐ Monitor the client's condition for adverse reactions to the antipyretic drug.

☐ Request a change in orders from the physician when adverse reactions to the antipyretic drug develop.

☐ Instruct clients who receive antipyretics as outpatients to adhere to the medications as prescribed. Warn against discontinuing therapeutic

Example of nursing process and antipyretic treatment

The clients are a mother and her 9-year-old daughter, who is brought to a pediatrician's office after developing a fever of 39.6°C (103.2°F). The girl is complaining of a "sore throat," difficulty in swallowing, thirst, feeling "hot and aching all over," and "being tired." Her dress appears wet between her shoulder blades and in the axillary region. Her face is flushed and perspiration is visible on her forehead; her throat is red and swollen.

The physician diagnoses acute pharyngitis and orders a throat culture, penicillin, and acetaminophen 300 mg PO q4h for fever of 39.4°C or higher.

When questioned by the nurse, the mother demonstrates a good understanding of the use of antipyretics in the control of fever and of antibiotics in the treatment of acute infection in children. She states, however, that she does not know what else to do to make her daughter more comfortable.

Assessment data	Nursing diagnosis	Intervention	Goals and outcome criteria
Acute pharyngitis Complaints of sore throat, difficulty in swallowing, thirst, feeling hot, aching, and being tired	Altered comfort: feelings of excessive warmth, increased perspiration, fatigue, thirst, and malaise related to fever and inflammation secondary to pharyngitis	**Administer** the first dose of acetaminophen immediately. Encourage the child to drink a full glass of fluid with the medication. **Loosen** and, if possible, remove some of the child's clothing to facilitate heat loss through evaporation of perspiration. **Encourage** the child to lie down and rest until she and her mother are ready to go home.	The child will state that she feels cooler and more comfortable; visible perspiration will subside. Before the child leaves the office, her temperature will be at or below 39.4°C.
Fever of 39.6°C	High risk for fluid volume deficit related to high fever secondary to pharyngitis	**Medicate** the client for fever as noted above. **Encourage** fluid intake of 1,500 to 2,000 ml daily.	The child will not become dehydrated from high temperature.
Statement by the mother that she does not know "what else" she can do to make her daughter more comfortable	Knowledge deficit on the mother's part related to comfort measures effective in fever and sore throat	**Develop** and implement a plan for teaching the mother comfort measures: bed rest, light clothing and bedding, frequent bathing, ample fluid intake (3,000 ml daily), and soft diet. Teach mother to assess temperature at least four times a day and to return to the physician if the fever does not decline or if it persists after the course of penicillin therapy. **Verify** that the mother can read a thermometer and that she understands procedures for controlling fever.	Before leaving the office, the mother will state that she understands what was taught and she will repeat the directions accurately. During the course of the illness, the child's temperature will drop below 39.3°C.

medications before the prescribed course is completed and also against exceeding the recommended dosage for palliative drugs, including antipyretic analgesics.

☐ Advise clients who employ herbal medicines to use willow bark instead of cinchona bark for antipyresis.

References

Wong D. (1989). Clinical news: From sites to sensors: Taking infants' temperatures. *American Journal of Nursing, 89(3)*, 321.

Bibliography

*Griffin JP. (1986). Fever: When to leave it alone. *Nursing 86, 16(2)*, 58–61.

*Gurevich I. (1985). Fever: When to worry about it. *RN, 49(12)*, 14–18.

*Guyton AC. (1986). *Textbook of medical physiology*, 7th ed, pp 849–860. Philadelphia: WB Saunders.

*Thomas DO. (1985). Fever in children. *RN, 49(12)*, 18–19.

*Weissman G. (1991). Aspirin. *Scientific American, 264(1)*, 84–90.

* Recommended for further reading.

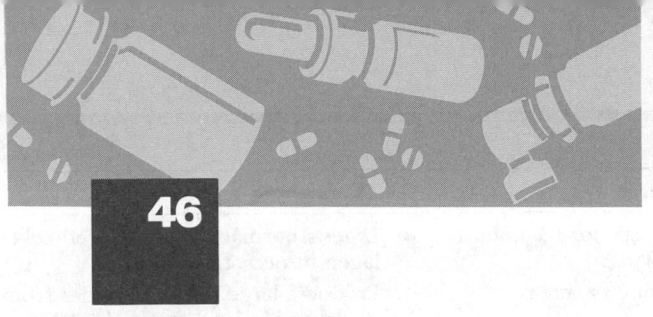

46

Agents used in debridement of wounds

Drug agents
  Anti-infectives
  Hydrogen peroxide
  Proteolytic enzymes
  Absorptive beads
    Nursing management
      Nursing implications
      Nursing process
        Client education

Wounds do not heal readily in the presence of tissue debris or purulent exudate. Such material promotes the growth of infectious organisms and stimulates inflammation in adjacent tissues. Mechanical methods are often used to remove necrotic material from wounds (surgical debridement, whirlpool baths, irrigation, suction drainage, wet-to-dry dressings; however, these methods can further traumatize tissues and increase the client's pain. Chemical agents can supplement or in some cases supplant mechanical methods.

Drug agents

Anti-infectives

Chemical agents that suppress the growth of pathogenic microorganisms cause inflammation and exudation to decrease as the infection subsides. Both systemic administration of antibiotics and topical applications of antiseptics are often effective in "cleaning up" an infected wound. This action is not directly related to the medication but is an indirect secondary effect. (With the exception of hydrogen peroxide, this chapter does not discuss antimicrobials in relation to

wound debridement. See Chapters 41, 42, 43 and 44, which discuss drugs used for infections.)

Hydrogen peroxide

Hydrogen peroxide has a long history of use in cleansing wounds.

Pharmacodynamics. An oxidizing agent, hydrogen peroxide combines with organic material in wounds, subsequently breaking down large molecules and liquefying solid matter. When hydrogen peroxide solution contacts organic material that contains catalase, oxygen is liberated rapidly enough to cause effervescence, which provides a mechanical cleansing effect. This action is especially helpful in grossly contaminated wounds or open cavities that have areas that are difficult to penetrate, such as jagged wounds with extensive tissue damage. (Saline irrigations are of limited effectiveness in such wounds.) The antiseptic or germicidal action is brief and ends with the completion of oxygen release, evidenced by the subsidence of visible foaming.

Pharmacokinetics. Hydrogen peroxide is applied topically only and is not absorbed in an active form. The compound breaks down rapidly, liberating free oxygen and leaving a residue of plain water.

Therapeutic uses. Available for purchase without a prescription, hydrogen peroxide solution (3% hydrogen peroxide in water) is commonly stocked in household medicinal supplies and is used to cleanse small wounds. It is also used as a mouthwash and to bleach hair.

Medically, this solution can be used undiluted for the initial cleansing of wounds. However, it is diluted 1:2 or 1:4 when used as a mouthwash.

Adverse reactions. Hydrogen peroxide may cause some tingling discomfort on initial application, when the effervescent action is greatest.

Long-term use of peroxide in the mouth can cause hypertrophy of the filiform papillae of the tongue ("hairy tongue"). When peroxide use is discontinued, the tongue reverts to its normal state.

Precautions. Hydrogen peroxide is rarely used alone because its effect is limited. Despite the visual appearance of deep penetration, hydrogen peroxide has a high surface tension, and its penetrating power is low. Moreover, the solution is quite unstable and rapidly loses its efficacy with exposure to light and air. Only fresh solutions protected in tightly closed light-resistant containers should be used. Solutions that do not produce effervescence should be discarded; they probably have decomposed and have no more effect than plain water.

The gaseous oxygen produced by the reaction between peroxide and organic matter must be allowed to escape from the tissues. The solution is never injected

Table 46-1. Proteolytic enzymes

Drug name	Preparation	Source	Therapeutic action
collagenase (Santyl)	Topical ointment	Cultures of *Clostridium histolytica*	Digests normal and denatured collagen in necrotic tissue
deoxyribonuclease	Topical ointment	Bovine pancreas	Produces large polynucleotides from nuclear proteins; attacks the DNA
papain (Panafil)	Topical ointment	Papaya fruit	Dissolves protein of purulent exudate and tissue debris only in the presence of activators (sulfhydryl groups) made accessible by the addition of urea
sutilains (*Travase*)	Topical ointment	Cultures of *Bacillus subtilis*	Dissolves nonviable or undenatured protein and purulent exudate
trypsin (Granulex, Parenzyme, Tryptar)	Topical spray	Bovine pancreas	Dissolves protein of purulent exudate and tissue debris
Combination product			
fibrinolysin and deoxyribonuclease (*Elase*)	Topical ointment	Bovine plasma	Dissolves fibrin and polynucleotides of exudate and tissue debris

into closed cavities with no exit, because gas may enter the circulation from the site, causing an embolus.

Proteolytic enzymes

A number of proteolytic enzymes produced by microorganisms have been isolated, purified, and marketed for medicinal use (Table 46-1).

Pharmacodynamics. Enzymes are themselves proteins that interact with organic compounds in such a way as to hydrolyze proteins or depolymerize DNA.

Therapeutic uses. Proteolytic enzymes are applied topically to wound surfaces to promote debridement. Some are also administered systemically in an attempt to resolve intravascular clots or to promote the reabsorption of hematomas. Their efficacy in such situations is not fully established.

Proteolytic enzymes are applied to wounds as ointments, sprays, or irrigating solutions.

Adverse reactions. As foreign proteins, enzymes are highly antigenic. The topical route of administration is the one most likely to induce allergic hypersensitivity. Allergy is likely to be manifested by increased inflammation in the tissues that surround the treated wound.

Proteolytic enzymes promote bleeding from the site of application, because the fibrin of existing clots may be broken down by the drug's action. The fibrinolytic action of these drugs reduces the body's natural barriers to the spread of infection.

Pain after application of sutilains (Travase) ointment has been reported.

Precautions and contraindications. Because they are protein substances, proteolytic enzymes must be protected from heat and agitation, which may denature them. Fresh solutions should be prepared daily.

Ointment preparations should be stored in cool environments, and agitation of liquids should be avoided.

When infection is present in the wound, particularly cellulitis, anti-infective therapy is required. Infection is likely to spread rapidly when proteolytic enzymes are used, increasing the risks of systemic bacterial infections and bacteremia.

Proteolytic enzymes are contraindicated for individuals allergic to them.

Drug interactions. Proteolytic enzymes tend to be inactivated by extremes of pH. Collagenase is active at pH levels of 6 to 8, papain at pH levels of 3 to 12, and sutilains at pH levels of 6 to 6.8 (Box 46-1). These enzymes are also inactivated by oxidizers such as hydrogen peroxide, by heavy metals such as silver and mercury, by detergents, and by iodine, nitrofurazone, and hexachlorophene. If any of these substances are used in wound treatment, they must be removed thoroughly by repeated flushings with normal saline before proteolytic enzymes are applied.

Absorptive beads

Another agent for the debridement of wounds is a preparation of small spherical beads of dextran macromolecules, dextranomer (Debrisan). Because the

Box 46-1. Optimum pH for proteolytic enzymes

Debriding agent	Range for optimum pH
collagenase	6–8
papain	3–12
sutilains	6–6.8

beads are only 0.1 to 0.3 mm in diameter, the material resembles a powder. Dextranomer is poured into wet surface ulcers or wounds. Highly porous and intensely hydrophilic, the beads act by physical absorption and capillary action to continuously cleanse the wound surface.

Substances with a molecular weight below 5,000 are absorbed by the beads, which can swell to four times their original size, resulting in removal of plasma protein, fibrinogen, bacteria, and inflammatory exudates from the surface of the wound. This action continues as long as unsaturated beads or paste are present.

Dextranomer may reduce tissue edema and inflammation; it inhibits infection because its suction effect removes fluid, microorganisms, and prostaglandins from the wound surface.

Dextranomer is not absorbed systemically; its action is local, and it leaves the wound by shedding from the site.

It should always be applied to a moist, freshly cleansed wound using aseptic technique.

Dextranomer appears to be nonantigenic, chemically inert, and free from toxic effects. Some clients experience a transient mild discomfort when the powder is applied because of its suction effect. The drug should not be used in dry areas or on ischemic ulcers.

Enrichment experience 46-1

Pour a small amount of Debrisan into your hand and note the texture of the material.

Place an ounce of water tinted with food coloring in a cup. Add measured amounts of Debrisan until no free liquid is apparent when the cup is tilted. How much Debrisan was required to absorb the liquid?

■ **Summary**

Drugs used to decrease exudation from wounds include anti-infectives, hydrogen peroxide, proteolytic enzymes, and dextranomer beads. Anti-infectives reduce the number of pathogens in the tissues and the production of debris in the wound. In addition to its anti-infective action, hydrogen peroxide liquefies dead tissue and exerts a mild mechanical cleansing action. Proteolytic enzymes liquefy the exudate, improving drainage. Dextranomers absorb liquid tissue debris and produce a mild suction effect in the wound.

Hydrogen peroxide, dextranomer, and some proteolytic enzymes can cause mild pain when applied to wounds. Proteolytic enzymes are antigenic and may increase inflammation if allergic sensitivity develops. In addition, they increase the risk of hemorrhage and the spread of infection to tissues adjacent to the wound.

Nursing management

Nursing implications

Agents used for wound debridement are applied topically to the wound surface. Dosage varies with the size of the wound and the amount of necrotic material present.

The treatment of a number of clients with necrotic wounds is complicated by the precursor diabetes mellitus. These clients need aggressive treatment of both the wound and the metabolic imbalance. Inflammation and infection act as stressors, stimulating hormones that antagonize the action of insulin, thus destabilizing the client's metabolic status. High glucose levels in the client's body fluids inhibit the action of leukocytes and impair the immune response to infection. This condition creates a vicious cycle that can be resolved only by simultaneous treatment of both problems.

Nursing process

Assessment Wounds should be regularly assessed for change in size, amount of exudate, and inflammation. Ulcers or craters should be measured for diameter (or size) and depth. The color, consistency, and volume of exudate should be recorded. The wound and the surrounding tissues should be assessed for indications of inflammation (redness, swelling, and pain).

The client should be assessed for factors that affect wound healing (physical activity, nutrition and hydration, tissue oxygenation, and local perfusion at the wound site). In addition, stress levels should be determined, because undue or poorly managed stress delays healing and inhibits general resistance to infection. Attention should also be given to the general physical health of the client. If diabetes is present, the blood sugar level should be monitored. Circulatory problems, including varicosities that lessen blood flow to the area, should be noted. Burns, trauma, postoperative areas, or decubiti must be observed for inflammation and infection.

Before initiating proteolytic enzyme therapy, the nurse should assess the client for allergic tendencies and risk of bleeding. The wound should be old enough so that healing has had a chance to seal off damaged blood vessels in the tissues.

If the situation is not a critical one, the nurse should also assess the client's knowledge of wound care.

Nursing diagnosis Nursing diagnoses likely to be made for clients treated with proteolytic enzymes include the following:

High risk for infection related to necrotic wound
Potential for impaired tissue integrity: inflammation related to allergic reaction to debriding agents

Impaired skin integrity: wound (decubitus)
Impaired physical mobility related to wound
(skin graft)
Body-image disturbance related to large
wound (draining wound)
Self-esteem disturbance related to disfiguring
wound (odors, drainage)
Pain related to wound (infection)
Knowledge deficit related to wounds, their
prevention, and their treatment

Planning Goals of treatment include healing the wound (decreasing the amount of exudate in the wound, decreasing the size of the wound), alleviating or preventing pain, promoting a positive self-image in the affected client, promptly detecting and treating any adverse reactions to debridement agents, and teaching the client how to treat and prevent recurrences of infected wounds.

Intervention Nursing interventions include treating the wound with debriding agents, promoting circulation to the affected area, administering analgesics, fostering a positive self-image in the client, controlling stress levels in the client, and monitoring the client for adverse drug reactions.

Drug agents used to debride wounds are most effective if the affected area is as clean as possible before application. Mechanical removal of loose debris can reduce the organic matter present in the wound, thereby increasing the efficacy of a given amount of solution or ointment. Wounds should be irrigated with saline solution before application of each debriding agent. In addition, if hydrogen peroxide and proteolytic enzymes are both used in the wound, the hydrogen peroxide must be completely removed before the enzyme preparations are applied, because hydrogen peroxide inactivates the enzymes. Wounds should be kept wet during treatment, because enzymes and dextranomers cannot act in a dry environment.

Proteolytic enzymes dissolve clots and proteins that act as interstitial barriers. They should not be used in fresh or bleeding wounds and are never applied to fresh arterial clots. These agents should be discontinued if hemorrhage occurs, if infection spreads, or if severe allergic reaction develops.

Nurses should avoid contact with debridement agents, especially preparations applied as sprays. All of these substances are harmful to delicate tissues such as the eyes. Skin contact with proteolytic enzymes can stimulate allergic sensitivity. Care should be taken not to inhale sprays or dextranomer beads, both of which could damage the lungs.

Tissues that surround the wound must be protected from contact with exudate, which can be irritating and infectious. Devices such as karaya rings and ostomy pouches may be used to create barriers between exudates and susceptible tissues.

When open wounds are being treated with any irrigating solution or medicinal preparation, strict aseptic techniques should be observed. In such conditions, the wounds may have been grossly contaminated at the time of injury and infection may be apparent. This possibility does not reduce the need for sterile asepsis, the purpose of which is to prevent the introduction of additional organisms from the environment. Treatment and dressing changes may be required several times a day and are unavoidably demanding of nursing time and energy. The care with which the procedure is carried out may determine the rate at which the wound clears and healing takes place.

Clients with diabetes mellitus need increased insulin to maintain normal blood glucose during treatment of necrotic lesions. This need fluctuates but should gradually subside to normal when the wound is healed. Usually, insulin is ordered according to protocols that provide for a sliding scale of dosage, depending on (fingerstick) blood sugars.

Circulatory problems should be managed with techniques to increase blood flow to the area (exercise, massage, frequent changes of position, not crossing the legs when sitting). The client with limited mobility should be helped to change position frequently and pressure areas massaged to prevent further tissue breakdown. The skin should be kept scrupulously clean and inspected regularly to detect any breaks, blisters, or reddened areas.

Client education. Warn the client that application of debriding agents can cause discomfort. Instruct the client who is receiving enzyme sprays to turn the head aside to protect the eyes from accidental contact with the medication. If clients are to carry out the treatment, tell them to take an analgesic medication to minimize discomfort before using the debriding agent. Teach them to store these medications where they are secure from access by children (preferably in a locked container). Describe signs and symptoms of allergic reactions and direct the client to report these to a health care professional promptly if they develop. Teach the client self-care measures to promote healing of the infected wound and to prevent recurrence of such wounds.

Evaluation Data required for evaluation include measurements of the open area of the wound, the amount of exudate, the degree of inflammation, reports by the client of changes in comfort level, comments by the client that reflect self-image and self-esteem, the promptness with which any adverse drug reactions are detected and treated, the ability of the client to relate back to the nurse self-care measures that promote healing and prevent recurrence of infected wounds, the client's compliance with the treatment regimen, and whether or not a healed lesion recurs (see Example of Nursing Process and Treatment of Sacral Decubitus).

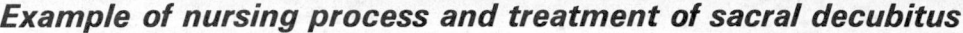

Example of nursing process and treatment of sacral decubitus

The client is a 58-year-old-female resident of a skilled nursing facility. She has had lower limb paralysis for 3 years, as a result of neurologic deficits from multiple sclerosis. Six months ago, the skin over the sacrum began to break down. The lesion has progressed to its present size: an open cavity about 4 by 6 cm in area and 1–2 cm deep. Thick grayish-green exudate partially fills the cavity (estimated volume 15–20 ml). At the perimeter of the wound, the exudate has dried, forming crusts. A ring of reddened, swollen, soft tissue extends 1–2 cm from the perimeter.

The client dislikes wound treatments because they cause pain and consume time that she prefers to spend in activities.

Two weeks ago, the client ran a low-grade fever and complained of fatigue and malaise. She was given cefaclor for 10 days with improvement in these symptoms, but the ulcer did not improve.

The physician has ordered care "as per institutional protocols." The nursing home has separate protocols for the use of hydrogen peroxide, sutilains, or dextranomer for decubitus care.

Assessment data	Nursing diagnosis	Intervention	Goals and outcome criteria
Deep decubitus ulcer Grayish-green purulent exudate	Impaired tissue integrity: sacral decubitus related to impaired physical mobility secondary to multiple sclerosis	**Question** the client to determine if she has ever used sutilains; if she has, ascertain her reaction to it. If the client is not allergic to sutilains, select this agent as the least painful to begin treating the decubitus; follow the protocol established by the nursing facility. If sutilains cannot be used, use one of the other protocols; administer an analgesic 20 to 30 minutes before the treatment. **Explore** with the client ways to improve her nutrition; reduce pressure on the sacrum. **Take** measures to reduce stressors that affect the client, and work with the client to improve her ability to manage stress. **Promote** activity by the client. **Place** the client on a stretcher in the activity areas when side-lying is necessary during activity periods. Consult with the physician and other staff members to plan rehabilitation aimed at crutch-walking.	Within a week, a measurable decrease in the size of the decubitus will be apparent. The client will state that the decubitus treatments are not painful.

(Continued)

Example of nursing process and treatment of sacral decubitus (Continued)

Assessment data	Nursing diagnosis	Intervention	Goals and outcome criteria
Dislike of treatments because they "waste time" Lack of active participation in treatment measures	Knowledge deficit concerning wounds and their treatment	**Prepare** and implement a teaching plan that covers the following: the prognosis for decubiti (which are a leading cause of death in paraplegics and quadriplegics); the factors that contribute to the development of infected decubiti (immobility, local pressure, malnutrition, excessive stress); the relation of pain and other stressors to general resistance to infection and the healing process; treatment and self-care measures that promote healing of decubiti (frequent changes in position, nutritional diet, adequate hydration, stress reduction). During convalescence, complete the teaching plan by covering self-care measures that will reduce the risk of recurrent decubiti. **Administer** an analgesic before beginning wound treatments. If a plan for crutch-walking materializes, inform the client of this prospect.	The client will cooperate in the treatment procedure; she will comply willingly with treatment measures.

Checklist of nursing actions

- ☐ Do not introduce hydrogen peroxide into closed cavities.
- ☐ Protect proteolytic enzyme preparations from heat or agitation.
- ☐ Clean wounds thoroughly before application of enzymes.
- ☐ Do not use proteolytic enzymes near the eyes.
- ☐ Do not use proteolytic enzymes in the presence of active hemorrhage.
- ☐ Do not apply proteolytic enzymes to fresh arterial clots.
- ☐ Assess clients for signs and symptoms of allergic sensitivity to the foreign protein preparations.
- ☐ Instruct clients who are receiving enzyme sprays to turn the head aside to protect the eyes during application.
- ☐ Instruct clients who are using proteolytic enzymes in the home about the proper storage of these medications.
- ☐ Instruct clients to promptly report any signs and symptoms of allergic sensitivity.
- ☐ Before initiating dextranomer treatments, warn clients that the drug can cause discomfort when first applied.
- ☐ Medicate clients with analgesics before carrying out painful debridement treatments.

Bibliography

Cassell BL. (1986). Treating pressure sores stage by stage. *RN, 49(1),* 36–41.

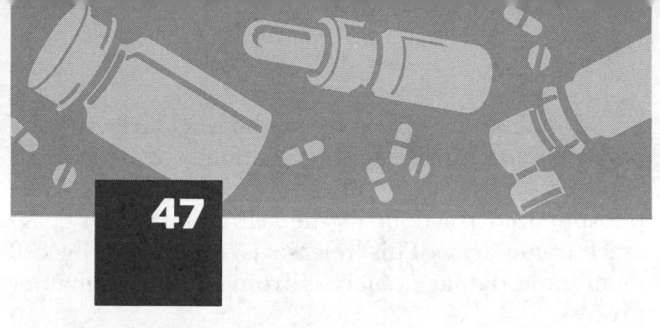

47

Anti-inflammatory and related agents

Pathophysiology of inflammation

The inflammatory process comprises multiple physiologic responses to a stimulus (McCance & Huether, 1990). The process of inflammation is not undesirable; it is a protective mechanism essential for survival (Fig. 47-1). The affected person lacks adequate protection if the process is not sufficient to combat the stimulus. On the other hand, in certain situations, the inflammation process may cause the person considerable harm. For example, in a young child, inflammatory edema in acute laryngitis could cause asphyxiation.

Inflammation should not be confused with infection. Box 47-1 highlights information on the inflammatory process.

Many diverse stimuli may initiate the inflammatory process but the process is not individual to the stimulus. The stimulus may be thermal (heat or cold); chemical (foreign substances, foreign organisms, drugs); or mechanical (trauma).

The cardinal signs of localized inflammation are redness, heat, swelling, pain, and loss of function (or, in Latin, *rubor, calor, tumor, dolor,* and *functio laesa*). Fever is an example of a systemic response that frequently accompanies many local inflammatory processes, noninfectious as well as infectious.

The most important activator of the inflammatory response is the mast cell, which indicates inflammation by releasing biochemical mediators (*eg*, histamine, chemotactic factors) from preformed cytoplasmic granules and synthesizing other mediators (*eg*, prostaglandins, leukotrienes) in response to a stimulus.

Prostaglandins are believed to contribute significantly to the inflammatory process. In 1936, while studying the activity of reproductive glands, Euler in Sweden identified a lipid-soluble acid, which he named prostaglandin.

Prostaglandins are 20-carbon unsaturated carboxylic acids with a cyclopentane ring. The different prostaglandins fall into several main classes: E, F, A, B, C, D. Although similar, there are subtle differences between the different prostaglandins that relate to the tissues from which they originate.

Prostaglandins have been detected in almost every tissue and body fluid. They produce a remarkably broad spectrum of effects, such as contraction of the pregnant uterus, relaxation of bronchial and tracheal muscles (PGEs), contraction of bronchial and tracheal

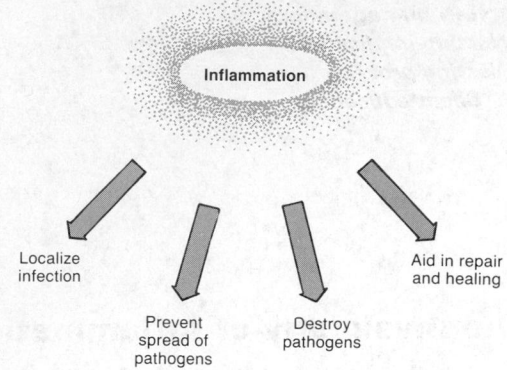

Figure 47-1. The purposes of inflammation.

muscles (PGFs), inhibition of gastric secretion (PGE_1 and E_2), increase in capillary permeability, and inhibition of platelet aggregation (PGE_1).

It has now been established that prostaglandins are released when cells are damaged and exist in increased concentrations in inflammatory exudates (for example, prostaglandins are present in high concentrations in the synovial fluid of inflamed joints). All available evidence indicates that cells do not store prostaglandins and that their release is dependent on biosynthesis. They are produced from arachidonic acid by the action of the enzyme prostaglandin synthetase (also known as cyclo-oxygenase). Arachidonic acid is a dietary unsaturated fatty acid that circulates in plasma as a free acid.

Box 47-1. The inflammatory process

Purposes of inflammation

- To neutralize and destroy noxious agents at site
- To prevent dissemination of noxious agents
- To establish conditions necessary for repair and resolution

Stimuli that initiate the process

- Thermal (heat or cold)
- Chemical (foreign substances, organisms, drugs)
- Mechanical (trauma)

Cardinal signs

- Redness (*rubor*)
- Heat (*calor*)
- Swelling (*tumor*)
- Pain (*dolor*)
- Loss of function (*functio laesa*)

Prostaglandins are associated particularly with the pain that accompanies inflammation.

Most cells can synthesize prostaglandins. The phospholipid fractions of the cell membrane release arachidonic acid. This release is stimulated by cell membrane damage, such as from the inflammatory process.

Normally, prostaglandin synthetase catalyzes the conversion of arachidonic acid to its unstable intermediate. It appears that various medications with an anti-inflammatory action inhibit the conversion of arachidonic acid by inhibiting the release of prostaglandin synthetase or by interfering in some other manner with the synthesis of prostaglandins. Individual medications have differing modes of inhibitory activity on the prostaglandin synthetase. For example, aspirin acetylates a serine at the active site of the enzyme. The inhibition of prostaglandin synthetase leads to a decrease in the inflammatory process and, subsequently, to symptom (pain) relief.

Nonsteroidal anti-inflammatory agents

This chapter features medications whose pharmacologic actions intervene at certain points in the inflammatory process. These medications are used when the inflammatory process has had or would appear to be causing a deleterious effect on a client.

Pharmacodynamics. In 1986, 100 million prescriptions were written for anti-inflammatory drugs. As a group, these drugs have anti-inflammatory, analgesic, antipyretic, and platelet-inhibitory action. They do differ chemically and pharmacokinetically but it is still unclear how significant these differences are (Brooks & Day, 1991).

The nonsteroidal anti-inflammatory drugs (NSAIDs) are classified by chemical group and include the carboxylic acids, the pyrazoles, and the oxicams. The carboxylic acids include the salicylates, acetic acids, propionic acids, and fenamates.

The major mechanism of action of this group of drugs is the inhibition of prostaglandin synthetase activity. The mode of inhibition of the enzyme varies among the NSAIDs. Normally, prostaglandin synthetase catalyzes the conversion of arachidonic acid to its unstable intermediate. The inhibition of prostaglandin synthetase leads to a decrease in the inflammatory process (see discussion of pathophysiology of inflammation) and, subsequently, to symptom (pain) relief.

It is now being suggested that these drugs have additional mechanisms of action that help account for their anti-inflammatory effect. For example, it is now noted that sodium salicylate, a weak inhibitor of prostaglandin synthetase, appears as effective as acetylsalicylic acid (ASA) in clients with rheumatoid arthritis.

Acetylsalicylic acid is a potent inhibitor of prostaglandin synthetase (Brooks & Day, 1991).

The other processes that are apparently influenced by the NSAIDs include leukotriene synthesis (both diclofenac and indomethacin decrease the production of leukotrienes); superoxide generation (piroxicam but not ibuprofen inhibits the generation of hydrogen peroxide from neutrophils); lysosomal enzyme release; neutrophil aggregation and adhesion; cell-membrane functions (*eg*, enzyme activity, transmembrane anion transport, oxidative phosphorylation, uptake of arachidonate); lymphocyte function; rheumatoid factor production; and cartilage metabolism.

Therapeutic uses. These drugs are used primarily for the anti-inflammatory effects in the treatment of musculoskeletal disorders like rheumatoid arthritis, osteoarthritis, and ankylosing spondylitis. With their analgesic effect, they are effective against pain of low-to-moderate intensity and they lack the unwanted effects of the opioids on the central nervous system (CNS). They are used with pain of dysmenorrhea and in some postoperative pain situations.

Adverse reactions. In addition to sharing similar therapeutic effects, the NSAIDs share several adverse effects including gastrointestinal (GI) effects (dyspepsia, gastric erosion, peptic ulcer formation, perforation and hemorrhage, inflammation, and change in the permeability of the intestine and lower bowel), renal dysfunction, and fluid and electrolyte imbalances.

Gastrointestinal effects. The NSAIDs' toxicity to the GI system probably occurs because of depletion of gastric prostaglandins, especially PGI_2 and PGE_2 (Gilman, et al, 1985), which promote the secretion of a protective mucus in the intestine. Inhibition of their synthesis appears to render the stomach more susceptible to damage.

Adverse effects of NSAIDs on the GI system are especially associated with older females. Physical changes occur in the elderly, including thinning of the gastric mucosa. Elderly women, after menopause, no longer have the beneficial stimulating effect of estrogens and progestogens on gastric mucosa and this fact may contribute to the association of NSAID gastropathy with women 75 years and older. Estimates suggest that NSAID-associated gastropathy accounts for 2,600 deaths and 20,000 hospitalizations each year in the United States in clients with rheumatoid arthritis alone (Brooks & Day, 1991).

Attempts have been made to combat the NSAID gastropathy using histamine H_2 receptor antagonists, and they appear to reduce the incidence of gastroscopically diagnosed NSAID-induced duodenal ulcers. They have not proven adequate to reverse gastropathy if NSAID therapy is continued. In addition,

some of these antagonists interfere with the use of other drugs and they are also expensive.

Sulcralfate and omeprazole are also used with NSAIDs, and these drugs and the histamine H_2 receptor antagonists are discussed in detail in Chapter 30.

Renal effects. NSAIDs induce a variety of renal side effects. NSAIDs can cause reversible impairment of glomerular filtration, acute renal failure, edema, papillary necrosis, chronic renal failure, and hyperkalemia (Brooks & Day, 1991). Individuals especially at risk for renal function deterioration or failure include those with hypovolemic states and pre-existing renal impairment due to age, atherosclerosis, or hypertensive renal disease. The NSAIDs can decrease renal blood flow and the rate of glomerular filtration in clients with these disorders. They (especially fenoprofen) have been known to produce acute interstitial nephritis and acute tubular necrosis.

Fluid and electrolyte imbalance. Sodium retention is the most universal side effect of NSAID therapy. There appears to be more than one mechanism underlying this. One mechanism is the decreased renal plasma flow that may occur with NSAID use. Also, prostaglandins normally inhibit both the reabsorption of chloride and the action of antidiuretic hormone. The use of NSAIDs reduces this inhibition and enhances tubular reabsorption of sodium chloride. Increased capillary permeability may also contribute to sodium retention. These effects may cause edema in some clients and may reduce the effectiveness of antihypertensive regimens.

NSAIDs raise serum potassium, sometimes to a marked degree (in excess of 6 mEq/L). Those with conditions known to interfere with renal potassium excretion should only use NSAIDs under carefully supervised conditions. Clients at risk include those with spontaneous or drug-induced hypoaldosteronism, and clients receiving potassium-sparing diuretics, angiotensin-converting enzyme inhibitors, or cyclosporine.

Drug interactions. Because elderly people are the most likely to have multiple organ dysfunction and since NSAIDs are commonly used in this group, it is at risk for interactions between other drugs and NSAIDs. Some interactions have been identified that occur with a specific NSAID but most can occur with any NSAID.

All NSAIDs reduce digoxin clearance, increase plasma digoxin concentration, and increase the risk of digoxin toxicity in those with reduced renal function. If renal function is normal, there is no problem with this combination. All NSAIDs also lower aminoglycoside clearance and increase plasma aminoglycoside concentration in those with reduced renal function.

The NSAIDs (probably all except possibly sulindac and aspirin) inhibit the renal excretion of lithium, increasing lithium concentration and the risk of toxicity. Probably all NSAIDs reduce the clearance of methotrexate by an unknown mechanism, increasing plasma methotrexate concentration and the risk of toxicity. This interaction is seen with the antineoplastic dose levels of methotrexate but not with the rheumatologic doses of methotrexate.

Antacids exert variable effects on the NSAIDs. The rate and extent of absorption of indomethacin is reduced by aluminum-containing antacids but its absorption is increased by sodium bicarbonate. The rate of absorption of other NSAIDs can be slowed by antacids.

There is a reduction in the metabolism and renal clearance of NSAIDs when probenecid is used concurrently causing a concomitant increase in the plasma concentration of the NSAID.

Anion-exchange resins (*eg*, cholestyramine) bind NSAIDs in the intestine, reducing the rate and possibly the extent of absorption. This has been observed with naproxen; the concept probably applies to the others. This potential interaction can be managed by separating the dosing times of the two agents by 4 hours and possibly by increasing the dose of the NSAID.

The NSAIDs (probably all except sulindac) cause a reduction in antihypertensive effect of beta-blockers and angiotensin-converting enzyme inhibitors. This is probably related to inhibition of prostaglandin synthesis in the kidneys (producing retention of salt and water) and inhibition of prostaglandin synthesis in the blood vessels (producing increased vasoconstriction). NSAIDs should be avoided in clients receiving these agents if possible.

Interaction between NSAIDs (except possibly sulindac) and diuretics produces a reduction in the effects of the diuretic, which may lead to an exacerbation of congestive heart failure in the client predisposed to such a complication. If the diuretic is the potassium-sparing variety, there may be potassium retention and consequent hyperkalemia. Use of indomethacin with triamterene potentiates the likelihood of nephrotoxicity, even in clients with normal renal function (*ie*, this combination is contraindicated).

NSAIDs should generally be avoided by clients on oral anticoagulant therapy, including warfarin (Coumadin) and dicumarol. With concurrent use of NSAIDs and anticoagulants, there is increased risk of GI bleeding. There is direct damage to the GI tract mucosa, inhibition of platelet aggregation, displacement of the anticoagulant from plasma protein-binding sites with consequent potentiation of the anticoagulant action, and a tendency toward reduced plasma prothrombin. Enteric-coated ASA preparations may minimize gastric erosions but platelets would still be inhibited.

Salicylates

The medicinal effect of the bark of willow has been known to several cultures for centuries. Salicin, the active ingredient in willow bark, was discovered in 1827. Acetylsalicylic acid (aspirin) was introduced in 1899. The word *salicylate* is derived from the Latin name for the willow tree, *salix*. The group of medications now known as the salicylates include ASA, salsalate, sodium salicylate, salicylic acid, methyl salicylate, and diflunisal. The information on the salicylates is summarized on Table 47-1.

Acetylsalicylic acid

Acetylsalicylic acid (aspirin, ASA) has anti-inflammatory, analgesic, antipyretic, antiplatelet, and antithrombotic properties. The name aspirin is said to have derived from *Spiraea*, the plant species from which salicylic acid was once prepared.

Pharmacodynamics. The anti-inflammatory action of ASA is caused by its action in the inhibition of prostaglandin synthetase.

Acetylsalicylic acid also has an analgesic effect. The salicylates relieve pain by both peripheral and CNS effects but ASA mainly acts peripherally in the inhibition of prostaglandin synthetase. The hypothalamus is believed to be the site of action of the ASA in the CNS. Acetylsalicylic acid is ineffective as an analgesic in noninflamed tissues.

The antipyretic effect of ASA is the result of its action to inhibit prostaglandin biosynthesis within the brain.

The antiplatelet effect of ASA is the result of inhibitory action on blood platelets that prevents the formation of thromboxane A2, which *induces* platelet aggregation. In vascular endothelial cells, ASA prevents the synthesis of prostacyclin, which *inhibits* platelet aggregation. Therefore, ASA is potentially either antithrombotic or thrombogenic but, to date, the clinical evidence is overwhelming that the antithrombotic effects predominate.

Pharmacokinetics. Acetylsalicylic acid taken orally is absorbed partly from the stomach but mostly from the upper small intestine. The rate of absorption depends on many factors, including dosage form, gastric and intestinal *p*H, gastric emptying time, and the presence of food in the stomach. There is little difference between the rates of absorption of pure and buffered ASA. The presence of food delays oral absorption. Rectal absorption does occur but it is slower, incomplete, and unreliable.

Acetylsalicylic acid is distributed throughout most body tissues and can be detected in synovial, spinal, and peritoneal fluid, in saliva, and in human milk. It crosses the placental barrier readily and the blood–brain barrier slowly.

Table 47-1. Nonsteroidal anti-inflammatory agents

Drug names	Preparations	Usual dosage/PC	Adverse reactions
Salicylates			
acetylsalicylic acid (aspirin) (Alka Seltzer, Arthritis Pain Formula, ASA, Ascriptin, Aspergum, Bayer Aspirin, Buffer-in, Easprin, Empirin, Measurin, Zorprin)	Capsules Tablets Timed-release and enteric-coated preparations Rectal suppositories	Oral, adult, for analgesia and anti-pyresis; 300–900 mg q4h–q6h (not to exceed 4 g/d); child: 65 mg/kg/d in 4–6 divided doses PC: D	Allergic hypersensitivity, GI side effects (dyspepsia, nausea and vomiting, ulceration of stomach or duodenum), nephrotoxicity, effects on platelet function, prolongation of gestation and labor
choline magnesium trisalicylate (Trilisate)	Tablet Liquid	Oral, adult: 435–870 mg q4h, in rheumatoid arthritis or osteoarthritis 1,500 mg bid or 3,000 mg qd at hs; each 500 mg tablet is equivalent in salicylate content to 10 g aspirin	GI side effects (nausea, vomiting, indigestion, heartburn, epigastric pain, diarrhea, constipation), tinnitus, hearing impairment, headache, light-headedness, dizziness, drowsiness, lethargy
choline salicylate (Arthropan, *Can:* Teejel)	Liquid	Oral, adult: 870–1740 mg qid	GI side effects (nausea, vomiting, diarrhea, heartburn, anorexia, bleeding), rash
diflunisal (Dolobid)	Tablets	Oral, adult, for analgesia: 1,000–1,500 mg bid PC: C	GI side effects (nausea, dyspepsia, abdominal pain, diarrhea), allergic hypersensitivity, sedation, weakness, tinnitus
magnesium salicylate (Magan, Mobidin)	Tablets	Oral, adult: 600 mg tid or qid, not to exceed 4,800 mg qd	GI side effects (nausea, vomiting, diarrhea, anorexia, heartburn, bleeding), rash
salsalate (Disalcid, Mono-Gesic, Salflex)	Capsules Tablets	1 g initially, then 500 mg q8–q12 h	Tinnitus, hearing impairment, nausea, vertigo, rash
Acetic acids			
diclofenac (Apo-Declo, Novo-difenac, Voltaren, Voltarol)	Enteric-coated tablets	Oral, adult, for osteoarthritis: 100–150 mg qd in divided doses, for rheumatoid arthritis, 150–200 mg qd in divided doses PC: B	GI side effects (abdominal pain, dyspepsia, heartburn, diarrhea, bleeding), liver function test abnormalities, headache, dizziness, pruritus, fluid retention, tinnitus, allergic hypersensitivity, hypertension
indomethacin (Amuno, Indocid, Indocin, Indomee, Metacen)	Capsules Sustained-release capsules Suspension Rectal suppositories IV	Oral, adult: analgesia, 25 mg bid or tid (increased as needed until total daily dose is 150–200 mg); child: 2–4 mg/kg/d in 2–4 divided doses; adult, sustained-release: 75 mg qd or bid (not to exceed 150 mg qd) PC: UK	Frontal headache, dizziness, vertigo, lightheadedness, drowsiness, somnolence, memory lapses, confusion, psychosis, hallucinations, depression, GI side effects (anorexia, nausea, vomiting, abdominal pain, diarrhea, bleeding, ulceration, perforation), allergic hypersensitivity, neutropenia, thrombocytopenia, aplastic anemia, hematuria, nosebleeds, vaginal bleeding, mouth sores, sore throat, fever, chills, tinnitus, hearing loss, nephrotoxicity
ketorolac tromethamine (Toradol)	IM IV	30–60 mg IM initially, followed by 15–30 mg q6h	GI side effects (dyspepsia, GI pain, nausea, vomiting, diarrhea), drowsiness, dizziness, edema, headache, sweating
sulindac (Clinoril, Novo-sudac)	Tablets	150–200 mg bid (maximum daily dose 400 mg) PC: UK	GI side effects (abdominal pain, nausea, vomiting, anorexia, diarrhea, constipation; but less frequent than with indomethacin), nervousness, dizziness, headache, sedation, pruritus, allergic skin rash, tinnitus, hypertension

(Continued)

Table 47-1. Nonsteroidal anti-inflammatory agents (Continued)

Drug names	Preparations	Usual dosage/PC	Adverse reactions
tolmetin (Tolectin)	Tablets Capsules	Oral, adult: 400 mg tid (maximum daily dose 2 g); child: 20 mg/kg/d in 3–4 doses	GI side effects (abdominal pain, dyspepsia, nausea, vomiting, diarrhea, constipation, ulceration), nervousness, anxiety, insomnia, sedation, headache, dizziness, weakness, tinnitus, visual disturbances, pruritus, allergic skin rash, hypertension
Propionic acids			
carprofen (Rimadyl)		300 mg/d in 2–3 divided doses PC: C	Skin reactions, liver function test abnormalities, GI side effects
fenoprofen (Fenopron, Nalfon, Nalgesic)	Capsules Tablets	300–600 mg tid or qid; maximum dose 3,200 mg qd PC: B	GI side effects (nausea, vomiting, anorexia, mild stomach distress, diarrhea, constipation), dizziness, weakness, sedation, anxiety, insomnia, tachycardia, tremors, increased sweating, sore and dry mouth, hives, allergic skin rash, tinnitus, visual changes
flurbiprofen (Ansaid, Froben, Ocufen)	Tablets Ophthalmic solution	50 mg q4–q6h; in ophthalmic use, 1 gtt q½ h 2 hr before surgery (4 gtts total) PC: C	GI side effects (mild abdominal discomfort, dyspepsia), headache, dizziness, drowsiness; ophthalmic preparation may cause burning, stinging in eye, bleeding or redness
ibuprofen (Actiprofen, Advil, Amersol, Brufen, Medipren, Motrin, Novoprofen, Nuprin, Rufen, Trendar)	Tablets	300–600 mg tid or qid, maximum dose of 3,200 mg in osteoarthritis and rheumatoid arthritis and 2,400 mg in dysmenorrhea PC: UK	GI side effects (epigastric pain, nausea, vomiting, anorexia, heartburn, abdominal discomfort, "fullness," constipation, diarrhea), thrombocytopenia, pruritus, allergic skin rashes, headache, dizziness, nervousness, sedation, hypertension, edema, ocular effects
ketoprofen (Orudis)	Capsules	150–300 mg qd in 3–4 divided doses PC: B	GI side effects (dyspepsia, nausea, abdominal pain, diarrhea, constipation, flatulence)
naproxen (Naprosyn), naproxen sodium (Anaprox)	Tablets Suspension	Naproxen, 500 mg initially, 250 mg q6–q8h; naproxen sodium, 550 mg initially, 275 mg q6–q8h PC: C	GI side effects (dyspepsia, abdominal pain, heartburn, nausea, vomiting, constipation, diarrhea, bleeding), CNS effects (drowsiness, dizziness, headache, fatigue, depression, ototoxicity), increased sweating, allergic skin rash, respiratory difficulties, increased bleeding, increased thirst, sores in mouth
Fenamates			
mefenamic acid (Ponstel)	Capsules	Oral, adult: 500 mg initially, followed by 250 mg q6h (not to exceed 7 days of therapy) PC: C	GI side effects (nausea, vomiting, abdominal pain, diarrhea), dizziness, sedation, headache, allergic skin rash
meclofenamate (Meclomen)	Capsules	200–400 mg qd in divided doses PC: UK	GI side effects (nausea, vomiting, anorexia, abdominal pain, diarrhea, constipation, ulceration or perforation), dizziness, headache, sedation, tinnitus, sore and dry mouth, sores in mouth, hives, pruritus, allergic skin rash, edema, hypertension

(Continued)

Table 47-1. Nonsteroidal anti-inflammatory agents (*Continued*)

Drug names	Preparations	Usual dosage/PC	Adverse reactions
Pyrazoles			
phenylbutazone (Apo-Phenbutazone, Azolid, Butagen, Butazolidin, Ecobutazone, Novobutazone, Phenbuff)	Capsules Tablets	300–600 mg qd; with gout initial dose is 400 mg, then 100 mg q4h; use for short periods PC: C	GI side effects (nausea, vomiting, dyspepsia, abdominal discomfort, diarrhea, ulceration, bleeding, stomatitis), cutaneous reactions, vertigo, insomnia, euphoria, nervousness, blurred vision, sodium retention, edema, cardiac decompensation, allergic hypersensitivity, hepatitis, blood dyscrasias (leukopenia, agranulocytopenia, aplastic anemia), nephrotoxicity, hematuria, hypothyroidism
oxyphenbutazone (Iridil, Oxalid, Oxybutazone, Tanderil)	Tablets	100–200 mg tid or qid	GI side effects (see phenylbutazone), nephrotoxicity, blood dyscrasias
Oxicams			
piroxicam (Feldene, *Can:* Novopirocam)	Capsules	20 mg qd PC: UK	GI side effects (nausea, epigastric distress, abdominal pain, anorexia, indigestion, flatulence, diarrhea, bleeding, ulceration), edema, headache, malaise, dizziness, somnolence, rash, anemia, leukopenia, thrombocytopenia, eosinophilia

KEY: PC = pregnancy risk category. (The validity of pregnancy risk categories has not been established. See Chapter 16, p 216.)

Biotransformation of ASA takes place in the liver, where five metabolic products are formed. These are excreted mainly by the kidneys. Urinary pH has a significant effect on elimination; alkaline urine favors excretion.

Therapeutic uses. One systemic use for ASA is antipyresis for clients in whom fever may be harmful. The relationship between fever and the immune process is not yet understood but it is believed that fever has a protective physiologic role (see Chapter 45, Antipyretics). The use of ASA does not influence the course of the disease that causes the fever.

A second use for ASA is as an analgesic for relieving low-intensity pain, such as headache, neuralgia, myalgia, dysmenorrhea, arthralgia, and other pains arising from integumental structures rather than viscera. Chronic use of ASA for pain relief does not lead to tolerance or addiction.

Acetylsalicylic acid is used in rheumatic fever to suppress the acute inflammatory process of the disease. After 24–48 hours of therapy, there is considerable relief of pain, swelling, immobility, local heat, and redness of involved joints. Fever and pulse are lowered and the client feels subjectively better. Cardiac complications, chorea, encephalopathy, subcutaneous nodules, and other aspects of the disease are not prevented or benefited.

Acetylsalicylic acid is also used in rheumatoid ar-

thritis to reduce inflammation in joint tissues and surrounding structures and to provide pain relief. The analgesia produced allows for more effective exercise. There seems to be an improvement in appetite and a feeling of well-being. Hypoalbuminemia may occur in rheumatoid arthritis. If this is present, there will be a higher level of salicylate in the plasma because the salicylate normally binds to albumin.

Many clinical trials have examined the use of ASA for its antithrombotic effect. Given the available data, the use of ASA is advocated in a dose of 160 to 325 mg/d in clients with clinical manifestations of coronary disease, if no specific contraindications are present. In the studies, ASA has reduced this risk by more than 50% as compared to placebo (Fuster, Cohen, & Halperin, 1989). In addition, ASA appears to be beneficial in the prevention of a first myocardial infarction, at least in men over the age of 50. It has its largest effect in those with uncontrolled risk factors for the development of coronary events. Other studies indicate that ASA reduces recurrent transient ischemic attacks in clients of both sexes who have experienced transient ischemia of the brain due to fibrin platelet emboli but it may prevent stroke in men only (*Drug evaluations annual*, 1990).

Dosage and administration. Acetylsalicylic acid is available in tablets ranging from 65 to 650 mg, 300-mg capsules, and 65 to 1,300 mg rectal suppositories.

Timed-release and enteric-coated tablets are also marketed.

The route of administration is oral or rectal. Oral doses should be taken with a full glass of water to minimize gastric irritation. Absorption from enteric-coated tablets is sometimes incomplete. Preparations of aspirin containing alkali or buffer can be better tolerated but these may cause alkalinization of urine, which can shorten the plasma half-life of salicylates by enhancing excretion of the drug.

The usual dosage is 300–900 mg every 4 hours. In rheumatic fever and rheumatoid arthritis, higher doses are used.

Adverse reactions. The adverse reactions of acetylsalicylic acid are summarized in Table 47-1.

Certain individuals display an intolerance to ASA and most aspirin-like medications. The underlying mechanism is unknown. It is seen usually in those with a previous allergic hypersensitivity to other chemicals, asthma, chronic urticaria, or the presence of nasal polyps. The signs of this intolerance range from rhinitis with profuse watery secretions and urticaria to laryngeal edema, bronchoconstriction, hypotension and shock, and complete vasomotor collapse.

Acetylsalicylic acid has a tendency to cause the gastrotoxicity described in the introductory section about the NSAIDs. These range from mild dyspepsia to nausea and vomiting to ulceration of stomach or duodenum. Salicylates injure the gastric mucosa by more than one mechanism. Local irritation allows diffusion of acid back into the mucosa and results in injury to submucosal capillaries, with subsequent necrosis and bleeding. An inhibition of the synthesis of prostaglandins normally produced by the gastric mucosa also results in the stomach being more susceptible to damage. There may be an increased bleeding tendency due to the salicylate effect on platelets.

In one study, daily ingestion of 4 or 5 g of ASA for about 1 month resulted in an average daily fecal blood loss of 3 to 8 ml. The fecal blood loss for individuals not receiving the ASA was 0.6 ml/day (Gilman, et al, 1985).

Acetylsalicylic acid also has been responsible for ototoxicity, including tinnitus, a feeling of fullness in the ear, and hearing loss. The mechanism of this reaction is not fully known but it may be due to effects on the synthesis of prostaglandins; reduction of serum calcium levels; interference with membrane ion transport and with energy-demanding functions of hair cells; an inhibition of oxidative enzymes in the cochlea; or increased labyrinthine pressure. The hearing loss is usually bilateral and is reversible within a few days after the medication is discontinued.

Epidemiologic evidence suggests an association between the use of ASA to treat fever in children during the prodromal phase of varicella (chickenpox) or influenza B or A infections and the subsequent development of Reye's syndrome. Reye's syndrome is characterized by an inflammatory encephalopathy, with fatty infiltration of the liver. Twenty to forty percent of cases of Reye's syndrome have been fatal. It is recommended that acetaminophen be substituted for ASA if antipyretic effect is needed in children and adolescents with fever.

Acetylsalicylic acid may also negatively affect renal function, as described in the introductory section on NSAIDs.

Because of the effect of ASA on platelet function, its use should be avoided in clients with severe hepatic damage, hypoprothrombinemia, vitamin K deficiency, or hemophilia. Acetylsalicylic acid therapy should also be stopped at least 1 week prior to surgery.

Prolongation of gestation and of spontaneous labor have been demonstrated with ASA use (Gilman, et al, 1985). Prostaglandins of the E and F series are potent uterotropic agents. Their biosynthesis increases dramatically in the hours before childbirth so it is hypothesized that they have a major role in the initiation and progression of labor and delivery (Gilman, et al, 1990). Inhibitors of prostaglandin biosynthesis have been shown to reduce contractions of the uterus in premature labor.

Drug interactions. Acetylsalicylic acid binds to plasma proteins, especially albumin and thus may displace other drugs from the binding sites. It is felt ASA displaces methotrexate from its protein-binding sites. As described in the introductory section on NSAIDs, NSAIDs reduce the renal clearance of methotrexate by an unknown mechanism. Thus, by two different mechanisms, the serum methotrexate level is increased. These interactions, with antineoplastic doses of methotrexate, increase the risk of methotrexate toxicity.

Aspirin inhibits the metabolism of sodium valproate and increases plasma valproate concentration. Plasma valproate concentrations should be monitored

---

Enrichment experience 47-1

Prepare a mini questionnaire to administer to your friends about their use of acetylsalicylic acid and acetaminophen. Determine the reasons why they use these agents, how frequently they use them, and under what conditions the agents are taken. Identify by trade name the variations of these agents they use. Visit a drug store and obtain prices for each agent identified. Compare the amounts of acetylsalicylic acid and acetaminophen in each of the agents identified. Write up your findings and share them with your classmates.

closely if other NSAIDs are used; aspirin should not be used.

Caffeine increases the rate of absorption of aspirin. Use of metoclopramide and aspirin has led to increased rate and extent of absorption of the aspirin in clients with migraine.

Toxicity. Because it is widely used in medicine and is easily available to lay people over-the-counter, ASA is connected with a high incidence of toxic reactions. The fatal dose varies but death in adults has occurred after 10 to 30 g of ASA (Gilman, et al, 1985).

Mild salicylate intoxication is called salicylism, which usually occurs after repeated administration of large doses. This syndrome is characterized by headache, dizziness, tinnitus, decreased auditory acuity, dimness of vision, mental confusion, lassitude, drowsiness, sweating, thirst, hyperventilation, nausea, vomiting, and (occasionally) diarrhea.

More severe intoxication is characterized by CNS disturbances, skin eruptions, and marked alterations in acid-base balance. The CNS effects include an accentuation of the signs and symptoms seen in salicylism, as well as restlessness, garrulity, incoherent speech, apprehension, vertigo, tremor, diplopia, delirium, hallucinations, convulsions, and coma. Fever may occur, especially in children. Gastrointestinal symptoms also occur and include epigastric distress, nausea, vomiting, and anorexia. Dehydration often occurs as the result of hyperpyrexia, sweating, vomiting, and the loss of water vapor during hyperventilation.

As poisoning progresses, CNS stimulation is replaced by CNS depression, manifested as stupor and coma. Cardiovascular collapse and respiratory insufficiency may ensue. Terminal asphyxial convulsions and pulmonary edema can occur. Death usually results from respiratory failure after a period of unconsciousness.

Diflunisal

Diflunisal (Dolobid) is a difluorophenyl derivative of salicylic acid which has anti-inflammatory and analgesic properties. It does not have antipyretic effects.

Pharmacodynamics. Diflunisal does inhibit prostaglandin synthetase.

Pharmacokinetics. It is rapidly and completely absorbed from the GI tract. Its onset of action is within 60 minutes with a peak in 2 to 3 hours and a duration of action of 8 to 12 hours. It is excreted in urine.

Therapeutic uses. Diflunisal is used on an acute or long-term basis for mild to moderate pain; it is effective in the symptomatic management of osteoarthritis and rheumatoid arthritis. It is about three to four times more potent than ASA.

Dosage and administration. Consult Table 47-1 for preparations and usual dosages. Administration

with meals or milk is suggested, and tablets should be swallowed whole, not crushed or chewed.

Adverse reactions. The most frequent type of side effect is GI and includes nausea, dyspepsia, abdominal pain, and diarrhea. Diflunisal seems to cause fewer and less intense GI effects and antiplatelet effects than ASA. Other side effects include allergic skin rash, sedation, weakness, and tinnitus.

Salsalate

Pharmacodynamics. Salsalate (Disalcid, Mono-Gesic) is a salicylate which has anti-inflammatory, analgesic, and antipyretic properties. It does not inhibit platelet aggregation.

Pharmacokinetics. Salsalate is well absorbed after oral administration. Consult Table 47-1 for preparations and usual dosages. Alleviation of symptoms is gradual and benefits may not be evident for 3–4 days. It is metabolized by the liver.

Therapeutic uses. Salsalate is used for mild-to-moderate pain associated with rheumatoid arthritis, juvenile rheumatoid arthritis, and osteoarthritis.

Dosage, administration, and adverse reactions are summarized in Table 47-1.

Salicylic acid and methyl salicylate

Much of what has been said about ASA also applies to salicylic acid and methyl salicylate. Salicylic acid is a component of benzoic and salicylic acid ointment, as well as zinc oxide and salicylic acid paste. These agents are applied topically as keratolytic agents. Salicylic acid is used (10% to 20% in collodion) for the removal of warts and corns. It is prescribed in talc form for hyperhidrosis.

Methyl salicylate is also called sweet birch oil, wintergreen oil, gaultheria oil, and betula oil. It is a colorless, yellowish, or reddish liquid. Found in ointments or liniments, it is used externally as a counterirritant for painful muscles and joints. Absorption through the skin can occur, and death has resulted from systemic poisoning due to local misapplication of methyl salicylate. Poisoning with this salicylate has also occurred when children have mistaken the aromatic oil for candy. In such a situation, the odor of the drug can be detected on the breath and in the urine and vomitus.

Acetic acids

The acetic acids include indomethacin, sulindac, tolmetin, diclofenac, and ketorolac. The information on the acetic acids is summarized on Table 47-1.

Indomethacin

Pharmacodynamics. Introduced in 1963, indomethacin has anti-inflammatory, analgesic, and antipyretic properties. It is a methylated indole derivative and one of the most potent inhibitors of prostaglandin synthetase. It also inhibits motility of polymorphonuclear leukocytes and it impairs platelet function.

Pharmacokinetics. Indomethacin is absorbed almost completely from the GI tract and has an onset of action within 30 minutes. The peak plasma concentration is reduced within an hour, but may be delayed when the medication is taken after meals. The concentration in synovial fluid is equal to the plasma concentration within 5 hours of administration. Indomethacin's half-life averages 3 hours, and it is excreted in urine and feces.

Therapeutic uses. Indomethacin relieves pain, decreases the length of morning stiffness, increases grip strength, and reduces swelling and tenderness of joints with clients with ankylosing spondylitis, osteoarthritis, rheumatoid arthritis, and gout. Estimates of its potency indicate it is 10 to 40 times more potent than salicylates.

It has been used successfully with uveitis, pleurisy, pericarditis, pericardial effusion, dysmenorrhea, and following ophthalmic surgery.

Indomethacin has been used as an alternative to surgical ligation for "pharmacologic closure" of patent ductus arteriosus in infants, especially premature infants. A typical regimen would be 0.1 to 0.2 mg/kg every 12 hours for three doses. It has been given intravenously, through a retention enema, or through a nasogastric tube. Indomethacin's greatest limitation is its potential renal toxicity. Therapy is stopped if the output of urine drops below 0.6 ml/kg per hour. This use of indomethacin is felt to be contraindicated in the face of renal failure, enterocolitis, thrombocytopenia, or hyperbilirubinemia.

Indomethacin has been used as an antipyretic in Hodgkin's disease when the fever has been refractory to other agents.

Dosage and administration. Consult Table 47-1 for preparations and usual dosages. Special considerations related to the administration of this drug include administering with meals, milk, or antacids to minimize gastric irritation.

Administering the sustained-released form at bedtime with milk allows the client to sleep better and also reduces morning stiffness. The side effects seem better tolerated when the medication is given at night.

Adverse reactions. Up to 50% of persons who receive indomethacin experience side effects, the most common of which is severe frontal headache.

The CNS side effects appear somewhat more prominent with this NSAID than with others. Dizziness, vertigo, lightheadedness, drowsiness or somnolence, memory lapses, and mental confusion are common. Psychosis, hallucinations, and depression can also occur.

GI side effects include anorexia, nausea, abdominal pain, and diarrhea. Gastrointestinal bleeding, ulceration, and perforation have also occurred. Sources of blood loss have included diarrhea, vomiting, hematuria, nosebleeds, and vaginal bleeding.

Neutropenia, thrombocytopenia, and even aplastic anemia have been observed. Mouth sores, sore throat, fever, and chills should be reported. Individuals allergically sensitive to ASA may also be sensitive to indomethacin.

Tinnitus and hearing loss have been reported.

Drug interactions. Indomethacin antagonizes the diuretic and antihypertensive effects of furosemide and the antihypertensive effects of thiazide diuretics, beta-adrenergic blocking agents, or angiotensin-converting enzyme inhibitors. The nephrotoxic potential of indomethacin appears to increase when triamterene is administered concurrently.

Indomethacin does inhibit platelet aggregation like other NSAIDs; the effect appears dose-related and may be of shorter duration than that seen with ASA. Indomethacin may also displace the anticoagulant from plasma binding sites. Concomitant administration of indomethacin and an anticoagulant should be carried out with caution. The ulcerogenic action of indomethacin may also complicate the interaction.

Concurrent use of indomethacin and ASA appears to reduce plasma concentration of indomethacin, possibly by interfering with its absorption. There seems to be no benefit to this combination and the combination could lead to additive GI toxicity.

Interactions with lithium and methotrexate are documented (see section on Drug Interactions of NSAIDs).

Sulindac

Sulindac (Clinoril) is less than half as potent as indomethacin.

Pharmacodynamics. Sulindac, itself, is apparently not active; rather, its sulfide metabolite is responsible for its pharmacologic activity. The sulfide metabolite is more than 500 times more potent than sulindac as a prostaglandin synthetase inhibitor.

Pharmacokinetics. Sulindac is almost completely absorbed after oral administration and has an onset of action within 1 hour. Its peak action is reached in 2 hours. When taken with meals, absorption is delayed and peak plasma concentration is attained more slowly. Its duration of action ranges from 7 to 16 hours, and it is finally excreted in urine and feces.

Therapeutic uses. Sulindac is used for clients with ankylosing spondylitis, osteoarthritis, and rheumatoid arthritis. It has also been used for gout. Its analgesic and anti-inflammatory effects at 400 mg/d are comparable to those achieved with ASA (4 g/d), ibuprofen (1200 mg/d), indomethacin (125 mg/d), and phenylbutazone (400–600 mg/d) (Gilman, et al, 1985).

Dosage and administration. Consult Table 47-1 for preparations and usual dosages. The drug is usually administered with food to reduce GI side effects.

Adverse reactions. Gastrointestinal side effects of sulindac include abdominal pain, nausea, vomiting, anorexia, diarrhea, and constipation. GI side effects, however, occur less frequently with sulindac than with indomethacin, possibly because the active part of the drug, the sulfide metabolite, is not in contact with the gastric mucosa.

Other side effects include dizziness, headache, nervousness, sedation, pruritus, allergic skin rash, tinnitus, and hypertension.

Tolmetin

Pharmacodynamics. Tolmetin (Tolectin) has anti-inflammatory, analgesic, and antipyretic properties. It inhibits prostaglandin synthetase.

Pharmacokinetics. Administered orally, tolmetin is absorbed rapidly and almost completely. Accumulation of tolmetin in synovial fluid begins within 2 hours and lasts up to 8 hours after a dose. It is approximately 99% bound to plasma proteins. The drug is metabolized in the liver and excreted in urine.

Therapeutic uses. Tolmetin is used in treating adult and juvenile rheumatoid arthritis, osteoarthritis, and ankylosing spondylitis. Its effects (0.8 to 1.6 g/d) compare with ASA (4 to 4.5 g/d) or indomethacin (100 to 150 mg/d) and it may be somewhat better tolerated than ASA.

Dosage and administration. Consult Table 47-1 for preparations and usual dosages. The medication may need to be taken with meals, milk, or antacids to minimize gastric irritation.

Adverse reactions. Gastrointestinal side effects are the most common and include abdominal pain, dyspepsia, nausea, vomiting, diarrhea, and constipation. Ulceration has occurred. Other side effects include nervousness, anxiety, insomnia, sedation, headache, dizziness, weakness, tinnitus, visual disturbances, pruritus, allergic skin rash, and hypertension.

Diclofenac

Pharmacodynamics. Diclofenac sodium (Voltaren) is a phenylacetic acid derivative. It has anti-inflammatory, analgesic, and antipyretic properties.

Pharmacokinetics. It is well absorbed from the GI tract after oral administration. When administered with food its onset of action may be delayed and its peak concentration decreased. The peak action is usually reached within 2 to 3 hours with an action duration of 4 to 6 hours. It is approximately 99% bound to plasma proteins. It is metabolized in the liver and excreted via bile and urine.

Therapeutic uses. Diclofenac sodium has been used for rheumatoid arthritis, osteoarthritis, and ankylosing spondylitis. It may also be used for short-term treatment of acute musculoskeletal injury, postoperative pain, and dysmenorrhea.

Dosage and administration. Consult Table 47-1 for preparations and usual dosages.

Adverse reactions. The adverse reactions of diclofenac are summarized in Table 47-1.

Ketorolac tromethamine

Pharmacodynamics. Ketorolac tromethamine (Toradol) is a pyrrole acetic acid derivative that exhibits anti-inflammatory, analgesic, and antipyretic properties.

Pharmacokinetics. Ketorolac tromethamine is completely absorbed after intramuscular administration and begins to act in 10 minutes. The peak action is reached in 50 minutes. The half-life is 3.8 to 5 hours in young adults, but is more prolonged in elderly clients, with a range of 4.7 to 8.6 hours. Ketorolac is excreted in urine and feces.

Therapeutic uses. Ketorolac tromethamine has been used for short-term management of pain, such as after dental surgery and orthopedic and gynecologic surgeries.

Dosage and administration. Consult Table 47-1 for preparations and usual dosages. It is available in 15-, 30-, and 60-mg Cartrix syringes.

Adverse reactions. The adverse reactions are summarized in Table 47-1.

Propionic acids

The propionic acids include ibuprofen, fenoprofen, flurbiprofen, ketoprofen, naproxen, and carprofen. See Focus on propionic acid derivatives: similarities and differences. These preparations all inhibit prostaglandin synthetase. These medications seem to be better tolerated than ASA, indomethacin, and pyrazoles. However, they share many of the negative qualities of these medications. The information on the propionic acids is summarized on Table 47-1.

Therapeutic uses. The propionic acids appear comparable to ASA in the control of symptoms of rheumatoid arthritis and osteoarthritis.

The propionic acids are used for pain associated with soft tissue injury, such as postpartum pain and pain that follows dental, ophthalmic, and other types of surgery. Acute tendonitis and bursitis have been treated with propionic acids.

The release of prostaglandins by the endometrium during menstruation may be a cause of severe cramps and other symptoms of primary dysmenorrhea. Treatment of severe cramps and other symptoms of primary dysmenorrhea with NSAIDs has met with

Propionic acid derivatives: similarities and differences

Similarities	Differences

Similarities

Pharmacodynamics

These agents inhibit prostaglandin synthesis and inhibit platelet aggregation and prolong bleeding time.

Pharmacokinetics

These agents are rapidly and completely absorbed from the GI tract. They are mostly bound to plasma proteins and are metabolized by the liver and excreted in the urine.

Therapeutic uses

These agents are used to treat pain of soft tissue injury, rheumatoid arthritis, osteoarthritis, dysmenorrhea and in the symptomatic relief of mild to moderate pain and inflammation.

Adverse reactions

These include: (CNS) headache, dizziness, drowsiness; (EENT) blurred vision, toxic amblyopia, tinnitus; (CV) tachycardia, palpitations; (GI) dyspepsia, heartburn, epigastric distress, nausea, abdominal pain, GI bleeding, anorexia; (GU) flank pain, nephrotoxicity, fluid retention, hematuria, urinary tract infection, elevated BUN, frequency, oliguria; (HEMA) thrombocytopenia, prolonged bleeding time, elevated liver enzymes; (SKIN) rash; (OTHER) edema.

Contraindications

These agents are contraindicated in persons with renal insufficiency, known hypersensitivity and in whom asthma, rhinitis or urticaria is precipitated by aspirin or other nonsteroidal agents.

Precautions

These agents should be used cautiously in persons with peptic ulcer disease, GI bleeding, impaired renal or hepatic function, hypertension, and compromised cardiac function.

Differences

• **Fluribiprofen** decreases migration of leukocytes into inflamed tissue and depresses monocyte function. Topically it induces or reduces miosis. • **Ketoprofen** inhibits leukotriene synthesis and has antibradykinin activity and lysosomal membrane-stabilizing activity. • **Carprofen** retards polymorphonuclear leukocyte motility and affects lysosomal enzyme release and activity.

• **Fenoprofen** has an onset of action of 15–30 minutes, peaking in 2 hours with a duration of 4–6 hours and a plasma half-life of 2.5–3 hours. • **Ibuprofen** has an onset of 1 hour, peaking in 2–4 hours with a duration of 6–8 hours and a plasma half-life of 2–4 hours. • **Ketoprofen** peaks in $1/2$–2 hours with a plasma half-life of 2–4 hours. • **Naproxen** peaks in 2–4 hours with a half-life of 10–20 hours. • **Fluribiprofen** peaks in 1–2 hours with a half-life of 6 hours.

• **Fenoprofen** may cause lassitude and confusion. • **Ketoprofen** may cause diarrhea, constipation, flatulence, photosensitivity. • **Naproxen** may cause sweating, fatigue, depression, ototoxicity, cystitis, hypotension, and excitation. • **Carprofen** may cause elevated alkaline phosphatase. • **Fluriprofen** (Opth) may cause transient burning or stinging. • **Ibuprofen** may cause reduced creatinine clearance.

• **Fluriprofen** (Opth) is contraindicated in persons with active epithelial herpes simplex keratitis.

• **Ketoprofen** should be used cautiously in persons who may be affected by prolonged bleeding times and in persons with heart failure.

(continued)

Focus on

Propionic acid derivatives: similarities and differences (Continued)

Similarities	Differences
Nursing considerations	
Instruct in disease, treatment, drug regimen, adverse reactions, and compliance; administer 30 minutes before or 2 hours after meals with a full glass of water; give with meals if GI upset occurs; assess pain level prior to administration and then afterward to determine relief; monitor for signs and symptoms of infection; assess vital signs especially temperature and pulse for changes; assess for signs and symptoms of bleeding; assess eye and ear function prior to starting therapy and periodically thereafter for changes indicative of possible toxicity; obtain lab studies, including complete blood count, platelets, coagulation studies, renal and hepatic function studies for changes; institute safety measures if CNS effects occur; assess cardiopulmonary status for signs of possible fluid retention; check weights and monitor intake and output; instruct client in need for follow-up lab work.	Administer **ketoprofen** capsules with food or antacids. Monitor clients taking **fenoprofen** for CNS effects. When administering **fluriprofen** ophthalmic, do not touch eye dropper to eye and keep container tightly closed.

considerable success. Both ibuprofen and naproxen are more effective than ASA for relief of pain from dysmenorrhea (Gilman, et al, 1990). Ibuprofen has been shown to reduce elevated levels of prostaglandin in menstrual fluid and to reduce resting and active intrauterine pressure, as well as the frequency of uterine contractions.

Drug interactions. The discussion on the Drug Interactions of NSAIDs with lithium, methotrexate, probenecid, antihypertensives, diuretics, and oral anticoagulants applies to the propionic acids.

Concurrent use of propionic acids and ASA appears to reduce plasma concentrations of the propionic acid and decrease the effectiveness of the propionic acid. The protein binding of the propionic acid was decreased and the renal clearance of the propionic acid is increased.

Additive adverse GI effects may be noted when a propionic acid is used with ASA, other nonsteroidal anti-inflammatory agents, glucocorticoids, or alcohol.

Ibuprofen

Pharmacodynamics. Ibuprofen (Motrin, Rufen) has anti-inflammatory, analgesic, and antipyretic properties. It was the first propionic acid to be widely used.

Pharmacokinetics. Ibuprofen is administered orally and is absorbed rapidly. It is highly bound to plasma proteins and freely crosses the placenta. It passes into the synovial spaces and seems to remain there after the concentration in plasma has declined. It reaches its peak action in 1 to 2 hours, and has a duration of action of 2 to 4 hours. Ibuprofen is metabolized in the liver and excreted in the urine.

Therapeutic uses. Ibuprofen is as effective as aspirin and certain other agents in rheumatoid arthritis. It may be administered with maintenance doses of gold salts for additional symptomatic relief and it may also be given with corticosteroids. It is as effective as ASA and certain other agents in osteoarthritis. It has been reported to be useful in ankylosing spondylitis and gouty and psoriatic arthritis. It may be useful as an alternative in Reiter's syndrome.

Dosage and administration. Consult Table 47-1 for preparations and usual dosages.

Adverse reactions. Gastrointestinal side effects include epigastric pain, nausea, vomiting, anorexia, heartburn, abdominal discomfort, sensations of "fullness," constipation, and diarrhea. The incidence of these side effects is lower than with ASA or indomethacin.

Other common side effects include thrombocytopenia, prolonged bleeding time, pruritus, allergic skin rashes, headache, dizziness, nervousness, sedation, hypertension, and edema. Development of ocular side effects such as blurred vision and toxic amblyopia mandates discontinuing the use of ibuprofen.

Drug interactions. See discussion under Drug Interactions of NSAIDs. It appears that ibuprofen is one of the safer NSAIDs for concurrent use with anticoagulants if they are necessary.

Fenoprofen

Pharmacodynamics. Fenoprofen (Nalfon) has anti-inflammatory, analgesic, and antipyretic properties.

Pharmacokinetics. Fenoprofen is administered orally and is 85% absorbed. Its onset of action is 30 minutes with a peak action of 1 to 2 hours and a duration of 5 hours. It is excreted in urine.

Therapeutic uses. Fenoprofen is effective as initial therapy or as an alternative to aspirin in rheumatoid arthritis and osteoarthritis. 2.4 g/d of fenoprofen in rheumatoid arthritis was approximately equivalent to aspirin 3.9 g/d; in osteoarthritis 1.2 to 1.8 g daily offered benefit similar to that obtained with 2 to 3 g aspirin.

Dosage and administration. Consult Table 47-1 for preparations and usual dosages.

Adverse reactions. Adverse reactions include nausea, vomiting, anorexia, mild stomach distress, dizziness, and constipation.

Other side effects include dizziness, weakness, sedation, anxiety, insomnia, tachycardia, tremors, and increased sweating. Sore and dry mouth, hives, allergic skin rash, tinnitus, and visual changes have also been reported.

Drug interactions. See discussion under Drug Interactions of NSAIDs.

Flurbiprofen

Pharmacodynamics. Flurbiprofen (Ansaid) has analgesic, anti-inflammatory, and antipyretic properties. Besides inhibiting prostaglandin synthesis, it decreases migration of leukocytes into inflamed tissues and depresses monocyte function.

Pharmacokinetics. Flurbiprofen is rapidly absorbed after oral administration. Administration with food lowers peak plasma concentration but does not change total amount of drug absorbed. Almost all (over 99%) of the drug is bound to albumin. Its half-life is 6 hours and it is excreted in the urine. A solution for ophthalmic use is also available.

Therapeutic uses. Flurbiprofen is effective as initial therapy or as an alternative to salicylates or other NSAIDs for management of rheumatoid arthritis and osteoarthritis. 100 mg of flurbiprofen was equivalent to naproxen 250 mg bid in rheumatoid arthritis.

Dosage and administration. Consult Table 47-1 for preparations and usual dosages. A therapeutic re-

sponse should occur in 1 to 2 weeks. To decrease night pain, improve the quality of sleep, and decrease the duration of morning stiffness, 100 mg has been given at bedtime to clients with rheumatoid arthritis. Acute gout has been successfully treated with a 400-mg loading dose administered in the first 24 hours (*eg*, 100 mg every 6 hours), followed by 200 mg/d.

Adverse reactions. The adverse reactions are summarized in Table 47-1. Gastric mucosal changes with flurbiprofen are similar to those observed with ibuprofen and naproxen and fewer than those with indomethacin or tolmetin. Duodenal changes after flurbiprofen were fewer than those after indomethacin, naproxen, and tolmetin. Headache, dizziness, and drowsiness are reported by less than 5% of clients.

Drug interactions. See discussion on the Interaction of NSAIDs.

Flurbiprofen attenuates the antihypertensive response to propranolol but not atenolol. The diuretic action of furosemide is reduced when used concurrently with flurbiprofen.

Ketoprofen

Pharmacodynamics. Ketoprofen (Orudis) is one of the newer propionic acids. It has anti-inflammatory, analgesic, and antipyretic properties. Besides inhibiting prostaglandin synthesis, it inhibits leukotriene synthesis, has antibradykinin activity, and has lysosomal membrane-stabilizing action.

Pharmacokinetics. It is rapidly absorbed after oral administration. When administered with food, its rate of absorption is slowed. Its usual peak action is reached in 2 hours. It is excreted in the urine. There are no known active metabolites of ketoprofen.

Therapeutic uses. Ketoprofen is effective for the treatment of rheumatoid arthritis, osteoarthritis, ankylosing spondylitis, and acute gout.

Dosage and administration. Consult Table 47-1 for preparations and usual dosages. For dysmenorrhea, the usual dose is 25 to 50 mg every 6–8 hours.

Adverse reactions. The adverse reactions are summarized in Table 47-1. The most frequent side effects are GI. Upper GI symptoms are more common than lower GI symptoms. Gastrointestinal effects include dyspepsia, nausea, abdominal pain, diarrhea, constipation, and flatulence. Attempts to minimize these effects have included administration of ketoprofen with meals, milk, or antacids.

Drug interactions. See discussion under introduction to propionic acids.

The addition of ketoprofen to diuretic therapy increases the risk of renal failure. Administration of hydrochlorothiazide and ketoprofen reduced urinary potassium and chloride excretion more than hydrochlorothiazide alone.

There is increased risk of photosensitivity when ketoprofen is used with other agents known to be photosensitizing.

Naproxen

Pharmacodynamics. Naproxen (Naprosyn) has anti-inflammatory, analgesic, and antipyretic properties. It is 20 times more potent than ASA in its inhibition of prostaglandin synthetase. All NSAIDs have some activity as inhibitors of leukocyte migration. Naproxen appears to exert a particularly prominent inhibitory effect on the migration of leukocytes. This may contribute to its efficacy in the treatment of acute attacks of gout (Gilman, et al, 1990).

Pharmacokinetics. Naproxen is administered orally and is completely absorbed. Its onset of action is 1 to 2 hours with a peak action of 2 to 4 hours and a duration of action of 7 hours. In elderly clients, the half-life may be increased up to 28 hours and the dosage may need to be adjusted. It is excreted in the urine.

Therapeutic uses. Naproxen is effective in the symptomatic treatment of rheumatoid arthritis, juvenile rheumatoid arthritis, ankylosing spondylitis, osteoarthritis, and acute gouty arthritis. It may be useful as an alternative agent in the treatment of psoriatic arthritis and Reiter's syndrome. Studies show naproxen is equally or more effective than ibuprofen, fenoprofen, or indomethacin in rheumatoid arthritis.

Dosage and administration. Consult Table 47-1 for preparations and usual dosages.

Adverse reactions. Gastrointestinal side effects of naproxen include dyspepsia, abdominal pain, heartburn, nausea, vomiting, constipation, diarrhea, and gastric bleeding. Central nervous system side effects, which are about the same incidence as GI side effects, include drowsiness, dizziness, headache, fatigue, depression, and ototoxicity. Increased sweating, allergic skin rash, respiratory difficulties, increased bleeding episodes, increased thirst, and sores in the mouth have also been reported.

Drug interactions. See discussion under introduction to propionic acids.

The rate of naproxen absorption is decreased slightly by magnesium and aluminum hydroxide and is increased by sodium bicarbonate.

Naproxen is highly bound to plasma proteins and may displace albumin-bound drugs from their binding sites (such as oral anticoagulants, sulfonylureas, and hydantoins). Nevertheless, it appears that naproxen is one of the safer NSAIDs for concurrent use with anticoagulants if they are necessary.

There is increased risk of photosensitivity when naproxen is used with other agents known to be photosensitizing.

Carprofen

Pharmacodynamics. Carprofen (Rimadyl) is one of the newer propionic acids. It has anti-inflammatory, analgesic, and antipyretic properties. Besides inhibiting prostaglandin synthesis, it retards polymorphonuclear leukocyte motility and affects lysosomal enzyme release and activity.

Pharmacokinetics. It is well absorbed after oral administration with a peak action of 1 to 3 hours. When administered with food, its onset of action may be delayed and the peak concentration may be decreased. It distributes rapidly into synovial fluid, and is metabolized in the liver. Its half-life ranges from 6 to 17 hours and it is excreted in urine and feces.

Therapeutic uses. Carprofen is used in acute and chronic rheumatoid arthritis and osteoarthritis and in acute gouty arthritis.

Dosage and administration. Consult Table 47-1 for preparations and usual dosages. In the case of gout, 600 mg/d in divided doses is used for 2 days. If a satisfactory response occurs, treatment is continued with 300 mg/d for 8 days. If a satisfactory response does not occur, the drug should be discontinued.

Adverse reactions. The adverse reactions are summarized in Table 47-1. Skin reactions and elevated transaminase and alkaline phosphatase levels may occur more frequently with carprofen than with other NSAIDs. Major GI adverse reactions, however, may occur less frequently.

Drug interactions. See discussion on Interactions of NSAIDs.

Fenamates

This group of medications includes mefenamic acid and meclofenamate. The fenamates do not seem to have any clear advantages over other NSAIDs. The information on the fenamates is summarized on Table 47-1.

Mefenamic acid

Pharmacodynamics. Mefenamic acid (Ponstel) has anti-inflammatory, analgesic, and antipyretic properties.

Pharmacokinetics. It is well absorbed after oral administration. Administration with food may minimize adverse GI effects.

Therapeutic uses. Mefenamic acid is used to relieve moderate pain, such as that occurring with soft-tissue injuries and musculoskeletal conditions. It has also been used to manage dysmenorrhea.

Dosage and administration. Consult Table 47-1 for preparations and usual dosages. Mefenamic acid should not be used for pain relief for more than a week. With dysmenorrhea, the described dosage is started at the onset of bleeding and associated symptoms, and continued for 2 or 3 days.

Adverse reactions. Side effects include nausea, vomiting, abdominal pain, diarrhea, dizziness, sedation, headache, and allergic skin rash.

Meclofenamate

Pharmacodynamics. Meclofenamate (Meclomen) has anti-inflammatory, analgesic, and antipyretic properties.

Pharmacokinetics. Meclofenamate exhibits rapid and complete absorption from the GI tract. Its peak action is within 2 hours. The presence of food in the stomach delays the drug's absorption. It is excreted in urine and feces.

Therapeutic uses. Meclofenamate is used to relieve the symptoms of acute and chronic rheumatoid arthritis and osteoarthritis.

Dosage and administration. Consult Table 47-1 for preparations and usual dosages. Administering the drug with meals or milk may decrease or prevent GI side effects. Concomitant administration of aluminum or magnesium hydroxide antacids does not seem to interfere with meclofenamate absorption.

Learning experience 47-1

Interview clients who have osteoarthritis and rheumatoid arthritis. Identify other health problems the clients have. Take a medication history from each client. Assess their psychological reaction to long-term drug therapy for the arthritis. Determine what methods of pain relief they use in addition to the medications prescribed for the arthritis. Identify special problems they have encountered in relation to medications and how they solved these problems.

Adverse reactions. Side effects include nausea, vomiting, anorexia, abdominal pain, diarrhea, constipation, and GI ulceration or perforation. Other side effects include dizziness, headache, sedation, tinnitus, sore and dry mouth, sores in the mouth, hives, pruritus, and allergic skin rash. Edema and hypertension have been reported.

Pyrazoles

This group of medications includes phenylbutazone and oxyphenbutazone (Table 47-1).

Phenylbutazone

Introduced in 1949, phenylbutazone (Butazolidin, Azolid) has analgesic and anti-inflammatory effects but because of potentially severe adverse reactions, it is not used routinely. It shows mild uricosuric activity. In the animal world, its prominent anti-inflammatory effects have been employed to enhance the performance of race horses.

Pharmacodynamics. It is theorized that the anti-inflammatory effect of this agent may be due to inhibition of factors involved in the inflammatory process, including prostaglandin synthesis and leukocyte migration, as well as either the release or the activity of lysosomal enzymes, or both.

Pharmacokinetics. Phenylbutazone is absorbed rapidly and completely from the GI tract. Its peak action is reached in 2 hours, but its duration of action ranges from 3 to 5 days. Concentrations may remain in the joints up to 3 weeks after treatment is completed. The drug has a long half-life of 50 to 65 hours, is metabolized in the liver, and is excreted in the urine.

Therapeutic uses. Phenylbutazone is used to treat acute gout and can control an attack usually within 36 hours. It appears to be more reliable than colchicine when gout treatment has been delayed.

Phenylbutazone has also been used for acute exacerbations of rheumatoid arthritis, ankylosing spondylitis, and osteoarthritis but it is not considered the drug of choice for any condition and should be used only after other drugs have failed.

Dosage and administration. Consult Table 47-1 for preparations and usual dosages. Phenylbutazone should be used only after a careful assessment of the risks involved for the individual client and then only for short periods of time (*eg*, 1 week). This medication is taken with meals, milk, or antacids to lessen gastric irritation.

Adverse reactions. The adverse reactions are summarized in Table 47-1. Anywhere from 10% to 45% of clients treated with phenylbutazone suffer some side effects.

Phenylbutazone causes a significant retention of sodium and chloride, a reduction in urine volume, and an increase in plasma volume. Because of these effects, edema, cardiac decompensation, and acute pulmonary edema have occurred.

Peptic ulcer or its reactivation with hemorrhage or perforation, allergic reactions, ulcerative stomatitis, hepatitis, and nephritis also have occurred. Hematologic disorders, including bone marrow depression, are the most serious complications, and deaths have occurred from aplastic anemia and agranulocytosis. The side effects seem more severe in elderly clients, and its use in this group is not advised.

Drug interactions. Phenylbutazone is an example of a drug that is highly protein-bound. Other medications may be displaced from protein-binding sites by phenylbutazone, resulting in increased pharmacologic or toxic effects of the displaced drug.

Displacement of the plasma protein-bound thyroid hormone by phenylbutazone complicates the interpretation of thyroid function tests.

Phenylbutazone will cause an increased anticoagulant response when given concurrently with warfarin, and hemorrhagic crises have occurred. In this case, besides the displacement phenomenon, phenylbutazone also inhibits the metabolism of S-warfarin.

Phenylbutazone inhibits the metabolic inactivation of sulfonylurea drugs (oral hypoglycemic agents), an effect that can cause profound hypoglycemia. It can also increase the effect of insulin. The combination of phenylbutazone and oral hypoglycemic agents should be avoided if possible, but if not, blood glucose level must be monitored closely.

Administering phenylbutazone with phenytoin may increase the serum levels and toxicity of phenytoin through inhibition of the metabolism of the phenytoin.

Microsomal enzymes that metabolize digitoxin in the liver are stimulated by phenylbutazone, which will lower digitoxin serum levels.

If barbiturates and phenylbutazone are used together, there is increased metabolic clearance of the phenylbutazone, which could require higher doses of phenylbutazone.

Oxyphenbutazone

Oxyphenbutazone (Oxalid or Tandearil) is a metabolite of phenylbutazone and it has the same therapeutic uses, interactions, and toxicity. Oxyphenbutazone is believed to cause somewhat less gastric irritation than phenylbutazone and is administered in the same dosage schedule.

Oxicams

Piroxicam

Pharmacodynamics. Piroxicam (Feldene) has analgesic, anti-inflammatory, and antipyretic activity. It inhibits synthesis of prostaglandins. The information on piroxicam is summarized on Table 47-1.

Pharmacokinetics. Piroxicam is well absorbed after oral administration. Neither food nor antacids alter the rate or extent of absorption. As a result of its long half-life, plasma concentrations of the drug increase gradually for about 7–12 days and then reach a steady-state level. At this level, the concentrations in plasma and synovial fluid are approximately equal. Piroxicam is 99% bound to plasma proteins. It is metabolized by the liver and excreted in urine and feces.

Therapeutic uses. Piroxicam appears equivalent to ASA, indomethacin, and naproxen for long-term management of rheumatoid arthritis or osteoarthritis, and it may be better tolerated than ASA or indomethacin. Piroxicam is also used in treating ankylosing spondylitis, acute gouty arthritis, and acute musculoskeletal disorders. It is used to relieve postoperative or postpartum pain and dysmenorrhea.

Dosage and administration. Consult Table 47-1 for preparations and usual dosages. Maximal therapeutic effect will not be evident for 2 weeks but improvement in symptoms should be noted in 7–12 days. It may be administered with food to decrease any GI side effects.

Adverse reactions. The most frequent adverse reactions are GI disturbances, specifically nausea, epigastric distress, abdominal pain, anorexia, indigestion, flatulence, diarrhea, GI bleeding, and ulceration. Other adverse reactions include edema, headache, malaise, dizziness, somnolence, and rash. Hematologic changes have been observed to include reduced hemoglobin and hematocrit and, rarely, after long-term therapy with piroxicam, anemia, leukopenia, thrombocytopenia, and eosinophilia. It does interfere with the function of platelets.

Drug interactions. Piroxicam may increase the effects of oral anticoagulants. It may cause increased toxicity symptoms of diazepam, propranolol, phenylbutazone, and lithium.

Related agents

Para-aminophenol derivatives

Para-aminophenol derivatives include phenacetin and its active metabolite, acetaminophen (Table 47-2). Phenacetin was introduced for therapy in 1887 and acetaminophen in 1893. Acetaminophen's popularity has grown greatly since 1950.

Pharmacodynamics. The analgesic and antipyretic properties of phenacetin and acetaminophen are significant. Acetaminophen is, however, only weakly anti-inflammatory. Acetaminophen can inhibit prostaglandin synthetase only in an environment that is low in peroxides (*eg*, the hypothalamus). Sites of inflammation usually contain high concentrations of peroxides that are generated by leukocytes (Gilman, et al, 1985).

Therapeutic uses. The para-aminophenol derivatives are good analgesic or antipyretic substitutes for ASA when ASA is contraindicated or when its side effects pose a significant disadvantage. They do not produce the gastric irritation of the salicylates and they

Table 47-2. Related agents for inflammatory processes

Drug names	Preparations	Usual dosage/PC	Adverse reactions
Para-aminophenal derivatives			
phenacetin (example of combination: earlier composition of Fiorinal: butalbital 50 mg; aspirin 200 mg; phenacetin 130 mg; caffeine 40 mg)	Tablets Capsules	Fiorinal: 1–2 tabs or caps q4h	Allergic hypersensitivity, rash, implicated in analgesic abuse nephropathy
acetaminophen (Abenol, Atasol, Datril, Exdol, Panadol, Paralgin, Robigesic, Tempra, Tralgon, Tylenol, Valadol)	Tablets Chewable tablets Capsules Elixir Syrup Rectal suppositories	Oral, adult: 325–1,000 mg q4h (not to exceed 4 g/d); child: 10 mg/kg q4–q6h PC: B	Allergic hypersensitivity, rash, hyperchloremic acidosis
Gold compounds			
gold sodium thionalate (Myochrysine) aurothioglucose (Solganal)	IM	IM, test dose of 10 mg first week, then 25–50 mg every week until cumulative dose of 1,000 mg reached, follow this with maintenance regime PC: C	Cutaneous lesions (from erythema to exfoliative dermatitis, gray to blue pigmentation of skin and mucous membranes), lesions of mucous membranes (stomatitis, gingivitis, glossitis, pharyngitis, tracheitis, gastritis, colitis, vaginitis), metallic taste or itching of oral mucosa, blood dyscrasias, proteinuria and nephrotic syndrome, nitritoid reaction. Solganal has fewer nitritoid reactions
auranofin (Ridaura)	Capsules	6 mg qd in single or divided doses PC: C	See above, perhaps less toxic than parenteral preparations but high incidence of diarrhea, abdominal cramping

KEY: PC = pregnancy risk category. (The validity of pregnancy risk categories has not been established. See Chapter 16, p 216.)

have no effects on platelets, bleeding time, or uric acid excretion. Acetaminophen is usually preferred to phenacetin because it seems to have less overall toxicity.

The para-aminophenol derivatives have been used to relieve muscular aches and pains of various kinds.

Phenacetin

Pharmacokinetics. About 80% of phenacetin is metabolized to acetaminophen. Its plasma concentration peaks in 1 hour, and the acetaminophen derived from it peaks in 1–2 hours. Phenacetin is converted to about a dozen metabolites.

Dosage and administration. Phenacetin is usually available only in analgesic mixtures. It is frequently mixed with acetylsalicylic acid and caffeine (*eg*, APC or aspirin, phenacetin, caffeine tablets/capsules). A typical combination would contain 200 mg to 250 mg of acetylsalicylic acid, 120 mg to 150 mg of phenacetin, and 15 mg to 30 mg of caffeine. The combination approach is based on belief that administering these drugs in fractional rather than full doses should de-

crease adverse reactions. However, it cannot be said with any conviction that the combinations provide better analgesia than acetylsalicylic acid alone or that adverse reactions are fewer. There is also no real evidence that the caffeine added in the current amount of 30 mg contributes to pain relief. (Alexander and Spencer, 1986, p 18).

The addition of codeine or oxycodone to mixtures of acetylsalicylic acid and phenacetin does, on the other hand, result in greater relief of pain.

It is suggested that the use of phenacetin combinations should be discouraged, because other satisfactory analgesics and antipyretics exist with less serious adverse reactions.

Adverse reactions. Allergic reactions occur occasionally, including skin rashes.

The abuse of analgesic mixtures has been linked to the development of analgesic abuse nephropathy, causing drug-related chronic renal failure (Clive & Stoff, 1984). Methemoglobinemia and hemolytic anemia may also occur.

Severe hemolytic anemia, intravascular hemolysis,

hemoglobinuria, and acute anuria may occur in clients with glucose-6-phosphate dehydrogenase deficiency in erythrocytes or as an immunologic reaction.

Lethal doses of phenacetin are associated with cyanosis, respiratory depression, and cardiac arrest.

Acetaminophen

Pharmacokinetics. Acetaminophen is absorbed rapidly and almost completely from the GI tract. Its plasma concentration peaks in 30 to 60 minutes. Binding of the drug to plasma proteins ranges from 20% to 50%. It is metabolized by hepatic enzymes and excreted through the kidneys.

Dosage and administration. Consult Table 47-2 for preparations and usual dosages. A list of products containing acetaminophen appears in Box 47-2.

Adverse reactions. Acetaminophen is usually well tolerated. Allergic reactions, including skin rashes, occur occasionally.

Drug interactions. Repeated doses of acetaminophen may slightly increase the hypoprothrombinemic response to oral anticoagulants, and an occasional client may develop a more marked increase. However, unlike ASA, acetaminophen does not inhibit platelet function or cause gastric erosions. Thus, acetaminophen is probably safer than ASA.

Toxicity. Acute poisoning can occur because acetaminophen is available without prescription. The toxic effects of acetaminophen in acute poisoning are associated with its metabolism. Acetaminophen is normally conjugated in the liver with glucuronic acid. A small portion of acetaminophen undergoes cytochrome P450-mediated N-hydroxylation to form N-acetyl-benzo-quinoneimine. At usual therapeutic doses of acetaminophen, this metabolite normally reacts with glutathione. However, after overdoses of acetaminophen, this metabolite is formed in amounts sufficient to deplete the glutathione. The metabolite then bonds to hepatic cells and eventually causes liver necrosis (Gilman, et al, 1990).

Adults can develop hepatotoxicity after ingesting 150 to 250 mg/kg of acetaminophen (about 10 g for a 70-kg adult). Clients who have been on drugs, such as phenobarbital and phenytoin (Dilantin), that stimulate the cytochrome P450-mediated system, are more likely to develop hepatotoxicity. Prior stimulation of the system increases the rate at which the acetaminophen entering this system is metabolized to the toxic substance.

Box 47-2. Products that contain acetaminophen

Actifed Plus Caplets

Allerest Sinus Pain Formula

Anacin-3 Maximum Strength and Regular Strength

Congespirin for Children, Aspirin-Free Chewable Cold Tablets

Contac Sinus Tablets, Maximum Strength Non-Drowsy Formula

Coricidin Tablets

Datril Extra Strength Analgesic Tablets and Caplets

Dristan Decongestant/Antihistamine/Analgesic Coated Tablets

Drixoral Plus Extended-Release Tablets

Excedrin Extra Strength Analgesic Tablets and Caplets

Excedrin P.M. Analgesic/Sleeping Aid Tablets, Caplets, and Liquid

Liquiprin Children's Elixir

Maximum Strength Midol PMS, Premenstrual Syndrome Formula

Ornex Caplets

Junior Strength Panadol

Pyrroxate Capsules

Sinarest Tablets and Extra Strength Tablets

Sine-off Maximum Strength Allergy/Sinus Formula Caplets

Singlet Tablets

Sinutab Maximum Strength Caplets and Tablets

Sominex Pain Relief Formula

St. Joseph Nighttime Cold Medicine

Sudafed Sinus Caplets and Tablets

TheraFlu Flu and Cold Medicine

Triaminicin Tablets

Children's Tylenol Cold Liquid Formula and Chewable Tablets

Tylenol Cold Medication No Drowsiness Formula Caplets

Unisom Dual Relief Nighttime Sleep Aid/Analgesic

Vicks Daycare Daytime Cold Medicine Liquid

Vicks NyQuil Nighttime Colds Medicine—Original and Cherry Flavor

Derived from *Physicians' desk reference for nonprescription drugs.* (1991).

Early diagnosis of the overdosage is vital. Vomiting should be induced or gastric lavage carried out, followed by oral administration of activated charcoal. These measures are most likely to be of value when instituted within 4 hours of drug ingestion.

The principal antidotal treatment is the use of a sulfhydryl compound called acetylcysteine (Mucomyst), if less than 24 hours has passed since the acetaminophen was ingested, although treatment is even more effective if less than 10 hours has passed (Gilman, et al, 1985; Smilkstein, Knapp, Kulig, & Rumack, 1988).

Gold compounds

The observation that gold inhibited *Mycobacterium tuberculosis in vitro* led to the trial of it in arthritis and lupus erythematosus, which were thought by some to be manifestations of tuberculosis (Gilman, et al, 1985). It was first used with arthritis in the 1930s.

The benefits of gold therapy (or chrysotherapy) are still debated. The Empire Rheumatism Study showed significant improvement in clients after 36 months of treatment. The gold-treated group exhibited a greater improvement in functional capacity, grip strength, number of joints involved, analgesic medications used, subjective sense of well-being, rheumatoid factor, sedimentation rate, and anemia (Baker & Rabinowitz, 1986). Gold appears to be an agent that can arrest the progress of the disease and induce remission in some. The general consensus seems to be that gold is beneficial in clients who can tolerate it over the extensive therapy period (Box 47-3).

Pharmacodynamics. Gold compounds have many actions but which effect or group of effects is precisely responsible for a beneficial result in rheumatoid arthritis remains unclear. Gold does inhibit maturation and function of mononuclear phagocytes, suppressing immune responsiveness. Decreased concentrations of rheumatoid factor and immunoglobulins have been seen in clients treated with gold (Gilman, et al, 1985).

Box 47-3. Gold compounds

- Gold compounds are used for rheumatoid arthritis.
- Oral and parenteral preparations of gold are available.
- Prolonged or permanent remission occurs in about 15% of clients treated with gold.
- Six to eight weeks of therapy is usually needed before improvement is noted.
- Side effects will be experienced by 25% to 50% of clients; careful monitoring is required.

Pharmacokinetics. The two most widely used parenteral gold preparations are aurothioglucose and gold sodium thiomalate. A new triethylphosphine gold compound (auranofin) is reasonably well absorbed after oral administration. The information on gold compounds is summarized on Table 47-2.

Initially, the gold is highly bound to albumin. Later, it is found in the synovial fluid and many body tissues. As further doses are given, half-life lengthens to weeks and months. After a cumulative dose of 1 g of gold, about 60% of it is retained in the body.

Therapeutic uses. Gold compounds are used for rheumatoid arthritis. Gold is considered to be a second line of therapy for use in disease that is unresponsive to NSAIDs, rest, and intra-articular injections of steroids. It is estimated there may be prolonged remission in about 15% of clients treated with gold, improvement of symptoms in 60% to 70% of clients, need to discontinue therapy because of toxicity in 15% to 20% of clients and about 10% to 15% of clients who do not respond (Gilman, et al, 1990). It may be most effective in early rheumatoid arthritis but gold can also be useful in later-stage rheumatoid arthritis. See Example of Nursing Process and Aurothioglucose Treatment for Rheumatoid Arthritis.

Gold has also been used in juvenile rheumatoid arthritis, palindromic rheumatism, psoriatic arthritis, Sjögren's syndrome, nondisseminated lupus erythematosus, and pemphigus.

Dosage and administration. Consult Table 47-2 for preparations and usual dosage.

One approach when using Solganal and Myochrysine is to give at least a test dose of 10 mg the first week, followed by weekly injections of 25 to 50 mg until a cumulative dose of 1,000 mg is reached. Following this, clients proceed to a maintenance regimen, which is established by increasing the interval between injections to every second week for 3 months, every third week for 3 months, and, finally, every fourth week for an indefinite period (St. Clair & Polisson, 1986). Therapeutic effects occur slowly and several weeks of therapy is usually required before improvement is noted.

Since Solganal is administered in a sesame oil vehicle, there may be inexact dosing, large lumps at the site of injections, and more painful injections because larger bore needles are necessary (Baker & Rabinowitz, 1986).

Approximately 25% of an orally administered dose of auranofin (Ridaura) is absorbed. Therapeutic response is achieved in 3–6 months. If the response is inadequate after 6 months, the dosage may be increased to 9 mg/d. If the response is still inadequate after 3 months on 9 mg/d, the drug should be discontinued.

Example of nursing process and aurothioglucose treatment for rheumatoid arthritis

The client is a 48-year-old housewife who has had rheumatoid arthritis for 15 years. She is seropositive for the rheumatoid factor. She experiences fatigue and muscle pain and aching, as well as joint pain and stiffness. She lost 30 pounds since the initial diagnosis. Her knees are severely involved, as are her feet, hands, and wrists. Her range of motion in the affected joints is decreased, and she has to depend on a wheelchair whenever she is outside her home.

The client was maintained on aspirin until she experienced severe epigastric pain and nausea that was not relieved until the aspirin was discontinued. She has been admitted to the hospital for a re-evaluation of her drug regimen. She is going to be started on aurothioglucose injections at 50 mg/wk.

The client and her husband live in a city apartment with their three children, aged 12, 15, and 18. The client is unable to work outside the home but tries to maintain her own household. Her husband has a new boss at work and seems very unhappy with him. The husband has been going out more recently, almost every evening (bowling, playing pool, or playing cards with friends). The 15-year-old daughter was recently arrested for shoplifting; the 18-year-old son has been going out every weekend to parties with an older friend where alcohol is served; and the 12-year-old son has not been doing well in school, most recently getting a D in English. The client has made reference to these problems and how overwhelmed she feels because of them.

Assessment data	Nursing diagnosis	Intervention	Goals and outcome criteria
Diagnosis of rheumatoid arthritis. Admitted to hospital for re-evaluation of medication regimen. No longer able to use aspirin. Client is to be started on aurothioglucose 50 mg IM weekly.	Knowledge deficit concerning introduction of new therapeutic agent	**Explain** to client that a complete blood count and urinalysis are obtained prior to each injection to detect evidence of any hematologic or nephrotoxic complication. **Teach** client to watch for a variety of dermatologic complications, and explain that a rash needs to be reported to her physician so therapy can be temporarily interrupted until the rash subsides. **Explain** the nitritoid reaction which is less likely with aurothioglucose than with GST but still might occur.	The client will verbalize signs and symptoms of complications that must be reported to physician. The client will have complete blood count and urinalysis done before coming to receive gold injections.
Husband is unhappy at work; he is out of the house most evenings. The 18-year-old son is attending many parties. The 15-year-old daughter was arrested for shoplifting. The 12-year-old son is having difficulties in school. Client feels overwhelmed.	Ineffective family coping: disabling, related to stress of chronic illness and situational stressors of family members	**Encourage** client's participation in decisions about care needed. **Listen** empathetically and use therapeutic touch, as appropriate. **Assist** client and significant others in verbalizing their needs, fears, and feelings. **Allow** client and significant others to express their anger about demands placed on them.	The significant others will cope more successfully, as evidenced by fewer inappropriate behaviors. The significant others will demonstrate improved support of client, as evidenced by spending quality time with client and assisting her with daily activities.

(Continued)

Example of nursing process and aurothioglucose treatment for rheumatoid arthritis (*Continued*)

Assessment data	Nursing diagnosis	Intervention	Goals and outcome criteria
		Assist client and significant others in identifying community sources of support able to assist them in coping.	
		Encourage significant others to spend time with client.	
Diagnosis of rheumatoid arthritis for 15 years. Experiences muscle pain and aching, as well as joint pain and stiffness.	Chronic pain related to inflammation of joints secondary to rheumatoid arthritis	**Assess** for factors that seem to alleviate and aggravate pain.	The client will experience decreased discomfort as evidenced by verbalizing that pain is tolerable and by exhibiting relaxed facial expression and body positioning.
		Provide nonpharmacologic measures for pain relief (*eg*, back rub, position change, relaxation techniques, guided imagery, hot packs as ordered, restful environment, diversional activities).	
		Monitor for therapeutic and nontherapeutic effects of analgesic, antiinflammatory agents as ordered.	

Adverse reactions. Anywhere from one-fourth to one-half of clients who use gold will experience adverse reactions. There is no agreement about the relationship of adverse reactions to such factors as total content of gold in the body, remission, rate of elimination of gold from body, and gold concentration in plasma.

Cutaneous lesions and lesions of the mucous membranes are the most common adverse reactions. Skin lesions range from erythema to exfoliative dermatitis. The mucous membrane lesions include stomatitis, gingivitis, glossitis, pharyngitis, tracheitis, gastritis, colitis, and vaginitis.

Blood dyscrasias including eosinophilia, thrombocytopenia, leukopenia, agranulocytosis, and aplastic anemia may occur. Proteinuria is a common complication, occurring in 25% of clients receiving 50 mg/wk of gold.

Other severe reactions, including encephalitis, peripheral neuritis, hepatitis, and pulmonary infiltrates do occur.

A vasomotor (nitritoid) reaction resembling an anaphylactoid effect may occur with gold sodium thiomalate. The symptoms of the nitritoid reaction are fainting, dizziness, flushing, and perspiring. This response is usually more frightening than harmful.

In certain comparative studies, auranofin was less toxic than parenteral gold preparations. However, au-ranofin does cause a high incidence of GI disturbances, such as frequent or loose stools, often associated with abdominal cramping.

Drugs used in the management of gout

Gout may be classified as primary or secondary. Primary gout represents a group of inborn metabolic disorders. Although the inborn defects are different, the end result is hyperuricemia and the deposition of sodium urate crystals in joints. Secondary gout occurs in certain diseases in which there is an increased breakdown of nucleic acids, producing hyperuricemia, or in clients who have an interference with renal excretion.

With urate deposits in joints, there is local infiltration of granulocytes that will phagocytize the urate crystals. There is high production of lactate in the leukocytes associated with the inflammatory process that favors a decrease in pH. This decrease in pH further increases uric acid deposition.

Gout usually has an abrupt onset with severe arthritic pain in a peripheral joint. It is treated with colchicine, allopurinol (Table 47-3), and uricosuric agents.

Colchicine

Colchicine is an alkaloid of a plant called *Colchicum autumnale* (or autumn crocus). Benjamin Franklin, who suffered from gout, was supposedly responsible

Table 47-3. Drugs used in the management of gout

Drug names	Preparations	Usual dosage/PC	Adverse reactions
colchicine	Tablets IV	Oral, adult, for acute gout, 1–1.2 mg initially, then 0.5–0.6 mg every hour or 1–1.2 mg every 2 hr until pain is relieved or diarrhea occurs (total dose should not exceed 10 mg); prophylactic with gout, 0.5–2 mg qd or qod; IV 1–3 mg initially, then 0.5 mg q6h until response (total daily dose not over 4 mg) PC: oral, C; IV, D	Nausea, vomiting, diarrhea, abdominal pain, extravasation (after IV use), fluid and electrolyte disturbances, renal failure, sepsis, disseminated intravascular coagulation
allopurinol (Alloprin, Bloxanth, Caplenal, Foligen, Lopurin, Novopurol, Purinol, Zyloprim, Zyloric)	Tablets	Oral, adult: prophylactic with gout client, 100 mg qd and increase at weekly intervals to 300 mg qd (maximum dose 800 mg qd) PC: C	Allergic hypersensitivity, rash, headache, vertigo, drowsiness, nausea, vomiting, diarrhea, abdominal discomfort, metallic taste, hepatic effects, allopurinol toxic syndrome
Uricosuries			
probenecid (Benemid, Benuryl, Probalan)	Tablets	Oral, adult, for gout: 250 mg bid for 1 wk, then 500 mg bid; adjunct therapy with antibiotic, 2 g qd in divided doses PC: UK	GI side effects (anorexia, nausea, vomiting, diarrhea), headache, lightheadedness, sore gums, allergic hypersensitivity
sulfinpyrazone (Anturan, Anturane, Inturidin, Enturen, Lovopyrazone)	Tablets Capsules	Oral, adult, for gout: 200–400 mg qd, may be increased over 1 wk period to up to 800 mg qd PC: UK	GI side effects (nausea, vomiting, dyspepsia, abdominal pain), blood dyscrasias, rashes

KEY: PC = Pregnancy risk category. (The validity of pregnancy risk categories has not been established. See Chapter 16, p 216.)

for introducing colchicine in the United States for gout therapy in 1763.

Pharmacodynamics. Colchicine is a unique medication because it is relatively selective for gout. It is an antimitotic agent and by virtue of its ability to bind to microtubular protein (tubulin), it interferes with function of mitotic spindles and causes depolymerization and disappearance of fibrillar microtubules in granulocytes. It inhibits the migration of granulocytes into the inflamed area; reduces the release of lactic acid and proinflammatory enzymes that occur during phagocytosis; breaks the cycle that leads to the inflammatory response (Gilman, et al, 1985); and decreases the inflammatory response and, hence, the pain.

Pharmacokinetics. Colchicine is rapidly absorbed after oral administration with a peak action within 2 hours. It has a plasma half-life of 20 minutes and a half-life in white blood cells of 60 hours. It is excreted in urine and feces. Large amounts of colchicine and its metabolites enter the intestinal tract in the bile and intestinal secretions. This may account for the intestinal manifestations of toxicity.

Therapeutic uses. Colchicine is used to treat acute attacks of gout, as well as to prevent or abort acute attacks. If colchicine is given promptly following an attack, pain, swelling, and redness will be relieved within 12 hours and will completely clear in 48–72 hours. See Example of Nursing Process and Colchicine Treatment.

Other less common conditions where colchicine is used include familiar paroxysmal polyserositis, amyloidosis, primary biliary cirrhosis, multiple sclerosis, psoriasis, and Behçet's syndrome.

Dosage and administration. Consult Table 47-3 for preparations and usual dosages. Tablets should be protected from exposure to light in special containers. Because of the possibility of cumulative toxicity, colchicine should not be given again for 3 days (oral), once a 10-mg total dose is achieved.

When given intravenously, a total dose of 4 mg should not be exceeded. The medication should not be given again for 7 days.

Colchicine may be used prophylactically to prevent acute attacks of gout precipitated by surgery.

Adverse reactions. Nausea, vomiting, diarrhea, and abdominal pain are common GI side effects of colchicine. These effects may be unavoidable during the client's first therapeutic use of the medication.

Gastrointestinal side effects occur with less frequency after IV administration than after oral administration. Other reactions include tissue necrosis from local extravasation (after IV administration),

Example of nursing process and colchicine treatment

The client is a 79-year-old woman who has had osteoarthritis for about 30 years, and who has had two attacks of acute gout. Her gout is considered secondary to the use of thiazide diuretic during 15 years of antihypertensive therapy. She is currently receiving allopurinol 300 mg/d for the gout, Lopressor 50 mg bid and Dyazide 1 capsule daily for the hypertension, and sulindac 150 mg bid for the osteoarthritis.

Several years ago, she had total bilateral hip replacements. She is dependent on two canes for ambulation and spends the majority of her day sitting in a recliner in her living room. She rarely leaves the house because negotiating stairs and climbing in and out of a car are very difficult for her.

She and her 83-year-old husband live in their own home in a small village. They have four children but the nearest one lives about 1½ hours north of their home. The client manages all of the couple's meals but has a housekeeper who comes in once a week for a few hours to do the housecleaning.

Today, the client and her husband are in an ophthalmologist's office, where they have been referred by the client's general practitioner. The client will need to undergo cataract surgery in the city hospital's outpatient department. The city is about 25 miles north of the client's home, and neither the client nor her husband has been to the out-patient department before.

The ophthalmologist has a very busy practice and has not met the client before. A nurse works with him and is responsible for implementing client-education plans. She also prepares a suggested plan of care for each client to share with the hospital out-patient nurses because the nurses do not see clients until the time of surgery.

Assessment data	Nursing diagnosis	Intervention	Goals and outcome criteria
Diagnosis of long-standing osteoarthritis Uses two canes Rarely leaves home Requires sulindac Age 79 years. First visit to ophthalmologist's office.	High risk for injury: falls related to unfamiliar environment, weakness and pain in weight-bearing extremities, and advancing age	**Include** client and husband in planning and implementing measures to prevent injury. **Accompany** client during ambulation in office and at outpatient department. **Do not rush** client; allow time for trip to bathroom. **Avoid** unnecessary clutter in office examination room. **Keep** canes and pocketbook within easy reach during office visit. **Encourage** client to request assistance when needed in office and at outpatient department.	The client will not experience falls.
Has not had cataract surgery before. Has not been to city hospital's outpatient department before. Husband will be primary caregiver after surgery.	Knowledge deficit related to inexperience with upcoming surgery	**Instruct** client and husband in ways to prevent postoperative complications **Teach** husband how to administer ordered eye drops and ointment and how to apply shield to affected eye at bedtime. Emphasize need for good handwashing before treatment is carried out. **Encourage** questions and allow time for clarification of information provided.	The client and husband will state signs and symptoms of complications that must be reported to ophthalmologist. The client and husband will verbalize an understanding of and a plan for adhering to the follow-up care plan.

(Continued)

Example of nursing process and colchicine treatment (Continued)

Assessment data	Nursing diagnosis	Intervention	Goals and outcome criteria
History of two attacks of gout. Receives allopurinol 300 mg/d.	High risk for pain related to exacerbation of gout secondary to surgery	**Secure** order from ophthalmologist for colchicine 0.5 mg tid for 3 days before and 3 days after surgery. **Explain** to client the rationale for using colchicine. At the time of eye surgery, **confirm** that client has taken the ordered doses of colchicine for the previous 3 days. **Instruct** client to immediately report to physician any signs and symptoms of a gout attack after surgery.	The client will verbalize an understanding of the use of colchicine. The client will comply and take colchicine as ordered. The client will remain free of signs and symptoms of acute gout attack postoperatively.

volume depletion related to diarrhea, hyponatremia, hypocalcemia, renal failure, sepsis, and disseminated intravascular coagulation. Cumulative toxicity occurs.

Colchicine metabolism and excretion are impaired in renal or hepatic disease. It is felt administration of IV colchicine to clients with hepatic and renal disease should be approached very conservatively and it seems that clients with both hepatic and renal disease should not receive colchicine at all (Roberts, Liang, & Stern, 1987).

Elderly clients should be given no more than 2 mg of intravenous colchicine per attack, with at least 21 days between courses of the medication.

Toxicity. Acute poisoning and fatalities have occurred. In acute poisoning, the diarrhea becomes a hemorrhagic gastroenteritis with severe loss of fluid and electrolytes, and may lead to shock, kidney damage, muscle paralysis, and death.

Allopurinol

Allopurinol (Zyloprim, Lopurin) inhibits the final steps of uric acid biosynthesis.

Pharmacodynamics. Uric acid is formed by the xanthine oxidase-catalyzed oxidation of hypoxanthine and xanthine. Allopurinol inhibits the xanthine oxidase. This inhibition reduces plasma concentration and urinary excretion of uric acid and increases plasma concentration and renal excretion of uric acid precursors.

Pharmacokinetics. Allopurinol is fairly well absorbed after oral administration. It reaches its peak action within 2 hours, and its duration of action ranges from 18 to 30 hours. It is excreted in feces and urine.

Therapeutic uses. Allopurinol is used for treatment of primary and secondary gout. Hyperuricemia may be secondary to polycythemia vera, leukemias, and lymphomas, especially when antineoplastic or radiation therapy is used, and is sometimes induced by thiazide diuretics.

Dosage and administration. Consult Table 47-3 for preparations and usual dosages. In gout, the objective is to have the client's uric acid level at 6.0 mg/dl. Allopurinol should not be started during an acute gout attack. Acute attacks can increase in frequency or severity during early months of treatment with allopurinol because urate is mobilized from affected joints. Colchicine may be used in conjunction with the allopurinol prophylactically or, if necessary, in therapeutic doses if an attack occurs.

Dosage must be reduced if the client has renal impairment. If the glomerular filtration rate (GFR) is 10 to 50 ml/min, 50% of the usual dosage is given (perhaps 150 mg/d). When the interval extension method is used, at a GFR of 10 to 50 ml/min, 12 to 24 hours between doses of the usual size are recommended. If the GFR is 10 to 25 ml/min, 10% to 25% of the usual dosage is given or 48 to 72 hours between doses should be the guideline.

To prevent hyperuricemia secondary to chemotherapy for neoplasms, the adult dosage is 600 to 800 mg/d for 2 or 3 days before initiation of therapy. For children, the dosage would be 150 to 300 mg once daily.

When allopurinol is given, clients must be well hydrated. Fluid intake should be sufficient to maintain daily urine volume above 2,000 ml. Alkalinization of the urine is also desirable. These actions are taken to minimize the risk of xanthine stone formation during the allopurinol therapy.

Adverse reactions. Allopurinol is a medication that is well tolerated by most clients. *Allopurinol toxic syndrome,* has been described, which is associated with hypersensitivity. Manifestations include a diffuse, erythematous, desquamating skin rash, pruritus, GI distress, diarrhea, fever, eosinophilia, hepatic dysfunction, and renal dysfunction. Most clients who developed this syndrome were taking about 200 to 400 mg/d for a few weeks and had renal insufficiency. The causative factor seems to be allopurinol's active metabolite, oxipurinol, since the long half-life is prolonged further in clients with impaired renal function. If a rash and/or fever develop in clients receiving allopurinol, it should be discontinued.

Some clients recovered from manifestations of the syndrome spontaneously after drug withdrawal; some required steroids; some required hemodialysis; and some died. It was felt that one important factor in reducing the incidence of the syndrome is reducing the dose of the drug in clients with renal insufficiency (*Drug evaluations annual,* 1990). Other side effects include headache, drowsiness, nausea, vomiting, vertigo, diarrhea, and gastric irritation.

Uricosurics

A uricosuric agent is a drug that increases the rate of uric acid excretion. The uricosuric agents discussed are probenecid and sulfinpyrazone (see Table 47-3).

Probenecid

Probenecid was developed as an agent to depress the normally rapid tubular secretion of penicillin, so the available supply of penicillin might be used more thoroughly by the body.

Pharmacodynamics. Probenecid inhibits the transport of organic acids across epithelial barriers, primarily in the renal tubule. The only important endogenous compound whose excretion is increased by probenecid is uric acid. Probenecid increases the urinary excretion of uric acid by inhibiting its reabsorption.

Some degree of renal impairment may be present in clients with gout and probenecid may not be effective in chronic renal insufficiency when the GFR is reduced. Conditions in the kidney, such as an alkaline or acidic urine, may also alter the effects of probenecid.

Pharmacokinetics. Probenecid is rapidly absorbed after oral administration and it reaches a peak action in 2 to 4 hours. When probenecid is used as adjunct therapy with penicillin, penicillin serum levels will persist for 8 hours after a dose. It is excreted in the urine.

Therapeutic uses. Probenecid is used to treat gout and as adjunct therapy to penicillin. If penicillin and probenecid are given together, there are higher and more prolonged concentrations of the antibiotic in the plasma than when the penicillin is given alone. Probenecid has also been used as an adjunct with some of the cephalosporins. The concept has been important in the treatment of sexually transmitted diseases such as gonorrhea, acute pelvic inflammatory disease, and neurosyphilis.

Dosage and administration. Consult Table 47-3 for preparations and usual dosages.

Probenecid and colchicine may be used together. When probenecid is first used, acute attacks of gout may increase in frequency or severity because urates are mobilized. Colchicine may then be added to the regimen. A preparation called ColBenemid is available as tablets containing 0.5 g of probenecid and 0.5 mg of colchicine. The recommended dosage is one tablet daily for 1 week, followed by one tablet twice a day. ColBenemid can be used in treating chronic gout when it is complicated by frequent, recurrent acute attacks of the disease.

During the initial treatment stages of gout, there is also the possibility of precipitating renal calculi due to to the mobilization of urates. A large amount of fluids should be given to prevent this complication. In addition, uric acid tends to crystallize out of an acid urine. Therefore, alkalinization of the urine is recommended and may be accomplished through the daily use of 3–7.5 g of sodium bicarbonate or 7.5 g of potassium citrate. Alkalinization of the urine is recommended until the serum urate level is returned to normal, whereupon it may be decreased.

Adverse reactions. Probenecid is usually well tolerated. In a very small percentage of clients, particularly those receiving higher doses, GI side effects occur, such as anorexia, nausea, and vomiting. Headaches, lightheadedness, sore gums, and hypersensitivity reactions have also occurred.

Drug interactions. When probenecid is being used to treat gout, ASA or any salicylate should not be used simultaneously. The net effect of simultaneous administration is a decrease in elimination of uric acid.

Probenecid inhibits renal excretion and may increase plasma levels of methotrexate, sulfonamides, indomethacin, naproxen, ketoprofen, meclofenamate, nitrofurantoin, rifampin, lorazepam, and other medications.

Sulfinpyrazone

Sulfinpyrazone (Anturane, Aprazone) is chemically related to phenylbutazone but it lacks the same anti-inflammatory and analgesic properties of that drug.

Pharmacodynamics. Sulfinpyrazone decreases serum uric acid levels by inhibiting the renal tubular reabsorption of uric acid and subsequently increasing its urinary excretion.

It also inhibits thromboxane synthesis so it decreases platelet aggregation and has been studied as an antithrombotic agent.

Pharmacokinetics. Sulfinpyrazone is well absorbed after oral administration and has a peak action of 1 to 2 hours. After a duration of action of 4 to 10 hours, it is excreted in the urine.

Therapeutic uses. Sulfinpyrazone is used to treat chronic gout. It is chosen primarily for clients with normal renal function whose 24-hour urinary uric acid excretion is less than 800 mg (*Drug evaluations annual,* 1990). It is of no immediate value in acute attacks of gouty arthritis and is not usually used in those over 60 years of age.

Dosage and administration. Consult Table 47-3 for preparations and usual dosage. Special considerations related to administration of this drug include the following: the medication is given with meals, milk, or antacids. Increased fluid intake and alkalinization of the urine are recommended to minimize the renal deposition of urate during the first few weeks of therapy to prevent renal calculi. The drug should be used with caution in clients with impaired renal function or a history of renal calculi. It should not be used if the GFR is known to be less than 50% of normal.

Adverse reactions. The most common side effects are GI irritation, manifested as abdominal pain, nausea, vomiting, and dyspepsia. Since reactivation or exacerbation of peptic ulcer has been reported, the drug should be used cautiously in clients with a history of peptic ulcer. Blood dyscrasias have been reported as well, although rarely.

Drug interactions. Salicylates and some of the other NSAIDs diminish the uricosuric effect of sulfinpyrazone and should not be used concomitantly. This interaction should be explained to the client for it is documented as a definite cause of treatment failure.

Sulfinpyrazone may potentiate the actions of insulin and oral hypoglycemic agents. The antiprothrombin activity of oral anticoagulants may be enhanced.

■ Summary

The inflammatory process consists of multiple physiologic responses to a stimulus. Anti-inflammatory agents are used when this process has caused or appears to be causing deleterious effects to a client. Many of the agents have anti-inflammatory, analgesic, and antipyretic properties. The primary mechanism by which they create their effects is the inhibition of prostaglandin synthetase. The main NSAIDs are the salicylates, acetic acids, propionic acids, fenamates, pyrazoles, and oxicams. Related agents include para-aminophenol derivatives and gold compounds. Gout is a disorder related to the deposition of urate crystals in joints that may be treated with colchicine, allopurinol, probenecid, or sulfinpyrazone. Some of the agents used for inflammation, namely ASA and acetaminophen, are easily available to the public. Because their availability makes them widely used, there is a high incidence of problems experienced with them, ranging from side effects to toxicity from overdosage.

Nursing management

Nursing implications

Many anti-inflammatory agents have serious or toxic side effects. It is evident from a review of the drugs that the vast majority of them tend to share two common adverse effects to a greater or lesser degree: disturbances of the GI and renal systems.

Nursing process

Assessment Because there have been hypersensitive reactions to NSAIDs, the nurse should assess the client for a history of sensitivity to the prescribed medication or similar medications. Individuals sensitive to ASA, for example, might be sensitive to any of the NSAIDs. Equally important is the need to determine whether the client has a history of GI or renal complaints. A full understanding is necessary of what other medications the client may be receiving (such as ulcerogenic drugs or drugs known to interact with the prescribed medication).

When the client is on a prolonged drug regimen, as in circumstances where the drugs are being used for chronic conditions, it may be advisable to regularly perform certain laboratory tests. For example, salicylate levels may need to be checked. Clients receiving oral anticoagulants should expect to have frequent prothrombin time assessments when any NSAIDs are used. Likewise, in those clients with pre-existing renal disease, periodic renal function tests (*eg,* blood urea nitrogen and serum creatinine) would be warranted. Additionally, if a drug is known to have caused bone marrow depression, determination of the client's hematologic profile (*ie,* white blood cell count, hemoglobin, hematocrit) may be warranted.

Nursing diagnosis Many clients receiving anti-inflammatory drugs would be medically diagnosed as having osteoarthritis or rheumatoid arthritis. Nursing diagnoses that might apply would include the following:

Chronic pain
Activity intolerance

Impaired physical mobility
High risk for injury
Self-care deficit related to (specify the joints affected)
Sleep pattern disturbance
Self-esteem disturbance
Altered sexuality patterns
Ineffective individual coping
Altered family processes
Knowledge deficit concerning the disease process and medication therapy
Impaired home maintenance management
High risk for ineffective management of self-care regimen
Pain: gastrointestinal related to side effects of medication

A common collaborative problem that should be differentiated from the nursing diagnoses is

Potential complication: renal related to adverse effects of medication

Planning In preparing a plan of client care, the nurse should set goals to reach certain client outcomes: diminished pain; increased tolerance for activity; achievement of maximum physical mobility; performance of self-care activities within physical limitations; attainment of optimal amounts of sleep; adaptation to changes in body function and level of independence; perception of self as sexually adequate and acceptable; use of effective coping skills; adjustment of family to disruption of family process, and ability to discuss medications—their purpose, dosage prescribed, adverse effects, and any information relevant to the treatment regimen.

Intervention Because of the adverse effects of NSAIDs on the GI system, certain nursing interventions are necessary. As a general rule, the medications should be given with milk or food, or immediately after meals. The client should be advised to inform the nurse or physician if GI complaints occur or persist (*eg,* diarrhea, nausea, vomiting, evidence of GI bleeding, such as blood in the stool or tarry stools, or abdominal pain). The physician may reduce the dosage, change the specific preparation the client is receiving, or order antacids in certain cases.

Diabetic clients receiving some of these agents may require adjustment in the dosage of their insulin or oral hypoglycemic agent. These clients should perform glucose assessment tests daily and report to the nurse or physician changes in these tests, as well as any episodes of hypoglycemia.

Client education. Clients with arthritis need to be advised that their symptoms may not immediately improve because it may take several days or even weeks for the drug to produce its therapeutic effect.

Clients need to be educated to the various problems concerning anti-inflammatory and related drugs, namely side effects and toxicity, safe storage of the drugs, and advertising claims of over-the-counter drugs. (Over-the-counter drugs are discussed in Chapter 21.)

These medications frequently cause renal side effects. Adverse reactions are more likely to occur in those clients with pre-existing renal dysfunction. The client will need an explanation of the reason for any renal function tests that are ordered. The client should be advised to inform the nurse or physician if he or she experiences edema, dysuria, hematuria, or other urinary symptoms.

These medications may cause CNS side effects; the client should be taught to watch for these. If such neurologic effects as drowsiness or dizziness occur, the client should be advised to avoid driving and other activities that require alertness. Insomnia sometimes occurs.

Because of the high incidence of intoxication and poisoning with some of these agents, the nurse should take particular care in educating clients fully to this potential danger. Also, proper storage to prevent small children from gaining access to the preparation should be stressed.

Some of these drugs, such as ASA and acetaminophen, are available without a prescription (see Box 47-2). The danger exists that clients will misuse these preparations or use them inappropriately. Education is essential to prevent these possibilities. Specifically, clients should be advised to seek a physician's assistance when a symptom for which they are using one of these drugs persists for more than a few days. The client will also probably have misconceptions or questions about the advertising claims for these products. The nurse can help improve the client's knowledge in this area.

Evaluation The nurse must evaluate the client to determine drug efficacy and to observe for evidence of adverse reactions to the drugs. Data that would indicate drug efficacy include verbalization of pain relief, relaxed facial expression and body positioning, increased participation in activities, statements of feeling rested, and absence of frequent yawning and irritability. Examples of data that would indicate the drug was not causing adverse reactions include absence of diarrhea, nausea, vomiting, blood in the stool, and abdominal pain, as well as normal blood urea nitrogen, serum creatinine, white blood cell count, hemoglobin, and hematocrit. (See the accompanying Example of Nursing Process and Colchicine Treatment, and Example of Nursing Process and Aurothioglucose Treatment for Rheumatoid Arthritis.)

Checklist of nursing actions

☐ Assess clients for hypersensitivity or allergy to the selected NSAID or any NSAID.
☐ Determine if client has asthma, a history of GI

problems, a history of renal disease, or other medical problems. Some conditions may be exacerbated or worsened by the use of NSAIDs.

☐ Ascertain what other medications the client is currently taking. Many drugs interact with the NSAIDs (*eg*, anticoagulants, beta-adrenergic blocking agents, antacids, probenecid, cholestyramine, diuretics, angiotensin-converting enzyme inhibitors, lithium, methotrexate, digoxin, aminoglycosides, and others).

☐ Discuss compliance with the drug regimen, explaining that regular intake of the drug is necessary to sustain the anti-inflammatory effects of a NSAID.

☐ Advise taking the NSAID with a full glass of milk or with meals to reduce gastric irritation.

☐ Advise client that the therapeutic effects of the NSAID in many cases will take weeks to be achieved.

☐ Remind clients to tell other health care providers of the NSAID being taken to avoid having prescriptions written that would interact unfavorably with NSAIDs.

☐ Teach the client about adverse reactions that may be encountered.

☐ Advise client to report to the health care provider any symptoms of GI irritation not relieved by adhering to the prescribed GI-protective protocol or changes in GU functioning (*eg*, changes in voiding pattern, edema).

☐ Discuss the need for regular medical supervision so that dosage can be adjusted on basis of client's condition and drug response. Certain laboratory tests should be performed on a regular basis (*eg*, renal and hematologic studies).

☐ Teach client about proper use of any NSAIDs that are secured as over-the-counter preparations. Discuss advertising claims with the client.

References

Alexander D, Spencer R. (1986). Over-the-counter analgesics, antipyretics, and anti-inflammatories: The nurse's role in selection and use. *J Community Health Nurs, 3*, 11–23.

Baker DG, Rabinowitz JL. (1986). Current concepts in the treatment of rheumatoid arthritis. *J Clin Pharmacol, 26*, 2–21.

Brooks PM, Day RO. (1991). Nonsteroidal antiinflammatory drugs—differences and similarities. *N Engl J Med, 324(24)*, 1716–1723.

Clive DM, Stoff JS. (1984). Renal syndromes associated with nonsteroidal anti-inflammatory drugs. *N Engl J Med, 310(9)*, 563–571.

Drug evaluations annual. (1990). Department of Drugs, Division of Drugs and Toxicology. Milwaukee, WI: American Medical Association.

Fuster V, Cohen M, Halperin J. (1989). Aspirin in the prevention of coronary disease. *N Engl J Med, 321(3)*, 183–185.

Gilman AG, et al, eds. (1985). *Goodman and Gilman's the pharmacological basis of therapeutics*, 7th ed. New York: Macmillan.

McCance KL, Huether SE. (1990). *Pathophysiology, the biological basis for disease in adults and children.* St. Louis: C V Mosby.

Roberts WN, Liang MH, Stern SH. (1987). Colchicine in acute gout . . . reassessment of risks and benefits. *JAMA, 257*, 1920–1922.

Roth SH. (1988). NSAID and gastropathy: A rheumatologist's review. *J Rheumatol, 15*, 912–919.

Smilkstein MJ, Knapp GL, Kulig KW, Rumack BH. (1988). Efficacy of oral N-acetylcysteine in the treatment of acetaminophen overdose. *N Engl J Med, 319*, 1557–1562.

St. Clair EW, Polisson RP. (1986). Therapeutic approaches to the treatment of rheumatoid disease. *Med Clin N Am, 70(2)*, 285–301.

Bibliography

Abramson SB, Weissman G. (1989). The mechanism of action of nonsteroidal antiinflammatory drugs. *Arthritis Rheum, 32*, 1–9.

Brater DC, Anderson SA, Brown-Cartwright D, Toto RD. (1986). Effects of nonsteroidal anti-inflammatory drugs on renal function in patients with renal insufficiency and in cirrhotics. *Am J Kid Dis, 8(5)*, 351–355.

Carson JL, Strom BL, et al. (1987). The relative gastrointestinal toxicity of the nonsteroidal antiinflammatory drugs. *Arch Intern Med, 147*, 1054.

Cooke TDV, Scudamore RA. (1989). Studies in the pathogenesis of rheumatoid arthritis. *Br J Rheumatol, 28*, 243–250, 330–340.

Dukes MNG, Beeley L. (1990). *Side effects of drugs annual 14.* Amsterdam, Netherlands: Elsevier Science.

Forrest M, Brooks PM. (1988). Mechanism of action of non-steroidal anti-rheumatic drugs. *Clin Rheumatol, 2*, 275–294.

Lamy PP. (1986). Possible gastrotoxicity of NSAIDs in the elderly. *Journal of Gerontological Nursing, 12*, 32–33.

Lewis AJ, Furst DW, eds. (1987). *Nonsteroidal antiinflammatory drugs. Mechanisms and clinical use.* New York: Marcel Dekker.

Lombardino JG, ed. (1985). *Nonsteroidal antiinflammatory drugs.* New York: John Wiley and Sons.

Oates JA, FitzGerald GA, Branch RA, Jackson EK, Knapp HR, Roberts LJ. (1988). Clinical implications of prostaglandin and thromboxane A2 formation, Part I. *N Engl J Med, 319*, 689–698.

Oates JA, FitzGerald GA, Branch RA, Jackson EK, Knapp HR, Roberts LJ. (1988). Clinical implications of prostaglandin and thromboxane A2 formation, Part II. *N Engl J Med, 319*, 761–767.

Pinsky PF, Hurwitz ES, Schonberger LB, Gunn, WJ. (1988). Reye's syndrome and aspirin: Evidence for a dose-response effect. *JAMA, 260*, 657–661.

Reilly IAG, Fitzgerald GA, (1988). Aspirin in cardiovascular disease. *Drugs, 35*, 154–176.

Roth SH. (1988). Salicylates revisited: Are they still the hallmark of anti-inflammatory therapy? *Drugs, 36*, 1–6.

Sandler DP, Smith JC, Weinberg CR, Buckalew VM, Dennis VW, Blythe WB, Burgess WP. (1989). Analgesic use and chronic renal disease. *N Engl J Med, 320,* 1238–1243.

Schiff E et al. (1989). The use of aspirin to prevent pregnancy-induced hypertension and lower the ratio of thromboxane A2 to prostacyclin in relatively high risk pregnancies. *N Engl J Med, 321,* 351–356.

Shapiro SS. (1988). Treatment of dysmenorrhea and premenstrual syndrome with nonsteroidal anti-inflammatory drugs. *Drugs, 36,* 475–490.

Situnayake RD, Grindulis KA, McConkey B. (1987). Long-term treatment of rheumatoid arthritis with sulphasalazine, gold, or penicillamine: A comparison using life-table methods. *Ann Rheum Dis, 46,* 177–183.

Stevenson DD, Lewis RA. (1987). Proposed mechanisms of aspirin sensitivity reaction. *J Allergy Clin, 80,* 788–790.

Symposium. (1987a). Arachidonic acid metabolism and inflammation. Therapeutic implications. *Drugs, 33(Suppl):1,* 1–66.

Vane J, Botting R. (1987). Inflammation and the mechanism of action of anti-inflammatory drugs. *FASEB J, 1,* 89–96.

Ward JR. (1988). Role of disease-modifying antirheumatic drugs versus cytotoxic agents in the therapy of rheumatoid arthritis. *Am J Med, 85,* 39–44.

Drugs used for neoplastic disease

12

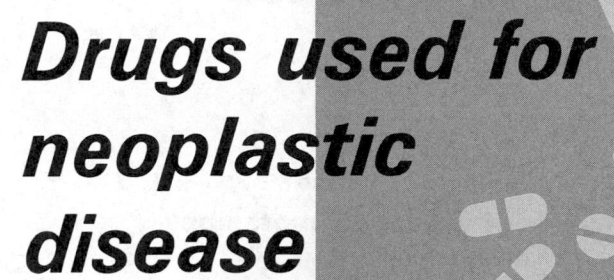

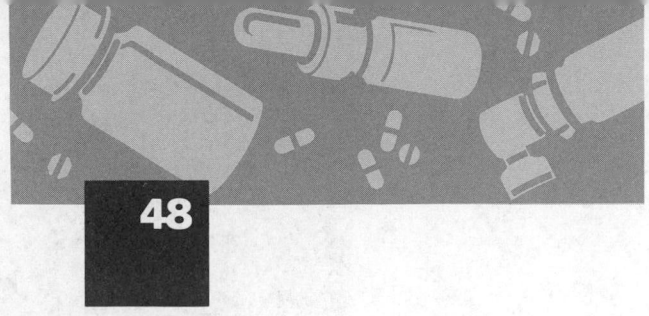

48

Chemotherapeutic agents: alkylating agents and antimetabolites

Pathophysiology of cancer

Cancer is a disorder of cell differentiation and replication. It is not a single disease and it can originate in almost any organ (Fig. 48-1). Cancer is the second leading cause of death in the United States. Although it strikes more frequently with advancing age, it causes more deaths in children between the ages of 3 and 14 than any other disease. It is estimated by the American Cancer Society that one out of four Americans develops cancer during their lifetimes. Four out of every ten Americans who get cancer today remain alive 5 years after diagnosis; in the 1930s, less than one in five had survived 5 years after diagnosis.

Cancer cells have characteristics that set them apart from normal cells. They do not undergo normal cell differentiation and replication, do not function normally, and do not die on schedule.

Normal cell proliferation is regulated so the number of cells actively dividing is equivalent to the number dying. Cancer cells multiply in a disorderly, uncontrolled, incessant way. They divide and duplicate without regard for the tissues they serve.

The term carcinogenesis refers to the process by which a normal tissue is transformed into cancerous tissue. Many mechanisms may contribute to this transformation (*eg*, heredity; oncogenes and oncogenic viruses; chemical and physical carcinogens, such as asbestos, vinyl chloride, cigarette smoke, and diethylstilbestrol; and immunologic system defects).

The term neoplasm refers to "new growth" and both benign and malignant neoplasms exist. Malignant neoplasms serve no useful purpose and they continue to grow at the expense of the host. Because of their rapid growth, they compress blood vessels and outgrow their blood supply, causing ischemia and tissue necrosis. They rob normal tissues of essential nutrients. They may elaborate enzymes that break down proteins and contribute to the invasiveness of the cancer. They may elaborate toxins that destroy both tumor tissue and normal tissue (Porth, 1990).

Principles of cancer chemotherapy

Three principle ways to treat cancer are used: surgery, radiotherapy, and antineoplastic drug therapy. Because each method has its advantages and disadvan-

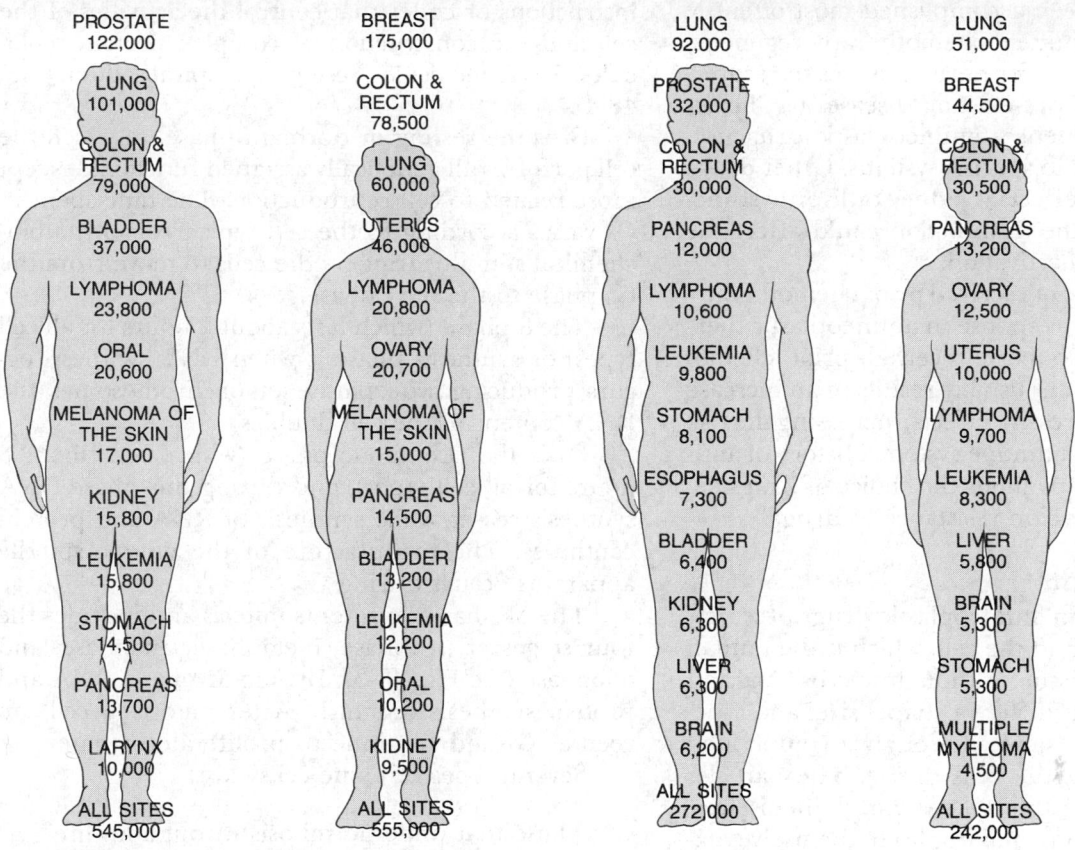

CANCER INCIDENCE BY SITE AND SEX*

PROSTATE 122,000	BREAST 175,000
LUNG 101,000	COLON & RECTUM 78,500
COLON & RECTUM 79,000	LUNG 60,000
BLADDER 37,000	UTERUS 46,000
LYMPHOMA 23,800	LYMPHOMA 20,800
ORAL 20,600	OVARY 20,700
MELANOMA OF THE SKIN 17,000	MELANOMA OF THE SKIN 15,000
KIDNEY 15,800	PANCREAS 14,500
LEUKEMIA 15,800	BLADDER 13,200
STOMACH 14,500	LEUKEMIA 12,200
PANCREAS 13,700	ORAL 10,200
LARYNX 10,000	KIDNEY 9,500
ALL SITES 545,000	ALL SITES 555,000

CANCER DEATHS BY SITE AND SEX

LUNG 92,000	LUNG 51,000
PROSTATE 32,000	BREAST 44,500
COLON & RECTUM 30,000	COLON & RECTUM 30,500
PANCREAS 12,000	PANCREAS 13,200
LYMPHOMA 10,600	OVARY 12,500
LEUKEMIA 9,800	UTERUS 10,000
STOMACH 8,100	LYMPHOMA 9,700
ESOPHAGUS 7,300	LEUKEMIA 8,300
BLADDER 6,400	LIVER 5,800
KIDNEY 6,300	BRAIN 5,300
LIVER 6,300	STOMACH 5,300
BRAIN 6,200	MULTIPLE MYELOMA 4,500
ALL SITES 272,000	ALL SITES 242,000

*Excluding nonmelanoma skin cancer and carcinoma in situ.

Figure 48-1. Cancer incidence and death by site and sex: 1991 estimates. (Courtesy of American Cancer Society)

tages, choosing the appropriate therapy depends on the specific situation. A combination of treatment modalities is frequently used in cancer management. Cancer treatment can be curative or palliative, and all three types of treatment can be used with either intent. Surgery is considered the best method of treatment if the cancer is localized and metastasis has not occurred. Only the pharmacologic aspects of treatment are discussed here.

Several factors or principles affect whether or not antineoplastic therapy is used to treat cancer and, if so, which agents are selected. These factors include type of malignancy, client's status, the cell cycle concepts, growth fraction, first-order kinetics, pharmacologic considerations, and resistance.

Antineoplastic drugs are commonly classified into several pharmacologic groups. Alkylating agents and antimetabolites are discussed in this chapter; natural products, antibiotics, hormones, biologic response modifiers, and miscellaneous agents are discussed in Chapter 49.

Type of malignancy

The type of malignancy greatly affects decisions about antineoplastic drug therapy. Some malignancies respond favorably to drugs in nearly all cases. Other types of malignancies respond only a small fraction of the time (*eg*, renal, pancreatic, colorectal, non–small cell lung carcinomas). Malignancies that respond to antineoplastic drug therapy almost to the point that they can be considered cured are choriocarcinoma and Burkitt's leukemia. Acute leukemias of childhood and Hodgkin's disease also have a high response rate to antineoplastic drug therapy.

Client's status

A client's overall physiologic status affects the use of antineoplastic therapy. The client's immune status, particularly cell-mediated immunity, is an important factor in client response to chemotherapy; immunocompetent individuals respond more favorably than immunocompromised clients. Most antineoplastic drugs are immunosuppressive because of their effects on bone marrow. Generally, maintenance of immunocompetence has been accomplished most often by using intensive intermittent chemotherapy regimens, in which time is allowed for normal tissues to recover.

The presence of pre-existing diseases (*eg*, heart, liver, or kidney) influences antineoplastic drug use. Some drugs are toxic to specific systems. Other drugs have increased toxic effects if kidney or liver dysfunction exists, because the dysfunction could affect the drug's excretion or inactivation.

Clients who have not received prior chemotherapy usually show a better response to antineoplastic therapy than clients who have received prior chemotherapy. Prior treatment usually results in an increase in bone marrow suppressive effects, increasing the risk of compromising the immune system. History of antineoplastic drug therapy limits the choice of drugs because cancer cells develop resistance to drugs.

Cell cycle concepts

To understand certain antineoplastic drugs, it is first necessary to understand the cell, which is the human body's basic unit of tissue. Although microscopic and highly organized cells differ in shape, size, and type, basic structure is the same. Through a complicated process called *mitosis*, the cells divide. The particles within the nucleus of the cell rearrange themselves, divide into two portions, and duplicate themselves exactly in new cells called daughter cells (Fig. 48-2).

Five phases in a cell's cycle of biochemical activity exist, and the entire cycle takes from 16 to 10,000 hours (Fig. 48-3). The cycle represents the interval from the midpoint of mitosis to the end point in mitosis in a daughter cell. Interphase is a term used to include four of the phases (G_0, G_1, S, and G_2).

G_1 is the first postmitotic phase during which deoxyribonucleic acid (DNA) synthesis ceases, ribonucleic acid (RNA) and protein synthesis increases, and cell growth occurs. DNA molecules carry the genetic instructions or codes that control the activities of the cell and the construction of complex protein molecules. DNA molecules resemble a spiral ladder (Fig. 48-4).

G_0 is the resting or dormant phase, in which the cell performs all genetically assigned functions, except those related to cell reproduction. The time spent in G_0 varies according to the cell type. Probably, a biochemical stimulus triggers the cells to move from the G_0 phase to the next phase.

The S phase (which lasts about 2 hours for all cell types) or synthesis phase is when DNA synthesis occurs, producing two separate sets of chromosomes (the DNA content of the cell doubles).

G_2 is the premitotic phase (which lasts about 8 hours for all cell types), and during this phase DNA synthesis ceases while synthesis of RNA and protein continues. The manufacture of the mitotic spindle apparatus occurs during G_2.

The M phase represents mitosis and includes the four stages of prophase, metaphase, anaphase, and telophase (see Fig. 48-3). During M phase, RNA and protein synthesis diminish. After mitosis, a cell can reenter G_1 and continue to proliferate or enter G_0.

Several types of tissue cells exist:

Those that undergo mitosis throughout life (*eg*, bone marrow stem cells, skin cells)

Those that are unable to reproduce themselves after their initial organ formation (*eg*, nerve cells of the central nervous system [CNS])

Those that are resting but can reproduce themselves if appropriately stimulated (*eg*, liver cells, thyroid gland cells)

Several antineoplastic drugs are effective primarily during a specific phase of the cell cycle, and one way

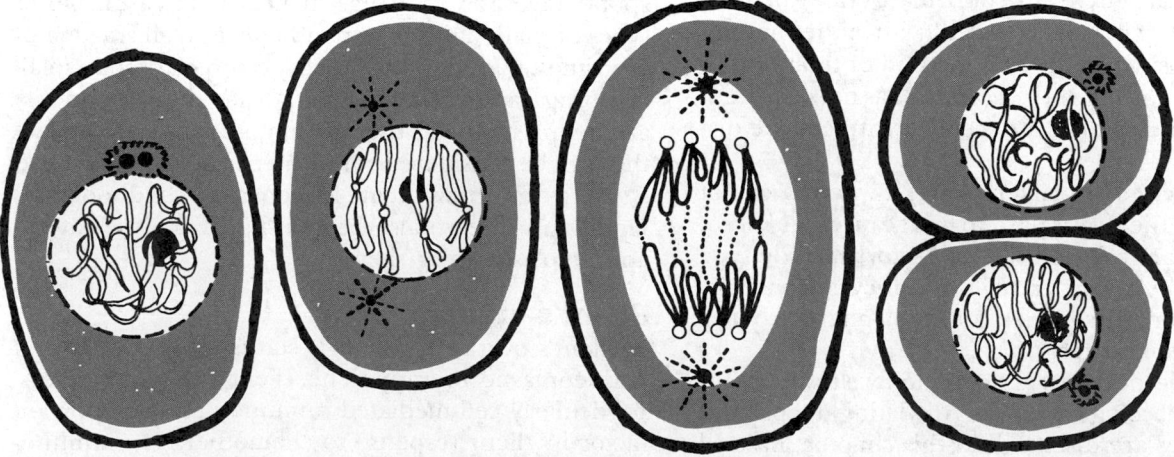

Figure 48-2. Simplified sequence of mitosis. The centrosome divides, the chromatin material of the nucleus changes into rod-shaped chromosomes, and two daughter cells form within the cell membrane.

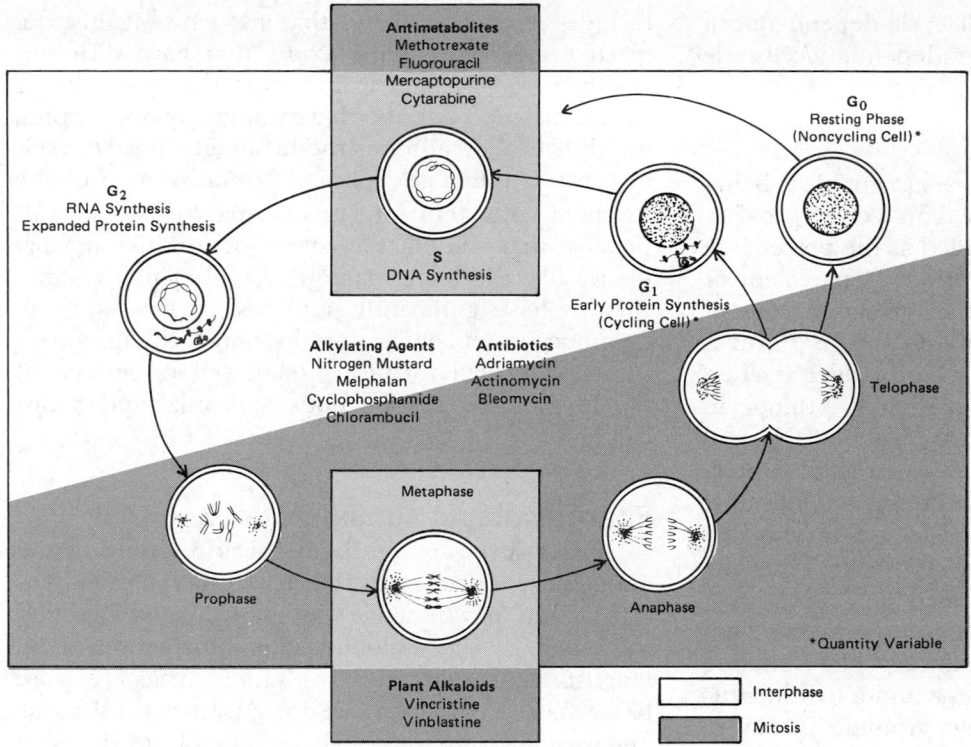

Figure 48-3. Drugs are identified in terms of where in the cell cycle they exert their distinctive tumor-killing effect. The antimetabolites are particularly effective during the period when a large proportion of tumor cells are in the S phase. Similarly, the plant alkaloids are most effective during phase M. Neither of these drug classes is as effective (on a relative dose basis) as the alkylating agents during the resting phase (G_0). No effort has been made in the diagram to indicate the relative time spent by the cell in each phase of the cycle. (Drawing by NL Gahan, from Lokich JJ. [1976]. Managing chemotherapy-induced bone marrow suppression in cancer. *Hosp Pract* 11, 63.)

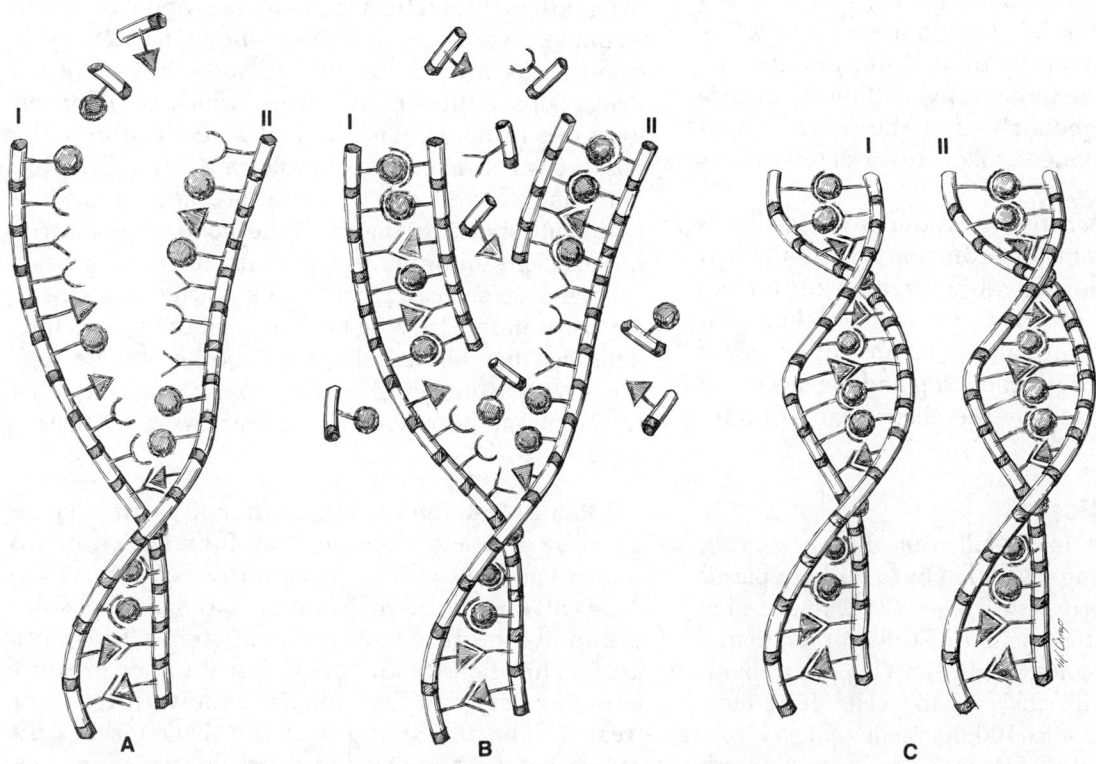

Figure 48-4. Schematic representation of the replication of DNA. (*A*) Before cell division, the bonds between the nitrogenous bases are broken, the two strands separate, and each strand takes with it the bases attached to its side. (*B*) The bases attached to each single strand attract free-floating nucleotide units and pair off, adenine with thymine, guanine with cytosine. (*C*) The end result is two exact replicas of the original DNA molecule, and the cell is ready to undergo division.

to classify the drugs is as cell cycle-dependent/cell cycle phase specific or cell cycle-independent/cell cycle phase nonspecific.

Growth fraction

Rapidly growing cancers are more susceptible to being killed by antineoplastic agents than slower growing cancers. Growth fraction is defined as the percentage of viable cells in active cell division (Department of Drugs, 1990). Tumors in which a large percentage of cells are actively making DNA and dividing over a short time span are said to have a high growth fraction and are more susceptible to drug action than tumors in which a small percentage of cells are making DNA and dividing. Unfortunately, certain normal cells like bone marrow, hair follicles, and cells of the gastrointestinal (GI) tract also have a high growth fraction; this fact explains why these tissues experience the most toxicity when antineoplastic drugs are used.

If tumors are small when therapy is begun, chemotherapy effectiveness is enhanced. The doubling time of a tumor—the time it takes a tumor to double its volume—increases as the tumor volume increases. Therefore, larger tumors have longer doubling times and slower growth fractions.

These principles have provided rationale for removing large tumors by surgery and following this action with adjuvant chemotherapy (*ie*, assuming any remaining tumor cells will be stimulated into active division with the bulk of the tumor gone and then be more susceptible to chemotherapy). Adjuvant chemotherapy is used immediately after the surgery. This therapy requires prolonged follow-up of clients to fully evaluate its success.

Another approach that is under investigation is the use of neoadjuvant (or induction) chemotherapy before surgery or radiotherapy. Potential advantages to this approach include the fact that chemotherapy is administered before any alteration in tumor vascularity caused by surgery or radiation and the fact that it may be better tolerated by the client than adjuvant chemotherapy is.

First-order kinetics

Antineoplastic drugs do not kill every tumor cell; they kill a certain percentage. Cell kill by an antineoplastic agent occurs in accord with first-order kinetics. That is, they kill a constant fraction of cells rather than a fixed number (this concept also applies in antibiotic use). If the drug kills 99% of the cells, it reduces 1,000,000 cells to 10 and 100,000 cells to 1.

Thus, cancer cells remain after antineoplastic agents have been used. Any remaining cancer cells may replicate and eventually kill the client. Combination chemotherapy is one way to deal with the residual cancer cells. In general, combinations of drugs are proving superior to single agents. Principles involved include selection of drugs that are active against the given tumor when used alone, that have different mechanisms of action to minimize the possibility of drug resistance, and that have minimally overlapping toxicities to allow administration of high doses to result in greater tumor cell kill and administration of the drugs at consistent intervals (*ie*, narrowest intervals possible that still allow recovery of sensitive normal tissues like the bone marrow). Combination chemotherapy has significantly improved survival in acute lymphocytic leukemia, certain non-Hodgkin's lymphomas, testicular cancer, small cell carcinoma of the lung, acute myelogenous leukemia, and breast carcinoma.

Pharmacologic considerations

Broad-spectrum vs. tissue-specific. Some of the antineoplastic drugs available have broad spectrums of activity and may be active with many hematologic and solid cancers (*eg*, cyclophosphamide, methotrexate, vincristine, and doxorubicin). Other drugs are more tissue-specific (*eg*, mitotane for adrenocortical tissue and streptozocin for the beta cells of the islets of Langerhans).

Drug distribution. The distribution of a drug within the body may influence the drug therapy. Some drugs are excluded from certain areas of the body. For example, because of the blood–brain barrier, brain tumor cells are inaccessible to most antineoplastic drugs. Most antineoplastic drugs, which are relatively insoluble in lipids, have limited access to the brain; passage is restricted to molecules that are fat soluble. Nitrosoureas and procarbazine are among the few antineoplastic drugs that cross the blood–brain barrier in sufficient amounts to be useful in treating brain tumors. In some cases, the CNS has acted as a sanctuary for tumor cells, a fact that contributed to relapse. This fact has helped shape chemotherapeutic regimens with acute lymphocytic leukemia to include intrathecal methotrexate as well as systemic methotrexate.

Route of administration. Although a drug may be given by a variety of routes, careful selection of the route of administration, taking into account the given drug and the specific malignancy, may make it possible to improve the drug's efficacy. For example, with intra-arterial infusion the drug is pumped under pressure into an artery that flows directly into the area to be treated. The full strength of the drug reaches the tumor before it enters the general circulation. Low blood flow to a large tumor can prevent adequate drug penetration of the tumor. In another example, for cancer cells in pleural or peritoneal cavities, intracavitary chemotherapy may provide high local concentrations and produce death of the cancer cells.

Dosage calculation. Doses of antineoplastic drugs are frequently not calculated on the basis of milligrams per kilogram. Instead, the client's body surface area is determined in square meters through the use of nomograms found in a reference book. Blood levels of drug correlate better with drug doses on the basis of body surface area, rather than on the basis of milligrams per kilogram.

Toxicity. One of the greatest problems with antineoplastic drugs is their nonselective toxicity to other normal tissue. The ideal antineoplastic drug would not be toxic to normal tissue, but no such drug exists. As pointed out above, bone marrow cells, with their high growth fraction, are very susceptible to antineoplastic drugs. The client must be monitored by laboratory data during and after antineoplastic drug therapy because the bone marrow suppression is asymptomatic until severe damage has occurred.

The time of maximum toxicity for a given adverse effect is referred to as the nadir. For example, the nadir for bone marrow suppression with a given drug may be 10 days; that is, about 10 days after antineoplastic drug therapy is started, the client's hemoglobin, hematocrit, leukocyte count, and platelet count will reach their lowest values.

Resistance

Cancer cells may develop resistance to a given antineoplastic agent or they may develop multiple drug resistance through several mechanisms. The cancer cell may become more capable of preventing a drug's activation, more able to deactivate the drug, more able to repair DNA damage, or less permeable to the drug's active form. When a tumor is large, greater heterogeneity within the tumor cell population increases the potential for drug resistance. Cancer cells may become cross-resistant to even structurally unrelated compounds with different mechanisms of action.

To avoid drug resistance, combination therapy is often used.

Alkylating agents

Two primary types of cytotoxic compounds are useful in treating cancer: the ones that interfere with the synthesis of DNA precursors and ones that interact with DNA itself. The alkylating agents interact with DNA itself. The major types of alkylating agents are the nitrogen mustards, the ethylenimines and methylmelamines, the alkyl sulfonates, the nitrosoureas, the triazenes, and the platinum complexes.

Pharmacodynamics. The alkylating agents are cell cycle-independent because they may act on cells at any phase of the cycle. Nevertheless, some do seem more cytocidal to cells in particular phases of the cell cycle (*eg*, nitrousoureas in G_1 or G_2).

The alkylating agents as a group affect a wide variety of cellular functions. They produce intermediates that readily form covalent bonds with negatively charged cellular substances. One reaction is alkylation of the 7-nitrogen of guanine in DNA, which can lead to miscoding and cross-linking between two DNA strands, preventing replication.

Alkylation of a single strand of DNA can often be repaired easily by the DNA repair system found in most cells. However, alkylating agents may attack DNA in double-stranded form, forming cross-links or chemical bonds between the strands. Because these strands must unwind and separate during replication, cross-linking blocks replication. Cross-linkages formed at low doses of these agents may also be corrected, but higher doses lead to the breakdown of DNA.

Most of the agents in this group are considered polyfunctional alkylating agents because they contain more than one alkylating group.

Nitrogen mustards

Nitrogen mustards were first synthesized in 1854 and were studied for use in chemical warfare during World Wars I and II. The nitrogen mustards include chlorambucil (Leukeran), cyclophosphamide (Cytoxan, Neosar), ifosfamide (Ifex), mechlorethamine (Mustargen), and melphalan (Alkeran; see Focus on Nitrogen Mustards: Similarities and Differences).

Chlorambucil

Pharmacodynamics. The pharmacodynamics of chlorambucil are discussed under the introductory section to alkylating agents.

Pharmacokinetics. Chlorambucil is well absorbed from the GI tract and often is administered on a daily basis. Its half life is 1.5 hours and it is excreted in the urine.

Therapeutic uses. Chlorambucil (Leukeran) is the slowest acting and least toxic nitrogen mustard. It is the medication of choice for the long-term management of chronic lymphocytic leukemia. It is also effective in Hodgkin's disease, non-Hodgkin's lymphomas, multiple myeloma, and primary (Waldenstrom's) macroglobulinemia. It has also been used in ovarian cancer, testicular cancer, and choriocarcinoma.

It has been used to treat vasculitis as a complication of rheumatoid arthritis and autoimmune hemolytic anemias.

Dosage and administration. Consult Table 48-1 for usual dosages.

Adverse reactions. The adverse reactions are listed in Table 48-1.

Alkylating agents have been positively implicated in the development of secondary tumors, including

Focus on

Nitrogen mustards: similarities and differences

Similarities

Pharmacodynamics

These agents act at any phase of the cell cycle and target nucleic acids and produce intermediates that readily form covalent bonds with negatively charged cellular substances. They interfere with DNA replication and RNA transcription by forming cross linkages.

Pharmacokinetics

These agents are well absorbed after oral administration. They are metabolized by the liver and excreted in the urine.

Therapeutic uses

These agents are used in the treatment of chronic lymphocytic leukemia, Hodgkin's disease, non-Hodgkin's lymphoma, multiple myeloma, ovarian and testicular carcinoma, and choriocarcinoma.

Adverse reactions

These include: (CNS) anxiety; (RESP) pulmonary fibrosis; (EENT) sore throat; (GI) nausea, vomiting, diarrhea, stomatitis; (GU) cystitis; (REPRO) gonadal suppression; (HEMA) bone marrow depression, leukopenia, thrombocytopenia, hyperuricemia; (SKIN) alopecia, redness, pain at injection site, rash; (OTHER) peripheral edema, fever, chills, flank and joint pain.

Contraindications

These agents are contraindicated in people with known hypersensitivity.

Precautions

These agents should be used with caution in people with myelosuppression or infection, renal impairment, hematologic compromise, or those with recent exposure to cytotoxic agents or radiation therapy.

Differences

• **Mechlorethamine** possesses some weak immunosuppressant activity.

• **Chlorambucil** has a half-life of 2 hours. • **Cyclophosphamide** is given orally or IV and is distributed throughout the body, with a half-life of 4 to 6 hours. • **Ifosfamide** is given by IV push or by intermittent infusion, with a half-life of 14 hours. • **Mechlorethamine**, because it is irritating to the tissue, is given IV or intracavitarily. • **Melphalan** is incompletely absorbed by the GI tract and has a biphasic half-life; 1st phase is 8 minutes, 2nd phase is 1/2 to 2 hours.

• **Melphalan** is used intraperitoneally for ovarian cancer and in the treatment of osteogenic sarcoma. • **Cyclophosphamide** is used to treat glomerular nephrotic syndrome in children, for immunosuppression after transplants, for treatment of rheumatoid disorders, sarcoma, breast, head, neck and lung cancers, and for neuroblastoma and retinoblastoma. • **Chlorambucil** is used to treat vasculitis as a complication of rheumatoid arthritis and autoimmune hemolytic anemia. • **Mechlorethamine** is used to treat breast and lung cancer, polycythemia vera, pleural or pericardial effusions secondary to tumor metastasis, and topically for the treatment of mycosis fungoides.

• **Chlorambucil** may cause seizures. • **Cyclophosphamide** may cause cardiotoxicity, thrombophlebitis, bladder fibrosis, hemorrhagic cystitis, hydronephrosis, and hyperpigmentation of the skin and nails. • **Cyclophosphamide** and **ifosfamide** may cause nephrotoxicity. • **Ifosfamide** may cause lethargy, confusion, dysuria, frequency, and elevated liver enzymes. • **Mechlorethamine** may cause tinnitus, metallic taste, oligomenorrhea, amenorrhea, azospermia, delayed spermatogenesis, and severe irritation if extravasation occurs.

• **Mechlorethamine** is contraindicated in people with chronic or suppurative inflammations.

• **Cyclophosphamide** should be used with caution in young men and women of childbearing age, pregnant and lactating females, people with infection, and those sensitive to tartrazine.

(continued)

Focus on

Nitrogen mustards: similarities and differences (Continued)

Similarities	Differences

Similarities

Nursing considerations

Instruct in disease, treatment, drug therapy regimen, adverse reactions, and compliance; assess cardiopulmonary status, including heart rate, rhythm, and breath sounds, for changes; monitor vital signs for changes; monitor nutritional status; encourage diet high in protein and calories; encourage adequate fluid intake; monitor intake and output; offer frequent mouth care; instruct client in mouth care and dietary needs; monitor lab studies, including complete blood cell count and platelets, frequently; avoid any IM injections if platelet count drops below 100,000/mm^3; assess for signs of occult bleeding, including checking stool and urine and watching for bruising, petechiae, and gingival bleeding; instruct client in signs of occult bleeding and need to report to physician; monitor renal and hepatic function studies for changes; avoid giving client any immunizations and instruct client to avoid contact with any people with infection; offer emotional support; explain that hair loss is temporary; offer suggestions to cope with hair loss, such as wigs, turbans, scarves; monitor uric acid levels; if increased, be aware that physician may order allopurinol; administer anticoagulants and aspirin products cautiously and monitor closely for signs of bleeding; instruct client to avoid use of over-the-counter products that contain aspirin; instruct client in signs and symptoms of infection and need to notify physician.

Differences

Administer **melphalan** on an empty stomach to enhance absorption. Instruct clients who are taking **cyclophosphamide** to practice contraception during and for 4 months after therapy. Encourage the client who is receiving **cyclophosphamide** to drink plenty of fluids and to void frequently to prevent hemorrhagic cystitis. Administer cyclophosphamide by IV push or infusion with normal saline or 5% dextrose and water. Avoid contact of **mechlorethamine** with skin, wear gloves when preparing; if extravasation occurs, apply cold compresses. When giving mechlorethamine intracavitarily, turn client side to side every 15 minutes to 1 hour to distribute the drug; administer by IV push or infusion within 20 minutes of reconstitution.

---

acute myeloid leukemias, myelodysplasia syndromes, and solid tumors. Survival from the time of diagnosis of secondary malignancies is usually brief.

Chlorambucil has been associated with the development of acute myelogenous leukemia. The risk appears to be increased with prolonged therapy and large cumulative doses, but the unsafe cumulative dose has not been adequately defined.

Drug interactions. No significant drug interactions have been identified with the use of chlorambucil.

Cyclophosphamide
Attempts to alter the chemical structure of mechlorethamine to increase its selectivity for neoplastic tissues led to the synthesis of cyclophosphamide (Cytoxan, Neosar).

Pharmacodynamics. The pharmacodynamics of cyclophosphamide are discussed under the introductory section to alkylating agents.

Pharmacokinetics. Cyclophosphamide is absorbed after oral administration or it may be given intravenously. It reaches a peak action in 1 hour, with a duration of action of 72 hours. Its half life ranges from 4 hours to 6 hours and it is excreted in urine and feces.

Therapeutic uses. Cyclophosphamide is probably the most commonly used antineoplastic drug. Cyclophosphamide itself does not have alkylating activity; it is a prodrug that is metabolically activated in the liver by the cytochrome P450 mixed-function oxidase system before it can alkylate cellular components. Its first metabolite is hydroxycyclophosphamide, and its cytotoxic metabolites are probably phosphoramide mustard and nor-nitrogen mustard.

Table 48-1. Alkylating agents

Drug name	Preparation	Usual dosage/PC	Adverse reactions
Nitrogen mustards			
chlorambucil (Chloraminophene, Leukeran)	Oral tablets	Adult: 1–3 mg/m² qd or 15–20 mg/m² and repeat every 2 weeks; Child: 0.1–0.2 mg/kg/day or 4.5 mg/m²/day PC: D	GI discomfort, rash, fever, urticaria, gonadal suppression, bone marrow suppression (BMS), occasional liver dysfunction, pulmonary fibrosis/toxicity with long-term use, hyperuricemia
cyclophosphamide (Cytoxan, Endoxan, Neosar, Procytox)	Oral tablets IV	Adult: oral 60–120 mg/m²; IV, 500–1.5 g/m² at 2–4 wk intervals; Child: oral or IV, 2–8 mg/kg/day or 60–250 mg/m² PC: D	Anorexia, nausea and vomiting, alopecia, hyperpigmentation of skin and nails, cardiotoxicity, hemorrhagic colitis, stomatitis, hepatic dysfunction, gonadal suppression, pulmonary fibrosis, hypersensitivity, hemorrhagic and non-hemorrhagic cystitis, nephrotoxicity, renal and bladder tumors, water retention, leukopenia
hexamethylmelamine (Altretamine, Hexistat, HMM)	Oral tablets	12 mg/kg qd for 21 days with 4-week rest periods between regimens PC: D	Nausea, BMS, skin rashes and pruritus, alopecia, and neurotoxicity
ifosfamide (Ifex)	IV Oral	Adult: 1.2 g/m² qd for 5 days or 1.5–1.8 g/m² every day for 5 days, repeat every 3 or 4 weeks PC: D	Cerebellar dysfunction, seizures, altered mental status (*eg*, somnolence, confusion, hallucinations, occasional coma), nausea and vomiting, hemorrhagic cystitis, alopecia, BMS, cranial nerve dysfunction, reversible hepatic dysfunction
mechlorethamine (Caryolysin, Cloramin, Erasol, Mustargen)	IV Intra-cavitary Topical	Adult: IV, 6 mg/m² on days 1 and 8 as part of MOPP, repeat q28d or 10–15 mg/m² at 4–6 week intervals PC: D	Anorexia, nausea and vomiting, BMS, menstrual irregularities, lacrimation, diarrhea, diaphoresis, vesication, thrombophlebitis, necrosis at injection site, hyperuricemia
melphalan or L-sarcolysin (Alkeran)	Oral tablets IV (investigational)	Adult: oral, 6–8 mg/m² for 4 days every 6 weeks PC: D	BMS, nausea and vomiting, rash, alopecia, delayed pulmonary fibrosis and infiltrates
Ethylenimines and methylmelamines			
triethylenethiophosphoramide (thiotepa)	IV, sub-cutaneous, IM Oral Intravesical, intra-cavitary, intrathecal Intra-arterial	Adult: IV, 6 mg/m² qd for 5 days every 4 wks; intravesical, 60 mg in 30–60 ml distilled water, instilled and retained for 2 h; intrathecal, 1–10 mg/m² PC: D	BMS, pain at injection site, nausea and vomiting, dizziness, headache, amenorrhea, interference with spermatogenesis
Alkyl sulfonates			
busulfan (Busulphan, Mielucin, Myleran, Sulfabutin, Mustargen)	Oral tablets	Adult: 2–6 mg/m² qd until white blood cell count is 10,000/μl, then dose adjusted to maintain white blood cell count between 10,000 and 20,000/μl Child: 0.06–0.12 mg/kg/day or 1.8–4.6 mg/m²/day PC: D	BMS, nausea and vomiting, diarrhea, hyperuricemia and associated nephropathy, ovarian suppression, testicular atrophy, gynecomastia, cataracts, pulmonary fibrosis, addisonian-like state (characterized by hyperpigmentation, weakness, hypotension, nausea and vomiting, weight loss but without abnormalities in adrenal function), transient increase in liver enzymes

(Continued)

Table 48-1. Alkylating agents (Continued)

Drug name	Preparation	Usual dosage/PC	Adverse reactions
Nitrosoureas			
carmustine/BCNU (BiCNU)	IV Topical Intra-arterial	Adults: IV, 200 mg/m^2 over 1–2 h period every 6 wk or 100 mg/m^2 on 2 successive days every 6 weeks; topically, 0.5–3 mg/ml in an aqueous solution with 30% alcohol Child: IV, 200 mg/m^2 every 6 weeks or 75–100 mg/m^2 every day for 2 days every 6 weeks PC: D	Nausea and vomiting, flushing of skin and suffusion of conjunctiva, esophagitis, diarrhea, hepatotoxicity, delayed BMS, burning pain after IV injection
lomustine/CCNU (CeeNu)	Oral	Adult: 130 mg/m^2 every 6 weeks PC: D	Nausea and vomiting, stomatitis, pulmonary fibrosis, disorientation, lethargy, ataxia, dysarthria, delayed onset of nephrotoxicity including renal failure, alopecia, BMS, stomatitis, transient increase in liver function tests
streptozocin (Zanosar)	IV	Adult: 1–1.5 g/m^2 weekly for 4–6 weeks PC: C	Nausea and vomiting, nephrotoxicity, abnormalities of glucose tolerance, abnormal liver function tests, burning sensation after IV injection
Triazenes			
dacarbazine (DTIC-Dome)	IV	Adult: IV, 250 mg/m^2/day for 5 days every 3 to 4 weeks; as part of ABVD combination 375 mg/m^2/day on days 1 and 15, repeat every 4 weeks PC: C	Anorexia, nausea and vomiting, BMS, alopecia, rashes, facial flushing, facial paresthesia, anaphylaxis, influenza-like syndrome (fever, myalgia, malaise), abnormal liver function tests, pain at infusion site and necrosis if extravasation
Platinum complexes			
carboplatin (Paraplatin)	IV	Adult: IV, 360 mg/m^2 over 15 min every 4 weeks PC: D	Nausea and vomiting, BMS, alopecia, abnormal liver function tests, hypersensitivity, stomatitis, mucositis, influenza-like syndrome
cisplatin (Neoplatin, Platinex, Platinol)	IV	Adult: IV, 60–120 mg/m^2 once every 3 to 4 weeks; with vinblastine or etoposide and bleomycin, 20 mg/m^2 every day for 5 days every 3 weeks for 4 courses	Nausea and vomiting, BMS, anaphylaxis, nephrotoxicity, ototoxicity, peripheral neuropathies, loss of taste, electrolyte disturbances

KEY: PC = pregnancy category. (The validity of pregnancy risk categories has not been established; see Chapter 16, p 216.)

Cyclophosphamide is used in Burkitt's lymphoma, non-Hodgkin's lymphomas, multiple myeloma, breast cancer and small cell lung carcinomas, soft tissue sarcomas, and pediatric solid tumors, such as embryonal rhabdomyosarcoma, Ewing's sarcoma, and neuroblastoma.

Most conditioning ("purging" of bone marrow) regimens for bone marrow transplantation use cyclophosphamide because of its potent immunosuppressive properties. It is also used in rheumatoid arthritis, nephrotic syndrome in children, and in Wegener's granulomatosis because of these properties.

Dosage and administration. Consult Table 48-1 for usual dosages.

Adverse reactions. The major adverse reactions appear in Table 48-1. An unusual side effect is hemorrhagic cystitis, caused by the metabolite acrolein that irritates bladder walls. The cystitis is particularly common in high-dose chemotherapy or with prolonged periods of oral therapy and may produce significant blood loss and inappropriate water retention. Systemic intravenous (IV) administration of a new drug, 2-mercaptoethane sodium sulfonate (MESNA), is proving the most helpful with the problem of hemorrhagic cystitis.

Cyclophosphamide also causes bladder fibrosis, hydronephrosis, hemorrhage and clot formation in the renal pelvis, vesicoureteral reflux, and secondary urothelial malignancies. Transitional cell carcinoma of the bladder occurs, generally in clients who previously developed the hemorrhagic cystitis, and may not be detected for several years after treatment.

FD and C Yellow No. 5 dyes in cyclophosphamide preparations may cause allergic-type reactions, including asthma, most frequently seen in people sensitive to aspirin.

More than 50% of clients who receive intensive or prolonged therapy with cyclophosphamide experience alopecia, which is usually reversible.

Cyclophosphamide causes dose-dependent hepatic injury, probably because of impaired metabolism of acrolein. This presents as raised serum aminotransferase levels and may be precipitated by prior exposure to azathioprine (Dukes & Beeley, 1990).

Drug interactions. Increased bone marrow depression may occur if cyclophosphamide is given to the client who is receiving other bone marrow depressants or radiation. A decrease in drug dosage may be indicated.

Hyperuricemia and gout may occur if cyclophosphamide is given with probenecid or sulfinpyrazone. The physician may adjust the antigout medication. Allopurinol may increase the bone marrow toxicity of cyclophosphamide.

Increased risk of infection and further development of neoplasms exists when cyclophosphamide is given with immunosuppressant agents, including adrenocorticosteroids, azathioprine, chlorambucil, cyclosporine, and mercaptopurine.

Live viral vaccines should be avoided if possible when cyclophosphamide is used, to avoid a decrease in antibody response along with an increase in adverse reactions.

Additive cardiotoxicity may be caused by concurrent use of doxorubicin. Concurrent use of cyclophosphamide with insulin increases hypoglycemia, with anticoagulants increases the anticoagulant effect, and with thiazide diuretics increases leukopenia.

Since cyclophosphamide is activated in the liver, its metabolism can be affected by drugs that induce (*eg*, phenobarbital) or inhibit (*eg*, allopurinol) enzymes of the mixed-function oxidase system. Although the half-life of cyclophosphamide is altered by such drugs, its antitumor activity does not change.

Ifosfamide

Ifosfamide (Ifex) is a synthetic analogue of cyclophosphamide.

Pharmacodynamics. The pharmacodynamics of ifosfamide are discussed in the introductory section to alkylating agents. Like cyclophosphamide, it is activated in the liver by the cytochrome P450 mixed-function oxidase system. It is activated at a slower rate than cyclophosphamide so larger doses are used.

Pharmacokinetics. Ifosfamide is absorbed from the GI tract or it may be given intravenously. Its half life ranges from 7 hours to 15 hours and it is excreted in urine and feces.

Therapeutic uses. Like cyclophosphamide, ifosfamide has a broad spectrum of activity. It has been used with lung, breast, testicular, gastric, bladder, pancreatic, head and neck, cervical, and ovarian tumors, certain sarcomas, Hodgkin's disease, and non-Hodgkin's lymphomas.

Dosage and administration. Consult Table 48-1 for usual dosages.

Adverse reactions. The adverse reactions are listed in Table 48-1. As with cyclophosphamide, clients must be well hydrated before the use of ifosfamide. In addition, concurrent systemic IV administration of MESNA is proving the most helpful with the problem of hemorrhagic cystitis.

Some differences in toxicity between cyclophosphamide and ifosfamide may relate to differences in their metabolism. For example, CNS toxicity is unique to ifosfamide. Severe encephalopathy has been seen in children treated with ifosfamide alone. Electroencephalogram abnormalities and seizures were reversible despite prolonged coma.

Ifosfamide should be used cautiously in clients with decreased renal function or known compromised bone marrow reserve. Bone marrow suppression is common, especially if ifosfamide is given with other antineoplastic agents. The main concern is leukopenia and, to a lesser extent, thrombocytopenia.

Drug interactions. No significant drug interactions have been identified with the use of ifosfamide.

Mechlorethamine

Pharmacodynamics. The pharmacodynamics of mechlorethamine are discussed in the introductory section to alkylating agents.

Pharmacokinetics. Mechlorethamine is given intravenously and its onset of action is within minutes. It is excreted in the urine.

Therapeutic uses. Mechlorethamine (Mustargen) was the first alkylating agent used clinically. It has been significant in treating Hodgkin's disease and other lymphomas. When Hodgkin's disease is localized, radiation may be the treatment of choice, because fewer complications occur with radiation than with chemotherapy and because these neoplasms are highly radiosensitive. However, when Hodgkin's disease is more generalized, chemotherapy is preferable to radiation. The treatment of choice for stages III and IV of Hodgkin's disease is mechlorethamine with other agents in the MOPP regimen, which is the regimen of mechlorethamine, Oncovin (vincristine), procarbazine, and prednisone (Table 48-2).

Mechlorethamine is also used in chronic myelocytic and lymphocytic leukemias, polycythemia vera, and

Table 48-2. MOPP regimen for Hodgkin's disease

Agent	Dosage	Route
Mechlorethamine	6 mg/m², days 1 & 8	IV
Vincristine	1.4 mg/m², days 1 & 8	IV
Procarbazine	100 mg/m², days 1–14	Oral
Prednisone	40 mg/m², days 1–14	Oral

cutaneous lymphomas (mycosis fungoides and Sezary syndrome). It has been used for ablating the pleural space in clients with pleural or pericardial effusion caused by tumor metastasis.

Dosage and administration. Mechlorethamine should be injected into the IV tubing of a rapidly flowing 5% dextrose solution to prevent thrombophlebitis and thrombosis, because it is a powerful vesicant. When extravasation into the subcutaneous tissues occurs, a severe tender induration persists for some time at the parenteral site. Tissue sloughing may occur.

Adverse reactions. The adverse reactions are listed in Table 48-1. A course of mechlorethamine may be repeated in about 6 weeks. This interval is primarily due to the suppression of bone marrow function by mechlorethamine, including lymphocytopenia, granulocytopenia, and decrease in platelets and erythrocytes. Bone marrow function is usually completely restored by 4 to 6 weeks. When the bone marrow function has recovered, more mechlorethamine may be given.

Alkylating agents have been positively implicated in the causation of secondary tumors. Survival from the time of diagnosis of secondary malignancies is usually brief.

Drug interactions. The drug interactions described under cyclophosphamide in relation to bone marrow depressants, radiation, probenecid, sulfinpyrazone, and live viral vaccines may all occur if these agents are used concurrently with mechlorethamine. In addition, the concurrent use of mechlorethamine and amphotericin B increases the possibility of the client developing blood dyscrasia.

Melphalan

Melphalan, a phenylalanine derivative of nitrogen mustard, is a bifunctional alkylating agent that causes interstrand, intrastrand, and DNA-protein cross-links.

Pharmacodynamics. The pharmacodynamics of melphalan are discussed under the introductory section to alkylating agents.

Pharmacokinetics. Melphalan is absorbed from the GI tract. It has a duration of action of 6 hours. Its half life is 1 hour to 2 hours. Twenty percent to fifty percent is excreted in the feces and the rest is excreted in the urine.

Therapeutic uses. Melphalan (Alkeran) was conceived as a compound that would localize in tumors that actively used phenylalanine (such as melanin-producing malignancies). It has been used for arterial infusion of extremities affected by malignant melanoma and for multiple myeloma, ovarian cancer, breast cancer, and lymphomas.

Because melphalan does not irritate peritoneal surfaces and does not require hepatic activation, it has been used for treatment of intraperitoneal malignancies, like ovarian cancer, by direct intraperitoneal instillation. It is also used in conditioning regimens for bone marrow transplantation.

Dosage and administration. Consult Table 48-1 for usual dosage.

Adverse reactions. Melphalan should be used cautiously in clients with decreased renal function. It appears more carcinogenic than cyclophosphamide. Secondary acute myelogenous leukemia has been observed in clients with multiple myeloma or ovarian cancer after treatment with melphalan.

Drug interactions No significant drug interactions have been identified with the use of melphalan.

Ethylenimines and methylmelamines

This group of alkylating agents includes triethylenethiophosphoramide and the investigational agent hexamethylmelamine.

Triethylenethiophosphoramide

Therapeutic uses. Triethylenethiophosphoramide (thiotepa) has been used in the palliative management of cancer of the breast and ovary, but other agents are usually preferred.

Intracavitary instillation may control pleural or peritoneal effusions. Intravesical instillation is sometimes useful in superficial papillary carcinomas of the bladder. It is absorbed through the bladder wall.

It has been used in carcinomatous meningitis. It is lipophilic and therefore does cross the blood–brain barrier.

Adverse reactions. Thiotepa must be used cautiously at reduced doses with clients with renal failure.

Hexamethylmelamine

It is not clear that hexamethylmelamine (HMM) functions as an alkylating agent, but it is classified here because of its structural relationship to other alkylating agents. It is considered a restricted drug, and information about it may be obtained from the Investigational Drug Branch, National Cancer Institute.

Therapeutic uses. HMM appears useful in refractory ovarian carcinoma. It also has been used in various lymphomas.

Adverse reactions Adverse reactions include nausea, bone marrow suppression, skin rashes and pruritus, alopecia, and neurotoxicity.

Alkyl sulfonates

Busulfan

Pharmacodynamics. The pharmacodynamics of busulfan are discussed under the introductory section to alkylating agents.

Pharmacokinetics. Busulfan is absorbed after oral administration. It has a half life of 2.5 hours and is excreted in the urine.

Therapeutic uses. Busulfan (Myleran) is frequently used in the palliative treatment of chronic myelogenous leukemia. It also may be useful in polycythemia vera and myelofibrosis with myeloid metaplasia.

Dosage and administration. Consult Table 48-1 for usual dosage.

Adverse reactions. The myelosuppression with busulfan can be prolonged and severe. Busulfan should be used cautiously in clients with compromised bone marrow reserve.

A rare but potentially fatal complication is the busulfan lung syndrome (also referred to as interstitial pneumonitis). It is characterized by persistent cough and progressive dyspnea caused by intra-alveolar exudation of fibrin. Pulmonary fibrosis results, and death may occur 1 to 10 years after treatment with busulfan. Large doses of corticosteroids may be beneficial.

Hyperuricemia also occurs, reflecting the rapid cellular destruction and release of purines that are oxidized by xanthine oxidase. Hyperuricemia and hyperuricosuria can lead to secondary gout from urate deposition and the formation of renal calculi from urate precipitation, which then can lead to renal damage.

Drug interactions. Concurrent use of busulfan and thioguanine may cause esophageal varices and abnormal liver function tests.

Nitrosoureas

The nitrosoureas include carmustine/BCNU, lomustine/CCNU, and streptozocin. These agents cross the blood–brain barrier, unlike most other alkylating agents. Many nitrosoureas have been tried, in attempts to improve therapeutic index and decrease bone marrow toxicity (see Focus on Nitrosoureas: Similarities and Differences).

Carmustine

Carmustine/BCNU (BiCNu) was the first nitrosourea used.

Pharmacodynamics. Carmustine undergoes spontaneous chemical degradation to a carbonium ion intermediate that alkylates DNA (DNA cross-linking occurs) and an isocyanate intermediate that carbamoylates proteins, such as DNA repair enzymes. RNA synthesis is also inhibited. Carmustine is considered cell cycle phase nonspecific but shows a selectivity for cells in G_1 or G_2.

Pharmacokinetics. Carmustine is often given intravenously (intra-arterial and topical routes are also used). Its half life is 5 minutes to 15 minutes and it is excreted in the urine.

Therapeutic uses. Carmustine is useful with Hodgkin's disease, non-Hodgkin's lymphomas, malignant melanoma, multiple myeloma (with prednisone), and GI tumors. It is highly lipid-soluble and crosses the blood–brain barrier and has been used to treat various brain tumors.

Intra-arterial carmustine has been used with glioblastoma, although ocular complications can occur. Supraophthalmic injection can lead to brain necrosis.

A topical solution has been used to treat cutaneous T cell lymphomas. It is also used experimentally in conditioning regimens for bone marrow transplantation.

Dosage and administration. Consult Table 48-1 for usual dosage.

Adverse reactions. The adverse reactions are listed in Table 48-1. Delayed onset bone marrow suppression is a dose-limiting toxicity. Platelet nadirs occur 4 to 5 weeks and leukocyte nadirs occur 5 to 6 weeks after treatment is started. Thrombocytopenia (low platelet count) is usually more severe, but both are considered dose limiting. Complete blood cell counts should be carried out for at least 6 weeks after each dose.

The bone marrow suppression is cumulative in nature. After initial use of carmustine, the subsequent dosage is determined by hematologic response to the preceding dose. The course should not be repeated until the platelet count is more than 100,000 and the leukocyte count is more than 4,000.

Persistent testicular damage and infertility may occur. Transient hyperpigmentation may occur with accidental skin contact with carmustine.

Drug interactions. Concurrent use of carmustine and cimetidine has caused additive bone marrow suppression.

Concomitant use with digoxin has led to decreased serum levels of digoxin and, thus, decreased digoxin effect. Likewise, use of carmustine and phenytoin has yielded decreased serum levels of phenytoin and decreased phenytoin effect.

Lomustine

Lomustine/CCNU (CeeNu) has a mechanism of action like that of carmustine. Unlike carmustine, it has good oral bioavailability.

Pharmacodynamics. Lomustine/CCNU (CeeNu) has a mechanism of action like that of carmustine.

Pharmacokinetics. Unlike carmustine, lomustine has good oral bioavailability, so it is administered orally. Its half life ranges from 16 hours to 48 hours and it is excreted in the urine.

Therapeutic uses. Lomustine has been used to treat primary and metastatic brain tumors and in combination regimens to treat small cell lung cancer. It has also been used in melanoma, Hodgkin's and non–Hodgkin's lymphomas, breast cancer, non–small lung cancer, and colorectal carcinomas.

Dosage and administration. Consult Table 48-1 for usual dosage.

Adverse reactions. The adverse reactions include bone marrow suppression, which is delayed, dose related, dose limiting, and accumulative. Thrombocytopenia develops about 4 weeks and leukopenia about 6 weeks after a dose. Hepatotoxicity is seen with lomustine.

Focus on

Nitrosoureas: similarities and differences

Similarities	**Differences**
Pharmacodynamics	
These agents cross-link strands of DNA, inhibiting DNA and RNA synthesis.	
Pharmacokinetics	
These agents have varying absorption after oral administration. They are widely distributed and cross the blood–brain barrier. Their metabolites are found in breast milk. They are rapidly metabolized and excreted in the urine as metabolites.	• **Carmustine** and **streptozocin** are given IV. • **Streptozocin** is not active orally and its distribution is unknown. • **Lomustine** is rapidly absorbed from the GI tract and does not appear to cross the blood–brain barrier; it has a biphasic half-life, with an initial half-life of 6 hours and a second half-life of 1 to 2 days. • **Carmustine** is also excreted in the feces and as respiratory carbon dioxide. • **Streptozocin** has a biphasic half-life, with an initial half-life of 5 minutes and a second half-life of 35 to 40 minutes.
Therapeutic uses	
These agents are used for the treatment of brain tumors, Hodgkin's disease, malignant lymphomas, and myeloma.	• **Lomustine** is used for the treatment of small cell lung cancer. • **Streptozocin** is used to treat islet cell cancer of the pancreas, carcinoid syndrome, pancreatic adenocarcinoma, and for palliative treatment of metastatic colorectal cancer.
Adverse reactions	
These include: (GI) nausea, vomiting, stomatitis, hepatotoxicity; (GU) nephrotoxicity; (HEMA) bone marrow depression, leukopenia, thrombocytopenia; (SKIN) hyperpigmentation, alopecia; (OTHER) pain at infusion site.	• **Carmustine** can cause flushing, esophagitis, and pulmonary fibrosis. • **Lomustine** can cause lethargy, ataxia, and arrhythmia. • **Streptozocin** can cause elevated liver enzymes and hypoglycemia or hyperglycemia.
Contraindications	
These agents are contraindicated in people with a known hypersensitivity.	• **Streptozocin** is contraindicated when other nephrotoxic agents are used.
Precautions	
These agents should be used with caution in people who are receiving myelosuppressants, those with infection, renal or hepatic dysfunction, or those who have recently been exposed to cytotoxic agents or radiation therapy.	• **Streptozocin** should be used cautiously in people with renal impairment.

(continued)

Focus on

Nitrosoureas: similarities and differences (Continued)

Similarities

Nursing considerations

Instruct in disease, treatment, drug therapy regimen, adverse reactions, and compliance; monitor vital signs for changes; monitor nutritional status; encourage diet high in protein and calories; encourage adequate fluid intake; monitor intake and output; offer frequent mouth care; instruct client in mouth care and dietary needs; monitor lab studies, including complete blood cell count and platelets, frequently; avoid any IM injections if platelet count drops below 100,000/mm³; assess for signs of occult bleeding, including checking stool and urine and watching for bruising, petechiae, and gingival bleeding; instruct client in signs of occult bleeding and need to report to physician; administer antiemetic before giving drug; avoid giving client any immunizations and instruct client to avoid contact with any people with infection; offer emotional support; explain that hair loss is temporary; offer suggestions to cope with hair loss, such as wigs, turbans, scarves; administer anticoagulants and aspirin products cautiously and monitor closely for signs of bleeding; instruct client to avoid use of over-the-counter products that contain aspirin; instruct client in signs and symptoms of infection and need to notify physician.

Differences

Administer **streptozocin** by IV push or infusion; wear gloves when preparing drug; wash skin immediately if skin comes in contact with drug; keep 50% dextrose available in case of possible hypoglycemia. Administer **lomustine** 2 to 4 hours after meals. Wear gloves when preparing **carmustine** and use only glass containers to administer it; do not mix **carmustine** with other drugs; if extravasation occurs, stop the infusion and infiltrate the area with liberal injection of 0.5 mEq/ml sodium bicarbonate solution; administer as a dilute solution slowly to avoid pain on infusion.

Drug interactions. No significant drug interactions have been identified with the use of lomustine.

Streptozocin

Streptozocin (Zanosar) is a naturally occurring antibiotic, originally derived from *Streptomyces achromogenes*. It is a nitrosourea, but its structure does differ from the others, so its properties differ.

Pharmacodynamics. Streptozocin has alkylating activity, but it cannot cross-link DNA. It does inhibit precursor incorporation into DNA. It is cell cycle phase nonspecific, but cells in the S phase seem the most sensitive.

Pharmacokinetics. Given intravenously, streptozocin has a duration of action of 24 hours. Its half life is 35 minutes and it is excreted via the urine and feces and also through the lung.

Therapeutic uses. Streptozocin's major use has been pancreatic islet cell carcinomas (including insulin-secreting and non–insulin-secreting beta cell and nonbeta cell tumors). It has also been shown to be effective in malignant carcinoid tumors and in some regimens for Hodgkin's disease.

Dosage and administration. Consult Table 48-1 for usual dosage.

Adverse reactions. Renal dysfunction is the major toxicity, involving both renal tubules and glomeruli. Signs include glycosuria, aminoaciduria, acetonuria, proteinuria, and hypophosphatemia. Dosages should be decreased 50% to 75% if renal failure is present in the client. Nephrotoxicity can occur with a single dose, but it is more common with repeated doses and develops in most clients who receive prolonged treatment. Mild renal function abnormalities may be reversible when the drug is discontinued, but irreversible damage occurs if treatment is continued.

Drug interactions. Concurrent use of streptozocin and nephrotoxic drugs is contraindicated because the combination increases streptozocin's nephrotoxicity.

Use of streptozocin with phenytoin should be avoided in clients with pancreatic tumors because the combination decreases streptozocin's cytotoxic effect.

Concurrent use with doxorubicin prolongs the half-life of doxorubicin, and its dose should be reduced.

Triazenes

Dacarbazine

Dacarbazine (DTIC-Dome) is an imidazole carboxamide derivative and is a structural analogue of a purine.

Pharmacodynamics. Dacarbazine was originally considered to be an antimetabolite, but its alkylating activity now appears to be its most important action. The drug inhibits RNA and protein synthesis more significantly than DNA synthesis.

Pharmacokinetics. Given intravenously, dacarbazine has a half life of 5 hours and is excreted in the urine.

Therapeutic uses. Dacarbazine is used in the treatment of malignant melanoma, soft tissue sarcomas, and in combination with other agents (it is a component of the ABVD regimen—Adriamycin [doxorubicin], bleomycin, vinblastine, and dacarbazine—which is an alternate to the MOPP regimen) for Hodgkin's disease, neuroblastoma, and islet cell cancer.

Dosage and administration. Consult Table 48-1 for usual dosages.

Adverse reactions. Nausea and vomiting occur in 90% of clients. They usually occur 1 to 3 hours after administration of the drug. Many clients develop tolerance to the nausea and vomiting, and the symptoms may abate after 2 to 3 doses of the drug.

Single-dose dacarbazine has been reported to be hepatotoxic, presenting as acute liver necrosis with hepatic venous thrombosis, which is often fatal.

Drug interactions. No significant drug interactions have been identified with the use of dacarbazine.

Platinum complexes

Cisplatin

Cisplatin (Platinol) is a heavy metal compound that contains a central atom of platinum surrounded by two chloride atoms and two ammonia molecules.

Pharmacodynamics. Cisplatin's cytotoxic properties are similar to those of bifunctional alkylating agents; it produces interstrand and intrastrand cross-links in DNA and is probably cell cycle nonspecific (although some cells seem more sensitive during G_1). The consequences of its action on DNA include changes in DNA conformation and inhibition of DNA synthesis.

Pharmacokinetics. Cisplatin is administered intravenously. It has a biphasic half life (25 minutes to 49 minutes and 58 hours to 73 hours). It is excreted in the urine.

Therapeutic uses. Cisplatin is one of the most active antineoplastic drugs against testicular tumors. It is effective against disseminated seminomatous and nonseminomatous testicular cancer in combination with vinblastine and bleomycin (PVB regimen).

It is used in metastatic ovarian carcinoma in a combination that includes cisplatin, doxorubicin, and cyclophosphamide. It also been used against bladder and cervical carcinoma, head and neck cancer, osteogenic sarcoma, non–small cell lung, esophageal, and gastric carcinomas, glioblastoma, and medulloblastoma (see Example of Nursing Process and Cisplatin and Cyclophosphamide Therapy To Treat Cancer of the Ovary).

Direct intrapericardial instillation of cisplatin daily for 5 days for malignant pericardial effusion is well tolerated with only mild nausea. Constrictive pericarditis is not produced.

Cisplatin given by regional limb perfusion has been advocated for melanoma and soft tissue sarcoma of the extremities.

Dosage and administration. Because of its nephrotoxic potential, protocols of hydration and diuresis are used. Adequate hydration decreases drug exposure in the renal tubules. One approach is to precede cisplatin administration with a 4- to 6-hour period of prehydration in conjunction with the use of mannitol. Administering mannitol prevents the immediate platinum binding onto renal tubular proteins. Furosemide is also used in different protocols. Mannitol and furosemide do not appear to alter cisplatin's pharmacokinetics. Another approach is to administer 250 ml of normal saline per hour for 12 hours before and 12 hours after cisplatin.

Cisplatin has been administered by intraperitoneal instillation in clients with intraperitoneal malignancies such as ovarian cancer. Systemic toxicity can be prevented by simultaneous administration of sodium thiosulfate. Consult Table 48-1 for further dosage information.

Adverse reactions. The adverse reactions are listed in Table 48-1. The nephrotoxicity is due to a direct toxic effect on renal tubules. Electrolyte abnormalities occur and include hypomagnesemia and hypocalcemia.

Any use of the drug with known renal dysfunction should be guided by the creatinine clearance ability of the kidney. Some suggest renal function must return to normal before any subsequent doses of cisplatin are given (as measured by a serum creatinine level below 1.5 mg/dl or the BUN level below 25 mg/dl). Impairment of renal function may be manifest for at least 6 months after treatment has been completed.

Cisplatin is associated with a sensory peripheral

Example of nursing process and cisplatin and cyclophosphamide therapy to treat cancer of the ovary

The client, Mary Strom, is a 63-year-old nulliparous woman who has been diagnosed as having cancer of the ovary with extension of the tumor to the uterus (stage IIa). She has had an abdominal hysterectomy and bilateral salpingo-oophorectomy, at which time the liver was biopsied and no metastasis was identified.

Mary will undergo a course of chemotherapy, which will include the use of cisplatin and cyclophosphamide.

Assessment data	Nursing diagnosis	Intervention	Goals and outcome criteria
Receiving cyclophosphamide	Potential complication: hemorrhagic cystitis*	**Encourage** minimum daily fluid intake of 2500 ml. **Encourage** client to void every 2 hours and before going to bed to prevent stasis of drug in bladder. **Tell** client to report any dysuria or hematuria to physician.	The client will not develop hemorrhagic cystitis as evidenced by absence of dysuria, urinary frequency or urgency, and hematuria.
Receiving cisplatin	Potential complication: nephrotoxicity*	**Prehydrate** client with 200 ml/h for 6 to 24 hours before administration of cisplatin. **Maintain** IV fluids as ordered during administration of cisplatin and for 24 hours after therapy. **Monitor** for therapeutic and adverse effects of mannitol or furosemide when administered. **Monitor** and report signs of renal dysfunction.	The client will maintain adequate renal function as evidenced by blood urea nitrogen below 25 mg/dl and serum creatinine level below 1.5 mg/dl and urine output at least 30 ml/h.
63-year-old woman receiving cyclophosphamide	Self-esteem disturbance related to changes in appearance (eg, alopecia, nail changes) secondary to cyclophosphamide therapy	**Inform** client that hair loss can be expected about 2 weeks after chemotherapy begins and that it may be partial or complete. **Reassure** client that hair loss is usually temporary and regrowth usually occurs 2 to 3 months after treatment is completed. **Explain** that regrowth may be a different color and texture. **Encourage** client to use a wig if desired and to use it before hair loss to facilitate integration of wig into body image. **Inform** client that her nails may undergo noticeable changes during treatment (eg, thicken, develop ridges, darken).	The client will demonstrate beginning adaptation to change in appearance by accepting the use of a wig or hair piece and my making as many positive as negative statements relating to self-image.

*Although potential complications generally are not included in the Examples of Nursing Process, in this situation the identification of this collaborative problem is critical to the outcome for this client and illustrates the broad range of nursing responsibilities.

neuropathy. It may be age-related, as it has not been recognized in children treated with cisplatin for neuroblastoma. It may be more apt to occur with prolonged treatment or high-dose therapy and may be reversible.

Cisplatin causes IgE-mediated hypersensitivity reactions, including flushing, pruritus, erythema, urticaria, dyspnea, bronchospasm, diaphoresis, vomiting, and hypotension. Pretreatment use of antihistamines and corticosteroids may be warranted.

Ototoxicity, including tinnitus or high-frequency hearing loss, is common in very young and very old clients. Hearing loss may be unilateral or bilateral and tends to become more severe with repeated doses; it is irreversible. Audiometric analysis should be performed before and during therapy and may be an indicator for withholding subsequent doses.

Sexual function may be compromised in men after treatment with the PVB regimen, including diminished libido and ejaculatory dysfunction.

Cisplatin given by regional limb perfusion has resulted in compartment syndrome, which has necessitated fasciotomies with permanent loss of dorsiflexion. Local adverse effects also include cellulitis and wound infections and are probably secondary to the technique rather than to the drug itself.

Resistance to cisplatin does develop and its mechanisms are not clear. Platinum compounds are not cross-resistant with nitrosoureas or classic alkylating agents.

Drug interactions. The drug interactions described under cyclophosphamide in relation to bone marrow depressants, radiation, probenecid, sulfinpyrazone, and live viral vaccines may all occur if these agents are used with cisplatin.

Concurrent or sequential use of cisplatin and nephrotoxic drugs (*eg*, aminoglycosides or amphotericin B) or ototoxic drugs (*eg*, aminoglycosides or loop diuretics) should be avoided. The risk of nephrotoxicity and ototoxicity, as described under adverse reactions, is increased with such combinations.

Concurrent use of cisplatin and phenytoin has yielded decreased phenytoin effect because of decreased serum levels of phenytoin.

Carboplatin

Carboplatin (Paraplatin) is a second-generation platinum analogue.

Pharmacodynamics. Carboplatin generates both interstrand and intrastrand cross-links in DNA. Cross-links appear more slowly after carboplatin than after cisplatin.

Pharmacokinetics. Given intravenously, carboplatin has a half life of 2.6 hours to 5.9 hours and is excreted in the urine.

Therapeutic uses. Carboplatin is used with ovarian cancer and testicular cancer. It has been used for palliative treatment of recurrent ovarian carcinoma, including for clients who previously received cisplatin. Initial trials of carboplatin have suggested modest activity in endometrial, cervical, bladder, and brain tumors and in refractory acute leukemia.

In advanced squamous cell head and neck cancer, the regimen of choice has been a combination of cisplatin and fluorouracil administered every 3 weeks. Studies in which carboplatin replaced cisplatin in this regimen have yielded similar results (Krasnow, 1990).

In small cell lung cancer, carboplatin is highly active as a single agent in previously untreated clients and modestly active in previously treated clients.

Dosage and administration. Aluminum can react with carboplatin, resulting in precipitation and decreased potency. Thus, aluminum needles or IV sets with parts that contain aluminum cannot be used. Consult Table 48-1 for further dosage information.

Adverse reactions. The major advantage to carboplatin over cisplatin is a different toxicity; it appears less nephrotoxic, less ototoxic, less neurotoxic, and less emetogenic.

A delayed type of myelosuppression is the primary toxicity. Thrombocytopenia is the predominant effect, with platelet nadirs occurring between 2 and 3 weeks and recovery by the 4th week after treatment. Leukopenia and anemia occur, but less frequently and to a less severe degree. The thrombocytopenia seems to be dose-related, to be higher in older clients, and to be greater in clients with renal dysfunction or a history of antineoplastic therapy.

In contrast to cisplatin, renal tubular secretion of carboplatin has not been reported, a fact that may account for its lower nephrotoxicity. Prehydration is not required. Carboplatin-induced nephrotoxicity is seen at high doses (more than 800 mg/m^2) and after prior cisplatin therapy.

Cross-resistance exists between cisplatin and carboplatin.

Drug interactions. No significant drug interactions have been identified with the use of carboplatin.

Summary

The alkylating agents as a group affect a wide variety of cellular functions. The basis for their therapeutic use against cancers is the process of alkylation by which they cause interstrand and intrastrand cross-linkages in DNA, blocking replication. Alkylating agents are cell cycle phase nonspecific, although in some cases cells appear more sensitive in one phase than another. The alkylating agents used as antineoplastic agents are the nitrogen mustards, the ethylenimines and methylmelamines, an alkyl sulfonate, the nitrousoureas, a triazene, and the platinum complexes. Of these, chlorambucil is the medication of choice for the management of chronic lymphocytic leukemia, cyclophosphamide is probably the most widely used antineoplastic drug, ifosfamide is a new drug, mechlorethamine was the first alkylating agent used and has been significant in treating Hodgkin's disease, busulfan is used in the palliative treatment of chronic myelogenous leukemia, the nitrosoureas are lipid soluble and can be used with various brain tumors, cisplatin is one of the most active antineoplastic drugs against testicular tumors, and carboplatin is a new cisplatin analogue. All of these drugs cause serious adverse reactions.

Antimetabolites

The antimetabolites include a folic acid analogue, the pyrimidine analogues, and the purine analogues (Table 48-3).

Folic acid analogues

Methotrexate

Pharmacodynamics. Folic acid and its derivatives are critical to the metabolism of proliferating cells. Methotrexate is an analogue of folic acid. It competitively inhibits dihydrofolate reductase, the enzyme that reduces dihydrofolic acid to tetrahydrofolic acid. Tetrahydrofolic acid is converted to various coenzymes required for several one-carbon transfer reactions. The reaction most sensitive to a lack of a coenzyme is the conversion of 2-deoxyuridylate (dUMP) to thymidylate (dTMP), an essential component of DNA.

Thus, as a result of the inhibition of dihydrofolate reductase, methotrexate causes an accumulation of cellular folates in the inactive oxidized form and leads to inhibition of dTMP, DNA, RNA, and protein synthesis.

Methotrexate, and all the antimetabolites, are cell cycle specific for the S phase.

Pharmacokinetics. Methotrexate may be administered orally, intravenously, intramuscularly, and intrathecally. Its half life is 2 hours to 4 hours and it is excreted in the urine.

Therapeutic uses. Methotrexate is used in the treatment of acute leukemia for maintenance therapy and for CNS prophylaxis (used intrathecally and with cranial irradiation). It is an agent of choice in combination with mercaptopurine.

Tumors sensitive to methotrexate include head and neck cancer, bone and soft tissue sarcomas, trophoblastic neoplasms (choriocarcinoma, chorioadenoma destruens, and hydatidiform mole), rhabdomyosarcoma, medulloblastoma, glioma, melanomas, testicular cancer, and bladder and cervical carcinomas.

It is a component of combination regimens used to treat non-Hodgkin's and Burkitt's lymphomas and breast and ovarian carcinomas.

Oral methotrexate has been used to treat psoriasis,

which is a non-neoplastic skin disease characterized by abnormally rapid proliferation of epidermal cells. It is used to treat mycosis fungoides, rheumatoid arthritis (when it has been refractory to other second-line drugs), and systemic lupus erythematosus. For these disorders, the drug is usually administered in a low dose of 7.5 to 15 mg weekly. Side effects of pancytopenia, GI toxicity, skin rash, headache, hepatotoxicity, and pulmonary toxic effects have all been reported at the low dose and are usually mild; the effects remain constant with prolonged use.

Methotrexate is used as an immunosuppressive agent to prevent graft-vs.-host disease after allogeneic bone marrow transplantation.

Dosage and administration. Consult Table 48-3 for usual dosages. The biochemical effects of methotrexate can be reversed by the administration of leucovorin calcium (or folinic acid or citrovorum factor). Leucovorin calcium is a folate coenzyme that does not need reduction by dihydrofolate reductase. When leucovorin calcium is supplied to cells, the methotrexate-induced block of tetrahydrofolic acid synthesis is bypassed. Using this "rescue" agent allows for recovery of normal tissues or prevention of toxicity to the bone marrow and GI epithelium. For example, side effects of mucositis, skin rashes, and altered taste sensation have been shown to be reduced by the administration of leucovorin calcium, and renal failure may be prevented.

In the use of leucovorin calcium, it is important to obtain serial methotrexate concentrations to determine at what point it is safe to discontinue the leucovorin calcium. After 24 to 48 hours of methotrexate therapy, the methotrexate level is measured and the leucovorin calcium is continued until concentrations of methotrexate fall below 500 mmol/L. The cytotoxic effects of methotrexate are irreversible after 42 to 48 hours without adequate rescue (Black, Livingston, 1990).

A typical way to administer the methotrexate and leucovorin calcium (Jaffe regimen) would be to give 50 to 250 mg/kg of methotrexate as an infusion over 6 hours. Leucovorin calcium administration begins 2 hours after the end of the drug infusion at a rate of 15 mg/m^2 intramuscularly (IM) every 6 hours for 7 doses.

Due to the potential nephrotoxicity of methotrexate, adequate hydration and alkalinization of the urine (using sodium bicarbonate or acetazolamide) are recommended to enhance excretion of methotrexate. Methotrexate is a weak dicarboxylic acid and precipitates in acid urine.

An example of prehydration may include, in the 12 hours before methotrexate treatment, 1.5 liters/m^2 D5W with 100 mEq HCO_3^- and 20 mEq KCl/liter. The urine pH should be tested at the time of drug infusion to be sure it is 7 or more.

Table 48-3. Antimetabolites

Drug names	Preparation	Usual dosage/PC	Adverse reactions
Folic acid analogues			
methotrexate sodium (Mexate, Folex, Rheumatrex)	Oral tablets IV IM Intrathecal	Adult: oral, 2.5–5 mg qd; IM or IV, 25 mg/m^2 once or twice weekly; high-dose IV, 1.5 g/m^2 with leuco-vorin rescue q 3 weeks; intrathecal, 5–10 mg/m^2 q2–5d until CSF cell count returns to normal PC: D	Arachnoiditis (on intrathecal use in first 48 hours), stomatitis, anorexia, nausea and vomiting, mucositis, BMS, nephropathy, hepatic fibrosis with long-term oral therapy, neurotoxicity with intrathecal use (motor dysfunction of extremities, cranial nerve palsies, sei-zures, coma), diarrhea (progressing to hemorrhagic enteritis and intestinal perforation), hypersensitivity-mediated pulmonary reaction, desquamative dermatitis
Pyrimidine analogues			
floxuridine (FUDR)	Intra-arterial	Intra-arterial, 5–20 mg/m^2/24 h continuously for 14–21 days, with infusion pump PC: D	Anorexia, nausea and vomiting, diarrhea, stomatitis, enteritis, gastritis, duodenal ulcer, glossitis, pharyngitis, dermatologic reactions, BMS, elevated liver function tests, acute and delayed CNS toxicity, complications of regional infusion, including arterial aneurysm, is-chemia, and thrombosis or bleeding, leaking, and infection at site
fluorouracil or 5-FU (Adrucil, Amethopterin)	IV Intra-arterial	IV, loading dose of 400–500 mg/m^2 every day for 4 successive days, fol-lowed by weekly mainte-nance dose; intra-arterial, 800 mg/m^2/day for 14–21 days PC: D	Anorexia, nausea and vomiting, stomatitis, esopha-gopharyngitis, diarrhea, BMS, alopecia, dermatitis, hyperpigmentation, acute and chronic conjunctivitis, excess lacrimation, cerebellar dysfunction, hand-foot syndrome, myocardial ischemia
fluorouracil (Efudex)	Topical cream and solution	PC: X	Pain, pruritus, hyperpigmentation and burning at application site; allergic contact dermatitis, scarring, soreness, tenderness, suppuration, scaling and swelling
cytarabine or cytosine arabinoside (Cytosar-U, Ara-C, Tarabine, Udacil)	IV Subcutaneous Intrathecal	Conventional IV, 200 mg/m^2/24 h for 5–7 days with an anthracycline, repeat course once in 1 week; sub-cutaneous, 50 mg/m^2/bid for 21 days; intrathecal 5–75 mg/m^2 in 10 ml nor-mal saline solution 1 to 3 times per week PC: D	BMS, nausea and vomiting, diarrhea, stomatitis, at high doses neurotoxicity (cerebellar and cerebral; ataxia, confusion, seizures, dysarthria, dysdiadocho-kinesia), acute painful swollen erythematous hands and soles (syndrome may be referred to as palmar–plantar erythrodysesthesia), keratoconjunctivitis, pancreatitis in those treated earlier with asparaginase, pulmonary toxicity (ARDS), hepatotoxicity, urticaria, anaphylaxis, alopecia, thrombophlebitis, and cellulitis at injection site
Purine analogues			
mercaptopurine (Purinethol)	Oral tablets	Adults and children over 5 yrs: for induction of remis-sion, 100 mg/m^2 every day for 4 weeks or 500–700 mg/m^2/day for 5 days with other drugs; children: for maintenance of remission in ALL, 50 mg/m^2 every day PC: D	BMS, GI toxicity, cholestatic injury and jaundice, pan-creatitis, pulmonary fibrosis, hepatic dysfunction
thioguanine (Lanvis)	Oral tablets	Adults and children: 80 mg/m^2 every day for 4 weeks; for induction of remission in AML with daunorubicin and cytarabine, 100 mg/m^2 q12h on days 1 through 7 PC: D	BMS, GI toxicity, cholestatic injury and jaundice, hepatic dysfunction
pentostatin			Acute renal failure, CNS effects (lethargy, coma, sei-zures), hepatic dysfunction, keratoconjunctivitis, nausea and vomiting

KEY: PC = pregnancy category. (The validity of pregnancy risk categories has not been established; see Chapter 16, p 216.)

Adverse reactions. The adverse reactions are listed in Table 48-3. Three distinct patterns of toxicity have been observed with intrathecal methotrexate. The acute form is a chemical arachnoiditis that begins shortly after the drug is administered and resolves in 1 to 5 days. The subacute form of toxicity develops over a period of a few weeks and is characterized by motor dysfunction of the brain or spinal cord. This form is probably related to a continuously elevated level of cerebrospinal fluid (CSF) methotrexate, which may occur when clients receive multiple injections per week. The third form of toxicity is associated with months or years of intrathecal methotrexate. It is a necrotizing demyelinating leukoencephalopathy characterized by progressive neurologic deterioration, including dementia, dysarthria, ataxia, spasticity, seizures, and coma (Black, Livingston, 1990). Serial electroencephalograms in clients who receive high-dose methotrexate may be used to predict the leukoencephalopathy entity.

Chronic brain injury appears to occur in many children with acute lymphocytic leukemia who receive CNS prophylaxis with intrathecal methotrexate and cranial irradiation. In these children, computed tomography reveals intracerebral calcification, hypodensities, thinning of cerebral cortex, and ventricular dilatation (DeVita, et al, 1989). Some studies indicate reduced doses of methotrexate and cranial irradiation will reduce CNS sequelae and others suggest using high-dose systemic methotrexate rather than intrathecal methotrexate.

Methotrexate may be distributed into the pleural or peritoneal cavities. If ascites or pleural effusion is present, these cavities may act as storage sites for methotrexate, subsequently releasing the drug and causing further adverse reactions. Therefore, pleural effusions and ascites should be evacuated before methotrexate administration.

Reactivation of sunburn has been reported after intermediate-dose methotrexate. It was not prevented by concurrent leucovorin administration.

Interaction with other drugs, renal impairment, or an idiosyncratic response may explain the cases of pancytopenia that have occurred with methotrexate.

Hepatic dysfunction may occur. Elevated aspartate aminotransferase levels are common in clients on long-term methotrexate therapy. These may be indicative of liver fibrosis or cirrhosis. Liver biopsy is the most reliable method of documenting actual liver damage.

Acute life-threatening pneumonitis has been reported after use of methotrexate in the treatment of rheumatoid arthritis. The possibility of an increased susceptibility to methotrexate pneumonitis in rheumatoid clients is under consideration.

Resistance to methotrexate may develop as a result of more than one mechanism, including increased levels of dihydrofolate reductase, sequestration of dihydrofolate reductase in a site inaccessible to the drug, decreased sensitivity of dihydrofolate reductase to methotrexate, defective transportation of methotrexate into malignant cells, or reduced conversion of methotrexate to active metabolites within malignant cells.

Drug interactions. Cellular uptake of methotrexate is decreased by concomitant use of penicillin, hydroxyurea, mercaptopurine, neomycin, kanamycin, corticosteroids, bleomycin, and asparaginase.

Methotrexate may be displaced from plasma albumin by sulfonamides, salicylates, tetracyclines, chloramphenicol, and phenytoin. This displacement may result in greater methotrexate toxicity.

In addition, salicylates and probenecid inhibit tubular secretion of methotrexate. Salicylates are contraindicated in the client who is receiving methotrexate because methotrexate effect can be increased by two different mechanisms with this group of drugs.

Concurrent use of alcohol or known hepatotoxic drugs with methotrexate increases the risk of hepatotoxicity. Such combination should be avoided if possible. Etretinate for psoriasis should be avoided for this reason.

Concurrent administration of methotrexate and nonsteroidal anti-inflammatory agents may result in severe methotrexate toxicity and should be viewed as a possible fatal interaction.

Administration of oral aminoglycosides decreases absorption of oral methotrexate.

Neurologic complications may occur with the use of the combination of intrathecal methotrexate and acyclovir. Vincristine and vinblastine impair methotrexate elimination from CSF.

Asparaginase may attenuate methotrexate toxicity if the timing of administration is correct. It is suggested that asparaginase be given 9 to 10 days before or within 24 hours after the methotrexate.

Pretreatment with cytarabine may enhance methotrexate cytotoxicity; cytarabine increases the cellular uptake of methotrexate.

Administered before fluorouracil, methotrexate promotes the conversion of this drug to fluorodeoxyuridylate (FdUMP), its active metabolite. This conversion could enhance the cytotoxicity of fluorouracil, but to date this interaction has not been used to clinical benefit. Administered in reverse order, fluorouracil inhibits dTMP synthetase, an action that could inhibit methotrexate cytotoxicity.

Pyrimidine analogues
See Focus on Pyrimidine Analogues: Similarities and Differences.

Fluorouracil
Fluorouracil (5-FU, Adrucil) is a fluorinated pyrimidine.

Pyrimidine analogues: similarities and differences

Similarities

Pharmacodynamics

These agents are cell cycle specific antimetabolites for the S phase of cell division. They interfere with the enzymes in the metabolic pathways, thereby inhibiting DNA and RNA synthesis.

Pharmacokinetics

These agents are unpredictably and poorly absorbed after oral administration and are therefore given parenterally. They are rapidly and widely distributed to tissues and cross the blood–brain barrier. They are metabolized by the liver and excreted by the kidneys as unchanged drug or as metabolites.

Therapeutic uses

These agents are used as adjuvant therapy for the palliative treatment of clients with solid tumors, including breast, colon, rectal, bile duct, pancreatic, liver, gastric, ovarian, cervical, and esophageal cancers.

Adverse reactions

These include: (CNS) ataxia, vertigo, nystagmus, drowsiness, euphoria, depression, hemiplegia, hiccups, and lethargy; (EENT) blurred vision, photophobia; (GI) nausea, vomiting, diarrhea, stomatitis, cramps, anorexia, paralytic ileus; (HEMA) bone marrow depression, thrombocytopenia, leukopenia, anemia; (SKIN) rash, erythema, alopecia; (OTHER) flulike symptoms, redness, pain at injection site.

Contraindications

These agents are contraindicated for people with known hypersensitivity, poor nutritional status, depressed bone marrow function, those with potentially serious infections, or those who have had major surgery within the previous month.

Precautions

These agents should be used with caution in people who have previously received high-dose pelvic irradiation or alkylating agents and those with impaired liver or kidney function.

Differences

• **Cytarabine** has little effect on RNA synthesis. It can suppress humoral and cell-mediated immune responses.

• **Floxuridine** is catabolized to **fluorouracil** and is administered by continuous intra-arterial infusion. • **Floxuridine** and **fluorouracil** are excreted primarily through the lungs as carbon dioxide. • **Fluorouracil** is given IV and topically; the onset of the topical form is 2 to 3 days; it has a plasma half-life of 16 minutes (IV). • **Cytarabine** is given IV, but it can be given IM, subcutaneously, and intrathecally; it is also metabolized by the kidneys, GI mucosa, and granulocytes; it has a terminal half-life of 1 to 3 hours.

• **Cytarabine** is used for remission induction in the treatment of leukemias, especially acute myelogenous leukemia. Topical **fluorouracil** is used in the treatment of premalignant skin lesions and superficial basal cell carcinoma.

Topical **fluorouracil** may cause an inflammatory response, burning, rash, itching, and photosensitivity. • **Cytarabine** may cause cerebellar dysfunction, neurotoxicity, dizziness, neuritis, peripheral neuropathy, hepatotoxicity, hyperuricemia, chest pain, shortness of breath, anaphylaxis, fever, sepsis, and headache. • **Fluorouracil** may cause mild angina, electrocardiographic changes, nail changes, pigmented palmar creases, lacrimation, weakness, malaise, epistaxis. • **Floxuridine** may cause cholangitis, jaundice, and elevated liver enzymes.

• **Fluorouracil** is contraindicated in pregnant females.

Topical **fluorouracil** should be used with caution in people with hemorrhagic ulcerated tissues and pre-existing dermatoses.

(continued)

Focus on

Pyrimidine analogues: similarities and differences (Continued)

Similarities

Nursing considerations

Instruct in disease, treatment, drug therapy regimen, adverse reactions, and compliance; assess cardiopulmonary status, including heart rate, rhythm, and breath sounds, for changes; monitor vital signs for changes; monitor nutritional status; encourage diet high in protein and calories; encourage adequate fluid intake; monitor intake and output; offer frequent mouth care; instruct client in mouth care and dietary needs; encourage client to avoid alcohol and cigarettes; administer antiemetic before giving drug; monitor lab studies including complete blood cell count and platelets, frequently; avoid any IM injections if platelet count drops below 100,000/mm^3; assess for signs of occult bleeding, including checking stool and urine and watching for bruising, petechiae, and gingival bleeding; instruct client in signs of occult bleeding and need to report to physician; monitor renal and hepatic function studies for changes; avoid giving client any immunizations and instruct client to avoid contact with any person with infection; assess infusion site and patency of infusion line, checking for any signs of redness, pain, or swelling; offer emotional support; explain that hair loss is temporary; offer suggestions to cope with hair loss, such as wigs, turbans, scarves; instruct client to use mild protein-base shampoo and cream rinse every 3 to 5 days; administer anticoagulants and aspirin products cautiously and monitor closely for signs of bleeding; instruct client to avoid use of over-the-counter products that contain aspirin; instruct client in signs and symptoms of infection and need to notify physician.

Differences

When administering **topical fluorouracil**, do not cover with an occlusive dressing to prevent possibility of increased inflammatory reaction; avoid applying it near eyes, nose, and mouth, wear gloves when applying. Assess neurologic status in the client who is receiving **cytarabine**; monitor for cerebellar dysfunction; institute safety precautions to prevent injury. When client is receiving **floxuridine** intra-arterially, assess the perfused area and arterial insertion site for problems; check the line for bleeding, blockage, displacement, or leakage. Monitor intake and output closely if the client is receiving **cytarabine**; encourage high fluid intake and monitor serum uric acid levels; be prepared to give allopurinol if hyperuricemia develops. Administer infusion of **fluorouracil** slowly over 2 to 8 hours to lessen toxicity.

Pharmacodynamics. The cytotoxicity of fluorouracil is probably related to several of its biochemical actions. Fluorouracil was developed because it has been observed that certain tumor cells used uracil, a pyrimidine base, after conversion of it to thymidine, for synthesis of DNA.

Metabolism of fluorouracil produces fluorodeoxyuridylate (FdUMP). FdUMP inhibits dTMP synthetase, which catalyzes methylation of dUMP to dTMP, an essential component of DNA. Thus, with this inhibition, a DNA precursor is not available, and DNA synthesis is prevented.

Metabolism of fluorouracil also produces fluorouridine-5'-triphosphate (FUTP), which is incorporated into RNA and interferes with its function.

FdUMP, dTMP synthetase, and N^{5,10}-methylene-tetrahydrofolate form a stable complex. Tumor sensitivity may correlate with the degree of inhibition of dTMP synthetase, which in turn correlates with the stability of the complex. It is possible to enhance this stability by exogenously adding reduced folates, such as calcium folinate; this concept has been used in treatment protocols to improve efficacy of the fluorouracil (Black, Livingston, 1990).

Fluorouracil is cell cycle specific for the S phase.

Pharmacokinetics. Fluorouracil has a half life of 8 minutes to 20 minutes and it is excreted in the urine and via the lungs as carbon dioxide.

Therapeutic uses. Fluorouracil is only useful in solid tumors. It is used in the palliative treatment of colorectal cancer. It is a component of the FAM regimen (fluorouracil, doxorubicin, mitomycin) used in the palliative management of gastric adenocarcinoma. The effectiveness of fluorouracil against colorectal and gastric adenocarcinomas is enhanced when calcium folinate is administered concomitantly.

Fluorouracil is a component of the CMF (cyclophosphamide, methotrexate, and 5-fluorouracil) or CAF regimens (cyclophosphamide, doxorubicin, fluorouracil) for breast cancer. It is also used with cancer of the ovary, bladder, cervix, endometrium, prostate, head and neck, pancreas, esophagus, and liver.

Dosage and administration. Consult Table 48-3 for usual dosages. Clients with colon cancer with liver metastasis or clients with primary liver tumors may be treated by hepatic arterial infusion of fluorouracil or other agents (*eg*, cisplatin, mitomycin, doxorubicin).

Systemic toxicity with this methodology is mild, but other complications occur (*eg*, catheter dislodgment, sepsis, and "local toxicity").

If the catheter slips into the gastroduodenal artery, necrosis of the intestinal epithelium, hemorrhage, or perforation may result. Signs of this complication include sudden onset of epigastric pain or ileus.

An erythematous blistering skin rash that corresponds to the distribution of the selected artery has occurred with fluorouracil and usually subsides 1 to 2 months after treatment is stopped, but a residual pigmentation is left. Persistent neck and shoulder pain has been reported and was abolished by the injection of long-acting local anesthetic through the infusion catheter. This pain is believed to be referred from the diaphragm.

Duodenal ulcers (fatal in some clients) have been reported in relation to hepatic artery chemotherapy with fluorouracil, appearing 5 to 7 months after initial administration of the fluorouracil.

Adverse reactions. Acute and chronic conjunctivitis occur and may lead to tear duct stenosis and ectropion. Discontinuing the drug may correct the acute inflammatory response; however, if tear duct stenosis develops, surgical correction may be needed.

GI disturbances are common with fluorouracil. GI damage can occur at any level, and lesions similar to those seen with stomatitis can be seen in the stoma of colostomies. Repeated episodes of watery diarrhea for several days may lead to dehydration, sepsis, and death, so dosage adjustments are usually indicated when diarrhea occurs.

Cardiac toxicity has been increasingly reported with fluorouracil. One variation is constrictive anginal chest pain during infusion. Outcome is favorable if the drug is stopped. Reintroduction of the drug has been associated with fatal outcome at times and is not recommended. Another example of cardiac toxicity is sudden death, apparently due to ventricular fibrillation. A syndrome of chest pain, serum enzyme elevations consistent with myocardial necrosis, and electrocardiogram findings consistent with myocardial ischemia has been identified.

Acute painful swollen erythematous hands and soles have been reported after protracted fluorouracil infusion. Some authors use the term *palmar–plantar erythrodysesthesia* for this syndrome. Fluorouracil also commonly causes other mucocutaneous effects, such as hyperpigmentation and multiple pigmented macules.

Cerebellar signs (including ataxia) may occur and may be dose-related. They may occur at any time during therapy, usually after several months, and may persist for several weeks after discontinuing the drug.

Resistance to fluorouracil could result from deletion of enzymes required for its activation or from an increase in dTMP synthetase activity.

Drug interactions. Synergistic toxicity from the use of fluorouracil and cisplatin together has been considered. What has been seen is an acute dilated cardiomyopathy with left ventricular dysfunction. With drug discontinuation, recovery occurred.

The interaction between fluorouracil and methotrexate has been discussed under methotrexate.

The concurrent use of fluorouracil and allopurinol may decrease fluorouracil toxicity.

The drug interactions described under cyclophosphamide in relation to bone marrow depressants and radiation may occur if these agents are used with fluorouracil.

The administration of any live virus vaccine concurrently with fluorouracil should probably be avoided. Fluorouracil suppresses the client's normal defense mechanisms and thus may increase replication of the virus and cause adverse effects in the client. It is usually recommended that live virus vaccines not be administered until months after chemotherapy has been discontinued. People in close contact with the client should not receive immunization with the oral polio virus vaccine because the live virus is excreted by the person receiving it, and it can be transmitted to an immunocompromised client.

Topical fluorouracil

Therapeutic uses. Topical fluorouracil is available as a solution at concentrations of 1% (Fluroplex) or 2% and 5% (Efudex) or as a cream at concentrations of 1% (Fluroplex) or 5% (Efudex).

The 2% or 5% preparation is used on multiple premalignant actinic keratoses of the head and neck, while the 5% preparation is used on keratoses of the body. For isolated lesions, curettage or cryosurgery is usually preferred.

In the 5% strength, it can be used in the treatment of superficial basal cell carcinomas when more usual treatment methods are impractical, such as with multiple lesions or difficult treatment sites. Carcinoma *in situ* of the vulva also has been treated successfully with a topical approach.

Dosage and administration. A specific regimen for the topical use of fluorouracil is indicated by the physician. Tight occlusive dressings are probably not advised because their use is associated with irritation to healthy tissue that surrounds the lesions being treated. A loose gauze dressing for cosmetic purposes may be used.

Gloves should be worn when applying the preparation, and a metallic applicator is not to be used. The preparation is applied twice daily to the affected area. Mucous membranes, scrotum, eyes, and intertriginous areas should be avoided. Application is continued for 2 to 4 weeks until the inflammation response progresses from erythema and vesiculation to erosion, ulceration, and necrosis. After cessation of therapy, healing may take 6 to 8 weeks. On the body, this healing phase can be accelerated by applying a topical corticosteroid, such as betamethasone valerate cream 0.1% (Valisone), twice daily to the affected area. On the face, 1% hydrocortisone cream can be used in the same manner.

Occasionally, with keratoses little or no inflammation develops. In this case, the period of treatment may be prolonged, or concomitant therapy with 0.1% tretinoin cream may be used (the tretinoin cream appears to aid penetration by fluorouracil). With basal cell carcinomas, the period of treatment may range from 3 to 12 weeks.

Clients need to know that treated areas may be unsightly during therapy and that healing of lesions may not be complete for 1 to 2 months after cessation of therapy. Restoration of skin color and texture is usually satisfactory, and scars usually do not occur.

Exposure to sunlight during and for 1 or 2 months after treatment should be minimized.

Floxuridine

Floxuridine (FUDR) is the deoxyriboside derivative of fluorouracil. Intra-arterial floxuridine is used for palliation of GI malignancies and liver metastases from these sites. Some of the difficulties with intra-arterial therapy have been identified under the discussion of fluorouracil.

Cytarabine

Cytarabine/cytosine arabinoside (ara-C) is one of several arabinose nucleosides first isolated from the sponge *Cryptothethya crypta*. Since its discovery, other similar preparations have been isolated or synthesized and tested as antitumor agents, but none are in general use at present. Two nucleosides (5-azacytidine/5-aza-C and 3-deazauridine) have undergone clinical trials.

Pharmacodynamics. Ara-C's cytotoxic capabilities are due to its metabolite, arabinofuranosylcytosine triphosphate (ara-CTP), which blocks DNA synthesis by competitively inhibiting DNA polymerase. It is incorporated into DNA, leading to a marked slowing of the elongating chain of DNA and a defect in ligation of fragments of newly synthesized DNA (DeVita, et al, 1989).

Entry into cells is an important determinant of sensitivity to ara-C. A strong correlation exists between the number of transport sites and the formation of the ultimate toxic metabolite (ara-CTP). Ara-C penetrates cells best by a carrier-mediated process; it can also enter cells by passive diffusion, but this is a less efficient mechanism.

Ara-C is subject to deamination by cytidine deaminase, an enzyme found in plasma and in granulocytes. This deaminating enzyme is believed to be a factor in limiting drug action and possibly in the development of resistance.

Ara-C is cell cycle specific for the S phase, but exposure of cells during other phases may lead to chromatid deletions and to a failure to repair strand breaks induced by other agents.

Pharmacokinetics. Ara-C has an onset of action within minutes and a duration of action of 2 hours. Its half life is 7 minutes to 20 minutes and it is excreted in the urine.

Therapeutic uses. Ara-C is used for treatment of acute myelogenous leukemia. Remission rates approach 75% to 85% in this disease with the use of ara-C and an anthracycline. It is also used in the blastic crisis phase of chronic myelogenous leukemia, as secondary treatment of acute lymphocytic leukemia, and in combination regimens for non-Hodgkin's lymphomas.

Ara-C is one of the few antineoplastic agents to cross the blood–brain barrier.

Dosage and administration. Three dosing schedules are used. Low-dose ara-C used for the treatment of myelodysplasia is typically a 20 mg/m²/day, continuous IV infusion for 14 to 21 days.

Conventional-dose ara-C given in combination with an anthracycline for acute myelogenous leukemia is commonly 200 mg/m²/day by continuous infusion for 5 to 7 days.

High-dose ara-C administration for refractory leukemia to overcome tumor cell resistance is 3 g/m² IV over 1 hour every 12 hours for 8 to 12 doses (Black, Livingston, 1990).

The cytotoxicity of ara-C depends not only on the cell cycle phase but also on the rate of DNA synthesis. Cytotoxicity is greatest if cells are exposed during periods of rapid DNA synthesis, for example during the recovery phase after treatment with an initial dose of ara-C. A study demonstrated a marked increase in DNA synthesis in residual leukemia cells 1 week after an initial dose of ara-C, and the study recommends the use of sequential ara-C doses 1 week apart to take advantage of this observation (DeVita, et al, 1989).

When administered by IV infusion, concentrations in the CSF reach 50% of simultaneous plasma levels after 2 hours of continuous infusion. Ara-C may also be administered intrathecally for treatment of meningeal leukemia or carcinomatosis. Deamination is minimal in the CSF, and cytotoxic concentrations are maintained for 24 hours. It has been substituted for methotrexate in clients who experience neurotoxicity, but, unfortunately, it is capable itself of neurotoxic effects.

Adverse reactions. The adverse reactions are listed in Table 48-3. The major dose-limiting adverse reaction is bone marrow suppression.

In the study of the use of high-dose ara-C in acute myelogenous leukemia, additional adverse reactions that were identified include cerebellar neurotoxicity, progressive hepatic failure, and adult respiratory distress syndrome.

Acute painful swollen erythematous hands and soles have been reported after the use of ara-C for induction therapy for acute myelogenous leukemia (the palmar–plantar erythrodysesthesia mentioned by some authors and also mentioned in connection with fluorouracil).

Resistance may result from impaired cellular uptake, decreased activation secondary to decreased kinase activity, or enhanced metabolism from increased cytidine deaminase activity.

Drug interactions. Ara-C has shown synergistic interaction with many other antineoplastic agents. It enhances cyclophosphamide and amsacrine. Methotrexate given before ara-C enhances formation of ara-CTP. Hydroxyurea also enhances ara-C cytotoxicity.

Enhancement of ara-C cytotoxicity is observed when clients are pretreated with tetrahydrouridine, which is a cytidine deaminase inhibitor. Tetrahydrouridine prolongs the plasma half-life of ara-C. This concept is not used in clinical practice yet, but the combination is expected to have synergistic activity against cells with high cytidine deaminase levels, as found in some clients with acute myelogenous leukemia.

Absorption of digoxin may be impaired when ara-C is used with other antineoplastic agents.

Purine analogues

The purine analogues include mercaptopurine, thioguanine, and pentostatin.

Mercaptopurine

Pharmacodynamics. Mercaptopurine (6-mercaptopurine, 6-MP, Purinethol) is a prodrug and an inactive compound in its native state. It is an analogue of the purine hypoxanthine, and it requires activation to the nucleotide level by the enzyme hypoxanthine-guanine phosphoribosyltransferase. The nucleotide inhibits purine biosynthesis at its first step and blocks the conversion of inosinic acid to adenylic acid or guanylic acid. Nucleotide metabolites are incorporated into DNA, a fact that may also be involved in the cytotoxic effects of the drug. Metabolites of the drug may also inhibit RNA synthesis.

Mercaptopurine is cell cycle specific for the S phase.

Pharmacokinetics. Mercaptopurine reaches its peak action in 2 hours with a duration of 8 hours. Its half-life is 20 minutes to 45 minutes.

It is excreted in the urine. Two pathways for the metabolism of mercaptopurine exist. One involves methylation and the subsequent oxidation of methylated derivatives. The second is its oxidation by xanthine oxidase, which is present in large amounts in the liver. An attempt to modify this second pathway of metabolic inactivation led to the important development of allopurinol, which is a potent inhibitor of xanthine oxidase. Allopurinol is also used in several common medical situations.

Therapeutic uses. Mercaptopurine is used to induce remission in adults and children with acute lymphocytic leukemia. However, better results are obtained with combination regimens. The major role of mercaptopurine is maintenance therapy in acute lymphocytic leukemia, most often in combination with methotrexate (see Example of Nursing Process and Methotrexate and Mercaptopurine Maintenance Therapy for Acute Lymphocytic Leukemia).

Mercaptopurine and a derivative of mercaptopurine, azathioprine (Imuran), are used for immunosuppression of cell-mediated immunity. They are used to suppress rejection of transplanted organs or to treat autoimmune diseases like Crohn's disease, ulcerative colitis, or rheumatoid arthritis. Therapeutic immunosuppression occurs at doses of 100 mg/day, and this dosage causes only a small decrease in the number of leukocytes.

Dosage and administration. Consult Table 48-3 for usual dosages.

Adverse reactions. Mercaptopurine has been implicated in liver vascular disorders, peliosis hepatitis, and hepatic veno-occlusive disease. During therapy, determinations of serum bilirubin, serum alkaline phosphatase, and aspartate aminotransferase should be made. With acute hepatic toxicity, elevations in a pattern are similar to those seen with cholestatic jaundice. The signs and symptoms of hepatotoxicity may appear 1 to 2 months after therapy is started, are reversible, and may occur more frequently with higher doses of the drug.

Bone marrow suppression is the major adverse reaction, but it usually develops more slowly with mercaptopurine than with folic acid analogues. Anorexia, nausea, and vomiting are frequently seen, but more often in adults than in children.

Hyperuricemia occurs frequently because of rapid cell lysis.

Biochemical resistance to mercaptopurine has been attributed to the absence of hypoxanthine-guanine phosphoribosyltransferase in tumors. In human leukemic cells, resistance is also associated with an increased concentration of a degrading enzyme.

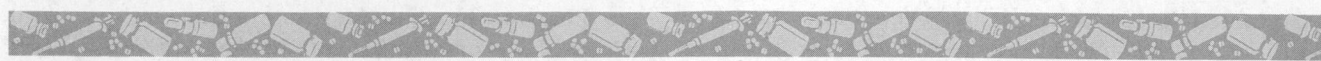

Example of nursing process and methotrexate and mercaptopurine maintenance therapy for acute lymphocytic leukemia

The client, Jack Cell, is a 5-year-old boy with acute lymphocytic leukemia. His lymphoblasts are of the L₁ subtype, and he is considered to be one of the better-risk clients. He is placed in a treatment program, which in the induction phase combined vincristine, prednisone, and daunorubicin. He is now beginning the maintenance phase. He is receiving oral dosages of methotrexate 30 mg/m² twice a week and mercaptopurine 1.5 mg/kg/day.

His initial signs and symptoms included anorexia, pallor and fatigue, petechiae, lymphadenopathy, and hepatosplenomegaly. He is much less active than usual.

Jack is one of two children (he has an identical twin) whose mother is studying for her baccalaureate degree in nursing. His father is a career Air Force officer, and they live on the local air base. The twin has shown no signs of leukemia to date.

Assessment data	Nursing diagnosis	Intervention	Goals and outcome criteria
Receiving methotrexate and mercaptopurine; earlier use of vincristine, prednisone, and daunorubicin. Diagnosis of acute lymphocytic leukemia	High risk for infection related to lowered natural resistance and neutropenia secondary to cytotoxic drug therapy	**Monitor** results of complete blood cell count and differential every 3 days. **Obtain** culture specimens as ordered. **Observe** for signs and symptoms of infection (skin, blood, sputum, urine). **Use** good hand-washing technique, and teach client and parents to do same. **Maintain** optimal nutritional status. **Avoid** invasive procedures; if necessary, maintain meticulous aseptic technique. **Carry out** actions to prevent respiratory infection (turn, cough, and deep breathe every 2 hours; increase activity as tolerated). **Carry out** actions to prevent urinary tract infection (teach client and parents proper perineal hygiene). **Place** client on protective precautions in private room.	The client will remain free of infection.
Receiving methotrexate and mercaptopurine; earlier use of vincristine and daunorubicin. Diagnosis of acute lymphocytic leukemia.	Potential complication: thrombocytopenia*	**Monitor** coagulation test results (platelet count, prothrombin time, partial thromboplastin time) every 3 days. **Observe** client for evidence of unusual bleeding (multiple bruises, petechiae, bleeding gums, melena, hematuria, epistaxis).	The client will not experience unusual bleeding or hemorrhage.

(Continued)

Example of nursing process and methotrexate and mercaptopurine maintenance therapy for acute lymphocytic leukemia (Continued)

Assessment data	Nursing diagnosis	Intervention	Goals and outcome criteria
		Avoid parenteral injections or invasive procedures like rectal temperatures.	
		Apply prolonged pressure at venipuncture sites.	
		Instruct client and parents to try to avoid cuts, bruises, and falls.	
		If hemorrhage occurs, monitor for therapeutic and nontherapeutic effects of agents that may be administered (*eg*, blood products, vitamin K).	
Receiving methotrexate and mercaptopurine.	High risk for altered oral mucous membranes related to cell injury secondary to methotrexate and mercaptopurine therapy	**Inspect** client's mouth daily for signs of stomatitis (erythema of mucous membrane, small white blisters) and check him for complaint of burning sensation in mouth.	The client will maintain a healthy oral cavity.
		Reinforce importance of and assist client with oral hygiene after meals and snacks.	
		Have client rinse mouth with warm-saline rinses and use soft bristle toothbrush for dental care.	
		Encourage client to use an artificial saliva product if his mouth is dry.	
		Lubricate lips with lip-care product.	
		Maintain optimal nutritional status with soft bland diet.	

*Although potential complications are generally not included in the Examples of Nursing Process, in this situation the identification of this collaborative problem is critical to the outcome for this client and illustrates the broad range of nursing responsibilities.

Tumor cells resistant to mercaptopurine usually are cross-resistant to thioguanine.

Drug interactions. Mercaptopurine is partly metabolized by xanthine oxidase to 6-thiouric acid. Because of allopurinol's ability to inhibit xanthine oxidase, the concurrent administration of allopurinol and mercaptopurine diminishes the catabolism of mercaptopurine and potentiates its cytotoxicity. If they must be given concurrently, the dose of mercaptopurine must be reduced to 25% of the usual dose.

Interaction between mercaptopurine and cyclophosphamide has been identified under cyclophosphamide. Concurrent use of mercaptopurine and trimethoprim-sulfamethoxazole increases the risk of bone marrow suppression because of the mercaptopurine.

Thioguanine

Pharmacodynamics. Thioguanine is also activated by hypoxanthine-guanine phosphoribosyltransferase. After activation, it is incorporated into DNA in place of guanine. Thioguanine metabolite incorporation into DNA leads to strand breaks, the frequency of which correlates with cytotoxicity.

Thioguanine is cell cycle specific for the S phase.

Pharmacokinetics. Thioguanine reaches its peak action in 6 to 8 hours. It has a half-life of 80 minutes to 90 minutes and is excreted in the urine.

Therapeutic uses. Thioguanine is used with clients with acute leukemias. The combination of ara-C and thioguanine is effective in adults with acute myelogenous leukemia, but the combination of ara-C and an anthracycline is usually more effective. Thioguanine is often employed as a third drug in these regimens. Thioguanine is also active in the blast crisis of chronic myelogenous leukemia and in acute lymphocytic leukemia.

Thioguanine has also been used as an immunosuppressant agent.

Dosage and administration. Consult Table 48-3 for usual dosages.

Adverse reactions. Adverse reactions include bone marrow suppression and GI symptoms, but fewer of the latter may occur with thioguanine than with mercaptopurine.

Drug interactions. The inactivation of thioguanine is different from that of mercaptopurine, and thioguanine is not metabolized by xanthine oxidase. Thus, no reduction in thioguanine dose is needed if allopurinol is used.

No significant drug interactions have been identified with the use of thioguanine.

Pentostatin

Pentostatin was isolated in 1974 from culture bottles of *Streptomyces antibioticus*. This purine analogue is considered a restricted drug, and information about it may be obtained from the Investigational Drug Branch, National Cancer Institute. It is also classified as an adenosine deaminase inhibitor.

Pharmacodynamics. Pentostatin is an inhibitor of adenosine deaminase, an enzyme that has its greatest activity in lymphoid tissues. Inborn deficiency of adenosine deaminase is highly toxic for T lymphocytes; this observation led to interest in the enzyme or enzyme inhibition as a treatment for T-cell tumors. Adenosine deaminase functions to control intracellular adenosine levels through the irreversible deamination of adenosine and deoxyadenosine. Clients treated with pentostatin thus accumulate deoxyadenosine and deoxyadenosine 5-triphosphate. Accumulation of deoxyadenosine 5-triphosphate correlates with cell death. Possible cytotoxic mechanisms include inhibition of DNA or RNA synthesis, impairment of DNA integrity, or disruption of adenosine triphosphate–dependent cellular processes (Black, Livingston, 1990).

Therapeutic uses. Pentostatin is used in the treatment of hairy cell leukemia. This disease had been resistant to chemotherapy but now responds to interferon-alpha and pentostatin. Complete remission rate seems higher with pentostatin. It is unclear if an advantage exists to one of these agents over the other for initial treatment of hairy cell leukemia, but pentostatin is active in clients resistant to interferon. Clients treated first with other agents for chronic lymphocytic leukemia respond to pentostatin.

Adverse reactions. The toxicity of pentostatin is dose-related. Acute renal failure and CNS side effects (*eg*, lethargy, coma, seizures) have been reported. Myelosuppression appears to relate more to the underlying disease than to the use of pentostatin. Other side effects reported include hepatic dysfunction, keratoconjunctivitis, and mild nausea and vomiting.

Drug interactions. No significant drug interactions have been identified with the use of pentostatin.

■ Summary

Antimetabolites are cycle-dependent antineoplastic drugs that are effective in phase S of the cell cycle. The antimetabolites include folic acid analogues, pyrimidine analogues, and purine analogues. Specific agents include methotrexate and mercaptopurine, significant in managing acute lymphocytic leukemia.

Nursing management

Nursing process

Assessment It is important for the nurse to assess the overall physical status of each client before the chemotherapy program begins. These baseline data become essential in the nurse's subsequent monitoring of the client for therapeutic and nontherapeutic drug actions.

The nurse should also determine whether the client is using other medications that may interfere with the chemotherapy program.

It is the nurse's responsibility to monitor the results of a variety of laboratory tests; which tests are necessary depend on what drugs are part of the chemotherapeutic program. For example, if the drug is likely to cause bone marrow suppression, culture reports (*eg*, urine, vaginal, rectal, mouth, sputum, blood, and skin), complete blood cell counts and differentials, and coagulation tests (*eg*, platelet count, prothrombin time, and partial thromboplastin time) need to be reviewed. For the client who is receiving a cardiotoxic drug, the nurse needs to assess heart sounds, venous pressure, intake and output, and weight, as well as to monitor electrocardiograms. If the drug is likely to cause nephrotoxicity, the nurse needs to assess urine output and specific gravity and to monitor serum plasma concentration of urea, creatinine, uric acid, and the electrolytes (Na, K, Mg, Ca). For the client who is receiving a neurotoxic drug, the nurse needs to assess musculoskeletal and neurologic systems. If an ototoxic drug is being administered, the nurse needs to assess the client's ability to hear (*eg*, whisper test, watch test, Weber and Rinne tests). For a client who is receiving a drug that may be hepatotoxic, the nurse needs to monitor the results of serum bilirubin and alkaline phosphatase tests.

Nursing diagnosis   Most clients who receive anti-neoplastic agents have cancer. Because of the nature of neoplastic disease, almost any of the recognized nursing diagnoses may apply to the client. For the cancer client who is being treated specifically with chemotherapy, the most applicable diagnoses include:

> *Anxiety related to life-threatening disease*
> *Knowledge deficit related to the diagnosed malignancy and its treatment*
> *Body image disturbance related to malignancy of body cells or to alopecia (weight loss, other body changes) secondary to chemotherapy*
> *Anticipatory grieving related to life-threatening disease or a poor prognosis*
> *Ineffective individual coping related to debility (perceived threat to life, inability to fulfill role functions, anxiety) secondary to malignant disease or chemotherapy*
> *High risk for infection related to bone marrow suppression secondary to chemotherapy*
> *Potential for impaired tissue integrity related to irritation and sloughing secondary to extravasation of vesicant drugs (see Chapter 49)*
> *Constipation related to adverse reactions to chemotherapy*
> *Diarrhea related to adverse reactions to chemotherapy*
> *Impaired physical mobility (activity intolerance, self-care deficit) related to malignancy or adverse reaction to chemotherapy*
> *Altered oral mucous membranes related to cell injury secondary to chemotherapy*
> *Pain related to malignancy or tissue injury secondary to chemotherapy*
> *Altered nutrition: less than body requirements related to anorexia, nausea, and vomiting secondary to chemotherapy*
> *High risk for fluid volume deficit related to chemotherapy*

Common collaborative problems that should be differentiated from the nursing diagnoses include

> *Potential complication: nephrotoxicity*
> *Potential complication: neurotoxicity*
> *Potential complication: ototoxicity*
> *Potential complication: hemorrhage*

Planning   In preparing a plan of client care, the nurse should set goals to achieve specific client outcomes. These outcomes include a decrease in anxiety, verbalization of understanding of the chemotherapeutic program, adaptation to changes in body appearance and function, progression through the grieving process, use of effective coping skills, absence of the variety of injuries that potentially could occur, absence of diarrhea or constipation, achievement of maximum physical mobility and activity tolerance, performance of self-care activities within physical limitations, maintenance of integrity of oral mucous membranes, diminished discomfort, maintenance of optimal nutritional status, and maintenance of fluid and electrolyte balance.

Interventions   The nursing interventions for clients who receive chemotherapy focus on five of the nursing diagnoses listed previously. These were chosen because they occur so frequently and because they emphasize the caring aspects of nursing management for an illness that has a great emotional impact on the client.

Body image disturbance.   The client with cancer who receives antineoplastic agents is frequently at risk for alopecia, causing the client to experience a disruption in their perception of their body image. Alopecia serves as a visible reminder of the cancer and its treatment and makes it difficult to deny the reality of the cancer. The antineoplastic drugs that can cause a great deal of hair loss include cyclophosphamide, ifosfamide, mechlorethamine, hexamethylmelamine, busulfan, streptozocin, dacarbazine, methotrexate, fluorouracil, floxuridine, and ara-C (discussed in this chapter), as well as bleomycin, daunorubicin, doxorubicin, etoposide, mitomycin-C, vinblastine, vincristine, and vindesine (see Chapter 49). Other drugs also have the potential to cause alopecia (*eg*, certain antibiotics, anticoagulants, anticonvulsants, hormones, and others).

Antineoplastic agents damage the DNA of the stem cells, resulting in atrophy of the hair follicle, producing weak brittle hair that either breaks off at the surface of the scalp or is spontaneously released from the hair follicle. The dose and length of drug exposure determine the degree and duration of hair loss. Alterations in a client's physiologic status (*ie*, contact dermatitis, hormonal dysfunction, herpes zoster, secondary or tertiary syphilis, pernicious anemia, and protein malnutrition) can increase the degree and duration of alopecia.

Clients must be informed when alopecia is probable. Alopecia varies from thinning to partial or complete baldness and affects all body hair. Hair loss usually occurs 2 or 3 weeks after chemotherapy begins; loss may be gradual or sudden.

Clients should be reassured that when the antineoplastic agent is discontinued, their hair will grow again but may be of a different color and texture. Scalp hair usually grows about a half inch each month.

The use of wigs or toupees, hats, scarves, and turbans should be explored with clients. Purchase of a wig before the hair falls out allows clients to match their own hair color and style.

The client should be referred to the American Cancer Society. In some regions, the Society provides new or used wigs free of charge. A wig is a tax-deductible medical expense. Some insurance companies reimburse cancer therapy recipients for the cost of their wigs because the purchase is directly related to medical treatment. The physician is asked for a prescription for "cranial hair prosthesis" and a statement of diagnosis. These are submitted with a copy of the receipt for the wig with a completed insurance form.

If a wig is not worn, the head needs to be covered in the summer to prevent sunburn and in the winter to prevent heat loss. A visit to a makeover specialist is helpful to learn eyebrow and eyelash application and eyeliner use. Dark-rimmed eyeglasses may be worn to conceal the loss of eyebrows and eyelashes.

The client should be taught interventions that minimize hair loss, such as using a mild protein-based shampoo and a cream rinse or hair conditioner every 3 to 5 days, avoiding hair dryers, curling irons, electric curlers, or bristly rollers, braids, ponytails, elastic bands, clips, barrettes, bobby pins, hair spray, hair dye, and permanent solutions.

In an attempt to prevent alopecia, many techniques, such as scalp tourniquets, scalp sphygmomanometers, and various turbans and caps for scalp hypothermia, have been tried. Since the scalp is supplied by superficial blood vessels from the subcutaneous tissues and the external carotid arteries, these methods decrease the blood circulation by causing vasoconstriction, or, if the drug is temperature-sensitive, the amount of drug absorbed. This then minimizes contact between the drug and the dividing hair follicle stem cells. These methods, since introduction in the 1960s, have not been recommended for certain cancers (such as hematological malignancies). In addition, many inconsistencies in study methodologies have limited conclusions that could be drawn about client benefit from these techniques.

Then in 1990 it became evident that the hypothermia caps were being marketed without fulfilling the requirements set forth in the Federal Food, Drug, and Cosmetic Act. Furthermore, it appears that microscopic scalp metastases may receive an inadequate dose of chemotherapy when such devices are used and that such metastases may have been responsible for certain deaths. Thus, the commercial sale of all scalp cooling devices has been halted. It is not known how long it will take for manufacturers to provide sufficient data to meet Federal Food, Drug, and Cosmetic Act regulations.

The client who is experiencing alopecia should be encouraged to share concerns, fears, and perceptions of the impact of alopecia on the client's life, spouse, children, friends, and coworkers. Significant others need to have opportunities to share feelings and fears.

High risk for infection related to the development of bone marrow suppression. Bone marrow suppression or myelosuppression in clients with cancer can result from tumor invasion of the bone marrow, chemotherapy, or radiotherapy. Anemia, thrombocytopenia, and neutropenia are the three most clinically significant complications that result from bone marrow suppression. Although anemia and thrombocytopenia can produce serious clinical problems, transfusions (*eg*, packed red blood cells and platelets) can usually correct or minimize related complications.

Neutropenia may be manageable, but at its worst it can progress to septicemia and septic shock. The longer the neutrophil count remains low, the more susceptible clients become to infection from endogenous and exogenous microbial flora. The risk of infection increases as neutropenia becomes more pronounced; a severe risk of infection occurs when the number of neutrophils is less than $500/mm^3$. It is estimated that 80% of the infections that occur in clients with cancer arise from endogenous microbial flora, with more than half of these occurring during hospitalization (Rostad, 1991).

All chemotherapeutic agents discussed, except vincristine, bleomycin, mithramycin, asparaginase, and mitotane (see Chapter 49), create a high risk of generalized bone marrow suppression, including neutropenia. In addition to the risk of infection associated with the antineoplastic agent, clients may also be exposed to infection by the presence of invasive devices, such as urinary catheters or venous access devices.

A variety of organisms may be the source of infection in the neutropenic client. Bacterial pathogens constitute the most frequent cause of infection and include the gram-negative organisms, *Escherichia coli*, *Klebsiella pneumoniae*, *Enterobacter* species, and *Pseudomonas aeruginosa*, and the gram-positive organisms, *Staphylococcus aureus*, *Staphylococcus epidermidis*, and *Streptococcus* organisms. The sites of infection usually are the lungs, urinary tract, skin wounds, IV or urinary catheter sites, the perianal and rectal area, the pharynx, and the mouth.

Other pathogens include *Candida albicans* and *Aspergillus* and *Cryptococcus* species. These fungal infections commonly occur in clients who have prolonged neutropenia and who receive protracted courses of antibiotics.

Viral and parasitic infections are observed, including infection with *Pneumocystis carinii* and herpes viruses (herpes simplex virus, varicella-zoster virus, and cytomegalovirus). Infection with *P. carinii*, usually transmitted through the air, is identified by a low fever, a dry nonproductive cough, dyspnea, x-ray evidence of pulmonary infiltrates, and hypoxemia.

Clients with neutropenia are often at home. Home is usually regarded as a safer environment than the hospital when considering sources of infection, but education is necessary to make home care of the client maximally effective. Education of the client and family about white blood cells and normal immunologic function, neutropenia and its relationship to the client's situation, signs and symptoms of infection, and measures to prevent or manage infection is a nursing responsibility.

Signs and symptoms associated with infection may be less apparent in immunocompromised clients as compared to immunocompetent clients. Inhibition of phagocytic cells minimizes the signs and symptoms of inflammation and infection. Nevertheless, the body's ability to generate fever in response to infection usually remains intact (Rostad, 1991). However, it should be noted that although fever may be the most reliable indicator of infection it could also be due to other causes, such as transfusion reaction or tumor lysis. In the home setting, clients should know how to take their temperature and what to report to whom; the nurse should check the client's skill at reading a thermometer. They should also be instructed how to maintain a record of the temperature and to take this record to each hospital, clinic, or doctor visit. Fever patterns may help to identify the cause of infection. For example, a pattern of intermittent fevers is often seen with gram-negative septicemia, while a slowly rising temperature that remains elevated may indicate a fungal infection. Two or three low-grade fevers (38°C) or a single elevation above 38.5°C in clients with neutropenia are indications to notify the physician so appropriate action can be taken.

At home clients should follow strict hand-washing procedures. They should be taught the importance of hand-washing before eating, as well as after urination and defecation. Clients with neutropenia can get an infection from an organism being transferred from one part of their body to another (endogenous organisms).

The client should be advised to limit contact with family and friends who have an infectious illness or who are potentially infected. Clients should wear a mask when out of the protective environment of the home. Sources of environmental contaminants (*eg*, stagnant water, pet litter, and potted plants) should be eliminated. Specific measures should be explained to try to avoid infection at common sites, such as pulmonary exercises (lungs); copious fluids, frequent voiding, and avoidance of douches and tampons (genitourinary tract); aseptic contact lens care (eyes); oral care regimen (mouth); antimicrobial soap and avoidance of injury (skin); meticulous care (existing wounds or sites of invasive devices).

With the hospitalized client, the client may be placed in a private room, screening is undertaken to avoid client contact with infected or potentially infected visitors and staff, and strict hand-washing procedures are followed. These steps constitute the simplest approach to protective precautions. Sometimes a total protective environment is used, including a laminar airflow room, with sterilization of the entire room and its contents and of every item brought into the room. The client may be "decontaminated" through use of oral nonabsorbable antibiotics, skin antiseptics, and antibiotic sprays and ointments.

Preventing infection in clients with neutropenia may include immunoprophylaxis (with IV gamma globulin) and immunomodulation (with various agents, including lithium carbonate and vaccines).

Oral nonabsorbable antibiotics have been used in regimens designed to reduce the amount of exogenous GI flora. Drugs used include vancomycin, gentamycin, polymyxin, and nystatin. However, lack of palatability, nausea, vomiting, and diarrhea may limit compliance with the ordered drug regimen.

The best prevention against viral and fungal infection is minimizing client contact with sources of these pathogens. Drugs that may be used prophylactically for these organisms include amantadine (against influenza A) and acyclovir and vidarabine for infections by herpes viruses. The use of amphotericin B, miconazole, clotrimazole, and ketoconazole have been tried for antifungal prophylaxis. Susceptible fungi are eradicated, but an overgrowth of more resistant fungi (*eg*, *Aspergillus* organisms) frequently occurs. Amphotericin B is associated with serious side effects, including nephrotoxicity, hepatotoxicity, and electrolyte imbalance.

If the client does acquire an infection, combination therapy with broad-spectrum antibiotics are used, including penicillins, cephalosporins, and aminoglycosides. However, with the third-generation cephalosporins and others, single-agent regimens may be more likely in the future. Some antibiotics and antineoplastic agents are incompatible; the client usually has one IV line for the chemotherapeutic agent and one for the antibiotic. Because early symptoms of fungal infection are not easily detected, diagnosis is difficult. If the client is still febrile and neutropenic, even with antibiotic therapy, an antifungal agent may be added. Treatment of a fungal infection is prolonged.

The neutropenic client who experiences septicemia that is not controlled becomes at risk for septic shock. The mortality rate from septicemia ranges from 10% to 40% and as high as 70% in clients with multiple pathogens (Rostad, 1991). The signs of early septic shock are fever with or without chills, warm, dry skin, confusion, tachypnea, and tachycardia. Late findings in septic shock include irritability and restlessness, cold clammy skin, rapid shallow breathing, thready pulse, and oliguria. Clients with septic shock are critically ill and unless treatment is immediate and aggressive irreversible organ damage and death occur.

The risk of infection goes down as the white blood cell count goes up, and some clients have been given granulocyte transfusions. However, this treatment has not been as effective as hoped and is not usually advocated.

High risk for injury (nephrotoxicity) related to chemotherapy. Several antineoplastic drugs pose a threat to the client's urinary tract, such as cyclophosphamide (which causes a severe hemorrhagic cystitis) and cisplatin (which causes renal toxicity with damage to the proximal tubules). Antineoplastic drugs that are nephrotoxic include cisplatin, methotrexate, streptozotocin, nitrosoureas, cyclophosphamide, vincristine, asparaginase, adriamycin, mithramycin, and mitomycin C. Other treatment-related entities that indicate urinary tract damage include radiation nephritis, hyperuricemic nephropathy, tumor lysis syndrome, and obstruction from ureteral or bladder tumors or retroperitoneal fibrosis.

Monitoring for nephrotoxicity may be difficult because a 75% to 80% loss of renal function may occur before significant laboratory changes or client symptomatology develop. Measures of BUN, serum creatinine, and 24-hour creatinine clearance can be monitored by the nurse, as well as urine color, *p*H, specific gravity, urinary concentration and acidification capacity, and absence or presence of glucose, proteins, blood, or ketones. The nurse is also able to compare the results of current laboratory data with the initial assessment data, including any pre-existing medical disorders that affect renal function and prescription or nonprescription medication. Allergic reactions to drugs, dyes, or blood components should also be noted because they can result in renal damage.

Monitoring for nephrotoxicity includes evaluation of fluid and electrolyte status by checking vital signs, fluid intake and output, weight, edema, skin turgor, and cognitive changes. Changes in vital signs can reveal dehydration or fluid overload, infection, and hypertension. Weight loss may indicate dehydration, nausea and vomiting, or anorexia, whereas weight gain in excess of 2.2 lb may be a reliable indicator of edema. Other reliable signs of fluid overload include dyspnea, neck vein distension, elevated blood pressure, pitting edema, or periorbital edema. Cognitive changes such as decreased ability to concentrate, lack of coordination, and increase in fatigue can also be signs of renal impairment.

Altered oral mucous membranes. The antineoplastic drugs that commonly cause alterations in oral mucous membranes (such as stomatitis) include cyclophosphamide, lomustine, methotrexate, fluorouracil and floxuridine, and ara-C (discussed in this chapter), as well as bleomycin, dactinomycin, daunorubicin and doxorubicin, mitomycin, and hydroxyurea (see Chapter 49).

Cells in the oral mucosa have one of the highest proliferation rates in the body, making them more susceptible to chemotherapy than cells in other kinds of healthy tissue. Younger cancer clients tend to have more oral complications than adults because the mitotic index of oral mucosa is highest in younger people.

Normal mucosal cells live 10 to 14 days. The rate of cell formation stays the same, even if the rate of cell death increases. When antineoplastic drugs are used, oral mucosa atrophies and thins out. Minor trauma can disrupt the remaining thin layer of mucosa and produce ulceration. Damage to the oral mucosa reverses itself unless problems occur, such as secondary infection. Bone marrow suppression with thrombocytopenia and neutropenia, simultaneously caused by the chemotherapy, increases the potential for secondary infection by opportunistic agents such as gram-negative bacteria, fungi, and viruses.

The nurse must encourage meticulous oral hygiene to try to prevent oral mucosa complications. Teeth should be brushed at least twice a day with a soft-bristle toothbrush and nonabrasive toothpaste. Unwaxed dental floss should be used daily but gently. A water pick may be used at a low setting.

Various agents have been used for oral care. Generally, the mouth should be rinsed three to four times a day. Normal saline may be used. A nonirritating mouthwash that can be made at home consists of 1 tsp baking soda and 1 tsp salt in 1 cup of warm water. Commercial rinses that contain a lot of salt or alcohol (*eg*, Listerine) must be avoided.

Flossing and even brushing may need to be discontinued when thrombocytopenia exists. If the teeth cannot be brushed, the nurse should clean the client's mouth with a 2-inch gauze pad soaked in solution and wrapped around a tongue blade. Do not use lemon and glycerin swabs; glycerin absorbs water and dries out the mucosa.

Dentures, partial dentures, and orthodontic devices should be removed for cleansing twice a day and may need to be removed entirely or for certain periods of time during the day. All mouth lesions should be cultured. To prevent or treat candidiasis, nystatin oral suspension, 500,000 to 1,000,000 U, may be swished and swallowed four to six times a day. It also comes as a vaginal troche that can be dissolved orally or as a powder that is reconstituted and frozen. Use should be continued for 48 hours after the resolution of lesions.

One way to prepare the nystatin in frozen form is as nystatin ice cups. The ingredients include 60 million U of nystatin powder, 300 ml black cherry concentrate, and 1,800 ml of sterile water. The nystatin powder is mixed with 300 ml of sterile water to make a solution, black cherry concentrate is added, and further sterile water is added to make a total volume of 1,800 ml. The mixture is stirred or shaken well and poured into 30 ml unit-dose cups (it makes 60 cups, 1 million U nystatin each). The cups are frozen and then one cup is eaten four times a day, using a spoon (Yasko, 1986).

If pain becomes a problem, topical anesthetic solutions may be used. Gargling 15 to 20 minutes before meals may help a client feel more comfortable. All topical anesthetic solutions have advantages and disadvantages. An example of one frequently used solution is Xylocaine Viscous 2%. This agent does decrease pain that occurs with swallowing, but the effect is brief, the taste is unpleasant to some people, and others dislike the feeling of numbness.

It may be necessary to adjust the diet. Have clients avoid foods with citric acid because it causes mucosa to "burn." Pear and peach nectars, warm tea (not hot), liquid gelatin, custards, and yogurt may be tolerated. Rough foods and very hot foods should be avoided. Spicy foods that contain pepper, chili powder, and nutmeg may bother the mouth more than spices like cinnamon, garlic, and oregano. Carbonated beverages and ices, such as Popsicles, are usually well tolerated. Sauces and gravies can be added to solid foods, and foods may be pureed.

Cigarette smoking and drinking alcohol should be discouraged; both irritate mouth tissues.

Altered nutrition: less than body requirements related to anorexia, taste changes, nausea, and vomiting due to chemotherapy. Anorexia, nausea, and vomiting are common adverse reactions to chemotherapy. They often produce a compromised nutritional status

that can lead to physical debilitation. The presence of nausea and vomiting may cause a client's treatment regimen to be delayed, altered, or discontinued. Some agents have a higher likelihood of causing emesis than others (Table 48-4).

Some authors have defined the emetogenic potential of antineoplastic agents as high, moderate, or low as a way to classify the agents. An agent with high emetogenic potential is defined as one with which more than 90% of clients experience nausea and emesis within 1 to 6 hours after the agent is administered (*eg*, cisplatin). An agent with moderate emetogenic potential (*eg*, cyclophosphamide, nitrogen mustard) causes moderate to severe nausea or emesis in 30% to 90% of clients with an onset of 2 to 12 hours after chemotherapy is started. Low emetogenic potential is defined as when less than 30% of clients experience nausea or mild to moderate emesis with the standard dosage (*eg*, fluorouracil, methotrexate; Wickham, 1989).

The onset and duration of emesis also varies among the agents. Some agents are associated with a delay between administration of the drug and the onset of the emesis. Differences in the degree of nausea and vomiting occur among agents, among individuals, and even among treatment courses in the same individual. When combinations of antineoplastic drugs are used, more than one of the various possible emetic pathways may be stimulated simultaneously, resulting in severe nausea and vomiting. An important concept about chemotherapy-induced nausea and vomiting is the absence of a negative feedback loop within the

Table 48-4. Emetogenic potential of selected neoplastic agents

Agent	% of time that agent induces emesis	Onset of emesis (hr)	Emesis duration (hr)
cisplatin (Platinol)	more than 90	1–6	24–48
dacarbazine (DTIC-Dome)	more than 90	1–3	1–12
mechlorethamine (Mustargen)	more than 90	0.5–2	8–24
carmustine (BCNU)	60–90	2–4	4–24
cyclophosphamide (Cytoxan)	60–90	4–12	4–10
dactinomycin (Actinomycin D)	60–90	2–6	12–24
plicamycin (Mithramycin)	60–90	4–6	12–24
daunorubicin (Cerubidine)	30–60	2–6	24
doxorubicin (Adriamycin)	30–60	4–6	6
fluorouracil (Adrucil)	30–60	3–6	—
mitomycin (Mitomycin-C)	30–60	1–4	48–72
bleomycin (Blenoxane)	10–30	3–6	—
cytarabine (ara-C)	10–30	6–12	3–5
etoposide (Vepesid)	10–30	3–8	—
methotrexate (Mexate)	10–30	4–12	3–12
vinblastine (Velban)	10–30	4–8	—
vincristine (Oncovin)	less than 10	4–8	—

(Adapted from: Martin Jr. JK and Norwood MB. (1988). Pharmacist management of antiemetic therapy under protocol in an oncology clinic. *American Journal of Hospital Pharmacy*, 45, p. 1327.)

emetic system. Thus, even with an empty stomach, protracted uncontrolled vomiting and retching can occur.

Learning experience 48-1

Assess a client who is experiencing anorexia, nausea, and vomiting due to antineoplastic drug therapy. Take a thorough dietary history. Prepare a detailed care plan to help the client cope with these side effects. Consider the client's food likes and dislikes, meal patterns, food associations, and environmental factors.

Other causes of nausea and vomiting in clients with cancer include GI obstruction, stimulation of the vagal nerves as a result of gastric distention or pain, hypercalcemia, hyponatremia, renal dysfunction, biliary obstruction, high anxiety levels, and radiation therapy to the chest, abdomen, back, or hypothalamus.

The nurse's assessment of factors that place the client at increased risk of developing anticipatory nausea or vomiting is used when developing interventions. These factors include a history of nausea or vomiting in response to stressful events, history of a "nervous stomach," age of 40 years or less, history of motion sickness, and previous experience with cancer therapy-related nausea or vomiting (Yasko, 1986).

The best intervention for nausea and vomiting is prevention. Studies have shown that a combination of antiemetic drugs with different mechanisms of action, higher doses, and round-the-clock administration are all more effective than single agents and as-needed dosage schedules.

The antiemetics most commonly used for chemotherapy-induced nausea and vomiting are classified as dopamine antagonists (*eg*, prochlorperazine [Compazine], metoclopramide [Reglan], and droperidol [Inapsine]) and nondopamine antagonists (*eg*, dexamethasone [Decadron], lorazepam [Ativan], and dronabinol [Marinol]).

Of the dopamine antagonists, prochlorperazine (Compazine) is the most frequently used phenothiazine. It blocks the dopamine receptors of the chemoreceptor trigger zone. The usual dose is ineffective in controlling chemotherapy-induced nausea and vomiting. Higher doses achieve better control of nausea and vomiting (*ie*, 20 to 40 mg every 30 minutes before and 3 and 6 hours after the start of chemotherapy). Also, prochlorperazine as Compazine Spansules 30 mg seems especially effective against delayed-onset nausea and vomiting. The usual dosage is 30 mg orally three times a day on day 1, 30 mg orally twice a day on day 2, and then 15 mg orally twice a day on days 3 to 5.

Metoclopramide (Reglan) is useful, although its duration of action is only 2 to 3 hours, so it must be administered frequently. It blocks dopamine and acts peripherally to enhance gastric emptying. Metoclopramide should be administered at 2 to 3 mg/kg. Metoclopramide often causes diarrhea as a result of its direct effect on GI motility. This side effect may be prevented by antidiarrheal medications administered the day before, the day of, and the day after chemotherapy (Peters, 1989).

Droperidol (Inapsine) is a butyrophenone related to haloperidol (Haldol). It has not been used as widely, so its dosage is less standardized, ranging from 1 to 15 mg.

The antiemetic mechanisms of action of the nondopamine antagonists are less clear. Steroids such as dexamethasone (Decadron) and methylprednisolone (Solu-Medrol) decrease emesis. Steroids may be used IV before and during chemotherapy for acute emesis and orally after chemotherapy for delayed and persistent nausea and vomiting. It has been proposed that the steroids provide antiemetic effects by interference with the permeability of the chemoreceptor trigger zone to chemical input or by affecting prostaglandin activity in the glial cells (Wickham, 1989).

The anxiolytic lorazepam (Ativan) is the benzodiazepine usually used because of its anterograde amnesic properties (*ie*, dose-related memory loss) and its sedative effects. It decreases the response of the true vomiting center to a variety of afferent stimuli. Administering lorazepam sublingually before administration of IV chemotherapy had the advantages of reducing anticipatory symptoms, avoiding hepatic first-pass effect, providing high serum levels, and being able to be administered in a small dose initially.

Several combination regimens have been used, including the following:

Regimen 1

Prochlorperazine: 30 to 40 mg in 50 ml D5W for 20 minutes before chemotherapy and 3 hours after

Diphenhydramine: 50 mg IV before prochlorperazine

Dexamethasone: 20 mg IV before chemotherapy and 8 mg orally qid for 2 days and 4 mg orally qid for 2 days

Prochlorperazine: 30 mg spansules tid for 2 days and bid as needed

Regimen 2

Metoclopramide: 1 to 2 mg/kg IV 30 minutes before and every 2 hours for 3 doses

Dexamethasone: 20 mg IV 30 minutes before chemotherapy

Lorazepam: 0.04 mg/kg IV 30 minutes before chemotherapy and every 4 hours orally for two doses after chemotherapy as needed

Diphenhydramine: 50 mg IV before first dose of metoclopramide (Peters, 1989)

The cannabinoids, dronabinol (Marinol) and nabilone (Cesamet), are two other nondopamine antagonists. Dronabinol has been shown to be as effective as low-dose prochlorperazine, but it is not generally used as a first-line antiemetic. The cannabinoids were tried because of reports of decreased emesis in clients who used marijuana while they received chemotherapy.

All drugs have side effects. The side effects most commonly caused by antiemetics are sedation, hypotension, and extrapyramidal symptoms. Sedation may be viewed as a positive side effect, but some clients do not like to be sedated. Oversedation may occur if the drugs are given to elderly clients with liver or renal damage or to clients who are receiving narcotics or other CNS depressants.

Extrapyramidal symptoms occur with metoclopramide, butyrophenones, and phenothiazines. Younger clients (younger than age 30) are more likely to experience extrapyramidal symptoms. Akathisia or uncontrolled motor restlessness is the most common. Dystonia is characterized by spasms in muscle groups, usually the muscles of the neck or jaw (trismus or torticollis). The recommended treatment for akathisia is 0.5 to 2 mg of a benzodiazepine such as lorazepam. Dystonia can be reversed with diphenhydramine (Benadryl) IV or IM or with benztropine (Cogentin) (Wickham, 1989).

Various authors point out that dietary adjustments do not make any significant difference in the degree of anorexia, taste changes, nausea, and vomiting a client experiences. Clients may become conditioned to dislike certain foods as "sick" foods or dislike "reward" foods if these foods are consistently associated with nausea and vomiting. These are learned food aversions. So that a client does not develop an aversion to favorite foods, it may be wise not to offer those foods at the time of chemotherapy sessions. Interventions that help relieve nausea during pregnancy, other illness, or times of stress should be used.

Clients with cancer may report changes in taste perception that contribute to their anorexia. These changes seem to be related to both the disease process and its therapy. Commonly reported taste alterations include hypogeusia, ageusia, dysgeusia, a decreased threshold for the bitter taste sensation that manifests as a constant or intermittent bitter taste sensation or an aversion to foods with high amino acid levels, an increased threshold for the sweet taste sensation (*ie*, more sugar is needed to achieve the pre-illness sweet taste sensation), an aversion to sweet foods, and metallic or medicinal taste sensation that manifests as a continuous or intermittent taste sensation unrelated to food intake (Yasko, 1986).

Clients who experience alterations in taste sensations such as an aversion to meats may find the taste less offensive if the meats are offered cold rather than hot. Chicken or ham in a salad or roast beef in a sandwich may be more acceptable, partly because the odor tends not to be as strong as when they are served hot. Use of plastic rather than metal utensils may reduce the bitter taste. Meats can be marinated in soy sauce or fruit juice and cooked with fruit to improve their taste.

If the meat aversion seems to increase throughout the day, a high-protein breakfast should be encouraged. Eggs and cheese should be encouraged because they are usually not rejected.

If zinc therapy has been prescribed in relation to the changes in taste sensation, the nurse should instruct the client to take the medication toward the middle of a meal and with a snack at bedtime to minimize potential GI symptoms.

Cold foods or room temperature foods are usually better tolerated than warm or hot foods for the client with anorexia, taste changes, nausea, or vomiting.

If the oral mucosa is dry, water, saline, or artificial saliva may be sprayed on the mucous membranes as often as necessary. Artificial saliva is commercially prepared and available by prescription. Suggested products include OREX Oral Lubricant and Xero-Lube. Lips can be lubricated with K-Y Jelly, cocoa butter, or Chapstick. In this situation, the client should be advised to chop meat or dry food that is difficult to swallow and serve it with gravy or broth. Salad dressings or mayonnaise may be added to vegetables to increase the ease of swallowing them.

The client should be advised to add to foods to increase food value of what is eaten. For example, nonfat dry milk powder may be added to milk, beaten eggs may be added to fruit juices, condensed soups can be diluted with milk instead of water, and extra sugar may be put on cereal.

Clients should avoid greasy foods because they take longer to leave the stomach. Carbohydrate-containing foods (*eg*, noodles or rice) leave the stomach more quickly. The volume in the stomach can be reduced by avoiding liquids at mealtimes and by drinking them 1 hour before or after eating. If the client "craves" a certain food, this should be provided if at all possible, because clients seem to tolerate foods they crave.

Clients may find it best not to cook themselves because the odors may contribute to their nausea. Clients should sit in another room or take a walk while the food is being cooked. Seeing food can decrease the appetite. Clients can be advised to keep foods out of sight except when eating.

Use of a liquid diet may be helpful with anorexia, taste changes, nausea, or vomiting. Liquids such as apple juice, cranberry juice, lemonade, fruit ades, broth, Gatorade, ginger ale, 7-Up, Popsicles, gelatin, tea, or cola are usually well tolerated. Liquids should be sipped slowly.

Sour foods such as lemons, sour pickles, hard sour candy, or lemon sherbet may be experimented with. The mouth can be rinsed with a mixture of lemon juice and water (if stomatitis is not present). Sugar-free mints or sugar-free gum may be used to mask unpleasant taste sensations.

Various eating patterns may be experimented with. Nausea that occurs in association with chemotherapy is usually not consistently severe throughout the day. It may be intermittent and occur more at one time of day than another. It is possible to identify periods when nausea is at a minimum so that food may be provided then, even if it is not consistent with the usual dietary routine. Some clients avoid eating or drinking for 1 to 2 hours before and after chemotherapy. Some follow a clear liquid diet for 1 to 12 hours before chemotherapy and for 1 to 24 hours after chemotherapy. Some eat a large meal 3 to 4 hours before therapy and then eat lightly for the rest of the day. Some eat frequent light meals throughout the day and find it helpful if hospital-provided meals are not laden with food. Trays should be simplified, containing smaller servings and even smaller dishes. Six small meals are better than the usual three. The three in-between meals should be composed of high-calorie, high-protein foods.

Stimuli such as sights, sounds, or odors that can initiate nausea (unpleasant odors, strong perfume, or other people who are nauseated or vomiting) should be avoided. Bedpans and urinals should be out of sight at meal time. Ostomy care, dressing changes, and other unpleasant treatments should not be scheduled too close to meal time.

Proper positioning in a semi-Fowler's or high Fowler's position accommodates digestion. Mouth care before meals may help increase appetite by eliminating unpleasant tastes. Washing the client's hands and face before meal time is important. Company (provided by the family or by having a group of clients eat together) makes the meal more normal and may help to increase the client's intake. Distractions like enjoyable music or a favorite television program may help. Techniques such as relaxation techniques with or without positive visual imagery may be helpful.

Client education. The nurse should provide information and literature about the specific type of cancer to the client and family, and the anticipated results of the selected antineoplastic drugs should be explained.

The nurse should provide the client and family with information and literature about the antineoplastic drugs being used. The types of adverse reactions that clients may be expected to experience must be identified for the client and family. The nurse should identify how and where to contact their health care providers to report any adverse reactions, ask questions, or to request clarification of instructions. The importance of complying with all aspects of the therapeutic regimen should be stressed.

The nurse needs to identify interventions that may be used to cope with specific adverse reactions. With the drugs discussed in this chapter, alopecia, bone marrow suppression with anemia, thrombocytopenia, and neutropenia, nephrotoxicity, stomatitis, anorexia, taste changes, nausea, and vomiting are the likely adverse reactions that will be experienced. Specific interventions for these adverse reactions are outlined in the sections on nursing process. In some situations, the client needs to take additional medications (such as with nausea and vomiting). Details of the protocol for additional medications need to be explained to the client and family.

Some of the antineoplastic drugs mandate that the client be monitored with a variety of laboratory tests. The client and family need to know when and where they need to go to have the laboratory work done. The results of the laboratory tests may need to be explained to the client and family.

The local cancer support groups and their specialized functions in the respective community should be explained to the client and family, and specific information should be given about how to contact them.

Evaluation The nurse must evaluate the client to determine drug efficacy and to observe for evidence of adverse reactions. Data that indicate efficacy include a reduction in fear and anxiety, verbalization of understanding of the chemotherapeutic program, adaptation to changes in body appearance and function, verbalization of feelings about the diagnosis of cancer and chemotherapy, expression of grief, use of available support programs, verbalization of ability to cope with chemotherapy and its effects, and identification of stressors and ways to cope with them. Other factors are absence of diarrhea, constipation, bone marrow suppression, cardiotoxicity, nephrotoxicity, neurotoxicity, and ototoxicity, maintenance of an optimal level of physical mobility and an increased tolerance for activity, increased ability to carry out activities of daily living, maintenance of healthy gums and oral mucous membranes, verbalization of relief of discomfort, maintenance of weight within normal range and normal skin turgor (see the previous Examples of Nursing Process to Treat Cancer of the Ovary and to Treat Acute Lymphocytic Leukemia).

Checklist of nursing actions

☐ Monitor laboratory data for evidence of side effects (*eg*, neutropenia, thrombocytopenia, anemia, hepatotoxicity, nephrotoxicity).

☐ Teach clients about the drugs—what to report to the physician and what to do if adverse reactions occur.

☐ When adverse reactions are experienced, follow suggested nursing interventions.

☐ When alopecia will occur, inform the client, help the client to find a wig or beauty consultants, assist the client to pursue financial assistance with wig if available, and teach the client what interventions to follow to minimize hair loss.

☐ When neutropenia occurs, monitor laboratory data, obtain physical assessment data, teach strict hand-washing procedures, advise client on interventions to follow to minimize development of infection, carry out protective precautions or total protective environment concepts, and administer antibiotics and other antimicrobial agents as ordered.

☐ When nephrotoxicity is likely to occur, monitor laboratory data, obtain physical assessment data, and carry out prehydration and post-hydration protocols as ordered.

☐ When stomatitis occurs, obtain physical assessment data following designated assessment instrument, encourage meticulous oral hygiene, help client carry out oral care protocol as ordered, and adjust diet appropriately.

☐ When anorexia, taste changes, nausea, or vomiting occur, carry out antiemetic protocol as ordered and adjust diet with client to facilitate appropriate intake.

References

Black DJ, Livingston RB. (1990). Antineoplastic drugs in 1990: A review (Part I). *Drugs, 39(4)*, 489–501.

Black DJ, Livingston RB. (1990). Antineoplastic drugs in 1990: A review (Part II). *Drugs, 39(5)*, 652–673.

Department of Drugs, Division of Drugs and Toxicology. (1990). *Drug Evaluations Annual*. Milwaukee, WI: American Medical Association.

DeVita Jr. VT, Hellman S, Rosenberg SA, eds. (1989). *Clinical Pharmacology of Cancer Chemotherapy*, 3rd ed. Philadelphia: JB Lippincott.

Dukes MNG, Beeley L. (1990). *Side Effects of Drugs Annual 14*. Amsterdam, Netherlands: Elsevier Science Publishers B. V.

Evans S. (1991). Nursing measures in the prevention and treatment of renal cell damage associated with cisplatin administration. *Cancer Nurs, 14(2)*, 91–97.

Goodman M. (1987). Cisplatin: Outpatient and office hydration regimens. *Semin Oncol Nurs, 3*(Suppl.), 36–45.

Kenny SA. (1990). Effect of two oral care protocols on the incidence of stomatitis in hematology patients. *Cancer Nurs, 13(6)*, 345–353.

Krasnow SH. (1990). Carboplatin: Current uses in oncology. *Drug Therapy*, 63–65 (Dec).

Lydon J. (1989). Assessment of renal function in the patient receiving chemotherapy. *Cancer Nurs, 12(3)*, 133–143.

Metheny NM. (1987). *Fluid and electrolyte balance: Nursing considerations*. Philadelphia: JB Lippincott.

Peters CA. (1989). Myths of antiemetic administration. *Cancer Nurs, 12(2)*, 102–106.

Porth CM. (1990). *Pathophysiology: Concepts of altered health states*, 3rd ed. Philadelphia: JB Lippincott.

Rostad ME. (1991). Current strategies for managing myelosuppression in patients with cancer. *Oncology Nursing Forum, 18*(Suppl. 2), 7–15.

Wickham R. (1989). Management of chemotherapy-induced emesis. In *Oncology Nursing Perspectives, Proceedings of a Symposium* (pp 4–10).

Yasko JM, ed. (1986). *Nursing management of symptoms associated with chemotherapy*. Columbus, OH: Adria Laboratories.

Bibliography

Anderson JL. (1989). The nurse's role in cancer rehabilitation. *Cancer Nurs, 12(2)*, 85–94.

Averette HE, Boike GM, Jarrell MA. (1990). Effects of cancer chemotherapy on gonadal function and reproductive capacity. *CA, 40(4)*, 199–209.

Cassileth BR, Berlyne D. (1989). Counseling the cancer patient who wants to try unorthodox or questionable therapies. *Oncology, 3(4)*, 29–34.

Check WA. (1990). Lessons from MOPP: 26 years old and still first-line. *Oncology Times, 12(5)*, 6–8.

Dunne CF. (1989). Safe handling of antineoplastic agents. *Cancer Nurs, 12(2)*, 120–127.

Gilman AG, et al, eds. (1990). *Goodman and Gilman's the pharmacological basis of therapeutics*, 8th ed. New York: Pergamon Press.

Goodman H. (1989). Managing the side effects of chemotherapy. *Semin Oncol Nurs, 5*(2, Suppl. 1), 29–52.

Gullatte MM, Graves T. (1990). Advances in antineoplastic therapy. *Oncology Nursing Forum, 17(6)*, 867–876.

Karp JE, Merz WG, Dick JD, Saral R, Burke PJ. (1990). Management of infectious complications of acute leukemia and antileukemia therapy. *Oncology, 4(7)*, 45–54.

Lanning RM, von Roemeling R, Hrushesky WJM. (1990). Circadian-based infusional FUDR therapy. *Oncology Nursing Forum, 17(1)*, 49–56.

Low AW. (1990). Prevention of pressure sores in patients with cancer. *Oncology Nursing Forum, 17(2)*, 179–184.

Lerman C, Rimer B, Blumberg B, Cristinzio S, Engstrom PF, MacElwee N, O'Connor K, Seay J. (1990). Effects of coping style and relaxation on cancer chemotherapy side effects and emotional responses. *Cancer Nurs, 13(5)*, 308–315.

Mahon SM. (1989). Signs and symptoms associated with malignancy-induced hypercalcemia. *Cancer Nurs, 12(3)*, 153–160.

Moss RW. *The cancer industry: Unravelling the politics*. New York: Paragon House.

Noyes DD, Mellody P. (1988). *Beauty and cancer*. Los Angeles: AC Press.

Poe CM, Taylor LM. (1989). Syndrome of inappropriate antidiuretic hormone: Assessment and nursing implications. *Oncology Nursing Forum, 16(3)*, 373–381.

Saba MT, Magolan JM. (1991). Understanding cerebral edema: Implications for oncology nurses. *Oncology Nursing Forum, 18(3)*, 499–505.

Steiner I, Siegal T. (1989). Muscle cramps in cancer patients. *Cancer, 63*, 574–577.

Sticklin LA, Dubbelde K, Larson E. (1989). Nursing care of the patient receiving subcutaneous low-dose ara-C therapy. *Oncology Nursing Forum, 16(3)*, 365–369.

Travaglini J, Nevidjon B. (1990). Complications related to cancer therapy. *Clinical Advances in Oncology Nursing, 2(2)*, 1–7, 11–13.

Wickham R. (1989). Managing chemotherapy-related nausea and vomiting: The state of the art. *Oncology Nursing Forum, 16(4)*, 563–574.

Winningham ML, MacVicar MG. (1988). The effect of aerobic exercise on patient reports of nausea. *Oncology Nursing Forum, 15(4)*, 447–450.

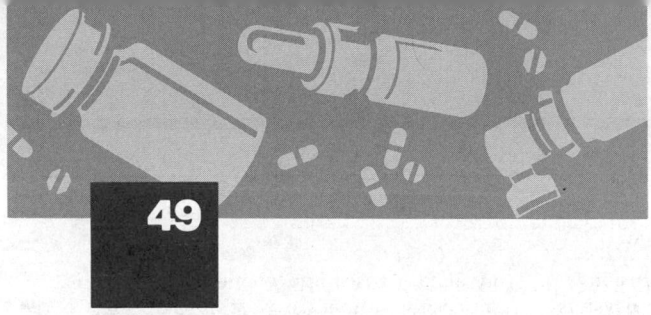

49

Other antineoplastic agents

Natural products

Natural products used in antineoplastic therapy include plant alkaloids, antibiotics, and enzymes.

Plant alkaloids

Vinca alkaloids

Table 49-1 summarizes material on the plant alkaloids.

The properties of the periwinkle plant, *Vinca rosea*, have been described in medicinal folklore. Owing to the purported hypoglycemic effects, the plant was studied in the laboratory, but no significant ability to lower glucose could be documented. However, it was discovered that the plant caused suppression of bone marrow function. This information led to the development of vinca alkaloids, vinblastine and vincristine. Structurally, they are very similar; the only difference is that vinblastine substitutes a methyl group for the formyl group in vincristine. However, their adverse reactions are very different. A third analogue, vindesine (Eldesine) is categorized as an investigational drug (see Focus on Vinca Alkaloids: Similarities and Differences).

Pharmacodynamics. Both vinblastine and vincristine bind to tubulin, a key component of macrotubules and the mitotic spindle. They prevent assembly of the microtubular components of the mitotic spindle, leading to arrest of cell division in metaphase.

Since microtubules are also involved in other cellular processes, the vinca alkaloids may affect other functions as well. For example, they inhibit the secretion of some hormones (*eg*, glucose-induced insulin release and thyrotropin-mediated thyroid hormone secretions; *Drug Evaluations Annual, 1990*).

Vinblastine

Pharmacokinetics. Vinblastine is poorly absorbed when given orally. About 80% of the drug is bound to plasma proteins. Multiphasic plasma clearance occurs, with the first half-life 0.06 hour, the second half-life 1.6 hours, and the third half-life 25 hours. Most vinblastine is excreted by the liver into the biliary system, with about 30% excreted in stool and 21% excreted in urine. Vinblastine penetrates the blood–brain barrier poorly.

Table 49-1. Plant alkaloids

Drug name	Preparation	Usual dosage/PC	Adverse reactions
Vinca alkaloids			
vinblastine (Velban)	Powder for preparing solutions for IV infusion	Continuous IV infusion, 2 mg/m²/day for 5 days; as part of VBP regimen 4–8 mg/m² days 1 and 2, repeat cycle q 21–28 d PC: D	Myalgia, nausea and vomiting, leukopenia, mucositis, stomatitis, glossitis, alopecia, Raynaud's phenomenon, neurotoxicity, extravasation causes tissue damage
vincristine	Solution for IV infusion	Adult: 1.4 mg/m²/week; maximum dose 2 mg/m² Child over 1 yr: 2 mg/m²/week for 4 weeks PC: D	Neurotoxicities (*eg*, decreased DTRs, paresthesia, ataxia, slapping gait, footdrop, cranial nerve deficits; constipation, abdominal pain, paralytic ileus, bowel obstruction), SIADH, alopecia, extravasation causes tissue damage
Epipodophyllotoxins			
bleomycin (Blenoxane)	Powder for preparing solutions for IV, IM, subcutaneous, intracavitary, intravesical, and intraarterial injection	10–20 U/m² once or twice weekly for total dose of 300–400 U PC: D	Pulmonary toxicity, cutaneous toxicity (*eg*, erythema, pruritus, thickening, desquamation, hyperpigmentation, hyperesthesia, ulceration), alopecia, stomatitis, Raynaud's phenomenon, hypertension, hypersensitivity reactions, idiosyncratic reaction in lymphoma clients

KEY: PC = pregnancy category. (The validity of pregnancy risk categories has not been established; see Chapter 16, p 216.)

Therapeutic uses. Vinblastine is used in many combination regimens (such as CVPP, VBC, VDP; doxorubicin, bleomycin, vinblastine, and dacarbazine (ABVD); MVAC, vinblastine, bleomycin, and cisplatin (VBP); see Example of Nursing Process and VBP Therapy). In the VBP combination, it is used as the agent of choice in disseminated nonseminomatous testicular cancer. It is a component of the ABVD regimen, which is an effective alternative to the combination of mechlorethamine, Oncovin, procarbazine, and prednisone (MOPP) in the treatment of Hodgkin's disease (see Chapter 48).

It is also used for non-Hodgkin's lymphomas, breast cancer, non–small cell lung cancer, neuroblastomas, head and neck cancer, cutaneous T cell lymphoma, histiocytosis X (Letterer-Siwe disease), and Kaposi's sarcoma. Vinblastine has been used effectively when a lymphoma has been refractory to alkylating agents and when choriocarcinoma has become refractory to methotrexate.

Dosage and administration. Vinblastine may be administered by continuous intravenous (IV) infusion (2 mg/m²/day for 5 days) or by IV bolus. Dosage is decreased with hepatic dysfunction because of the liver's role in vinblastine excretion. A reduction of 50% is recommended in clients with bilirubin levels above 3 mg/100 ml. No reduction is recommended for clients with impaired renal function (DeVita, et al, 1989).

A typical dosage of the VBP regimen for testicular cancer is 4 to 8 mg/m² IV on days 1 and 2, with the cycle repeated every 21 to 28 days. Due to the potential damage from extravasation, the correct technique

must be used when administering vinblastine (see discussion under Nursing Management).

Adverse reactions. Side effects with vinblastine include myalgia, mild to moderate nausea and vomiting, and bone marrow suppression. Leukopenia is usually dose-limited, with the nadir occurring in 5 to 10 days and recovery in 7 to 14 days. With higher doses, the white blood cell count may not return to normal for 3 weeks. Thrombocytopenia and anemia are uncommon.

High doses can cause mucositis, stomatitis, and glossitis. Raynaud's phenomenon has been reported with vinblastine and bleomycin in testicular cancer. Alopecia occurs but is less common than with vincristine, and it is reversible.

Vinblastine causes neurotoxicity (*ie*, paresthesia, loss of deep tendon reflexes, peripheral neuritis, mental depression, headache, and seizures). Extravasation can cause profound local tissue damage.

Resistance to the vinca alkaloids may result from mutations in tubulin. Cross-resistance between the vinca alkaloids does not seem to occur.

Drug interactions. As mentioned, the combination of bleomycin and vinblastine may produce signs of Raynaud's disease in clients who are being treated for testicular cancer.

The combination of vinblastine and mitomycin C has resulted in severe bronchospasm with shortness of breath.

Concurrent use of vinblastine and glutamic acid or tryptophan inhibits the effect of the vinblastine.

The use of phenytoin with vinblastine decreases the effect of the phenytoin because of decreased plasma levels of phenytoin.

Vincristine

Pharmacokinetics. Vincristine is poorly absorbed when given orally. It is extensively bound to tissues, but it does not penetrate the central nervous system (CNS). As is the case with vinblastine, a multiphasic plasma clearance occurs for vincristine, with the first half-life 0.08 hour, the second half-life 2.3 hours, and the third half-life is 85 hours. Elimination is primarily via the biliary system, with about 70% of a dose excreted in the feces and 12% in the urine.

Focus on

Vinca alkaloids: similarities and differences

Similarities	**Differences**
Pharmacodynamics	
These agents arrest cells in the metaphase portion (M phase) of the cell cycle by crystallizing the microtubular proteins. They are thought to inhibit nucleic acid and protein synthesis.	
Pharmacokinetics	
These agents are unpredictably absorbed from the GI tract and are therefore given parenterally. They are rapidly and widely distributed to the tissues and cross the blood–brain barrier. They are metabolized by the liver and excreted in bile. They have a triphasic half-life.	• **Vinblastine** has an initial half-life of .07 hours, a second half-life of 2.25 hours, and a terminal half-life of 85 hours. • **Vincristine** has an initial half-life of 4 minutes, a second half-life of 1.6 hours, and a terminal half-life of 25 hours; small amounts of **vincristine** are excreted by the kidneys.
Therapeutic uses	
These agents are used to treat lymphomas, Hodgkin's disease, and neuroblastomas.	• **Vinblastine** is used to treat choriocarcinoma, breast, cervical, testicular cancers, and Kaposi's sarcoma. • **Vincristine** is used to treat lymphocytic leukemias, lymphosarcomas, reticular cell sarcoma, rhabdomyosarcoma, and Wilms' tumor.
Adverse reactions	
These include: (CNS) depression, paresthesia, peripheral neuropathy, loss of deep tendon reflexes, muscle pain, weakness; (RESP) acute bronchospasm; (GI) anorexia, nausea, vomiting, constipation, stomatitis, abdominal pain, cramps; (GU) urinary retention, uric acid nephropathy; (HEMA) bone marrow depression, leukopenia; (SKIN) reversible alopecia, dermatitis; (OTHER) tissue necrosis, cellulitis at injection site if extravasation occurs.	• **Vincristine** may cause neurotoxicity, vocal cord paralysis, and inappropriate antidiuretic hormone secretion. • **Vinblastine** may cause oligospermia and aspermia.
Contraindications	
These agents are contraindicated in people with severe leukopenia and bacterial infections.	• **Vincristine** is contraindicated in people with the demyelinating form of Charcot-Marie-Tooth syndrome.
Precautions	
These agents should be used with caution in people with hepatic dysfunction or jaundice.	• **Vincristine** should be used with caution in people with pre-existing neuromuscular disease and those who are receiving radiation therapy through ports, including the liver. • **Vinblastine** should be used with caution in people with ulcerated skin lesions and those with cachexia.

(continued)

Focus on

Vinca alkaloids: similarities and differences (Continued)

Similarities	Differences

Similarities

Nursing considerations

Instruct in disease, treatment, drug therapy regimen, adverse reactions, and compliance; assess pulmonary status, including respiratory rate and breath sounds, for changes; have supportive equipment available in case of severe bronchospasm; monitor vital signs for changes; monitor nutritional status; encourage diet high in protein and calories; encourage adequate fluid intake; monitor intake and output; evaluate urinary and bowel status for changes; administer stool softener, laxative agent as ordered; offer frequent mouth care; instruct client in mouth care and dietary needs; administer antiemetic before giving drug; monitor lab studies, including complete blood cell count and platelets, frequently; avoid any IM injections if platelet count drops below $100,000/mm^3$; assess for signs of occult bleeding, including checking stool and urine and watching for bruising, petechiae, and gingival bleeding; instruct client in signs of occult bleeding and need to report to physician; monitor renal and hepatic function studies for changes; avoid giving client any immunizations and instruct client to avoid contact with any person with infection; offer emotional support; explain that hair loss is temporary; offer suggestions to cope with hair loss, such as wigs, turbans, scarves; monitor uric acid levels, if increased be aware that physician may order allopurinol; administer anticoagulants and aspirin products cautiously and monitor closely for signs of bleeding; instruct client to avoid use of over-the-counter products that contain aspirin; instruct client in signs and symptoms of infection and need to notify physician; administer by IV push or infusion into a central venous catheter; treat extravasation with injection of hyaluronidase into site followed by warm or cold compresses; assess neurologic status, including complaints of numbness, tingling of extremities, and signs of foot drop; check reflexes and gait; institute safety precautions as necessary.

Differences

Assess fluid balance if client is receiving **vincristine**; monitor intake and output and weights for fluid retention; institute fluid restrictions as necessary and be prepared to administer diuretics as ordered.

Therapeutic uses. Because it does not produce serious bone marrow suppression, vincristine is used in many combination regimens (such as DVP [daunorubicin, vincristine, prednisone], AVDP [asparaginase, vincristine, daunorubicin, prednisone], COAP [cyclophosphamide, vincristine, cytarabine, prednisone], COPE [cyclophosphamide, cisplatin, etoposide, vincristine], COP [cyclophosphamide, vincristine, prednisone], COPP [cyclophosphamide, vincristine, procarbazine, prednisone], VAD [vincristine, doxorubicin, dexamethasone], and MOPP). When vincristine is combined with prednisone, complete remissions are induced in up to 90% of children with acute lymphocytic leukemia. Vincristine has also been used for induc-

Example of nursing process and VBP therapy

The client is a 30-year-old man with a diagnosis of advanced-stage testicular non-seminoma. His symptoms include the presence of a testicular mass and a feeling of heaviness. The VBP program is to be followed for his treatment (vinblastine 6 mg/m^2 IV, days 1 and 2; bleomycin 30 U IV weekly; and cisplatin 20 mg/m^2 IV days 1 through 5). This pattern will be repeated every 21 days.

The client has been married for 3 years; he and his wife have recently started thinking about having a family.

Assessment data	Nursing diagnosis	Intervention	Goals and outcome criteria
Receiving bleomycin	Potential complication: fibrosis and inflammation of lung tissue*	**Monitor** for signs and symptoms of inflammation (*eg*, dry, hacking, persistent cough, tachypnea, dyspnea, rales). **Monitor** blood-gas values, chest x-ray reports, and pulmonary function studies. If signs and symptoms of inflammation and fibrosis occur, be prepared to administer antibiotics, corticosteroids, and bronchodilators. **Carry out** interventions to improve gas exchange (*eg*, positioning, coughing and deep breathing, inspiratory exerciser).	The client will not experience signs and symptoms of pulmonary inflammation and fibrosis; if they occur, they will be promptly detected and treated.
Receiving vinblastine, bleomycin, and cisplatin	Knowledge deficit concerning adverse effects of chemotherapy	**Monitor** for therapeutic and nontherapeutic effects of the three antineoplastic drugs. **Inform** client of various possible side effects and urge him to report any evidence of them to physician immediately. **Allow** time for questions and clarification. **Stress** importance of keeping appointments for laboratory tests that monitor for possible side effects.	If bone marrow suppression, nausea and vomiting, mucositis, glossitis, Raynaud's phenomenon, or neurotoxicity develop, they will be promptly detected and treated.
Married for 3 years He and wife had started thinking about having a family Infertility is usual during PVB therapy, but fertility may return years later	Self-esteem disturbance: expected infertility related to chemotherapy	**Clarify** physician's explanation about fertility. **Provide** information about possibility of sperm banking and testicular implants. **Discuss** alternate methods of parenthood. **Include** wife in discussion and encourage her continued support of client.	The client will demonstrate adaptation to changes in body functioning as shown by comments that indicate acceptance of alternative plans for parenthood that are realistic in relation to the side effects of antineoplastic therapy.

*Although potential complications generally are not included in the Examples of Nursing Process, in this situation the identification of this collaborative problem is critical to the outcome for this client and illustrates the broad range of nursing responsibilities.

tion in acute myelogenous leukemia and for chronic lymphocytic leukemia.

Other uses of vincristine include malignant lymphomas (Hodgkin's disease and non-Hodgkin's and Burkitt's lymphoma), small cell lung carcinoma, breast carcinoma, cervical carcinoma, multiple myeloma, neuroblastoma, Wilms' tumor, and certain sarcomas (*eg*, Ewing's sarcoma, embryonal rhabdomyosarcoma).

Dosage and administration. Vincristine is available in vials as a powder to be reconstituted. Methods of administration are the same as those for vinblastine.

When used in combination therapy with children older than 1 year of age to induce remission in acute lymphocytic leukemia, the usual dose is 2 mg/m² of body surface on a weekly basis for 4 weeks. The therapeutic effect does not appear to be dose-related, and adverse reactions increase significantly without increased benefit with larger doses. Dosage is decreased with hepatic dysfunction.

Intrathecal administration is absolutely contraindicated because it has been known to cause coma, seizures, and death.

Adverse reactions. Vincristine's adverse reactions are primarily neurologic, affecting the peripheral nervous system, the CNS, and the autonomic nervous system (ANS). Neurotoxicity is significantly greater than that of vinblastine, possibly because of its longer half-life, which prolongs its contact with nerve tissue that contains high concentrations of tubulin.

Loss of the Achilles tendon reflex is usually the first sign of peripheral neuropathy. Manifestations of peripheral neuropathy include loss of the Achilles tendon reflex, a decrease in other deep tendon reflexes, paresthesia of the upper and lower extremities, ataxia, slapping gait, and foot drop. The primary muscle groups involved are the dorsiflexors of the hands and the extensors of the feet. More advanced neurotoxicity may include cranial nerve deficits (*eg*, ptosis, diplopia, abducens nerve palsy, and vocal cord paralysis). Optic atrophy and blindness have been reported.

At higher doses, involvement of the ANS causes constipation, obstipation, abdominal pain, paralytic ileus, and bowel obstruction.

Because of the neurologic complications, vincristine should be used with caution for clients with preexisting neuromuscular disease (*eg*, Charcot-Marie-Tooth disease, Friedreich's ataxia), in combination with other neurotoxic drugs, and with clients predisposed to neurologic complications (*eg*, those with diabetes or peripheral vascular disease). In some individuals with Charcot-Marie-Tooth disease, quadriplegia occurred when vincristine was used.

The syndrome of inappropriate secretion of antidiuretic hormone (SIDH) has also been observed with use of vincristine. Fluid overload, hyponatremia, and hemodilution can result.

Extravasation of vincristine produces profound local tissue damage. Vincristine also causes reversible alopecia.

Drug interactions. Mitomycin C, phenytoin, and glutamic acid, if used with vincristine, interact in the same way as has been described under vinblastine.

Use of calcium channel blocking drugs with vincristine results in increased accumulation of vincristine in the cells. Vincristine decreases the effect of digoxin. The combination of methotrexate and vincristine may cause hypotension.

When asparaginase and vincristine are given concurrently, asparaginase decreases liver clearance of vincristine, and an increase in neurotoxicity from vincristine may result.

Concurrent use of vincristine with doxorubicin and prednisone has resulted in an increase in bone marrow depressant effects; this combination should be avoided.

Concurrent use of vincristine with probenecid or sulfinpyrazone may result in hyperuricemia and gout. Live viral vaccines should be avoided if possible when vincristine is used.

Plant alkaloids

Epipodophyllotoxins

Etoposide

Podophyllotoxin, an extract of the mandrake plant, *Podophyllum peltatum*, was used as a folk remedy by American Indians and early colonists for a variety of purposes (*eg*, catharsis, conception promotion, and treatment of poisoning, parasites, and warts). It was found to have antitumor properties, but it was too toxic for clinical use. However, two derivatives, VP-16 and VM-26, have been synthesized and have important antineoplastic applications. These derivatives differ only in a single substitution and have many similarities. Etoposide (Vepesid, VP-16) is in full use, but teniposide (VM-26) is used only on an investigational basis.

Pharmacodynamics. The mechanism of action is incompletely understood, but cells are arrested in the late S or G₂ phase of the cell cycle. These derivatives may bind with an enzyme called *topoisomerase-II* to produce cytotoxicity through single and double-strand breaks in DNA.

Pharmacokinetics. Etoposide is highly (94%) bound to serum proteins. Despite its high lipid solubility, it does not readily cross the blood–brain barrier. Concentrations of etoposide in cerebrospinal fluid range from 1% to 10% of the simultaneous value in plasma. Etoposide is eliminated predominantly in urine, largely as unchanged drug (40%) but also as metabolites.

Therapeutic uses. Etoposide is used mainly for

the treatment of testicular tumors in combination with bleomycin and cisplatin. It exhibits activity in small cell lung carcinoma and is used in combination regimens in this disease (average response rate is 40%).

It is also active against non-Hodgkin's lymphomas, acute myelogenous leukemia, choriocarcinoma, and Kaposi's sarcoma and exhibits some activity with carcinoma of the breast and with non–small cell lung carcinoma.

Dosage and administration. Etoposide is available as a solution (20 mg/ml) for IV administration and as 50-mg liquid-filled capsules for oral use. The IV dose for testicular tumors is 50 to 100 mg/m² daily for 5 days or 100 mg/m² on alternate days for three doses. Cycles of therapy are usually repeated every 3 to 4 weeks. When given orally, the dose should be doubled. Dosage by any route should be reduced in proportion to reductions in creatinine clearance.

When given IV, the drug should not be given by IV push but should be administered slowly via a 30- to 60-minute infusion (diluted in 5% dextrose injection or 0.9% sodium chloride injection) to avoid hypotension and bronchospasm. These reactions are believed to be due to solvents used in the drug's formulation.

Adverse reactions. Bone marrow suppression is the major adverse reaction to etoposide. The leukopenia is the dose-limiting feature, with a nadir of 10 to 14 days and recovery by 3 weeks. Thrombocytopenia occurs less frequently and is less severe.

Nausea and vomiting, stomatitis, and diarrhea occur in about 15% of clients treated IV and in about 55% of clients treated orally.

Alopecia is common and reversible. Fever, chills, and allergic reactions including anaphylaxis have been observed.

Mild peripheral neuropathy occurs, but this may be severe and cumulative in clients previously treated with a neurotoxic agent like vincristine. Acute neurologic dysfunction with exacerbation of pre-existing neurologic deficits was reported when high-dose etoposide was used with autologous bone marrow transplantation. This reaction occurred 9 to 10 days after etoposide treatment was initiated and did resolve after therapy with steroids.

Drug interactions. No significant drug interactions have been identified with the use of etoposide.

Antibiotics

Several antibiotics, natural products of certain soil fungi, are used in chemotherapy. They produce their effects by forming complexes with DNA, thereby inhibiting DNA activities. The antibiotics used in chemotherapy include bleomycin, dactinomycin, daunorubicin, doxorubicin, mitomycin, mitoxantrone hydrochloride, and plicamycin. Table 49-2 summarizes material on the antibiotics (see Focus on Antibiotic Antineoplastic Agents: Similarities and Differences).

Bleomycin

Bleomycin (Blenoxane) was first isolated in 1962 from *Streptomyces verticillus* obtained from a soil sample in a Japanese coal mine. More than 200 congeners of bleomycin exist.

Pharmacodynamics. The cytotoxic action of bleomycin results from its ability to fragment DNA.

Bleomycin first binds to DNA. Ferrous iron is bound to nitrogen-containing groups of bleomycin. The bleomycin-ferrous iron complex catalyzes reduction of molecular oxygen to superoxide or hydroxyl radicals, causing DNA strand breaks and inhibition of DNA synthesis (Department of Drugs, 1990). Bleomycin seems most active during the G_2 phase of the cell cycle.

Pharmacokinetics. Bleomycin is not absorbed orally and therefore must be administered parenterally. It concentrates particularly in the skin, lung, kidney, peritoneum, and lymph nodes, but it does not enter the cerebrospinal fluid. The half-life is 2 to 4 hours, and 45% to 70% is recovered in the urine as active drug.

Deactivation of bleomycin is apparently due to the enzyme bleomycin hydrolase, which is found in normal and most malignant cells of certain tissues and is especially prominent in the liver. The enzyme, however, is found in low concentration in the lung and skin.

Therapeutic uses. Because it does not produce serious bone marrow suppression, bleomycin is used in several combination regimens. The combination of VBP is a combination of choice in disseminated non-seminomatous testicular cancer and is also effective with disseminated seminomatous testicular cancer. The combination of ABVD is an effective alternative to MOPP (see Chapter 48) in the treatment of Hodgkin's disease.

Bleomycin has been used for non-Hodgkin's lymphoma, squamous cell carcinomas of the head and neck (*eg*, buccal mucosa, tongue, tonsil, and pharynx), cervix, and esophagus.

Bleomycin has been administered intravesically to treat recurrent bladder tumors (although this use has caused severe cystitis), intracavitarily to manage malignant pleural or peritoneal effusions, and intra-arterially.

Dosage and administration. Bleomycin is available in ampules as a powder. For intramuscular (IM) or subcutaneous use, the ampule contents are dissolved in 1 to 5 ml of sterile water for injection, sodium chloride injection, or 5% dextrose injection. For IV use, the ampule contents are dissolved in 5 ml or more of sodium chloride injection or 5% dextrose injection and

Table 49-2. Antibiotics

Drug name	Preparation	Usual dosage/PC	Adverse reactions
dactinomycin (Actinomycin D, Cosmegen)	Powder for preparing solutions for IV infusion	Adult: 10–15 µg/kg IV/day for 5 days, repeat every 3–4 weeks Child: 100–400 µg/day for 10–14 days PC: C	Leukopenia, thrombocytopenia, anorexia, nausea, vomiting, abdominal pain, diarrhea, stomatitis, cheilitis, glossitis, proctitis, cutaneous toxicity, alopecia, interactive reaction with radiation, hypersensitivity reactions, extravasation causes tissue damage
etoposide (VP-16, Vepesid)	Oral capsules, and concentrated solutions for dilution and IV infusion	50–100 mg/m²/day IV for 5 days PC: D	Leukopenia and thrombocytopenia, nausea, vomiting, stomatitis, diarrhea, alopecia, hypersensitivity reactions, peripheral neuropathy
Anthracyclines			
daunorubicin (Cerubidine)	Powder for preparing solutions for IV infusion	30–60 mg/m²/day for 3 days, repeat at 3- to 6-week intervals PC: D	Leukopenia, thrombocytopenia, stomatitis, alopecia, GI disturbances, cutaneous toxicity, cardiotoxicity, extravasation causes tissue damage
doxirubicin	Powder for preparing solutions for IV infusion	20 mg/m²/week PC: D	Cardiotoxicity (acute and delayed), leukopenia, thrombocytopenia, stomatitis, esophagitis, nausea, vomiting, alopecia, facial flushing, conjunctivitis, lacrimation, "adriamycin flare," hypersensitivity reactions, extravasation causes tissue damage
mitomycin (Mitomycin-C, Mutamycin)	Powder for preparing solutions for IV infusion	10–20 mg/m² every 6 to 8 weeks PC: D	Myelosuppression, anorexia, nausea, vomiting, stomatitis, alopecia, skin rashes, pulmonary toxicity, cardiomyopathy, nephrotoxicities
Mitoxantrone hydrochloride (Novantrone)	Concentrated solutions for dilution and IV infusion	For induction with ANLL, 12 mg/m² every day on days 1 to 3, with cytarabine given as a continuous infusion over 24 h on days 1 to 7 PC: D	Nausea, vomiting, diarrhea, alopecia, mucositis, stomatitis, bone marrow suppression, fever, GI bleeding, cardiotoxicity
plicamycin (Mithracin)	Powder for preparing solutions for IV infusion	Hypercalcemia: 25 µg/kg given over period of 4–6 h, daily for 3–4 days, repeated at weekly intervals; testicular tumors: 25–30 µg/kg every day or every other day for 8–10 doses or until toxicity intervenes PC: X	Anorexia, nausea, vomiting, diarrhea, stomatitis, bleeding syndrome, fever, hyperpigmentation, acneiform rashes, drowsiness, lethargy, malaise, headache, depression, abnormal liver function tests, abnormal renal function tests

KEY: PC = pregnancy category. (The validity of pregnancy risk categories has not been established; see Chapter 16, p 216.)

administered slowly over 10 minutes (IV bolus method). Continuous IV infusions may be used, but glass bottles should be used because plastic containers may absorb the drug.

One milligram has been defined as 1 U of activity. A typical dose is 10 to 20 U/m² once or twice weekly to a total dose of 300 to 400 U. Dosage modifications (decreases of 50% to 75%) are required in clients with impaired renal function.

Clients with a lymphoma-like non-Hodgkin's lymphoma appear to be at risk for an idiosyncratic reaction when bleomycin is used, and some have recommended that the client receive a test dose of 1 to 2 U before administration of a therapeutic dose.

Intracavitary dosage for pleural effusion is 15 to 240 U diluted in 100 ml of normal saline, with instillation after thoracostomy tube drainage.

Adverse reactions. Bleomycin causes minimal bone marrow suppression and minimal nausea and vomiting.

As mentioned above, lung tissue contains low concentrations of the bleomycin hydrolase, which deactivates bleomycin. The low concentrations of this enzyme can result in pulmonary toxicity which will limit the dosage of bleomycin that can be used. Clients especially at risk for this toxicity are those 70 years of age or older, those who are receiving a total dose of 400 U or more of bleomycin, those who have received pulmonary or mediastinal irradiation, and those with under-

Focus on

Antibiotic antineoplastic agents: similarities and differences

Similarities

Pharmacodynamics

These agents interfere with the growth of malignant cells and inhibit DNA and RNA synthesis. They inhibit protein synthesis by inhibiting DNA-dependent RNA synthesis, by directly inhibiting RNA synthesis, by altering DNA and inhibiting RNA synthesis, or reacting with DNA to cause strand breakage. They appear to act by intercalation between base pairs, inhibiting DNA and RNA synthesis by template disordering and steric obstruction.

Pharmacokinetics

These agents are poorly absorbed orally and therefore are given parenterally. They are widely distributed. They are metabolized by the liver and excreted primarily in bile.

Therapeutic uses

These agents are used to treat tumors associated with Hodgkin's disease, non-Hodgkin's lymphoma, testicular and gastric cancer, and sarcoma.

Adverse reactions

These include: (CNS) anxiety, confusion, headache; (GI) nausea, vomiting, diarrhea, sore throat, stomatitis, anorexia; (HEMA) bone marrow depression, leukopenia; (SKIN) reversible alopecia, erythema, desquamation, hyperpigmentation; (OTHER) fever, chills redness, pain at injection site.

Differences

- **Bleomycin** affects G_2 and M phases of cell division.
- **Dactinomycin** and **daunorubicin** are cell cycle nonspecific.
- **Doxorubicin** is cell cycle specific for the S phase of cell division. • **Mitomycin** is cell cycle nonspecific and causes cross-linking of DNA, inhibiting DNA and, to a lesser extent, RNA synthesis. • **Plicamycin** lowers serum calcium concentrations, but the exact mechanism is unknown.

- **Bleomycin** is excreted unchanged in the urine and its metabolism is unknown; it has a terminal half-life of 2 hours.
- **Dactinomycin** is minimally metabolized by the liver, and only small amounts are excreted in urine; it has a plasma half-life of 36 hours. • **Daunorubicin** is excreted in small amounts in the urine and has a terminal half-life of 18.5 hours. • **Doxorubicin** is excreted in small amounts in the urine and has a terminal half-life of 16.5 hours. • **Mitomycin** is also metabolized by the kidneys, brain, and heart; it is excreted primarily in the urine with small amounts excreted in bile and feces; it has a terminal half-life of 50 minutes. • **Plicamycin** is distributed mainly to the Kupffer cells of the liver and renal tubular cells; it crosses the blood–brain barrier; its metabolism is unknown, and it is primarily excreted by the kidneys.

- **Plicamycin** is used to treat hypercalcemia and hyperuricemia associated with neoplasms. • **Dactinomycin** is used to treat squamous cell carcinoma, melanomas, and trophoblastic tumors. • **Daunorubicin** is used for remission induction for acute nonlymphocytic leukemia. • **Doxorubicin** is used to treat bladder, kidney, cervical, ovarian, and brain cancer. • **Mitomycin** is used to treat pancreatic, colon, and head and neck cancer.
- **Doxorubicin** and **mitomycin** are also used to treat breast and liver cancer.

- **Bleomycin** may cause hyperesthesia of the scalp and fingers, vesiculations, hardening and discoloration of the palmar and plantar surfaces, fine crackles, dyspnea, cough, and pulmonary fibrosis. • **Dactinomycin** may cause abdominal pain and severe damage to soft tissues. • **Doxorubicin** and **daunorubicin** may cause irreversible cardiomyopathy, electrocardiographic changes, arrhythmias, pericarditis, myocarditis, nephrotoxicity, and transient red urine. • **Doxorubicin**, **daunorubicin**, and **mitomycin** may cause severe cellulitis, ulceration, or tissue sloughing if extravasation occurs. • **Mitomycin** may cause paresthesia. • **Plicamycin** may cause lethargy, metallic taste, proteinuria, elevated blood urea nitrogen and creatinine levels, decreased serum calcium, potassium, and phosphorus, and irritation and cellulitis if extravasation occurs.

(continued)

Focus on

Antibiotic antineoplastic agents: similarities and differences (Continued)

Similarities

Contraindications

These agents are contraindicated in people with a history of hypersensitivity, severe infection, and impaired bone marrow function.

Differences

• **Dactinomycin** is contraindicated in people with chicken pox or herpes zoster, and in pregnant and breastfeeding females, infants less than 6 months of age, and those with renal and hepatic impairment. • **Doxorubicin** and **daunorubicin** are contraindicated in people with severe myelosuppression, pre-existing cardiac disease, and hepatic or renal dysfunction. • **Mitomycin** is contraindicated in people with white blood cell counts of less than 3,000/mm³, platelets less than 75,000/mm³, serum creatinine greater than 1.7 mg/100 ml, and those with coagulation disorders and prolonged prothrombin times. • **Plicamycin** is contraindicated in people with thrombocytopenia, coagulation disorders, and electrolyte imbalances.

Precautions

These agents should be used with caution in people with renal impairment.

• **Bleomycin** should be used with caution in people with pulmonary impairment. • **Dactinomycin** should be used with caution in people with metastatic testicular tumors, people who have received cytotoxic drugs or radiation therapy within 6 weeks, or people with a history of gout or hematologic compromise. • **Plicamycin** should be used with caution in people with hepatic dysfunction and those who have received abdominal or mediastinal radiation.

Nursing considerations

Instruct in disease, treatment, drug therapy regimen, adverse reactions, and compliance; monitor vital signs for changes; monitor nutritional status; encourage diet high in protein and calories; administer antiemetic 30 minutes before giving drug; encourage adequate fluid intake; monitor intake and output; offer frequent mouth care; instruct client in mouth care and dietary needs; monitor lab studies, including complete blood cell count and platelets, frequently; avoid any IM injections if platelet count drops below 100,000/mm³; assess for signs of occult bleeding, including checking stool and urine and watching for bruising, petechiae, and gingival bleeding; instruct client in signs of occult bleeding and need to report to physician; monitor renal and hepatic function studies for changes; avoid giving client any immunizations and instruct client to avoid contact with any person with infection; offer emotional support; explain that hair loss is temporary; offer suggestions to cope with hair loss, such as wigs, turbans, scarves; administer anticoagulants and aspirin products cautiously and monitor closely for signs of bleeding; instruct client to avoid use of over-the-counter products that contain aspirin; instruct client in signs and symptoms of infection and need to notify physician; assess IV site and catheter patency frequently during infusion.

Prepare **bleomycin** for infusion in glass bottles; administer **bleomycin** by intracavitary, intra-arterial, or intratumoral routes or instill directly into the bladder; premedicate client with aspirin, steroids, and diphenhydramine to decrease fever and possible anaphylaxis; assess pulmonary status, including respiratory rate, breath sounds, and chest x-ray, for changes. When giving **daunorubicin** and **doxorubicin**, watch for red streaking along vein or facial flushing, which indicate too rapid infusion; warn client that urine may turn red; monitor cardiac status, including electrocardiogram and heart rate and rhythm; apply cold compresses to infusion site if extravasation occurs; discontinue infusion if tachycardia develops and obtain an electrocardiogram after infusion; never give IM or subcutaneously. Treat extravasation of **dactinomycin** with topical dimethyl sulfoxide and cold compresses. Monitor coagulation blood studies when giving **mitomycin** and **plicamycin**. If **plicamycin** IV infiltrates, stop infusion and apply ice; monitor liver enzymes, blood urea nitrogen, creatinine, calcium, potassium, and phosphorus levels; assess client for signs of calcium imbalance.

lying lung disease. Toxicity can occur at lower than the total dose of 400 U in those treated with combination therapies, such as bleomycin and cyclophosphamide (which can independently cause pulmonary toxicity).

The development of pulmonary toxicity is usually delayed and may occur 4 to 10 weeks after initiation of therapy. Symptoms include cough, dyspnea, and fever. The first signs are insidious and include rales, rhonchi, and occasionally pleural friction rubs. These signs and symptoms often precede changes identifiable by radiography.

The radiographic appearance is typical of interstitial pneumonitis and may progress to that of pulmonary fibrosis. Identifiable damage often includes bibasilar pulmonary infiltrates. Computed tomography scans and gallium scans may detect drug-induced effects before chest radiographs do. The drug should be discontinued immediately if lung reaction is detected. It should be noted that the toxicity can be potentiated by the administration of oxygen.

Some suggest that pulmonary fibrosis can be prevented with the use of corticosteroids. When bleomycin therapy is discontinued, resolution of abnormalities may or may not occur. One percent of individuals treated with bleomycin have died of this pulmonary toxicity.

The skin also lacks significant amounts of bleomycin hydrolase, so bleomycin frequently produces skin reactions. About 50% of clients develop erythema or pruritic erythema, thickening and desquamation of fingers and palms (peeling), and hyperpigmentation of skin creases with a general darkening of the skin. The changes may begin with swelling and hyperesthesia of the hands or ulcerating lesions over elbows, knuckles, and other pressure areas of the body.

Other less frequent side effects include alopecia, stomatitis, Raynaud's phenomenon, and hypertension. Hypersensitivity reactions may occur.

A peculiar idiosyncratic reaction has been observed in clients with lymphomas. It is characterized by hypotension and hyperthermia. It does not appear to be a classic anaphylactic reaction and may be related to release of an endogenous pyrogen (Gilman, et al, 1990). This has occurred in about 1% of lymphoma clients and has resulted in deaths.

Drug interactions. Bleomycin may decrease plasma levels and renal excretion of digoxin.

Dactinomycin

Dactinomycin or actinomycin D (Cosmegen) is derived from *Streptomyces parvullus*. It is the only member of a large class of similar drugs with a significant clinical use.

Pharmacodynamics. This antibiotic intercalates between adjacent quanine-cytosine base pairs of DNA, and subsequently the transcription of DNA by RNA polymerase is blocked. In addition, the drug causes single-strand breaks in DNA, possibly as a result of action with topoisomerase-II. The drug is probably cell cycle phase-nonspecific, but activity may be maximal in G_1.

Pharmacokinetics. Dactinomycin is poorly absorbed orally and thus is administered IV. Clearance of the drug from the plasma is initially rapid, but the terminal half-life is 36 hours because of slow release from tissue stores. Most of the drug is excreted unchanged in bile and urine. Dactinomycin does not cross the blood–brain barrier or enter the cerebrospinal fluid.

Therapeutic uses. The most important use for dactinomycin is the treatment of Wilms' tumor. Effective therapy of this pediatric cancer requires multiple approaches, including surgery, radiation therapy, and combination chemotherapy with dactinomycin and vincristine.

Dactinomycin is also used to treat embryonal rhabdomyosarcoma, Ewing's sarcoma, osteosarcoma, and Kaposi's sarcoma. Advanced choriocarcinoma has also been sensitive to dactinomycin.

Dactinomycin has been helpful with chlorambucil and methotrexate in clients with metastatic testicular carcinoma, but this combination is not as satisfactory as the VBP regimen.

Dactinomycin has been used as an immunosuppressant in surgical transplant procedures.

Dosage and administration. Dactinomycin is supplied as a powder to be reconstituted. One dose schedule is 10 to 15 μg/kg IV for 5 days. If no toxic manifestations occur, additional courses may be given at intervals of 3 to 4 weeks.

Daily injections of 100 to 400 μg have been given to children for 10 to 14 days. Another regimen is 3 to 6 μg/kg for a total of 125 μg/kg and weekly maintenance doses of 7.5 μg/kg. It is best to inject the medication into the IV tubing of a flowing infusion because of its vesicant property.

Adverse reactions. Bone marrow suppression (leukopenia, thrombocytopenia) is the most common dose-limiting toxicity. The nadir is usually 1 to 2 weeks after a course of the drug, and thrombocytopenia is often seen first.

Anorexia, nausea, and vomiting usually occur 4 to 5 hours after the drug is administered. Abdominal pain and diarrhea may occur. Stomatitis, cheilitis, glossitis, and proctitis are common and may be dose-limiting. Oral and gastrointestinal (GI) ulceration may develop.

Cutaneous reactions include dactinomycin folliculitis (an acneiform eruption), erythema, desquamation, and hyperpigmentation. Alopecia may occur, occurring 7 to 10 days after treatment and continuing for 2 to 4 weeks.

Combining dactinomycin and radiation leads to accelerated skin and GI toxicities. Erythema, progressing sometimes to necrosis, has been noted in areas of skin exposed to radiation therapy before, during, or after administration of dactinomycin.

Damage from extravasation may occur when dactinomycin is used. Anaphylactic reactions have also been reported.

Drug interactions. If the client who is receiving dactinomycin receives radiation as well, skin or GI reactions from the radiation are potentiated or could be reactivated if the radiation was used before the dactinomycin.

Anthracyclines

Daunorubicin and doxorubicin are anthracycline antibiotics. Daunorubicin (Daunomycin, Cerubidine) is produced by a strain of *Streptomyces coeruleorubidus* and doxorubicin (Adriamycin, Rubrex) is isolated from cultures of *Streptomyces peucetius*, var *caesius*.

Pharmacodynamics. Although significant differences in the clinical use of these two agents exist, their chemical structures differ only by a single hydroxyl group on C 14. The mechanism of action is not precisely clear, and at least three actions may contribute to cytotoxicity. These compounds can intercalate between strands of the DNA double helix. DNA intercalation does appear to trigger DNA cleavage by topoisomerase-II. Single and double-strand breaks occur. Maximum toxicity occurs during the S phase of the cell cycle. At low concentrations of drug, cells proceed through the S phase and die in G_2.

Cytochrome P450 reductase, xanthine oxidase, and cytochrome B-5 reductase all can reduce daunorubicin and doxorubicin to free radicals that, in turn, can react with molecular oxygen to yield superoxide, hydrogen peroxide, and the hydroxyl radical. It has been shown that this process kills human breast cancer cells *in vitro* (DeVita, et al, 1989). Iron plays a significant role in complexing with doxorubicin to catalyze free radical reactions such as the conversion of hydrogen peroxide to the hydroxyl radical.

Daunorubicin and doxorubicin can also react with cell membranes at low concentrations, and the resultant alterations in membrane function could help explain their cytotoxicity.

Daunorubicin

Pharmacokinetics. Daunorubicin is poorly absorbed orally and is administered IV. It is extensively tissue bound and does not cross the blood–brain barrier.

Therapeutic uses. Daunorubicin is part of the DVP combination regimen used to induce remission in acute lymphocytic leukemia in children and in the AVDP combination that may be used for relapse in this leukemia. It is used for induction with other drugs in acute myelogenous leukemia. It has shown activity with neuroblastomas, but it has not been found useful in solid tumors in adults.

Dosage and administration. Daunorubicin is available as a powder in 20-mg vials. The recommended dosage is 30 to 60 mg/m² daily for 3 days, repeated at 3- to 6-week intervals. It is generally believed that dosage should be decreased with hepatic dysfunction because of the liver's role in its metabolism. Because the renal clearance of anthracyclines is minor, dosage decreases are not necessary with renal dysfunction.

Clients should be advised that this drug may color urine red.

Daunorubicin should be administered through the tubing of a flowing IV infusion because of its vesicant nature.

Adverse reactions. The toxic manifestations of daunorubicin include bone marrow suppression, GI disturbances, and skin reactions. The bone marrow suppression is a dose-limiting factor. Leukopenia is usually more significant than the thrombocytopenia, and its nadir is between 10 and 14 days with recovery over 1 to 2 weeks. Nausea and vomiting can be mild or severe. Stomatitis occurs. Alopecia occurs and often has a sudden onset after 3 to 4 weeks of therapy, but it is usually reversible.

The cardiotoxicity parallels that described under doxorubicin.

Extravasation of daunorubicin produces profound local tissue damage. Erythema and pain usually develop within 24 hours and can progress over weeks, resulting in deep ulceration that can reach tendon and bone. The lesions heal slowly and are difficult to skin graft. Multiple measures have been tried to manage the reaction, including ice packs and local injection of steroids, bicarbonate, or saline solution (DeVita, et al, 1989).

Drug interactions. Previous or concurrent cyclophosphamide, doxorubicin, or chest irradiation potentiate daunorubicin's cardiotoxicity. If potentiation occurs, daunorubicin dose is decreased.

Doxorubicin

Pharmacokinetics. Doxorubicin is poorly absorbed orally and is administered IV; it does not appear to cross the blood–brain barrier. Rapid uptake of the drug occurs in the heart, kidney, lung, liver, and spleen. It exhibits multiphasic plasma clearance with elimination half-lives of 11 minutes, 3 hours, and about 30 hours. Doxorubicin is metabolized to doxorubicinol and others derivatives and is eliminated in bile and urine.

Therapeutic uses. Doxorubicin is used in acute leukemias and in malignant lymphomas, but, in contrast to daunorubicin, it is also active in solid tumors such as breast cancer.

Doxorubicin is often used in combination with other agents. For example, used with cyclophosphamide, vincristine, and procarbazine, it is a successful treatment for Hodgkin's disease and non-Hodgkin's lymphomas. With cyclophosphamide and cisplatin it has been used with cancer of the ovary.

Doxorubicin has been helpful with osteogenic sarcoma, Ewing's sarcoma, and rhabdomyosarcoma. It may be the best agent for managing metastatic thyroid carcinoma. It has been used with carcinomas of the endometrium, cervix, testes, prostate, head and neck, stomach, lung pancreas, and bladder. It has also been used with neuroblastomas, Wilms' tumor, and plasma cell myeloma.

Dosage and administration. Doxorubicin is available as a red-orange powder and as solutions in 5- to 100-ml containers for injection. The recommended dose is 20 mg/m² repeated every week. Dosage should be decreased with hepatic dysfunction because of the liver's role in doxorubicin metabolism.

Earlier recommendations were for IV bolus administration, but continuous infusion over 96 hours or weekly administration of doses may be the least cardiotoxic approaches to administration. These newer administration approaches may be accompanied by increased GI toxicity.

Clients should be advised that the drug may discolor urine red.

Adverse reactions. One of the most unusual aspects of the anthracyclines daunorubicin and doxorubicin is the ability of these agents to cause cardiomyopathy; it seems that the free-radical formation contributes to this toxicity. Heart tissue is able to activate doxorubicin to a free radical at multiple sites, including the mitochondria and sarcoplasmic reticulum. It is believed that free radical–induced cardiac injury results from the reaction between doxorubicin, iron, and peroxide. Thus, a cardioprotective agent has been identified, an iron chelator, but this experimental agent is not yet widely available. In addition, heart tissue has low levels of catalase, an enzyme needed in the detoxification of hydrogen peroxide. Doxorubicin also destroys glutathione peroxidase activity, a major mechanism of peroxide removal (DeVita, et al, 1989).

Two forms of cardiac toxicity occur: acute and delayed. Acute toxicity is characterized by electrocardiographic abnormalities, including ST-T wave alterations and arrhythmia.

Delayed toxicity is manifested by congestive heart failure that is unresponsive to digitalis.

Doxorubicin also produces other adverse reactions. Myelosuppression is a major dose-limiting factor, with leukopenia reaching a nadir 10 to 15 days after the initial dose with recovery occurring by the 4th week. Thrombocytopenia and anemia follow a similar pattern but may not be as severe.

Stomatitis, esophagitis, nausea and vomiting, and alopecia are common but reversible. Regrowth of hair is usually complete 2 to 5 months after treatment ends.

Erythematous streaking near the infusion site (*adriamycin flare*) is a local allergic reaction and considered benign. Fever, chills, and urticaria have been observed, and anaphylaxis may occur.

Facial flushing, conjunctivitis, and lacrimation do occur. Doxorubicin may cause a recurrence of radiation-induced skin reaction and exacerbates tissue changes due to irradiation in mucous membranes and in the liver.

Extravasation of doxorubicin produces profound local tissue damage.

Drug interactions. Increased bone marrow depression may occur if doxorubicin is given to the client who is receiving either other bone marrow depressants or radiation. A decrease in drug dosage may be indicated.

Hyperuricemia and gout may occur if doxorubicin is given with probenecid or sulfinpyrazone. Live viral vaccines should be avoided if possible when doxorubicin is used.

Previous or concurrent cyclophosphamide, daunorubicin, or chest irradiation potentiate doxorubicin's cardiotoxicity. If the client has received previous chest radiation or other cardiotoxic drugs, the maximum recommended dose for doxorubicin is reduced. Doxorubicin may decrease plasma levels and renal excretion of digoxin.

Previous or concurrent use of cyclophosphamide with doxorubicin increases the risk of hemorrhagic cystitis. Concurrent use of doxorubicin and mercaptopurine increases the risk of hepatotoxicity, and concurrent use of doxorubicin and barbiturates increases the plasma clearance of doxorubicin.

Mitomycin

Mitomycin (Mitomycin C, Mutamycin) is an antibiotic that was first isolated from *Streptomyces caespitosus* in 1958.

Pharmacodynamics. Mitomycin's molecular structure is different from the alkylating agents described in Chapter 48; however, after intracellular activation, mitomycin basically functions as an alkylating agent. It can cause interstrand and intrastrand cross-linking of DNA, which results in inhibition of DNA synthesis. In high doses, it also decreases RNA and protein synthesis. It is cell cycle nonspecific but appears to be most active in the late G_1 and early S phases.

Pharmacokinetics. Mitomycin is not absorbed orally, making parenteral administration necessary. Clearance of the drug is rapid after IV administration. The drug is widely distributed throughout body tissues, except the CNS. It is metabolized primarily in the liver.

Therapeutic uses. Mitomycin is used in the palliative treatment of various solid tumors. It is part of the fluorouracil, doxorubicin, mitomycin (FAM) regimen used in gastric adenocarcinoma. Other uses include non–small cell cancer of the lung and cervical, colorectal, breast, bladder, pancreatic, head and neck, and esophageal carcinomas. In these cases, responses to the drug are usually brief and complicated by adverse reactions. It has also been used for lymphomas and leukemias, especially chronic myelocytic leukemia.

Intraperitoneal mitomycin has been suggested for use with relapsed gynecologic cancers that involve the abdomen. Mitomycin is also used intravesically at a dose of 40 mg in 40 ml for treatment of superficial bladder cancer.

Ophthalmic solution has been used as an adjunct to surgical excision to treat primary or recurrent pterygia.

Dosage and administration. Mitomycin is available as deep blue-violet crystals in vials to be reconstituted. It is administered through the tubing of a flowing IV infusion because of its vesicant nature. A typical dose is 20 mg/m^2 given in a single dose. Toxicity includes myelosuppression that is cumulative in nature so the client must be reevaluated before such a dose can be repeated in 6 to 8 weeks. Another dose should not be administered until the leukocyte count has returned to 3,000 and the platelet count to 75,000.

Adverse reactions. The major dose-limiting toxicity of mitomycin is myelosuppression, both delayed and cumulative. Leukopenia persists for 1 to 2 weeks, and thrombocytopenia persists for 2 to 3 weeks, with recovery of the blood count in about 74% of clients within 8 weeks (Department of Drugs, 1990).

Anorexia, nausea, vomiting, and stomatitis occur frequently, Alopecia, skin rashes, and cardiomyopathy have been reported.

Pulmonary fibrosis occurs occasionally and can be severe. It manifests as interstitial pneumonitis, presenting with dyspnea, nonproductive cough, and fever. It has been suggested that steroid administration at the time of mitomycin therapy may prevent this toxicity (Black, Livingston, 1990). The incidence of this toxicity is higher in those who are receiving both mitomycin and a vinca alkaloid or doxorubicin.

Renal failure, often associated with microangiopathic hemolytic anemia can occur in a syndrome called the *hemolytic-uremic syndrome.* Both hemolysis and renal failure appear to be precipitated by renal vascular endothelial injury from the drug. This syndrome seems to be dose-related and seems more likely to occur when mitomycin is used with fluorouracil.

Glomerular sclerosis has been reported after several months of therapy and is manifested by increased levels of blood urea nitrogen and serum creatinine and often severe hypertension.

Drug interactions. Concurrent use of vinca alkaloids and mitomycin causes severe bronchospasm and shortness of breath.

Mitoxantrone hydrochloride

Mitoxantrone hydrochloride (Novantrone) was originally synthesized as a structural analogue of doxorubicin. Mitoxantrone hydrochloride is classified as an anthraquinone. As a synthetic compound it is not a true antibiotic, but some of its actions resemble those of many antibiotics.

Pharmacodynamics. The mechanism of action is not definitively understood, but mitoxantrone hydrochloride does inhibit both RNA and DNA synthesis. An electrostatic mode of DNA binding is thought to be involved in the generation of DNA strand breaks in cells treated with mitoxantrone hydrochloride. It is not cell cycle specific, but it seems most active in the late S phase of cell division.

Pharmacokinetics. Mitoxantrone hydrochloride is rapidly and extensively distributed in tissues after administration, except that distribution to the brain, spinal cord, cerebrospinal fluid, and eyes is low. It is highly bound to plasma proteins. The drug is excreted through both the feces (via the bile) and the urine. It has a half-life of both 12 to 15 minutes and of 1 to 2 days (the latter probably reflects release of the drug from tissue binding sites).

Therapeutic uses. Mitoxantrone hydrochloride is used in a variety of combination regimens for therapy of acute nonlymphocytic leukemia and acute myelogenous, promyelocytic, monocytic, and erythroid leukemias in adults.

It also has produced some response in clients with metastatic breast cancer and malignant lymphoma (primarily non-Hodgkin's).

Dosage and administration. The drug comes in an aqueous solution that must not be frozen and that must be diluted before use with a minimum of 50 ml of either 5% dextrose injection or 0.9% sodium chloride injection. The diluted solution is given into a freely running IV infusion of 5% dextrose or 0.9% sodium chloride over 3 minutes. Care should be taken to avoid extravasation, of course, but it does not appear to be a vesicant. It should not be mixed in the same infusion as other drugs (*eg,* precipitation may occur with heparin).

Adverse reactions. Clients should be informed that mitoxantrone hydrochloride may color urine, sclera, and skin a greenish-blue color for 24 hours after therapy. Sometimes the vein used for administration develops a bluish discoloration, but this resolves within a few hours. Painful onycholysis has occurred in those treated with mitoxantrone hydrochloride. Blue discoloration of nails and reversible loss of fingernails have been reported.

Rapid lysis of tumor cells may cause hyperuricemia and may require concurrent administration of allopurinol.

Myelosuppression is the major adverse reaction. The nadir occurs in 1 to 2 weeks, and recovery is noted by the 3rd week. The major effect is leukopenia, with anemia and thrombocytopenia occurring relatively infrequently.

Other adverse reactions include nausea, vomiting, mucositis, fever, and alopecia. Hepatic and renal reactions also may occur. Cardiovascular reactions that resemble those seen with daunorubicin or doxorubicin may occur, including ST-T wave changes, decreased ejection fraction, arrhythmia, myocardial infarction, and congestive heart failure.

Drug interactions. No significant drug interactions have been identified with the use of mitoxantrone hydrochloride.

Plicamycin

Plicamycin (Mithramycin, Mithracin) is produced by *Streptomyces plicatus, Streptomyces argillaceus,* and *Streptomyces tanashiensis.*

Pharmacodynamics. Plicamycin inhibits RNA synthesis more than it affects DNA synthesis. It does bind tightly to DNA in the presence of magnesium or other divalent cations. It is cell cycle nonspecific, but shows some selectivity for the S phase.

Plicamycin affects calcium metabolism and decreases blood calcium by blocking the hypercalcemic effect of vitamin D, acting on osteoclasts that normally liberate calcium from bone and preventing the action of parathyroid hormone, which normally causes calcium release.

Pharmacokinetics. Plicamycin is poorly absorbed after oral administration, making parenteral administration necessary. The drug crosses the blood–brain barrier, and cerebrospinal fluid levels are comparable to those in the blood at 4 to 6 hours. It is cleared rapidly from the blood. It concentrates in liver cells, renal tubular cells, and along formed bone surfaces. Forty percent is excreted via the urine after 15 hours.

Therapeutic uses. The major antineoplastic use of plicamycin is embryonal cell carcinoma of the testes, but it is a secondary drug because it is toxic and other effective drugs are available (such as the VBP regimen).

Lower doses have been helpful in severe hypercalcemia and hypercalciuria when associated with advanced or metastatic cancer that involves bone or produces parathyroid hormone-like substance. Its effects in this type of situation last for 7 to 21 days. In most cases, specific therapy directed against the specific neoplasm is necessary for permanent control of the serum calcium to be achieved.

Dose and administration. Plicamycin is available in vials as a powder to be reconstituted. The preparation also contains mannitol 100 mg and sufficient disodium phosphate to adjust to pH 7. For antineoplastic therapy, it is given IV in doses of 25 to 30 $\mu g/kg/day$ of body weight or on alternate days for eight to ten doses. It is diluted in 1 liter of 5% dextrose in water and administered by IV infusion over 4 to 6 hours because of its vesicant nature. In responsive tumors, some degree of regression is usually seen within 3 to 4 weeks of initial therapy. Additional courses of therapy can be given at monthly intervals.

For hypercalcemia and hypercalciuria that have not responded to conventional treatment, doses of 25 $\mu g/kg$ of plicamycin are given daily for three to four doses. This treatment may be repeated at 1-week intervals, or a single dose may be given on a weekly basis, a schedule that seems to make toxicity less of a problem.

Adverse reactions. The most important form of toxicity is a dose-related bleeding syndrome, manifested by thrombocytopenia, prolonged prothrombin time, and depressed clotting factors II, V, VII, and X. The first symptom may be an episode of epistaxis that may or may not progress to death due to uncontrolled GI hemorrhage. Plicamycin is contraindicated in clients with thrombocytopenia or coagulation disorders.

Other adverse reactions include anorexia, nausea, and vomiting, which may begin 1 to 2 hours after initiation of therapy and persist for 12 to 24 hours. Diarrhea, stomatitis, fever, hyperpigmentation, acneiform rashes, drowsiness, lethargy, malaise, headache, depression, abnormal liver function tests, and abnormal renal function tests (*eg*, proteinuria, increased serum creatinine, increased blood urea nitrogen) may occur occasionally.

A reversible "flushing" reaction has been seen in clients who receive multiple courses of the drug. Diffuse head and neck erythema progresses to edema and coarsening of facial features.

Drug interactions. No significant drug interactions have been identified with the use of plicamycin.

Enzymes

Asparaginase

Asparaginase is an enzyme derived from cultures of either *Escherichia coli* or *Erwinia carotovora* (a plant parasite). It has a mechanism of action quite different from that of other antineoplastic agents, based on the concept of nutritional deprivation.

Pharmacodynamics. Asparaginase (L-asparaginase, Elspar), catalyzes the hydrolysis of the amino acid asparagine to aspartic acid and ammonia, thus depleting the amount of asparagine available to tumor cells. Most normal tissues synthesize whatever asparagine they need. The lymphoblast in acute lymphocytic leukemia appears to lack asparagine synthetase and cannot convert aspartic acid to asparagine, but it does require asparagine for growth purposes. The asparagine-depleting action interferes with the synthesis of protein, DNA, and RNA in tumor cells. Asparaginase is probably cell cycle specific for the G_1 phase (Department of Drugs, 1990).

Leukemic cells can become resistant to asparaginase because of the emergence of strains that make asparagine synthetase or produce a mutated form of the enzyme.

Pharmacokinetics. Asparaginase is not absorbed from the GI tract and must be administered IM or IV. The plasma half-life varies from 8 to 30 hours and varies among preparations and individuals, but it is usually stable in a single individual.

The vast majority of the drug is confined within the body's vascular system because of the large molecular size. The inactivation of asparaginase is probably carried out by the immune and reticuloendothelial systems.

Therapeutic uses. Asparaginase is usually used with vincristine and prednisone to induce remission in acute lymphocytic leukemia in children.

Dosage and administration. Asparaginase is available in vials as a powder to be reconstituted. The preparation contains 80 mg of mannitol. For IM use, 2 ml of sodium chloride injection is added, and, for IV use, 5 ml of sterile water for injection or sodium chloride injection is added. When administered IV, it should be injected into the tubing of a flowing infusion of sodium chloride injection or 5% dextrose and water over a period of 30 minutes.

When given in the regimen with vincristine, the vincristine should be given before the asparaginase since administration of asparaginase may impair hepatic clearance of vincristine.

For a child, the dose schedule is 1,000 IU/kg/day for 10 successive days, beginning on day 22 of the treatment cycle, or 6,000 IU/m² on days 4, 7, 10, 13, 16, 19, 22, 25, and 28.

Adverse reactions. It was originally thought asparaginase exploited a unique difference between normal and leukemic cells, but now it is known that many normal tissues are sensitive to asparaginase. Thus, various adverse reactions to asparaginase may occur.

As a foreign protein, asparaginase is antigenic. About two-thirds of clients experience immediate side effects, including nausea, vomiting, chills, and fever. Hypersensitivity reactions that range from urticaria to anaphylactic shock occur in up to 40% of clients and can be fatal. The incidence of anaphylactic reactions is greater with IV administration than with IM administration. An intradermal skin test with 2 U of drug is recommended before the initial dose and before each subsequent dose if a week or more has elapsed (although even this step is not completely able to predict allergic reactions; allergic reactions have followed negative skin test results).

The neurotoxic reactions observed are believed to be caused by inhibition of protein synthesis in the brain. About 25% of clients exhibit a decreased level of consciousness, ranging from confusion to coma. This encephalopathy is reversible.

Both thrombosis and hemorrhage have occurred with asparaginase, possibly related to inhibition of protein synthesis.

Pancreatitis has been observed and may progress to severe (even fatal) hemorrhagic pancreatitis. Biochemical evidence of hepatic dysfunction occurs (such as elevation of liver enzymes), but these abnormalities are usually reversible with discontinuation of therapy. Acute renal insufficiency, which can be fatal, has been reported.

The drug does not result in alopecia or stomatitis. It is rarely associated with bone marrow suppression.

Drug interactions. Vincristine and asparaginase interact (see discussion under vincristine). Asparaginase should be administered after vincristine is administered to reduce the possibility of increased vincristine toxicity from this combination.

When asparaginase and methotrexate are used concurrently, the effect of methotrexate is diminished, so this combination is not recommended (see discussion under methotrexate).

When used with prednisone, the toxicity of asparaginase is increased, but administering asparaginase after prednisone may reduce this effect.

■ **Summary**
Natural products used in antineoplastic drug therapy include plant alkaloids, antibiotics, and enzymes. Vincristine's toxic effects are largely neurologic, affecting the CNS, ANS, and peripheral nervous system. Bleomycin may cause a pulmonary toxicity that may be fatal. Daunorubicin and doxorubicin both may cause cardiotoxicity, acute or delayed in nature. Mitomycin may cause two types of kidney damage among other adverse reactions, whereas plicamycin may cause a bleeding syndrome. Asparaginase has a unique mechanism of action but may also induce serious adverse reactions.

Hormones

Hormones used in antineoplastic therapy include adrenocorticosteroids, androgens, estrogens, antiandrogenic compounds, antiestrogenic compounds, progestins, synthetic estrogen antimetabolites, synthetic analogues of luteinizing hormone-releasing hormones, and synthetic analogues of somatostatin.

Adrenocorticosteroids

The adrenocorticosteroids are a group of steroid hormones produced by the adrenal cortex with similar chemical structure but varied physiologic effects. Chapter 32 provides an in-depth discussion of this group of hormones. The major adrenocorticosteroids used in antineoplastic therapy are dexamethasone (Decadron) and prednisone.

Pharmacodynamics. The precise mechanism of action of the adrenocorticosteroids is not completely understood. However, in some cancers (*eg*, breast, lymphoid, and probably endometrial), the effectiveness of adrenocorticosteroids depends on the presence of specific steroid receptor proteins in the cytoplasm or nucleus of the tumor cells. For the adrenocorticosteroid to act on lymphoblasts, binding of the hormone to the receptor is necessary. The adrenocorticosteroid interferes with mitosis in lymphocytes and lymphoid proliferation and induces cell death. The effects may result from a decrease in use of energy due to glucose deprivation (Department of Drugs, 1990). Adrenocorticosteroids are cycle-dependent and are active in phase G_1.

Therapeutic uses. In acute lymphocytic leukemia in children, an adrenocorticosteroid is used in combination with vincristine, with or without daunorubicin or asparaginase, for induction of remission. Adult leukemia has not responded to adrenocorticosteroids, but the adrenocorticosteroids are helpful in management of hemorrhagic complications of thrombocytopenia that frequently accompany malignant lymphomas and chronic lymphocytic leukemia. They can also assist in the management of frank hemolytic anemia.

Adrenocorticosteroids are components of the MOPP regimen for Hodgkin's disease, the CVP (cyclophosphamide, vincristine, prednisone) regimen in non-Hodgkin's lymphomas, and the CHOP (cyclophosphamide, doxorubicin, vincristine, prednisone) regimen in non-Hodgkin's lymphoma.

Adrenocorticosteroids are sometimes used in radiation therapy. When certain regions of the body are irradiated, adrenocorticosteroids are needed to reduce radiation edema (*eg*, in the mediastinum, brain, and spinal cord).

Adrenocorticosteroids are sometimes indicated for specific medical complications, such as hypercalcemia. Adrenocorticosteroids are used in antiemetic regimens when chemotherapeutic agents have caused nausea and vomiting. They are also used for palliation and symptomatic improvement by temporarily decreasing pain and fever while increasing appetite, strength, and a sense of well-being. If the client's physical condition improves, it then may be possible to proceed with additional antineoplastic drug therapy.

Dosage and administration. A typical daily dosage of prednisone would be 10 to 100 mg. With the induction regimen for acute lymphocytic leukemia, the dosage of the prednisone is 40 mg/m² daily in divided doses for 4 to 6 weeks.

Clients who receive long-term steroid therapy are more susceptible to infection, and sudden withdrawal of the drug or development of stress may result in acute adrenocortical insufficiency. To minimize the likelihood of these types of complications, dosage of adrenocorticosteroids should be tapered off and eventually discontinued in most cases.

Dexamethasone (Decadron) is chosen when an adrenocorticosteroid is combined with radiation therapy. The drug may be given orally, IM, or IV, and a usual dosage is 4 to 16 mg/day in divided doses.

Adverse reactions. Some adverse reactions to adrenocorticosteroids may occur with short-term use, including sodium and water retention, potassium loss, psychosis, and exacerbation of diabetes. Other reactions are more likely to occur with prolonged use, such as myopathy, osteoporosis, aseptic necrosis of bone, peptic ulceration, pancreatitis, pseudotumor cerebri, glaucoma, cataracts, hypertension, obesity, hyperlipidemia, immunosuppression, impaired wound healing, infection, striae of the skin, growth failure, amenorrhea, and suppression of the hypothalamic-pituitary-adrenal axis.

Androgens and estrogens

A detailed discussion of estrogens and androgens is given in Chapters 32 and 36. The discussion in this chapter is confined to the use of estrogens and androgens in antineoplastic therapy; this information is summarized in Table 49-3.

The rationale for using estrogens and androgens in antineoplastic therapy is based on the fact that some tumors, such as those of the breast and prostate, are hormone-sensitive. It is possible to change the course of the neoplastic process to some degree by changing the hormonal environment of such tumors.

Androgens

Therapeutic uses. Androgens can be used in the palliative management of estrogen receptor-positive metastatic breast carcinoma in postmenopausal women. Androgens have induced objective responses in up to 50% of such clients, and these responses have lasted 12 to 14 months. Soft tissue metastases are the most responsive, followed by bone metastases. Metastases to the viscera are the least responsive.

Adverse reactions. The most frequent adverse reaction to androgen therapy is masculinization of clients. This includes hirsutism, deepening of the voice, acne, clitoral enlargement, increased libido, and amenorrhea. The extent of virilization is related to the specific androgen, the dose, and the duration of treatment. Testolactone (Teslac) seems to produce the least masculinization.

Table 49-3. Hormones

Drug name	Preparation	Usual dosage/PC	Adverse reactions
Estrogens			
chlorotrianisene (TACE)	Oral capsules	12–25 mg every day PC: X	Sodium and water retention (edema), nausea and vomiting, thromboembolic complications, hypertension, congestive heart failure, hypercalcemia, changes in libido, anxiety, and insomnia
conjugated estrogens (Premarin)	Oral tablets, solutions for IV infusion, and vaginal cream	Oral, for breast carcinoma, 10 mg tid for 90 days; for prostate carcinoma, 3.75–7.5 mg every day PC: X	*In women:* aggravation of chronic cystic mastitis, uterine fibroids, endometriosis, migraine, breast tenderness and pigmentation of nipples and areola, stress incontinence, uterine bleeding (with high doses or on withdrawal of drug), sensitization to the drug's oil carrier
diethylstilbestrol diphosphate (Stilphostrol)	Oral tablets and solution for IV infusion	For prostate carcinoma, oral, 50–200 mg tid; IV, 1 g every day for 5 days followed by 250–500 mg once or twice a week PC: X	*In men:* feminization, as evidenced by gynecomastia and testicular atrophy, impotence
esterified estrogens (Estratab)	Oral tablets, suspension for IM injection, and vaginal cream	For breast carcinoma, 10 mg tid; for prostate carcinoma, 1.25 mg or more tid PC: X	
ethinyl estradiol (Estinyl)	Oral tablets, suspension in oil for IM injection, dermal patch, and vaginal cream	For breast carcinoma, 0.5–1 mg tid; for prostate carcinoma, 0.15–0.3 mg every day PC: X	
polyestradiol phosphate (Estradurin)	Powder and diluent for preparing solutions for IM injection	For prostate carcinoma, 40 mg every 2–4 weeks, up to 80 mg	
stilbestrol (Diethylstilbestrol/ DES)	Oral tablets and concentrated solution for dilution for IV infusion	For breast carcinoma, 5 mg tid with range of 5–15 mg every day; for prostate carcinoma, 1–3 mg every day PC: X	
Androgens			
dromostanolone propionate (Drolban)	Solution in oil for IM injection	For breast cancer, 100 mg three times per week	Fluid retention, hypercalcemia, masculinization (clitoral enlargement, hirsutism, deepening of voice, increased libido, acne), alopecia, erythrocythemia, cholestatic jaundice (with oral therapy) hepatocellular neoplasms (long-term therapy), increased appetite and weight gain (or anorexia and nausea and vomiting at high doses)
fluoxymesterone (Halotestin)	Oral tablets	For breast cancer, 15–30 mg every day PC: X	
methyltestosterone	Oral tablets, powder, and buccal tablets	For breast cancer, oral, 200 mg in divided doses; buccal, 100 mg in divided doses PC: X	
testolactone (Teslac)	Solution in oil for IM injection	For breast cancer, 250 mg qid PC: C	
testosterone propionate in oil (Malogen)	Oral tablets	For breast cancer, 100 mg 3 times a week PC: X	

KEY: PC = pregnancy category. (The validity of pregnancy risk categories has not been established; see Chapter 16, p 216.)

Androgens may also produce fluid retention, cholestatic jaundice, hypercalcemia, alopecia, and erythrocythemia. If hypercalcemia develops, the androgen should be discontinued immediately (see discussion under estrogen therapy and hypercalcemia).

Androgens have also caused a rare condition called *peliosis hepatis* (blood-filled cysts in the liver), hepatic adenomas, and hepatomas.

Antiandrogenic compounds: flutamide

Pharmacodynamics. Flutamide (Eulexin) acts either to inhibit uptake of androgen or to inhibit nuclear binding of androgen in target tissues. Thus, the effect of androgen in androgen-sensitive tissues is decreased.

Pharmacokinetics. Flutamide is absorbed through the GI system after oral administration. It is highly bound to plasma proteins and rapidly metabolized in the liver, and its metabolites are mainly excreted in the urine. The half-life is 6 hours.

Therapeutic uses. Flutamide is used in combination with leuprolide acetate (a luteinizing hormone-releasing hormone analogue; see below) to treat stage D_2 metastatic prostatic carcinoma. Treatment must be initiated simultaneously with both drugs for maximum benefit.

Dosage and administration. Flutamide is available as 250 mg capsules and it is given every 8 hours for a total daily dose of 750 mg.

Adverse reactions. Since flutamide and leuprolide acetate are given concomitantly, it is difficult to distinguish side effects between the two drugs. However, the diarrhea seems more attributable to the flutamide. Hot flashes, impotence, and other reactions occur.

Estrogens

Pharmacodynamics. The rationale for the use of estrogen for breast cancer in the postmenopausal women and for prostatic tumor in men is based on changing the hormonal environment of the tumor.

Estrogen receptor and progesterone receptor determinations should be made on all breast cancer clients. If the breast cancer is positive for receptors for both estrogen and progesterone, the chances of response to hormonal manipulation are greater.

In prostatic cancer, androgen-control therapy does not result in cure, but it produces relief of pain, increased appetite, weight gain, and a sense of well-being.

Pharmacokinetics. Estrogens are well absorbed from the GI tract after oral administration. They are metabolized in the liver. They are primarily excreted in the urine, although small amounts are also eliminated through the bile in feces.

Therapeutic uses. Estrogens can be used in the palliative management of estrogen receptor-positive metastatic breast carcinoma in postmenopausal women and in the palliative management of advanced carcinoma of the prostate.

Estrogen therapy for breast cancer is contraindicated in premenopausal women, because evidence indicates that estrogen in premenopausal women may accelerate the neoplastic process. Clients should be at least 5 years postmenopausal before they receive estrogen therapy.

The use of estrogen in the postmenopausal woman whose cancer contains estrogen receptors changes the hormonal environment and has produced objective tumor responses in 50% to 60% of treated clients. Positive responses involve metastatic disease in soft tissues and bone and last from 6 to 12 months or even for years. It may take 8 to 12 weeks before the effectiveness of the hormonal therapy can be satisfactorily gauged. If hormonal therapy is beneficial, it should be continued until the symptoms recur. At the time of exacerbation, discontinuing the hormone may produce another remission.

Despite this positive discussion of their use, the antiestrogenic compound tamoxifen citrate is often used instead of an estrogen preparation.

Prostate carcinoma is the most common male cancer in the United States. While orchiectomy and administration of estrogens remove 90% of circulating testosterone, orchiectomy is often psychologically troubling. Diethylstilbestrol (DES) is frequently the agent of choice to change the hormonal environment of the prostatic tumor. It is inexpensive and effective by oral administration, and its rate of activation is relatively slow, allowing small doses to be given once a day. If the client is older than 75 years of age, another form of endocrine therapy may be considered because of the cardiotoxicity related to DES.

Dosage and administration. Dosages and routes of administration for estrogens and androgens are summarized in Table 49-3. Several are given orally.

Adverse reactions. Adverse reactions do not usually mandate that hormonal treatment be discontinued. However, fluid retention may become severe, especially in clients with cardiovascular, liver, or renal disease. Death from cardiac complications has occurred. The liver inactivates estrogens, so toxic effects may be more severe in the presence of hepatic damage.

Gynecomastia occurs frequently in males. In rare instances, carcinoma of the male breast has occurred in clients given estrogen for prolonged periods of time. Some oncologists order a modest dose of radiation for the male breasts before estrogen therapy to prevent nipple tenderness, but it does not necessarily prevent the gynecomastia (Holleb, et al, 1991).

Because of the possibility of hypercalcemia, plasma

calcium levels should be routinely monitored during estrogen therapy. If an elevated serum calcium level is found, a high fluid intake should be maintained. The combination of hormone and bone metastasis may result in significant hypercalcemia, which can cause renal calculi, polyuria, neurologic changes, and cardiac arrhythmias.

Hypercalcemia may be life-threatening. In this case, the hormone is discontinued until resolution of the hypercalcemia.

Drug interactions. No known significant drug interactions exist.

Antiestrogenic compounds

Tamoxifen citrate

The development of this nonsteroidal antiestrogenic agent has been a fairly recent event. Various compounds have been tested, and tamoxifen citrate (Nolvadex) has become the drug of choice for palliative treatment of advanced breast cancer in premenopausal and postmenopausal women with estrogen receptor-positive tumors.

Pharmacodynamics. Tamoxifen citrate's effects appear to be related to the drug's ability to compete with estradiol for binding to estrogen receptors. Tamoxifen citrate forms a stable complex with the estrogen receptor in the nucleus of receptor-positive cells. This binding leaves cells refractory to further estrogen stimulation, leading to impaired tumor growth.

Tamoxifen citrate may inhibit replication by additional mechanisms, including effects on transforming growth factor expression.

Pharmacokinetics. Tamoxifen citrate is absorbed after oral administration. Peak concentration in the blood occurs between 4 and 7 hours. An initial half-life of 7 to 14 hours occurs with a terminal half-life of 4 to 7 days. After metabolism, tamoxifen citrate's metabolites are slowly excreted in the feces.

Therapeutic uses. Tamoxifen citrate is used for advanced breast cancer in premenopausal and postmenopausal women. Response rates that range from 4 to 40 months have been cited. Metastatic soft tissue and osseous lesions respond better than do visceral lesions. Previous hormonal therapy with other agents does not preclude a response to tamoxifen citrate.

Dosage and administration. Tamoxifen citrate is administered orally in two divided doses for a total daily dose of 20 to 40 mg. Objective responses may occur in 4 to 10 weeks or may be further delayed in clients with bone metastases.

Adverse reactions. Adverse reactions occur less frequently and are milder with tamoxifen citrate than with estrogens or androgens. The most common reactions are nausea or vomiting and hot flashes (see Example of Nursing Process and Side Effects of Anti-neoplastic Therapy). Vaginal bleeding, vaginal discharge, and menstrual irregularities do occur. Transient decreases in platelet and white blood cell counts have been noted. Other side effects include rash or dermatitis, edema, anorexia, pruritus vulvae, depression, dizziness, lightheadedness, headache, and pulmonary embolism.

A few cases of serious retinal or corneal damage have been reported and seem related to use of large doses (120 to 160 mg twice a day for over a year).

Drug interactions. An interaction between tamoxifen citrate and warfarin has been identified, occasionally resulting in life-threatening bleeding episodes. This interaction is probably related to the displacement of warfarin from protein binding sites by tamoxifen citrate and necessitates close monitoring of prothrombin times when this combination is used.

Synthetic estrogen antimetabolite

Estramustine phosphate sodium

Estramustine phosphate sodium is an antineoplastic agent that combines estradiol and nor-nitrogen mustard.

Pharmacodynamics. The intact molecule of estramustine phosphate sodium acts as a weak alkylating agent by promoting microtubule disassembling, and, after hydrolysis, the released estrogen exerts an antigonadotropin effect.

Pharmacokinetics. Estramustine phosphate sodium is well absorbed after oral administration. Peak plasma concentrations are reached in 2 to 3 hours. The half-life is multiphasic with a terminal half-life of about 20 hours. The majority of the drug is apparently excreted into the biliary tract and eliminated in the feces.

Therapeutic uses. Estramustine phosphate sodium is used for the palliative management of clients with advanced prostatic carcinoma who have become refractory to estrogen therapy. The response rate in those clients previously treated with hormones is about 35%, with a duration of response of 3 to 36 months.

Dosage and administration. Doses range from one to ten capsules daily in three or four divided doses (14 mg/kg/day). Response may be evident in 2 weeks or therapy may need to be continued for 30 to 90 days before response is evident. Therapy is continued as long as a favorable response occurs. Capsules need to be refrigerated and protected from light.

Adverse reactions. A variety of adverse reactions have been reported and most seem related to the estrogenic component. Gynecomastia is the most common side effect, and breast tenderness occurs. Fluid retention is common, and the drug should be used with caution in clients with cardiovascular disease. Hyper-

Example of nursing process and side effects of antineoplastic therapy

The client is a 71-year-old woman who had a mastectomy 5 years ago. The cancer has recurred, and her pelvic bones and left femur are involved. She has had chemotherapy and radiation therapy. No additional radiation therapy is considered possible. She is discharged to her daughter's home on a drug regimen of Zantac, MS Contin every 8 hours, Dulcolax tablets, and tamoxifen 10 mg tid.

The client eats very little. She has lost 8 pounds in the last 4 weeks. Her daughter purchased special foods to tempt her appetite. She complains of nausea and an inability to "swallow one more bite." She does take water and coffee in small amounts.

Her daughter is the primary caregiver. After a few weeks, the client begins to require total care. The services of a public health nurse and home health aide are obtained. A hospice volunteer visits. The client is unable to get out of bed with only one assistant. She is continent, but the movement necessary to use a bedpan causes some pain. She has not had a bowel movement in 2 days.

Except for when using the bedpan, the client does not appear to have any pain. However, over the past 3 days she has become increasingly confused, disoriented, and somnolent. Several times it was apparent that she was experiencing a paranoid hallucination, and one episode of severe agitation occurred.

Assessment data	Nursing diagnosis	Intervention	Goals and outcome criteria
Nausea Inability to "swallow one more bite" Receiving Zantac, MS Contin, and tamoxifen (all known to cause nausea for some clients)	Altered nutrition: less than body requirements related to elevated metabolic rate secondary to malignant process and decreased oral intake due to nausea associated with use of Zantac, MS Contin, and tamoxifen	**Monitor** percentage of meals eaten. **Provide** oral hygiene before and after meals. **Provide** small, frequent, low-fat meals. **Provide** liquid nutritional supplement. **Have** client rest with head of bed elevated after eating. **Consult** with physician about possible use of antiemetic drug.	Client will have improved nutritional status as shown by cessation of weight loss.
Over last 3 days, increasingly confused, disoriented, and somnolent Experiencing paranoid hallucinations One period of extreme agitation	Altered thought processes related to CNS changes secondary to morphine therapy	**Consult** with physician about possible reduction in morphine dosage. **Reorient** client to person, place, and time as necessary. **Repeat** instructions using clear, simple language. **Implement** measures to protect client from injury.	Client will attain improved thought processes as evidenced by orientation to person, place, and time as well as absence of agitation.
Has not had a bowel movement in 2 days Decreased oral intake Receiving Zantac and MS Contin (both known to cause constipation for some clients) Unable to get out of bed with only one assistant	Constipation related to decreased oral intake, use of Zantac and MS Contin, and decreased mobility	**Monitor** and record bowel movements. **Administer** Dulcolax tablets. **Carry out** measures to increase fluid and food intake. **Place** on commode for bowel movements, if possible. Before placing on commode, offer warm liquid to stimulate peristalsis. If client has not had bowel movement in 2 days, administer Fleet enema.	Client will not develop impaction.

calcemia is serious but uncommon. Altered liver function tests are common and caution should be exercised if estramustine phosphate sodium is being administered to clients with hepatic dysfunction.

Progestins

Therapeutic uses. About 80% of localized endometrial cancer is cured by surgery and radiotherapy. Clients with more widespread inoperable disease or with recurrent disease after local treatment are often treated with progestins. In about 35% of these clients, positive responses are seen, with remissions in pulmonary, bone, hepatic, intra-abdominal, and pelvic metastases. Some remissions have lasted for years, and even clients who do not experience objective regression usually have periods of time when pain is relieved, and they have an increased sense of well-being. It appears that response to progestins depends on the presence of progesterone receptors in the tumor. Treatment is continued until the disease recurs.

Progestins have also shown activity in breast cancers, prostate cancer, and ovarian cancer.

Dosage and administration. Many progestins are available, including medroxyprogesterone acetate (Provera), hydroxyprogesterone caproate (Delalutin), and megestrol acetate (Megace). Hydroxyprogesterone caproate is usually given IM in a dose of 1 g twice weekly or up to 5 g/week. A dose of 40 to 320 mg/day (usual dosage, 160 to 320 mg/day) of megestrol acetate is given in divided doses for endometrial carcinoma. At least 2 months of continuous treatment with megestrol acetate is necessary to determine its efficacy.

Adverse reactions. Adverse reactions to progestins are usually minimal. They may cause menstrual irregularities, edema, weight gain, rash, embolic disorders, depression, and pain at the injection site. Hypercalcemia may develop if osseous metastases exist.

Synthetic analogues of luteinizing hormone-releasing hormones

Leuprolide acetate and goserelin acetate

Leuprolide acetate (Lupron) and goserelin acetate (Zoladex) are synthetic analogues of luteinizing hormone-releasing hormone (LHRH) and offer an alternative method for the treatment of prostate cancer.

Pharmacodynamics. Leuprolide acetate and goserelin acetate have greater potency than the natural LHRH. Lupron and Zoladex reduce the amount of testosterone available for conversion, thereby inhibiting the growth of prostate cancer.

Initial doses of leuprolide acetate or goserelin acetate increase luteinizing hormone (LH) and follicle-stimulating hormone (FSH) production in the pitui-

tary gland, resulting in transient increases in testosterone and dihydrotestosterone in males and estrone and estradiol in premenopausal females. Prolonged administration has the effect of "downregulating" LH and FSH receptors in the pituitary gland, thereby eventually decreasing gonadotropin secretion and ultimately decreasing testosterone to castration levels in males (Department of Drugs, 1990). Castration levels of testosterone persist for up to 3 years.

Therapeutic uses. Leuprolide acetate and goserelin acetate are effective in the palliative treatment of advanced prostate cancer when alternative treatment such as orchiectomy or estrogen is not indicated or is unacceptable to the client.

Goserelin acetate is being evaluated in conjunction with radiation therapy for the treatment of early prostate cancer and for disease that involves the pelvic lymph nodes (stage D_1). It has also been used in advanced breast cancer, endometriosis, and uterine fibroids.

Dosage and administration. Leuprolide acetate is available as a solution for injection; 1 mg as a single daily injection is the usual dose.

Goserelin acetate is available in prefilled, single-use, disposable syringes. It is a depot preparation that contains 3.6 mg of goserelin in a biodegradable matrix and is injected into the upper abdominal wall for continuous release over 28 days.

Adverse reactions. Initial stimulation of gonadotropin release and sex steroid production may cause disease flare-up during the first weeks of therapy. Hot flashes are common, but they decrease in frequency and severity over time. Gynecomastia, nausea and vomiting, edema, and thrombophlebitis are occasionally seen. Impotence and loss of libido may occur.

Synthetic analogue of somatostatin: octreotide acetate

Pharmacodynamics. Octreotide acetate (Sandostatin) exerts effects similar to the natural hormone somatostatin. It acts on the anterior pituitary to inhibit growth hormone and thyrotropin and on the pancreas to inhibit insulin and glucagon. It inhibits the release of serotonin and gastrin from the GI tract, decreases GI blood flow, motility, and carbohydrate absorption, and increases water and electrolyte absorption.

Pharmacokinetics. Octreotide acetate is rapidly absorbed from injection sites. Peak plasma levels are reached in 25 minutes, and plasma half-life is 1.5 hours. The duration of action is up to 12 hours. About one-third of a dose is excreted in the urine unchanged.

Therapeutic uses. Octreotide acetate is used in metastatic carcinoid tumors and vasoactive intestinal peptide-secreting tumors (VIPomas). The drug inhibits severe diarrhea in both situations and causes improvement in hypokalemia in VIPomas. It has demonstrated activity in pancreatic neoplasia and GI and pancreatic fistulas.

Dosage and administration. Administration should be by subcutaneous injection, but it may be given IV as a bolus in emergency. The initial dosage is 50 μg one to two times daily. For carcinoid tumors, 100 to 600 μg is given daily in two to four divided doses for the first 2 weeks. After that, the usual maintenance dose is 450 μg daily.

For VIPomas, 200 to 300 μg is given daily in 2 to 4 divided doses for the first 2 weeks, followed by maintenance doses of 150 to 750 μg daily. Ampules should be stored at 36°F to 46°F, but letting the solution reach room temperature before injection decreases the incidence of pain at the injection site.

Plasma clearance is reduced in clients with renal dysfunction, and a dosage reduction is recommended.

Adverse reactions. Octreotide acetate can cause a variety of adverse reactions, but they are generally mild to moderate in nature. The most frequent side effects are nausea, vomiting, dizziness, headache, diarrhea, abdominal pain, and weakness.

Drug interactions. Octreotide acetate has various effects on endogenous hormones, so clients who receive therapies for diabetes or thyroid conditions need to be monitored carefully. It seems to interfere with diazoxide, insulin, β-adrenergic blocking agents, and sulfonylureas.

■ Summary

A variety of hormones are used in antineoplastic therapy. Adrenocorticosteroids are used in combination with other agents or alone to treat complications or to act in palliative fashion. Estrogens and androgens are used to change the hormonal environment in prostate and breast carcinomas. Progestins may be beneficial with endometrial cancer. An antiestrogenic agent (tamoxifen citrate) is the drug of choice for palliative treatment of advanced breast cancer in premenopausal and postmenopausal women. Other newer agents include an antiandrogenic agent, a synthetic estrogen antimetabolite, and synthetic analogues of LHRH and somatostatin that are being used in a variety of ways as antitumor agents.

Biologic response modifiers

Biotherapy is a newer treatment modality for certain cancers. Included in the category of biologic response modifiers are interferons, colony-stimulating factors, interleukins, tumor necrosis factor, and monoclonal antibodies. Many of these agents are investigational agents. Some are being studied for use as single agents, and some are believed to have potential in combination with other antineoplastic agents or cancer treatment modalities.

Biologic response modifiers are immunomodulating agents; that is, they have the ability to enhance the body's immune responses. Certain disorders may be responsive to this approach, including cancer, immunodeficiency diseases, some types of viral and fungal infections, and certain autoimmune disorders. The agents work on the cellular or humoral immune aspects or both. They tend to be more effective when the disease entity or tumor mass is quantitatively small. For this reason, they may be used in combination with other agents or modalities.

Interferons

Interferons are glycoproteins that are produced and secreted by cells in response to viral infections. The first interferon was discovered in 1957 by two scientists, Drs. Isaac and Lindenmann.

Interferons are now known to be not one but a family of glycoproteins. Interferon-α is produced normally by leukocytes, interferon-β is produced normally by fibroblasts, and interferon-τ is produced normally by lymphocytes. Within the α class of human interferon, fourteen different subclasses are known, each differing slightly in amino acid sequence.

Experimentation with interferon was initially limited by prohibitive costs. In the early 1980s breakthroughs in genetic engineering, or recombinant DNA technology, led to the cloning of a human gene for interferon. Now interferons are produced by a recombinant DNA process that involves genetically engineered *Escherichia coli*, making possible the production of large quantities of purified interferon.

In 1985 the World Health Organization and United States Adopted Names Council recommended a uniform nomenclature. Interferon-α is to be spelled *alpha* when used in scientific classifications and *alfa* in reference to the generic name of a special commercial product. The subclass is to be identified by number, and subspecies by assigned letter (eg, Intron A is interferon alfa-2b, recombinant).

Pharmacodynamics. Several mechanisms are identified as typical of interferons. First, in response to viral challenge, interferon is synthesized and released by infected cells. This protects neighboring cells from infection with a second virus.

Interferons also have an antiproliferative effect. In *in vitro* studies, interferons have been shown to slow down the cycle of cell division of all cells; they interfere with the replication of DNA and protein synthesis. This effect is more pronounced with cancer cells.

Interferons have been shown to inhibit the expression of oncogenes, genes believed to be associated with the transformation of a normal cell into a malignant one.

Interferons augment the cytotoxicity of natural killer cells. They have been shown to alter the body's own immune defense system in a number of ways, including the stimulation of natural killer cells to attack and destroy tumor cells.

After exposure of cancer cells to interferons, changes have been observed in the appearance and behavior of malignant cells, so that they look and behave more like normal cells.

Therapeutic uses. Interferon-α has made a significant therapeutic impact in hairy-cell leukemia, both in previously splenectomized and nonsplenectomized clients, producing either complete remission or long-term remission. Interferon-α is also indicated for treatment of selected clients with AIDS-related Kaposi's sarcoma.

Interferon-α is used with juvenile laryngeal papilloma or papillomatosis, and condylomata acuminata (venereal warts).

It is also being studied for use with certain neurologic conditions and malignancies such as renal cell carcinoma, malignant melanoma, and multiple melanoma.

Dosage and administration. Because interferon is a protein, it is destroyed by digestive enzymes and must be administered IM or subcutaneously. Interferons are supplied as powder in vials that contain from 3 to 50 million IU per vial. Each vial of interferon alfa-2a is packaged with a diluent (that contains sodium chloride, albumin, and phenol). Alfa-2a and alfa-2b are not interchangeable. Interferon alfa-2b is diluted with sterile water for injection (stable for 24 hours) or bacteriostatic water for injection (stable for 1 month when stored between 36°F and 46°F). The reconstituted solution is clear, colorless to light yellow. When the diluent is added during reconstitution, the vial should not be shaken but swirled gently to dissolve the contents.

With hairy-cell leukemia, induction with alfa-2a is accomplished by using 3 million U/day IM or subcutaneously for 16 to 24 weeks. The maintenance dose is 3 million U IM or subcutaneously three times per week.

With Kaposi's sarcoma, induction may be achieved by the use of IM or subcutaneous administration of 36 million U/day for 10 to 12 weeks. Other protocols are also used.

With condylomata acuminata, 1 million U of alfa-2b are administered intralesionally per wart three times a week for 3 weeks.

A variety of dosage schedules have been used on an investigational basis for solid tumors and non-antineoplastic purposes.

Adverse reactions. Adverse reactions are predominantly mild to moderate, reversible on cessation of therapy, and noncumulative in nature. Generally they appear dose-related.

The most common adverse effect is a flulike syndrome, which includes fever and chills, aching muscles, headache, and possibly joint pain. These symptoms tend to decrease in severity and number as therapy continues. Fever and chills may possibly be prevented, or at least alleviated, by taking acetaminophen. Aspirin, nonsteroidal anti-inflammatory agents, and steroids should not be used because of the possibility that they may block enzyme production and thus inhibit the effectiveness of the interferon.

Additional common adverse effects include leukopenia, thrombocytopenia, cardiotoxicity (chest pain and supraventricular arrhythmia), neurotoxicity (confusion, memory loss, depression, and difficulty with concentration), unusual fatigue, and anorexia associated with nausea and vomiting.

Drug interactions. Concurrent use of alcohol or CNS depression-producing medications may enhance the CNS depressant effects of either those medications or the interferon.

Leukopenic and thrombocytopenic effects of interferon may be increased with concurrent or recent therapy of blood dyscrasia-causing medications. Dosage adjustment of interferon-α can be made based on blood counts. For example, severe leukopenia may result in clients who are taking azidothymidine (AZT) simultaneously with interferon-α.

Additive bone marrow depression may occur if radiation therapy is used concurrently or consecutively with interferon-α.

Colony-stimulating factors

Colony-stimulating factors (CSFs) are powerful new investigational agents that stimulate the growth of hematopoietic cells. The CSFs are a group of polypeptide hormones originally discovered by investigators who were studying the growth of granulocyte and mononuclear phagocyte colonies in semisolid bone marrow cultures. Four of the factors active on myeloid cells—granulocyte-macrophage colony-stimulating factor (GM-CSF), granulocyte colony-stimulating factor (G-CSF), macrophage colony-stimulating factor (M-CSF), and interleukin-3 (1L-3)—have been molecularly cloned, and the biosynthetic (recombinant) products have been introduced into pharmacotherapy. The largest clinical experience to date is with G-CSF and GM-CSF (Glaspy & Golde, 1990).

Pharmacodynamics. Hematopoiesis, or the formation and development of blood cells, begins in the bone marrow with the stem cell. The CSFs increase the production of granulocytes and monocytes by stimulating stem cell and precursor cell replication and maturation. The precise level at which the various CSFs act is not known. G-CSF primarily stimulates the production of mature neutrophils, but it is known to also have effects on early stem cells. GM-CSF stimulates monocyte, eosinophil, neutrophil, and megakaryocytic growth *in vitro*. Interleukin-3 appears to act earlier in stem cell development than GM-CSF; it stimulates platelet and basophil production *in vivo*. Macrophage CSF affects only mononuclear phagocyte development (Glaspy, Golde, 1990). The CSFs exert their biologic activity by interacting with specific cell surface receptors.

Pharmacokinetics. Subcutaneous administration of Neupogen (Filgrastim, G-CSF) resulted in maximum serum concentrations within 2 to 8 hours. The elimination half-life is about 3.5 hours.

Therapeutic uses. To date, the uses of CSFs have related to states of bone marrow dysfunction that are iatrogenically induced: antiviral therapy associated with AIDS treatment, myelosuppression associated with cancer chemotherapy and bone marrow transplantation, as well as states of intrinsic bone marrow dysfunction, such as myelodysplasia, congenital cyclic neutropenia, aplastic anemia, and other states of bone marrow infiltration, such as hairy-cell leukemia.

The goals of CSF use are meaningful and measurable benefits, such as reduction in inpatient hospital days, antibiotic use, febrile days, and transfusion requirements. These benefits are reflected in improvements in quality of life and in reduction in treatment costs (Garnick, 1990).

The CSFs have been used in conjunction with various cytotoxic regimens in certain malignancies like small cell lung cancer, urothelial cancer, breast or ovarian cancer, and neuroblastomas. CSFs have been administered after autologous bone marrow transplantation for solid tumors. Outcomes with CSF use have included less severe neutropenia of shorter duration and fewer febrile and infective events.

In AIDS, G-CSF is being administered in combination with erythropoietin (Epogen) and AZT to study their impact on the neutropenia associated with the myelosuppressive therapy of AIDS. Similar studies are underway with GM-CSF given in combination with ganciclovir (Cytovene) for AIDS clients with active cytomegalovirus infection.

Dosage and administration. To date, the preferred route of administration is the subcutaneous injection because of simplicity. G-CSF may be given IV by slow infusion over a period of 20 to 30 minutes. The line should be flushed with an appropriate sterile solution before and after administration.

G-CSF can be transported home unrefrigerated; however, in hot weather, it should be kept out of the sun and sent home in a cooler but not packed in dry ice because it will freeze. It should be stored in the refrigerator at 36° to 46°F to avoid freezing. A new vial is used for each injection; any vial that contains particulate matter or discolored liquid should be discarded, and the medication should not be shaken.

To date, G-CSF is administered no less than 24 hours after administration of cytotoxic chemotherapy to avoid killing the body's reserve pool of neutrophils and hematopoietic progenitor cells.

The white blood cell count should be monitored at least twice weekly when the client is receiving G-CSF. The G-CSF is discontinued when the absolute neutrophil count is calculated to surpass 10,000/mm^3 after the anticipated chemotherapy-induced absolute neutrophil count nadir.

Adverse reactions. G-CSF seems less toxic than GM-CSF. The toxicities of G-CSF include bone pain, exacerbation of pre-existing inflammatory conditions, and possibly increase in spleen size. The bone pain is relatively well tolerated, transient, and usually short in duration. It has responded to acetaminophen therapy.

Exacerbation of underlying inflammation was noted in clients with hairy-cell leukemic vasculitis and in one client with psoriasis. This complication responded to discontinuation of CSF therapy.

Toxicities of GM-CSF have included bone pain, rash, fevers, myalgia, fatigue, anorexia, phlebitis, thrombosis, and, at doses higher than 16 μg/mg/day, capillary leak syndrome with pericardial and pleural effusions and edema. In addition, eosinophilia has developed and may represent a toxicity.

Interleukin-2

Pharmacodynamics. One of the cytokines produced by leukocytes was identified as interleukin-2 around 1980.

Peripheral blood lymphoid cells from a client have been induced to proliferate *in vitro*, using a tissue culture that contains interleukin-2. This expanded population of cells has been injected back into the same client with the simultaneous IV administration of interleukin-2. Such treatment with interleukin-2-activated cells and interleukin-2 has produced definite regression in some cancers. Interleukin-2 stimulates lymphocytes, induces interferon-τ, and enhances the generation of both lymphokine-activated killer cells and natural killer cells. It supports the growth of macrophages as well as both B and T cells.

Therapeutic uses. Interleukin-2 is being studied in treatment of colon cancers, renal cell carcinoma, malignant melanomas, and tumors refractory to other therapies. In some clients with advanced melanoma or renal cell carcinoma, partial or complete regression of detectable metastatic lesions has been noted.

It is also being studied in combination with interferon-β in Kaposi's sarcoma, colon cancer, malignant melanoma; non–small cell carcinoma of lung, and renal carcinoma. It is used as an immunopotentiating agent in clients with AIDS.

Dosage and administration. Optimum dosages are still being identified. When used as a single agent, the maximum tolerated dose seems to be 1 million U/m^2 daily for a week via IV bolus or continuous IV infusion.

It may be used for a 1- or 2-week cycle with 2- to 6-week intervals between cycles.

Adverse reactions. The adverse effects are similar to those seen with interferon, including fever, nausea, vomiting, fatigue, malaise, and violent chills. Other side effects include flushing, diarrhea, rash, edema, and hypertension. High doses can cause supraventricular tachycardia or lead to myocardial infarction. Chronic effects seem to be anorexia and depression.

Tumor necrosis factor

Pharmacodynamics. In 1975 a factor was discovered in the sera of mice that had been primed with certain substances and subsequently challenged with bacterial endotoxin. This factor, named *tumor necrosis factor*, was found to induce hemorrhagic necrosis, growth inhibition, or regression in a variety of human and mouse tumors, both *in vivo* and *in vitro*. The major source of tumor necrosis factor was subsequently discovered to be monocytes, and study of it suggests it plays an important role in host response to inflammatory insults. Recombinant gene technology has made it possible for tumor necrosis factor to be cloned and mass produced.

Therapeutic uses. Tumor necrosis factor is still in early phases of development. Researchers believe a major use will be in combination with other biologic response modifiers or antineoplastic agents to produce the highest possible cell kill of malignant cells.

Dosage and administration. Different routes are being studied, including arterial therapy and intraperitoneal administration.

Adverse reactions. Acute adverse effects include fever and chills, headache, hypotension, arthralgia, anorexia, and diarrhea. Chronic effects include fatigue and malaise.

Monoclonal antibodies

Pharmacodynamics. Most monoclonal antibodies are murine proteins produced by the immunization of mice with an antigen (such as human cancer cells). Once monoclonal antibodies have been produced, they have been combined with selected entities (such as a biologic toxin or antineoplastic drug). The goal is to have the antibody carry the toxic agent to the tumor site or sites.

Therapeutic uses. It is believed that monoclonal antibodies may eventually have a role in the detection of cancer or cancer's metastatic sites (*ie*, by labeling the monoclonal antibody with a radioisotope like I[131]). Clinical trials of monoclonal antibody IV infusions have also been initiated to treat several tumors, including malignant melanoma, lymphomas, leukemias, and colorectal carcinomas. Tumor remissions have been noted in some clients.

■ **Summary**
Interferons, colony-stimulating factors, interleukins, tumor necrosis factor, and monoclonal antibodies are examples of biologic response modifiers; the use of these agents with cancer clients is currently being explored.

Miscellaneous agents

Several antineoplastic agents that do not fit under the established categories are listed as miscellaneous agents: aminoglutethimide, amsacrine/MAMSA, hydroxyurea, isotretinoin, levamisole hydrochloride, mitotane, and procarbazine. Table 49-4 summarizes information about the preparations, usual dosage, and adverse reactions of these agents. Their pharmacodynamics and therapeutic uses are described below.

Pharmacodynamics

Aminoglutethimide. Aminoglutethimide inhibits the enzymatic conversion of cholesterol to pregnenolone at the first step in adrenal corticosteroid biosynthesis, thereby reducing the synthesis of glucocorticoids, mineralocorticoids, and other steroids. In addition, it inhibits the aromatase enzyme that converts androstenedione to estrone and estradiol in extra-adrenal tissues. Because the adrenal gland is the principal source of estrogens in postmenopausal women, this dual inhibitory action lowers plasma estrogen levels to the same extent as surgical adrenalectomy (Department of Drugs, 1990, pp. 1793–1794).

Amsacrine. Amsacrine intercalates between strands of DNA and produces single-stranded and double-stranded breaks in DNA. Amsacrine forms a tight complex with topoisomerase-II, which is felt to be involved in amsacrine's cytotoxicity. The normal action of topoisomerase-II seems to be to break and reseal DNA at points of torsion, but in the presence of amsacrine, resealing of breaks does not take place. Cytotoxicity is greatest during the S phase of the cell cycle when topoisomerase-II levels within the cell increase to a maximum (DeVita, et al, 1989, p. 387).

Hydroxyurea. Hydroxyurea is representative of a group of compounds that have as their primary site of action the enzyme ribonucleoside diphosphate reductase. It inhibits the enzyme that normally catalyzes the conversion of ribonucleotides to deoxyribonucleotides and is crucial to DNA biosynthesis. There is little effect on RNA or protein synthesis. The drug is specific for the S phase of the cell cycle and causes cells to arrest at the G_1-S interface.

Isotretinoin. Vitamin A and its analogues (retinoids) are essential for epithelial cell differentiation. Deficiency of vitamin A promotes neoplasia in various animal models. In animal models retinoids have delayed the appearance, retarded the growth, and

Table 49-4. Miscellaneous agents

Drug name	Preparation	Usual dosage/PC	Adverse reactions
aminoglutethimide (Cytadren)	Oral tablets	250 mg bid for 2 wks increased to 250 mg qid PC: D	Lethargy, ataxia, skin rash, nausea, vomiting, anorexia, headache, tachycardia, myalgia, fever, pruritus, orthostatic hypotension, dizziness, weakness, masculinization and hirsutism in women, goiters, bone marrow suppression, elevated liver enzymes
amsacrine/MAMSA (Amsidyl)	Solution for IV infusion	100–150 mg/m²/d for 5 days, diluted in 500 ml 5% D/W	Bone marrow suppression, acute and chronic cardiotoxicity, mucositis, alopecia, nausea, vomiting, diarrhea, hepatic dysfunction, tissue damage on extravasation
hydroxyurea (Hydrea)	Oral capsules	(1) 80 mg/kg every third day or (2) 20–30 mg/kg every day for 6 weeks PC: D	Bone marrow suppression, nausea, vomiting, stomatitis, skin atrophy, hyperpigmentation of areas previously exposed to radiation, erythema, alopecia, drowsiness, headache, dizziness, disorientation, hallucinations, convulsions
isotretinoin (Accutane)	Oral capsules	40 mg/m² every day PC: X	Dry skin, dry mucous membranes, exfoliation, increased susceptibility to sunburn, cheilitis, conjunctivitis, corneal opacities, GI disorders, musculoskeletal disorders, pseudotumor cerebri, elevated liver enzymes, mild bone marrow suppression, lipid abnormalities
levamisole hydrochloride (Ergamisol)	Oral tablets	*Initially*, 50 mg q8h for 3 days starting 7–30 days after surgery; *maintenance*, 50 mg q8h for 3 days every 2 weeks for 1 yr PC: C	Nausea, vomiting, diarrhea, taste perversion, altered sense of smell, bone marrow suppression, arthralgia, myalgia, pruritus, skin discoloration, rash, alopecia
mitotane (Lysodren)	Oral tablets	8–10 g every day in 3–4 divided doses PC: C	Anorexia, nausea, vomiting, diarrhea, lethargy, somnolence, dizziness, vertigo, dermatitis, blurred vision, diplopia, lens opacities, retinopathy, albuminuria, hemorrhagic cystitis, flushing, hyperpyrexia, orthostatic hypotension, hypertension, hypersensitivity reactions
procarbazine (Matulane)	Oral tablets	2 to 4 mg/kg/day in single or divided doses for 1 week PC: D	Bone marrow suppression, anorexia, nausea, vomiting, stomatitis, dry mouth, dysphagia, diarrhea, constipation, paresthesia, peripheral neuropathies, weakness, unsteadiness, ataxia, footdrop, decreased DTRs, tremors, confusion, lethargy, drowsiness, convulsions, coma, pruritus, hyperpigmentation, flushing, alopecia, jaundice

KEY: PC = pregnancy category. (The validity of pregnancy risk categories has not been established; see Chapter 16, p 216.)

caused regression of cancers of the skin, GI tract, breast, and other tissues. Clinical trials evaluating the role of isotretinoin as a chemopreventive agent are in progress.

Levamisole hydrochloride. The mechanism of action of levamisole hydrochloride in combination with fluorouracil is unknown. Levamisole hydrochloride does have complex effects on the immune system. The drug appears to restore depressed immune function. It can stimulate formation of antibodies to various antigens, enhance T-cell responses by stimulating T-cell activation and proliferation, potentiate monocyte and macrophage functions, including phagocytosis and chemotaxis, and increase neutrophil mobility, adherence, and chemotaxis.

Mitotane. The exact mechanism of action of this agent is not known. It acts on the adrenal cortex, causing rapid reduction in the levels of corticosteroids and their metabolites in blood and urine.

Procarbazine. The mechanism of action of procarbazine is not clear; however, it appears that it requires activation and that the end product is an alkylating agent. The drug appears to inhibit DNA, RNA, and protein synthesis. It seems to be activated by the cytochrome P450 mixed-function oxidase system of the liver to a number of metabolites, with subsequent production of formaldehyde and hydroxyl-free radicals that produce changes in DNA similar to the effects of ionizing radiation and alkylating agents (Black & Livingston, 1990, p. 661). Procarbazine is cell cycle nonspecific.

Therapeutic uses

Aminoglutethimide. Aminoglutethimide is as effective as surgical adrenalectomy in the treatment of postmenopausal women with estrogen receptor-positive advanced breast cancer. Durations of response have averaged 14 to 30 months and occur primarily in soft tissue and bone metastases. In this situation it would be given with replacement hydrocortisone to prevent reflex ACTH hypersecretion from overcoming adrenal inhibition. Aminoglutethimide and hydrocortisone were compared to tamoxifen citrate in a trial, and the results were comparable. Tamoxifen citrate is the agent of choice because of its lower potential for toxicity, but the combination of aminoglutethimide and hydrocortisone is an alternative for clients who relapse with tamoxifen citrate.

Aminoglutethimide is also used in suppression of adrenal function in some clients with Cushing's syndrome.

Amsacrine. Amsacrine has activity against human acute nonlymphocytic leukemia. It seems particularly helpful because of its synergy with ara-C, its activity in clients resistant to anthracyclines, and its lower incidence of cardiotoxicity than the anthracyclines.

Hydroxyurea. Hydroxyurea is used in the management of myeloproliferative disorders, including chronic granulocytic leukemia (CGL). Myelosuppression is a major adverse reaction, but bone marrow recovery is prompt after stopping therapy, a feature that distinguishes hydroxyurea from busulfan, which is also used for the management of CGL.

It is also used in polycythemia vera and essential thrombocytosis.

It has produced temporary remissions with metastatic malignant melanoma and occasionally with solid tumors, including carcinomas of the head and neck and genitourinary system.

Since cells are highly sensitive to irradiation in the G_1 phase of the cell cycle, combinations of hydroxyurea and irradiation cause synergistic toxicity *in vitro*. Thus, it has been used in combination with radiotherapy in carcinomas of the cervix, head and neck, and lung.

Isotretinoin. Retinoids have been effective in severe acne and in the treatment of basal cell carcinomas and cutaneous T cell lymphomas.

Levamisole hydrochloride. This drug is used in combination with fluorouracil as adjuvant therapy to treat clients with Dukes' stage C colon cancer, after surgical resection.

Mitotane. Mitotane is used in the palliative management of inoperable carcinoma of the adrenal cortex. The mean duration of response is about 10 months.

Procarbazine. The primary use of procarbazine is in advanced Hodgkin's disease in combination with mechlorethamine, oncovin, and prednisone (MOPP regimen). Procarbazine has also shown activity in primary and metastatic brain tumors and small cell lung cancer.

It has been used as an immunosuppressant in clients with systemic lupus erythematosus (SLE) and for suppression of graft-versus-host disease in bone marrow transplantation.

Nursing management

The section on Nursing Management in Chapter 48 was designed to apply to Chapter 49 as well. Clients who are receiving the drugs discussed in this chapter have cancer and are experiencing the same actual or potential problems as discussed in Chapter 48 (see the Examples of Nursing Process). The management of extravasation of antineoplastic drugs is discussed here.

Nursing process

Assessment Early symptoms of extravasation are pain or a burning sensation at or above the IV site. Physical assessment of the site may reveal blanching, erythema, or swelling. The infusion may slow or stop without explanation, and blood return may be absent. The signs of extravasation may not be immediately evident but may be noted several hours later.

Nursing diagnosis One nursing diagnosis that applies to several agents discussed in Chapter 49 and a few discussed in Chapter 48 is the high risk for impaired tissue integrity related to administration of vesicant drugs. The drugs discussed in the two chapters that are vesicants are listed in Box 49-1.

Extravasation of an antineoplastic agent can be a serious problem. Vesicants can cause significant tissue damage, loss of function, infection, and tissue necrosis that requires surgery.

Planning In preparing a plan of client care for a client who is receiving a potential vesicant, one desirable client outcome is absence of the injury that could occur from extravasation.

Interventions Prevention of injury from a vesicant drug begins with the knowledge of how to administer the drugs properly or how to assist in their proper administration. Continuous infusions may be best administered through a central line. Vascular access devices may offer an appropriate alternative.

Vesicant push chemotherapy may be used; the

Box 49-1. Vesicants

amsacrine	mechlorethamine
carboplatin	mitomycin
dacarbazine	plicamycin
dactinomycin	vinblastine
daunorubicin	vincristine
doxorubicin	

procedure is defined as administering the agent via IV push over a period of time less than 30 minutes. This procedure includes establishing a running IV line with 5% dextrose and water or normal saline (as specified in printed information on the particular agent) and assessing the IV site before drug administration for patency, infiltration, and phlebitis. The vein's patency may be checked by instilling 5 to 7 ml of normal saline. The vesicant drug is administered via the side arm of the running IV, and the nurse must check for infiltration and patency every 1 ml of drug infusion. Tubing is flushed after completion of the drug infusion with 5 to 10 ml of normal saline. The drug must be administered at the specified speed to prevent untoward sensations.

If extravasation does occur, the infusion must be stopped. Each institution has its own set of subsequent procedures. Some interventions that may be specified include attempting to aspirate any remaining drug from the needle, injecting an appropriate antidote, using a specific topical ointment, and applying heat or cold to the site. A photograph of the site may be ordered as a reference to evaluate progression or resolution of the extravasation. Careful documentation in the client's chart is important.

Specific antidotes are recommended for certain agents. For example, 10% sodium thiosulfate is recommended as the antidote for mechlorethamine extravasation. If the 10% solution is not immediately available, the 25% solution may be used or diluted to a 10% solution status. It has been suggested that, if extravasation occurs with mitomycin, pain and necrosis may be diminished with local injection of pyridoxine (Dukes & Beeley, 1990). With the vinca alkaloids, local infiltration of hyaluronidase and warming of the area of infiltration are recommended. With daunorubicin or doxorubicin, topical applications of dimethyl-sulfoxide are mentioned.

Client education. The nurse should provide information and literature about the specific type of cancer to the client and family, and the anticipated results of the selected antineoplastic drugs should be explained.

The types of adverse reactions that clients may be expected to experience from the antineoplastic drugs must be identified for the client and family. The nurse should identify how and where to contact their health care providers to report any adverse reactions, ask questions, or to request clarification of instructions. The importance of complying with all aspects of the therapeutic regimen should be stressed.

The nurse needs to identify interventions that may be used to cope with specific adverse reactions. Some of the antineoplastic drugs mandate that the client be monitored with a variety of laboratory tests. The client and family need to know when and where to go to have the laboratory work done. The results of the laboratory tests may need to be explained to the client and family.

The local cancer support groups and their specialized functions in the respective community should be explained to the client and family, and specific information about how to contact them should be given.

Evaluation The nurse must evaluate the client for signs or symptoms of extravasation and, if extravasation occurs, for evidence of progression or resolution of the extravasation. The effect of any antidote or treatment used should be noted.

Checklist of nursing actions

☐ Monitor laboratory data for evidence of adverse reactions (*eg*, leukopenia, thrombocytopenia, anemia, hypercalcemia).

☐ Teach the client about the drug: what to report to the physician and what to do if adverse reactions occur.

☐ When adverse reactions are experienced, follow suggested nursing interventions for the given problem.

☐ With vincristine, observe for the early symptoms of CNS, ANS, and peripheral nervous system toxicity so that steps may be taken to prevent more serious adverse reactions.

☐ With vincristine, take actions to prevent or control hyperuricemia (*eg*, encourage high fluid intake, check with the physician about alkalinization of the urine and use of allopurinol).

☐ In assisting with the IV administration of amsacrine, dactinomycin, daunorubicin, doxorubicin, mithramycin, mitomycin, vinblastine, and vincristine, take appropriate precautions to avoid extravasation of the drug into subcutaneous tissues.

☐ Advise clients who receive daunorubicin and doxorubicin that their urine will be red for 8 to 48 hours after drug administration. Clients who receive mitoxantrone hydrochloride may experience greenish-blue urine, sclera, skin, or nails for 24 hours after drug administration.

☐ Observe for signs and symptoms of cardiotoxicity with doxorubicin, daunorubicin, mitoxantrone hydrochloride, and amsacrine.

☐ With asparaginase, observe for signs and symptoms of allergic reaction to the medication.

References

Black DJ, Livingston RB. (1990). Antineoplastic drugs in 1990: A review (Part I). *Drugs, 39(4),* 489–501.
Black DJ, Livingston RB. (1990). Antineoplastic drugs in 1990: A review (Part II). *Drugs, 39(5),* 652–673.

Brophy LR, Sharp EJ. (1991). Physical symptoms of combination biotherapy: A quality-of-life issue. *Oncology Nursing Forum, 18*(Suppl. 1), 25–30.

Department of Drugs, Division of Drugs and Toxicology. (1990). *Drug Evaluations Annual.* Milwaukee, WI: American Medical Association.

DeVita Jr VT, Hellman S, Rosenberg SA, eds. (1989). *Clinical pharmacology of cancer chemotherapy*, 3rd ed. Philadelphia: JB Lippincott.

Dukes MNG, Beeley L. (1990). *Side effects of drugs annual 14.* Amsterdam, Netherlands: Elsevier Science Publishers BV.

Garnick M. (1990). The article reviewed. *Oncology, 4(9)*, 32–33.

Gilman AG, et al, eds. (1990). *Goodman and Gilman's the pharmacological basis of therapeutics*, 8th ed. New York: Pergamon Press.

Glaspy JA, Golde DW. (1990). The colony-stimulating factors: Biology and clinical use. *Oncology, 4(9)*, 25–32.

Gulatte MM, Graves T. (1990). Advances in antineoplastic therapy. *Oncology Nursing Forum, 17(6)*, 867–876.

Holleb AI, Fink DJ, Murphy GP. (1991). *American Cancer Society textbook of clinical oncology.* Atlanta, GA: American Cancer Society.

Levine RR. (1990). *Pharmacology: Drug actions and reactions*, 4th ed. Boston: Little, Brown.

Bibliography

Averette HE, Boike GM, Jarrell MA. (1990). Effects of cancer chemotherapy on gonadal function and reproductive capacity. *CA, 40(4)*, 199–209.

Brogley JL, Sharp EJ. (1990). Nursing care of patients receiving activated lymphocytes. *Oncology Nursing Forum, 17(2)*, 187–193.

Cassileth BR, Berlyne D. (1989). Counseling the cancer patient who wants to try unorthodox or questionable therapies. *Oncology, 3(4)*, 29–34.

Dunne CF. (1989). Safe handling of antineoplastic agents. *Cancer Nurs, 12(2)*, 120–127.

Hahn MB, Jassak PF. (1991). Nursing management of patients receiving interferon. *Semin Oncol Nurs, 4(2)*, 95–101.

Hogan CM. (1991). Coping with biotherapy: Physiological and psychosocial concerns. *Oncology Nursing Forum, 18*(Suppl. 1), 19–23.

Mahon SM. (1989). Signs and symptoms associated with malignancy-induced hypercalcemia. *Cancer Nurs, 12(3)*, 153–160.

Moertel CG, Fleming TR, MacDonald JS, et al. (1990). Levamisole and fluorouracil for adjuvant therapy of resected colon cancer. *N Engl J Med, 322*, 352–358.

Pazdur R, et al. (1991). 5-Fluorouracil and recombinant interferon alfa-2a: Review of activity and toxicity in advanced colorectal carcinomas. *Oncology Nursing Forum, 18*(Suppl. 1), 11–17.

Poe CM, Taylor LM. (1989). Syndrome of inappropriate antidiuretic hormone: Assessment and nursing implications. *Oncology Nursing Forum, 16(3)*, 373–381.

Terebelo HR. (1991). Alpha interferon: Perspectives in the biotherapy of chronic myelogenous leukemia. *Oncology Nursing Forum, 18*(Suppl.), 5–9.

Nutritional supplements

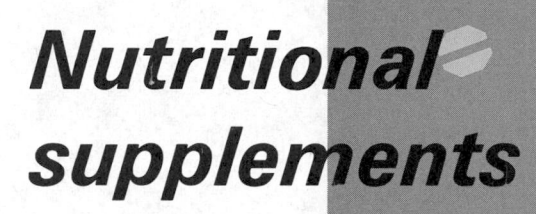

13

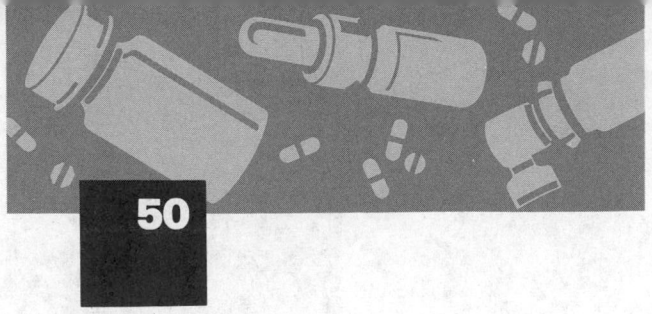

50

Oral supplements

Nutrition and the detection and correction of nutritional deficiencies has always been a major concern of nurses. With improvement in food supplies and education of the public to the risks of undernutrition, deficiency states have become uncommon. However, health food fads and the marketing of supplemental nutrients have provoked an increasing incidence of toxicity. Many clients can benefit from nutritional counseling.

The science of nutrition has shared in the scientific knowledge explosion of recent decades. Advances in this discipline are sophisticated enough to provide a basis for adaptation of diet to meet individual needs. Clients with unusual nutritional needs or severe nutritional imbalances should be referred to a nutritionist for expert diagnosis and treatment. The nurse may, however, screen clients for nutritional problems and advise them on diet and the use of nutritional supplements. Nurses who function as primary health care providers often become very knowledgeable about nutrition and are able to diagnose and treat a variety of nutritional problems.

A number of therapeutic agents are administered to prevent or correct nutritional deficiencies. These include vitamins, minerals, hematinics, injectable fluids, electrolytes, energy nutrients, and blood. Certain chemicals in these preparations are also employed for specific pharmacologic effect, thus acting as medicinal drugs. Although these agents are substances used by or produced in the body naturally during normal function, they can precipitate adverse reactions, especially when administered in high doses.

What follows is a discussion of the prophylactic and therapeutic uses of vitamins, minerals, and hematinics. For the most part, these substances are not classified as drugs and are not controlled by the U.S. Food and Drug Administration (FDA). The labels on these

---

Enrichment experience 50-1

Examine lay periodicals (such as *Prevention* magazine, published by Rodale Press) that feature nutrition and dietary supplementation. Are the data reported in the articles well documented? Are they accurate? Complete? What proportion of the writing is devoted to testimonials? How much advertising space is devoted to proprietary nutritional supplements?

Discuss with your classmates the following question: To what degree does the selling of advertising space for the purpose of promoting use of commercial nutritional supplements pose a conflict of interest for the publishers of a magazine devoted to promoting healthy living?

---

product packages rarely inform the consumer about use, safe dosage, or adverse reactions.

There is, however, an active lay press that discusses these supplements. Most publications convey enthusiasm for their use. Some also discuss adverse reactions and risks of overdose. Yet, nearly all these sources accept advertisements from firms that produce a variety of vitamin, mineral, and nutrient concentrates. This raises the issue of conflict of interest: can a publication deriving income from firms marketing nutritional supplements also provide unbiased advice to the consumer regarding their use?

Vitamins

Vitamins are organic chemicals found in foods that are essential in small quantities for growth, health, and the preservation of life. They perform vital functions in many biochemical processes of the body. Vitamins do not resemble each other chemically. Some are water-soluble and some are fat-soluble. Their molecules do not share common structures that are characteristic of vitamins as a group. They are distinguished only by the fact that deficiencies cause impaired health, delayed growth, or disease states.

Chemicals are classified as vitamins because they cannot be manufactured by the body and, hence, must be present in the diet for normal function. Chemicals required by specific species vary. A vitamin necessary to humans may be synthesized readily by other animals. Generally, a given vitamin is not required in a single chemical form. Rather, several similar molecules can be used by the body to produce the required biochemical.

Physiology. Most vitamins are necessary to metabolic processes that transform food into tissue or energy. They are used by the body to synthesize cofactors or coenzymes, which participate in essential metabolic processes in the body (Table 50-1). At least one, vitamin D, acts as a hormone.

Although much has been learned about the physiologic functions of vitamins, this area is still poorly understood. Vitamins are known to be necessary to normal growth, development, and body maintenance but the degree to which they may enhance health in people who show no overt signs or symptoms of deficiency remains controversial.

The dietary need for vitamins appears to assume a normal distribution. Requirements for most people lie within a fairly narrow range, and relatively few people need dosages that deviate markedly from this norm.

Pathophysiology. Vitamins were first discovered because they were capable of reversing the signs and symptoms of disease states caused by severe nutritional deficiencies. Diseases stemming from severe vitamin deficiencies include xerophthalmia, beriberi, pellagra, pernicious anemia, scurvy, rickets, osteomalacia, infantile hemolytic anemia, and hemorrhagic disease in the newborn (Table 50-2). Moderate deficiencies also produce symptoms of impaired health. The degree to which subtle deficiencies may contribute to minor problems, such as discomfort or fatigue, in people whose health is normal, has not been established.

Individual requirements for specific vitamins can be influenced by both genetic and environmental factors. Resistance to the effects of certain vitamins can be inherited. Some people do not absorb these nutrients readily. Hormone balance, growth, disease processes, and drugs can influence the function of vitamins, as well as the dietary requirement. Although the number of people so affected may be relatively low, it is important that the nutritional requirements of these people be met.

Vitamin deficiencies are relatively rare in the United States. When they do occur, they usually involve multiple rather than single deficiencies. For example, vitamin B deficiencies usually involve inadequate levels of all of the nutrients in this group. Special circumstances usually underlie single deficiencies (*eg*, pellagra in corn-eating populations, pernicious anemia after gastrectomy, and scurvy in elderly people subsisting on soft foods [milk, bread, eggs] who neglect to eat citrus fruits). Most often, poor dietary habits involve an inadequate intake of many nutrients, including all vitamins.

Pharmacodynamics. In addition to the physiologic effects on metabolism just described, vitamins administered for pharmacologic effect exert specific drug effects (Table 50-3). To achieve these effects, doses much larger than those recommended for nutritional maintenance are usually required.

Vitamin A ointment has been used successfully to treat dry eye syndrome (No more tears?, 1984). Its mechanisms of action are unknown but it acts to alleviate dryness, irritation, and light sensitivity. It also stimulates the development of goblet cells, which excrete tears, thus exerting a curative action.

Three derivatives of vitamin A (etretinate, tretinoin, and isotretinoin) are prescribed medicinally to treat specific diseases. These drugs regulate the proliferation and differentiation of epithelial tissue; suppress the synthesis of keratin within skin cells; reduce the size of sebaceous glands; inhibit production of sebum; and act as vesicants, causing peeling that removes excess cells and scar tissue in superficial skin layers.

Niacin's action also is unknown. In large doses, this vitamin lowers blood levels of cholesterol by about 10% and of triglycerides by about 25%. Large doses of niacin also dilate blood vessels.

Vitamin C, ascorbic acid, promotes the conversion

Table 50-1. Physiologic functions of vitamins

Vitamin	Metabolic function	Physiologic effects
Vitamin A (retinol, retinaldehyde, retinoic acid, retinyl esters)	Promotes mucin production in epithelial cells by an unknown mechanism	Is essential in the growth, development, and maintenance of epithelial tissue
	May play a role in cell membrane regulation as an enzyme cofactor; may function as an enzyme cofactor in steroid and mucopolysaccharide synthesis	Is essential in growth and reproduction
	Enhances resistance to carcinogenesis, possibly by destabilizing lysosomes, enhancing anti-tumor immunity, or direct cytotoxic action on abnormal cells	Reduces susceptibility to carcinogenesis
	Retinol is a component of the photosensitive pigments of the eye, rhodopsin, and iodopsin	Is essential for normal function of the retina
Vitamin B complex: Thiamine (vitamin B_1)	Functions as a coenzyme (thiamine pyrophosphate or TPP) in Krebs' cycle	Is essential for energy metabolism, especially that involving carbohydrates
	Plays a role in the transmission of impulses on nerve membranes, possibly by promoting sodium influx	Is essential for normal nerve function
Riboflavin (vitamin B_2, vitamin G)	Is a constituent of two coenzymes, flavin mononucleotide (FMN) and flavin adenine dinucleotide (FAD)	Is essential for the completion of several reactions in the energy cycle that produces ATP
	Is a component of amino acid oxidases and xanthine oxidase	Is involved in the oxidation of amino acids and hydroxy-acids to alpha-keto acids and the oxidation of a number of purines
Niacin (nicotinic acid, nicotinamide)	Is a constituent of two coenzymes, nicotinamide-adenine dinucleotide (NAD) and nicotinamide-adenine dinucleotide phosphate (NADP), which act as hydrogen acceptors in many metabolic reactions	Is essential for the synthesis of fatty acids and cholesterol and for the conversion of phenylalanine to tyrosine
Vitamin B_6 (pyridoxine, pyridoxal, pyridoxamine)	Is a constituent of pyridoxal phosphate, a coenzyme for many metabolic reactions involved in amino acid metabolism	Serves an important role in amino acid metabolism, including decarboxylation, transamination, transulfuration, and the conversion of tryptophan to niacin
		Is required for glycogenolysis, the synthesis of hemoglobin, and the formation of antibodies
		May be required for the conversion of linoleic acid to arachidonic acid
		Is necessary to the formation of norepinephrine, epinephrine, tyramine, dopamine, and serotonin
Folacin (folic acid, pteroylglutamic acid)	Forms coenzymes known as tetrahydrofolates involved in one-carbon transfers in metabolism	Is essential for DNA synthesis
		With cyanocobalamin, regulates the formation of red blood cells in the bone marrow
Pantothenic acid (calcium pantothenate, dexpanthenol)	Is a constituent of coenzyme A, which serves as a cofactor for reactions involving transfer of acetyl (two-carbon) groups	Is required for the oxidative metabolism of carbohydrates, gluconeogenesis, synthesis and degradation of fatty acids, and the synthesis of sterols, steroid hormones, and porphyrins
Vitamin B_{12} (cyanocobalamin, hydroxocobalamin, extrinsic factor)	Is a constituent of coenzymes involved in the demethylation of methylfolate and the maintenance of sulfhydroxyl groups of enzymes in a reduced state, the conversion of homocysteine to methionine and the maintenance of methyl-malonate-succinate isomerization	Is required for DNA synthesis in bone marrow; with folacin, regulates the production of red blood cells
		May be essential for the maintenance of the metabolic activity of folacin
Biotin	Is a constituent of a coenzyme for carboxylation and deamination reactions	Is required in the synthesis of fatty acids, the generation of the tricarboxylic acid cycle, and the formation of purines
Vitamin C (ascorbic acid, ascorbate)	Functions as a cofactor in hydroxylation reactions	Is necessary for the formation of collagen, the conversion of tryptophan to serotonin, and the conversion of cholesterol to bile acids

(Continued)

Table 50-1. *Physiologic functions of vitamins* (Continued)

Vitamin	Metabolic function	Physiologic effects
	Functions as an antioxidant	Protects vitamins A and E and polyunsaturated fatty acids from excessive oxidation
		Inhibits oxidation of crystallins (proteins in the eye lens), thereby delaying the formation of cataracts.
		May play a role in resistance to carcinogenesis and malignant tumor growth
		Promotes the absorption and use of iron
		Converts folacin to its active metabolite, folinic acid
		By as yet unknown mechanisms, is involved in clotting, the synthesis of adrenocortical hormones, and resistance to infection
Vitamin D (cholecalciferol, calcitriol, dihydrotachysterol, ergocalciferol, viosterol)	Is a constituent of a calcium-controlling hormone, calcitriol	Is necessary for the proper metabolism of calcium and phosphorus; promotes intestinal absorption of calcium and phosphorus, stimulates renal reabsorption of phosphate, and stimulates the release of calcium from bone tissue and bone resorption
Vitamin E (tocopherols of several types)	Functions as a biologic antioxidant	Has no proven function in humans
		May oppose pathologic conditions characterized by increased oxidation, particularly by free-radicals (cellular aging, oxygen toxicity, damage from air pollutants, and other degenerative biochemical transformations)
Vitamin K (menadione, phytonadione)	Is the lipid cofactor for membrane-bound peptide carboxylase	Is essential for the formation of prothrombin and other clotting proteins by the liver
		May participate in oxidative phosphorylation in the tissues

of methemoglobin to hemoglobin and reduces the pH of urine when excreted.

Dihydrotachysterol is converted by the body to the hormone calcitriol, which controls calcium and phosphorous metabolism. This hormone promotes a rise in blood levels of both minerals by facilitating their absorption in the gut; by enhancing their mobilization from bony tissues; and by reducing their excretion by the kidneys. By maintaining adequate blood levels of these minerals, dihydrotachysterol supports normal rates of bone formation.

The antioxidant properties of vitamin E are responsible for its therapeutic effect on premature infants with hemolytic anemia. The erythrocytes of these babies are abnormally susceptible to peroxide hemolysis, and their serums exhibit low concentrations of tocopherol. Alpha-tocopherol acts chemically to reduce peroxide, which prevents its damaging effects on the red blood cells.

Vitamin K is useful in warfarin toxicity because it competes with warfarin for participation in metabolic processes in liver microsomes that produce the clotting factors prothrombin (factor II), proconvertin (factor VII), plasma thromboplastin component (factor IX), and the Stuart factor (factor X). The competition between vitamin K and warfarin is a dynamic equilibrium reaction. Increasing the concentration of vitamin K at the cellular sites allows the liver to resume production of clotting factors despite the continued presence of warfarin, which tends to inhibit use of vitamin K by liver cells.

Pharmacokinetics. As constituents of the diet, vitamins enter the body normally through the digestive tract. They are widely distributed in the tissues and are found in high concentration in the liver. Some are destroyed by the metabolic processes in which they participate, whereas others are transformed and subsequently excreted in urine or feces. Because they are handled differently by the body, fat-soluble and water-soluble vitamins will be discussed separately (Box 50-1)

Fat-soluble vitamins. Natural forms of fat-soluble vitamins require digestible fat and bile salts for absorption in the small intestine. Conditions in which fat absorption is decreased, such as diarrhea or steatorrhea, cause reduced absorption of these nutrients. Nondigestible fats in the tract, such as mineral oil, carry the fat-soluble vitamins out of the body in feces. Synthetic forms of these vitamins that are water-miscible are available. These preparations do not require

Table 50-2. Physiologic manifestations of vitamin deficiencies

Vitamin	Signs and symptoms of deficiency	Deficiency disease
Vitamin A	Changes in the eyes progressing from night blindness to xerosis of the conjunctiva, xerosis of the cornea, loss of corneal substance, and scarring	Xerophthalmia
	Shrinking, hardening, and progressive degeneration of epithelial tissues and reduced resistance to invasion by infectious organisms	Keratomalacia
	Overgrowth of the bones with resultant nerve lesions	
	Growth retardation characterized by osteoblastosis, impaired protein synthesis, and loss of appetite	
	Vague apathy	
	Dry, rough skin	
	Increased risk of lung and GI infections leading to an increased death rate in children	
Thiamine	Mild deficiency: fatigue, weakness, lack of interest, irritability, depression, sleep disturbance, restlessness, emotional instability (aggressiveness, sensitivity to criticism, poor impulse control, mood swings), anorexia, and weight loss	Beriberi
	Moderate deficiency: Pallor, apathy, indigestion, constipation, headaches, nightmares, bruxism, insomnia, sweating, tachycardia after moderate exercise, muscle cramps, and paresthesias	
	Pronounced deficiency: muscle degeneration due to peripheral neuropathy, cardiomyopathy with congestive failure, emaciation, confusion, and loss of memory. In infants: pallor, facial edema, irritability	
	Abdominal pain, vomiting, loss of voice, and convulsions	
Riboflavin	Moderate deficiency: cheilosis, glossitis, greasy dermatitis (sebbhorea) in skin folds (nasolabial, scrotal, vulval), asthenia, vascularization of the cornea, and growth retardation in the young	
Niacin	Early signs: fatigue, muscle weakness, lassitude, depression, headache, backache, anorexia, indigestion, weight loss, mild skin eruptions, and loss of memory	Pellagra
	Late signs: asthenia, beefy-red glossitis, cheilosis, abdominal discomfort, nausea, vomiting, diarrhea, dermatitis (most pronounced in exposed areas), dementia, and, in children, growth retardation	
Vitamin B$_6$ (pyridoxine)	In adults: seborrheic dermatitis, peripheral neuritis, impaired immunity	
	In children: anemia, impaired immunity, vomiting, ataxia, weakness, abdominal pain, nervous irritability, and convulsive seizures	
	During pregnancy or use of oral contraceptives: possibly carbohydrate intolerance, depression, hypertriglyceridemia	
Folic acid	Pallor, asthenia, megaloblastic leukopenia and macrocytic anemia, reduced platelet levels, possibly glossitis and diarrhea. During pregnancy, an increased risk of spina bifida in the offspring	
Pantothenic acid	Malaise, vomiting, burning cramps, fatigue, tenderness in the heels, insomnia, diarrhea	
Vitamin B$_{12}$	Lemon yellow pallor, asthenia, anorexia, vomiting, diarrhea, hand and foot paresthesias, signs and symptoms of psychosis, megaloblastic macrocytic anemia and progressive neuropathy due to progressive demyelinization	Pernicious anemia
Biotin	Dermatitis, glossitis, lassitude, hyperesthesia, pallor, anorexia, nausea, loss of sleep, depression, muscle pains, and hypercholesterolemia	
Vitamin C	Early signs: intermittent joint pains, gum disease, dry skin, irritability, anemia, shortness of breath, poor wound healing, increased susceptibility to infection, petechiae due to increased capillary fragility, and, in children, growth retardation	Scurvy
	Late signs: anorexia, pain, tenderness and swelling of the joints, rough skin with dingy brown color, gingivitis, loss of teeth, anemia, petechial hemorrhages (progressing to spontaneous ecchymoses), muscle and cartilage degeneration. In infants: pallor, fever, diarrhea, vomiting, enlargement of the ends of the long bones, disinclination to move, and crying when handled	
Vitamin D	Unexplained cochlear deafness in middle age, demineralization of the teeth and bones with skeletal deformity, pretetany, bone pain	In children: rickets In adults: osteomalacia
	In infants: delayed closure of the fontanelles, softening of the skull, bossing of the forehead, enlargement of the ends of the long bones, bowing of the legs,	

(Continued)

Table 50-2. *Physiologic manifestations of vitamin deficiencies* (Continued)

Vitamin	Signs and symptoms of deficiency	Deficiency disease
	enlargement of the costochondral junction (the "rachitic rosary"), pigeon breast, scoliosis, narrowing of the pelvis, poorly developed muscles, weakness, restlessness, irritability, delayed dentition, malformed teeth, and retarded growth	
Vitamin E	Increased hemolysis of red blood cells, macrocytic anemia, increased capillary fragility	Hemolytic anemia in low–birth-weight infants
Vitamin K	Petechiae, ecchymoses, bleeding into the joints or muscles, GI bleeding, asthenia	Hemorrhagic disease in newborns

fat or bile salts for absorption but may be incompletely absorbed if peristalsis is excessive.

Retinoic acid, which is applied topically, is at least partially absorbed by the skin. The greater the degree of skin inflammation present, the greater the absorption. Because this derivative of vitamin A is used in high doses for the medical treatment of skin disease, significant levels of the drug are apt to enter the systemic circulation.

About 75% of a given dose of isotretinoin is degraded before it reaches the systemic circulation, apparently by biodegradation in the intestinal tract and in the liver during first-pass through. The drug does enter the entero-hepatic circulation.

Table 50-3. *Pharmacologic effects of vitamins used as drugs*

Vitamin	Pharmacologic effect(s)	Preparation	Therapeutic use(s)
etretinate (Tegison)	Regulates the proliferation and differentiation of epithelial cells	Oral capsules	Treatment of recalcitrant psoriasis (as a drug of last resort)
tretinoin (Retin-A)	Suppresses the synthesis of keratin; reduces the formation of comedones	Solution, cream, or gel for topical use	Treatment of acne, psoriasis, Darier's disease, and ichthyosis
isotretinoin (Accutane)	Reduces the size of sebaceous glands and the production of sebum	Oral capsules	Treatment of severe acne (Dosage: 0.5–1 mg/kg body weight daily, divided in two doses, for up to 20 weeks depending on response)
niacin	Reduces blood cholesterol and triglycerides	niacinamide (Diacin, Niac, Niacels, Nico-400, Nicobid, Nico-Span, Nicotym, Tega-Span): tablets and sustained-release tablets for oral use	Treatment of hypercholesterolemia and hyperbeta-lipoproteinemia
vitamin C (ascorbic acid)	Promotes the conversion of methemoglobin to hemoglobin	Ascorbic acid: tablets for oral use and solutions for injection	Management of idiopathic methemoglobin
	Reduces the *p*H of urine		Reduction of the rate of recurrent urinary tract infections in clients at high risk
dihydrotachysterol	Maintains calcium and phosphorus levels in bone and blood	Hytakerol: tablets, capsules, and solution in oil for oral use	Management of hypoparathyroidism
vitamin E	Reduces endogenous peroxidases	alpha-tocopherol acetate (Alpha-E-400, Aquasol E, CEN-E, Chew-E, E-Ferol, Eprolin, Epsilan-M, Pheryl-E, Tocopher-M, Tocopher-Plus, Tokols, Vita-Plus E, Viterra); tablets and capsules for oral use and solutions for injection	Treatment of hemolytic anemia in premature infants
vitamin K	Increased liver production of prothrombin	phytonadione; tablets for oral use and solution for injection	Treatment of warfarin toxicity Prevention of hemorrhagic disease in newborns

Box 50-1. Classification of vitamins

Fat-soluble
   vitamin A
   vitamin D
      cholecalciferol
      ergocalciferol
   vitamin E
      alpha-tocopherol
   vitamin K
      menadione

Water-soluble
   vitamin C (ascorbic acid)
   vitamin B complex
      thiamine (B_1)
      riboflavin (B_2)
      niacin (nicotinic acid)
      pyridoxine hydrochloride (B_6)
      pantothenic acid
      biotin
      choline; inositol; para-aminobenzoic acid
      folic acid*
      cyanocobalamine (B_{12})*

*B_{12} and folic acid are discussed in detail in the section on hematinics in this chapter.

Retinol, isotretinoin, and vitamin D bind to specific plasma globulins. Retinoic acid and isotretinoin bind to albumin; vitamin D binds to a specific α-globulin known as vitamin D-binding protein. Vitamin E in the bloodstream is associated with plasma lipoproteins. These complexations serve to prevent renal excretion of the vitamin molecules. Transport of vitamin A from body depots is dependent on the globulin carrier, and deficiency of the vitamin associated with protein deficiency cannot be corrected by administering the vitamin alone.

Vitamins A and D (but not retinoic acid or isotretinoin) tend to accumulate in the liver. (Animal livers are excellent dietary sources of these nutrients, and commercial preparations are derived from fish livers.) Some vitamin A is also deposited in the kidneys, lungs, adrenals, retinas, and intraperitoneal fat. Additional storage of vitamin D uses fat depots in the body. Vitamin K is not stored in large quantities in the body. Except in infants, vitamin E is widely distributed in large quantities in the tissues. The plasma tocopherol concentrations in newborns is only about one-fifth that of their mothers.

The precursors of vitamins A and D (beta-carotene and 7-dehydrocholesterol, respectively) accumulate in the skin. High levels of carotene in the skin impart a yellow or orange tinge to the skin that may be pronounced but appears to be physiologically harmless. The sclerae are not affected by this color change.

Precursors are transformed to active vitamin forms within the body. Vitamin D is produced by ultraviolet irradiation of 7-dehydrocholesterol. The deposition of this chemical in the skin is fortuitous because it is only in body tissues exposed to ultraviolet light that the conversion can occur. Beta-carotene is transformed to vitamin A in the wall of the small intestine.

Vitamins A, E, and K (including medical derivatives of vitamin A) are metabolized by the liver and enter the enterohepatic circulation. Eventually, metabolites are excreted in both feces and urine. Calcitriol is transformed in the kidneys and is excreted mainly in bile and feces. Vitamin A derivatives can persist in body tissues for up to 3 years after use of the drugs is stopped.

Water-soluble vitamins. Most of the water-soluble vitamins are well absorbed by the gastrointestinal (GI) tract. Folic acid and thiamine cross the intestinal membrane by active transport systems in specific areas of the small bowel. Adequate absorption of vitamin B_{12} requires hydrochloric acid and a specific gastric glycoprotein (intrinsic factor) for transport across the ileal mucosa. Passive diffusion of this vitamin is inadequate to maintain body stores unless concentrations in the intestinal lumen are extremely high. Niacin, pyridoxine, pantothenic acid, and vitamin C are absorbed readily from all areas of the GI tract and are widely distributed in the tissues.

Plasma binding of water-soluble vitamins appears to be minimal. Only folic acid and vitamin B_{12} are bound to a significant degree.

Vitamins of the B complex are stored in the liver to variable degrees. Although high concentrations of vitamin C are found in tissues such as the adrenals, there appear to be no significant depots of this nutrient, and regular daily intake is considered essential to good health.

Thiamine used by the body is completely degraded in the tissues. Other water-soluble vitamins are metabolized by the liver. All are excreted by the kidneys. Vitamin B_{12} also participates in the enterohepatic cycle, an important avenue for body losses when reabsorption is inadequate. This vitamin may be present in feces in large amounts.

Therapeutic uses. All vitamins are used to prevent and treat deficiency states. Because the underlying causes of deficiency in most clinical situations—inadequate dietary intake or malabsorption—affect most nutrients, attention must be given to total nutrition rather than to levels of individual nutrients. For this reason, vitamin supplementation usually involves administering multivitamins.

Multivitamin preparations for dietary supplementation are marketed in two strengths: maintenance and therapeutic. A daily dose of most maintenance preparations contains vitamin doses approximating the recommended daily allowances (Table 50-4). Vitamin A doses rarely exceed this allowance. Slight excesses of water-soluble vitamins may be included. Therapeutic formulas have much higher doses. They are used for treatment of existing deficiencies and for preventive treatment of persons deemed at high risk for deficiencies because of increased nutrient needs.

In some situations, individual needs for specific vitamins can be unusually high due to inborn errors of metabolism, or to environmental factors that increase tissue needs. In these cases, vitamin dosage must be tailored to meet the needs. Occasionally, as in pernicious anemia, a single vitamin is needed.

Pharmacologic uses of vitamins include the control of photosensitivity in porphyria; the treatment of certain skin diseases; the reduction of serum lipids; the management of parathormone deficiency; the treatment of premenstrual syndrome; the prevention of recurrent urinary tract infections; and the treatment of idiopathic methemoglobinemia, hemolytic anemia in newborns, and warfarin toxicity (see Table 50-3).

Table 50-4. Comparison of vitamin dosages used for various purposes

Vitamin	Recommended daily allowance*	Maximum dosage recommended for correction of deficiencies	Pharmacologic dose/PC
vitamin A	1,400–6,000 IU (one IU = 0.3 μg retinol; one retinol equivalent = 3.33 IU)	30 mg retinol (100,000 IU) daily, in a single dose	Topical solutions containing up to 100 mg retinoic acid per milliliter PC: A (X if >RDA)
thiamine	0.3–1.5 mg	90 mg daily in divided doses	Up to 4 g daily, in divided doses PC: A (C if >RDA)
riboflavin	0.4–1.8 mg	10 mg daily	10 mg daily for 10 days PC: A (C if >RDA)
niacin	5–20 mg	500 mg daily	2000 mg daily in divided doses PC: A (C if >RDA)
vitamin B$_6$	0.3–2.5 mg	100 mg daily	100–600 mg daily; for isoniazid toxicity, an amount equal to that of isoniazid ingested, usually several grams PC: A (C if >RDA)
folic acid	50–800 μg	1,000 μg daily	Up to 15 mg daily PC: A (C if >RDA)
folinic acid (Leucovorin)	Not used for nutrition	Not used for nutrition	IV: Weight equal to that of the folic acid antagonist (when used as an antidote for an antineoplastic folic acid antagonist) PC: C
pantothenic acid	10 mg	No recommendation available	250–500 mg q4h–q12h
vitamin B$_{12}$	0.3–4.0 μg	100 μg daily	Up to 5 mg daily PC: A (C if >RDA)
vitamin C	60 mg (100 mg for smokers)	500 mg daily	1,500 mg daily PC: A (C if >RDA)
vitamin D	400 IU (one IU = 0.025 μg pure crystalline vitamin D)	50,000 IU (malabsorption) 1,000 IU (uncomplicated deficiencies)	0.8–2.4 mg daily (dihydrotachysterol) PC: A (D if >RDA)
vitamin E	4–15 IU (one IU = 1 mg alpha-tocopherol)	100 mg daily	Up to 800 mg daily (in hemolytic anemia of newborns) PC: A (C if >RDA)
vitamin K	No recommendation available (estimated minimum daily requirement is 0.03 μg/kg of body weight or about 1.8–3 mg for adults)	10 mg daily	20–40 mg every 4 hours (in warfarin toxicity) Menadione (vitamin K3) PC: C (X if >RDA) Phytonadione PC: C

*As established by the Food and Nutrition Board, National Academy of Sciences—National Research Council (Specific recommendations vary with age, sex, and reproductive status).

KEY: RDA = recommended daily allowance; and PC = pregnancy risk category. (The validity of pregnancy risk categories has not been established. See Chapter 16, p 216.)

Adverse reactions. Theoretically, all vitamins are capable of producing adverse reactions. The margin of safety for water-soluble vitamins is wide, and toxic symptoms are rare. With the exception of vitamin E, fat-soluble vitamins are more toxic.

Hypervitaminosis A is the most frequent toxicity. The symptoms of this condition may be due, at least in part, to retinyl esters associated with plasma lipoproteins that act as surfactants. Dosages as low as twice the recommended daily allowance may produce toxicity if continued over time. Signs and symptoms include malaise, nausea desquamation, corneal opacities or erosion decalcification of bones, early epiphyseal closure, bone tenderness, lethargy, increased intracranial pressure, and coma. Death may occur. The vitamin is highly teratogenic, and congenital malformations are likely to develop in exposed embryos.

Isotretinoin (Accutane) can sometimes worsen acne, transforming crusted lesions into lesions resembling pyogenic granulomas. It can also cause cheilitis (lip inflammation) and conjunctivitis. High doses have caused gigantic bony overgrowth or skeletal hyperstosis. Isotretinoin and etretinate are also teratogenic (Scherer, 1987).

Drug therapy of skin diseases using retinoic acid may cause an increased sensitivity to the harmful effects of sunlight and ultraviolet light.

Concurrent use of thiazide diuretics and calcium and vitamin D supplements may result in hypercalcemia. Vitamin D enhances GI absorption of calcium, and thiazide diuretics reduce its excretion by the kidneys.

Vitamin E toxicity in preterm infants is characterized by respiratory distress, renal failure, liver disease, ascites, and thrombocytopenia.

Vitamin D toxicity may develop at dosages 12 times the recommended daily allowance. Signs and symptoms include weakness, fatigue, lassitude, headache, nausea, vomiting, diarrhea, renal impairment, or hypertension. Calcifications of soft tissues tend to develop. These are most dangerous when they occur in the kidneys. High calcium serum levels characteristic of vitamin D toxicity are especially dangerous to persons under treatment with digitalis because calcium excess increases the risk of toxicity of this medication. In children, hypervitaminosis D may cause cessation of growth for up to 6 months; some permanent stunting of stature may result. Persons who have experienced this toxicity may retain thereafter a permanent hypersensitivity to normal doses of the vitamin.

Although vitamin K is nontoxic in usual doses, large doses may cause problems in adults, and children are sometimes affected by moderate doses. The drug can cause hemolytic anemia, hyperbilirubinemia, and kernicterus in infants. It is irritating to skin and respiratory tract tissues. Rapid intravenous (IV) administration may cause flushing, dyspnea, chest pains, and, rarely, death. Administration of vitamin K to persons with severe hepatic disease may aggravate the liver disease.

Toxic syndromes have not been considered in the past to be a problem with most water-soluble vitamins. However, some toxic reactions have been recognized with pharmacologic doses, and several additional syndromes have been described recently.

Among the B vitamin complex, niacin in large doses produces vasodilation, flushing, and increased peristalsis. Pyridoxine (B_6) overdose causes neurologic problems characterized by paresthesias, numbness, and ataxia. Permanent physiologic dependence on large doses of the vitamin may develop following doses of 200 mg or more for over 30 days. Large doses of folic acid have caused recurrence of seizures in individuals using anticonvulsants with antifolate properties such as phenytoin, phenobarbital, and primidone. Vitamin B_{12} toxicity is characterized by polycythemia vera and peripheral vascular thrombosis. Very large doses are required for these effects.

Vitamin C in large doses may block the effect of copper, causing anemia. Exposure to large doses of the vitamin may increase body metabolism and excretion of this chemical. Abrupt withdrawal then causes a temporary hypovitaminosis C, despite adequate dietary intake. Rebound scurvy may occur; infants are particularly vulnerable. Vitamin C is also excreted as oxalate and can cause oxalate renal calculi.

Allergy to some vitamin preparations may represent reactions to extraneous chemicals in the medicinal preparation (*eg*, tartrazine). However, some allergic reactions appear to be true allergy to the vitamin molecule. Allergy may be manifested by itching, diarrhea, or anaphylaxis.

Precautions and contraindications. Vitamin supplements and pharmacologic dosages of vitamins should be discontinued if signs and symptoms of toxicity develop.

Large dosages of vitamin A, or use of its derivatives, are contraindicated during pregnancy. Women of childbearing age should practice reliable contraception while on these drugs and for a prolonged period after the therapy is withdrawn (2–3 years in the case of etretinate). Isotretinoin should not be used by individuals who are allergic to parabens, a preservative used in the formulation.

The dosage of vitamin D and calcium supplements should be reduced or discontinued in clients for whom thiazide diuretics are prescribed.

Dosages of pyridoxine supplements used for premenstrual tension should not exceed 100 mg/day. Clients for whom supplements are prescribed should be warned to report any signs or symptoms of neuropathy, such as numbness or unusual sensations.

Existing hypervitaminosis or allergic sensitivity

contraindicate use of the particular vitamin or vitamins involved. Prolonged use of large dosages should be avoided unless there is a demonstrated need for abnormally high doses. The fat-soluble vitamins are particularly dangerous.

Intravenous doses of vitamins should be given slowly to avoid acute reactions. (See Chapter 44 for more information on parenteral vitamins.)

To prevent toxicity, plasma levels of vitamin E used to treat premature infants should not exceed 3.5 mg/dl.

Folic acid supplements during pregnancy should not exceed 1 mg/d in dosage. This will prevent folate deficiency, even in individuals on antifolate anticonvulsants.

■ Summary

Vitamins are organic chemicals found in food that are essential in small quantities for health and normal growth. They cannot be synthesized by the body. Most are converted to metabolic coenzymes or cofactors by the body.

Although a well balanced diet provides adequate vitamins for most people, supplements may be needed by persons at high risk for developing deficiencies because of inadequate diet, malabsorption, or increased tissue needs. Certain vitamins are also administered in high doses to treat specific diseases.

Water-soluble vitamins and vitamin E have a wide therapeutic margin of safety. Other fat-soluble vitamins are more apt to cause toxicity, especially vitamins A and D.

Nursing management

Nursing implications

Vitamins are among the most frequently used nutritional supplements. Nutritionists decry the waste of money spent on unneeded vitamin preparations, contending that a well balanced diet furnishes all the vitamins needed by most consumers. Either the public is unwilling to act on this evaluation, or it does not believe that the average diet is sufficiently nutritious. The use of vitamin supplements is widespread and this use may ensure adequate intake at relatively low cost.

Administration   When oral vitamin preparations are prescribed, they should be administered with food. This will ensure secretion of adequate bile to promote absorption of fat-soluble vitamins. In addition, food will dilute the vitamin preparation. This may ameliorate the appetite-depressing effect experienced by some persons after ingesting vitamin preparations. (Vitamin preparations usually contain fish-liver oils and concentrated yeasts, which have strong odors and flavors. These can cause anorexia or nausea, partic-

ularly if eructation occurs after the tablet or capsule has dissolved.)

Parenteral forms of vitamins are usually injected intramuscularly (IM). Water-soluble vitamins (B and C) are often added to IV infusions.

Storage   Vitamin preparations are generally stable. However, ascorbic acid tablets are sensitive to light, heat, and moisture and should be stored in dry, cool environments. Darkened tablets are safe to use but a vinegar odor to the tablet or container indicates that the vitamin molecule has been chemically broken down.

Nursing process

Assessment   Basic assessment includes dietary analysis and physical assessment for signs and symptoms of both nutritional deficiency or excesses.

To determine dietary practices, clients should be questioned about their usual food intake. A listing of all foods consumed over the previous 24 hours often is revealing. It may corroborate the general diet history or raise questions about its accuracy.

Physical assessment should address the signs and symptoms of vitamin deficiency—abnormalities of skin and mucous membranes; delayed or abnormal skeletal development; defects in vision, such as night blindness; low energy levels; emotional lability; mental aberrations; poor resistance to infection; poor color; anorexia; bleeding gums; or petechiae. The presence of such symptoms in a person with good dietary habits may indicate malabsorption or a condition in which tissue needs for nutrients are abnormally high (see Table 43-2).

The history may reveal conditions that place the person at high risk for vitamin deficiencies. Pregnancy, use of oral contraceptives, high aspirin intake, smoking, habitual use of alcohol, rapid growth, and hyperthyroidism increase metabolic needs for vitamins. Dietary intake is apt to be reduced in the elderly person and in persons on rigorous weight-reduction regimens. A history of sprue, ulcerative colitis, or any other condition characterized by malabsorption may indicate that the person is not able to assimilate normal amounts of nutrients. People who have undergone gastric surgery or who have serious gastric disease are at high risk for pernicious anemia. Acute febrile illness with tissue-wasting increases, temporarily, the need for vitamins. Vitamins can also be lost from the system through dialysis or diuresis.

The detection of hypervitaminosis is as important as the detection of deficiencies. Excesses of vitamin intake are seen most commonly in children. Parents may administer toxic doses of vitamins by mistake. Sometimes they are overzealous in attempts to provide optimal nutrition. Typically, in such situations, various kinds of fortified foods are offered to children in addition to vitamin supplements. Fortified foods are dietary products to which have been added vitamin doses in excess of the nutrients that may have been destroyed or removed during the processing of the food. They contain, therefore, higher levels of vitamins or other nutrients than do the natural foods from which they were made. Dairy products (milk, margarine, cheese), cereal products, and syrups for flavoring milk drinks are sometimes fortified with vitamins A and D. Ingestion of large quantities of such products, especially if a multivitamin supplement is used, can lead to hypervitaminosis of these nutrients.

Signs and symptoms of hypervitaminosis from fat-soluble vitamins include lethargy, fatigue, skeletal abnormalities, bone tenderness, headache, nausea, vomiting, diarrhea, increased urine output, and soft-tissue calcification as shown by palpable lumps. In infants, fontanelles may bulge or cranial bones may soften. Coma may develop in very severe overdosage.

Nursing diagnosis   Nursing diagnoses may identify vitamin deficiencies, vitamin toxicity, or adverse reactions to pharmacologic doses of vitamins. Examples include the following:

> *Altered nutrition, less than body requirements: vitamin C deficiency related to inadequate dietary intake of foods rich in ascorbic acid*
> *Altered nutrition, less than body requirements: pyridoxine deficiency related to increased need for vitamin B$_6$ during the premenstrual period*
> *Altered nutrition, less than body requirements: multiple vitamin deficiency related to malabsorption due to ulcerative colitis*
> *Altered nutrition, more than body requirements: hypervitaminosis A related to concurrent use of high-dose vitamin supplements and vitamin A fortified foods*
> *Altered nutrition, more than body requirements: hypervitaminosis D related to simultaneous intake of calcium/vitamin D supplements and thiazide diuretics*

Planning   Goals for nursing care are specific to the nutritional problem diagnosed. For the diagnoses just listed, appropriate goals might include increasing intake of a deficient vitamin, referral to a physician for therapeutic or parenteral vitamin supplementation, reduction in intake of vitamins causing toxicity, and prevention of birth defects by withdrawal of a teratogenic drug prior to conception or (if necessary) during pregnancy.

Intervention   When hypovitaminosis is suspected, the client may need referral to a physician for definitive diagnosis and prescription. Clients under treatment for medical conditions contributory to nutritional problems should discuss this problem with their physicians. When faulty health habits pose a risk for

vitamin deficiency, however, the nurse may advise the client regarding the correction of these habits.

If the underlying health practices cannot be corrected immediately, specific suggestions may be made to reduce the risk of frank vitamin deficiencies. Smokers have an increased need for vitamin C and may need a multivitamin formula with extra ascorbic acid in the formula. The use of oral contraceptives or pregnancy increases tissue needs for vitamins C, B$_6$, B$_{12}$, and folic acid. Vitamin formulas specially prepared to meet these needs are available. The ingestion of alcohol increases the body's needs for B-complex vitamins. Clients with an alcohol problem should be advised to take high-potency B-complex vitamins. (Clients should be warned that vitamin therapy will not prevent all harmful effects of excessive alcohol use and will not eliminate the need to address and treat the problem of alcoholism.) Weight-reduction regimens should be analyzed to determine which nutrients are likely to be deficient. If carbohydrate allowances are low, as shown by a restricted allowance for "cereal" exchanges, B-complex deficiency is likely. A very low allowance of fat exchange may predispose to vitamin A and D deficiencies.

Clients deficient in intrinsic factor need supplementary doses of cyanocobalamin. If some gastric function remains, high doses of B$_{12}$ given orally may suffice. Some preparations contain powdered intrinsic factor from animal tissues that enhance their effectiveness. These tend to become less effective over time due to the development of antibodies to the foreign intrinsic factor. Persons who cannot maintain adequate levels of vitamin B$_{12}$ with oral supplementation need parenteral injections of this nutrient. (Vitamin B$_{12}$ is discussed later in this chapter.) Injectable vitamin preparations cannot be purchased without a physician's prescription. Unfortunately, even though a prescription is needed, the cost of the medicine is usually not covered by insurance prescription plans because it is a vitamin.

If frank symptoms of vitamin toxicity are present, the family should be referred for medical care. Vitamin supplementation and the use of fortified foods should be discontinued immediately.

Client education.   Nurses are often asked for advice on the use of vitamin supplements by persons with good dietary habits and normal health. This is a controversial question. Few people argue with the basic nutritional principle that a varied balanced diet is the best source of nutrients, including vitamins. However, actual dietary practices among large numbers of the population do not provide such a diet. American grocery products include many highly processed or highly caloric foods that may be relatively deficient in important nutrients. Because personal preference and emotional conditioning influence food selection, highly nu-

Learning experience 50-1

Prepare a *retrospective* list of all foods consumed in the last 24 hours. Compute the total amount of the following vitamins contained in your diet: vitamin A, thiamine, riboflavin, niacin, vitamin C, and vitamin D. Is your intake of any vitamin less than the RDA? More than 150% of the RDA?

If you take a vitamin supplement, add the dosages of the vitamins contained in that preparation to your dietary intake. How do these overall totals compare with the RDAs?

tritious diets may not be consumed by many people and may not be consistently used even by concerned people with considerable knowledge of nutrition. The idea of using supplemental vitamins as "insurance" against deficiencies is not devoid of merit.

Another question that remains unresolved is the issue of optimum nutritional levels. Recommended dietary allowances in present use derive, in part, from older "minimal daily requirements." The latter represented the amount of nutrient that was sufficient to eliminate overt signs and symptoms of frank deficiency. For the most part, recommended daily allowances are only slightly higher than these levels. Linus Pauling believes, as do other respected authorities in the field of biochemistry, that optimum levels may be considerably higher for many nutrients (Worthington-Roberts, 1981).

In some instances, vitamin supplements may be cheaper than the food items required to provide a specific nutrient. For example, the cost of an ascorbic acid tablet is usually considerably lower than the price of an orange. The fruit contains other nutrients that may be important but if it is purchased solely for its vitamin C content, the pure vitamin may represent a more prudent purchase. Persons on a severely restricted food budget may find that they are able to provide better overall nutrition by using part of that money to buy vitamin supplements.

In counseling clients regarding the use of vitamin supplements, the nurse should point out the importance of maintaining a good diet. Clients need information that will enable them to make a reasonable decision. This includes facts about the risks of hypervitaminosis. The difference between dosage levels of maintenance and therapeutic formulas should be explained clearly.

Conservation of nutrients in food. Clients may need instruction in techniques for conserving the nutrients present in food. Proper refrigeration or storage is important to prevent breakdown of nutrients before food

is cooked and consumed. High temperatures destroy vitamin C unless the pH of the food involved is low. Copper* also catalyzes the destruction of this vitamin. Dietary sources of this nutrient require care in handling to ensure that their nutrient content is not compromised.

Water-soluble vitamins tend to leach from food if large amounts of water are used in cooking. Steaming with small amounts of liquid may be recommended. If boiling is preferred, the pot liquor (the liquid remaining after cooking is completed) should be used in the preparation of food, such as soups or gravies, so that the nutrients will not be lost.

Other vitamin-related problems. Clients who habitually consume mineral oil are at high risk for fat-soluble deficiencies because this indigestible lipid carries these nutrients through the tract in an indigestible form. Mineral oil is used to prevent or relieve constipation. Unless the medication has been prescribed for a sound medical reason, the nurse should attempt to substitute an alternative regimen to maintain fecal elimination. Clients who are self-medicating may benefit greatly from instruction in health practices designed to promote bowel function. In consultation with the physician, alternatives to the drug prescription should be explored. If the mineral oil regimen cannot be changed, clients should be advised to take vitamins and oil at different times to minimize interaction in the gut. Higher than normal doses of fat-soluble vitamins may be needed because it may be impossible to schedule mineral oil medication at times when it will not be interacting with either food or vitamin supplements, and some loss of nutrients is likely.

Certain vitamins interfere with the therapeutic effect of specific drugs prescribed for the treatment of disease. In such situations, the dosage of the drug is adjusted to compensate for normal vitamin levels. Clients should be warned to maintain consistent levels of vitamins in such situations. (They should *not* be told to avoid the vitamins or the foods containing them because deficiencies could then develop.) The most common interactions of this type are those involving L-dopa and vitamin B_6, and coumarin anticoagulants and vitamin K.

Clients receiving retinoic acid treatment for skin disease should be cautioned about the increased sensitivity to skin damage from ultraviolet irradiation that commonly develops. This is particularly severe in people with light complexions. Clients should avoid exposure to sunlight and should not use lights designed to promote tanning.

---

* The use of copper utensils or of water that has absorbed the metal from copper pipes is enough to lower vitamin levels. If the water system is copper, running a faucet long enough to flush out standing water before drawing water to be used in preparing food will prevent destruction of vitamin C.

Megavitamin therapy. Some clients believe in the value of megavitamin therapy and consume large amounts of these nutrients. Although the risk of hypervitaminosis from water-soluble vitamins does not appear great, large doses of fat-soluble vitamins are dangerous. This risk should be clearly explained. Vitamin preparations should be assessed for total fat-soluble vitamin content. If dangerous levels are being consumed, specific suggestions may be made to moderate vitamin A and vitamin D consumption. Clients should be reminded that exposure to sunlight increases vitamin D levels in the body by converting biochemicals in the skin to the vitamin.

If clients are consuming large amounts of vitamin C, they should be advised not to discontinue such dosages abruptly. A temporary vitamin C deficiency can occur in such situations due to the enhanced metabolism and excretion of that chemical after prolonged use of large doses. Weaning off the megavitamin doses is advisable during pregnancy to avoid vitamin C deficiency in the fetus and newborn. Large doses of vitamin A are also undesirable in women of childbearing years because this vitamin is teratogenic.

Nurses working with clients who persist in using megavitamins may contribute to the ongoing investigation of the effects of such therapy. Careful client records may provide important data about the long-term health effects of such regimens.

Nutritional therapy sometimes masks the symptoms of medical conditions. Clients who rely on vitamins or other nutrients to alleviate multiple symptoms should be advised to seek definitive diagnosis of any underlying condition that may be the cause of these symptoms. A 4- to 6-week holiday from vitamin use may be needed to reveal the baseline condition so proper diagnostic and medical treatment measures can be taken.

Evaluation Data required for evaluation include the absence or incidence of signs and symptoms of nutritional imbalance, and signs and symptoms of the positive health benefits of optimum nutrition. When pharmacologic doses of vitamins or vitamin derivatives are employed for therapy, clients should be monitored for toxicity and therapeutic response.

Checklist of nursing actions

☐ Assess nutritional practices and the general health of clients to determine the risk of vitamin deficiency.

☐ Promote good dietary nutrition as the best source of vitamin nutrients.

☐ Teach clients about vitamins to enable them to make rational decisions about the use of vitamin supplements.

☐ Caution clients about the risks of toxicity from high doses of vitamins A and D.

☐ Monitor clients using megavitamin doses for toxic signs and symptoms.

☐ Advise clients taking large doses of vitamin C to wean themselves off these dosages rather than discontinue them abruptly.

☐ Advise women of childbearing age not to use extremely large doses of vitamins A or C.

☐ Refer clients with signs and symptoms of frank vitamin deficiency for medical care.

☐ Administer oral vitamin preparations with meals.

☐ Protect vitamin C preparations from air, light, heat, and contact with copper.

☐ To reduce the risk of fat-soluble vitamin deficiency, assist clients dependent on mineral oil to use alternative measures to promote bowel function.

☐ Advise clients receiving coumarin anticoagulants to maintain a steady dietary intake of vitamin K.

☐ Advise clients receiving L-dopa to maintain a steady dietary intake of vitamin B_6.

☐ Monitor clients receiving pharmacologic doses of vitamins for toxic signs and symptoms.

☐ Warn clients receiving retinoic acid for skin disease against excessive exposure to ultraviolet light, including sunlight.

☐ Warn women of childbearing age who receive drugs derived from vitamin A to prevent conception until after withdrawal of treatment and a drug-free period adequate for elimination of body stores of these substances.

Minerals

Minerals are inorganic chemicals used by the body for essential physiologic functions. They are ingested in the form of salts contained in the diet. Certain minerals—sodium, potassium, calcium, magnesium, phosphorus, and chlorine (chloride)—are electrolytes; that is, in solution, their salts dissociate into two charged particles or ions, which perform vital physiologic functions (*eg*, in the transmission of impulses). Other minerals function as components of enzymes and complex proteins such as hemoglobin. Certain minerals, called *trace minerals* are needed only in very small amounts. These trace minerals include cobalt, chromium, copper, fluorine (fluoride), iodine, iron, manganese, molybdenum, selenium, and zinc.

Some of the body's mineral needs have been long recognized. The compelling need for sodium chloride (table salt) led to the development of early trade routes, which were used for exchange between populations who could make salt from sea water and inland people whose local sources of salt were inadequate. Requirements for calcium and iron were also delineated fairly early. Only in recent decades has the need for many trace minerals become evident. These were first appreciated in relation to animal husbandry. Many were regarded only as toxic poisons until newer research techniques revealed them to be constituents of essential biochemicals.

Physiology. Minerals are involved in a wide variety of physiologic functions (Table 50-5). In the form of salts, they serve as structural materials in such tissues as bone, teeth, cell membranes, and connective tissue. They are components of biochemicals necessary for vital functions such as impulse transmission, oxygen transport in the blood, and cellular respiration. They are incorporated in many biologic enzymes. The electrolyte minerals also function to maintain osmotic pressure in the fluid compartments of the body and to buffer strong acids and bases.

Mineral metabolism is extremely complex. Many elements affect each other in both pharmacokinetics and pharmacodynamics. They sometimes compete with each other for absorption, biologic activity, and excretion. Two or more may be required to complete a physiologic function. For example, moderation of nerve and muscle impulses requires both calcium and magnesium; cholesterol metabolism is influenced by zinc and copper; and the production of red blood cells requires iron, copper, and cobalt (in the form of vitamin B_{12}).

Mineral nutrition is a rapidly expanding field of study, characterized by extensive research activity and a proliferating knowledge base. Only minerals for which dietary recommendations have been developed, or those used for pharmacologic purposes, will be discussed here. Other minerals known to play a role in physiology include silicon, cadmium, and nickel. Even the deadly poison arsenic has been found in certain bioenzymes. The student would be well advised to keep abreast of developments in this area because they are likely to affect greatly future developments in nutritional therapy.

Pathology. Inappropriate mineral nutrition is emerging as a serious health problem. Iron deficiency anemia, the most frequent mineral deficiency, is discussed in the following section on hematinics. Lack of calcium (especially in postmenopausal women) occurs frequently. The incidence of trace-mineral deficiencies is unknown but is suspected to be significant. These may arise from use of highly processed foods from which many mineral constituents have been removed. Enrichment and fortification replace some, but not all, of these elements. Malabsorption and unusually high physiologic requirements for minerals may also lead to deficiencies.

Recommended daily doses have not been established for most minerals. Daily dietary intake estimated to be safe and effective has been designated for some minerals for which recommended daily allowances are not yet available. However, methods for assaying mineral content have not been standardized, and optimum levels are still unknown.

The diagnosis of deficiency states requires analysis of dietary habits, urine or serum mineral levels, mineral content of hair, and a complete history and physical examination. Serum levels are often of questionable value because tissue reserves may be seriously depleted before blood levels decline. For some minerals, specific diagnostic procedures provide important data (*eg*, red blood cell count to detect iron deficiency anemia and x-ray examination to reveal bone thinning due to calcium deficiency).

Mineral toxicity can also be a problem. Minerals are constituents of many metallic and organochemical environmental pollutants. Some people ingest high doses of mineral supplements in an attempt to enhance nutritional status. The requirement for specific minerals is often extremely low, and there is a narrow margin of safety between therapeutic and toxic doses. The ability of the body to eliminate these chemicals is limited, and harmful levels may accumulate within a short time.

Physiologic effects of mineral imbalance vary with different elements (Table 50-6). In general, deficiencies impair growth and development; lead to tissue breakdown; or interfere with vital functions, such as circulation, oxygen transport, nerve and muscle function, or hormone balance. Symptoms of toxicity also vary with the specific chemicals involved.

Pharmacodynamics. Nutritional supplements of mineral nutrients replenish body stores and promote normal function. They correct many signs and symptoms of deficiency diseases but cannot reverse structural changes, such as bone deformities or scarring of organs due to tissue damage.

Mechanisms of action of pharmacologic doses vary with the mineral involved (Table 50-7). For example, potassium and calcium oppose each other's effects on myocardial contractility. Magnesium reduces nerve-cell irritability and may play a role in the inhibition of toxin production by bacteria responsible for toxic shock syndrome. Iodine stimulates respiratory secretion, causing production of a more dilute sputum that is easier to raise and expectorate.

Lithium and chromium are two minerals used medicinally whose normal dietary requirements are as yet unknown. Lithium alters sodium transport in nerve and muscle cells; the two minerals appear to compete for movement across the membrane. Chromium is believed by some people to enhance the cell's use of glucose.

Pharmacokinetics. Normally, mineral salts are ingested in food. Their absorption in the intestine is affected by binding and chelating agents that may

(*Text continues on p. 1265*)

Table 50-5. Physiologic functions of minerals

Mineral element	Representative functions
Sodium (Na)	Maintains osmotic pressure in the intravascular and extracellular fluids
	Plays an essential role in ion movement across cell membranes, which generate impulses in nerves and muscles
Potassium (K)	Maintains osmotic pressure in intracellular fluid
	Plays an essential role in ion movement across cell membranes, which generate impulses in nerves and muscles
	Is necessary to relaxation of cardiac muscle
	May exert a protective role in preventing blood vessel damage by hypertension
Calcium (Ca)	Is a structural component of bone and teeth
	Functions as an activator of certain enzymes (*eg*, coagulation factors)
	With magnesium, plays a role in the moderation of nerve and muscle impulses
	Is necessary to contraction of cardiac muscle
	Is a component of intracellular cement and cell membranes
	Blocks intestinal absorption of lead
	May play a role in preventing hypertension
Magnesium (Mg)	Is second only to potassium in concentration in intracellular fluid
	With calcium, moderates the transmission of stimulant impulses in nerves and muscles
	Is a component of many enzymes (*eg*, transfer enzymes)
	Aids in bone growth and regulation of the heart rhythm
	May play a role in preventing hypertension, especially during pregnancy
Phosphorus (P)	Aids bone growth and mineralization of teeth
	Is a component of molecules such as ATP that are essential for energy metabolism
	Maintains structural integrity of cells
	Plays a part in cellular immunity
Chloride (Cl) (chloride)	Is important to normal fluid shifts, normal pH of the blood, and the production of hydrochloric acid in the stomach
Iron (Fe)	Is a component of heme-containing enzymes (*eg*, cytochromes, catalase, peroxidase) and metalloproteins (*eg*, transferritin, xanthine oxidase, and hemoglobin)
Copper (Cu)	Plays a role in the production of red blood cells
	Is a component of microsomal enzymes (*eg*, ferroxidase, cytochrome oxidase, tyrosinase)
	Plays a role in the function of mitochondria, collagen metabolism, and melanin formation
	May help protect the heart from cardiomyopathy and angiopathy
	Acts as a cofactor in the use of iron by RBCs
Iodine (I)	Is a component of thyroid hormones, which control the rate of metabolic oxidation in cells
Fluoride (F)	Is an essential component for normal formation of dentin and tooth enamel
	Keeps skin, hair, and nails healthy
	May help prevent osteoporosis in older people
Zinc (Zn)	Is an essential component of many enzymes (*eg*, alcohol dehydrogenase, DNA polymerase, retinol dehydrogenase)
	Plays a role in healing, acuity of taste and smell, growth (especially of the immune system *in utero*), and sexual development
	May help protect the heart from cardiomyopathy and angiopathy
Manganese (Mn)	Is a component of enzymes (*eg*, pyruvate carboxylase)
	Plays a role in oxidative phosphorylation, fatty acid metabolism, and mucopolysaccharide synthesis
	Is required for normal bone growth and development, reproduction and cell functions
Cobalt (Co)	Is a component of vitamin B_{12}, a coenzyme necessary to red blood cell production
	Plays a role in biologic methylation
Chromium (Cr)	Is a component of glucose tolerance factor, which mediates insulin effects on cell membranes
Selenium (Se)	Is a component of enzymes (*eg*, glutathionine peroxidase)
	Appears to protect the body from toxic effects of mercury and cadmium
	Complements vitamin E to fight cell damage by oxygen
Molybdenum (Mo)	Is a component of flavoenzymes (*eg*, xanthine oxidase)
	Plays a role in xanthine and hypoxanthine metabolism

Table 50-6. Physiologic requirements for minerals and effects of imbalances

Mineral	Nutritional requirements	Effects of deficiencies	Toxic effects/PC
Sodium	115–3,300 mg daily* Normal serum level = 136–145 mEq/liter	Hypotension and tendency to develop circulatory shock If hydration is maintained, weakness and debility	Hypertension owing to hypervolemia Thirst In dehydration, irritability, delirium, and convulsions PC: C
Potassium	350–5,625 mg daily* Normal serum level = 3.5–5.0 mEq/liter	Weakness or paralysis of muscles Abdominal distention, paralytic ileus Prolongation of cardiac systole, cardiac arrest	Smooth muscle spasm, intestinal colic Skeletal muscle weakness Prolongation of cardiac diastole, cardiac arrest Increased secretion of glucagon Locally, vascular constriction PC: A (C for potassium acetate)
Calcium	360–1,200 mg daily† Normal serum levels = 4.5–5.5 mEq/liter or 9–11 mg/dl (Increased in individuals with high intake of caffeine and alcohol, and in heavy smokers)	Osteoporosis, periodontal disease Rickets in children When serum levels decline, tetany or convulsions	Anorexia, nausea, vomiting Headaches, seizures, coma Muscle weakness, lethargy, coma Calcification of soft tissues Renal lithiasis Prolongation of cardiac systole, cardiac arrest Locally, irritation to tissues Constipation Renal and gallstones Weight loss Slowed mentation Inappropriate behavior Bone pain Thirst Joint pain; exacerbation of rheumatoid arthritis PC: C
Phosphate	800–1,200 mg daily Normal serum levels: 2.7–4.5 mg/dl	Muscle weakness Encephalopathy Cardiomyopathy with congestion Hemolytic anemia Ventilating collapse GI and skin hemorrhages	Tachycardia Nausea, diarrhea Abdominal cramps Muscle weakness Hyperreflexia
Chloride	1,700–5,100 mg/d Normal plasma levels: 100–110 mEq/l or 350–390 mg/dl	Metabolic alkalosis	Increased risk of atherosclerosis Metabolic acidosis
Magnesium	50–450 mg daily† Normal serum levels = 1.5–2.5 mEq/liter	Increased muscle tone, irritability, convulsions	Flaccid paralysis Cardiac arrest in diastole Increased congenital defects in exposed embryos PC: B
Iron	10–60 mg daily† Normal serum levels = 105 ± 35 µg/100 mg	Iron deficiency anemia	Hematemesis, diarrhea, hypotension, coma Cellular damage; organ dysfunction PC: A
Copper	0.5–3.0 mg daily* Normal serum levels = 114 ± 14 µg/100 ml	Anemia, leukopenia, neutropenia	Damage to liver, kidneys, and other organs Possible mutagenesis or carcinogenesis PC: C

(Continued)

Table 50-6. Physiologic requirements for minerals and effects of imbalances (Continued)

Mineral	Nutritional requirements	Effects of deficiencies	Toxic effects/PC
Iodine	40–200 μg daily†	Goiter, thyroid imbalances	Goiter, thyroid imbalances PC: C
Fluorine	0.1–4.0 mg daily*	Abnormal dentin formation; soft tooth enamel	(During tooth formation) permanent discoloration of the teeth Abnormal bone and tooth structure PC: C
Zinc	50–200 μg daily	Retarded wound healing Growth retardation Hypogonadism Night blindness nonresponsive to vitamin A therapy Decreased acuity of taste Decreased resistance to infection Increased risk of heart disease During pregnancy, toxemia and increased incidence of fetal distress and congenital anomalies	Possible increase in the incidence of congenital anencephaly Decrease in high density lipoproteins and increased risk of myocardial infarction PC: C
Chromium	Unknown	Impaired glucose tolerance Diabetes mellitus characterized by high levels of circulating insulin	Hyperemia, emphysema, bronchitis, cancer of the respiratory tract (inhaled) PC: C
Cobalt	0.3–4.0 μg daily (as vitamin B_{12})	Macrocytic (pernicious) anemia	Polycythemia
Lithium	None available	Accelerated atherosclerosis and coronary artery disease Pronounced mood cycles	Polydipsia, polyuria, nephrogenic diabetes insipidus Allergic dermatitis and vasculitis Goiter Nausea, vomiting, diarrhea Ataxia, fine tremors, hyperreflexia Confusion, sedation Tremor, convulsions, coma, and death Increased incidence of cardiac anomalies in exposed embryos
Manganese	0.5–5.0 mg/d*	Defective growth Reproductive dysfunction Collagen problems CNS disorders	Possible mutagenesis or carcinogenesis PC: C
Molybdenum	0.03–0.5 mg/d*	Growth retardation (in animals) Dental disease	Molybdenum deposits in bone and soft tissue
Selenium	0.01–0.2 mg/d*	Poor wound healing Growth retardation, hypogonadism Uremic impotence	Weakness, lethargy, tremors, anorexia, nausea, vomiting, abdominal pain, profuse diaphoresis and garlicky breath Fatigue, irritability Nail changes PC: C

*Estimated safe and effective daily dietary intake recommended by the Food and Nutrition Board, National Academy of Sciences—National Research Council.

†Recommended Daily Allowance as established by the Food and Nutrition Board, National Academy of Sciences—National Research Council (Specific recommendations vary with age, sex, and reproductive status).

KEY: PC = pregnancy risk category. (The validity of pregnancy risk categories has not been established. See Chapter 16, p 216.)

either inhibit or facilitate their transfer across the intestinal membrane. Absorption may also be altered by other minerals, vitamins and hormones, and the oxidative state (valence) of the mineral (Table 50-8).

Except for the electrolytes and lithium, most minerals are protein-bound in the serum. In some cases, the protein is specific to one mineral (*eg*, transferrin, which binds iron, and ceruloplasmin, which binds copper). Protein deficiency can increase the loss of such minerals in urine because the unbound form is readily excreted in the kidneys. Minerals are distributed widely in tissues. Potassium uptake by the cells is enhanced by insulin. Lithium crosses the blood–brain barrier slowly but central nervous system concentrations eventually stabilize during long-term use. Most minerals also cross the placenta and appear in the milk of nursing mothers.

Minerals are stored in many tissue depots. Bone contains large amounts of calcium, magnesium, phosphorus, zinc, and fluorine. High levels of iron and cobalt are found in the liver; iodine is concentrated in the thyroid, copper in the intestinal mucosa, and iron in the spleen. Many metallic compounds are deposited in the kidneys.

Electrolytes, fluoride, and lithium are excreted by the kidneys. Adrenal mineralocorticoids control renal elimination of sodium and potassium, stimulating sodium reabsorption and potassium excretion. Calcium loss in urine is inversely related to parathormone and vitamin D levels. When potassium concentrations are excessive, the mineral is released by the gut and eliminated in feces.

Other minerals are excreted largely as metallic salts of bile acids. They participate in the enterohepatic cycle and are partially reabsorbed, thus conserving body supplies. Eventually, they are eliminated in feces. Excess concentrations of these minerals stimulate their renal excretion. Urinary elimination also may be increased by diuresis, injury, infection, and other stressors. Minerals present in the body in high concentrations are eliminated also by the sweat glands.

Therapeutic uses. Mineral salts are incorporated in many nonprescription nutritional supplements, often with vitamins. Many "one-a-day" preparations contain mineral doses equal to the recommended daily allowances* or estimated safe and effective daily dietary intake,* in addition to recommended daily allowances of vitamins. Preparations are available that contain iron, iron with vitamins, dicalcium phosphate with vitamin D, and various other combinations. In addition, proprietary preparations of less highly refined mineral sources are marketed, such as dolomite (mainly calcium) or kelp (rich in iodine).

---

* Categories established by the Food and Nutrition Board, National Academy of Sciences—National Research Council nutritional recommendations

Physicians prescribe minerals to replenish body supplies for the treatment of deficiency states. In addition, parenteral or oral preparations are used for many therapeutic purposes. Electrolyte solutions are employed to maintain hydration and proper chemical composition of body fluids in patients suffering excessive losses or in those unable to maintain adequate oral intake.

The dangerous cardiac effects of high concentrations of calcium may be ameliorated by administration of potassium salts, and vice versa. In addition, potassium can be used to reduce the toxic effects of high doses of digitalis. Parenteral calcium salts are administered to relieve the painful muscle spasms of tetany. Oral calcium is used in the treatment of osteoporosis.

Magnesium sulfate is the treatment of choice for convulsions due to eclampsia of pregnancy. Iodine salts are components of stimulant expectorants and radiopaque dyes. Zinc salts are administered to debilitated patients to promote the healing of decubiti and other wounds.

Lithium carbonate is used in the treatment of manic–depressive psychoses of both unipolar and bipolar types. These mental states have not been categorized as deficiency diseases but the mineral appears to produce favorable changes in brain-cell function and reverses many of their symptoms. Maintaining therapeutic levels of the mineral by regular prophylactic doses reduces the incidence of acute psychotic episodes in many clients. (See Chapter 26, Psychoactive Drugs, for more information on lithium.)

Iron is discussed in greater detail under Hematinics later in this chapter.

Dosage and administration. Preparations of minerals usually used for medical therapy are given in Table 50-7.

Adverse reactions. The margin of safety for mineral preparations is much narrower than for other nutritional components. Toxic signs and symptoms often appear with dosages only slightly above the recommended range. Persons with impaired liver or kidney function are likely to develop toxic reactions while receiving normal doses (see Table 50-6).

Unless balanced by water intake, *sodium* excess leads to hyperosmolarity of body fluids and a rise in concentration of the sodium ions. Hyperirritability of nerve and muscles follows. As toxicity increases, delirium, convulsions, and death can ensue. Sodium excesses in the presence of ample fluids cause hypervolemia and hypertension. This is the most common form of mineral toxicity in developed countries.

Excessive levels of *potassium* stimulate smooth muscle contraction and prolong cardiac diastole. Hyperkalemia is characterized by colicky abdominal pain, diarrhea, paresthesias, weakness, and cardiac arrhyth-

(Text continues on p. 1269)

Table 50-7. Mineral preparations used as drugs

Mineral	Preparations	Usual adult dosage	Pharmacologic effects	Therapeutic uses	Method of administration
Sodium	sodium chloride (table salt)	Sodium equivalent to 1–2 tsp of table salt daily	Increases blood volume	Prevention of hypovolemia in excessive perspiration, Addison's disease, and excessive sodium losses, such as ileostomy	Increase the amount used in cooking Ingest plain table salt Use electrolyte solution as beverage
	bicarbonate of soda	1 tsp	Increases blood volume; increases base buffer	Prevention and treatment of metabolic acidosis	Dissolve in 3–4 oz water; sip slowly; do not take on a full stomach
	saline solutions	50–150 ml/hr PC: C	Maintains blood volume	Prevention and treatment of dehydration	Administer orally or intravenously
Potassium (KaoChlor, Kay Ciel, Kaon, KCl, K-Dur, K-Lyte, K-Lor, Slow-K)	Flavored effervescent tablets containing potassium citrate and bicarbonate (K-Lyte)	25 mEq potassium once or twice daily	Replenishes potassium; prolongs diastole of the heart	Prevention or treatment of hypokalemia Prevention of digitalis toxicity due to hypokalemia	Dissolve tablet completely in 3–4 oz water and administer while still effervescing
	potassium chloride solutions for oral use	20–100 mEq potassium daily in divided doses			Dilute well and administer orally; give with meals
	potassium gluconate solution for oral use (Kaon)	20–100 mEq potassium daily in divided doses			Dilute well and administer orally; give with meals
	potassium chloride tablets	20–100 mEq daily, in divided doses PC: A			Administer orally; direct client to swallow tablet whole without chewing or dissolving tablet
	potassium chloride for injection	20–100 mEq daily, in divided doses			Infuse slowly, IV
Calcium (Apo-Cal, Caltrate, Citracal, Os-Cal)	calcium chloride for oral use	6–8 g daily in divided doses	Replenishes calcium	Treatment of calcium deficiency (osteomalacia)	Administer orally
	dibasic calcium phosphate with vitamin D	One wafer (equal to 0.35 g calcium) tid	Replenishes calcium losses	Treatment of calcium deficiency (rickets)	Instruct client to chew wafers before swallowing; give with meals
	calcium gluconate solution (10%) for injection	1.5–3.0 ml (equal to 7–14 mEq calcium); for tetany, up to 20 ml	Reduces nerve and muscle irritability	Treatment of hypocalcemic tetany	Infuse slowly, IV

	Preparations	Dosage	Action	Uses	Nursing implications
	calcium carbonate for oral use (eg, Tums)	1–2 g with meals PC: C	Replenishes calcium	Renal failure, weight reduction regimens, and other conditions with high potential for hypocalcemia	Administer orally
Magnesium (Magnesium Gluconate)	Antacid magnesium salts	Variable	Buffers gastric acid	Reduction in gastric acidity	Administer orally
	Laxative magnesium salts	Variable	Promotes fecal elimination by saline catharsis	Counteraction of the constipating effects of drugs such as aluminum or calcium antacids	Administer orally
	magnesium sulfate solutions for injection	0.5–3.0 g daily	Replenishes magnesium	Prevention of magnesium deficiency	Add to total parenteral nutrition solutions
	magnesium sulfate 10% solution for injection	Up to 4 g magnesium sulfate (40 ml)	Reduces muscle and nerve irritability	Termination of convulsions of eclampsia of pregnancy	Administer slowly IV infusion (1.5 ml/min or less)
	magnesium sulfate 20%, 25%, or 50% solutions for injection	4–5 g magnesium sulfate at 4-hour intervals PC: B	Same as above	Same as above	Administer IM injection
Iron (Femiron, Feosol, Fergon, Fer-In-Sol, Ferrous Gluconate, Mol-Iron)	ferrous sulfate enteric-coated tablets for oral use	100–1000 mg/day in divided doses	Provides iron for hemoglobin formation	Treatment of iron-deficiency anemia	Administer orally with fruit juice
	iron-dextran solution for injection (0.05%)	50–500 mg	Same as above	Treatment of iron-deficiency anemia when rapid response is required or iron cannot be taken orally	Inject intramuscularly, using Z-tract technique
	ferrous sulfate elixir for oral use	1–2 ml (equal to 220–440 mg ferrous sulfate) tid	Same as above	Treatment of iron-deficiency anemia when rapid response is required or iron cannot be taken orally	Mix with water or juice (*not* milk or alcoholic beverages), and administer by placing a straw well back in the mouth; avoid contact between solution and teeth
Copper	copper sulfate solutions for injection (no commercial preparations available)	Up to 0.05 mg/kg body weight (injected)	Replenishes copper	Prevention or treatment of copper deficiency in patients on chronic total parenteral nutrition	Inject as directed by the pharmacist

(Continued)

Table 50-7. Mineral preparations used as drugs (Continued)

Mineral	Preparations	Usual adult dosage	Pharmacologic effects	Therapeutic uses	Method of administration
Iodide	Iodide solution for oral use (Lugol's solution)	0.1–0.3 ml tid	Replenishes iodine Promotes storage of thyroid hormone and reduces vascularity of the thyroid gland	Treatment of simple goiter Preoperative preparation for thyroidectomy	Dilute and administer orally
	saturated solution of potassium iodide	0.3 ml or 0.6 ml (equal to 300 mg KI) 3–4 times daily	Stimulates sputum secretion	Treatment of respiratory infections	Dilute and administer orally
	Radiopaque dyes containing iodide	Varies with preparation	Blocks x-rays to outline structures upon x-ray film	Diagnosis of organ pathology	Inject IV or administer orally
Fluoride (EASYgel, Fluorinse, Fluoritab, Fluotic, Fluorodex, Pediaflor, Thera-Flur)	sodium silicofluoride	1 ppm in water supplies	Promotes formation of normal dentin and strong tooth enamel in children	Prevention of dental disease (caries)	Add to water supply
	sodium fluoride tablets for oral use	1.1–2.2 mg/day (depending on age)	See above	See above	Administer orally
	stannous fluoride (toothpaste)	QS for oral hygiene	See above	Desensitization of tooth enamel	Use in place of nonmedicated toothpaste
Zinc	zinc sulfate capsules and tablets for oral use (Zinc-220)	220 mg/day (equivalent to 80 mg of elemental zinc)	Replenishes zinc	Promotion of the healing of wounds in zinc deficiency	Administer orally with meals or milk
Cobalt	cyanocobalamin solution for injection	100 μg/wk	Promotes formation of red blood cells	Treatment of pernicious anemia	Administer subcutaneously or intramuscularly
Lithium (Lithane, Lithobid, Lithotabs, Priadel)	lithium carbonate tablets and capsules for oral use	300–600 mg tid (individualized to produce a serum level of 1.0–1.5 mEq lithium/liter)	Alters sodium transport in nerve and muscle cells	Treatment and prevention of manic episodes of manic–depressive psychosis Treatment of severe recurrent unipolar psychosis	Administer orally

KEY: PC = pregnancy risk category. (The validity of pregnancy risk categories has not been established. See Chapter 16, p 216.)

Table 50-8. Factors affecting pharmacokinetics of selected minerals

Mineral	Interacting factors	Effect on mineral levels
Calcium	Parathormone and vitamin D	Increases intestinal absorption and renal reabsorption
	Lactose	Increases intestinal absorption
	pH of body fluids	Alters ionization of calcium (relationship is inverse)
	Protein	In excess, reduces calcium levels in the body
	Weightbearing	Increases calcium deposition in bone
	Stress	Increases renal loss of calcium
	Phytates and oxalates	Binds calcium, reducing intestinal absorption
	Fluoride	Reduces calcium levels
Iron	Vitamin C and other acids	Increases intestinal absorption
	Cobalt, antacids, phytates, tannates, clay (geophagia), ethylenediaminetetraacetic acid (EDTA), and tea	Decreases intestinal absorption
Copper	Zinc	Displaces copper, reducing its absorption and increasing its excretion
	Iron	Decreases copper absorption in infants
Fluoride	Copper, iron	Decreases absorption
Zinc	Vitamin B$_6$	Increases absorption
	Copper	Decreases absorption
Manganese	Copper, phosphorus, iron	Decreases absorption
	Soy supplements	Decreases absorption
Cobalt	Intrinsic factor	Increases absorption

mias. The cardiac manifestations are most dangerous because ventricular fibrillation may occur. In addition, excessive potassium may stimulate secretion of glucagon and raise blood glucose. Local concentrations of the electrolyte may compromise circulation by causing pronounced vasoconstriction, leading to infarction.

Initially, high serum levels of *calcium* cause some degree of lethargy and muscle weakness. The electrolyte is excreted by the kidneys, and high levels in the urine predispose to renal calculi. Prolonged hypercalcemia often causes inappropriate calcification of soft tissues. Very high concentrations cause "calcium rigor" of the heart, a condition characterized by prolonged systole and inadequate filling time. Cardiac arrest in systole may ensue.

Magnesium excesses are most likely to occur in persons with impaired renal excretion. Muscle contractility decreases. Flaccid paralysis or cardiac arrest in diastole may develop. The mineral is also mutagenic and can cause anomalies in exposed embryos.

For a detailed discussion of systemic iron toxicity, see the section on Hematinics later in this chapter.

Copper excess in the body is damaging to the liver, kidneys, and other organs. The mineral is suspected of being both mutagenic and carcinogenic.

Iodine excesses, like iodine deficiencies, inhibit thyroid function. Enlargement of the thyroid (goiter) may develop in response to this effect. Acute poisoning by iodine solutions causes severe damage to the exposed tissues of the GI tract. (Concentrated iodine is a protoplasmic poison.) Circulatory collapse and death may

occur. Chronic iodism is characterized by increased secretions of the respiratory tract, a brassy taste, soreness of the oropharyngeal tissues, eye irritation, and GI irritation. Signs and symptoms include soreness of the teeth and gums, coryza, sneezing, swelling of the eyelids, enlargement and tenderness of the parotid and submaxillary glands, bloody diarrhea, fever, anorexia, and depression. Iodine allergy is a frequent problem, particularly in relation to organic preparations, such as those used as radiopaque dyes. Hypersensitive reactions are characterized by rash, angioedema, bronchospasm, thrombocytopenic purpura, or symptomatology similar to serum sickness (fever, joint pain, and lymph node enlargement).

Acute *fluoride* toxicity causes local symptoms similar to those of iodine: salivation, nausea, abdominal pain, vomiting, and diarrhea. Hyperirritability of the nervous system follows with paresthesias, hyperactive reflexes, and tetany. Hypoglycemia and convulsions can occur. Systemic symptoms may be delayed for several hours. Shock, cardiac failure, or respiratory paralysis may lead to death. Chronic fluoride toxicity is characterized by increased density and calcification of bone (osteosclerosis) and by mottling of tooth enamel that is in the process of formation.

Medicinal preparations of *zinc* are irritating to the stomach and may act as emetics in high doses. The introduction of zinc supplements is fairly recent, and there undoubtedly are toxic effects that have yet to be reported.

Manganese is suspected to have mutagenic or carcinogenic properties. Massive doses of *cobalt* (as vitamin B_{12}) overstimulate bone-marrow production of red blood cells and lead to polycythemia.

Lithium is a relatively toxic substance. Persons taking therapeutic doses of this mineral have developed fluid imbalances similar to diabetes insipidus. Goiter sometimes develops. Nausea, vomiting, and diarrhea are common manifestations. In toxic doses, effects of the mineral on the nervous system cause increased muscle irritability manifested by hyperreflexia, fine tremors, ataxia, convulsions, coma, and eventual death. Allergic reactions to this mineral include dermatitis and vasculitis. An increased incidence of cardiac anomalies in children exposed *in utero* has been reported.

Few adverse reactions have been reported as a result of *selenium* or *molybdenum* therapy. This is probably due to their limited use to date.

Precautions and contraindications. Precautions required during parenteral treatment of fluid and electrolyte imbalances are discussed in detail in Chapter 44. Solutions containing concentrations of minerals greater than those normally found in body fluids should be administered with great caution to avoid toxic responses.

Oral preparations of minerals are best administered with food or diluted with large amounts of fluids. Salt tablets are highly irritating to the gastric mucosa and are no longer recommended. Adding table salt to food is the safest and easiest way to provide additional sodium for the few people who require high intakes of this mineral.

Potassium salts are usually administered in liquid form and should be well diluted. High concentrations in the intestinal vasculature must be avoided because they produce vasospasm and intestinal infarction. Administration of potassium supplements with food provides further dilution. Slow-release forms of potassium salts have recently been introduced. Clients receiving these preparations should be monitored closely for abdominal symptoms to ensure that they are free of such toxicity.

Although iron is most efficiently absorbed when administered on an empty stomach, it is very irritating, and administration with meals may be necessary to control intestinal symptoms, such as nausea and diarrhea. Because total absorption may be reduced when the drug is given with food, dosages may have to be increased. Iron therapy is discussed in the next section, Hematinics.

Clients receiving lithium should have frequent tests to determine serum concentrations of the mineral. Adequate sodium levels must be maintained to minimize the risk of lithium toxicity.

Allergic sensitivity is a relative contraindication for mineral therapy. Allergy is most common in relation to iodine, especially organic preparations used as radiopaque dyes. Before such medications are administered, a careful history should be taken to rule out hypersensitivity.

All mineral preparations should be secured to prevent accidental ingestion, especially by children. They have a high toxic potential and can cause serious poisoning.

■ **Summary**
Minerals are inorganic chemicals that greatly influence fundamental physiologic processes such as internal respiration, impulse transmission, membrane transport, and enzymatic reactions. They are used medicinally to prevent and treat deficiency states and for selective treatment of certain diseases. Mineral preparations generally have a narrow therapeutic index and are capable of causing serious poisoning.

Nursing management

Nursing implications
Minerals in the environment. Cooking utensils may influence the mineral content of food significantly. Cast-iron utensils add some iron to the food cooked in them, especially when acid substances are present. Glass and enameled metal (if unchipped) appear to be inert and add nothing to the food prepared in them. According to recent reports, stainless steel utensils may release nickel into the food cooked in them. The degree to which aluminum leaches into food is unknown but the obvious erosion of the metal with prolonged use implies that significant amounts of the metal may be consumed.

Aluminum is presently under suspicion as a toxin because excessive accumulations of the metal in brain tissue have been associated with degenerative brain diseases, such as Alzheimer's disease. Aluminum utensils have been widely used for cooking for many years. Why only a small proportion of the people exposed to this metal develop brain damage is not known; possibly their bodies are unable to detoxify and excrete aluminum efficiently. Caution in the use of aluminum cooking materials and aluminum medicinals would seem reasonable until the pathogenesis of such conditions is better understood.

Environmental pollution with mineral chemicals imposes a heavy burden of metal salts on exposed populations. Persons with renal impairment are most vulnerable to trace-metal poisoning because they cannot eliminate metallic salts efficiently. Certain populations are exposed to high levels of pollution from mining and smelting operations or industrial processes involving metals. Whenever mineral poisoning is suspected, assessment for mineral levels should be carried out, including laboratory analysis of urine, serum, and hair for metal content.

Nursing process

Assessment An important nursing responsibility in relation to mineral deficiencies is casefinding and referral for treatment.

Iron deficiency anemia is the most prevalent mineral deficiency. This condition is discussed in detail in the next section, Hematinics.

Calcium deficiency is the second most prevalent mineral deficiency. At risk are both the very young and the elderly: growing children because they have a high need for calcium for skeletal growth, and older adults because they absorb calcium poorly and may ingest less in their diets. Postmenopausal women are especially vulnerable.

Sodium deficit is most likely to occur in warm environments because of excessive loss in perspiration. Susceptible persons include those engaged in strenuous physical exercise, ileostomates, those with draining fistulas, and those undergoing surgery (during the postoperative period). Persons taking diuretics and those with marginal or inadequate production of corticosteroids are also at risk. Sodium loss is accompanied in most cases by fluid loss. Hypovolemia results in hypotension, weakness, syncope, and general malaise. Such dehydration is usually accompanied by mild metabolic acidosis.

Potassium deficiencies are most likely to develop in persons subject to increased stress, those receiving potassium-wasting diuretics, and those losing large amounts of intestinal fluids as a result of diarrhea, and ileostomy or fistula drainage. Hypokalemia is particularly dangerous to clients receiving digitalis because it is the main physiologic antagonist to the action of this drug.

Risk factors for *magnesium* deficiency include alcoholism and diuresis. Hypomagnesemia occurs frequently in hospitalized clients but is not always diagnosed. Levels of this mineral are not measured by automated analyses of blood. Because magnesium is lost with other electrolytes, it should be measured whenever low serum levels of sodium, calcium, or phosphate are detected. Magnesia depletion is believed to be a contributing factor in the development of eclampsia during pregnancy.

Inadequate levels of *trace minerals* may be associated with an environmental deficiency. For example, communities with fluoride-poor water show a higher incidence of dental caries (a condition associated with fluoride deficiency) than do communities with naturally or artificially fluoridated water. Inland uplands tend to have poor levels of iodine in the soils, and iodine-deficient diseases (goiter and thyroid imbalances) are common unless iodine is added to the diet.

Trace mineral deficiencies are most likely to develop in persons whose diet is sharply limited, especially those relying entirely on parenteral fluids. Persons with intestinal malabsorption are at risk because ingested minerals may remain in the gut and be excreted in feces. Vegetarians may also develop mineral deficiencies unless care is taken to include mineral rich foods in the diet.

Sodium chloride excess is the most frequent mineral toxicity. The average intake of table salt among persons in developed countries is at least 10 times greater than physiologic need. Excess salt predisposes to hypertension and edema.

Clients at highest risk for developing *iron* toxicity are those receiving multiple transfusions of whole blood or packed cells. Excesses also may develop in clients taking high potency iron supplements.

Hyperkalemia (*potassium* excess) occurs much less frequently than hypokalemia. In most cases, this problem is related to disease (renal impairment, inadequately treated Addison's disease, crush syndrome), or the use of potassium-sparing diuretics.

Excess blood levels of *calcium* often indicate loss of calcium from the bone and depletion of body stores. Rarely, hypercalcemia will be caused by excessive dosages of calcium and vitamin D supplements.

Persons at risk for *magnesium* excess are those with renal impairment who cannot excrete the mineral efficiently. These clients may develop high blood levels of many minerals unless intake is controlled carefully.

Assessment for mineral imbalances begins with the history, important for identifying risk factors and symptoms. Physical examination should include observation to identify or rule out signs indicating imbalance (see Table 50-6). Imbalances may be substantiated with analysis of levels in serum, urine, and hair samples for mineral content.

Nursing diagnosis Nursing diagnoses are specific to the mineral imbalance present. Examples include the following:

Fluid volume excess related to excess intake of sodium chloride
Altered nutrition, less than body requirements: calcium deficiency related to impaired absorption secondary to postmenopausal estrogen deficiency and lack of weightbearing exercise
Altered nutrition, less than body requirements: iron deficiency secondary to blood loss and iron-poor diet

Many clients will have a

Knowledge deficit concerning mineral nutrition and self-care measures to enhance supply and use of mineral nutrients.

A common collaborative problem that should be differentiated from the nursing diagnoses is

Potential complication: hypokalemia

Planning Nursing goals are to alleviate or eliminate mineral imbalances and promote the absorption and use of mineral nutrients.

Intervention

Treatment of deficiencies. The treatment of iron deficiency is discussed in the next section, Hematinics. Treatment of *calcium* deficiency requires adequate intake of calcium plus vitamin D necessary for its absorption, and sufficient protein and phosphate for remineralization of body structures. Children are given additional milk when possible. An adequate diet is an important part of the treatment. When therapeutic minerals and vitamins are needed, multivitamin and mineral preparations high in calcium are often prescribed. Dicalcium phosphate with vitamin D or calcium-containing antacids, such as Tums, may be employed for selected clients. Absorption and use of calcium is enhanced by weightbearing exercise.

Calcium salts tend to be constipating, and clients should be monitored for difficulties with fecal elimination. The supplements must not be administered concurrently with drugs that form nonabsorbable complexes with divalent cations, such as tetracycline.

Sodium and water depletion produce dehydration and may proceed to hypovolemic shock, a medical emergency. If the dehydrated client is able to take oral fluids, a solution of sodium salts in water may be given as a first-aid measure (Box 50-2). As an alternative, saline may be administered IV. If the signs and symptoms do not subside promptly with fluid replacement, emergency medical aid should be summoned. If kidney function is normal, solutions administered in such situations should contain potassium salts in addition to the sodium compounds (Box 50-3). Oral mixtures may be mixed with fruit juices for better flavor.

Many clients maintain adequate *potassium* levels by dietary means alone. Foods of animal origin (meat, milk), orange juice, and bananas are rich sources of this mineral. Clients using potassium chloride as a salt substitute ingest extra potassium from this preparation also.

Medicinal preparations of potassium are pre-

Box 50-2. Electrolyte solution for replacement of sodium

1 teaspoon sodium chloride (table salt)

$1/2$ teaspoon sodium bicarbonate (baking soda)

Water to make 1 quart of solution

Box 50-3. Electrolyte solution for replacement of sodium and potassium

1 teaspoon sodium chloride (table salt)

$1/2$ teaspoon sodium bicarbonate (baking soda)

$1/3$ teaspoon potassium chloride (salt substitute such as Lite Salt)

Water or fruit juice to make 1 quart of solution

---

scribed for persons who are unable to maintain normal levels of this mineral by dietary means. These medications must be administered with ample fluids to dilute them thoroughly. They are best given with meals. Concentrated potassium in the intestine is highly irritating and causes smooth muscle spasm. If absorbed rapidly, concentrations in the intestinal blood vessels may reach toxic levels, causing vascular spasm that can compromise circulation and produce infarction.

Potassium solutions have a strong, brassy taste. Administration in fruit juices or milk may ameliorate but cannot completely disguise this. Effervescent tablets containing potassium chloride (K-Lyte) must be dissolved in water just before administration and given while still effervescing. This preparation is colored and flavored.

Potassium solutions must be used cautiously in persons with renal impairment because excess potassium will not be eliminated efficiently, and hyperkalemia may develop. They must also be used with caution in clients deficient in corticosteroids who tend to retain potassium.

Calcium solutions are injected IV to alleviate acute hypocalcemia characterized by tetany.

Iron and zinc are marketed in tablet form and may be prescribed in selected situations.

Deficiencies of *trace minerals* are best treated by ingestion of a variety of high quality foods. Wholegrain cereals and vegetables (especially their peels) are good sources of most minerals. Because these salts dissolve in water, pot liquors should be used to make soups or gravies that will be consumed so they are not lost from the diet. Hard water contains significantly more minerals than soft water and is preferable for drinking and cooking.

Treatment of toxic states. Treatment of toxic states requires that exposure to metallic pollutants be controlled and excretion of these substances from the body be promoted. For some minerals, fecal excretion can be increased by oral administration of ion exchange resins or chelating agents that prevent the reabsorption of minerals secreted in bile or intestinal juices. If renal function is adequate, diuretics may be given to promote urinary excretion. In severe or refractory toxicity, dialysis may be necessary to achieve rapid reduction of serum levels.

Pharmacologic use of minerals. Using minerals to treat disease involves doses close to the toxic level. Clients must be monitored carefully for early signs of toxicity. Drug dosages should be withheld when these appear.

Lithium is particularly dangerous, producing fluid imbalances, skin changes, GI upset, and central nervous system disturbances. Clients receiving this drug should be monitored for polydipsia, polyuria, rash, thyroid enlargement, nausea, vomiting, diarrhea, tremors, abnormal gait, lethargy, and confusion. Adequate sodium levels help to minimize lithium toxicity. Clients must be provided sufficient dietary salt to compensate for body losses. In warm environments, sodium loss through perspiration is increased, and additional salt will be needed.

Lithium is teratogenic and may cause congenital anomalies when administered to women in the early stages of pregnancy. A pregnancy test should be administered to women of childbearing years before drug therapy is initiated. Therapy may be delayed until the second trimester if pregnancy is discovered. Some method of contraception should be provided for nongravid women at risk who are to receive lithium.

Lithium and zinc are therapeutic agents introduced relatively recently. Clients treated with these preparations should be monitored closely for unexplained signs and symptoms that could be side effects or toxic manifestations. Such responses should be reported to the government agency responsible for gathering data on drug reactions (see Chapter 2).

Client education

Dietary sodium. High levels of dietary sodium are the most prevalent mineral excess occurring in developed countries. High sodium intake poses an increased risk of developing hypervolemia, hypertension, and cardiovascular disease.

Public health measures are important to educate the public to this health risk. Educational campaigns should stress the importance of controlling use of sodium compounds, such as table salt, baking soda, baking powder, and monosodium glutamate (*eg*, Accent). Processed food labels should be read carefully because large amounts of sodium compounds are used as preservatives and flavoring agents in most such products. To enhance flavors of unsalted food, the use of herbs and other low-sodium condiments should be promoted.

Persons at high risk for hypertension (in the United States, blacks and men) need help to develop low-sodium diets acceptable to them. Suitable flavoring agents for specific dishes favored by the client may be suggested. Cookbooks that address cooking with herbs contain helpful suggestions. The client may be referred to a nutritionist or dietitian for help with difficult problems. Compliance with a low-sodium regimen is unlikely unless the low-sodium diet is satisfying to the client.

Persons at high risk for sodium deficiency should be taught how to prepare an electrolyte solution for use as a beverage. Liberal use of table salt should be encouraged. Ileostomates or others losing large amounts of liquid feces should take some of their sodium as the bicarbonate to restore base bicarbonate. Some physicians advise the use of 1 teaspoon of baking soda in water once a week. Because sodium bicarbonate reacts with hydrochloric acid in the stomach to produce carbon dioxide gas, this solution should be sipped slowly to prevent rapid generation of gas and gastric distention.

Potassium. Clients at high risk for hypokalemia should be advised to increase their dietary intake of sources rich in this mineral. Fruits are recommended rather than meat to minimize calorie and fat intake. One banana a day provides an adequate supplement for many people. Orange juice and apricots are also good sources of the mineral. Citrus fruits other than oranges do not contain high levels of potassium.

Clients experiencing high stress levels need skills in stress management to minimize potassium-wasting induced by high levels of corticosteroids. The nurse should assist the client in developing effective coping strategies, including skills in relaxation techniques.

Clients receiving potassium supplements should be instructed to take these preparations with meals, with a full glass of water to prevent GI complications. If urinary output diminishes, the client should discontinue potassium dosage and seek immediate medical attention.

Other minerals. The use of medications containing *calcium* or *aluminum* compounds is likely to result in constipation. Unless medically contraindicated, the nurse should recommend fluid intake of 2,400 to 3,000 ml/d; regular exercise; a high-fiber diet; use of laxative foods, such as pears and prunes; prompt response to the defecatory impulse; and promotion of a regular daily habit of fecal elimination. Taking a glass of warm liquid (lemon juice or coffee) prior to the usual time of defecation tends to stimulate mass peristalsis. Tea should be avoided as it is constipating. If difficulty in fecal elimination does develop, the physician should be consulted to determine if a less constipating preparation can be substituted.

Clients taking medicines containing *magnesium* may have a tendency toward loose stools. They should consult the physician for a change in medication if diarrhea becomes a problem.

When *iron* supplements are prescribed, the client should be informed that the color of the stools will change to black or gray. Bowel habits may also change, and the client should be informed of measures to minimize both constipation and diarrhea because either can occur. The iron preparation may be taken with meals to minimize GI irritation. If this is not the schedule recommended by the physician, the doctor should be informed of the change because the dosage of iron may need to be increased to compensate for reduced overall absorption. Bloody stools or persistent abdominal discomfort should also be reported to the physician.

Client teaching relevant to *iodine* medication is discussed in Chapter 34. The use of iodine solutions as dietary supplements without prescription should be discouraged. The amounts used (usually one drop in a glass of water per day) are difficult to measure accurately and may raise total intake of the mineral to toxic levels, especially if iodized salt and multimineral preparations are used concurrently. The use of iodized salt by populations living in iodine-poor geographic areas (goiter belts) is recommended.

The nurse should recommend the use of fluoridated toothpastes by growing children. Nonprescription *fluoride* dietary supplements should not be used unless the fluoride content of the water used for drinking is clearly inadequate and other sources of fluoride are ruled out.

The use of *zinc* supplements by healthy persons should be discouraged. This is particularly important in women of childbearing years because the drug is suspected of increasing the incidence of congenital anencephaly in exposed embryos.

Minimizing mineral toxicity. To promote appropriate mineral intake and minimize the risk of mineral toxicity, the nurse may recommend the use of cast iron, glass, stainless steel, enameled or ceramic cooking utensils. Despite isolated reports of leaching of nickel, stainless steel is generally considered to be safe. Ceramic dishes used for food must be made with *lead-free* pigments and glazes. Use of aluminum cookware is probably innocuous for most people, although the possibility of aluminum toxicity in some persons cannot be ruled out.

Clients receiving lithium medications should be taught the toxic effects of the drug. These should be reported promptly to the physician. The importance of blood tests for serum concentrations and regular medical supervision should be stressed. Women of childbearing age must be informed of the increased risk of congenital anomalies in offspring if the drug is taken during pregnancy. Instruction in contraception techniques should be provided.

Clients receiving relatively new medications (those developed within the past 10–20 years), such as lithium and zinc, should be advised to report any unusual signs, symptoms, or change in health status because they could represent previously unrecognized side effects or toxic effects.

Evaluation Data required for evaluation relate to the incidence or absence of signs and symptoms of mineral deficiency or toxicity. Client education may be evaluated over the short term by the client's ability to relate accurately material conveyed during the teaching sessions. (See accompanying Example of Nursing Process and Estrogen Replacement Therapy with Calcium Supplement.)

Checklist of nursing actions

☐ Assess clients for signs and symptoms of mineral deficiency or excess.

☐ If signs and symptoms of mineral imbalance are present, refer clients for definitive diagnosis and treatment.

☐ Advise a high-quality diet containing whole-grain cereals, low fat dairy products, adequate protein sources, and vegetables as the best sources of adequate mineral intake.

☐ Discourage the use of high potency mineral preparations as dietary supplements by healthy people.

☐ Administer iron supplements with fruit juice; schedule drug doses between meals unless GI irritation causes client distress.

☐ If iron supplements cause abdominal distress, give the medication with meals; consult with the physician regarding the need to increase dosage to compensate for decreased absorption.

Enrichment experience 50-2

Visit a drug store and explore the section in which mineral and vitamin preparations marketed for dietary supplementation are displayed. List the various combinations of nutrients available. Determine whether: 1) labels on the products warn of toxic effects of excessive intake; 2) labels on such products as kelp, fish liver oil, and alfalfa indicate the constituent ingredients and their doses; and 3) labels indicate the percentage of recommended daily allowances provided by each dose of the medicine.

Hematinics

A hematinic is an agent that improves the quality of blood. For example, it might increase the hemoglobin level or the number of erythrocytes. Hematinics discussed here are iron, vitamin B_{12}, and folic acid. The daily requirements for each are given in Table 50-9.

Iron

The human body contains about 45 mg/kg body weight of iron (or about 5 g in the usual adult). A small

Example of nursing process and estrogen replacement therapy with calcium supplement

The client is a 50-year-old housewife who complains of having intermittent pain in the thoracic vertebrae and hips for the last 3 months. Her last menstrual period was a year ago. She states she has experienced no hot flashes or other signs and symptoms of "menopause."

During the history, the client states that none of the older women on her mother's side of the family developed spinal curvature but that all of her father's sisters (and her father, also) had typical "dowagers' humps" in their older years.

A chest x-ray reveals osteoporosis with moderate kyphosis. The physician has prescribed replacement estrogen therapy and supplemental calcium with vitamin D.

The client has led a sedentary life for years. When younger, she enjoyed swimming and bicycling. The client does not have dentures; most of her teeth are intact.

Assessment data	Nursing diagnosis	Intervention	Goals and outcome criteria
Menopause	Knowledge deficit concerning decreased calcium absorption resulting from estrogen deficiency secondary to menopause	**Explore** the client's knowledge of nutrition, especially calcium nutrition.	The client's bone pain will decrease and disappear.
Family history of "dowager's hump"		**Develop** and implement a teaching plan that covers: 1) recommendations for administering calcium with food, taking divided doses to promote absorption; 2) cautions regarding excessive vitamin D intake, which promotes calcium loss by bones; 3) and self-care practices to prevent constipation, which is likely to develop with high calcium intake.	The kyphosis will cease to progress.
Diagnosis of osteoporosis and moderate kyphosis			
Orders for estrogen replacement and calcium supplement		**Recommend** that the client undertake a gradually accelerated program of exercise that involves weight bearing activities (walking, bicycling, workouts with weights); inform the client that, although excellent exercise, swimming is not a weightbearing activity and will not promote recalcification of bone.	
	High risk for constipation, colonic, secondary to high calcium intake	**Recommend** an active life style including daily exercise	The client will not develop constipation
		Recommend a high fluid intake (at least 10 glasses daily)	
		Recommend high fiber intake in the diet (or a bulk "laxative" daily)	
	High risk for impaired tissue integrity: stomatitis related to excessive plaque formation secondary to high calcium concentrations in saliva	**Recommend** meticulous oral hygiene and professional cleaning every 3 months	The client will not develop stomatitis.

Table 50-9. Recommended daily allowances of hematinics

Hematinic	Population	Daily amount
iron	Infant 6 mo–1 yr	15 mg
	Child 4–6 yr	10 mg
	Child 11–14 yr	18 mg
	Pregnant woman	30–60 mg supplement
	Lactating woman	30–60 mg supplement*
	Menstruating female	18 mg
	Adult male	10 mg
vitamin B_{12}	Infant 6 mo–1 yr	1.5 µg
	Child 4–6 yr	2.5 µg
	Child 11–14 yr	3.0 µg
	Pregnant woman	4.0 µg
	Lactating woman	4.0 µg
	Menstruating female	3.0 µg
	Adult male	3.0 µg
folic acid	Infant 6 mo–1 yr	35 µg
	Child 4–6 yr	75 µg
	Child 11–14 yr	150 µg
	Pregnant woman	400 µg
	Lactating woman (first 6 months)	280 µg
	Menstruating female	180 µg
	Adult male	200 µg

* The iron needs during lactation are not substantially different from those of nonpregnant women but continued supplementation of the mother for 2–3 months after delivery is advisable to replenish stores depleted by pregnancy.
Adapted from *Recommended dietary allowances*, 10th ed., 1989.

amount, 80–180 mcg/dL for men and 60–160 mcg/dL for women, is found in the plasma bound to its transport carrier protein called transferrin, which delivers iron to specific receptors on cell membranes. The greatest amount, about 70%, occurs in red blood cells as a constituent of the heme portion of hemoglobin. Another 5% is in myoglobin, a muscle component. About 20% is stored as the protein-iron compound ferritin in the liver, spleen, and bone marrow. Storage as ferritin provides a stable storage form, which can be used as needed in synthesizing hemoglobin for red blood cells. Hemosiderin is a second, less soluble storage compound, an increase of which is usually seen in iron overload. The remaining 5% is distributed throughout the body cells and functions as a component of enzyme systems for oxidation of glucose to produce energy.

Iron is necessary for hemoglobin synthesis. As a component of hemoglobin, iron plays a crucial role in transport of oxygen for both the lungs and the peripheral cells. In muscle myoglobin, iron supplies oxygen for use in muscle contraction.

Iron requirements

Human iron requirements are the outcome of obligatory physiologic losses and needs imposed by growth. The recommended daily allowance for the adult male is 10 mg, whereas the menstruating female requires about 18 mg (Williams, 1989). Menstrual losses are influenced by the use of intrauterine devices. Loss is decreased by about one-half when oral contraceptives containing estrogen are used.

After birth, healthy infants have significant iron stores. Iron is transferred to the fetus from the mother in the last trimester of pregnancy. Some of this iron is stored in the liver. The fetus has a much higher hemoglobin level than is normally needed after birth. The hemoglobin level usually drops during the first 6–8 weeks of life. Iron from the breakdown of old red blood cells is stored for later use in the production of new red blood cells when the infant is 2–4 months old. The term infant uses up the iron stores by 4–6 months of age. The American Academy of Pediatrics Committee on Nutrition recommends that iron supplements from one or more sources be added to infants' diets by 6 months of age. Premature infants and infants whose mothers were anemic require iron supplements sooner because they were born with less adequate stores. Building up iron stores during infancy can help prevent iron deficiency during the preschool years, when it may be more difficult to provide for adequate intake.

In the last two trimesters of pregnancy, the mother's daily iron requirements increase to about 80 mcg per kilogram. This requirement is based on the need to maintain the increased number of red blood cells in an expanded circulating blood volume; the fact that the growing fetus draws from the mother's stores of iron; and the fact that normal blood loss during delivery further reduces iron stores. The mother needs 30–60 mg elemental iron daily during the last two trimesters, provided as ferrous salts. This recommended amount is so high that an iron supplement is necessary. Such a supplement should not be given during the first trimester, because iron may be capable of causing congenital malformations if taken during early fetal development.

The dietary content of iron in developed countries is about 6 mg per 1,000 calories. The iron content of selected foods appears in Table 50-10. It has also been found that cooking in iron cookware can increase the iron content of the diet. Foods low in iron (with less than 1 mg per 100 g) include milk, milk products, and most nongreen vegetables.

Absorption

Absorption is very important in determining body content of iron. The iron in food comes to the intestinal mucosa as either nonheme iron or heme iron. All the iron in grains and vegetables and about 60% of the

Table 50-10. Hematinic content of selected foods

	Amount of U.S. RDA
Iron	
3 oz. beef liver	42%
3 oz. beef patty	17%
3 oz. pork chop	15%
½ cup baked beans	13%
3 oz. fried chicken	11%
½ cup mustard, spinach, or turnip greens	8%
2 hard-cooked eggs	12%
Folic acid	
1 oz. ready-to-eat, fortified cereal	25%
½ cup cooked broccoli	10%–24%
½ cup cooked green peas	25%–39%
3 oz. calf liver	40% or more
½ cup diced chicken or turkey liver	40% or more
½ cup black-eyed peas	40% or more
½ cup cooked kidney beans	25%–39%
½ cup cooked lentils	40% or more

iron in meats is nonheme iron; about 40% of iron in meats is heme iron. Meat facilitates iron absorption by stimulating gastric-acid production. The heme protein in meat helps transport nonheme iron across the intestinal mucosa. In a vegetarian diet, nonheme iron is poorly absorbed because of the absence of the heme iron (no meat) and because of inhibitory action of dietary phosphates.

Nonheme iron, ingested in its nonheme food sources, is in the form of ferric iron. In the acidic medium of the stomach, it must dissociate and be reduced to the more soluble ferrous iron for absorption. As such, it then forms complexes with other compounds in the food mix.

Heme iron from animal sources remains unmetabolized and is delivered to the small intestine. Here, it is rapidly absorbed intact by the mucosal cells, then is broken down and the iron released within the cells.

Once in the small intestine, mainly the duodenum and also the proximal jejunum, the iron eventually is all in ferric form. It is bound by an intracellular carrier molecule, which delivers a portion to the cell mitochondria for metabolic needs. Intracellular carrier molecule then distributes the rest, depending on the person's current iron needs. Intracellular carrier molecule distributes some to apoferritin, the receptor with which the iron combines to form the immediate holding compound, ferritin. Intracellular carrier molecule also distributes some to apotransferrin, the blood's special protein receptor with which the iron combines to form its transport carrier protein, transferrin.

When all available apoferritin has been bound to iron to form ferritin, any additional iron is returned to the lumen of the intestine and eliminated via the feces. A means of calculating the bioavailability of iron, considering the factors that enhance its absorption, was determined and shows about 10%–30% of ingested iron is absorbed and about 70%–90% is eliminated.

A number of factors facilitate the absorption of iron. These include body need, calcium, ascorbic acid, and hydrochloric acid. The lower the reserve ferritin, the greater the body's need. An adequate amount of calcium helps bind and, remove agents such as phosphate and phytate, which if not removed would combine with iron and inhibit its absorption. Ascorbic acid helps increase the solubility of iron in the duodenum and thus aids in iron absorption. And, finally, hydrochloric acid in gastric secretions provides the optimal acid medium for the preparation of iron for use.

Other factors hinder iron absorption. These include binding agents, reduced gastric acid secretion, infection, and GI disease. Phosphate, phytate, and oxalate are binding agents that remove iron from the body so a diet high in any of these leads to a decrease in iron absorption. Tea and coffee also appear to have inhibitory effects on nonheme iron absorption.

A gastrectomy reduces the number of cells that secrete hydrochloric acid; therefore, the acid medium needed for iron reduction is not provided. Severe infection hinders absorption of iron. Malabsorption syndromes or any disturbance that causes diarrhea or steatorrhea will hinder iron absorption.

Iron in the body is used very efficiently; under normal circumstances, it is not used up or destroyed but is reused. The body recycles the iron when red blood cells are destroyed after their average lifespan of about 120 days. Some iron is excreted in sloughed cells from skin and the GI tract or in blood loss as from menstruation or GI tract loss.

Iron deficiency

Iron deficiency, more common than iron excess, is the most common cause of anemia throughout the world. In the United States, about 20% of women of childbearing age and about 2% of adult males are iron-deficient, as are up to 10% of preschool-age children (Braunwald, Isselbacher, Petersdorf, Wilson, Martin, & Fauci, 1987). Iron deficiency affects as many as 20% of the population in certain areas in the Middle East, North Africa, and Asia (Williams, 1989).

Iron deficiency can develop during periods of increased requirements (growth spurts and pregnancy); from inadequate dietary intake; from decreased intestinal absorption; and from blood loss (*eg*, menstrual, GI, or associated with parasitic infestations like hookworm) (see Box 50-4).

The general symptoms of iron-deficiency anemia include weakness, pallor, fatigue, headache, and pal-

Box 50-4. Iron deficiency

Iron deficiency may result from several situations including the following:

  inadequate dietary supply

  increased requirements

  postgastrectomy

  excessive blood loss (*eg*, hemorrhage)

  infestation of GI tract with hookworm

  malabsorption syndromes (*eg*, chronic diarrhea, sprue, celiac disease, steatorrhea)

Iron deficiency results in the following:

  hypochromic microcytic anemia

  koilonychia

  Plummer-Vinson Syndrome

  GI disturbances

pitations. If the anemia becomes more severe, there may be shortness of breath and cardiac hypertrophy.

The distinctive signs of iron-deficiency include koilonychia, Plummer-Vinson syndrome, and GI symptoms. Koilonychia is a condition in which nails appear spoon-shaped. In many clients with iron-deficiency anemia, the fingernails become brittle and flat and develop longitudinal ridges. In some cases, these changes progress to koilonychia.

About half the clients with iron deficiency have a papillary atrophy of the tongue, some have fissures at the corners of the mouth, the mouth may be sore, and difficulty in swallowing may occur.

Gastrointestinal findings include achlorhydria, gastric atrophy, symptoms of gastritis, anorexia, flatulence, epigastric distress, constipation, and the liver and spleen may be enlarged.

Some clients experience numbness and tingling of the hands and feet but this is more likely to be seen in pernicious anemia.

Laboratory findings include below normal hemoglobin level, reduced or increased red blood cell count, low hematocrit, low serum iron level, and above normal total iron-binding protein level.

The hemoglobin and hematocrit level are the routine screening measures used to detect the anemia. Oral administration of ferrous salts is the usual treatment. The use of oral iron supplements should be accompanied by nutritional counseling to emphasize selection of foods that are high in iron. To help counteract the relatively common problem of iron deficiency, some foods, including cereals, flour, breads, and infant formulas, are fortified with iron.

Iron overload

Once considered rare, iron overload is now felt to be common. Its causes include increased iron absorption from diets with normal amounts of iron. For example, hemochromatosis, which is an iron-storage disease sometimes referred to as bronze diabetes, is a genetic disease that occurs chiefly in males. In this disease, iron saturates body tissues with deposits chiefly in the liver, pancreas, skin, and joints. These deposits disrupt normal function of these organ systems and a bronze coloration, liver damage and hepatomegaly, cardiovascular disease, arthritis, and diabetes occur. Other reasons for increased iron absorption include iron-loading anemias (*eg*, thalassemia), chronic liver disease, porphyria, cutanea tarda, and hemosiderosis.

Diets with excessive amounts of iron can also be a factor. In Africa, for example, a traditional fermented maize beverage home-brewed in steel drums has been identified as the cause of iron overload (Gordeuk, Bacon, & Brittenham, 1987).

Another cause could be parenteral iron loading produced by repeated blood transfusion.

The body lacks an effective means to excrete excess iron. When the body's storage capacity for iron is exceeded, there is widespread damage to the liver, heart, pancreas, and other organs. Therapy for iron overload currently consists of phlebotomy and treatment with a chelating agent capable of sequestering iron and allowing its excretion from the body.

Iron poisoning

Poisoning and fatalities with iron have occurred. In adults, fatalities have been due to suicides; in children (between the ages of 12 and 24 months), accidental poisoning is the cause. The frequency of this problem is probably related to the ready supply of iron in the home. Also, the colored coating of certain preparations may remind children of candy, such as M&Ms.

Signs and symptoms of poisoning may occur within 30 minutes or may not appear for several hours. The nausea, vomiting, and abdominal pain caused by the corrosive action of iron may be followed by cardiovascular collapse and death. At times, the client appears to be recovering, and then death occurs 12 or 24 hours following ingestion of the iron. The injury to the stomach, if nonfatal, may result in pyloric stenosis or gastric scarring.

If the diagnosis is made early, vomiting should be induced. Iron in the upper GI tract should be precipitated by lavage with sodium bicarbonate or phosphate solution. An iron antidote, deferoxamine (Desferal), a chelating agent with specific affinity for ferric iron and low affinity for calcium, is used as necessary. This agent binds ferric ion into a stable, water-soluble chelate readily excreted by the kidneys. Its main effect is to remove iron from transferrin, ferritin, and hemosiderin.

For adults, the dosage would be 1 g IM followed by 500 mg every 4 hours for two doses. No more than 6 g should be used in a 24-hour period. For children, the dosage is 50 mg/kg every 6 hours or 15 mg/kg/hr by continuous IV infusion. Reconstituted solutions should be protected from light and should not be stored for any longer than 1 week.

Adverse reactions to this agent include blurred vision, tachycardia, dysuria, pruritus, and painful induration at the injection site.

Ferrous sulfate and other oral preparations

Ferrous sulfate is the oldest iron preparation and is probably the most commonly administered preparation. Other oral ferrous compounds include ferrous fulmarate and ferrous gluconate. The *Physicians' desk reference* (1987) lists over 20 ferrous sulfate preparations, 14 ferrous gluconate preparations, and 20 ferrous fumarate preparations. The *Physicians' desk reference for nonprescription drugs* (1987) lists 24 hematinic preparations which contain iron. Table 50-11 reviews the contents of a sample of preparations containing iron and Table 50-12 reviews dosage and adverse reactions of the most common iron preparations.

Dosage and administration. The therapeutic dose of iron is calculated according to the amount of elemental iron the preparation contains. Ferrous sulfate yields 20% elemental iron. One 300 mg ferrous sulfate tablet contains 65 mg of elemental iron. A typical total daily dosage would be 300–1,200 mg in divided doses.

Iron preparations are best absorbed in the duodenum by active transport and is absorbed most readily in its ferrous form. Absorption is optimal if the client is fasting (not having eaten in the last 2 hours and not planning to eat in the next 2 hours) when the ferrous sulfate is taken. If GI distress occurs, this is reported to the physician and enteric-coated tablets may be tried or tablets may be taken with a snack.

If liquid iron preparations are used, the solution is placed on the back of the tongue with a dropper or is given well diluted and sipped through a straw. The teeth should be brushed thoroughly after administration. These steps can prevent transient staining of teeth and damage to the enamel. The Feosol elixir can be mixed with water but cannot be mixed with milk, fruit juice, or wine. If the taste is not well tolerated, Fer-in-sol drops may be mixed in fruit juices or with any liquid. Sustained-release products cannot be crushed or chewed.

Substances have been added to iron in attempts to enhance its absorption. For example, ascorbic acid has been added and it does increase the absorption of the iron by about 10%. Ascorbic acid does help keep the iron in its ferrous form.

The duration of treatment depends on the individual circumstances. With a steady daily increase in hemoglobin, anemia can be resolved within a predictable period of time. If iron stores are to be rebuilt, however, this rebuilding may take many months. Chronic therapy might be necessary with the client who, for some reason, loses blood at a higher-than-normal rate.

To evaluate response, the hemoglobin and hematocrit are monitored. A measurable increase in hemoglobin and hematocrit should be evident after 3–7 days of treatment. If the hemoglobin had been decreased by more than 3 g/dl before treatment, an average increase of hemoglobin of 0.2 g/dl is usual. An increase of 2 g/dl or more in the hemoglobin in 3–4 weeks is considered to be a positive response.

Iron-combination preparations contain compounds that are therapeutic in their own right, and administration of such a preparation can make the client's response to iron therapy more difficult to interpret.

Drug interactions. Antacids will reduce absorption of ferrous sulfate if they are taken concurrently. Tea and coffee consumed with a meal or 1 hour after, and eggs and milk, can also inhibit iron absorption.

Tetracycline forms a relatively insoluble chelate with iron. Chloramphenicol delays iron clearance from plasma, delays iron incorporation into red blood cells, and interferes with erythropoiesis.

Parenteral iron preparations

Iron-dextran injection (Imferon) is a complex of ferric hydroxide with dextran in a sodium chloride solution; it is the major example of a parenteral iron preparation and serves as a source of supplementary iron.

Pharmacokinetics. When given IM, the majority of the preparation is well absorbed after injection within 72 hours and the remaining drug is absorbed over the next 3–4 weeks. Reticuloendothelial cells of the liver, spleen, and bone marrow separate the iron from the dextran complex and gradually release it and it then combines with transferrin for transport to the bone marrow. The half-life of the drug is 5–20 hours.

Therapeutic uses. Response to parenteral iron is not faster than response to a course of oral iron. However, iron stores may be more rapidly created parenterally than orally. Parenteral iron may be used when absorption of iron from the GI tract is not satisfactory (*eg*, extensive bowel surgery, ulcerative colitis, regional enteritis). When iron losses are great, when noncompliance with oral preparations is high, and when intolerance for oral preparations is great, parenteral iron could be used.

Table 50-11. Iron and iron-combination preparations

Name	Active ingredients	Preparations	Usual dosage
Chromagen	ferrous fumarate 200 mg ascorbic acid 250 mg cyanocobalamin 10 µg dessicated stomach substance 100 mg	Oral	Adults: 1 capsule daily
Feosol	Dried ferrous sulfate USP 200 mg (65 mg of elemental iron) equivalent to 325 mg of ferrous sulfate USP Also several inactive ingredients	Oral tablet; also available with slightly different formulations as elixir and targeted-release capsules	Adults: 1 tablet 3–4 times qd after meals and hs Children: 6–12 yr: 1 tablet tid pc Under 6 yr: use elixir
Feostat	ferrous fumarate 100 mg	Oral tablet (chocolate-flavored and chewable); also available as suspension and drops	
Ferancee	Iron (from ferrous fumarate) 134 mg, vitamin C 300 mg, also FD&C yellow No. 5 and other inactive ingredients	Oral chewable tablet; also available as Ferancee-HP, a high potency formulation with less iron and more vitamin C per tablet	Adults: 2 tablets qd Children: Over 6 yr: 1 tablet qd
Ferro-Sequels (time-release iron)	ferrous fumarate 150 mg docusate sodium 100 mg also several inactive ingredients	Oral tablet	Adults: 1 tablet 1–2 times/d

Niferex daily tablets	iron (as polysaccharide-iron complex)
	vitamin A 5,000 IU
	vitamin E 30 IU
	vitamin C 60 mg
	folic acid 0.4 mg
	B_1 1.5 mg
	B_2 1.7 mg
	niacinamide 20 mg
	pantothenic acid 10 mg
	biotin 0.3 mg
	B_6 2 mg
	B_{12} 6 mcg
	vitamin D 400 IU
	calcium 259 mg
	iodine 150 µg
	phosphorus 5.4 mg
	manganese 5 mg
	magnesium 100 mg
	zinc 15 mg
	copper 2 mg
		Oral tablet, elixir; other variations of product include
		  Niferex—150 capsules
		  Niferex with vitamin C tablets
		  Niferex—150 Forte capsules
		  Niferex Forte elixir
		  Niferex—PN tablets	

Dosage and administration. Iron-dextran injection is available in 10-ml vials for IM use and in 2-ml and 5-ml ampules for IM or IV administration. The strength is 50 mg/ml of elemental iron. The initial dose may be 1 or 2 ml. A 0.5-ml test dose should be given before a client receives the full therapeutic dose. Doses of up to 5 ml per buttock have been given but such large doses are not generally used because of local discoloration of the skin; long, continued discomfort at the injection site; and concern about possible malignant change at the injection site.

To determine the appropriate dose of Imferon, the following formula is followed:

$$0.3 \times \text{body wt in lb} \times \left(100 - \frac{\text{Hgb in g/dl} \times 100}{14.8}\right) = \text{mg iron}$$

Table 50-12. Iron preparations

Drug name	Preparation	Usual dosage	Adverse reactions
ferrous sulfate (Fer-in-sol) (contains 20% ferrous elemental iron)	Oral tablets Liquids Elixirs Drops Timed-release capsules	Adult: 300–1,200 mg in divided doses daily Child 6–12 yr: 120–600 mg/d in divided doses Child under 6 yr: 300 mg/d in divided doses	GI irritation, anorexia, nausea, vomiting, constipation/diarrhea, abdominal distress, dark-colored stools (green, black)
ferrous gluconate (Fergon) (contains 11.6% ferrous elemental iron)	Oral	Adult: 300–640 mg 1–3 times/d Child 6–12 yr: 300 mg 1–3 times/d Child under 6 yr: 100–300 mg/d in divided doses	Same as above but somewhat less GI irritation.
ferrous fumarate (Femiron, Ircon) (contains 33% ferrous elemental iron)	Oral	Adult: 200 mg 1–4 times/d Child under 6 yr: 100–300 mg/d in divided doses	Same as above.
iron dextran (Imferon) (1 ml = 50 mg elemental iron)	IM IV	About 250 mg/d for every gram hemoglobin is below normal, formula based on weight (see text)	Chills, fever, headache, joint pain, urticaria, convulsions, weakness, chest pain, hypotension, tachycardia, shock, anaphylaxis, flushing, local brown temporary or permanent discoloration at injection site, tumor at injection site after latent period.

The formula results in a figure for the total amount of iron in milligrams required to restore the hemoglobin to normal and to replenish iron stores. This figure is converted to dose in milliliters of Imferon by dividing it by 50. Applying the formula, it would be found that a 120-pound client with a current hemoglobin of 8.0 g/dL would need 33 ml of Imferon to restore the hemoglobin level and iron stores.

Oral iron should be discontinued if Imferon is to be used.

To cut down on skin discoloration, separate needles are used to withdrawn the solution from its container and to inject it. A 19–20 gauge 2- or 3-inch needle is recommended. The Z-track method is then used to avoid injection or leakage into subcutaneous tissue. The best site for administration of Imferon is the dorsal gluteal area of the buttocks; the client's arms must not be used.

Intravenous administration of iron-dextran injection (prepared without preservative) avoids local skin discoloration and deposition of the preparation in tissues. A 0.5-ml test dose is given to determine whether any signs or symptoms of anaphylaxis will appear (*eg*, chills, fever, headache, joint pain, or urticaria). Anaphylactic reactions would usually be evident within a few minutes. Nevertheless, it is recommended that an hour be allowed to elapse before further Imferon is given. Phlebitis is a common side effect of IV administration but this can be minimized by adding the calculated dose to 200- to 250 ml of normal saline and infusing the solution over 2 hours.

Intravenous administration has provoked acute exacerbation of joint pain and swelling in clients with rheumatoid arthritis and iron deficiency anemia. Peripheral vascular "flushing" (if the Imferon has been administered too rapidly) has been noted.

■ Summary

A normal, healthy adult has less than 5 g of iron, about 70% of which is found in hemoglobin. Yet, the body uses and stores those 5 g well. Human iron requirements are the outcome of obligatory physiologic losses and needs imposed by growth. Absorption is very important in determining how much iron the body contains. Because iron deficiency is prevalent worldwide, some foods are fortified with iron. Iron deficiency anemia is treated with oral ferrous sulfate or parenteral iron preparations.

Vitamin B$_{12}$

In 1948, vitamin B$_{12}$ was the last of the vitamins to be identified. It refers to a group of cobalt-containing compounds called cobalamins, several of which are found in foods and in the body. The recommended daily allowances are summarized in Table 50-9.

During gastric digestion in the presence of gastric acid, vitamin B$_{12}$ is released from the proteins to which it is bound. It forms a complex with a substance called intrinsic factor, which is produced by the parietal cells of the stomach. Intrinsic factor protects vitamin B$_{12}$ from being destroyed by digestive enzymes. The B$_{12}$-

intrinsic factor complex is adsorbed onto the mucosa of the distal ileum, an attachment that is calcium-dependent. During transport across the mucosa of the ileum, vitamin B_{12} is separated from intrinsic factor and is transported through the plasma by way of a transport protein called transcobalamin II. Most American adults absorb more vitamin B_{12} than they need and have a 2- to 5-year supply stored in the liver. It is also stored in minute amounts in the kidney, heart, muscle, pancreas, testes, brain, spleen, and bone marrow. Stores are very slowly depleted.

Vitamin B_{12} is needed to act as a coenzyme for deoxyribonucleic acid (DNA) synthesis and for formation of normal red blood cells. It is also essential for methylation reactions (the transfer of $-CH_3$ groups), as in the conversion of hemocystine to methionine and in the conversion of L-methylmalonyl-CoA to succinyl-CoA. Related to these reactions, deficiency in childhood can result in homocystinuria and methylmalonic aciduria.

Vitamin B_{12} deficiency

The development of B_{12} deficiency during adult life does not normally result from dietary deficiency. The ordinary diet easily provides the recommended daily allowance and more (for example, the recommended daily intake is 3.0 μg and 1 cup milk, 1 egg, and 4 oz. meat provide 2.4 μg). Vitamin B_{12} is unique among nutrients in that it is found almost exclusively in animal flesh. The only reliable sources are meats, eggs, fish, poultry, and dairy products. Lacto-ovo-vegetarians (who use milk, cheese, and eggs) are protected from deficiency. But strict vegetarians must use B_{12}-fortified soybean products or take B_{12} supplements to avoid a dietary deficiency.

A deficiency in vitamin B_{12} can occur because of lack of intrinsic factor (pernicious anemia); postgastrectomy; with diseases involving the ileum; with bacterial overgrowth of the intestine; and with inherited defects in the metabolism and use of the vitamin. In some populations, infestation of the GI tract with a particular fish tapeworm, which dissociates the B_{12} intrinsic factor complex, may precipitate the vitamin deficiency (see Box 50-5).

A deficiency triggers the defective synthesis of DNA. The earliest sign of deficiency is megaloblastic anemia. The defective DNA synthesis results in the formation of megaloblasts. Megaloblasts are abnormal, large, nucleated, immature cells that form macrocytes, which are abnormally large erythrocytes that have a relatively short life span. It is very important to establish the precise cause of megaloblastic anemia because folic-acid deficiency can also cause megaloblastic anemia. Vitamin B_{12} and folic acid share close metabolic interrelationships. Vitamin B_{12} normally affects hemopoiesis by providing an activated reduced form of

---

Box 50-5. Vitamin B_{12} deficiency

Vitamin B_{12} deficiency does not normally occur in adults from inadequate dietary supply. It may result from the following:

 lack of intrinsic factor (*ie*, pernicious anemia)

 postgastrectomy

 diseases involving ileum

 bacterial overgrowth of intestine

 infestation of GI tract with a specific fish tapeworm

Vitamin B_{12} deficiency results in the following:

 megaloblastic anemia

 GI disturbances

 cardiovascular symptoms

 neurologic symptoms

---

folate. A deficiency in vitamin B_{12} actually causes secondary folate deficiency.

Besides causing megaloblastic anemia, vitamin B_{12} deficiency causes GI symptoms (sore tongue, anorexia, diarrhea, and moderate weight loss), circulatory symptoms (dyspnea, palpitations, weakness, precordial pain), and neurologic symptoms (vertigo, tinnitus, paresthesia, diminution of vibratory and position senses, deep tendon reflex changes, incoordination, and mental disturbances). Neurologic complications can be irreversible, which requires that every effort be made to make the diagnosis before neurologic involvement. Signs or symptoms that have been present for only a few months disappear rapidly after treatment is started but a defect present for years may never be fully corrected.

The combination of multisystem involvement due to vitamin B_{12} deficiency is called *pernicious anemia*. Pernicious anemia is caused by the failure of parietal cell function, which, in turn, results in the failure of intrinsic factor production. The etiology of pernicious anemia is unclear; heredity may be a factor. Pernicious anemia occurs most often in middle-aged persons. Elderly clients who infrequently receive medical care or follow-up may present with pernicious anemia that has been producing symptoms for quite some time. It has even been associated with overt psychosis in the elderly. Before vitamin B_{12} was isolated and the disease understood, untreated pernicious anemia was fatal because it caused progressive nervous system degeneration.

A combined deficiency of B_{12}, iron, and folate is common in clients with anemia following gastric resection. Clients who have had a total gastrectomy invariably will develop malabsorption of vitamin B_{12}. Megaloblastic anemia due to vitamin B_{12} deficiency is rare after partial gastrectomy but reduced serum vitamin B_{12} levels have been observed in about 14% of these clients (Braunwald, et al, 1987). Two reasons the anemia is rare are that the stomach secretes intrinsic factor approximately 100 times in excess of need, and the resected portion of the stomach is almost always principally antrum, which contains few parietal cells. However, some clients after peptic resection do develop decreased serum vitamin B_{12} levels. The reason is not exactly clear but it may be due, in part, to rapid emptying of gastric contents and reduced efficiency of intrinsic factor binding of the vitamin.

Clients with gastric resection also malabsorb dietary iron but have normal absorption of oral iron preparations. Folate deficiency may result from either reduced dietary intake or impaired folate absorption. The development of anemia after peptic ulcer surgery is gradual, usually appearing several years after surgery.

Because of the interdependence of vitamin B_{12} and folic acid, the hematopoietic evidence of pernicious anemia can appear to improve with therapy with folic acid. However, the neurologic symptoms would not respond to folic acid therapy. This explains why is it so very important to establish the precise cause of a megaloblastic anemia so that treatment will be specific. As indicated in relationship to gastric resection, therapy might need to include all three hematinics.

Vitamin B_{12} preparations

Two preparations of vitamin B_{12} are available (Table 50-13). These preparations are cobalt-containing substances produced from *Streptomyces griseus* or obtained from human liver. It is possible to have a cobalt hypersensitivity and if this is suspected, an intradermal test dose may be given before therapy is begun.

Pharmacodynamics. Parenteral vitamin B_{12} does not need to go through the regular route of absorption; it bypasses the absorption defect. Consequently, it provides the client with usable vitamin B_{12}, even in the absence of intrinsic factor.

Therapeutic uses. Vitamin B_{12} is used for any of the conditions that result in the vitamin's deficiency or when requirements are increased. It has also been tried in a number of conditions, such as multiple sclerosis, without apparent success.

Dosage and administration. Vitamin B_{12} is administered by IM injection in doses of 1–100 μg. The injection is usually given daily for 1 week, then three times a week for up to 2 months, followed by a maintenance dose of 100 μg once a month for life. Doses larger than 100 μg have been tried but it is felt by most that larger doses provide no greater benefit since they are rapidly cleared from the plasma and excreted in the urine.

The client should have blood counts taken every 3–6 months to determine the accuracy of therapy. Refractoriness to therapy can develop. The hemoglobin and hematocrit should return to normal after 6–8 weeks of therapy. The reticulocyte response normally appears in 2 or 3 days.

Vitamin B_{12} is available for oral administration and could be given in combination with other vitamins and minerals for possible dietary deficiency. However, oral administration is not effective in the event of intrinsic factor deficiency or ileal disease.

Drug interactions. Cimetidine impairs absorption of vitamin B_{12}. Neomycin, colchicine, para-aminosalicylic acid, potassium, and alcohol may cause malabsorption of the vitamin.

■ Summary

Vitamin B_{12} is essential in the human diet and is found in most foods of animal origin. Only strict vegetarians who avoid all meats and animal products are likely to develop a dietary deficiency. Pernicious anemia causes a variety of symptoms involving many body systems and is caused by the failure of parietal cell function, which, in turn, results in the failure of intrinsic factor production. Intrinsic factor is required for the absorption of vitamin B_{12}. The earliest sign of deficiency of vitamin B_{12} is megaloblastic anemia. Untreated pernicious anemia can be fatal because of progressive nervous system degeneration.

Table 50-13. Vitamin B_{12} preparations

Drug name	Preparation	Usual dosage	Adverse reactions
cyanocobalamin (Betalin 12)	IM	Adult: 100–1,000 μg/d for 6–7 days, then 100–1,000 μg monthly Child: 100 μg weekly to monthly	Optic nerve atrophy, anaphylaxis, diarrhea, pruritus, urticaria, pain at injection site.
hydroxocobalamin (Alpharedisol)	IM	Adult: 1,000 μg/mo Child: 100 μg/mo	Same as above.

Folic acid

Folate is a generic term for the many different forms of this water-soluble vitamin. In the 1940s, a substance was isolated from spinach leaves and named *folic acid* from the Latin word *folium* meaning leaf. Later in the 1940s, folate was chemically synthesized and available commercially.

The reduced form of folic acid is folinic acid, first called *citrovorum factor* because it supplies an essential growth factor of a bacterium called *Lactobacillus citrovorum* (Williams, 1989). Folinic acid has found a special function in chemotherapy with certain cancer clients (see Chapter 48).

The primary dietary form of the vitamin is the conjugated polyglutamate form, which must be converted to the monoglutamate form before absorption in the jejunum. The vitamin is first converted to the monoglutamate form by a hydrolytic enzyme (conjugase) located in the membrane of the intestinal mucosal cells. This form is then absorbed by an active transport, carrier-mediated uptake system. The absorption process is sensitive to changes in pH in the jejunum and to factors that interfere with the activity of conjugase. Absorption is facilitated in a slightly acid environment. After absorption, dietary folates are transported in plasma as monoglutamate derivatives primarily bound to albumin (Bailey, 1990).

The synthetic pharmaceutical form of the vitamin is called pteroylglutamic acid, which becomes biochemically active after it has undergone reduction. This commercial form is basically the monoglutamate form, with one glutamic acid residue (the polyglutamate form has up to seven glutamic acid residues). When this pharmaceutical form is consumed as a vitamin supplement or added to food such as fortified breakfast cereals, it can be absorbed directly.

The liver is the primary storage site for the vitamin and the amount normally stored in the entire body ranges from 5 to 10 mg. The concentration of folate in the bile is about five times that of serum. Enterohepatic recirculation from the intestine to the liver is important in the maintenance of serum folate levels.

The primary biochemical function of folate is in the transfer and use of one-carbon units in a variety of essential reactions involved in amino acid interconversions, biosynthesis of the nucleic acids, purines, and pyrimidines, and certain methylation reactions. A folate deficiency can lead to alterations in the pattern of cell replication, such as in the synthesis of DNA. Rapidly dividing cells would be most affected by a deficiency. Folic acid is needed for the production of normal red blood cells and some studies have documented impaired immune responses associated with a folate deficiency.

The recommended daily allowance for folate is 200 µg for a 70-kg adult male and 170 µg for a 60-kg adult nonpregnant, nonlactating woman. Folic acid requirement is increased during pregnancy and lactation, during disease, during growth, and with women using oral contraceptive agents. These requirements are summarized in Table 50-9.

Concentrated dietary sources of folate include green leafy vegetables such as raw spinach, asparagus, legumes (peas, black-eyed peas, red kidney beans, lentils), citrus fruit, and liver (beef, calf, chicken, and turkey especially). Methods of preparation make a difference in the amount of folate available since there is a certain amount of destruction caused by heat and loss caused by leaching of the vitamin into the cooking water. A person absorbs only 25%–50% of dietary folates ingested.

Folic acid deficiency

Folic acid deficiency has three stages: stage I or negative balance, stage II or tissue depletion, and stage III or functional changes (Bailey, 1990). The type of anemia caused by a folate deficiency is different from an iron deficiency anemia but the same as a vitamin B_{12} deficiency. A deficiency of folic acid produces a macrocytic anemia associated with megaloblastic arrest in red blood cell production. Megaloblasts are described in the section on vitamin B_{12} deficiency. Also found in folate deficiency are hypersegmented neutrophils relating to the impaired DNA synthesis.

Folate deficiency can result from several situations, including inadequate dietary supply, pathology of the jejunum, or increased metabolic demands (*ie*, pregnancy, lactation, infancy, adolescence) (see Box 50-6).

Environmental considerations may affect folate status. For example, folate depletion is associated with alcoholism. Alcohol negatively affects folate absorption and increases urinary folate excretion. With hepatic disease, there may be interference with the flow of folate into bile for reabsorption and transport to tissues (the enterohepatic cycle).

Box 50-6. Folic acid deficiency

Folic acid deficiency may result from several situations including the following:
- inadequate dietary supply
- pathology of jejunum
- renal failure
- alcoholism
- hepatic disease
- nontropical sprue
- tropical sprue
- use of certain medications

Folic acid deficiency results in the following:
- megaloblastic anemia
- growth retardation
- GI disturbances

Folate blood levels have been found to be lower in smokers than in nonsmokers. The lower blood folate levels in smokers are associated with increases in preneoplastic changes, such as bronchial metaplasia and chromosome fragility. Folate levels have been found to improve in smokers treated with folate and vitamin B_{12} supplements.

Nontropical and tropical sprue are also common causes of folate deficiency.

Drug use increases the chance of developing a folate deficiency due to specific effects of certain drugs on folate metabolism. Drugs that negatively affect folate status include estrogen, aspirin, methotrexate, sulfasalazine (Azulfidine), cimetidine, aluminum hydroxide, and sodium bicarbonate. Sulfasalazine is reported to cause a decrease in serum folate levels and may produce symptoms of folic acid deficiency. Oral contraceptives may impair folate metabolism but the effect is said to be too mild to cause anemia. An increase in seizure frequency and a decrease in serum phenytoin concentration to subtherapeutic levels have been reported in clients receiving folic acid with diphenylhydantoin. This appears related to an increased metabolism of the diphenylhydantoin.

The general symptoms of folic acid-deficiency anemia include weakness, pallor, degeneration of surface mucosal tissue resulting in ulceration and secondary infection, sore tongue, and GI disturbances, such as diarrhea.

Folic acid preparations

Many folic acid preparations, with and without additional ingredients, are available.

Pharmacokinetics. Folic acid is absorbed after oral administration. It is stored primarily in the liver and excreted by urine. Its onset of action is rapid with a peak of 30–60 minutes and a duration of 12–24 hours.

Therapeutic uses. Folic acid is used to correct its deficiency or it may be given prophylactically with certain drug therapy or when the need is known to be increased.

Dosage and administration. Tablets contain 0.1–1 mg of pteroylglutamic acid. Oral administration of folate is satisfactory unless the client is acutely ill with megaloblastic anemia. Usually 1 mg is given two or three times per day but doses up to 20 mg/d may be given. Children up to 4 years would receive 0.3 mg/d and infants would receive 0.1 mg/d.

Folic acid is also available as folic acid injection, an aqueous solution of the sodium salt of pteroylglutamic acid. It is available in multidose vials at 5 mg/ml and 10 mg/ml. The vials should be kept in the dark and be refrigerated. It can be given IM or IV. The use of folinic acid in chemotherapy with certain clients with cancer is discussed in Chapter 48.

Adverse reactions. There have been reports of reactions to parenteral injections of folic acid but these have been rare. Folic acid in its oral form is not toxic at the usual therapeutic doses.

■ Summary

Folic acid is essential in the diet. It is found in most foods. However, because it is unstable to heat, protracted cooking can destroy 90% of the folate content in foods.

Nursing management

Nursing process

Assessment The nurse has a role in the identification of persons who may be deficient in iron, vitamin B_{12}, or folic acid. A thorough client history may elicit clues that should alert the interviewer to the possibility of deficiencies. For example, the client's previous medical history might reveal a history of a partial or total gastrectomy. The family history might identify a repeated incidence of anemia. For example, relatives of clients with pernicious anemia show an increased incidence of the disease (Braunwald, et al, 1987).

When discussing the living and working environment, exposure to toxic substances that may affect hematopoietic status could be identified. Drugs that cause hematologic toxicity (*eg,* agranulocytosis, aplastic anemia, hemolytic anemia, megaloblastic anemia, or thrombocytopenia) include antimalarials, antithyroid drugs, cephalosporins, chloramphenicol, chlorpropamide, diphenylhydantoin, folic acid antagonists, gold salts, mephenytoin, methyldopa, nitrofurantoin, phenothiazines, phenylbutazone, sulfonamides, and thiazides. A careful and detailed diet history may reveal a vegetarian diet, a diet deficient in a certain type of food, or cooking practices that rob foods of their nutritional value.

In the review of the systems, signs that could indicate chronic blood loss, such as tarry stools, blood in the stools, smokey urine, or frequent nosebleeds may be elicited. Menstrual difficulties may be a clue to excessive blood loss. Symptoms of a decrease in available oxygen may be cited, such as vertigo, tinnitus, weakness, easy fatigability, faintness, drowsiness, headache, loss of libido, or shortness of breath.

Physical examination may elicit a rapid heart rate that increases significantly with mild exercise, a heart murmur, or an accentuated S_1. Respiratory rate may be elevated. The skin, especially the mouth and face, will be pale; mucous membranes, conjunctiva, and nailbeds will be pale. The tongue may be glossy in appearance.

Nursing diagnosis Clients receiving hematinics would be likely to have a medical diagnosis of anemia.

Nursing diagnoses that might apply include the following:

> Impaired gas exchange
> Altered nutrition: less than body requirements
> Altered oral mucous membrane
> Activity intolerance
> Impaired physical mobility
> Fatigue
> Altered thought processes
> High risk for infection

(See Example of Nursing Process and Hematinic Therapy.)

Planning In preparing a plan of client care, the nurse should set certain client outcome goals (*eg*, adequate tissue oxygenation, improved nutritional status, healthy oral cavity, increased tolerance for activity, maximum physical mobility, participation in activities, improved thought processes, and a minimized risk of infection.

Intervention During the assessment period, various diagnostic tests will be performed (*eg*, red blood cell counts and indices, hematocrit, hemoglobin, serum iron and folate levels, total iron-binding capacity, reticulocyte count, vitamin B_{12} and folic acid levels, and serum ferritin and transferrin levels). The Schilling Test and bone marrow examination may be performed. Following diagnosis and during administration of a hematinic, the hemoglobin and hematocrit will be measured periodically, as well as other laboratory tests perhaps. The nurse needs to explain these tests to the client, monitor the results, and discuss them with the physician.

With the anemic client, the nurse should maintain a comfortable room temperature and provide the client with adequate clothing and blankets because cold causes vasoconstriction, which impairs tissue perfusion. Measures to promote rest, improve activity tolerance, and reduce risks of injury and infection should also be implemented.

If the client has glossitis and stomatitis from the anemia, the nurse should assist the client with oral hygiene and apply special measures as needed (*eg*, normal saline mouth rinses, lip lubricants, topical anesthetic solutions).

If an injectable iron preparation is used (*eg*, Imferon), the nurse must adhere carefully to the recommended methods of drawing the medication into the syringe and administering the medication using the Z-track method (see discussion of Imferon for details) to avoid skin discoloration.

If a liquid iron preparation is used, a method of administration must be followed that will avoid staining of the teeth. One way would be to use a dilute solution and administer it through a straw, followed by a thorough brushing of the teeth.

Client education. The nurse should explain the importance of diet therapy in the treatment of anemia. Obtain a dietary consultation to assist the client in menu planning if appropriate.

Explain the rationale for, side effects of, and importance of taking the medications prescribed. If discharged on an iron preparation, the client should be instructed to take the iron on an empty stomach for best absorption (if difficulties are encountered with this approach, the physician is consulted). The client should increase intake of vitamin C or take a vitamin C preparation to increase iron absorption. The client should be advised that feces may be green or black while a person is on iron medication and that this is not a sign of GI bleeding. Bowel habits may also change, and the client should be informed that either constipation or diarrhea can occur. The client should be told to keep the iron preparation out of the reach of children.

If clients are discharged on parenteral vitamin B_{12} and it is planned that they will self-administer it, then the nurse will have to explain correct technique. The nurse should allow time for questions, clarification, and return demonstration.

If discharged on a folic acid preparation, the client should be instructed in foods high in folic acid content and cautioned that cooking foods containing folic acid for more than 15 minutes will destroy their content of folic acid. The client should be told of the problems encountered when taking certain medications with folic acid and advised to report any need to take such medications to the physician.

Instruct the client in ways to reduce the risk of infection and injury. Reinforce the importance of keeping follow-up appointments with the physician and for laboratory studies. Explain the need to adhere to planned rest periods and avoid strenuous activity until the anemia has improved. Use measures to improve client compliance, such as including significant others in the teaching sessions and providing instructions in writing.

Evaluation The nurse must evaluate the client to determine drug efficacy and to observe for evidence of adverse reactions. Data indicating drug efficacy would include increased hemoglobin and hematocrit levels; weight within normal range for client's age, height, and build; healthy gums and oral mucous membranes; improved strength and activity tolerance; verbalization of less fatigue and participation in desired activities at level of ability; improved thought processes (*eg*, better memory, longer attention span, absence of confusion); and absence of signs and symptoms of infection.

Checklist of nursing actions

☐ Assess clients at high risk for iron, vitamin B_{12}, and folic acid deficiencies for signs and symptoms of anemia.

- ☐ Keep anemic clients warm to promote peripheral perfusion.
- ☐ Provide special mouth care for clients experiencing altered oral mucous membranes.
- ☐ Promote rest for anemic clients.
- ☐ Implement nursing measures to reduce risk of infection and trauma for anemic clients.
- ☐ Administer oral iron preparations with client fasting.
- ☐ Use Z-track methodology to administer IM iron solutions.
- ☐ Teach clients receiving hematinics how to manage their drug regimens.
- ☐ Teach clients treated for anemia how to improve dietary intake of hematinic nutrients.

(See Example of Nursing Process and Hematinic Therapy.)

Health food products

The health food industry offers many nutrient concentrates for the lay public. In most cases, these substances are marketed as single ingredient preparations but combinations of two or more are also available. In addition to various vitamin and mineral formulations, substances such as single amino acids, phospholipids, fatty acids, flavor essences, vinegar, and kelp are marketed. These products are not classified as drugs and do not fall under control of the FDA. Directions for their use, including recommended dosages (which tend to be generous), usually do not appear on the labels but are available from salespersons or in writing as "take home" leaflets. For the most part, there is little or no scientific proof of the efficacy of these substances, nor is there controlled testing for adverse effects. Selected health food products are discussed below as examples.

Amino acids

The amino acid *L-tryptophan* has been heralded in the lay literature as a natural sleep aid. It is found in abundance in milk and milk products and is believed to be the sedative agent in milk taken warm at bedtime for sleep. There is considerable evidence that this substance does indeed promote sleep. Some physicians have been advising clients, especially those with autoimmune diseases such as rheumatoid arthritis and scleroderma, to use it in lieu of other hypnotic drugs. The usual dosage was 500–1,000 mg taken at bedtime.

One study (Nemzer, Arnold, Votolato, & McConnell, 1986) reported that tryptophan improves the behavior of hyperactive children, in some cases producing greater improvement than d-amphetamine.

When L-tryptophan is taken concurrently with certain antidepressants, it can cause acute psychotic signs and symptoms: restlessness, anxiety or depression, inability to concentrate, and exacerbation of obsessive–compulsive disorder (Steiner & Fontaine, 1986).

Currently, L-tryptophan has been withdrawn from the United States market because a serious neuromuscular disorder, eosinophile myalgia, developed among recipients of the drug. Adverse effects included paralysis and death. Due to this, the federal FDA banned the sale of L-tryptophan (FDA seeks recall . . . , 1988). A contaminant in a batch of drugs is now suspected of being the real cause of the eosinophile myalgia. If this proves to be the case, the drug may again be approved for sale, either over-the-counter or by prescription.

L-Glutamine is sold as a brain stimulant and cognitive aid. A report of two men using large dosages of this substance indicated that glutamine may have stimulant properties. Both men exhibited manic behavior, which resolved with discontinuation of the drug. L-Glutamine is not recognized as a therapeutic drug by the medical profession.

Tyrosine has been used successfully in the treatment of depression when other therapies fail. Tyrosine is a precursor of the neurotransmitters norepinephrine and dopamine (Cerrato, 1988).

The above effects of specific amino acids cannot be achieved by increasing dietary intake of protein because amino acids compete for transfer across the blood–brain barrier. Only an increase in the proportion of a single amino acid to other amino acids will produce therapeutic levels in the brain.

Lipids

Linoleic acid is an essential fatty acid recommended by health food proponents for preventing cardiovascular degeneration. This acid is known to play a role in biomembrane structure and production of prostaglandins. It has been found to be helpful in delaying and ameliorating relapses in the early stages of multiple sclerosis. Linoleic acid is unproved, however, as a cardiovascular protectant. This substance has the same caloric value as other fatty acids.

Lecithin is, according to health food advocates, also believed to protect the cardiovascular system. Lecithin is a phospholipid with a high linoleic acid content. Studies have not substantiated its purported hypocholesterolemic effect. Preliminary evidence suggests that it does improve the HDL/LDL ratio in the blood, especially in women. High doses of either linoleic acid or lecithin can significantly increase calorie intake.

Unrefined products

One flavoring element available in capsule form is *garlic*, which is under study for hypotensive effects. Perhaps some component of this substance will eventually be accepted as a helpful drug. However, its pharmacologically active component appears to be removed during the processing of garlic; the capsules are reported to exert no helpful pharmacologic effects.

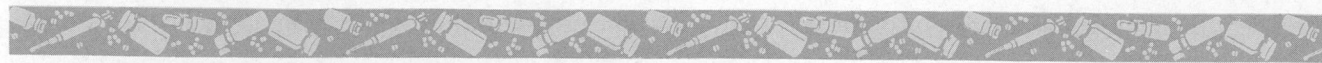

Example of nursing process and hematinic therapy

The client, Jackson Pale, is an 80-year-old man who had a subtotal gastric resection for a peptic ulcer when he was 60 years old. At the time of his ulcer surgery, he was a mechanical engineer for a large manufacturing company. He has had no recurrence of ulcer symptoms since his surgery. He has been on a regular diet, although he by choice did not eat highly spiced foods.

Currently, he exhibits lassitude, weakness, and fatigue. He complains of headaches, dizziness, palpitations, and a sore tongue. On examination, he was found to be pale, have a rapid pulse, and his tongue was smooth and redder than normal. His hematocrit is 20, the serum level of vitamin B_{12} is 100 pg/ml, and the serum level of folic acid is 4 ng/mL. He is anorexic and has lost weight; currently he is 5'10" and weighs 154 lbs.

A diagnosis of deficiencies of iron, vitamin B_{12}, and folic acid is made. He will be receiving ferrous sulfate 325 mg tid, cyanocobalamin 30 mcg/d intramuscularly for 10 days (followed by 100 mcg/mon), and folic acid 1 mg/d.

Mr. Pale's wife, Agnes, died 2 years ago. They had been married 51 years and lived alone in their own home. They had three children, only one of them lives in the city where they reside. Mr. Pale has seemed apathetic and irritable lately. He has no interest in the future and has withdrawn from friends and neighbors. He often behaves as if his wife died yesterday. In the past, he was busy every day on some task of maintenance of their home but has done no work on the house since her death. His children are beginning to feel nursing home placement might be more appropriate than living alone but Mr. Pale is opposed to this idea.

Assessment data	Diagnosis	Intervention	Goals and outcome criteria
Anorexia Has lost weight; is under the normal weight for his height Has a sore tongue Exhibits other symptoms of anemia Exhibits laboratory data consistent with diagnosis of anemia.	Altered nutrition: less than body requirements (iron and folate) related to inadequate intake of nutritious foods	**Monitor** percentage of meals eaten. **Serve** small portions of nutritious foods/fluids that appeal to client. **Allow** adequate time for meals; reheat food if necessary. **Instruct** and assist client to select foods/fluids that are high in iron, vitamin C, vitamin B_{12}, and folic acid. **Administer** ferrous sulfate, cyanocobalamin, and folic acid as ordered and monitor for therapeutic/nontherapeutic effects.	The client will have an improved nutrition/status.
Lassitude, weakness, and fatigue Dizziness. Diagnoses of deficiencies of iron, vitamin B_{12}, and folic acid Apathetic. No work on home maintenance in 2 years.	Activity intolerance related to altered nutritional status	**Carry out** interventions relating to improving nutritional status. **Encourage** progressive activity and increased self-care as allowed and tolerated. **Instruct** client in energy-saving techniques such as shower chair for showering and sitting to do other parts of personal hygiene like brushing teeth, combing hair. **Provide** adequate rest periods between periods of activity.	The client will demonstrate an increased tolerance for activity.

(Continued)

Example of nursing process and hematinic therapy (*Continued*)

Assessment data	Diagnosis	Intervention	Goals and outcome criteria
Anorexia and weight loss. Wife died 2 years ago. Had been married 51 years. Apathetic and irritable. No interest in the future and has withdrawn from friends and relatives. Often behaves as if his wife died yesterday. No work on the house since wife's death.	Dysfunctional grieving related to loss of wife	**Permit** and encourage review of life's achievements and experiences. **Support** past achievements, current strengths, and coping skills. **Use** active listening and encourage exploration of feelings and thoughts about wife. **Work through** emotional reaction (apathy, hopelessness). **Encourage** client to seek assistance from friends, relatives, professionals, and/or self-help groups.	The client will experience less or no dysfunctional grieving.

Kelp is available in concentrated form from drug store counters and health food stores. This substance is rich in iodine but has no other known pharmacologic agent.

Vinegar is another component of certain supplement capsules. Ingested vinegar is not accepted as a medicinal substance. It has no known therapeutic effect. Like the iodine in kelp, the main ingredient of vinegar, acetic acid, is available in foodstuffs (pickles and liquid salad dressing).

■ Summary

Most concentrated nutrients marketed by the health food industry are not controlled by the FDA. These products generally contain no instructions or cautions on their labels. Instructions for their use are disseminated by word of mouth, anonymous printed material, or in publications largely supported by advertisements featuring proprietary preparations of these products. Some products have been recognized and used by the medical care system but others have no proven value and some have proved to be toxic.

Nursing management

Nursing implications

To advise clients on the merits of health foods, the nurse needs to have some knowledge of nutritional research. By studying the literature in this discipline, the nurse can advise knowledgeably and specifically on individual products.

In the absence of expertise in this area, the nurse should caution clients about the pitfalls that may await them if they use products of unproved worth that are not controlled by the FDA.

References

Bailey LB. (1990). The role of folate in human nutrition. *Nutrition Today,* 12–19.

Braunwald E, Isselbacher K, Petersdorf R, Wilson J, Martin J, Fauci A, eds. (1987). *Harrison's principles of internal medicine,* 11th ed., pp 1249, 1498–1504, 1632–1635. New York: McGraw-Hill.

Cerrato PL. (1988). Nutritionist on call: The most overlooked aspect of nursing. *RN, 51,* 85–88 (September).

FDA seeks recall of L-tryptophan supplements. (1990). *American Journal of Nursing, 90,* 88 (April)

Gordeuk VR, Bacon BR, Brittenham GM. (1987). Iron overload: Causes and consequences, in Olson RE, ed. *Annual review of nutrition.* Palo Alto, CA: Annual Reviews.

Gralla RJ, Tyson LB, Kris MG, Clark RA. (1987). The management of chemotherapy-induced nausea and vomiting. *Med Clin N Am, 71(2),* 289–301.

Nemzer ED, Arnold LE, Votolato NA, McConnell H. (1986). Amino acid supplementation as therapy for attention deficit disorder. *J Am Acad Child Adolesc Psychiatry, 25,* 509–513.

Physicians' desk reference, 41st ed. (1987). Oradell, NJ: Medical Economics.

Physicians' desk reference for nonprescription drugs, 8th ed. (1987). Oradell, NJ: Medical Economics.

Scherer P. (1987). Hands-on experience, part 2: Antipsoriatic etretinate. *American Journal of Nursing, 87,* 645–646 (May).

Steiner W, Fontaine R. (1986). Toxic reaction following the combined administration of fluoxetine and L-tryptophan: Five case reports. *Biol Psychiatry, 21,* 1067–1071 (September).

Williams SR. (1989). *Nutrition and diet therapy,* 6th ed. St. Louis: Times Mirror/Mosby College Publishing.

Worthington-Roberts BS. (1981). *Contemporary developments in nutrition.* St. Louis: CV Mosby.

Bibliography

Al + fluoride = Bad mix for cooks? (1987). *Science News, 131*, 73.

Albin R, et al. (1987). Acute sensory neuropathy-neuronopathy from pyridoxine overdose. *Neurology 37*, 1729–1732 (November).

Aloia J, et al. (1988). Calcitriol in the treatment of post-menopausal osteoporosis. *Am J Med, 84*, 401 (March).

*Anderson BJ. (1986). Tube feeding: Is diarrhea inevitable? *American Journal of Nursing, 83*, 704–706.

Anderson D, Gustafson C. (1987). Health foods: Are they worth the extra money? *Privileged Information, 3(2)*, 6 (January 15).

Another challenge to coffee's safety. (1990). *Science News, 138*, 253.

Arieff A. (1986). Hyponatremia, convulsions, respiratory arrest, and permanent brain damage after elective surgery in healthy women. *N Engl J Med, 314*, 1529.

Baker C. (1989). Is it drug toxicity—or something else? *Nursing 89, 19(4)*, 86 (April).

*Barta MA. (1987). Correcting electrolyte imbalances. *RN, 50(2)*, 30–33.

Beck W. (1988). Cobalamin and the nervous system (editorial). *N Engl J Med, 318*, 1752–1754 (June 30).

Beil L. (1988). Boning up on fluoride. *Science News, 134*, 134 (August 27).

Bittiner S, et al. (1988). A double-blind, randomized, placebo-controlled trial of fish oil in psoriasis. *Lancet, 1*, 370–380 (February 20).

*Blanchard DS. (1990). What women can do to protect against osteoporosis. *RN, 53(10)*, 60–64 (October).

Calcium may block lead poisoning. (1985). *RN, 48(9)*, 76.

Cameron H. (1988). Calcium supplements and arthritis. *Can Med Assoc J, 138*, 208 (February 1).

*Cerrato PL. (1985). Hidden malnutrition in geriatric patients. *RN, 48(7)*, 60–62.

*Cerrato PL. (1985). Can vitamins cure your psych patient's symptoms? *RN, 48(12)*, 51–52.

*Cerrato PL. (1986). How diet helps the skin fight pressure sores. *RN, 49(1)*, 67–68.

*Cerrato PL. (1986). When your patient is eating for two. *RN, 49(6)*, 67–68.

*Cerrato PL. (1986). Would you miss these clues to a vitamin C deficiency? *RN, 49(9)*, 69–71.

*Cerrato PL. (1986). Why some patients suffer a zinc deficiency. *RN, 49(10)*, 69–70.

*Cerrato PL. (1986). When your patient needs extra calcium. *RN, 59(8)*, 51–53.

*Cerrato PL. (1987). Does that patient need extra vitamins? *RN 50(1)*, 123–124 (October).

*Cerrato PL. (1989). Spotting the patient who looks healthy but isn't. *RN, 52(3)*, 81 (March).

Cooper BA, Rosenblatt DS. (1987). Inherited defects of vitamin B_{12} metabolism. *Annual review of nutrition*, 291–320. Palo Alto, CA: Annual Reviews.

Dagnelie PC, van Staveren WA, van den Berg H. (1991). Vitamin B-12 from algae appears not to be bioavailable. *Am J Clin Nutr, 53*, 695–697.

Do you know where your patient's feeding tube is? (1990). *RN, 53(3)*, 125–126 (March).

*Drinking Water. (1988). *Harvard Medical School Health Letter 14(1)*, 1–5 (November).

Edwards DD. (1985). Diet allowances to slim down? *Science News 128(13)*, 199 (September 28).

Fackelmann KA. (1988). Tretinoin: Lasting results, lingering doubts. *Science News, 134*, 375 (December 10).

Fackelmann KA. (1990). Magnesium eases diabetic blood pressure. *Science News, 138*, 189 (September 22).

Fackelmann KA. (1990). Beta carotene may slow artery disease. *Science News, 138*, 308 (November 17).

*Flynn KT, et al. (1987). Enteral tube feeding: Indications, practice and outcome. *Image: Journal of Nursing Scholarship, 19(1)*, 16–19 (Spring).

Flynn W, et al. (1988). Potential neurotoxicity of tryptophan. *Ann Intern Med, 108*, 312–313 (February).

Food and Nutrition Board, National Academy of Sciences. (1990). *Nutrition during pregnancy*. Washington, DC: National Academy Press.

Food and Nutrition Board, National Research Council. (1989). *Recommended dietary allowances*, 10th ed. Washington, DC: National Academy Press.

*Gaffney J. (1987). Helping a patient manage tube feedings at home. *RN, 50(5)*, 70 (May).

*Gever LN. (1987). Large-dose potassium. *Nursing 87, 17(1)*, 90.

Glauber H, et al. (1988). The adverse metabolic effect of omega-3 fatty acids in non-insulin-dependent diabetes mellitus. *Ann Intern Med, 108*, 663–668 (May).

Goldberg M. (1987). Calcium supplements—a reply. *Journal of Enterostomal therapy, 14*, 179 (August).

Grobbee D, Hoffman A. (1986). Effect of calcium supplementation on diastolic blood pressure in young people with mild hypertension. *Lancet, 2*, 703 (September 27).

Hallberg L, Brune M, Erlandsson M, Sandberg A-S, Rossander-Hulten L. (1991). Calcium: Effect of different amounts on nonheme- and heme-iron absorption in humans. *Am J Clin Nutr, 53*, 112–119.

Heading off malnutrition. (1989). *Nursing 89, 19(4)*, 23–24 (April).

*Helping a patient manage tube feedings at home. (1987). *RN, 50(5)*, 70.

Hernandez O, et al. (1988). Obligate nasal breathing in an elderly woman: Increased risk of nasogastric tube feeding. *Journal of Parenteral and Enteral Nutrition 12*, 531 (September/October).

Hoyt R. (1986). Hyperkalemia due to salt substitutes (Letter). *JAMA, 256*, 1726.

In osteoporosis, fluoride giveth but also taketh away. (1990). *RN 53(6)*, 117 (June).

*Irwin M. (1987). "Encourage oral intake"—Yes, but how? *American Journal of Nursing, 87*, 100–106.

Kremer J, et al. (1987). Fish-oil fatty acid supplements in active rheumatoid arthritis. *Ann Intern Med, 106*, 497 (April).

Lippman SM. (1987). Treatment of advanced squamous cell carcinoma of the skin with isotretinoin. *Ann Intern Med, 107*, 499 (October).

*Lockhart JS, Griffin CW. (1988). Tetany. *Nursing 88, 18(8)*, 33 (August).

Low-calorie allergy. (1986). *Science News, 129*, 26.

*Magnesium: A pregnancy problem? (1986). *Science News, 129*, 376.

*Mahon SM. (1987). Symptoms as clues to calcium levels. *American Journal of Nursing, 87*, 354–356.

McLeod E. (1986). Treating iron toxicity. *Nursing 86, 16(8)*, 74.

Minerals: Fact and fancy. (1986). *University of California, Berkely Wellness Letter 2(4)*, 5 (January).

Moore MC. (1987). Do you still believe these myths about tube feeding? *RN, 50(5)*, 51–54.

Muir A, Kalnins D. (1987). False advertising resulting in infant malnutrition. *Can Med Assoc J, 136*, 1274 (June 15).

Paccione P, et al. (1987). Pill-induced intramural esophageal hematoma (letter). *JAMA, 257*, 929 (February 20).

*Pauly-Oneill S. (1990). Critical questions (number 1). *American Journal of Nursing 90*, 94 (September).

Perry R. (1986). Salt substitute as potassium replacement in hypertensive patients. *Clin Pharm, 5*, 155–159.

Peters EA. (1987). A better way to give meds through a feeding tube. *RN 50(3)*, 95 (March).

Picciano MF, Stokstad EL, Gregory JF, eds. (1990). *Folic acid metabolism in health and disease.* New York, NY: Wiley Liss.

Postop hyponatremia: An overlooked menace. (1986). *RN, 49(11)*, 87–88.

Potassium slow-release. (1986). *American Journal of Nursing, 86(10)*, 98 (October).

Quinn N, Marsden CD. (1986). Lithium for painful dystonia in Parkinson's disease (Letter). *Lancet, 1*, 1377.

Raloff J. (1986). Diet, metals and hidden heart disease. *Science News, 130*, 201.

Raloff J. (1987). Copper: What a difference sex makes. *Science News, 131*, 70–71.

Raloff J. (1987). Does fetal zinc affect later immunity? *Science News, 131*, 375.

Raloff J. (1988). Boosting immunity in the elderly. *Science News 134*, 351 (November 26).

Raloff J. (1989). Revised RDAs add a few good nutrients. *Science News 136*, 277 (October 28).

Raloff J. (1989). Carotenoids: Colorful cancer protection. *Science News, 136*, 294 (November 4).

Reid I, Ibbertson H. (1986). Calcium supplements in the prevention of steroid-induced osteoporosis. *Am J Clin Nutr, 44*, 287–290.

Root vegetables. (1986). *University of California, Berkeley Wellness Letter 2(4)*, 8 (January).

Rossander-Hulten L, Brune M, Sandstrom B, Lonnerdal B, Hallberg L. (1991). Competitive inhibition of iron absorption by manganese and zinc in humans. *Am J Clin Nutr, 54*, 152–156.

*Rupp SL. (1986). Vitamin B6 controversy. *American Journal of Nursing, 86(6)*, 652 (June).

Safai-Kutti S, Kutti J. (1986). Zinc supplementation in anorexia nervosa. *Am J Clin Nutr, 44*, 581 (October).

Schectman G, et al. (1989). Can the hypotriglyceridemic effect of fish oil concentrate be sustained? *Ann Intern Med, 110*, 346–352 (March 1).

Schilling R. (1986). Nitrous oxide and B_{12} deficiency. *JAMA, 255*, 1605 (March 28).

*Schwartz MW. (1987). Potassium imbalances. *American Journal of Nursing, 87(10)*, 1292 (October).

Silberner J. (1987). A fish (oil) story? *Science News, 131*, 89 (February 7).

Something to remember. (1988). *Nursing 88, 18(4)*, 17 (April).

Spätling L, Spätling G. (1988). Magnesium supplementation in pregnancy: A double-blind study. *Br J Obstet Gynecol, 95*, 120–125 (February).

Steiner W, Fontaine R. (1986). Toxic reaction following the combined administration of fluoxetine and L-tryptophan: Five case reports. *Biol Psychiatry 21*, 1067–1071 (September).

Strauss A, Trujillo M. (1986). Lithium-induced goiter and voice changes (Letter). *J Clin Psychopharmacol, 6*, 120–121.

Strom B, et al. (1987). Upper gastrointestinal tract bleeding from oral potassium chloride. *Arch Intern Med, 147*, 954 (May).

Summer K, Iles CA, James C, Thompson RP. (1987). Are iron-folate supplements harmful? *Am J Clin Nutr, 45*, 122–125.

Suter P, Russell R. (1987). Vitamin requirements of the elderly. *Am J Clin Nutr, 45*, 501 (March).

*Toto KH. (1987). When the patient has hypokalemia. *RN, 50(3)*, 38–41.

Vitamin A effects of PCBs and dioxins. (1986). *Science News, 130*, 360 (December 6).

Vitamin C at work in the eye. (1986). *Science News, 129*, 26.

Vitamins may reduce neural tube defects. (1988). *Science News, 134*, 380.

*Walter J. (1987). Which of your patients is starving to death? *RN, 50*, 45–47.

What's too much vitamin A? (1986). *RN, 49(1)*, 6.

Wickelgren I. (1989). Revealing the finicky functions of fish oil. *Science News 135*, 183 (March 25).

Wickelgren I. (1989). Water-soluble vitamin A shows promise. *Science News, 135*, 204 (April 1).

*Worthington-Roberts BS. (1981). *Contemporary developments in nutrition.* St. Louis: CV Mosby.

*Wrap-up: Minerals. (1986). *University of California, Berkeley Wellness Letter, 2(4)*, 4–5.

*Wrap-up: Sodium. (1986). *University of California, Berkeley Wellness Letter, 2(7)*, 4–5.

Yankelson S. (1987). Distilled water: A simple solution? *Nutrition Support Services 7*, 8 (January).

* Recommended for further reading.

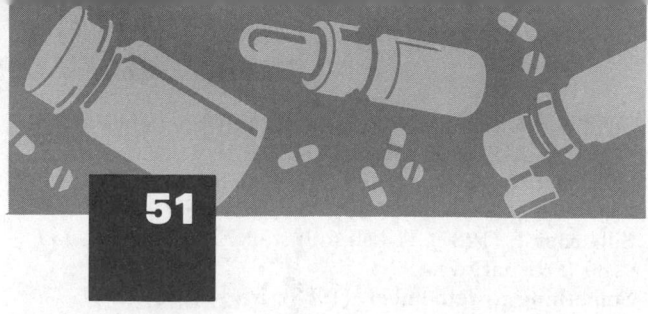

Parenteral supplements

Parenteral fluids

Whenever food and fluids cannot be taken orally, or when sudden, large losses of body fluids occur, fluids and nutrients may need to be given parenterally. Depending on the nature of the disease, clients may require water, electrolytes, vitamins, minerals, calories, plasma volume expanders, or blood. Although some clear fluids with osmolarity close to that of body fluids can be administered subcutaneously or intramuscularly, most of these solutions are given by intravenous (IV) infusion.

Physiology. The composition of blood and other body fluids is maintained within a narrow range in normal persons. A multitude of compensatory mechanisms adjust osmolarity, mineral levels, and pH to maintain homeostasis despite variations in the rate of intake, metabolism, or excretion of chemical constitu-

ents. Proper balance is necessary for the normal function of individual cells, organ systems, and the organism as a whole.

Pathology. Whenever fluid and nutrient intake is inadequate to meet body needs, or sudden losses occur, homeostasis is disturbed. Blood volume drops, fluids shift among body compartments, tissue breaks down to provide energy, and electrolyte and acid–base balance are disrupted. Proper physiologic function cannot be maintained; illness and death may follow.

Parenteral fluid therapy is the major treatment used to maintain a proper chemical environment in the body until the underlying disruptive condition can be corrected. The degree of correction required and the duration of therapy depends on the severity of the problem and the response of the client to treatment. If the underlying condition cannot be corrected, parenteral solutions are administered palliatively to maintain hydration, nutrition, and a reasonable level of function and comfort for as long as possible.

Clear solutions

Clear solutions for parenteral administration contain a number of components in a variety of combinations for use in appropriate clinical situations. Water is the solvent for all solutions. Solutes include salts of sodium, potassium, calcium, and ammonia; sugars; and synthetic carbohydrate polymers (Table 51-1).

Pharmacodynamics. Parenteral fluids maintain or replenish body levels of essential chemicals. Water provides hydration. Sodium, potassium, and calcium maintain cation electrolytes necessary for normal nerve and muscle function. Chloride and bicarbonate act as buffers to correct acid–base imbalance. Sugars in concentrations of 10% or less provide carbohydrate calories. All molecular solutes increase osmotic tonicity of the solution and help preserve proper osmotic pressure in the intravascular compartment and other fluid compartments of the body. Hypertonic solutions cause immediate fluid shift into the intravascular compartment and stimulate osmotic diuresis.

Pharmacokinetics. Clear parenteral solutions are administered by subcutaneous (SC), intramuscular (IM), or IV injection. Large volumes are given by slow infusion over long periods of time. They may be injected into SC or muscle tissue by means of hypodermoclysis equipment, infused into a peripheral vein, or delivered directly into the vena cava through a central venous (CV) catheter. Peripheral veins are most commonly used.

Absorption is least rapid by the SC route because the movement of fluid through the tissues is opposed by increasing extracellular hydrostatic pressure as the fluid is administered. Dispersion through the tissues can be accelerated by injecting hyaluronidase, an enzyme that breaks down the tissue cement (hyaluronic acid) that binds cells together. However, because there are relatively few blood vessels in SC tissue, movement into the intravascular space is still somewhat slow. When hypodermoclysis needles are placed in muscle tissue, absorption is more rapid. Increasing hydrostatic pressure within engorged vessels remains a limiting factor to the speed of absorption. Poor local perfusion reduces absorption significantly by both routes.

Intravenous administration delivers the solution directly into the vascular compartment. Absorption is virtually instantaneous and complete.

Distribution of water (the solvent component) of IV solutions depends on their osmolarity. *Isotonic* solutions (those whose osmotic pressures are equal to those of body fluids) triggers the least movement of water from the intravascular compartment into or out of the interstitial and intracellular compartments. The administration of *hypotonic* solutions causes water to leave the intravascular compartment and enter, successively, the interstitial and intracellular compartments. *Hypertonic* solutions draw water from the interstitial and intracellular compartments into the intravascular space.

Solute components of clear solutions are widely and rapidly distributed throughout the body.

Distribution and metabolism of specific components vary (Table 51-2). The kidneys are the major excretory pathway for most components of parenteral solutions, including the fluid content.

Adverse reactions. Rapid infusion of IV fluids can produce toxicity from excesses of any or all of the constituent chemicals. Fluid excesses produce circulatory overload and hypertension. Congestive heart failure and pulmonary edema may result. Excesses of solute components produce characteristic signs and symptoms (Table 51-3).

Rapid infusion of solutions by hypodermoclysis or extravasation of IV fluids produces painful local tissue swelling. If interstitial hypertension is severe and prolonged, local tissue perfusion is compromised, and tissue damage can occur.

Tissue cells can be irritated or injured by several other mechanisms during IV therapy. Unless solutions have an osmotic tonicity close to that of normal body fluids or are rapidly diluted, cells are likely to suffer injury. Hypotonic fluids cause swelling and lysis of cells; hypertonic fluids crenate or shrink them (Box 51-1). When IV infusion is used, the cells most often affected are the erythrocytes. If such solutions are administered by clysis or infiltrate from an IV line, extravascular cells are vulnerable. Tissue necrosis and sloughing can result.

Solutions containing electrolytes in concentrations greater than normal serum levels are irritating to the tissues or veins into which they are introduced. Phle-

---

Box 51-1. Osmolarity of IV solutions

1. *Isotonic solutions* are equal in osmolarity to physiologic (intravascular, interstitial, and intracellular) fluids; when administered IV they increase intravascular volume but cause minimal changes in volumes of the interstitial and intracellular compartments.
2. *Hypotonic solutions* tend to increase interstitial and intracellular volumes; when administered into small blood vessels at a rapid rate they can destroy (lyse) blood cells by causing rupture of the cell membrane
3. *Hypertonic solutions* tend to pull water from the interstitial and intracellular compartments into the vascular system; when administered into small blood vessels at a rapid rate they can rapidly dehydrate (crenate) blood cells.

---

bitis may occur. If the solutions infiltrate, local tissue damage is likely.

Some people develop an allergic sensitivity to dextrans, hetastarch, or nickel, a contaminant in some solutions. Nickel also tends to increase coronary artery resistance and has an oxytoxic effect on the uterus.

The injection or infusion of parenteral solutions breaches the natural barriers against microbial invasion and predisposes to infection. This is a particularly serious complication when the IV route is used because the invading organism is introduced directly into the blood. Septicemia results with pronounced systemic symptoms, such as chills, fever, and septic shock.

Precautions. Intravenous infusions must be monitored closely to maintain proper rate of flow and correct placement of the needle or intracatheter. If the infusion infiltrates (delivers or leaks fluid into the extravascular extracellular compartment, it should be discontinued and restarted in another vein.

Parenteral fluids must be administered with careful regard for fluid, electrolyte, and acid–base status so that treatment will not exacerbate imbalances.

Caution is required when sodium solutions are administered to clients with circulatory insufficiency, liver disease, kidney dysfunction, hypoproteinemia, and concurrent corticosteroid therapy. Clients receiving dextrose solutions must be monitored for hyperglycemia and glucosuria.

Before administering potassium solutions, hydration and adequate renal function must be ensured. Dextrose in water or in another solution low in electrolytes is commonly given before potassium solutions are infused. Renal function should be assessed carefully during this hydration phase. Once potassium solutions are started, the rate of administration should be kept

(*Text continues on p. 1296*)

Table 51-1. Clear solutions commonly used for parenteral therapy

Solution	Osmotic tonicity (total mEq/liter, cations plus anions)	Method of administration	Usual adult dosage	Mechanisms of action	Therapeutic uses
Saline					
0.45% NaCl in water	Hypotonic (154)	IV infusion	90–125 ml/hr	Helps maintain osmotic pressure in extracellular fluid; helps maintain blood volume; sodium is necessary for impulse transmission in nerves and muscles; chloride buffers alkaline chemicals in the body and tends to lower *pH*.	Replacement of sodium, chloride, and water losses; prevention of sodium, chloride, and water deficits in persons experiencing vomiting or nasogastric suction.
0.9% NaCl in water	Isotonic (308)	IV infusion	90–125 ml/hr		
3.0% NaCl in water	Hypertonic (1027)	IV infusion	Up to 80 ml/hr		
5.0% NaCl in water	Hypertonic (1700)	IV infusion, preferably into a central vein	Up to 50 ml/hr		Treatment of hypovolemic shock due to addisonian crisis or severe sodium depletion.
Dextrose (D-glucose)					
5.0% dextrose in water (D$_5$W)	Isotonic	IV, SC, or IM infusion	90–125 ml/hr (maximum dose 650 ml/hr)	Provides fluid and calories for energy (200 calories/liter of D$_5$W)	Maintenance of fluid levels when electrolytes are not needed or contraindicated; provision of calories to those unable to eat
2.5% dextrose in half normal saline	Isotonic	IV, SC, or IM infusion	90–125 ml/hr	Provides fluid, electrolytes, and calories for energy	Treatment of shock due to diabetic ketoacidosis
10% dextrose in water	Hypertonic	IV infusion	45–65 ml/hr	Provides calories with minimal fluid intake	Treatment of persons needing extra calories who cannot tolerate fluid overload
20% dextrose in water	Hypertonic	IV infusion	90–125 ml/hr	Raises intravascular osmotic pressure and induces osmotic diuresis	Promotion of fluid loss through osmotic diuresis
5% dextrose in 0.9% NaCl; 5% dextrose in 0.45% NaCl	Hypertonic	IV infusion	90–125 ml/hr	Provides fluid, electrolytes, and calories for energy; increases osmotic pressure in the intravascular compartment	Treatment of shock Replacement of fluid loss
Fructose					
10% fructose in water	Hypertonic	IV infusion	90–125 ml/hr	Provides energy without the need for insulin to promote intracellular use of the sugar	Replacement or supplementation of food and water
Potassium chloride					
0.15% KCl in D$_5$W; 0.3% KCl in D$_5$W	Hypertonic (cannot be used undiluted)	IV infusion, diluted in 500–1,000 ml of electrolyte or dextrose solution for IV infusion.	Up to 20 mEq/hr (potassium concentration in IV fluids should not exceed 40 mEq/liter)	Provides the actions of chloride listed above; potassium helps maintain intracellular osmotic pressure, is necessary to impulse transmission in nerves and muscles, and promotes cardiac diastole	Maintenance or replenishment of potassium levels in adequately hydrated persons with good renal function, especially surgical patients and those experiencing fluid losses from the lower intestinal tract

Preparation	Tonicity (mOsm)	Route	Dosage	Action	Use
Ringer's solution 0.86% NaCl, 0.03% KCl, and 0.033% $CaCl_2$ ($2H_2O$) in water	Isotonic (311)	IV infusion	90–125 ml/hr	Provides fluid and the actions of saline and potassium listed above; calcium modifies impulse transmission in nerves and muscles and promotes cardiac systole	Maintenance or restoration of levels of fluid, sodium, chloride, potassium, and calcium in persons with actual or potential deficits of moderate degree. (Potassium concentration is inadequate to correct severe hypokalemia.)
Lactated Ringer's solution 0.6% NaCl, 0.03% KCl, 0.02% $CaCl_2$ ($2H_2O$) and 0.31% Na lactate in water	Isotonic (273)	IV infusion	90–125 ml/hr	Provides the actions of Ringer's solution listed above plus lactate, which is metabolized in part to bicarbonate, which buffers acid in the body, raises the pH, and alkalinizes urine; the remainder of the lactate is metabolized to glycogen, which provides carbohydrate calories for energy	Maintenance or restoration of fluid and electrolytes; treatment of dehydration accompanied by mild acidosis (especially ketoacidosis); alkalinization of urine in sulfonamide therapy
Ammonium chloride 2.14% NH_4Cl	Hypertonic	IV infusion	In accordance with chloride deficit as calculated from carbon dioxide combining power	Provides the actions of chloride listed above; ammonia is metabolized by the liver and excreted as urea, which stimulates osmotic diuresis and helps mobilize edema fluid	Treatment of metabolic alkalosis, tetany due to metabolic alkalosis and chloride depletion
Bicarbonate 5% $NaHCO_3$ in water	Hypertonic	IV infusion	In accordance with plasma CO_2 levels or dyspnea and hyperpnea owing to acidosis	Buffers acids in the body and raises pH	Treatment of severe acidosis accompanied by dyspnea and hyperpnea
Synthetic carbohydrate polymers 10% dextran 40 with 0.9% NaCl (or with 5% dextrose) in water (Rheomacrodex) 6% dextran 70 with 0.9% NaCl (or with 5% dextrose) in water (Macrodex) 6% hetastarch with 0.9% NaCl in water	Hypertonic	IV infusion	30–60 g d, depending on degree of fluid volume loss and hemoconcentration	Increase the osmotic pressure of circulating blood, causing a fluid shift into the intravascular compartment; increase blood volume and reduce the hematocrit; may coat the red blood cells, reducing bonding forces and aggregation; may reduce red blood cell rigidity, facilitating movement through small blood vessels	Restoration of circulation in hypovolemic shock due to burns, hemorrhage, or sepsis; priming solutions for plasmapheresis procedures

Table 51-2. Distribution, metabolism, storage, and excretion of components of parenteral solutions

Component	Distribution	Metabolism/Storage	Excretion
Sodium	Distributes widely in the extracellular fluid compartment (interstitial and intravascular spaces)	Sodium remains primarily in the extracellular compartment	Sodium is excreted mainly through the kidneys and sweat glands.
Potassium	Moves quickly through the extracellular space and is actively transported into cells	Dextrose, insulin, and oxygen facilitate movement of potassium into cells.	Excretion is primarily renal, by active secretion in the distal tubule, a process stimulated by corticosteroid hormones secreted by the adrenal cortex; small amounts excreted by the skin
Calcium	Binds to plasma proteins; crosses the placenta and appears in fetal circulation in higher concentrations than in maternal blood	Ions in excess of normal blood levels are stored in bony structures. (Nonionized calcium compounds in the blood are physiologically inactive.)	Excesses are excreted largely in feces by way of bile and pancreatic juices: kidney excretion is proportional to serum concentration of ionized mineral, parathyroid hormone, and vitamin D; also secreted in breast milk and by sweat glands
Chloride	Distributes widely in body tissues	Chloride combines with alkaline salts, reducing base reserve.	Chloride is excreted by kidneys and sweat glands.
Dextrose	Distributes widely in the extracellular space	Dextrose requires insulin for use by most body cells; it is oxidized for energy, producing water and carbon dioxide.	Excesses are excreted by the kidneys.
Fructose	Distributes rapidly throughout the tissues	Fructose does not require insulin for use by the cells; it is oxidized for energy.	Excesses are excreted by the kidneys.
Lactate	Distributes widely throughout the tissues	The levo form is oxidized to bicarbonate; the dextro form is converted to glycogen and stored.	Excess salts are excreted by the kidneys.
Ammonium	Distributes widely throughout the tissues	Ammonia is metabolized by the liver to urea with release of hydrogen ions, which combine with bicarbonate to produce water and carbon dioxide.	Water is eliminated through the kidneys; carbon dioxide is eliminated through the lungs.
Bicarbonate	Distributes widely throughout the tissues	Bicarbonate combines with hydrogen ions to produce water and carbon dioxide.	Water is eliminated through the kidneys; carbon dioxide is eliminated through the lungs.
Dextrans	Remain in the intravascular compartment initially (about 70% of dextran 40 and 50% of dextran 70 are excreted within 24 hours)	Molecules of molecular weight greater than 15,000 are degraded slowly to glucose and are metabolized for energy.	Molecules of molecular weight less than 15,000 are rapidly excreted by the kidneys; small amounts are excreted in feces by the bile.
Hetastarch	Remains in the intravascular compartment initially (about 40% of hetastarch is excreted within 24 hours)	Molecules of molecular weight greater than 50,000 are slowly degraded to smaller molecules; some are metabolized as glucose.	Molecules of molecular weight less than 50,000 are excreted by the kidneys.

below the level of approximately 20 mEq of potassium per hour; elderly persons or clients with renal impairment should receive one-quarter to one-half as much. Serum potassium level should remain below 6 mEq/liter.

Before ammonium chloride solutions are administered, acid–base balance must be determined. Carbon dioxide combining power should be measured before fluid therapy is begun and again after one-half of the solution has been administered. Ammonium chloride solutions must be administered slowly because they tend to deplete base bicarbonate and lower blood pH. Clients should be watched for signs and symptoms of potassium imbalance. Temporary hyperkalemia can

Table 51-3. Adverse reactions to excesses of specific components of parenteral fluids

Component	Toxic effects	Treatment of toxic state
Sodium	Hypervolemia and fluid overload; edema Cellular dehydration with weakness and disorientation indicative of hypernatremia Excessive potassium loss by the kidneys with distention, anorexia, nausea, and depressed respirations Oliguria and increased blood urea nitrogen may develop	Discontinuation of sodium solutions; supportive care until excess sodium is eliminated; administration of diuretics
Potassium	Locally, tissue irritation; causes smooth muscle spasm and vasoconstriction; can compromise circulation Nausea, vomiting, cramping abdominal pain, prolonged cardiac diastole, and reduced response to the stimulus of cardiac pacemakers indicative of hyperkalemia	Administration of dextrose and insulin or bicarbonate to stimulate movement of extracellular potassium into the cells; in extreme toxicity, administration of calcium salts to restore normal cardiac function
Calcium	Locally, tissue irritation; phlebitis or extravascular tissue necrosis Upon rapid administration, vasodilation, hypotension, bradycardia, cardiac arrhythmias, syncope, and cardiac arrest With excessive doses, increased risk of calcium renal stone formation	Administration of fluids to promote dilution of the urine and diuresis; in extreme toxicity, administration of potassium to restore normal cardiac function
Chloride	Hyperchloremic acidosis as shown by acid urine, dyspnea, and hyperpnea, and by a reduction in body fluid pH Hyperkalemia and depletion of intracellular potassium	Administration of lactate or bicarbonate to increase alkaline reserve
Dextrose	Hyperglycemia, glucosuria, and hyperosmolar nonketotic coma	Slowing of infusion rate; administration of insulin to promote metabolism of glucose
Fructose	Hyperosmolarity, especially with rapid administration	Slowing of infusion rate; administration of hypotonic solutions
Lactate	Metabolic alkalosis; tetany	Bag rebreathing and administration of calcium to relieve tetany; giving chlorides to reduce alkaline reserve
Ammonia	Hyperammonemia as shown by CNS abnormalities (headache, tremor, hyperreflexia, confusion, electroencephalogram changes, stupor alternating with excitement and coma) Azotemia, metabolic acidosis and hyperkalemia if kidney function is impaired Depletion of intracellular potassium Skin rash	Discontinuation of infusion and providing supportive care; Hemodialysis for severe toxicity
Bicarbonate	Metabolic alkalosis; tetany	Bag rebreathing and administration of calcium to relieve tetany; giving chlorides to reduce alkaline reserve
Synthetic carbohydrate polymers	Increased bleeding time and hemorrhage	Measures to control bleeding; transfusion if blood loss is severe
	Hypervolemia, hypoproteinemia, and congestive failure	Slowing or discontinuation of polymer infusion; administration of diuretics and digitalis
	Allergic reactions (urticaria, nasal congestion, wheeze, mild hypotension, and rare anaphylaxis), especially with dextran	Discontinuation of polymer infusion; administration of epinephrine, antihistamines, and glucocorticoids
	In dehydrated persons, renal tubular stasis, tubular obstruction, renal failure	Diuresis or hemodialysis

develop due to displacement of potassium by hydrogen ions. Potassium is excreted by the kidneys, resulting in a net loss of the electrolyte.

In general, only clients with severe or refractory acidosis require bicarbonate solutions. During treatment, blood gases are monitored as a guide to therapy. Clients receiving bicarbonate should be watched for signs and symptoms of alkalosis (shallow respirations, paresthesia, cramps) because overcorrection of the acid–base disorder can develop quickly. Caution must be exercised when bicarbonate solutions are administered to persons with congestive failure or edema because significant amounts of sodium will be given.

Adequate hydration and renal function should be established before plasma expanders are administered. During therapy with dextran or hetastarch, urinary output and specific gravity must be monitored. Both should increase as elimination of the solution is established. If the amount and density of urine do not rise, the polymer solution should be discontinued. However, the IV line must be maintained because further parenteral medication will probably be required.

Monitoring of CV pressure is recommended when plasma volume expanders are administered. The infusion should be slowed or discontinued if CV pressure rises above normal.

Coagulation or bleeding time should be evaluated before plasma-expander therapy is begun. These solutions should be given with caution to persons at risk for hemorrhage because the risk of bleeding is increased by synthetic polymers.

Contraindications. Infusions of large amounts of fluid are contraindicated in persons experiencing circulatory overload or edema, as in cardiac, renal, or liver failure. Potassium must be given cautiously when urinary excretion is impaired. Liver or renal impairment are contraindications for ammonium chloride administration. Pulmonary edema or known allergic hypersensitivity to components in the solutions precludes treatment with dextran or hetastarch.

■ Summary

Clear parenteral fluids can be lifesaving when administered to maintain or restore fluid, electrolyte, and acid–base balance. They also provide minimal carbohydrate calories for energy. These solutions are administered most often by IV infusion but can sometimes be delivered to SC or muscle tissue by hypodermoclysis. Solutions infused directly into the vascular system enter systemic circulation directly and are distributed rapidly. Overdosage (or overcorrection of imbalances) must be avoided because once the medication enters a vein, the dose can neither be retrieved nor its absorption delayed.

Learning experience 51-1

Examine the labels of solutions used for parenteral therapy in the hospital. Note the chemical constituents of the solutions and their concentrations. Which solutions are isotonic? Hypertonic? Hypotonic? How do the concentrations of individual electrolytes compare with their concentrations in normal serum? Which of the solutions has the greatest toxic potential if administered at a rapid rate of infusion?

Parenteral therapy can cause toxic responses such as excess fluid and high serum concentrations of sodium, potassium, calcium, ammonia, and glucose, or acid–base imbalance (metabolic acidosis or alkalosis). Dextran and hetastarch can cause allergic reactions.

Nursing management

Nursing implications

Whenever parenteral therapy is in progress, the client is vulnerable to infection, extravasation, and other complications of infusion.

The order in which solutions are administered is often critical. Preparations must be given in succession as specified by the physician. Often a client must be hydrated to establish good renal function before solutions containing potentially toxic components can be administered. Changing the order of administration can have disastrous consequences. For example, the administration of potassium salts to a dehydrated client with poor renal function may cause cardiac arrest.

Nurses should be aware that the results of certain laboratory tests are altered by the presence of dextran in the blood. During therapy with this type of plasma expander, blood sugar, blood cross matching by proteolytic enzymes, and bilirubin assays using alcohol will be unreliable.

Nurses responsible for parenteral therapy need a thorough understanding of physiology, especially in relation to fluid, electrolyte, and acid–base balance. They must be able to evaluate the risks of such therapy and recognize the early signs and symptoms of adverse reaction. Considerations relative to specific components of common solutions are outlined in Table 51-4. Although nurses do not prescribe fluid therapy or change the medical regimen outlined by the physician, they may discontinue treatment judged to be detrimental to the client, and they must be able to judge when consultation with the physician for a change in orders is needed.

Table 51-4. Nursing considerations in relation to parenteral administration of specific solution components

Solution component	Factors increasing the risk of therapy	Signs and symptoms of complications	Precautions/corrective treatment
Sodium	Cardiac or renal impairment	Hypertension, edema, cough, or dyspnea indicative of circulatory overload Elevated serum sodium levels	Place client in high Fowler's position to facilitate breathing. Administer diuretics when ordered to eliminate sodium and fluid.
Chloride	Acidosis	Hyperpnea and dyspnea indicative of acidosis Elevated serum chlorine levels	Administer lactate or bicarbonate when ordered to raise *p*H.
Dextrose	Hyperglycemia; diabetes mellitus	Hyperglycemia; glucosuria	Slow the infusion rate and administer insulin when ordered to reduce serum glucose.
Potassium	Dehydration	Oliguria	Mix potassium additives thoroughly with diluting solutions.
	Renal impairment with oliguria, anuria, or azotemia	Elevated serum potassium levels	Administer solutions at a slow rate of speed (20 mEq potassium or less/h).
	Recent crush injury	Elevated serum potassium levels	Limit potassium content of solution to 40 mEq/liter.
	History of hyperkalemic familial periodic paralysis	Decreased serum calcium levels	Administer dextrose and insulin, bicarbonate, or Kayexalate as ordered to reduce serum potassium.
	Heat cramps	Weak cardiac contraction Cardiac arrhythmias	Administer digitalis as ordered to strengthen cardiac contraction.
Calcium	Digitalis therapy	Cardiac arrhythmias	Administer solutions slowly.
	Renal or cardiac impairment	Elevated serum calcium level	Maintain good respiratory function. Administer potassium when ordered to restore cardiac function.
	Sarcoidosis Cor pulmonale Respiratory acidosis Respiratory failure Hypercalcemia	Lethargy	
Lactate	Alkalosis Low serum calcium	Shallow respirations Paresthesias, tetany	Bag rebreathe to relieve paresthesias or tetany.
Bicarbonate	Alkalosis Hypertension Cardiac or renal impairment	Elevated base excess Alkalosis Edema Hypertension	Administer chlorides when ordered to relieve alkalosis.
Ammonium	Pulmonary insufficiency Cardiac or renal impairment Pronounced hepatic impairment	Abnormal CNS function (confusion, lethargy alternating with excitement, coma) Elevated serum levels of ammonia or urea	Have carbon dioxide combining power measured before initiating therapy and when half the ordered solution has been administered. Administer solutions very slowly.
Synthetic carbohydrate polymers	Pregnancy History of allergic reaction to the solution ordered Dehydration	Hypertension Dyspnea, cough Abnormal bleeding Hematocrit less than 30% Elevated CV pressure	Observe client closely for first half-hour of treatment. Have epinephrine available for prompt treatment of allergic reactions should they occur.

Nursing process

Assessment Before initiating treatment with IV fluids, the nurse should assess the client to determine cardiac and renal function, as well as fluid, electrolyte, and acid–base balance. The client's emotional reaction to the ordered therapy should also be assessed. (Anxiety or fear can predispose to hypervolemia by activating hormone-regulated mechanisms of sodium and fluid retention.) The very old, the very young, individuals with small body size, and those with renal impairment are at increased risk for complications.

Nursing diagnosis Nursing diagnoses for clients receiving IV solutions could include the following:

Fluid volume deficit related to inadequate oral intake secondary to nausea and vomiting
Fluid volume deficit related to excessive fluid losses secondary to diarrhea
Fluid volume deficit related to loss of plasma secondary to burn wound
High risk for fluid volume deficit related to cessation of oral intake and surgery

Common collaborative problems arising from the possibility of adverse reactions to IV fluids that should be differentiated from the nursing diagnoses include

Potential complication: pulmonary edema
Potential complication: cardiac arrest
Potential complication: metabolic acidosis

Planning The goal of nursing care is to restore and maintain homeostasis, including fluid, electrolyte, and acid–base balance.

Intervention Parenteral fluid therapy may be initiated by the nurse if fluids are to be administered by hypodermoclysis, or if the nurse is qualified by training to perform venipuncture.

Persons receiving parenteral fluids must be monitored carefully for early signs and symptoms of circulatory overload, a serious complication of parenteral therapy. To prevent hypervolemia, fluid administration must be controlled to prevent excessive rates of flow. Volume-controlled pumps deliver measured doses most reliably. Clients should be assessed at least every 4 hours and more often if their condition is unstable.

If pumps or mechanical flow monitors are not available, the infusion should be checked three to four times hourly and adjusted as necessary to ensure an appropriate rate of flow. Solutions containing components that are hazardous at high serum levels are best administered with a small bore needle into a large vein to prevent rapid rates of infusion and to promote rapid dilution. The client's general condition and respiratory function are noted with each contact. Output and specific gravity of urine should be measured regularly.

If sugar solutions are used, blood or urine is tested for glucose also.

If fluid flow is impeded and the rate of administration is below that specified in the physician's order, the client must never be flooded with solution in an attempt to "catch up." If the client's condition indicates that a more rapid administration could be needed, the physician should be consulted for a change in the rate ordered. Excessive flow rates can be especially dangerous for clients with cardiac or renal impairment and when solutions contain ammonium, potassium, magnesium, or calcium salts.

Clients under treatment for "heat exhaustion" or hypovolemic shock due to a sodium and water deficit could have an underlying corticosteroid deficiency. If blood pressure does not stabilize at an adequate level, the physician should be notified promptly so that alternative therapy can be considered.

The nurse should carefully evaluate laboratory data from blood studies. Electrolyte levels, blood glucose, blood gases, and blood urea nitrogen are all significant. Movement of these values toward normal usually indicates positive response to treatment.

Client education. Parenteral fluid therapy is an invasive procedure that stimulates stress and anxiety in most clients. Immediately before infusion, the client should be told about the procedure; informing the client too early causes anxiety levels to rise. Information offered should describe what the client will experience, the expected benefits of therapy, and the alternatives to this method of treatment.

Clients should be instructed to keep the dressing over the insertion site dry and to avoid manipulation of the tubing. The nurse should caution clients against putting pressure on the tubing or sharp flexion of the involved extremity, which could impede solution flow. The client is encouraged to ambulate with assistance and maintain as many activities of daily living as possible.

For some clients, total parenteral nutrition is a treatment that will be needed for life. For others, it is a temporary measure prescribed to sustain them through a limited period when eating and drinking are proscribed. As soon as gastrointestinal function resumes, the nurse should encourage these clients to resume oral intake, stressing the need for beverages and foods rich in electrolytes and other nutrients. Ice chips, tea, or ginger ale are usually tolerated better than is plain water. The usual progression is from clear liquids to full liquid, then to soft diet and full diet, as tolerated.

Clients on long-term parenteral therapy may need to manage their own therapy at home. These clients or their families will need detailed instruction in techniques for preparing and administering parenteral solutions.

Example of nursing process and treatment of IV side effects

The client is a 45-year-old housewife who has been in the recovery room for 2 hours following a hysterectomy. An IV infusion is running in her left forearm at 100 ml/hr. Examination of the infusion site reveals swelling of the tissues and increased luminosity of the site, as compared with the corresponding tissues in the right arm.

Assessment data	Nursing diagnosis	Intervention	Goals and outcome criteria
IV infusion running at 100 ml/hr Swelling and increased luminosity of tissues at the infusion site.	Altered tissue perfusion at the infusion site related to extravascular infiltration of parenteral fluids	**Discontinue** IV infusion; apply a dry sterile dressing to the venipuncture site. **Elevate** the affected limb. **Apply** warmth to the site. **Encourage** the client to exercise the affected limb **Monitor** the site for signs and symptoms of inflammation or tissue necrosis.	The swelling will decrease and disappear; signs and symptoms of inflammation or tissue necrosis will not develop.

Evaluation Data required for evaluation include information related to fluid, electrolyte, and acid–base balance. Teaching success may be evaluated by the client's ability to cooperate in procedures related to the infusion and by the client's adherence to the instructions and cautions conveyed during the teaching session. (See accompanying Example of Nursing Process and Treatment of IV Side Effects.)

Checklist of nursing actions

☐ Inform clients about parenteral therapy just prior to initiating infusions.

☐ Carry out strict surgical asepsis to minimize the risk of infection in clients receiving parenteral fluids.

☐ Maintain infusion flow at the rate specified.

☐ Administer solutions in the order specified.

☐ Monitor clients receiving parenteral solutions for circulatory overload and symptoms of toxic blood concentrations of solutes being administered.

☐ Monitor clients to assess therapeutic response to treatment.

☐ Administer solutions containing potassium, calcium, ammonium, or bicarbonate at a slow rate.

Total parenteral nutrition

The parenteral solutions previously described cannot provide all the nutrients needed to produce energy and build tissue. Therefore, clients who cannot take oral nourishment continue to break down body tissues to meet these needs. To reverse this catabolic state, sufficient calories, proteins, and fats must be supplied to sustain metabolism and tissue repair.

Preparations

Parenteral nutrition sufficient to provide for normal metabolism, tissue growth, and weight gain requires preparations containing concentrated sugars, amino acids, and lipids. Few formulas can contain all necessary nutrients because certain combinations tend to be unstable. Often, lipid emulsions and combinations of dextrose, amino acids, vitamins, and minerals are infused at different times or through different venous lines because of compatibility problems. Formulas are tailored to meet individual needs, using a combination of ingredients (Table 51-5).

Pharmacodynamics. Nutrients administered IV replace those that normally would be absorbed from the intestinal tract.

Pharmacokinetics. Nutrients administered IV are introduced directly into the blood vessels and are subsequently metabolized and degraded as are nutrients normally absorbed from the intestinal tract.

Therapeutic uses. Parenteral nutrition is used to stabilize and improve the condition of cachectic or debilitated persons who cannot take adequate oral nutrition. It is used frequently to prepare such clients for surgery. Through use of these preparations, it is now possible to restore full nutrition to persons with severe intestinal malfunction. Parenteral nutrition can be used as a temporary measure to improve the prognosis

Table 51-5. Components of solutions used for parenteral nutrition

Component	Composition	Usual concentration and calorie content	Osmotic tonicity	Usual adult dosage
Protein hydrolysates (Amigen, Aminosol, Hyprotigen, Parentamine, Travamin)	Amino acids and short chain peptides that reflect the nutritive value of the natural protein (casein, lactalbumin, plasma, fibrin, or others) from which it is derived by hydrolytic processes, sometimes modified by partial removal or addition of specific amino acids	Concentration and calorie content vary with preparation	Hypertonic	50–100 g in 5–6 hr (1 g/kg of body weight/ day)
Amino acids (*Aminosyn*, Branch Amin, Freamine, Travasol, Veinamine)	Approximately 15 amino acids in varying proportions. Both essential and nonessential amino acids	Concentration and calorie content vary with preparation	Slightly hypertonic (can be administered in a peripheral vein)	1 g/kg or body weight/day
Essential amino acids (Nephramine)	Eight essential amino acids in a solution virtually free of electrolytes		Hypertonic (must be diluted with hypotonic glucose for administration in a peripheral vein)	Individualized in accordance with renal function (the preparation is used in the treatment of patients with renal failure)
Vitamins	Injectable preparations of essential vitamins	Concentration depends on diluent. Calorie content: 0	Dependent on tonicity of diluent	Equal to or greater than the recommended daily allowances, depending on degree of deficiency present
Minerals	Injectable preparations of electrolytes and trace minerals	Concentration depends on diluent. Calorie content: 0	Dependent on tonicity of diluent	Equal to or greater than the recommended daily allowances, depending on degree of deficiency present
Fat				
Intralipid	Soy bean oil, egg yolk phospholipids, and glycerin	Calorie content: 450 per 500 ml	Isotonic	500 ml/day (maximum of 2.5 g/kg of ideal weight)
Safflower oil	Safflower oil	Calorie content: 450 per 500 ml	Isotonic	500 ml/day

of debilitated clients who need corrective therapy, such as surgery, or as long-term therapy to maintain clients with chronic debilitating intestinal malfunction.

Adverse reactions. Parenteral formulas containing sugars and amino acids are concentrated and cannot be infused into peripheral veins because their high osmotic tonicity would damage erythrocytes and other cells, as well as the vessels themselves. To provide rapid dilution to normal tonicity, these fluids are infused directly into the largest veins, such as the vena cava, by means of a central venous (CV) catheter. Air embolism may occur during insertion of a CV catheter.

Amino acid and protein hydrolysate solutions tend to aggregate and form solid particles that can cause emboli. Lipid emulsions can also form emboli if the emulsion separates, forming fat globules.

Metabolic imbalances that can develop during total parenteral nutrition include hypophosphatemia, hyperammonemia, and trace mineral deficiencies. Glycosuria occurs commonly when therapy is initiated but tends to subside with continued administration as endogenous insulin response is re-established. Although solutions for parenteral nutrition are formulated to provide complete nourishment, they do not always meet individual needs completely. Optimum levels of some nutrients and variations in individual needs cannot always be determined accurately.

Administration of lipid emulsions sometimes causes nausea.

Parenteral nutrition induces gallstones in some children; it can be hepatotoxic for premature infants. Long-term parenteral nutritional therapy is associated with a crippling bone disease affecting the weightbearing joints.

Parenteral nutrition solutions are rich media for microbial growth, and infection is a serious complication.

Precautions. Special precautions are required during insertion of the CV line and whenever the system must be opened to air to prevent air embolus and pneumothorax. Strict surgical asepsis is required to maintain sterility of tubing and solutions. Because the infusion rate must be carefully controlled, IV pumps should be used for administration. Medications are not administered through the hyperalimentation port because they tend to be incompatible with hypertonic solutions.

Fat emulsions should be administered through tubing that has a low phthalate concentration in the plastic because fat may extract this chemical from the tubing.

■ **Summary**

Total parenteral nutrition involves the administration of hypertonic solutions through a CV line, and of lipid solutions through either a central or a peripheral venous line. These solutions can support anabolic metabolism, tissue repair, and weight gain. They are used to build up debilitated individuals and to maintain nutrition in those who cannot absorb nutrients via the intestinal route. Complications include infection (most frequently); electrolyte imbalance; trace mineral deficiencies; and emboli of air, fat, or protein aggregates.

Nursing management

Nursing implications

Parenteral nutrition through CV lines presents some risks not inherent in the usual IV therapy. Air or fat embolism may occur, and septicemia is more likely to develop. Clients are completely dependent on parenteral nutrients and usually ingest little or no food or fluids.

Nursing process

Assessment Before parenteral nutrition is instituted, the client should be assessed for fluid, electrolyte, acid–base, and nutritional status. The nurse

should also assess the client's (and family's) knowledge about this treatment, as well as emotional reaction to it.

Nursing diagnosis Nursing diagnoses may include the following:

> *Altered nutrition: less than body requirements related to inability to eat secondary to esophageal obstruction or nausea and vomiting*
> *Altered nutrition: less than body requirements related to malabsorption secondary to inflammation of the small intestine*

Diagnoses arising from hyperalimentation therapy include the following:

> *High risk for infection: septicemia related to introduction of pathogens through a CV line*
> *Altered nutrition, less than body requirements: trace mineral deficiency related to inadequate intake or absorption*
> *Anxiety related to inability to ingest or absorb nutrients and to parenteral nutritional therapy*
> *Knowledge deficit concerning hyperalimentation therapy*

Common collaborative problems that should be differentiated from the nursing diagnoses include

> *Potential complication: pulmonary embolism*
> *Potential complication: lipid embolism*
> *Potential complication: hyperglycemia*
> *Potential complication: hyperammonemia*

Planning Goals of nursing care include improvement of nutrition; maintenance of fluid, electrolyte, acid–base, and trace mineral balance; prevention of, or prompt detection and treatment of IV aspiration of air; prevention of, or prompt detection and treatment of septicemia; emotional acceptance of the therapy by client and family; and their education to parenteral nutrition and the procedures required for its administration.

Intervention Before parenteral nutrition is initiated, the client should be informed about the procedure. Clients and their families should be encouraged to ask questions about the therapy and to express their feelings about its implications.

Central venous lines usually introduce solutions into the vena cava through jugular or subclavian veins. If parenteral nutrition will be long-term, the line and a sealed reservoir may be implanted surgically. Temporary lines will enter the vein transdermally.

To prevent aspiration of air into the circulation, the CV line is established with the client in the Trendelenberg position. When the vein is entered, the client is instructed to perform the Valsalva maneuver to increase intrathoracic pressure. If air embolism occurs despite these precautions, the client should be placed immediately on the left side, trapping air in the right ventricle. Intracardiac aspiration or cardiac massage may be attempted by the physician to remove or disperse the air bubble.

Whenever the system must be opened for tubing changes, the client should perform the Valsalva maneuver to minimize the risk of air entering the system. Tubing changes should be completed quickly to minimize the risk of air embolism.

Central venous catheters are anchored with a stay suture to prevent displacement. Normal saline is infused initially until proper placement of the catheter has been confirmed by x-ray.

Fluids are administered through implanted lines by a special needle shaped at a 90° angle and terminating with a heparin lock. This is inserted into the reservoir transdermally and remains in place for several days. Solutions are commonly infused during sleep, with the tubing removed from the heparin lock for the rest of the day. When a transdermal CV line is employed, infusions are often continuous.

Parenteral nutrient solutions containing amino acids may form microscopic aggregates in the bag, bottle, or tubing. Such degraded fluids must not be administered because they can cause massive emboli. To prevent infusion of such material, microscopic filters are required in the IV tubing. Such filters cannot be used when lipid emulsions are administered because the fat molecules are too large to pass through them. These preparations are best administered through a double-lumen Hickman catheter in a central vein or by infusion into a peripheral vein. They are not mixed with other solutions. The preparations are isotonic and can be administered safely peripherally.

When infusion of fat emulsions is initiated, the rate should not exceed 1 ml/min for adults. Children should receive 0.1 ml/min. For the first half-hour, the client should be observed closely for dyspnea, cyanosis, allergic reaction, headache, flushing, nausea, vomiting, or pain in the chest and back. Should these reactions occur, the infusion should be discontinued and the physician notified.

Fat emulsions should be handled carefully to minimize the risk of separation. The container should never be agitated. The fluid should appear cloudy but uniform in color and density. Fluids that have separated or are not homogeneous in appearance should not be used.

Infusion of a daily dose of lipids requires 4–6 hours. Administration must be scheduled at a time when blood need not be drawn for analysis for at least 4 hours after completion of the infusion because high lipid levels in the serum can alter some blood values. Usually, fat infusions are begun immediately after early morning blood specimens have been collected.

Because rapid administration of hypertonic solutions does not allow dilution to normal tonicity, the rate of administration of such fluids must be carefully controlled. Physical signs and symptoms and laboratory data must be monitored closely to detect metabolic imbalances early and to guide adjustments in the formulation of succeeding solutions for infusion. If hyperammonemia develops, the nitrogenous (amino acid) content of the solution is reduced. Hyperglycemia is controlled with insulin injections to prevent excessive water loss through osmotic diuresis. Phosphate should be administered when parenteral therapy is prolonged.

Medications are not administered in the CV line where these solutions are given because they tend to be incompatible with total parenteral nutrition formulations. Lipid emulsions are also administered without addition of other drugs but the peripheral line used for lipid administration is available for long periods of time for the administration of other substances because only a few hours are required for the infusion of the daily allotment of this solution.

Because concentrated solutions used for parenteral nutrition are good media for microbial growth, precautions to prevent contamination of the solutions and equipment are particularly important.

Strict surgical asepsis must be maintained throughout the duration of parenteral nutrition to reduce the risk of infection. Once exposed to room temperatures, solutions must be infused within 24 hours or discarded. Microfilters will remove most particulate matter and bacteria for a day but rapid bacterial proliferation may develop if the solution is continued beyond that period (Masoorli, 1985). Additives should be mixed with solutions using strict surgical asepsis. This procedure is best carried out under a laminar flow hood by personnel wearing surgical masks. In many institutions, the pharmacist is responsible for preparing the solutions.

If the solution is significantly colder than room temperature when administered, multiple small bubbles tend to form in the tubing, some of which will be below the microfilter. To prevent this, solutions should be exposed to room temperatures for 30–60 minutes prior to infusion. If bubbles do form in the tubing, the equipment should not be agitated to coalesce them because they cannot be forced back through the microfilter. Instead, the tubing should be disturbed as little as possible. Small bubbles tend to adhere to the tubing and, therefore, do not usually coalesce or move into the client's vascular system.

Clients receiving parenteral nutrition should be monitored for signs and symptoms of fluid, electrolyte, acid–base, and trace mineral imbalance, infection (especially septicemia), and nutritional status. Weight should be monitored daily. Blood specimens are collected periodically to verify homeostasis. The physician should be informed of abnormal laboratory data,

Example of nursing process and parenteral nutrition

The client is a 67-year-old retired railroad engineer who had had metastatic stomach cancer for 7 months. He has been hospitalized because of a progressive inability to eat, dehydration, and weight loss. His physician has ordered 1 liter of D_5W at the rate of 120 ml/hr, to be followed by a liter of dextrose in saline. He plans to order supplemental potassium according to electrolyte levels. A permanent CV catheter will be surgically implanted when the client's condition is stabilized; parenteral nutrition will be administered indefinitely. The client and his family will be informed about the requirements for treatment.

Assessment data	Nursing diagnosis	Intervention	Goals and outcome criteria
Diagnosis of metastatic stomach cancer Inability to eat Order for parenteral nutrition of indefinite duration by implanted CV catheter	High risk for knowledge deficit concerning parenteral nutrition and the equipment and procedures required for its administration	**Explore** with the client and his family their knowledge about and emotional reaction to the proposed treatment. **Prepare** and implement a teaching plan that covers: the benefits to be derived from the treatment; sterile aseptic technique as it applies to IV infusions; thorough explanation of parenteral nutrition and the procedures necessary for its administration; supervised practice in the procedures required for administration of this therapy; and signs and symptoms of adverse reaction to the treatment, specifying those that require notification of healthcare personnel. **Refer** the client and his family to a community nursing service that offers care to clients receiving parenteral nutrition; inform this nursing service of the care plan used during the hospital stay and the response of the client and his family to it.	The client and his family will be able to demonstrate proper technique when carrying out procedures required for administration of parenteral nutrition. The client and family will state that nursing care and support have continued without interruption during the illness.

rapid changes in weight, fever, or other signs and symptoms indicating inadequate therapeutic response or adverse reaction.

Evaluation Data required for evaluation include signs and symptoms of fluid, electrolyte, acid–base, or trace mineral balance or imbalance; absence or incidence of signs and symptoms of infection; client participation in procedures required for the treatment; the ability of clients and families to manage parenteral nutrition therapy in the home; and emotional acceptance of the treatment by the client and family. (See accompanying Example of Nursing Process and Parenteral Nutrition.)

Checklist of nursing actions

☐ Provide emotional support for clients (and their families) during parenteral nutrition.

☐ Explain parenteral nutrition to the client and family prior to initiation.

☐ Position clients in Trendelenberg's position for insertion of CV catheter; instruct them to perform the Valsalva maneuver during insertion of the catheter.

☐ If air enters the CV catheter, place the client immediately on the left side in Trendelenberg position and inform the physician.

☐ Use IV tubing with in-line microfilters to administer concentrated solutions containing amino acids or protein hydrolysates.

☐ Use low-phthalate tubing without microfilters to administer fat emulsions.

☐ Handle containers of fat emulsions without agitation to minimize risk of separation.

☐ Inspect fat emulsions for homogeneity before administration.

☐ Begin infusion of fat emulsions slowly and monitor the client closely for the first half-hour of treatment for signs and symptoms of adverse reaction.

☐ Use strict aseptic technique when handling equipment used for parenteral nutrition.

☐ Monitor clients receiving parenteral nutrition for fluid, electrolyte, acid–base, and trace mineral balance.

☐ Monitor clients for changes in nutritional status.

☐ When parenteral nutrition is administered at home, teach the client and family how to manage the therapy.

Blood

Blood is the ideal parenteral fluid because it contains all of the constituents necessary for maintenance of homeostasis in circulation: cells, proteins, electrolytes, and nutrients. Because blood is a natural liquid tissue, transfusions are a kind of tissue transplant. Infusions of blood or blood components can restore homeostasis in many conditions not amenable to other therapeutic approaches.

The recipient of blood and blood products is at high risk for serious, life-threatening reactions, some of which cannot be ruled out for 2 years following treatment. For this reason, there is renewed interest in developing synthetic substances that can perform some or all of the functions of blood. As early as 1965, a perfluorochemical called Fluosol-DA was known to support internal respiration (Weiss, 1987). It later was developed to the phase of clinical human trials but its efficacy could not be proven as required by federal Food and Drug Administration regulations. Research continues with the goal of producing a safe, effective blood substitute.

Physiology. To maintain a proper chemical milieu in the tissues, blood contains water, electrolytes, plasma proteins (albumin, globulins, and fibrinogen), nutrients, respiratory gases, hormones, antibodies, enzymes, clotting factors, red blood cells, white blood cells, and platelets. This mixture performs many vital functions in the tissues. It transports oxygen and nutrients to the cells and removes carbon dioxide and other metabolic wastes. It distributes hormones and enzymes throughout the tissues and conveys antibodies and white blood cells to sites of infection, injury, or inflammation. Its viscosity and volume contribute to the hydraulic factors that sustain adequate circulation.

Pathology. The need for blood arises because of hemorrhage, accelerated destruction of certain constituents, or inadequate replenishment of components lost through normal attrition. In addition, in certain diseases, harmful components accumulate in the blood, and large proportions of the circulating blood must be replaced by fresh blood to prevent permanent injury or death.

Pharmacodynamics. Transfusions of whole blood or its components usually act to replenish blood constituents deficient in the client. Occasionally, blood is administered to replace large volumes of the client's blood, which are removed to eliminate one or more dangerous components, such as antibodies. Blood is also used as the priming medium for heart–lung machines used for bypass perfusion. In addition to the physiologic components unique to blood, transfusions provide calorie nutrients, electrolytes, vitamins, minerals, amino acids, and buffer salts.

Pharmacokinetics. Blood and blood derivatives are administered by injection. Whole blood, packed cells, plasma, platelets, and albumin are infused directly into the venous vascular system. Clotting factors and gamma globulins may be injected IM; they are absorbed into the circulation from these sites and eventually enter the systemic circulation. Blood components are handled by the body just like the corresponding constituents of the client's blood; they are eventually metabolized by or eliminated from the body.

Therapeutic uses. Transfusions are used as therapy for a number of clinical conditions not amenable to treatment by other parenteral fluids (Table 51-6). Blood or blood products can temporarily correct deficiencies in erythrocytes, white blood cells, platelets, clotting factors, plasma proteins, and antibodies. They are used to treat such conditions as bone marrow depression, hemolysis, protein wasting by the kidneys or intestines, impaired liver function, and clotting disorders.

The life span of transfused erythrocytes is somewhat less than the life span (averaging 120 days) of normal red blood cells produced by the client's bone marrow.

Table 51-6. Therapeutic uses of blood and blood components

Blood or blood component	Disease condition	Therapeutic effect
Whole blood	Hemorrhage	Restoration of blood volume
Replacement transfusion of whole blood	Erythroblastosis neonatorum	Removal of maternal antibodies from the baby's circulation and substitution of Rh negative blood for Rh positive blood with consequent reduction in hemolysis due to antigen–antibody reaction
Packed cells	Anemia	Replenishment of erythrocytes
Leukocyte-poor packed red blood cells	Anemia in persons with high levels of antibodies against white cells	Replenishment of erythrocytes without administering cells with antigens to which the recipient's antibodies will react
Platelets	Platelet deficiency as in aplastic anemia, leukemia, lymphomas, infection, drug toxicity, antineoplastic chemotherapy, consumptive coagulopathy, or immune destruction of platelets	Provision of platelets to promote coagulation
Blood plasma	Nephrosis, protein-wasting intestinal disease	Replenishment of blood proteins
Specific clotting factors	Clotting disorders such as hemophilia	Provision of clotting factors to promote coagulation
Gamma globulins	Potential infection due to known exposure, such as contact with hepatitis virus	Provision of temporary passive immunity, which will prevent development of active infection

Adverse reactions

Componential imbalances. Like other parenteral fluids, blood can produce excesses of one or more of its components in the client. Hyperkalemia is most likely to develop when banked blood is used because stored blood gradually releases the potassium from its erythrocytes into the plasma. Circulatory overload can also develop,, particularly when more than one unit of whole blood is administered.

Banked blood tends to lower serum levels of ionic calcium and can cause hypocalcemic tetany or prolongation of coagulation time. This effect is caused by the citrate added to the blood to prevent clotting. Citrate binds calcium, changing it from the ionic form to a physiologically inactive salt.

Allergic reactions. Allergic reactions to blood arise because of the presence in donor blood of antibodies to such materials as milk, eggs, chocolate, or pollens. Initial signs and symptoms include urticaria, itching, and wheals. In some persons, laryngeal edema or bronchospasm can occur. Symptoms can be controlled by treatment with antihistamines, epinephrine, and corticosteroids. If possible, infusion of the suspect blood should be discontinued and another unit substituted. Allergic reactions are as likely to occur with the administration of plasma as with whole blood. Anaphylaxis can occur.

Infectious disease. Blood can also transmit infectious disease present in the donor at the time the blood was collected. Banking of blood eliminates the risk of some diseases (*eg*, syphilis, cytomegalovirus infection) because the causative organisms cannot survive prolonged exposure to refrigeration. The transmission of most other diseases by blood is a rare occurrence, probably because persons harboring the causative organisms are likely to be overtly ill and obviously unsuitable as donors. The major exceptions are hepatitis, which accounts for most instances of transfusion-transmitted infection, and acquired immunodeficiency syndrome (AIDS).

The onset of hepatitis is signaled by general malaise and fatigue followed by jaundice. Various degrees of liver malfunction develop during the period of acute illness. Convalescence can be prolonged. The incubation period varies from weeks to months. Treatment of the disease is supportive. The illness can be severe and at times fatal.

The cause of AIDS is a retrovirus that suppresses the immune system, leading to serious infections and malignant tumors. At present, there is no curative treatment for AIDS. Certain antiviral anti-infectives appear to delay the progress of the disease, and attempts are underway to develop a vaccine against the virus.

Incompatibility reactions. A serious complication of blood therapy comes from antigen–antibody reactions due to tissue incompatibility. Although there are a number of antigenic systems characterizing blood types, most do not cause significant clinical problems. The ABO and Rh systems can induce serious reactions, however.

Blood types of the ABO system are inherited as

single autosomal traits. Either antigen A, antigen B, or both may be present on the erythrocytes of a person, giving rise to four different blood types: A, B, AB, or O (the absence of both antigens). Antibodies against these antigens are present naturally in any person whose erythrocytes lack them (Table 51-7).

All persons receiving blood of a type different from their own are at risk for some degree of antigen–antibody reaction. The most common type of reaction is hemolysis, which can cause serious disruption of circulation and damage to organ systems, especially the kidneys. The severity of the reaction is influenced by the degree of mismatching and by the source of the antibodies (whether donor or recipient) (Table 51-8).

The most serious reactions occur when the plasma of the recipient contains antibodies against the antigens of transfused erythrocytes. The plasma in donated blood of types A, B, or O contains small amounts of antibodies that will react with the B, A, or A and B antigens, respectively, if they are present on the recipient's erythrocytes. Such reactions are normally of such small magnitude that they produce no clinical signs or symptoms. Repeated or massive transfusions of this type may produce a cumulative effect that is clinically significant, however. The risk of such complication can be reduced by removing most of the plasma from donated blood and administering it in the form of packed cells.

Although persons of type AB are considered "universal recipients" and those of type O "universal donors," some degree of antigen–antibody reaction occurs whenever transfused blood is not identical in type to that of the recipient.

Blood for transfusion is always in short supply. A given unit must be used within 3 weeks of collection or processed for blood products with a longer shelf-life. Although exact matching of blood types is carried out whenever possible, often the types of blood available do not correspond to the types needed. It has been necessary, therefore, to use blood with a potential for reaction between donor antibodies and recipient antigens. A new process for removing the antigens of type B blood, converting it to a B antibody-free type O blood, promises to facilitate the matching of blood types. If a similar process can be developed for treating type A blood, all donated blood could be freed of antigens of the ABO type, and transfusions could be made much safer.

The Rh factor involves erythrocyte antigens designated as D antigens. Inheritance of these traits is determined by three pairs of autosomal genes. There appears to be more than one type of D antigen with varying degrees of potency in producing allergic reactions. One D antigen (D^u) reacts with some anti-D sera but not others. The person with this type of blood must be treated as Rh negative when receiving blood but Rh positive when donating.

Antibodies against D antigens do not occur naturally but arise as a result of a sensitizing exposure of Rh-negative persons to Rh-positive blood either through transfusion or transplacental passage of red cells from an Rh-positive fetus. These antibodies can cause hemolysis if a second transfusion of Rh-positive blood is attempted. They also cross the placenta during subsequent pregnancies and can cause hemolytic disease in the fetus with Rh-positive blood type.

Immunosuppression. Transfusion may weaken the recipient's protective immune systems. Some researchers have found that clients receiving blood are not as likely as others to reject organ transplants but have an increased risk of relapse following treatment for malignant neoplasms. The evidence is controversial since the results are not supported by other studies.

Precautions. Blood used for transfusions must be tested for compatibility with the blood of the potential recipient. Laboratory tests for compatibility involve typing for both ABO and Rh systems. Samples of donated blood of a suitable type are then mixed with the recipient's blood and observed for abnormal changes. If no adverse reaction occurs, the blood is considered suitable for the person tested. When the transfusion is begun, care must be taken to verify that the unit of blood given is identical to the unit tested and approved for administration to the recipient.

During transfusion, the recipient must be monitored carefully for signs and symptoms of transfusion reaction. Should these occur, the transfusion must be stopped immediately. The IV line should be kept open because emergency treatment may be needed if the reaction is severe.

During blood administration, the recipient should also be monitored for signs and symptoms of circulatory overload, hyperkalemia, hypocalcemia, and abnormal bleeding.

The incidence of adverse reactions to transfusion can be reduced by careful screening of potential donors. Blood should not be accepted from persons who are acutely ill, are taking drugs (whether therapeutic or nonmedicinal), or have a history of jaundice. It has been found that blood collected from volunteers is

Table 51-7. ABO antigens occurring naturally in plasma of various blood types

ABO blood type	Antibodies contained in the plasma
A	B antibodies
B	A antibodies
AB	No antibodies of ABO type
O	Both A and B antibodies

Table 51-8. Possible ABO antigen–antibody reaction from transfusions

Blood type of recipient	Blood type of donor	Type of reaction	Relative severity of reaction
A	A	None	
	B	B antibodies of recipient's plasma react with B antigens on donor's erythrocytes and A antibodies of transfused plasma react with A antigens on recipient's erythrocytes.	Severe
	AB	B antibodies of recipient's plasma react with B antigens on donor's erythrocytes.	Severe
	O	A antibodies of transfused plasma react with A antigens on recipient's erythrocytes	Negligible unless repeated or massive transfusions are given
B	A	A antibodies of recipient's plasma react with A antigens on donor's erythrocytes and B antibodies of transfused plasma react with B antigens on recipient's erythrocytes.	Severe
	B	None	
	AB	A antibodies of recipient's plasma react with A antigens on donor's erythrocytes.	Severe
	O	B antibodies of transfused plasma react with B antigens on recipient's erythrocytes.	Negligible unless repeated or massive transfusions are given
AB*	A	B antibodies of transfused plasma react with B antigens on recipient's erythrocytes.	Negligible unless repeated or massive transfusions are given
	B	A antibodies of transfused plasma react with A antigens on recipient's erythrocytes.	Negligible unless repeated or massive transfusions are given
	AB	None	
	O	B antibodies of transfused plasma react with B antigens on recipient's erythrocytes and A antibodies of transfused plasma react with A antigens on recipient's erythrocytes.	Negligible unless repeated or massive transfusions are given
O†	A	A antibodies of recipient's plasma react with A antigens on donor's erythrocytes.	Severe
	B	B antibodies of recipient's plasma react with B antigens on donor's erythrocytes	Severe
	AB	A antibodies of recipient's plasma react with A antigens on donor's erythrocyte and B antibodies of recipient's plasma react with B antigens on donor's erythrocytes.	Severe
	O	None	

* The so-called universal recipient.

† The so-called universal donor.

generally safer than that purchased from professional donors.

Diphenhydramine (Benadryl) is sometimes injected into the IV tubing before blood is infused. This tends to reduce the incidence and severity of allergic reactions to transfusions.

Blood should not be transfused through a CV line unless large amounts of blood are required quickly. The injection of cold blood directly into the heart can cause cardiac arrhythmias, especially in neonates.

Whenever possible, autotransfusions should be used. When the need for blood or a blood component can be predicted, many clients are now encouraged to bank their own blood. The required components may be separated from the blood unit and the remainder reinfused into the client. The generation of red blood cells may be accelerated in between donations by administration of a bone marrow stimulant.

Numerous precautions are taken to ensure the safety of banked blood. These include testing blood for hepatitis B organisms, and for HIV antibodies indicative of exposure to the AIDS retrovirus. Screening for

AIDS antibodies is believed to have an error rate of approximately one in 10,000.

Contraindications. Blood containing ABO or Rh antigens (A, B, AB, or Rh⁺ types) should never be administered to clients whose blood contains specific antibodies to these antigens (*eg*, O or Rh⁻ type blood) (see Table 51-8).

■ Summary

Transfusions of blood or blood components are administered to maintain or replenish blood constituents that cannot be duplicated or provided by synthetic substitutes. Blood is also used to replace blood that must be removed from the body to eliminate one or more toxic elements and to prime heart–lung machines prior to bypass perfusion.

Although blood transfusions provide unique therapeutic benefits, adverse reactions can be catastrophic. Because of its dangers, blood should never be administered unless absolutely necessary, and precautions designed to reduce its risks must be strictly observed.

Nursing management

Nursing implications

Blood is highly perishable and must be kept refrigerated until it is administered. It should not be allowed to freeze. If blood or platelets is to be warmed, remove it from the refrigerator and allow it to stand at room temperature for up to 1 hour before using. *Never* attempt to warm it by any method that could warm any part of it above body temperature.

Nursing process

Assessment When a transfusion is to be administered, the client's general condition should be appraised and the condition that mandates transfusion identified.

Clients who are to receive transfusions must give informed consent for the procedure. Some clients will not accept transfusions because of religious proscriptions. Others fear blood-borne infection. As with any other treatment, clients have the right to refuse therapy.

The client who is to receive blood or blood products by IV should be assessed for signs and symptoms of allergy or systemic infection resembling transfusion reaction. If present, these symptoms should be recorded as accurately and quantitatively as possible so that they will not be mistaken for transfusion reaction. Any increase in these symptoms should be interpreted as possible transfusion reaction until proven otherwise.

Nursing diagnosis Nursing diagnoses for the client receiving blood products include the following:

> *Fluid volume excess related to IV administration of large volumes of blood*
> *High risk for altered comfort: itching related to urticaria secondary to allergic reaction to blood*

Common collaborative problems that should be differentiated from the nursing diagnoses include

> *Potential complication: cardiac arrest*
> *Potential complication: hyperkalemia*
> *Potential complication: tetany*
> *Potential complication: anaphylaxis*
> *Potential complication: hemolysis*

Planning Goals of nursing care are prevention of administration of mismatched blood; correction of the condition for which blood is used; and prevention or prompt detection and treatment of adverse reactions to blood or blood products.

Intervention Proper matching of the designated unit of blood with the client is crucial because the administration of the wrong type blood can be fatal. Acute-care facilities in which blood is used generally designate specific procedures to be followed when blood is given. Each unit of blood is identified by a multicopy label bearing the name and number of the donor; blood expiration date; ABO and Rh types; the results of tests for the presence of infectious pathogens; and the name and address of the blood bank that processed the unit. When a client's blood is matched, one copy of this information from each unit of blood used is placed in the client's chart. Before initiating the transfusion, two nurses (or a nurse and a physician) should verify independently all identifying information, matching the label attached to the blood container with its copy in the chart and the client's identification band. Unless all information corresponds, the blood must not be used and should be returned to the laboratory.

Blood must be administered through tubing with a special blood filter and a needle with a large bore (18 gauge or larger). The system is primed with normal saline or other solution compatible with blood. Dextrose is not used because it promotes cell aggregation. Medication must not be administered in the system containing blood because drugs might injure the red cells.

Blood should be started at a slow flow rate of 1 ml/kg of body weight per hour or less. Clients should be closely monitored for signs and symptoms of transfusion reaction for the first half-hour of the infusion. Early signs and symptoms include anxiety, restlessness, chest or back pain, flushing, and increased pulse and respirations. These reactions may be followed by shaking chill, fever, and cyanosis. The transfusion must be stopped at the first sign of a reaction. To prevent the absorption of even small amounts of additional blood, the infusion bottles should be lowered below the level of the infusion site to induce a flashback. The tubing can then be disconnected at the injection site, flushed with priming solution, and reconnected to restore flow of priming solution through the IV needle. It is essential that the IV line be kept open because it may be needed for emergency medications.

The physician must be notified immediately when any reaction to blood occurs. The nurse should be prepared to institute measures to treat the reaction, including medications that may be ordered.

The client with urticaria should be instructed to press on itching sites and to avoid scratching. Excessive clothing or bedding should be removed so that the client is comfortably cool because heat increases itching.

A thorough investigation must be made of all transfusion reactions to determine the cause. The blood container and fresh samples of blood from the client are sent to the laboratory with a description of the reaction. The most frequent cause of such reactions is the administration of blood to the wrong person, a fact that emphasizes the importance of accuracy in matching blood to the client at the time of administration.

Client education. The client or, if the client is incompetent, a family member must be informed of the plan for transfusion before blood is administered. Although written permission for the procedure is not always required, the use of blood is proscribed by some religions (notably Jehovah's Witness), and fear of blood-borne disease has increased since the dangers of AIDS have been recognized. An opportunity must be provided for refusal of treatment.

The need for a transfusion provokes anxiety for most people. It is well known that using blood is somewhat hazardous, that blood is scarce, and that it is not used unless absolutely necessary. Therefore, transfusion implies that the illness is grave. The need for blood therapy should be explained to the client or family in as reassuring a manner as possible.

During the initial period of transfusion, when constant monitoring of the client is necessary, the nurse should maintain a calm, matter-of-fact demeanor. Productive use of time with the client for nursing care will deemphasize the critical nature of this interval. Before leaving, the nurse should instruct the client to report promptly any discomfort.

Education of the public regarding blood and its medical uses is important to promote donations and to maintain adequate supplies. Persons between the ages of 18 and 65 who are in good health and at low risk for harboring AIDS should be encouraged to donate regularly.

Evaluation Data required for evaluation relate to incidence or absence of signs and symptoms of adverse reaction to the transfusion. The client should be assessed for fluid, potassium and calcium balance, as well as for circulation and tissue perfusion.

Checklist of nursing actions

☐ Before initiating a transfusion, assess clients for signs and symptoms of conditions that resemble transfusion reaction.

☐ Inform clients about the transfusion and verify that the treatment is acceptable to them.

☐ Verify with another health professional that the unit of blood to be used is properly matched with that of the recipient.

☐ Observe the client continuously for signs and symptoms of adverse reaction until at least 50 ml of blood have been absorbed.

☐ Administer blood at a slow rate.

☐ If signs and symptoms of adverse reaction develop, discontinue the transfusion immediately; maintain a patent IV line for administration of medications.

☐ When transfusion reactions occur, save the blood container and send to the laboratory to facilitate tests required to determine the reason for the reaction.

References

Weiss R. (1987). Sanguine substitutes. *Science News 132*, 200–202 (September 26).

Bibliography

*Atkins JM. (1986). A nurse's guide to TPN. *RN, 49(6)*, 20–24.

*Birdsall C. (1985). How should parenteral nutrition be tapered? *Am J Nurs, 87*, 582.

Brown P. (1989). Consult stat: Filters for blood transfusions. *RN 52(8)*, 70 (August).

*Butler S. (1989). Current trends in autologous transfusion. *RN 52(11)*, 44–54 (November).

*Carr P. (1986). When the patient needs TPN at home. *RN, 49(6)*, 25–29.

*Cerrato PL. (1986). Will IV feeding endanger your patient? *RN, 49(121)*, 59–61.

*Choosing the correct port for hyperalimentation. (1987). *RN, 50(3)*, 78–79.

Clinical news: Red blood cell transfusion risks. (1989). *American Journal of Nursing, 89(1)*, 14 (January).

Corcoran E. (1989). The burden of proof: Donated blood runs a costly gauntlet of tests. *Sci Am, 260(4)*, 79–80 (April).

* Recommended for further reading.

Drug news: Erythropoietin: Eliminating transfusions. (1989). *Nursing 89, 19(11)*, 85 (November).

Drug news: Fluosol: Improving angioplasty. (1990). *Nursing 90, 20(7)*, 82 (July).

*Gasparis L, et al. (1989). IV solutions: Which one's right for your patient? *Nursing 89, 19(4)*, 62–64 (April).

Guarda NP, Peterson JZ. (1986). Screening for HIV antibodies. *Nursing 86, 16(11)*, 28–29.

Hahn K. (1989). Monitoring a blood transfusion. *Nursing 89, 19(10)*, 20–21 (October).

Hennessy KA. (1988). Now TPN therapy begins at home. *RN, 51(6)*, 81–84 (June).

Hutchison R, et al. (1989). Beneficial effect of brief pre-transfusion incubation of platelets at 37°C. *Lancet, 1*, 986 (May 6).

Jenks S. (1989). Case builds against transfusions. *Medical World News, 30*, 28 (December 11).

*Johndrow PD. (1988). Making your patient and his family feel at home with TPN. *Nursing 88, 18(10)*, 65–69 (October).

*Johnson JJ. (1987). AIDS Update: How safe is the blood supply? *Nursing 87, 17(12)*, 26–27 (December).

Johnson-Querin J. (1988). Consultation: Blood transfusions and CMV. *Nursing 88, 18(3)*, 76 (March).

Kresevic DM. (1990). Understanding therapeutic plasma exchange. *Nursing 90, 20(4)*, 68 (April).

*The latest protocols for blood transfusions. (1986a). *Nursing 86, 16(10)*, 34–41.

*McCormac M. (1990). Managing hemorrhagic shock. *American Journal of Nursing, 90(8)*, 22 (August).

McVan BW. (1987). RN at home: How we give blood transfusions at home. *RN, 50(8)*, 79–80 (August).

*Metheny NM. (1990). Why worry about IV fluids? *Am J Nurs, 90(6)*, 50–57 (June).

NIII consensus panel recommendations for red cell transfusion. (1988). *Internal Medicine Alert, 10*, 93 (December 29).

Philips A. (1987). Are blood transfusions really safe? *Nursing 87, 17(6)*, 63–64 (June).

Rutman RC. (1989). Add two transfusion steps? (letter) *American Journal of Nursing, 89(12)*, 1612.

*Rutman RC, et al. (1989). Blood transfusions. *American Journal of Nursing, 89(4)*, 486–489.

Sanders MK. (1989). Nursing consult: Autologous transfusions: Safer and easier. *Nursing 89, 19(8)*, 66 (August).

*Transfusions precautions. (1986). *Nursing 87, 17(3)*, 6.

Weiss R. (1987). Sanguine substitutes. *Science News, 132*, 200–201 (September 26).

*Recommended for further reading.

Miscellaneous drug families

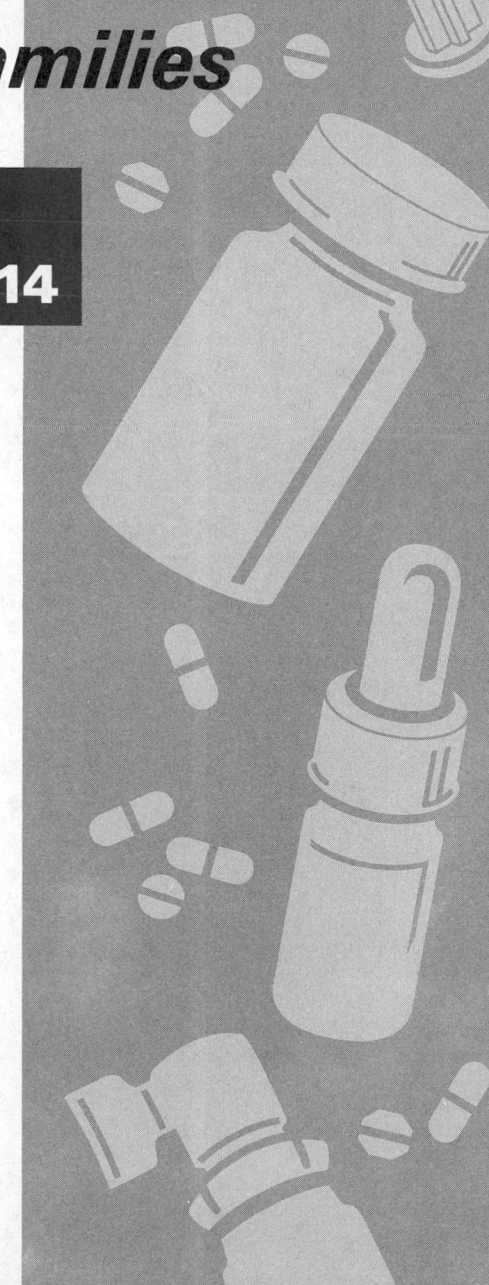

14

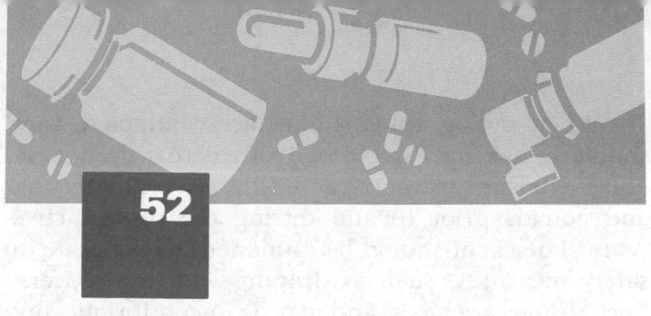

Diagnostic agents

Pharmacologic agents are frequently used to carry out diagnostic procedures to determine the underlying cause of illness. These agents fall into four general categories:

1. Radiopaque materials that serve as contrast media for x-ray photography;
2. Markers that can be measured in tests designed to determine the concentration, volume, or rate of flow of body fluids;
3. Radioactive isotopes that reveal the tissue concentration of certain chemicals when scanned for radiation; and
4. Provocative agents that stimulate measurable body responses indicative of the presence or absence of disease.

Although these agents are not administered therapeutically, all exert pharmacologic actions and cause toxic effects and side effects. Before a decision is made to carry out diagnostic tests, the potential risks and benefits should be weighted. When tests are ordered, they must be conducted as carefully as any therapeutic measure to ensure that reliable diagnostic data will be generated with the least risk to the client.

Radiopaque contrast media

Although plain x-rays reveal much about the shape, density, and integrity of dense tissues such as bone, the shadows cast by soft tissues are vague and difficult to interpret. Some structures, such as blood vessels, cardiac chambers, and ductal systems are not revealed at all. Visible organs generally project only a vague outline. Radiopaque chemicals inside such structures add contrast to films, clearly outlining their internal silhouettes. These drugs, in conjunction with fluoroscopy or cinematography, also allow study of the kinetic function of specific organs. Data from such radiographic studies are critical in making definitive diagnoses in many areas of medicine.

Although the benefits of radiography are undeniable, it is not without significant risk. X-rays are one form of ionizing radiation, exposure to which causes cumulative effects over a person's life span. Such radiation has been associated with increased risk of birth defects, infertility, increased risk of malignant neoplasm, and tissue changes characteristic of aging. Although the body's repair processes seem capable of reversing some of the effects of radiation, no standards have been established for safe levels of exposure. Many authorities believe that there is no "safe" level. For this reason, diagnostic radiography should be kept to a minimum and should never be used unless absolutely necessary.

Nursing management

Nursing implications

Modern radiographic equipment is designed to minimize exposure to ionizing rays. Low-voltage emissions, narrow beams, and shielding screens help confine radiation to the target area and keep it at a low level. Nevertheless, each radiogram taken adds to the cumulative load imposed on a person.

Nursing process

Assessment An attempt should be made to assess total exposure to radiation prior to the planned diagnostic study. A history of exposure to radiography and radioactive drugs or tracers, as well as nonmedicinal exposure to ionizing radiation, should be taken. The reproductive status of women should be determined.

The client's knowledge about the procedure, and his or her emotional reaction to it and to the implied presence of an, as yet, undiagnosed health problem should be explored.

Nursing diagnosis Probable diagnoses for clients about to undergo diagnostic tests involving ionizing radiation include the following:

> Knowledge deficit related to exposure to radiation and its use in diagnostic procedures
> Anxiety related to the threat of an, as yet, undiagnosed illness

A potential complication is damage to the fetus if frequent x-rays are performed during early pregnancy.

Planning Goals of nursing care are to prevent excessive exposure to ionizing radiation, to prevent birth defects, to educate clients to the risks of exposure to radiation, and to alleviate anxiety.

Intervention The physician and radiologist should be notified if the client is pregnant, or has a history of radiation sickness or frequent exposure to ionizing radiation. Tests performed on women of childbearing age should be scheduled for the first half of the menstrual cycle, when the likelihood of pregnancy is minimal.

Clients undergoing diagnostic tests should be given emotional support. Without giving false assurances, the nurse should encourage client trust in the skill and concern of health care personnel and express hope for a favorable outcome of diagnosis and treatment.

Client education. Clients should be discouraged from requesting diagnostic x-rays for trivial reasons. They should be fully informed of the health risks of exposure to ionizing radiation and should be involved in the decision-making process when studies requiring radiation are contemplated.

When radiographic studies are conducted, care should be taken to shield body areas that do not require exposure to the x-ray beam, especially fetuses and gonads prior to and during the reproductive years. The client should be cautioned to cooperate in safety measures, such as draping with lead covers. Such drapes are heavy and may be uncomfortable but usually are required only for a short time.

A complete list of known exposure to ionizing irradiation should be part of every individual health record.

Evaluation Data required for evaluation include the incidence or absence of elective diagnostic procedures involving exposure to irradiation; the incidence or absence of birth defects attributable to *in utero* exposure to irradiation; and the incidence or absence of illness attributable to excessive exposure to irradiation. Client teaching is evaluated according to the incidence or absence of signs and symptoms of anxiety; the client's ability to cooperate with x-ray personnel during the diagnostic procedures; and client statements indicating an awareness of the risk of exposure to ionizing radiation.

Checklist of nursing actions

- [ ] Assess cumulative exposure to ionizing radiation prior to radiographic studies. Report excessive or unusual exposure promptly to the physician.
- [ ] Determine the reproductive status of women of childbearing years about to undergo diagnostic tests involving ionizing radiation.
- [ ] Schedule tests involving exposure to radiation for the period immediately following menstruation for women of childbearing age.
- [ ] Provide emotional support for clients with undiagnosed illness.
- [ ] Act as an advocate to ensure client involvement in the decision-making process.
- [ ] Instruct the client about safety measures used to reduce exposure to radiation.
- [ ] Teach clients to include a history of exposure to ionizing radiation in their personal health records.

Learning experience 52-1

Care for a client undergoing diagnostic radiography that requires use of radiopaque contrast media. Observe the procedure, taking care to avoid personal exposure to ionizing radiation. Afterward, interview the client to determine his or her reaction to the testing procedure.

Barium sulfate

Barium sulfate* is an insoluble, nonabsorbable, opaque powder that is also radiopaque. It must not be confused with other salts of barium (barium sulfide or barium sulfite) that are soluble, readily absorbed, and highly toxic.

Pharmacodynamics. The function of barium sulfate depends on its distribution and concentration in the organs to be studied. Barium casts a shadow on radiographic films capable of outlining the lumen of structures in the gastrointestinal (GI) tract. Space-occupying lesions within the tract will show up on films as filling defects, and ulcerations or discontinuities of the mucosa appear as outward deviations of the lumen.

Pharmacokinetics. Barium sulfate is administered orally or rectally as an aqueous suspension. It is not absorbed and passes through the tract to be eliminated in feces.

Diagnostic uses. Barium sulfate is commonly used as a contrast medium in radiographic examinations of the esophagus, stomach, duodenum, and colon (barium swallow, upper GI radiogram, and barium enema). When necessary, as orally administered material progresses through the tract, serial films can be taken for a complete study of the small intestine.

Adverse reactions. The most common side effect of barium sulfate is constipation. The substance produces a hard stool. Obstipation and intestinal obstruction have occurred following its use. Barium can remain in the appendix, providing a nidus for the formation of fecaliths; acute appendicitis with rupture can follow.

Although practically inert within the GI tract, barium sulfate is irritating to peripheral tissues. Leakage outside the tract through perforations or fistulas can produce inflammation and symptoms of peritonitis or mediastinitis.

The elderly are at increased risk for adverse reactions such as fluid imbalance, hypotension, and changes in mental states (Tests hazardous to elderly, 1985).

Anaphylactic reactions associated with barium enemas appear to be caused by hypersensitivity to latex rubber used to make cuffed enema tips. (Severe adverse reactions to barium enema procedures, 1990)

Precautions and contraindications. Barium sulfate should not be administered to clients with known intestinal obstruction, GI perforations, or fistulas.

Ample hydration before the procedure reduces the risk of hypovolemia and hypotension. For clients with a history of latex allergy, barium enemas should be administered via a nonlatex enema tip.

Following radiographic studies using barium, measures to prevent constipation should be instituted. A laxative such as milk of magnesia is often prescribed.

■ Summary

Barium sulfate is a chemical used as a radiopaque contrast medium in radiography of the GI tract. It is not absorbed systemically. It is contraindicated for clients with perforations or fistulas because it is irritating to the tissues. Barium produces a hard stool and can cause serious constipation.

Nursing management

Nursing implications

Barium studies are among the most frequently used diagnostic tools. They are helpful in identifying abdominal strictures, obstructions, ulcers, polyps, and tumors.

Nursing process

Assessment Clients scheduled for GI radiography should be carefully assessed for history of allergy, particularly sensitivity to latex signs and symptoms of intestinal obstruction or perforation, such as abdominal pain, rigidity, or pronounced distention. Bowel status should be evaluated to determine the relative need for poststudy catharsis.

The client's knowledge about the planned procedure and emotional reaction to the threat of illness as yet undiagnosed should be explored.

Nursing diagnosis Probable nursing diagnoses for clients undergoing barium studies include the following:

> *High risk for constipation, obstipation or obstruction related to barium ingestion (or barium enema) secondary to diagnostic studies*
> *Knowledge deficit related to diagnostic procedures involving barium preparations*
> *Anxiety related to diagnostic procedures and the threat of an as yet undiagnosed illness*

Planning Nursing care goals are to prevent complications such as hypotension, constipation, obstipation, or obstruction; to promptly detect and treat adverse reactions to barium; to improve clients' ability to collaborate in the diagnostic procedures; and to alleviate anxiety.

Intervention Physicians and radiologists should be notified of risk factors revealed during the initial nursing assessment by clients scheduled for barium studies.

---

* Trade names for barium sulfate include Colobar-100, Esobar, Esophocat, E-Z-Cat, E-Z-HD, E-Z-Jug, E-Z-Pague, Liqui-Jug, Polibar, Readi-Cat, Recto Barium, Ultra-R, and Unibar-100.

The need for and safety of radiographic studies can then be re-evaluated. If barium is inadvisable, an iodine contrast medium may be substituted.

When clients are instructed to fast prior to barium studies, they should also be urged to drink water freely before the procedure to maintain hydration.

Throughout contact with the client, the nurse should promote confidence in the competence and concern of the health care team, and, without giving false assurances, should foster hope for a favorable outcome of diagnosis and treatment.

After studies are completed, the nurse should encourage consumption of ample fluids to reduce the risk of constipation.

Barium enema solutions are drained from the colon after radiographic studies are completed, and the client is encouraged to defecate immediately to eliminate as much of the residual suspension as possible. Following upper GI studies involving ingested barium, the client's bowel status must be monitored carefully and measures taken to promote bowel elimination. Laxatives are administered if ordered.

Client education. Clients should be instructed to fast the night before GI barium studies.

Do not tell the client to take nothing by mouth (NPO); water should be taken freely prior to the test. On the morning of the test, a bowel-cleansing regimen (laxative or enema) is usually required to prepare for barium enemas. Inadequate preparation may result in poor quality films and the need to repeat the series.

Clients having upper GI studies should be informed at the beginning of the test that they will be asked to swallow a suspension resembling a thick milkshake. Clients scheduled for colonic studies need to know that an enema will be administered in the x-ray department.

Various positions are used for serial exposures; clients will be required to hold their breath when exposures are made. Clients who have been adequately informed are likely to make fewer errors during the procedure, reducing the need for repeated exposures. They will also experience less anxiety than poorly prepared persons.

The client should be informed that barium colors the stools a pale clay gray. Stools should be monitored until the barium has passed and normal fecal color is resumed. Unless contraindicated, a laxative should be recommended to clients subject to constipation.

Evaluation Data required for evaluation include incidence or absence of hypotension during the test; constipation, obstipation, obstruction, or inflammation of parenteral tissues after the test; and incidence or absence of signs and symptoms of anxiety. Client teaching can be evaluated by the effectiveness of bowel cleansing (when conducted by the client); the ability of clients to cooperate with x-ray personnel during the procedure; and statements by clients indicating they felt well prepared for the procedure.

Checklist of nursing actions

- [ ] Prior to barium studies, assess the client for latex hypersensitivity, intestinal perforation, fistula, or obstruction, and tendency toward constipation.
- [ ] Instruct clients to fast and to take ample amounts of water before the test.
- [ ] Follow protocols for diagnostic studies carefully to ensure the generation of useful data without the need for repeated studies.
- [ ] To reduce anxiety, instruct the client about procedures to be followed during the study.
- [ ] Provide emotional support for clients who have undiagnosed health problems.
- [ ] Teach clients what will be expected of them during the procedure.
- [ ] Monitor clients closely during studies for hypovolemia, hypotension, and mental changes such as confusion.
- [ ] Warn clients that stools containing barium will be clay-colored.
- [ ] Following barium studies, administer laxatives as required by test protocols or physician's order. Recommended a laxative to noninstitutionalized clients prone to constipation.

Iodinated contrast media

A variety of iodine compounds with radiopaque properties are used as contrast media in diagnostic radiographic procedures. Their function depends on their distribution, concentration, and excretion within the body, rather than on their pharmacologic effects. Pharmacologic effects of iodinated contrast media are, therefore, considered side effects.

Pharmacodynamics. Contrast media are opaque to x-rays and cast shadows on x-ray film. These substances can be injected into the body to produce images that illustrate the distribution and flow of body fluids such as blood, bile, and urine.

Pharmacokinetics. Routes of absorption, distribution, and excretion vary with different preparations and are related to their diagnostic uses (Table 52-1). Oral preparations not readily absorbed by the GI tract are used for radiographic examination of this tract. (However, variable amounts of these preparations *will* be absorbed systemically.) Preparations readily absorbed in the GI tract and subsequently concentrated and excreted by the biliary or urinary tracts are used in examining these systems. Injectable solutions are often administered directly into the structures to be studied (arteries, veins, cardiac chambers, joints) and must be absorbed systemically prior to elimination. Most radio-

Table 52-1. Iodinated x-ray contrast media

Drug name	Preparations	Usual adult dosage	Diagnostic uses/additional information
Aqueous injectable agents			
diatrizoate Meglumine (Cardiografin, Cystographin, Hypaque-Cysto, Hypaque Meglumine, Reno-M, Urovist)	Solutions for injection or instillation (30%, 60%, 76%, 85%)	Varies with the test to be done	Diatrizoate meglumine is employed in various procedures including angiography, phlebography, cardiography, IV and retrograde urography, direct cholangiography, and enhancement of computed tomography of the brain.
diatrizoate sodium (Hypaque)	Solutions for injection or instillation (25%, 41.66%, 50%) Solutions for instillation (20%, 41.66%)	Varies with the test to be done	Diatrizoate is employed in various procedures including hysterosalpingography. It is used in preference to barium for GI radiography when perforation or obstruction is suspected.
iodamide meglumide (Renovue)	Solutions for injection (24%, 65%)	Varies with the test to be done	Iodamide is employed for IV urography and contrast enhancement of computerized tomography of the brain.
iodipamide meglumine (Cholografin, Meglumine)	Solutions for injection or instillation (10.3%, 52%)	Varies with the test to be done	Iodipamide is employed for IV cholecystography and cholangiography.
iophendylate (Pantopaque)	Solution for intrathecal injection (305 mg iodine/ml)	Varies with the test to be done	Iophendylate is employed in myelography, especially in the lumbar region. It is usually aspirated from the CSF following the procedure.
iothalamate meglumine (Conray, Cysto-Conray)	Solutions for injection or instillation (30%, 43%, 60%) Solutions for instillation (17.2%, 43%)	Varies with the test to be done	Iothalamate meglumine is employed in various procedures including IV urography, cerebral arteriography, peripheral arteriography, and venography.
iothalamate sodium (Angio-Conray, Conray-400)	Solutions for injection (54.3%, 66.8%, 80%)	Varies with the test to be done	Iothalamate sodium is employed for IV urography, angiocardiography, contrast enhancement of computerized tomography of the brain, and aortography; it is not suitable for cerebral angiography.
metrizamide (*Can:* Amipaque)	Solutions for instillation	Varies with the test to be done	Metrizamide is employed for myelography, cisternography, and ventriculography
Oils			
ethiodized oil (Ethiodol)	Oil containing 370 mg iodine/ml for instillation or intralymphatic injection	Varies with the test to be done	Ethiodized oil is employed for lymphography and hysterosalpingography; it is not suitable for administration intravenously, intra-arterially, intrathecally, or by way of the bronchial tree.
propyliodone (*Can:* Dionosil)	Suspension for instillation	Varies with the test to be done	Propyliodone is employed for bronchography and laryngography
Oral agents			
iocetamic acid (Cholebrine)	Tablets for oral use	3–4.5 g	Iocetamic acid is employed for oral cholecystography; it may be used for children older than 12 years of age.
iopanoic acid (Telepaque)	Tablets for oral use	3 g	Iopanoic acid is employed for oral cholecystography.
ipodate (Oragrafin, Bilivist)	Capsules and powder for preparing suspension for oral use	3 g	Ipodate is employed for oral cholecystography; suspensions should be prepared with lukewarm water and used promptly because they are unstable. Both calcium and sodium salts are available.
tyropanoate sodium (Bilopaque)	Capsules for oral use	3 g	Tyropanoate is employed for oral cholecystography.

KEY: *Can* = Canadian trade name.

paque compounds are excreted in large part by the kidneys, with lesser amounts eliminated in bile and feces.

Diagnostic uses. Iodinated contrast media are used to produce or enhance film images in many diagnostic studies, as indicated in Box 52-1. When sufficiently concentrated in body fluids, they serve to outline the structures (blood vessels, joints, cerebrospinal space) in which they are contained or the ducts and tubules (urinary or biliary) by which they are excreted. Their presence in tissues also enhances the images produced by computed tomography.

Dosage form and route of administration must be chosen in relation to the area to be visualized, as well as the equipment and method employed. Dosage and concentration are individualized and proportional to the size of the area to be studied, the anticipated dilution, and the degree of contrast required.

Adverse reactions. Side effects from iodinated contrast media can affect many systems of the body and can range in severity from mild to life-threatening. Some effects are transitory, whereas others produce permanent sequelae (Table 52-2).

Vasomotor reactions affect up to half the clients receiving contrast media. These reactions may include flushing, warmth, tingling sensations, vertigo, nausea, and a metallic taste. The reactions tend to be mild and rarely require treatment (Bush, Mullarkey, & Webb, 1980).

Allergic reactions to iodinated contrast media include skin rashes and anaphylaxis. Anaphylactoid reactions may be manifested by urticaria, sneezing, chest tightness, bronchospasm, angioedema, hypotension, and tachycardia. Incidence among clients with a history of iodine allergy is about 4%; incidence among clients with a history of a previous anaphylactoid reaction to iodinated contrast dyes is about 35%. Ana-

Table 52-2. Adverse reactions to iodine contrast media

Type of reaction	Signs and symptoms
Idiosyncratic/ allergic	Anaphylaxis
Cardiovascular	Increased osmolarity in fluid compartments, hypotension or hypertension, bradycardia or tachycardia, hemodynamic shifts and thrombophlebitis, (rarely) shock, fibrillation, cardiac arrest, disseminated intravascular coagulation
Respiratory	Rhinitis, dyspnea, cough, sneeze, bronchospasm, laryngospasm, pulmonary edema, cyanosis (with oil lymphography), pulmonary embolism
Gastrointestinal	Metallic taste, salivation, salivary gland swelling, nausea, vomiting, retching
Neurologic	Restlessness, confusion, apprehension, anxiety, headache, dizziness, tremor, agitation, visual disturbances, convulsions, stroke, coma, paraplegia, permanent visual field defects
Dermatologic	Flushing, warmth, urticaria, pruritus, rash, edema, pallor, petechiae, diaphoresis; necrosis has been reported following extravasation during injection
Hematopoietic	Neutropenia
Renal	Acute renal failure, oliguria, anuria, proteinuria
General	Chills, fever, flushing, warmth

phylactoid reactions can be serious. Treatment includes vasopressors, IV fluids, oxygen, antihistamines, and steroids. Pretreatment (with glucocorticoids and antihistamines) of clients at high risk may reduce the severity of reaction.

Apprehension, restlessness, hypotension, and bradycardia indicate a vagal reaction to contrast media, requiring treatment with atropine and IV fluids.

Radiopaque iodine compounds are irritating to tissues. Pain can occur at injection sites.

Pulmonary embolism is so common following lymphography that it is considered usual. Fortunately, this reaction is usually asymptomatic.

Toxicity of iodine contrast media is influenced by many factors. The type of cation in the molecule is significant; for example, meglumine salts are better tolerated than sodium salts. Factors directly related to toxicity include osmolarity, volume, concentration, viscosity, and rate of the drug's administration. The route of administration affects the type of reaction likely to occur. For example, neurotoxic reactions are most likely to occur in cerebral angiography when the drugs are delivered directly to the brain by carotid injection. Reactions are most likely with repeated tests over a short time and in clients who are dehydrated.

Box 52-1. Diagnostic radiographic tests in which iodinated contrast media are used

Angiography, venography, lymphography

Cardiography, aortography

Urography (IV and retrograde)

Arthrography, discography, myelography

Cholecystography (direct, IV, and oral)

Gastrointestinal radiography (when barium is contraindicated)

Hysterosalpingography

Computer tomography (especially cerebral)

Precautions and contraindications. Iodine contrast media are contraindicated for clients with a history of severe reaction to any drug of this type. Other contraindications vary, depending on the type of test desired. For example, cerebral angiography is contraindicated if cranial subarachnoid hemorrhage is suspected or in the presence of active migraine; IV urography is contraindicated in anuria.

Caution must be used with clients who have a history of mild reaction to these agents, a history of migraine, or a personal or family history of allergy, especially asthma.

A number of medical conditions increase the risk of adverse reaction because they slow elimination of the drugs or predispose the client to injury to specific organs. Caution should be used when giving contrast media to persons with renal or hepatic impairment, hemocystinuria, congestive heart failure, multiple myeloma, thrombosis, phlebitis, ischemia, or diabetic nephropathy. Extreme caution is required if pheochromocytoma is known or suspected because severe hypertension may occur. Serial studies within a short time increase the risk of reaction.

Before studies using these agents are undertaken, clients should be well hydrated. Vasopressor drugs should not be given before the test. When the drugs are injected, care should be taken to deliver them to the desired site. Blood vessels should be flushed immediately after injection with an IV solution.

Supportive equipment must be readily available to treat serious reactions, such as anaphylaxis. Clients should be monitored for signs and symptoms of adverse reaction for 30–60 minutes following drug administration. Because pretests for sensitivity can produce severe reactions, they are generally not recommended.

■ Summary

Radiopaque iodine compounds are employed as contrast media in many types of diagnostic radiographic studies, including computed tomography. Dosage, route, and time of administration vary depending on the test required. Although serious adverse reactions are uncommon, these drugs can produce many toxic and side effects.

Nursing management

Nursing implications

Although x-ray personnel are responsible for administering radiopaque dye and completing the study, the nurse is usually responsible for preparing clients and monitoring for delayed adverse reactions.

Nursing process

Assessment Clients scheduled for diagnostic studies involving iodine contrast media should be assessed carefully for hypersensitivity to iodine, especially for previous reaction to contrast media. Previous exposure to ionizing radiation and iodine contrast media should be documented. Clients should also be evaluated for fluid balance.

The client's knowledge about the planned procedure and emotional reaction to it should be explored.

Nursing diagnosis Nursing diagnoses for client undergoing diagnostic studies involving iodinated contrast media include the following:

> High risk for altered comfort: flushing, warmth, nausea, vertigo, dyspnea, apprehension, and restlessness related to adverse reaction to iodinated contrast media
> Knowledge deficit concerning iodinated contrast media and their use in diagnostic procedures
> Anxiety related to diagnostic procedure and an as yet undiagnosed health problems

Planning Nursing goals for clients scheduled for diagnostic procedures requiring iodinated contrast media include preventing adverse reactions to the radiopaque dyes; promptly detecting and treating adverse reactions should they occur; alleviating anxiety; and educating the client to the planned procedure and to the implications of exposure to radiopaque dyes.

Intervention The physician and radiologist should be informed promptly if dehydration, a history of drug reaction, recent use of iodine compounds, or excessive exposure to radiation is found upon initial assessment. Clients scheduled for diagnostic studies involving radiopaque dyes should be encouraged to drink ample water prior to the test. If necessary, an IV infusion should be requested to ensure adequate hydration.

Throughout contact with the client, the nurse should provide emotional support, promote trust in the competence and concern of the health care team, and, without giving false assurances, encourage hope for a favorable outcome of diagnosis and treatment.

Protocols for test procedures must be followed carefully to ensure the generation of useful data without repeated studies. Fasting is often required. Bowel cleansing is necessary prior to most abdominal studies. Sedation may be ordered for clients undergoing procedures that require instrumentation such as cystoscopy. Oral radiopaque drugs administered prior to the test must be timed correctly to ensure optimum results.

Following diagnostic tests, clients should be monitored for adverse drug reaction such as skin rash, changes in vital signs, or dyspnea. Reactions are most likely to occur following parenteral administration of contrast media. Nursing personnel should be prepared to treat anaphylaxis with sympathomimetic vasopressors such as epinephrine or to treat vagal reactions with atropine. Oxygen may also be required. Clients should be monitored for 30–60 minutes following treatment to ensure against recurrence of symptoms.

Client education. Clients should be informed about the usual procedure for carrying out the planned test. They should be told what will be expected of them during the procedure.

Clients who are to receive parenteral preparations should be informed that they will feel a sensation of warmth when the contrast medium is injected. All clients should be instructed to report any unusual response, especially difficulty in breathing or faintness.

Clients who have experienced adverse reactions to contrast media should be instructed to report this whenever radiographic studies are proposed involving similar agents. If the reaction was anaphylactic, a medical identification device should be carried warning of hypersensitivity to iodine contrast media.

Evaluation Data required for evaluation include absence or incidence of signs and symptoms of anxiety; the promptness of detection and treatment of adverse drug reaction; and the absence or incidence of serious sequelae following exposure to radiopaque contrast media. Client education can be evaluated by the client's ability to cooperate in conducting the diagnostic test and by client comments indicating they felt well prepared for the experience. (See accompanying Example of Nursing Process and Treatment of Radiopaque Dye Reaction.)

Checklist of nursing actions

☐ Prior to radiographic studies involving iodine contrast media, assess client for hypersensitivity to these agents, previous exposure to ionizing radiation, recent use of iodine compounds, and tissue hydration.

☐ Explain procedures to clients to reduce anxiety and promote valid test results.

☐ Provide emotional support to clients with undiagnosed health problems.

☐ Promote adequate hydration before the study is carried out.

☐ Follow test protocols carefully to ensure valid test data without repeated studies.

☐ Be prepared to treat serious adverse reactions, including anaphylaxis, should they occur.

☐ Inform clients they will feel a sensation of warmth when contrast media are injected.

☐ Monitor clients carefully for adverse reactions following administration of iodine contrast media.

☐ Urge clients who have experienced adverse reactions to contrast media to carry a medical identification device.

Agents used for volumetric diagnostic tests

Chemicals with characteristic distribution and excretion patterns can be used to assess physiologic processes by which they move through the body. Rates of uptake, distribution, storage, and excretion reflect the function of organs involved in their pharmacokinesis and can be used to measure flow rates, diffusion, and volumes of various body fluids. Chemicals that are relatively inert pharmacologically are preferred in such diagnostic studies because they induce minimal side effects and adverse reactions. The compounds used must be measurable by chemical assay, colorimetric analysis, or radioactivity monitoring.

Nonradioactive compounds

Physiology/pathology. The processes by which chemicals and fluids are distributed, metabolized, and excreted by the body can be monitored by tracer chemicals whose presence can be detected and measured. Once norms are established for a process, diagnostic tests can be developed to detect problems indicative of impairment or abnormality.

Preparations. Nonradioactive diagnostic agents are substances that can be detected by chemical or color measurements. They include polysaccharides and dyes (Table 52-3).

Pharmacodynamics. The use of volumetric diagnostic agents depends on the ways in which the compounds are distributed, metabolized, and excreted rather than on pharmacologic activity of the drugs.

Pharmacokinetics. Most volumetric agents are administered by IV injection and enter the extracellular fluid compartment. They are poorly or only temporarily bound to plasma proteins. They are usually taken up rapidly by the specific organ whose function is under study. Most are excreted by the liver or kidneys.

Diagnostic uses. Polysaccharides, phenolsulfonphthalein, and aminohippurate are used to assess kidney function. Indigotindisulfonate serves to locate the ureteral orifices and mark abnormal fluid passage from damaged ureters. The sulfobromophthalein (Bromsulphalein) test is a sensitive indicator of early liver impairment.

Adverse reactions. Side effects of polysaccharides include increased circulatory volume and diuresis sec-

Example of nursing process and treatment of radiopaque dye reaction

The client is a 43-year-old man with a history of headaches and changes in visual fields, who has been admitted to the hospital for a series of diagnostic studies. This morning he has undergone a brain scan during which a radiopaque dye containing iodine was injected by IV. In the early afternoon, he tells the nurse that his lower back and hips are itching. The affected skin is covered with various sized wheals; several scratch marks are also present.

Assessment data	Nursing diagnosis	Intervention	Goals and outcome criteria
Complaint of itching	Impaired tissue integrity: skin rash possibly related to allergic reaction to radiopaque dye	**Bathe** the affected area with cool water; apply a soothing lotion.	No new scratch marks will appear on the affected area.
Urticaria		**Advise** the client to keep the area cool to reduce itching.	The rash will gradually fade and disappear.
Scratch marks		**Advise** the client to apply pressure to itching areas rather than to scratch.	
		Take measures to reduce the client's stress level to minimize the allergic reaction.	
		Notify the physician of the adverse reaction; request antiallergy medication such as an antihistamine.	
		Provide the client with diversion to distract his attention from the itching stimuli.	

ondary to the osmotic effects of these compounds. Aminohippurate is administered in such large doses that hypervolemia also occurs initially. Large doses of indigotindisulfonate impart a temporary blue discoloration to the skin.

Among adverse reactions to these agents are nausea, vomiting, urticaria, pruritus, malaise, fever, hypotension or hypertension, and bronchoconstriction. Hypersensitivity reactions, including anaphylaxis, may occur. The compounds tend to be irritating, and extravasation during administration may cause tissue necrosis. Aminohippurate can also induce cramps and a desire to void or defecate; D-xylose can cause abdominal bloating, cramping, abdominal discomfort, and diarrhea.

Precautions and contraindications. These agents are contraindicated for clients with a history of hypersensitivity to them. They should be administered with caution to allergic clients, especially asthmatics. Equipment, supplies, and trained personnel to treat allergic

reactions, including anaphylaxis, must be available when tests are conducted.

These agents are contraindicated during pregnancy, especially in the early stages.

Compounds used for kidney function tests should be avoided when renal function is severely impaired or the recipient is dehydrated. Polysaccharides and aminohippurate are not given when pulmonary edema or active intracranial bleeding is present. These drugs must be administered with caution to clients with limited cardiac reserve because they increase blood volume. Central venous pressure should be monitored and the test discontinued if it rises.

■ Summary

Nonradioactive volumetric diagnostic agents are used to measure the concentration and movement of chemicals through the body and to ascertain volumes, flow, and diffusion of body fluids and organ function. They are commonly used to assess kidney and liver function. Serious

Table 52-3. Substances used for volumetric diagnostic tests

Drug name	Preparations	Tissue distribution	Usual adult dosage/PC	Diagnostic use
Polysaccharides				
mannitol (D-Mannitol, *Can:* Isotol, Osmitrol)	Solutions for injection (5%, 10%, 15%, 20%, or 25%)	Freely filtered by kidney glomeruli	200 mg/kg body weight PC: C	Measure glomerular filtration rate
inulin (Alantin, Starch Alant, Dahlin)	Solution for injection (100 mg/ml in 0.9% NaCl)	Freely filtered by kidney glomeruli	50 mg/kg body weight (priming dose); 18.8 mg/m² body surface area per minute (following priming dose)	Measure glomerular filtration rate
Dyes				
indigotindisulfonate (Indigo Carmine)	Solution for IM or IV injection (8 mg/ml)	Excreted by the kidneys, appearing in urine	40 mg IV; 50–100 mg IM	Localize ureteral orifices during cystoscopy and ureteral catheterization
				Identify severed ureters and fistulous communications
indocyanine green (Cardio-green)	Powder for preparing solution for IV injection	Highly bound to plasma proteins	0.5–5 mg/kg body weight	Measurement of cardiac output
		Excreted unchanged in bile		Test of hepatic function and measurement of hepatic blood flow
phenolsulfonphthalein (Phenol Red, PSP)	Solutions for IM or IV injection	Partially bound to plasma proteins	6 mg	Evaluate renal blood flow
		Excreted primarily by the kidneys		Assess urinary retention and total kidney function
sulfobromophthalein (Bromsulphalein, BSP)	Solution for IV injection	Rapidly taken up and stored by liver parenchyma	5 mg/kg body weight to maximum of 500 mg	Detect cirrhosis, acute hepatitis, and liver cell damage
Miscellaneous				
aminohippurate sodium (Sodium para-aminohippurate, PAH)	Solution for IV infusion (200 mg/ml)	Rapidly excreted from the kidneys by proximal tubular secretion and (to some extent) glomerular filtration	2 g; adjusted in accordance with plasma concentration	Estimate effective renal plasma flow
				Assess tubular secretion
sodium dehydrocholate (Decholin)	Solution for IV injection	Circulated by the blood to the tongue where it stimulates the taste buds	3–5 ml of 20% solution	Measure arm-to-tongue circulation time by counting seconds between injection and taste sensation
D-xylose (wood sugar)	Powder for oral administration	Absorbed in the GI tract and subsequently passed through the blood to the kidneys where it is excreted	25 g	Assess intestinal absorption and diagnose malabsorptive states

KEY: PC = pregnancy risk category. (The validity of pregnancy risk categories has not been established. See Chapter 16, p 216.)
Can = Canadian trade name.

reactions, including anaphylaxis, may occur during the course of such tests. These agents are not used for clients with a history of adverse reaction to them. Staff must be prepared to deal with serious adverse reactions when tests are undertaken.

Nursing management

Nursing process

Assessment Before beginning volumetric diagnostic tests, a careful history should be taken to determine whether the client has been exposed previously to the drug agent. Adverse reaction to such exposure is particularly significant. A history of allergy, especially asthma, is also pertinent. The client should be evaluated for circulatory homeostasis, as well as for cardiac and kidney function.

The client's knowledge about the scheduled test and emotional reaction to it should be explored.

Nursing diagnosis Nursing diagnoses for the client scheduled to undergo a volumetric diagnostic test may include the following:

Anxiety related to volumetric diagnostic tests and threat of an undiagnosed health problem
High risk for altered comfort: nausea, vomiting, itching, malaise, vertigo, dyspnea, and abdominal cramping related to adverse reaction to volumetric diagnostic agents
Diarrhea related to adverse reaction to D-xylose
Knowledge deficit concerning volumetric agents and their use in diagnostic procedures

Common collaborative problems that should be differentiated from the nursing diagnoses include

Potential complication: anaphylaxis
Potential complication: hypovolemia
Potential complication: hypotension

Planning Nursing goals include maintaining fluid balance, alleviating anxiety, increasing comfort, maintaining normal bowel elimination, preventing adverse drug reactions, promptly detecting and treating adverse reactions should they occur, and increasing the client's ability to cooperate in the diagnostic test.

Intervention The physician and radiologist should be notified of any risk factors apparent during the initial nursing assessment of the client. This information may include previous exposure and adverse reaction to the diagnostic agent used in the planned diagnostic test; history of asthma or other allergy; dehydration or circulatory overload; and cardiac or renal impairment.

The nurse should provide emotional support to the client. Trust in the health care team's competence and concern should be promoted. Without giving false assurances, the nurse should foster hope of a favorable outcome of diagnosis and treatment.

If the intended drug preparation contains crystals, it may be warmed and agitated gently for redissolution. Test protocols must be followed precisely. Reliability of test results depends on accurate dosage and timing of specimen collection. If a specimen collection is inadvertently delayed, the exact time it is obtained must be recorded so that proper adjustments may be made in the test calculations.

Clients must be monitored for adverse reaction to the diagnostic agent for at least 1 hour following completion of the test. Blood pressure and respirations should be monitored when agents that affect circulatory volume are used. Central venous pressure should be monitored for early detection of undesirable increases when polysaccharides or aminohippurate are used. Equipment, supplies, and trained personnel must be readily available to treat anaphylaxis, should it develop during the test.

Client education. To allay anxiety, clients should be informed of the test in terms that reflect the subjective experience they will perceive. The client's cooperation should be sought to ensure accurate completion of the test. Clients who experience a bluish skin discoloration after receiving indigotindisulfonate should be reassured that this is temporary.

Evaluation Data required for evaluation include absence or incidence of fluid imbalance (either hypovolemia or hypervolemia), diarrhea, urticaria, hypotension, soft tissue necrosis, and signs and symptoms of anxiety. Client education can be evaluated by the clients' ability to participate in the test procedure and by comments indicating that they knew what to expect during the procedure.

Checklist of nursing actions

When volumetric diagnostic tests are scheduled
- ☐ Assess clients for increased risk of adverse reaction to the drug agent (history of adverse reaction to the compound, allergy [especially asthma], cardiac or kidney impairment).
- ☐ Assess fluid balance; report to the physician any evidence of dehydration or circulatory overload.
- ☐ Describe to clients what they will experience during the test.
- ☐ Provide emotional support to clients with undiagnosed health problems.
- ☐ Follow test protocols precisely to ensure accuracy and test reliability.
- ☐ Monitor clients receiving agents that affect circulatory volume for evidence of altered circulation.
- ☐ Monitor clients for adverse reaction during and following the test procedure.

Radioactive tracers
Radioactive drugs are compounds containing atoms that disintegrate by emission of electromagnetic radiation. They may be naturally occurring radionuclides or substances prepared in particle accelerators. They are useful in diagnosis because their movements through the body can be monitored or "traced" by methods that reveal or measure radioactivity.

Box 52-2. Units used for measuring radiation

Curie	The quantity of radioactivity emitted from a radionuclide, equal to 3.7×10^{10} transformations per second
Roentgen	The quantity of X or gamma radiation in air
Rad	The dose of any ionizing radiation absorbed per unit of mass of material
Rem	Roentgen-equivalent-man; the estimated biologic effect relative to a dose of one roentgen of x-rays
MPL	Maximal permissible limit; the recommended limit of accumulated exposure to ionizing radiation at any age

The National Council of Radiation Protection and Measurements recommends the following limits: for radiation workers, 5 rems multiplied by the number of years beyond age 18, or MPL = 5(N − 18) rems. In any consecutive 13 weeks, exposure should not exceed 3 rems. For the general population, limits are one-tenth of these,

$$MPL = \frac{5(N - 18) \text{ rems}}{10}$$

Levels of radioactivity can be defined in several ways, depending on the attribute or effect in question. Definitions of terms used in measuring radiation are given in Box 52-2.

Physiology/pathology. The body handles chemicals in characteristic ways: transporting, storing, metabolizing, and excreting them so as to provide substrate for vital life processes and to eliminate toxic substances. Radionuclides allow some of these biochemical processes to be studied. Abnormalities in the distribution and concentration of radioactive chemicals reflect pathologic changes in the functions of organs containing them.

Choice of the specific chemical used in a given situation is influenced by the biochemistry of the organ or system studied. For example, radioiodine is used to study the thyroid gland because this element is used by the gland in large amounts. The concentration and distribution of radioiodine in thyroid tissue as shown on scintiphotographs yield useful information about the organ's size, integrity, and function.

Preparations. Diagnostic radionuclides include several classes of compounds used medicinally in nonradioactive forms. These may be diuretics, vitamins, dyes, or iodides (Table 52-4). Dosage is measured in curies, which are units of radioactivity. Because radioactive substances are constantly decaying (losing radioactivity), dosage must be computed according to the age of the drug. The volume or mass of drug required for a given dose of radioactivity will increase as the preparation ages.

Pharmacodynamics. Radioactive tracers emit energy particles that can be detected or measured by photography, scintiscopy, scintiphotography, monitoring with Geiger counters, or other techniques for measuring radioactivity.

Pharmacokinetics. Radioactive compounds are handled by the body in the same way as normal chemicals. They are administered orally or parenterally. Distribution, storage, metabolism, and excretion are identical to the compound in its nonradioactive form.

Radiation effects at any given time depend not only on tissue concentration but on residual radioactivity in the drug as well. Tissue concentration of the chemical depends on distribution and biologic half-life of the compound. It decreases as the compound is deactivated and excreted by the body. Concurrently, radioactive decay reduces the ionizing activity of the drug residues as decay proceeds. Radioactivity declines in inverse proportion to radioactive half-life of the chemical.

Diagnostic uses. Radionuclides are used as radioactive tracers in three types of diagnostic procedures: biochemical concentration, dilution techniques, and flow or diffusion measurements. Concentration, commonly measured by scintiscope or scintiphotographs of the body area being studied, reflects organ or tissue function (Fig. 52-1). Dilution techniques are used to determine volume of whole blood, total body water, red blood cells, or other components. Cardiac output, pulmonary ventilation, and peripheral vascular circulation are among the measures taken by flow or diffusion tests.

Adverse reactions. Although they have the same potential for producing toxic effects and side effects as their nonradioactive counterparts, diagnostic radionuclides are administered in such small doses that adverse reactions are unlikely except with iodides, which can trigger allergic responses in some recipients (see previous section, Iodinated Contrast Media).

The radioactivity of these compounds is potentially toxic. Radiation emitted includes beta and gamma particles (Table 52-5). Because of their high radiation and low penetrating ability, substances emitting alpha particles are not used medicinally.

There is no evidence that clients incur measurable

harm from the doses usually given in diagnostic procedures. However, each exposure to ionizing radiation adds to the cumulative lifetime load. Excessive exposure is associated with increased risk of malignant neoplasms, congenital defects in offspring, and premature aging. Rapidly dividing cells are most vulnerable to the harmful effects of radiation.

Precautions and contraindications. Precautions pertinent to the nonradioactive form of the drug in use are appropriate (see previous discussion on iodides in this chapter). In addition, special precautions to control radioactive exposure are required when using radionuclides. All radiobiologic products are controlled by the Division of Biologics Standards of the United States Public Health Service. In Canada, radiopharmaceuticals are controlled by the Atomic Energy Control Board. Persons and institutions wishing to use radioactive substances in the United States must be licensed by the Atomic Energy Commission.

When radionuclides are used, precautions must be taken to control exposure of everyone in the area. Dosage of ionizing radiation is proportional to the time spent in proximity to the source of emissions and inversely related to the distance between subject and source. Shielding with lead barriers decreases exposure.

Clients most vulnerable to radiation damage are those with rapidly dividing cells (high growth rates). To prevent exposure of embryos, tests performed on women of childbearing age should be scheduled for the first half of the menstrual cycle. Testing of children and nursing mothers is avoided whenever possible (radioactive chemicals may be secreted in breast milk following the test).

Clients receiving tracer doses experience minimal exposure. Neither their bodies nor their excreta are considered significant sources of radiation. No special precautions need be taken by persons undergoing diagnostic tests with radionuclides. (This does *not* apply to recipients of *therapeutic* doses, which involve much larger amounts of radiation.)

Personnel working in nuclear medicine units are at greater risk than clients because they spend more time near radioactive materials. Operating procedures are designed to minimize exposure of personnel. All workers wear devices that measure radiation exposure. When individual exposure levels approach maximal permissible levels, the person must be assigned to other work until an appropriate time period has elapsed without further exposure.

■ Summary

Radioactive tracers are radionuclides used in small doses to assess the function of body organs or tissues and to measure fluid volume, flow, or diffusion. Although they emit beta and gamma radiation, these compounds add little to the cumulative radiation load of the client undergoing single tests. Clients exposed to repeated testing and personnel in nuclear medicine units receive greater doses. Use of radiopharmaceuticals is limited to personnel and institutions licensed by the Atomic Energy Commission.

Nursing management

Nursing implications

Radioactive compounds should be stored in lead containers to control ionizing emissions. In addition, storage must be appropriate to the chemical nature of the substance. Radiocyanocobalamin must be refrigerated. Solutions may darken with time but this does not alter efficacy.

Duration of radioactive emissions in the body is influenced by two variables: the biologic half-life of the compound and its physical half-life. Biologic half-life varies and depends on metabolic and excretory function. For this reason, clients with liver or kidney impairment receive more radiation than those with normal organ function. Physical half-life reflects the rate of decay of the radionuclide and is the same in all clients. Radioactivity declines by 50% in each half-life period. After seven half-lives have elapsed, radioactivity of any remaining material is less than 1% of the original level.

During procedures involving radionuclides, protocols for handling radioactive compounds must be followed carefully. Nurses working in nuclear medicine units must be trained in radiation control techniques.

Nursing process

Assessment Clients undergoing diagnostic tests should be assessed for risk of adverse reactions to the chemical to be used. If an iodide is to be administered, a history of past response to iodides must be carefully taken and any severe or repeated adverse reaction to these drugs must be reported to the physician. The nurse should initiate nursing measures to support the client and reduce discomfort from such reactions as nausea, vomiting, itching, or diarrhea. Exposure to ionizing radiation should also be assessed (see previous discussion in this chapter).

The client's knowledge of and emotional reaction to the proposed diagnostic test should be explored.

Nursing diagnosis Nursing diagnoses for clients undergoing radioactive tracer tests include the following:

Anxiety related to exposure to irradiation secondary to diagnostic procedure using radioisotopes

(Text continues on p. 1328)

Table 52-4. Radioactive tracer compounds

Drug name	Preparations	Usual adult dosage	Physical half-life	Whole body radiation exposure (for adult male of 70 kg)	Diagnostic uses
Mercurial diuretics					
chlormerodrin $^{Hg}197$ (Neohydrin-197)	Solution for IV injection	For kidney imaging: 100–150 μc; For brain imaging: 10 μc/kg body weight to a maximum of 1,050 μc	64.8 hours	17 mrad/μc administered	Assess the anatomic and functional integrity of the kidneys; Localize brain tumors
chlormerodrin $^{Hg}203$ (Neohydrin-203)	Solution for IV injection	For brain imaging: 10 μc/kg body weight to a maximum of 700 μc	46.6 days		Assess the anatomic and functional integrity of the kidneys; Localize brain tumors
Vitamins					
cyanocobalamin $^{Co}57$ (Rubratope-57, Racobalamin-57)	Capsules and solutions for oral use; Solution for IM or SC injection	Oral: 0.5 μc	270 days	9.6 mrad/μc administered	Assess GI absorption of cyanocobalamin; Differentiate pernicious anemia from other causes of cyanocobalamin malabsorption; Assess liver uptake of cyanocobalamin
Dyes					
rose bengal sodium $^{I}131$ (Radio-iodinated Rose Bengal, Robengatope)	Solution for IV injection	For nonscanning liver studies: 5–25 μc	8.08 days	1.47 mrad/μc administered	Assess liver function; Detect biliary obstruction
Iodides					
iodinated $^{I}125$ serum albumin (Albumotope I-125, Risa-125, IHSA-I-125)	Solution for IV injection	5–60 μc	60 days	0.4 mrad/μc administered	Measure blood or plasma volume
sodium iodide $^{I}125$ (Iodotope I-125)	Capsules and solution for oral use; Solution for IV injection	For thyroid uptake study: 50–100 μc; For protein bound iodine study: 25–50 μc	60 days	0.39 mrad/μc administered	Assess thyroid function
iodinated $^{I}131$ serum albumin (Albumotope I-131, IHSA-I^{131}, Risa-131)	Solution for IV injection	For blood and plasma volume determinations: 5–60 μc; For placenta location: 5–10 μc	8.08 days	1.7 mrad/μc administered	Measure blood or plasma volume; Placenta location

Name	Preparations	Usual dose	Half-life	Radiation	Use
iodinated I131 serum albumin, macroaggregated (Albumotope-LS, MAA131I, Macroscan-131)	Solution for IV injection	150–300 μc	8.08 days	0.67 mrad/μc administered	Assess arterial perfusion of the lungs
iodohippurate sodium I 131 (Hippuran I 131, Hipputope-131)	Solution for IV injection	For nonimaging renal function: 1–30 μc; For kidney imaging: 200–300 μc	8.08 days	0.03 mrad/μc administered	Assess kidney function
sodium iodide I131 (Radiocaps-131, Tracervial-131)	Capsules and solution for oral use; Solution for IV injection	For thyroid uptake test: 1–25 μc; For thigh–neck clearance test: 10–50 μc; For PBI and conversion ratio studies: 25–30 μc; For thyroid imaging: 50–100 μc	8.08 days	0.5 mrad/μc administered	Assess thyroid function; Localize thyroid tissue or tumors
Miscellaneous					
sodium pertechnetate Tc 99m (Pertechtin, Pertscan-99m)	Generators for producing solutions for oral or IV administration	For brain imaging: 5–15 mc; For cardiac blood pool imaging: 3–5 mc; For salivary gland imaging: 1–5 mc	6 hours	0.013 mrad/mc administered	Locate intracranial lesions; Assess salivary gland function; Assess cardiac blood pool
sodium phosphate P32 (Phosphotope)	Capsules and solution for oral use; Solution for IV injection	250–1,000 μc	14.3 days	1 mrad/μc administered during the first 3 days; after this time, exposure varies with the tissues involved	Locate ocular tumors; Locate cerebral tumors when other agents or techniques are unsuitable
technetium sulfide Tc 99m (Technetium Sulfide Tc 99m Colloid, Technetium Sulfur Colloid Tc 99m)	Generator for producing solutions for IV injection; Solutions for IV injection	1–3 mc	6 hours	16.7 mrad/mc administered	Produce images of the liver and spleen
sodium chromate Cr51 (Chromitope Sodium, Rachromate-51)	Solution for *in vitro* labeling of red blood vessels and subsequent IV administration	For estimating red blood cell volume: 15–20 μc; For estimating RBC survival time: 100 μc; For estimating GI blood loss: 150–200 μc	27.8 days	0.24 mrad/μc administered	Measure red cell or total blood volume, red cell survival time, and GI loss
thallium	Solution for injection	2 mc (given in conjunction with dipyridamole)	Not available	Not available	Detect the presence and assess the severity of coronary artery disease

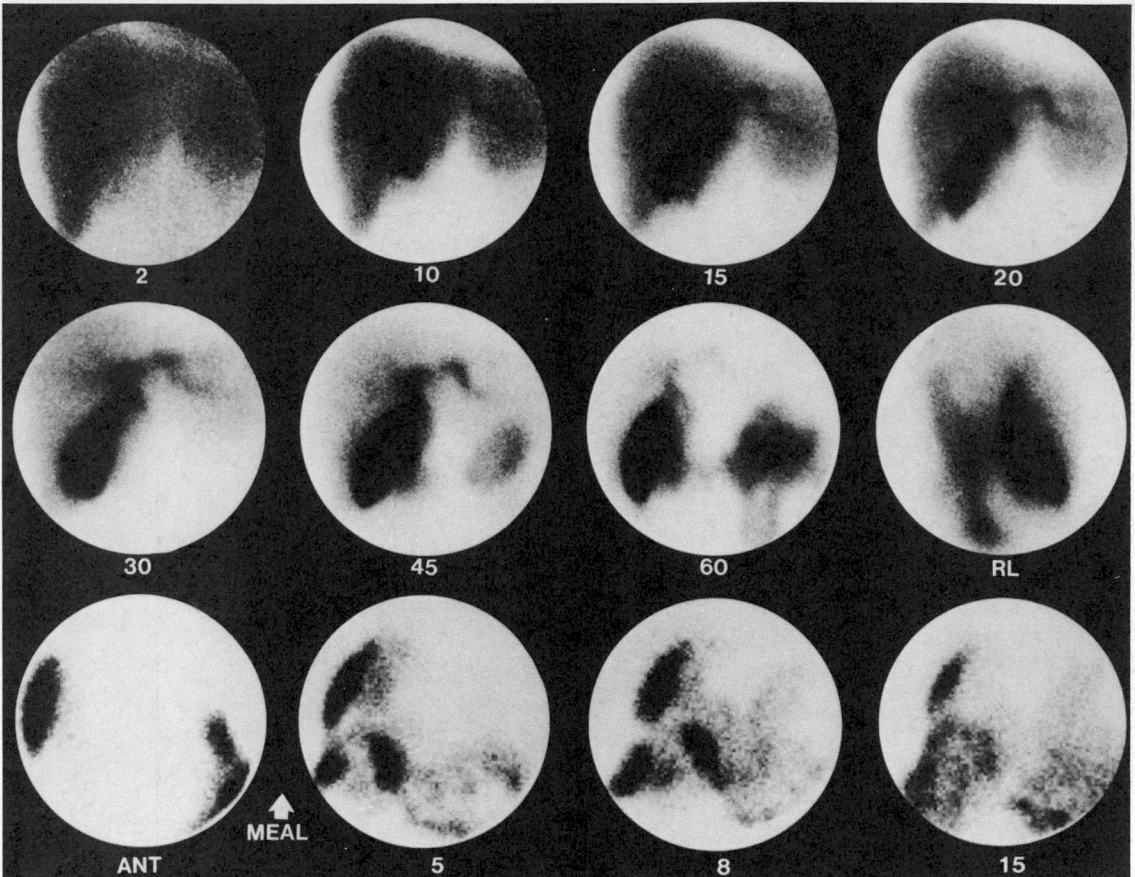

Figure 52-1. Serial images produced by a ^{99m}Tc-HIDA cholescintigram. Numbers under the images indicate the minutes elapsed since administration of the tracer. Normal features include rapid hepatic uptake of tracer; visualization of main biliary ducts by 10 minutes after administration; progressive gallbladder accumulation of tracer; and appearance of intestinal activity by 45 minutes. Anterior gallbladder location is demonstrated on right lateral (*RL*) view. Subsequent images with diverging collimator show normal response to orally ingested fatty meal with rapid reduction in gallbladder size and activity and markedly increased intestinal activity within 15 minutes. Rothfeld B. [1980]. *Nuclear medicine: Hepatorenal*, p 25. Philadelphia: JB Lippincott.)

Anxiety related to an undiagnosed health problem

Planning Nursing goals include alleviating anxiety and preventing or promptly detecting and treating adverse drug reactions.

Intervention The physician and radiologist should be notified of any history of adverse reaction to the chemical to be used for testing or of unusual exposure to ionizing irradiation.

Clients need emotional support during diagnostic procedures involving radionuclides. Not only are they threatened by an as yet unidentified disease process, but they are also often acutely aware of the risks inherent in exposure to ionizing radiation. Anxiety may be heightened by perception of the protective measures taken by personnel in the nuclear medicine unit.

Client education. Clients undergoing diagnostic studies involving radioactive tracers should be reassured that exposure to ionizing radiation in such tests is comparable to radiographic procedures. Although repeated exposure is undesirable, isolated or limited testing involves little risk. No undesirable effects have been detected as direct effects of tracer doses. No special precautions are required of the client undergoing such a study.

Evaluation Data required for evaluation include the incidence or absence of adverse reactions; the incidence or absence of serious sequelae following adverse reactions; and reports from the client indicating that discomfort was reduced by the nursing care given.

Checklist of nursing actions

☐ Assess clients for risk of adverse response to the chemical substance in use (*eg*, allergy to iodides).

Table 52-5. Types of radiation emitted by radionuclides

Type of radiation	Nature of particles emitted	Characteristics
Alpha	Positively charged helium ion (helium nucleus)	Has a relatively low velocity
		Has low penetrative capacity
		Is blocked by a thin sheet of paper
		Deposits a large radiation dose in short distances
		(Not used medicinally)
Beta	Negatively charged electrons	Is more penetrative than alpha rays
		Is blocked by tissue from 1 mm to more than 1 cm thick, depending on density
Gamma	Identical to x-rays except for differing wavelengths	Has high velocity and penetrative power

☐ Assess clients' exposure to ionizing radiation; report unusual histories to the physician.

☐ Provide emotional support during the procedure.

☐ Reassure clients that tracer doses of radionuclides carry no demonstrable risk of physical harm.

Provocative agents

Drugs used in provocative diagnostic tests are administered to induce a measurable response in the body, the magnitude of which is medically significant. Most drugs fall into one of two categories: secretagogues and agents that influence endocrine secretion or activity. Secretagogues act to stimulate exocrine secretion such as production of gastric acid, pepsin, and pancreatic enzymes, as well as contraction of the gallbladder. Agents affecting endocrine function include autocoids such as tropic hormones and histamine; hormone inhibitors such as metyrapone; competitive inhibitors of hormones such as saralasin; and chemicals that influence endocrine activity by as yet unknown mechanisms.

Preparations. Provocative agents are usually administered parenterally. Doses vary but tend to be very small for autocoids. (These physiologic constituents are produced in minute amounts by the body and are very potent.) Because they tend to be unstable, many injectable solutions must be refrigerated. Some are marketed in powder form and are freshly reconstituted at the time of administration (Table 52-6).

Pharmacodynamics. Many secretagogues and tropic hormones stimulate organ functions by the same mechanism as natural autocoids. Mechanisms of action of other drugs in this group vary. Metyrapone inhibits adrenal cortex production of cortisol, triggering the negative feedback mechanism that stimulates pituitary secretion of adrenocorticotropin. Anticholinesterases oppose the breakdown of acetylcholine by the enzyme cholinesterase, inducing a rise in tissue levels of the neurotransmitter. Saralasin decreases physiologic response to angiotensin II by competitive inhibition at its receptor site on smooth muscle of blood vessels.

Pharmacokinetics. Most provocative agents are administered systemically. After absorption into the circulation, they move to the target organ or tissue, where they induce a characteristic alteration of physiology. Metabolic deactivation, especially with autocoids, occurs rapidly.

Diagnostic uses. See Table 52-6 for diagnostic uses of specific provocative agents.

Adverse reactions. Because most secretagogues influence multiple body processes, they tend to produce multiple side effects. Pentagastrin increases GI motility, stimulates pancreatic and biliary secretion, inhibits water and electrolyte absorption from the ileum, and promotes sodium and chloride diuresis. It may produce cramping pain, nausea and vomiting, and borborygmi. Secretin stimulates duodenal and intestinal secretion, pepsinogen release in the stomach, and insulin release.

Secretagogues also affect the cardiovascular system. Side effects of pentagastrin include hypotension, palpitation, dizziness, faintness, or lightheadedness, and a feeling of tightness in the chest. Both this drug and betazole tend to produce tachycardia and a subjective feeling of warmth. Betazole also can induce flushing and diaphoresis. Drowsiness, blurred vision, fatigue, and headache have been reported with pentagastrin.

Secretagogues can produce acute symptoms of GI disease. Gallbladder stimulation tends to move stones into the common bile duct, where they can obstruct the flow of bile. Increased secretion of gastric acid and pepsin exacerbate the symptoms of peptic ulcer. Stimulation of pancreatic exocrine secretion increases symptoms of pancreatitis. As a result, tests may be followed by abdominal pain, nausea or vomiting, and increased risk of complications such as hemorrhage, perforation, and shock.

The sudden increase in hormone production induced by endocrine stimulants can produce toxic symptoms. Such reactions are most likely to occur in clients being evaluated for excess hormone production. For example, a histamine test is apt to produce a

Table 52-6. Provocative agents used for diagnostic tests

Drug name	Preparations	Mechanism of action	Usual adult dosage/PC	Diagnostic use
Secretagogues				
pentagastrin (Gastro-diagnost, Paptavlon)	Solution for SC injection	Stimulation of gastric acid secretion	6 μg/kg of body weight	Evaluation of gastric acid secretion
betazole hydrochloride (Histalog)	Solution for Im or SC injection	Stimulation of gastric secretion of hydro-chloric acid	0.5 mg/kg body weight	Testing of gastric secretory capabilities
secretin	Powder for preparing solutions for IV infusion	Stimulation of pan-creatic secretion	1 C.H.R. unit*/kg of body weight over 5 min	Diagnosis of chronic pancreatic dysfunction
sincalide (C8-CCK, Kinevac, OP-CCK)	Powder for preparing solutions for IV injection	Stimulation of gall-bladder contraction and evacuation. Stimulation of pan-creatic secretion	0.02 μg/kg body weight	Assessment of gall-bladder function in conjunction with cholecystography or bile aspiration. Assessment of pancre-atic exocrine function
Stimulants to endocrine secretion				
corticotropin (ACTH, Acthar, adrenocor-ticotropin hormone, Cortrophin)	Gel or solution for IM or IV injection	Stimulation of adrenal cortex secretion of glucocorticoids	10–40 units PC: C	Diagnosis of adreno-corticoid insufficiency
cosyntropin (Syn-Cortrosyn, Synacthen, Tetracosa-peptide, Tetracosactide, Tetracosactrin)	Powder for preparing solutions for IM or IV injection	Stimulation of adrenal cortex secretion of glucocorticoids	250 μg PC: C	Diagnosis of adreno-corticoid insufficiency
thyrotropin (Thytropar, T.S.H.)	Powder for preparing solutions for IM or SC injection	Stimulation of thyroid secretion of iodinated hormones (thyroxine and others)	10 IU	Differential diagnosis of primary thyroidal myxedema from pitui-tary myxedema
histamine	Solutions for IV injection	Stimulation of cate-cholamine release	10 μg of histamine base† initially	Diagnosis of pheochromocytoma
metyrapone (Metopirone)	Tablets for oral use	Stimulation of pitui-tary secretion of ACTH by inhibiting hydrocortisone secre-tion by the adrenal cortex	Orally, 750 mg q4h for 6 doses PC: C	Evaluation of hypo-thalamic pituitary function in the diagnosis of hypopituitarism. Differential diagnosis of primary from sec-ondary Cushing's syndrome
sodium tolbutamide (Orinase Diagnostic)	Powder for preparing solutions for IV injection	Stimulation of insulin secretion by beta cells of the pancreatic islets	1 g PC: C	Diagnosis of mild dia-betes mellitus, pancre-atic carcinoma, acute pancreatitis, and func-tional pancreatic islet-cell tumor
arginine hydrochloride (R-Gene 10)	Powder for preparing solutions for IV injection	Stimulation of pitui-tary secretion of GH	30 g infused over 30 minutes as a 10% solution. In children, 500 mg/kg of body weight	Evaluation of pituitary growth hormone reserve
Anticholinesterases				
edrophonium chloride (Enlon, Tensilon)	Solution for IV, IM, or SC injection	Inhibition of cholines-terase and subsequent accumulation of acetylcholine	10 mg PC: C	Diagnosis of my-asthenia gravis. Differentiation of cho-linergic crisis from myasthenia crisis

(Continued)

Table 52-6. Provocative agents used for diagnostic tests (Continued)

Drug name	Preparations	Mechanism of action	Usual adult dosage/PC	Diagnostic use
Anticholinesterases				
saralasin (Sarenin)	Solution for IV infusion	Competitive inhibition of angiotensin II at the receptor site	18 mg over 20–30 min *or* 0.05 µg/kg body weight/min, increased by 5, 10, and 20 µg/min at 10 min intervals.	Assess the function of endogenous angiotensin II in the regulation of blood pressure
Cholinergics				
methacholine	Metered dose inhaler	Bronchoconstriction	Five breaths	Diagnosis of asthma in the absence of clinically obvious asthma
Nutrient				
glucose	Flavored solution for ingestion	Hyperglycemia and insulin secretion	75 g	Diagnosis of diabetes mellitus and reactive hypoglycemia

* Crick-Harper-Raper unit.

† 1 mg histamine base is equivalent to 2.75 mg histamine phosphate.

KEY: PC = pregnancy risk category. (The validity of pregnancy risk categories has not been established. See Chapter 16, p 216.)

severe hypertensive reaction in clients with pheochromocytoma. By their very nature, provocative tests tend to produce exaggerated responses that can reach serious proportions.

Adverse reaction to saralasin is rare. Headache, hypotension, lightheadedness, nausea, and discomfort at the injection site have been reported. Clients who are severely sodium depleted prior to the test may experience an exaggerated depressor response, as well as signs and symptoms of circulatory shock.

Allergic reactions to provocative agents are fairly common. Some agents are proteins derived from animal material and are highly antigenic. Allergic manifestations include pruritic rashes, bronchospasm, and anaphylaxis.

Precautions and contraindications. Secretagogues that increase gastric acid secretion are contraindicated in clients with acute peptic ulcer disease. They should be used with caution in clients with pancreatic, hepatic, or biliary tract disease.

When tests of endocrine function are scheduled, the health care team must be prepared to treat toxic reactions characterized by sudden increases in hormone levels. Adrenergic blocking agents, such as phentolamine, are used to treat hypertensive crises following administration of histamine.

Edrophonium can cause cholinergic crisis, respiratory paralysis, or cardiac arrest. Although infrequent, such reactions must be treated vigorously. Before administration of edrophonium, atropine is often administered to clients who are over 50 years old to prevent muscarinic side effects. Atropine sulfate should always be available as an antagonist when edrophonium is used.

Although *mild* sodium depletion increases blood pressure response to saralasin, clients scheduled to undergo a saralasin infusion test should *not* be *severely* sodium depleted. If hypotensive shock occurs during the test, the saralasin infusion is discontinued and normal saline administered by IV. Blood pressure is monitored q15 min for 3 hours to detect continued hypotension or rebound hypertension.

Provocative agents are administered with caution to clients with a history of allergy, especially asthma. Skin tests may be administered prior to initiation of the test to detect allergic hypersensitivity. Equipment, supplies, and personnel trained in the treatment of acute allergic reaction such as anaphylaxis should be available when provocative tests are undertaken.

■ Summary

Provocative diagnostic agents include secretagogues and stimulants of endocrine secretion. They are used in tests to diagnose GI and endocrine disease and myasthenia gravis.

Because they manipulate physiologic processes, provocative tests carry an inherent risk. Exaggerated responses can be life-threatening. Tests designed to exaggerate symptoms characteristic of disease are most likely to produce severe reactions in diseased clients.

Provocative agents tend to be allergenic. Allergic reactions range from skin rashes to anaphylaxis.

Nursing management

Nursing implications

To yield reliable data, provocative tests must be conducted with meticulous attention to detail. Drug dosage must be accurately measured. Syringes or IV tubing should be rinsed and the washings administered to ensure delivery of a complete dose. Timing of drug administration and specimen collection are also crucial. If either is delayed, the exact times must be reported so that calculations can be adjusted accordingly and misinterpretations of data avoided.

Risk of toxic reaction depends on the nature of both the disease suspected to be present and the physiologic response to the drug agent. Whenever a provocative test is intended to increase signs or symptoms of the suspected disease, risk of serious reaction is high.

Nursing process

Assessment Before beginning provocative tests, the client should be assessed for increased risk of adverse reaction. A history of previous exposure and reaction to the intended drug agent and of allergic disease, personal and familial, should be taken.

The client's knowledge of and emotional reaction to the scheduled test should be explored.

Clients scheduled for tests involving secretagogues that increase hydrochloric acid secretion should be screened for peptic ulcer disease or other conditions associated with gastric hyperacidity. When a saralasin infusion test is planned, sodium balance should be determined; *mild* sodium depletion is desirable.

Nursing diagnosis Nursing diagnoses appropriate or clients undergoing provocative tests include the following:

> *High risk for altered comfort: itching related to toxic or side effects of provocative agents*
> *Anxiety related to provocative tests and undiagnosed health problem*
> *Knowledge deficit concerning provocative agents and the diagnostic tests in which they are used*

Planning Nursing goals for the client undergoing provocative diagnostic tests are to increase comfort; prevent adverse drug reactions; promptly detect and treat adverse drug reactions should they occur; reduce anxiety; and educate the person about provocative agents and their use in diagnostic procedures.

Intervention The nurse should report promptly to the physician any risk factors revealed during the initial nursing assessment. If a history of allergy is found, a skin sensitivity test should be ordered to rule out allergic hypersensitivity to the test agent.

Clients undergoing provocative diagnostic tests are uncertain of the outcome and are understandably apprehensive that serious disease may be discovered. Their anxiety is compounded by the nature of many tests, which often involve parenteral injections and precise timing. By working competently and expressing a warm concern for the client, the nurse promotes trust in the health care team, thus reducing client anxiety.

Before the test is begun, chemical antidotes and equipment must be readily available (Table 52-7). The

Table 52-7. Treatment measures for reactions to provocative tests

Test	Adverse reaction	Corrective action
Gastric acid secretion	Epigastric pain	Analgesics
	Increased risk of gastric hemorrhage	Nasogastric suction/transfusion/surgery
	Increased risk of perforation of peptic ulcer	Nasogastric suction/surgery
	Hypotension	Epinephrine
	Bronchospasm	Epinephrine
Pancreatic function	Pain and shock	Analgesics, nasogastric suction, IV fluid therapy
Gallbladder function	Acute symptoms of cholecystitis or biliary obstruction	Analgesics/surgery
Pheochromocytoma (histamine)	Hypertensive crisis	Phentolamine and other vasodilators
	Hypotension	Epinephrine
	Bronchospasm	Epinephrine
Myasthenia gravis	Cholinergic crisis	Atropine/assisted ventilation
methacholine	Marked bronchoconstriction	A beta-adrenergic agonist by inhalation
glucose tolerance test	Hypoglycemia	Sugar (sweetened fruit juice, candy, table sugar) or glucagon
All tests	Allergy/anaphylaxis	Epinephrine, antihistamines, corticosteroids

nurse assists in administering the provocative agent and in accurately observing the results. Timing is crucial to most tests. If a specimen or an observation is unavoidably delayed, the exact time it is performed should be recorded so that calculations using the data can be adjusted to correct for the delay.

During and following the test, clients should be closely monitored for signs and symptoms of toxicity or adverse reactions. Following a saralasin test with a positive result, clients should be monitored for rebound hypertension. Following a methacholine test, a beta-adrenergic agonist may be ordered to reverse bronchoconstriction.

Client education. Tests should be explained to clients in terms appropriate to their level of intellectual capacity and education. The subjective perceptions and sensations likely to occur should be described. Although the risks of the procedure must be explained, the client should be reassured that serious reactions are infrequent, and that skilled medical treatment is available.

Evaluation Data required for evaluation include incidence or absence of adverse reaction; incidence or absence of serious sequelae following the tests; and comments by clients indicating that their discomforts and anxieties were reduced. Client education can be evaluated according to the extent to which the client cooperates in the conducting of the test.

Checklist of nursing actions

☐ Assess clients for previous exposure or adverse reaction to the drug used and for allergy; report significant findings to the physician promptly.

☐ Explain the test procedure to clients in terms of the subjective sensations and perceptions they will experience.

☐ Ensure that equipment, supplies, and personnel to treat adverse reactions are readily available.

☐ Follow test protocols exactly to ensure accuracy of test results.

☐ Monitor clients closely to detect adverse reactions promptly.

☐ Provide emotional support to clients throughout the procedure.

Dermal reactivity indicators

Dermal reactivity indicators are substances used to determine the presence of antibodies by means of skin tests for hypersensitivity.

Preparations. Antigenic preparations used for skin testing include concentrates derived from microbial cultures and extracts from antigenic materials (Table 52-8). They are marketed as solutions for patch, scratch, or intradermal tests. Testing materials for sensitivity to some pathogens are also marketed in the form of solution-coated tines for multipuncture skin tests. These preparations should be protected from heat because most are proteinaceous. Materials for tine testing are not refrigerated, however, because moisture within the sealed package may condense, causing a loss in potency.

Pharmacodynamics. Antigenic material induces an antigen–antibody reaction, producing local inflammation proportional to the client's degree of hypersensitivity. The substance is applied to the skin or injected intradermally; the area of erythema or induration is measured after a specified time. Skin tests for sensitivity to infectious pathogens require hours (up to 2 days) for the reaction to appear. Tests for allergic sensitivity are read within minutes.

A positive response to microbial extracts indicates previous exposure to the pathogen but does not necessarily mean that active infection is present. Positive reactions indicate the need for further diagnostic studies to rule out active disease. A negative response does not rule out disease in symptomatic clients. Severe infections can overwhelm the body's immune defenses, depleting antibody titers to levels too low to produce a skin reaction.

Pharmacokinetics. Dermal reactivity indicators are applied to the skin, where they induce a local response. The material is absorbed systemically and sometimes reacts with antibodies in the tissues. The antigen–antibody complexes are assimilated by phagocytosis.

Diagnostic uses. See Table 52-8 for diagnostic tests specific to each dermal reactivity indicator.

Adverse reactions. Local reactions to skin tests include ulceration and necrosis in response to microbial extracts and itching after skin tests for allergy. Systemic allergic reactions can occur, although these are rare because of the low doses used.

Precautions and contraindications. Using dermal reactivity indicators to diagnose infectious disease is contraindicated in clients who have previously exhibited a severe local reaction to the specific antigen. For example, anyone who has developed tissue breakdown following an old tuberculin test should not be subjected again to skin testing for tuberculosis. When a high degree of sensitivity is suspected, an initial test with extremely dilute solutions should be used.

■ Summary

Dermal reactivity indicators are allergenic materials used in skin tests to evaluate sensitivity to infectious pathogens or allergenic substances.

Table 52-8. Dermal reactivity indicators used in skin tests

Drug name	Preparations	Usual adult dosage	Diagnostic test
Microbial extracts			
coccidioidin	Solution for intradermal injection (1:100 and 1:10)	0.1 ml of 1:100 dilution	Sensitivity to the organism that causes coccidioidomycosis or to assess the status of cell-mediated immunity
histoplasmin	Solution for intradermal injection (1:100) Tine test (1:100)	0.1 ml 1 dosage unit	Sensitivity to the organism that causes histoplasmosis or to assess the status of cell-mediated immunity
tuberculin old tuberculin (OT)	Tine test (multipuncture device)	1 dosage unit	Sensitivity to the tubercle bacillus
purified protein derivative (PPD)	Solutions for intradermal injection—1 TU*/0.1 ml, 5 TU/0.1 ml, 250 TU/9.1 ml Tine test (multipuncture device)	0.1 ml (of 5 TU/0.1 ml) 1 dosage unit	Sensitivity to the tubercle bacillus
mumps skin test antigen	Suspension for intradermal injection	0.1 ml	Sensitivity to the mumps virus or to assess the status of cell-mediated immunity
Allergic extracts			
Extracts of material from virtually any allergenic substance can be prepared for skin testing purposes. Common extracts used for allergy testing include ragweed, grasses, molds, animal danders, and food substances.	Suspensions for intradermal injection of varying dilutions	0.1 ml	Allergic sensitivity to foreign antigens

*Tuberculin units.

They are applied to the skin by patch, scratch, or intradermal techniques. The development of local inflammation indicates a positive response. The reaction is proportional to antibody levels.

Systemic allergic reactions can occur following skin tests, although they are rare because of the low doses used. Health care personnel involved in such tests must be prepared to treat both systemic and local reactions if they occur. Local reactions may also be severe in highly sensitive clients, producing ulceration or necrosis.

Nursing management

Nursing implications

Skin testing for allergy can precipitate an acute systemic allergic reaction. For this reason, medical treatment, including a physician, should be readily available.

Nursing process

Assessment A history of previous skin testing and reactions to allergenic substances should be taken before dermal reactivity indicators are administered.

Any systemic or severe local reaction should be reported to the physician. An initial test with a dilute solution (commonly one-tenth the usual concentration) may be desirable.

Nursing diagnosis Nursing diagnoses appropriate for the client undergoing dermal sensitivity testing include the following:

Altered comfort: itching related to antigen–antibody reaction secondary to exposure to allergenic extracts
High risk for injury: falls related to dizziness or loss of consciousness secondary to use of saralasin

Planning Nursing goals for the client undergoing skin testing are to prevent or promptly detect and treat adverse reaction to the allergens used, alleviate itching, and restore tissue perfusion.

Intervention The nurse should report promptly to the physician any risk factors revealed during the nursing assessment. An initial test using a very dilute (usually 1 : 10) solution of antigen should be performed if the client's history indicates likelihood of an exaggerated response to the usual preparations.

Skin testing for sensitivity to infectious pathogens

is commonly performed by nursing personnel, often in a public health agency or other community setting. Systemic reactions to these solutions are unlikely. The tine test is increasingly used because of its convenience and low level of trauma.

When intradermal tests are ordered, care must be taken to avoid piercing the internal layers of the skin; subcutaneous penetration may produce a false-positive reaction. Tuberculin syringes are used for such tests because the volumes to be administered are very small (0.01–0.1 ml).

Clients undergoing skin tests for allergy must be observed for systemic reactions. Signs and symptoms include sneezing, rhinorrhea, itching in areas other than the test site, and difficulty in breathing. Anaphylaxis may occur. Epinephrine and antihistamines should be readily available to treat such reactions.

Client education. Before skin tests are performed, the nature of the test should be explained to the client. The possible results (and their significance) should also be described.

To relieve discomfort, clients should be advised to apply pressure or cold compresses to test sites that itch.

Evaluation Data required for evaluation include incidence or absence of signs and symptoms of adverse reaction; incidence or absence of serious sequelae from adverse reactions; and comments by the client indicating that itching was promptly relieved.

Checklist of nursing actions

☐ Question clients who are to undergo skin sensitivity tests about previous tests of this nature and their responses to them; report systemic or severe local reactions to the physician.

☐ Measure doses of dermal reactivity indicators in tuberculin syringes for greater accuracy in dispensing small volumes.

☐ Avoid piercing the inner layers of the skin when performing intradermal tests.

☐ Observe clients receiving allergenic extracts for signs and symptoms of systemic reaction.

☐ Explain tests and the significance of the results to clients undergoing skin tests.

☐ Advise clients to apply pressure or cold compresses to skin sites that itch following completion of the tests.

References

Severe adverse reactions to barium enema procedure (1990). *FDA Drug Bulletin, October 1990*, p. 2.
Tests hazardous to elderly. (1985). *Nursing 85, 15(12)*, 15 (December).

Bibliography

Godwin C. (1985). Outpatient myelography. *Nursing 85, 15(12)*, 57.
Lam J, et al. (1988). Safety and diagnostic accuracy of dipyridamole-thallium imaging in the elderly. *J Am Coll Cardiol, 11(3)*, 585–589 (March).
McEvoy GK. *Drug information 91*, pp 1391–1477. Bethesda MD: American Society of Hospital Pharmacists.
Monroe D. (1989). Patient teaching for x-ray and other diagnostics. *RN, 42(12)*, 36–40 (December).
New drugs: Asthma diagnostic. (1987). *American Journal of Nursing, 87*, 646 (May).
Robertson C. (1988). What glucose tolerance test results mean. *RN, 51(6)*, 89–90 (June).
Schwab S, et al. (1989). Contrast nephrotoxicity: A randomized controlled trial of a nonionic and an ionic radiographic contrast agent. *N Engl J Med, 320*, 149–153 (January 19).
Winfield AG. (1989). Dipyridamole-thallium testing. *Nursing 89, 19(9)*, 85 (September).

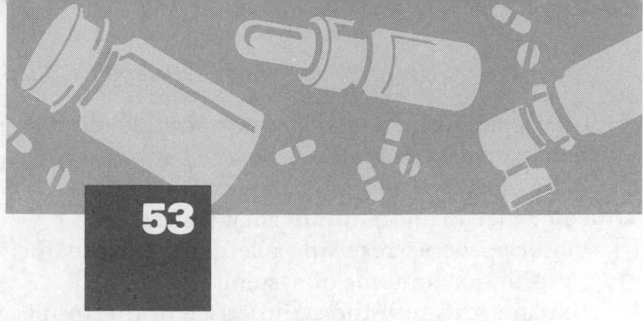

Enzymes and drugs affecting enzymes

Enzymes

Enzymes are protein or proteinlike substances that act as organic catalysts. According to the "one gene one enzyme theory," enzymes in the body are determined by genetic inheritance and are a major mechanism for expressing this inheritance. Enzymes performing the same function for different biologic sources are often chemically different.

As organic catalysts, enzymes act to initiate or speed up certain chemical processes. Most enzymes are produced in minute amounts and act within cells. Exceptions are the digestive enzymes, which are produced in relatively large amounts and act outside the cells in the lumen of the digestive tract.

Enzymes have promising potential as cancer drugs. Theoretically, every malignant growth no longer able to synthesize an amino acid (that is normally synthesized by body cells) could be treated by an enzyme that degrades the amino acid and decreases its concentration in body fluids. This form of therapy would capitalize on the differences in metabolism between normal cells, which can synthesize amino acids, and malignant cells, which require exogenous supplies of specific enzymes.

Successful enzyme replacement therapy could prevent or reverse many manifestations of genetic diseases in which enzyme action is usually intracellular. Current enzyme drug preparations rarely distribute to the intracellular space. If the problem of delivery to the site of action can be solved, treatment of such disorders with enzyme drugs has a bright future.

Enzyme drugs derive from plant sources (*eg*, papain); from animal sources (*eg*, pancreatic digestive enzymes); from bacterial cultures (*eg*, L-asparaginase); from human sources (*eg*, urokinase); or, increasingly, from human tissue cultures.

Pharmacodynamics. Most enzymes used as drugs either replace deficient digestive enzymes or act to break down protein, such as blood clots, purulent material, or protrusions and fragments of intervertebral disks.

Pharmacokinetics. When administered orally, most enzymes are destroyed by the digestive process. When used to replace digestive enzymes, large amounts are required to achieve the desired effect. In some instances, complexation of enzymes with chemical radicals protects them from degradation before absorption from the intestinal tract. Such preparations may not reach the systemic circulation, however, due to entrapment in the liver.

Many enzymes are administered by injection, mainly intravenously. Because their molecules are large, their distributions and uptake by cells tend to be limited. Enzymes do not cross the blood–brain barrier and, once inside the body, are degraded and excreted by the same mechanisms as endogenous enzymes. Their biologic half-lives tend to be short.

Therapeutic uses. Enzymes have been used medicinally as replacement therapy in genetic disorders; to promote fibrinolysis and proteolysis; to treat malignant tumors; to prevent infection; and to treat herniated nucleus pulposus.

Studies are underway to develop enzymes for use in correcting inborn errors of metabolism and to broaden their potential use in cancer chemotherapy (Table 53-1).

Adverse reactions. Enzymes, especially those produced by plants or animals, are extremely antigenic. Allergic sensitivity often severely limits the usefulness of enzyme drugs. Contaminants and endotoxins in parenteral enzyme preparations can also cause adverse reactions.

Certain enzymes (*eg*, L-asparaginase) may inhibit the synthesis of proteins, causing damage to the liver, pancreas, central nervous system, and kidneys. Other adverse effects include malaise, anorexia, nausea and vomiting, central nervous system changes, chills and fever, and liver impairment (Table 53-2).

Precautions and contraindications. Before enzymes are administered parenterally, the client's history of any prior use of enzymes must be taken. Some enzymes, such as chymopapain, cannot be used repeatedly because of the high incidence of subsequent allergic hypersensitivity. Skin tests can determine individual sensitivity prior to initiation of therapy. The incidence of allergic reactions to enzyme drugs can be reduced by using enzymes from human tissue cultures, ideally using the client's cells, instead of cells from animals or plants.

Parenteral enzyme preparations must be highly purified to eliminate contaminants that may act as allergens or endotoxins.

■ **Summary**

Enzymes are biologic proteins that act as catalysts to initiate or speed up specific organic chemical reactions. They are produced by plants, animals, and human tissues. Enzyme drugs are used for a variety of purposes, most involving the breakdown of specific biologic proteins. Except for digestive enzymes, most enzyme drugs must be administered parenterally.

Enzymes are useful in treating digestive enzyme deficiencies, intravascular thrombi, and malignant neoplasms. It is hoped that they will prove useful in treating genetic errors of metabolism, once the problem of intracellular distribution is solved.

Enzyme drugs are highly antigenic and repeated use may cause serious allergic reactions. Other adverse effects include damage to body organs due to inhibition of protein synthesis.

Table 53-1. Medical uses of enzymes

Therapeutic use	Enzyme(s)
Promotion of digestion (replacement therapy, cystic fibrosis, and postprandial abdominal distress)	pepsin
	Pancreatic enzymes (trypsin, chymotrypsin, lipase, amylase)
Dissolution of intravascular clots	streptokinase
	urokinase
Treatment of herniated nucleus pulposus	chymodiactin containing two proteolytic enzymes (from papaya latex)
Treatment of malignant neoplasms	L-asparaginase (from cultures of *E. coli* or *Erwinia carotovora*)
Conversion of B type blood to B antigen-free O type blood	α-galactosidase (from coffee beans)
Production of lactose-free milk for use by lactose-intolerant individuals	lactase (Lact-Aid, *Lactsid, Lactrose*)
Treatment of insect stings and bites	papain (Adolph's Meat Tenderizer)
Debridement of wounds	collagenase from cultures of *Clostridium histolytica* (Santyl)
	deoxyribonuclease from bovine pancreas
	papain from papaya (*Panafil*)
	sutilains from cultures of *Bacillus subtilis* (Travase)
	trypsin from bovine pancreas (Granulex)
	fibrinolysin and deoxyribonuclease from bovine tissues (Elase)
Acceleration of absorption of fluids administered by clysis infusions	hyaluronidase derived from mammalian testes (Wydase)
Control of one form of serious combined immunodeficiency disease ("bubble boy" disease)	pegademase bovine

Table 53-2. Adverse effects of selected enzyme drugs

Enzyme	Adverse effects
chymopapain (*chymodiactin*)	Anaphylaxis (in about 1% of recipients)
	Erythema, rash, urticaria, conjunctivitis, rhinitis, piloerection, and GI upset
	Muscle spasms, back pain, and stiffness
	Paresthesia, hypalgesia, numbness, pain, weakness or cramping in the legs
	Sacral burning
hyaluronidase (*Alidase, Diffusin, Hyalose, Hyazyme, Infiltrose, Wydase*)	Increased risk of infection in infused tissues
	Fluid volume excess due to rapid absorption of infused fluids
L-asparginase	Immediate hypersensitivity reactions
	Damage to liver, pancreas, CNS, and kidneys due to inhibition of protein synthesis
	Malaise, anorexia, nausea, vomiting, chills and fever, immunosuppression
enzymes used topically for wound debridement	Increased inflammation at the site of application
	Renewed bleeding or hemorrhage from the treated wound

Nursing management

Nursing implications

As protein substances, enzyme drugs require careful handling; they must be protected from excessive heat and agitation. To prevent allergic sensitization, nurses should avoid contact with enzymes.

Nursing process

Assessment Before initiating enzyme therapy, the nurse should question the client about previous exposure to the drug in question. Personal and family history of allergy should also be determined.

Nursing diagnosis Nursing diagnoses appropriate for clients receiving replacement digestive enzymes include the following:

> *Altered nutrition, less than body requirements related to malabsorption of nutrients secondary to deficiency of digestive enzymes due to cystic fibrosis*
> *Altered comfort: postprandial abdominal distress related to inadequate digestion secondary to digestive enzyme deficiencies of unknown origin*

A nursing diagnosis arising from enzyme therapy is

> *Impaired tissue integrity: inflammation related to antigen–antibody reaction due to enzyme therapy*

Planning Goals of nursing care are specific to the enzyme used and relate to improvement in the medical condition requiring enzyme therapy and to prevention or prompt detection of adverse drug reactions. In most situations, the prevention or prompt detection of allergic reactions is an important goal.

Intervention Nursing interventions vary with the specific enzyme used. With all enzyme preparations, however, clients must be monitored for signs and symptoms of allergic reaction. In some cases, this is manifested by increasing refractoriness to treatment due to enzyme deactivation or elimination by antibodies. In most cases, however, antigen–antibody reactions cause inflammatory conditions ranging from local erythema (with topical preparations) to serious systemic reactions, including anaphylaxis.

Client education. Clients need information about the drug that is prescribed, the regimen for its use, the therapeutic effects that are desired, and the most common and most serious adverse reactions it may cause. They should also be instructed to report to the primary health care provider any signs or symptoms of allergic reaction that may develop.

Evaluation Data required for evaluation include incidence or absence of signs and symptoms of therapeutic response and adverse drug reactions. Signs and symptoms of allergic reactions to enzyme preparations are always pertinent.

Checklist of nursing actions

☐ Before initiating enzyme therapy, determine previous exposure of the client to the particular enzyme, the client's response to that enzyme, and allergy history of the client and family.

☐ Monitor clients treated with enzymes for therapeutic response to treatment and for signs and symptoms of adverse reactions, especially allergic reactions.

☐ Handle enzyme drugs carefully to prevent degradation; protect from heat and agitation. Avoid direct contact with enzyme drugs.

(See Example of Nursing Process and Hyaluronidase Therapy.)

Example of nursing process and hyaluronidase therapy

The client is a 62-year-old housewife who has been comatose for 3 days following a stroke. She was admitted to a small, rural hospital. The physician has ordered a daily clysis of 2,000 ml of clear fluids with added vitamins. During the clysis yesterday, the fluid was absorbed slowly, the sites remained hard and swollen, and the client became restless. Hyaluronidase has been ordered for subsequent clyses.

Although the clysis fluids are being absorbed rapidly today, 2 hours after therapy began, the client's blood pressure rose above the desirable range established by her physician.

Assessment data	Nursing diagnosis	Intervention	Goals and outcome criteria
Clysis infusion absorbing well at a rapid rate Blood pressure above optimum levels	Fluid volume excess related to rapid absorption of clysis fluid	**Reduce** the fluid flow rate of the clysis to a keep-open rate (less than 1 ml/min). **Measure** blood pressure q 15 min. When blood pressure stabilizes within the desirable range, **resume** administration of clysis fluids at a slower rate than initially.	The client's blood pressure will drop to the desired range.

Specific enzyme preparations

For further information on specific enzyme drugs, refer to the following: Chapter 46, Agents Used in Debridement of Wounds (collagenase, deoxyribonucleasc, papain, sutilains, trypsin, and fibrinolysin); Chapter 29, Drugs Affecting Coagulation (streptokinase and urokinase); and Chapter 30, Agents Affecting the Upper Gastrointestinal Tract (pepsin, pancreatic enzymes, including trypsin, chymotrypsin, lipase, and amylase).

Chymopapain

Chymopapain, (Chymodiactin) a derivative of papaya latex, contains two proteolytic enzymes.

Pharmacodynamics. The exact mechanism of action of chymopapain is not known. The drug is believed to hydrolyze noncollagenous polypeptides within the chondromucoprotein of the nucleus pulposus. It does not appreciably affect collagen.

Pharmacokinetics. Chymopapain is administered by injection into injured intervertebral disks. It is highly concentrated in the disk and binds to protein molecules at the site. A portion escapes into the systemic circulation, where it appears to be inactivated by globulins in plasma. Only small amounts of the drug appear in urine.

Therapeutic uses. Chymopapain is used to treat herniated lumbar intervertebral disks. It has been used as an alternative to surgery when conservative therapy has been ineffective.

The procedure for chymopapain injection is involved and is usually carried out in the operating suite, often with a general anesthetic. Prior to administering the drug, the needle tip must be positioned within the herniated disk, using diskography and an image intensifier to ensure proper placement. Time must be allowed for dispersion and absorption of the contrast medium from the site before chymopapain is administered.

Dosage and administration. Chymopapain (Chymodiactin) is marketed as a powder for preparing parenteral solutions for lumbar intradiskal injection. The usual adult dose is 2,000–4,000 units per disk. The maximum dose per client is 10,000 units.

Adverse reactions. The most serious adverse reaction to chymopapain is anaphylaxis, which occurs in approximately 1% of clients. It may be immediate or delayed up to 1 hour following administration of the drug. Other allergic manifestations include erythema, rash, urticaria, conjunctivitis, rhinitis, piloerection, and gastrointestinal (GI) upset. Less severe but more common side effects of chymopapain include pain, stiffness, soreness, and muscle spasm in the back; nausea; paralytic ileus; urine retention; headache; dizziness; paresthesia; hypalgesia or numbness; pain, weakness, or cramping in the legs; and sacral burning.

Precautions and contraindications. The use of chymopapain should be limited to specially trained physicians with experience in treating lumbar disk disease. Chymopapain is administered only in hospital settings, where health care personnel must be capable of treating drug-related complications including anaphylaxis. Halothane anesthesia is not recommended during procedures with chymopapain because cardiac arrhythmias may occur if epinephrine is required to treat an anaphylactic reaction. Because exposure to the drug is likely to induce allergic hypersensitivity, chymopapain is used only once for each client.

Chymopapain is contraindicated for persons with allergy to papaya or papaya derivatives; for those who have previously been treated with chymopapain injections; and for persons with severe spondylolisthesis, severe progressing neurologic dysfunction with paralysis, or evidence of spinal cord tumor or cauda equina lesion. Safe use for children and pregnant women has not been established.

Nursing management

Nursing implications

When preparing chymopapain, the alcohol used to disinfect the top of the vial must be allowed to evaporate completely before needles are inserted because alcohol can inactivate the drug. Only sterile water for injection is recommended as a diluent; bacteriostatic water for injection must *not* be used.

Chymopapain is administered by the physician during surgery.

Nursing process

Assessment Clients about to receive chymopapain should be screened for allergy, particularly to papaya and papaya derivatives. The physician must be informed of positive findings. Risk of anaphylactic reaction is increased in clients prone to allergy, and the drug is not used to treat persons with specific papaya allergy.

Candidates for chymopapain therapy are clients who have experienced back pain and have undergone conservative therapy without lasting improvement. They know that chymopapain therapy cannot be repeated. For these reasons, they may be apprehensive about the procedure. The client's knowledge of and emotional reaction to the proposed therapy should be assessed.

Nursing diagnosis Nursing diagnoses appropriate for clients receiving papain therapy include the following:

Pain: back pain related to pressure of a disk on nerve roots secondary to a herniated intervertebral disk
Fear related to the back condition and the surgery required for its treatment
High risk for pain: back pain and stiffness related to papain therapy
Knowledge deficit concerning papain and its use in the treatment of back pain

A common collaborative problem that should be differentiated from the nursing diagnoses is

Potential complication: paralytic ileus

Planning Goals of nursing care are to increase comfort, alleviate fear, prevent or promptly treat adverse drug reactions, and to inform the client about papain and its medical use.

Intervention During the preoperative period, nursing measures should be instituted to reduce the client's pain from the back lesion. Sitting should be discouraged; standing or lying down does not compress the intervertebral space as much as sitting. Analgesics should be administered as ordered by the physician. Promoting muscle relaxation reduces pain due to spasm. Applying moist heat, reducing stressors, and promoting relaxation may be helpful.

Throughout the treatment period, the client requires emotional support. The nurse should encourage ventilation of feelings and reassure the client by competent management of nursing procedures and expression of concern for the client's welfare.

Postoperatively, the client should be monitored for back pain and stiffness, disrupted digestion, paresthesia or numbness of the legs, and other signs and symptoms of adverse reaction. Analgesics should be administered liberally to control pain, which can be severe. For optimum pain relief, the nurse may request an order for patient controlled analgesia

Client education. Before surgery, the client should be informed by the physician about papain, the risks of surgery, and alternative methods of treatment. Clients may not absorb or remember all the details they were told. The nurse may repeat the information and answer questions the client have about the procedure.

Clients about to undergo chymopapain therapy should be informed that they may experience back pain or muscle spasm in the lumbar region for several days postoperatively. Stiffness and soreness can persist for several months. Clients should be cautioned to report any signs and symptoms of allergic reactions, which may develop up to 15 days after treatment. During convalescence, measures to prevent further injury to the back should be reviewed, including proper techniques for lifting and the use of good body alignment for all muscular activities.

Example of nursing process and chymopapain side effects

The client is a 37-year-old housewife who has received chymopapain injections for an acute back injury 1 week ago. On being discharged from the hospital, she was given a prescription for pain medication. Since then she has had little pain but is experiencing persistent muscle stiffness in the legs, which the analgesic does not relieve. She asks a friend who is a nurse what to do about it.

Assessment data	Nursing diagnosis	Intervention	Goals and outcome criteria
History of disk injection with chymopapain Complaints of muscle stiffness	Altered comfort: muscle stiffness related to spasm secondary to chymopapain injection	**Inform** the client that analgesics are not effective in treating muscle stiffness. **Recommend** that the client report her symptoms to the physician for possible change in the drug regimen. **Advise** the client that muscle stiffness sometimes persists for some time following chymopapain injection but that it eventually subsides. **Recommend** self-care measures that may reduce the muscle stiffness: warm baths, stretching exercises, stress management techniques.	Tone in the affected muscles will decrease. The client will state that she is feeling more comfortable.

Evaluation Data required for evaluation relate to client statements about levels of fear and pain, as well as the incidence or absence of signs and symptoms of adverse drug reaction.

Checklist of nursing actions

☐ Assess clients scheduled for chemonucleolysis for allergic sensitivity to papaya and for previous exposure to chymopapain.

☐ Use nursing measures to control pain following chemonucleolysis; administer analgesics liberally.

☐ Provide emotional support to clients undergoing chemonucleolysis.

☐ Monitor clients treated with chymopapain for adverse reactions to the drug.

☐ Teach clients treated with chymopapain what to expect during convalescence.

☐ Teach clients measures to reduce discomfort during convalescence from chemonucleolysis. (See Example of Nursing Process and Chymopapain Side Effects.)

Hyaluronidase

Pharmacodynamics. Hyaluronidase hydrolyzes hyaluronic acid, a viscous polysaccharide that acts to bind soft tissue cells together.

Pharmacokinetics. Hyaluronidase acts locally in tissues into which it is injected. It then enters the metabolic pool and is metabolized like other proteins.

Therapeutic uses. Hyaluronidase is used as a dispersal agent to facilitate the absorption of fluids administered subcutaneously. It is often injected into the tubing used for hypodermoclysis infusions. It is also used to diffuse local anesthetics, particularly in nerve blocks. During eye surgery, hyaluronidase is injected subconjunctivally to decrease intraocular pressure.

Adverse reactions. Hyaluronidase is well tolerated; allergic reactions occur rarely.

Precautions and contraindications. Hyaluronidase should not be injected into or around infected tissues, acutely inflamed tissues, or cancerous areas. An intradermal sensitivity test may be performed before administering the drug, which is contraindicated for clients with an allergic sensitivity to it.

■ Summary

Hyaluronidase is an enzyme that hydrolyzes one of the substances that cements cells together into tissues. It is used to facilitate diffusion of clysis fluids and local anesthetics through the tissues and to decrease intraocular pressure during eye surgery. Because the drug is antigenic, clients previously exposed to the drug should be tested for allergic hypersensitivity.

Nursing management

Nursing implications

When large amounts of fluids are to be administered by hypodermoclysis, the nurse may suggest using hyaluronidase if it has not been ordered. The drug prevents pain at the site of injection due to local edema and increased tissue hydrostatic pressure.

Nursing process

Assessment   Before initiating an infusion with hyaluronidase, the nurse should assess the client's fluid balance and inspect the infusion sites for infection or inflammation.

Nursing diagnosis   Nursing diagnoses related to this drug include the following:

Pain at the site of infusion related to increased hydrostatic pressure and edema secondary to clysis infusion
High risk for infection related to decreased resistance to the spread of infection secondary to breakdown in hyaluronic acid
Impaired tissue integrity: increased inflammation related to diffusion of chemicals produced by injured cells secondary to use of hyaluronidase

Planning   Nursing care goals are to increase comfort during infusion, prevent infection, and contain inflammation by maintaining tissue cements that wall off inflammation.

Intervention   The nurse exercises judgment in using hyaluronidase. The drug should not be infused into inflamed tissues. The physician should be consulted if it is necessary to adapt clysis protocols.

Hyaluronidase is injected into the distal portion of the clysis tubing so that it enters the tissues before appreciable amounts of fluid are infused. During the infusion, the client's blood pressure should be monitored. If the infusion is absorbed rapidly, intravascular pressure may rise abruptly.

Client education.   The procedure for hypodermoclysis should be explained to the client before beginning the infusion.

Evaluation   Data related to evaluation include the rate of absorption of the clysis; the presence or absence of tissue edema at the site of infusion; the presence or absence of pain during infusion; and the incidence or absence of signs and symptoms of infection and inflammation.

Checklist of nursing actions

☐ Before initiating a clysis infusion with hyaluronidase, assess the sites for evidence of infection or inflammation; if present, do not use the enzyme.
☐ Administer a skin test to screen for allergic sensitivity to hyaluronidase.
☐ Inject hyaluronidase into the distal tubing so that it enters the tissues before large amounts of fluid are infused.
☐ Monitor the client for signs and symptoms of allergic reaction or for infection or inflammation at the infusion sites. (See Example of Nursing Process and Hyaluronidase Therapy.)

Lactose intolerance

Physiology.   Lactase is an enzyme normally present in the GI tract of milk-tolerant individuals. Its function is to break down lactose molecules into simpler sugars that can be absorbed from the gut.

Pathology.   Certain populations (mainly in cultures with no dairy industry or no dietary use of milk) lack the intestinal enzyme for lactose digestion. If a lactase-deficient individual ingests untreated milk, the lactose is not absorbed. Remaining in the chyle, it increases the osmolarity of the intestinal contents, causing water to move from the parenteral tissues into the gut. When this material reaches the large intestine, microorganisms in the bowel ferment lactose, causing flatulence. Lactase-deficient persons experience distention, flatulence, and diarrhea when they consume milk or milk-containing foods.

Lactase

Pharmacodynamics.   Lactase is an enzyme that breaks down the sugar in milk (lactose) into its monosaccharide components: glucose and galactose.

Pharmacokinetics.   Lactase is added to ordinary milk prior to consumption. It is broken down in the digestive tract and handled by the body in the same way as nutrients.

Therapeutic uses.   Lactase is used to convert ordinary milk into a product well tolerated by lactase-deficient persons. For the most part, the taste and palatability of milk are unchanged by the enzyme. To treat one quart of milk, 10 drops of lactase (Lact-Aid) are added. The milk is then refrigerated for 1 day before consumption.

Adverse reactions. Although lactase is well tolerated by most people, it can stimulate allergic hypersensitivity in susceptible persons.

Precautions and contraindications. Lactase is contraindicated for individuals with an allergic sensitivity to it.

■ **Summary**

Lactase is a food additive that converts milk to a product acceptable to lactase-deficient persons. It is well tolerated but can cause allergic sensitivity in susceptible individuals.

Nursing management

Nursing implications

The incidence of lactose deficiency is high among some ethnic minorities, including many adult black Americans.

Nursing process

Assessment When a dietary history is taken, clients should be questioned about food intolerances. Milk use should be evaluated and symptoms of milk intolerance described.

Nursing diagnosis Nursing diagnoses in milk intolerance include the following:

> *Altered nutrition, less than body requirements: protein and calcium deficiency related to omission of milk in the diet secondary to lactose intolerance*
> *Pain related to abdominal distention, flatulence, and diarrhea secondary to milk ingestion and lactase deficiency*
> *High risk for fluid volume deficit: increased fecal loss of fluid related to diarrhea secondary to lactose intolerance*

Planning Nursing care goals are to increase comfort, maintain fluid balance, and improve nutrition.

Intervention When dietary assessments reveal an absence of milk in the diet, the nurse should ask specifically about milk intolerance. Clients who do not use milk should be assessed carefully for signs and symptoms of protein and calcium nutrition.

Client education. The nurse should explain to clients the reason for milk intolerance. If clients like milk and wish to include it in their diets, the nurse should recommend treating milk with lactase (Lact-Aid) before consumption.

Evaluation Data required for evaluation relate to the client's statements about abdominal comfort after eating, general nutritional status, and absence or incidence of diarrhea.

Checklist of nursing actions

☐ When taking a dietary history, inquire specifically about use of milk and milk products and reaction to these foods.
☐ When milk is not a part of the diet, assess the client for protein and calcium deficiency.
☐ If lactase-deficient clients wish to include milk in their diet, advise them to pretreat the milk with lactase.

Adenosine deaminase deficiency

Adenosine deaminase plays a role in antibody production during the immune response to infection. A deficiency of this enzyme causes one-third of the cases of the genetic disease, severe combined immunodeficiency disease (SCID), also known as "bottle boy disease." Children affected by SCID must be completely isolated from all infectious organisms until or unless immune function can be provided through a bone marrow transplant or by enzyme therapy.

Pegademase bovine

Pegademase bovine is an orphan drug that acts similarly to adenosine deaminase. It has been approved by the federal Food and Drug Administration for the treatment of SCID. Although derived from bovine tissue, the substance is treated to alter the nonhuman DNA to render it less allergenic.

Pharmacodynamics. Treatment with pegademase bovine raises the blood levels of adenosine deaminase, thus initiating and sustaining antibody production and immune function. Children so treated experience fewer infections and grow more rapidly than untreated victims of SCID.

Pharmacokinetics. Pegademase bovine must be administered by injection. It is supplied as an injectable solution containing 250 units/ml. Details of its distribution are unknown. It is metabolized as are autogenous enzymes.

Therapeutic uses. Treatment with pegademase bovine is reserved for children with SDIC who are not candidates for bone marrow transplantation, or in whom a bone marrow transplant has failed. Weekly injections are required by the treatment regimen.

Adverse reactions. Pegademase bovine was approved in 1990 after trial in only 12 cases. At this writing, clinical data is so limited that little is known about reactions to the drug. Pain at the injection site or minor headaches have been reported by 3 of the 12 individuals treated (Hussar, 1990).

Precautions and contraindications. To date none are recommended.

■ Summary

Pegademase bovine is an enzyme used in the treatment of severe combined immunodeficiency disease, a relatively rare genetic disease. It controls the disease in some of the children who cannot be cured by bone marrow transplantation. The drug is very new and little is known about its risks.

Nursing management

Nursing implications

Although treated to reduce antigenicity, pegademase bovine is of animal origin and allergic hypersensitivity may develop in susceptible individuals. When handling the drug, the nurse should avoid direct contact with the solution.

Assessment Prospective recipients are limited to individuals affected by SCID who cannot be (or have not yet been) treated with bone marrow transplantation. Because the condition involves a failure of antibody production, the children will probably not have a history of allergic hypersensitivity. A family history should be taken to determine the relative risk of allergy, which could become apparent if the child responds favorably to enzyme therapy.

The nurse should assess family process, particularly parent–child bonding and the relationships between the affected child and others.

The nurse should ascertain how much the family knows about SCID and enzyme treatment for its control.

Nursing diagnosis Diagnoses likely to be made prior to treatment include the following:

> *High risk for infection related to immunodeficiency secondary to severe combined immunodeficiency disease (SCID)*
> *Fear of infection related to the diagnosis of SCID*
> *Altered family processes related to barriers to social interaction between the affected child and others secondary to the need for absolute protective (reverse) isolation*
> *Pain at the injection site related to irritation of the tissues by a potentially allergenic medication*

Many families will have a

> *Knowledge deficit about SCID and enzyme treatment for its control.*

Planning Goals of nursing care include an increase in antibody production and immune response; a decrease in fear; enhancement of interpersonal relationship within the family; alleviation of discomfort at injection sites; and education of the family about SCID and its treatment.

Intervention The administration of pegademase will be effective in some, but not all, recipients. The nurse should store and handle the drug carefully to maintain its potency. Because the drug is a protein, it should be refrigerated but never allowed to freeze. Agitation should be avoided; if frothing occurs, some of the drug probably has been denatured. To distribute the drug throughout the solution prior to drawing up a dose, the vial should be rotated gently.

The nurse cannot tell the family that enzyme therapy will be effective but should strive to foster hope and provide emotional support without false assurances. If a complete isolated environment (plastic bubble) is in use, the normal tactile interaction between child and others is impaired. The nurse should foster as normal interaction as possible. Referral for family counseling may be needed for some families.

The nurse can recommend cold applications to the injection site to relieve pain. Cuddling the child also reduces discomfort, even when performed through the plastic barrier of a bubble.

Client education. Because it is a rare condition, many nurses may know little about the disease or its treatment. The nurse is in a position, however, to obtain information and assist the family to learn about it. If the family has been referred to a specialist in genetic diseases, information will be readily available from the physician and the office nurses. If treatment is under the control of the family physician, the nurse may seek information from such specialists through a regional medical center.

Evaluation Data required for assessment include blood antibody levels; the absence or incidence of infection when isolation is relaxed; the absence or incidence of signs and symptom of fear; evidence of good family bonding and interpersonal relationships; and the absence or incidence of signs of pain at the injection site.

The effectiveness of the teaching plan can be judged by the ability of members of the family to explain the disease and the treatment accurately, and statements by them that they have received answers to their questions.

Checklist of nursing actions

☐ Store and handle vials of enzyme drug carefully to prevent denaturation of the protein.

☐ Provide emotional support for families of children affected by severe combined immunodeficiency disease.

☐ Promote child–parent bonding and good interpersonal relationships in the families of affected children; refer the family for counseling when appropriate.

☐ Recommend cold applications to relieve pain at the injection site.

☐ When necessary, contact specialists in genetic diseases and their treatment to obtain up-to-date information on SCID and its treatment. Carry out a plan for teaching the families of children with SCID about the disease and its treatment.

Enzyme inhibitors

Substances that interfere with enzyme action are called *enzyme inhibitors*. A number of drugs inhibit liver microsomal cells, which normally metabolize drugs into less active or inactive metabolites that are excreted by the kidneys. As a consequence, peak serum drug levels tend to persist; if doses are repeated, serum levels can increase to toxic levels. Microsomal enzyme inhibitors can delay their own elimination, as well as that of other drugs taken concurrently. (See Chapter 9, Drug Reactions and Interactions.)

Anticholinesterase inhibitors are the active agents in many insecticides, such as chlorophenothane (DDT), and in chemical warfare substances, such as nerve gas.

A number of enzyme inhibitors are used medicinally for specific effects on autogenous enzymes (see Table 53-1).

Pharmacodynamics. Enzyme inhibitors are compounds that interfere with enzyme action in the body. They increase concentrations in body fluids of the biochemicals normally broken down by the enzyme in question and decrease the biochemicals normally produced as a result of enzyme action. For example, monoamine oxidase inhibitors, which inhibit the oxidases that normally break down catecholamines in the body, act as antidepressants by raising the concentration of adrenergic neurotransmitters in the brain.

Pharmacokinetics. Enzyme inhibitors are administered orally. Some require weeks to produce a peak effect and dissipate slowly, whereas others are absorbed and excreted within hours. Excretion is usually through the urinary tract.

Therapeutic uses. Therapeutic uses for selected enzyme inhibitors are shown in Table 53-3.

Adverse reactions. Adverse reactions to enzyme inhibitors are specific to each drug. Toxic levels of the substrate degraded by the enzyme can accumulate, especially if the client ingests foods or beverages that increase substrate levels (Table 53-4).

Precautions and contraindications. Clients should be fully instructed regarding the adverse reactions possible during enzyme inhibitor therapy. They should be aware of precautions necessary to avoid toxic reactions.

■ Summary

Enzyme inhibitors are drugs that decrease the effect of one or a class of enzymes in the body. They cause an increase in the substrate nor-

Table 53-3. Selected enzyme inhibitors used as drugs

Enzyme inhibitor	Enzyme acted upon	Therapeutic use
allopurinol	Xanthine oxidase	Treatment of gout
alpha 1-PI (Prolastin)	An autogenous enzyme that attacks lung tissue	Treatment of one form of emphysema
captopril	Angiotensin converting factor	Treatment of hypertension
captothecin	Topoisomerase I, a metaboic enzyme synthesized by normal tissue but not by malignant cells	Investigational drug for the treatment of cancer (effective against leukemia and some malignancies in rats)*
disulfiram (Abstinyl, Antabuse)	Microsomal enzymes, including aldehyde dehydrogenase	Prevention of impulse drinking in alcoholism
enalapril	Angiotensin converting factor	Treatment of hypertension and control of thirst in people in renal failure who are treated with hemodialysis
hydrazines (iproniazid, isocarboxazid, phenelzine sulfate)	Monoamine oxidase	Treatment of depression
Sn-protoporphyrin	An (unknown) enzyme involved in the synthesis of bilirubin	Treatment of jaundice in the newborn
tranylcypromine sulfate	Monoamine oxidase	Treatment of depression

*Edwards DD. (1988). Hitting enzymes to kill cancer cells. *Science News, 133*, 358 (June 4).

Table 53-4. Adverse reactions to selected enzyme inhibitors

Enzyme(s)	Adverse reaction	Events that trigger adverse reactions
captopril (Capoten)	Asthma	Exposure to other allergens to which the individual is sensitive, or none
disulfiram (Abstinyl, Antabuse)	Disulfiram reaction	Exposure to alcohol in alcoholic beverages, added to foods after cooking, in medicine (*eg*, elixirs), and as vapor
Drugs that inhibit liver microsomal enzymes involved in the degradation of other drugs	Increase in serum level of drugs whose degradation is slowed; toxic states if dosage is not reduced	Concurrent use of an enzyme inhibitor and a drug degraded by those enzymes without adjustment of dosage
enalapril	Anuria in the newborn	Treatment of the mother during gestation
Monoamine oxidase inhibitors	Hypertensive crisis	Ingestion of foods processed through fermentation by certain microorganisms (*eg*, hard cheeses, Chianti wine) rich in tyramine

mally degraded by the enzyme. Toxic reactions can follow, especially if foods or beverages that further increase the substrate are ingested.

Nursing management

Nursing implications

Clients treated with enzyme inhibitors need careful instruction regarding what foods, beverages, and medicines to avoid to prevent adverse reaction to the inhibitor.

Data regarding adverse reactions to some drugs in this class are sometimes few, possibly because of underreporting of reactions to the federal Food and Drug Administration. For example, the writer has been told by a rheumatologist of "many adverse effects" of enalapril among his patients, but perusal of the current *ASHP Drug Information* shows little change over the last 4 years in the low incidence and few types of reactions reported for this drug. Nurses can take an active role in the gathering of these data; the FDA accepts reports from nonphysicians. (See Chapter 2 for the FDA Drug Experience Report form.)

Disulfiram

Disulfiram is an enzyme inhibitor used to treat chronic alcoholism.

Pharmacodynamics. Disulfiram is a nonspecific inhibitor of microsomal drug metabolism. One of the enzymes affected by disulfiram is aldehyde dehydrogenase, an oxidase responsible for converting acetaldehyde to acetate during normal alcohol catabolism. The accumulation of acetaldehyde or other chemical changes causes unpleasant symptoms in persons who consume alcohol (Box 53-1).

Pharmacokinetics. Disulfiram is administered orally and is rapidly but incompletely absorbed from the GI tract. The portion not absorbed (5%–20%) is eliminated unchanged in feces. Onset of action of the systemic drug occurs 3–12 hours after administration.

Disulfiram is slowly metabolized in the liver and excreted mainly in urine. A small portion may be excreted from the lungs as carbon disulfide. The drug has a long half-life; up to 20% of absorbed drug remains in the body 6 days after a single dose; drug effects may persist as long as 1–2 weeks.

Therapeutic uses. Disulfiram is used as a deterrent to alcohol in the treatment of chronic alcoholism,

---

Box 53-1. Signs and symptoms of disulfiram–alcohol reaction

Early manifestations

Flushing of the face, throbbing in the head and neck, throbbing headache

Hypotension

Dyspnea and hyperventilation

Nausea, vomiting, thirst

Chest pain, palpitation, tachycardia

Syncope and vertigo

Confusion and anxiety

Blurred vision

Sweating

Weakness

Late, severe manifestations

Respiratory depression

Cardiovascular collapse, arrhythmias, myocardial infarction, acute congestive failure

Unconsciousness, seizures

Death

primarily to assist in maintaining abstinence by discouraging impulse drinking.

Dosage and administration. Disulfiram (Antabuse) is marketed as oral tablets. Usual adult dosage is up to 500 mg daily for 1–2 weeks, followed by 250 mg daily for maintenance. The maximum daily dosage is 500 mg.

Adverse reactions. The disulfiram–alcohol reaction is precipitated by small amounts of alcohol (15 ml of 100 proof or 50% alcohol, or its equivalent). It will persist as long as alcohol remains in the blood. The intensity and duration of the reaction vary with the person, as well as the dose of both disulfiram and alcohol. Although most reactions are self-limiting and not life-threatening, others can be serious and deaths have occurred.

In the absence of alcohol, disulfiram can still produce adverse reactions. Manifestations include drowsiness, irritability, insomnia, abnormal gait, slurred speech, disorientation, confusion, polyneuritis, optic neuritis, delirium, seizures, bizarre behavior, personality changes, and psychoses. Preexisting electroencephalogram abnormalities may be aggravated. In addition, skin manifestations (dermatitis or acne), hepatitis, and blood dyscrasias can occur.

Because it inhibits liver metabolism, disulfiram interacts with many drugs degraded by the liver. It may increase blood concentrations and toxicity of such drugs as barbiturates, warfarin, paraldehyde, and phenytoin. Clients receiving disulfiram concurrently with metronidazole are at increased risk for acute psychoses and confusion. Using disulfiram with isoniazid may result in behavioral changes and incoordination. The addition of amitriptyline to a disulfiram regimen can enhance the disulfiram–alcohol reaction.

Precautions and contraindications. Candidates for disulfiram therapy must be carefully chosen. The person must be well motivated and should be participating in an active treatment program, which includes regular medical supervision. The client must be fully aware of the drug therapy and understand the disulfiram–alcohol reaction thoroughly.

Clients taking disulfiram must be warned to avoid alcohol in any form including beverages, medications, topical preparations, and foods. Alcohol must be avoided for at least 12 hours prior to the initial dose of disulfiram and for 2 weeks following its discontinuation. During disulfiram therapy, transaminase levels and blood cell counts should be monitored regularly.

Caution is advised when disulfiram therapy is used in treating clients with diabetes mellitus, hypothyroidism, seizures, cerebral damage, hepatic or renal impairment, abnormal electroencephalograms, or multiple drug dependence. The drug is contraindicated in alcohol intoxication, cardiovascular disease, psychoses, or allergic hypersensitivity to the drug or to other thiuram derivatives.

Clients receiving disulfiram should not be exposed to ethylene dibromide or its vapors because interaction between this substance and disulfiram has been shown to be tumorigenic in rats. Safe use of disulfiram during pregnancy has not been established.

Nursing management

Nursing implications

Disulfiram must never be given without the client's knowledge and participation. Serious reactions can occur if clients are unaware of receiving the drug and of the need to avoid all forms of alcohol while on disulfiram therapy.

Nursing process

Assessment Prospective clients for disulfiram therapy should be screened for contraindications (pregnancy, cardiovascular disease, psychoses, or allergy to thiuram drugs) and for factors that increase the risk of treatment (diabetes mellitus, hypothyroidism, seizure disorders, brain damage, abnormal electroencephalograms, and multiple drug dependence). If the client has ingested alcohol within the preceding 12 hours, the initial dose of disulfiram must be delayed for another 12 hours.

Nursing diagnosis The main nursing diagnosis related to disulfiram is

> *Knowledge deficit concerning disulfiram; its use in the control of impulse drinking; and the adverse reactions that develop when an individual taking disulfiram is exposed to alcohol*

Planning Goals of nursing care are to prevent adverse reactions to disulfiram by educating the client regarding the drug, its therapeutic use, and measures required to prevent adverse reactions.

Intervention The nurse should prepare and implement a teaching plan that includes facts about the drug, its therapeutic role, signs and symptoms of disulfiram reaction, and precautions required to prevent exposure to alcohol.

Client education. The treatment plan, action of the drug, and characteristics of the disulfiram–alcohol reaction should be fully explained to the client and family before therapy. The client should be cautioned against relying on the drug over other treatments, such as psychotherapy, group therapy, and continued medical supervision. The drug assists the client in preventing impulse drinking. Both family and client should be warned against using disulfiram as treatment for alcohol intoxication; life-threatening reaction could ensue. The client should understand that tolerance to disulfiram does not develop. On the contrary, sensitivity to alcohol increases with prolonged use of the drug. The deterrent effect persists up to 2 weeks after disulfiram is discontinued.

The client should be warned to avoid alcohol in all forms, including foods (*eg*, fruit cakes soaked in rum, creme de menthe on ice cream), medicines (*eg*, elixirs), and alcohol vapors (*eg*, from gasohol fuel).

Evaluation Data required for evaluation relate to absence or incidence of signs and symptoms of disulfiram reaction.

Checklist of nursing actions

☐ Before initiating disulfiram therapy, teach the client about disulfiram, its use in controlling impulse drinking, and the signs and symptoms that occur when recipients are exposed to alcohol.

☐ Caution the client to avoid alcohol in every form, not just in beverages.

☐ Warn the client that exposure to very small amounts of alcohol, such as vapors, can precipitate a reaction.

☐ Warn the client that severe reactions can be life-threatening.

Enzyme activators

Enzymes can be activated, as well as inhibited. Many therapeutic drugs are enzyme inducers; they activate liver microsomal enzymes, decreasing serum levels of other drugs taken concomitantly. (See Chapter 9 for a discussion of this phenomenon.) One therapeutic drug, pralidoxime chloride, acts as an enzyme reactivator.

Pralidoxime chloride

Pralidoxime chloride is a cholinesterase reactivator.

Pharmacodynamics. Pralidoxime reverses the chemical reaction by which certain organophosphates inactivate cholinesterase, thus reactivating the enzyme. Pralidoxime also detoxifies certain organophosphates directly and may interact with cholinesterase to protect it from the effects of these compounds. Pralidoxime reverses the nicotinic but not the muscarinic effects of anticholinesterase poisoning.

Pharmacokinetics. Although pralidoxime is effective when administered orally, absorption from the GI tract is variable. Parenteral (intramuscular or intravenous) administration is more reliable in producing the desired therapeutic plasma concentrations of 4 μg/ml or more. Following absorption, pralidoxime is distributed throughout the extracellular compartment. Whether it crosses the blood–brain barrier is

controversial. The drug does not bind readily to plasma proteins. Distribution in breast milk is unknown.

The metabolic fate of pralidoxime is not known, although a portion of the drug is metabolized, possibly in the liver. Both drug and metabolites are excreted in urine. Reported serum half-life is from 1.8 to 2.7 hours.

Therapeutic uses. Pralidoxime is used with atropine to treat poisoning caused by anticholinesterase medications and pesticides (Box 53-2).

Dosage and administration. Pralidoxime chloride (Protopam) is available as oral tablets and sterile powder for the preparation of solutions for injection. Ini-

---

Box 53-2. Toxins susceptible to pralidoxime treatment

Organophosphate pesticides

azodrin
bidrin
carbophenthion
co-ral
DFP
diazinon
dichlorvos
dichlorvos with chlordane
dicrotophos
dimethoate
disulfoton
EPN
guthion
isoflurophate
malathion
Metasystox 1 and fenthion
methyl demeton
methyl parathion
mevinphos
OMPA
parathion
parathion and mevinphos
phosdrin
phosphamidon
sarin
Systox
trithion
TEPP

Anticholinesterase medications

ambenonium
neostigmine
pyridostigmine

McEvoy GK. ed. (1984). *Drug information 84,* p 1601–1602. Bethesda: American Society of Hospital Pharmacists.

tially, adults are usually given 1–2 g parenterally (intramuscularly, by intravenous bolus over 5 minutes, or diluted with normal saline and infused over 15–20 minutes). This may be repeated in 1 hour if necessary. Alternatively, a continuous infusion of 500 mg/hr may be given. According to the manufacturer's recommendations, the drug may be given orally in dosages of 1–3 g q5h. The initial parenteral dose for children is 20–40 mg/kg body weight.

Adverse reactions. Although pralidoxime is generally well tolerated, adverse reactions occur depending on the route employed. When administered orally, the drug can cause anorexia, malaise, nausea, vomiting, and diarrhea. Intramuscular injection can produce mild pain at the injection site. Intravenous injection can cause hypertension, and rapid intravenous administration has caused tachycardia, laryngospasm, muscle rigidity, and transient neuromuscular blockade. Other signs and symptoms have developed but the degree to which they were caused by pralidoxime, or by the organophosphates and atropine present in the recipient, is not known. These effects include excitement, confusion, manic behavior, dizziness, blurred vision, diplopia and impaired accommodation, rash, and muscular weakness or rigidity.

Pralidoxime can accelerate atropine toxicity, signs of which sometimes appear earlier when pralidoxime is added to the regimen. When administered to persons with myasthenia gravis, myasthenia crisis may occur.

Precautions and contraindications. Close medical supervision is required during pralidoxime treatment. Blood pressure should be monitored to detect abnormal increases, and phentolamine mesylate may be required to treat pralidoxime-induced hypertension. Caution should be used when the drug is administered to clients with renal impairment or myasthenia gravis. Respiratory depressants, succinylcholine, theophylline, and aminophylline should not be given to clients with anticholinesterase toxicity.

Nursing management

Nursing implications

Treatment of anticholinesterase toxicity is usually an emergency procedure carried out in an acute-care setting. In addition to pralidoxime, atropine and other drugs may be administered, and general supportive measures, such as assisted respirations, may be instituted. The client and family need emotional support and reassurance that all possible measures to assist in recovery are being taken.

Nursing process

Assessment The client requiring pralidoxime will be in a life-threatening physiologic crisis characterized by seizures. Vital functions must be assessed quickly so that emergency life-support can be instituted.

Nursing diagnosis Nursing diagnoses likely to be made for the client requiring pralidoxime treatment include the following:

> *Anxiety related to life-threatening episode of chemical poisoning*
> *Knowledge deficit concerning safe use of poisonous substances, such as anticholinesterase insecticides*

Planning Nursing care goals are to restore respirations, alleviate seizures, and educate the client and family about the hazards of exposure to anticholinesterase compounds such as insecticides.

Intervention Emergency intervention is required to restore vital functions such as respiration. The nurse functions as a member of the emergency medical team. Vital signs must be monitored closely. Phentolamine should be available to treat hypertension, which may complicate pralidoxime therapy. Pralidoxime solutions are relatively unstable and must be used within a few hours after preparation. The drug should be administered slowly and the client watched closely for adverse reactions. The client and family need emotional support and reassurance that all possible measures to assist in recovery are being taken.

After resolution of the crisis, the nurse prepares and implements a teaching plan to educate the client and family about safe handling of anticholinesterase compounds (such as insecticides) and other poisons in common use.

Client education. Following recovery from an episode of anticholinesterase toxicity, the client and family should be assisted in identifying the cause of the episode. Safety practices related to the use of anticholinesterase medications or pesticides should be reviewed and corrective measures recommended when necessary. Following exposure to toxic levels of pesticides, clients should be cautioned against rapid weight loss. Toxins are stored in the body's fatty tissues, and their release can elevate serum levels and precipitate a recurrence of signs and symptoms of toxicity. Affected women of childbearing age should be cautioned to consult a physician before undertaking breast-feeding. Pesticide residues may be distributed in breast milk and could affect the nursing child. If breast-feeding is permissible, the mother should avoid losing weight during lactation.

Evaluation Data required for evaluation include statements by the client or family members indicating that the staff was supportive of them during the medical emergency. Client teaching can be evaluated by the absence or incidence of recurrent poisoning.

Checklist of nursing actions

☐ Quickly assess the vital functions of clients affected by anticholinesterase poisoning.

☐ Assist in emergency care to restore and maintain vital functions.

☐ After the crisis is resolved, educate the client and family regarding safe handling of poisonous substances.

References

Edwards DD. (1988). Hitting enzymes to kill cancer cells. *Science News, 133*, 358 (June 4).

Hussar DA. (1990). New drugs: Drug for SCID: Pegademase bovine. *Nursing 90, 20(12)*, 49 (December).

Bibliography

Goldner F, Danley D. (1985). Enzymatic digestion of esophageal meat impaction: A study of Adolph's Meat Tenderizer. *Dig Dis Sci, 30*, 456–459.

Murray M. (1987). Battling illness with body proteins. *Science News, 131*, 42.

Neonatal jaundice: Better than phototherapy. (1989). *Nursing 89, 19(9)*, 31 (September).

Oldenburg B, et al. (1988). Enalapril quenches dangerous thirst. *RN, 51(7)*, 80 (July).

Rodman MJ. (1988). What's new in drugs: Biological product forestalls rare COPD. *RN, 51(2)*, 97 (February).

Rodman MJ. (1990). Drug news: New product combats rare immune disorder in children. *RN, 53(8)*, 101 (August).

Schubiger G, et al. (1988). Enalapril for pregnancy-induced hypertension: Acute renal failure in a neonate. *Ann Intern Med, 108*, 215–216 (February).

Semple P, Herd G. (1986). Cough and wheeze caused by inhibitors of angiotensin-converting enzyme (letter). *N Engl J Med, 314*, 61 (January 2).

Sesoko S, Kaneko Y. (1985). Cough associated with the use of captopril. *Arch Intern Med, 145*, 1524 (August).

*Tompkins JS, Brown MD. (1985) Chemonucleolysis. *Nursing 85, 15(7)*, 47–49 (July).

*Turning their backs on chemolysis. (1986). *Nursing, 86(11)*, 18 (November).

*Recommended for further reading.

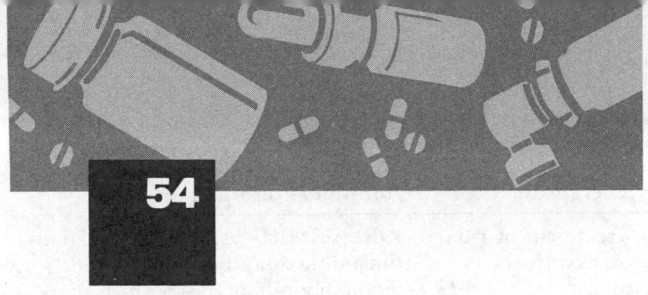

Complexes: chelators and ion-exchange compounds

Complexes

Complexes are chemical compounds that contain in their molecules one or more bonds that do not conform to the classic theories of valency between atoms. They may be classified as metal complexes (inorganic complexes, chelators, olefin complexes); molecular complexes (aromatic complexes, hydrogen-bonded complexes); no-bond complexes (clathrates, channel-lattice types, intercalation "compounds"); and ion-exchange compounds. Complexes used medicinally include chelators and ion-exchange compounds (Table 54-1).

Chelators

Pharmacodynamics. Chelators bind metallic ions, forming complexes that are easily eliminated from the body.

Pharmacokinetics. Most chelators are administered parenterally. Penicillamine is the exception; it is administered orally. Following absorption, most are widely distributed. The edetate preparations do not cross the blood–brain barrier in appreciable amounts. Dimercaprol and penicillamine are partially metabolized by the liver. All chelators are eliminated in urine. To prevent release of chelated metals in the kidneys, urinary pH should be alkaline during dimercaprol therapy. Ferriosamine (the complex formed by iron and deferoxamine mesylate) can be eliminated by dialysis.

Therapeutic uses. Chelators are used to remove toxic substances from the body (see Table 54-1).

Adverse reactions. Adverse reactions to chelators often affect the gastrointestinal (GI), renal, and hepatic systems. Effects are usually reversible with discontinuation of the drugs. Allergic reactions may also occur. Chelators tend to deplete the body's supply of trace metals; this effect may underlie their teratogenic properties. The drugs also tend to cause inflammation at the sites of administration. Under certain circumstances (using an inappropriate route of administration or choosing an inappropriate agent) chelators can increase the toxicity of heavy metals (see Table 54-1).

Precautions and contraindications. Prior to initiating chelator therapy, kidney function and proper hydration should be ensured. Parenteral solutions should be well diluted and infused slowly. Clients should be monitored closely for signs and symptoms of adverse reactions specific to the drug involved.

Chelators are generally considered to be contraindicated during pregnancy.

■ Summary

Chelators are chemical agents used medicinally to treat toxicity caused by heavy metals and certain other chemicals. Therapy should be initiated as early as possible. Adverse reactions include nephrotoxicity, hepatotoxicity, depletion of trace minerals, and teratogenic effects in exposed embryos. Chelators are contraindicated during pregnancy.

Nursing management

Nursing implications

Heavy metal poisoning may develop from occupational exposure to metals (particularly their vapors) and to their ingestion. Ideally, the way to prevent this disease is to eliminate metallic pollutants from the environment. Exposure to heavy metals ranges from lead in paint flakes and water (found in older houses), to cadmium in food (barbecued on makeshift grills made from old refrigerator shelves), to mercury contamination of water (from dumping of industrial wastes). The removal of lead from gasoline has elimi-

Table 54-1. *Chelators used as heavy metal antagonists*

Drug name	Preparations	Usual dosage	Therapeutic uses	Additional information
deferoxamine mesylate (Desferal, Desferin)	Powder for preparing solutions for IV infusion, IM injection, or topical application to the eye	Adults: 125 mg–2 g/d, divided in 2–6 doses Children: initially: 20 mg/kg body weight or 600 mg/m body surface; subsequently, 10 mg/kg body weight or 300 mg/m q4h for 2 doses Maximum daily dose: 6 g	Treatment of iron overload or toxicity Removal of rust rings from the eye following surgical removal of foreign bodies containing iron Treatment of aluminum-associated neurotoxicity Treatment of bone abnormalities in individuals undergoing dialysis	Adverse reactions: Allergic reactions (including anaphylaxis), blurred vision, abdominal discomfort, diarrhea, leg cramps, tachycardia, fever, ocular or otic toxicity, cataract formation, skeletal malformations in fetuses exposed *in utero*, and inflammation at the sites of administration Contraindications: severe renal impairment and pregnancy
dimercaprol (BAL in oil, Sulfactin)	Oily solution for deep IM injection 5% ointment for topical application 5%–10% oil solution for ophthalmic use	2.5–3 mg bid 6 times daily (initial doses are highest, with succeeding doses declining progressively)	Treatment of arsenic, lead, mercury, or gold toxicity	Adverse reactions (usually mild and transitory): hypertension with tachycardia, nausea, vomiting, seizures, stupor, coma, strong mercaptan-like odor to the breath, a burning sensation of lips, mouth, throat, eyes, and penis, tooth pain, blepharal spasm, conjunctivitis, lacrimation, rhinorrhea, salivation, inflammation at the sites of administration, and pain and sterile abscesses at injection sites The drug may terminate gold-induced remissions of rheumatoid arthritis. Precautions: Maintain an alkaline urine, exercise caution in renal impairment and hypertension Contraindications: renal failure, hepatic impairment, and pregnancy
edetate calcium disodium (Calcium Disodium Versenate)	Solution for parenteral injection	Varies with severity of lead toxicity 0.5–1.5 g/m body surface	Treatment of heavy metal poisoning involving chromium, lead, manganese, nickel, zinc, and radioactive and nuclear fission products	Adverse reactions: renal tubular necrosis, anorexia, nausea, vomiting, headache, paresthesias, bone and joint pain, hypercalcemia, hypotension, depletion of trace minerals, and inflammation at the site of administration Precautions: establish renal function and proper hydration prior to therapy, monitor renal and cardiovascular function Contraindications: anuria, pregnancy
edetate disodium (Disotate, Endrate)	Concentrated solution for dilution and IV infusion	40–70 mg/kg body weight Concentration of solutions must be no greater than 30 mg/ml (3%)	Treatment of hypercalcemia, digitalis toxicity	Adverse reactions: hypocalcemia, nephrotoxicity, nausea, vomiting, diarrhea, paresthesias, headache, hypotension, fever and chills, anemia, glycosuria, hyperuricemia, skin rash, and inflammation at the site of administration Precautions: determine cardiovascular and renal function before initiating treatment, amply dilute and slowly administer infusions, monitor cardiovascular status

(Continued)

Table 54-1. Chelators used as heavy metal antagonists (Continued)

Drug name	Preparations	Usual dosage	Therapeutic uses	Additional information
				Contraindications: Hypocalcemia, renal impairment, active or arrested tuberculosis, seizure disorders, intracranial lesions, and advanced atherosclerosis
penicillamine (Cuprimine, Depen, Distamide)	Oral capsules and tablets	Adults: 250 mg–1 g/d, in divided doses administered ac Children: 20 mg/kg body weight/d	Treatment of Wilson's disease, nephrolithiasis due to cystinuria, rheumatoid arthritis, primary biliary cirrhosis, and poisoning caused by the metals arsenic, organic mercury, copper, and lead	Adverse reactions: allergic reactions (skin rash), nephrotoxicity, hepatotoxicity, blood dyscrasias, skin and mucous membrane lesions, GI upset, hypogeusia, and depletion of iron and zinc stores
				Precautions: monitor for skin and mucous membrane lesions, and for renal or liver impairment
				Contraindications: pregnancy, inorganic mercury poisoning

nated a major source of lead contamination from exhaust vapors.

Treating heavy metal poisoning is not effective unless the affected person is protected from further exposure to the offending metal. Treatment is most effective during the early stages of poisoning; delay may result in irreversible damage to body systems, especially the central nervous system (CNS).

Nursing process

Assessment Before initiating chelation therapy, clients should be assessed for impaired nervous, renal, and hepatic systems and for signs and symptoms attributable to heavy metal poisoning. In women of childbearing age, pregnancy should be ruled out. An appraisal of trace mineral nutrition should also be made.

Nursing diagnosis Nursing diagnoses during chelation therapy will be specific to the drug used. They may include the following:

Altered comfort: anorexia, nausea, and vomiting related to irritation of the intestinal tract secondary to chelator therapy
Fluid volume deficit related to diarrhea secondary to chelator medication
Impaired tissue integrity: skin rash related to antigen–antibody reaction secondary to allergy to a chelator preparation
Altered nutrition, less than body requirements: trace mineral deficiency related to depletion of body stores secondary to chelation therapy
Knowledge deficit concerning pollution and poisoning by heavy metals and the treatment of poisoning by chelation therapy

Common collaborative problems that should be differentiated from the nursing diagnoses include

Potential complication: liver impairment
Potential complication: renal impairment

Planning The goals of therapy are to eliminate exposure to heavy metals, eliminate heavy metals from the body, and prevent or promptly detect and treat adverse drug reactions, as well as to educate the client regarding heavy metal poisoning and its treatment.

Intervention Before chelation therapy begins, the nurse should inform the physician of risk factors for adverse reaction, such as pregnancy or signs and symptoms of trace mineral deficiency.

Treatment by chelator drugs is often carried out in acute-care facilities. The nurse is responsible for administering parenteral preparations. Intravenous drugs must be adequately diluted and administered at a slow rate of infusion. Rapid infusion may cause serious adverse reactions.

Clients receiving chelators should be closely monitored for signs and symptoms of adverse drug reactions and trace mineral depletion. Signs and symptoms of renal, liver, or CNS impairment should be reported promptly to the physician. If signs and symptoms of GI disturbance develop, nursing measures should be instituted to decrease nausea, vomiting, and diarrhea. In addition, an order for antiemetic or antidiarrheal medication may be requested from the physician.

Client education. Clients who are at risk for heavy metal poisoning should be warned to avoid exposure. For example, clients using makeshift equipment for barbecuing (specifically racks taken from refrigerators made from cadmium during the 1940s) should never place food directly on the grill. Food may be cooked in containers such as frying and sauce pans using the grill as a stove top. Clients in occupations at high risk for exposure to metallic vapors should follow all safety precautions recommended by the Occupational Safety and Health Administration.

If water pipes in the client's home are made of lead, they should be replaced by pipes made of other materials. The leaching of metal from pipes into water has risen steadily as the acidity of ground water (caused by acid rain) has increased. Also, old paint used in interiors should be replaced with a leadless paint.

Before beginning chelation therapy, steps should be taken to eliminate further absorption of the metal causing the poisoning. Clients should be informed of the sources of exposure and safety practices required for their control.

Clients should be given information about the specific chelator chosen for therapy, the treatment regimen, and signs and symptoms that should be reported promptly to the nursing staff.

More broadly speaking, the public should be educated to the harmful potential of heavy metal pollution. Measures to reduce the risk of poisoning include proper disposal of materials containing heavy metals (including colored dyes in magazines or newspapers and industrial wastes containing mercury, lead, or arsenic). Colored papers should not be burned or incorporated in compost that will be applied to the soil.

Evaluation Data required for evaluation include blood levels of the heavy metal affecting the client, and absence or incidence of signs and symptoms of adverse drug reactions.

Checklist of nursing actions

☐ Assess clients who are to receive chelator drugs for renal, liver, and CNS impairment, as well as for trace mineral nutrition; determine reproductive status of women of childbearing age.

☐ Inform the physician of pregnancy or other contraindications for therapy.

☐ Determine the source of exposure to the metal causing toxicity.

☐ Take measures to protect the client from further absorption of the metal causing toxicity.

☐ When preparing parenteral solutions of chelating agents, dilute the solution adequately.

☐ Administer intravenous agents slowly.

☐ Monitor the client for signs and symptoms of adverse drug reaction, including trace mineral depletion.

☐ Educate the client and general public in measures to reduce environmental pollution by heavy metals.

☐ Teach the client self-care measures that reduce exposure to poisonous metals.

Ion-exchange compounds

Ion-exchange compounds are capable of inactivating ions to which they are exposed by binding them to exchange sites on the surface of their molecules. This action continues until all exposed sites have been used. Although ion exchange compounds include natural substances such as clay, zeolites, and ultra-marines, most are synthetic substances designed for a specific purpose. Ion-exchange compounds are used in processes, such as the softening of water, the purification of drug products, and the conversion of potassium salts to sodium salts. Medicinal uses include the removal of ionic calcium from the blood; the removal of bile acids from the intestinal tract; the neutralization of stomach acids; and the removal of waste materials in impaired kidney function.

Pharmacodynamics. Ion-exchange compounds act by binding the ion that is to be removed or inactivated to the surface of their molecules, releasing at the same time a radical or ion of like charge. The resulting complex is then usually excreted from the body.

Pharmacokinetics. Ion-exchange compounds are administered orally. They react with the substance to be removed from the body within the GI tract and are subsequently eliminated in feces. Reduction of intestinal concentration of a substance reduces concentration within the body because less is reabsorbed from the gut, and additional amounts are secreted into the gut through bile or intestinal secretions.

Therapeutic uses. Ion-exchange compounds are used to treat gastric hyperacidity, hyperkalemia, and hypercholesterolemia (Table 54-2).

Adverse reactions. Ion-exchange compounds tend to disrupt electrolyte and acid–base balance. Their use is often accompanied by GI disturbances (nausea, distention, discomfort, and constipation or diarrhea), skin rash, and (with cholestyramine) asthmatic reactions in individuals allergic to tartrazine.

Precautions and contraindications. Clients receiving ion-exchange compounds should be monitored for signs and symptoms of electrolyte and acid–base imbalances. Drugs containing aluminum, calcium, or magnesium should not be used concurrently with sodium polystyrene sulfonate because this ion-exchange compound will bind them and render them ineffective. Clients receiving cholestyramine should reduce their chloride intake because this ion-exchange compound releases chloride ions in the GI tract, increasing their absorption.

Cholestyramine and sodium polystyrene sulfonate should be avoided during pregnancy and lactation.

■ Summary
Ion-exchange compounds are used medicinally to remove from the GI tract certain ions or

Table 54-2. Medicinal ion-exchange compounds

Drug name	Preparations	Usual dosage	Therapeutic uses	Additional information
sodium poly-styrene sulfonate (Kayexalate, SPS)	Suspensions or powder for pre-paring suspensions for oral or rectal administration	Adults: *Oral:* 15 g once to four times daily; *Rectal:* 30–50 g q1–q6h as needed Children: 1 g/mEq of potassium to be eliminated	Treatment of hyperkalemia	Adverse reactions: gastric irritation, constipation, sodium retention, hypo-calcemia, and (when taken with mag-nesium or calcium compounds) metabolic alkalosis Precautions and contraindications: monitor for electrolyte imbalances, use a mild, *non–magnesium-containing* laxative (sorbitol) to prevent or treat constipation, withdraw aluminum, cal-cium, or magnesium-containing drugs Contraindications: pregnancy
cholestyramine (Cholybar) (Cuemid, Questran)	Chewable bar Powder for pre-paring oral suspensions	Adults: 12 g, divided in 2–3 doses, adminis-tered ac Children: 8–16 g/d, divided in 2–3 doses, admin-istered ac	Treatment of hypercholes-terolemia charac-terized by elevated low density lipoprotein levels	Adverse reactions: GI upset (constipa-tion, distention, bloating, flatulence, heartburn, biliary colic steatorrhea), hyperchloremic acidosis, depletion of body calcium, skin rash, allergic reac-tion (to the tartrazine content) Precautions: reduce chloride intake, monitor electrolyte levels Contraindications: complete biliary obstruction, pregnancy, lactation
Antacids	Oral tablets Oral suspensions	Varies with specific preparation (See section on antacids in Chapter 30.)	Neutralization of excess gastric acidity	Adverse reactions: altered bowel func-tion (diarrhea or constipation) depending on cation content, meta-bolic alkalosis

compounds whose levels in the body are exces-sive. These drugs are not absorbed but exert their action in the intestinal tract and are ex-creted in feces. They tend to cause electrolyte and acid–base imbalances and intestinal upsets. (For additional information, see Chapters 28 and 30).

Nursing management
Nursing implications

Some ion-exchange compounds (cholestyramine and sodium polystyrene sulfonate) are marketed as dry powders from which a suspension is prepared. When preparing these drugs, the nurse should avoid per-sonal contact with the powder, especially inhaling its dust. Exposure causes respiratory embarrassment and allergic sensitization.

Nursing process

Assessment Clients who are to receive ion-ex-change compounds should be assessed for electrolyte and acid–base balance, and bowel function.

Nursing diagnosis Nursing diagnoses for clients re-ceiving ion-exchange compounds include the fol-lowing:

Altered bowel function: constipation (or diarrhea) related to changes in fecal composition secondary to use of ion-exchange compounds
Altered comfort: abdominal distention and discomfort related to use of ion-exchange compounds
Impaired gas exchange related to bronchospasm secondary to allergy to tartrazine in cholestyramine
Knowledge deficit concerning the use of ion exchange compounds and their effects on the body

A common collaborative problem that should be differentiated from the nursing diagnoses is

Potential complication: allergic reaction

Planning Nursing goals include maintaining electro-lyte and acid–base balance, maintaining normal bowel function, preventing or promptly detecting and treat-ing bronchospasm, alleviating or eliminating discom-fort, and educating clients regarding their drug regi-mens and their effects.

Intervention Nursing measures to maintain normal bowel function and prevent GI upset should be initi-ated at the same time as the ion exchange therapy.

Example of nursing process and sodium polystyrene sulfonate therapy for hyperkalemia

The client is a 50-year-old man with progressive renal impairment for the last 10 years due to glomerulonephritis. He has developed hyperkalemia. To postpone the need for dialysis treatments, the physician has ordered sodium polystyrene sulfonate treatment to lower serum potassium.

The client has no known allergies.

Assessment data	Nursing diagnosis	Intervention	Goals and outcome criteria
Renal failure Hyperkalemia	Potential complication: cardiac arrhythmias*	**Explore** the client's knowledge of nutrition, specifically food content of potassium. **Advise** the client to decrease dietary potassium intake. **Identify** for the client foods that are rich and others that are poor in potassium content; explain cooking techniques that will lower potassium intake.	The client will not develop cardiac arrhythmias due to hyperkalemia.
Order for sodium polystyrene sulfonate therapy (Sodium polystyrene therapy can cause constipation.)	High risk for constipation, colonic, related to sodium polystyrene sulfonate therapy	**Advise** the client of self-care measures to prevent or alleviate constipation: ample hydration, exercise, increased fiber intake, habit of daily defecation.	The client will report that constipation has not developed, or that it responds to self-care measures and does not become severe.

* Although potential complications generally are not included in the Examples of Nursing Process, in this situation the identification of the collaborative problem is critical to the outcome for this client and illustrates the broad range of nursing responsibilities.

Throughout therapy, the client should be monitored for signs and symptoms of electrolyte and acid–base imbalance, GI upset, and allergic reaction characterized by bronchospasm.

Client education. Clients should be taught the nature of the drug they are receiving, and the signs and symptoms of adverse reaction to it. Appropriate measures to maintain normal GI function should be recommended. Clients should also be warned to avoid inhaling the powder or dust of cholestyrene or sodium polystyrene sulfonate medications when they are prepared.

Evaluation Data required for evaluation include serum levels of the substances causing toxicity; absence or incidence of signs and symptoms of adverse drug reaction; severity of adverse drug reactions; and reports from the client indicating comfort levels and knowledge of the drug regimen. (See accompanying Example of Nursing Process and Sodium Polystyrene Sulfonate Therapy for Hyperkalemia.)

Checklist of nursing actions

☐ Before initiating therapy using ion exchange compounds, assess the client's bowel function and electrolyte and acid–base balance.

☐ When preparing medications from dry powders, avoid inhalating the drug powder or dust.

☐ Monitor clients receiving ion exchange compounds for electrolyte and acid–base imbalance and GI upset.

☐ Teach clients about their medications and their effects. Advise clients of self-care measures that can minimize adverse reactions to ion exchange compounds.

Bibliography

Gilman AG, et al, eds. (1985). *Goodman and Gilman's the pharmacological basis of therapeutics*, 7th edition, pp 1605–1628. New York: Macmillan.

McEvoy GK, ed. (1991). *Drug information 91*, pp 1517–1521, 1798–1808. New York: Macmillan.

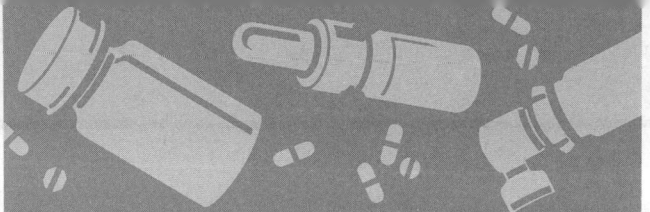

Appendix

Client's name _____

Date _____

Pharmacist _____

Pharmacy _____

Pharmacy telephone _____

Physician _____

Physician's telephone _____

To the pharmacist: Use this form in counseling the client about his medications.

To the client: Use this form to assist in asking for information about your medications.

Adapted from "The Right Drug To The Right Patient," copyright 1977, American Pharmaceutical Association. Prepared in cooperation with APhA. Adapted with permission.

⬭42   Stock No. 320119

Prescription No. _____

Name of drug _____

Purpose for taking
this drug is _____

Prescription can be renewed _____ times

Take _____ every _____
        (Amount)   (How Often)

By _____ for _____
        (Route or Method)   (How Long)

Circle hours the drug is to be taken.

AM clock   PM clock

Physical description of the drug _____

_____

This drug should
not be taken with _____

This drug should
be taken with _____

Possible side-effects _____

Contact your physician or pharmacist
if the following side-effects occur _____

_____

Special instructions _____

_____

_____

_____

Prescription No. _____

Name of drug _____

Purpose for taking
this drug is _____

Prescription can be renewed _____ times

Take _____ every _____
        (Amount)   (How Often)

By _____ for _____
        (Route or Method)   (How Long)

Circle hours the drug is to be taken.

AM clock   PM clock

Physical description of the drug _____

_____

This drug should
not be taken with _____

This drug should
be taken with _____

Possible side-effects _____

Contact your physician or pharmacist
if the following side-effects occur _____

_____

Special instructions _____

_____

_____

_____

(Continued)

Prescription No._____

Name of drug_____

Purpose for taking
this drug is_____

Prescription can be renewed_____ times

Take_____ every_____
    (Amount)   (How Often)

By_____ for_____
  (Route or Method)   (How Long)

Circle hours the drug is to be taken.

AM clock / PM clock

Physical description of the drug_____
_____

This drug should
not be taken with_____

This drug should
be taken with_____

Possible side-effects_____
_____

Contact your physician or pharmacist
if the following side-effects occur_____
_____

Special instructions_____
_____
_____

Prescription No._____

Name of drug_____

Purpose for taking
this drug is_____

Prescription can be renewed_____ times

Take_____ every_____
    (Amount)   (How Often)

By_____ for_____
  (Route or Method)   (How Long)

Circle hours the drug is to be taken.

AM clock / PM clock

Physical description of the drug_____
_____

This drug should
not be taken with_____

This drug should
be taken with_____

Possible side-effects_____
_____

Contact your physician or pharmacist
if the following side-effects occur_____
_____

Special instructions_____
_____
_____

Prescription No._____

Name of drug_____

Purpose for taking
this drug is_____

Prescription can be renewed_____ times

Take_____ every_____
    (Amount)   (How Often)

By_____ for_____
  (Route or Method)   (How Long)

Circle hours the drug is to be taken.

AM clock / PM clock

Physical description of the drug_____
_____

This drug should
not be taken with_____

This drug should
be taken with_____

Possible side-effects_____
_____

Contact your physician or pharmacist
if the following side-effects occur_____
_____

Special instructions_____
_____
_____

DEPARTMENT OF HEALTH AND HUMAN SERVICES
PUBLIC HEALTH SERVICE
FOOD AND DRUG ADMINISTRATION
ROCKVILLE' MD 20857

FORM APPROVED: OMB NO. 0910-0002

FDA CONTROL NO.
ACCESSION NO.

DRUG EXPERIENCE REPORT

I. REACTION INFORMATION

1. PATIENT ID/INITIALS (In Confidence)	2. AGE	3. SEX	4. WGT.	5. HT.	6. REPORTING DATE			7. REACTION ONSET DATE		
					MO	DA	YR	MO	DA	YR

8. DESCRIBE SUSPECTED REACTION(S)

9. OUTCOME OF REACTION TO DATE
☐ Alive with sequelae
☐ Recovered
☐ Still under treatment for reaction
☐ Died (Give cause/date)

10. TESTS/LABORATORY DATA CONFIRMING REACTION (Include biopsy and/or autopsy results)

11. WAS OUTPATIENT TREATMENT FOR REACTION REQUIRED?
☐ Yes ☐ No

12. WAS HOSPITAL TREATMENT FOR REACTION REQUIRED?
☐ Yes ☐ No

II. SUSPECT DRUG(S) INFORMATION

13. SUSPECT DRUG(S) - TRADE/GENERIC NAME(S), MANUFACTURER, IND/NDA NO.

14. TOTAL DAILY DOSE

15. ROUTE OF ADMINISTRATION

16. INDICATION(S) FOR USE	17. THERAPY DATES (From/To)	18. THERAPY DURATION

19a. WAS TREATMENT WITH SUSPECTED DRUG REDUCED IN DOSAGE? ☐ Yes ☐ No OR: ☐ Discontinued	19b. DID REACTION ABATE? ☐ Yes ☐ No	20a. WAS DRUG REINTRODUCED OR DOSE INCREASED? ☐ Yes ☐ No	20b. DID REACTION REAPPEAR? ☐ Yes ☐ No

III. RECENT/CONCOMITANT DRUGS AND MEDICAL PROBLEMS

21. OTHER DRUGS	TOTAL DAILY DOSE	ROUTE	DATES/DURATION OF ADMINISTRATION	INDICATIONS

22. DESCRIBE OTHER RELEVANT MEDICAL HISTORY (i.e., allergies, environmental or occupational exposure, previous drug reactions, pregnancy with gravidity/parity, ethnic origin.)

Your cooperation is needed to insure comprehensive, accurate, and timely use and interpretation of these data.

23. MFR NAME/ADDRESS	24. Check one ☐ Initial Report ☐ Follow-up Report	25. REPORTER'S NAME AND ADDRESS (In confidence)
MFR CONTROL NO.	DATE SENT TO FDA	

NOTE: Required of manufacturers by 21 CFR 310.300, 310.301 and 431.60. Manufacturers may attach additional clinical material and product analyses at their discretion.

26. MAY THE SOURCE OF THIS REPORT BE RELEASED TO THE ARMED FORCES INSTITUTE OF PATHOLOGY? ☐ Yes ☐ No

FORM FDA 1639 (1/82) PREVIOUS EDITIONS ARE OBSOLETE.

Examples of drug level ranges expressed in conventional and Systeme International (SI) units

Drug	Blood component*	Conventional units	SI units
acetaminophen	P		
Therapeutic		0.2–0.6 mg/dL	13–40 µmol/L
Toxic		>5.0 mg/dL	>300 µmol/L
Barbiturate, therapeutic: see Phenobarbital	S		
bromide, toxic	S		
As bromide ion		>20 mg/dL	>15 mmol/L
As sodium bromide		>150 mg/dL	>15 mmol/L
		>15 mEq/L	>15 mmol/L
carbamazepine, therapeutic	P	4.0–10.0 mg/L	17–42 µmol/L
chlordiazepoxide	P		
Therapeutic		0.5–5.0 mg/L	2–17 µmol/L
Toxic		>10.0 mg/L	>33 µmol/L
chlorpropamide, therapeutic	P	76–250 mg/L	270–900 µmol/L
citrate (as citric acid)	B	1.2–3.0 mg/dL	60–160 µmol/L
corticotropin (ACTH)	P	20–100 pg/mL	4–22 pmol/L
cyanocobalamin (vit. B_{12})	S	200–1000 pg/mL	150–750 pmol/L
desipramine, therapeutic	P	50–200 ng/mL	170–700 nmol/L
diazepam	P		
Therapeutic		0.1–0.25 mg/L	350–900 nmol/L
Toxic		>1.0 mg/L	>3510 nmol/L
digoxin, therapeutic	P	0.5–2.2 ng/mL	0.6–2.8 nmol/L
		0.5–2.2 µg/L	0.6–2.8 nmol/L
diphenylhydantoin, therapeutic	P	10–20 mg/L	40–80 µmol/L
doxepin, therapeutic	P	50–200 ng/mL	180–720 nmol/L
epinephrine (radioenzymatic procedure)	P	31–95 pg/mL	170–520 pmol/L
Estrogens (as estradiol)	S		
Female		20–300 pg/mL	70–1100 pmol/L
Peak production		200–800 pg/mL	750–2900 pmol/L
Male		<50 pg/mL	<180 pmol/L
ethchlorvynol, therapeutic	P	>40 mg/L	>280 µmol/L
ethosuximide, therapeutic	P	40–110 mg/L	280–780 µmol/L
folate (as pteroylglutamic acid)	S	2–10 ng/mL	4–22 nmol/L
		mg/dL	nmol/L
fructose	P	≤10 mg/dL	≤0.55 mmol/L
glucagon	S	50–100 pg/mL	50–100 ng/L
glucose	P	70–110 mg/dL	3.9–6.1 mmol/L
glutethimide	P		
Therapeutic		<10 mg/L	< 46 µmol/L
Toxic		>20 mg/L	>92 µmol/L
gold	S	300–800 µg/dL	15.0–40.0 µmol/L
imipramine, therapeutic	P	50–200 ng/mL	180–710 nmol/L
insulin	P,S	5–20 µU/mL	35–145 pmol/L
		5–20 mU/L	35–145 pmol/L
		0.20–0.84 µg/L	35–145 pmol/L
Iron	S		
Male		80–180 µg/dL	14–32 µmol/L
Female		60–160 µg/dL	11–29 µmol/L
isoniazid	P		
Therapeutic		<2.0 mg/L	<15 µmol/L
Toxic		>3.0 mg/L	>22 µmol/L
Lithium, therapeutic	S	0.50–1.50 mEq/L	0.50–1.50 mmol/L
		µg/dL	mmol/L
		mg/dL	mmol/L
Magnesium	S	1.8–3.0 mg/dL	0.80–1.20 mmol/L
		1.6–2.4 mEq/L	0.80–1.20 mmol/L

(Continued)

Examples of drug level ranges expressed in conventional and Systeme International (SI) units (Continued)

Drug	Blood component*	Conventional units	SI units
meprobamate	P		
Therapeutic		<20 mg/L	<90 µmol/L
Toxic		>40 mg/L	>180 µmol/L
methsuximide, therapeutic	P	10–40 mg/L	50–210 µmol/L
norepinephrine (radioenzymatic procedure)	P	215–475 pg/mL (at rest for 15 min)	1.27–2.81 nmol/L
phenobarbital, therapeutic	P	2–5 mg/dL	85–215 µmol/L
phenylbutazone, therapeutic	P	<100 mg/L	<320 µmol/L

potassium	S	3.5–5.0 mEq/L
		      mg/dL
			3.5–5.0 mmol/L
			      mmol/L

primidone	P		
Therapeutic		6–10 mg/L	25–45 µmol/L
Toxic		>10 mg/L	>46 µmol/L
procainamide	P		
Therapeutic		4.0–8.0 mg/L	17–34 µmol/L
Toxic		>12 mg/L	>50 µmol/L
propoxyphene, toxic	P	>20 mg/L	>5.9 µmol/L
propranolol hydrochloride (Inderal), therapeutic	P	50–200 ng/mL	190–770 nmol/L
pyruvate (as pyruvic acid)	B	0.3–0.9 mg/dL	35–100 µmol/L
quinidine	P		
Therapeutic		1.5–3.0 mg/L	4.6–9.2 µmol/L
Toxic		>6.0 mg/L	>18.5 µmol/L
salicylate (salicylic acid)	S	Toxic >20 mg/dL	>1.45 mmol/L
Sulfonamides, all as sulfanilamide, therapeutic	B	10.0–15.0 mg/dL	580–870 µmol/L
theophylline, therapeutic	P	10.0–20.0 mg/L	55–110 µmol/L
thiocyanate (nitroprusside toxicity)	P	10 mg/dL	1.75 mmol/L
thyroxine (T$_4$)	S	4–11 µg/dL	51–142 nmol/L
trimethadione, therapeutic	P	<50 mg/L	<350 µmol/L
trimipramin, therapeutic	P	50–200 ng/mL	170–680 nmol/L
vitamin B$_2$ (riboflavin)	S	2.6–3.7 µg/dL	70–100 nmol/L
vitamin B$_6$ (pyridoxal)	B	20–90 ng/mL	120–540 nmol/L

vitamin B$_{12}$ (cyanocobalamin)	P,S	200–1000 pg/mL
		      ng/dL
			150–750 pmol/L
			      pmol/L

vitamin E (alpha tocopherol)	P,S	0.78–1.25 mg/dL	18–29 µmol/L

*P = plasma; B = blood; S = serum.

Adapted from Metric Commission Canada, Sector 9.10 Health and Welfare: *The SI Manual in Health Care*, Ottawa, Canada, 1981.

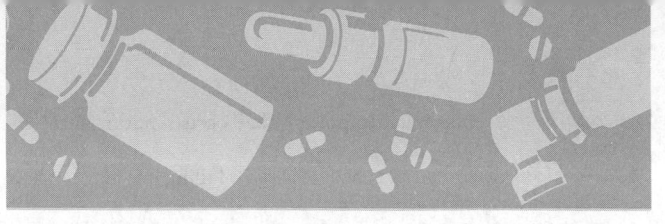

Glossary

absorbent   Capable of reception by molecular or chemical action

absorption   The movement of a substance into body fluids and tissues by passage through some entry. Except for direct injection, absorption involves passage through some surface or membrane barrier such as the skin or gastrointestinal mucosa

abuse (of drugs)   Persistent inappropriate use of drugs

acid   A molecule or ion that acts as a proton or hydrogen ion donor; a substance that ionizes in solution to form hydrogen ions; any substance that contains hydrogen capable of being displaced by basic radicals

acidifier, systemic   A drug used to lower internal body pH

acidifier, urinary   A drug used to lower the pH of urine

acidosis   A physiologic state characterized by a shift in chemical balance toward acidity; a relative reduction in base buffers, a relative increase in acid salts, or an actual reduction in the pH of body fluids

acupuncture   Therapeutic insertion of needles

addiction   A behavioral state characterized by loss of power to control a drive or craving for a substance; also see *dependence*

addition   Summation; when two drugs, acting simultaneously, elicit the same mechanism of action, and their combined effect is equal to the added sum of both drugs

adrenergic   A drug whose effect on living systems is similar to that of epinephrine (Adrenalin) or the stimulation of sympathetic nervous tissue

adrenergic blocking agent   A drug that inhibits responses to adrenergic nerve stimulation and to sympathomimetic drugs

adsorbent   An agent that binds chemicals to its surface

adsorption   Adhesion of a substance to the surface of a solid

aerosol   A colloidal solution that is dispensed in the form of a mist

affinity   A measure of the effectiveness of the interaction of a drug and its receptor; the greater the affinity of the drug, the greater its propensity to bind with its receptor and the smaller the concentration of drug needed to produce a given response

agent of choice   The drug preparation generally regarded by physicians as the best choice for treatment of a given clinical condition

agonist   A substance having a specific cellular affinity that produces a predictable response; a chemical capable of stimulating a cell membrane receptor

agranulocytosis   A marked reduction in the number of granular leukocytes

akathisia   Extreme restlessness, mental turbulence, and increased motor activity

akinesia   Impaired or absent motor function

alkalizer, systemic   A drug used to raise internal body pH

alkaloid   One of a class of basic nitrogenous organic chemicals occurring in natural materials

alkalosis   A physiologic state characterized by a shift in chemical balance toward alkalinity; a relative increase in base buffers, a relative decrease in acid salts, or an actual rise in pH of body fluids

allergen   A substance that can elicit a specific immunologic response; an antigen

allergenic extract   A suspension of antigenic chemicals prepared from the natural substance to which a person is allergic and which is administered to that person in gradually increasing doses for the purpose of decreasing the allergic response on subsequent exposure

allergic response   An adverse response to a chemical due to the presence in an organism of immune bodies whose production was stimulated by previous exposure to that chemical

alopecia   Loss of hair, baldness

amblyopia   Dimness of sight

amebicide   A drug used to destroy *Entamoeba histolytica*, the organism that causes amebic dysentery

ampules   Sealed glass containers for powdered or liquid drugs

anabolic   An agent that promotes body processes of repair and growth; a drug that promotes anabolism

anabolism   Constructive metabolism; the building up of body tissue

analeptic   A potent central nervous system stimulant, especially one that stimulates respiration and wakefulness

analgesic   An agent that relieves pain without producing loss of consciousness

anaphylactoid reaction   An immediate and serious physiologic response characterized by bronchospasm, vasospasm, and severe hypotension; usually fatal unless treated promptly

androgen   A hormone that stimulates and maintains male secondary sex characteristics

androgenic   Producing or promoting masculine characteristics

anesthetic   An agent that causes reversible loss of feeling or sensation

anesthetic, general   An anesthetic that not only causes loss of sensation but also loss of consciousness

anesthetic, local   An anesthetic which causes loss of sensation only in the particular area where it is applied, by blocking out nerve impulses from the affected area

angioneurotic edema   Large hives due to reflex nervous vasodilation

anhydrotic   A drug that checks perspiration flow systemically; an antiphoretic

anodyne   A medicine that relieves pain

anorexia   Loss of appetite

anorexiant   A drug that reduces appetite

antacid   A substance that neutralizes acids; a drug taken to counteract symptoms caused by gastric hydrochloric acid produced in excessive amounts or present in an inappropriate body location, as in esophageal reflux

antagonism   An interaction between two drugs in which the combined effect of the two agents is less than the sum of the effects of the drugs acting separately

antagonist   A drug that reduces the physiologic effect of another drug, often a chemical that can occupy a cell membrane receptor without stimulating it and thereby block the action of agonists that interact with that receptor

anthelmintics   Drugs used to rid the body of worms

antiadrenergic   A drug that prevents response to sympathetic nervous system stimulation and adrenergic drugs; sympatholytic or sympathoplegic drugs

antiarrhythmic   A drug used in the prevention and treatment of disorders of cardiac rhythm

antibacterial   A drug that kills or inhibits pathogenic bacteria

antibiotic   A chemical substance or metabolic product of living cells of molds, bacteria, or other plants that destroys or prevents the growth of microorganisms

antibodies Substances in the tissues or fluids of an organism that act to antagonize specific foreign bodies and are produced by the immune system in response to an initial exposure to the specific foreign body or antigen

anticholesteremic A drug that lowers blood plasma cholesterol level

anticholinergic A drug that decreases the activity of cholinergic nerve fibers or the physiologic effects of cholinergic nerve activity; parasympatholytic, parasympathoplegic

anticoagulant A drug that decreases blood coagulability and reduces the extension of blood clots already present but does not dissolve clots already formed

anticonvulsant A drug that selectively prevents epileptic seizures

antidepressant A psychotherapeutic drug that elevates mood

antidiarrheic A substance that reduces the production of frequent, watery stools and the intestinal cramping that accompanies diarrhea

antidote A chemical agent used to overcome the action or the effects of another chemical agent

antiemetic A drug that decreases nausea and vomiting

antigen A substance that can elicit a specific immunologic response; an allergen

antihistamine A drug that prevents response to histamine, including histamine released by allergic reactions

antihypertensive A drug that reduces blood pressure

anti-infective A drug used to treat infections

anti-inflammatory A drug that reduces the inflammatory response

antimuscarinic A substance that blocks the stimulating effect of muscarinic autocoids and drugs on the postganglionic receptors of the parasympathetic nervous system

antineoplastic A drug used to reduce the size of or the growth rate of a malignant tumor

antiplatelet A substance (drug) that delays coagulation by inhibiting platelet aggregation

antipruritic A drug that prevents or relieves itching

antipsychotic A drug used in the treatment of mental illness

antipyretic A drug used to reduce an abnormally high body temperature

antirheumatic A drug that alleviates inflammatory symptoms of arthritis and related connective tissue diseases

antiseptic A chemical agent that inhibits the growth of microorganisms but does not necessarily kill them

antisialogogue A drug that diminishes the flow of saliva

antispasmodic A drug that reduces the spasms of muscles, especially involuntary smooth muscle

antitoxin A biologic drug containing antibodies against the toxic principles of a pathogenic microorganism and used for passive immunization against the associated disease

antitussive A drug that suppresses coughing

anuria Lack of urinary output

aphasia Loss or impairment of speech

aplastic anemia Anemia due to impairment of the bone marrow

astringent A mild protein precipitant that diminishes secretions and toughens tissue

ataxia Lack of normal muscular coordination, especially the inability to coordinate voluntary movements

atomizer A device that breaks drugs into comparatively large particles for inhalation

atopy An allergy (usually manifested by bronchial asthma, vasomotor rhinitis, and chronic urticaria) for which there is a genetic predisposition

autocoid A chemical compound that occurs naturally in the body

bactericide An agent capable of rapidly killing microorganisms; disinfectant; germicide

bacteriostatic A substance that arrests the growth of bacteria

base A molecule or ion that acts as an acceptor of protons or hydrogen ions; a substance that ionizes in solution to form hydroxyl ions; any substance that has the property of neutralizing acids to form salts; any substance that can replace the hydrogen of an acid

binders Substances that give adhesiveness to a powdered drug

bioassay A procedure for determining the quantitative relationships between a dose of a drug and the intensity of the biologic response it evokes; used to determine the relative potencies of more than one drug or used as a standard of purity for the preparation of drugs

bioavailability The rate and extent to which a drug enters the circulation and reaches the site of action; the rate and extent to which the active drug ingredient is absorbed from a pharmacologic product and becomes available at the site of drug action (as defined by Federal Drug Administration [FDA] regulations)

bioavailable dose A dose available to an organism by virtue of the concentration of drug in the blood or at the active site

bioequivalent drug products Pharmaceutical equivalents, that is, drugs whose rate and extent of absorption do not show a significant difference when administered at the same molar dose under similar experimental conditions

biofeedback A process by which biologic changes normally unsensed by a person are converted to stimuli that provides sensory information about these changes

biotransformation Chemical changes in drugs that occur by virtue of physiologic processes in the body; metabolism

biotransport The translocation of a solute from one side of a biologic barrier to the other side

bronchodilator A drug that can dilate the lumina of air passages in the lungs

buffered Containing a substance that tends to preserve a proper hydrogen ion concentration

capsule A gelatin case for administering drugs in oral doses

capsule, time-release Capsule containing small beads of the active drug, some of which are treated to delay absorption by the gastrointestinal tract

carcinogenic Capable of causing cancer

cardiotonic A drug that increases the force of the heart muscle's contraction; a cardiac stimulant

carminative An aromatic or pungent drug that mildly irritates the gastrointestinal tract and is useful in the treatment of flatulence and colic

catecholamine A compound characterized by a catechol molecule combined with the aliphatic portion of an amine that mimics the effects of sympathetic nervous system stimulation when administered as a drug

cathartic A drug that causes defecation, usually by enhancing peristalsis or by softening or lubricating feces

caustic A topical drug that destroys tissue on contact and is suitable for removing abnormal tissue growth

ceiling effect The maximum intensity of a specific effect that can be produced by a given drug, no matter how large a dose is administered

central depressant A drug that decreases the functional state of the central nervous system

central stimulant A drug that increases the functional state of the central nervous system

chemical name A name that indicates the actual chemical composition of a drug, often designating the chemical atoms or radicals in the molecule and their placement in the drug molecule

chemotherapy The use of chemical agents that have a toxic effect on the disease-causing agent; specifically the use of drugs capable of destroying invading organisms or malignant tumor cells without destroying the host

cholagogue A drug that stimulates the emptying of the gallbladder and the flow of bile into the duodenum

cholinergic A drug that enhances the response of or the physiologic effects of cholinergic nerve fibers; parasympathomimetic

chrysotherapy Treatment (as in arthritis) by injection of gold salts

CNS Central nervous system

coagulant A drug that replaces a deficient blood factor necessary for coagulation; clotting factor

compartment A kinetically distinguishable pool in the body in terms of drug concentration profile

compendium A collected body of information on drugs, especially their strength, purity, and quality

compliance The degree to which advice (including prescriptions) is followed accurately and completely by the client

compounding The preparation of a medicinal substance by combining two or more ingredients

concomitant Associated with; taking place at the same time

concurrent Taking place at the same time

congener A drug that belongs to a group of chemical compounds having the same parent compound

contraceptive A drug used to prevent pregnancy

contraindication A condition or fact that makes a course of action, such as the use of a drug, inadvisable

corticoid A substance, natural or synthetic, that has actions similar to hormones of the adrenal cortex

coulomb The quantity of electricity that flows across a surface when a steady current of 1 ampere flows for 1 second

counterirritant An agent that irritates the part to which it is applied and thereby produces vasodilation and an increase in blood supply in that part

cycloplegic A drug that paralyzes accommodation of the eye

cytotoxic A drug used to treat tumor growths; antineoplastic

deaggregation Dispersal of the particles of a whole

decongestant A drug that reduces congestion caused by an accumulation of blood

demulcent An agent that soothes and protects

dependence A condition in which the user of a drug has a compelling desire to continue taking the drug, either to experience its effects or to avoid the discomfort of its absence

dependence, physical An altered or adaptive physiologic state produced in a person by repeated administration of a drug (formerly termed *addiction*)

dependence, psychologic An emotional or mental drive, characterized by a compulsion to continue taking a drug (formerly termed *habituation*)

depressant A drug that temporarily slows some functional activity or process

detergent An emulsifying agent useful for cleansing wounds, ulcers, or skin

diaphoretic A drug used to increase perspiration; hydrotic; sudorific

diffusion The movement of molecules from a region of high concentration to one of lower concentration. Movement across the membrane may occur because the substance dissolves in its lipid portion, or because it attaches to a substance in the membrane which transports it to the opposite side (*facilitated diffusion*) where it is released

diffusion gradient The relative difference between concentrations of molecules from one region to another, which is directly related to the rate of diffusion

digestant A drug that promotes the process of digestion in the gastrointestinal tract

diluent A substance used to increase the bulk of a drug

disinfectant An agent capable of rapidly killing pathogenic microorganisms; especially used for killing microorganisms on inanimate objects; germicide

disintegrator A substance, such as starch, added to a dry drug to facilitate dissolution of the finished tablet in water

dissolution Solution in a liquid substance

distribution The movement of a chemical through the fluids and tissues of the body, usually in characteristic patterns and concentrations

diuretic A drug that promotes renal excretion of electrolytes and water, thereby increasing urine volume

dosage The regulated administration of doses expressed in terms of a quantity per unit of time

dose The quantity of drug to be administered at one time or the total quantity to be administered

drug Any chemical agent that affects living organisms, especially one used in the treatment, diagnosis, or prevention of disease, or one that poses a high risk of harmful effects

ecbolic A drug used to stimulate the gravid uterus to expel the fetus or to cause uterine contraction; oxytocic

ecology The branch of biology dealing with the relations between organisms and their environment

eczema An inflammatory disease of the skin with infiltrations, watery discharge, scales, and crusts

effector Organ or cell that responds in a characteristic manner to a stimulus

effervescent Bubbling, sparkling, giving off gas bubbles

elixir An aromatic, sweetened, alcoholic preparation

emetic A drug that induces vomiting, either locally by gastrointestinal irritation or systemically by stimulating receptors in the central nervous system

emollient A topical drug, especially a fat or oil, used for its local protective or softening action

empiric Dependent on experience or observation alone without regard to science or theory

emulsion Suspension of fats or oils in water with the aid of an emulsifying agent (surface tension reducer), often stabilized by acacia or gelatin

endorphins See *enkephalins*

enkephalins Autogenous peptides that act as agonists on opioid receptors in the body; endorphins

enteral, enteric Pertaining to the intestinal tract

enteric coating A layer of material placed on the outer surface of a tablet or capsule to prevent dissolution in the stomach. Enteric coating may be used to protect the drug from the effect of gastric secretions or to protect the stomach from irritation by the drug

environmental medicine That branch of medicine dealing with the effect of the environment, especially pollutants, on the health of humans

enzyme A protein produced by living cells that accelerates biochemical reactions

equipotency The property of having equal strength, force, or power

essence A concentrated alcoholic solution of a volatile substance; spirits

estrogen A hormone that stimulates female secondary sex characteristics and functions in the menstrual cycle to promote uterine gland proliferation

excipient An inert substance used to give a pharmaceutical preparation a suitable form or consistency

excretion The physiologic elimination of substances from the body

expectorant   A drug that increases secretion of respiratory tract fluid, making it less viscous, reducing its cough-inducing irritancy, and promoting its ejection

extracellular compartment   The sum of the fluid-filled spaces of the body that are outside cell membranes (include both *interstitial* and *intravascular* compartments)

extracts   A concentrated preparation of pharmacologic substances obtained from vegetable or animal materials by dissolving the active ingredients of the drug in a suitable solvent then evaporating all or part of the solvent

extravasation   The leakage of fluid into surrounding tissue, especially that of a vesicant or irritant drug, resulting in necrosis, pain, and tissue sloughing

fibrolytic   A drug that dissolves the fibrin of blood clots

fluidextracts   Alcoholic liquid extracts of vegetable drugs in 100% strength (*ie*, 1 ml of fluidextract contains 1 g of drug)

folk remedy   A traditional familial practice related to health beliefs and customs in a specific cultural group, which has been passed on from generation to generation

forensic medicine   The branch of medicine dealing with legal questions arising from illness, such as homicide, suicide, or accidental injury

galactorrhea   Excessive flow of breast milk; inappropriate production of milk not associated with childbirth and nursing

galenical   A medicinal prepared by extracting one or more active constituents of a plant

gels   Aqueous suspensions of insoluble drugs in hydrated form

generic name   A name indicating the origin of a drug; a name established by an authority, such as the Committee on International Nonproprietary Names (of the World Health Organization) to designate a single drug that may be marketed under various trade names

germicide   Disinfectant; an agent capable of rapidly killing pathogenic microorganisms, especially one used for killing microorganisms on inanimate objects

glucocorticoid   One of a class of hormones produced by the adrenal cortex, which exerts pronounced effects on the body's metabolism of carbohydrates by increasing gluconeogenesis

habituation   See *dependence, psychologic*

half-life (t1/2)   The time it takes for one half of an observed change to occur; serum half-life is the time it takes for one-half of a drug to disappear from the serum, or the time it takes for serum concentration to drop by half. (Serum half-life may be characterized by distinct phases: [1] the distribution phase during which the drug leaves the blood and enters the tissues, including tissue depots, [2] the phase during which the drug is simultaneously undergoing excretion and also moving from tissue depots to the blood, and [3] the elimination phase during which drug levels are influenced only by excretion; when serum half-life is termed *triphasic* figures are given for all three phases, when it is termed *biphasic*, figures are usually reported for the distribution and elimination phases.)

Radioactive half-life is the time it takes for the loss of one-half of the radioactive particles emitted by a radionuclide, or the time required for the radioactive emissions of the radionuclide to decline by half.

hapten   A relatively simple compound that, although not itself a stimulant of antibody formation, reacts with specific antibodies after they have been produced

hematinic   A medicine that promotes hemoglobin formation by supplying a factor essential for its synthesis

hematopoietic   A drug that stimulates formation of red blood cells, especially by supplying deficient vitamins

hemostatic   A locally acting drug that arrests hemorrhage by promoting clot formation

herb   A plant with a soft stem containing little wood, especially one that contains aromatic constituents used as flavoring agents or medicines

herbal medicine   The practice of using plants that contain active constituents known to be useful in the prevention or treatment of an illness

holoprosencephaly   Birth defect involving facial bones

homeostasis   The maintenance of the body's optimal internal environment

hormone   A specific chemical substance secreted by cells in one part of a living organism that influences the growth, development, or behavior of other cells remote from the source of the hormone

hydrolysis   A chemical reaction in which a compound is cleaved by the addition of a molecule of water

hyperglycemic   A drug that elevates blood glucose level, especially for the treatment of hypoglycemic states

hyperosmotic   Pertaining to solutions that have a higher osmotic pressure than a reference standard (usually physiologic fluids) and that cause a reduction of cell volume; hypertonic

hyperresponsivity   Hypersensitivity

hypersensitivity   A state in which a drug dose produces a response quantitatively greater than usual for that dose; hyperresponsivity

hypersensitivity, allergic   A state characterized by the presence of antibodies that react with a given substance to produce an allergic reaction

hypertonic   See *hyperosmotic*

hypnotic   A drug that induces a clinical state resembling sleep

hypnosis   A condition or state of consciousness that can be artificially induced and is characterized by strong susceptibility to suggestion and loss of sensation

hypodermic   Beneath the skin, as in a hypodermic injection, which delivers drugs to the subcutaneous tissue

hypodermoclysis   The introduction of large amounts of fluid into subcutaneous tissue

hypoglycemic   A drug that promotes glucose metabolism and lowers the blood sugar level

hyposmotic   Pertaining to solutions that have a lower osmotic pressure than a reference standard (usually physiologic fluids) and that increase cell volume; hypotonic

hypotensive   A drug that diminishes pressure or tension to lower blood pressure

hypotonic   See *hyposmotic*

hypovolemia   Diminished blood supply in the body

iatrogenic   Arising from or caused by medical treatment

idiosyncratic response   An abnormal response to a drug that takes the form of extreme sensitivity to low doses, extreme insensitivity to high doses, or a response that is qualitatively different from the usual response

immune serum   A biologic drug containing antibodies for a pathogenic microorganism; useful for passive immunization against a disease

immunity   Resistance to disease by the presence of antibodies

immunizing agent, active   An antigenic preparation (toxoid or vaccine) used to induce the formation of specific antibodies against a pathogenic microorganism, thus providing delayed by permanent protection against a disease

immunizing agent, passive   A biologic preparation (antitoxin, antivenom, or immune serum) containing specific antibodies against a pathogenic microorganism

infection   The presence of living organisms within the tissues

inflammation   A local response to cellular injury, protective in nature, characterized by capillary dilation, leukocyte infiltration, swelling, heat, and pain

inhaler   A device used to spray liquid or powder in a fine mist into the lungs during inhalation

inscription   The part of a prescription that states the name of the drug, the drug's dose form, and the amount of the dose

interstitial compartment   The sum of the fluid-filled spaces of the body that are outside cell membranes and also outside blood vessels

intra-arterial   Into an artery, as in an intra-arterial injection, which delivers drug to the blood in the arterial circulation

intracellular compartment   The sum of the fluid-filled spaces inside cell membranes

intradermal   Intracutaneous, as in an intradermal injection, which is made into the upper layers of the skin

intramuscular   Into the muscle, as in an intramuscular injection, which introduces a drug into muscle tissue

intraperitoneal   Into the peritoneal space

intrapleural   Into the pleural space

intrathecal   Into the spinal fluid, as in an intrathecal injection; the introduction of a drug into the spinal fluid, usually by means of a lumbar puncture (not administered by nurses unless they have received special training in the technique, as in the case of nurse-anesthetists)

intravascular compartment   The sum of the fluid-filled blood vessels (including the heart chambers, arteries, capillaries, and veins)

intravenous   Into a vein, as in an intravenous injection, which delivers drug into the blood of the venous circulation

inunction   A drug or medication administered by rubbing into the skin

ionic bond   The chemical bond formed between two atoms by the outright transfer of one or more electrons from one atom to the other

ionizing radiation   Forms of radiant energy that tend to dissociate compounds into their constituent ions

irritant   Property of a drug whose administration causes pain and may be accompanied by inflammation

isotonic   Pertaining to solutions that have the same osmotic pressure as the reference standard (usually physiologic fluids) and that do not cause any volume changes in cells; iso-osmolar

keratolytic   A drug that softens the superficial keratin-containing layer of skin to promote exfoliation

laxative   A gentle purgative medicine; a mild cathartic

lichenification   Leathery hardening of the skin

liniments   Liquid suspensions or dispersions intended for external application, often containing oil, soap, alcohol, or a rubefacient in addition to one or more active ingredients

lipid   A broad term used to include all the ethersoluble, water-insoluble substances obtained from plant and animal sources; included are esters of fatty acids and alcohols (fats, oils, waxes, phospholipids, glycolipids, fatty acids, glycerols, sterols, and alcohols)

lipotropic factor   A drug that prevents the abnormal accumulation of fat in the liver by promoting the transportation and utilization of fats

lotions   Liquid suspensions or dispersions intended for external use

lozenges   Flat, round, or rectangular preparations held in a cavity (mouth or vagina) until they dissolve, liberating the drug or drugs involved; troches

lubricant   A substance added to a dry drug to prevent the formed tablet from sticking to the tablet-making machinery; a drug that acts by reducing friction

lysis   Cellular destruction

magmas   Bulky suspensions of insoluble preparations in water

materia medica   The substances used in the composition of remedies for the treatment of disease; also the branch of medical science that deals with the sources, nature, and properties of drugs

median effective dose   The smallest dose required to produce a stated effect in 50% of a population; ED_{50}; also median therapeutic dose (TD_{50})

median lethal dose   The smallest dose required to produce death in 50% of a population; LD_{50}

medication   The administration of drugs for the purpose of treating illness

medicine   A substance administered for the purpose of treating illness

metabolism   The changing of a substance by chemical processes in the body

metabolite   A substance produced as a result of chemical transformation of another substance in the body. A given chemical often gives rise to a number of different but related metabolites

mineralocorticoid   One of a class of hormones produced by the adrenal cortex with marked effects on metabolism of minerals, such as sodium and potassium

miotic (myotic)   A substance that constricts the pupils

mists   Medications administered in the form of cloudlike aggregations of minute particles

misuse (of drugs)   The occasional inappropriate use of drugs, including nonmedical use, inappropriate medical use, or appropriate use in improper doses

mixture   A solid material suspended in a liquid; also any preparation of several drugs for internal use

mucolytic   A drug that reduces the thickness and stickiness of pulmonary secretions (usually administered by aerosol inhalation)

muscarinic   A substance that, like muscarine, stimulates the postganglionic receptors of the parasympathetic nervous system

mutagenic   Capable of causing genetic mutation

mydriatic   A drug that dilates the pupils

narcotic   A drug that induces sleep or stupor; legally: marijuana, cocaine, or a drug with morphinelike properties

narcotic analgesic   A drug with both an analgesic and a sedative action

nebulizer   A device for producing a fine spray or mist

neuroeffector junction   A junction between a neuron and an effector organ or cell, such as smooth muscle or a gland cell

neuromuscular junction   A junction between a somatic motor neuron and a skeletal muscle fiber

nonpolar compound   A substance whose molecular centers of positive and negative charges almost coincide, so that no permanent dipole moments are produced (nonpolar molecules do not ionize or conduct electricity)

nonprescription drug   A medicine that is sold without a prescription; over-the-counter drug

nosocomial   Acquired during hospitalization; of, or pertaining to, a hospital

nucleic acids   A group of complex compounds of high molecular weight that occur in all plant and animal cells and in viruses; the chemical compounds that form deoxyribonucleic acids (DNA) and ribonucleic acids (RNA)

official drugs   Preparations listed in pharmacopeiae that have been adopted by a government as pharmaceutical standards

ointments   Semisolid preparations of medicinal substances in a base, such as petrolatum or lanolin, intended for application to the skin or mucous membranes

ointments, ophthalmic   Sterile ointments for use in the eye

opiate   A derivative of opium; a drug obtained from the opium poppy, *Papaver somniferum*

opioid   A drug that resembles opium or morphine in its properties

osmotic effect   The net movement of water across a semipermeable membrane when it separates two solutions of unequal concentration of solutes, or unequal osmotic pressure

over-the-counter drug Nonprescription drug; a medicine sold directly to the public without requiring a prescription; usually a well-known substance of mixture taken for minor symptoms that is judged safe for use without medical supervision

oxidation A chemical reaction in which oxygen is added to a compound or the proportion of oxygen in a compound is increased by the removal of other groups

oxytocic A drug that selectively stimulates uterine motility and is useful in obstetrics

palliative A drug used for the control, rather than the cure, of a disease; suppressant

paradoxical reaction A physiologic response to a drug opposite to that which is usually seen (*eg*, restlessness and wakefulness following the administration of a hypnotic)

parasympatholytic A substance that tends to decrease the action of parasympathetic nerves or their effect on the body; anticholinergic

parasympathomimetic See *cholinergic*

parenteral Pertaining to the administration of drugs into any part of the body other than the gastrointestinal tract; although including topical applications and inhalation administration, in common usage applies only to administration by injection

paste A stiff ointmentlike preparation suitable only for external application

patent medicine A proprietary drug whose process of manufacture is controlled by patents granted to the developer; in common usage, used primarily to designate drugs advertised for self-use by the public

pathognomonic Indicative or characteristic of and specific to a disease

pharmaceutical chemistry The science dealing with the synthesis of new drugs either as modifications of older or natural drugs or as entirely new chemical entities

pharmacodynamics The science and study of the actions and effects of chemicals on living material

pharmacogenetics The science and study of genetic factors that account for individual differences in responses to drugs

pharmacognosy The science that deals with natural (animal and plant) sources for drugs

pharmacokinetics The science and study of the factors that determine the amount of a pharmacologic substance present at biologically effective sites at various times after its application to a biologic system

pharmacology The science and study of all aspects of the interactions of chemicals and living organisms

pharmacopeia A book, especially one published by an authority, that lists drugs and medicines and describes their preparations, properties, and uses

pharmacotherapeutics The use of drugs in the prevention, treatment, or diagnosis of disease and their use in the conscious alteration of normal functions

pharmacy That branch of pharmacology concerned with the preparing, compounding, and dispensing of drugs

pills Mixtures of a drug or drugs with a cohesive material, subsequently molded into globular, oval, or flattened bodies convenient for swallowing

pinocytosis The process whereby a particle is enveloped by the outer layer of a membrane, encased in the sac so formed, and transported to the inner layer of the membrane where it is released from the sac (the sac then merges with the inner layer of membrane)

placebo An inert substance used in place of a drug for its psychological effect and the physiologic changes that are triggered by the psychological response

placebo effect An actual biologic response to an inert substance believed to be caused by the power of suggestion

plasma The liquid part of blood or lymph

plasma clearance (renal) The volume of plasma needed to supply the amount of a specific substance excreted in urine in 1 minute

plasters Solid preparations that serve as simple adhesives or counterirritants

poison Any substance that impairs health or destroys life, especially one that exerts these effects in small doses

polar compound A compound that exhibits polarity, or local differences, in electrical properties; included are all electrolytes, most inorganic substances, and many organic ones

polarity The existence of opposing qualities; in relation to chemicals, the existence of electrical charges on a molecule or ion

pollutant An impurity

polypharmacy The concurrent use of two or more drugs

population A collection of items defined by a common characteristic

potency A comparative expression of drug activity measured in terms of the dose required to produce a particular effect of given intensity relative to a given or implied standard; strength, force, power

poultices Soft, moist preparations applied to the skin to exert osmotic pressure on fluids in the tissues (or to supply moist heat when warmed)

powders Finely divided solid drugs or mixtures of drugs for internal or external use

prescription A written formula given to the pharmacist by a physician, dentist, veterinarian, or other person legally permitted to prescribe medicine

prescription drug A drug whose purchase requires a prescription, because it has been judged to be unsafe for use except under supervision; a legend drug

prophylactic A remedy that prevents disease

proprietary drugs Preparations whose use is protected by patent or trademark to allow secrecy and monopoly in their manufacturing and sale

protectant A topical drug that remains on the skin and serves as a physical barrier to the environment

proteolytic enzyme An enzyme used to liquefy fibrinous or purulent exudates

psychoactive See *psychotropic*

psychoprophylaxis A technique of psychophysical training aimed at modifying the perception of painful sensations associated with normal childbirth

psychosomatic Pertaining to the interrelationship of the mind and body

psychotherapeutic A drug or interaction that modifies the behavior and emotional state of a person

psychotropic Affecting behavior, experience, or the function of the mind; psychoactive

purgative An agent that causes watery evacuation of the intestinal contents

rad Acronym for *radiation absorbed dose*; the quantity of ionizing radiation absorbed per unit mass of matter

radionuclide Atoms that disintegrate by emitting electromagnetic radiation

receptor A specialized area on a cell membrane that interacts with a drug substance

reduction A chemical reaction in which oxygen is removed from a compound or in which the reaction leads to a decrease in the proportion of oxygen in a compound

relaxant, muscle A drug that reduces muscle tension, especially in voluntary muscles

rem Acronym for *roentgen equivalent* (in) *man*; the estimated biologic effectiveness of one roentgen of radiation

resistance (In a host) the capability of an organism to counteract or destroy harmful agents or processes; a state of decreased response or a complete lack of response to drugs that ordinarily produce a biologic response

roentgen Unit for describing exposure dose of x or y radiation, with one unit representing the liberation of ions carrying positive and negative charges of 2.58×10^{-4} coulombs per kilogram of air

rubefacient A drug that reddens the skin; a counterirritant that increases circulation of blood in a specific part of the body

safety margin The relative distance between therapeutic and toxic doses of a given drug

sanitizer An agent that promotes health by its cleansing action

sciences, physical The fields of knowledge dealing with material phenomena

sciences, social The fields of knowledge dealing with psychosocial phenomena

scintiphotograph A graphic record of the scintillations emitted by radioactive tracers used to determine the outline and function of organs and tissues in which the radionuclide collects or by which it is secreted

sclerosing agent An irritant suitable for injection into varicose veins to induce their fibrosis and obliteration

secretogogue A chemical that simulates secretion by glandular organs

sedative A drug that exerts quieting or soothing effects

selectivity The capacity of a drug to produce one particular effect instead of multiple effects

semisynthetic Of or pertaining to a substance that is produced by a combination of natural and artificial processes or materials, often a natural substance that is chemically manipulated to modify its pharmacologic properties

sensitivity The ability of a member of a population, in comparison with other members of the same population, to respond in a qualitatively normal fashion to a particular drug dose

serum The clear, pale-yellow liquid that separates from the clot in the coagulation of blood; containing all the constituents of plasma except those involved in clot formation

side effect Any physiologic effect other than that for which a given drug is administered

signature The part of the prescription that gives directions for its use to the client who is to take the medicine

skeletal muscle relaxant A drug that inhibits contraction of voluntary muscles, usually by interfering with their innervation

smooth muscle relaxant A drug that inhibits contraction of involuntary (*eg,* visceral) muscles, usually by acting on their contractile elements

solution A homogenous dispersal of one substance in another without chemical change, usually that of a solid in a liquid

solution, true Nonvolatile substances dissolved in water

spasmolytic An agent that relieves spasms and involuntary contraction of a muscle; an antispasmodic

specificity The capacity of a drug to manifest its effects by a single mechanism of action; selectivity

spinnbarkeit Ability to spin cervical mucus into a long thread at the time of ovulation

spirits Concentrated alcoholic solutions of volatile substances; essences

standard safety margin The percentage by which the dose effective in virtually all (99%) of the population has to be increased to produce a lethal effect in a minimum percentage (1%) of the population

sterilization The elimination of all life forms

stereoisomers Two substances of the same composition and constitution that differ in the relative spatial position of their constituent atoms or groups in that one is the mirror image of the other

stimulant A drug that temporarily quickens some vital process or functional activity

stomachic A drug used to stimulate appetite and gastric secretion

subcutaneous Within the tissue lying between the skin and muscle, as in a subcutaneous injection, which is the introduction of a drug by hypodermic into the subcutaneous tissue or the pocket between subcutaneous and muscle tissue

sublingual Beneath the tongue

subscription The part of a prescription that contains the directions to the pharmacist

summation The simultaneous action of two drugs that is the algebraic sum of their individual effects

superinfection An infection developing during antimicrobial treatment of another infection. The secondary infection is often caused by an organism that is resistant to the treatment agent and that grows more readily in the absence of the organisms suppressed by the treatment agent

superscription The part of the prescription that includes the client's name, age, and address; the date; and the symbol ℞ (an abbreviation for "recipe," meaning "take thou")

suppositories Mixtures of a drug with a firm base that can be molded into shapes suitable for insertion into a body cavity, melting at body temperature to release the drug

suppressant See *palliative*

surfactant A surface active agent that decreases the surface tension between two miscible liquids

suspension A combination of a solid and a fluid in which the particles of the former are mixed with but not dissolved in the latter

sympatholytic A drug that decreases the activity of the sympathetic nervous system, or the physiologic effect of sympathetic nervous activity

sympathomimetic A drug that produces a physiologic effect similar to that of sympathetic nervous activity

synapse The junction between two neurons

synergism When the combined effects of two drugs acting simultaneously are greater than the sum of the individual effects of these drugs

synthetic Of or pertaining to a substance that is produced by an artificial rather than a natural process or material

syrup Aqueous solution of sucrose (85%) used as a vehicle and preservative for drugs

tablet A preparation of powdered drug that is compressed or molded into small disks; usually containing in addition to the drug a diluent, a binder, a disintegrator, and a lubricant

tachyphylaxis A significant decrease in effectiveness of a drug following repeated administration

teratogen A substance that induces abnormal fetal development when administered to a pregnant animal

teratogenic Property of developing abnormal structures in an embryo resulting in fetal deformities

therapeutic index The ratio between the median lethal dose and median effective dose; computed according to the formula: $TI = LD_{50}/ED_{50}$

therapeutics The treatment of disease

threshold dose The dose of a drug barely sufficient to produce any preselected intensity of effect

tinctures Alcoholic or hydroalcoholic solutions of the active principles of drugs

tocolytic A drug used to inhibit uterine contractions

tolerance A condition of decreased responsiveness acquired after a single or repeated exposure to a given drug or one closely allied in pharmacologic activity

tonic An agent used to restore tone to muscle tissue; to laymen, a remedy that improves general body function

toxic effect A drug effect that is deleterious to the organism, especially an effect characteristic of high doses

toxicology The study of the toxic or harmful effects of chemicals as well as the mechanisms and conditions under which these harmful effects occur

toxicology, economic The study of the toxic effect of chemicals intentionally administered to a living organism to achieve a specific purpose; including therapeutic agents, food additives, cosmetics, insecticides, and herbicides

toxicology, environmental The study of toxic agents that influence health and safety in the work environment, in the atmosphere, and in ingested nutrients; the effects of these toxic elements on the human organism

toxicology, forensic The study of poisoning (intentional and accidental) and the legal aspects of the relationship between exposure and the harmful effects of chemicals

toxoid A modified bacterial toxin, less toxic than the original form, used to induce active immunity to bacterial pathogens

tracer A radioactive isotope that can be incorporated into compounds whose course through the body can be followed or traced by measuring the radioactivity of body tissue or fluids

tranquilizer A drug that reduces mental and emotional tension

transport Movement or transfer of substances in a biologic system; especially across cell membranes

transport, active Transfer of a substance across a membrane by means of carrier systems that require energy for their function; active transport systems often move substances against the diffusion gradient, from areas of low concentration to areas of high concentration

transport, passive Diffusion

troches Flat round or rectangular preparations that are held in a cavity (the mouth or vagina) until they dissolve, liberating the drug or drugs involved; lozenges

unction The rubbing of medication into the skin

uricosuric A drug that increases the excretion of uric acid in the urine (useful in treating gout)

vaccine A suspension of either attenuated or killed microorganisms administered for the prevention of infectious diseases by the induction of active immunity

vasoconstrictor A drug used to constrict blood vessels and reduce tissue congestion

vasodilator A drug that relaxes vascular smooth muscles, especially for the purpose of improving peripheral or coronary blood flow

vasopressor A drug used systemically to constrict blood vessels and raise blood pressure

vertigo Dizziness, giddiness

vesicant An agent that causes blistering and the formation of vesicles when applied to the tissues

vesiculation Formation of small sacs filled with fluid

vials Glass containers with rubber stoppers containing one or more doses of a drug

waters Solutions (saturated unless otherwise stated) of volatile oils or other aromatic substances in distilled water

Index

Page numbers followed by *f* indicate figures; those followed by *t* indicate tabular material; those followed by *d* indicate a display; those followed by *b* indicate boxed material. Generic drug names are indicated by boldface; trade names are indicated by small capital letters; Canadian trade names are followed by (Can).

AAP. *See* American Academy of Pediatrics
ABACTRIM. *See* **co-trimoxazole-sulfamethoxazole-trimethoprim** combination
ABBOCIN. *See* **oxytetracycline**
ABBOKINASE. *See* **urokinase**
abbreviations
  for drugs, 83, 181*t*
  for orders, prescriptions, and labels, 178–179, 180*t*
  that are easily misread or misinterpreted, 179, 181*t*
ABENOL. *See* **acetaminophen**
ABO antigen–antibody reaction, from blood transfusion, 1308, 1309*t*
ABO system of blood type(s), 1307–1308, 1308*t*
absence seizures, treatment of, 469, 478
absorbable gelatin, 624
  notes on use of, 620*t*
  preparations, 620*t*
  usual dosage, 620*t*
absorbent, definition of, 1363
absorption. *See also* drug absorption
  definition of, 1363
absorptive beads, 1142–1143
ABSTINYL. *See* **disulfiram**
abuse. *See also* substance abuse
  definition of, 1363
ABVD chemotherapy regimen, 1193, 1218, 1223
Account of the Foxglove and Some of Its Uses: With Practical Remarks on Dropsy and Other Diseases, An (Withering), 534
ACCUTANE. *See* **isotretinoin**
acebutolol, 565
  adverse reactions to, 563*t*, 599*t*
  effects on fetus and breast-fed neonate, 222*t*
  pharmacodynamics of, 566*d*
  pharmacokinetics of, 566*d*
  preparations, 563*t*, 599*t*
  therapeutic use of, 566*d*, 604
    nursing considerations with, 567*d*
  usual dosage, 563*t*, 599*t*
ACETA. *See* **acetaminophen**
ACETAGESIC. *See* **acetaminophen**
acetaminophen, 1163
  adverse reactions to, 94*t*–95*t*, 1133*t*, 1164*t*, 1165

as antipyretic, 1132
  dosage and administration of, 1134
  client education about, 1138
  contraindications to, 305
  dosage and administration of, 293*t*, 932*t*, 1133*t*, 1138, 1164*t*, 1165
  drug interactions, 305, 1165
  effects of, 932*t*
    on fetus and breast-fed neonate, 222*t*, 226*t*
  hepatotoxicity, 1165–1166
  notes on use of, 932*t*
  pharmacodynamics of, 1163
  pharmacokinetics of, 1165
  plasma levels, expressed in conventional and Systeme International (SI) units, 1361*t*
  preparations, 1133*t*, 1164*t*
  products containing, 1165*b*
  safety of, during lactation, 246, 247*t*
  therapeutic use of, 1163–1164
  toxicity, 1165–1166
acetazolamide
  adverse reactions to, 984*t*, 987
  as anticonvulsant, 484
  contraindications to, 987
  drug interactions, 987
  effects on fetus and breast-fed neonate, 224*t*
  notes on use of, 473*t*
  pharmacodynamics of, 987
  pharmacokinetics of, 987
  precautions with, 987
  preparations, 473*t*, 984*t*
  safety of, during lactation, 247*t*, 249
  therapeutic use of, 984*t*, 987
  usual dosage, 473*t*, 984*t*
acetic acid(s), 1155–1159
acetohexamide
  approximate time of onset (hours), 786*t*
  contraindications to, 788*d*
  duration of activity (hours), 786*t*
  peak action (hours), 786*t*
  pharmacokinetics of, 788*d*
  plasma half-life (hours), 786*t*
  pregnancy risk category, 786*t*
  usual adult dosage, 786*t*
acetophenazine
  indications for, 497*t*
  pharmacokinetics of, 503*d*
  usual daily dosage, 501*t*
acetophenetidin, hemolytic anemia caused by, 844

ACETOSPAN. *See* **triamcinolone acetonide**
acetylation, 75
acetylcholine, 316, 318*f*, 343–344, 495
  pharmacokinetics of, 345*d*
  preparations, 342*t*
  therapeutic use of, 342*t*, 345*d*
    nursing considerations with, 345*d*
  usual dosage, 342*t*
acetylcysteine
  adverse reactions to, 912
  dosage and administration of, 912
  inhalation, 72*t*
  notes on use of, 913*t*
  pharmacodynamics of, 912
  precautions with, 912
  preparation, 913*t*
  storage of, 912
  usual adult dosage, 913*t*
N-**acetylprocainamide,** 568–569
  adverse reactions to, 565*t*, 569
  pharmacodynamics of, 568
  pharmacokinetics of, 568–569
  therapeutic use of, 569
acetylsalicylic acid. *See also* **aspirin**
  adverse reactions to, 1151*t*, 1154
  as analgesic, 1153
  antiplatelet effect of, 1150
  as antipyretic, 1132, 1153
  antithrombotic effect of, 1153
  dosage and administration of, 1153–1154
  drug interactions, 1154–1155
  effects on labor and delivery, 1154
  gastrotoxicity of, 1154
  generic name for, 82
  ototoxicity of, 1154
  pharmacodynamics of, 1148–1150
  pharmacokinetics of, 1150–1153
  preparations, 1151*t*
  and Reye's syndrome, 1154
  therapeutic use of, 1153
  toxicity, 1155
  usual dosage, 1151*t*
Achillea millefolium. *See* yarrow
achlorhydria, 69
ACHROMYCIN. *See* tetracycline(s)
ACHROMYCIN V. *See* tetracycline(s)
Achyranthes bidentata, ethnopharmacologic use of, 137*t*
acid, definition of, 1363
acid–ash foods, 111
  alteration of urinary *p*H with, 1065–1067

definition of, 1363
drug preparations, 743
effects of
on fetus and breast-fed neonate, 227*t*
on prepubertal males, 743–745
on sexual response, 943–950, 947*t*
on women, 743
nursing implications, 746
nursing process and, 746–751
pharmacodynamics of, 743, 947*t*
pharmacokinetics of, 743
physiology of, 741–743
precautions and contraindications, 746
in pregnancy, 743
preparations, 1234*t*
replacement therapy
client education about, 749
nursing process and, 749
similarities and differences, 747*d*–748*d*
therapeutic use of, 743, 947*t*
toxic effects of, 746
usual dosage, 1234*t*
androgenic, definition of, 1363
ANDROID. *See* **methyltestosterone**
ANDROID-T. *See* **testosterone**
ANDRO L.A. *See* **testosterone enanthate**
ANDROLAN. *See* **testosterone propionate**
ANDRONATE. *See* **testosterone cypionate**
androstenedione, 722
ANDRYL. *See* **testosterone enanthate**
ANDURACAINE. *See* **procaine**
ANECTINE. *See* **succinylcholine chloride**
anemia, 1285. *See also* aplastic anemia;
hemolytic anemia; iron-deficiency
anemia; pernicious anemia
after gastric resection, causes of,
1282–1283
client education about, 1286
in drug reactions, 844
of folic acid deficiency, 1285
intervention with, 1286
megaloblastic, with vitamin B$_{12}$ deficiency, 1282
nursing diagnoses with, 1285–1286
with plumbism, 47–48
signs and symptoms of, 96*t*
ANERGAN. *See* **promethazine**
anesthesia. *See also* general anesthesia;
local anesthesia
alternative regimens for, 421*t*, 421–422
definition of, 401, 402*b*
means of producing, 401*b*
stages of, characteristics of, 404*t*
anesthetic(s), 400–422
classification of, 400
definition of, 1363
effects of
on fetus and breast-fed neonate, 226*t*
on personnel, 191*t*
hazardous vapors from, 50
inhalant, 71, 72*t*
intravenous
notes on use of, 403*t*
preparations, 403*t*
nonprescription, 303*t*
anesthetic gases
exposure to, of hospital personnel, 78
reproductive hazards from, 219
angel dust. *See* **phencyclidine**
Angelica sinensis, ethnopharmacologic use
of, 137*t*
anger, effects on drug therapy, 125, 126*f*

angina pectoris, 588
pathophysiology of, 588
treatment of, 588, 593
ANGIO-CONRAY. *See* **iothalamate sodium**
angioedema, 841–842
drug-related, 842*t*
treatment of, 842
angioneurotic edema, definition of, 1363
angiotensin-converting enzyme inhibitor(s), 602
for congestive heart failure, 554
drug interactions, with NSAIDs, 1150
similarities and differences, 603*d*–604*d*
angiotensin I, 602
angiotensin II, 602
ANHYDRON. *See* **cyclothiazide**
anhydrotic, definition of, 1363
ANACIN-3. *See* **acetaminophen**
anileridine, 197
administration, 209*t*
dependence, 209*t*
duration of effects, 209*t*
overdose, 209*t*
tolerance, 209*t*
uses and effects of, 209*t*
withdrawal, 209*t*
animal models, advantages and disadvantages of, 18, 18*t*
animals, as source of drugs, 85, 85*t*
anion-exchange resin(s), drug interactions,
with NSAIDs, 1150
anise, 143*t*
ethnopharmacologic use of, 134*t*
anisindione, 631
notes on use of, 631*t*
preparations, 631*t*
usual dosage, 631*t*
anisotropine methylbromide
preparations, 354*t*
therapeutic use of, 354*t*
usual dosage, 354*t*
anistreplase, 641
ankylosing spondylitis, treatment of, 1149,
1156–1157, 1160–1163
anodyne, definition of, 1363
anorectic(s)
amphetamines as, 370
effects on fetus and breast-fed neonate,
226*t*
nutrient deficiency caused by, 120*t*
anorexia
in chemotherapy, nursing management
of, 1211–1214
definition of, 1363
drug-induced, 94*t*, 118
management of, 105–106, 106*t*
anorexiant, definition of, 1363
ANOREXIN. *See* **phenylpropanolamine
hydrochloride**
anorgasmia, drug-induced, 95*t*
ANS. *See* autonomic nervous system
ANSAID. *See* **flurbiprofen**
ANSPOR. *See* **cephradine**
ANTABUSE. *See* **disulfiram**
antacid(s), 671–674
administration of, 676
adverse reactions to, 93*t*, 673, 673*t*,
1355*t*
aluminum-containing, adverse reactions
to, 93*t*, 673, 673*t*
calcium-containing, adverse reactions to,
673, 673*t*

client education about, 676–677
definition of, 671, 1363
drug interactions, 98, 104*t*, 673–674
with NSAIDs, 1150
magnesium-containing, adverse reactions to, 673, 673*t*
nonprescription, 303*t*
notes on use of, 1355*t*
nutrient deficiency caused by, 120*t*
pharmacodynamics of, 671
pharmacokinetics of, 671
precautions and contraindications, 673
preparations, 1355*t*
properties of, 672*t*
sodium-containing, adverse reactions to,
673, 673*t*
therapeutic use of, 673, 1355*t*
nursing process and, 678
usual dosage, 1355*t*
antagonism, definition of, 1363
antagonist, definition of, 65, 1363
ANTEPAR. *See* **piperazine**
ANTHATEST. *See* **testosterone enanthate**
anthelmintic(s)
adverse reactions to, 1121
agents used for, 1113–1121
client education about, 1121
contraindications to, 1120–1121
definition of, 1363
nursing implications of, 1120
nursing process with, 1120–1121
traditional, 1119–1120
Anthemis nobilis. See camomile
anthracene, 702
anthracycline antibiotics, 1228–1229
adverse reactions to, 1224*t*
antidote for, 53*t*
pharmacodynamics of, 1228
preparation, 1224*t*
usual dosage, 1224*t*
anthraquinone(s), 702
adverse reactions to, 702
notes on use of, 699*t*
pharmacodynamics of, 702
pharmacokinetics of, 702
precautions and contraindications, 702
preparations, 699*t*
therapeutic use of, 702
usual dosage, 699*t*
antiadrenergic(s)
definition of, 1363
effects on sexual response, 948*t*, 950
pharmacodynamics of, 948*t*
therapeutic use of, 948*t*
antiandrogen(s). *See also* male hormone
antagonist(s)
in antineoplastic therapy, 1235
antianxiety drug(s), 507–512
classification of, 508
client education about, 511–512
effects on sexual response, 944*t*
indications for, 497*t*–498*t*
nursing process and, 511–512
pharmacodynamics of, 508, 944*t*
precautions, 508
therapeutic use of, 944*t*
usefulness of, 507
in various conditions, 507*t*
antiarrhythmic(s), 554–572
class I, 556–562
examples, 556*t*
mechanism of action, 556*t*

therapeutic use of, 946t
  nursing considerations with, 521d
  usual dosage, 515t
phenelzine sulfate
  drug interactions, 306
  enzyme acted upon, 1345t
  therapeutic use of, 1345t
PHENERGAN. See **promethazine**
phenindione, 631
  notes on use of, 631t
  preparations, 631t
  safety of, during lactation, 246, 247t
  usual dosage, 631t
pheniramine, effects on fetus and breast-
    fed neonate, 220t
phenmetrazine
  administration, 210t
  adverse reactions to, 372d
  dependence, 210t
  duration of effects, 210t
  effects on fetus and breast-fed neonate,
    226t
  overdose, 210t
  precautions with, 372d
  preparations, 369t
  therapeutic use of, 369t
    nursing considerations with, 373d
  tolerance, 210t
  uses and effects of, 210t
  usual dosage, 369t
  withdrawal, 210t
phenmetrazine hydrochloride, 203
phenobarbital, 447
  adverse effects of, 477, 479d
    on children, 486t
  allergic hypersensitivity to, 477
  as anticonvulsant, 240, 475–478
  dosage and administration, 475
  drug interactions, 99, 477–478, 1083
  duration of action, 200t
  effects of
    and age, 477
    on fetus and breast-fed neonate, 223t
  notes on use of, 471t
  for pain relief during labor, 234t
  pharmacodynamics of, 475, 479d
  pharmacokinetics of, 475, 479d
  placental transfer of, 475
  plasma levels, in conventional and Sys-
      teme International (SI) units,
      1362t
  precautions and contraindications, 478,
      480d
  preparations, 471t
  safety of, during lactation, 246, 247t,
      475
  side effects of, 486t
  therapeutic use of, 475, 479d
  tolerance, 477
  toxic effects of, 486t
  uses and effects of, 209t
  usual dosage, 471t
phenobarbital-substitution technique, to
      treat benzodiazepine addiction,
      202
phenol
  adverse reactions to, 414
  preparations, 416t
  therapeutic use of, 416t
  usual dosage, 416t
phenol(s)
  for antifungal therapy, 1079–1080
  toxic risk from exposure to, 51

PHENOLAX. See **phenolphthalein**
phenolphthalein, 702
  notes on use of, 699t
  nutrient deficiency caused by, 121t
  preparations, 699t
  safety of, during lactation, 248t, 250
  usual dosage, 699t
PHENOL RED. See **phenolsulfonphthalein**
phenolsulfonphthalein
  diagnostic uses of, 1322t
  preparations, 1322t
  tissue distribution, 1322t
  usual adult dosage, 1322t
  for volumetric diagnostic tests, 1320
phenothiazine(s), 500–502, 501t
  action of, 500
  adverse reactions to, 94t, 500
  agranulocytosis caused by, 844
  agranulocytosis with, 502
  aliphatic, 501t
  as antiemetics, 680
    mode of action, 681t–682t
    notes on use of, 681t–682t
    preparations, 681t–682t
    usual dosage, 681t–682t
  antipsychotic action of, 500
  behavioral effects of, 500
  classification of, 500
  dosage and administration, 500
  drug interactions, 500, 502
  effects of
    on fetus and breast-fed neonate, 227t
    on sexual response, 496, 945t
  extrapyramidal effects of, 500–502
  eye and skin reactions to, 500
  history of, 500
  indications for, 497t
  with narcotic analgesics, 502
  orthostatic hypotension with, 500–501
  pharmacodynamics of, 500, 945t
  piperadine, 501t
  piperazine, 501t
  safety of, during lactation, 248t, 249
  sedative action of, 500
  side effects of, 502
  similarities and differences, 503d–504d
  therapeutic use of, 500, 945t
  usual dosage, 501t
phenoxybenzamine, 335
  adverse reactions to, 335, 598t
  effects on sexual response, 948t
  as male contraceptive, 953
  pharmacodynamics of, 335, 948t
  pharmacokinetics of, 335
  precautions and contraindications, 335
  preparations, 598t
  therapeutic use of, 335, 602, 948t
  usual dosage, 598t
phenoxybenzamine hydrochloride
  preparations, 333t
  therapeutic use of, 333t
  usual dosage, 333t
phenprocoumon
  notes on use of, 631t
  preparations, 631t
  usual dosage, 631t
phensuximide
  notes on use of, 472t
  preparations, 472t
  usual dosage, 472t
phentermine, 203
  administration, 211t

adverse reactions to, 372d
dependence, 211t
duration of effects, 211t
overdose, 211t
preparations, 369t
therapeutic use of, 369t
  nursing considerations with, 373d
tolerance, 211t
uses and effects of, 211t
usual dosage, 369t
withdrawal, 211t
phentolamine, 335
  adverse reactions to, 335, 598t
  effects on sexual response, 948t
  pharmacodynamics of, 948t
  pharmacokinetics of, 335
  precautions and contraindications, 335
  preparations, 598t
  therapeutic use of, 335, 602, 948t
  usual dosage, 598t
phentolamine mesylate
  preparations, 333t
  therapeutic use of, 333t
  usual dosage, 333t
PHENTROL. See **phentermine**
PHENURONE. See **phenacemide**
PHENYLAZO. See **phenazo-pyridine**
phenylbutazone
  adverse reactions to, 94t, 1133t, 1152t,
      1162–1163
  dosage and administration of, 1162
  drug interactions, 99, 1163
  pharmacodynamics of, 1162
  pharmacokinetics of, 1162
  plasma levels, expressed in conventional
      and Systeme International (SI)
      units, 1362t
  preparations, 1133t, 1153t
  therapeutic use of, 1162
  thrombocytopenia caused by, 844
  usual dosage, 1133t, 1152t
phenylephrine, 328
  metabolism, inhibition of, 100–101,
      102t
phenylephrine bitartrate
  clinical uses of, 322t
  mode of action, 322t
  preparations, 322t, 900t
  usual dosage, 322t, 900t
phenylephrine hydrochloride
  clinical uses of, 322t
  mode of action, 322t
  preparations, 322t
  usual dosage, 322t
β-phenylisopropylamine. See
      amphetamine(s)
phenylpropanolamine, metabolism, inhi-
      bition of, 100–101, 102t
phenylpropanolamine hydrochloride
  clinical uses of, 322t
  mode of action, 322t
  preparations, 322t
  usual dosage, 322t
phenytoin, 559–560
  administration, 474, 560
  adverse effects of, 94t–95t, 474, 476d,
      559t, 560
    on children, 486t
  for alcohol detoxification, 203
  as anticonvulsant, 473–475
  drug interactions, 99, 101, 102t, 104t,
      474–475, 560, 798, 1084, 1163

North American Nursing Diagnosis Association (NANDA)
Approved Nursing Diagnoses

Activity Intolerance
Activity Intolerance, High Risk for
Adjustment, Impaired
Airway Clearance, Ineffective
Anxiety
Aspiration, High Risk for
Body Image Disturbance
Body Temperature, High Risk for Altered
Breastfeeding, Effective
Breastfeeding, Ineffective
*Breastfeeding, Interrupted
Breathing Pattern, Ineffective
*Caregiver Role Strain
*Caregiver Role Strain, High Risk for
Communication, Impaired Verbal
Constipation
Constipation, Colonic
Constipation, Perceived
Decisional Conflict (Specify)
Decreased Cardiac Output
Defensive Coping
Denial, Ineffective
Diarrhea
Disuse Syndrome, High Risk for
Diversional Activity Deficit
Dysreflexia
Family Coping: Compromised, Ineffective
Family Coping: Disabling, Ineffective
Family Coping: Potential for Growth
Family Processes, Altered
Fatigue
Fear
Fluid Volume Deficit
Fluid Volume Deficit, High Risk for
Fluid Volume Excess
Gas Exchange, Impaired
Grieving, Anticipatory
Grieving, Dysfunctional
Growth and Development, Altered
Health Maintenance, Altered
Health-Seeking Behaviors (Specify)
Home Maintenance Management, Impaired
Hopelessness
Hyperthermia
Hypothermia
Incontinence, Bowel
Incontinence, Functional
Incontinence, Reflex
Incontinence, Stress
Incontinence, Total
Incontinence, Urge
Individual Coping, Ineffective
*Infant Feeding Pattern, Ineffective
Infection, High Risk for
Injury, High Risk for